*Primary
Health Care
of Infants,
Children, &
Adolescents*

Primary Health Care of Infants, Children, & Adolescents

Second Edition

Edited by

Jane A. Fox, EdD, RN-CS, PNP
Clinical Associate Professor, Parent Child Health
School of Nursing
State University of New York at Stony Brook
Stony Brook, New York
President and Founder
Fox Educational Systems, Inc.
Southampton, New York

With 85 illustrations

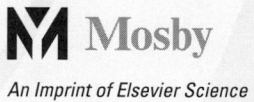 Mosby

An Imprint of Elsevier Science

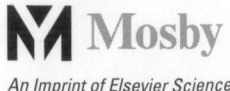

An Imprint of Elsevier Science

Vice President and Publishing Director, Nursing: Sally Schrefer
Executive Editor: Barbara Nelson Cullen
Managing Editor: Sandra Clark Brown
Developmental Editor: Stacy Welsh
Publishing Services Manager: Catherine Jackson
Project Manager: Clay S. Broeker
Designer: Amy Buxton

SECOND EDITION

NOTICE

Pharmacology is an ever-changing field. Standard safety precautions must be followed, but as new research and clinical experience broaden our knowledge, changes in treatment and drug therapy may become necessary or appropriate. Readers are advised to check the most current product information provided by the manufacturer of each drug to be administered to verify the recommended dose, the method and duration of administration, and contraindications. It is the responsibility of the licensed prescriber, relying on experience and knowledge of the patient, to determine dosages and the best treatment for each individual patient. Neither the publisher nor the editor assumes any liability for any injury and/or damage to persons or property arising from this publication.

Mosby, Inc.
An Imprint of Elsevier Science
11830 Westline Industrial Drive
St. Louis, Missouri 63146

Printed in the United States of America

International Standard Book Number 0-323-01335-X

02 03 04 05 06 GW/MVY 9 8 7 6 5 4 3 2 1

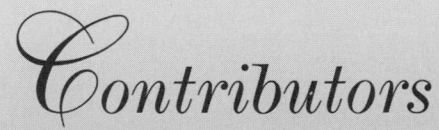
Contributors

Nancy E. Alfieri, MSN, RN-CS, PNP
Pediatric Nurse Practitioner
Division of Developmental and Behavioral Pediatrics
Schneider Children's Hospital
North Shore–Long Island Jewish Health System
New Hyde Park, New York

Linda C. Andrist, PhD, RNC, WHNP
Associate Professor and Coordinator
Women's Health Nurse Practitioner Program
Graduate Program in Nursing
MGH Institute of Health Professions
Boston, Massachusetts

Catherine Ascher, MSN, RN
Clinical Nurse Specialist
Department of Pediatric Neurology
Schneider Children's Hospital
New Hyde Park, New York

Stephanie Bonney, MS, RN, CPNP
Pediatric Nurse Practitioner
St. Mary's Hospital for Children
Bayside, New York

Marie Scott Brown, PhD, RN, PNP, CNM
Professor
Department of Family Nursing
Oregon Health Sciences University
Portland, Oregon

Fern Campbell, MSN, RN, FNP-C
Pediatric Urologic Nurse Practitioner
Department of Urology
University of Virginia
Charlottesville, Virginia

Jennifer Piersma D'Auria, PhD, RN, CPNP
Associate Professor and Director of Master's Programs
The University of North Carolina at Chapel Hill
School of Nursing
Chapel Hill, North Carolina

Barbara Jones Deloian, PhD, RN, CPNP
Pediatric Nurse Practitioner
Child Development Unit
Program Evaluator
Nursing Research
The Children's Hospital
Denver, Colorado

Loren O'Connor Dempsey, RN, MA, CPNP
Pediatric Nurse Practitioner
Hempstead High Health Center
Department of Pediatrics
Winthrop University Hospital
Mineola, New York

Susan M. DeVivio, MPH, RN, CPNP
Pediatric Nurse Practitioner
Division of Pediatric Infectious Diseases
Nassau University Medical Center
East Meadow, New York

Catherine J. Dillon Dolan, MS, RN, CPNP
Clinical Instructor
School of Nursing
State University of New York at Stony Brook
Stony Brook, New York

Susan Dulczak, MSN, RN-CS, PNP
Nurse Practitioner
Department of Urology
Children's Hospital of Philadelphia
Philadelphia, Pennsylvania

Theresa M. Eldridge, MS, RN, CPNP
Nurse Practitioner
Surgical Services
The Children's Hospital
Denver, Colorado

Barbara A. Elliott, PhD
Professor and Director of Clinical Research
Department of Family Medicine
University of Minnesota–Duluth
Duluth, Minnesota

Christie Sandra Ehle Erickson, MA, RN, CFNP
Family Nurse Practitioner and Clinical Coordinator
TeenLife Center Health Services
University of Minnesota–Duluth
Duluth, Minnesota

Jane C. Evans, PhD, RN
Professor and Director
Center for Nursing Research and Evaluation
Medical College of Ohio School of Nursing
Toledo, Ohio

Carolyn D. Farrell, MS, CNP, CEC
Director, Clinical Genetics Service
Department of Cancer Genetics
Roswell Park Cancer Institute
Buffalo, New York

Jane A. Fox, EdD, RN-CS, PNP
Clinical Associate Professor, Parent Child Health
School of Nursing
State University of New York at Stony Brook
Stony Brook, New York
President and Founder
Fox Educational Systems, Inc.
Southampton, New York

Bonnie Gance-Cleveland, PhD, RNC, PNP
Assistant Professor
School of Nursing
University of Colorado
Denver, Colorado

Miriam Gilday, MSN, CRNP
Pediatric Nurse Practitioner, Hematology
Department of Hematology
St. Christopher's Hospital for Children
Philadelphia, Pennsylvania

Linda Gilman, EdD, RN, CPNP
Associate Professor of Nursing and Director, Pediatric Nurse
  Practitioner Major
Indiana University School of Nursing
Indianapolis, Indiana

Barbara Golden, MSN, RN, CPNP
Pediatric Nurse Practitioner
Pediatric Neurology
Schneider Children's Hospital
New Hyde Park, New York

Mikel Gray PhD, CUNP, CCCN, FAAN
Nurse Practitioner and Professor
Department of Urology
School of Nursing
University of Virginia
Charlottesville, Virginia

Elizabeth F. Gunhus, MSN, RN, CPNP
Pediatric Nurse Practitioner
Aspen Medical Group
Pediatric and Adolescent Medicine
St. Paul, Minnesota

Susan Hagedorn, PhD, RN, PNP
Pediatric Nurse Practitioner and Women's Health Nurse
  Practitioner
School of Nursing, Health Sciences Center
University of Colorado
Denver, Colorado

Susan M. Heffernan, MSN, RN, CPNP
Pediatric Nurse Practitioner
Women and Children Care Center
New York Presbyterian Hospital
New York, New York

Marilyn J. Hockenberry, PhD, RN-CS, PNP, FAAN
Professor of Pediatrics
Section of Hematology/Oncology
Baylor College of Medicine
Houston, Texas
Director of Pediatric Nurse Practitioner Program
Texas Children's Cancer Center
Texas Children's Hospital
Houston, Texas

Judith Bellaire Igoe, MS, RN, FAAN
Associate Professor and Director
Office of School Health
University of Colorado Health Sciences Center
Denver, Colorado

Jacqueline G. Ioli, MSN, RN-CS, CRNP
Advanced Practice Nurse, Hematology
St. Christopher's Hospital for Children
Philadelphia, Pennsylvania

Arlene E. Johnson MA, RN, CPNP
Assistant Professor
Department of Nursing
The College of St. Scholastica
Pediatric Nurse Practitioner
Department of Pediatrics
SMDC Duluth Clinic
Duluth, Minnesota

Barbara R. Kelley, EdD, MPH, RN, CPNP
Associate Professor
School of Nursing
Northeastern University
Boston, Massachusetts

Kathleen M. Kenney, MS, RN-CS, PNP
Coordinator, Advanced Practice Nursing Pediatrics
Division of Nursing
New York University
Steinhardt School of Education
New York, New York

John C. Kirchgessner, MSN, RN, PNP
Assistant Professor
School of Nursing
University of Virginia
Charlottesville, Virginia

Nancy E. Kline, PhD, RN, CPNP
Assistant Professor of Pediatrics
Baylor College of Medicine
Pediatric Nurse Practitioner
Texas Children's Hospital
Houston, Texas

Linda M. Kollar, MSN, RN
Associate Director for Clinical Services
Division of Adolescent Medicine
Children's Hospital Medical Center
Cincinnati, Ohio

Mary Koslap-Petraco, MS, RN-CS, CPNP
Coordinator, Child Health
Suffolk County Department of Health Services
Hauppauge, New York
Clinical Assistant Professor
State University of New York at Stony Brook
School of Nursing
Stony Brook, New York

Kimberly L. LaMar, MSN, RNC, CNNP
Department of Perinatal Medicine
University of Michigan
Ann Arbor, Michigan

Maureen Leahey, PhD, RN
Manager, Outpatient Mental Health Program, and Director,
 Family Therapy Training Program
Calgary Health Region
Adjunct Associate Professor
Faculties of Nursing and Medicine (Psychiatry)
University of Calgary
Calgary, Alberta, Canada

Anne Marie C. Levac, MN, RN
Advanced Practice Nurse, Child Psychiatry Program
Centre for Addiction and Mental Health
Toronto, Ontario, Canada
Lecturer, Faculty of Nursing
University of Toronto
Toronto, Ontario, Canada

Marie Ann Marino, EdD, RN, PNP
Clinical Associate Professor
School of Nursing
State University of New York at Stony Brook
Stony Brook, New York
Pediatric Nurse Practitioner and Forensic Medical Examiner
Child Advocacy Center
Central Islip, New York

Phyllis K. Marion, MS, RN, CPNP
Pediatric Nurse Practitioner
Division of General Pediatrics and Adolescent Medicine
Children's Medical Center
State University of New York at Stony Brook
Stony Brook, New York

Margaret A. McCabe, DNSc, RN, PNP, DNSc
Nurse Manager
Mallinckrodt General Clinical Research Center
Massachusetts General Hospital
Boston, Massachusetts

Clare McLaughlin, RD
Pediatric Clinical Dietitian
Department of Nutrition
Clarian Health Inc.
Methodist Hospital
Indianapolis, Indiana

Susanne Meghdadpour, MSN, RN, FNP
Clinical Associate
Department of Pediatrics, Pulmonary Division
Duke University
Durham, North Carolina

Mary E. Muscari, PhD, RN, CRNP, CS
Associate Professor
Nursing Department
University of Scranton
Scranton, Pennsylvania

Susan Nordberg, MS, RN-CS, CPNP
Pediatric Nurse Practitioner
Medical Clinical/Foster Care
St. Christopher—Ottilie, Services for Children and Families
Brentwood, New York

Kathleen R. Pitzen, MSN, RNC
Metro Nurse Manager
Neonatal Services
Mercy Children's Hospital, St. Vincent Mercy Medical Center
Toledo, Ohio

Cynthia A. Prows, MSN, RN
Clinical Nurse Specialist, Genetics
Department of Patient Services, Division of Human Genetics
Children's Hospital Medical Center
Cincinnati, Ohio

Joyce Pulcini, PhD, AN, CS-PNP, FAAN
Associate Professor
Boston College School of Nursing
Chestnut Hill, Massachusetts

Marijo Ratcliffe, MN, ARNP
Pediatric Nurse Practitioner
Pulmonary Center
University of Washington
Pediatric Nurse Practitioner
Pulmonary Department
Children's Hospital and Medical Center
Lecturer, Family and Child
School of Nursing
University of Washington
Children's Hospital and Regional Medical Center
Seattle, Washington

Virginia E. Richardson, DNS, RN, CPNP
Assistant Dean for Student Affairs and Associate Professor
Indiana University School of Nursing
Indianapolis, Indiana

Kathy H. Rideout, EdD, RN-CS, PNP
Pediatric Advanced Practice Nurse and Assistant Professor
 of Nursing
School of Nursing
University of Rochester, Children's Hospital at Strong
Rochester, New York

Kathleen A. Shea, MS, RN, CPNP
Pediatric Nurse Practitioner
Park Slope Family Health Center of Lutheran Medical Center
Brooklyn, New York

Katherine E. Simmonds, MSN, MPH, RNC
Clinical Instructor
Department of Women's Health
MGH Institute of Health Professions
Boston, Massachusetts

Sharon L. Sims, PhD, RN-CS
Associate Professor and Chairperson
Family Health Nursing
Indiana University School of Nursing
Indianapolis, Indiana

Arleen Nast Steckel, PhD, RN, CPNP
Clinical Associate Professor, Parent Child Health,
  and Assistant Dean, Clinical Placements
School of Nursing
State University of New York at Stony Brook
Stony Brook, New York

Debbie Thompson, BSN, RNC, CCRN
Staff Development Coordinator and Perinatal Outreach
  Coordinator
Department of Newborn Intensive Care
St. Vincent Mercy Medical Center
Toledo, Ohio

Christina Trout, MSN, RN
Clinical Nurse Specialist
Department of Pediatrics
University of Iowa
Iowa City, Iowa

Victoria Vecchiariello, MA, RN, CPNP
Pediatric Nurse Practitioner
Department of Pediatrics
Bellevue Hospital
New York, New York

Peggy Vernon, MA, RN, CPNP
Nurse Practitioner and Practice Administrator
Leslie Capin, MD
Parker, Colorado

Amy Verst, MSN, RN, CPNP, ATC
Assistant Professor
Bellarmine University
Louisville, Kentucky

Ericka K. Leibold Waidley, MSN, RN
President and Chief Executive Officer
EKW and Associates
Laguna Beach, California
Faculty
Department of Nursing
California State University, Fullerton
Fullerton, California

Susan M. Watson, MSN, RN, CPNP
Pediatric Nurse Practitioner
Developmental and Behavioral Pediatrics
Schneider Children's Hospital
New Hyde Park, New York

Marty Witrak, PhD, RN, CS
Associate Professor and Chairperson
Health Sciences Division
Department of Nursing
The College of St. Scholastica
Duluth, Minnesota

Lorraine M. Wright, PhD, RN
Director, Family Nursing Unit, and Professor, Faculty
  of Nursing
University of Calgary
Calgary, Alberta
Canada

Contributors to the First Edition

Deborah Arnold, RN, MSN, CPNP MPH
Kathryn Ballenger, RN, MSN, CCRN
Maryanne E. Bezyack, RN, MSN, CPNP
Janice F. Bistritz, RN, MSN, PNP
Sue Ann Boote, RN, MS, CPNP
Maura E. Byrnes, RN, MA, PNP
Barbara Carty, RN, EdD
Lisa M. Clark, RN, MS, CPNP
Marilu Dixon, RN-CS, MSN, PNP
Emily E. Drake, RNC, MSN
Ann Ford Fricke, RN, BSN
Patricia A. Gardner, RN, MA, PNP
Lynn Howe Gilbert, RN, PhD, CPNP
Bonnie Gitlitz, RN, MSN, CPNP
Denise Gruccio, RN, MSN, PNP
Leah Harrison, RN, MSN, CPNP
Sandra P. Hellerman, RN, MSN, CPNP
Vicki Young Johnson, RN, MSN

Susan Carol Kay, RN, MS, CPNP
Susan Kennel, RN, MSN, CPNP
Ellen M. McCabe, RN, MSN, CPNP
Bernadette Mazurek Melnyk, RN-CS, PhD, PNP
Julie C. Novak, RN, DNSc, CPNP
Ann M. Orth, RN, MSN, CPNP
Julie K. Osterhaus, RN, MA, CPNP
Jeanne Peacock, RNC, MSN
Gloria A. Perez, RN, MSN, PNP
Maura E. Porricolo, RN, MS, MPH, CPNP
Linda J. Ross, RN, MA, PNP
Pam Scheibel, RN, MSN, CPNP
Esther Seibold, RN, MSN, PNP-CS
Teresa Stables-Carney, RN, MS, CPNP
Janet F. Sullivan, RN, C, PhD, CPNP
Elizabeth D. Tate, RN, C, MN, FNP
Jo Ann Thomas, RN, MSN, CPNP

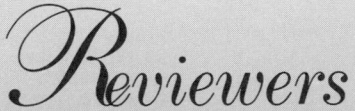Reviewers

Elissa Emerson, PhD, RN, CS, CRNP
Family Nurse Practitioner Program
University of Maryland, Baltimore
School of Nursing
Baltimore, Maryland

Deborah Kiley, MN, RN, CS, FNP
Assistant Professor
University of Alaska Anchorage
School of Nursing
Anchorage, Alaska

Elaine O'Leary, MSN, RN, CPNP
Associate Professor
University of Texas at Austin
School of Nursing Graduate Program
Austin, Texas

To Jack, my best friend and husband.
To Thatcher and Ibsen, our retired guide dogs.

Preface

It is a pleasure to introduce the second edition of *Primary Health Care of Infants, Children, & Adolescents*. As with the first edition, this book is written to provide a comprehensive clinical reference text for nurse practitioners (NPs), students, and others who provide primary care to infants, children, adolescents, and their families. It is a joint effort by more than seventy expert clinicians and educators, most of whom are pediatric nurse practitioners (PNPs) from the United States and Canada. Although the book is written by PNPs for PNPs, advanced practice nurses (APNs), students, educators, public health and community health nurses, family nurse practitioners (FNPs), neonatal nurse practitioners (NNPs), school nurse practitioners (SNPs) and school nurses, pediatric nurses, camp nurses, and others who provide primary care to infants, children, and adolescents should find this book particularly useful. It is important to note that all chapters were reviewed by at least one and often two colleagues.

This book is divided into five major sections. *Section 1: Health Promotion and Well Child Care* provides a comprehensive overview of the foundation of clinical practice (i.e., history and physical examination, genetics, counseling and teaching, ethics) and the context in which is takes place (i.e., family, culture). All aspects of well-child care, including immunizations, injury prevention, screening, and nutrition (including common parenting concerns), are covered in this section. Tables are included throughout. Two important chapters have also been added to this section. *Providing Primary Health Care to Children* discusses the history of the PNP role and current issues that affect NPs and the care they provide. *Common Adolescent Concerns* has also been included to address the unique health promotion needs and concerns of adolescents.

Section 2: Families with Special Parenting Needs discusses parenting situations commonly encountered in clinical practice, including divorce, adoption, foster care, gay parenting, and so on. It is often the practitioner who identifies and addresses the unique concerns and issues these families face. An overview, incidence, risk factors, suggestions on information to gather in the history, pertinent areas to assess in the physical examination, primary care issues and concerns, and management are all included. Pertinent resources, including Internet sites, are identified.

Section 3: Common Presenting Symptoms and Problems addresses the common presenting complaints seen in daily practice. A symptom approach is used because it is most relevant to clinical practice. Children do not present with a medical diagnosis but rather with a symptom or problem that the practitioner must then diagnose. Books using a medical diagnosis approach assume the practitioner or student already knows the diagnosis, which is often not the case. This section is unique in stressing the diagnostic process and management and is organized by body system, with common presenting symptoms and problems also listed alphabetically. Each body system section begins with an overview discussing general risk factors, health promotion strategies (including counseling and interventions), and subjective (history) and objective (physical examination) data specific for a problem within that body system. A description of diagnostic tests and procedures that may be ordered is also included.

Next the commonly presented symptoms and problems are listed in alphabetical order. Each symptom begins with an *Alert* describing situations that may require a consult or referral to another professional or physician. *Etiology* discusses the possible causes for the symptoms or problems, with *Incidence* and *Risk Factors* following. *Differential Diagnosis* includes a narrative on each diagnosis to be considered, including a brief definition and pertinent subjective and objective findings. A table for quick reference and easy comparison is usually included, comparing the possible diagnoses using subjective and objective criteria (including laboratory tests). ICD-9 codes are also included in the differential diagnosis tables. *Management* is presented for each diagnosis and includes treatments and medications, counseling and prevention, follow-up, and consultations and referrals. Helpful resources and Internet sites are included at the end of each section.

Section 4, Families with Children Requiring Long-Term Management is divided into three chapters: *Diseases and Problems, Developmental Difficulties,* and *Social Disorders*. It is often the practitioner who identifies such problems and is responsible for meeting the primary care needs of these children and their families, though these children are usually managed in consultation with a physician and other professionals. Each disease or problem is discussed in a similar format as Part Three, using *Alert, Etiology, Incidence, Risk Factors, Subjective Data, Objective Data, Primary Care Implications,* and *Management* sections. Resources for both the professional and the family are provided, including Internet sites.

Section 5, Emergencies and Preparation for Hospitalization consists of two chapters. The first, *Managing Pediatric Emergencies in a Primary Care Setting,* presents in outline format the assessment and management of common pediatric emergencies. The second, *Preparation for Painful Procedures, Hospitalization, and Surgery,* offers a developmental approach to preparation. Identification of children who may be at risk for problems during hospital stays and specific interventions aimed at these problems are discussed.

The *Appendixes* include growth and measurement charts, developmental and other screening tests, and laboratory tests, including normal values and interpretation of results. An appendix on radiologic tests discusses commonly ordered tests and provides a developmental approach to preparation of a child. The appendixes on telephone triage and protocols and CPT and ICD-9 codes will also prove helpful to health care practitioners. A new appendix, *General Health, Pediatric, and Nurse Practitioner Internet Sites*, has been included to help practitioners identify excellent Internet resources to assist in providing evidence-based care.

Jane A. Fox

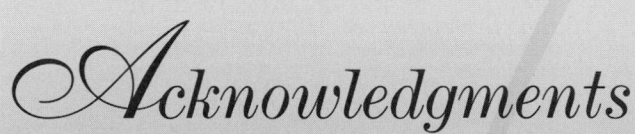

Acknowledgments

To all the contributors who have generously shared their knowledge and expertise in their chapters and to the reviewers who have offered helpful suggestions and insights, I offer a heartfelt thanks.

I am most appreciative to Sandy Brown, Stacy Welsh, Barbara Cullen, Clay Broeker, and all the staff at Mosby who worked so hard to bring this project to completion. I am grateful for their encouragement and patience.

Many students and colleagues offered suggestions that were incorporated into this edition. Thank you.

Last, but not least, a sincere thanks to my family and friends for their support and encouragement.

Contents

Section 1
Health Promotion and Well-Child Care, 1

1 **Providing Primary Health Care to Children,** 3
Linda Gilman and Virginia E. Richardson

2 **Children and Families: Models for Assessment and Intervention,** 10
Anne Marie C. Levac, Lorraine M. Wright, and Maureen Leahey

3 **Parenting,** 20
Theresa M. Eldridge

4 **Cultural Diversity in Clinical Practice,** 35
Barbara R. Kelley

5 **Genetic Evaluation and Counseling,** 44
Carolyn D. Farrell and Cynthia A. Prows

6 **The Ethics of Practice,** 69
Barbara A. Elliott

7 **Pediatric Pain Assessment and Management,** 74
Kathy H. Rideout

8 **Prenatal Interview,** 82
Jane A. Fox

9 **Health History and Physical Examination,** 86
Marie Scott Brown and Judith Bellaire Igoe

10 **Newborn Assessment,** 107
Jane C. Evans, Kimberly L. LaMar, Kathleen R. Pitzen, and Debbie Thompson

11 **Developmental Assessment,** 137
Margaret A. McCabe

12 **Screening Tests,** 146
Barbara Jones Deloian

13 **Immunizations,** 157
Mary Koslap-Petraco

14 **Injury Prevention,** 186
Theresa M. Eldridge

15 **Nutritional Assessment,** 208
Clare McLaughlin

16 **Dental Health,** 220
Linda Gilman

17 **Issues of Sexuality,** 229
Susan Hagedorn

18 **Assessing School Readiness,** 235
Joyce Pulcini

19 **Common Parenting Concerns,** 245
Jane A. Fox

Breath-Holding, 245

Bullies and Victims, 247

Child Care, 249

Circumcision, 251

Discipline, 252

Fears, 253

Fighting, 254

Latchkey Children, 255

Lying, Stealing, and Cheating, 256

Masturbation, 257

Separation Anxiety, 258

Sleep Problems, 260

Sibling Rivalry, 262

Stranger Anxiety, 263

Temper Tantrums, 264

Thumbsucking and Digit-Sucking, 265

Toilet Training, 266

20 **Common Adolescent Concerns,** 268
Linda M. Kollar

Section 2

Families With Special Parenting Needs, 281

21 **Children with Addicted Parents,** 283
Bonnie Gance-Cleveland

22 **Adoptive Families,** 287
Marty Witrak and Arlene E. Johnson

23 **Childhood Loss,** 293
Peggy Vernon

24 **Divorce,** 296
Jane A. Fox

25 **Foster Care,** 300
Susan Nordberg

26 **Gay or Lesbian Parenting,** 305
Sharon L. Sims

27 **The Gifted Child,** 309
Theresa M. Eldridge

28 **The Addicted Infant,** 315
Phyllis K. Marion

29 **The Premature Infant,** 322
Barbara Jones Deloian

30 **The Stepfamily,** 331
Marty Witrak

31 **The Violent Family,** 335
Jane A. Fox

Section 3

Common Presenting Symptoms and Problems, 339

32 **Cardiovascular System,** 341
Kathleen Kenney

Chest Pain, 343

Congenital Heart Defects, 346

Heart Murmurs, 350

Hyperlipidemia, 353

Hypertension, 356

33 **Endocrine System,** 360
Jane A. Fox

Delayed Puberty, 363

Precocious Puberty, 365

Short Stature, 366

Thyroid Disorders, 369

34 **Eyes and Ears,** 373
Jane A. Fox and Amy Verst

Cerumen: Impacted or Excessive, 378
Jane A. Fox

Ear Pain and Discharge, 379
Jane A. Fox

Ear Trauma and Foreign Body, 386
Jane A. Fox

Hearing Changes or Loss, 387
Jane A. Fox

Blindness and Visual Impairment, 389
Amy Verst

Eye Deviations, 393
Amy Verst

Eye Injuries, 396
Amy Verst

Infections of the Eyelid and Orbit, 400
Amy Verst

Red Eye, 402
Amy Verst

35 **Gastrointestinal System,** 409
(Chapter overview by Catherine J. Dillon Dolan)

Abdominal Pain, 412
Marie Ann Marino and Susan M. DeVivio

Constipation and Fecal Impaction, 420
Jane A. Fox

Diarrhea and Loose Stool, 425
Catherine J. Dillon Dolan

Hernias: Inguinal, Scrotal, and Umbilical Bulges, 434
Arleen Nast Steckel

Infantile Colic, 441
Theresa M. Eldridge

Mouth Sores, 447
Elizabeth F. Gunhus

Nausea and Vomiting, 452
Jane A. Fox

Perianal Itch and Pain, 458
Jane A. Fox

Stool Odor, Color, and Consistency Changes, 462
Jane A. Fox

36 Hematologic System, 468
(Chapter overview by Jacqueline G. Ioli)

Anemia, 471
Jacqueline G. Ioli

Jaundice in the Newborn, 480
Jacqueline G. Ioli

Pallor, 483
Jennifer Piersma D'Auria

Petechiae and Purpura, 486
Jacqueline G. Ioli

37 Integumentary System, 490
*(Chapter overview by Jane A. Fox and
Lauren O'Connor Dempsey)*

Abscesses (Boils), 496
Loren O'Connor Dempsey

Acne, 499
Jane A. Fox

Birthmarks, 504
Jane A. Fox

Bites: Insect, Animal, and Human, 508
Jane A. Fox

Corns and Calluses, 513
Jane A. Fox

Diaper Rash, 514
Jane A. Fox

Hair Loss, 518
Victoria Vecchiariello

Heat Rash, 520
Victoria Vecchiariello

Hives (Urticaria), 521
Victoria Vecchiariello

Lice (Pediculosis), 522
Jane A. Fox

**Minor Trauma: Abrasions, Lacerations, Bruises,
and Puncture Wounds,** 525
Jane A. Fox

Nail Injury and Infection, 526
Loren O'Connor Dempsey

Rash, 528
Jane A. Fox

Scaly Scalp, 533
Victoria Vecchiariello

Sunburn, 535
Loren O'Connor Dempsey

Warts (Verrucae), 537
Loren O'Connor Dempsey

Weeping Lesions (Impetigo), 540
Victoria Vecchiariello

38 Musculoskeletal System, 544
Amy Verst

Athletic Injuries, 556

Back Pain, 559

Disturbance in Gait: Limp, 561

Disturbance in Gait: Toeing-In, 566

Foot Deformity and Pain, 568

Growing Pains, 569

Hip Pain and Click, 569

Joint Pain and Swelling, 570

Leg Deformity, 572

Spine Deformity, 574

39 Neuropsychiatric System, 576
(Chapter overview by Nancy E. Alfieri)

Depression, 584
Susan M. Watson

Headaches, 587
Barbara Golden

Large Head and Small Head, 590
Catherine Ascher

Seizures, Breath-Holding Spells, and Syncope, 595
Catherine Ascher

Suicide Attempts and Suicide, 605
Susan M. Watson

Tics, 607
Barbara Golden

40 Reproductive System, 611
(Chapter overview by Margaret A. McCabe)

Ambiguous Genitalia, 616
Margaret A. McCabe

Breast Masses and Changes, 616
Margaret A. McCabe

Genital Lesions, 618
Margaret A. McCabe

Menstrual Irregularities, 621
Linda C. Andrist

Penile Discharge, 625
Margaret A. McCabe

Penile Irritation, 627
Margaret A. McCabe

Pregnancy, 628
Katherine Simmonds

Undescended Testes (Cryptorchidism), 632
Margaret A. McCabe

Vulvovaginal Symptoms, 634
Margaret A. McCabe

41 **Respiratory System,** 642
Jennifer Piersma D'Auria

Breathing Difficulty, Stridor, and Wheezing, 645

Cough, 653

Nasal Bleeding (Epistaxis), 656

Nasal Congestion and Obstruction, 659

Sore Throat (Pharyngitis), 664

Voice Changes, 667

42 **Urinary System,** 670
Mikel Gray and Fern Campbell

Abdominal Mass, 675

Bladder and Urethral Anomalies, 676

Blood in the Urine (Hematuria), 677

Diurnal Incontinence and Altered Patterns of Urine Elimination, 679

Nocturnal Enuresis, 684

Painful Urination, 686

Protein in the Urine (Proteinuria), 690

43 **Nonspecific Complaints and Problems,** 694

Allergies, 694
Linda Gilman

Failure to Thrive, 699
Kathleen Kenney

Fever, 704
Jennifer Piersma D'Auria

Irritability, 710
Nancy E. Alfieri

Lymphadenopathy, 714
Kathleen Kenney

Obesity, 718
Elizabeth F. Gunhus

44 **Infectious Diseases,** 723
Nancy E. Kline

Diphtheria, 723

Fungal Infections (Superficial), 724

Influenza, 727

Lyme Disease, 728

Meningitis, 730

Mumps, 731

Parasitic Diseases, 731

Pertussis (Whooping Cough), 735

Poliovirus Infections, 737

Reye Syndrome, 738

Roseola, 738

Rubella (German Measles), 739

Rubeola (Measles), 740

Scabies, 741

Tetanus, 742

Tuberculosis, 743

Varicella-Zoster Virus, 745

Viral Hepatitis, 746

Section 4
Families with Children Requiring Long-Term Management, 749

45 **Diseases and Problems,** 751

Anorexia and Bulimia, 751
Mary E. Muscari

Asthma, 757
Marijo Ratcliffe

Cystic Fibrosis, 770
Suzanne Meghdadpour

Diabetes Mellitus, 778
John C. Kirchgessner

Hemophilia and Bleeding Disorders, 787
Jacqueline G. Ioli

Human Immunodeficiency Virus and Acquired Immune Deficiency Syndrome, 796
Susan Heffernan and Kathleen A. Shea

Neoplastic Disease, 815
Susan Dulczak and Marilyn J. Hockenberry

Rheumatic Fever, 826
Kathleen Kenney

Sickle Cell Anemia, 829
Jacqueline G. Ioli and Miriam Gilday

46 Developmental Difficulties, 841

Autism, 841
Stephanie Bonney

Cerebral Palsy, 844
Stephanie Bonney

Down Syndrome, 850
Stephanie Bonney

Duchenne (and Becker) Muscular Dystrophy, 856
Carolyn D. Farrell and Christina Trout

Developmental Difficulties, 862
Stephanie Bonney

Mental Retardation, 867
Stephanie Bonney

Spina Bifida, 869
Stephanie Bonney

47 Social Disorders, 877

Barbara A. Elliott and Christie Sandra Ehle Erickson

Fetal Alcohol Syndrome and Alcohol-Related Neurologic Disorder, 877

Lead Poisoning (Plumbism), 879

Physical Abuse and Neglect, 882

Poverty and Homelessness, 884

Sexual Abuse, Incest, and Rape, 886

Substance Abuse, 889

Section 5
Emergencies and Preparation for Hospitalization, 895

48 Managing Pediatric Emergencies in a Primary Care Setting, 897
Jane A. Fox

Acute Foreign-Body Aspiration (Choking), 897

Acute Hemorrhage, 898

Acute Respiratory Arrest, 898

Airway Obstruction, 899

Burn Injury, 900

Coma and Loss of Consciousness, 901

Frostbite, 902

Head Injury, 903

Hyperthermia, 904

Near Drowning, 904

Orthopedic Fractures, 906

Shock, 906

49 Preparation For Painful Procedures, Hospitalization, and Surgery, 908
Theresa M. Eldridge

Appendixes

A Growth Charts and Developmental Screening Tools, 917
Jane A. Fox

B Age-Appropriate Reference Chart for Well-Child Care Visits, 937
Barbara Jones Deloian

C Laboratory Tests, 946
Kathleen Kenney

D Radiologic Tests, 953
Ericka K. Leibold Waidley

E CPT and ICD-9 Codes, 961

F General Health, Pediatric, and Nurse Practitioner Internet Sites, 975
Jane A. Fox

G Telephone Triage and Protocols, 977
Susan M. Watson

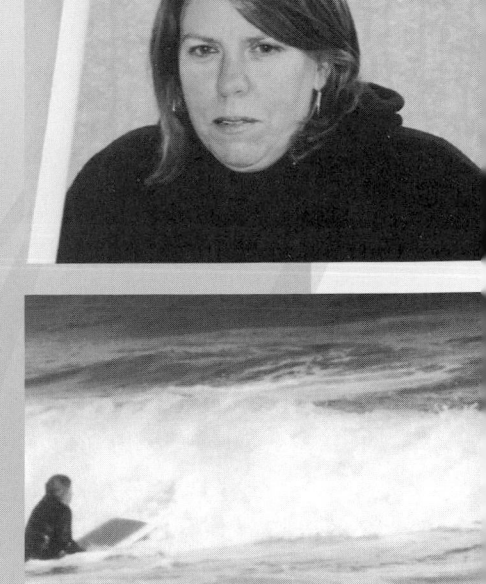

Section 1
Health Promotion and Well-Child Care

*I*n the 25 years that have passed since I graduated as a pediatric nurse practitioner (PNP), I have witnessed the profession grow in number and expand in scope of practice. Although much has changed for NPs, many issues remain unresolved, including autonomy, third-party reimbursement, and professional recognition.

I received my BSN from Cornell University, New York Hospital School of Nursing, after completing a BA in Communication Arts from a small women's college. After graduation I worked as a staff and home care nurse at New York Hospital. Next, I was hired as a pediatric nurse by the Community Health Program of Queens-Nassau, one of the very first health maintenance organizations (HMOs). While there I learned about the role of NP and was accepted into the PNP certification program at Babies Hospital Columbia Presbyterian Medical Center in New York City. This was a wonderful 12-month program developed by Dr. Catherine DeAngelis, a nurse and pediatrician. I continued my education at Columbia University Teachers College where I earned MA, MEd, and EdD degrees.

Over the years I have tried to combine academia and clinical practice. I have had faculty appointments at several universities including Pace University, C.W. Post Center Long Island University, and New York University. Presently I'm serving as a Clinical Associate Professor at the State University of New York at Stony Brook. My clinical practice has encompassed working as a PNP in various settings including a hospital-based clinic, a community-based clinic, an HMO, home care, a school-based clinic, and a privately-owned NP practice. In the past few years, I have participated as a PNP in short-term missions to the Dominican Republic and Guatemala, providing primary health care to children and families in the rural areas of these countries. Future trips are being planned for Cuba and El Salvador.

My first book, *Primary Health Care of the Young*, was published by McGraw-Hill in 1981. The first edition of *Primary Health Care of Children* was published by Mosby in 1997. In 2001, I coauthored *Pediatric Nurse Practitioner Certification Review* with Linda Gilman, a book also published by Mosby. In addition, I have contributed to other texts on the role of the NP. I have presented at various national conferences and am particularly interested in evidenced-based practice and documentation of clinical practice and the unique expertise of NPs. Over the past year I have been working to develop Fox Educational Systems, Inc., a company devoted to offering certification and other courses on-line for advanced practice nurses (APNs).

As I have crossed the half-century mark, I have taken up surfing and yoga. I live near the ocean and try to surf every day during the summer. Although I still struggle to stand up on the board, I am forging ahead and enjoying the challenge. I have a great husband named Jack and am an avid tennis player (much better at tennis than surfing) and animal lover (with two yellow labs). I also look forward to traveling on various medical missions to foreign countries in the future.

Jane A. Fox

Chapter 1 *Providing Primary Health Care to Children*

Linda Gilman & Virginia E. Richardson

Nurse Practitioner History

The first nurse practitioner (NP) program was developed and implemented at the University of Colorado School of Nursing in 1965. Dr. Henry Silver, a pediatrician in the School of Medicine, and Dr. Loretta Ford, a faculty member in the School of Nursing, were the forerunners of the NP movement. The initial program was designed to expand the role of nurses to provide access to health care for children and adolescents because of the shortage of pediatricians and physicians as providers of primary care. The nurses in their new role were to practice in private pediatricians' offices and in public health facilities in urban and rural low-income neighborhoods.

The initial program consisted of a 4-month course of intensive theory and practice in pediatric primary care at the University of Colorado Medical Center. Nurses increased their knowledge and skills in assessing and managing the well child. They were prepared to manage a variety of well, acute, and chronic disorders that together form the majority of problems seen in office practices. At the completion of the 4-month course, students were awarded a certificate. It was not until the 1980s that NP programs moved to the master's degree level. With the shift to graduate education, a more independent nursing role evolved as NPs provided health and illness care to children and adolescents and families. Most NPs now work collaboratively with physicians and other health care providers as primary care providers (PCPs). Many hold hospital privileges to provide inpatient services as well as outpatient primary health care services. Several states such as Alaska recognize the ability of NPs to practice independently. Other states (e.g., Utah) may require collaboration only with prescriptive authority. NPs now have title protection in all states, but licensure laws specific to NP licensure vary from state to state.

Certification

The trend has been to require the master's degree as the educational preparation level and national certification in the specialty area as entry requirements into NP practice. National certification for pediatric nurse practitioners (PNPs) is offered through two nursing organizations, the National Certification Board of Pediatric Nurse Practitioners and Nurses (NCBPNP/N) and the American Nurses Credentialing Center (ANCC). Certifying examinations are offered in such specialty areas as *family nurse practitioner, adult nurse practitioner,* and *women's health nurse practitioner*. Recertification involves proof of continuing education or a certification maintenance program. *Certified nurse practitioners* may use a *C* either in front of or behind their credentials. Some NPs may use the credential *advanced practice nurse* (APN). The term *APN* covers a broad category of APNs that includes the *clinical nurse specialist,*

certified nurse midwife, nurse anesthetist, and *nurse practitioner*. NPs, as APNs, have demonstrated themselves (through multiple studies) to be affordable, accessible, and cost effective and to deliver quality health care within their scope of practice and standard of care.

Multi-State Nurse Licensure Compact

The National Council of State Boards of Nursing in 1997 approved a proposal for a single licensing system in which nurses have one license and are permitted to practice in any state that is identified as a party to the compact state. States participating in the compact would require nurses to be licensed by their state of residence rather than the current situation in which nurses are licensed in the state where they practice. This type of licensure compact evolved because of the rapid expansion of services across state lines through multimedia communication technology. The stated goal of the compact is to facilitate a reduction in the barriers for nurses to practice in more than one state at the same time. For this type of licensure to work, all states need to have the same licensure standards and requirements to practice. A major concern for the compact is education and standards for practice in individual states that may be lower in some states than in others; this would lower the minimum licensure standards to the lowest common denominator.

Reimbursement and Billing

Reimbursement for health care services provided is dictated by federal, state, and local policies of insurers and managed care units. Some states allow NPs to be reimbursed by certain insurers; other states do not allow for or provide for NP reimbursement and do not designate NPs as providers. Reimbursement may be secured on an individual basis as provided by the policy of local insurance companies and managed care organizations.

The major means by which an NP is reimbursed for services rendered in a primary health care setting is *fee for service*. Fee schedules are based on a complex system such as the *Current Procedural Terminology* (CPT) and *International Classification of Disease* (ICD-9) codes, which were developed by the American Medical Association. Reimbursement services for fees using the CPT codes may vary from different locations and different providers. NPs may be reimbursed at 85% of the physician fee schedule under the Medicare program. Under a fee-for-service system, the more services that are provided, the more reimbursement is generated for the office practice. The billing for services rendered is based on a system of resources used. The system was developed by the Health Care Financing Administration (HCFA) and is known as the *relative based value scale* (RBVS), which is administered by Medicare. The components of RBVS are practice expenses, work performed, and malpractice insurance. The RBVS determines the amount Medicare will reimburse.

NPs working in a *rural health professional shortage area* and delivering health and medical services may be covered at the same rate as physicians. Billing is through a direct billing system such as a hospital, physician group practice, or rural clinic. The services are limited to those services legally authorized by the nurse practice act for the state in which the NP resides or practices.

Incidence to Service

Incidence to service is also referred to as *indirect billing* and is a term meaning billing for services furnished as an integral, though incidental, part of the physician's professional services in the course of diagnosis or treatment of an illness or injury. To qualify under this definition, nonphysician providers must render services under a physician's direct personal supervision and be employees of a physician or physician group. Services must be furnished during a course of treatment where a physician performs an initial service and subsequent services are frequent enough to indicate that the physician has active participation in the management of this patient.

Risk Management

Risk management is commonly defined as a style of practice that reduces the risk of legal liability by recognizing and avoiding problem areas in the delivery of primary health care. The process of minimizing the risk of liability should occur through implementing a practice based on standards of care and functioning within the scope of practice as defined by the discipline. A risk management program has three components: risk involving patients, risk involving personnel, and risk involving equipment. A risk management program should decrease the likelihood of exposure to a professional liability claim for the NP. If the program does not decrease or prevent a lawsuit, it should minimize the chance of liability.

The most effective way to decrease exposure to professional liability claims is the maintenance of a good relationship with the patient, parent, or child. Communication is the key. An explanation of proposed treatments, a diagnosis of conditions, and a description of the procedures indicated and the risks associated with each procedure are aspects known to decrease liability. In addition, the NP must communicate the expected outcomes when describing alternative courses of treatment, benefits, and risks.

As the health care industry is continually changing, NPs must practice risk management in their day-to-day practice to reduce the potential for professional liability claims.

Negligence and Malpractice Issues

NPs are accountable for their own actions in the delivery of health care. To determine whether conduct is negligent, a standard of care exists that describes what a reasonable, prudent NP would do in the same or similar circumstances. Negligence is the failure to act in accord with this standard of care. An NP who deviates from the acceptable standard of nursing practice may be found negligent and thus liable for harm.

Failure to obtain consent for a given treatment leaves the NP open for battery. *Battery* by definition is the absence of consent for the NP to touch a child.

The NP must conform to the concept of *duty to consult*. This concept is described as the NP recognizing that a health or medical situation is beyond the NP's skill, knowledge, or scope of practice. The NP is obligated to consult with a health care provider who has expertise and knowledge of the condition in question. Without consultation, the NP is practicing outside the *scope and standard of practice*.

Failure to refer is a concept based in all health care professions and may result in negligence. Failure to refer is when the NP fails to refer a patient to a health care provider when the condition or situation falls outside the NP's scope or standard of practice. The duty to refer arises when the NP discovers that the treatment is beyond the NP's existing skill or knowledge.

A *tort* is a civil wrongdoing, a breach of a standard of care. A tort might not be deemed a crime, but it is an event that is severe enough to make the wrongdoer financially liable for injuries suffered by the victim. The most common kind of tort is *negligence,* in which a failure to meet a duty of care occurs; this failure must result in injury or harm sustained by the victim for a civil action to occur. *Respondeat superior* ("let the master answer") is a legal doctrine in which an employer is responsible for torts committed by an employee while the employee is acting in the course and scope of employment.

Written policies, procedures, and protocols provide for documentation of the appropriate standard of care that indicates when to consult and refer. Policies, procedures, and protocols must be continually updated and be realistic to the situation. They are essential documents that outline what a reasonable and prudent NP would do in a similar situation to prevent professional liability. In a lawsuit, the breach of a standard of care is an essential issue.

Vicarious liability is a legal term in which an NP may be legally responsible for the action of others if the NP has employed the other health care–related employees. The NP is liable for failure to properly supervise the care given. An example would be the incorrect administration of immunizations by a medical assistant.

Personal Malpractice Insurance

NPs purchase professional liability insurance to provide protection against payments of judgments and legal expenses if a claim for professional negligence should occur. Liability insurance covers the NP in a case of injury (tort) resulting in a lawsuit. It also shifts the risk of liability from the NP to the insurance company for defense purposes; the insurance carrier provides both an attorney to represent the NP's defense and financial coverage in the event that a court decision awards fault or injury.

Elements of malpractice that must be proved by the plaintiff include:
- The NP owed the plaintiff a duty, and that duty was not adequately performed.
- The NP conducted the delivery of care, and that delivery of care fell below the standard of care.
- The NP failed the duty to consult as a result of this action or conduct, and an injury to the plaintiff occurred.

There are two types of professional liability insurance policies: occurrence policies and claims-made policies. *Occurrence policies* provide for coverage of events of alleged malpractice that occur during the effective period of the policy. *Claims-made policies* provide coverage only for those claims actually filed during the policy period. *Tail coverage* may be needed to cover the risk for the period not covered by the policy.

Whistle-blower laws are laws that provide protection to those who speak out about patient care issues. Federal legislation is in process to offer additional protection.

Scope and Standards of Practice, and Nurse Practice Acts

Scope of practice documents are an outgrowth of the standards of practice. The *scope of practice* specifies activities that govern the services provided to patients, whereas the standards cover qualifications, process of care, the environment in which the care is delivered, collaborative responsibilities, documentation of care provided, quality assurance, and research. In general, the NP role is to provide primary health care services to individuals, families, and groups of patients that is characterized by an emphasis on health promotion, disease prevention, and risk reduction. The role involves diagnosis and management of common acute illnesses or injuries and stable chronic diseases. Key components of the NP role involve educating and counseling individuals and their families regarding healthful lifestyle behaviors. The NP's scope of practice traditionally includes these main categories: assessment of health status, collaboration, diagnosis, referral, and case management.

NPs are responsible for recognizing the limits of their knowledge and experience and practicing within the scope of practice based on their specialty certification. *Consultation* and *referral* are an integral part of the scope of practice statement. Scope of practice may be defined by the state legislature. Many state legislatures incorporate the scope of practice and standards of practice from the discipline into the practice acts or administrative law.

The term *expanded role of the nurse* is in many state nurse practice acts. The expanded role definition tends to mean a process of role change in the health care system. The authority for expansion rests on the body of knowledge that constitutes the nurse's preparation for practice; the expanded role requires specialized knowledge, judgment, and skill but may not require or permit medical diagnosis. Inherent in the definition of advanced practice is the use of independent judgment and collaboration with other health care professionals when indicated.

Collaboration, as outlined in the state practice acts, varies from state to state, and states indicate if collaboration is required. If a collaboration agreement is required or if activities are legally delegated by a physician or must be directly supervised by a physician, this agreement is usually adopted through rules and regulation of the respective state in which the nurse resides. NPs should review the language of the state nurse practice act regarding their scope of practice. Qualifications to practice as an NP vary from state to state and may include a master's degree or national certification.

Managed Care and Insurance

The health care industry and the insurance industry have changed and evolved over the past decade to control health care costs. A *managed care organization* is a health care organization that provides or finances medical care using a provider payment mechanism that encourages cost containment and imposes control on the utilization of health care services. Managed care organizations employ a network of providers, physicians, and NPs to provide these health care services. Managed care organizations should provide accessible, affordable, quality health care for members; however, reports have surfaced about denial of necessary care, underfunding of public health and preventive services, lack of accountability, members losing their choice of health care providers, inadequate access to specialist care, abuses in marketing health care plans, and lack of consumer information about health care plans.

One type of managed care organization is the *health maintenance organization* (HMO), a prepaid system of health and illness benefits. An HMO combines financing and delivery of health and illness care for patients enrolled in the organization. In HMOs, NPs may sit on the provider panel and be designated as PCPs; they have demonstrated the ability to move patients through the managed care system (with consideration for both cost and consumer satisfaction) while still providing quality health care.

Indemnity insurance carriers pay for services rendered but do not provide for those services. Indemnity insurance carriers have fee schedules based on what "reasonable and customary" charges should be. If the fee is more than what the insurance carrier considers reasonable and customary, the patient is responsible for the difference.

Preferred provider organizations (PPOs) are systems of hospitals and network providers receiving a predetermined rate of reimbursement for a patient's health and medical services. There are incentives in place to encourage patients to use providers on the PPO list. When patients use providers outside of those in the PPO network, higher copayments for services are charged.

Capitation is a fee paid to a health care provider each month for each patient in a specific health plan. Capitated fees for primary care services typically vary from $5 to $35 per member per month. The federal health insurance Medicaid is an example of capitation, but how Medicaid is implemented at the state level varies and is determined by each state.

Utilization Review

Utilization review is a procedure designed to evaluate the necessity, appropriateness, and efficacy of the use of medical services and facilities. The challenge for utilization review is to ensure that decisions made concerning patients are based on clinical, not financial, reasons. An NP's role in the utilization process is in the areas of health education, wellness, risk reduction, and prevention of disease.

Prescriptive Authority

Prescriptive authority is granted to an NP by the state in which the NP practices. States have various administrative rules and regulations (through nurse practice acts) that allow NPs to prescribe medications, and depending on the individual state, there may be limited authority subject to medical supervision. Some states have a formulary that identifies drugs that NPs may prescribe and under what conditions they may prescribe them (e.g., a practice agreement between the physician and the NP).

Tele-Health/Medicine

Tele-health/medicine is the use of computer technology, video conferencing, telecommunication, and other new technologies in response to the health care needs of rural America and the world. The increasing computerization of health data has created vast opportunities to expand services to medically underserved populations and improve their access to health care. Tele-health/medicine may be as simple as two health professionals discussing a case over the phone or as sophisticated as using satellite technology to broadcast a consultation between providers at facilities in two countries using video conferencing equipment or two-way interactive television.

There are many advantages to the use of tele-health/medicine. It makes specialty care more accessible to underserved rural and urban populations, and it is projected to cut the cost of medical care for those in rural areas, since travel to larger areas with the needed health services may be prohibitive.

Barriers to the practice of tele-health/medicine are associated with licensure, insurance rules, and privacy of information. Many states will not allow out-of-state providers to practice unless licensed in that state, and some private insurers will not reimburse for services performed outside a given state. The Health Care Financing Administration (HCFA) reimburses for teleradiology and telepathology but not for specialty consultation for patients receiving Medicare benefits. Licensure is also of concern, since a provider is frequently not licensed in the state in which a patient resides. Licensure across state lines in the United States continues to be of concern as the health industry expands in the area of computerized medicine.

The Telecommunication Reform Act of 1996 allows rural education and health care networks to be connected and have rates similar to those charged in urban areas. Many tele-health/medicine projects have been awarded federal funds to help pay for the installation of telephone lines, wiring, or other necessary access equipment for rural areas. In the future, this form of consultation will be just another way to "visit" a health professional.

Federal Health Programs

Federal health programs began in 1912 with the creation of the Children's Bureau, and Title V legislation was enacted by Congress in 1935 as part of the Social Security Act. Title V is the only federal legislation dedicated to promoting and improving the health of the nation's mothers and children. Major changes and developments have occurred over the years; however, the aim of the legislation has not changed.

Medicaid (Title XIX)

Medicaid (Title XIX) was enacted in 1965 as part of the Social Security Act. It is a federal and state matching entitlement program (an insurance program) that pays for medical assistance for vulnerable and needy individuals and families with low incomes. It is a joint cooperative venture between federal and state governments to assist the states in furnishing such medical assistance. Medicaid contains provisions for categorically needy eligible groups, such as individuals eligible for the Aid Families Dependent Children (AFDC) program; children under 6 years of age whose family's income is at or below 133% of the federal poverty level (FPL); pregnant women whose family income is below 133% of the FPL; recipients of adoption or foster care assistance under Title IV of the Social Security Act; special protected groups; all children born after September 30, 1983 who

are under the age of 19 years; and families with incomes at or below the FPL. The program is a "phase in coverage," so that by the year 2002 all poor children under 19 years of age will be covered; certain Medicare beneficiaries may be included. States have the option of including coverage for other categorically related groups such as special-needs children.

Services under state Medicaid programs generally include:
- Inpatient services
- Outpatient services
- Prenatal care
- Vaccines for children
- Physician services
- Rural health clinic services
- Laboratory and x-ray services
- Early and periodic screening, diagnostic, and treatment services (EPSDT) for children under 21 years of age

Special Supplemental Nutrition Program for Women, Infants, and Children

The Special Supplemental Nutrition Program is commonly referred to as the *Women, Infants, and Children (WIC) program* and is administered by the Department of Agriculture through state health departments. It provides money to states for supplemental foods, health care referral, and nutritional education for low-income pregnant, breastfeeding, and non-breastfeeding postpartum women and to infants and children who are found to be nutritionally at risk. The WIC program provides participants with supplemental foods, nutrition education and counseling, nutrition screening, and referrals to welfare and social services.

Eligibility is based on family income at or below 185% of the FPL guidelines or can be determined automatically if patients are eligible for such programs as Medicaid, food stamps, or temporary assistance for needy families. Nutritional risk is determined by a health professional. Other food programs such as the Child and Adult Care Food Program provide meals and snacks to children in eligible day care centers and to school lunch and breakfast programs for low-income children at a reduced price or for free. The Summer Food Service Program offers free meals and snacks to needy children during the months when school is not in session

School Lunch Program

The National School Lunch, School Breakfast, and Special Milk Program was authorized in 1966. It provides cash and commodity assistance to help schools to make nutritious, low-cost or free meals and milk available to all school children. To qualify for free or reduced-cost meals, households must be at or below 130% of the FPL guidelines. A school can obtain information directly from the local food stamp program, and those families receiving food stamps are automatically eligible for free meals or milk.

Children's Health Insurance Program

The Children's Health Insurance Program (CHIP) program (Title XXI) provides funding to states to develop comprehensive health insurance coverage for children not covered by Medicaid or employer-sponsored health insurance. It began as part of the Balanced Budget Act of 1997, in which Congress provided states the opportunity to expand health care coverage for children living at up to 200% of the FPL. This 5-year program offered states the flexibility to design their own children's health insurance program at an enhanced federal match rate of $2 to every $1 the states provided.

Family Planning Grants (Title X)

These grants, furnished through the Social Security Act, provide funds for comprehensive family planning and reproductive health. This legislation and funding is important for adolescent and young adults, since the funding provides for services frequently not provided for by health care providers

Title XX of the Social Security Block Grant

This grant provides funds for but not limited to child care services, protective services for children, foster care for children, services related to managing and maintaining home care, transportation, family plan services, mental retardation, physical handicap, and emotionally handicapped children.

Head Start is a child development program that has served low-income children and their families since 1965. Children between 3 and 5 years of age from families that meet the FPL guidelines are eligible for the services. There is a requirement that 10% of Head Start enrollments be offered to children with disabilities. Early Head Start programs are available to serve low-income pregnant women and families with infants and toddlers. This program is an extension of Head Start.

Clinical Laboratory Improvement Amendments

The Clinical Laboratory Improvement Amendments (CLIA) have most recently been transferred from Communicable Disease Control (CDC) to the Federal Drug Administration (FDA). Beginning in 1988, CLIA has set standards designed to improve the quality of laboratory testing; included in the CLIA standards are quality control, quality assurance, and personnel and proficiency testing. CLIA standards apply to all laboratory testing, even if basic tests are performed as part of the physical examination. Some simple tests (e.g., urine dipstick, spun hematocrit) may be waived, though if tests are to be waived, there needs to be a certificate of waiver to exempt the tests from specific CLIA requirements. Proficiency testing is required for all personnel who perform the testing.

Food Stamps

The Food Stamp Program is authorized under the Food Stamp Act of 1977 and administered by the United States Department of Agriculture (USDA). The program helps low-income families purchase food. Households meeting the income and resource standard set forth by the USDA may purchase food stamps or an electronic benefit card that can be used like cash at most grocery stores. The program is operated through local county government offices. The USDA gives as much as $122 a month in food stamps to a person living alone or having no income. Households with more than one person receive less for each person; for example, a household of four persons could receive up to $408 a month. It is projected that a household should use about 30% of their income for food. Families do not need to be U.S. citizens to be eligible to receive food stamps.

Maternal and Child Health Services Block Grant (Title V)

This grant provides for funding to states for prenatal care for women and primary and preventive care for children. It has as a general purpose the improvement of the health of mothers and children in keeping with the national health objectives established by the Public Health Service Act for the year 2010. The Title V Block Grant Program requires that every $4 of federal Title V money must be matched by at least $3 of state and local money. The program also requires that a minimum of 30% of federal money be used to support services for children with special health care needs and to provide preventive and primary care services for children. State maternal and child health programs are usually housed in state departments of health and meet the Title V Block grant responsibilities by offering a wide range of programs with specific goals. One such goal is to reduce morbidity and mortality by ensuring that pregnant women, infants, children, and adolescents have full access to good-quality, community-based preventive and primary care. Other significant activities supported by a Title V Block Grant would be genetic services and hemophilia diagnostic and treatment centers.

Civilian Health and Medical Program Uniformed Services

TRICARE is the government's health insurance program for all seven of the uniformed services. Eligibility for TRICARE/CHAMPUS is determined by the individual services, and members must be enrolled in the Defense Enrollment Eligibility Reporting System. Members on active duty, their families, retirees, and retirees' families and survivors may participate in at least one of the three TRICARE options. Military personnel are required to go to military hospitals if the service is available. If the patient lives 40 miles from a military hospital and the hospital does not have the needed services, patients may be referred to a civilian hospital.

The three TRICARE options for health care are:
1. TRICARE Prime (an HMO)
2. TRICARE Standard (previously known as CHAMPUS)
3. TRICARE Extra (the Department of Defense Preferred Provider Pool)

Public Law 94-142

Public Law 94-142, the Education for Handicapped Children Act (commonly known as the *Mainstreaming Law*), is a federal law passed in 1975 and reauthorized in 1990 that mandates all children receive a free and appropriate public education regardless of the level of severity of their disability. The law requires states to complete an Individual Education Plan (IEP) based on the unique needs of a child in the least restrictive environment possible, and there is a due process procedure to ensure that the child's needs are adequately met. School districts must test the child to assess the actual ability of sensory, motor, or language impairment. A multidisciplinary team evaluates the abilities and develops an IEP. This becomes a legal document that describes the special education and related services to be provided to the child or student. The local school district is then responsible for the implementation of the IEP.

Public Law 101-476

Public Law 101-476, known as the *Individuals with Disabilities Education Act* (IDEA), is a federal law that encourages states to provide educational opportunities for all children, from birth to 21 years of age, with disabilities. Services such as speech therapy, physical therapy, medical services, counseling and training of parents, transportation, psychologic care, social work, and fair assessment of disabled children are covered. A nondiscriminatory educational evaluation must be done before a child receives educational services and at least every 3 years thereafter. (Though not initially covered, infants and toddlers were included through Public Law 99-457. This legislation expands the opportunity for and benefits of early intervention for preschool services to support families with infants and toddlers with disabilities.)

Research

The primary research areas in NP practice have been research utilization and the comparison of NP and physician clinical practice. The use of research through utilization by NPs has influenced thinking, clinical decisions, knowledge about disease processes, and the application of the scientific process in delivering health care.

Early research studies in primary care found that NPs provided an equivalent quality of care to that provided by physicians. The results of these studies describe relationships and processes but not causes of relationships with patients and families. Researched focus areas involving an NP's practice include productivity, resources used, decision making, patient satisfaction, and burnout. Traditional measures of outcome research have been morbidity and mortality, length-of-stay rates in hospitals, rates of hospital readmissions, and complications of illness. These studies have yet to capture the contributions NPs have made in primary health care. The future of research should be the outcomes of care and services delivered by NPs. This will allow NPs to focus on higher quality care and service and to influence health policy through existing credible data. NPs use the scientific method of identifying the presence of a problem or knowledge need and searching and evaluating the existing literature to determine if there is adequate data for research. If there is insufficient existing research, an NP would consult with experts in the field of interest (e.g., physiology, social science) for the appropriate theory data base. Formulating a research design, collecting and analyzing data, and interpreting the results are the remaining steps in the investigation of a problem or knowledge need in NP practice.

Evidence-Based Practice

Evidence-based practice is the application of the best available research evidence to identify clinical problems; it uses published research of random controlled trials and meta-analysis. It also involves tracking the best external evidence with which to answer a clinical question. Evidence-based practice is not restricted to using research; the emphasis is on dissemination of information so that the research results may be used in clinical practice. Decisions are made by practitioners, who use available evidence to determine what interventions are appropriate to specific clinical situations. Clinical decision making is a key component of the practice of evidence-based nursing. Evidence-based practice begins with asking an expert for help, checking references, finding relevant articles, and using a database bibliography to identify or solve clinical questions. There are times the necessary evidence will come from the basic sciences (e.g., genetics, immunology). Currently, the Agency for Health Care Practice is gathering data regarding the use of evidence-based practice for dissemination to clinical practitioners.

Healthy People 2010

The first set of national public health goals was described in 1979 in *Healthy People: The Surgeon General's Report on Health Promotion and Disease.* This report set the target for the health status to be achieved in five major stages of life: infants (below 1 year of age), children (1 to 14 years), adolescents and young adults (15 to 24 years), adults (25 to 64 years), and older adults (65 years of age and older). It was clear that the age groups faced very different issues as primary determinants of their health.

Healthy People 2010 is an extension of the national prevention initiative to improve the health status of all Americans. This new draft has continued many of the objectives from the earlier *Healthy People* document. In fact, 138 objectives were maintained, 96 objectives were revised, and 297 new objectives were introduced. New areas include school health, health provider activities, and worksite health. Broad goals in the new draft include an increase in the lifespan of Americans, reduction of disparities among Americans, and achievement of access to preventive services for all Americans. This document is the most comprehensive public health document of its kind in the United States and provides a framework for measuring performance outcomes. It is a strategic management tool for the federal and state governments, communities, and private sector partners. Success is measured by positive changes in health status or risk reduction, as well as improved provisions of health services. States have been active in developing public health goals for their citizens to mirror the national goals.

Clinical Practice Guidelines

Clinical practice guidelines define a standard of care. These guidelines represent the highest practice standard based on current and extensive scientific research and other available evidence. However, clinical practice guidelines cannot take into consideration every variable in a clinical situation a patient may encounter, and the guidelines may not be appropriate for every patient with a clinical diagnosis.

Providers must clearly document why any variation from a practice guideline is appropriate and in a patient's best interest. An example of this type of variation would be the use of a specific antibiotic not listed as an option in the treatment for a specific diagnosis. Clinical practice guidelines must be updated annually (more often if appropriate). Guidelines should include documentation of interventions or instructions, patient understanding of the recommended treatment, and when or if referral is indicated. These guidelines should involve conscientious, planned, judicious use of state-of-the-art practice and research to assist providers in making clinical decisions about the health care of patients. Clinical practice guidelines must also be signed and dated by all practice providers.

Resources

Websites

Advance (www.advancefornp.com)
American Academy of Nurse Practitioners (www.aanp.org)
American College of Nurse Practitioners (www.nurse.org/acnp/)
American Nurses Credentialing Center
      (www.nursingworld.org/ancc)
Evidence-Based Practice Centers of the Agency for Healthcare Research and Quality (www.ahcpr.gov/clinic/epc/)
Medscape Nursing (www.medscape.com/nursing)
National Association of Pediatric Nurse Associates and Practitioners (www.napnap.org)
National Certification Board of Pediatric Nurse Practitioners and Nurses (NCBPNP/N) (www.pnpcert.org)
N.P. Central (www.nurse.net.np)
University of Sheffield (www.shef.ac.uk)

Bibliography

American Academy of Pediatrics, Committee on Bioethics. (1995). Informed consent, parental permission and assent in pediatric practice. *Pediatrics, 95,* 314-317.

Baucher, H. (1999). Evidence-based medicine: A new science or an epidemiologic fad? *Pediatrics, 103,* 1029-1031.

Buppert, C. (2000). Measuring outcomes in primary care practice. *The Nurse Practitioner, 25*(1), 88-98.

Buppert, C. (1999). Legal scope of nurse practitioner practice. *Nursing Management, 8,* 5-9.

Buppert, C. (1999). Nurse practitioner's business practice and legal guide. Gaithersburg, MD: Aspen.

Buppert, C. (1998). Reimbursement for nurse practitioner services. *The Nurse Practitioner, 23,* 69-81.

Burns, M., Moores, P., & Breslin, E. (1996). Outcome research: Contemporary issues and historical significance for nurse practitioners. *Journal of the American Academy of Nurse Practitioners, 8,* 107-112.

Gardner, S. & Hagedorn, M. (1997). *Legal aspects of maternal child nursing practice,* Menlo Park, CA: Addison-Wesley.

Haas, S. (2000). Update on multistate licensure. *Focus on the Federation: National Federation for Specialty Nursing Organizations Newsletter,* 10.

Hill, D.T., Cohen, S.S., & Mason, D.J. (1998). Managed care for NPs. *The Nurse Practitioner. 24,* 15-16.

McKibbon, A. (1999). *PDQ: Evidence-based principles and practice.* St Louis, MO (Hamilton, Ont.): B.C. Decker.

Melnyk, B., Stone, P., Fineout-Overhold, E., & Ackerman, M. (2000). Evidence-based practice: The past, the present, and recommendations for the millennium. *Pediatric Nursing, 26*(1), 77-80.

Sharp, N. (1998). From "incident" to telehealth: New federal rules and regulations. *The Nurse Practitioner 24,* 68-69.

Talbott, S.W. & Leavitt, J.K. (1999). *Policy and Politics for Nurses: Action and change in the workplace, government; organization and the community* (3rd ed.), 349-383. Philadelphia: W.B. Saunders.

Werk, L.N., Bauchner, H., & Chessare, J. (1999). Medicine for the millennium: Demystifying EBM. *Contemporary Pediatrics, 16*(12), 87-107.

Chapter 2 *Children and Families: Models for Assessment and Intervention*

Anne Marie C. Levac, Lorraine M. Wright, & Maureen Leahey

The family is considered to have the most profound and lasting influence on a child's development and subsequent life cycle. When the identified patient is a child, it is imperative that practitioners embrace the concept that "illness and health concerns are a family affair," thereby including the child's family in health care discussions and practices. When families are viewed as the unit of care, practitioners may better understand the child's needs and devise interventions to promote positive and desired change both within the child and the family and between practitioners and families. Wright and Leahey (2000) recommend the following:

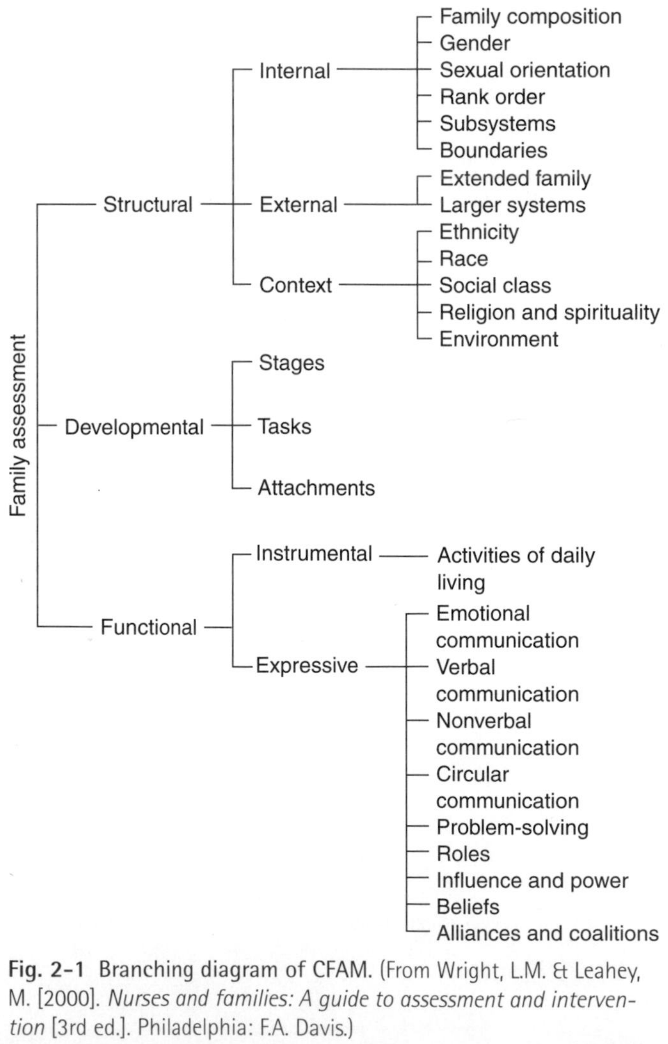

- The nursing of families should focus on the whole family system (versus its individual parts), relationships, patterns, and interactions.
- When practitioners "think interactionally," they raise the delivery of health care from an individual to a family (interactional) level. They are also are able to conceptualize and respond to the effect of a health problem or illness on the family *and* the effect of the family on the health problem or illness.
- The practitioner-family relationship has a significant influence on the child and the family's functioning.

This chapter describes and applies Wright and Leahey's Calgary Family Assessment Model (CFAM) (Fig. 2-1) and Calgary Family Intervention Model (CFIM) to families with children experiencing health problems. These models provide a systematic framework for working with families.

Theoretical Foundations for the Calgary Family Assessment and Intervention Models

Drawing from systems, cybernetics, communication and change theory, as well as postmodernism and a theory of biology, Wright and Leahey (2000) outline a theoretical foundation for assessing and intervening with families:

- Individuals are best understood within their larger context, which is usually the family.
- A circular/systemic perspective guides the practitioner to understand the reciprocity between family relationships and health status. Unlike a linear perspective, which focuses on the individual, the circular/systemic perspective emphasizes relationships and the reciprocal effects that individuals have on each other.
- A change in one family member affects all others. For instance, a child's diagnosis of "attention deficit disorder" affects the parent-child relationships as well as other family subsystems, such as sibling, marital, and possibly extended family relationships. It also affects community relationships, such as the family-school relationship.
- All form of communication is relevant. There is no such thing as not communicating—silence *is* communication.
- Reality is subjective, not fixed or true, and cannot be imposed. Therefore each family member's perspective is

Fig. 2-1 Branching diagram of CFAM. (From Wright, L.M. & Leahey, M. [2000]. *Nurses and families: A guide to assessment and intervention* [3rd ed.]. Philadelphia: F.A. Davis.)

valid and legitimate and deserves to be heard. Negative labels such as *dysfunctional family, noncompliant patient,* or *resistant mother* are observer (subjective) perspectives and are disrespectful of families. They do not stimulate thoughts of how to help families change. Rather, they inhibit creativity.

- Practitioners are not change agents but rather facilitators of change. By creating a context of collaboration and mutual trust with families, the knowledge, expertise, and strengths of both the practitioner and family are honored and exemplified (Leahey & Harper-Jaques, 1996).

Family Assessment

Family is "who the family say they are" (Wright & Leahey, 2000). Family assessment is a continuous process of evaluating patterns of interaction between family members relevant to the child's health issue or problem; it is an organized framework for conceptualizing and documenting observable or reported family data.

Indications

Whenever a child or adolescent is the identified patient or whenever a family is experiencing emotional, physical, or spiritual disruption related to developmental or situational crises, family assessment is needed.

Goal

The goal is to assess family structure, development, and functioning and identify family strengths as they relate to the health problem. Specific family nursing interventions are then formulated to effect the desired changes.

Planning

Before initiating a family assessment the practitioner needs to:
- Ascertain the purpose and benefit of a family assessment from the family's perspective.
- Explain why a family assessment may be beneficial to the family.
- Determine who in the family agrees that a problem exists and who might be willing to come to a family meeting.
- Mutually determine with the family when and where a meeting could take place (e.g., home, office, school).
- Read literature about working with families experiencing similar health problems to better understand the issues, concerns, and lived experiences of that specific population.

- Begin to formulate hypotheses (explanations about the family's behaviors that connect the family system and the particular problem).
- Prepare linear and circular questions that will elicit relevant data about family structure, development, and functioning. (See the discussions of CFAM and CFIM in this chapter for examples of questions.)

Engagement

Engagement is the first stage in developing a therapeutic relationship with a family, and it begins with the first contact, whether it is in person or by telephone.

Engagement has several purposes:
- To promote a positive practitioner-family relationship by developing an atmosphere of comfort, mutual trust, cooperation, and collaboration between the practitioner and the family
- To recognize that the family members bring strengths and resources to this relationship that may have previously gone unnoticed by health care practitioners
- To prevent potential practitioner-family misunderstandings or problems later on in the therapeutic relationship

Important *ABCs* for the engagement of families with children are outlined in Table 2-1.

The following are examples of questions used to promote engagement and provide an implicit message to the family that the practitioner cares about them and to give the family an opportunity to voice concerns or clarify expectations:
- Can you tell me about any past experiences that you have had with health care professionals?
- If you become frustrated with our work, would you be open to having a conversation with me about your concerns?
- On a scale of 1 to 10 (with 1 being very low and 10 being very high), how well do you think I understand your situation?
- In what ways was our discussion useful to each of you?

The following are examples of questions that the practitioner may ask himself or herself as a means of promoting and maintaining engagement with the family through self-awareness within the therapeutic relationship:
- In what ways am I creating a safe, collaborative, and therapeutic culture for the child or children and the family?
- How well am I adjusting the conversation to the developmental stages of the child or children in the family and balancing "adult talk" with "child talk"?

Table 2-1 The ABCs of Engaging Families

A	B	C
Assume an active, confident approach.	Begin by providing structure to the meeting (e.g., time frame, orientation to the context).	Create a context of mutual trust.
Ask purposeful questions that draw forth family assessment data.		Clarify expectations about your role within the family.
Address all who are present, including small children.	Behave in a curious manner and take an equal interest in all family members, whether present or not.	Collaborate in decision making, health promotion, and health management.
Adjust the conversation to children's developmental stages.	Build upon family strengths by offering commendations to the family.	Cultivate a context of racial and ethnic sensitivity.
	Bring relevant resources to the meeting (e.g., list of agencies, phone numbers, pamphlets).	Commend family members.

- How am I inviting family members' ideas, opinions, and concerns and coevolving mutually agreed-upon goals with them?
- To what extent am I routinely conveying to the family my perceptions of their strengths?

Calgary Family Assessment Model

Wright and Leahey's CFAM is a comprehensive, multidimensional framework that assists practitioners in collecting, organizing, and categorizing observational and family reported data. CFAM includes three major categories—structural, developmental, and functional—and several subcategories (see Fig. 2-1). Because each family is unique, a practitioner may sometimes need to assess some subcategories in more depth than others.

It is important to recognize that a family assessment is based on the practitioner's perspective; thus it is influenced by the practitioner's experience and history. It should not be considered *the* truth about the family but rather as one perspective at a particular point in time.

Structural family assessment. Structural family assessment explores who is in the family and the connections between family members and between the family and the community. It comprises three dimensions: internal structure, external structure, and context.

Internal structure. Family composition refers to who is a member of the family. There are many family forms besides the two-parent nuclear family (e.g., single-parent families, adoptive families, gay families, stepfamilies). Significant changes in family composition over time need to be assessed because these changes may affect family functioning. It is also important to explore losses by death and the nature of any lost relationship, especially if the death occurred as a result of violence.

Gender plays a significant role in family relationships and child and family health care. Family roles are often gender based, and gender differences in relation to parent roles with an ill child may exist. For example, most health care concerns and referrals are made by mothers, and they tend to assume stronger caregiving responsibilities than fathers. Assessment of gender is particularly important when there are societal, cultural, or family beliefs about male and female roles that are creating family stress.

Sexual orientation refers to gay, lesbian, heterosexual, transsexual, and bisexual relationships. It is important to assess how family members respond to differences in sexual orientation that may exist within the family. In much the same way, a practitioner needs to reflect on his or her own attitudes toward sexual orientation, particularly being attentive to any discrimination, stereotyping, and insensitivity toward others whose sexual orientation may be different.

Rank order refers to the position of children with respect to age and gender. Generally, firstborn children are expected to become more responsible earlier than children who hold the youngest child position in the family. Assessment of rank order may provide hypotheses about parental expectations of children at various family life-cycle stages.

Subsystems are parts of larger systems. Every system can be divided into subsystems. The larger sociocultural context may comprise smaller subsystems, such as school, community, child protective services, church, and so on. The two-parent nuclear family system can be divided into subsystems such as the marital, parental, and sibling subsystems. An important

question is: What subsystem is most affected by this problem and how?

Boundary relates to family rules about who participates in the family system and how they participate. Boundaries can be very closely and richly connected at the expense of individual autonomy, or they can be diffuse, ambiguous (unclear and confusing), or clear. Assessment of the boundaries between parents and children may be particularly useful when one is assessing child rearing–related concerns.

Box 2-1 provides possible questions to ask to gather information about internal structure.

External structure. Extended family comprises the family of origin, the family of procreation, the present generation, and steprelatives. Special relationships and social support systems may exist within these relationships, even at a great geographical distance. Conflictual and painful relationships may also exist within the extended family, creating intrafamilial stress. Assessment of the extended family and its contact and type of

---

Box 2-1 Examples of Questions to Assess Internal Structure

Family Composition

Who do you consider to be in your family? Are there any family members who don't live with you or who are not blood related that you would consider to be "family"? Has anyone recently entered or left your family?

Gender

How do you respond to Allison differently than to Daniel when both come in late for their curfew? How did it come to be that Mother would assume more responsibility for the tube feedings than Father?

Sexual Orientation

When your sister told your parents that she was a lesbian, how did they respond? How has your relationship with your son changed since he revealed that he is gay?

Rank Order

Starting from the eldest, could you tell me the names and ages of your children? If Francois were the youngest child instead of the eldest, how might your expectations of him be different? When Hank moved in with his kids and you suddenly became the youngest child in the house, how did it feel?

Subsystems

Parent-child—How has your relationship with Dacarla changed since her diagnosis of learning disability?
Marital—How much couple time is set aside each week that does not involve discussing the children?
Sibling—On a scale of 1 to 10, with 10 being the happiest, how happy are you to have a new baby brother?
To parent—How does Hector show his happiness about being a big brother?

Boundary

Who is the boss at your house? Whose job is it to implement the rules, your mom's or your older sister's? When your big brother drinks, does your dad get mad or does he drink with him?

relationship with the family can provide a practitioner with insight about the quality and quantity of family support systems.

Larger systems refer to systems outside the family system, such as the practitioner's office or clinic, school, child-protective services, the women's shelter, the place of parental employment, and church. The use of computer networks and the Internet as a larger system can positively or negatively influence family functioning. Family relationships with larger systems may range from unclear or unstable to quite clear, stable, and helpful. Therefore these relationships must be assessed to understand family behavior in this context. Practitioners should assess their relationships with the family because they are a "larger system" (i.e., the health care system) in relation to the family and need to avoid potential family-practitioner pitfalls and conflicts.

Box 2-2 provides possible questions to ask to gather information about external structure.

Context. Context encompasses the whole situation or background relevant to some event or personality. It includes five subcategories:

Ethnicity includes family culture, history, race, and religion. Family functioning may be subtly or obviously shaped by ethnicity; thus the practitioner needs to assess how ethnicity influences the family and how the family influences ethnicity.

Race is a basic construct referring to biologic and genetic differences between people. Racial and cultural differences must be considered in family assessment. In assessing ethnicity and race, practitioners should examine their own beliefs and assumptions and be willing to change their own ethnic and racial filters. This area of assessment helps the practitioner to show racial and cultural sensitivity and understand how family beliefs and behaviors may be influenced by ethnicity and race.

Social class is depicted by occupation, educational achievement, economic status, and the interplay between these variables. A family's social class is probably the prime molder of family lifestyle, family values, and family members' views of the world. Assessment of social class assists the practitioner in understanding family stressors and resources and recognizing that social class differences between practitioners and families may invite differences in approaching health promotion and management.

Religion and *spirituality* influence family members' beliefs about illness and coping strategies. A religious place of worship can represent a safe haven, one rich with instrumental, emo-

tional, and spiritual support in times of crisis. Religious beliefs can also induce a wide range of emotions (e.g., peace, fear, guilt, relief, anger, hope) and behaviors. Dietary restrictions and habits, weekly rituals, and alternative health care practices may be directly or indirectly related to religious beliefs. Assessment of religion is most critical at the time of diagnosis of a chronic or life-shortening illness; when one is working with families experiencing life-shortening illnesses (e.g., cancer, trauma) and grief; and when the members of a family offers information about their religious beliefs. The concept of spirituality is more encompassing than religion and includes how people orient their lives in light of an inner awareness. Wright (1999) describes how suffering becomes transposed to an issue of spirituality as family members try to find meaning about an illness or crises.

Environment encompasses aspects of the larger community, the neighborhood, and the home. Practitioners need to assess the accessibility of schools, day care, health services, recreation, and public transportation; family mobility; adequacy of the home (because children belong to the fastest growing homeless population in North America); and the home environment (e.g., family hygiene; sleep patterns; adequacy of space, privacy, and safety).

Box 2-3 provides possible questions to ask to gather information about context.

Box 2-2 Examples of Questions to Assess External Structure

Extended Family

To parent—Are your parents living? Do they live close by? In what ways do they show support of you (e.g., instrumental, emotional, financial)? Since your remarriage, do the children have more, less, or the same contact with their paternal grandparents?

Larger Systems

With what agencies has your family had previous involvement? What has been the best and worst advice you've been given from the social worker, teacher, or minister about this problem? What agency will you continue to stay involved with and for what purpose? How are we doing in our working relationship these days?

Box 2-3 Examples of Questions to Assess Context

Ethnicity

As a second-generation Chinese family, how do you suppose your health care practices are different from or the same as those of your grandparents? Does your community and social network support your practices? How are your beliefs about child rearing, diet, and medication influenced by your Cuban culture?

Race

I am aware that we are of different races. Help me to understand what I might need to know about your race that will assist me to be most helpful to you.

Social Class

How did Jorge's job influence your family and relationships? What free community resources might you use? How has being a practitioner yourself helped or not helped you as a parent of a child with special needs?

Religion and Spirituality

How do your religious or spiritual beliefs help you cope with Pedro's illness? How has your faith helped you during this difficult time? What has been the effect of this illness on your spiritual life?

Environment

On a scale of 1 to 10, with 10 being the most comfortable, how comfortable are you in your neighborhood and your home? What would make you more comfortable? Who does Francesca share a room with? How many schools has Tanya attended since kindergarten? In the last 3 years, how many times has your family moved?

Genogram

- The genogram is a tool for family assessment, a family tree that depicts the internal family structure (using symbols and lines as outlined in Chapter 5).
- It is a useful engagement tool to apply during the first interaction or meeting with the family.
- It provides rich data about family relationships over time.
- It can be used simultaneously to elicit information about other subcategories of a family assessment (developmental and functional, in addition to structural).
- It may include data about health status, occupation, religion, ethnic background, and migration date.
- It acts as a continual visual reminder for the practitioner to "think family" when it is placed on the child-family chart.

Helpful hints for constructing a genogram. To construct a genogram, priorities for construction should be determined based on the family situation. A three-generational genogram should be constructed when the child's health problem (physical or emotional) is influenced by family functioning in a problematic way or when grandparents are involved in health care management. A briefer two-generational genogram may be sufficient for a family that has preventive health care needs (e.g., immunizations) or minor health concerns (e.g., sports injury, flu).

The family may be engaged in an exercise to complete the genogram. Children, in particular, often engage easily when asked to help the practitioner draw the genogram.

- Use the genogram to "break the ice," provide structure, and introduce purposeful conversation.
- Invite as many family members to the initial meeting or visit as possible to obtain each family member's view and to observe family interaction.
- Ask others how an absent significant member might answer a question.
- Avoid discussion that is negative or blameful of family members, particularly absent ones.
- Take an interest in each family member and be sensitive to developmental differences.
- Tailor questions to children's developmental stages so that they remain active participants.

If some members (such as adolescents) are shy or uninterested in directly participating, ask other family members about them.

The genogram should be drawn (with tools such as the genograph, designed by Duhamel and Campagna [2000]) by beginning with questions about individuals, followed by a broader exploration of subsystems.

- Ask concrete, easy-to-answer questions of individuals about age, occupation, interests, health status, school grades, and teachers to increase their comfort level.
- Move the discussion about individuals to subsystems that target relational family data. Inquire about parent-child or sibling relationships depending on the presented concerns.
- With stepfamilies, ask questions about contact with the noncustodial parent, custody, the children's satisfaction with visits, and stepfamily relationships.
- Observe family interactions.
- During genogram construction, observe the content (what is said) and the process (how it is said) and write down observational notes.
- Pay particular attention to nonverbal cues and verbal comments of children during the conversation.

Discussion may move from the present family situation and the immediate household to questions about extended family relationships (e.g., Are Fatima's paternal and maternal grandparents living?, Mrs. Teves, you are the eldest of five. Who follows you?).

While discussing generations, practitioners may take the opportunity to ask about psychosocial family health history (i.e., Is there a history of alcohol abuse/violence/learning problems/mental illness in your family?). Practitioner questions should be tailored to the particular area (or potential area) of concern.

Ecomap

- The ecomap is another tool for family assessment and portrays the family's connections to larger systems, such as the social network, community services, church, agencies, institutions, and the workplace.
- It depicts the flow of energy and the nature of relationships between the family and the larger systems (Fig. 2-2).
- It assists the practitioner in developing hypotheses about family functioning.

Helpful hints for drawing an ecomap. To begin drawing an ecomap, questions should be posed that explore the family's connections to other individuals or groups external to the family.

- What community agencies are you involved with now? What agencies have you been involved with in the past? Which was most or least helpful?
- How would you describe your relationship with school staff?
- How did you first become involved with Child Protective Services, and what is the nature of your current agreement with them?

Family connections to outside agencies should also be drawn (see Fig. 2-2).

Developmental assessment. It is useful for a practitioner to have an understanding of family life cycles because the child's individual life cycle takes place within the family life cycle, the primary context for human development. The practitioner needs to view each family with flexibility and acknowledge the existence of various family forms before being able to thoroughly understand the issues and tasks of this family's current developmental stage.

Wright and Leahey (2000) make useful distinctions between family development and family life cycle:

Family development is the unique path that families construct. It is shaped by both predictable and unpredictable events, such as illness, divorce, death, and societal trends (e.g., more women in the workforce, lower birth rates, later marriages).

Family life cycle encompasses the typical, predictable life cycle events that families encounter (e.g., births, child's entry into school, launching, marriages, retirement).

According to Carter and McGoldrick (1999), two of the six stages of the family life cycle are: (1) families with young children and (2) families with adolescents. The authors also distinguish specific phases, emotional responses, and developmental issues associated with the divorce, postdivorce, and remarried-family life cycles.

Families with young children

Adjustment of the marriage to make space for children. The birth of a child often challenges the marital subsystem because there is less time for socializing, personal space, couple intimacy, and sexual relations. "Marital friendship" (Shapiro, Gottman, & Carrere, 2000) acts as a buffer against marital dissatisfaction and the stresses associated with having a child. Marital friend-

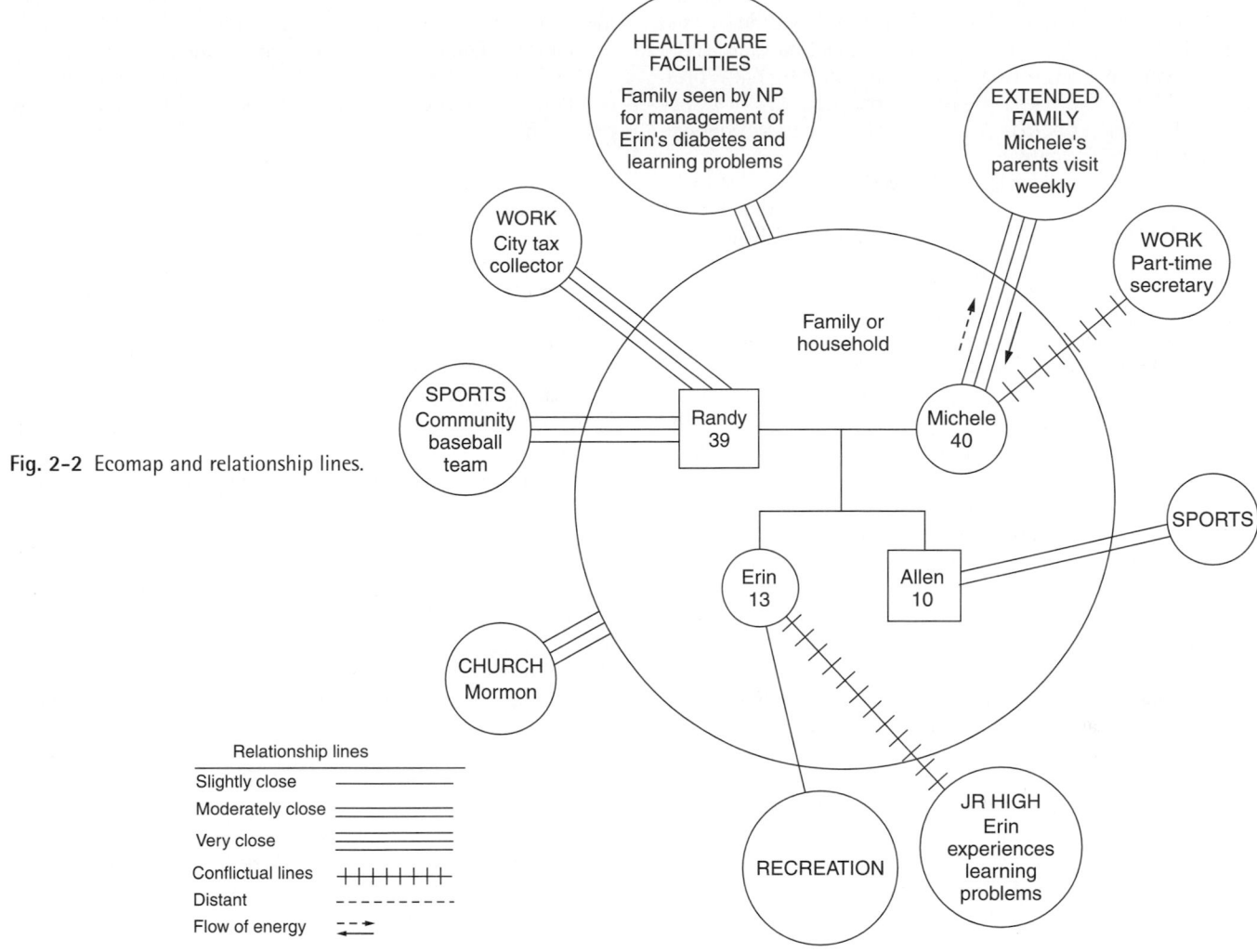

Fig. 2-2 Ecomap and relationship lines.

ship involves the "level of awareness each spouse has of their relationship, their spouse, and their spouse's life" and the fondness each spouse has for the other.

Joining in child-rearing, financial, and household tasks. Balancing finances, work, and family and home life become paramount tasks for families with young children. Children begin to socialize outside the home as school and community connections develop. Teachers and other community leaders may identify psychosocial and developmental problems not previously distinguished by the family as problematic.

Realignment of relationships with extended family members to include parenting and grandparenting. Husbands and wives integrate their new roles as mothers and fathers while new extended family roles are created. The extended family can prove to be a great support for the family during these years. With increased technology, families are more able to keep in contact by e-mail, digital photographs, and websites. However, when generational differences emerge, intervention may be required.

Families with adolescents

Shift of parent-child relationships to permit adolescents to move into or out of the system. Families may experience feelings of loss as adolescents connect with peers and show less dependence on the parental subsystem. Parents may become overwhelmed and respond either by attempting to control their adolescents arbitrarily or by giving up control completely. The once-held parental role of *protector* moves to that of *preparer* for adulthood, where boundaries need to be made more flexible to allow for adolescent autonomy.

Refocus on midlife, marital, and career issues. As the socially and sexually maturing adolescent challenges family values and traditions, parents are faced with evaluating their own marital and career issues. Depending on many factors, this may be a time of either positive growth or of painful, disruptive loss.

Beginning of shift toward joint caring for the older generation. At a time when parents are experiencing the growing independence of their adolescent children, they (especially women) are negotiating new roles with grandparents who may be growing more dependent. With the growing trend of parents having children later in life, this double demand for attention may grow even greater.

Divorced, postdivorced, and remarried families. In addition to the previously discussed transitions experienced by families with young children or adolescents are the added issues superimposed on those families who experience divorce, single parenting, or remarriage. Critical nursing implications include exploring a child's responses to divorce, supporting single parents in their expanded roles, promoting positive sibling relationships, and encouraging effective coparenting of the children. This last task begins with the transformation of the spousal relationship to a parental team, which is characterized by flexible boundaries, clear and direct communication, and a lack of overt criticism of the other parent in the child's presence. Children should never be placed in a position where they believe that loving one parent will hurt the other (McDonough & Barton, 1999). (See also Box 24-1.)

Helpful hints for collecting family developmental data. The practitioner may ask linear and circular questions (as outlined in the discussion of interventive questions) about the family life-cycle stage:

• How has your new marriage affected your relationship with your teenage sons or daughters?
• Now that your child is an adolescent, how have you noticed that your parenting style has changed?

The practitioner may also ask linear and circular questions about family development (e.g., marriages, divorce, death, family stressors) as it pertains to the current family situation or the child's health problem:

• Who in the family needs the most emotional support to deal with the diagnosis of autism right now?
• What has been the most significant difference in each of the children since the separation?

Attachment diagrams should be drawn to depict the nature of the attachment between family members. An attachment diagram and attachment symbols are outlined in Fig. 2-3.

Functional assessment. Functional assessment explores interactions between family members and family functioning and explores the reciprocal relationship between the family and illness. It comprises instrumental functioning and expressive functioning.

Instrumental functioning. Instrumental functioning includes the activities of daily family living (such as eating, sleeping, and health care regimens [e.g., taking temperatures, giving injections and medications]). It can change drastically when a child develops a health problem.

Expressive functioning. Expressive functioning focuses on the interaction between family members and assists a practitioner to assess the family strengths and limitations.

Emotional communication refers to the range and types of emotions or feelings that are expressed or observed by the practitioner.

Verbal communication refers to the meaning of an oral (or, less frequently, written) message between those involved in the interaction. Verbal communication may be direct and clear or masked and unclear. Experts in child behavior management encourage parents to "say what you mean and mean what you say" so children receive clear, direct communication versus mixed messages or masked communication.

Nonverbal communication includes all other forms of communication that are not verbal in nature, such as body posture (e.g., slumped, fidgeting, open, closed), eye contact (e.g., intense, minimal), touch, facial movements (e.g., grimacing, staring, yawning), and personal space between family members. Nonverbal communication is closely linked to emotional communication. It may be particularly important to inquire about the meaning of nonverbal communication when it is incongruent with verbal communication.

Circular communication refers to the reciprocal communication that may be illustrated by a *circular pattern diagram* (CPD) (Fig. 2-4). A circular pattern diagram has the following characteristics:

• It illustrates a reciprocal positive or negative communication cycle between individuals.
• It outlines the thoughts, feelings, and behaviors of each person within an interaction and his or her effect on another's behavior.
• It may be applied to relationships between family members or between the practitioner and the family (because the practitioner and the family also mutually influence each other).

Fig. 2-3 Sample attachment diagram and attachment symbols. (Adapted with permission from Wright, L.M. & Leahey, M. [2000]. *Nurses and families: A guide to assessment and intervention* [3rd ed.]. Philadelphia: F.A. Davis.)

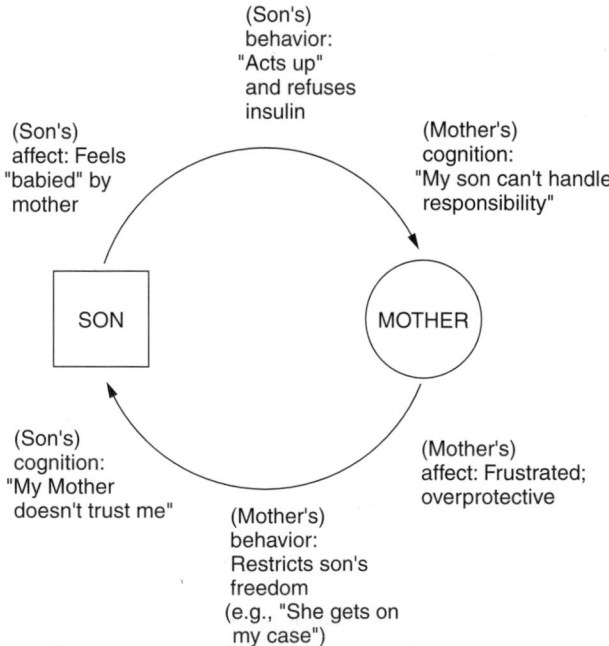

Fig. 2-4 Circular pattern diagram.

- It invites the practitioner to think interactionally about problems and to help the family think interactionally.
- Using circular questions, one can draw it with the family to illuminate problematic cycles and then generate possible solutions with the family (Table 2-2; see also Fig. 2-4).

Problem-solving refers to the family's ability to solve its problems. Family problem-solving is strongly influenced by the family's beliefs about its abilities and past successes. It may be useful to explore who identifies the problem, who attempts to solve the problem, and how much influence each member of the family believes he or she has on the problem. The family's choice of solution may be perpetuating the problem, or families may use solutions that were previously helpful to assist them with the current crisis.

Roles are established patterns of relating to others within the family. Roles may be formal (e.g., husband, grandmother, friend) or informal (e.g., class clown, black sheep, peacemaker). It is helpful to learn how the family roles evolved, how the assigned and informal roles affect family functioning, and whether the roles need to be altered or can be highlighted to help cope with the health problem.

Influence refers to behavior used by one person to affect another's behavior. This is a significant area to assess in the parent-child subsystem. One of the biggest tasks for families with children is how to effectively discipline or influence a child. Wright and Leahey (2000) outline several measures used by individuals to influence others, including instrumental control (e.g., positive or negative behavior reinforcements), psychologic control (e.g., use of feelings, talking, threatening), and corporal control (e.g., hugging, spanking, hitting).

Beliefs, as Wright, Watson, and Bell (1996) maintain, are the blueprints of people's lives, and a belief about the problem is the problem. Beliefs drive behaviors: "we think (believe); therefore we do"—and, reciprocally, behaviors affect beliefs. Beliefs are one of the most significant areas of assessment. A practitioner may focus on beliefs about etiology, treatment, prognosis, role of the family, and role of the practitioner. The reciprocal relationship between family beliefs and the health problem should be assessed.

Alliances and *coalitions* focus on the directionality, balance, and intensity of relationships between family members or between practitioners and families. When one family member becomes strongly aligned with another, it may create problems for a third person and that individual's relationships with the other two. Coalitions can also be positive, as when family members join in a cooperative effort to help another family member stop smoking or stop drinking alcohol; they collectively voice their concerns to the individual and their intent to provide support and help.

Box 2-4 provides possible questions to ask to gather information about expressive functioning.

Helpful hints to organize and document family assessment data

- Identify and document a list of presenting problems and family strengths.
- Create a CFAM document that lists each category and subcategory. Enter reported and observed data in relevant categories or subcategories. Note information gaps to be filled at a future date.
- Include a genogram, an ecomap, brief family life cycle and family development data, and an attachment diagram for a significant family relationship.
- Formulate systemic hypotheses.
- Formulate an intervention plan.
- Continue to update the family assessment, using progress notes to document family changes and the effect of family nursing interventions.

Table 2-2 Examples of Circular Questions to Change the Cognitive, Affective, and Behavioral Domains of Family Functioning

QUESTION TYPE	COGNITIVE	AFFECTIVE	BEHAVIORAL
Difference Question Explores differences among people, relationships, time, ideas, and beliefs	What information would be helpful to you about managing Ming's night fears?	Who is most worried that Ming won't outgrow the night fears?	Now that you are leaving the light on and his door open at bedtime, what difference is it making?
Behavioral Effect Question Explores the effect of one family member's behavior on that of another	When your Mom is "getting on your case," what do you think?	When you think that your Mom doesn't trust you, how do you feel?	What do you do when you feel "babied" and that your Mom doesn't trust you?
Hypothetical or Future-Oriented Question Explores family options and alternative actions or meaning in the future	What would be the worst thing that could happen if someone is not closely watching baby Sandra?	If your husband spent more time playing with Sandra, how would you feel?	What might you do in the future to prevent accidents from happening at home?
Triadic Question Posed to a third person to explore the relationship between two others	How does your Dad know that your sister needs his support right now?	When your dad shows support to your sister, how does your Mom feel?	What do you think your father needs to do to prepare for your sister and her baby coming to live with you?

Adapted with permission from Wright, LM & Leahey, M. (1994). Nurses and families: a guide to assessment and intervention, (3rd ed.). Philadelphia: F.A. Davis.

Family Intervention

Family intervention is any action or response by a practitioner, which includes the practitioner's overt therapeutic actions and internal cognitive and affective responses occurring in the context of a practitioner-patient relationship, to affect individual family or community functioning, for which the practitioner is accountable. Thus "relationships are not just central to care, they are care" (Robinson, 1996).

Box 2-4 Examples of Questions to Assess Expressive Functioning

Emotional Communication

When Mom is sad, how does she show it? How were feelings expressed differently between Mom and Dad before the accident? Who has the most trouble showing sadness about Lucy's autism?

Verbal Communication

Does Dad usually talk about what bothers him? Who is the one in the family who gives you the bottom line? Do you ever get confused about what Mom really wants from you?

Nonverbal Communication

You seem preoccupied today and not wanting to talk; can you help me understand my observations? When you begin to cry, Leslie, what are you thinking?

Circular Communication

When your husband doesn't talk, what do you do? When you get mad at him for not talking, what does he do?

Problem-Solving

Who identified Dustin's anxiety? Whom do you go to when you are worried? Do you usually try to deal with the problems by yourselves or do you like to get outside help? What solutions have you tried? How were they helpful?

Roles

Who usually changes the baby's diapers? Who talks about sadness the best in your family? If there is one person in your family you would consider the peacemaker, who would it be? Whose job is it to make sure that you get lunch when you come home at noon from school?

Influence and Power

What helps Emmanuel follow your directions? When he disobeys the rules, what do you do? When you show pride in Emmanuel's accomplishments, what does he do? How much control do you feel you have over this problem?

Beliefs

What do you believe about the diagnosis? The prognosis? The treatment and your roles in it? My role in helping your family? (Wright, Watson, & Bell, 1999)

Alliances and Coalitions

When your husband agrees with your teenage son that he should move out, what effect does that have on your marriage? When Mom and Linda talk privately in the bedroom, what does Jessica do?

Indications

Whenever a child's health is influencing or being influenced by family functioning in a detrimental way, family intervention is indicated.

Goal

The goal of family intervention is to effect positive change in the child or the family.

Helpful hints and interventions

- Interventions are the core of clinical work with families.
- They should be devised with sensitivity to the family's ethnic and religious background.
- They can only be *offered* to families, since a practitioner cannot direct change but can create a therapeutic context for change to occur.
- They are offered in the context of collaborative conversations as the practitioner and family together devise solutions so that they can find the most useful fit.
- When the practitioner's ideas are not a good fit for the family, the practitioner should be open to offering other ideas rather than becoming blameful of self or the family because the intervention was not chosen.

Calgary Family Intervention Model

The field of family nursing is moving beyond assessment toward family nursing intervention. A recent development in family nursing is the emergence of the CFIM, a companion model to CFAM. The CFIM focuses on promoting, improving, or sustaining effective family functioning in three domains: cognitive (thoughts), affective (emotions), and behavioral (actions). It also assists practitioners in determining which domain of family functioning most needs to be changed and then devising interventions to target that domain.

Wright and Leahey (2000) describe a variety of family systems nursing interventions, including asking interventive questions, providing commendations, offering information or opinions, validating emotional responses, "storying" the illness experience, drawing forth family support, encouraging family members as caregivers, encouraging respite, and devising rituals. The first three of these family interventions are discussed here.

Interventive questions. Interventive questions are powerful questions to elicit family assessment data while simultaneously triggering change in the family system by the information the questions implicitly offer. They can be developed to target any one of the three domains of family functioning (Table 2-2). Linear and circular questions are two types of interventive questions.

Linear questions are used to obtain history or factual information in the form of effective data. They have the following characteristics:

- Investigative in nature
- Help define problems
- Draw forth cause and content

Examples include: How is Mike? What is the problem you are struggling with? When did it start?

Circular questions explore relationships and differences and change as they relate to the presenting concerns of the child and family. These questions:

- Focus on patterns, relationship dynamics, interactions, and circularity.
- Require the practitioner to be curious and neutral to all family members.

- Evoke a reflective response by family members because the family begins thinking about new connections (e.g., about relationships, family functioning, the health problem).
- Often assist families in pursuing different explanations for problems.

Examples include: How are you today compared to when I last saw you? When you talk about AIDS, what does your Mom do? What is the most difficult adjustment to Clara's seizures?

Four types of circular questions are difference, behavioral effect, hypothetical/future oriented, and triadic (Table 2-2).

Commendations. Commendations are "observations of patterns of [constructive] behavior and interactions that occur across time" (Wright & Leahey, 2000). They:

- Are statements made by the practitioner to family members about individual and family strengths, abilities, and resources.
- Are powerful when they counteract negative family beliefs.
- Often empower families and create a context for change.
- Are most often targeted to the cognitive domain of family functioning because they invite family members to think differently.
- May invite feelings of relief, validation, and affirmation.
- May simultaneously trigger changes in the affective and behavioral domains of family functioning.

Examples include: I have noticed how you each respect each other despite your differences. Your persistence in dealing with the temper tantrums is most impressive. Other mothers could really benefit from your knowledge about managing diaper rashes.

Helpful hints about offering commendations

- Be a "family strengths" detective, looking for opportunities to commend families.
- Ensure that sufficient evidence for the commendations are provided; otherwise they may sound insincere and ingratiating.
- Use the family's language and integrate important family beliefs to strengthen the validity of the commendation.
- Offer commendations within the first 10 minutes of meeting with a family to enhance the practitioner-family relationship and to increase family receptivity to later ideas.
- Routinely include commendations to families at the end of an interaction or meeting, before an opinion is offered.

Offering information and opinions. The need for information constitutes the most significant need for families experiencing health care problems. Families need to gather and integrate information about developmental issues, health promotion, and illness management.

Helpful hints about offering information and opinions

- Use language that is relevant, clear, and specific.
- Provide easy-to-read literature; write out key points on a small card.
- Inform families of community support groups and resources. Determine if they have been helpful to families who have used them and how.
- Build on family abilities by encouraging them to independently seek resources. Inquire about the family's reactions after seeking resources.

- If possible, take a brief break (10 minutes) from the family meeting and return with some ideas for them written on paper. Families appreciate when practitioners write down their reflections because this signifies individual attention and caring.
- Offer ideas, information, or reflections in a spirit of learning and wondering (e.g., "*I wonder* what would happen if you tried a slightly different approach to talking with Lourdes about sex and birth control. *Perhaps* you might…").
- Do not be invested in the outcome; if the family does not apply the teaching materials, be curious about what did not fit for them rather than becoming judgmental and angry with the family.

Conclusion

Working with families is essential in pediatric health care. Children cannot be viewed in isolation from their families, and thus family assessment and family intervention are imperative components of pediatric health care.

Resources

Websites
Family Nursing Resource Center (www.efamilynursing.com)
Family Nursing Unit, University of Calgary
  (www.ucalgary.ca/NU/fnu.html)

Bibliography

Carter, B. & McGoldrick, M. (Eds.). (1999). *The expanded family life cycle: Individual, family and social perspectives* (3rd ed.). Boston: Allyn & Bacon.

Duhamel, F. & Campagna, L. (2000). *Family genograph.* Montreal: Université de Montréal, Faculty of Nursing.

Leahey, M. & Harper-Jaques, S. (1996). Family-nurse relationships: Core assumptions and clinical implications. *Journal of Family Nursing, 2*(2), 133-151.

McDonough, H. & Bartha, C. (1999). *Putting children first: A guide for parents breaking up.* Toronto: University of Toronto Press.

McGoldrick, M., Gerson, R., & Shellenberger, S. (1999). *Genograms: Assessment and intervention* (2nd ed.). New York: W.W. Norton.

Robinson, C.A. (1996). Health care relationships revisited. *Journal of Family Nursing, 2*(2), 152-173.

Shapiro, A.F., Gottman, J.M., & Carrere, S. (2000). The baby and the marriage: Identifying factors that buffer against the decline of marital satisfaction after the baby first arrives. *Journal of Family Psychology, 14,* 59-70.

Tomm, K. (1980). Towards a cybernetic systems approach to family therapy at the University of Calgary. In Freeman, D. (Ed.). *Perspectives on family therapy.* Vancouver: Butterworth.

Tomm, K. (1988). Interventive interviewing. Part 3: Intending to ask lineal, circular, strategic, or reflexive questions? *Family Process, 27*(1), 1-15.

Wright, L.M. (1999). Spirituality, suffering and beliefs: The soul of healing with families. In Walsh, F. (Ed.). *Spiritual resources in family therapy.* New York: Guilford.

Wright, L. M. & Leahey, M. (2000). *Nurses and families: A guide to assessment and intervention* (3rd ed.). Philadelphia: F.A. Davis.

Wright, L.M., Watson, S.L., & Bell, J.M. (1999). *Beliefs: The heart of healing in families and illness.* New York: Basic Books.

Chapter 3 *Parenting*

Theresa M. Eldridge

Parenting is one of the most complicated, challenging, and potentially rewarding tasks that a family or an individual can perform. It is a learned behavior whereby individuals provide for the safety and physical and emotional well-being of a child. It is also the process by which a child is socialized to the dominant values of the parent's culture. Frequently, parenting skills are developed by trial and error.

Parents are individuals first and parents second. They have their own needs and problems and are in various developmental stages themselves. Parents may develop appropriate or inappropriate parenting skills. Parents who have successfully completed their own developmental tasks can contribute to well-developed and successful children. Parents who lack parenting skills and who have poor self-esteem may be unable to promote the behaviors and skills children need to become successful and independent adults.

Raising children has far-reaching and serious consequences for the family and society. Societal and economic stresses today have caused many changes in the family and parenting, and many believe that children are worse off today than in previous years. In 1988 a survey of parents showed that 20% of children 13 to 17 years of age had one or more developmental, learning, or behavioral disorders. Rates of child abuse tripled between 1976 and 1986, and homicide rates and teenage suicide rates doubled.

The numbers of divorced, single, and adolescent parents have increased. It has been reported that the percentage of children living in households with only one adult has tripled in the last 30 years. The proportion of children living in homes where all adults work outside the home has also sharply increased. These changes present multiple challenges for today's parents. The demands of daily living often leave parents depleted with little time or energy for parenting. It is no wonder many parents feel frustrated and ill equipped to meet the daily challenges of parenting.

Many parents equate loving their children with effective parenting. Love is critical for effective parenting, but love alone does not make one an effective parent. Effective parenting comes from education, practice, patience, and a sense of humor. The most important role of parenting is to provide nurturing of the child's personality and development in a climate of love and security.

Tasks of Parenting

Parenting is really a form of leadership. As leaders, parents are responsible for accomplishing certain tasks and goals. They achieve these in different ways, depending on their culture, individual characteristics, and available resources. In general, the ultimate goal of parenting is to raise healthy, productive individuals who are self-regulating, successful, contributors to society. To accomplish this goal parents need to complete the tasks of parenting by providing for basic needs, teaching social skills and behaviors, and assisting children in developing cultural values and beliefs. Additionally, parental tasks include

sharing customs and traditions, fostering skills for economic survival, promoting interpersonal and communication skills, and helping children become self-regulatory, productive and self-actualized.

According to Maslow (1968), after meeting the basic needs of survival, safety, and security, individuals begin to search for ways to meet their needs for a sense of belonging, affection, self-esteem, self-respect, and self-actualization. Parents can foster their children's journey to self-actualization by the positive promotion of the development of the child's personality and independence. After the physical needs of their children are met, the intellectual, emotional, social, and spiritual needs remain. Erickson's (1963) psychologic theory identifies the eight stages of man as a lifelong struggle for emotional-social equilibrium. These stages have their own tasks to be mastered and unresolved issues from previous stages to be resolved. Parents as well as their children are in these various stages of development. Parents who have successfully mastered the developmental tasks are better prepared to assist their children in attaining successful mastery. For example, parents who do not have a sense of autonomy and self-esteem will find it difficult to parent a toddler who is attempting to achieve autonomy. Effective parents need a variety of skills to accomplish parenting tasks.

Six Stages of Parenthood

Galinsky (1987) states that, "Stages are periods of time in which one's emotional and intellectual energy is primarily focused on one major psychosocial task or issue to be resolved." She identifies these tasks as having related issues and themes and as being present from the beginning of parenthood. Since parents may have children of different ages, they may be going through several stages concurrently. She views parental growth as an "interactive process with the development of the child influencing the development of the parent." The six stages of parenthood are summarized in Table 3-1.

According to Galinsky, images are based on memories and experiences and influenced by circumstances and culture. Parents have images and expectations of their roles and their partner's roles. If these images of child-rearing practices are in conflict, they can be a source of later dissension. Parents may expect or imagine a sweet, cuddly baby. The reality might be a child who resists being held and is fussy.

During the various stages of parenthood, parents continue to reconcile images and realities. When the images and expectations of parents fit reality, there is a balance and absence of conflict. When the reality and the images conflict, it is an opportunity for growth; growth can occur when there is an attempt to resolve conflict. Growth of the parents is on a continuum, just as growth of their children is.

Galinsky identifies subsets of parenting tasks and various issues and themes that occur during each of the parenting stages. These issues recur during each stage, manifested by the changes and growth that the child is experiencing. The issues

20

and themes identified in the stages of parenthood demonstrate the polarities of two feelings that form a continuum. Although contradictory, they exist together. In all stages the goal is to develop consistency and congruency and to reconcile fantasy and reality while the parent is adapting to an ever-changing child.

Common Issues Occurring during Parenting Stages

Control versus *loss of control* occurs when images and realities collide. Parents must learn to come to grips with the child's ever-increasing demands for control: the toddler wants to do it himself; the school-age child wants to stay overnight at a

Table 3-1 Stages of Parenthood

STAGE	APPROXIMATE AGE	PARENTAL TASKS	ISSUES/THEMES
Image-making	During pregnancy	Form images of parenthood and future roles Accept separateness of baby Prepare for change in roles Develop feelings for baby Evaluate, identify, and differentiate selves from their own parents Prepare for change in relationship with partner Prepare for birth	Control/lack of control Giving/getting Independence/ dependence Nostalgia/impatience
Nurturing	Birth to 18-24 months	Reconcile actual birth with imagined birth Form attachment to new baby Reconcile image of child with actual child Accept new baby Answer self-doubts and uncertainties about ability to care for child Become attached Enlarge family to include grandparents, siblings and friends Redefine relationship with partner Redefine identity as parent and individual	Control/lack of control Affinity/dissimilarity Separateness/ connectedness Push/pull feelings Holding on/letting go
Authority	2-5 years	Accept authority over child Determine scope of authority Communicate and enforce authority Determine how to handle conflicts between children Develop skills to change as child changes; avoid battles of will Establish ways to work with partner and others (e.g., grandparents, teachers) in autonomous relationship with child Gain distance from child; accept feelings of separateness; child is not an extension of parents Reevaluate images of "perfect" parent and "perfect" child Become an authority and determine how to protect child and how to expose child to realities Respond to queries about origins of life and sexuality	Control/lack of control Time for self and time for children Push/pull feelings Separateness/ connectedness Issues of power Shaping self-concepts
Interpretive	Preschool to preadolescence	Evaluate past years of parenthood; reinterpret and revise theories of child-rearing practices and parenthood Form images of the future Interpret world to child Interpret and develop child's self-concept Accept child's individuality Help child develop skills and values Reconcile images of child with actual child Assimilate and reconcile other people's perceptions of child Decide what morals, values, and beliefs to promote Reconcile child's self-evaluation with parents' own Decide on time for family, self, work and partner Define changing relationship with child	Separateness/ connectedness Sharing/withholding Telling/listening Control/lack of control Holding on/letting go
Interdependent	Teenage years	Redefine relationship with almost-adult child Redefine authority relationship Revise and develop new communication patterns Set limits and give guidance Accept child's sexuality Deal with the distance between self and child and create new ties Prepare for changes in self and family when child leaves home	Authority/dissimilarity Separateness/ connectedness Control/lack of control Images/reality
Departure	Children leave home	Evaluate years of parenthood Prepare for child's departure Redefine sense of identity Loosen control Accept child's separate identity and maintain connectedness	Images/reality Separateness/ connectedness Control/lack of control

Modified from Galinsky, E. (1987). The six stages of parenthood. *New York: Addison-Wesley.*

friend's house; the teen wants to drive to a concert. How much control is enough but not too much, and how much control does a parent really have?

Separateness versus *connectedness* issues emerge again and again during parenthood. Parents often view their child as a part of themselves and must learn to see the child as a unique individual. During each stage parents must seek to define and redefine their individual identities and accept their child as a separate individual while maintaining the connectedness between parent and child.

Giving versus *getting* demonstrates the desire to provide (give) the child material things, such as spending money, dance lessons, and enrollment in scouts, all while getting the child to act responsibly.

Independence versus *dependence* issues are also found throughout parenthood. Infants are very dependent initially, but as they grow and develop, they become more independent and autonomous. Toddlers learn to walk, feed themselves, dress themselves, and later control their bodily functions. Teens stay home alone, drive cars, date, and select their own clothes. Each new skill presents a challenge for parents. How much involvement should they have? When do they let their child be independent and make mistakes? How do they determine the limits? Parents must answer these and many other questions throughout each parenting stage. Many of these issues are being experienced by parents not only in their relationship with their child, but also in their relationships with each other and with their own parents. Many of the issues of independence versus dependence are also closely related to holding on versus letting go and separateness versus connectedness.

Many parents experience *nostalgia* versus *impatience*. Initially, parents experience impatience for the birth of their child or impatience for the child to "grow up." As the child grows, however, the parents become nostalgic for the past. The parent of a rebellious 2-year-old may be nostalgic for the infant who slept all night and was less mobile. The parents of a school-age child may be nostalgic for the period when their child was more dependent on them and spent more time with them. Parents of teens often eagerly anticipate the adolescent's departure from home but experience depression when it actually occurs.

In the beginning period of parenthood, *affinity* versus *dissimilarity* is the feeling of attachment for the baby. Later, parents interpret their child's behavior in relationship to their individual characteristics. Parents may feel an affinity for the child who is perceived as having assertive behaviors if the parents themselves are assertive. However, the assertive parents may be disappointed or feel a dissimilarity when their child is shy and reluctant to try new activities. Parenting is an ongoing process of accepting the individuality of the child and reconciling images of the child with the actual child.

Parenting provides many opportunities to experience *push* versus *pull* feelings. There may be feelings of possessiveness toward the new infant or jealousy and resentment when a child prefers the company of others. All parents experience the full range of human emotions toward their child. A working mother might resent the demands for her time when she comes home from a difficult day at work. A father might be envious of the attention his child is receiving from his partner.

Parenthood presents a challenge for parents to continually examine and integrate the images they have of themselves, their child, and parenting with the realities. Parents are constantly changing and growing as their child changes and grows. The issues identified by Galinsky are experienced by all parents at one time or another. Resolution of the conflictual feelings and successful accomplishment of the parenting tasks contribute to the child's development of a positive self-concept. Many factors, however, can influence the successful development of parents and children.

Parenting Styles

Parenting style is a characteristic of the parent that is influenced by many factors and has significant effects on the child's development. Baumrind (1971) describes three distinctive styles of parenting: authoritative, permissive, and authoritarian.

Darling and Steinberg (1993) further define three separate aspects of parenting: the parental goals of socialization; parenting practices used by parents to achieve these goals; and the parenting style, which is a reflection of parental attitudes and emotional climate. Thus parenting style encompasses parental behaviors through which parents directly assist their child in attaining their socialization goals and the parents' attitude toward their child and the emotional climate in which these socialization goals are achieved.

The parenting styles summarized in Table 3-2 reflect the three methods identified by Baumrind. They are not intended to be all-inclusive. Although there are different effects of parenting practices on child development, no one parenting style has been proved to be more effective than another.

Cultural beliefs about the socialization agenda of children, the role of parents, and the accepted norms of behavior greatly influence parenting styles and patterns. In the European-American culture parenting techniques traditionally stress achievement, autonomy, independence, and self-control. In this context, the authoritative parenting style is perceived as the most desirable approach to successful parenting. Many ethnic minorities, however, stress interdependence and cooperation as a primary socialization goal for children and may perceive the nonauthoritarian style as the most appropriate method of achieving these goals.

Parents may not fit one style but have a blend of styles. They may use a variety of parenting techniques based on the situation, the age of the child, and the individual characteristics of that child. Studies have shown that parents select strategies that are directed at preparing their children to be successful in the society where they will work, marry, and live as adults. No matter what parenting style is used, unless it is used in the extreme and is of some harm to the child, studies have shown that parents who are sensitive and accepting versus those who are rejecting and inconsistent have the best success in rearing successful, competent adults. The methods they use to attain those goals, however, may vary based on culture and a variety of other factors.

Factors Affecting Parenting

Many factors affect parenting styles: the parents' intellectual and social level, individual characteristics and temperament of the parents and the child, cultural values and beliefs, the environment, the availability and quality of community resources, and the type of parenting situation.

Culture has a significant influence on child-rearing practices. Table 3-3 describes the differences between the "mainstream" North American/Anglo-European culture and other

Table 3-2 Three Parenting Styles

STYLE	PARENTING CHARACTERISTICS	TECHNIQUES USED TO SOCIALIZE CHILD	CHILD OUTCOMES
Democratic/ authoritative	Responsive to child's needs Controlling/demanding Warm Rational Receptive to child's communication High control and positive encouragement of child's autonomous and independent behaviors	Clear expectations Negotiation of limits Gives reasons Employs positive reinforcement Finds mutually acceptable alternatives	Socially competent Self-reliant Self-control Explorative Content For boys: Friendly Cooperative Socially responsible For girls: Achievement oriented Purposeful Dominant
Restrictive/ authoritarian	Not responsive to child's needs Demanding Less warm Expect obedience and respect Have high maturity demands Power replaces authority Fear and anger replace respect Evaluate child's behavior in accord with set standards	Employs punitive measures often physical and psychologic Employs negative reinforcement Uses orders or commands and threats to motivate	Discontent Withdrawn Distrustful For boys: Hostile Resistive For girls: Lack independence and dominance
Permissive	Responsive to child's needs Noncontrolling Nondemanding Relatively warm Few limits Limited guidance Value child's individuality and verbal expressiveness	Uses reason Seldom uses punitive measures Sometimes employs positive reinforcement Usually ignores or tolerates noncompliance Emphasis placed on child being the decision-maker	Least self-reliant Least explorative Least self-controlled Resistive Less achievement oriented For boys: Socially responsible For girls: Less assertive and less independent

Modified from Baumrind, D. (1971). Current patterns of parental authority (Monograph 4). Developmental Psychology, 1(2):1-103.

common cultures. The clinical implications of culture on discipline, child care, socialization, and parental teaching are identified. Many cultural beliefs affect parenting, and further information about this area can also be found in Chapter 4.

Socioeconomic factors also have significant influence on parenting. Middle-class parents are more likely to work in jobs that require self-direction and autonomy, and so they often place a high value on self-control for their children. In the lower socioeconomic class, parents are more likely to value conformity and external authority, since they often have jobs that require taking orders from others. The parents' choice of parenting and disciplinary style may help prepare the child for the occupational atmosphere the parents experience every day and the one that the parents anticipate the child will eventually also experience.

The relationship between poverty and parenting is not clear, but it is known that more than 20% of children in the United States live in poverty, with double that rate for minority children. Being poor means having insufficient resources, with poor families more likely to lack some of the elements that are fundamental to good child outcomes, such as literacy, stimulation, appropriate toys and books, role models, and

higher expectations. Poverty is also associated with higher rates of single parenthood, divorce, family violence, and school dropouts, all of which place children at risk for poor outcomes. Families living in poverty may not lack love and affection, but they do lack the availability and quality of resources that increase the success of parenting and socialization of children.

Other factors also have significant influence. The cognitive level of the parents is important. Parents with a higher cognitive level are able to problem solve and to assist in teaching their children to use problem solving in everyday activities. Parents with a higher cognitive level are also able to reinforce behaviors and have a variety of strategies that they can use in their parenting. They tend to have a better understanding of growth and development and appropriate developmental tasks.

Parents are products of their childhood. For a parent raised in a loving home, raising a child in an atmosphere of love and security may not be difficult. If, however, a person experienced an unloving or insecure childhood, successful parenting may be more difficult. There is a high correlation between parents who were abused and parents who are abusers. An effective parent needs to understand the importance of giving

Table 3-3 Cultural Characteristics Related to Parenting

AREAS OF CHILDREARING	ANGLO-EUROPEAN/ AMERICAN	AFRICAN-AMERICAN	HISPANIC/LATINO	ASIAN-AMERICAN	NATIVE AMERICAN	CLINICAL CONSIDERATIONS
Cultural family values and characteristics	Stresses importance of early attachment of mother and infant Later stresses: independence, individualism Two-parent nuclear family is the ideal Equal sex rights Less respect for elders	Extended family Interdependence with other African Americans Extensive social network and shared child care Family is matrifocal (women centered) often with grand-mother as major decision-maker and primary caregiver Many three-generation family homes Religion valued Folk care practices Parents may fear that showing too much attention to child will "spoil" the child and not adequately prepare child for the harsh realities of life	Extended family Interdependence with family Family centered Patriarchal (machismo) High respect for older adults Godparents significant to family and are coresponsible for child's upbringing and religious education Many three-generation family homes Folk care practices	Extended family Family centered Reliance on family members Value self-reliance and self-restraint Self-expression repressed; value harmony, self-sacrifice, and respect for older adults Sharing of emotions discouraged Folk care practices Respect for authority	Extended family, includ-ing the village and tribal elders May have multiple grand-parents and cousins, aunts, and uncles who are all part of the extended family and part of the child care and decision making Value harmony between land, people, and the environment Stoic in presence of pain or emotional distress Quiet, reserved, avoid eye contact with strangers Little physical touch Use folk healers Value children and elders May be patriarchal (e.g., Apache, Cherokee) or matriarchal (e.g., Navajo, Hopi, Crow)	Practitioner can be more effec-tive in working with diverse cultures in the following ways: Accept a broad definition of family Involve extended family members in the health care of the child (including decision making) Include extended family as part of the assessment process and interventions Do not make assumptions or have biased expectations of any family regardless of culture Make accurate assessment and plan interventions based on the unique needs of the family Consider the context in which families must parent Develop interventions based on the existing social and cultural structures if appropriate
Discipline	Some families value nonphysical, firm authoritative disci-pline; others value more strict discipline Emphasis on explana-tions and giving reasons for parental action Children raised with firm control in infancy; increased freedom and choice as child gets older Expectations for behavior determined by parents but with respect for child's autonomy and indi-viduality	Emphasis on obedi-ence and parent-defined rules Physical punishment often employed Discipline and parent-ing often parent-focused Expect child to "be good"	Children taught to obey and respect parents Often use corporal pun-ishment to ensure obedience Families from lower socioeconomic group may be less authori-tarian and less restrictive	Child's behavior is a reflec-tion of the family Respect for elders and acceptance without ques-tioning or talking back is expected and taught early Verbal approval or disap-proval used Also use rewards (candy, toys) for desired behavior Use ridicule or threaten abandonment if child misbehaves Children obey and honor their parents (filial piety) Often permissive with young child; increasing responsibility as child becomes older Often expects adult child to take care of parents	Ignore misbehavior Also shame, tease, ridicule child's behavior Use quiet voice to tell child what is expected Rare physical punishment May be permissive and nondemanding (Note that there are over 500 Native American tribes in the United States, with many sub-cultures and each tribe having different expec-tations and behaviors. These are very general guidelines)	Acknowledge and respect indi-vidual parenting and discipline styles Provide appropriate alternatives Evaluate the context of the par-enting situation (e.g., strict structure may be needed to protect children from chaotic and dangerous environment) Involve family in a mutually agreed-upon plan for discipline that acknowledges the differ-ences and similarities of prac-titioner's and family's culture Provide for the safety and well-being of the child within the context of the culture

Socialization issues	Achievement/competition oriented Work oriented Oriented toward development of child's self-esteem, autonomy, and independence	Relationships of family and kin important with more orientation toward interdependence and cooperation Obligation, reciprocity, and sharing part of the social interactions See child as attached to the family, household, and community	Traditionally, men are economic providers and key decision-makers Males considered big and strong (machismo) Children valued highly and taken everywhere Social status of females attained by childbearing, especially a male child to carry on the family name	Self-reliance and self-restraint valued Cooperative, patient, expects self-sacrifice for the good of the family Females submissive to males Males valued more highly Achievement for the good of the family is emphasized Respect for authority	Maintaining culture and traditions important Males have more prestige Respect for children and older adults	Various socialization methods and family values may be in conflict with those of mainstream culture and the practitioner. To achieve effective health care, the practitioner may: Encourage programs that are congruent with the cultural values of the family Explore the motivational processes of child and family before trying to effect behavior change Involve family in negotiation of mutually acceptable goals
Parental teaching	Emphasis on early learning associated with later competence Parents have largest number of instructional loops, most frequent elaborate instructions, and fastest pacing in their teaching Teaching perceived as one of the roles of the mother High use of early vocal interactions Encourages early dependence with gradual achievement of independence and autonomy	Importance of early learning and later competence less emphasized Less vocalization with child Average number of teaching loops with moderate pacing and few reasons given to child Emphasis on developing survival skills and education to achieve success	Individual responsibility less emphasized Relationship-oriented Feelings and expressions encouraged Respect for authority Needs of family supersede individual needs Mother-child interactions frequently nonverbal in early infancy Fewest teaching loops, with slower pacing by taking more time to complete teaching loops High percentage of adults working Uses verbal and nonverbal instruction More negative feedback and less praise Mothers perceive themselves as mothers, not teachers	Teach restraint early ("If you fall, don't cry") Very specific instruction with positive feedback Regular formal instruction seen as part of maternal role Group oriented; infant seen as extension of parent Teach child humility Tend to model behaviors Nurture infant, then train older child to bring honor to family Education valued	Mothers tend to be more passive Use of storytelling by elders to teach about culture, heritage, traditions, and values Emphasize observation, living, and learning by decisions Teach respect for tradition and honor wisdom	Develop teaching strategies and interventions based on: • Cultural beliefs • Child and parents' cognitive level • Role modeling Foster cognitive development by teaching parents and other family members cognitive growth–fostering activities to do with their child Encourage early preschool and school involvement Encourage the family and child to identify and support education as a route to success Support parents who wish to further their education

Modified from Andrews, M.M. & Boyle, J.S. (1995) Transcultural concepts in nursing care. Philadelphia: J.B. Lippincott; Clark, A.A. (1981). Culture and childrearing. Philadelphia: F.A. Davis; Giger, J.N. & Davidhizar, R.E. (1995). Transcultural nursing: Assessment and intervention. St Louis: Mosby; and Yoos, H.L., et al. (1995). Childrearing benefits in the African-American community: Implications for culturally competent pediatric care. Journal of Pediatric Nursing, 10, 343-353.

love and guidance in an atmosphere of love and security. Nurturing the personality and development of the child is one of the more critical tasks of parenting. However, adults who are lacking in self-esteem and self-efficacy may find it difficult to promote those behaviors in their children. Other parenting experiences also can contribute to effectiveness and successful parenting. Parents who have parented other children or who have come from families where they had an opportunity to experience ancillary parenting skills (e.g., helping to raise siblings) often bring a different set of skills and values to their parenting situation. The type of communication that was experienced in their families of origin and the attitudes regarding different roles in the family contribute to how parents perceive their current parenting situation. The expectations and philosophies of parenting as previously described also influence parenting effectiveness.

Just as permissiveness and restrictiveness refer to the degree of autonomy that parents allow their children, warmth and hostility refer to parental affection and the degree to which the affection is expressed. The amount of affection may vary considerably among families, based on cultural factors and individual differences in personality and temperament of both parents and children. Parents who are described as warm and nurturing often praise and encourage their child and limit their criticisms, punishments, and signs of disapproval. Parents who came from homes where they were loved and accepted are generally cooperative and more emotionally stable; they are much more likely to form satisfactory relationships with others. Hostile, cool, and rejecting parents may have grown up in homes where they experienced cool and rejecting parenting. These parents may criticize, belittle, and punish their children and limit their expressions of affection or approval. Children who feel rejected often develop feelings of insecurity and inferiority; they believe they are unworthy of love and have no value.

Parents who display realistic standards and expectations and who demonstrate warmth and nurturance generally produce children with high self-esteem who are self-reliant, assertive, content, and successful in society. Children who experience unrealistic expectations and frequent rejection become either hostile and aggressive or withdrawn and submissive. Rejection may be manifested as neglect, belittling, or emotional or physical abuse. Often, rejecting parents either overtly or covertly indicate that the child is unwanted or unloved. The desirability of parenthood, whether planned or unplanned, may contribute to these attitudes toward parenting.

The environment in which the family lives also can affect the parenting attitudes and style. Urban parents tend to be more authoritarian as a result of the increased safety hazards typical of urban living. Families living in crowded apartment buildings with few or no play areas may experience increased stress and difficulties with parenting.

The individual temperament and personality traits of the child and the parents may have a significant effect on parenting. Temperament is often defined as the style of behavior that a child or a person uses to cope with the demands and expectations of their environment. Children are very different and have their own responses to life's challenges and experiences. Parents also differ with regard to their parenting, based on their individual temperament. Chess and Thomas (1996) identify nine temperament variables, which are summarized in Box 3-1. These variables make up three distinctive temperament styles that have been studied by Chess and Thomas for over 40 years. They do not represent either good or bad characteristics but rather a way to look at the individual characteristics of both parents and children.

These temperament categories have been identified in children of all races and cultures. Children from European countries, Canada, Japan, Israel, and many other countries have all exhibited these temperament characteristics. Although temperament is one of the important factors that help shape personalities, its influence is varied, depending on the other factors that are operating at the time of the child's development. Longitudinal studies on temperament demonstrate that children's temperaments actively influence the attitudes and behavior of the parents and the other individuals with whom they interact. Their responses, in turn, shape children's behavior and development.

A *goodness of fit* exists when the demands and expectations of the parents are compatible with a child's temperament, abilities, and other characteristics. When there is a goodness of fit, the parent-child relationship is positive and the child's development is healthy. A *poorness of fit,* however, exists when demands and expectations are excessive and not compatible with a child's temperament, abilities, and other characteristics. With a poorness of fit, the child is more likely to experience stress and have a poor parent-child relationship with potentially less positive developmental outcomes.

In Box 3-2, parenting responses to individual temperaments are listed. One of the first steps that parents need to accomplish is learning to understand their child's temperament and its relationship to behavior. To promote a positive parent-child relationship, parents need to adjust their expectations and perceptions to fit the individual differences of their child. As previously discussed, parents who have an image of the ideal baby who cries little, sleeps through the night, and is cuddly and responsive may need to readjust their image when their child does not meet these expectations.

Chess and Thomas (1996) propose interventions to promote a goodness of fit, thereby facilitating smooth and positive development. Attempting a goodness of fit does not alleviate

---

Box 3-1 Temperament Characteristics

Activity level—Motor component of activity and the proportion of active versus inactive periods

Rhythmicity—Predictability versus the unpredictability of biologic functions (e.g., sleep, hunger, bowel elimination)

Adaptability—Long-term response to new or altered situations

Approach or withdrawal—Initial response to new situations or stimuli

Sensory threshold—Intensity level of stimulation needed to produce a response from the child (e.g., touch, sounds, light)

Intensity of reaction—Energy level of response, either positive or negative

Quality of mood—Amount and quality of mood expression (e.g., joyful, crying, friendly or unfriendly behavior)

Distractibility—Effectiveness of extraneous stimuli in interfering with or changing the direction of a child's behavior

Persistence and attention span—Continuation of an activity in the face of obstacles and the length of time an activity is continued without interruption

Modified from Chess, S. & Thomas, A. (1996). Know your child: An authoritative guide for today's parents. Northvale, NJ: Jason Aronson.

stress or problems; it merely provides opportunities for positive psychologic development and family harmony. Parents also have their individual temperament attributes that influence their response to the individual characteristics of their children. Families with more than one child may have a variety of temperament traits. They may have an easy child and a difficult child. To be effective parents, they need to be flexible and use different techniques to respond to the individual characteristics of each child.

A healthy, positive self-esteem is critical for a child to meet the daily challenges of life with confidence and master them successfully. Children with poor self-esteem have low opinions of themselves and their abilities to function and master challenging tasks. The goodness of fit between the environment and a child's temperament can either positively or negatively affect their self-esteem. A positive goodness of fit stimulates the strong development of self, whereas a poorness of fit often undermines the child's self-confidence and self-esteem.

Box 3-2 Guidelines for Adapting Parenting to a Child's Temperament

Easy Child

High rhythmicity
Positive mood
High adaptability
High intensity
Positive approach
Approximately 40% of the population

- Remember that this child adapts to almost any parenting approach and is easy to manage if expectations are clearly defined, consistent, and not incongruent with what the child finds in the outside world.
- Keep in mind that this child seldom develops behavior problems. If behavior problems do occur, it is because there is conflict between home-taught values and those of the outside world. Because of this child's easy adaptability, it is important not to initiate any practice or ritual that is undesirable to continue over time, as the child will quickly incorporate this practice into his or her own living pattern.
- Spend separate time with this child who may be overlooked because he or she is so "easy."
- Because this child is highly adaptable, keep in mind that the child may always do what others wish, even if it is not in his or her own best interest.
- Teach this child how to discriminate and develop his or her own rules.
- Teach this child caution, because the child is generally positive in approach and may not use caution when meeting strangers and get into dangerous situations.

Slow-to-Warm Child

Low activity
Low adaptability
High intensity
Low rhythmicity
Negative mood
Withdrawal
Approximately 15% of the population

- Use a patient, relaxed, persevering approach. New situations or rules should be presented gradually but repeatedly, without pressure. Because of some common elements in the traits of the difficult and slow-to-warm personality types, some management guidelines apply to both types.
- Refuse to compete with the child or to demand strict adherence to every rule in the home. Such actions only increase negative displays of behavior.
- Try not to explode at the child, because fury only exaggerates inappropriate behavior.
- Clearly identify on a regular basis what behaviors are acceptable or unacceptable. Help this child in identifying what behaviors are contingent to the situation at hand. This clarification should

occur at times when the child is not misbehaving because if tense, the child may not hear the rules. Be consistent in enforcing established limits. A democratic approach is least overwhelming for this child; however, an autocratic approach may also work as long as it is not extreme.

- Remember that this child learns slowly, so repeat rules often.
- Build in daily successes for this child.
- Maintain established routines while this child is mastering a rule or behavioral expectation.
- Remember key words to management (e.g., firmness, repeated exposure, consistent reinforcement, patience).

Difficult Child

Low rhythmicity
Negative mood
Withdrawal
Low adaptability
High intensity
Approximately 10% of the population

- Remember that a firm, consistent approach that emphasizes the positive is most effective with this temperament style. Those aspects of a child's temperament that may have undesirable consequences if allowed unrestricted expression should be controlled and limited in a calm but firm and consistent manner.
- Be patient, as this is essential. Parents need to exert an active effort to avoid a negative parent-child relationships that may arise out of this child's constant stressful behaviors.
- Keep in mind that parents of a child of this temperament cope best if they take turns and give each other a daily chance to get away from the child. Certain activities may predictably cause negative behaviors, but it is important to persist in introducing the child to these situations or expectations so that he or she can eventually learn control. Parents may especially wish to take turns handling the child during these experiences because they take a great deal of energy.
- Provide gradual and repeated reinforcement, both positive and negative, for expected behaviors so that this child can internalize them. Problems in behavior usually arise from conflict between the child and almost any aspect of the environment, whether it be parents, new situations, or the world outside.
- Give a minimal number of rules at a time (e.g., one to three). The rules need to be straightforward and unencumbered by explanations or choices.
- Provide constructive avenues for this child's excess emotions and energy.

Mixed-Temperament Child

Respond to whichever of the other three personality types seems to predominate in this child.

Modified from Chess, S. & Thomas, A. (1996). Know your child: An authoritative guide for today's parents. Northvale, NJ: Jason Aronson.

Later in this chapter are some suggestions for parents for adapting to the three types of temperament identified by Chess and Thomas (1996).

Parenting Situations

Parenting is a demanding role even under the most ideal circumstances, but many families experience situations that may increase the potential for family disruption and deficits in parenting (see Section 2, Families with Special Parenting Needs). Children are brought up in many family situations. Some are raised in a tight nuclear family with a mother, a father, and perhaps one or two siblings. Other children live in an extended family with several siblings, grandparents, and perhaps aunts, uncles, and cousins living in the same house or nearby. Many children in an extended family spend large quantities of time with caregivers who are family members or friends, and there is much shared parenting.

There are families in which the mother and the father work outside the home and others in which the mother or the father stays at home and provides the majority of care. Some parents (mother or father) may devote all their time to child-rearing and do not work outside the home until the children are grown, if at all. Recent years also have seen the emergence of a group of self-supporting single women who voluntarily choose to have a child through artificial insemination, adoption, or contractual agreement and to raise the child without a father in the home.

A person may become a single parent through divorce, death, incarceration of a spouse or significant other, or voluntary self-selection. There are also homosexual women who become pregnant through heterosexual relationships, artificial insemination, or adoption. They may be either single parents or part of a two-parent, same-sex parenting relationship. Many single, never-married parents are teenagers who may reside with their parents or relatives after becoming pregnant. Often these women are poor, undereducated, immature, and ill equipped to raise children and could be considered children themselves. Because many young single pregnant women do not seek prenatal care, they have a higher incidence of premature babies.

Single parents often require additional support systems, such as an additional caregiver or an acceptable child care facility, to cope with the demands of child-rearing. Substantial research demonstrates that a child is not necessarily at risk for psychologic harm if a "mother" or "father" figure is lacking. There is evidence, however, that the stresses and conflicts within the family situation can cause more emotional harm and potential behavior problems than the lack of one parent. A single teenage mother or father who is on welfare, living in a crowded apartment, and a high school dropout poses a much higher risk for parenting problems than a mature, educated woman who voluntarily chooses single parenthood. The parenting tasks, goals, and styles are the same for single parents, dual parents, and extended families, but the issues, intrinsic strengths, and potential problems vary with each family situation. Many children seen by a practitioner may come from nontraditional nuclear families. It is generally not the specific type of parenting situation that leads to problems for children; it is conflict within the family. The practitioner should assess each parenting situation for its strengths, vulnerabilities, and family stressors and intervene as early as possible to assist parents in all types of situations to achieve their optimal effectiveness.

Discipline

Although the term *discipline* is often used to denote punishment, it actually refers to teaching, as in the word *disciple*. Flexible but firm discipline fosters responsible and self-confident development (see also the discussion of discipline in Chapter 19). Parents teach their children their values, ethics, and rules of conduct to help socialize the child into the family and society. Rules and setting limits provide a child with predictable boundaries, which increases the child's security and reinforces trust. As children master the rules of conduct, they experience a sense of confidence and self-worth that contributes to their independence and self-regulation.

Rules provide children with guidelines as to what is acceptable and unacceptable behavior. They are needed to assist children in learning what actions are never acceptable because they are immoral, illegal, dangerous, or antisocial. The practitioner can assist parents in establishing clear, realistic rules that have clear consequences for noncompliance. Consistency in implementing rules and discipline are important parenting skills. Although consistency is important, it is even more critical for parents to provide discipline in a nurturing environment. (Box 3-3 provides questions that the practitioner may wish to ask to assess consistency in discipline and parenting rules.)

Children are natural imitators— they imitate how parents act, communicate, and solve problems. Parents need to practice what they preach. If it is a rule that everyone wears a seat belt, parents should model the appropriate behavior and not expect compliance from their child if they are not wearing seat belts themselves. Caregivers should agree on the rules and the methods of enforcement and make a commitment to follow through with the details of discipline. Discipline strategies should reflect the developmental level and characteristics of the child and the circumstances. Biting a child to discipline the unacceptable behavior of biting a sibling shows incongruency because the child is unable to problem solve the inconsistencies; the child does not learn an acceptable behavior or internalize the rule "Thou shalt not bite" when this method of discipline is involved. (Disciplinary methods used to decrease undesired behavior and set limits [rules] are summarized in Box 3-4; see also the discussion of discipline in Chapter 19.)

Louise Hart (1993) discusses ways that parents effect self-esteem in their children in her book *The Winning Family*. She

---

Box 3-3 Assessment of Consistency in Parenting Rules

Do parents practice what they preach?
Are the rules realistic for the child's age, temperament, and circumstances?
Do parents follow through by enforcing rules?
Have parents communicated rules to other caregivers?
Do parents agree on the rules to be enforced and the methods for enforcement?
Is enforcement promptly enacted?
Is the rationale shared with the child an age-appropriate one?
Are enforcement methods congruent with the rule involved?
Does the child show signs of developing respect for rules?
Do parents give choices?
Do parents respect the rights of the child?

describes four basic types of parenting responses: nurturing and structuring responses that increase self-esteem and "marshmallowing" and criticizing responses that tear down self-esteem. Nurturing responses encourage self-responsibility and are based on love, respect, and support. Structuring responses are also based on respect and serve to protect, set limits, and demand performance. Marshmallowing responses remove responsibility from the child and invite dependence and encourage failure, while ridicule, putdowns, blaming, fault finding, and labeling are examples of criticizing responses. Marshmallowing and criticizing responses are damaging to a child's self-esteem and result in anger, dependence, and powerlessness. (A situation with examples of the various responses is found in Box 3-5.)

Regardless of the type of discipline used, certain principles are necessary to promote self-esteem and help children learn and develop self-discipline and self-responsibility. Strategies such as rewards, behavior modification, and others listed may be used by parents to discipline and set limits, but none of these strategies is as effective as natural and logical consequences. The use of natural consequences, such as the child not having favorite blue jeans to wear, provides a method for a parent to allow the child to learn the natural order of events. The parent allows the child to discover without outside interference the advantages of respect for the natural order of the physical world. The child then learns to respect order not because of fear of punishment but because of developed self-discipline and internal motivation. Parents should be firm and kind, inform a child once of the natural consequences, and must not allow serious harm to come to the child. Parents may allow a child to touch a warm oven door so that they may learn the cause and effect of "hot" but should not allow the child to be burned. Instead of nagging or threatening children to place their dirty clothes in the laundry hamper, the parent lets them know that any dirty clothes not put in the hamper will not be washed; children who do not put their dirty laundry in the hamper will not have clean clothes to wear.

Logical consequences are structured situations that allow children to learn the consequences of their behavior. They are not punishments but rather rational consequences that are related to the misbehavior or situation. They are nonjudgmental and permit a choice. For example, the children may be fighting in the back seat of the car while riding to their grandmother's house. A parent using logical consequences might respond by pulling off the road, stopping the engine, and quietly explaining that the noise is too distracting and the trip cannot continue until it is quiet. The children might be quiet for a few minutes but then resume their fighting. After several stops along the road, the children learn the connection between cause and effect (fighting and yelling causes the parent to pull off the road). When children know what is expected and do not comply with the rules, they learn the consequences of their behavior; when children know what is expected and comply with the rules, they experience a sense of accomplishment and increased self-esteem. With natural and logical consequences, children are responsible for their own behavior and are allowed to make their own decisions and learn from their successes and mistakes. Using a logical and natural consequence-oriented approach to discipline teaches *self*-discipline, *self*-direction, and *self*-responsibility. (Parents must still model the behaviors they want to see in their children.) Using consequences and nurturing and structuring responses in parenting promotes increased self-esteem and empowers children and adults to be independent, responsible, and competent.

Box 3-4 Methods Used to Decrease Undesirable Behavior

Punishment—The "price" for not adhering to the established rules. Physical punishment is generally considered a retaliation by parents instead of a teaching tool, and it may be injurious to the child.

Disapproval—Verbal or nonverbal. Disapproval may be learned at a very early age.

Privilege withdrawal—Often effective for older children. Specifics should be predetermined (e.g., watching television contingent on completion of chores).

Isolation—Timeout is a form of isolation. Isolation should be limited to 1 minute per year of age for a young child and up to 1 hour for an older one.

Substitution—Generally used for infants and toddlers. Substitution is to remove the child from the situation that is prompting misbehavior and divert his or her attention with another activity or toy.

Reasoning—An explanation of why a behavior is wrong, with provision of a rationale. Best used for older children.

Positive reinforcement—Rewards (e.g., tokens, hugs, activities) for desired behavior.

Negative reinforcement—Ignoring of behavior.

Natural consequences—Experiences that allow a child to learn from the natural order (e.g., a child who doesn't put dirty clothes in the laundry hamper will not have clean clothes to wear).

Logical consequences—Structured situations based on mutual respect. A consequence is logically related to the misbehavior and is sensible. The reality of the social order and parental choice are also emphasized. (If a parent states, "I'm not washing any clothes not put in the laundry hamper," a child who does not place dirty clothes in the laundry hamper will not have clean clothes to wear.)

Box 3-5 Parenting Responses that Affect Self Esteem

The situation is that Ryan (8 years old) won't clean his room and says, "I hate you, Mom."

Nurturing response—"Ryan [mother touches him], I know you don't want to clean your room and that you're mad at me. That's okay. I still love you. Let's both clean our rooms at the same time, and when we finish, we'll go outside and play."

Structuring response—"We're all part of the family, Ryan, and we all have chores to do. Cleaning your room is an important way of being part of our team."

Marshmallowing response—"Don't hate me. You're right. It is too hard for you. I'll do it for you so we can be pals. Maybe when you get bigger you'll be able to do something by yourself, poor thing."

Criticizing response—"You bad boy! Get in your room right now and don't come out until it's perfect! And just wait until your father gets home!"

Reprinted with permission from Hart, L. (1993). The winning family: Increasing self-esteem in your children and yourself. Berkeley, CA: Celestial Arts. Available from your local bookstore, or by calling (800) 841-2665 or visiting www.tenspeed.com.

Box 3-6 Parental Strengths and Vulnerabilities

Strengths

Enjoys the child
Praises the child and promotes self-esteem
Projects warmth, understanding, and honesty
Good communication skills
Teaches appropriate social skills and behaviors
Understands and responds appropriately to the child's developmental needs
Provides emotional support and comfort
Promotes healthy habits
Has extended support systems and resources
Is emotionally and physically healthy
Models with competent, healthy adult behaviors
Encourages independence, maturity, and achievement
Able to set limits and discipline appropriately
Aware of and responsive to individual temperament of the child
Provides safe, nurturing environment

Vulnerabilities

Unrealistic expectations of themselves and child
Extreme parenting style
Disturbed relationship with child (e.g., controlling, domineering, intrusive)

Poor communication skills
Poor self-esteem
Lack of parental presence
Inadequate parenting skills
Marital or relationship problems
Depression
Substance abuse
Inability to model healthy, competent adult behaviors
Family violence, abuse, or neglect
Family stressors:
• Divorce
• Family or parent emotional or physical illness
• Death of a family member
• Change in family situation (e.g., remarriage, mother or father going to work, loss of job, moving)
• Social isolation
• Lack of resources
• Homelessness
Too distant or "cold"
Inappropriate reactions to child's temperament and developmental level
Child with special needs (e.g., chronic illness, disability, emotional or behavioral problems)

Assessment

No family is perfect, and no parent is perfect. The majority of parents do more than an adequate job of raising their children to be successful adults, sometimes against tremendous odds. All parents make mistakes and may learn and grow from those mistakes. Practitioners can assist parents in achieving their optimal level of parenting by performing an adequate assessment of the parents' level of parenting abilities, strengths, and flaws. Assessment can begin before the child is born by assessment of the parents' readiness to parent, their level of preparation for the child, the plans they have made for the birth, and what expectations and perceptions they have of parenting (see Chapter 8). At each well-child visit, a practitioner can also observe and assess for parental strengths and vulnerabilities (Box 3-6).

There are multiple assessment tools for parenting, many of which are used to identify parents at risk for abuse of their children. However, many of these tools are not designed for the short health supervision visits in a busy primary care practice or may address only one specific aspect or risk factor for parenting, and tools that attempt to address the full scope of parenting values, beliefs, expectations, and behaviors are too unwieldy to administer on a consistent basis. A practitioner not only must identify the extreme parenting behaviors that place children at risk for emotional and physical injury but also must assess parents at all points on the continuum. Box 3-7 provides trigger questions practitioners can use to assess parenting capabilities and potential areas of concern at each visit.

An overall assessment of the parent can also provide important clues for the practitioner. Box 3-8 provides a general assessment format.

Interventions can then be structured to meet the individual needs of parents and families. Baseline data on the cultural background of the family, number of family members, parent-

ing situation, parental employment, socioeconomic status, special health needs, educational background, and any stress factors should be obtained as soon as possible. Parents' knowledge of normal growth and development and their expectations, temperament, and parenting and disciplinary style should also be assessed. At each visit there should be an ongoing assessment of the parenting process and its effect on the child. The practitioner can help parents increase their awareness and understanding of their child's developmental level and temperament and its influence on their parenting behaviors.

Assessment of support systems is also critical in assisting parents in developing effective parenting skills. Helping parents identify their available resources, both personal and professional, and evaluate the positive or negative effect of their support systems should be a major focus of the practitioner. If support systems are not being supportive or are inadequate, the practitioner should assist the parent in developing resources that can strengthen those they already have or should create additional ones.

The parent-child relationship is a vital piece of the assessment process. Parents who are unable to describe the personality traits of their child, the child's types of activities, and the child's typical daily routine may not be emotionally attached to that child. It is critical when one is gathering these data that open-ended questions be asked in a nonjudgmental way. The trigger questions found in Box 3-7 facilitate open communication between the parent and the practitioner and provide opportunities for parents to express concerns. Observation of the parent-child interaction is also an essential part of the health care examination (Box 3-9).

The physical examination offers an opportunity not only to evaluate the normal growth and development of the child for medical and genetic problems but also to identify children

Box 3-7 Trigger Questions to Ask Parents to Assess Parenting Capabilities and Vulnerabilities

How are you today?

How are things going at home?

Have there been any major stresses or changes in your family since your last visit?

How are you balancing your roles of partner and parent?

Have you ever been in a relationship where you have been hurt, threatened, or treated badly?

What are some of the things you do together as a family?

What are some of the main hassles in your life right now? Transportation? Money? Family problems? Housing? Personal safety?

How do family members interact and play with your child?

What ties does your family have to the community?

How were things for you when you were growing up?

Who helps you with the baby?

When are you planning to return to work? To school? Have you thought about child care arrangements?

How do you and your partner feel about your child's behavior?

What do you enjoy most about your child?

What seems most difficult?

Do you and your partner tend to agree or differ in your ideas about discipline?

How is your health?

Is there anyone in the family about whom you are worried?

Do you plan to raise your child the way you were raised or somewhat differently?

What would you change?

Do you smoke? Do you drink? Have you taken any drugs? Does your partner take drugs?

Are you concerned about being able to afford food or supplies for your baby?

What are your child's achievements?

Whom do you turn to when you need help?

What do you find most rewarding about your child?

What do you do when your child wants something he or she shouldn't have?

What do you do when you become angry and frustrated with your child?

Have you ever been worried someone was going to hurt your child?

Has your child ever been abused? Were you ever abused as a child?

How are you setting limits for your child and disciplining him or her?

What about your child makes you proud?

Do you talk with your child about sensitive subjects such as sex, drugs, and drinking?

How is your child doing in school?

What concerns do you have?

From Green, M. (Ed.). (2001). Bright futures: Guidelines for health supervision of infants, children, and adolescents (2nd ed.). Arlington, VA: National Center for Education in Maternal and Child Health, supported by the Maternal Child and Health Bureau and the Medical Bureau.

Box 3-8 Assessment of the Parent

General appearance

Parental developmental level (e.g., cognition, ability to read and write, ability to follow directions, problem-solving ability)

History:
- Parent abused as a child
- Type of parenting parent received as child
- Planned or unplanned pregnancy
- Self-awareness of temperament and personality traits
- Knowledge of normal growth and development
- Expectations and philosophies of parenting

Steps taken to prepare for the child (e.g., providing a room, bed, and clothes; taking time off from work; seeking child care)

Available support systems:
- Personal (e.g., family, friends)
- Professional (e.g., practitioner, physician)
- Social (e.g., assistance programs, housing, medical)

Level of parenting ability

Box 3-9 Observation of the Parent-Child Interaction

How do the parent and child interact?

Does the parent pay attention to the child's behavior and intervene appropriately? (E.g., Does the parent of a 6-month-old infant leave the infant alone on the examination table and sit across the room?)

How does the parent talk to and about the child?

How does the parent provide for safety? What disciplinary style is used for misbehavior in the clinic?

Does the parent have eye contact with the child and vocalize or talk with the child?

Does the parent allow the child to answer questions?

How does the parent provide support for stressful situations?

not receiving adequate parenting. Box 3-10 outlines a brief assessment of the child. There are many reasons why children may be failing to thrive or may be developmentally delayed, but the practitioner should be aware that these may be symptoms of parenting deficits. Box 3-11 lists potential risk factors that might lead to parenting deficits. The results of these deficits may include childhood behavior problems, perpetual inappropriate behavior, child neglect, failure to thrive, developmental delays, or child abuse. As the child becomes older, being questioned alone without the parents in the

room allows the child an opportunity to express feelings and concerns.

Early assessment of parenting capabilities and vulnerabilities allows for early intervention to promote family strengths and relationships and parent effectiveness. The practitioner can assist parents and children in developing mutually enjoyable and satisfying parent-child interactions and community ties. Many parents need assistance in learning how to promote the healthy growth and development of their child and accomplish their parenting tasks and goals.

Box 3-10 Assessment of the Child

Physical Examination

General appearance of child
Natural growth parameters and failure to thrive
Evidence of physical trauma or neglect
Developmental examination and evidence of delays

Child-Parent (Caregiver) Relationship

Infant vocalizes to, has eye contact with, and is responsive to parent.
Child has positive, age-appropriate descriptions of activities, discipline, and the rules of the house.
Child is able to discuss concerns with parents.
Child seeks a parent for comfort and support.
Child demonstrates and communicates a positive self-esteem.

Note whether the child is doing well in school, has friends, and is involved in age-appropriate activities.
Observe sibling interactions or ask questions about siblings.

Box 3-11 Potential Risk Factors for Parenting

Child neglect and abuse experienced by parents during their own childhoods
Parental depression
Parental alcoholism
Marital problems
Poor parent-child bonding
Stressors (e.g., finances, housing, loss of job, homelessness)
Family illness
Family violence
Negative support systems or lack of support systems
Lack of parental self-esteem
Poor family communication
Children with chronic or debilitating diseases or developmental, physical, or emotional delays
Family changes (e.g., divorce, illness, death, parent returning to work outside of the home)

Consultations and Referrals

A practitioner should refer for the following:

- Financial assistance
- Home visitor programs
- Support groups
- Substance abuse
- Family and mental health counseling
- Child care
- Housing

A practitioner should also consult or refer if there are extreme parenting styles or conflicts that have a negative effect on the child. The practitioner may need to involve a multidisciplinary team.

Promoting Effective Parenting

The practitioner can promote effective parenting in the following ways:

- Assist parents by assessing and identifying parenting strengths, risk factors, and parenting skills and by providing appropriate interventions when necessary.
- Provide information and counseling concerning normal growth and development, identification of the unique characteristics and needs of each child, and child-rearing practices.
- Help parents identify, develop, and modify parenting capabilities according to their own style and the needs of the child.
- Demonstrate appropriate role model behaviors to the parents.
- Encourage parents to participate in parenting classes that include information on normal growth and development, child rearing, and discipline and in parenting groups that can provide support and information.
- Help parents identify their expectations of their children and of parenthood and assist them in analyzing these expectations to see if they are appropriate and realistic.
- Have parents identify their support systems and resources and how best to utilize them.

- Counsel parents regarding their parenting skills, strengths, and vulnerabilities.
- Assess significant stresses for parents and children and assist in developing acceptable solutions and resources to deal with stressful events and situations.
- Use multiple intervention strategies to assist parents in developing effective parenting skills and reinforce their existing skills. The key is to start early.
- Counsel parents-to-be about preparations, expectations, and parenting goals.
- Observe at health supervision and illness visits for parenting style, the child's temperament and behavior, and parent-child interaction. This assessment should be ongoing and provide opportunities for parents to discuss concerns and problems.
- Recognize parents for their strengths as well as their vulnerabilities and deficits.
- Provide parents with educational handouts and videos, group sessions, and information on resources within the community (e.g., parenting classes).
- Assist parents in being effective, free from unjustified guilt, and self-confident in their parenting skills.
- Help parents find a compromise between what they expect of themselves and their children and what is realistic.
- Reinforce those attitudes and behaviors in parents and children that promote healthful socialization.
- At each visit help parents identify important issues and concerns and target behaviors that may need intervention.
- Recognize that good parenting can be accomplished in a variety of ways. Acknowledgment and validation of the emotions of parents and children can facilitate a strong therapeutic relationship.
- Assist families in identifying their feelings of guilt, hurt, regret, and sadness and refer family members to trained therapists if needed.
- Listen and help families discover their own solutions to their concerns, based on their individual needs and circumstances.

Box 3-12 Positive Parenting Strategies

Model acceptable and desirable behaviors (e.g., using a calm voice instead of shouting).

Use effective communication skills (e.g., "I" messages, active listening). ("You" messages denote blame [e.g., "You'd better pick that up," versus the "I" message "I don't like seeing these toys all over the floor"].)

Teach positive practices (e.g., apologizing) and how to repair the results of a misdeed (e.g., paying for a broken window).

Initiate discipline as soon as the child misbehaves and always disapprove of the behavior, not the child.

Respect the rights of children; treat them as you would guests. (Would you scream at a guest for spilling a drink on the carpet?)

Administer discipline in private to avoid shaming the child in front of others.

Once the discipline is administered, consider the child to have a "clean slate" and avoid lecturing or repeatedly bringing up past misbehaviors.

Give choices and, whenever possible, allow the child to have power and control.

Avoid lose-lose and win-lose conflicts; try to develop win-win situations whenever possible.

Follow through and do not make empty threats; set limits and rules that can be enforced.

Use positive statements (e.g., "Put the glass down") instead of negative ones (e.g., "Don't play with that glass").

Keep cool and calm; if you become angry, cool down and discuss the situation later.

Set clear expectations.

Modify the environment to minimize unacceptable behaviors.

Use natural and logical consequences.

Encourage mutual respect.

Promote a positive self-esteem.

Reinforce positive behaviors.

- Focus on parents' unique strengths and capabilities and facilitate the development of additional parenting skills as needed.
- Promote positive parenting practices (Box 3-12).
- Many health care practitioners believe that teaching children how to parent in school is an effective way to change cycles of battering and abuse. Many middle and high schools have courses on growth and development and parenting that may assist children in developing positive parenting practices in the future.

Conclusion

Parenting is both challenging and rewarding, with many factors affecting the level of parenting abilities. Working with such a broad range of lifestyles, child-rearing practices, and cultural beliefs is often difficult, and health care practitioners' own values, beliefs, and culture influence how they perceive and react to various parenting situations. It is essential for practitioners to attempt to understand and acknowledge their own values and beliefs about parenting and various parenting situations. This does not mean agreement with the choices others have made in child rearing, but it does mean focusing on each family's strengths and capabilities and responding to the

unique needs of each family. The emphasis should be on mutual respect and acceptance of the unique characteristics of parents and children. Practitioners should accentuate the positive and assist parents in being successful and effective parents who can enjoy, learn, and grow along with their children.

Resources

Organizations

Active Parenting, Inc, 810 Franklin Court, Suite B, Marietta, GA 30067; (770) 429-0565 or (800) 825-0060

Parents Without Partners, 1650 South Dixie Highway, Suite 500, Boca Raton, FL 33432; (800) 637-7974

Single Mothers by Choice, PO Box 1642, Gracie Square Station, New York, NY 10028; (212) 988-0993

Publications

American Academy of Child and Adolescent Psychiatry. (1998). *Your adolescent—what every parent needs to know: What's normal, what's not, and when to seek help.* New York: HarperCollins.

American Academy of Child and Adolescent Psychiatry. (1998). *Your child—what every parent needs to know: What's normal, what's not, and when to seek help.* New York: HarperCollins.

American Academy of Pediatrics. (1999). *Caring for your school-age child: Ages 5 to 12.* New York: Bantam.

American Academy of Pediatrics. (1998). *Caring for your baby and young child: Birth to age 5.* New York: Bantam.

American Academy of Pediatrics. (1991). *Caring for your adolescent: Ages 12 to 21.* New York: Bantam.

Brazelton, T.B. (1972). *Infants and mothers: Differences in development.* New York: Dell.

Brazelton, T.B. (1974). *Toddlers and parents: A declaration of independence.* New York: Dell.

Brazelton, T.B. (1992). *Touchpoints: Your child's emotional and behavioral development.* New York: Addison-Wesley.

Dinkmeyer, D., et al. (1997). *The parent's handbook: STEP systematic training for effective parenting.* Circle Pines, MN: American Guidance Service.

Green, M. (Ed.). (2001). *Bright futures: Guidelines for health supervision of infants, children and adolescents* (2nd ed.). Arlington, VA: National Center for Education in Maternal Child Health.

Levine, S.B. (2000). *Father courage: What happens when men put family first.* New York: Harcourt.

Phelan, T.W. (1995). *1,2,3, Magic.* Glen Ellyn, IL: Child Management.

Powell-Hopson, D. & Hopson, D. (1990). *Different and wonderful: Raising Black children in a race-conscious society.* New York: Prentice-Hall.

Schiff, E. (Ed.). (1987). *Experts advise parents: A guide to raising loving, responsible children.* New York: Delacorte.

Websites

ABCs of Parenting (www.abcparenting.com/)

American Academy of Pediatrics (www.aap.org)

Bright Futures (www.brightfutures.org)

Parents Place (www.parentsplace.com)

PedInfo (lhl.uab.edu/pedinfo/miscellaneous.html)

Resources for Nurses, Children, and Families (pegasus.cc.ucf.edu/wink/home.html)

Bibliography

Baumrind, D. (1971). Current patterns of parental authority (Monograph 4). *Developmental Psychology, 1*(2), 1-103.

Bornstein, M. (Ed.). (1991). *Cultural approaches to parenting.* Hillsdale, NJ: Lawrence Erlbaum Associates.

Chess, S. & Thomas, A. (1996). *Know your child: An authoritative guide for today's parents.* Northvale, NJ: Jason Aronson.

Coleman, W. & Taylor, E. (Eds.). (1995). Family-focused pediatric issues, challenges, and clinical methods. *Pediatric Clinics of North America, 42,* 1-304.

Darling, N. & Steinberg, L. (1993). Parenting style as context: An integrative model. *Psychological Bulletin, 113*(3), 487-496.

Erickson, E. (1963). *Childhood and society.* New York: W.W. Norton.

Fuchs, V. & Reklis, D. (1992). America's children: Economic perspectives and policy options. *Science, 255,* 41-46.

Galinsky, E. (1987). *The six stages of parenthood.* Reading, MA: Addison-Wesley.

Gellerstedt, M.E., et al. (1995). Beyond anticipatory guidance: parenting and the family life cycle. *Pediatric Clinics of North America, 42,* 65-78.

Green, M. (Ed.). (2001). *Bright futures: Guidelines for health supervision of infants, children, and adolescents* (2nd ed.). Arlington, VA: National Center for Education in Maternal and Child Health.

Gross, D. & Conrad, B. (1995). Temperament in childhood. *Journal of Pediatric Nursing, 10,* 146-151.

Hart, L. (1993). *The winning family: Increasing self-esteem in your children and yourself.* Berkeley, CA: Celestial Arts.

Maslow, A.H. (1968). *Toward a psychology of being.* Princeton: Van Nostrand.

McClowry, S.G. (1995). The influence of temperament on development during middle childhood. *Journal of Pediatric Nursing, 10,* 160-165.

Regaldo, M.G. & Halfon, N. (1998). Parenting: Issues for the pediatrician. *Pediatric Annals, 27,* 31-37.

Smetana, J.G. (Ed). (1994). Parenting styles and beliefs about parental authority. *New Directions for Child Development, 66,* 1-95.

Sturner, R. (1998). The child health supervision visit as an opportunity address parenting issues during infancy. *Pediatric Annals, 27,* 44-50.

Yogman, M.W. & Kindlon, D. (1998). Pediatric opportunities with fathers and children. *Pediatric Annals, 27,* 16-22.

Yoos, H.L., Kitzman, H., Olds, D.L., et al. (1995). Childrearing beliefs in the African-American community: Implications for culturally competent pediatric care. *Journal of Pediatric Nursing, 10,* 343-353.

Chapter 4 *Cultural Diversity in Clinical Practice*

Barbara R. Kelley

The provision of health care is a reciprocal process that involves giving and taking advice and sharing ideas and beliefs. This process requires an understanding of a patient's belief system and health care practices. Practitioners do not necessarily share the same concerns and beliefs as their patients about children or their well care, sick care, nutrition, stimulation, and discipline. To be helpful to culturally diverse families and children, practitioners need to become more knowledgeable about cultural differences, values, beliefs, and practices. Understanding what is meaningful and important to parents and families enables practitioners to support cultural integrity as families adapt to the demands of the dominant culture.

Primary care providers (PCPs) are often the first health care professionals encountered by people from another culture. Seeking health care in a strange environment from people who are different can be an overwhelming experience. Practitioners must take care not to create additional stress within a family by giving health and child care advice that is not culturally acceptable. People from other countries come to the United States with preconceived notions of America and Americans. They may believe that all Americans are rich; that everyone has it easy; that American youth are spoiled, use drugs, and are violent; and that parents have no authority over their children. Ideas such as these may be reinforced when families have children, especially teens, attending school. Individuals from other cultures who are concerned about American values and behaviors may not be ready to listen to advice or believe practitioners, the majority of whom are Caucasian and represent the mainstream culture. Helping people cope with the stress of acculturation in addition to the anxiety of an illness requires that practitioners be open and sensitive to their patients' belief systems and health care practices. The provision of culturally congruent, acceptable health care requires an understanding of a practitioner's own values and beliefs, the acceptance of the relativity of these values, and an awareness of areas of possible conflict when assisting someone from another culture.

Multiculturalism

Multiculturalism has long been a hallmark of the United States. Today more than ever, increasing numbers of people from diverse backgrounds are moving to the United States to live and raise families. One striking characteristic of these newer immigrants is their desire to maintain their cultural identity. The U.S. Bureau of the Census (2000) indicates that the population of the United States is more than 280 million people and that one in every three Americans is from a minority group. Foreign-born people represent 10.4% of the total U.S. population. Many immigrants choose to live in East Coast and West Coast cities, with increasing numbers moving to the South. The fastest-growing group is described as Hispanic or of Hispanic origins. (The most recent ethnic breakdown of the U.S. population is displayed in Table 4-1.)

Table 4-1 2000 Census Data

People	281,421,906	
Families	70,920,749	
Households	102,503,262	
RACE		**PERCENTAGE OF TOTAL POPULATION**
Caucasian	211,460,626	75.1%
African American	34,658,190	12.3%
Native American and Alaska Native	2,475,956	0.9%
Asian	10,242,998	3.6%
Native Hawaiian and Other Pacific Islander	398,835	0.1%
Hispanic	35,305,818	12.5%
HISPANICS (PLACE OF ORIGIN)		**PERCENTAGE OF HISPANIC POPULATION**
Mexico	23,337,145	66.1%
Puerto Rico	3,177,523	9%
Cuba	1,412,232	4%
Central and South America	5,119,343	14.5%
Other	2,259,572	6.4%

Terms

Culture defines a person's beliefs and behaviors, whereas genetics defines an individual's basic inherited human characteristics. The concept of culture is derived from anthropology (the study of human beings) and sociology (the study of groups). It supports the understanding of individual behavior within a collective identity. Culture is the sum total of knowledge, attitudes, and habitual behavior patterns shared and transmitted by the members of a particular society. It includes art, morals, laws, customs, language, gestures, religions, and philosophical systems. A culture constitutes whatever it is one has to know or believe to operate in a manner acceptable to its members.

Cultural embeddedness refers to the extent to which an individual uses cultural guidelines or share cultural beliefs with another person of the same culture. Cultural embeddedness is influenced by education, socioeconomic status, immigration status, age, country of origin, rural versus urban upbringing, religion, and degree of acculturation.

Race refers to group members who share distinguishing physical characteristics such as skin color, hair texture, or genetic code patterns. A person's race is often readily apparent, but it may not define that individual's sense of belonging.

Ethnicity or *ethnic categorization* refers to a person's identity with a racial or national subgroup that shares characteristics such as language, eating habits, religion, and customs. These attributes give a sense of distinctiveness to the group.

Minority is a term used to describe a group of people who, regardless of their numerical status, are singled out in their society for differential and unequal treatment. The term *emerging majority* is currently being suggested as a replacement for *minority*.

Ethnocentrism is the belief in the superiority of one's own ethnic group.

Stereotypes are based on the belief that people from the same cultural background share identical values and behavior.

Health Care Values and Beliefs

Cultural values are internalized and socially transmitted through a system of beliefs, customs, and behaviors. These values, based on an integral worldview of how and why things happen, are so pervasive and subconscious that individuals are often unable to use them as an explanation for their behavior. When asked why specific behaviors or activities occur, the common response is simply that things have always been done in this fashion or that everyone has always done it this way.

Health care is that set of practices that has evolved over time to sustain life and support the well-being of individuals within a belief system. A practitioner's responsibility is to examine health care behaviors in an effort to understand the cultural assumptions underlying them. To do this, individuals must examine their own set of assumptions and be aware of what formed these health care beliefs and cultural biases. For example, rapid technologic advances in the United States support the future-oriented notion that individuals are in control of their destiny. This value orientation is in direct conflict with the orientation toward the past of many cultural groups, who see their destiny controlled by a predetermined fate. Table 4-2 provides a comparison of common cultural values.

American Values and Beliefs

In the United States the prevailing view of health is not just the absence of disease. It is a sense of well-being, an ability to re-

Table 4-2 Comparison of Common Values

ANGLO-AMERICAN	OTHER ETHNOCULTURAL GROUPS
Mastery over nature	Harmony with nature
Personal control over environment	Fate
Doing (activity)	Being
Dominance of time	Dominance of personal interaction
Human equality	Hierarchy, rank, and status
Individualism and privacy	Group welfare
Youth	Elders
Self	Birthright inheritance
Competition	Cooperation
Future orientation	Past or present orientation
Informality	Formality
Directness, openness, and honesty	Indirectness, ritual, and "face"
Practicality and efficiency	Idealism
Materialism	Spiritualism and detachment

From Randall-David, E. (1990). Strategies for working with culturally diverse communities and clients. Washington, DC: Association for the Care of Children's Health.

spond to one's environment, and an ability to develop and pursue a personal view of "health." Moreover, many Americans believe that healthful living includes an environment that does not put individuals at risk. This inclusive, individualistic view of health derives from the cultural values and belief system that have evolved over time in the United States, including:

- A long history of public health practices and laws recognizing the need for a healthful environment, the common good, and the individual
- Industrialization and unionization resulting in child labor laws, workplace safety requirements, and benefits in the form of health insurance
- Social concerns valuing individual autonomy, self-reliance, and independent thinking
- Judeo-Christian beliefs promoting social justice
- Reliance on science and technology to develop new knowledge and solve problems

Contrasting Cultural Values and Beliefs

People often come to the United States from more traditional or less affluent parts of the world where health is viewed as simply the absence of disease. This is a functional value—if one is able to get up and perform the routine of daily activities, one is healthy. In many cultural groups, both in the United States and other parts of the world, health care practices are centered around the relief of an individual's symptoms to support a normal, daily routine. A large number of immigrants to the United States come from small villages or rural areas where health practices are a result of the following:

- Traditional beliefs and practices handed down from generation to generation with little outside influence
- Subsistence-level living, where the availability of food influences dietary habits and the existence of medicinal plants and herbs supports health practices (Table 4-3)
- Social concerns that necessitate mutual dependence, collective responsibility, and identity within a family structure
- A belief that events in the current life are a prelude to the next life

Table 4-3 Examples of Medicinal Uses of Food

CULTURE	FOOD	SPECIAL PREPARATION	MEDICINAL USE
Hispanic	Lemon juice	Added to water or hot tea	Thought to cure colds
	Garlic		Used fresh as an antibiotic and topically on insect bites
			Thought to lower blood pressure
	Raw onions	Chopped with honey	Believed to be good for a cold or other respiratory infection
Vietnamese	Oregano tea	Served hot with salt instead of sugar	Given for an upset stomach
	Rice porridge		Considered standard food for sick people
Taiwanese	"Tonic" herbs	Cooked slowly	Believed to increase blood circulation
Caribbean, Filipino	Chayote and papayas		Used as a treatment for hypertension
	Soup	Prepared with cow's feet and viandas	Believed to restore strength
	Porridge	Prepared with grated green plaintain (peel included)	Believed to cure anemia
	Beet juice		
Iranian	Liver, beets, and pomegranates		Believed to increase blood
American	Chicken soup		Believed to cure anything

From Eliades, D.C. & Suitor, C.W. (1994). Celebrating diversity: approaching families through their food, *Arlington, VA: National Center for Education in Maternal and Child Health.*

- A reliance on magic and superstition as protection against unseen, powerful forces

These cultural practices mean that many people come to the PCP having already treated themselves or having sought advice from their family members, traditional healers, and spiritual advisors. Furthermore, in addition to traditional health beliefs, there are other major influences that practitioners must consider when providing culturally appropriate health care.

Major Culturally Based Influences

Spirituality

Spirituality is an important healing mode in many cultures. It may take the form of an organized religion such as Christianity, Buddhism, Judaism, or Islam. Within a cultural system the practice of religion may have been combined with more traditional, animistic forms of worship, making it unrecognizable to outsiders. Because these spiritual beliefs prescribe how one is to behave in this life and what to expect in the next, they have much influence over acceptable health care practices.

In some belief systems, suffering may be viewed as an inescapable human condition; therefore an illness becomes something to bear. Furthermore, a belief in an afterlife that is attained through human suffering may prevent an individual from seeking health care early in the course of an illness. One following such health care advice must consider such views if recommendations are to be acceptable.

Magic

Magic serves as an explanation for incomprehensible occurrences for many of the world's peoples. Superstitions and folk beliefs often mingle with religious beliefs, and protection against unseen and powerful forces often takes the form of amulets and charms worn on the body. For example, Cambodian babies wear a metal amulet, often inscribed with religious scripture, suspended from a string around the neck or wrist. Cambodian children and adults may wear a knotted string, usually red, around the waist to keep out a bad wind or a bad spirit. For women who have undergone spontaneous abortion, this type of amulet is used to ensure a successful pregnancy. Cambodian males are inscribed with elaborate tattoos of Buddhist scripture and holy drawings as a means of protection, especially in war. The Puerto Rican and Dominican cultures believe in the "evil eye," or *mal ojo*. To protect their babies, parents wrap the baby's wrist with a red or black string with a small red horn or black hand. In addition to these magical practices, many parents pin a medal of the Blessed Virgin to their infant's clothing because of their Catholic background. The Haitian culture also has a strong traditional belief in magic and voodoo. A distinction is made between black magic, which is sorcery, and white magic, which is medicine.

Balance of Opposing Forces

Many cultural groups adhere to a philosophy of harmony or balance within the universe. The body operates in harmony with nature. There is a delicate balance between two basic equal and opposing forces: *yin* and *yang,* or light and dark, male and female. These opposite elements also have the connotation of "hot" and "cold," which is a description of the properties of the substance rather than the temperature. Health is the perfect equilibrium of hot and cold elements. An excess in either direction may lead to discomfort and illness. Acupuncture and herbal medicines are typical Chinese treatments that follow the *yin* and *yang* principle. The Chinese also categorize diseases into *yin* and *yang,* which they treat with the appropriate opposing "hot" or "cold" food (Table 4-4). Many Asian cultures have incorporated Chinese medicine into their care beliefs. Other cultures that believe to some degree in the "hot" and "cold" theory of bodily imbalance are the Mexican, Puerto Rican, Central and South American, and Caribbean and the Tamils from India. It is often difficult to obtain specific information from a patient regarding the occasions that require particular foods and which foods are to be taken or avoided at those times. This is information often known only by elderly members of the group or by traditional healers.

Table 4-4 Yin and Yang Health Conditions and Foods

	YIN	YANG
Conditions		
	Cancer	Constipation
	Lactation	Infection
	Menstruation	Sore throat
	Postpartum condition	Upset stomach
	Pregnancy	Venereal Disease
Foods		
	Bean sprouts	Beef
	Boiled foods	Chicken
	Broccoli	Eggs
	Cold (in temperature) foods	Fatty meats
	Fish (some types)	Fried foods
	Fruit (some types)	Garlic
	Milk	Hot (in temperature) foods
	Pork	Liquor
	Water	Red foods
	White foods	Spicy foods

Adapted from Ludman, E.K. & Newman, J.M. (1984). Yin and Yang in the health-related food practices of three Chinese groups. Journal of Nutrition Education, 16, 1.

Box 4-1 Explanatory Model Questions

What do you call your problem? What name does it have?
What do you think caused your problem?
Why do you think it started when it did?
What is your sickness doing in your body? How does it work?
How severe is it? Will it have a short or long course?
What do you fear most about your sickness and its treatment?
How has this sickness affected your life? What problems has it caused you?
What kind of treatment do you think you should receive?
What are the most important results you hope to receive from the treatments?
What have you done so far to treat your sickness?

From Kleinman, A., Eisenberg, L., & Good, B. (1978). Culture, illness, and care. Annals of Internal Medicine, 88, 251-258.

Values and beliefs about the meaning of life and an individual's place within it are powerful motivators for health care practices. By being open and understanding the importance of an individual's belief system, practitioners are in a position to offer choices within an acceptable framework. In addition to recommending a restricted diet or a medication for a patient, the practitioner can also support the use of folk remedies, the burning of incense before a spirit altar, the completion of a novena, or the wearing of special clothing as part of a treatment plan.

Culturally Congruent Care

In the provision of culturally congruent health care, it is not always possible to have a great deal of culture-specific information. It is essential, however, that the practitioner be willing to suspend the ethnocentric notion that the biochemical model of health care practiced in the United States is superior or the only effective way to provide health care. Culturally congruent care requires an acceptance of multiple realities, an understanding of differences, and an open, sensitive, inquiring manner.

Cultural Assessment

Cultural assessment is an ongoing process that provides practitioners with an opportunity to understand and appreciate an individual's culturally unique lifestyle and life choices. Information obtained through the cultural assessment process enables practitioners to support individuals and families in clarifying needs and setting priorities. This information lays the groundwork for providing culturally appropriate health care and advice and negotiating culturally acceptable modifications.

An exhaustive cultural assessment is impractical for busy practitioners. It is important, however, to gather information in the following areas:

- Country of origin
- Length of time in the United States
- Native language literacy (i.e., reading and writing skills)
- English language proficiency
- Religion (e.g., beliefs, practices, superstitions, magic)
- Tradition (e.g., beliefs, customs, folklore)
- Family (e.g., roles, interaction, child-rearing)
- Foods, both dietary and medicinal
- Time orientation
- Living arrangements
- Health care practices and practitioners

Kleinman, Eisenberg, and Good (1978) have devised a set of questions to elicit the meaning an illness or event has to the individual (Box 4-1). Such understanding is necessary to avoid ineffective treatment or inappropriate advice. Giger and Davidhizar (1995) have developed a transcultural assessment model to help with planning and implementing care that is unique for each patient. Their model comprises six essential cultural phenomena to be considered when one is addressing a person's cultural values, beliefs, and behaviors (Table 4-5).

Framework for Assessment

In addition to the use of questions and assessment tools, the following categories provide a framework of inquiry for practitioners.

Family structure. Family structure and definition, which varies among cultures, is generally a result of adaptation to the external environment. Changes in family patterns often occur as cultural groups attempt to adapt to life in the United States. Available housing, geographical location, and local housing and public health regulations may impose significant changes in cultural and family living arrangements. Since these changes may be a source of concern and stress, family assessment is a necessary function of the practitioner. Practitioners should consider: (1) matriarchal or patriarchal living arrangements, (2) the individual's role and status within the family, and (3) hierarchical versus shared decision making.

The care provided to a family whose culture values self-reliance and individual autonomy differs from one whose culture values interrelatedness and mutual dependence. Advice and treatments given to an American patient generally result in

Table 4-5 Quick Reference Guide to Cultural Assessment

NATIONS OF ORIGIN	COMMUNICATION	SPACE	TIME ORIENTATION	SOCIAL ORGANIZATION	ENVIRONMENTAL CONTROL	BIOLOGIC VARIATIONS
Asian China Hawaii Philippines Korea Japan Southeast Asia (Laos, Cambodia, Vietnam)	National language preference Dialects, written characters Use of silence Nonverbal and contextual cuing	Noncontact people	Present	Family: hierarchical structure, loyalty Devotion to tradition Many religions, including Taoism, Buddhism, Islam, and Christianity Community social organizations	Traditional health and illness beliefs Use of traditional medicines Traditional healers: Chinese doctors, herbalists	Liver cancer Stomach cancer Coccidioidomycosis Hypertension Lactose intolerance
African West Coast (as slaves) Many African countries West Indian Islands Dominican Republic Haiti Jamaica	National languages Dialect: Pidgin, Creole, Spanish, and French	Close personal space	Present over future	Family: many female, single parent Large, extended family networks Strong church affiliation within community Community social organizations	Traditional health and illness beliefs Folk medicine tradition Traditional healer: root worker	Sickle cell anemia Hypertension Cancer of the esophagus Stomach cancer Coccidioidomycosis
Europe Germany England Italy Ireland Other European countries	National languages Many learn English immediately	Noncontact people Aloof Distant Southern countries: closer contact and touch	Future over present	Nuclear families Extended families Judeo-Christian religions Community social organizations	Primary reliance on modern health care system Traditional health and illness beliefs Some remaining folk medicine traditions	Breast cancer Heart disease Diabetes mellitus Thalassemia
Native American 170 Native American tribes Aleuts Eskimos	Tribal languages Use of silence and body language	Space very important and has no boundaries	Present	Extremely family oriented Biological and extended families Children taught to respect traditions Community social organizations	Traditional health and illness beliefs Folk medicine tradition Traditional healer: medicine man	Accidents Heart disease Cirrhosis of the liver Diabetes mellitus
Hispanic Spain Cuba Mexico Central and South America	Spanish or Portuguese primary language	Tactile relationships Touch Handshakes Embracing Value physical presence	Present	Nuclear family Extended families *Compadrazzo:* godparents Community social organizations	Traditional health and illness beliefs Folk medicine tradition Traditional healer: *curandera, espiritista, partera, señora*	Diabetes mellitus Parasites Coccidioidomycosis Lactose intolerance

Compiled by Specter, R. In Potter, P.A. & Perry, A.G. (2001). Fundamentals of nursing: concepts, process, and practice (5th ed.). St Louis: Mosby.

the individual accepting the information and returning home to inform others what needs to be done. However, cultures in which the individual functions as part of a group may need to discuss health care information or advice with elders or those in authority before acting on it. For example, the decision to hospitalize a Cambodian child requires a discussion with parents, grandparents, and other adults in the household. Practitioners may greatly increase an Asian patient's anxiety by being direct or confrontational in an encounter or by encouraging independence from the family or individual expression of feelings. In cultures where the male is the head of the family, decision maker, and money handler, children may not, for example, receive dental care if the father does not agree that it is a priority.

Group cohesiveness and family loyalty can greatly support immigrants in a new land. It is important to remember that family orientation can also work against individuals, particularly women and children, who may be subject to abuse or domestic violence. For example, in the traditional Vietnamese culture, the family is the primary source of social identity and is responsible for all decisions. The family structure is also patriarchal, with the senior male heading the household. Traditionally a Vietnamese woman lives with her husband's family after marriage and is expected to be dutiful and respectful toward her husband and his parents throughout the marriage. In the United States, Vietnamese women who remain home while their husbands work and their children attend school are not in a position to acquire a new language and gain new skills. In situations such as this, women become isolated at home and grow more dependent on the family to meet their needs.

Marriage and parenting. The tradition of marriage is culturally dependent. It serves many purposes, the least of which is the love relationship seen in Western cultures (Table 4-6). In many Middle Eastern and Asian cultures and in some African cultures, marriages are arranged, and bartering for the bride is customary. The family's reputation and the bride price are dependent on the young girl's virginity. Unmarried Cambodian women who become pregnant are a source of shame and embarrassment and an indelible blot on the goodness of the whole family. Caribbean, Mexican, and Central and South American cultures with Catholic traditions have strong religious sanctions against premarital sex. Marriage therefore becomes a prerequisite for pregnancy and parenting.

However, even culturally approved marriages may not necessarily be legally sanctioned. Meeting civil requirements before a traditional ceremony has more to do with the econom-

ics and geographical location of the couple and family. Information about the circumstances of a marriage and pregnancy is also important. If indeed the pregnancy is culturally unacceptable, little support may be available to the young woman and her future child.

Childbearing. Attitudes toward children are dependent on cultural values and norms. Children serve many purposes. They: (1) bring status and respect to their mother, (2) afford power and authority to their father, and (3) are potential contributors to the family workload. Practitioners should be aware that the need to produce children may preclude the use of contraceptives for both men and women. Contraception and abortion counseling, when appropriate, must be culturally sensitive. The gender of the child also may be a source of cultural conflict. For example, in northern India, poor girls and women are becoming increasingly marginalized. Because of this, poor families attempt to maximize male survival as insurance against old age and poverty. Wealthy families may even use genetic screening to abort females and bring male fetuses to term.

Pregnancy and childbirth. Pregnancy and childbirth occur across cultures but are accomplished in different ways by different groups of people. Many cultures view pregnancy and parenthood as a transitional step into adulthood. The Buddhist belief in reincarnation indicates that pregnancy is a way of bringing back to this life dead relatives or fetuses that were spontaneously aborted. Rural Turkish culture defines *procreation* as an aspect of divine creation; a man's godlike power and authority is based on his power to generate life.

Birth is a rite of passage that is invested with much cultural tradition. Beliefs and practices are categorized into those that pertain to the mother and those regarding the newborn.

Maternal care. Because the immediate postpartum period is a vulnerable time for mothers, many cultures have developed elaborate and extensive rituals designed to minimize maternal mortality and support the mother in her recovery period. Traditional rituals are designed to prevent the "bad" postpartum blood from building up inside the body and allow the mother's internal organs to return to their normal body position. Covering orifices prevents "bad spirits" from entering her body to do harm. Enforced rest ensures an adequate recovery period. (Table 4-7 lists other selected postpartum practices.) Many

Table 4-6 Purposes of Marriage

CULTURE	PURPOSES OF MARRIAGE
Arabic/Islamic	Marriage cements the bond between two families.
	A son is highly desired to ensure the male lineage.
Buddhist	Marriage occurs to produce children.
	Children pray for and accumulate merit for parents in their afterlife.
	Children are expected to care for parents in their old age.
Roman Catholic	Marriage is a religious sacrament designed for procreation.
Jewish	Marriage produces children to carry on Jewish traditions.

Table 4-7 Selected Postpartum Practices

CULTURE	POSTPARTUM PRACTICES
Cambodian	New mothers must be cared for in order to conserve their energy. They must: Rest in bed Avoid sitting for long periods Avoid any unnecessary lifting Avoid loud noises and arguments
Vietnamese, Cambodian	Mothers are periodically placed over hot coals to keep their bodies warm ("mother roasting"). Mothers must be well wrapped, especially their head and ears.
Haitian	Mothers must become healthy and "clean" by: Taking baths, drinking teas, and using vapor inhalations Dressing warmly Mothers use abdominal binders and bed rest to close the "open" bones of pregnancy.

"standard" newborn care practices, such as the first-week follow-up visit and expectations of maternal-infant bonding behavior (e.g., feeding, holding), may interfere with traditional cultural practices and create anxiety in the mother and family.

Newborn care. The newborn period is fraught with dangers. Infant mortalities in the first month of life range from a high of 157.1 per 1000 births in Sierra Leone to a low of 2.6 per 1000 births in Iceland. (The U.S. infant mortality is 7 per 1000.) Care of the newborn is centered around sustaining life by preventing outside interference from infection, malevolent spirits, or bad winds and by encouraging growth. An individual's or group's beliefs in God, deities, saints, magic, fate, destiny, or biomedicine define appropriate caregiving practices (Table 4-8). Parental support requires an understanding of the beliefs surrounding cultural practices. The practice of praising parents for their efforts and pointing out all the positive aspects of their newborn may offend or frighten some parents and not prove helpful for them.

Childhood. Parents support and nurture their children's growth and development in a variety of culturally specific ways designed to produce culturally acceptable adult behavior. Table 4-9 outlines environmental factors that contribute to specific cultural practices. For example, toilet training is an important achievement of American children. However, because of the surrounding environment and group behavior, children's toileting behavior may be of little or no concern in some cultures. Another important consideration is that behaviors such as constant holding of a baby, carrying a child to work, or community sleeping provide children with the social security and sense of community that is consistent with their later life. An understanding of the rationale for child-rearing practices can provide the basis for cultural negotiation and acceptable cultural adaptation.

Discipline. As children grow and move into the larger society, they are expected to conform to acceptable cultural behavior. Practitioners need to explore methods of setting limits and realistic expectations with parents. This is particularly important as school-age children become influenced by peer pressure. In many cultures, behavior that brings shame, embarrassment, and dishonor to the family is a matter for punishment. Discipline is seen as a parental responsibility and "face-saving" measure. Punishment may take the form of scolding, screaming, spanking, or isolation. In the United States corporal punishment is not regarded by many child care advocates as the best method of discipline. When spanking, paddling, and the use of a switch or belt are the cultural norm, an open and sensitive attitude on the part of the practitioner can be helpful in negotiating alternative methods of discipline.

Disease prevention. Disease prevention is a concept that requires a belief in control over one's destiny. This concept, prevalent in future-oriented societies, is based on scientific knowledge regarding cause and effect. For example, members of Western cultures believe in the practice of childhood immunizations and understand the part cholesterol plays in cardiovascular disease.

Cultural groups whose explanatory system for natural phenomena and life experiences is based on magic, destiny, or fate include disease causation within this framework. The avoidance of disease is dependent on luck, charms, and the propitiation of the proper spirits. The older, wiser members of the group possess the traditional healing knowledge, which is passed from generation to generation. Because the future is not within a person's control, the present becomes the important time concept. Treatment of disease is relegated to the treatment of symptoms as they appear. This means symptoms must be explored for their cultural meaning. (Table 4-10 offers cultural explanations for some common symptoms.)

Understanding cultural causation and somatization is key to treatment. For example, the treatment of a Latino baby's sunken fontanel, or *caída de la mollera,* includes pushing up on the roof of the mouth, holding the infant upside down over water, or restricting fluids, the opposite of the Western treatment for dehydration.

This kind of information is critical for the practitioner to be able to support beneficial cultural practices and modify harm-

Table 4-8 Selected Newborn Practices

CULTURE	NEWBORN PRACTICES
Navajo	Ceremonies and taboos ensure health, prosperity, and well-being and place newborns "in tune" with the Holy people charged with watching over the Navajos.
	Newborns are gently shaken and massaged to stimulate breathing.
	Newborns heads are turned toward the hogan fire, a sacred symbol of life.
Haitian	"Belly bands" are used to help newborns develop a nice form, a strong body, and a sense of balance.
	Purgatives made from the *maskreti* plant, boiled water, sugar, salt, and nutmeg are given to clean newborns' "insides."
	Newborns must be kept warm, especially their heads, which are covered with bonnets.
Cambodian	Newborns' anterior fontanels are protected with a paste made from bakers' yeast mixed with herbs.
	Newborns must be well wrapped, with their heads and ear openings covered.
	Bathing is not done by immersion; water should never enter newborns' ears.
Vietnamese, Cambodian	News of the birth of newborns is to be kept hidden from jealous spirits who might steal them, so babies are dressed in old clothes and praise is avoided.

Table 4-9 Environmental Factors Contributing to Behaviors

ENVIRONMENT	BEHAVIOR
Safety	
Child crawling or falling from house built on stilts	Child held or placed in a hammock
Dangerous ground insects and animals	Child carried in a backpack or hip sling
Night dangers or "evil spirits"	Child sleeps in the same bed or room as parents
Toilet Training	
Tropical climate	Child goes without clothing
Lack of toileting facilities	Designated toileting areas easy to reach
Communal living	Child sees and imitates siblings and adults

Table 4-10 Cultural Explanations for Symptoms

CULTURE	SYMPTOMS	EXPLANATION
Haitian	Description of child's appearance: • Looks very sick • Looks very sad • Does not develop normally • Looks sick and fragile • Fever drying up child's body • Illness bringing on other things	Description of whole body effect a result of Haitian ethnomedical belief that entire body is involved with any apparent symptoms of illness
Cambodian	Complaint of a weak, fussy baby	Fear that a spell was placed on the infant
	Complaint that the new infant cries too much	Fear that the mother from a previous reincarnation is returning to claim her child
Hispanic	Description of a fallen fontanel or *caida de la mollera* accompanied by vomiting, diarrhea, and symptoms of dehydration	Dislocation of the internal organs caused by sudden withdrawal of the nipple from the baby's mouth or by the baby falling

ful ones. Southeast Asian practices include "coin rubbing," in which an older family member or a traditional healer applies a eucalyptus-based ointment to an area of the body. This area is then vigorously rubbed with a coin or metal object in long, downward strokes, resulting in reddened, bruiselike marks. Coin rubbing is done to relieve the body of bad spirits or bad winds believed to be the cause of the illness. This practice, though startling to see, is not harmful. In fact, it is a way of providing human contact through hands-on care.

In contrast to coin rubbing is a form of Chinese medicine called *moxibustion*. This practice, based on the therapeutic value of heat, involves the use of heated, pulverized wormwood being applied directly to the skin along specified meridians. The Cambodians have adopted this practice and refer to it as *circular burning*. It is used as a treatment for diarrhea, stomachache, malaria, back pain, knee pain, or hernia. Strategic locations around the umbilicus are measured out and heated herbs or plants are placed on these locations, causing circular burns approximately $\frac{1}{2}$ inch in diameter. However, in the United States, burning a baby's abdomen is not an acceptable practice. Practitioners must understand that this practice is done to be helpful, not abusive. An explanation to the parents must be given in a way that will not make them fearful to return for follow-up care.

Use of Interpreters

The ability to communicate ideas, thoughts, concerns, and fears is a culturally constructed human function that is taken for granted until cultures clash. As a translator of languages as well as cultures, an interpreter becomes a necessary third party to culturally congruent health care. In the process of asking questions, it is the interpreter who must translate the words, ideas, and concepts. Interpreters become "culture brokers," explaining the Western health care system and practices to the individual seeking care and pointing out the meaning of traditional practices and beliefs to the provider. Interpretation is much more than word-for-word translation; it serves as the basis for appropriate and acceptable health care.

Because the process of interpretation is a dynamic one with constant shifting of emphasis among data gathering, problem solving, therapy, and education, interpreters working in tandem with health care providers often take on the function of PCPs. It is their job to put new and often confusing advice and directions into a culturally understandable for-

mat, and it is the interpreter who is quizzed by the practitioner when the parent or child does not understand or has not followed through with the treatment plan. On the other hand, it is also the interpreter who is asked by the patient why the practitioner is asking so many unnecessary questions. The interpreter-practitioner relationship must be one of mutual trust and collaboration in which both are free to discuss the nuances of the interaction.

The nature of interpreting requires bilingual proficiency and substantial knowledge regarding the health care beliefs and practices of at least two cultures. People seeking health care do so for sensitive and personal reasons. This means that interpreting should be done by an individual who is well respected within the cultural community, one who is educated and trained for this position. A last resort as an interpreter is a family member, an individual from the same cultural background who may work in the laboratory or the housekeeping department, or an employee who may have basic knowledge of the patient's language. When this becomes necessary, the practitioner must be aware that information obtained in this manner is subject to misinterpretation and is often incomplete.

Resources

Websites
Children's Defense Fund (www.childrensdefense.org)
Ethnomed (www.ethnomed.org)
Health Resources and Services Administration, Office of Minority Health (www.hrsa.gov/omh/omh/disparities)
Southern Poverty Law Center (Teaching Tolerance) (www.splcenter.org/teachingtolerance/tt-index.html)
United Nations' Children's Fund, Innocente Research Centre (www.unicef-icdc.org)
U.S. Census Bureau (www.census.gov)

Bibliography

1995 World population sheet. Washington, DC: Population Reference Bureau.

Babington, L.M., Kelley, B.R., Patsdaughter, C.A., Soderberg, R.M., & Kelley, J.E. (1999). From recipes to *recetas*: Health beliefs and health care encounters in the rural Dominican Republic. *Journal of Cultural Diversity, 6*(1), 20-25.

Barnes, L.L., Plotnikoff, G.A., Fox, K., & Pendleton, S. (2000). Spirituality, religion, and pediatrics: Intersecting worlds of healing. *Pediatrics, 106*(Suppl 4), 899-908.

Eliades, D.C. & Suitor, C.W. (1994). *Celebrating diversity: approaching families through their food,* Arlington, VA: National Center for Education in Maternal and Child Health.

Giger, J. & Davidhizar, R. (1995). *Transcultural nursing* (2nd ed.). St Louis: Mosby.

Kelley, B.R. (1996). Cultural considerations in Cambodian childrearing. *Journal of Pediatric Health Care, 10*(1), 2-9.

Kleinman, A., Eisenberg, L., & Good, B. (1978). Culture, illness, and care. *Annals of Internal Medicine, 88,* 251-258.

Ludman, E.K. & Newman, J.M. (1984). The health related food practices of three Chinese groups. *Journal of Nutrition Education, 16,* 4.

Manio, E. & Hall, R. (1987). Asian family traditions and their influence in transcultural health care delivery. *Children's Health Care, 15*(3), 170-177.

Martínez, R.A. (Ed.). (1978). *Hispanic culture and health care.* St Louis: Mosby.

Nguyen, D. (1985). Culture shock: A review of Vietnamese culture and its concepts of health and disease. *Western Journal of Medicine, 142*(3), 409-412.

Phillips, S. & Lobar, S. (1990). Literature summary of some Navajo child health beliefs and rearing practices within a transcultural nursing framework. *Journal of Transcultural Nursing, 1*(2), 13-20.

Randall-David, E. (1990). *Strategies for working with culturally diverse communities and clients.* Washington, DC: Association for the Care of Children's Health.

Rothbaum, F., Morelli, G., Pott, M., & Liu-Constant, Y. (2000). Immigrant-Chinese and Euro-American parents' physical closeness with young children: Themes of family relatedness. *Journal of Family Psychology, 14*(3), 334-348.

Satz, K. (1982). Integrating Navajo tradition into maternal-child nursing. *Image, 14*(3), 89-92.

Specter, R. (1993). Quick reference guide to cultural assessment. In Potter, P.A. & Perry, A.G. (Eds.), *Fundamentals of nursing: Concepts, process, and practice* (3rd ed.). St Louis: Mosby.

U.S. Bureau of the Census. (2000). *Census of the population, 2000.* Washington, DC: U.S. Government Printing Office.

Chapter 5 *Genetic Evaluation, Counseling, and Health Management*

Carolyn D. Farrell & Cynthia A. Prows

Role of Genetics in the Health of Children

Advances in genetics—scientific knowledge, technologic capabilities, and abilities for clinical evaluation—associated with fruition of the Human Genome Project have led to an increasing awareness of infant, pediatric, and adolescent disorders attributable to genetically determined or influenced factors; this awareness includes recognition of such information as:

- Major congenital malformations occur in about 2% of live births.
- Of these, nearly 80% are associated with a genetic cause and an increased risk of recurrence.
- Only 43% of congenital malformations are diagnosed in the neonatal period.
- Approximately 82% of congenital malformations are detected before 6 months of age.
- Genetic disorders account for 15% of pediatric admissions.
- Approximately 25% of medical disorders are attributable to a combination of genetic and nongenetic factors.

These figures underscore the necessity for practitioners to recognize persons and families at risk. A practitioner must have an understanding and appreciation of the presentations of various genetic disorders to facilitate prompt detection and diagnosis. Prompt diagnosis is critical to early intervention and implementation of treatment, which limits the extent of physical and mental involvement associated with the disorder, and permits timely education of the parents. In these ways both the practitioner and family can be prepared to make considered and informed decisions about management, treatment, lifestyle, and reproductive choices.

Thus genetics is increasingly affecting the health of children and the daily delivery of health care through: (1) the evaluation and diagnosis of chromosomal and single-gene disorders, with advances allowing broader ability and improved methods for testing and detection of additional disorders; (2) deoxyribonucleic acid (DNA)–based findings, which can be interpreted for clinical use in further evaluation and in treatment and management decisions; (3) improved understanding, diagnosis, and treatment of disorders not traditionally thought of as genetic, such as childhood obesity, hypertension, and hypercholesterolemia, which may be of a complex genetic nature; (4) developments in genetics-based pharmacology and technology that offer treatment options, reduction of risk, and realistic hope where previously little or none existed; (5) innovations in the area of reproductive, prenatal, or preconception assessments and alternatives for couples with a history of problematic genetic conditions or infertility; (6) research that has identified and will continue to identify susceptibility genes that allow for presymptomatic clinical testing for recognition of persons at increased risk, which is critical to providing individualized medical surveillance, options to confirm or rule out risk, and optimal interventions and management; (7) dilemmas that arise relating to legal, ethical, regulatory, psychosocial, and informed-consent issues; (8) directions for future-oriented therapies, such as immune therapy, cloning tissues for healing burns, the ability to deal with amputations, replacement of malfunctioning organ parts, and the treatment of complex disorders; and (9) recognition of genetics as a nursing specialty by the American Nurses Association (ANA), with established standards of practice for nurses at all levels (International Society of Nurses in Genetics, 1998).

Defining Genetics and Identifying Persons at Risk

The term *genetics* is used in both a broad and a specific context. In a strict scientific sense, genetics refers to the study of factors that deal with the underlying programmed coding components of cells. In the broader sense, genetics encompasses not only the traditional view of disorders associated with chromosome imbalances or the inheritance of a single gene or multiple genes, but also includes multifactorially determined conditions associated with a combination of several inherited and other (such as environmental) factors that collectively increase risk. Furthermore, genetics extends to a new realization that inherited nonpathologic variations influence susceptibility to disease, individual biochemical processes, and responses to drugs.

Six general categories of manifesting problems alert practitioners to a possible genetic disorder. These risk factors, along with potential genetic problems, rationales for increased risk, and available testing, are addressed in Tables 5-1 and 5-2.

Genetic Counseling: Purpose, Definition, and Essential Components

Genetic evaluation, consultation, and counseling are provided by a genetic specialist, specifically a clinical or medical geneticist, a genetic counselor, or a genetics nurse specialist (such as an advanced practice nurse [APN] in genetics). These genetics

Text continued on p. 52

Table 5-1 Indications for Genetic Evaluation

POTENTIAL GENETIC PROBLEM	RISK FACTOR	RATIONALE	AVAILABLE TESTING
Advanced age at reproduction	Fetal numerical chromosome abnormality	Maternal age greater than 35 and paternal age greater than 50 are associated with increased risk of a nondisjunctional chromosome error in germ cells (e.g., egg, sperm).	*Prenatal:* Chorionic villus sampling (CVS) and/or amniocentesis. *Prenatal screening:* Maternal serum alpha-fetoprotein (MSAFP) or "triple screen" (MSAFP, beta human chorionic gonadotropin (HCG), and estriol).
	Fetal autosomal dominant genetic disorder	Paternal age over 40 is associated with increased risk of new mutation for certain autosomal dominant disorders (e.g., achondroplasia).	Because autosomal dominant conditions often have structural effects, a level II ultrasound can be done at 18 to 20 weeks; however, normal results do not guarantee the fetus is free of genetic disorders.
History of spontaneous abortions or stillbirths	Fetal chromosome abnormality	Couples experiencing three or more spontaneous abortions are at increased risk that one member carries an unbalanced chromosomal rearrangement (translocation) that can predispose to spontaneous abortions or risk for mentally and physically impaired chromosomally unbalanced offspring.	Parental chromosome analysis (consider after two spontaneous abortions); if either parent has a translocation, then prenatal CVS and/or amniocentesis for fetal chromosome assessment and diagnosis. Chromosome analysis and pathology study should be done on products of conception (especially after one or more spontaneous abortions).
Previous offspring with birth defects, mental retardation, growth retardation, a neurologic condition, or a familial condition	Recurrence in future offspring	Congenital malformations, mental retardation, growth retardation, or neurologic abnormalities can occur as an isolated event, as part of a syndrome, or as a component of a genetic or chromosomal disorder.	Chromosome analysis of affected offspring (e.g., routine or prometaphase, depending upon suspected condition). Consult with genetics expert. *Prenatal:* AFP testing, ultrasonography, CVS and/or amniocentesis, if associated with a known detectable genetic or chromosomal disorder.
Family history of birth defects, mental retardation, or a familial condition	Recurrence in future offspring or inheritance of a single gene associated with increased susceptibility	Couple may be needlessly concerned when their risk is negligible or may inappropriately dismiss potential risk because of lack of information about the disorder, its associated problems, and its risk of inheritance.	May involve chromosome analysis, DNA testing, or enzyme analysis of affected, depending upon phenotype (physical manifestations) and suspected condition. If risk is for genetic susceptibility to a specific disease or condition, consult with genetics expert before proceeding. *Prenatal:* Ultrasonography, AFP testing; CVS, amniocentesis, depending on the nature of the condition.
Exposure to medications, infections, radiation, toxic chemicals, or illegal substances during pregnancy	Congenital malformations or mental impairment	Exposure to substances or viruses in pregnancy can be teratogenic (increase the risk for fetal abnormalities); risk is correlated with type of exposure, dosage, and stage of embryogenesis (see Fig. 5-6), and is interpreted in the context of gestational age and information known from human studies and animal research.	*Prenatal:* Ultrasonography; AFP testing, (e.g. if risk of neural tube defect). *Postnatal:* Dependent upon presenting signs.
Ethnic or racial background	Offspring with an autosomal recessive genetic disorder	Certain ethnic or racial groups are at an increased risk for carrier status for specific genetic disorders.	If possible, carrier testing of parents. *Prenatal:* CVS or amniocentesis if couple is at risk to have a child with a known detectable genetic disorder; adult-onset conditions warrant additional considerations before proceeding with testing.

Modified with permission from Farrell, C.D. (1989): Genetic counseling: The emerging reality. In Angelini, D. & Gives, R. (Eds.) Genetics. Journal of Perinatal and Neonatal Nursing, 2(4):24–25.

Table 5-2 Genetic Disorders and Phenotypic Presentations in the Pediatric Population

DISORDER AND INCIDENCE	PHENOTYPE (COMMON CHARACTERISTICS)	ETIOLOGY AND RECURRENCE RISKS	TESTING AND CONSIDERATIONS
Chromosomal Disorders			
Autosomal			
Down syndrome (trisomy 21) 1 in 700 newborns; risk increases with advanced maternal age (e.g., at maternal age 25, 1 in 1350; at age 35, 1 in 84; at age 45, 1 in 28)	Brachycephaly; oblique palpebral fissures; epicanthal folds; Brushfield spots; flat nasal bridge; protruding tongue; small, low-set ears; clinodactyly; single palmar crease; congenital heart defects; hypotonia; mild to moderate mental retardation; growth retardation; dry, scaly skin	Extra copy of number 21 chromosome (total of three copies): 94%—trisomy 21 (karyotype 47, +21)—three distinct number 21 chromosomes because of nondisjunction, (failure of chromosomal separation during meiosis); recurrence risk 1%, plus maternal age-related risk if over 35 (e.g., about 2% risk for chromosome abnormality at age 35) 4%—translocation Down syndrome—extra number 21 attached to another chromosome, usually number 13 or 14; half of these translocations are new occurrences while the other half are inherited from a parent 2%—mosaic Down syndrome—individual has two different cell lines, one with normal number of chromosomes and the other cell line trisomic for the number 21 chromosome; result of a nondisjunctional event during mitotic chromosomal division (after conception) in the affected individual	Recurrence risk for parents of affected are dependent on one or more of the following: chromosomal type of disorder, maternal age, parental karyotype, family history, sex of transmitting parent, and other chromosome involved (if translocation) Fetus may demonstrate nuchal thickening prenatally on ultrasound examination No phenotypic differences between trisomy Down syndrome and translocation Down syndrome Chromosome analysis should be performed for all persons with Down syndrome May be associated with low maternal serum AFP
Trisomy 13 (Patau syndrome) 1 in 5000 live births	Holoprosencephaly; scalp defect; microophthalmia or anophthalmia; cleft lip or palate, or both; rocker-bottom feet; postaxial polydactyly; seizures; severe mental retardation	Extra number 13 chromosome (total of three copies): Either trisomy form, because of nondisjunction, with less than a 1% recurrence risk; or translocation form, with recurrence risk dependent on the other chromosomes involved	Chromosome analysis indicated 44% die within the first month; 18% survive first year of life
Trisomy 18 (Edward syndrome) 1 in 6000 live births	Small for gestational age (may be detected prenatally); feeble fetal activity; weak cry; prominent occiput; low-set, malformed ears; short palpebral fissures; small oral opening (micrognathia); overlapping positioning of fingers (fifth digit over fourth, index over third); nail hypoplasia, short hallux; rocker-bottom feet; cardiac defects; inguinal or umbilical hernia; cryptorchidism in males; severe mental retardation	Extra number 18 chromosome (total of three copies); majority because of trisomy, with less than 1% recurrence risk	Chromosome analysis indicated Most trisomy 18 conceptions spontaneously abort; 90% of live-born die within first year of life Maternal serum screening tests may be outside the normal range

Disorder	Clinical features	Cause/genetics	Counseling and management
Sex chromosome			
Klinefelter syndrome 1 in 700 males 47,XXY abnormality in 90%; other 10% have more than two X chromosomes in addition to the Y chromosome or have mosaicism (about 2%)	Body habitus may be tall, slim, and underweight; long limbs; gynecomastia; small testes; inadequate virilization; azoospermia or low sperm count; cognitive defects; behavioral problems	Result of chromosomal nondisjunction during meiosis, except for cases of mosaicism, which are due to mitotic nondisjunction	Chromosome analysis indicated. No distinguishing features prenatally. Diagnosis may not be suspected before puberty. Diagnosis in childhood is beneficial in planning for testosterone replacement therapy and accurate understanding of learning or behavioral problems. Tend to be delayed in onset of speech and have difficulty in expressive language; may be relatively immature; may have history of recurrent respiratory infections
Turner syndrome (45,X) 1 in 2500 female births	Webbing of neck and short stature; lymphedema of hands and feet as newborn; congenital cardiac defects (especially coarctation of the aorta); low posterior hairline; cubitus valgus; widely spaced nipples; underdeveloped breasts; immature internal genitalia (e.g., streak ovaries); primary amenorrhea; learning disabilities, mild mental retardation, or normal intelligence	About 50% due to a nondisjunctional error during meiosis (karyotype 45,X); 20% are mosaic due to nondisjunction during mitosis; 30% have two X chromosomes but one is functionally inadequate (e.g., because of presence of abnormal genes); generally a sporadic occurrence	Chromosome analysis indicated. Webbing of neck and short stature may be detected prenatally by ultrasound. Early diagnosis enhances optimal health care management (e.g., planning for administration of growth hormone therapy, estrogen replacement). Psychosocial implications associated with short stature and delayed onset of puberty. Infertility associated with ovarian dysgenesis
Microdeletion/microduplication			
Fragile X 1 in 1200 males 1 in 2500 females	Motor delays; hypotonia; speech delay and language difficulty; hyperactivity; classic features including long face, prominent ears, and macroorchidism manifest around puberty; autism (about 7% of males); mental retardation in most males; learning disabilities or reluctance to make eye contact in social settings in some females who have the disorder	Mutation in the fragile X mental retardation gene (FMR-1) on X q27.3; represented as a large DNA expansion of a normally present trinucleotide CGG repeat. Carrier mother of an affected male has a 50% risk for future affected males and 50% risk to transmit the FMR-1 X chromosome to a daughter who would be a carrier and may either be unaffected or manifest features associated with the fragile X syndrome and has a 50% risk to transmit that gene to future offspring	Both chromosome testing for expression of the fragile X site and DNA analysis for the expansion available, but the latter superior. Fragile X should be considered in the differential diagnosis of any mentally retarded male who is undiagnosed; most common mental retardation in males. Phenotypic expression of this gene in males and females is variable; genetic mechanisms determining expression of this gene are very complex. Both females and males can carry the fragile X gene in a "premutation" state and have no symptoms, but they are at risk to have affected children or grandchildren; the premutation is susceptible to expansion

Continued

Modified from Farrell, C.D. & Campbell, J. Genetic and developmental nursing disorders. In Duso, S. (Ed). The Lippincott manual of nursing practice (ed. 6), Philadelphia: J.B. Lippincott.

Table 5-2 Genetic Disorders and Phenotypic Presentations in the Pediatric Population—cont'd

DISORDER AND INCIDENCE	PHENOTYPE (COMMON CHARACTERISTICS)	ETIOLOGY AND RECURRENCE RISKS	TESTING AND CONSIDERATIONS
Chromosomal Disorders—cont'd			
Prader-Willi syndrome Estimated incidence 1 in 25,000	Hypotonia and poor sucking ability in infancy; almond-shaped palpebral fissures; small stature; small, slow growth of hands and feet; small penis, cryptorchidism; insatiable appetite, behavioral problems beginning in childhood; below-normal intelligence or mental retardation	Cytogenetic microdeletion in chromosome 15 q11–13 identified in 50% to 70% of cases; deletion associated with paternally inherited number 15 chromosome Generally sporadic occurrence; empiric recurrence risk of 1.6%	Consider diagnosis in infants presenting with hypotonia and sucking problems when etiology is unknown Prometaphase chromosome analysis of chromosome 15 is indicated Another distinct entity, termed *Angelman syndrome*, is associated with a deletion of the maternal contribution in this same cytogenetic region; it is also associated with mental deficiency, but with different phenotypic presentation
Mendelian Disorders (Single Gene) ***Autosomal dominant***			
Achondroplasia 1 in 10,000 live births Increased incidence associated with advanced paternal age (> 40)	Megalocephaly; small foramen magnum and short cranial base with early spheno-occipital closure; prominent forehead; low nasal bridge; midfacial hypoplasia; small stature; short extremities; lumbar lordosis; short tubular bones; incomplete extension at the elbow; normal intelligence	Autosomal dominant inheritance; 80% to 90% because of a new mutation In those cases that are inherited, the parent with the gene has a 50% risk to transmit the gene to each child	Hydrocephalus can be a complication of achondroplasia and may be masked by megalocephaly Risk for apnea secondary to cervical spinal cord and lower brain stem compression because of alterations in shape of cervical vertebral bodies; respiratory problems are also a risk because of the small chest and upper airway obstruction Can be diagnosed prenatally by ultrasound, *not* chromosome analysis
Osteogenesis imperfecta (type 1) 1 in 15,000 live births	Blue sclerae; fractures (variable number); deafness may occur	Defect in the procollagen gene associated with decreased synthesis of a constituent chain important to collagen structure Can occur as a new mutation in that gene or can be inherited from a parent who has a 50% risk to transmit the gene; most severe cases represent a sporadic occurrence within a family	At least four general classifications of osteogenesis imperfecta, associated with varying clinical severity, presentation, and pattern of genetic transmission Genetic (DNA) testing is possible; consult with a genetics expert Treatment with calcitonin and fluoride may be beneficial in reducing number of fractures

Disorder			
Familial adenomatous polyposis (FAP) 1 in 5000–10,000 1% of inherited colorectal cancer	Normal appearance at birth; Classic Symptoms include appearance of hundreds to thousands of colon polyps (susceptible to malignant transformation). Polyps may present in childhood or as young adult; other FAP-associated features include desmoids (benign growths anywhere in body that may interfere with tissue or organ function); osteomas (jaw cysts); congenital hypertrophy of retinal pigment epithelium (CHRPE, or benign "freckling" of the retina); increased susceptibility to desmoids at surgical incision sites Attenuated "atypical" form of FAP may present with fewer than 10 polyps, especially if detected at a young age	Abnormal adenomatous polyposis coli (APC) gene located on chromosome 5q, poses increased susceptibility for associated features (gene penetrance is 98% by age 40) Majority of cases caused by an inherited mutation; however, 30% of cases arise as a new mutation	Genetic testing for clinical diagnosis possible at few laboratories; testing does not sequence the DNA of the gene, but instead analyzes for the presence of an abnormal protein product of the gene (method termed *protein truncation*) which detects abnormality in 50% to 80% of cases; thus, presence of altered gene product confirms diagnosis, but inability to detect an abnormality does not rule out this condition Although genetic testing for cancer-associated susceptibility genes is not generally recommended for children, it is a consideration in these families; children at risk should have flexible sigmoidoscopy at 10 or 12 years of age (consult a genetics expert)

Autosomal recessive

Sickle cell disease 1 in 400 live births of African-American ancestry	Physically normal in appearance at birth; hemolytic anemia and the occurrence of acute exacerbations (crises), resulting in increased susceptibility to infection and vascular occlusive episodes	Point mutation in the beta-globin gene resulting in an altered gene product; red blood cells susceptible to sickling at times of low oxygen tension Parents of an affected individual are both unaffected carriers of one abnormal copy of the sickle gene (sickle cell trait) and together have a 25% risk for recurrence in any offspring	Of African Americans 1 in 10 a carrier of the mutated sickle cell gene; screening is indicated for this population Healthy siblings of an individual with sickle cell disease have a 67% risk to be carriers (have one copy of the sickle cell gene) and should be screened Genetic (DNA) and prenatal testing available from blood specimens obtained during chorionic villi sampling or amniocentesis Health care management critical to minimizing frequency and severity of crises; early intervention in illness or injury
Cystic fibrosis (CF) 1 in 2000 live births (predominantly Caucasian)	Phenotypically normal at birth; may present with meconium ileus (10%) as neonate or later with persistent cough, recurrent respiratory problems, gastrointestinal complaints, abdominal pain, congenital bilateral absence of the vas deferens or infertility	Mutation of the cystic fibrosis transmembrane receptor gene (CFTR) on chromosome 7 results in an abnormality of a protein integral to the cell membrane Parents of an affected individual are both considered obligate carriers of one copy of the abnormal CF gene; thus, together they have a 25% recurrence risk with each conception	About 1 in 20 Caucasians a carrier of a CF gene mutation Hundreds of different mutations; various mutations may account for differences in symptoms and severity CF screening can identify about 85% of all CF mutations (95% in Jewish population) DNA analysis of the CFTR gene advised for affected individuals and their relatives
Tay-Sachs disease 1 in 3600 Ashkenazi Jews	Normal at birth; progressive neurodegenerative manifestations, including loss of developmental milestones and lack of central nervous system (CNS) maturation; cherry redspot on macula	Mutation in the gene for hexosaminidase A, an enzyme important to cellular metabolic processes, results in accumulation of metabolic byproducts within the cell (especially brain), impairing functioning and causing the neurodegenerative effects Parents of an affected individual are both considered obligate carriers of one copy of the Tay-Sachs disease gene; together they have a 25% risk of recurrence in their offspring	Genetic (DNA or enzyme) testing advised for persons of Ashkenazi Jewish (about 1 in 25 are carriers) and French-Canadian (about 1 in 17 are carriers) ancestry No treatment available, results in death in childhood Prenatal testing available

Continued

Modified from Farrell, C.D. & Campbell, J. Genetic and developmental nursing disorders. In Duso, S. (Ed). The Lippincott manual of nursing practice (ed. 6). Philadelphia: J.B. Lippincott.

Table 5-2 Genetic Disorders and Phenotypic Presentations in the Pediatric Population—cont'd

DISORDER AND INCIDENCE	PHENOTYPE (COMMON CHARACTERISTICS)	ETIOLOGY AND RECURRENCE RISKS	TESTING AND CONSIDERATIONS
Mendelian Disorders (Single Gene)—cont'd			
X-linked recessive			
Duchenne muscular dystrophy (DMD) 1 in 3500 males	Phenotypically normal at birth; dramatically elevated creatine kinase (CK) level (detectable as early as 2 days of age); hypertrophy of the calves; history of tendency to trip and fall (by about 3 years of age); Gower sign (tendency to push off oneself when getting up from a sitting position)	DNA mutation, generally a deletion, detectable in 70% of affected males Carrier females have a 25% risk with each pregnancy to have an affected male, a 25% risk to have a carrier female, a 25% chance to have a healthy male, and a 25% chance to have a healthy noncarrier female	1 in 1750 females is carrier of the DMD gene (dystrophin) In the case of an isolated male with DMD, the mother has a $^2/_3$ statistical risk that she is a carrier of the DMD gene and a $^1/_3$ chance that her son's disorder arose as the result of a new mutation in that gene (she is not a carrier) DNA testing is recommended for males with DMD; if gene mutation is identified, prenatal diagnosis and evaluation of potential female carriers can be carried out; may eliminate need for muscle biopsy DNA analysis may provide clues to expected clinical severity Becker muscular dystrophy is a milder phenotype presentation of DMD and involves the same gene
Hemophilia A 1 in 7000 males	Phenotypically normal at birth; bleeding tendency (ranging from frequent spontaneous bleeds, associated with the severe form, to bleeding only after trauma, associated with the mild form)	Deficiency of factor VIII (antihemophilic factor) because of abnormality in this gene located on the X chromosome Carrier females have a 25% risk with each pregnancy to have a son with hemophilia, a 25% risk for a carrier daughter, and a 25% chance each for a healthy non-carrier daughter or healthy son	Frequency of carrier females is about 1 in 3500 Severe form occurs in about 48% of cases Moderate cases account for 31% Mild form accounts for 21% of cases Genetic (DNA) testing available

Disorder	Description	Genetics/Cause	Counseling
Glucose 6-phosphate dehydrogenase (G6PD) 10%–14% of male live births of African-American origin	Phenotypically normal at birth; many remain asymptomatic through life; may manifest acute hemolysis associated with exposure to outside factors (e.g., certain medications)	Abnormality of the G6PD gene on the X chromosome Carrier females have a 25% risk with each pregnancy to have a male with G6PD, and 25% risk to have a carrier female	Be aware of drugs, such as antimalaria drugs or sulfonamides, or chemicals, such as phenylhydrazine (used in silvering mirrors, photography, soldering) associated with hemolysis in G6PD-deficient individuals Genetic (DNA) testing available
Multifactorial Disorders Neural tube defects (NTDs) 1 in 1000 live births	Abnormalities of neural tube closure, ranging from anencephaly to myelomeningocele to spina bifida occulta	For all multifactorial disorders, probably several genetic factors may predispose certain individuals, or families to susceptibility, but certain environmental (e.g., prolonged hyperthermia) and other unknown factors play an additive role in surpassing an arbitrary threshold, placing the developing fetus at risk Recurrence risk for isolated neural tube defects ranges between 1% and 5%	Recurrence risk for isolated neural tube defects dependent on the severity of the defect (i.e., a defect in neurulation [the cranial end] versus cannulation [the development of the caudal end of the spine]), and if there is a positive family history Maternal screening for a fetal NTD can be performed prenatally (after 14 weeks gestation) through AFP testing of maternal serum NTDs can be associated with chromosomal or genetic disorders Folic acid supplementation recommended for subsequent pregnancies of women who have had an infant with a NTD to reduce risk for recurrence
Cleft lip and/or cleft palate 1 in 1000 live births	Unilateral or bilateral; cleft lip and/or palate may occur together or in isolation	Failure of migration and fusion of the maxillary processes during embryogenesis Recurrence risk for first-degree relatives of a person with an isolated cleft lip and/or palate ranges between 2% and 6%	For isolated cleft lip and for cleft palate, no specific chromosome or genetic test Clefting can occur as an isolated congenital abnormality or be one component of a syndrome, genetic disorder, or chromosomal abnormality; these latter three are associated with a recurrence risk specific to that disorder (genetic testing may or may not be possible) Recurrence for isolated cleft lip and/or palate dependent on the type of cleft, sex of the affected individual, and family history

Modified from Farrell, C.D. & Campbell, J. Genetic and developmental nursing disorders. In Duso, S. (Ed). The Lippincott manual of nursing practice (ed. 6), Philadelphia: J.B. Lippincott.

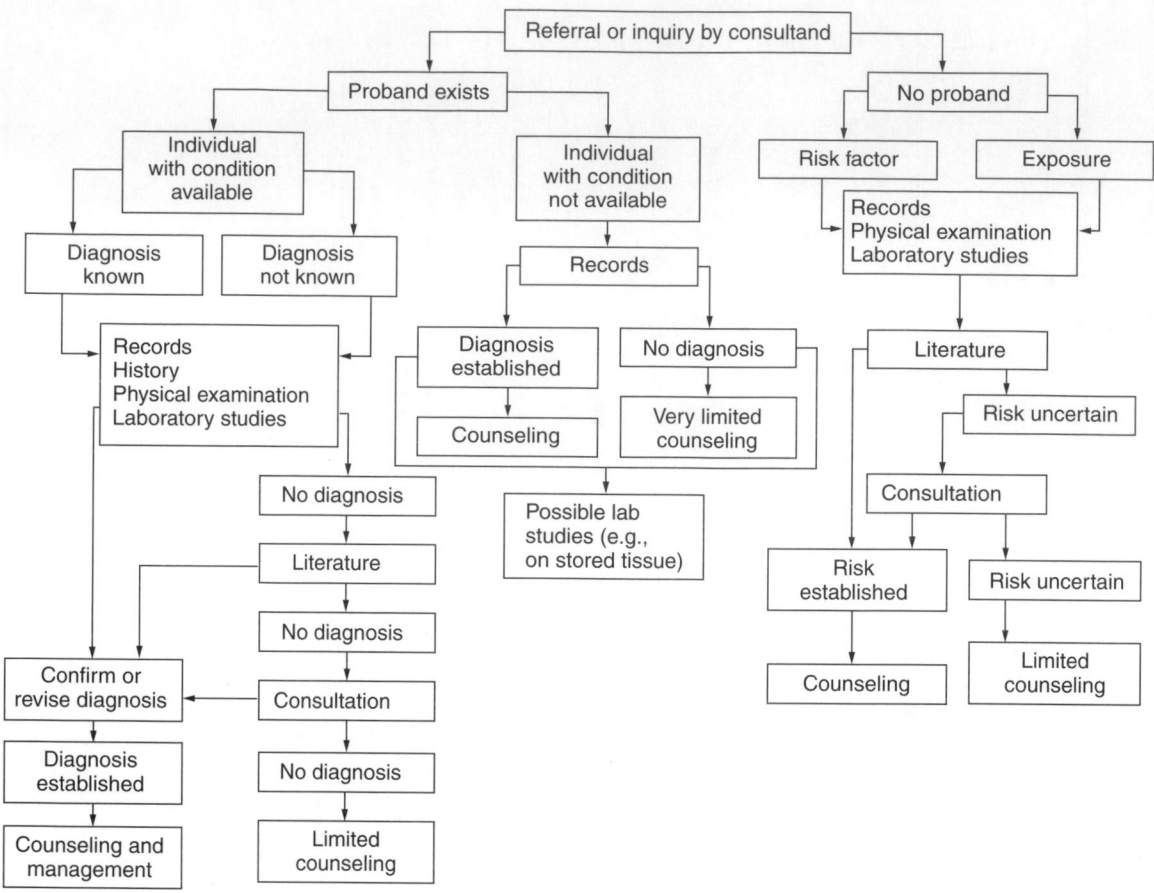

Fig. 5-1 The genetic counseling process. (Modified from Erbe, R.W. [1989]. Genetic counseling. In Kelly, W.R. [Ed.]. *Textbook of internal medicine.* Philadelphia: J.B. Lippincott.)

professionals also practice using the resources of other genetics experts (e.g., biochemical geneticists, cytogeneticists, molecular geneticists) and frequently use a multidisciplinary approach with other health care professionals.

Genetic counseling involves first and foremost a communication process. The manifesting problems or concerns are identified and explored from the perspectives of the referring health care provider, the consultand (the person seeking the information) or the proband (the person affected with the disorder), and the genetics professional. As defined by the American Society of Human Genetics and expanded here, the essential components of the genetic counseling process include the following (Fig. 5-1):

• Construction and evaluation of a family history pedigree (three-generation minimum)
• Assessment or confirmation of the manifesting condition, concern, and diagnosis by review of medical records, physical examination, and relevant laboratory and imaging studies and results
• Education about the diagnosis, diagnostic impression, or genetic risk factor, and the associated features and risks
• Provision of information about the mode of inheritance, if known, and the associated recurrence risk and risk to relatives
• Recommendations for additional evaluations, genetic tests, and risk management, as indicated
• Education about and discussion of options for case management, treatment, referral and resources (e.g., profes-

sional, support group), reproductive options, and health promotion/disease prevention strategies
• Support for individual and family choices
• Follow-up regarding risk factors and management

Genetic Screening Versus Testing: Principles, Limitations, and Considerations

Genetic Screening

The purpose for screening is to identify persons within a defined population who are at increased risk for specific disorders, for carrier status for specific genes, or for birth defects. *Genetic screening* refers to screening for genetically determined or influenced conditions or disorders. Principles underlying effective screening are discussed in Chapter 12.

Genetic screening is divided into three types: prenatal, newborn, and population.

Prenatal. Prenatal screening is used to identify pregnancies at potential risk for chromosome abnormalities, neural tube defects (NTDs), or other developmental abnormalities. It includes maternal serum alpha-fetoprotein (MSAFP) testing (elevated or reduced levels are associated with increased risk of neural tube defects or Down syndrome, respectively) and a "multiple screen" approach (Table 5-3).

Newborn. Newborn screening is used to identify infants with specific congenital disorders, as mandated by each state

Table 5-3 Prenatal Screening and Diagnosis: Methods, Genetic Studies, and Gestational Timing

METHOD	GESTATIONAL TIMING	STUDIES AVAILABLE (TISSUE)	DISORDERS TESTED/DETECTED/SUSPECTED
Chorionic villus sampling (CVS)	8-12 weeks	Chromosome (chorionic villi cells)	Chromosomal disorders: numerical (e.g., Down syndrome [trisomy 21], trisomy 13 or 18; translocations)
		Biochemical (chorionic villi cells)	Metabolic disorders, (e.g., Tay-Sachs disease [risk of maternal cell contamination])
		DNA (chorionic villi cells)	Cystic fibrosis, sickle cell disease, Duchenne muscular dystrophy; disorders wherein gene identified and DNA mutation detectable; cannot detect neural tube defects (NTDs)
Amniocentesis	Early at 11-14 weeks; 15-19 weeks for second trimester diagnosis	Chromosome (amniocytes)	Chromosomal, biochemical, and DNA, as for CVS
		Biochemical (amniocytes or amniotic fluid)	
		DNA (amniocytes)	
		AFP/triple screen (amniotic fluid)	NTDs (e.g., anencephaly, spina bifida); body wall defect (e.g., gastroschisis); defects can be associated with other abnormalities, possibly of chromosomal or genetic etiology (e.g., trisomy 13)
Ultrasound examination	Throughout pregnancy (fetal structures best viewed after 12 weeks)	Dating of pregnancy	Intrauterine growth retardation (IUGR), large for gestational age (e.g., gigantism)—can be associated with chromosomal or genetic disorder; abnormal head size (e.g., large: X-linked hydrocephalus, NTD; small: fetal chromosome abnormality); abnormality or disproportionate size of fetal structures (e.g., osteogenesis imperfecta, Apert syndrome, absent radius, hemihypertrophy)—can be associated with chromosomal or genetic disorder
		Assessment of fetal structures	
		Assessment of placenta	
		Assessment of amount amniotic fluid	
Alpha fetoprotein (AFP)	After 14 weeks' gestation	Maternal serum screening (MSAFP)—maternal serum	Elevated: fetal neural tube or body wall defect; low: associated with increased risk of fetus with Down syndrome; also associated with trisomy 18
	After 14 weeks (possibly earlier)	Amniotic fluid AFP amniotic fluid (AFAFP)	
Triple screen (AFP, beta human chorionic gonadotropin [HCG], estriol)	After 14 weeks' gestation	Maternal serum	Varied levels of each factor may indicate risk of Down syndrome, trisomy 18 (associated with low levels of all three), or other chromosome abnormalities
			Fewer false positives and false negatives than AFP alone
Acetylcholinesterase	After 14 weeks	Amniotic fluid levels	Elevated: neural tube defect
Fetoscopy	Second trimester	Fetal blood	Chromosomal, biochemical, and DNA, as for CVS
		Details of fetal structures	Subtle abnormalities associated with disorder (e.g., abnormal skin)
		Fetal transfusion or treatment	Blood group incompatibility (e.g., Rh)
Percutaneous umbilical blood sampling (PUBS)	Second trimester	Fetal blood (cord)	Chromosomal, biochemical, and DNA, as for CVS

(see Resources for the Centers for Disease Control and Prevention [CDC] Office of Genetics and Disease Prevention Weekly Update); these disorders include phenylketonuria (PKU), sickle cell disease, hypothyroidism, histidinemia, and maple syrup urine disease. Newborn screening is also used for prompt implementation of dietary modifications or treatment critical to prevention or minimizing risks associated with such a disorder.

Population. Population screening is used to identify carriers in a specific group at increased risk for a genetic condition. Examples of groups that might be tested include:

- Ashkenazi Jewish or French-Canadian populations for Tay-Sachs disease (through biochemical analysis for level of hexosaminidase A)
- People of Mediterranean ancestry for beta-thalassemia (through blood testing for mean corpuscular volume [MCV]; carriers have a MCV of less than 80)
- Caucasians for cystic fibrosis, because detection capabilities approach 95%, as in the Ashkenazi Jewish population (testing through DNA screening for the most common mutations)

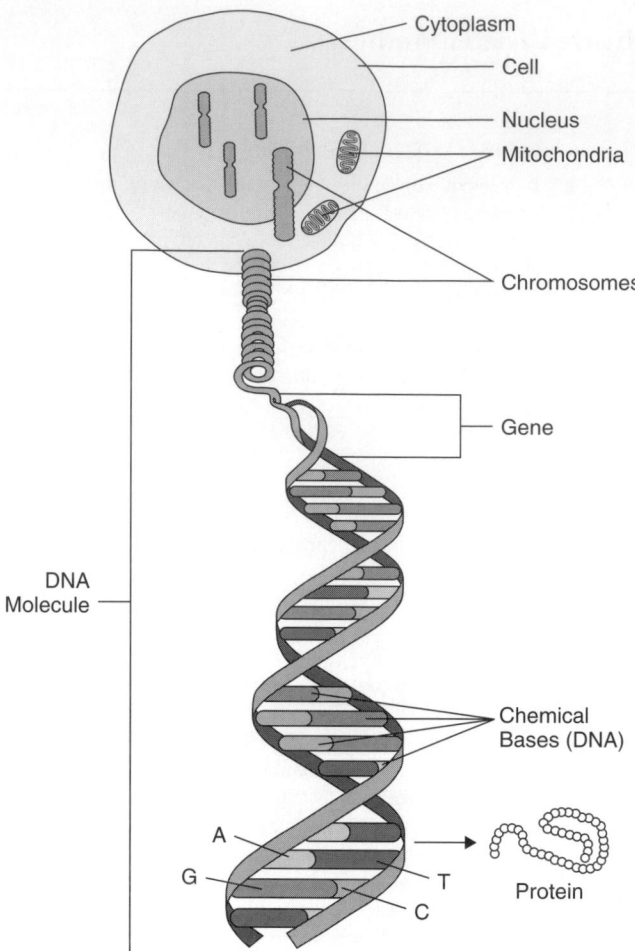

Cytoplasm

Cell

Nucleus

Mitochondria

Chromosomes

Gene

DNA
Molecule

Chemical
Bases (DNA)

A

G

T

C

Protein

Fig. 5-2 DNA, which carries the individual instructions (genes) that allow cells to make proteins, is made up of four chemical bases (A, T, G, C). Tightly coiled strands of DNA are packaged in units called *chromosomes* and housed in the cell's nucleus.

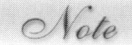

It is *critically important* that candidates for specific screening be counseled in advance about the nature of the screening test, what it can and cannot detect, the rate of detection, the risk for false negative and false positive results, and what further evaluations or recommendations may be indicated if the test result falls outside the defined "normal" range.

Box 5-1 Human Genetics at a Glance: Key Concepts

Cell Composition (See Fig. 5-2)
Cytoplasm—Contains cell structures important to function, including mitochondria
Nucleus—Separate cell compartment; contains chromosomes

Types of Cells
Somatic—All body cells except germline; contain 46 chromosomes; *not inherited*
Germline—Egg and sperm cells; contain 23 chromosomes; involved in conception and inheritance

Genetics
Chromosomes—Structures in the cell that carry genes
Gene—Basic unit of inherited material
- Approximately 30,000 nuclear genes total per cell (750 genes per chromosome, on average)
- Each gene codes to make a protein important to cell or body function and development
- Mitochondria also have some genes

Inheritance
Chromosomal disorders—Origin:
- New event in affected person; not inherited, but may be transmitted to offspring
- Inherited from unaffected parent who carries a balanced chromosomal rearrangement
- Inherited from a similarly affected relative

Genetic—Relating to single gene or pair of genes (see Table 5-5)
- Mendelian inheritance:
  - Autosomal dominant
  - Autosomal recessive
  - X-linked recessive
  - X-linked dominant
- Mitochondrial inheritance
- Multifactorial—Combination of several genes (polygenic) and additional nongenetic factors (e.g., environmental factors)

Screening provides a useful, practical approach to identify individuals or pregnancies that may be at increased risk for conditions associated with increased morbidity or mortality or that compromise individual health and well-being. To minimize the risk of false negatives, a screening test may purposely define a narrow "normal" range, therefore increasing the number of false positive results, as with MSAFP testing. This effect is diminished when one uses the triple screen approach that combines alpha-fetoprotein (AFP), beta human chorionic gonadotropin (HCG), and estriol measurements. However, screening does not result in

a diagnosis of a disorder; rather, screening identifies persons at risk for having, developing, or transmitting a specific condition. Thus further evaluation (e.g., ultrasonography, amniocentesis for a low MSAFP result) may be indicated (Box 5-1 and Fig. 5-2).

Genetic Testing

Genetic testing may be biochemical, cytogenetic, or molecular. These analyses, together with typical presentations and testing indicated, are elaborated in Table 5-4. *Biochemical* testing is the analysis of the quantity or quality of a protein product or enzyme activity, usually in serum, urine, or amniotic fluid. *Cytogenetic* testing is the analysis of the chromosomes in a cell (e.g., blood, skin, amniocyte, bone marrow) for numerical or structural abnormalities. Chromosomal microdeletions or microduplications may be detected by a special application of cytogenetic analysis, termed *prometaphase banding,* which arrests chromosomal condensation earlier in the cell cycle, thus allowing for higher resolution of more bands on a specific chromosome and region. Finally, DNA testing may be done by means of *molecular* techniques for detection of direct mutations in a gene or for linkage analysis. If the specific DNA se-

Table 5-4 Genetic Testing: Indications for the Pediatric Population

INDICATION AND PHENOTYPIC PRESENTATIONS	TESTING (METHOD AND TISSUE TYPE)	USE AND ABNORMALITY DETECTED	LIMITATIONS/RECOMMENDATIONS
Chromosomal abnormality: Birth defects, mental retardation or learning disabilities, developmental delay	Chromosome analysis: Routine (G banding, R banding) for general analysis of all 46 chromosomes; blood cells (lymphocytes), skin, cheek tissue (buccal swab)	Numerical or structural chromosomal abnormalities (e.g., trisomy, translocation as in Down syndrome, trisomy 13 or 18)	Routine chromosome analysis cannot detect microdeletions or microduplications. Method and extent of gene analysis and sensitivity and specificity are specific to each gene and may differ from one laboratory to another.
As above, but may present with more subtle dysmorphic features (e.g., when chromosome abnormality is partial or limited in region involved)	Chromosome analysis: Prometaphase analysis—extended banding of *one specific chromosome* for detection of deletions or duplications in smaller chromosomal regions	Chromosomal microdeletions or microduplications (e.g., 15q for Prader-Willi or Angelman syndrome)	Clinician must know which chromosome to study for the suspected disorder because each prometaphase chromosome analysis is a separate procedure. Analysis cannot detect single-gene abnormalities or chromosomal microdeletions or microduplications smaller than the banding resolution and does not provide information on other chromosomes. Consult with a genetics expert.
	Fluorescence in situ hybridization (FISH)—rapid method to identify specific chromosomal regions by use of a fluorescing probe	Presence or absence of specific chromosomal regions (e.g., for rapid prenatal diagnosis of numerical chromosomal abnormalities, submicroscopic deletions, X-linked chromosomal disorders)	Method does not detect single-gene disorders or chromosomal abnormalities not probed.
Specific single gene disorders. Examples: cystic fibrosis, Duchenne muscular dystrophy, fragile X syndrome, hemophilia, sickle cell disease, spinal muscular atrophy, Tay-Sachs disease, thalassemia (see Table 5-2) Phenotypic presentations different and dependent on each specific disorder but are frequently *not* associated with overt birth defects; intellectual functioning can range from normal to mental retardation	Molecular/DNA: Direct gene analysis (DNA sequence of gene, RNA transcript) to detect mutations (deletions, duplications, base pair changes) in the DNA sequence; can be done from various tissues (blood cells, skin, muscle) (if stored in a manner that preserves DNA) Molecular/DNA: Genetic linkage analysis of DNA segments in the region of a gene since adjacent genetic regions tend to be inherited with nearby genes	DNA deletions, duplications, or base pair changes in the specific gene tested Single-gene disorders wherein inheritance and chromosomal localization is known but the gene sequence itself has not been identified; provides a means to identify and track a specific chromosomal region in a family	Analysis cannot detect all mutations within a specific gene (actual likelihood of detecting a DNA mutation ranges between 60% and 99%, depending upon the specific gene, method of analysis, and technologic capabilities) and failure to detect a DNA mutation does not necessarily rule out that disorder. Genetic linkage analysis requires other family members. There is also the risk of genetic recombination between the disease gene and the linked genetic marker; in such cases, presence or absence of the linked marker would not provide accurate information about the actual disease gene (the more tightly linked the genetic marker to the actual disease gene, the less likely the risk of recombination).
Single-gene disorders for which molecular DNA analysis is not possible or for which biochemical analysis is the better approach (because of ease of analysis, lower cost, and so on). Presentation specific to specific genetic disorder; may include dysmorphic features, developmental delay, normal intelligence to mental retardation, short stature, failure to thrive, progressive deterioration in health status, seizures	Analysis of levels of a specific enzyme, amino acid, or other specific protein important to a biochemical pathway necessary for cellular functioning or metabolic processes	Deficient amount, abnormal functioning; disorders associated with suspected metabolic, biochemical, or amino acid abnormalities wherein the defective protein or enzyme is known, or there is abnormal product of biochemical pathway associated with specific genetic disorder (e.g., Tay-Sachs disease—hexosaminidase A; PKU—phenylalanine hydroxylase; mucopolysaccharidoses—several different enzymes involved in the different types)	The amount of enzyme activity necessary for normal functioning is variable in different disorders; a normal result, especially in a screening test (e.g., amino acid screening) does not totally exclude a possible biochemical disorder involving that pathway because in some cases levels can fluctuate and fall within the normal range, and not all enzymes in pathway can be tested.

quence and common mutations are known and testing provides reliable results, direct analysis of the DNA can be performed. The method and extent of gene analysis and sensitivity and specificity are specific to each gene and may differ from one laboratory to another. If the gene has not been sequenced, DNA linkage studies are employed to locate and track genetic markers associated with a known gene. The most common tissues used for DNA analysis are blood and amniocytes, but skin, muscle, bone marrow, hair, and other tissues are also used.

Prenatal Testing and Diagnosis

The purpose of prenatal testing is to establish a diagnosis of a specific fetal abnormality or disorder associated with increased morbidity or mortality (see Table 5-3). Early detection and diagnosis permits consideration of reproductive options, modification of health care management, planning for special needs at delivery, and initiation of education, information, and support aspects for the pregnant woman and her partner. Testing should be implemented based on an identified or suspected problem or a known genetic risk factor or condition and should be appropriate to detect or diagnose the problem of concern.

Pediatric Genetic Evaluation

For a practitioner to consider initiating any form of genetic evaluation, two components are critical: (1) the ability to elicit thorough individual and family medical and reproductive and

Instructions:
— Key should contain all information relevant to interpretation of pedigree (e.g., define shading)
— For clinical (non-published) pedigrees, include:
  a) family names/initials, when appropriate
  b) name and title of person recording pedigree
  c) historian (person relaying family history information)
  d) date of intake/update
— Recommended order of information placed below symbol (below to lower right, if necessary):
  a) age/date of birth or age at death
  b) evaluation
  c) pedigree number (e.g., 1-1, 1-2, 1-3)

	Male	Female	Sex unknown	Comments
1. Individual	b. 1925	30 y	4 mo	Assign gender by phenotype.
2. Affected individual	■	●	◆	Key/legend used to define shading or other fill (e.g., hatches, dots, etc.).
				With ≥ 2 conditions, the individual's symbol should be partitioned accordingly, each segment shaded with a different fill and defined in legend.
3. Multiple individuals, number known	5	5	5	Number of siblings written inside symbol. (Affected individuals should not be grouped.)
4. Multiple individuals, number unknown	n	n	n	"n" used in place of "?" mark.
5a. Deceased individual	d. 35 y	d. 4 mo		Use of cross (†) may be confused with symbol for evaluated positive (+). If known, write "d." with age at death below symbol.
5b. Stillbirth (SB)	SB 28 wk	SB 30 wk	SB 34 wk	Birth of a dead child with gestational age noted.
6. Pregnancy (P)	P LMP: 7/1/94	P 20 wk	P	Gestational age and karyotype (if known) below symbol. Light shading can be used for affected and defined in key/legend.
7a. Proband	P↗	P↗	P↗	First affected family member coming to medical attention.
7b. Consultand	↗	↗		Individual(s) seeking genetic counseling/testing.

Fig. 5-3 Common pedigree symbols, definitions, and abbreviations. (From Bennett, R.L., et al. [1995]. Recommendations for standardized human pedigree nomenclature. *American Journal of Human Genetics, 56*, 745-752.)

Family History

The practitioner should start with a thorough family and medical history. A genetic family history includes medical and health information about the proband, the index case (the first affected person), or the consultant. Vital history should include prenatal and perinatal history; the onset of the problem or disorder; the nature of the onset and initial symptoms; the progression of the condition; any medical management, tests, evaluations, and procedures; and the current status of the affected child or adult.

Genetic Pedigree

The minimum information necessary for a family history includes information about siblings (including those spontaneously aborted or stillborn), parents, aunts, uncles, nieces, nephews, first cousins, and grandparents. If the affected person has children, this information also should be included. The health and medical status of these persons should be noted, together with their current ages, information specific to symptoms, age at onset, physical or mental problems associated with the disorder in question (if the practitioner is unfamiliar with this information, it should be obtained), and the gestational age and abnormalities associated with spontaneous abortions. The practitioner may find it helpful to draw a genetic pedigree using the standardized format and symbols depicted in Figs. 5-3 to 5-5; the pedigree should incorporate the following:

- The oldest generation is placed at the top of the pedigree.
- Generations are designated by roman numerals; individuals within a generation are designated by Arabic numerals reading from left to right.
- Females are designated by circles, males by squares.
- Generally when a union (such as marriage) is depicted, the male is on the left and the female is on the right.
- Siblings within a generation are listed in birth order from left to right, except that the proband or consultand is usually placed at one end of the sibship or the other to facilitate diagramming and visual clarity.
- Individuals with the condition are depicted by a filled-in symbol with specific symptoms listed below the symbol.
- Individuals who are carriers of the condition are depicted by a half-filled symbol (if an autosomal disorder) or by a smaller filled-in circle within the open circle (if a woman is an unaffected female carrier for an X-linked disorder).
- A key to the symbols is boxed in a corner of the pedigree.

The pedigree should also indicate the ethnic origin of the person or segment of the family, the status concerning other medical or genetic conditions (if known), and the age and cause of death of deceased persons. All this information may be helpful in clarifying a diagnosis, understanding if the condition could be genetic, determining whether a particular phenotype (physical manifestation) is a distinct entity or part of a greater syndrome present in the family, ascertaining if couples are related to each other (consanguineous) or have a common ethnic ancestry, and identifying a potential pattern of inheritance. Each mode of inheritance is associated with a different risk of recurrence. The characteristics of these modes, including the horizontal or vertical distribution of affected individuals in the family, designation of carrier status, and sex distribution associated with each of these patterns, is depicted and described in Table 5-5. This approach helps the practitioner discern clues about the condition, prognosis, and management and identify relatives at risk.

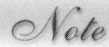

Note

If individuals in a couple are related to each other, there is a greater risk of rare autosomal recessive disorders in their offspring. The statistical risk depends on the degree of the relationship but is generally not significant if the relationship is more distant than third cousins.

Instructions:
—Symbols are smaller than standard ones, and individual's line is shorter. (Even if sex is known, triangles are preferred to a small square/circle; symbol may be mistaken for symbols 1, 2, and 5a/5b of Fig. 5-3, particularly on hand-drawn pedigrees.)
—If gender and gestational age known, write below symbol in that order.

	Male	Female	Sex unknown	Comments
1. Spontaneous abortion (SAB)	Male	Female	ECT	If ectopic pregnancy, write ECT below symbol.
2. Affected SAB	Male	Female	16 wk	If gestational age known, write below symbol. Key/legend used to define shading.
3. Termination of pregnancy (TOP)	Male	Female		Other abbreviations (e.g., TAB, VTOP, Ab) not used for sake of consistency.
4. Affected TOP	Male	Female		Key/legend used to define shading.

Fig. 5-4 Pedigree symbols and abbreviations for pregnancies not carried to term. (From Bennett, R.L., Steinhaus, K.A., Uhrich, S.B., O'Sullivan, C.K., Resta, R.G., et al. [1995]. Recommendations for standardized human pedigree nomenclature. *American Journal of Human Genetics, 56,* 745-752.)

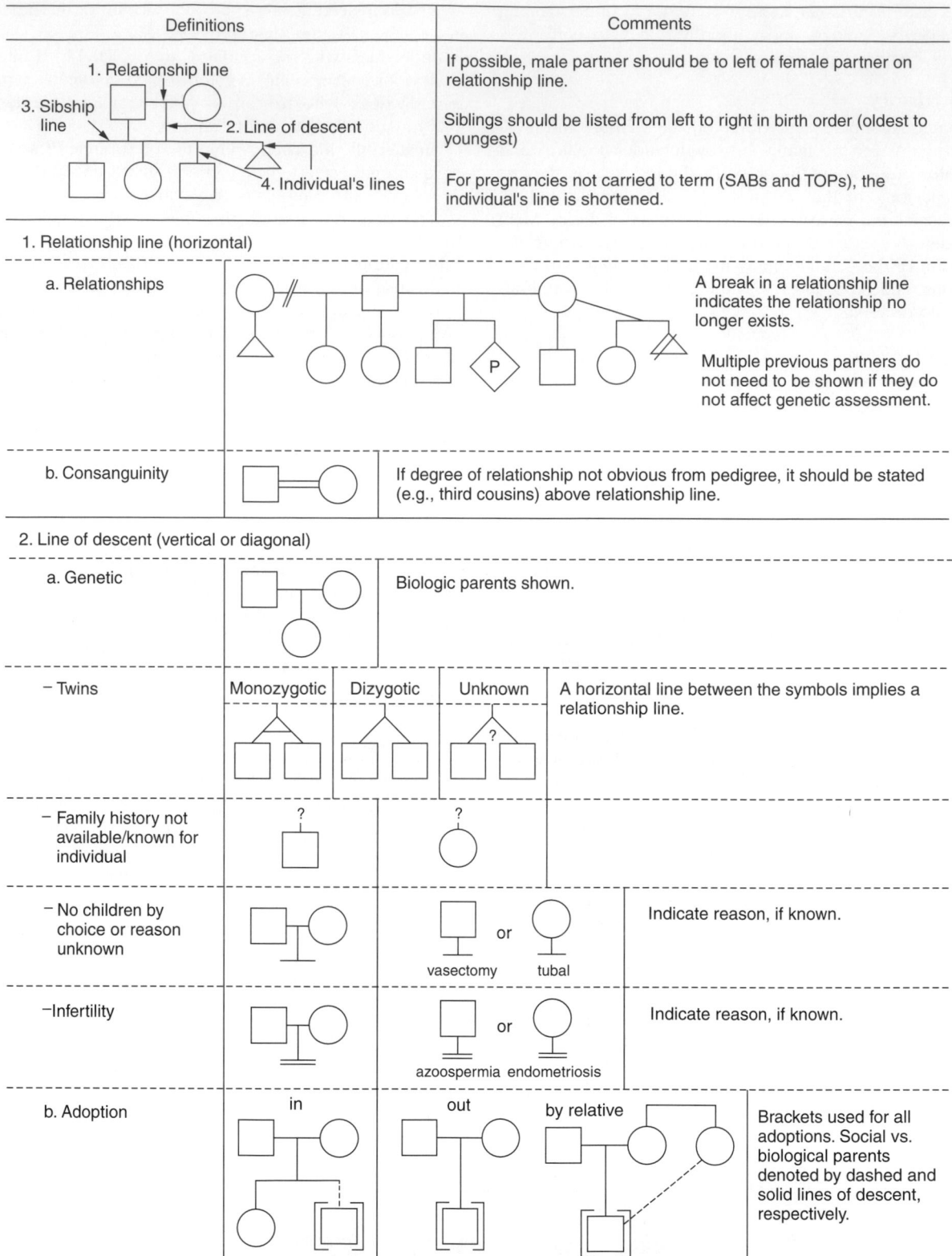

Definitions	Comments
1. Relationship line 3. Sibship line 2. Line of descent 4. Individual's lines	If possible, male partner should be to left of female partner on relationship line. Siblings should be listed from left to right in birth order (oldest to youngest) For pregnancies not carried to term (SABs and TOPs), the individual's line is shortened.

1. Relationship line (horizontal)

a. Relationships	A break in a relationship line indicates the relationship no longer exists. Multiple previous partners do not need to be shown if they do not affect genetic assessment.
b. Consanguinity	If degree of relationship not obvious from pedigree, it should be stated (e.g., third cousins) above relationship line.

2. Line of descent (vertical or diagonal)

a. Genetic	Biologic parents shown.
– Twins (Monozygotic, Dizygotic, Unknown)	A horizontal line between the symbols implies a relationship line.
– Family history not available/known for individual	
– No children by choice or reason unknown (vasectomy, tubal)	Indicate reason, if known.
– Infertility (azoospermia, endometriosis)	Indicate reason, if known.
b. Adoption (in, out, by relative)	Brackets used for all adoptions. Social vs. biological parents denoted by dashed and solid lines of descent, respectively.

Fig. 5-5 Pedigree line definitions. (From Bennett, R.L., Steinhaus, K.A., Uhrich, S.B., O'Sullivan, C.K., Resta, R.G., et al. [1995]. Recommendations for standardized human pedigree nomenclature. *American Journal of Human Genetics, 56,* 745-752.)

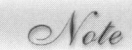

Note

Two favorite genetic questions often result in significant information and may be helpful to practitioners:
- Is there anything that tends to "run in the family"?
- Do you have any other questions or concerns about your family's health or history?

Genetic Assessment

Evaluation of a newborn or infant. If an infant is born with an obvious congenital malformation, the practitioner should obtain a thorough prenatal and family history and perform a complete physical examination (see Chapter 10). It is important for the practitioner not only to recognize but also to be able to articulate the variations from normal and the characteristics that raise clinical concern. The use of correct terminology and descriptive information facilitates appropriate testing and accurate diagnosis. The key is to look for subtle differences; the major abnormalities are generally noticed anyway.

Presentation. Presentations in a newborn that are suggestive of a chromosomal or genetic disorder (see Table 5-2) include the following major and minor malformations:
- Abnormal head size: macrocephaly or microcephaly
- Small forehead
- Ears: low set or abnormally rotated; skin tags; pits (perform hearing test [evaluate kidneys, since kidneys form at same time as ears, by renal ultrasound examination; abnormality will not be detected by routine urinalysis])
- Eyes: microophthalmia: close set; slanted palpebral fissures (openings for the eyes)

Table 5-5 Characteristics of Common Genetic Disorders

PATTERNS OF INHERITANCE	CHARACTERISTICS	COMMON DISORDERS
Mendelian Inheritance Patterns Autosomal dominant 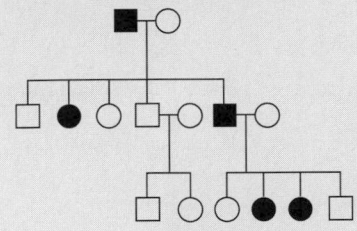	The initial case in a family occurs as a new mutation, and depending on genetic fitness of the individual has a risk to either be transmitted to next generation or end with this person. Males and females are equally affected. Requires only one copy of the abnormal gene to manifest the condition. Each offspring of the affected person has a 50% chance of inheriting the abnormal gene. Unaffected persons do not transmit the disorder to the next generation. However, it is possible that an apparently unaffected individual carries the mutated gene but does not exhibit obvious manifestations (this is called nonpenetrance) or manifestations are subtle (low expressivity). Transmission of the mutated gene occurs from one generation to the next (vertical transmission). Affected children usually have one affected parent (except in achondroplasia—80 to 90% of cases are because of new mutation) The physical manifestations that are associated with a specific condition vary in their expression. New mutations for certain disorders have been associated with advanced paternal age.	Achondroplastic dwarfism Huntington chorea Marfan syndrome Neurofibromatosis Retinoblastoma Tuberous sclerosis Myotonic dystrophy Hemochromatosis

Autosomal recessive
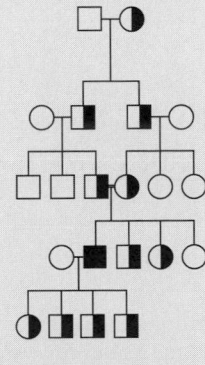
	Males and females are equally affected.
	Requires two copies of the abnormal gene to manifest the disorder.
	Affected persons usually have unaffected parents who are carriers of the gene for that disorder.
	Each conception of carrier parents has a:
	  25% chance of being affected
	  50% chance of being a carrier
	  25% chance of being an unaffected non-carrier
	Affected persons whose mates do not carry this gene will have children who will all be unaffected carriers of the gene (obligate carriers).
	Affected persons generally appear in one generation (horizontal pattern).
	Consanguinity (individuals who share common ancestor and gene pool) increases the risk for autosomal recessive disorders (especially those that are rare).
		Tay-Sachs disease
		Cystic fibrosis
		Sickle cell anemia
		Phenylketonuria
		Adrenogenital syndrome
		Albinism
		Diastrophic dwarfism
		Spinal muscular atrophy

Modified from Richards T: Genetic evaluation. In Fox, J.A. (Ed.). (1981). Primary health care of the young. New York: McGraw-Hill.
● ■ = Affected female, male. ○ □ = Unaffected female, male. ◐ ◧ = Carriers of recessive gene.
◖■ = Consanguineous first-cousin marriage (both carriers). ⊙ = Female carrier of X-linked recessive trait.

Continued

Table 5-5 Characteristics of Common Genetic Disorders—cont'd

PATTERNS OF INHERITANCE	CHARACTERISTICS	COMMON DISORDERS
Mendelian Inheritance Patterns—cont'd		
X-linked recessive	Affected males have one abnormal X-linked recessive gene. They are affected because they have no corresponding normal gene on their Y chromosome. They are hemizygous (have only one copy) for all genes on the X chromosome. The abnormal X-linked recessive gene in a male can be inherited from a carrier mother, or the gene defect may have occurred as a new mutation in that male. Each male child of a female carrier has a 50% risk of inheriting the abnormal gene and being affected and a 50% chance of inheriting the normal gene and being unaffected. Each female child has a 50% risk of being a carrier and a 50% chance of being a non-carrier. There is no male-to-male transmission because the father transmits his Y chromosome to sons. Female offspring of affected males are all obligate carriers; they inherit their father's only X chromosome which has the defective recessive gene. Transmission occurs from one generation to the next through carrier females; generally only males are affected. In rare situations, females can be affected (e.g., father was color-blind and mother was a carrier of an X-linked gene for color-blindness). The disorder may "skip" a generation if only females inherit the recessive gene, the males are unaffected, or there are no males born.	Hemophilia Duchenne muscular dystrophy Lesch-Nyhan syndrome Hurler syndrome Agammaglobulinemia Color-blindness G6PD
X-linked dominant	There is no male-to-male transmission because the father gives his Y chromosome to sons. Twice as many females are affected as males, if affected males can reproduce; may be a genetic lethal in male conceptus. The affected male who reproduces will have no affected sons; all daughters will be affected. The affected female's offspring will have a 50% chance of being affected whether male or female. There is positive family history where the gene is transmitted from one generation to the next unless it represents a new mutation.	Vitamin D–resistant rickets Incontinentia pigmenti
Mitochondrial	Matroclinal (maternal) inheritance, *not* Mendelian: abnormal gene is contained in mitochondria located in the cytoplasm, not the nucleus (see Fig. 5-2). Almost all mitochondria are inherited from the mother's egg cell (comprised of cytoplasm and nucleus with chromosomes) in contrast to sperm cell (almost exclusively nucleus). Males and females are equally affected, but only females transmit the abnormal gene. Any number of children can be affected. The degree to which an individual is affected is dependent upon the number of mitochondria inherited with the genetic defect, and their distribution in body tissues.	Mitochondrial myopathies

Modified from Richards T: Genetic evaluation. In Fox, J.A. (Ed). (1981). Primary health care of the young. New York: McGraw-Hill.
● ■ = *Affected female, male.* ○ □ = *Unaffected female, male.* ◑ ◪ = *Carriers of recessive gene.*
◑=◪ = *Consanguineous first-cousin marriage (both carriers).* ⊙ = *Female carrier of X-linked recessive trait.*

- Mouth: cleft lip or cleft palate, high arched, narrow palate; unusual shape (such as "tented" mouth associated with poor muscle tone in an infant with myotonic dystrophy)
- Small or recessed jaw
- Short or webbed neck
- Extremities and digits: disproportionate length (compared to neonatal size and gestational age); abnormal shape (rocker-bottom feet) or positioning (overlapping digits)
- Spine: curvature; tuft of hair
- Shape of chest: abnormal spacing of nipples; small chest of a size inconsistent with head circumference

Table 5-6 Minor Anomalies (Examples of Associated Disorders)

	MINOR ANOMALIES	ASSOCIATED DISORDERS
Head		
	Unusual shape	Dolichocephaly, seen in trisomy 18
	Low-set or posteriorly rotated ears	Brachycephaly, seen in trisomy 21
	Malformed ears	Chromosomal abnormalities
	Ear tags or pits	Treacher Collins syndrome
	(Always evaluate hearing and consider possibility of associated renal problems)	Ear tags seen in facioauriculovertebral spectrum
		Ear pits seen in branchiootorenal syndrome
Face		
	Synophrys	Cornelia de Lange syndrome
	Short palpebral fissures (below average distance between inner and outer canthi)	Velocardiofacial syndrome or fetal alcohol syndrome
	Epicanthal folds	Trisomy 21
	Upward slanting palpebral fissures	Trisomy 21
	Downward slanting palpebral fissures	Treacher Collins syndrome
	Hypertelorism	Opitz-Frias syndrome
	Telecanthus	Waardenburg syndrome
	Hypotelorism	Trisomy 13
	Blepharophimosis	Blepharophimosis syndrome
	Brushfield spots	Trisomy 21
	Anteverted nares	Williams syndrome
	Micrognathia	Treacher Collins syndrome; Stickler syndrome
	Prognathism	Fragile X
	Flattened facial profile	Stickler syndrome; Treacher Collins syndrome
Extremities		
	Single transverse flexion palmar crease	Trisomy 21
	Brachydactyly	Trisomy 21
	Arachnodactyly	Marfan syndrome; connective tissue disorders
	Clinodactyly with or without single interdigital crease	Trisomy 21
	Camptodactyly	Trisomy 18
	Hypoplastic or absent nails	Ectrodactyly-ectodermal dysplasia-clefting syndrome
	Syndactyly	Smith-Lemli-Opitz syndrome
	Polydactyly	Trisomy 13 (postaxial)
	Rocker-bottom feet	Trisomy 13; trisomy 18
Skin		
	Café au lait spots	Neurofibromatosis
	Hypopigmented macules	Tuberous sclerosis
	Soft, elastic skin	Ehlers-Danlos syndrome
	Lymphedema	Turner syndrome

- Genitalia: small or absent penis, testes, or vulvar structures; hypospadias
- Imperforate anus
- Neurologic abnormalities: abnormal reflexes (e.g., startle, sucking, Moro, Babinski); altered muscle tone (rule out hypotonia and spasticity); seizures; poor feeding ability
- Skin: hyperpigmentation or hypopigmentation; elasticity; scarring and healing

Assessment. Assessment includes prenatal, perinatal, health, medical and family histories, and careful examination of both obvious malformations and features that are variations of normal, are minor anomalies, or are not obvious (e.g., hypotonia).

Minor anomalies can include physical features that do not require cosmetic, surgical, medical, or developmental interventions. They may be indicators of altered development that are either part of a pattern of features consistent with a genetic condition or are isolated variations inherited from one or both parents.

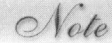
Note

The identification of one congenital malformation or minor anomaly should prompt suspicion that another malformation, albeit subtle, may exist.

Table 5-6 lists minor anomalies assessed during the physical examination. It may also be helpful to refer to Hall's *The Handbook of Physical Measurements* (1989). A practitioner should remember that a specific diagnosis requires evidence of more features than the one minor anomaly with which it is listed.

Major malformations are suggestive of a chromosomal or genetic disorder (Table 5-7) and require surgical, medical, or developmental intervention. Affected infants require a thorough

Table 5-7 Major Anomalies (Examples of Associated Disorders)

MAJOR ANOMALIES	ASSOCIATED DISORDERS
Abnormal head size: macrocephaly or microcephaly	X-linked hydrocephalus; basal cell nevus syndrome; trisomy 18
Cleft lip and/or palate: Assess nature of cleft:	
High-arched, narrow, unusual shape (e.g., "tented" mouth)	Myotonic dystrophy
Unilateral	Stickler syndrome
Central with holoprosencephaly	Agenesis of corpus callosum; trisomy 13
Small or recessed jaw	Robin sequence
Short or webbed neck	Turner syndrome
Spine: curvature; tuft or hair	Spinal defect
Shape of chest: abnormal spacing of nipples; small chest, size inconsistent with head circumference	Turner syndrome; chromosomal abnormality
Genitalia: small or absent penis, testes, or vulvar structures; inguinal hernias secondary to undescended testes; hypospadias; ambiguous genitalia	Androgen insensitivity; congenital adrenal hyperplasia (risk for masculinization of external female genitalia)
Imperforate anus	Congenital adrenal hyperplasia
Neurologic abnormalities: abnormal reflexes (startle, sucking, Moro, Babinski); altered muscle tone (rule out hypotonia, spasticity); seizures; poor feeding ability	Chromosomal abnormality; spinal muscular atrophy; muscular dystrophies; Prader-Willi syndrome

genetic physical assessment together with investigation for less obvious or "hidden" malformations. Other organs developing at the same gestational timing as that of the manifesting problem should be evaluated. (Fig. 5-6 illustrates what other anomalies are to be considered.)

Other conditions that should alert the practitioner to a possible genetic condition in a newborn or infant include:

- Intrauterine growth retardation or failure to thrive (FTT)
- Abnormal muscle tone (hypertonia or hypotonia)
- Abnormal cry
- Congenital or early-onset sensory deficits
- Developmental delay
- Seizures

The ability to distinguish a single birth defect from a clustering of manifesting features in a newborn, coupled with family history and prenatal history information, provides relevant clues for classifying a chromosomal, genetic, or nongenetic cause and for deciding what tests or treatments are most likely to produce optimal results (Table 5-8).

The presence of a congenital malformation is a sign that a disturbance occurred prenatally; this may have had an underlying genetic cause. It is important to distinguish whether the birth defect is the result of a deformation, malformation, or disruption because this understanding has relevance to cause, prognosis, treatment, and recurrence. The practitioner should evaluate the nature of the abnormality with an understanding of embryonic development (see Figs. 5-6 and 5-7).

A *deformity,* such as a clubfoot, demonstrates that a physical structure is present and intact but that some event or situation altered it. Thus a deformity is often not genetically determined, because the structure did undergo normal development biologically. Rather, a separate condition, such as oligohydramnios, constrained fetal movement and positioning, which resulted in the clubfoot deformity. Management and treatment are specific to proper alignment and improvement of the function and mobility of the feet. Prognosis is dependent on the ability to correct or modify the physical problem.

In contrast, a *malformation,* such as bilateral absence of the radii, demonstrates that a normal structure was never present

and that absence occurred symmetrically in the body. This absence of normal development and bilateral involvement are consistent with a genetically determined cause involving the gene or genes of every cell. Prognosis is related to the underlying genetic disorder and its associated problems. The risk for recurrence is dependent on the genetic disorder and mode of inheritance.

Alternatively, unilateral absence of a structure, such as a missing digit on a hand where the other four digits are present and normal, indicates that some *disruption* may have interfered with an otherwise normal and present structure. Intrauterine amputation from vasoconstriction associated with amniotic bands is not the result of a genetic disorder in general, is not associated with other congenital abnormalities, and does not pose an increased risk for recurrence.

Management. If the anomaly is truly an isolated defect in the absence of other physical abnormalities, the cause of the problem is most likely multifactorial or sporadic, with a relatively low recurrence rate. Treatment and prognosis are dependent on the limitations associated with that physical defect.

On the other hand, if other anomalies are present, the practitioner should suspect an underlying chromosomal or genetic disorder and observe and examine the infant or child for other congenital anomalies (as listed previously) and altered mental status. (Table 5-2 enumerates the specific characteristics associated with the more common disorders in the pediatric population and may also be helpful to the practitioner.) In these cases, genetic evaluation is indicated and genetic testing should be considered (see Table 5-4). Genetic consultation should be requested before genetic testing. Chromosome analysis, either routine or prometaphase banding of a specific chromosome, is generally ordered to rule out this type of cause, which is typically associated with birth defects and mental retardation. Pending the exclusion of a chromosomal abnormality, testing for a specific single-gene disorder is dependent on the particular clustering of manifesting physical problems, the prenatal and family history, and knowledge of the breadth and extent of genetic disorders and syndromes included in a differential diagnosis. Again, the management and prognosis are specific to the nature and extent of physical in-

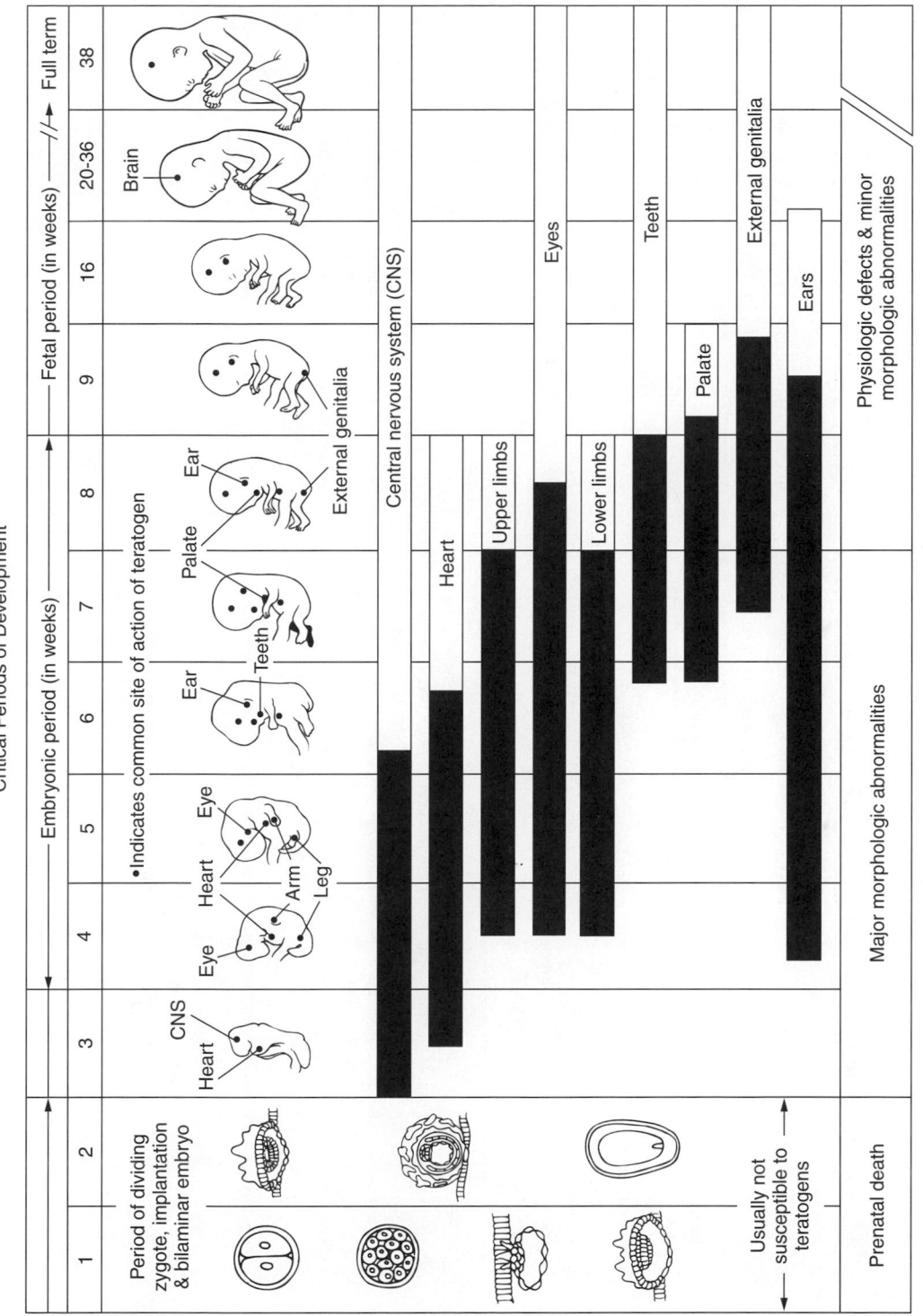

Fig. 5-6 Critical periods of embryonic development. Solid black denotes highly sensitive periods. (From Moore, K.L. [1993]. *The developing human* [5th ed.]. Philadelphia: W.B. Saunders.)

Table 5-8 Classification of Genetic Disorders: General Characteristics

ASSESSMENT AND MANAGEMENT	CHROMOSOMAL ABNORMALITY	SINGLE GENE ABNORMALITY	MULTIFACTORIAL DISORDER	TERATOGEN
Presentation at birth	Two or more congenital abnormalities: dysmorphic, (e.g., low-set ears, unusual shape of head, low forehead, eyes slanted, small for gestational age, congenital defects [e.g., cardiac, cleft], subtle differences in hands, fingers, feet, toes—position, creases, and so on)	Usually normal appearance (e.g., metabolic disorder) but can be dysmorphic (e.g., with autosomal dominant structural gene defect such as achondroplasia, osteogenesis imperfecta)	Isolated birth defect (e.g., NTD [spina bifida, anencephaly], cleft lip and/or palate, cardiac abnormality)	Physical manifestations range from subtle facial differences (e.g., small palpebral fissures, long philtrum, thin upper lip—associated with fetal alcohol syndrome) to overt abnormalities (e.g., limb reduction associated with thalidomide exposure)
Intellectual development	Mental retardation associated with autosomal aneuploidies; may be learning disability in persons with sex chromosome abnormality	Usually normal; may become mentally retarded if untreated biochemical disorder (e.g., PKU)	Usually normal	Normal (e.g., thalidomide) to learning disabled (e.g., fetal alcohol syndrome) to mental retardation (e.g., can be associated with primary CMV infection)
Family history	Can be positive (e.g., recurrent spontaneous abortions, mental retardation)	Frequently negative if autosomal recessive disorder (both parents unaffected carriers); positive or negative if autosomal dominant disorder	Usually negative (e.g., cardiac defects occur in 1% of live births) but can be positive (e.g., family history of cleft)	Usually negative, but can be positive, (e.g., recurrence of fetal hydantoin syndrome)
Genetic testing	Cytogenetic—chromosome analysis for extra or missing chromosomes, duplications, deletions, or rearrangements	DNA analysis of specific gene, if sequence is known, or by linkage with DNA markers in a family, if possible; chromosome analysis is not indicated (would be normal)	Chromosome and DNA analyses would be normal; ultrasound examination prenatally, if defect is detectable (e.g., NTD)	Chromosome and DNA analyses not indicated (would be normal); ultrasound may detect overt abnormality; amniocentesis for antigen levels, but limited interpretability
Treatment	Cannot correct chromosome abnormality (exists in all cells); supportive and preventive (e.g., physical therapy, infant stimulation program, early antibiotic treatment for respiratory infection)	Preventive in some cases (e.g., low phenylalanine diet in PKU to prevent mental retardation; gene therapy via inhalant in cystic fibrosis [experimental]) Symptomatic (e.g., treatment during sickle crisis; management of fracture with osteogenesis imperfecta)	Specific to defect (e.g., surgery to repair cleft, NTD) refer to specialists; supportive	Supportive; palliative; preventive with regard to education before next pregnancy

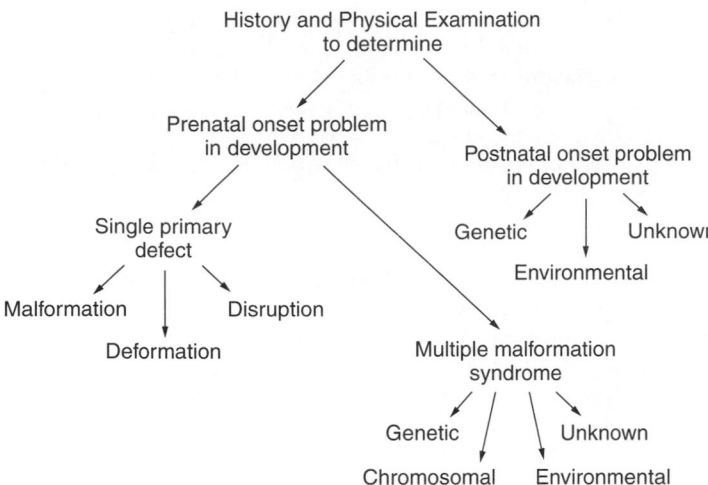

Fig. 5-7 Approach to a child with structural defects. (From Jones, K.L. [1988]. *Smith's recognizable patterns of human malformation* [4th ed.]. Philadelphia: W.B. Saunders.)

volvement and mental status. In general, physical defects such as a cleft or heart valve abnormality can be surgically corrected, physical and developmental delays associated with mental retardation can be managed and maximum potential enhanced through early intervention programs, and families can be offered support and guidance through support groups and referrals (both professional and lay). However, the underlying chromosomal or genetic defect present in all cells cannot yet be corrected.

Intervention. Refer to the discussion of interventions later in this chapter.

Evaluation of a child (age 1 year through preschool)

Presentation. A child with a genetically determined disorder that does not appear until childhood may have any combination of the following:
- Mental retardation or learning difficulty
- Developmental delay
- Growth retardation
- Hypotonia
- Small stature
- Eating disorder (e.g., compulsive, insatiable)
- Failure to thrive
- Behavioral problems
- Seizure disorder
- History of nonspecific medical illness

It is often difficult to begin to determine the cause of the problem, especially if the disorder may be of a metabolic or biochemical nature. Symptoms may be nonspecific or intermittent, various treatment and medication regimens may obscure symptoms or alter presentation, or medical evaluations and tests may have been incomplete, inconsistent, or conflicting.

Assessment. Normal growth in the first year of life is reassuring, but a child with a genetic disorder may not have significant problems within that time. If evaluations are not begun until the child is symptomatic (older), it is difficult to try to understand the true onset and progression of the problem.

Every child should be evaluated for height, weight, and head circumference at every visit. The practitioner should record and plot this information on the growth chart appropriate to the child's age, race, and sex and note it in the medical record. Growth charts also exist for children with disorders associated with short stature, such as Down syndrome, achondroplasia, and Turner syndrome. (See Resources at the end of this chapter.)

For a child with any of the previously described problems, the best approach by the practitioner is to:
- Methodically review the medical, health, and developmental histories from the intrauterine period through the present.
- Note the chronologic sequence and progression of physical or intellectual problems.
- Obtain specific information and results about previous testing and treatments.
- Explore the family history in detail, especially to look for similarly affected individuals (pictures may be helpful).

The family and medical history may be extremely helpful or, at a minimum, provide the ability to exclude certain known inherited disorders. If the child has growth retardation, the cause may be chromosomal (e.g., Down syndrome, Turner syndrome) (see Table 5-4) or genetic (e.g., achondroplasia, metabolic disorders).

If the child is mentally retarded or has a learning difficulty and has evidence of dysmorphology, a chromosomal abnormality should be considered in the differential diagnosis. Some such children are not detected at birth because their physical anomalies are subtle or minimal; these features only become more apparent as the children grow. They may have a chromosomal abnormality involving only part of a chromosome (e.g., a microdeletion), or they may have fragile X syndrome (see Table 5-2).

A child manifesting a loss of milestones is a likely candidate to have a progressive autosomal recessive or X-linked recessive (in a male) genetic disorder. The involved gene or genes may be important to metabolic, biochemical, or cellular functioning. Thus screening for an amino acid or carbohydrate disorder or performing other metabolic testing should be considered because it may provide some clue in determining cause, potential treatment, or need for further testing. The practitioner should be alert to signs of abnormal metabolism or storage that may be subtle or difficult to distinguish from abnormal development, as with a mentally retarded child, or secondary to medication effects, as with some anticonvulsant medications. These features include the following:
- Thick tongue
- Coarse facies (caused by cellular storage of abnormal metabolic byproducts): prominent forehead; thickened eyebrows; broad nose; gingival hypertrophy; facial hair; general hirsutism

- Shortness or thickening of the fingers or toes
- Liver or spleen enlargement
- Below-normal intelligence (though it can be in normal range)
- Bony abnormalities
- Unusual odor of urine
- Seizures

The first five manifestations listed above are present to varying extents in children with disorders of carbohydrate metabolism, such as Hurler, Hunter, or Scheie syndrome. The variable phenotypes are attributable to different mutations in genes, which affect the nature and extent of the disruption of a specific defective enzyme important to a particular biochemical pathway.

Other biochemical disorders, such as one affecting amino acid or purine metabolism, may have any or all of the following symptoms:

- FTT, weight loss, or inability to gain weight
- Growth retardation
- Intermittent seizures
- Behavioral problems
- Progressive decline in developmental or intellectual capabilities
- Concurrent illnesses (some may resolve with or without treatment)
- Unusual odor of urine
- Serum abnormalities
- Positive family history

The pattern and the extent of manifesting problems in these metabolic disorders are extremely variable, depending on the severity and the metabolic function of the underlying biochemical defect. Thus some such disorders present in an infant or toddler as metabolic and developmental demands increase, whereas others may appear later in childhood or adolescence because of the additional stress of concurrent illness or pubertal changes.

Clues to an autosomal recessive metabolic disorder include:

- Progressive deterioration (not usually static)
- Evidence of previously listed symptoms
- Family history of similarly affected siblings but unaffected parents
- Abnormal screening test results (e.g., amino acid screening)

Management. The primary considerations in the differential diagnosis of a child with a combination of these manifestations are a chromosomal cause or a biochemical genetic disorder. Although hundreds of proteins or enzymes are necessary for various cellular functions, an appropriate screening test can detect abnormal levels of the more common enzymes in many of these disorders. However, it is important for the alert practitioner to recognize that these are only screening tests, and thus a "normal" level does not necessarily exclude the diagnosis of this type of disorder. A genetic consultation should be requested. Referral to another specialist, such as a neurologist, a developmental specialist, or a metabolic or endocrine specialist may also be indicated for further evaluation.

Intervention. Refer to the discussion of interventions later in this chapter.

Evaluation of an adolescent

Presentation. The most common manifesting symptoms in an adolescent with a genetically determined disorder include the following:

- Mental retardation or learning difficulty
- Developmental delay
- Deviation from normal growth and development
- Delayed puberty
- Alterations in normal pubertal development
- Weakness or altered motor ability
- Dietary intolerance

It is not uncommon that only one of the above manifestations is present; this finding does not rule out the possibility of a chromosomal or genetic disorder.

Assessment and management. Abnormalities involving the sex chromosomes (see Table 5-2) are not associated with the moderate to severe mental retardation found in autosomal chromosome disorders; instead the child or adolescent may have mild retardation or only learning difficulties.

A female with Turner syndrome (45,X) may show symptoms of primary amenorrhea and short stature. Females suspected of having this condition should have a chromosome analysis and be assessed for neck webbing, history of pedal edema, and cardiac abnormalities. (Coarctation of the aorta is one associated feature.) Referral for an endocrine evaluation may also be indicated. Males with Klinefelter syndrome (47,XXY) may not come to medical attention until the expected time of puberty or later; they may or may not have experienced voice changes or nocturnal emission, and their habitus is more similar to that of a female. In rare instances, some affected males are not detected until a couple shows a history of infertility, since most males with Klinefelter syndrome are azoospermic or have oligospermia. Males who are being evaluated for Klinefelter syndrome should be checked for variation in the distribution of pubic hair (which is more consistent with that of a female), gynecomastia, and testosterone levels.

Another genetic disorder that may not be apparent before puberty is the androgen insensitivity syndrome. An apparently normally developed female's manifesting symptom is primary amenorrhea. In this disorder, the phenotypic female is actually cytogenetically a male, having a 46,XY karyotype. An abnormality in the gene important to androgen receptors on male genital cells causes these cells to be unreceptive to the effects of androgens. It is important to remember that these individuals are healthy phenotypic females. Personal perception and psychosocial considerations are extremely important in all genetic conditions but are more directly apparent in these cases. Since these females usually have testes in the inguinal canal, it is not uncommon for them to appear in childhood with inguinal hernias. This diagnosis should be kept in mind in a child with such symptoms. There are variations in the androgen-insensitivity syndrome, probably the result of different mutations within the gene, associated with complete or partial androgen insensitivity. This diagnosis also has important ramifications for the family, its dynamics, and issues of recurrence.

The fragile X syndrome is another genetically determined disorder that can appear in childhood or adolescence, initially as a learning difficulty problem. The practitioner should investigate further for the presence of subtle phenotypic manifestations such as large prominent ears, a long narrow face, increased testicular volume, and the features listed in Table 5-2.

Summary of the Approach to Pediatric Assessment in Consideration of Genetic Cause

1. Obtain a full description of the manifesting problem or symptom, including the age of onset, progression, and associated features.
2. Obtain a thorough three-generation family history, including spontaneous abortions and stillbirths, and note the

health status and medical problems of first- and second-degree relatives. (Specifically ask about the presence of features similar to those in the proband.)

3. Analyze the above two components, then evaluate and determine the differential diagnosis.
   - If mental retardation and physical abnormalities are present, suspect a chromosomal disorder.
   - If the family history is positive for a similar condition, suspect a genetically determined or influenced condition, which can be chromosomal, caused by a single gene (or pair of genes), or multifactorial in nature.

4. Consider if additional physical examination (e.g., dysmorphology), evaluation, or testing is indicated. Consult with or refer to a clinical geneticist, a genetic counselor or clinical genetics nurse specialist, a development specialist, a neurologist, an endocrinologist, and so on, as appropriate.

5. Explain and discuss considerations of this initial evaluation and history, inform and educate about potential considerations, answer individual or family questions, and provide options, recommendations (confer with relevant resources), and referral.

6. Determine a plan of action.

7. Consider genetic testing, if indicated (e.g., chromosome analysis [routine versus prometaphase], metabolic screening, fragile X testing). Consult with a genetics professional in advance of genetic testing to ensure accurate evaluation of the suspected diagnosis, the particulars of the tissue to be analyzed, the type of blood tube or specimen container, and the appropriateness of specific testing. Facilitate informed consent.

8. Plan for management, coordination of specialty services, and follow-up evaluation.

9. Provide ongoing evaluation, education, reinforcement of correct genetic information, and assessment of individual and family health care management and psychosocial needs and facilitate counseling or support as needed.

Intervention

1. Provide information about known genetic and teratogenic risk factors. Educate, counsel, and advise patients.

2. Implement appropriate prenatal counseling, education, and screening to promote optimal maternal and fetal well-being.

3. Identify populations at risk and discuss options for screening.

4. Follow up abnormal or inconclusive screening or test results.

5. Implement medical management and treatment to optimize health, promote early identification of anticipated risks, and time interventions appropriately. For example:
   - Prompt institution of special diet (e.g., to prevent brain damage in PKU)
   - Evaluation for children with growth retardation and treatment with growth hormone (depending on cause or condition)
   - Consideration of gene-based therapy (for conditions such as cystic fibrosis and autoimmune deficiency disorder)
   - Genetic testing to rule out or confirm genetic disorder or susceptibility associated with increased risk (for conditions such as hemochromatosis, hypercholesterolemia, familial adenomatosis polyposis)

6. Advocate for optimal patient and family care, including consultations, referrals, and addressing the concerns of relatives at risk. Be aware of advances in genetics that allow for future evaluation or testing not currently available, such as DNA banking.

7. Consult with or refer for genetic evaluation, risk assessment, counseling, and discussion of options.

8. Promote and facilitate informed consent.

9. Promote educational opportunities about genetics for the child, other nurses, and health care professionals through contact with resources, networks, and support groups.

Ethical, Legal, Psychosocial and Professional Issues Associated With Genetic Services and Testing

1. Understand the difference between categories of testing: clinical (ability to use information for medical management purposes), investigational (some restrictions to clinical application), or research (anonymous specimen; prohibited for clinical use).

2. Understand the type of genetic testing considered, including sensitivity, specificity, and limitations.

3. Ensure that the laboratory and director used for clinical diagnostic genetic testing have appropriate certifications and gene-specific permits.

4. Be aware that individual and family psychosocial issues arise in conjunction with genetic testing; these include confidentiality, privacy, self-perception, and family relationships.

5. Remember that informed consent is a process involving communication, education about risks and benefits, and awareness of potential issues or sequelae that may occur as a result of testing. Furthermore, in testing for genetic susceptibility rather than actual diagnosis of a disorder (e.g., cancer), the value, limitations, concerns, and effect of testing on unaffected persons at risk must be seriously evaluated before testing. This involves concerns related to health insurance, life insurance, employment, discrimination, and access to genetic information about the individual and family members.

6. Remember that genetic testing of children is appropriate for diagnosis of specific chromosomal and known genetic disorders. However, it is not a standard recommendation for identification of susceptibility genes (e.g., those associated with increased risk for cancer in adulthood). Genetic testing for susceptibility genes is appropriate in children when these cancers can occur in childhood (e.g., multiple endocrine neoplasia) or when invasive medical interventions are indicated because the child is assumed to be at risk (e.g., familial adenomatous polyposis).

7. Be aware of ethical issues and related recommendations for patients receiving genetic services and testing, (e.g., the *International Guidelines on Ethical Issues in Medical Genetics and Services* (see Resources).

8. Remember that genetic risk assessment, diagnosis, and testing may require the involvement of a psychologist and coordination and collaboration with other health care professionals, experts, resources, and the individual and family.

9. To assess unaffected persons at risk in a family, keep in mind that it is frequently necessary to first test an affected close relative to confirm and define a genetic mutation, thus allowing for appropriate testing and interpretation of results in the unaffected individual.

10. Keep in mind that professional standards exist for nurses related to genetics knowledge and clinical practice at both basic and advanced practice levels.
11. Remember that genetics factors will increasingly be identified as contributing to or modifying the risk associated with the more common conditions occurring in children and their families. Thus, every nurse may be dealing with genetic tests or "DNA on a chip" technology to test for certain susceptibilities or genetic factors that may influence the choice of medications or likelihood of adverse reactions and to identify potential health risks to engender early and proactive health promotion behaviors.

Resources

Organizations
International Society of Nurses in Genetics; (603) 643-5706; nursing.creighton.edu/isong

March of Dimes Birth Defects Foundation, 1275 Mamaroneck Avenue, White Plains, NY 10605; (914) 428-1700; www.modimes.org

National Organization of Rare Disorders (NORD); (800) 999-6673

Websites
American Cancer Society (www.cancer.org)

American College of Medical Genetics (www.faseb.org/genetics/acmg/acmgmenu.htm)

Association of Women's Health, Obstetric and Neonatal Nursing (www.awhonn.org)

CDC Office of Genetics and Disease Prevention Weekly Update (www.cdc.gov/genetics/update/current.htm)

Evaluation of the Newborn with Single or Multiple Congenital Anomalies: A Clinical Guideline (www.health.state.ny.us/nysdoh/apprd/index.htm)

Gene Clinics (www.geneclinics.com)

Genetic Alliance (www.geneticalliance.org)

Great Plains Genetic Services Network Bulletin Board (www.unmc.edu/mrimedia/gpgsn/edresnur.html)

International Guidelines on Ethical Issues in Medical Genetics and Services (www.who.int/ncd/hgn/docline.htm)

Mendelian Inheritance in Man (Online) (www.ncbi.nlm.nih.gov/Omim/)

The National Center for Human Genome Research, and National Human Genome Research Institute (NHGRI) (www.nhgri.nih.gov/)

National Society of Genetic Counselors (www.nsgc.org)

Oncology Nursing Society, including Genetics Special Interest Group (www.ons.org)

Organization of Teratology Information Service (orpheus.ucsd.edu/otis/)

Secretary's Advisory Council on Genetic Testing (www.4.od.nih.gov/oba/sacgt.htm)

World Health Organization Document: Proposed International Guidelines on Ethical Issues in Genetics and Genetic Services (www.who/hdp/gl/eth/98.1)

Bibliography

Ad Hoc Committee on Genetic Counseling of the American Society of Human Genetics: Genetic counseling. (1975). *American Journal of Human Genetics, 27,* 240-242.

American Society of Human Genetics & American College of Medical Genetics. (1995). *ASHG/ACMG report: Points to consider—ethical, legal, and psychosocial implications of genetic testing in children and adolescents.* Atlanta: American Society of Human Genetics.

Bennett, R.L., Steinhaus, K.A., Uhrich, S.B., O'Sullivan, C.K., Resta, R.G., et al. (1995). Recommendations for standardized human pedigree nomenclature. *American Journal of Human Genetics, 56,* 745-752.

Brenner, S. & Miller, J.H. (Eds.). (2001). *Encyclopedia of Genetics.* Academic Press. Available online at www.academicpress.com/genetics.

Cronk, C., Crocker, A.C., Pueschel, S.M., et al. (1988). Growth charts for children with Down syndrome: 1 month to 18 years of age. *Pediatrics, 81,* 102-110.

Erbe, R.W. (1989). Genetic counseling. In Kelley, W.R. (Ed.). *Textbook of internal medicine,* Philadelphia: J.B. Lippincott.

Farrell, C.D. (1999). Genetic testing—an ethical practice issue. *Nursing Spectrum, 11A,* NJ4.

Farrell, C.D. (1989). Genetic counseling: The emerging reality. *Journal of Perinatal and Neonatal Nursing, 2*(4), 21-33.

Farrell, C.D. & Campbell, J. (1996). Genetic and developmental disorders. In Duso, S. (Ed.). *The Lippincott manual of nursing practice* (6th ed.), Philadelphia: J.B. Lippincott.

Hall, J.G., Froster-Iskenius, U.G., & Allanson, J.E. (1989). *The handbook of physical measurements,* Oxford, UK: Oxford University Press.

Hanson, J.W. & Thomson, E.J. (2000). Genetic testing in children: Ethical and social points to consider. *Pediatric Annals, 29*(5), 285-291.

Harper, P.S. (1998). *Practical genetic counseling* (5th ed.). London: The Wright Group.

International Society of Nurses in Genetics, Inc., and American Nurses Association. *Statement on the scope and standards of genetics clinical nursing practice.* (1998). Kansas City, MO: American Nurses Association.

Jones, K.L. (1988). *Smith's recognizable patterns of human malformation* (4th ed.). Philadelphia: W.B. Saunders.

Jones, K.L. & Robinson, L. K. (1983). An approach to the child with structural defects. *Journal of Pediatric Orthopedics, 3,* 238-244.

Lea, D.H., Jenkins, J.F., & Francomano, C.A. (1998). *Genetics in clinical practice: New directions for nursing and health care.* Boston: Jones & Bartlett.

Moore, K.L. (1982). *The developing human* (3rd ed.). Philadelphia: W.B. Saunders.

Regemorter, M.D., et al. (1994). Congenital malformations in 10,000 consecutive births in a university hospital: Need for genetic counseling and prenatal diagnosis. *Journal of Pediatrics, 104*(3), 86-390.

Richards, T. (1981). Genetic evaluation. In Fox, J.A. (Ed.). *Primary health care of the young.* New York: McGraw-Hill.

Rimoin, D.L., Connor, J.M., & Pyeritz, R.E. (2001). *Emery and Rimoin's principles and practice of medical genetics* (4th ed.). New York: Churchill Livingstone.

Scriver, C.R., et al. (2001). *The metabolic and molecular bases of inherited disease* (8th ed.). New York: McGraw-Hill.

Seashore, M.R. (2000). Genetic screening and the pediatrician. *Pediatric Annals, 29*(5), 272-276.

Chapter 6 *The Ethics of Practice*

Barbara A. Elliott

An ethical framework provides important insights for every profession and for pediatric nurse practitioners (PNPs); it defines ethical behavior for the practitioners of the discipline, acknowledges the limits of personal integrity for individual practitioners, and offers a way to approach dilemmas that present themselves in practice. An ethical framework for health care providers is founded on the core values of bioethics that provide guidance for all health professionals who interact directly with patients. To specify the ethical framework for PNPs, these values are enhanced with an understanding of the defining values of the field of nursing and interpreted in light of the PNP's scope of practice.

Core Values

The four core values of bioethics—beneficence, nonmaleficence, justice, and autonomy—have relevance in every patient-family-practitioner interaction. Each concept has philosophic roots but also has specific application in the clinical setting. Each of these concepts raises a unique question that should be considered with every patient encounter (Box 6-1).

Beneficence and Nonmaleficence

The concept of *beneficence* describes the core value that all practitioners desire to benefit their patients in the contacts and interventions that are prescribed. Beneficence is often balanced with the ethical concept of *nonmaleficence,* which represents the goal of all practitioners to do nothing that harms a patient. All clinical work needs to be a careful, considered balancing of the potential benefits and harm that can result; this is an ethical issue.

Justice and Autonomy

Two additional core values can also serve to balance each other. *Justice* refers to the concept that decisions regarding health care need to represent the best use of the family's, health providers', and society's resources. Although decisions about the use of society's resources should not and cannot be made at the bedside, a family's and providers' resources (e.g., energy, skills, transportation, finances) play into every decision. These issues are often balanced by the issues raised by the concept of autonomy. *Autonomy* represents the value that each person has the right to make decisions about health care for and by himself or herself. For adults this means that every person can decide what she or he wants for health care, regardless of what may seem to be the best choice in the larger context. For pediatric patients who are immature and often not able to participate in the decisions, this concept becomes more complicated.

Parental informed permission. Health care decisions for pediatric patients are rarely made by the patients themselves, since American society has determined that people are not mature enough to know what is best for themselves until they reach the age of maturity (18 years of age in all states). Instead, the authority to make health decisions for children is given to parents, with the assumption that the parents make these decisions in a child's best interest after becoming informed about the options (informed consent). This responsibility to act in the child's best interest is taken seriously. When parents provide care that harms their child or make decisions that are not in the child's best interest, the society in which they live can take their authority away. As a part of this process, practitioners are mandated to identify parents who hurt their children to the authorities, at which time the courts decide whether to assign guardianship to others.

Case example. The example of well-child care (including immunizations) for a young child offers a clinical example of the role of justice and autonomy as concepts in everyday clinical practice. Immunizations are an appropriate recommendation to families for preventive care and public health reasons. This represents the concept of justice, which defines the best care as that which provides the greatest benefit for the largest number of citizens given the expense. However, despite the recommendation, there are families who choose not to immunize their children for personal, religious, financial, and neglectful reasons, among others. The principle of autonomy would dictate that the person receiving the immunization would decide whether to get the vaccine; however, it is impossible to know what the children would choose for themselves because of their young age. When a parent decides not to provide care that is recommended, it is important for the practitioner to reflect on why the parents are making that decision and to respond accordingly. Parents do have the authority to refuse care for a child, given good reasoning and the appropriate legal paperwork, but "they are not free to make martyrs of their children" (Justice Holmes, *Prince v. Massachusetts,* 1944).

Age of assent and age of discretion. Working in pediatrics adds several other important dimensions to the ethical concept of autonomy as it pertains to clinical decision making. As children mature, they become more capable of participating in making decisions about their own health care and behaviors (see Chapter 20). Commonly, children reach a cognitive level ("age of assent"), usually before 10 years of age, when they need to be informed about and assent to treatments.

Box 6-1 The Four Core Values

Beneficence—How will what I am doing or recommending provide a benefit to the patient and/or family?

Nonmaleficence—How will what I am doing or recommending harm this patient and/or family?

Justice—Is what I am doing or recommending a good use of limited resources?

Autonomy—Is the decision the family and I are making for this child in the child's best interest?

As they mature further, the law recognizes that children achieve an "age of discretion" in participating in health decisions before they reach maturity at 18 years of age. This achievement is usually recognized once adolescents reach 14 years of age and can both understand and participate in their health care decisions. At this time it is appropriate to provide information to them and include their preferences for care as a part of the decision-making process. Their opinions are valid and important and should be legally honored as such. However, at these ages, their opinions remain only one part of the decision. The parents' opinions and those of the practitioners are also part of the process. Until the child reaches 18 years of age, parents are the decision makers, unless one or more of the legal exceptions described subsequently also apply.

Minors' treatment statutes. In working with children, another legal issue influences the role of parents' decision making in a youth's health care. Statutes in each state define the health care issues about which youth of any age can make their own decisions. In most states, these issues include any health care decisions involving the youth's drug abuse or any sexually transmitted diseases; in some states, youths' decision-making capacity also includes the health issues of contraception, abortion, and mental illness. When youth seek health care concerning these issues, they have the legal right as mature minors to make the decisions without their parents' or guardians' participation. In fact the parents or guardians learn about these health issues only if the youth chooses to include them in the discussions.

Emancipated minors. Some adolescents have been deemed *emancipated minors* by the courts, legally conferring the status of full independence from their parents or other guardians. These adolescents are treated as legal adults in all settings, including health care. Emancipated minors are: (1) self-supporting or not living at home, (2) pregnant or a parent, (3) married, (4) in the military, or (5) declared emancipated by the courts.

Baby Doe laws. There is an additional issue that affects the decisions that families and practitioners can make while caring for a child. Since young patients cannot tell others their preferences, federal and state laws limit and specifically define when health care interventions can be withdrawn or not offered to a child patient. These laws began as the federal *Baby Doe laws* (Federal Register, 1985) and are now written into every state's child abuse directives. In addition, the Americans with Disabilities Act has further emphasized the same point: parents and health care providers must provide care to children regardless of a child's handicaps or health status. Only when (1) a child is living in chronic and irreversible coma, (2) the treatment would prolong the dying process, or (3) the treatment would be inhumane, can aggressive, life-sustaining interventions be withheld or withdrawn.

Values of Nursing

The aforementioned four core values of bioethics are acknowledged by and relevant to every discipline that serves the health needs of others. Each of these disciplines also has its own set of defining values—principles of the profession that guide practitioners in their behaviors and relationships with patients. Over time, the general public comes to expect that all the practitioners of a discipline will portray the specific values of the profession in their practice of it. Thus the values become the expectations of the public and define the field too.

Nursing is one of the disciplines with its own set of defining values. When the values of the nursing profession are added to the core values of bioethics, they define the ethical framework of the nursing profession. In clinical settings, practitioners often experience tension when these values are not in balance with each other. Commonly, practitioners have to make recommendations and decisions that favor one value over another.

Unconditional and Universal Acceptance
Nurses define their work as "patient-centered care," meaning that nurses provide care to patients, whatever the patients' or families' circumstances and values. This principle of compassion and tolerance is an important defining value of the profession. However, by necessity it has limits. At times patients' requests for care or refusals of care are not consistent with the science of appropriate nursing. At times practitioners are asked by patients or families to negotiate care plans that not only compromise ideal care but may indeed achieve less than adequate care. When this happens, the frustration experienced by a practitioner is the result of a conflict of values. The professional value of acceptance is in conflict with the core values of providing benefit to patients or families and avoiding harm to them. The practitioner believes that his or her care is being compromised. Resolution follows when either the care plan is renegotiated or the relationship is ended.

Honesty with Patients and Colleagues
Another defining value of the nursing profession is that as professionals, nurses are honest with patients, families, colleagues, and themselves. The information that is exchanged is assumed to be truthful and candid. However, at times, the limits of the prognosis; the circumstances of the discussion; the personalities, ages, and abilities of the people involved; and numerous other conditions can limit the possibilities for honesty in an exchange. Also there are times when it may be professionally impossible to be honest (e.g., when it is not appropriate to inform about a diagnosis, since it is in another professional's or the family's purview to do that). Nonetheless there is a strong value of honesty that needs to be managed as part of the professional identity.

Patient Advocacy
Advocating the needs of patients and families is another defining value of the nursing profession. People who are patients and related to patients are to be respected, and their choices are to be respected and honored. Nurses recognize that it is their role to help adult patients achieve their autonomous choices in their health care, to maintain confidentiality, and to help family members who are making decisions be heard by other members of the health care team. When practitioners are advocating for child patients, they are helping the patients achieve their best interests, maintaining confidentiality, and coordinating family participation in decision making while managing continuing care and negotiating the health care system.

Without the value of advocacy for child and family needs and choices, these tasks could not be achieved. The limits of the advocacy value for nurses become evident when the life choices of a child or family are not consistent with ideal or even adequate nursing practice. This tension evolves because of differences between the nursing value of advocacy and the core values of providing benefit and not causing harm with provided health care services.

Competence and Commitment to Excellence

Another defining value of the profession of nursing is professional competence. Nurses are expected to be competent in their professional work, with a commitment to excellence that assumes that a nurse's practice will incorporate new information, skills, and science as they become available. Nurses are expected to be diligent in their acquisition of new information and to be capable in the practice of the profession. Practitioners are also expected to be adding to the skills, science, and research that provide the basis for their specialty.

Accountability

The nursing profession has its own scientific base, skills, and methods of meeting and providing care to children and families. Nurses are accountable for knowing their profession; for providing appropriate, confidential care; and for making decisions within the limits of the job descriptions. Nurse practitioners (NPs), as independent practitioners, place a special value on accountability for their own decisions, for the consequences of their own decisions, and for the limits of their knowledge and care. Since no other practitioner is responsible for the care an NP provides and there is no institution that will accept that responsibility (e.g., a hospital), accountability as a value becomes defined legally as *liability*.

Professional Autonomy

Professional autonomy is a currently voiced concern of the nursing profession, especially of the NP specialties (and it is also obviously related to the accountability value). Becoming a profession with autonomous practitioners is a goal and an ongoing effort being pursued by the nursing profession. PNPs are among the specialists in the nursing field who have varying amounts of independence in their practices around the country. It is the intention of the profession that professional autonomy for nurses be further recognized, honored, and established. This value is being publicly debated in legal and policy discussions about supervision, prescribing, and reimbursement, among other topics.

Duties of the Practitioner

The core values of bioethics, complemented by the values of the nursing profession, begin to define the ethical framework within which practitioners work, and the responsibilities and duties that make up the scope of a practitioner's practice are described in Chapter 1. These duties define the settings within which the values are enacted by practitioner-child-family groups. The goal of these interactions for the practitioner is to make decisions that are clinically and technically sound, suitable for the specific problems of the particular child and family being treated, and morally appropriate in that they represent the best interests of the child.

The NP's duties imply that practitioners, working independently: (1) make accurate determinations of a patient's condition, (2) inform and educate the child and family about the health condition, (3) recommend and formulate a care plan, (4) discuss the benefits and the risks of the options included in the plan, (5) discuss the prognosis, and (6) use skill and contacts to achieve the care plan. All of this is to be done while the practitioners are skillfully working with children and their families, individualizing decisions to their needs, preferences, and circumstances.

Practitioner Integrity

Each individual practitioner practices the profession by integrating personal values with the profession's values and core bioethics values in his or her daily clinical work. The decisions that are made or recommended reflect what the practitioner personally thinks should happen, given the circumstances. The practitioner's values may or may not be consonant with the profession's values.

Many times, clinical work demands that choices be made that emphasize one value over another. The choices each person makes reflect the importance of that person's values relative to the other values. This pattern of preferences is a reflection of the practitioner's integrity, or personal ethical identity. How well an individual's own values actually reflect those of the profession and the core bioethics values indicates that person's integrity. The general public also has expectations about professional work and how professionals in a field relate to the public when they are patients or family members. How the public sees professional work and personal integrity allows them to form an impression of how ethical (or unethical) the work is.

There are times in every profession when an individual practitioner cannot provide the requested services or care that a patient desires. When this happens, each practitioner needs to acknowledge the limits that personal values (integrity) place on the practice and respectfully decline to provide further care in that circumstance. It is then appropriate to refer the child and family to other providers whose values allow them to provide that care. Examples of times when this can happen include, but are not limited to, the following: requests by teenagers for abortion services, families who are noncompliant with a negotiated care plan, and cases where the child and family care plan does not meet the practitioner's expectations of adequate care or safety.

Analyzing Ethical Dilemmas

Every case that a practitioner encounters can be analyzed from a variety of perspectives. One is the nursing perspective, another is the medical perspective, and a third is the ethical perspective. Practitioners automatically use the nursing perspective when approaching a case; alternatively, practitioners will appeal to a pediatrician and acquire the medical interpretation of what might be occurring when a troubling case presents itself. Another approach when "there is something wrong" in a case is to use the case method for ethics analysis described subsequently. It is a way to sort out the values that often cause the troublesome issues attached to a case. The medical perspective may be able to explain the anatomic, physiologic, or pharmacologic issue, and the nursing perspective may be able to add the personal, social, and contextual issues that inform a method of achieving a goal. The ethics analysis provides insight into why a solution is difficult at its most basic level, exploring the values that are in conflict and thus interfere with achieving the care plan. Whenever a case or a situation related to a case "feels bad" or leaves a practitioner with a "knot in the stomach," it is time to investigate the issues using ethics analysis.

The case method shown in Box 6-2 can provide a template for considering the most specific issues, as well as those that seem very complex and convoluted. The first and most basic issue is defining the problem, as indicated in the first step. All the confusion that emotion brings can be set aside once the problem to be addressed is clearly stated. For example, ethical problems may be expressed similar to the following: Should

Box 6-2 Case Method for Ethics Analysis

1. Define the problem using a sentence that includes the verb *ought* or the verb *should*.
2. What are related concerns, including family, prognosis, physiologic, and legal issues?
3. Who is the decision-maker and is he or she making appropriate decisions given the circumstances?
4. What are the decision-maker's values as they pertain to this case?
5. What are the practitioner's (and other providers') values as they pertain to this case?
6. What are the pros and cons of each option available to resolve the dilemma? Which one is the best option?
7. What constraints (e.g., legal, financial) need to be considered in the implementation of the best choice?
8. Implement and evaluate the resolution.

narcotic pain relief be prescribed for this teenage addict with a broken leg? Ought I tell this adolescent's mother about her sexual activity? Should I continue to work with this pediatrician whose values do not allow me full PNP practice? As these potential questions indicate, this approach can be used with a variety of issues in practice.

The second step is the opportunity to list all the contextual issues that can influence the child's and families' outcomes and create difficulties for practitioners.

The third step can be a critical one in pediatrics; it pertains to who makes the decision and whether the best interests of the child are represented fairly by that identified decision maker.

The fourth and fifth steps are often the most revealing and challenging steps in an ethics case analysis. The differences between the providers' values and the child's and family's values are the essence of an ethical dilemma. Providers value maximizing function, curing when possible, and managing symptoms when they can. Children and families may value doing everything possible to keep the child alive, to keep the child at home, or to not have the child placed in medical foster care. These differences can make managing a case very problematic unless a common goal can be found. Often this happens only when common values are identified as the basis for the care plan.

The sixth step is taking stock of the options and each of the pros and cons associated with them and then making a choice. With ethical dilemmas there rarely is a right choice; usually it is the best choice among less-than-optimal options. The best choice is the one in which common goals or values are most clearly identified.

The seventh step is (once the first choice is made) determining whether there are any constraints that limit the implementation of the best choice. As examples, it may be possible that there is no funding to obtain a certain treatment, or it may be likely that a malpractice liability suit will be filed if a certain decision is pursued. These issues need to be recognized and anticipated as consequences of any decisions that are made.

Finally, the remaining "best choice" is then implemented and reevaluated as it progresses.

Case Example

Your best friends, John and Sue, have three children. The oldest one, Sally (17 years of age), has come to your office be-

cause she has not felt well for nearly 3 weeks and is now complaining of abdominal pain. Her mother has brought her to the office, but as usual you see Sally alone. After you have taken the history and examined Sally, it is evident that she is pregnant and in the process of a spontaneous abortion. Sally tells you that her parents do not know about her sexual activity or pregnancy and asks you not to tell them anything. She was afraid she was pregnant and is relieved she is having a spontaneous abortion. You advise her about what to expect over the next 24 hours and ask her to call if any worrisome symptoms occur. You then schedule another appointment to see her in a week, both to check on the spontaneous abortion and to talk more with her.

Case Method for Ethics Analysis

1. Make a simple "ought" statement of the major ethical problem.
   - Ought I keep Sally's confidence? Who ought to tell these parents about their daughter's sexual activities, if anyone?
2. List considerations (facts and options) that are important to making a good decision.
   - Sally is currently miscarrying, which may or may not need further medical intervention. She does not yet need a dilatation and curettage (D&C), and she may not need one at all.
   - Sally is likely to continue being sexually active, and I hope that she will use birth control in the future.
   - Sally's parents are "reasonable people"; when they learn of her sexual activity, they will have concerns, but I do not expect major family disorganization.
   - Options:
     A. I could keep the confidence with Sally.
     B. Sally could tell her parents.
     C. Sally and I could tell her parents together.
     D. I could tell her parents (with Sally's permission).
3. Who is the decision maker in this case?
   - Sally was competent and speaking clearly for herself when she made the request for confidentiality.
   - By state law, Sally is an "emancipated minor" with regard to her pregnancy and sexuality issues. That means her request is legally supported; her pregnancy makes her a legal adult, and all of her medical conversations and records about the pregnancy are not available to anyone else—even her parents—without her permission.
4. Identify relevant patient values that are involved.
   - Sally is 17 years of age and both frightened and relieved; she is at the appropriate developmental level and does not want to tell or involve her parents in her independent activities. This developmental task is the basis for Sally's stated value of not informing her parents. Her sexual behavior expresses her developmental level too. Her request is both an expression of this need and of her fear of her parents' reaction.
5. Identify relevant health professional values that are important.
   - Nearly all the health promotion goals and societal health care values might be applied in this circumstance. The confidentiality value is the specific value in question in this case, but each of the others provides a rationale to consider the options that broaden the one Sally requests.

6. Propose and test solutions.
   - One option is to agree with Sally's request now and honor it. This would respect her preferences but would upset her parents greatly in the future when or if they learn of her activities and my silence.
   - Another option is to agree with her request now and plan to talk with her at the next appointment about her telling her parents (or at least about the birth control I am hoping she will take). This honors her preferences now and leaves the door open for family communication, support, and development later.
   - A third option is to agree with her request now and talk with her at the next appointment about us talking with her parents. This honors her preferences now and offers the opportunity to talk with her parents with professional (and personal) support.
   - It would be inappropriate to ignore her request and break the confidence unless she says she has changed her mind.
7. Identify constraints that need to be addressed.
   - The following constraints need to be addressed:
     A. *(A personal issue)* The friendship I have with her parents and the expectations of honesty that are the basis for a true friendship will need consideration and planning.
     B. *(A business issue)* The bill to the insurance company indicates the diagnosis (i.e., pregnancy, spontaneous abortion). It is important to make sure that information is not on the copy of the bill that goes to the family home.
     C. *(A doctor-patient issue)* If Sally has a medical emergency as a result of this spontaneous abortion or needs a D&C, I will need to explain the circumstances to her parents. What would she want me to say to them?

Resources

Websites

American Academy of Nurse Practitioners (www.aanp.org)

American Nurses Association Center for Ethics and Human Rights (www.nursingworld.org/ethics/chcode.htm)

American Society of Law, Medicine & Ethics (www.aslme.org)

College of Nurse Practitioners (www.nurse.org/acnp)

Ethics Links on the Internet (www.mcw.edu/bioethics/bioweb)

Nurse Practitioner Central (www.nurse.net)

Nursing Ethics Network (NEN) (jmrileyrn.tripod.com/nen/ethic-slinks.html)

Bibiliography

Beauchamp, T. L. & Childress, J. F. (2001). *Principles of biomedical ethics* (5th ed.). New York: Oxford University Press.

Child abuse and neglect prevention and treatment in rural communities: Two approaches. (1978). Washington, DC: U.S. Department of Health, Education, and Welfare, Office of Human Development Services, Administration for Children, Youth, and Families: Children's Bureau, National Center for Child Abuse and Neglect.

Elliott, B. (2001). *Case method for ethics analysis.* Duluth, MN: Ethics Curriculum, University of Minnesota at Duluth, School of Medicine.

Federal Register. (1985, April 15). *Child abuse and neglect prevention and treatment.* 45 CFR 1340.15.

Leiken, S. (1982). Minor's assent or dissent in medical treatment. In President's Commission for the Study of Ethical Problems in Medicine and Biomedical and Behavioral Research. *Making health care decisions. A report on the ethical and legal implications of informed consent in the patient-practitioner relationships.* Washington, DC: U.S. Government Printing Office.

Lo, B. (2000). *Resolving ethical dilemmas: A guide for clinicians* (2nd ed.). Baltimore: Williams & Wilkins.

Chapter 7 Pediatric Pain Assessment and Management

The management of pain in the pediatric patient begins with an accurate understanding of the physiology of pain, careful attention to the myths and truths about pediatric pain, and a thorough, developmentally appropriate assessment of pain that factors in all possible contributors to the pain experience. The information that follows is based on the assumption that pain is both physiologically and psychologically harmful to children and it is the health care provider's ethical responsibility to properly and accurately assess and manage that pain.

In 2000, the Joint Commission on Accreditation of Healthcare Organizations (JCAHO) developed formal standards of care for the assessment and management of pain. Since the JCAHO views pain management as a particularly integral component of care, it expanded the scope of its pain management standards. Although pain is a common finding in many diseases, injuries, and conditions, it does require specific and explicit attention.

The JCAHO (2000) standards apply to all age groups. All health care organizations must:

- Recognize the right of individuals to appropriate assessment and management of pain.
- Assess the existence and, if present, the nature and intensity of pain in all patients and residents.
- Establish policies and procedures that support the appropriate prescribing or ordering of effective pain medications.
- Educate patients, residents, and their families about effective pain management.
- Address the individual's needs for symptom management in the discharge planning process.
- Incorporate pain management into the organization's performance measurement and improvement program.

Research on Pain in Children

There has been significant improvement in the assessment and management of pain in infants and children since the 1970s. At that time, research indicated that infants and children were not assessed or medicated adequately for their pain, particularly in comparison with similar procedures for adults. During this past decade:

- A paradigm shift has occurred with the recognition that not only does pain exist in children it is also a significant cause of morbidity and can contribute to mortality.
- Multiple assessment scales have been developed and validated to assess pain in all pediatric age groups (from premature babies to adolescents).
- Pain management algorithms have been developed for use with specialized groups of pediatric patients, including cases of postoperative neonatal and pediatric cardiac

surgery, sickle cell disease, neonatal circumcisions, and general postoperative pain management.

- Pharmacologic interventions for pain management in children now include new administration methods for opioids (transdermal and transmucosal), use of neuraxial analgesia, and increased use of patient-controlled modalities (peripheral and epidural).
- Nonpharmacologic interventions, such as hypnosis and biofeedback, have been recognized as effective in pain and anxiety management.
- Safety and efficacy of medications used for sedations for painful or anxiety-producing procedures have been validated.

Despite these unprecedented advances in pain management over the past decade, some clinicians remain reluctant to incorporate new concepts and therapies into the care of children. Concern related to the developmental differences in children, side effects of medications, and difficulty in assessing pain in children are the major reasons for this continued trend. The prevalence of inaccurate beliefs and myths about children's pain and lack of understanding about different types of pain, rather than scientific evidence, however, remain the most significant roadblocks to effective management.

Truths about Pediatric Pain

For decades many myths existed about pediatric pain that ultimately influenced the way pain was managed. Although at times appearing trivial, the myths outlined below need to be expounded on because not all health care providers are convinced of their significance.

All pain is real. Regardless of whether the provider believes there is a physiologic cause for the pain, all complaints of pain must be taken seriously. Treatment for pain must never be denied because of the belief that the child's pain is not "true pain" or is "all in the child's head."

Infants and children do feel pain. In preterm infants as young as 24 weeks of gestation, sufficient elements of the central nervous system have developed to transmit painful stimuli.

Children of all ages do have memory of pain. By the age of 6 months, infants have been found to actually avoid a painful stimulus they have experienced in the past, validating their memory of the prior experience.

The activity level of the child cannot be used as a single factor in determining the degree of pain a child is experiencing. Some children may lie very still to prevent pain from increasing, whereas other children may subconsciously increase their activity level to try to "get away from the pain." Clinicians must be alert to changes in the normal pattern of activity level for the individual child to assist in this aspect of assessment.

Children will not always tell the truth about the presence or intensity of their pain. They may have fears or misperceptions about the cause of their pain (e.g., "I must be bad to feel so bad") or may fear pain management itself (e.g., "If I say I hurt, they might make me take medicine that tastes bad or makes me hurt even more," "I don't want a shot. I'll just tough it out"). Adolescents may deny their pain for fear that the pain medicine prescribed may lead to addiction; many adolescents are proud to be "drug free" and do not want to risk this achieved status.

Children do not become addicted to pediatric analgesics more easily than adults do. The assumption that narcotics used by pediatric patients will lead to addiction is significantly flawed; there are no data to support this myth. Children are not at an increased risk of developing physical dependence or addiction from brief courses of opioids for acute pain management.

Narcotics can safely be given to infants and children. Careful attention always must be given to the dosage prescribed, and monitoring for side effects must be diligent.

Pain Definitions

McCaffery's (1999) definition is very broad and defines pain "whatever the experiencing person says it is, existing whenever the experiencing person says it does." Merskey and Bogduk (1994) define pain as "an unpleasant sensory and emotional experience associated with actual or potential tissue damage, or described in terms of such damage or both." Both definitions are well accepted and recognize the subjective nature of the pain experience. Pain can be defined further according to its duration, location, and cause, that is, acute versus chronic, malignant versus nonmalignant.

Pain may also be classified according to the site of pain origination. This classification is important not only in the assessment of the origin of pain, but also in the choice of pain management.

- *Somatic pain* originates in bone, skin, ligament, and muscle and is generally well localized. Somatic pain is generally described as aching, throbbing, or gnawing.
- *Visceral pain* originates in solid or hollow organs, is initiated by distension, traction, or ischemia, is generally poorly localized, and can be referred to other areas. Visceral pain is generally described as cramping, pressure, deep aching, or squeezing.
- *Neuropathic pain* stems from dysfunction or lesions of the central or peripheral nervous systems and may be associated with neurologic deficit or altered sensation. Neuropathic pain is generally described as burning, electrical shock, hot, stabbing, shooting, numbing, itching, or tingling sensations.

Although it may be difficult to assess the type of pain a person is experiencing, especially in the very young, nonverbal, or cognitively impaired, it is important to differentiate between these various types of pain whenever possible. Different types of pain necessitate different methods or medications for management. For example, somatic and visceral pain responds better to opioids and nonsteroidal antiinflammatory drugs (NSAIDs), whereas neuropathic pain responds best to antidepressants, anticonvulsants, and other adjuvant medications.

Other terms that are critical to define because of common misunderstanding about their meaning are:

- *Tolerance*—A need for escalating doses of a drug to maintain an analgesic effect without an increase in nociception.
- *Physical dependence*—A biologic response to chronic opioid administration characterized by onset of withdrawal symptoms upon opioid cessation or antagonist administration. Withdrawal symptoms include sweats, chills, tremors, increased pain, diarrhea, nausea, vomiting, and runny nose.
- *Addiction*—Concomitant behavioral pattern of drug use characterized by craving for a drug and overwhelming involvement in obtaining and using a drug for reasons other than pain control. Actual risk for addiction in medical use is less than 1%.
- *Pseudoaddiction*—Undermedication for pain leads to some behaviors that mimic addiction. These behaviors subside when pain is adequately treated.

Conducting a Pediatric Pain History

Conducting a thorough pain history is the important first step in the assessment of pain. Standardized pain history forms have been developed for both parents and children, and their use is recommended by the Agency for Health Care Policy and Research (AHCPR). Regardless of the method or form used, the environment where the history is conducted needs to be relaxed, safe, and supportive for the patient and the patient's family. Several issues need to be addressed when one is obtaining a history of prior pain experience and of the current pain complaint.

History of Previous Pain
- Any previous history of pain (if yes, when and type: procedural versus surgical, acute versus chronic versus episodic)
- Child's communication of pain (or lack of communication: verbal versus nonverbal)
- Behavioral response to pain ("curls up into ball" versus "wild flailing arms")
- Agreement to treatment ("I want to tough it out" versus "Help me now!")
- Effective versus ineffective therapies (pharmacologic versus nonpharmacologic)
- Adverse response to therapies

History of Current Pain Complaint
- *Onset of pain*—When did it begin? What was the child doing before the pain began?
- *Description of pain*—Can you describe the type of pain (e.g., sharp, dull, stabbing, burning)? The duration? Location? Intensity and frequency? Is there any radiation?
- *Temporal pattern*—Is the pain constant or intermittent? If intermittent, what is the frequency and duration of episodes? Does the pain change with the time of day (better or worse during day or night)?
- *Aggravation or alleviating factors*—What has helped the pain to feel better? Worse? Has the pain been relieved at all since it began? What factors increase or elicit the pain? Has the child taken or been given any medication to attempt pain relief?
- *Associated symptoms*—Does the child have nausea, vomiting, dizziness, lightheadedness, diarrhea, or difficulty ambulating?
- *Effect on daily living*—Is the child unable to go to school? Needing to be held all the time? Having difficulty eating? Unable to get out of bed? Not wanting to play?

When the information obtained from the history indicates a medical or surgical emergency (such as an acute abdomen), no further information is necessary before treatment. Assessment of the following factors may be considered after treatment has been provided and when postoperative or postprocedural pain is the issue.

- *Age and developmental level of the child*—The child's ability to understand the pain may contribute to the pain experience.
- *Temperament of the child and the family*—Wide variations in temperament affect the impression of the pain experience and may cloud the initial assessment of the type of pain and any accompanying symptoms.
- *Cultural, ethnic, or religious background of the child or family*—Different groups of people incorporate their personal values and beliefs into the pain experience differently. Some groups believe the pain should be a sacrificial offering to God and medications for relief should not be

taken, whereas others may believe that pain is a punishment or should be used for character building. The influence of these values and beliefs on the child's physical and emotional health must always be considered and appropriate action taken.

- *Previous pain experience*—A positive or negative pain experience in the past definitely influences the current experience. A discussion of past pain experiences or lack of pain experiences may affect management.

Mnemonics for Pain Assessment

Two mnemonic methods have been developed for the assessment of chronic pain, and they can easily be adapted to acute pain as well. Both of these mnemonic methods should be considered in the assessment of acute pain reports, in addition to recurrent episodes of pain or chronic pain.

Table 7-1 Developmental Considerations in Pain Assessment

AGE GROUP	PHYSIOLOGIC	BEHAVIORAL	AVAILABLE ASSESSMENT TOOLS
Premature infants	Vital sign changes Bradycardia, sustained tachycardia, periods of apnea, tachypnea, irregular respirations, changes in blood pressure Decrease in oxygen saturation	Crying or cry face: bulging brow, eyes squeezed shut, nasolabial furrow, stretched mouth, taut/cupped tongue, quivering chin Gross motor movement: very rigid, increased motor activity, or completely flaccid/limp	Neonatal Infant Pain Scale (NIPS) CRIES (cries, oxygen saturation, heart rate and blood pressure, expression, sleeplessness) Scale
Infants-2 years	Vital sign changes Hiccoughing Chin quivering Pursed lips	Crying/hyperalertness Lethargy/total exhaustion Rocking/increased restlessness Regression Disturbed sleep (increase in non-rapid eye movement [REM] sleep) Increased thumbsucking Aggressive behavior	Children's Hospital of Eastern Ontario Pain Scale (CHEOPS) Face, Legs, Arms, Cry, and Consolability (FLACC) Scale
2-5 years	Vital sign changes Pupil dilation Flushing of skin	View pain as punishment May deny they are having pain Refusal of everything Physically resist Loud verbal response Withdrawal (exhaustion) Increased clinging behavior Disinterest in play General regression	Faces Rating Scale Eland Color Tool CHEOPS Poker Chip Tool Oucher Scale FLACC Scale
5-12 years	Vital sign changes Clenched fist or teeth Rigid posture	Plea bargain Overt resistance/aggression Detachment/withdrawal Increased sleep Hyperactivity/passivity General regression	Faces Rating Scale Numerical Rating Scale Word Graphic Rating Scale Poker Chip Tool Visual Analogue Scale Global Rating Scale Oucher Scale
12-18 years	Vital sign changes	Focus on self "Personality change" Overt resistance/aggression Compliant Withdrawal/depression Manipulative Changes in hygiene/appearance	Numerical Rating Scale Word Graphic Rating Scale Visual Analogue Scale

Modified from McCready, M., MacDavitt, K., & O'Sullivan, K.K. (1991). Children and pain: easing the hurt. Orthopedic Nursing, 10(6), 33-42.

MPQRST

M Meaning of the pain for the patient and the family
P Provocative or palliative factors
Q Quality
R Region and radiation
S Severity
T Temporal factors

PAIN

P Physical aspects or causes for the pain (e.g., nerve damage, infection)
A Anxiety, either past or present, that may be affecting the pain experience
I Interpersonal problems the child or family may be having (e.g., loss of peers, isolation, family stress) that could directly or indirectly influence the pain experience in a variety of ways
N Nonacceptance of what has caused the pain or the effects of the pain (which has been referred to as the "spiritual pain")

Variables Included in Pediatric Pain Assessment

Three variables must be included in all pain assessments: physiologic signs, behavioral cues or responses, and subjective or verbal reports. For the preverbal or developmentally delayed child, the physiologic signs and behavioral cues may be emphasized more, though the importance of the parents' report is recognized.

As noted earlier in reference to conducting a pain history, the age and developmental level of children also affect their expression of the pain experience (Table 7-1). The wide variation in the expression of pain necessitates a thorough physical examination.

To quantify pain in children, many standardized and validated pain assessment tools have been developed. Standardizing pain assessment by incorporation of the use of a validated pain assessment tool is recommended by the AHCPR guidelines, regardless of the pain tool selected (Table 7-2).

Management of Pain in Children

Quantifying the pain assessment through the use of a standardized tool can assist in the management of pain. Practitioners can develop either a mental or written algorithm for pain management based on their pain assessment (Fig. 7-1).

In developing an algorithm, one should categorize the degree of pain assessed for ease of management: such as mild, moderate, severe; a little, a lot, unbearable. All factors obtained in the pain history described previously need to be considered when one is categorizing the pain, recognizing that the pain experience is very individual. Attention must also be given to determining whether the symptoms described are predominantly pain or anxiety. (Standardized anxiety assessment scales that are similar to the pain assessment scales have not been developed to quantify the degree of anxiety experienced, thereby making the assessment of anxiety very complicated.) Although this differentiation may be very difficult to make, treatment for each will vary, and combination therapy may be indicated.

Table 7-2 Pain Assessment Tools

TOOL	INDICATIONS	SPECIFIC CONSIDERATIONS FOR USE
Neonatal Infant Pain Scale (NIPS) (Lawrence et al, 1993)	Recommended for preterm neonates (gestational age less than 37 weeks) and full-term neonates (gestational age of 37 weeks up to 6 weeks after birth)	None noted.
CRIES Scale (Krechel and Bildner, 1995)	Recommended for use in neonates	Specifically designed to assess postoperative pain.
CHEOPS (McGrath et al, 1985)	Recommended for children 1-7 years of age	None noted.
Faces Rating Scale (Wong and Baker, 1988)	Recommended for children ages 3 years and above	Need to recognize the child's temperament profile and cultural norms, because child's facial expression may not change with pain.
FLACC Scale (Merkel et al, 1997)	Recommended for children ages 2 months-7 years	None noted.
Eland Color Tool (Eland, 1985)	Recommended for children ages 4 years and above	Child needs to have developed color recognition skills.
Poker Chip Tool (Hester, 1979)	Recommended for children ages 4-8 years	Child needs to have developed rank ordering of number skills.
Oucher Scale (Beyer, 1988; Beyer et al, 1992)	Recommended for children ages 3-12 years	Recently developed tool that includes attention to various cultures; need to continue to consider child's temperament and cultural norms for facial expressions.
Numerical Rating Scale (Whaley and Wong, 1987)	Recommended for children ages 5 years and above	Child needs to have developed rank ordering of number skills.
Glasses Rating Scale (Whaley and Wong, 1995)	Recommended for children ages 6 years and above	Child needs to have developed an understanding of proportionality.
Word Graphic Rating Scale	Recommended for children ages 5 years and above	Child needs to be able to read simple words, with accurate comprehension of words used.
Visual Analogue Scale	Recommended for children ages 5 years and above	Child needs to have developed an understanding of proportionality.

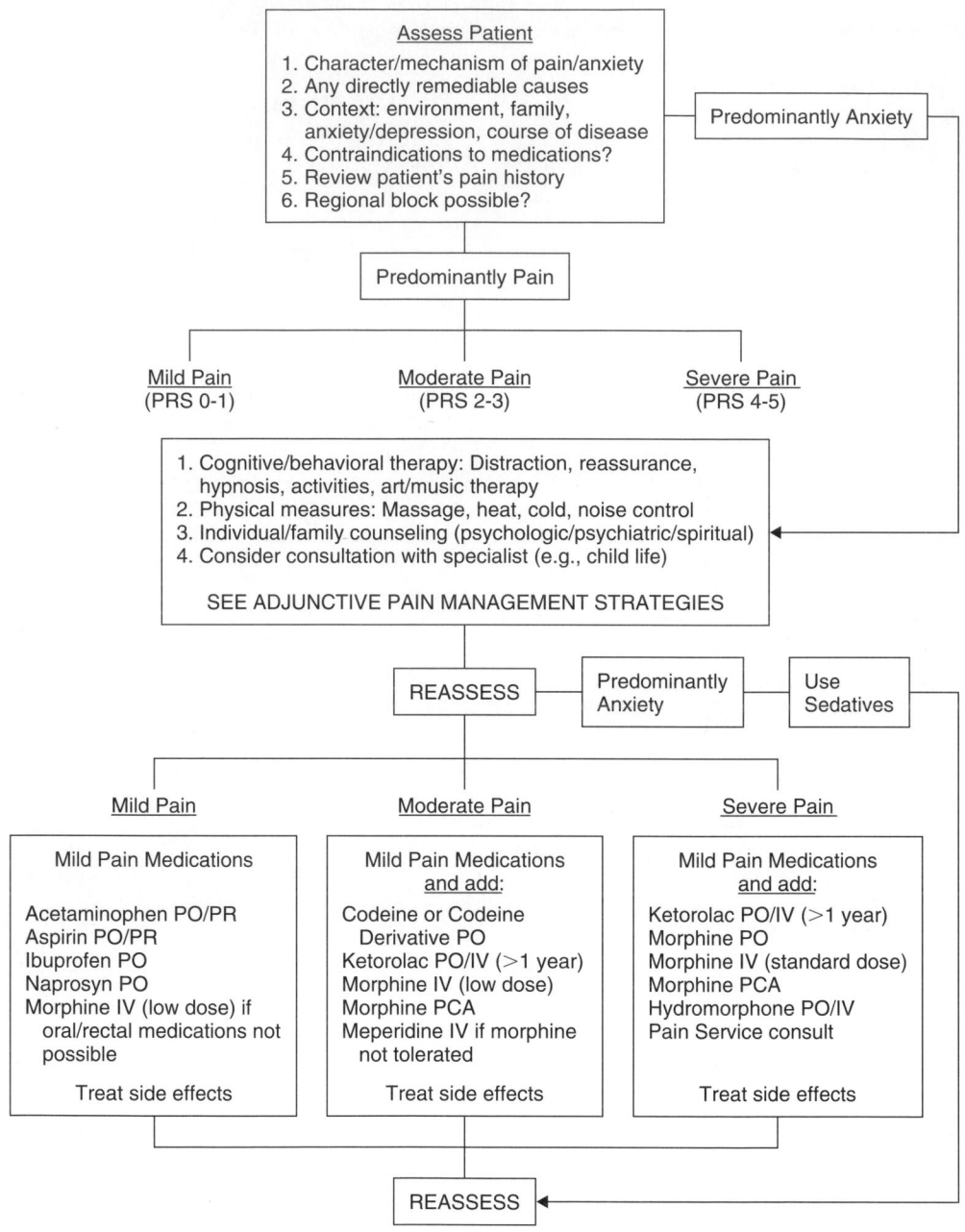

Fig. 7-1 Pediatric pain management algorithm. *PRS*, Pain rating scale.

Box 7-1 Frequently Used Medications Recommended for Pediatric Pain Management

Mild Pain

Acetaminophen

Ibuprofen

Naproxen

Aspirin (when pain is not associated with viral illnesses, influenza, or varicella infections)

Moderate Pain

(These medications may be used in addition to or in combination with those used for mild pain.)

Codeine

Ketorolac

Hydrocodone

Morphine (oral and low-dose)

Oxycodone

Severe Pain

(Practitioner may not initially be able to manage treatment of severe pain in an outpatient setting and may need to refer for invasive devices [e.g., intravenous, subcutaneous, or epidural route; regional anesthesia].)

Fentanyl

Hydromorphone

Morphine

Alert

When prescribing medications containing a combination of Tylenol (acetaminophen) and an opioid (e.g., Vicodin, Percocet), remember that Tylenol amounts cannot exceed 1000 mg per dose and 4000 mg per day.

Pharmacologic Pain Management Strategies

Pharmacologic pain management strategies vary according to the cause of the pain, intensity of the pain, the age and developmental level of the child, and the existence of any comorbidities. Examples of frequently used medications that are recommended for pediatric pain management are described in Box 7-1.

Procedural Pain Management Strategies

Many procedures performed in the pediatric office or clinic setting are both painful and anxiety producing for children. Briefly, some key issues of concern for all practitioners include:

- Before any procedure, both the parent and child must be prepared truthfully about the amount, intensity, and duration of pain expected from the procedure.
- Parents should be encouraged to be present during painful procedures. They should be taught simple distraction and relaxation techniques to use with their child during the procedure.
- Nonpharmacologic pain management strategies should be incorporated for both nonpainful and painful procedures (Table 7-3).

Box 7-2 EMLA

EMLA (eutectic mixture of local anesthetics [lidocaine and prilocaine]) is an approved topical anesthetic for procedure-related pain management in children. Children undergoing the following procedures may benefit from it:

- Venipuncture or phlebotomy
- Arterial puncture
- Accessing of intravenous devices
- Lumbar puncture
- Bone marrow aspiration or biopsy

Some considerations for the cream's use include:

- It should be used with children over 1 month of age. Studies are currently examining its use in newborns, especially for circumcisions.
- For full anesthetic effect, it must remain intact on the skin for at least 1 hour before the procedure. A placebo effect has been observed within minutes of application for some children.
- It can be used only on intact skin.
- It is contraindicated for patients with congenital or idiopathic methemoglobinemia, patients with known sensitivity to local anesthetics, and patients less than 1 year of age who are receiving methemoglobinemia-inducing medications (e.g., sulfonamide, phenytoin, phenobarbital, nitroprusside).

- Analgesics (topical or systemic) should be used for painful procedures in addition to possible use of an anxiolytic (Box 7-2).
- If conscious or deep sedation is necessary to perform the procedure, the guidelines developed by the American Academy of Pediatrics need to be carefully followed.

Table 7-3 Adjunctive Pain Management Strategies

AGE LEVEL	PREPARATION	RELAXATION	FOCUSED ATTENTION	IMAGERY*
Birth–2 years	Prepare parents Review history of strategies that have worked in the past Explain role of parental anxiety to reduce its transmission to the child	Oral stimulation Sucking Rhymes Rocking Massage Holding personal comfort items Singing Talking	Cause-and-effect toys Singing Rattles Music Pop-up toys and books	Not beneficial in this age group
Preschool (2–5 years old)	Review history of strategies that have worked in the past Prepare just before a procedure History of temperament and coping abilities Discuss sensory aspects Use teaching dolls and transitional objects	*This age rarely uses physical relaxation to cope; it may be counterproductive.* Holding Massaging Singing Nursery rhymes Holding personal comfort items Breathing rhythm, with focus on exhalation	Pop-up toys and books Stories Videotapes and games Counting ABCs Manipulatives Blowing Massage Eye fixation	Use of external, concrete stimuli Pop-up books Stuffed animals Puppets Videotapes or audiotapes
School age (6–11 years old)	Prepare as early as 1 day in advance of procedure Use teaching dolls and transitional objects Discuss sensory objects Offer choices of strategies Use medical play Rehearse strategies Discuss parents' roles with child	Preschool methods Eye fixation Progressive relaxation Relatively indirect methods more effective than suggestions to "relax"	Preschool methods Audiotapes and video tapes Humor	"Favorite place" Enjoyable memories "Dimmer switch" Revivify anesthetic experiences (e.g., cold, gloves) Dissociation Use pain scale Peer demonstration
Adolescent (11–18 years old)	Prepare in advance Use body outlines Use correct terminology Give written material Offer choices of strategies Rehearse strategies Discuss parents' role	Talking Music Videotapes Audiotapes Massage Eye fixation Progressive relaxation	School-age methods that are of appropriate sophistication	Elaboration upon school-age techniques Music tapes Books on tape Peer demonstration

Used with permission of Kane, T. & Sugarman, L. (1995). Adjunctive pain management strategies: Summary table *(unpublished document)*. Rochester, NY: University of Rochester Medical Center.
Clinicians require training in clinical hypnosis to employ advanced forms of imagery.

Resources

Publications

Agency for Health Care Policy and Research. (1992). *Acute pain management in infants, children, and adolescents: Operative and medical procedures* (AHCPR Pub. No. 92-0019). Rockville, MD: US Department of Health and Human Services.

Duff, L. (1998). *The recognition and assessment of acute pain in children: Recommendations.* London: Royal College of Nursing Institute.

Kuttner, L. (1996). *A child in pain: How to help, what to do,* Point Roberts, WA: Hartley & Murks.

McGrath, P., Finley, G.A., & Ritchie, J. (1994). *Pain, pain, go away: Helping children with pain,* Rockville, MD: Association for the Care of Children's Health.

Websites

American Academy of Pain Medicine (www.painmed.org)

American Association of Pain Management (www.aapainmanage.org)

American Board of Pain Managers (www.abpm.org)

American Chronic Pain Association (www.theacpa.org)

Pediatric Pain Discussion List (to subscribe, send message to mailserv@a.dal.ca; in the message, type the following: subscribe. pediatric-pain [your first name] [your last name]; send list mail to pediatric-pain@ac.dal.ca)

Pediatric Pain Professional Resources (www.pedspain.nursing.uiowa.edu)

Bibliography

American Academy of Pediatrics. (1992). Guidelines for monitoring and management of pediatric patients during and after sedation for diagnostic and therapeutic procedures. *Pediatrics, 59,* 1110-1115.

Beyer, J.E. (1988). *The Oucher: A user's manual and technical report.* Denver: University of Colorado.

Beyer, J.E., Denyes, M.J., & Villarruel, A.M. (1992). The creation, validation, and continuing development of the Oucher: A measure of pain intensity in children. *Journal of Pediatric Nursing, 7*(5), 335-346.

Boughton, K., Blower, C., Chartrand, C., Dircks, P., Stone, T., Youwe, G., & Hagen, B. (1998). Impact of research on pediatric pain assessment and outcomes. *Pediatric Nursing, 24*(1), 31-35.

Cote, C.J., Karl, H.W., Notterman, D.A., Weinberg, J.A., & McCloskey, C. (2000). Adverse sedation events in pediatrics: Analysis of medications used for sedation. *Pediatrics, 106*(4), 633-644.

Eland, J.M. (1985). The child who is hurting. *Seminars in Oncology Nursing, 1*(2), 116-122.

Feldon-Sinkin, L., Tesler, M., & Savedra, M. (1997). Word placement on the word-graphic rating scale by pediatric patients. *Pediatric Nursing, 23*(1), 31-34.

Franck, L.S. (1997). The ethical imperative to treat pain in infants: Are we doing the best we can? *Critical Care Nurse, 17*(5), 80-87.

Furdon, S.A., Pfeil, V.C., & Snow, K. (1998). Operationalizing Donna Wong's principle of atraumatic care: Pain management protocol in the NICU. *Pediatric Nursing, 24*(4), 336-342.

Golianu, B., Krane, E.J., Galloway, K.S., & Yaster, M. (2000). Pediatric acute pain management. *Pediatric Clinics of North America, 47*(3), 559-587.

Hester, N.K.O. (1979). The preoperational child's reaction to immunization. *Nursing Research, 28*(4), 250-255.

Joint Commission on Accreditation of Healthcare Organizations. (2000). *Pain assessment and management: An organizational approach.* Illinois: Joint Commission on Accreditation of Healthcare Organizations.

Kane, T., & Sugarman, L. (1995). *Adjunctive pain management strategies: Summary table* (unpublished document). Rochester, NY: University of Rochester Medical Center.

Krechel, S.W. & Bildner, J. (1995). CRIES: A new neonatal postoperative pain measurement score: Initial testing of validity and reliability. *Pediatric Anaesthesia, 5,* 53-61.

LaFleur, C.J. & Raway, B. (1999). School-age child and adolescent perception of the pain intensity associated with three word descriptors. *Pediatric Nursing, 25*(1), 45-55.

Lawrence, J., et al. (1993). The development of a tool to assess neonatal pain. *Neonatal Network, 12*(16), 59-65.

Litman, R.S. (1995). Recent trends in the management of pain during medical procedures in children. *Pediatric Annals, 24*(3), 158-163.

McCaffery, M. & Pasero, C. (1999). *Pain: Clinical manual.* St. Louis: Mosby, Inc.

McGrath, P.J., Rosmus, C., Camfield, C., Campbell, M.A., & Hennigar, A.W. (1998). Behaviours caregivers use to determine pain in non-verbal, cognitively impaired individuals. *Developmental Medicine and Child Neurology, 40,* 340-343.

McGrath, P., et al. (1985). CHEOPS: A behavioral scale for rating postoperative pain in children. In Fields, H.L., Kubner, R., & Cervero, F. (Eds.). *Advances in pain research and therapy* (vol. 9) (proceedings of the Fourth World Congress on Pain). New York: Raven.

McRae, M.E., Rourke, D.A., Imperial-Perez, F.A., Eisenring, C.M., & Ueda, J.N. (1997). Development of a research-based standard for assessment, intervention, and evaluation of pain after neonatal and pediatric cardiac surgery. *Pediatric Nursing, 23*(3), 263-271.

Merskey, H. & Bogduk, N. (Eds.). (1994). *Classification of chronic pain: Descriptions of chronic pain syndromes and definition of pain terms* (2nd ed.). Seattle: International Association for the Study of Pain Press.

Merkel, S.I., Voepel-Lewis, T., Shayevitz, J.R., & Malviya, S. (1997). The FLACC: A behavioral scale for scoring postoperative pain in young children. *Pediatric Nursing, 23*(3), 293-297.

Schechter, N.L., Berde, C.B., & Yaster, M. (1993). Pain in infants, children, and adolescents: An overview. In Schechter, N. L., Berde, C. B., & Yaster, M. (Eds.). *Pain in infants, children, and adolescents.* Baltimore: Williams & Wilkins.

Shapiro, B.S. (1995). Treatment of chronic pain in children and adolescents. *Pediatric Annals, 24*(3), 148-156.

Storey, P. (1995, June). *Pain management and hospice care* (presented paper). Rochester, NY: University of Rochester Pain Conference.

Sugarman, L.I. (2001). Self-regulation therapies: Hypnosis and biofeedback. In Hoekelman, R.A. (Ed.). *Primary pediatric care* (4th ed.). St Louis: Mosby.

Tobias, J.D. (2000). Weak analgesics and nonsteroidal anti-inflammatory agents in the management of children with acute pain. *Pediatric Clinics of North America, 47*(3), 527-543.

van der Jagt, E. (1995). *Pediatric pain management algorithm* (unpublished document). Rochester, NY: University of Rochester Medical Center.

Whaley, L. & Wong, D.L. (1995). *Nursing care of infants and children.* St. Louis: Mosby.

Wong, D.L. & Baker, C.M. (1988). Pain in children: Comparison of assessment scales. *Pediatric Nursing, 14*(1), 9-17.

Yaster, M., Kost-Byerly, S., Khandwala, R.S., & Maxwell, L.G. (2001). Management of acute pain in children. In Hoekelman, R.A. (Ed.). *Primary pediatric care* (4th ed.). St Louis: Mosby.

Zempsky, W.T. & Schechter, N.L. (2000). Office-based pain management. The 15-minute consultation. *Pediatric Clinics of North America, 47*(3), 601-615.

Chapter 8 *Prenatal Interview*

Jane A. Fox

The American Academy of Pediatrics (AAP) encourages making prenatal interviews part of pediatric practice and recommends more involvement with anticipatory guidance during the prenatal period. This interview offers the practitioner a unique opportunity to obtain important baseline information, identify risk factors (Box 8-1) or potential problems, and initiate anticipatory guidance. It should be scheduled no later than the seventh or eighth month of pregnancy, the ideal time being 4 to 8 weeks before birth. Both parents should be invited to participate at a convenient time for all and when the practice may be quiet (e.g., late morning, early afternoon). About 30 minutes should be scheduled for the visit, and two comfortable adult chairs should be provided so that eye-to-eye contact is possible. The parents should complete a history form, and it should be reviewed with them. The visit also provides the expectant parents an opportunity to meet the practitioner before their infant's birth, if they are not already acquainted. Expectant parents have many questions, and this visit provides an opportunity to have questions addressed and answered. Another option is to offer group prenatal visits. These sessions offer an opportunity to answer questions, to review the philosophy of the practice, and to provide information. If a group format is initiated, individual private time should be available with each couple to address their particular concerns and begin to establish an individual relationship.

Box 8-1 Perinatal Medical Risk Factors

History of previous pregnancy loss or infertility
Previous preterm delivery or threatened preterm delivery
Pregnancy complications (e.g., infections, bleeding, trauma, high blood pressure)
Occupational exposures and risks
Drug exposure (prescribed and illicit)
Smoking
Alcohol use
Unusual or highly restricted diet; malabsorption syndrome
Thyroid disease; diabetes mellitus
Hepatitis B or HIV (disease or carrier status or unknown status)
Poor weight gain
Inherited disease (e.g., hemoglobinopathies, neurologic disorders)
Prenatal identification of concerns (e.g., low alpha-fetoprotein)
Prenatal ultrasound abnormalities, including abnormal growth
Family history or perinatal or early neonatal illness or death
Previous birth interval less than 18 months
Multiple fetuses (e.g., twins, triplets)
Maternal age less than 15 or older than 35 years
Maternal chronic illness (e.g., renal disease, cardiac disease, colitis)
Breast abnormalities, past surgeries, or past difficulties with breastfeeding

From Dixon, S.D. & Stein, M.T. (2000). Encounters with children: Pediatric behavior and development. *St. Louis: Mosby.*

Subjective Data

Ideally both expectant parents should be included in the interview (Table 8-1). Information to obtain includes:

- General health of the parents
- Whether the father of the baby is involved
- Parental ages
- History of the current pregnancy
  - Planned or unplanned?
  - When did the mother first receive prenatal care? How many prenatal visits did she attend?
  - How do the parents feel about this pregnancy? This child? Their future expectations?
  - Any prenatal nutrition (e.g., vitamin supplements, prenatal iron supplements)?
  - Any medications taken during the pregnancy?
  - Any substance abuse during the pregnancy (e.g., of alcohol, cigarettes, illegal drugs)?
  - Any problems during the pregnancy (e.g., infections, high blood pressure, diabetes, other illnesses)?
  - Have the parents taken childbirth classes? Do they plan to?
  - Have the parents cared for an infant before? What was that like?
  - Any episodes of physical violence, abuse, or threats? (This should be asked only if the mother is alone.)
- Other children
  - Ages and sexes
  - Pregnancy, birth, and neonatal period details for each
  - Health problems and problems in infancy
  - Developmental progress
  - Difficulties the parents had adjusting to the child
  - Children's reaction to the pregnancy
  - Preparation of other children for the birth
  - Arrangements made for the older child or children when new baby is born
  - Parental anticipation of the response of sibling or siblings to the new baby
- Plans to feed the baby and preparation for nursing (if applicable)
- Circumcision (if child is a boy)
- Family health history, both maternal and paternal (include all chronic and genetic diseases)
- Environmental and social history
  - Length of time the family has lived in the area
  - Location of the extended family live
  - Available help for after the baby arrives
  - Living conditions for the apartment or house
  - Walk-up or elevator
  - Number of rooms
  - Condition (e.g., peeling paint, window guards, mice, bugs, smoke detectors, covered electric sockets)
  - Heat; hot water
  - Neighborhood
  - Guns, matches, and tools present in the house and where kept

- Smokers in the home; pets in the home; persons living in the home with the child (e.g., mother, father, siblings, grandparents, other relatives, nonrelatives)? Who is the head of the household?
- Primary caregiver during the day
- Educational level of the parents

- Sources and amount of income, type of employment, and hours of work
- Medical insurance
- Does the mother plan to work outside of the home after the birth of the child? If so, when does she plan to return to work? Attend school? Plans made for infant's care?

Table 8-1 Questions to be Asked in Prenatal Visit

QUESTION	OBJECTIVE
How are you feeling?	Lay the territory to include parents' well-being; assess response to the situation overall.
Ask how the pregnancy has gone; expand to cover medical events, life stresses, and so on, as noted on the medical history form and your own individual outline (i.e., a pregnancy history from a pediatric standpoint)	Gather data for objective risk factors and the parents' perception of them; assess general response to the pregnancy and the perception of the pregnancy as high risk (whether it is by medical criteria or not).
Turn to the father and ask how the pregnancy has gone for him.	Assess the father's perceptions and concerns about his wife and baby and his own adjustment to the pregnancy.
Was this a planned pregnancy?	Assess the place of the child in the relationship, parents' adjustment to pregnancy, and degree and nature of adjustment for child's health.
Do you have other children at home? What are their ages and sexes? Have you cared for an infant before? What was that experience like?	Assess the family structure; note the child's place in it; assess experience and expectations for infant care; note locus of control (i.e., do parents see themselves in control of this event?); assess preparedness and give general information on the subject; open opportunity to give information or your own preferences about the delivery event, which may tap in on particular anxieties or fears in the third trimester; assess unrealistic or rigid expectations; when appropriate, assert that you think that the parents are in charge.
How do you plan to feed the baby? (Expand to include a diet history during pregnancy, preparation for nursing.)	Assess realistic planning for the baby and advise; reaffirm parents' control of this option; emphasize the importance of nurture in general; offer the opportunity for parents to say how they feel about the situation; assess maternal nutrition vis-à-vis the infant; assess specific breastfeeding preparations; do not push a decision if the family is not ready.
If the infant is a boy, will you have him circumcised? (Address this question to the father).	Assess individuation of the baby; bring the father into the decision-making process; open this topic for a two-way discussion, providing objective information on circumcision (i.e., the lack of clear medical indications) and the procedure itself.
Have you purchased a carseat?	Show interest in safety and caretaking; assess the parents' anticipation of the needs of the infant.
How long have you lived in this area? Where do most of your family live? Who will be available to help you after the baby comes?	Assess family support systems; assess the realignment of old relationships; tap in on parents' relationship to their own feelings.
Do you have other responsibilities outside the family?	Assess the mother's other areas of responsibility and stress; assess what realignment of these areas is anticipated; discuss areas of ambivalence and concern.
Are both of you working outside your home? What are your job plans? Do you have any ideas about the time you will return to work? Are you attending school? Have you made plans for the infant's care?	Assess the psychosocial situation of the family; assess parents' perceptions of their roles in career or education and as parents; assess realistic planning for infant care.
Do you have any worries about your infant? Most parents do have some concerns about the child. Would you like to share any of those with me? Is there anything in your past history that makes you think you have some special worries about your child?	Open discussion of concerns directly; but also use this setting to discuss normalcy of feelings and perhaps deeper concerns; provide information about common fears, fantasies, and dreams during a normal pregnancy.
How are your other children reacting to your pregnancy? What things have you done to prepare them for the birth? Most parents have some worries about how they'll manage to have enough time and love for more than one child. Do you share any of these concerns? What are the specific arrangements you've made for the older child at the time of the baby's birth?	Assess the realignment of family relationships; assess the plans for readjustment around the care of the infant; assess maternal and paternal feelings toward the attachment to their children who have already been born.
Do you have any questions?	Set a model for pediatric visits (i.e., you are open to questions and waiting for parents to take the lead).

From Dixon, S.D. & Stein, M.T. (2000). Encounters with children: pediatric behavior and development. St. Louis: Mosby.

Box 8-2 Prenatal Risk Factors for Attachment

Recent death of a loved one
Previous loss of or serious illness in another child
Previous removal of a child
History of depression or serious mental illness
History or infertility or pregnancy loss
Troubled relationship with parents (i.e., the grandparents)
Financial stress; job loss
Marital discord or poor relationship with the other parent
Recent move or no community ties
No friends or social network
Unwanted pregnancy
No good parenting model
Experience of poor parenting
Drug and/or alcohol abuse
Extreme immaturity

From Dixon, S.D. & Stein, M.T. (2000). Encounters with children: Pediatric behavior and development. St. Louis: Mosby.

- Do the parents have any specific worries about the infant?
- How do the parents think the baby will change their lives?
- How were things for the parents growing up? Do they plan to parent the same? What changes will they make?
- Any questions from the parents?

Identification of Attachment Risk Factors

- Identify risk factors that may place a family at risk for attachment problems (Box 8-2).
- Assess the readiness to parent (see Chapter 3).

Management

Provision of Anticipatory Guidance

- Discuss with parents how to set priorities for what is most important to do in the prenatal period.
- Discuss plans made for the arrival of the new infant.
  - Feeding method should be selected. Encourage breastfeeding (see Chapter 15).
  - Discuss circumcision (see Chapter 19).
  - Review questions that the family has about pregnancy, labor and delivery, and childrearing.
  - Identify a supportive person to help the mother after the birth (e.g., father of infant, relative, friend, hired assistant).
  - Explain the delivery room and nursery procedures for all types of deliveries and the rationale for the procedures.
  - Plan sleeping arrangements for the infant.
  - Review how to purchase a car seat.
  - Discuss the equipment needed at home for the infant (Box 8-3).
  - Keep in mind that parents may need to complete or enroll for classes on infant care.
- If parents or other household members smoke, encourage cessation.
- Discuss methods and plans for childrearing and discipline.
- Advise parents to anticipate a sibling response (see Chapter 19).

Box 8-3 Newborn Equipment and Supplies

The following is a list of possible equipment and supplies parents may need for their newborn. This list should be individualized based on the needs and financial resources of the family.
Crib: Slats no more than $2\frac{3}{8}$ inches apart
    No cutouts in the headboard or footboard
    (See Chapter 14)
Crib mattress: Firm and covered with material that can be easily cleaned
Crib bumpers: Remove when the child can stand
Bedding for the crib: Flannel-backed, waterproof mattress cover, two fitted sheets, and a quilt or soft full-size blanket; no pillow
Changing table: Place on a carpet and against a wall
    Put shelves for diapers, pins (for cloth diapers), and other changing equipment within immediate reach
Diaper pail with deodorizer: If cloth diapers are to be used
Large plastic washtub: For bathing the baby
Thermometer
Car seat: Required by law (see Chapter 14)
Clothes: Buy big (at least "size 3 months"); flame-resistant; easy-open crotch for diaper changes

3-4 pajama sets, with feet	4-6 receiving blankets
6-8 T-shirts	1 set of baby washcloths
3 newborn sacques	and towels
2 sweaters	3-4 dozen newborn-size
1 sleeping bag or bunting	diapers (diaper pins and
2 bonnets	elastic pants if using cloth)
4 pairs of socks or booties	

Intercom: Especially if the child sleeps in another room
Accessories for feeding (e.g., breast pump, nursing bottles, nipples, pacifiers, bibs)

- Advise parents about what to expect of the new infant.
  - Discuss behavior (e.g., crying, sleeping, noises, grimaces, feeding, individuality, Temperament).
  - Discuss physical appearance and changes throughout the first 2 weeks.
- Counsel the mother about postpartum depression. Depression and feelings of vulnerability after the birth of a baby are not uncommon. The mother may lose interest in her surroundings, cry frequently, and feel withdrawn. These feelings usually pass but encourage the mother to talk about her feelings if concerned.
- Discuss the role of the father. Support active involvement with the infant in holding, diapering, and feeding. Help the parents negotiate a plan for sharing care of the infant, if desired. Encourage the father to assist the mother with household tasks.
- Introduce the parents to other health team members of the practice (if possible) and give information about the practice.
  - Inform the parents how soon after the birth their baby will be seen.
  - Discuss when the baby's examinations should be scheduled.

- Inform the parents about the practice's telephone hours in regard to answering questions.
- Share with the parents information on which hospital the practice is affiliated with and how coverage works.
- Discuss with the parents what they should do in case of an emergency.
- Review the fee schedule.
- Review what to bring to an office visit (e.g., immunization card, insurance card, diapers, formula).
- Discuss immunization schedules.
- Refer to Chapter 3 for additional information.

Follow-Up

Request referral from the nursery or have the parent or parents call after the child is born. Determine if problems exist. Schedule the first well-child visit at 2 weeks of age. (In some practices the first visit may be at 1 month of age.)

Consultations and Referrals

For social problems, refer to a social worker, Visiting Nurse Service (VNS), or public health nurse.

Refer parents for prepared childbirth, breastfeeding, or parenting classes, if indicated:

- *Breastfeeding*—Refer to a lactation specialist or the La Leche League.
- *Bottle-feeding*—Refer to infant care programs for free formula, if such programs are available and if the need exists.

Resources

Publications
For Parents
(See also Chapter 3)
Brazelton, T.B. (1992). *Touchpoints.* Redding, MA: Addison-Wesley.
Eisenberg, A., Murkoff, H.E., & Hathaway, S.E. (1991). *What to expect when you're expecting.* New York: Workman.
Profet, M. (1995). *Protecting your baby-to-be.* Redding, MA: Addison-Wesley.
Shelov, S.P. & Hannerman, R.E. (2001). *Caring for your baby and young child: Birth to age 5* (2nd ed.). New York: Bantam.
For Professionals
American Academy of Pediatrics, Committee on Psychosocial Aspects of Child and Family Health. (1996). The prenatal visit. *Pediatrics, 97,* 141.
Dixon, S. & Stein, M. (2000). *Encounters with children* (3rd ed.). St Louis: Mosby.
Green, M. (2001). *Bright futures: Guidelines for health supervision of infants, children, and adolescents* (2nd ed.). Arlington, VA: National Center for Education in Maternal and Child Health.

Websites
For Parents
American Baby (www.americanbaby.com)
Baby Center (www.babycenter.com)
Baby Zone (www.babyzone.com)
National Parent Information Network (www.npin.org)
Top Parenting Sites (www.100topparentingsites.com)
For Professionals
Bright Futures (www.brightfutures.com)

Chapter 9 *Health History and Physical Examination*

Marie Scott Brown & Judith Bellaire Igoe

This chapter delineates the information to be obtained during the course of a health history and a physical examination. The practitioner, in performing these functions, is identified as: (1) a decision-maker with regard to the health status of children and youth, (2) a health educator, and (3) an inquirer into the health practices and beliefs of consumers. The health evaluation as conducted by a practitioner can be a meaningful experience. The overall health status of a child is clarified, active participation is encouraged, and disease prevention and health promotion plans are derived from the preferred health practices and beliefs of the child and family involved.

A special set of guidelines for history-taking and physical examination are found in Tables 9-1 and 9-2. This information is designed to assist the examiner with health evaluations by providing direction in three areas:

1. Outlining the component parts of the history and physical (i.e., "what to ask," "what to examine").
2. Presenting practical advice with respect to the actual conduct of the evaluation to enhance the quality of the practitioner's clinical performance (i.e., "practical hints").
3. Offering various ideas for health education and counseling to accompany the evaluation of different body parts.

Table 9-1 Guidelines for History-Taking

WHAT TO ASK ABOUT	PRACTICAL HINTS	EDUCATION AND COUNSELING
Introduction	It's important to take enough time during the introduction to make sure the parent and child or adolescent are comfortable with you. Be sure to introduce yourself to all members of the family who are present.	Introduce the family to what you will be doing, including the purpose of your history and physical examination. You may want to alert them to the fact you will be using it as an opportunity for teaching. Then find out the nature of the complaint and what they expect from the encounter. Occasionally expectations are unrealistic (e.g., recovery from a strain or sprain in time for a sporting event) and clarification is necessary. The result you are seeking is a mutual problem-solving relationship so that people will follow through with treatment plans.
Chief Complaint—What to Include	The chief complaint is not necessarily a complaint. It may just be recorded as "here for well-child visit." Nevertheless it is important to find out what parents expect will be the outcome of the evaluation. You may need to point out that certain immunizations and laboratory tests are due. In addition, you may need to point out that the numbers of topics and questions they wish to cover are beyond the time limit of one visit and prioritize what must be addressed during this visit.	Find out how knowledgeable the informants are regarding the chief complaint.
Past History **Birth** ***Prenatal*** Chronologic order of this pregnancy; any other births, stillbirths, therapeutic abortions, or spontaneous abortions; length of gestation; known family history of genetic defects; prenatal care, including when and where; health of mother during pregnancy: bleeding, high blood pressure, illness, cigarettes, alcohol or drugs taken during pregnancy, infection, vomiting, fever, rashes, medications, accidents, hospitalizations, diet, weight gain; blood type, hepatitis B, group B streptococci, HIV/AIDS (father also)	A common notation in this part of the history is the use of *G* for gravida (the number of times a woman has been pregnant), and *P* for para (the number of pregnancies that terminated in the birth of one or more viable fetuses). In this notation system the first digit after the *P* indicates the number of babies born at term (after 36 weeks), the second indicates the number of premature infants (between 28 and 36 weeks), the third indicates the number of pregnancies ending in either spontaneous or therapeutic abortions (before 28 weeks), the fourth indicates the number of children now alive, and the fifth indicates the number of pregnancies resulting in multiple birth. For instance, a G6P24241 is a woman who delivered one live-term birth, one full-term stillbirth, one premature live birth, and premature triplets of whom two lived and one died; she also had two abortions.	Explanation for the relationship between such prenatal events as nutrition, drug ingestion, and exposure to infectious diseases and x-rays can be important to the parents in terms of preventive care for future pregnancies and often alleviation of guilt for things the parents did or did not do during this child's gestation that may be unrelated to the current problem. Of prime importance is a discussion of rubella and hepatitis, stressing the need for rubella and hepatitis immunizations between pregnancies for unprotected women. When the conversation involves school-age children and adolescents, the prenatal portion of the history often catches their attention. Take advantage of their curiosity to explain the relationship of their present health and prenatal beginnings. For adolescent girls, they may soon be making decisions regarding their own pregnancies.

Continued

Table 9-1 Guidelines for History-Taking—cont'd

WHAT TO ASK ABOUT	PRACTICAL HINTS	EDUCATION AND COUNSELING
Birth—cont'd **Natal** Length of labor and difficulty, breech or cephalic, Apgar score, analgesia, anesthesia, hospital, birth weight, birth injuries, conditon of baby (e.g., cry, color, incubator, oxygen)	Except in the case of a very young infant, this information may be difficult for parents to remember. A form mailed out beforehand may help parents sort through memories before coming to the office. For an adolescent, this affords an opportunity to obtain the information from the parents, often an ideal situation for sex education.	Explanation of the relation of length and type of labor, drugs, and anesthesia may be helpful preventive counseling for the next pregnancy; again, this section of the history offers anticipatory guidance opportunities if the examiner is dealing with adolescents.
Postnatal Any problems in the nursery, whether baby went home with mother, twitching, cry, jaundice, cyanosis, feeding problems, rashes, weight gain, excessive mucus, paralysis, convulsions, hemorrhage, fever, congenital anomalies, difficulty in sucking	In some situations, a request for medical records from the hospital may be necessary. Be sure to phrase questions in terms of signs and symptoms that parents will remember rather than a medical diagnosis that a physician or nurse would remember (e.g., "Was your child's skin yellow?" rather than "Was your baby jaundiced?").	This information may provide an opportunity to clear up misconceptions about early infancy care for future children or to allay guilty feelings about early care. It is also highly relevant to adolescents.
Allergies Specific allergies, reactions, and timing (food, medications, insects, animals, seasons); history of rashes		Education regarding avoidance of specific allergens and care for allergic reactions (e.g., "home remedies" such as cornstarch baths for itching versus recognizing serious reactions that require immediate or eventual medical treatment or emergency intervention) may be indicated. In highly allergic children, counseling regarding how to keep life as "normal" as possible may be necessary. Teaching the child directly about developing an awareness of the body and its reactions to certain allergies and related self-care measures is important for older children. Counseling regarding the need for specialized care may be indicated.
Accidents When, where, what happened; treatment, both immediate and long-term; follow-up; child's reaction; residual affects	Particularly with very traumatic accidents, there is usually a period of amnesia for the accident itself and often for subsequent events. This amnesia could be permanent or temporary. It is more common for the child, but may involve the parents also. Be alert to "accident-prone" children; this may be a symptom of psychologic problems within the child or family. Be alert to the possibility of child abuse when there are inadequate explanations for many accidents.	Preventive safety education (e.g., about car seats and seat belts, locked medicine cabinets, ipecac, burn prevention, swimming classes, sports, firearm safety, bicycle helmets) may be indicated. Education needs to be developmentally appropriate for children and youths. The Bibliography included with this chapter will assist you in developing your own collection of teaching aids. Discussion of behavior or problems to be expected after major traumas and developmentally appropriate ways of "working through" these residual effects (e.g., "talking it out" for the adolescent; "playing it out" through puppet, dramatic, or artistic play for the preschooler) are important.

Illnesses

Childhood diseases (e.g., measles, rubella, roseola, mumps, chickenpox, whooping cough, RSV, undiagnosed rashes, fever); numerous ear infections; any other illnesses or infections; adolescent illnesses (e.g., mononucleosis, sexually transmitted diseases [STDs]); when, where, severity, treatment, follow-up, response to follow-up

For a child over 10 years of age, the memory of both parents and child may be vague. Again, results may be better if the parents or the child has been alerted beforehand that these questions will be asked. Ask in terms of signs and symptoms as well as diagnosis. Explain why it is important to remember if there were any reactions (this usually improves recall). For adolescents, a written history form filled out beforehand may help handle embarrassment about sensitive areas such as STDs. Confidentiality must be specifically addressed.

Recognition of the importance of home care for various "childhood diseases" may be appropriate, as may be counseling on fever control, pruritis control, control of infection in the home by isolation, and handwashing. Counseling parents concerning immunization may be appropriate. Suggestions of particularly good self-care books are also worthwhile, though it is important to evaluate the style and content of each book to be sure it is compatible with the child's level of understanding. Certain early problems may alert to possible current difficulties (e.g., the relationship between numerous early ear infections and current speech and hearing problems).

Operations

What happened, when, where, why, outcome, child's reactions, temporary or permanent residual effects, including cosmetic effects

It may be necessary to get a consent for release of information to be sent to the operating hospital. Fears or phobias, particularly fear of the dark and castration anxieties, are common in preschoolers. Their problems and fears usually relate to body image and health care.

Discussion of any residual effects of a specific type of surgery is important. For the young child, parental education concerning the normal childhood response to parental separation and surgery as well as appropriate methods of helping the child work through these reactions is essential. (Reliving it through "play-acting" allows a chance for catharsis and a chance for parents to clear up childhood misinterpretations.) Children very often feel operations or hospitalizations are punishments because they are "bad."

Hospitalizations

What happened, when, why, where, follow-up, child's reaction; temporary, permanent physical, or psychologic residual effects, including cosmetic effects

It may be necessary to get a consent for release to be sent to the hospital to receive details of the problem. Fears or phobias, particularly fear of the dark and castration anxieties, are common in preschoolers. Younger children's problems and fears may relate more specifically to body image and health care. Fears of separation from parents may also remain.

Education may be indicated related to the reason for hospitalization. With a young child, the normal reaction to hospitalization and ways to handle this are important (e.g., reliving it through play-acting). Numerous programs for familiarizing children with the hospital environment before hospitalization are now available and should be utilized (see Chapter 49).

Immunization and Tests

Immunization status; type and timing of tests; location of injection and reactions; tuberculosis (TB) test, x-ray examinations, laboratory tests; other screening tests for vision, speech, hearing, and development; lead screening and results

Most clinics and offices now provide parents with a copy of the immunization record, which simplifies changes from one health facility to another. Some states have immunizations recorded on a statewide computer network. Other screening tests, however, are usually not included.

Parents should be taught to hold the child during or immediately following an immunization, because this has been shown to significantly reduce the stress of the situation. Explanations of the need for immunizations and watching for and handling untoward effects (e.g., recognition and control of fever) are important. School-age children and adolescents are in many instances mature enough to carry their own immunization record and should be encouraged to do so and to be aware when boosters are needed.

Dental Care

See Chapter 16 for recommended ages for visits to the dentist

See Chapter 16 for suggestions on how to prepare children for dental visits.

Continued

Table 9-1 Guidelines for History-Taking—cont'd

WHAT TO ASK ABOUT	PRACTICAL HINTS	EDUCATION AND COUNSELING
Family History *Family members* Mother's age and state of health, father's age and health, siblings, other family members ("Who is at home with you?")	This information may be recorded in graphic form on a "family tree." In many cultural groups, the extended family or even good friends can be as important as or more important than the nuclear family. Be sure to inquire about non-nuclear relatives living in or coming often to the house. Remember the possibility of communes or other living arrangements.	This may be an opportunity to discuss safety issues for which family members provide child care.
Family health history Any of the following conditions: Eyes, ear, nose, and throat (EENT): Nosebleeds, sinus problems, glaucoma, cataracts, myopia, strabismus, other problems related to EENT Cardiorespiratory: TB, asthma, hay fever, hypertension, heart murmurs, heart attacks, strokes, anemia, rheumatic fever, leukemia, pneumonia, emphysema, high cholesterol levels ("Has anyone in the family died suddenly from heart disease before the age of 50?"), other problems Gastrointestinal: Ulcers, colitis, vomiting, diarrhea, other problems Genitourinary: Kidney infections, bladder problems, congenital abnormalities, bedwetting Musculoskeletal: Congenital hip or foot problems, muscular dystrophy, arthritis, other problems Neurologic: Convulsions, seizures, epilepsy, nervous disorders, mental retardation, mental problems, comas, other problems Chronic disease: Diabetes, jaundice, cancer, tumors, thyroid problems, congenital disorders Special senses: "Is anyone deaf or blind?" Miscellaneous: "Any other medical problems not mentioned?"	It may be useful to take this in a *review of systems* format so that all diseases are covered systematically. The primary purpose is to discover genetic diseases that may have an effect on the child at a particular time (e.g., juvenile onset of diabetes in the case of an adolescent). To elicit complete information it is often helpful to begin with a general question (e.g., "Are there any neurologic problems in the family?") and follow with specific ones (e.g., "like epilepsy or headaches?"). Common synonyms as medical terms should be included (e.g., "Does anyone have convulsions? Fits? Seizures?" "Does anyone have hypertension? High blood pressure?"). In addition to revealing potential diseases related to family genetics, these questions may also elicit factors of psychosocial concern (e.g., if a family member is very ill or handicapped, the child is likely to be affected in some way; the child may worry or be frightened or feel guilty; normal childhood experiences may be more limited than usual). If a form or checklist is filled out beforehand by the child or caregiver, it must be discussed in detail during the visit; written forms related to family history are frequently misunderstood. Always explain to the informant that these questions (like all other questions in the history) are standard and not unique to this informant's particular circumstances. All too often parents and children worry that a certain condition is suspected because the examiner says, "Does anyone have diabetes?" Frequently children with learning disabilities or attention deficit disorders have a relative with a similar problem. Nocturnal enuresis commonly occurs in a number of family members rather than just in the designated patient.	The genetic potential for all the diseases found in the family history needs to be discussed. In those where early detection can provide remediation (e.g., myopia) appropriate screening or diagnostic studies should be encouraged. Genetic counseling may be appropriate if future pregnancies are being considered or for adolescents anticipating their future as parents (see Chapter 5). Discussion of how serious illness or handicaps in important family members can affect children, and how to handle these (e.g., direct discussions with the older child, perhaps with the help of primary caregiver; doll play, play-acting, or drawing to elicit the younger child's feelings and interpretations) is important, particularly when there is serious mental illness in the family. Certain children's books may be suggested for older children. Mental health prevention measures for a child may be appropriate. Counseling regarding how to ensure adequate childhood experiences is appropriate if the child's caregivers have major health problems. Children 10 years of age or older should know their own family history as one means of assuming personal responsibility for their own health. Efforts should be made to facilitate this type of learning.

Social history

Residence: Apartment or house size, yard, stairs, proximity to transportation and shopping, safe neighborhood, city water. For adolescents, are they living with their parents or separately? Is homelessness an issue?

Financial situation: Who works, where, occupation, income, welfare, food stamps, spending habits, debts, major expenditures, health insurance

Outside help: Babysitters, daycare center, preschool, teen center

Family interrelationships: Happy, cooperative, antagonistic, chaotic, multiproblematic, violent

School: Chronology of school experiences (including number of schools attended) beginning with pre-school and child or adolescent response to learning. What were strengths and weaknesses developmentally? Any need for special services at school? History of absenteeism, discipline problems, bullying or victimization frequent use of the health room, and long periods of time expended for transportation to and from school. For adolescents, is school providing them with preparation for college or the work force? If pregnant or an adolescent parent, are educational needs being met?

Review of Systems (for the Child)

EENT

Eyes ever cross? Unilateral tearing? Foreign object in eye? Redness? Burning? Earaches, ear infections, colds, strep throats, nosebleeds, postnasal drip, sneezing, sore throat, stuffy nose, snoring, adenitis, or mouth breathing?

Teeth

Age of eruption of deciduous and permanent; number at 1 year; comparision with siblings

Cardiorespiratory

Heart murmurs, blue baby, asthma, pneumonia, frequent upper respiratory tract infections, cystic fibrosis, congenital heart defect, rheumatic fever, trouble breathing, turning blue, tiring easily, cough (when, where, what position, wet or dry)

Gastrointestinal

Diarrhea, constipation, vomiting, abdominal pain, bloody stools, bleeding from rectum, fissures, ulcer, pyloric stenosis, jaundice

Genitourinary

Urinary system: period of dryness (urine); color, odor, and frequency; pain, bleeding; menstruation: how often, regularity, problems (pain, increased flow, etc.); age at first menses, urinary tract infection (UTI), enuresis, dysuria, frequency, polyuria, pyuria, hematuria, character of stream; vaginal discharge, menstrual history; bladder control; abnormalities of penis or testes

---

Some of this information may be considered personal, and it may not be appropriate to elicit it until the rapport of several visits has been established. When eliciting, it is often helpful to justify the need for it (e.g., "In taking care of your child, it is helpful for me to know a little about the persons outside the family with whom he has contact. Do you use a babysitter? A daycare home?" "It is also helpful if I understand the kinds of places where your child plays. Do you have a backyard? Is it fenced?" "It is also helpful for me to understand how things are going in your family. Do you feel that Jimmy and his dad get along pretty well?").

Some of this information (e.g., occupation, address) may be filled out by the parents or child before the visit on a form mailed beforehand or given out in the waiting room. It should be read before the visit and clarifying or elaborating information then sought.

A useful technique is beginning with a general question (e.g., "Has Jimmy had any trouble with his bones or joints?") and then proceeding to specifics (e.g., "Has he had painful joints, sprains?"). Questions using both the names of diseases and a description of the symptoms are helpful (e.g., "Has Jimmy ever had a urinary tract infection? Have you ever noticed that there have been times when it seems to hurt him or make him cry when he passes water? Or times when he wets his bed or pants when you can't explain or that he wets his bed or pants when you don't expect it?").

Children over 10 years of age can usually be asked these questions directly with some assurance that their memories are accurate enough that they can be considered reliable informants. At even earlier ages, the examiner should encourage the child's participation in his or her own health care by including the child in the questioning process (e.g., "Mrs. Jones and Jane, do either of you recall if Jane has had frequent nosebleeds?"). Initiating this practice as young as the preschool years is most important in promoting the development of active (as opposed to passive) health consumer roles.

Counseling concerning the safety hazards of particular residences may be indicated (e.g., traffic, drinking water, structural problems, high lead content).

Referrals to appropriate community resources may be indicated if a precarious financial situation is endangering the child's health.

Guidelines for choosing caregivers, daycare homes, or preschools are often important (see Chapter 20).

This is an excellent opportunity to point out the interrelatedness of health and social events. Discussion of suggestions about the health of various kinds of individual and family activities, including sports, hobbies and use of the Internet, may be important here.

A significant amount of counseling regarding how family interrelationships (parent-parent, parent-child, child-child) affect the child's mental health and how good relationships can be fostered is often important.

Discussion of particular diseases diagnosed is indicated.

Knowledge is important concerning how to recognize various diseases, when home remedies may be appropriate, and what signs, symptoms, or circumstances indicate a need for eventual or immediate medical intervention.

Counseling regarding disease prevention may be appropriate (e.g., not propping a milk bottle for children with frequent otitis media, diet modifications for children with frequent diarrhea or constipation, early precautions for children with seizure disorders).

Explanations of disease causes may be of interest to some parents.

Children are interested in different parts of their bodies at different ages. Hence the examiner should choose to discuss and explain those sections of the review of systems segment of the history about which the child is most curious.

Continued

Table 9-1 Guidelines for History-Taking—cont'd

WHAT TO ASK ABOUT	PRACTICAL HINTS	EDUCATION AND COUNSELING
Review of Systems (for the Child)—cont'd		
Genitourinary		
History of sexual activity: Has the child had sexual activity (voluntarily or otherwise) or been thinking about it? Does the child have a history of sexual abuse? If so, when? How has it been dealt with? Is adolescent aware of sexual attractions to same- or other-sex people? Is this attraction a concern? Is adolescent aware of how to protect against pregnancy and STDs? Have there been any symptoms of STDs (e.g., vaginal or penile discharge, itching, dysuria, dyspareunia, genital rashes, or groin lymph nodes)? Have young women had their first pelvic examination?	Children (and their parents) are likely to be quite uncomfortable with this discussion. History sheets given out beforehand can be helpful. Separate sheets need to be given to parents and teens. They should be given an opportunity to answer each question or cross it out, indicating they do not wish to discuss it. Then discussion on those answers of concern can be initiated by the practitioner rather than forcing the teenager to start the discussion. Issues of confidentiality between parents and child must be addressed at the outset.	Teaching about sexuality, menses, and wet dreams is important, as are breast and testicular self-examination. This may be done more appropriately without the parent being present, depending on the family. The choice should be made in conjuction with them. Good pamphlets are available and often helpful. Diagrams are also helpful. Information about contraception and protection from venereal disease is important for adolescents who are considering becoming or are sexually active. Many adolescents at this age are concerned about same-sex attraction, and this needs to be addressed.
Neurologic		
Convulsions, fainting, tremors, twitches, blackouts, dizziness, headaches, and their frequency		
Skeletal		
History of fractures, sprains, painful joints, swelling or redness around joints; posture and exercise tolerance; gait	Discussions of sports interests and involvement can provide an opportunity for teaching.	Teaching about the use of helmets and other sports safety issues, including pre-play stretching, is important to older children.
Endocrine		
Diagnosed thyroid or adrenal problems or diabetes		
Senses		
Do parents and the child think child can see and hear well? Is the child clumsy? Uncoordinated? Does muscle strength seem adequate for age? Any numbness? Any difficulty in seeing blackboards? Does the child sit too close to the television or radio? Does the child "ignore" voices, not react to loud sounds?		
Habits		
Diet		
If formula, what kind, how much, how mixed, frequency of feedings, how much in 24-hour period; if taking solids, look for sources of vitamin C, calcium, protein, and iron in diet; what size portions, frequency of snacks; self-help skills; use of a cup, spoon, knife, fork; how messy; what kind of vitamins, how often, how much; likes and dislikes; meal pattern or constant snacking; food attitude: use as a symbol for love or as a reward; food deprivation as a punishment; vitamin supplements	There are two general categories of information important in a diet history; one pertains to nutrient intake and one to diet habits and attitudes. Nutrients most likely to be lacking are iron, calcium, vitamins A and C, and protein. It is helpful to ascertain vitamin C intake in a typical day and the rest in a typical week. If a child is getting sufficient milk, then calcium and protein intake are usually adequate. Iron and vitamins A and C may be taken separately; a system based on the basic food groups is also sometimes useful. Discussion of appetite and education about it must be developmen-	Education regarding nutrition is one of the foundations of well-child care. Discussion is needed about appropriate intake of required nutrients, avoidance of empty calories, and formation of good food habits. Discussion of methods of recognizing and dealing with normal developmental problems and changes in eating habits is important (e.g., the nursing infant's 2-week and 2-month appetite spurt that may temporarily outstrip the mother's milk supply, the 1-year-old's decrease in appetite, the toddler's need for finger food, the adolescent's need to learn to blend good nutrition with peer socialization).

tally appropriate. (These questions should be asked separately and viewed in a context of the family meal, food habits, and attitudes.)

Instruction about nutritional sources of iron is frequently important. Discussion about avoiding high-carbohydrate foods, which predispose to caries and obesity, is appropriate.

Discussion of regulation of bowel movements by dietary measures rather than by enemas or laxatives is important. Anticipatory guidance may be needed regarding toilet training (see Chapter 19).

If there is suspicion of an eating disorder, one may refer to Chapter 45.

Discussion of sports diets may be useful.

Elimination

Bowel patterns: frequency, consistency, color, discomfort; when toilet trained, any accidents, by day or night or both

For some cultural groups or certain individuals, questioning in this area may cause embarrassment. Tact and an explanation of why this information is needed may be important. Many synonyms are used when talking to the child directly, so words like "wee wee," "poop," and "tinkle" may be needed. (This is also true for some adults.)

Knowledge of "normal" daytime or nighttime accidents is indicated for toddlers, preschoolers, and early school-age children.

Wiping from front to back should be mentioned to young girls. Counseling related to toilet training may be done at this time.

It is important to help parents avoid conveying to their children the idea that this part of them is "dirty."

There is a need to help new mothers understand the meaning of words "constipation" and "diarrhea."

Exercise

Sports, hobbies, tolerance for exercise, amount of exercise, school-related activities

Parental expectations for the child in sports are important to determine.

Leg cramps are a common complaint among children with a habit of constantly exercising, more so than for children who take intermittent rest periods.

Exercise is an important area to explore when a child is labeled "hyperactive." How purposeful is exercise and activity?

Explore social relationships connected with exercise.

Physical fitness plans should begin in infancy through parental instruction and example.

Adaptive physical education plans should be encouraged for children with motor problems. These programs allow the child to experience success at the child's own individual rate of development, thereby promoting a positive response to physical exercise.

These programs will, one hopes, reduce situations in which children are ridiculed for poor motor performance by peers and consequently grow up to become very sedentary adults at risk for numerous health problems.

Sleep

When to bed, sleep through night, frequency of awakening during night, what does parent do; nightmares, night terrors; naps: when, how long, where does child sleep, number of hours slept in 24 hours, tired during the day; sleep position

Research has not yet validated the idea that early feeding of solids helps the average baby sleep through the night, although this may work for individual children.

It may be helpful to get a baby over 6 months old out of the parents' room if the child has slept there since birth. For some families, however, such a sleeping arrangement works fine.

Discussion is important regarding normal developmental patterns of sleep (e.g., the toddler's refusal to go to bed). The practitioner should also:

Determine if there are sleep problems (e.g., nightmares, night terrors, bruxism).

Discuss the need for adequate sleep and sleeping arrangements.

Discuss the fact that children vary greatly in the amount of sleep they need. The best indicator of getting enough sleep is probably daytime behavior.

Emphasize sleeping in the supine position to prevent sudden infant death syndrome (SIDS) for young infants.

Continued

Table 9-1 Guidelines for History-Taking—cont'd

WHAT TO ASK ABOUT	PRACTICAL HINTS	EDUCATION AND COUNSELING
Habits—cont'd		
Development		
Ordinal position compared with siblings, age when developmental tasks achieved (e.g., rolled over, sat alone, stood, walked, talked); if in school, what grade, does child like it, playmates, what activities does child enjoy in school or after school; what special services at school utilized by child (e.g., speech, counseling). Is the adolescent preparing for further schooling or a job? Learning to handle money? Having good relations with peers? One or more close friends? Is the adolescent comfortable with their sexuality?		Counseling about family relations and parenting is often important.
Personality		
Self-image; relationships with peers, parents, and siblings; hallucinations, obsessions, and delusions; fears, anxieties, and sensitivities; depression, acting out, or withdrawal; temper tantrums; recent changes in behavior	Data is best obtained from both the parents and the child. Children under 10 years of age best express themselves through play, drawings, or telling stories about pictures presented.	It is important for the parents to have an awareness of the child's personality. The examiner is in a position to stimulate awareness through discussion.
	For young adolescents who are uncomfortable with their bodies, it may be easiest for them to express themselves through writing poems or stories or interpreting favorite movies.	Schools have staff psychologists and counselors who are capable of providing psychosocial evaluations. Many parents are unaware this service is available to their child. The child needs awareness of his or her own personality strengths. These can be identified during the evaulation and positively reinforced.
	Any child having personality changes or whose personality is consistently incompatible with others may have fears of being "crazy."	Parents need to help in identifying and consistently reinforcing those strengths within the child's personality.
	Depression is increasing in children and adolescents.	
	Do not take threats by children to harm themselves lightly.	

Table 9-2 Guidelines to Physical Examination

WHAT TO EXAMINE	PRACTICAL HINTS	EDUCATION AND COUNSELING
Vital Signs Temperature, pulse rate, and respiratory rate; blood pressure; weight, height, and head circumference	The height, weight, and head circumference of the child should be compared with standard charts and the approximate percentiles recorded. Multiple measurements at intervals are of much greater value than single ones because they give information regarding the pattern of growth that cannot be determined by single measurements. During the child's first years of life many parents prefer to take a child's temperature rectally. The child should laid face down across the parent's lap and held firmly with the parent's left forearm placed flat across the child's back. With the thumb and index finger the parent can then separate the buttocks and insert the lubricated thermometer with the right hand. Axillary temperatures are also useful. The parents should carefully follow the directions for the specific thermometer. This is also true for ear thermometers. Rectal temperature may be 1° F higher than oral temperature. A rectal temperature up to 100° F (37.8° C) may be considered normal in a child. Apprehension and activity may elevate the temperature.	It may be important that some parents be taught how to take and read an infant's temperature. As the child gets older, parents should be taught to take the temperature orally. Later the child should be taught. Parents should be taught how high a temperature should be allowed to go before calling for medical help. Fever control measures (e.g., antipyretics, sponge baths) should be taught. If baby acetaminophen or ibuprofen is used, poison prevention measures should be included (see Chapter 43). Advise parents to avoid giving aspirin.
General Appearance Child appearing well or ill; degree of prostration, cooperation, comfort, nutrition, and consciousness; abnormalities; gait, posture, and coordination; estimate of intelligence; reaction to parents, examiner, and examination; nature of cry and degree of facial activity and facial expression.	Specifics listed by area.	Specifics listed by area.
Skin Color: cyanosis, jaundice, pallor, and erythema; texture: eruptions, hydration, edema, hemorrhagic manifestations, scars, dilated vessels and direction of blood flow, hemangiomas, café au lait areas and nevi; Mongolian (blue–black) spots, pigmentation, turgor, elasticity, and subcutaneous nodules; striae and wrinkling (perhaps indicating rapid weight gain or loss); sensitivity, hair distribution and character, and desquamation; tattooing and body piercing to be noted and discussed	Loss of turgor, especially of the calf muscles and skin over the abdomen, is evidence of dehydration. The soles and palms are often bluish and cold in early infancy; this is of no significance. The degree of anemia cannot be determined reliably by inspection because pallor (even in the newborn) may be normal and not a result of anemia. To demonstrate pitting edema in a child, it may be necessary to exert prolonged pressure. A few small pigmented nevi are commonly found, particularly in older children. Spider nevi occur in about one sixth of children under 5 years of age and almost half of older children.	Parents of infants are particularly likely to be interested in skin care. Should they use baby powder? Baby ointment? How often should they bathe their babies? Discussion of these subjects is often useful to parents. Parents are also very interested in any unusual or different markings on their infants. Are they serious? Will they disappear? Do they mean disease? Very common markings such as milia, miliaria, or stork bites will cause these concerns, as will slightly less common markings such as cavernous hemangiomas, port-wine stains, and café au lait marks. Adolescents are attentive audiences concerning skin care.

Continued

Table 9-2 Guidelines to Physical Examination—cont'd

WHAT TO EXAMINE	PRACTICAL HINTS	EDUCATION AND COUNSELING
Skin—cont'd	Mongolian spots (large flat black or blue-black areas) are frequently present over the lower back and buttocks; in noncaucasion children they have no pathologic significance; be sure to distinguish them from the ecchymosis of child abuse. Cyanosis will not be evident unless at least 5 g of reduced hemoglobin is present; therefore, it develops less easily in an anemic child. Carotenemic pigmentation is usually most prominent over the palms and soles and around the nose, sparing the conjunctivas; it is absent in the sclerae; conversely, jaundice is present in the sclerae. Note birthmarks.	
Hair Texture, distribution, and parasites	Normal infants may lose their hair around 3 months of age; this is of no significance. Familial balding may begin in adolescence. See Chapter 40 for Tanner staging of axillary and pubic hair.	How and with what to shampoo an infant's hair is a frequent concern of parents. Most adolescents are very interested in hair care measures. Appearance of axillary, facial, and pubic hair in adolescents warrants anticipatory guidance and reassurance about the normality of the body changes that will occur.
Lymph Nodes Location, size, mobility, and consistency; routine attempts to palpate suboccipital, preauricular, anterior cervical, posterior cervical, submaxillar, sublingual, axillary, epitrochlear, and inguinal lymph nodes	Enlargement of the lymph nodes occurs much more readily in children than in adults. Small inguinal lymph nodes are palpable in almost all healthy young children. Small, mobile, nontender shotty nodes are commonly found as residua of previous infections. Adolescent girls frequently have slightly enlarged lymph nodes in the axilla because of infections from shaving. When a node is enlarged, remember to look above the swollen lymph node for the source of infection.	Older children, both school-age and adolescent, are frequently surprised to feel a lymph node someplace in their bodies. A discussion of its normality and the purpose of the lymphatic system may be very helpful.
Head Size, shape, circumference, asymmetry, cephalohematoma, bosses, craniotabes, control, molding, bruit, fontanel (size, tension, number, abnormally late or early closure), sutures, dilated veins, scalp, face, and transillumination	The head is measured at its greatest circumference, which is usually at the midforehead anteriorly and around to the most prominent portion of the occiput posteriorly. The ratio of head circumference of the chest or abdomen is usually of little value. Fontanel tension is best determined with the child quiet and in the sitting position. Slight pulsations over the anterior fontanel may occur in normal infants. Although bruits may be heard over the temporal areas in normal children, the possibility of an existing abnormality should not be overlooked.	Parents of infants are often interested to learn more about the baby's "soft spot." Many parents are unduly concerned about the vulnerability of this spot and will even avoid washing the hair over it. Counseling about this can be very helpful. Discuss the importance of always wearing a proper fitting helmet when cycling, rollerblading, or skateboarding. Discussion of when various sinuses first develop and the problem of sinusitis may be helpful (see Chapter 41).

Face

Symmetry, paralysis, distance between nose and mouth, depth of nasolabial folds, bridge of nose, distribution of hair, size of mandible, swellings, hypertelorism, Chvostek's sign, and tenderness of sinuses

Craniotabes may be found in normal newborns (especially the premature) and for the first 2 to 4 months, but they may also indicate rickets.

A positive Macewen's sign ("cracked-pot sound" when skull is percussed with one finger) may be present as long as the fontanel is open.

Transillumination of the skull can be performed by means of a flashlight with a sponge rubber collar so that it forms a tight fit when held against the head; this should be done in a completely dark room; several minutes should be allowed for the examiner's eyes to accomodate to the dark.

Many infants with chromosomal abnormalities have recognizable facial characteristics (e.g., widely spaced eyes, low-set ears).

Eyes

Photophobia, visual acuity, muscular control, nystagmus, mongolian slant, Brushfield's spots, epicanthal folds, lacrimation, discharge, lids, exophthalmos or enophthalmos, and conjunctivas; pupillary size, shape, and reaction to light and accommodation; corneal opacities, cataracts, fundi, and visual fields (in older children)

The newborn infant usually will open the eyes if placed prone, supported with one hand under the abdomen, and lifted over the examiner's head.

Occasionally, one pupil is normally larger than the other. This sometimes occurs only in bright or in subdued light.

"Hippus" (a phenomenon in which the pupils alternately constrict and dilate when a light is shined on them) can be a normal finding.

Vision evaluation is essential in all children.

Dark blotches are commonly present in the sclerae of African-American children.

The retinas of African-American children are darker than those of Caucasian children.

Asian-American children often have some degree of epiblepharon; as long as it does not irritate the cornea, it should be considered normal.

Parents of newborns are always interested to find out when and how much their babies can see. They are often interested in receiving counseling in regard to how they can stimulate their baby's vision through the use of brightly colored mobiles at a distance of approximately 14 inches. They will probably also be interested a few weeks later in helping their baby learn to follow by tracking objects (or their own faces) slowly from one side to the other.

There are many myths in this country that too much reading or reading in a car can damage the eyes. Parents are often interested in discussing these myths.

Parents of infants often ask when their babies will achieve their final eye color. (About 50% do so by 6 months of age; over 90% do so by 1 year.)

Questions of the inheritability of eye disease and vision problems can provide very important opportunities for counseling. As children who wear glasses become adolescents, a variety of questions arise about the possibility of contact lenses. Because children's eyes continue changing shape as they mature, the new laser surgeries for myopia are not appropriate.

Nose

Exterior, shape, mucosa, patency, discharge, bleeding, pressure over sinuses, flaring of nostrils, septum, and turbinates

A head mirror and nasal speculum or the largest otoscope speculum may aid visualization.

Pushing the nose tip with a thumb so that it flattens against the face also aids visualization.

Education concerning how to stop a nosebleed (by pinching at the base of the nose without releasing or holding ice at this point, the point of Kiesselbach's area) is important for some children and their parents.

Continued

Table 9-2 Guidelines to Physical Examination—cont'd

WHAT TO EXAMINE	PRACTICAL HINTS	EDUCATION AND COUNSELING
Mouth Lips (thinness, down-turning, fissures, color, cleft), teeth (number, position, caries, mottling, discoloration, notching, malocclusion or malalignment), mucosa (color, redness of Stensen's duct, exanthems, Bohn's nodules, Epstein's pearls), gums, palate, tongue, uvula, mouth breathing, and geographic tongue (usually normal) Gums Teeth	Many parents are concerned that their baby is tongue tied. If the tongue can be extended as far as the alveolar ridge, there will be no interference with nursing or speaking.	Dental hygiene is important, because caries is the leading childhood disease. Tooth cleansing should begin with the eruption of the first tooth, with the parent using a washcloth to cleanse the tooth. Brushing by the child becomes possible later, but for the job to be done well, the parent must at least finish it after the child has begun until about age 7; children below this age are not manually dexterous enough to do a complete job. Flossing also must be done by the parent until the child is about age 10 to 11 years, when the child can be taught. Topical, systemic, and water supply fluoride are also topics of educational importance. A healthy preparation of a child for dentist visits is important. There are many good children's books written to help with this preparation. Teething control is an important area for health education until all primary teeth have erupted (by about 2 to 2½ years). The contribution of high-carbohydrate foods to caries must be stressed. Emergency care for tooth evulsion may be appropriate in certain cases. See Chapter 16 for a chart of dental eruption times. This is often of interest to parents of young children.
Throat Tonsils (size, inflammation, exudate, crypts, inflammation of the anterior pillars), mucosa, hypertrophic lymphoid tissue, postnasal drip, epiglottis, and voice (hoarseness, stridor, grunting, type of cry, speech)	Before examining a child's throat it is advisable to examine the mouth first and permit the child to handle the tongue blade, nasal speculum, and flashlight to help overcome fear of the instruments. Then ask the child to stick out the tongue and say "Ah" louder and louder. In some cases this may allow an adequate examination. In others, if the child is cooperative enough, you may ask the child to "pant like a puppy"; while the child is doing this, the tongue blade is applied firmly to the rear of the tongue. Gagging need not usually be elicited to obtain a satisfactory examination. Many small babies will cry after their ears are examined. Often such a cry results in a mouth wide open and easily seen without a tongue blade. In still other cases, it may be expedient to examine one side of the tongue at a time, pushing the base of the tongue to one side and then to the other. This may be less unpleasant and is less likely to cause gagging. Young children may have to be restrained to obtain an adequate examination of the throat. Eliciting a gag reflex may be necessary if the oral pharynx is to be adequately seen.	Education concerning tonsils is frequently appropriate. Many parents want children's tonsils pulled out, thinking this will stop frequent colds. The way a child is handled for this type of procedure can provide the practitioner an opportunity to give parents an example of the appropriate way to handle things that are unpleasant but necessary for the child. An age-appropriate brief explanation, followed by a firm but quick examination, and ending with a chance for the child to express feelings in an age-appropriate manner is important. Respect for the child and the child's feelings must be maintained, and cuddling or other age-appropriate reassurance should be given after the examination.

Continued

A small child's head may be restrained satisfactorily if the parent's hands are placed at the level of the child's elbows while the child's arms are held firmly against the sides of the head.

If the child can sit up, the parent is asked to hold the child erect in her or his lap with the back against the parent's chest. The child's left hand is then held in the parent's left hand and the right hand in the parent's right hand. The parent places them against the child's groin or lower thigh to prevent the child from slipping down from the lap. If the throat is to be examined in natural light, the parent faces the child. If a flashlight is to be used, the parent sits with her or his back to the light. In either case, the practitioner uses one hand to hold the child's head in position and the other to manipulate the tongue blade. Young children seldom complain of sore throats even in the presence of significant infection of the pharynx and tonsils. The present of a clean tongue blade to bring home and use on a doll is usually appreciated by preschoolers.

Ears

Pinnas (position, size), canals, tympanic membranes (landmarks, mobility, perforation, inflammation, discharge), mastoid tenderness and swelling, hearing

An evaluation of hearing is an important part of the physical examination of every child.

The ears of all sick children should be examined.

Before actually examining the ears, it is often helpful to place the speculum just within the canal, remove it and place it lightly in the other ear, remove it again, and proceed in this way from one ear to the other, gradually going farther and farther, until a satisfactory examination is completed.

In examining the ears, as large a speculum as possible should be used, and it should be inserted no farther than necessary, to avoid both discomfort and pushing wax in front of the speculum so that it obscures the field. The otoscope should be held balanced in the hand by holding the handle at the end nearest the speculum. One finger should rest against the head to prevent injury resulting from sudden movement by the child. Pneumoscopy may be useful if a tympanogram is not available. The most common difficulty in getting the tympanic membrane to move is failing to get an airtight seal because the speculum used is too small. The sound of air whistling back out the canal indicates this is the case.

A child may be restrained most easily when he or she is lying on the abdomen.

Low-set ears are present in several congenital syndromes, including several that are associated with mental retardation. The ears may be considered low set if they are below an imaginary line drawn from the lateral angle of the eye to the external occipital protuberance.

Congenital anomalies of the urinary tract are frequently associated with abnormalities of the pinnas.

Cleaning of the ears is a subject that often comes up, particularly if a child's ears must be curetted. It is important to help the parents realize that the wax being removed is not dirt and the fact that it is there does not indicate they are doing a poor job cleaning their child's ears. Careful instruction to avoid putting pointed and small objects such as cotton swabs and bobby pins in the ear is important because damage to the tympanic membrane is possible. Hydrogen peroxide is occasionally suggested if the child has bothersome wax; otherwise removal of the wax is not really necessary.

Again, a good example of how to handle a child during a potentially uncomfortable experience can be very helpful to parents.

Older children are interested in seeing pictures or models of what is being looked at in their ears. School-age children often have many misconceptions about this part of their anatomy. Discussion of how to protect hearing may be appropriate to adolescents interested in loud music.

Table 9-2 Guidelines to Physical Examination—cont'd

WHAT TO EXAMINE	PRACTICAL HINTS	EDUCATION AND COUNSELING
Ears—cont'd	To examine the ears of an infant it is usually necessary to pull the auricle backward and downward; in an older child the external ear is pulled backward and upward. "Examining" the parent's or a doll's ears first is often very helpful in allaying a child's fears; so is allowing handling of the instruments and "blowing out" the light.	Older schoolchildren are often interested in the anatomy of the thyroid and larynx.
Neck Position (torticollis, opisthotonos, inability to support head, mobility), swelling, thyroid (size, contour, bruit, isthmus, nodules, tenderness), lymph nodes, veins, position of trachea, sternocleidomastoid (swelling, shortening), webbing, edema, auscultation, movement, and tonic neck reflex	In an older child, the size and shape of the thyroid gland may be more clearly defined if the gland is palpated from behind. Asking the child to swallow will help in discerning movement. Full range of motion is elicited in an infant most easily by getting the child to follow an object with the eyes. Pushing the head from side to side often elicits the rooting reflex or resistance.	
Thorax Shape and symmetry, veins, retractions and pulsations, and beading; Harrison's groove, flaring of ribs, pigeon chest, funnel shape, size and position of nipples and breasts, length of sternum, intercostal and substernal retraction, asymmetry, scapulas, and clavicles	At puberty in normal children, one breast usually begins to develop before the other. In both sexes, tenderness of the breasts is relatively common. Gynecomastia is not uncommon in boys. Some male or female newborns will have engorged and occasionally secreting breasts. This occurs because of passage of maternal hormones and generally lasts only a day or so. Appropriate draping is important for adolescent girls. See Chapter 40 for a discussion of Tanner staging of the breasts.	Breast development in girls and gynecomastia in boys are extremely important topics of health education for adolescents. They are frequently too embarrassed to ask questions, and the examiner should take the initiative in this discussion. Reassurance of the normality of this development is vital. Teaching adolescent girls self–breast examination is important. Parents of newborns with breast engorgement also need to be reassured that this is normal and that "milking" the breasts will not stop the secretion.
Lungs Type of breathing, dyspnea, prolongation of expiration, cough, expansion, fremitus, flatness or dullness to percussion, resonance, breath and voice sounds, rales or crackles, and wheezing	Breath sounds in infants and children are normally more intense and more bronchial than in adults, and expiration is more prolonged. Most of a young child's respiratory movement is produced by abdominal movement; there is very little intercostal motion. Allowing the child to listen to his or her own lungs often helps rapport tremendously. A preschooler will often understand the analogy between the stethoscope and listening on a telephone. Placing the bell of the stethoscope first on the child's hand and "listening" may help allay fears. Allowing the child to listen to a parent's heart first will often put the child at ease. The fearful child should always be allowed to touch and handle the stethoscope first. Having a preschooler blow a pinwheel or Kleenex makes breath sounds easier to auscultate.	Parents of young infants are likely to be interested in learning the early signs of respiratory infections, what measures they can take at home, and when they should call for professional help concerning such problems. They are also likely to be interested in learning what measures to take to prevent the spread of such infections. Parents may also be interested in discussing what effect their own smoking or living in polluted areas has on the health of their children's respiratory systems. Adolescents are highly conscious of their bodies. Those interested in sports are particularly motivated to learn how to keep their lungs in good condition. Avoidance of smoking is an important topic at this time. By school age, children are becoming more interested in the inner workings of their bodies and are able to understand simple cause-and-effect relationships. This is an ideal time to discuss the basic workings of the lungs and how to prevent their injury by avoiding habits such as smoking.

Continued

Heart

Location and intensity of the apex beat, precordial bulging, pulsation of vessels, thrills, size, shape, and auscultation (rate, rhythm, force, quality of sounds, including murmurs [location, position in cycle, intensity, pitch, effect of change of position, transmission, effect of exercise])

Many children normally have sinus arrhythmia. The child should be asked to hold his or her breath to determine its effect on the rhythm. If the arrhythmia disappers when the breath is held, it was a normal sinus arrhythmia.

Extrasystoles are common in childhood.

The heart should be examined with the child erect, recumbent, and turned onto his or her left side.

In certain situations, parents are interested in discussing the inheritability of diseases of the respiratory tract that may exist in their family tree (e.g., asthma, hay fever, cystic fibrosis).

Parents of newborns are very interested in their infants' bodies and are often delighted to have the opportunity to listen to their children's hearts.

Preschoolers are interested in listening to their own hearts. At this age they can learn some very basic concepts about their hearts (e.g., the fact that the heart pumps blood around the body).

By the school years, a child becomes much more interested in the parts of the body that cannot be seen (toddlers and preschoolers are more interested in the surface characteristics of their bodies) and can learn a great deal about the heart's functions. Plastic models kept in the examining room for explanations may help in this teaching. Children of this age also enjoy listening to their hearts.

School-age children are good candidates for learning about the effect of diet and exercise on the well-being of their hearts; they are old enough to begin to understand this kind of cause-and-effect reasoning, and they are usually highly motivated in learning to care for their bodies.

Adolescents are highly concerned about all parts of their bodies. Constant reassurance is necessary. This is particularly true if any concerns are elicited from the patient; adolescents are often frightened, for example, by the pounding of their hearts or other sensations they feel are associated with their hearts. If an innocent murmur is found and mentioned, it must be made very clear that this does *not* mean anything is wrong. Teaching about the effect of such things as smoking, diet, and exercise on the health of the heart can be very effective with adolescents.

Abdomen

Size and contour, visible peristalsis, respiratory movements, veins (distention, direction of flow), umbilicus, hernia, musculature, tenderness and rigidity, tympany, shifting dullness, tenderness, rebound tenderness, pulsation, palpable organs, or masses (size, shape, position, mobility), fluid wave, reflexes, femoral pulsations, and bowel sounds

The abdomen may be examined while the child is lying on his or her back in the mother's lap. Older children are usually flattered to get on the "big girl (or boy) table." These positions may be particularly helpful when a tenderness, rigidity, or mass must be palpated. In an infant the examination may be aided by having the child suck on a pacifier or bottle.

Light palpation, especially for the spleen, often will give more information than deep palpation.

Umbilical hernias are common during the first 2 years of life. They usually disappear spontaneously. "Let me feel what you had for breakfast" often helps make this part of the examination a game and allay the child's fears.

Distraction and the use of the child's own hand to palpate may avoid the ticklish reaction many children have.

Older school-age children are often interested in learning the location and function of their liver and spleen.

Table 9-2 Guidelines to Physical Examination—cont'd

WHAT TO EXAMINE	PRACTICAL HINTS	EDUCATION AND COUNSELING
Rectum and Anus Irritation, fissures, prolapse, and imperforate anus; rectal examination should be performed with the little finger (inserted slowly); note muscle tone, character of stool, masses, tenderness, and sensation; examine stool on gloved finger (gross, microscopic, culture, guaiac) as indicated		Education concerning hygiene may be indicated for parents of diaper-age children. Questions about diaper rash, wiping from front to back, and care of diapers may come up. For older children, teaching about washing hands after bowel movements and wiping from front to back may be appropriate. Helping parents avoid conveying the idea of "dirtiness" to their young children concerning any part of the body is important. This is particularly troublesome if it is directed toward bowel movements because children may generalize this to their genitals because of the proximity. Everything "down there" may become associated with dirt. Discussion related to potty training may be very important and may come up naturally during this part of the physical examination.
Extremities *General* Deformity, hemiatrophy, bowlegs, knock-knees, paralysis, gait, stance, and asymmetry	Children can seldom understand directions about how to move their bodies; it is generally easiest to demonstrate and play the "just like me" game.	Parents of young toddlers are often not aware of the normal stages of bowleggedness occurring at this age. It is often helpful to point this out to them.
Joints Swelling, redness, pain, limitation of motion, tenderness, rheumatic nodules, carrying angle of elbows, and tibial torsion	When observing the gait of a toddler, remember that the toddler won't walk *away* from the parents, but will walk *toward* them; pick the child up and put him or her down several yards from the parent. Feet commonly appear flat during the first 2 years.	Parents of preschoolers are frequently not aware that in this stage children are often naturally knock-kneed and that most will outgrow it. Reassurance is often helpful. Parents of newborns are sometimes concerned about the normal hyperflexibility of joints (a newborn's wrist can be flexed flat against the forearm, for example). Reassurance that this is normal may be useful.
Hands and feet Extra digits, clubbing, simian lines, curvature of little finger, deformity of nails, splinter hemorrhages, flat feet, abnormalities of feet, dermatoglyphics, width of thumbs and big toes, syndactyly, length of various segments, dimpling of dorsa, and temperature	Intrauterine position results in many contortions of the limbs, particularly of the feet: generally if one can passively overcorrect an abnormal position, the child will outgrow it.	Children are often interested in their own growth patterns (i.e., how much more they will grow). Children of later school age are often very interested in first aid for such things as fractures. Advice on posture may be appropriate for school-age children and adolescents. Discussion of the normal "flat feet of infancy" or defects from intrauterine position is often important for parents of infants. Discuss injury prevention (see Chapters 14 and 38).
Peripheral vessels Presence, absence, or diminution of arterial pulses		
Spine and Back Posture, curvatures, rigidity, webbed neck, spina bifida, pilonidal dimple or cyst, tufts of hair, mobility, and Mongolian spot; tenderness over spine, pelvis, or kidneys	African-American children normally have an exaggerated lumbar curve. If an apparent scoliosis corrects itself when the child bends over, it is functional; if it does not, it is organic.	

Male Genitalia

Circumcision, meatal opening, hypospadias, phimosis, adherent foreskin, size of testes, cryptorchidism, scrotum, hydrocele, hernia, and pubertal changes

In examining a suspected case of cryptorchidism, palpation for the testicles should be done before the child has fully undressed, become chilled, or had the cremasteric reflex stimulated. If the cremasteric reflex has been activated and the testes have retracted out of the scrotum into the abdomen, it may be helpful to examine the child while sitting in a warm bath. The boy should also be examined while sitting in a chair holding his knees with his heels on the seat; the increased intraabdominal pressure may push the testes into the scrotum.

To examine for cryptorchidism, start above the inguinal canal and work downward to prevent pushing the testes up into the canal or abdomen.

In an obese boy, the penis may be so obscured by fat as to appear abnormally small. If this fat is pushed back, a penis of normal size is usually found.

With questions of sexual abuse, remember that tissue in the genital area heals quickly; lack of visible injury does not prove lack of abuse.

The following applies to both male and female genitalia in the physical examination:

Infancy and toddlerhood: Parents may need education regarding hygiene of the genital areas, including wiping from front to back in little girls to prevent urinary tract infections, and gradual retraction of the foreskin of little boys. (Authorities differ on the best time to retract the foreskin of infant boys, but once it is retracted, it is important to continue to retract it to prevent it from becoming adherent to the shaft because of adhesions.)

Parents of infants need to understand that infants often play with their genitals in much the same way that they play with their ears or hands. This is not true masturbation.

Preschoolers and school-age children: Parents may need help realizing that their own reactions to their children's genitals will form the foundation for the children's reactions to them now and to their sexuality now and later.

Parents need to know that masturbation, "playing doctor," and concerns of the boy that his penis will be cut off and of the girl that she has already had a penis cut off are all normal as long as the child is not totally preoccupied with these activities. Parents may need help in handling these matters. This may be a perfect opportunity to help children learn about "good touch and bad touch." Helpful statements may be things such as "Now we know that your heart is healthy and your tummy is healthy. Now we'll find out if your private parts are healthy. Do you know why it's okay for me to look at your private parts and touch your private parts? It's because I'm not telling you it's a secret. If anybody looks at your private parts or touches your private parts and tells you it's a secret, that's not okay and you need to tell an adult you trust. Who could you tell?" It is important not to say that it is okay because you're a nurse or doctor (that's what some perpetrators say) or "because Mommy and Daddy are here" because many perpetrators are parents.

Adolescents: This age group needs a great deal of education and counseling concerning changing genitals and changing sexuality.

The sequence of changes in the bodies of adolescents is often of interest to them; examination provides an opportune time for anticipatory guidance.

Continued

Table 9-2 Guidelines to Physical Examination—cont'd

WHAT TO EXAMINE	PRACTICAL HINTS	EDUCATION AND COUNSELING
Female Genitalia *External genitalia* Pattern of hair growth, lice, and size and shape of labia majora, minora, and vestibule; swelling, edema, cysts, inflammation, irritation, discoloration, varicosities, tenderness, lesions, condylomata, chancre, herpes vesicles, hymen, discharge, and swelling or discharge of Skene's and Bartholin's glands	Pelvic examinations can be very traumatic for young women. They are seldom warranted for those not sexually active, and many practitioners are willing to start young women on contraceptives even without a pelvic examination if they are particularly frightened. Good preparation and a comfortable, relaxed attitude and environment are essential. Explaining the entire procedure, using a speculum and model and including all the steps, at the time of the examination or during the preceding visit is helpful. Remember that in the questions of sexual abuse, healing occurs very rapidly and unless one sees a child immediately after the abuse, there may be no indications of the abuse. Also, many types of sexual abuse do not involve damage to the genitalia. Recent research indicates that some of the changes in the hymen that examiners used to believe were evidence of abuse are actually typical of normal growth and development of the hymenal tissue.	Education in preparation for the examination is important, as is education related to sexuality, contraception, and sexually transmitted disease protection, signs, and symptoms. Many good pamphlets are also available on these topics. Questions of sexual abuse may emerge related to this part of the examination.
Internal genitalia Vaginal vault integrity and muscle tone, color, position, eversion, ectopy, friability of cervix, nabothian cysts, growths, cervicitis, bleeding, and size and shape of os	Absence of hymenal tissue between 6 o'clock and 9 o'clock is still the most worrisome physical red flag of sexual abuse. Many young girls want an ongoing discussion of what is being done while it is being done; some prefer you simply get it done as quickly as possible.	
Bimanual examination Size, shape, consistency, mobility, and tenderness and position of uterus; size, shape, tenderness, and consistency of ovaries; presence of masses	Girls should be allowed to have someone with them (e.g., mother, friend, boyfriend, person of their choice). Some clinics keep a teddy bear that can be held; teenagers like them too. Warming the speculum, using a small speculum, and exerting pressure with the left forefinger on the posterior vaginal wall and then sliding the speculum gently over it are all methods of easing the discomfort. A metal speculum is often more comfortable than a plastic one. The speculum should always be inserted at an angle rather than horizontally. If a Papanicolaou (Pap) smear is to be done, warm water may help lubricate the speculum. Otherwise, speculum jelly should be used.	
Neurologic Examination *Cerebral function* General behavior, level of consciousness, intelligence, emotional status, memory, orientation, illusions, hallucinations, cortical sensory interpretation, cortical motor integration, language, ability to understand and communicate, auditory/verbal and visual/verbal comprehension, recognition of visual object, speech, ability to write, and performance of skilled motor acts	Because this part of the examination can so easily be made into a game, doing it at the beginning before the child undresses can help establish a rapport for the rest of the examination. A 4-year-old can be expected to repeat three digits or words after the examiner; a 5-year-old can do four; a 6-year-old, five. Familiar words (e.g., cat, dog, pig) often hold the younger child's interest better than numbers.	The nervous system is one of the last systems of the body with which children become familiar. Usually their interest in this system peaks around 9 years of age; at this time, explanations of what you are doing and why you are doing it during the neuromuscular examination are usually well received. Children's interest in mental health also peaks around 9 years of age, or fourth grade, and they will often associate this with

Cranial nerves

I (*olfactory*): identification odors; disorders of smell

II (*optic*): visual acuity, visual fields, ophthalmoscopic examinations, and retina

III (*oculomotor*), IV (*trochlear*), and VI (*abducens*): ocular movements, ptosis, dilatation of pupil, nystagmus, pupillary accommodation, and pupillary light reflexes

V (*trigeminal*): sensation of face, corneal reflex, masseter and temporal muscles, and maxillary reflex (jaw jerk)

VII (*facial*): wrinkle forehead, frown, smile, raise eyebrows, asymmetry of face, strength of eyelid muscles, and taste on anterior or portion of tongue

VIII (*acoustic*): cochlear portion—hearing lateralization, air and bone conduction, and tinnitus; vestibular—caloric tests

IX (*glossopharyngeal*), X (*vagus*): pharyngeal gag reflex and ability to swallow and speak clearly; sensation of mucosa of pharynx, larynx, and soft palate; autonomic functions

XI (*accessory*): strength of trapezius and sternocleidomastoid muscles

XII (*hypoglossal*): protrusion of tongue, tremor, and strength of tongue

Cerebellar function

Finger to nose, finger to examiner's finger, rapidly alternating pronation and supination of hands, ability to run the heel of one foot down the shin of the opposite leg and to make a requested motion with foot, ability to stand with eyes closed, walk, heel-to-toe walk, tremor, ataxia, posture, arm swing when walking, and nystagmus abnormalities of muscle tone or speech

Motor System

Muscle size, consistency, and tone; muscle contours and outlines, muscle strength, myotonic contraction, slow relaxation, symmetry of posture, fasciculations, tremor, resistance to passive movement, and involuntary movement

Reflexes

Deep reflexes: biceps, brachioradialis, triceps, patellar, and Achilles tendon; rapidity and strength of contraction and relaxation

Superficial reflexes: abdominal, cremasteric, plantar, and gluteal

Pathologic reflexes: Babinski, Chaddock, Oppenheim, and Gordon

Bottlecaps, coins, and buttons often work well when testing a young child for stereognosis.

Schoolchildren can usually identify the numbers 0, 7, 3, 8, and 1 when testing graphesthesia; preschoolers do better with squares and circles or parallel and crossing lines.

When testing the kinesthetic sense using the up/down position of the toes, the examiner must be sure to hold the sides of the toes; not the top and bottom; otherwise the pressure sensation may give the answer away.

Hand claps and bells work well with young children when testing auditory recognition.

Folding a piece of paper is a good test for a young child when testing for motor integration.

Orange peel and peanut butter rather than coffee smell are more likely to be recognized by a young child when testing the first cranial nerve.

The "let's-make-a-face" game for the seventh cranial nerve and the "tell-me-where-the-goblin-touches-you" game for testing sensations are examples of how this part of the examination can be made interesting to a young child.

Young children do not have enough sense of direction to be able to perform Weber's test accurately.

Remember that an infant's cry may be a danger sign related to neurologic problems; high-pitched shrieking may indicate intracranial damage, a "cat's cry" is associated with the cri-du-chat syndrome, a hoarse cry may indicate cretinism, and a weak cry may indicate neurologic problems.

If two adults are present, visual fields may be more accurately assessed from behind.

When testing for cerebellar functions, it is useful to know that a 4-year-old can stand on one foot for about 5 seconds; a 6-year-old can stand on one foot with arms crossed for 5 seconds; and a 7-year-old can do it with eyes closed for 5 seconds.

the brain, so questions about mental health and mental illness as well as mental retardation may occur during this examination. It is a very useful time to help children begin to understand these very complex ideas and some preventive mental health concepts in relation to handling emotions.

Questions about sensations are likely to occur during the sensory part of the examination, and children can be encouraged to use their senses fully and appreciate the information brought to them by their senses.

Certain infantile reflexes may cause concern. One example is the Moro reflex. Infants with a very strong Moro reflex often alarm their parents. Education as to the normality and healthfulness of this response can also be useful.

Learning about the expected times of the appearance and disapperance of certain reflexes can add to parents' understanding of and interest in their growing baby.

A developmental examination is often considered the best neurologic examination at this age. Parents are usually highly interested in their baby's development, and counseling about what kinds of developments are expected and what kinds of developmental stimulation are appropriate can be very important.

Resources

Organizations

The Health PACT Program, Office of School Health, School of Nursing, University of Colorado Health Sciences Center at Fitzsimons, PO Box F-541, Aurora, CO 80011; (800) 669-9954; (303) 724-090 (fax); www.uchsc.edu/schoolhealth.com

Bibliography

Algranati, P.S. (1992). *The pediatric patient: An approach to history and physical examination.* Baltimore: Williams & Wilkins.

Baretich, D.M., Stephenson, P., & Igoe, J. (1989). Using art to understand children's perception of roles in physicians office visits. *Pediatric Nursing, 15*(4), 355-360.

Engel, J. (2002). *Pocket guide to physical assessment* (4th ed.). St. Louis: Mosby.

Igoe, J.B. (1991). Empowerment of children and youth for consumer self-care. *American Journal of Health Promotion, 6*(1), 55-64.

Igoe, J.B. (1993). Healthier children through empowerment. In Barnett, J.W. & Clark, J.M. (Eds.). *Research in health promotion and nursing.* London: MacMillan.

Koster, M.K. (1983, April). Self-care: health behavior for the school age child. *Topics in Clinical Nursing,* 29-40.

Lewis, M. & Lewis, C. (1990). Consequences of empowering children to care for themselves. *Pediatrician, 17,* 63-67.

Mezey, M. & McGivern, M. (Eds.). (1998). *Nurses, nurse practitioners: Evolution to advanced practice* (3rd ed.). New York: Springer.

Chapter 10 *Newborn Assessment*

Jane C. Evans, Kimberly L. LaMar, Kathleen R. Pitzen, & Debbie Thompson

Assessment and management of a newborn depends on the age at which the newborn is first examined. The practitioner may assess the newborn in the nursery or birthing room, or the initial visit may occur days or weeks after birth. Many practitioners have contact with the family during the prenatal period, especially when there are other children in the family. The earliest possible contact with the family and infant is desirable.

Newborn assessment includes prenatal and natal history, health history of the newborn and both parents within the context of family assessment, and physical examination. Physical assessment without knowledge of the parental history, parental perceptions of the newborn, and home conditions can be likened to an examination of an artistic masterpiece through a keyhole. Accurate diagnoses arise from analysis of the total context within which one views physical evidence.

Assessment of a newborn may not progress in as orderly a fashion as assessment of an older child or adult. Much of the assessment can be conducted before one touches the newborn, and it is important to remember that a moderately firm, not light, touch is preferred. If the newborn is asleep or quiet, the practitioner may begin the examination with observation and auscultation of the chest to enable accurate assessment before crying obscures the heart, breath, and abdominal sounds. The sequence of the examination depends on the infant's response and the skill of the practitioner in establishing rapport with the infant. If newborns are unable to quiet themselves when they become fussy, the practitioner may try a pacifier or place a hand firmly over the infant's abdomen. If the newborn fails to regain control, the practitioner can progress to holding one or both arms firmly across the chest. If the newborn still remains fussy, the practitioner can also hold the legs firmly near the buttocks until the infant becomes calm and the examination can proceed. This sequence of adding containment is often soothing because it provides limits similar to those in the womb and facilitates self-regulation. A parent (if present) may hold the infant or provide a pacifier for comfort and talk softly for distraction.

Prenatal Management and Postnatal Protocol

Prenatal Management

Management of a normal newborn begins before birth with the assessment of parental acceptance of the pregnancy and of the individuality of the fetus after quickening. A thorough prenatal and birth history is important for early identification of problems (see Chapter 8), and Fig. 10-1 provides a suggested format to help obtain such a history. Prenatal acceptance and preparedness lay the foundation for a successful relationship with the baby and the development of a healthy child.

The primary developmental tasks of pregnancy for both parents include:
- Accepting the pregnancy (by both parents and other important people)
- Developing a relationship with the fetus as a part of self and then identification of the fetus as a separate being
- Adjusting to physical and emotional changes in self and spouse
- Adjusting to changes in couple and family relationships
- Preparing for the birth process and the responsibilities of parenthood

Early identification of maternal and paternal behaviors is helpful so that interventions may be instituted to prevent abuse of the fetus. Early identification of attachment behaviors that may be detrimental to continuation of the pregnancy provides more time for intervention and counseling. Some rejection behaviors constitute abuse of the fetus and may be followed by abuse of the newborn.

Prenatal psychologic care. The primary causes of rejection behaviors in parents are related to stress. Concerns for the health and survival of their infant or their own survival interfere with their ability to form and express an attachment to the infant. If the parents believe that they or their infant may not survive the birth process, they are afraid to invest much emotional energy in attachment. Any source of stress that causes the parents to feel unloved or unsupported also interferes with their ability to form an attachment. Sources of stress that may lead to the expression of rejection behaviors include:
- Geographic change of residence
- Death of a close friend or relative
- Previous abortions
- Loss of previous children or multiple pregnancies
- Age of mother being either very young or over 35 years
- Lack of successful coping mechanisms
- Financial problems
- Lack of support system (e.g., friend or supportive family member, preferably same sex)
- Poor state of health (e.g., weak from anemia or malnutrition, having babies too close together, excessive fatigue, sleep deprivation)
- Unwanted pregnancy
- Ambivalence about assuming the responsibilities of parenthood
- Changing sexual patterns or relationships
- Concerns about ability to parent

Parents who experienced poor or abusive relationships with their own parents or emotional deprivation during childhood, as well as those with unresolved grief over the death of a previous child, may not be able to develop a healthful attachment to their infant unless they receive counseling.

Prenatal intervention
- Identify the source or sources of stress.
- Counsel and support the mother and father psychologically toward acceptance of the pregnancy and of the fetus as an individual.
- Discuss feelings and explore stress.
- Reassure parents that their feelings are normal in view of stresses.

Mother's name _____ Father's name _____
Address _____
Date of delivery _____ Hour _____ Sex _____ Race _____

Paternal History

Age _____ Educational level _____ Health status _____
Blood type _____ Rh: ☐ Positive   ☐ Negative
Congenital anomalies/familial disorders _____

Chronic illness/surgical events _____

Maternal History

Age _____ Educational level _____ Health status _____
Parity _____ Gestation _____ Weeks _____ EDC _____
Blood type _____ Rh: ☐ Positive   ☐ Negative

Antibodies	☐ Negative	☐ Positive	Date of last titer _____
Chlamydia	☐ Negative	☐ Positive	Date of last culture _____
HSV type 2	☐ Negative	☐ Positive	Date of last culture _____
GBS	☐ Negative	☐ Positive	Date of last culture _____
Syphillis	☐ Negative	☐ Positive	
HIV	☐ Negative	☐ Positive	
HPV	☐ Negative	☐ Positive	
GC	☐ Negative	☐ Positive	
Hepatitis	☐ Negative	☐ Positive	

If positive: Type _____   ☐ No Rx   ☐ Rx Date

Prenatal care provider (e.g., midwife, friend, physician) _____

Number (%) of prenatal/counseling visits actually kept _____

Substance use during pregnancy e.g.,
(e.g., aspirin, steroids, alcohol, marijuana, tobacco, number smokes/day) _____

Congenital anomalies/familial disorders _____

Chronic illness/surgical events _____

Domestic violence _____

Fig. 10–1 Prenatal and delivery history form.

Continued

- Grant parents' desire in fantasy (e.g., "Pretend..." or "How would you feel if...").
- Discuss problems and explore possible solutions and alternatives.
- Promote discussion with other parents if such discussion is desired and appropriate.
- Emphasize positive parenting skills.
- Provide anticipatory guidance about anticipated physical, emotional, and relationship changes.
- Discuss talking to the fetus and keeping a record of fetal movements.
- Discuss the need for preparation of siblings and reinforcement of previous parenting successes.

- Discuss the limited-time nature of the anticipated changes.
- Provide appropriate reading materials.
- Mobilize additional support for parents with family, friends, or community groups.

Feelings of rejection or ambivalence toward a fetus are common during the first trimester of pregnancy. However, rejection behaviors that persist or appear beyond the first trimester should be followed closely and may warrant counseling (Box 10-1). Mood swings, physical complaints, and concern over physical appearance are normal for all women. When the practitioner deems these behaviors excessive, intervention may be appropriate.

No	Lenght of labor	Anesthesia/ sedation	Route of delivery	Complications	Birth weights	Problems during first week of life (e.g., jaundice, sepsis, RDS)	Place of birth (e.g., home, hospital)
1.							
2.							
3.							
4.							
5.							

Labor History

Membranes ruptured _____ ☐ Spontaneous   ☐ Artificial
(date and time)

Duration of labor _____ (Stage 1 _____ Stage 2 _____ Stage 3 _____)

Complications _____

Delivery History

Position _____ Analgesia (type, time, dose, and route) _____

Anesthesia (type and duration) _____

Abnormality of placenta (e.g., too large, too small, infarcts, previa) _____

Color of amniotic fluid _____

Type of delivery _____
(e.g., spontaneous, C-section, vacuum,
vaginal birth after C-section [VBAC])

Forceps used   ☐ No   ☐ Yes

Vitamin K administered   ☐ No   ☐ Yes _____
(Time and date)

Eyes treated   ☐ No   ☐ Yes _____
(Name of medication)

Apgar score _____ 1 minute _____ 5 minute

Complications _____

Fig. 10-1—cont'd

Crucial Principles of Parent-Infant Attachment after Birth

- The first minutes and hours of life are a sensitive period during which it is necessary that the mother and father have close contact with their newborn for later development to be optimal.
- Specific responses to the infant are exhibited by human mothers and fathers when they are first given their newborn (e.g., unwrapping baby, exploring infant's body with a finger).
- The attachment process is structured so that the father and mother become optimally attached to only one infant at a time. (This creates problems in the case of multiple births.

During the process of parental attachment to the infant, it is essential for the newborn to respond to the parents by some signal such as body or eye movements. This is sometimes described as, "You can't love a dishrag."
- People who see the birth process become strongly attached to the newborn.
- It is difficult to become attached to a newborn while simultaneously going through the process of detachment, or grief (i.e., to develop an attachment to one person while mourning the loss or threatened loss of the same or another person). For example, the death of a parent or close friend or a premature birth may interfere with the ability to attach. Also, maternal grief over the loss of a

Box 10-1 Prenatal Parental Rejection Behaviors (after the First Trimester)

Maternal

Strong *negative* self-perception and body image (e.g., anger over "fat," facial changes)

Preoccupation with physical appearance (e.g., makeup, clothes)

Excessive mood swings or emotional withdrawal

Excess physical complaints (e.g., excessive fatigue, aches, pains)

Lack of response or negative response to quickening (e.g., does not touch abdomen or respond to kicking, bruises abdomen by hitting the baby when it kicks)

Absence of any preparatory behavior during the last trimester (e.g., no purchase of equipment or clothes for the baby). Note that some religious groups discourage buying articles for the baby before birth, and financial constraints for low socioeconomic parents may be normal behavior rather than a rejection behavior

Violent accidents or physical abuse of her body (e.g., falling down stairs, ramming soda bottles up her vagina)

Lack of desire for knowledge of labor and delivery or excessive anxiety and fear of labor and delivery

Paternal

Negative self-perception (e.g., feels unqualified and unable to meet societal and own expectations of being a father)

Negative preoccupation with partner's physical appearance (e.g., "She's too fat and ugly")

Emotional withdrawal from partner (e.g., anger at lack of attention from her, failure to meet her dependency needs)

Excessive physical complaints (e.g., low back pain, fatigue, abdominal cramps)

Unwillingness to touch the mother's abdomen and no desire to feel fetal movements

Refusal to attend prenatal classes and to allow partner to make preparatory purchases

Unwillingness to accept responsibility (e.g., excessive drinking with male cronies, excessive purchase of personal or household items that are not infant related, resignation from job)

Insistence on repeated intercourse near delivery date

Physical abuse of partner directed toward abdomen

"fantasy" child and the loss of a body part, fetus, or placenta may interfere initially with attachment. A parent may experience guilt because he or she is *expected* to love the newborn but is not yet ready to feel love. Parents may question whether in fact this is really their newborn.

- Early events may have long-lasting effects. Anxieties about the well-being of a newborn with a temporary disorder (e.g., premature birth) may result in persistent concerns that may adversely shape the development of the child. Parents may stereotype a premature infant as "sickly and delicate" and treat the child that way for life.

Newborn Physical Assessment Techniques

A great deal of emphasis has been placed on the clinical expertise of practitioners in the physical assessment of newborns as a valuable means of detecting abnormalities and ill health

and providing preventive intervention. Skills in expert assessment of newborns have improved radically in the last one or two decades, and care of newborns has improved accordingly. Table 10-1 provides a sample newborn assessment guide.

Neonatal Resuscitation Program

The Apgar Score developed by Virginia Apgar has been used to determine a neonate's overall condition at the time of birth, but this score is no longer used to determine the need for resuscitation of the newborn. The American Academy of Pediatrics (AAP) and the American Heart Association have devised a program for anticipating, preparing for, and intervening with neonates at risk. The Neonatal Resuscitation Program, implemented in 1987, provides a systematic method of resuscitation based on an action/evaluation/decision cycle. Resuscitation interventions at the time of birth are based on immediate evaluations of respirations, heart rate, and color. Apgar Scores are still reported at 1 and 5 minutes and still may be used in the assessment of the effectiveness of the resuscitative measures. Retrospective use of Apgar Scores to evaluate birth history may not be sufficient in the current legal environment.

Gestational Age

The New Ballard Score (NBS) is the most commonly used instrument for the assessment of gestational age. This instrument (see Appendix A) has reported an interrater reliability of 0.95. The concurrent validity reported for the NBS, with the gestational age determined by either the last menstrual period or by ultrasonography, ranges between 84% and 97% depending on gestational age. This instrument is accurate for newborns between 20 and 42 weeks of gestational age when used within 12 hours of birth.

Rapid assessment of gestational age may be accomplished by measurement of foot length and intermamillary distance with a right-angled ruler calibrated in millimeters. Foot length is measured from right heel to first toe. Intermamillary distance is measured between the nipples at the end of respiration. Significant correlations were found between the NBS and foot length, $r = 0.62$ ($p < 0.001$), and intermamillary distance, $r = 0.67$ ($p < 0.001$). Mean foot length or intermamillary distance for newborns ranges from 53.7 mm at 26 weeks of gestation to 67.2 mm at 35 weeks of gestation, increasing approximately 2 mm per week of gestation.

Behavioral States

States of consciousness in newborns and the newborns' ability to transition from sleep to waking states are highly correlated with autonomic and central nervous system (CNS) integrity and maturity. The premature neonate may have only three states: sleeping, waking, and indeterminate, whereas the full-term newborn should have six: two sleeping and four waking. Behavioral states are characterized by the following:

Sleep

- *Deep or quiet*—Regular respirations, no eye movements, and not easily aroused by environmental noise; represents 35% to 45% of the total sleep
- *Active (rapid eye movement, or REM)*—Irregular respirations, eye movements, and aroused by unusual noises (but returns quickly to sleep); represents 45% to 50% of total sleep

Alert

- *Drowsy or semidozing*—Mild starts, with eyes opening and closing

Table 10-1 Newborn Assessment Guide

	NORMAL	ABNORMAL	COMMENTS
Date of initial assessment:			
I. General			

A. Birth weight _____kg _____(%)
    Today's weight _____kg _____(%)
  B. Birth length _____cm _____(%)
    Today's length _____cm _____(%)
  C. T _____ P _____
    R _____ BP _____
  D. Age
    Date of birth _____
    Gestational age _____(at birth)
    Corrected postconceptual age _____
  E. Position/posture (flexion, rigidity)
  F. Activity level/seizures, tremors
  G. Appearance/body proportion/symmetry
  H. Cry quality			

II. Skin			

A. Color
  B. Texture
  C. Opacity
  D. Lanugo
  E. Vernix
  F. Pigmentation
  G. Wrinkling/peeling/redundant
  H. Vesicles/lesions			

III. Head			

A. Circumference _____cm _____(%)
  B. Shape/symmetry
  C. Size: Anterior
    fontanel
  D. Size: Posterior
    fontanel
  E. Head lag
  F. Hair distribution
    1. Whorls
    2. Fine or electric
  G. Centimeters of transillumination
    Anterior _____
    Parietal _____
    Posterior _____			

IV. Ears			

A. Shape/symmetry
  B. Alignment with eyes
  C. Rotation
  D. Cartilage development
  E. Tympanic membrane
  F. Adherent lobes/pits			

V. Face			

A. Symmetry/feature placement
  B. Shape
  C. Expression/movement
  D. Depth nasolabial fold			

Continued

Table 10-1 Newborn Assessment Guide—cont'd

	NORMAL	ABNORMAL	COMMENTS
VI. Eyes			
A. Size/slant			
B. Placement/symmetry			
C. Color: sclera/conjunctiva			
D. Cornea clarity/luster			
E. Pupil reaction			
F. Blink reflex			
G. Eyelids/lashes			
H. Discharge/tearing			
I. Muscular control			
VII. Nose			
A. Patent nares/symmetry			
B. Milia			
C. Discharge			
D. Septum			
E. Breadth of bridge			
VIII. Mouth			
A. Size/symmetry			
B. Shape of hard and soft palate			
C. Rooting reflex			
D. Strong suck			
E. Saliva			
F. Lip margins			
G. Mucous membranes			
H. Tonsils			
IX. Tongue			
A. Size/grooves			
B. Color/coating			
C. Mobility			
D. Tongue extrusion			
X. Neck/chin			
A. Shape/size			
B. Masses			
C. Movement/lag			
D. Flexion			
E. Chin size and distance from lips			
XI. Chest			
A. Circumference			
B. Shape/symmetry			
C. Pulsations			
D. Retractions (intercostal/substernal)			
E. Nipple size/position/distance between			
F. Length of sternum			
XII. Heart			
A. Heart sounds, regularity/split/gallop			
B. Murmurs—present/absent/quality/ intensity/duration/location			
C. PMI			
D. Femoral/brachial pulses			
E. Perfusion/capillary refill			
F. Edema—present/absent			
G. Cyanosis—present/absent/circumoral/ acrocyanosis/central			
H. Precordium—active/quiet			

Table 10-1 Newborn Assessment Guide—cont'd

	NORMAL	ABNORMAL	COMMENTS
XIII. Lungs			
A. Breath sounds—clear/rales or crackles/ wheezing/transmitter			
B. Aeration—good air entry/diminished			
XIV. Abdomen			
A. Shape/size			
B. Peristalsis			
C. Tension/pulsations			
D. Umbilicus/hernia			
E. Organs			
XV. Genitalia			
A. Female			
1. Labia size/symmetry			
2. Discharge			
B. Male			
1. Meatus			
2. Foreskin/circumcision			
3. Size/color scrotum			
4. Testes descended			
XVI. Anus—patent			
XVII. Extremities			
A. Range of motion, hip click			
B. Length/symmetry			
C. Dermatoglyphics			
D. Number of digits			
E. Nail quality			
F. Movement/tremors			
G. Gluteal folds even			
XVIII. Back			
A. Symmetry/curvature			
B. Alignment of scapulae			
C. Mobility			
XIX. Reflexes/symmetric responses			
A. Plantar/palmar grasp			
B. Gag			
C. Sucking			
D. Rooting			
E. Blink			
F. Tonic neck			
G. Moro			
H. Stepping			
I. Babinski			
J. Ankle dorsiflexion			
K. Scarf sign			
XX. Other			
A. Stools			
1. Number per day			
2. Color/consistency			
3. Odor			
B. Urine/voidings			
1. Number per day			
2. Color/odor			

Continued

Table 10-1 Newborn Assessment Guide—cont'd

	NORMAL	ABNORMAL	COMMENTS
XX. Other—cont'd			
C. Feedings			
1. Number per day			
2. Formula			
a. Kind			
b. Preparation			
3. Breast—length of feeding at each breast			
4. Calories per day			
5. Fluid per day			
6. Beikost (solid food)			
D. Sleep pattern/facilities			
1. Hours of sleep per day			
E. Disposition/temperament			
1. Happy			
2. Fussy			
3. Sleepy			
F. Drugs			
1. Vitamins			
2. _____ (sleep)			
3. _____ (diarrhea/colic)			
4. _____ (other)			
G. Lab data			
1. WBC _____			
2. Hgb _____			
3. Hct _____			
4. Metabolic screening			

- *Alert or wide awake*—Eyes open and able to follow and fixate on objects or face
- *Active alert*—Eyes open, thrusting extremity movements, and high activity level
- *Crying*—"Cry face" and jerky motor movements

Preterm Developmental Care Protocols

Preterm infants are assessed for interaction of autonomic, motor, state, and attention systems. Instability and stability cues used by an infant to signal distress or comfort are identified, along with each infant's tolerance for stimuli. Practitioners provide environmental interventions (e.g., reducing noise and lighting to signal rest periods). Responding to infant cues, they also provide developmentally sensitive interventions (e.g., position support, transitioning facilitation between states). Further interventions include alerting parents to infant cues and increasing parental confidence and satisfaction in caregiving. Preterm graduates of developmental care nurseries are expected to have less severe developmental delays than their counterparts who received neonatal intensive care before developmentally appropriate care was instituted (see Chapter 29).

Neonatal intensive care survivors may present unique problems to pediatric caregivers. Some of the issues these former premature infants face after discharge include growth delays, nutritional deficits, chronic lung disease, hearing disturbances, retinopathy of prematurity (ROP), and developmental delays. Premature infants are known to lag in growth and then spurt in growth to catch up at 36 to 40 weeks of postconceptual age (PCA), dependent on the degree of prematurity and the severity of illness encountered. If growth does not catch up by 40 weeks of PCA, it should parallel below the curves for the first year of life. Head growth may be slowed; however, a head circumference 2 standard deviations below the mean is associated with mental retardation and should warrant a closer look. Premature infants have an increased caloric need for energy and growth while notoriously being difficult to feed. Caloric intake should equal at least 120 kcal/kg/day for a normal growing premature and as much as 160 kcal/kg/day for infants with concurrent difficulties such as small for gestation, chronic lung disease, or cardiac disease.

Chronic lung disease is defined as oxygen dependency at 36 weeks PCA. The management of chronic lung disease is multidisciplinary and includes pulmonary technicians, nutritionists, and pediatricians. Medical management involves oxygen and monitoring at home and medications such as diuretics, methylxanthines, steroids, and inhaled bronchodilators. Hearing loss is a risk associated with not only prematurity but also with the many treatments and diseases encountered by infants in the intensive care setting. These include aminoglycosides, furosemide, bacterial meningitis, hyperbilirubinemia, asphyxia, intracranial hemorrhage, congenital infection, craniofacial abnormalities, pulmonary hypertension, and hyperventilation. Graduates of intensive care should have a hearing screening before discharge and again at 6 months.

Retinopathy of prematurity (ROP) involves an abnormal growth of the blood vessels from the retina that, if left untreated, could lead to retinal detachment and blindness. Premature infants are followed by ophthalmology and, if ROP progresses, will be treated with laser surgery or cryosurgery to prevent further vessel growth. Even in simple ROP that has regressed without requiring surgery, there are potential long-term effects such as myopia, strabismus, glaucoma, and, rarely, retinal detachment. This means all premature infants should be followed by an ophthalmologist until the retina is fully vascularized. If ROP is diagnosed, it must be followed diligently by an ophthalmologist until it is resolved or treated with surgery. The vision of a premature infant may also be affected by a CNS insult such as intraventricular hemorrhage or periventricular leukomalacia. Parents should be instructed to recognize cues for hearing and vision disturbances.

Some developmental delay is expected in premature infants. Infants with delays should be followed by a multidisciplinary team trained in the diagnosis and treatment of these delays.

Kangaroo care is one example of developmentally appropriate care that has been used in intensive care nurseries since the beginning of the 1990s. Kangaroo care consists of placing a diaper-clad infant on the parent's bare chest and then covering the infant and parent with a blanket. The preterm infant remains on the parent's chest for as long as is mutually tolerable. Skin-to-skin contact along with the social interaction and bonding that takes place is vitally important to the preterm infant's incorporation into the family unit. Optimally, kangaroo care occurs at least daily, and parents are incorporated into the care of their preterm infant from the first day. Practitioners can expect graduates of this type of caregiving to be more confident parents and have better parent-infant relationships.

Pain Assessment

Although infants cannot verbalize pain, they can and do communicate their pain through physiologic and behavioral responses (see Chapter 7). Pain can be inferred from behavioral, physiologic, and contextual indicators. Facial expressions and some body movements are valid indicators of pain, but they are also manifestations of stress. Researchers prefer multidimensional measures of pain that include: (1) some physiologic measures (e.g., heart rate, respiratory rate, vagal tone, oxygen saturation), (2) behavioral measures (e.g., cry, facial activity, body movements), and (3) situational or contextual variables (e.g., state of consciousness, age, previous experiences with pain, temperament). Multidimensional tools are considered more accurate because pain is measured from more than one perspective or assessment approach. One-dimensional tools such as the Neonatal Facial Coding System measure pain from only one approach (e.g., facial expressions). The argument is that many conditions such as hunger could elicit facial expressions. Several valid and reliable pain multidimensional measures are available for assessment of acute pain in term and preterm neonates. However, for practical use in an office situation, three multidimensional measures of acute pain are recommended because they have been found to be clinically useful. Each tool has demonstrated interrater reliability and internal consistency. Each tool also has demonstrated content, construct and criterion, or concurrent validity.

The *Neonatal Infant Pain Scale* (NIPS) is used to measure pain before, during, and after intrusive procedures and includes six indicators: respiratory pattern, facial expressions, state of arousal, cry, movement of arms, and movement of legs. The scale was developed for use with infants and children up to 7 years of age. Each behavior is rated on a 2-point scale (0 for no; 1 for present) except for the cry behavior, which is rated on a 3-point scale (0 for no cry, 1 for whimper, or 2 for vigorous cry). This scale can be used repeatedly at 1-minute intervals before, during, and after a procedure. Scores are totaled on the bottom of each column for each 1-minute interval and range from 0 to 7 for each 1-minute interval. This scale provides objective measures of pain intensity, and may therefore be used to evaluate pain relief measures. It can be used with full-term and preterm infants.

The *CRIES* is used to measure postoperative pain and includes five indicators that make up the approximate acronym for the name: cries, oxygen saturation, heart rate and blood pressure (BP), expression, and sleeplessness. Each indicator is rated on a 3-point scale, (0, 1, or 2) that is summed for a total score between 0 and 10. This is a single score for any given point in time. However, it can be used sequentially to determine the effectiveness of pain management.

The *Riley Infant Pain Scale* (RIPS) is also used to measure postoperative pain and has five indicators: facial expressions, body movement, sleep, crying or vocalizations, consolability, and response to movement or touch. Each indicator is rated on a 4-point scale (0 for no pain to 3 for severe pain) and summed for a total score of 0 to 15. However, the most common use of the scale is for observers to simply choose the column score that is most representative of the infants overall behaviors (i.e., 0 for no pain and up to 3 for severe pain). This scale can also be used sequentially to determine the effectiveness of pain management.

Physical Assessment Techniques and Measurements

Weight, height, and head circumference. Postnatal growth charts can be used to compare the infant's growth at repeated intervals with standardized norms. Newer charts include preterm infants. The average weight of a full-term newborn is 3000 g at birth. Birth weight is doubled by 4 to 6 months of age and tripled by 12 months. The average total length is approximately 49.6 cm but varies with gender. Sitting height, or crown-rump length, should compose 70% of total height at birth and should be roughly equivalent to head circumference. Head circumference is measured around the largest point of the occiput and the forehead, just over the eyebrows and above the ears. Circumference ranges from 31 to 38 cm in full-term females and from 34 to 36 cm in males.

The ratio of weight to length (ponderal index) may be calculated with the following formula, if growth charts are not available:

$$\frac{100 \times \text{Weight in grams}}{\text{Length in centimeters}^3} = \text{Ponderal index}^3$$

An average ponderal index is 2.54; an index of 3 indicates that the newborn is heavy for length, whereas an index of 2.21 indicates that the newborn is light for length. The growth profile is more important than any individual measurement in determining whether the newborn is maintaining growth between the 3rd and 97th percentiles on standardized charts. Sudden drops or large increases in ponderal index are suggestive of the nutritional pattern, and the genetic heritage should be evaluated.

Temperature. Many sites can be used for temperature measurement. Axillary measurements are the most commonly used site and are both safe and practical. Tympanic measurement of temperatures is replacing axillary measurement for the newborn because it is quicker and less disruptive. The tympanic site may be 0.5° to 0.7° F higher than axillary measurements, just as rectal and axillary mean readings differ. The important fact is to record the route of temperature measurement as well as the results. The normal tympanic temperature range for neonates is 97.6° to 99° F, or 36.5° to 37.2° C. Rectal temperature measurements are used primarily when no other route or device can be used because of the risk of vagal stimulation or rectal perforation.

Blood pressure. The measurement of BP has become routine in infant assessment because hypertension may be present. The "flush method" may be used in early infancy, or systolic measurement may be obtained by palpation of the radial pulse, with the first pulsation roughly 10 cm below the true systolic pressure.

Both oscillometric and ultrasound Doppler BP measurement devices are accurate means of measuring neonatal systolic BP. The oscillometric mean BP is the least variable indirect BP measurement; however, systolic BP measurements can be erroneous and misleading. Ultrasound Doppler BP measurements of systolic BP were more accurate than direct measures of BP in pediatric intensive care settings, especially when the patients were hemodynamically unstable. The advantage of oscillometric measurement is that it detects pressure oscillation rather than sound, which is more valuable in newborns and small children because the Korotkoff sounds may be too weak to provide accurate sound detection.

Skin. Simply stroking the skin gently over the abdomen, back, or chest with a fingernail can provide diagnostic information. *Tache cerebrale,* an early sign of meningitis (particularly during the neonatal period), is a red streak flanked by pale, thin margins that develops within 30 seconds of the stroking and lasts several minutes. Dermatographism is a white or pale line with red margins that is produced by stroking. This wheal is common in those with fair skin, vasomotor instability, or urticaria pigmentosa.

Head. Transillumination of the skull is easier now that special hand-held devices are available. A special flexible black "collar" may be attached to a flashlight to eliminate light leakage around the cone, if better equipment is not available.

Starting with the frontal area of the head, one finger breadth (1 to 2 cm) of transillumination should be visible in the frontal area. Slide the light toward the occipital area; normally transillumination is 1 cm or less in the parietal and temporal areas and 0.5 cm or less in the occipital area. Each hemisphere should be visualized in this fashion. The transillumination area is increased in premature infants and in congenital anomalies of the brain; a sharply delineated area of increased light transmission may indicate a subdural hygroma, subdural hematoma, or effusion.

Anteroposterior and lateral measurements of both fontanels are recommended and recorded as a mean and actual fontanel size. Mean fontanel size may be defined as length and width divided by 2, whereas the actual fontanel size is measured from apex to apex for both lateral and anteroposterior measurements. The range for mean anterior fontanel size in the newborn is 1 to 3.5 cm. Mean fontanel diameters greater than 3.5 cm indicate skeletal disorders, chromosomal disorders, or conditions such as malnutrition, rubella, progeria, hypothyroidism, Russell-Silver syndrome, or Hallermann-Streiff-François syndrome. Disorders associated with small-for-age fontanels include craniosynostosis, hyperthyroidism, microcephaly, and a high calcium/vitamin D ratio in pregnancy.

With severe or unusual molding, the head diameter should be measured with calipers so that the resolution of the molding can be monitored. Measurements should be taken both anteroposteriorly and side to side at the same level.

Ears. The tragus of the ear should be level with the eye as measured by an imaginary line drawn from inner canthus to outer canthus of the eye. If the ears are lower than this imaginary line or are rotated backward more than 20 degrees from perpendicular, eponymic or chromosomal anomalies or renal anomalies should be suspected. Peaking of the upper helix or other malformations of the ear may indicate possible congenital renal anomalies; however, these malformations occur as "variants of normal" in many otherwise healthy infants.

Universal hearing screening. The National Institutes of Health (NIH) in 1993 and the AAP policy statement in 1999 recommended a goal of 100% identification of hearing loss before hospital discharge for all newborn infants. This early identification fosters opportunities for intervention in the prevention of speech, language, and cognitive developmental delays.

At this time, universal hearing screening for infants has been adapted and placed into law in 13 states, with numerous others states currently involved in legislation to mandate the program.

The NIH recommendation offers otoacoustic emissions (OAE) testing as the first screen. Those infants who fail the OAE should be retested with auditory brainstem response (ABR) or ALGO. If the infant fails again, referral should be made for diagnostic evaluation and treatment.

Eyes. Interpupillary and inner canthal distances should be measured to confirm the presence of hypotelorism and hypertelorism, which is useful in syndrome identification. The normal distance between the center of each pupil ranges from 1.4 to 1.75 cm, whereas the normal distance between the inner canthi is 1.5 to 2.5 cm.

Face. The average width of the face in the newborn is 8 cm. The length of the face is approximately 9 cm (5 cm from the top of the skull to the upper margin or orbit and 4 cm from the upper orbit margin to the lower edge of the mandible). Prominent, narrow, flat, round, or depressed faces are associated with chromosomal anomalies. The distance between the nose and lips and the depth of the nasolabial fold should be noted. Short or long distances between the nose and lips or deep nasolabial folds may signal chromosomal anomalies. A shallow or absent philtrum may indicate the presence of fetal alcohol syndrome (FAS).

Mouth. Observe particularly high, narrow arches of the palate, which are associated with several identified eponymic syndromes. Fusion of the lips may signal genetic disorders, whereas agenesis of oral structures or labial tubercles present on the lips may indicate teratogenic injury. Macroglossia, or large tongue, may be related to genetic disorders. A hypertonic suck may indicate drug withdrawal, whereas a weak, uncoordinated suck may indicate asphyxia or neuromuscular disorders.

Neck. Clavicles should be carefully palpated, especially in a neonate weighing more than 4 kg. An effective palpation method is to place the fingers over the lateral and medial ends of the clavicle and "wiggle" them. Crepitus usually occurs with this maneuver in the presence of a fractured clavicle. Observe if there is a short or long neck, and check for bruits over the thyroid and carotid arteries. Bilateral carotid artery bruits are normal, but a unilateral bruit is suggestive of an anomaly. Presence of a mass in the neck may indicate cystic hygroma. Webbing of the neck may indicate the presence of Turner syndrome in females.

Chest. Increased anteroposterior diameter is suggestive of an aspiration syndrome. Note that a wide sternum may occur before the anteroposterior chest diameter increases in infants with a left-to-right cardiac shunt and pulmonary hypertension. The intermamillary index is the distance between the nipples in centimeters multiplied by 100 and divided by the circumference of the chest in centimeters; an index above 28 indicates a chromosomal anomaly.

Extremities. The average distance from hip joint to extended heel is 16.5 cm in neonates. The average ankle-to-knee measurement is 7.5 cm. The average length of the upper extremities is roughly the same as that of the lower extremities, 16.5 cm. Short extremities, small hands or feet, incurving or hypoplasia, broad toes, polydactyly, or syndactyly indicate chromosomal anomalies.

Hands, feet, fingers, and toes. The average foot length is 6.5 cm. The hand measures roughly the same from the heel of the palm to the tip of the middle finger. The length of the middle finger averages about 2.2 cm. Observe whether there are long, short, large, broad, clawlike, overlapping, tapering, or unusually placed fingers or toes or wide spaces between fingers and toes.

To test feet that seem out of alignment, rest the feet in the palms of your hands and notice their position. If the malposition is corrected by spontaneous movement, it is probably attributable to the fetal position and will correct itself spontaneously. However, if spontaneous movement increases the defect, further evaluation is required. If there is little improvement after 3 months, treatment is required. Early detection of common orthopedic abnormalities such as metatarsus adductus, calcaneovalgus, and talipes equinovarus requires early treatment that enables the child to reach maximum potential with minimal difficulty. Observe the feet from the bottom. In both metatarsus adductus and clubfoot, the soles of the feet form a set of parentheses when viewed from the bottom: ( ). Differentiation between the two can be made because of the limited dorsiflexion and the valgus position of the heel in clubfoot, whereas in metatarsus adductus there is no limitation of dorsiflexion or heel valgus. Calcaneovalgus feet form reverse parentheses when viewed from the bottom of the soles:) (. The foot can be dorsiflexed, and the heel is valgus.

Nails. Nail color, length, convexity, concavity, pitting, and so on should be noted because increasing correlations have been determined between nail abnormalities and chromosomal and systemic disorders.

Dermatoglyphics and creases. Dermatoglyphics for the neonate is difficult. The easiest method is to take handprints and footprints while the neonate is in deep sleep and study them with a magnifying glass. A magnifying glass can be used with a strong light to study the fingers themselves. This is an especially important feature of the examination when other signs of chromosomal anomalies have been detected.

Hip instability. Assessment of the hips for congenital dislocation or instability is usually conducted by use of either the

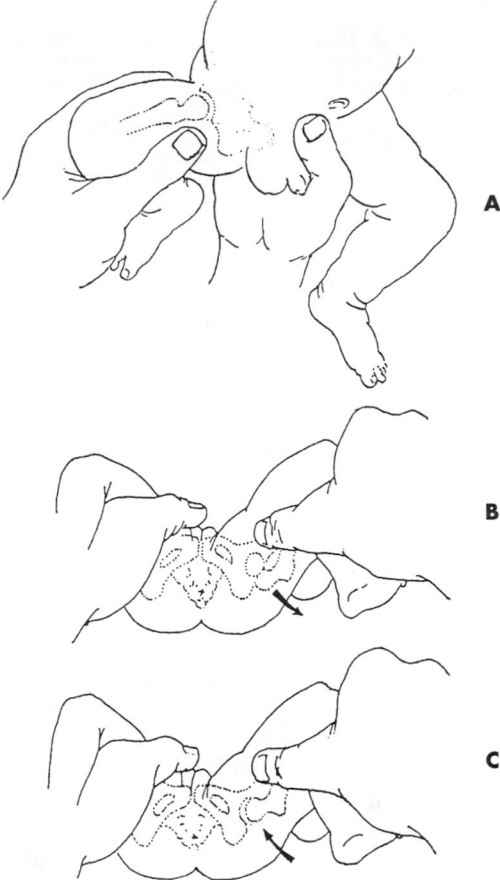

Fig. 10-2 Barlow and Ortolani tests, the definitive tests for unstable hip. **A,** Position. Examine only one hip at a time, with one hand around flexed thigh. Feel the greater trochanter with the fingertips. **B,** The Barlow test causes dislocation by adduction and axial pressure. Note the sudden "clunk." **C,** The Ortolani test causes reduction by abduction and traction. Note the "clunk" with reduction. (From Seidel, H.M., Rosenstein, B.J., & Pathak, J. [2001]. *Primary care of the newborn* [3rd ed.]. St Louis: Mosby.)

Ortolani or the Barlow technique. Either of these techniques is valid in infants up to 6 weeks of age. Both the Ortolani and Barlow techniques of hip assessment are conducted with the newborn in the supine position with the knees flexed at a 90-degree angle to the hips. Holding the knee with the thumb and the middle or index finger is placed over the greater trochanter. The hip is gently abducted and lifted without force while one is pressing down on the knee at the same time. The practitioner may feel a click or pop as the femoral head slides into the socket. This is a positive Ortolani sign. The Barlow test involves pressing down on the knee with the thumb while using the middle finger to check for dislocation. If the hip dislocates out of the socket, it is considered unstable. Additionally, the height of the knees can be measured to detect whether one knee is shorter than the other. Gluteal folds may be unequal when the infant is placed prone or suspended in an upright position if a hip dislocation is present. Fig. 10-2 illustrates the Barlow and Ortolani test positions and motions.

Table 10-2 gives a complete list of physical norms and abnormalities in the newborn and infant.

Text continued on p. 130

Table 10-2 Reference Table for Physical Norms and Abnormalities

PHYSICAL EXAMINATION	NORMAL	ABNORMAL
General		
Gestational age	Use New Ballard (1991) scale for estimation of gestational age	
Weight	Average: 3400 g	Less than 2500 g (premature)
	Range: 2500-4300 g	Over 4300 g (diabetes, postmature)
	Percentage of weight loss more important than actual weight loss	Loss of 3% birth weight during first 24 hours or loss > 6% of birth weight during first 13 days (small cleft palate, congenital heart disease, infection, stress)
	Stabilized by age of 4 days	
Length	Average: 49.6 cm	Less than 45 cm (premature)
	Range: 48-54 cm	Long (Marfan's syndrome)
		Short (dwarfism, osteogenesis imperfecta)
Vital signs		
• Axillary temperature	97.7°-98.6° F (36.5°-37.2° C)	Too high or low (cold, severe infection, CNS injury)
• Pulse	Apical/femoral pulse 120-140 per minute	Above 160 per minute (cardiac or respiratory distress; metabolic, hematologic, or infectious disease)
		Below 100 per minute (hypoxia, heart block, intracranial disorders)
		Wide bounding pulse (aortic regurgitation)
		Narrow thready pulse (severe aortic stenosis or congestive failure)
• Respiration	Abdominal; irregular in depth and rate; transient tachypnea normal	Below 30 per minute (alkalosis, drug intoxication, brain tumor, anoxia, impending failure)
	Rate: 30-50 per minute	Weak, slow, or very rapid (brain damage)
	Ratio of respiration to pulse = 1:4	Above 60 per minute without retractions (congenital heart disease, BPD)
	Respiratory increase with fever = 4 respirations per 1° above normal	Above 60 per minute sustained (pneumonia, fever, heart failure, aspirin poisoning, shock, meningitis, RSV)
		Deep sighing respirations (acidosis)
		Weak, groaning respirations (hypoxia)
		Grunting, rapid respirations (anemia, distended abdomen, severe lung, heart, or brain disease)
		Stridor (laryngeal malacia, floppy epiglottis)
		Decreased abdominal respirations (distended abdomen, pulmonary disease)
		Thoracic breathing/asymmetric chest motion (diaphragmatic hernia, massive atelectasis, phrenic nerve paralysis)
		Head rocking, nasal flaring, retractions, sudden increase in heart rate (impending failure)
• Blood pressure	Average blood pressure according to birth weight (Versmold, Kitterman, & Phibbs, 1981) (12 hours to 5 days old)	

Birth Weight	Mean	Systole	Diastole
1000-2000	50	30	38
2001-3000	59	35	42
Over 3000	66	41	50

PHYSICAL EXAMINATION	NORMAL	ABNORMAL
		Premature: 70 systolic (hypertension/hypernatremia, hypoxia)
		Full term: 89 systolic (coarctation of aorta, renovascular problems or intracranial hemorrhage, hypoxia)
	Range: 60/20 to 90/60 ± 16	
	Thigh and arm systolic pressure equal	45/20 or lower (shock, hemorrhage, hypoxia)
		Wide pulse pressure (aortic regurgitation, patent ductus arteriosus, complete heart block)
		Persistent high systolic with a wide pulse pressure (hyperthyroidism or cardiovascular problems)
	Normal pulse pressure: $\frac{1}{2}$ systolic pressure; range of 20-50 mmHg	Narrow pulse pressure (aortic stenosis, pericardial tamponade)
		Thigh systolic pressure 10 mmHg below arm pressure (coarctation)
Position/posture	Tense with flexion or partial flexion of extremities ("frog" position); muscle tone consistent and firm; assumes fetal position for comfort	Opisthotonus (CNS infection, tetanus)
		Spasticity, flaccidity, extension of extremities (CNS injury, illness)
		Head held to one side (torticollis, dislocation, spasm nutans)

Table 10-2 Reference Table for Physical Norms and Abnormalities—cont'd

PHYSICAL EXAMINATION	NORMAL	ABNORMAL
General—cont'd		
Activity level/ disposition	Spontaneous movement; newborn tremors Happy, quiet, and content	Lethargic or absent movement (infection, CNS lesions) Jittery (hypocalcemia, hypoglycemia, CNS damage, drug withdrawal, hypoxic encephalopathy) Irritable (meningitis, increased intracranial pressure, drug withdrawal, CNS damage) Increased muscle tone (significant CNS damage, cerebral palsy) Hypotonic, perhaps "floppy" (hypermagnesemia, hypoxia, hypothyroidism, hypoglycemia, myasthenia gravis neonatorum, Down syndrome, myotonic dystrophy, Werdnig-Hoffman disease, CNS anomalies, or cerebral hepatorenal syndrome) Convulsions (hyperbilirubinemia, CNS injury, hyperthermia, allergy, abuse, shaken baby syndrome) Fussy or crying and cannot soothe (pain somewhere) Quiet, sad expression, no eye contact (autism, bonding problem) Fatigue with slight exertion (congenital heart disease, respiratory disease)
Appearance and body proportion/ symmetry of body parts	Trunk longer than extremities, arms longer than legs, and head ¼ of total length Short neck or no neck appearance	Asymmetry (birth trauma, congenital defects) Flattened face (Down syndrome, fetal alcohol syndrome [FAS]) Continuous eyebrows, thin upper lip (Cornelia de Lange syndrome) Paralysis (birth trauma, abuse) Cretinism
Cry	Vigorous, especially after stimulation; tone and pitch moderate Quiets when left alone; no tearing; crying periods average 3.7 minutes before consoling measures are necessary	Absent or continuous at birth (brain injury) Weak (seriously ill infant) Hoarse (laryngitis, foreign body, epiglottitis, hypothyroidism, hypocalcemic tetanus, heart disease, tracheomalacia, stenosis, tumor, laryngeal paralysis) Low raucous cry (hypothyroidism) Growling cry (Cornelia de Lange syndrome) Hoarse cry at 2-5 days of age (hypocalcemic laryngospasm) Too strong (pain) Sharp, whining cry (intussusception, peritonitis, or severe GI disturbance) High-pitched, piercing (CNS disorder) Excessive (parental anxiety, colic, maladjustment) Infrequent (hypothyroidism, Down syndrome) "Cat cry" (cri-du-chat syndrome, 5P) Moaning (meningitis) Grunting (respiratory distress) Two-tone cry (congestive heart failure, congenital anomaly of larynx)
Skin		
Color	Pink, acrocyanosis (normal first week only) Transient harlequin pattern or transient mottling Occasional petechiae	Dusky color, circumoral cyanosis (hypoxia, respiratory or cardiac in origin) Circumoral pallor with red chin and cheeks (hypoglycemia, scarlet or rheumatic fever) Generalized cyanosis (severe cardiopulmonary distress) Overly red (hypoglycemia, immature vasomotor reflexes, cardiac anomaly, or cord was "milked") Multiple petechiae, ecchymosis (birth trauma, infection, congential apillary fragility, drugs, hemorrhagic disease, thrombocytopenia) Pale yellow-orange tint to palms, nasolabial folds (carotenemia) Jaundice: Before to 48 hours (blood incompatibility, hepatitis) After 48 hours (physiologic, hepatic lesion or obstruction, bruising, breastfeeding)

Continued

Table 10-2 Reference Table for Physical Norms and Abnormalities—cont'd

PHYSICAL EXAMINATION	NORMAL	ABNORMAL
Skin—cont'd		
Color—cont'd		Pallor (circulatory failure, edema, shock)
		With tachycardia (anemia)
		With bradycardia (anoxia)
		> 7 café au lait patches (fibromas, neurofibromatosis)
	Telangiectasia	Spider nevi on chest and shoulders (liver disease)
		Multiple hemangiomas (congenital vascular anomalies, Sturge-Weber disease)
		Tache cérébrale (meningitis, febrile illnesses, hydrocephalus)
Texture	Thin, delicate, soft and smooth with evidence of fat pads	Firm (cold stress, shock, infection)
		Hard (sclerema)
		Lacks "baby fat" (premature, malnutrition, retarded intrauterine growth—susceptible to cold stress)
	Resilient, elastic; good turgor	Perspiring (neonatal narcotic abstinence, CNS injury)
		Hyperelastic (Ehlers-Danlos syndrome)
		Nonresilient (dehydration, inadequate nutrition)
		Edema (anemia, RDS, heart failure)
		Nonpitting edema (cretinism)
	Dry and peeling, third day	Excessively dry (dehydration)
		Shagreen patches (adenoma sebaceum)
		Massive peeling (generalized edema, postmaturity, prematurity, congenital ichthyosis, diabetic mother, kidney disfunction, blood incompatibility, "scalded skin" syndrome)
		Profuse scaling on palms, soles (scarlet fever)
Opacity	Opaque	Very thin, translucent (prematurity)
Lanugo/hair distribution	Back, face, shoulders covered in fine downy hair	Pronounced in premature
Dermatoglyphics	Whorls common to thumbs and ring finger	Radial loops on fourth/fifth finger (trisomy 21)
	Radial loops and arches on index finger	Simian crease, arches and whorls or ulnar loops on all ten fingers (trisomy 21)
	Ulnar loop on little finger	Simian crease and distorted patterns, large thenar patterns (trisomy 13)
		Arches on all 10 fingers (trisomy 18)
		Large fingertip loops and whorls (Turner syndrome)
		Small fingertip patterns with lower ridge count (Klinefelter syndrome)
Vernix caseosa	White, cheesy protective coating on skin, especially in creases	Absence (postmature)
		Excessive (premature)
		Yellow vernix (hyperbilirubinemia)
		Meconium stained (intrauterine distress)
Pigmentation	Mongolian spots (common to dark-skinned neonates)	
	Normal only over sacrum, buttocks, shoulders, and back	
Lesions	Birth marks; milia	Port-wine stain
	Telangiectasia ("stork bites")	Widespread bruising (hemorrhagic disease, abuse, birth trauma, bleeding disorders)
	Erythema toxicum rash	Localized bruises (underlying fracture, abuse, bleeding disorders)
	Red-mauve blotches	Hemangioma
	Xanthomas	Pustules (impetigo, herpes)
	Red diaper rash	Bruises (underlying fracture, abuse)
		Blueberry muffin rash (rubella)
		Rash (*candida* dermatitis, infection)
Head		
Circumference	Range: 32-38 cm (40 weeks gestational age)	
	Average male: 34.5-35.5 in	

Table 10-2 Reference Table for Physical Norms and Abnormalities—cont'd

PHYSICAL EXAMINATION	NORMAL	ABNORMAL
Head—cont'd		
Circumference—cont'd	Average female: 33.5-34.5 in	> 35.5 cm (hydrocephaly, tumor, increased intracranial pressure)
	Average: In occipitofrontal circumference (OFC)/week during first 8 weeks of life	< 31 cm (microcephaly, anencephaly, congenital infections, polymicogyria, trisomies 13 to 15, 18)
	Gestational age = Head growth	Head circumference below 3rd percentile for age = mental retardation
	38-40 wk: 0.5 cm/week	> 95% or < 3% = intracranial disorder
	34-37 wk: 0.8 cm/week	
	30-33 wk: 1.1 cm/week	
	"Sick" premature: 0.25 cm/week	
	Head 1-2 cm larger than chest	
Shape/symmetry	Molded up to 4 weeks; caput succedaneum	Cephalohematoma (possible fracture)
		Conical shape (oxycephaly)
	Intermittent, movable nodes	Nonmovable nodes (tumors, hematoma, cysts)
		Small, shallow, conical pits (rickets)
		Broad, short cephalic index 81.0-85.4 (brachycephalia)
		Long, narrow cephalic index 75.9 or less (dolichocephaly)
		Flat occiput (Down syndrome)
		Craniotabes (premature, syphilis, hydrocephalus, osteogenesis imperfecta, etc.)
Fontanels	Open, soft, flat; may see slight pulsation	Anterior fontanel closed or small, less than 1 cm (cranial synostosis, microcephaly, high calcium to vitamin D ratio in pregnancy, hyperthyroidism)
	Average size	Large anterior: greater than 5 cm fontanel (hydrocephaly, achondroplasia, hypothyroidism, malnourishment)
	Anterior fontanel: 4-6 cm anterior/posterior and lateral measurement	Bulging, tense (meningitis, encephalitis)
	Posterior fontanel: 0.5-1 cm	Depressed (dehydration, inanition)
		Strong pulsation (increased intracranial pressure, venous sinus thrombosis, patent ductus arteriosus, obstructed venous return)
		Third fontanel (possible Down syndrome)
		Large posterior fontanel (hypothyroidism)
Transillumination	Frontal transillumination of 1 cm or less decreasing to minimal or none in occipital area (premature has periosteal thinning and will look anencephalic)	No transillumination (craniosynostosis)
		Increased transillumination > 1 cm (anencephaly, microcephaly, gross CNS disorders)
		Asymmetric transillumination (brain anomalies)
Bruit	Normal in 50% of infants	Bruit (meningitis, subdural effusion, thyrotoxicosis, cerebral aneurysm, intracranial pressure, fever, anemia)
		Percussion dullness near sagittal sinus (subdural hematoma)
Hair	Coarse, evenly distributed, and growing toward face and neck	Fine, electric (premature 27-38 weeks)
		Hair won't comb down (chromosomal anomalies)
		Silky hair (premature 37-41 weeks)
		Uneven distribution (CNS disorder, chromosomal anomalies)
		Hair growing toward crown (chromosomal anomalies)
		Diffuse hair loss (induced by drugs, malnutrition, anemia, high fever)
		Scalp hair on cheeks (Treacher Collins syndrome)
		Very brittle, dry, coarse (hypothyroidism)
		Alopecia with scaling (fungus)
		Alopecia with scarring (trauma, Darier's disease, ichthyosis, sarcoid, lupus)
		Alopecia (Hutchinson-Gilford syndrome, ringworm, monilethrix, piliatorti, ectodermal dysplasia, progeria)
		White forelock (Waardenburg syndrome, deafness)
		Low-set hairline (Turner syndrome)
		Two-color hair: red and regular color (Kwashiorkor)
Scalp	Smooth, intact, and free from lesions and crusting	Abrasions or bruising (trauma)
		Scalp defects (trisomy 13)
		Cradle cap
		Dandruff, lice

Continued

Table 10-2 Reference Table for Physical Norms and Abnormalities—cont'd

PHYSICAL EXAMINATION	NORMAL	ABNORMAL
Head—cont'd		
Scalp—cont'd		Scaliness, especially over anterior fontanel with rash elsewhere (seborrhea)
		Dimples (hemangiomas, dermal sinus)
		Dilated scalp veins (hydrocephalus, tumors, subdural hematoma, congenital vascular anomalies)
		Scalp pain (cerebral hemorrhage, trauma, hypertension)
		Occipital tenderness, pain (brain tumor, abscess)
Ears		
Alignment/shape	Symmetric, aligned with eyes, well-developed cartilage, ruddy earlobes	Large or low-set ears (trisomies or renal anomalies)
		Malformed, asymmetrical, large or small ears (renal anomalies, chromosomal anomalies)
	> 2.5 cm in size	Associated with Down syndrome
		Soft, pliable ears (chromosomal anomalies)
		Failure to respond to loud environmental sounds or awaken or move in response to speech in quiet room (hearing loss)
		Defects of pinnae, nose, lips, or palate (hearing loss)
		Dimples or periauricular skin tags (sinus, chromosomal anomalies 4, 5, 22)
		Sagging of posterior canal wall (mastoiditis)
		Discharge (external otitis, otitis media or perforation)
		Pale lobes (anemia)
		Adherent lobes (chromosomal anomalies)
Tympanic membrane	Pearly gray, translucent, light reflex present, mobile	Redness, induration or bulging, short light reflex, perforation, discharge (otitis media)
		Opaque, yellow, or blue light reflex, malpositioned landmarks, perforation, occasionally cholesteatoma (serous otitis media)
		Immobile or jerky movement (fluid in middle ear)
Hearing	Blinking or Moro reflex reaction to loud noise at a distance of 12 in or 30.5 cm	No response (deafness, syphilis, kernicterus, full ear canals)
Face		
Symmetry/shape/facial expression	Symmetric, regular features; average size = 8 cm wide; alert, interested	Prominent forehead (chromosomal anomalies 7q+, 8+, 9p−, 11p+, 13)
		Narrow forehead (chromosomal anomalies 13+, 13q+, 15q+)
		Flat forehead (chromosomal anomalies 9, 13, 15, 21)
		Facial asymmetry (low birth weight, molding, Silver syndrome, cranial nerve V injury); infants with facial nerve injuries usually not asymmetrical at birth, except during crying and feeding
		Scalp hair on cheeks (Treacher Collins syndrome)
		Dysmorphic features (chromosomal anomalies)
		Flat, round, or depressed face (chromosomal anomalies)
		Anxious (respiratory, emotional problems)
		Sloping (Noonan syndrome)
Eyes		
	Corneal reflex; ability to follow to midline or 60 degrees	Delayed pupil reaction (CNS injury, possible emergency)
		No blink reflex (impaired vision)
	Blink reflex to light, or pupils reacting to light	Microphthalmia (chromosomal anomalies 4, 10, 13, 14)
Sclerae/iris color	Sclerae	Jaundice (hyperbilirubinemia, liver disease)
	Bluish tint	Schleral hemorrhage (trauma)
		Blue sclera (osteogenesis imperfecta, Ehlers-Danlos syndrome)
	Iris	Brushfield spots (trisomy 21)
	Caucasian—grayish blue	Hyphema (blunt trauma, leukemia, hemophilia, retrolental fibroplasia, retinoblastoma, iritis, retinoschisis, hyperplastic vitreous)
	Other races—grayish brown	Coloboma (chromosomal anomalies 4, 13, 22)
		Palpebral hematoma "black eye" (trauma, nasal or skull fracture)
		Scleral protrusion (trauma, increased intraocular pressure)

Table 10-2 Reference Table for Physical Norms and Abnormalities—cont'd

PHYSICAL EXAMINATION	NORMAL	ABNORMAL
Eyes—cont'd		
Distance between	Normal interpupillary distance: 1.4-1.75 cm Normal inner canthal distance: 1.5-2.5 cm	Increased interpupillary or inner canthal distance = hypertelorism (Apert syndrome, Pyle's disease, hypertelorism-hypospadias syndrome, otopalatodigital syndrome, chromosomal anomalies 4, 5, 9, 13, 18, 21, 22) Hypotelorism (chromosomal anomalies 13, 15, 21) Mongoloid slant (chromosomal anomalies 9, 15, 21) Antimongoloid slant (chromosomal anomalies 4, 5, 10, 11, 15, 21, 22) Narrow palpebral fissures (trisomy 18)
Movements	Nonparalytic strabismus, incoordinate eye movement. Doll's eye movements Strabismus up to 6 months	Nystagmus (chromosomal anomalies 11, 18, 21, or may represent seizures) Paralytic strabismus (brainstem lesion and increased intracranial pressure) Setting sun (hydrocephalus)
Optic disc	Red reflex	White disc (optic atrophy, neurofibroma of optic nerve, optic neuritis, methyl alcohol poisoning) Gray stippling around disc (lead poisoning) Unilateral papilledema with contralateral atrophy (Foster Kennedy syndrome, frontal lobe tumor)
Cornea/lens	Clear, bright, and shiny	Cataract, dull, hazy (rubella, Hurler syndrome, Lowe's syndrome, congenital hypoparathyroidism, chromosomal anomalies 15 and 21)
Eyelashes	Medium length, upward curved; very long eyelashes perhaps familial	Long incurved lashes (chromosomal anomaly 13) Very long eyelashes (chronic illness, degenerative disease) Absence of lower lashes (Treacher Collins syndrome)
Eyebrows		Arched and widespread (trisomy 10) Bushy, confluent eyebrows (Cornelia de Lange syndrome)
Eyelids	No ptosis; symmetric blink Lid edema with facial presentation Irritation from eye-drop prophylaxis at birth	Ptosis, asymmetric blink (cranial nerve III damage) Edema beyond 1 week (contact dermatitis, early indication roseola infantum) Pustule (sty) Unilateral enophthalmos (trauma, inflammation) Bilateral enophthalmos (chromosomal anomalies 9, 11, 15, 18; inanition; dehydration; cervical spine; brachial plexus; brain damage) Unilateral exophthalmos (cellulitis, abscess, hemangioma, gumma, neoplasm, fracture, mucocele, hyperthyroidism) Bilateral exophthalmos (glaucoma, congenital acromegaly, lymphomas, hyperthyroidism, leukemia, oxycephaly)
Conjunctiva	Dark pink and moist	Pale (anemia) Red (conjunctivitis) Purulent discharge (obstructed duct, gonorrhea) Tearing before 2 months of age (narcotic withdrawal syndrome)
Nose		
	Patent, low, broad, and relatively long Average length: 18-19 mm Greatest width: 1.1 cm Height: 1.4 cm	Edema (rhinitis, allergy) Obstructed nares (choanal atresia, tumor, foreign body, trauma, encephalocele, deviated septum, inflammation) Nosebleed (syphilis, trauma, hypertension, kidney disease, tuberculosis)
Shape/placement	Located centrally in middle to upper section of face; septum straight	Peak shape (chromosomal anomalies 1 or 4) Broad nose (chromosomal anomalies 5, 9, 11, 22) Small nose (trisomies 7, 10, 18, 21)
Bridge		Broad nasal bridge (chromosomal anomalies 4, 5, 9, 13, 21) Flat nasal bridge (chromosomal anomalies 9, 14, 18, 22)
Tip of nose		Depressed nasal bridge (chromosomal anomalies 10, 18, 21; syphilis fracture) Broad or notched tip (Warfarin exposure)
Nasolabial space	Vertical groove	Absence of nasolabial philtrum (fetal alcohol syndrome)

Continued

Table 10-2 Reference Table for Physical Norms and Abnormalities—cont'd

PHYSICAL EXAMINATION	NORMAL	ABNORMAL
Mouth		
Symmetry/size	Symmetric grimace	Asymmetry, paralysis of mouth alone (peripheral trigeminal nerve lesion)
Reflexes	Strong suck and rooting reflex	Weak suck (prematurity, cardiopulmonary problems, CNS depression—drugs, anorexia, or CNS defects)
Palate	Arched palate, short, wide	Cleft palate
	Average size: 2.3 cm long × 2.2 cm wide	Exceptionally high narrow arch (Treacher Collins syndrome, Ehlers-Danlos syndrome, Turner syndrome, Marfan syndrome, arachnodactyly)
Tonsils	No tonsils, scant saliva, teeth may be present, tumors, epulis, retention cysts, ulcers, Epstein's pearls, pink mucous membranes	Profuse saliva (tracheoesophageal fistula, cystic fibrosis, tracheal aspiration)
		Drooling (esophageal atresia)
		Flat, thick white plaques (thrush)
		Pale mucous membranes (anemia)
		Enlarged stensen's duct (mumps)
		Brown/black/blue spots (Addison's disease, intestinal polyposis)
	Uvula midline	Black line around gums (metal poisoning)
		Purple, bleeding gums (scurvy, leukemia, poor hygiene)
		Uvula deviates to one side with gag reflex (cranial nerve IX, X injury)
Lips	Moist, pink, smooth	Cleft lip
		Scaly patches at corner (vitamin nutritional deficiencies)
		Gray-blue lips (cardiopulmonary problems, methemoglobinemia, poisons, or anoxia)
		Bright red lips (acidosis, ingestion of aspirin, diabetes, carbon monoxide poisoning)
Odor	Not remarkable	Halitosis (any illness, foreign body, sinusitis, poor hygiene)
		Sweet, acetone (dehydration, diabetic acidosis, malnourishment)
		Ammonia odor (kidney failure)
Mandible	In proportion with face	Small mandible, or micrognathia (birdface syndrome, Pierre Robin syndrome, juvenile rheumatoid arthritis, chromosomal anomalies)
		Large mandible (Crouzon's disease, chondrodystrophy)
Tongue		
Size/grooves	Congenital transverse furrows	Large and protruding (cretinism, Down syndrome, Beckwith syndrome, tumor)
	Average size: 4 cm long, 2.5 cm wide, 1 cm thick	Glossoptosis with micrognathia (Pierre Robin syndrome)
		Protruding, snake tongue (brain damage)
		Atrophy (Möbius syndrome, injury to cranial nerves VI and VII)
Color/coating	Pink, no coating, geographic tongue	Dry without furrows (Sjögren syndrome, mouth breathing)
		Dry with furrows (dehydration)
		Desquamation with longitudinal furrows (syphilitic glossitis)
		Coated tongue (infection, *Candida albicans*)
		Hairy, black tongue *(Aspergillus niger)*
		Magenta cobblestone tongue (riboflavin deficiency)
		Canker sores (food allergy, herpes simplex)
Mobility	Symmetric fasciculations with cry	Asymmetrical (damage to XII cranial nerve)
		Unequal fasciculation (degenerative disease)
		Fasciculations at rest (Werdning Hoffmann disease, Pompe's disease)
Reflexes	Gag and swallow reflex present	Absent (jaundice, prematurity, damage to cranial nerves IX and X)
Throat	Pink with no swelling	Dull red throat, some edema (viral inflammation)
		Bright, red, swollen, swollen uvula studded with white or yellow follicles (streptococcal or staphylcoccal infection)
		Dull red with white, gray, or yellow patch membrane (diphtheria)

Table 10-2 Reference Table for Physical Norms and Abnormalities—cont'd

PHYSICAL EXAMINATION	NORMAL	ABNORMAL
Neck/Chin		
Shape/size/movement	Not visible in supine position; short, straight, has complete range of motion, flexes easily	Mastoid skinfolds (gonadal dysgenesis)
		Webbing of neck or excess skin on posterior area of neck (Turner syndrome)
		Stiff neck (meningitis, torticollis, pharyngitis, trauma, arthritis)
		Wry neck (congenital torticollis, trauma)
		Very short, poor range of motion (Klippel-Feil syndrome)
Masses		Distended neck veins (mass in pneumomediastinum or chest, or congestive heart disease, pulmonary disease, liver problems)
		Mass in the lower third of the sternocleidomastoid muscle (congenital torticollis)
		Midline mass (thyroglossal duct, cyst, congenital goiter)
		Clavicular mass
		Soft (cystic hygroma)
		Hard (fracture)
		Crepitus over clavicle (fracture, air leak from lung complication)
		Bronchial cyst
		Generalized adenopathy (leukemia, Hodgkin's disease, serum sickness)
		Absence of lymph nodes (agammaglobulinemia)
		Occipital or postauricular node enlargement (scalp infection, external otitis, varicella, pediculosis, rubella)
		Periauricular node enlargement (sties, conjunctivitis)
		Cervical adenopathy (infection of throat, mouth, teeth, ears, sinuses)
Reflex	Tonic neck present	Absence (CNS damage)
Bruit	None	To and fro bruit over thyroid (enlarged thyroid)
		Unilateral bruit over carotid (vascular insufficiency)
Chest		
Size/shape/symmetry	Circular, 1-2 cm smaller than head circumference, symmetric	Increased A-P diameter (aspiration syndrome)
	Sternum: 5 cm long	Depressed sternum (respiratory distress syndrome, funnel chest, atelectasis)
Inspection		Retractions (respiratory distress, usually upper airway obstruction)
		Asymmetry (pneumothorax, emphysema, tension cysts, pleural effusion, pneumonia, pulmonary agenesis, diaphragmatic paralysis or hernia)
		Abnormal ribs (chromosomal anomalies 4, 7, 8, 10, 13, 14, 18)
		Wide sternum (pulmonary hypertension, L→R shunt, cystic fibrosis, emphysema)
		Funnel breast (rickets, Marfan syndrome)
		Short sternum (trisomy 18)
	Protruding xiphisternum with pectus carinatum is a normal variation	Pigeon chest and pectus excavatum (rickets, Marfan syndrome, upper airway obstruction, or Morquio's disease)
		Barrel chest (asthma, cystic fibrosis, emphysema, pulmonary hypertension with L→R shunt)
		Left parasternal bulge (ventricular hypertrophy)
		Precordial bulge (biventricular hypertrophy)
		Visible pulse in suprasternal notch (aortic insufficiency, patent ductus arteriosus, or coarctation of the aorta)
		Harrision's groove (rickets, congential syphilis)
		Active precordium (congenital heart disease)
Palpation	Fremitus	Rachitic rosary (vitamin C deficiency, hypophosphatasia, chondrodystrophy)
		Increased fremitus (atelectasis, pneumonia)

Continued

Table 10-2 Reference Table for Physical Norms and Abnormalities—cont'd

PHYSICAL EXAMINATION	NORMAL	ABNORMAL
Chest—cont'd		
Palpation—cont'd	No thrills	Decreased or absent fremitus (pneumothorax, asthma, emphysema, bronchial obstruction, pleural effusion)
		Pleural friction rub or crepitation (fractured rib, lung puncture)
		Suprasternal thrill (aortic stenosis, patent ductus, pulmonary stenosis, coarctation)
		Other thrills (ventricular septal defect, aortic or pulmonary stenosis)
		Epigastric pulsations (ventricular hypertrophy)
		Tap sensation (right ventricular hypertrophy)
		Heaving sensation (left ventricular hypertrophy)
Percussion	Resonant	Hyperresonance (pneumothorax, diaphragmatic hernia, emphysema, pneumomediastinum, asthma, pneumonia)
		Decreased resonance (pneumonia, atelectasis, empyema or respiratory distress syndrome, hernia, neoplasm, pleural effusion)
Breath sounds	Easy air entry	Delayed or barely audible air entry (pneumonia, atelectasis)
	Bilateral bronchial breath sounds; rub sounds are common; rales may be present with normal newborn atelactasis	Peristaltic sounds in chest (diaphragmatic hernia)
		Expiratory grunt (pneumonitis, [L] heart failure or respiratory distress syndrome)
		Amphoric (pneumothorax, pleural effusion, bronchopleural fistula)
		Absent or decreased (bronchial obstruction, diaphragmatic hernia, fluid or air in pleura, thickened pleura)
		Wet rales (pneumonia, bronchitis, bronchiectasis, atelectasis, pulmonary edema, heart failure)
		Dry rales (edema, bronchospasm, foreign body, asthma, bronchitis)
Heart sounds	S_1 louder than S_2	Distant heart sounds (cardiac failure, pneumothorax, CNS injury, pneumomediastinum, congenital heart disease)
	S_2 shorter and pitched higher than S_1	Varying rhythm (cerebral defects, anoxia, increased intracranial pressure)
	S_3 normal	
	Sinus arrhythmia normal; otherwise rhythm is normal	Cracking sounds with heart beat (mediastinal emphysema)
	Low systolic murmurs may be normal; venous hum may be normal	Murmur (congenital heart disease)
	Apex heart (PMI) at fourth intercostal space, left of midclavicular line	PMI fifth or sixth intercostal space and farther left of midclavicular line (left ventricular hypertrophy, diabetic mother, erythroblastosis fetalis, von Gierke's disease)
		PMI in back (dextrocardia)
		PMI farther "R" or "L" (dextrocardia, atelectasis, pneumothorax)
Breasts	Full areola, 5-10 mm bud	Asymmetric placement (fractured clavicle)
	Symmetric placement (distance between)	Wide-set nipples (Turner syndrome, chromosomal anomalies 4, 18)
	Some breast engorgement normal	Low-set nipples (chromosomal anomaly 22)
	Milk after 3 days normal	Dark nipples (adrenogenital syndrome)
	Extra nipples	Redness or firmness around nipples (abscess, mastitis)
Abdomen		
Shape/size/symmetry	Same as chest circumference	Absent femoral pulses (coarctation of the aorta)
	Cylindrical with slight protrusion, symmetric	Distension (lower bowel obstruction, paralytic ileus, peritonitis, tracheoesophageal fistula, omphalocele, Hirschsprung's disease, atresia, imperforate anus, prune belly)
	Bowel sounds within 2-3 hours of birth	Localized flank bulging (Wilm's tumor, enlarged kidneys, hydronephrosis)
	Femoral pulses present	Engorged abdominal vessels (pylephlebitis, peritonitis)
		Reverse filling of abdominal veins (vena cava obstruction)
		Visible peristalsis (intestinal obstruction)
		Peristaltic waves from "L→R" (pyloric stenosis, malrotation of bowel, urinary tract infection, gastrointestinal allergy, duodenal ulcer or stenosis)
		Flat abdomen (tracheoesophageal fistula)

Table 10-2 Reference Table for Physical Norms and Abnormalities—cont'd

PHYSICAL EXAMINATION	NORMAL	ABNORMAL
Abdomen—cont'd		
Shape/size/symmetry—cont'd		Scaphoid abdomen (if bowel sounds in chest—diaphragmatic hernia, malnutrition)
		Ascites (liver or kidney disease, ruptured viscus, necrotizing enterocolitis, obstruction portal vein, urethral obstruction, peritonitis)
		Tympanitic, distended, tender, silent (peritonitis)
		Pulsating (aortic aneurysm)
		Venous hum (umbilical or portal vein anomalies, liver hemangioma)
		Umbilical area murmur (renal artery anomaly)
		Mass with plastic feel (megacolon)
		Sausage-shaped mass (intussusception)
		Rubbery or hard masses (meconium ileus)
		Other masses (tumors, localized hemorrhage, cysts, fecal impaction, pyloric stenosis)
		Purple scars (adrenal problems)
		Friction rub (peritoneal obstruction, inflamed spleen, or liver with a tumor)
Umbilicus	Translucent or dry; no bleeding	Bruit (aneurysm; dilated, distorted, or constricted vessel)
	Two arteries and one vein	One artery (kidney or cardiovascular problems; CNS, GU or GI anomalies)
	Ventral hernias and diastasis recti may be present	Large, flabby umbilicus (patent urachus)
	Normal umbilical hernia: 2-5 cm	Presence of granuloma
		Blue umbilicus—Cullen's sign (intraabdominal hemorrhage)
		Green, yellow, or meconium stained (fetal distress)
		Wet, red odiferous stump (omphalitis)
		Serous or serosanguineous discharge (granuloma)
		Cord present after 2 weeks and/or drainage after 3 weeks (sinus or urachal cyst)
		Umbilical fecal discharge (Meckel's diverticulum, omphalomesenteric duct, ileal prolapse)
		Dark red with mucoid discharge (umbilical polyp)
		Pus (urachal cyst or abscess)
Liver/spleen	Liver palpable 2-3 cm below right costal margin	Enlarged liver/spleen (sepsis, HIV, erythroblastosis fetalis, trauma, syphilis, hemolytic icterus, biliary atresia, infants of diabetic mothers, Riedel's lobe, glycogen storage disease, rubella, cytomegalic inclusion disease)
	Spleen tip is palpable after 1 week of age	Left side liver (situs inversus)
		Systolic liver pulsations (cardiac anomalies)
		Tenderness (abscess, hepatitis, mononucleosis)
Kidney/bladder	Kidneys may or may not be palpable; bladder palpable 1-4 cm above symphysis pubis	Enlarged kidneys (Wilm's tumor, neuroblastoma, hydronephrosis, polycystic kidneys; unilateral = renal vein thrombosis)
		Distended bladder (bladder neck obstruction, urethral obstruction, spina bifida)
Genitalia		
Female	Hymenal tag, large clitoris in premature, mucoid or sanguineous vaginal discharge, large labia minora (2.5 mm thick)	Dark pigmentation in Caucasians (adrenal hyperplasia)
	Vaginal orifice: 0.5 cm	Epispadias (hermaphroditism)
		Very large clitoris (pseudohermaphroditism, adrenal hyperplasia, small penis)
		Imperforate hymen (hydrocolpos)
		Vaginal atresia
		Ulcerations (venereal disease, chancres, granuloma, herpes)
		Red swollen labia (vulvitis, vulvovaginitis, cellulitis)
		Foul discharge (gonorrhea, *Trichomonas*, foreign body)
		Fecal urethral discharge (fistulas)
		Masses (condyloma latum or acuminatum, neoplasms, inguinal hernia)
		Lymphedema (lymphatic obstruction)
		Hematoma (trauma)

Continued

Table 10-2 Reference Table for Physical Norms and Abnormalities—cont'd

PHYSICAL EXAMINATION	NORMAL	ABNORMAL
Genitalia—cont'd		
Female—cont'd		Varicosities (tumors, enlarged organs)
		Bartholin's or Skene's enlargement (gonorrhea, infection)
		Adhesions
		Grape-like growth (sarcoma botryoides)
Male	Slender penis 2.5 cm long and 1 cm wide	Penis < 2 cm in length (hermaphroditism, chromosomal anomalies 9, 15, 18, 21)
	Scrotum length 3 cm by 2 cm wide	Absent or undescended testis (cryptorchidism, intersex chromosomal anomalies 4, 9, 13, 14, 15, 18, 21)
	Testes should be descended and average 10 mm in length and 5 cm in width at birth	Enlarged scrotum (hydrocele, orchitis, hernia, hematocele, chylocele)
	Glans should be tapered at the tip with the meatal opening in the center	Fecal-urethral discharge (fistula)
	Foreskin may not retract easily	Ventral meatus (hypospadias)
	Erection and priapism may occur	Dorsal meatus (epispadias)
		Phimosis/stenosis/meatal atresia
		Preputial adhesions
		Ulceration of meatus (circumcision, balanitis)
		Unilateral dark swollen testis (infarction)
		Red, edematous glans (infection, balanoposthitis)
		Urethritis, conjunctivitis, arthritis (Reiter syndrome)
		Warts (condyloma acuminatum or latum)
		Swollen penis with soft midline mass (diverticulum)
		Mass in Littré's follicle (periurethral abscess)
		Inflamed glans with palpable cord in shaft (dorsal vein thrombosis)
		Varicosities/cavernositis (thrombosis, septicemia, leukemia, infection, or trauma)
		Priapism (lesions of spinal cord or cerebrum, neoplasms, hemorrhage, inflammation, thrombosis)
		Red, shiny scrotum (orchitis)
		Very dark scrotum in Caucasians (adrenal hyperplasia)
		Epididymal mass (retention cyst, spermatocele, neoplasm)
		Epididymal nodules (syphilis)
		Scrotal nodules (tuberculosis)
		Epididymitis
		Thick vas deferens (inflammation, syphilis, tuberculosis)
		Boggy mass (hematoma)
		Sausage bulge over testes (hydrocele of cord)
		"Bag of worms" mass (varicocele)
		Inguinal hernias
Anus	Patent	Imperforate anus or fistula
		Urine or fecal drainage (fistula)
		Anal atresia (chromosomal anomalies 13, 22)
		Hematoma or bruising (trauma)
Extremities		
Arms	Full range of motion (ROM)	Limited ROM (fracture, dislocation, paralysis, osteogenesis imperfecta)
Hands/fingers		Polydactyly (trisomy 13)
		Extended, pronated (brachial plexus, injury)
		Inability to flex or abduct (Erb's palsy, Klumpke's palsy, C5-7, T1 injury)
		Syndactyly (chromosomal anomalies 5, 22)
		Camptodactyly (trisomy 4, 8, 10, 13, 18)
		Thumbs absent (chromosomal anomaly 13)
		Thumbs located distally (trisomy 18)
		Thumbs located proximally (trisomy 10, 18)
		Short fingers (myositis ossificans, pseudohypoparathyroidism)
		Short, broad, clawlike hand (Hurler syndrome, gangliosidoses, Scheie syndrome, Hunter syndrome type II)

Table 10-2 Reference Table for Physical Norms and Abnormalities—cont'd

PHYSICAL EXAMINATION	NORMAL	ABNORMAL
Extremities—cont'd		
Hands/fingers—cont'd		Short, broad, equal length of three middle fingers and space between first three fingers (chondrodystrophy)
		Large fingers (neurofibromatosis)
		Incurved fifth finger (chromosomal anomalies 13, 21, 22)
		Short fifth finger (trisomy 8, 15, 21)
		Fingers overlapping (trisomy 10, 13, 18)
		Long tapering fingers (trisomy 1, 18)
		Cortical thumb with extension of index and middle finger (decreased non–protein bound calcium)
		Hypoplastic phalanges (trisomy 8, 9, 13, 21)
		Wide wrists (rickets)
Fingernails/toenails	Pink, convex, length to edge of fingers	Long nails, yellow beds (postmaturity)
	Possible cyanosis during first hours of life	Absence or defect of nails (ichthyosis, ectodermal dysplasia)
		Hyperconvex nails (trisomy 4, 13)
		Square, round nails (cretinism, acromegaly)
		Nail hypoplasia (trisomy 8, 9, 13, 21)
		Long narrow nails (Marfan syndrome, hypopituitarism)
		Pitted nails (fungal infections)
		Paronychia
		Dark nail beds (porphyria)
		Clubbing (pulmonary disease, cardiac disease, chronic obstruction, jaundice, hyperthyroidism)
		Concave nails (hypochromic anemia, iron deficiency, syphilis, rheumatic fever)
		Nailbed splinter hemorrhages (trichinosis, subacute bacterial endocarditis)
		White proximal nail beds
		80% bed white (hepatic cirrhosis)
		50% bed white (renal disease)
		Red lunulae (cardiac failure)
		Light-blue lunulae (Wilson's disease)
		Blue-green (*Pseudomonas* infection)
		Brown-black (fungal infection)
		Brown-yellow (phenindione ingestion)
		Blue-gray (argyria)
Legs	Full ROM, slightly bowed legs, positional deformities corrected with ROM	Limited ROM (fracture, dislocation, paralysis, osteogenesis imperfecta)
	Average length is 16.5 cm	Patella absent (trisomy 8)
		Hyperextensible joints (trisomy 15, 21, 22)
		Hip click (dislocated hips, trisomy 7, 9, 13, 18)
		Pes cavus (chromosomal anomalies 5, 7)
		Tibial torsion
		Scissoring or bicycling motion (cerebral palsy)
		Metatarsus valgus/varus
Feet/toes	Foot length averages 6.5 cm from heel to tip of big toe	Pes valgus or varus
	Width averages 1 cm	Edema hands and feet (Milroy's disease, Turner syndrome)
		Pretibial edema (hypothyroidism)
		Syndactyly (trisomy 10, 22)
		Polydactyly (trisomy 13)
		Rocker bottom feet (trisomy 13, 18)
		Wide spaces between toes (trisomy 10, 21)
		Third toe equal to or longer than second toe (chromosomal anomaly)
		Short feet (trisomy 15)
Back	No curve or slight lumbar lordosis	Nevus flammeus on spine (underlying defect)
	Sacral dimple without hair tufts or nevus flammeus are usually benign	Cysts, dimple, tufts of hair, discoloration over coccygeal area (spina bifida, spina bifida occulta)
		Scoliosis
		Pilonidal sinus

Continued

Table 10-2 Reference Table for Physical Norms and Abnormalities—cont'd

PHYSICAL EXAMINATION	NORMAL	ABNORMAL
Reflexes (See Table 39-3)	Moro, rooting, sucking, gag, tonic neck, stepping, palmer and plantar grasp Tonic neck reflex frequently absent or incomplete in normal infants	Moro reflex present at birth but disappears shortly (cerebral hemorrhage) Moro reflex slow or absent (severe CNS injury, debilitation) Tonic plantar grasp (hypoxia, hypertonia) Slow or absent grasp reflex (cervical or spinal cord lesions, malformations, hypertonia, lower brachial plexus injury, or lumbosacral plexus injury) Absent cremasteric reflex (spinal cord lesion) Weak, absent rooting (infant just fed, bulbar lesion, sleepy infant) Continuous tonic neck position (CNS injury)

Box 10-2 Early Rejection Behaviors of Postpartum Mother or Father

Attempts to avoid or is indifferent to arrival of infant for feeding

Holds infant away from body

Is repulsed by infant's excretory processes

Talks very little to or about infant

Discusses infant *excessively* (e.g., "supermother")

Exhibits depression or little or no sensitivity in handling infant or meeting infant's needs

Is disturbed unduly by infant's crying

Is upset by idea of being alone with infant

Does not think infant is better than others or perceives infant as ugly or unattractive

Holds infant so that eye contact with infant is not possible

Suspects (*without* evidence) that infant has an illness or defect and cannot be reassured when none is found

Exhibits conflicting attitudes and inconsistent behaviors toward infant

---

Psychosocial Assessment of the Newborn

Psychosocial assessment is as important as physical assessment in detecting the infant at risk. Multiple clues have been identified to assist in early intervention with rejection, potential for child abuse, and emotional disturbances. Fatigue, pain, anxiety, and lack of experience are common parental feelings that may result in the expression of one or more of the rejection behaviors found in Box 10-2. A diagnosis of parental rejection should be made only after an interview to rule out temporary conditions such as fatigue. The presence of multiple rejection behaviors is more likely to represent true rejection feelings than a single observation of a single behavior.

Categories of Maladaptive Parenting Behaviors

Feeding behaviors
- Provides inadequate types or amounts of food for the infant
- Does not hold the infant or holds in an uncomfortable position during feeding
- Does not burp the infant
- Prepares food inappropriately
- Offers food at a pace too rapid or slow for the infant's comfort

Infant's stimulation behavior
- Provides no verbal stimulation or aggressive verbal stimulation for the infant during the visit
- Does not provide tactile stimulation or only that of aggressive handling of the infant
- No evidence of age-appropriate toys
- Frustrates infant during interactions (e.g., excessive tickling, bouncing)

Infant rest
- Does not provide a quiet environment or schedule rest periods according to the child's need
- Does not attend to the infant's needs for food, warmth, or dryness before sleep

Perception
- Shows an unrealistic perception of the newborn's ability
- Demonstrates unrealistic expectations of condition
- Has no awareness of the infant's development
- Shows unrealistic perception of own parenting

Initiative
- Shows no initiative in attempts to meet the infant's needs or to manage problems; does not follow through with plans

Recreation
- Does not provide positive outlets for own recreation or relaxation

Interaction with other children
- Demonstrates hostile or aggressive interaction with other children in home (e.g., sarcasm, passive-aggressive behavior)

Parenting role
- Expresses dissatisfaction with parenting

Behavioral Patterns or Structures Known to Cause Maltreatment of Children
- Documented drug or alcohol addiction of one or both parents
- Documented neurosis, psychosis, or mental deficiency in one or both parents
- History of domestic violence or child abuse or neglect
- Authoritarian, highly structured, and inflexibly disciplined family

- Emotionally immature parents with loose, ill-defined structure
- Poor mother-infant bonding

Infant Indices of Emotional Maladjustment during the First Year of Life

The presence of the following infant indices after organic or physical causes have been ruled out is suggestive of potential emotional maladjustment during the first year of life:
- Vomiting (excessive)
- Insomnia (less than 16 hours of sleep a day)
- Crying (excessive)
- Head rolling or banging
- Sadness or apathy
- Hyperactivity or inactivity, apprehension, or irritability
- Resistance to cuddling (e.g., stiffens when held or fails to respond to being held)
- Lack of clinging behavior (e.g., arms in the air like a puppet)
- Absence of smiles or few smiles
- Feeding problems (e.g., poor suck, resisting food, rumination, deriving no pleasure from feeding [i.e., remains fussy after adequate feeding])

In relation to these cues, many tools are available to assist the practitioner in a systematic evaluation of an infant's psychosocial uniqueness, the parental perception of the infant, and the parental-infant interactions, thereby determining the potential or actual risk to the infant and to the relationship.

Some of the tools, such as the Neonatal Perception Inventories and the Infant Temperament Questionnaire, are concerned with the mother's perception of her infant or his or her temperament. These are important because research indicates that the mother's perception of her infant at 1 month of age is a *critical* variable associated with the need for later intervention for the child. The mother should perceive her infant as generally better than other infants by 1 month of age.

Other tools, such as Brazelton's Neonatal Behavioral Assessment Scale (NBAS) and Erickson's Parent-Infant Care Record, are more objective and based on the infant's behavior. These are particularly helpful to the practitioner and the mother in helping the mother identify and cope with the unique personality of her infant. These tools also assist the practitioner in identifying the mother's need for support and reassurance regarding her mothering skills.

Neonatal Behavioral Assessment Scale

Brazelton's NBAS is an extremely valuable tool for use with parents of newborns. This tool enables practitioners to assess and describe individual strengths and needs along with cues for interpreting each newborn's behavioral means of communication. Research indicates that use of the NBAS in primary care promotes parent confidence, enhances parent-infant bonding, and can mitigate potentially dysfunctional patterns of parent-infant bonding before they become well established.

At the 2-week examination of the newborn the NBAS should be performed, with the parents watching. Demonstrate for the parents how their newborn indicates fatigue or overstimulation, how the newborn prefers to be comforted, and how well he or she is able to tune out noise and bright lights. Educational handouts, such as *Getting to Know Your Newborn: The Brazelton Neonatal Assessment,* provide the parents and other home caregivers important information for interacting with the newborn.

See the Brazelton Institute website at the end of this chapter for materials for home study for parents and information on training sessions. Home-study programs that prepare the practitioner to use the NBAS as a tool for parent teaching are available on videotapes and in books.

The NBAS covers 37 infant behavioral responses and 18 neurologic reflexes. The following are representative categories:
- *Habitation*—The length of time it takes for the infant to diminish the response to light, sound, and heel pinch
- *Orientation*—How much and when the infant attends to, focuses on, and gives feedback in response to auditory and visual animate or inanimate stimuli
- *Motor maturity*—The degree and organization of coordination and control of motor activity
- *Variation*—The amount and rate of change during alert periods and states, including activity, color, and peaks of excitement throughout the examination
- *Self-quieting activities*—How soon, how much, and how effectively the infant quiets and consoles self when distressed
- *Social behaviors*—Smiling and cuddling behaviors of the infant

The NBAS demonstrates the uniqueness of each individual at birth, including the infant's patterns of response and attempts to control his own environment. Research demonstrates the NBAS is especially useful with couples at risk for parenting dysfunction. The greater the risk of parenting dysfunction, the greater are the potential benefits achieved by teaching the parents how to interpret their infant's needs and behaviors. Parents of premature or newborns oversensitive to stimulation need to modulate their approach to prevent maladaptive interaction, poor bonding, and exhaustion from overstimulation. Overstimulation and exhaustion waste precious calories that could be used for growth and healing.

Assessment of Preterm Infant Behavior

The Assessment of Preterm Infant Behavior (APIB) is a refinement of the NBAS used with preterm infants. It covers essentially the same areas and provides parents with information about the preterm developmental level of their infant. This information provides a guide so that parents know what type of stimulation their infant tolerates best (e.g., tactile only, verbal with tactile and visual) and how the infant can best be consoled. Table 10-3 compares the NBAS, APIB, and a neurobehavioral assessment scale.

The number of psychologic, behavioral, and social assessment tools for parents and infants is enormous. Tools are available for measuring psychosocial behaviors from preconception through pregnancy, including childbirth, paternal assessments, sibling behaviors, and beyond.

Management of the Normal Newborn

The average length of stay in the hospital after delivery has decreased during the 1990s. Provision of comprehensive quality perinatal and neonatal care is virtually impossible, and time to provide information to new mothers on bodily changes, developmental tasks associated with becoming a new parent, and normal newborn care is extremely limited. Additionally, this is an adverse time to attempt education with new parents. Labor may have induced sleep disruptions and fatigue for mothers, and excitement for sharing the newborn with other family members is high. Retention of information

Table 10-3 Neurobehavioral Assessment Tools

TOOLS	AUTHOR (YEAR)	DISCUSSION	ADMINISTRATION TIME	SCORING TIME	RELIABILITY REPORTED
Neonatal Behavioral Assessment Scale (NBAS)	Brazelton & Nugent (1995)	Scores infant's interactive behavior with environment; normal newborn	30 minutes	15 minutes	Test-retest interrater
Assessment of Premature Infant Behavior (APIB)	Als et al. (1982)	Systematically identifies the infant's relative standing in terms of differentiation and modulation of behavioral sub-systems	90-180 minutes	60 minutes	Extensive inter-rater training; validity reported
Neurobehavioral Assessment Scale	Medoff-Cooper & Brooten (1991)	Evaluates neurologic integrity, developmental maturity, behavioral organization	Not reported	Not reported	Not reported

shared at this time is low. Internet sites and video or written information should be given to parents so that they can access the information when they are ready. (See Resources at the end of this chapter.)

Practitioners must assess the level of the parent's retention of necessary child-care information from the discharge plan. Major concerns for parents of infants discharged early include feeding, sleeping, crying, and management of jaundice.

Major concerns of new parents and other caregivers

- *Feeding*—Parents need to know much food, how often, what kind of food, and what amount and type of vitamins are desirable. (See Chapter 15.)
- *Sleeping*—An interruption of parental patterns and loss of sleep are to be expected. Parents need reassurance that infants do learn to sleep through the night, usually by 3 months of age. A thorough examination and evaluation should be performed on any infant not sleeping through the night after 5 months.
- *Crying*—Parents may need advice about how to interpret and handle crying and how to cope with it. The practitioner may observe the infant and teach the parents about the infant's unique personality, consoling patterns, and so on. Use of the NBAS with parents is very helpful in teaching them how to interpret their infant's cries and the best ways of consoling the child.
- *Elimination*—The number of wet diapers to be expected may vary between bottle-fed and breastfed infants. Parents need to know that at least six to eight wet diapers per day is normal. Infants should have bowel movements at least once a day, but breastfed infants may have bowel movements every other day.
- *Jaundice*—Jaundice developing within the first 48 hours after birth may signal blood incompatibility or hepatitis. Jaundice developing 48 hours after birth is usually considered physiologic. Breastfeeding of a newborn is often more associated with physiologic jaundice than bottle-feeding. (Pathologic causes to be ruled out include hepatic lesions, obstructions, and bruising.) Sunlight or other home bilirubin treatment equipment is available (see Chapter 36).

Counseling. Parents need counseling and support to reinforce parenting skills and promote better parent-child relations. The sooner consonance is developed between parental perceptions and expectations and their infant's unique abilities, the sooner more positive infant development occurs. Also, the more confident a parent is with parenting skills, the more secure the infant is, and the faster the infant will develop. Using the information gathered from the psychosocial assessment tools, discuss the following with the parents *before discharge* and as needed thereafter:

- Teach the parents about the infant's temperament and behavior patterns and discuss an individualized approach to what the infant's crying means, when to hold and console the crying infant, when to reduce or present stimuli to the infant, the position the infant likes best, feeding techniques, and how the infant responds to caregiving activities (e.g., bathing).
- Discuss the infant's attachment behaviors.
- Provide an opportunity for the parents to discuss perceptions and concerns.
- Orient the parents to the infant's positive attributes.
- Reinforce parenting skills.
- Reinforce and encourage parents to maintain a consistent approach.
- If the parental perception of the infant is negative or the infant is difficult, discuss the following with the parents:
  - When did they begin to view the baby this way?
  - What are the reasons they view the baby as not better than average?
  - What do they think would make it easier to tolerate the crying, feeding, or other major problem?
  - What do they think would help the infant with the problem?
  - What do they expect of the infant at this time?
  - What particular things about the infant have they noticed since the concern first arose?
- Explore the parents' feelings and reassure appropriately:
- Suggest that the parents keep a diary or log of the infant's undesirable behavior for 4 to 5 days, noting the difficulties experienced, how long they last, how often they occur, and what they do to alleviate the situation.
- Reassure the parents regarding their ability to keep records, the importance of these observations, the fact that change is possible, and that they can discuss any further concerns that may arise.
- Use records to validate parental concerns, support the parents, and give assistance in trying various techniques to alter the infant's behavior.

Table 10-4 Home/Environmental Assessment Tools

TOOLS	AUTHOR (YEAR)	DISCUSSION	ADMINISTRATION TIME	SCORING TIME	RELIABILITY REPORTED
Health Behavior Questionnaire	Albrecht (1990)	Selected health behaviors among pregnant women who smoke	133 questions	Test-retest	Not reported
Nursing Child Assessment Satellite Training (NCAST) scales	Barnard (1989)	Provides information and support to parents, documents parent-infant behaviors, provides predictability of behaviors, and supports positive behavior	3 types: NCASA (sleep-activity), NCAFS (feeding scale), NCATS (teaching scale); each has a different number of questions and observations	Not reported	Not reported
Home Observation for Measurement of the Environment (HOME)	Caldwell & Bradley (1978)	Measures home environment, and ability to support cognitive, emotional, and social systems; uses animate and inanimate environment	Observation and interview; 45 questions	Internal consistency interrater	Content, construct, criterion

- Use records to reinforce parenting skills (e.g., if parents believe that they are not good parents, point out how quickly the infant is consoled, how well the infant sleeps).
- Mobilize resources to support the parents of difficult infants, because an exhausted parent cannot cope well.
- Use a questionnaire (such as the Nursing Child Assessment Satellite Training [NCAST] feeding assessment tool, Neonatal Perception Inventory [NPI], or a practitioner-designed questionnaire) as a base for *mutual* problem-solving with the parents to develop intervention techniques and illuminate the parental role in changing or responding to their newborn's unique behavior.

If the mother is exhibiting rejection behaviors or if the infant is abused or displaying maladjustment behaviors, the practitioner should:

- Assess the infant for physical, developmental, or psychologic delays.
- Assess the parent-infant attachment.
- Explore the parents' feelings and reinforce appropriately.
- Counsel the parents, depending on what are perceived to be the causative factors.
- Draw parents out about their expectations for this child, reasons for such expectations, perceptions, and so on.
- Where appropriate, point out the infant's assets and positive attributes.
- Suggest alternative methods of achieving changes in undesirable behavior.
- Reassure parents that change is possible.
- See also Chapter 31 and the section on physical abuse and neglect in Chapter 47.

Postpartum depression in mothers is a significant behavior that could have severe adverse effects on the mother and her relationship with significant others, as well as the child's emotional and psychologic development. Key identifiers include:

- Abnormal sleep disturbances (e.g., hyposomnia, hypersomnia)
- Uncharacteristic appetite changes (e.g., anorexia, bingeing)
- Persistent personality variation that represents a change from preceding characteristic patterns
- Obvious confusion and mood changes

- Lack of affect displaying interest or pleasure
- Recent history of alcohol or substance abuse or dependence
- Display of atypical feelings of anxiety or panic
- Poor relationship or connection to own mother
- Unexpected failure to keep follow-up appointments

If an assessment tool is needed to determine postnatal depression, the Edinburgh Postnatal Depression Scale is useful. The scale is a 10-item, self-rated instrument that is easily and quickly scored. A threshold score of 12.5 has been shown to detect major depression, with a sensitivity of 100% and a specificity of 95.5%.

Follow-up. The extent of follow-up care is determined by the individual needs of the parents and infant.

Consultations and referrals. As necessary, refer parents to the following:

- Agency social worker
- Child welfare organization
- Parents Anonymous
- Adoption agency
- Counseling or psychotherapy

Environmental Assessment

Enriching an infant's environment promotes the child's development and is particularly beneficial to the infant at risk in reaching his or her full developmental potential. However, it is important that the stimuli provided for each infant be neither excessive nor deficient for that child's individual needs. Tools that may be of assistance in assessing an infant's environment and identifying problem areas are Erickson's Assessment of the Infant's Animate and Inanimate Environment and Caldwell's Home Observation for Measurement of the Environment (HOME). Research using HOME has shown that an optimal environment during a child's first year of life has a dramatic influence on that child's cognitive performance at 3 years of age. The NCAST is extremely useful in assessing the parents' sensitivity to their infant's needs and readiness cues. This tool enables the practitioner to objectively observe the mother in interaction with her infant during a feeding. (Environmental assessment tools are compared in Table 10-4.)

Environmental Management to Enhance Development

- Use observations as guidelines to provide verbal support for parents regarding their provision of appropriate and inappropriate stimuli. Parents want to know if they are doing the right things for their child.
- Encourage and reinforce parental sensitivity to the developmental needs of the infant.
- Educate parents regarding the developmental needs of the infant *based on the parents' value system* (e.g., if the parents value intelligence, stress how appropriate stimuli improve intellectual development) (see Chapter 11).
- Stress the positive aspects of the infant's development.
- Assist parents in relaxing if they are trying "too hard" to provide the right stimuli at the right time. Praise positive efforts.
- Provide anticipatory guidance in relation to safety hazards (see Chapter 14).
- If a good environment is lacking, discuss positive findings first, reinforce parenting skills, and then ask parents appropriate questions related to such areas as:
  - Have they thought about the kinds of toys they select, the variety, and so on?
  - Have they noticed how they respond to their infant?
  - Would they like to change anything about the environment, and what is their first priority for change?
  - Have they thought of ways to change the environment to benefit their child or themselves?
- Discuss setting limits and reassure parents that this is a common problem.
- Discuss parental concerns and assist parents to differentiate concerns and set priorities.
- Repeat HOME on a routine basis to monitor changes when change is recommended.
- Encourage parents to identify alternative ways of dealing with problems.

Management and Counseling for Parents with Atypical Newborns

The birth of an atypical child (a premature child or a child with an anomaly) represents loss to the parents: loss of a desired goal (i.e., delivery of a perfect newborn), loss of the fantasized "perfect" infant, loss of self-esteem, and loss of satisfaction in the birth process. This precipitates a grief response, an overwhelming sense of failure in both parents, and a subsequent crisis reaction. Since attachment cannot take place in the presence of such grief, atypical infants are at high risk of rejection by parents and siblings.

The initial reactions of parents to a premature birth or to the birth of a child with a congenital anomaly are essentially the same. However, the degree of reaction is greater in parents of infants with visible congenital defects. Mothers tend to experience two periods of pronounced anxiety; the first is immediately after birth and the second occurs when she returns home with the infant.

Initial Reactions of Parents to Premature Birth

Anxiety and guilt are the two most prominent emotional reactions of parents to the premature birth of a child (see Chapter 29). The following reactions may also be observed:
- Disbelief, shock, and disorganization
- Grief over the loss of a "perfect" baby

- Inability to absorb explanations
- Fear of being alone when seeing the child for the first time
- Impaired perceptions as a result of a high anxiety level, focusing on detail rather than on the whole (e.g., can only see only the baby's leg with an intravenous tube or the baby's heaving chest)
- Fear that touching the infant might cause the child to stop breathing and die
- Fear of leaving the hospital because if anything happens they "wouldn't be there"

Concerns of Parents of Premature Infants after the Infant's Outlook Improves

- What kind of long-term complications will there be?
- Will the infant be mentally retarded?
- Could the infant be blind?
- Will the infant ever catch up in growth and development?
- Will the baby ever be "normal"?
- Is there anything else wrong with the baby?
  Maternal anxieties and guilt. The mother may:
- Feel heightened concern over whether the baby will live
- Feel lonely and lost, "unable to do anything"
- Expect to hear at any moment that the baby has died
- Feel she is an inadequate mother or a failure because she did not carry the infant to term (or because the infant has a defect)
- Feel a loss of self-esteem
- Feel anxious and guilty that nurses care for the infant better than she does
- Worry whether the child will love her
- Feel angry that the infant "belongs" to the nurses and doctors and guilty because she feels that way
  Paternal anxieties and guilt. The father may:
- Feel guilty about his involvement in the child's prematurity or defect
- Worry about what he could have done differently
- Feel guilty because he is the father but cannot help his child
- Feel premature delivery or defects reflect on his masculinity
- Be jealous of the infant because of diminished attentions from his wife
- Fear the social stigma of the "defect," which may influence the responses of others to him
- Be concerned over an inability to meet the financial responsibility for the infant
- Feel guilty about the revulsion he feels when he sees the defect
- Fear that the mother will be unable to care for the baby at home
- Feel guilty about the revulsion the mother experiences when she sees the defect

Counseling for Parents of Premature Infants or Infants with Congenital Birth Defects

Parents of premature infants or infants with congenital birth defects experience similar levels of shock and grief. They are afraid the infant will die, and they grieve over the loss of the "perfect" baby they had desired and envisioned. However, parents of children with congenital defects may be unable "to resolve their acute grief and may progress into chronic sorrow.

Marital discord is much more pronounced after the birth of a child with a congenital birth defect than it is after a premature birth. Depending on the parents' level of emotional maturity and self-esteem, there is a great tendency to blame each other for the anomaly. In fact, more than 50% of marriages in families of children with a birth defect end in divorce within 2 years of the birth. Supportive counseling from a practitioner, or in severe cases from psychiatrists or marriage counselors, can do much to assist parents in coping with children who have birth defects.

Parental responses to an infant with congenital birth defects. The first responses are the same as those for a premature infant; then the following responses are more specific:

- Shock or disbelief, verbal and nonverbal denials, and withdrawal
- Anger (e.g., "Why did this happen to me?"), rarely directed toward the infant but sometimes turned toward others
- Grief, depression, anger turned inward, decreased self-esteem, and shame
- Constant anxiety over the cause (e.g., "What did I do to cause this?", "Maybe if I hadn't taken aspirin"
- Initial revulsion, shame, and unwillingness to "claim" the infant (e.g., no claiming behaviors, such as "He looks just like..." or "He definitely has your eyes and nose")
- Twice as much expression of interest in the infant's functional ability as in appearance
- Each new development (e.g., hospitalization, surgery) perhaps precipitating another crisis and grief response
- Fear that the child will be mentally retarded
- If parents knew of a genetic risk, a feeling of tremendous remorse (i.e., "What have we done to you?")
- Hopelessness about the future of children
- Fear of establishing a bond with the infant because the baby might die
- Escalation of maternal fear responses during the first 3 months of life
- Acute sensitivity to the attitudes of others
- Possible resentment, isolation, or alienation

Counseling parents of infants with congenital birth defects. Practitioners must be aware of their own feelings because they normally experience the same shock, disbelief, and anger as parents do. Talk to the parents *together*, assisting each to appreciate, understand, and deal with the other's feelings. Practitioners must create an environment in which parents feel free to express their feelings, both positive and negative. The practitioner should:

- Express warmth, concern, and caring (perhaps through touch, just "being there," or tears) in whatever way feels best.
- Help parents to realize that their feelings are accepted and that their feelings are normal; this relieves some guilt and hastens resolution.
- Help parents to feel they are not alone.
- Reply to hostility with understanding (e.g., "You must feel dreadfully hurt and disappointed that this has happened to you").
- Provide hope through factual information rather than reassurance with platitudes and clichés. However, if there is no hope, do not instill false hope.
- Recognize that many parents tend to blame each other for the defect.
- Recognize that parents need to proceed at their own pace. They may need to withdraw, to not see or handle their baby for a while. However, consultation is indicated if parents show little progress toward acceptance and adaptation after a reasonable period.
- Encourage parents to participate in the care of the infant as soon as possible. Facilitate this, and give constant feedback to the parents about the infant when care cannot be given by them. The feedback can be manifested as information about weight gain, what the baby looks like, the quality of feeding, what tests have been done, who is caring for the infant, what care has been given, and the baby's unique characteristics. Such information reassures the parents that care is being given and progress is being made.
- Compliment parents on positive care provided by them and reinforce parenting skills. This is particularly important after discharge.
- Assess family strengths and weaknesses and mobilize outside support (e.g., friends, relatives, church groups, community organizations) when necessary.
- After parents begin to ask questions about the defect, arrange for them to talk with other parents who have had similar experiences.
- Suggest genetic counseling and make appropriate referrals.
- If parents seem overly concerned about mental retardation, discuss it with them. Explore the ramifications. Give pointers about what to look for in infant development.
- Discuss childrearing practices. There is often little or no transference of childrearing practices suitable for the normal child to the atypical child. Special guidance or instruction from a professional may be needed.
- Inform parents about available community resources and the services they provide.
- Encourage parents to find capable babysitters. (Perhaps an older relative may want to make a contribution.) The parents need time together alone.

Resources

Pain Assessment Tools

Grunau, R. & Craig, K. (1987). Pain expression in neonates: Facial action and cry. *Pain, 28,* 395-410.

Grunau, R.V., Johnston, C.C., & Craig, K.D. (1990). Neonatal facial and cry responses to invasive and noninvasive procedures. *Pain, 42,* 295-305.

Krechel, S.W. & Bildner, J. (1995). CRIES: A neonatal postoperative pain measurement score. Initial testing of validity and reliability. *Pediatric Anesthesia, 5,* 53-61.

Lawrence, J., Alcock, D., McGrath, P., et al. (1993). The development of a tool to assess neonatal pain. *Neonatal Network, 12*(6), 59-66.

Websites

For Parents

Babycenter (www.babycenter.com)

Harriet Lane Links (www.med.jhu.edu/peds/neonatology/poi2.html)

Parentcenter (www.parentcenter.com)

Parenthood.com (www.parenthood.com)

Pediatrics at About.com (pediatrics.about.com)

Score Learning, Inc. (www.escore.com)

Working Moms Refuge (www.moms-refuge.com)

For Practitioners

American Academy of Pediatrics (www.aap.org)

The Brazelton Institute, including the Brazelton Neonatal Behavioral Assessment Scale (www.childrenshospital.org/brazelton)

The Newborn Individualized Developmental Care and Assessment Program (NIDCAP) (fhdno2.tch.harvard.edu/www/nidcap) (www.jfkpartners.org/nidcap.asp)

Bibliography

Alexander, M. & Kuo, K.N. (1997). Musculoskeletal assessment of the newborn. *Orthopedic Nursing, 16*(1), 21-31.

Als, H., Lester, B., Tronick, E., & Brazelton, T. (1982). Toward a research instrument for the assessment of preterm infants' behavior (APIB). In Fitzgerald, H., Lester, B., & Yogman, M. (Eds.). Theory and research in behavioral pediatrics (vol. 1). New York: Plenum.

Ballard, J.L., Khoury, J.C., Wedig, K., Wang, L., Eilers-Walsman, B.L., & Lipp, R. (1991). New Ballard Score, expanded to include extremely premature infants. *Journal of Pediatrics, 119*(3), 418-423.

Barlow, T.G. (1962). Early diagnosis and treatment of congenital dislocation of the hip. *Journal of Bone and Joint Surgery, 44,* 292.

Bernstein, S., Heimler, R., & Sasidharan, P. (1998). Physical assessment: Approaching the management of the neonatal intensive care unit graduate through history and physical assessment. *Pediatric Clinics of North America, 45*(1), 79-105.

Bodurtha, J. (1999). Assessment of the newborn with dysmorphic features. *Neonatal Network, 18*(2), 27-30.

Brazelton, T.B. & Nugent, J.K. (1995). *Neonatal Behavioral Assessment Scale* (3rd ed.). London: MacKeith.

Brown, G.A. & Swenson, D.R. (2000). A descriptive system for lower extremity evaluation in children: data for the newborn infant. *Orthopedics, 23*(2), 111-115.

Dodd, V. (1996). Gestational age assessment. *Neonatal Network, 15*(1), 27-36.

Epperson, C. (1999). Postpartum major depression: Detection and treatment. *American Family Physician, 59*(8), 2247-2254.

Fernbach, S.A. (1998). Common orthopedic problems of the newborn. *Nursing Clinics of North America, 33*(4), 583-594.

Fowles, E.R. (1999). The Brazelton Neonatal Behavioral Assessment Scale and maternal identity. *Maternal Child Nursing, 24*(6), 287-293.

Graham, J. (1988). *Smith's recognizable patterns of human deformation* (2nd ed.). Philadelphia: W.B. Saunders.

Hall-Johnson, S.H. (1986). *Nursing assessment and strategies for the family at risk: High-risk parenting*. Philadelphia: J.B. Lippincott.

Holditch-Davis, D. (1998). Neonatal sleep-wake states. In Kenner, C., Brueggemeyer, A., & Gunderson, L. (Eds.). *Comprehensive neonatal nursing* (2nd ed.). Philadelphia: W.B. Saunders.

Johnson-Crowley, N. (1998). Systematic assessment and home follow-up: A basis for monitoring the neonate's integration into the family unit. In Kenner, C., Brueggemeyer, A., & Gunderson, L. (Eds.). *Comprehensive neonatal nursing* (2nd ed.). Philadelphia: W.B. Saunders.

Jones, K. (1988). *Smith's recognizable patterns of human malformation* (4th ed.). Philadelphia: W.B. Saunders.

Katatwinkel, J. (2000). *Textbook of neonatal resuscitation* (4th ed.). Washington, DC: American Academy of Pediatrics and American Heart Association.

Korner, A. & Thom, V.A. (1991). *Neurobehavioral assessment of the preterm infant*. New York: The Psychological Corporation.

Lawhon, G. & Melzar, A. (1988). Developmental care of the very low birthweight infant. *Journal of Perinatal and Neonatal Nursing, 2*(1), 56-65.

Ortolani, M. (1937). Un segno poco noto e sua importanza per la diagnosi percoce de prelussazione dell'anca. *La Pediatrica, 45,* 129.

Thompson, D., Evans, J., Pitzen, K., Koch, H., & Lemon, B. (1995, March). *Comparison of tympanic, electronic and mercury in glass measures of temperature in newborn infants over 2000 grams*. Presentation at the MCN Convention. Atlanta.

Versmold, H.T., Kitterman, J.A., & Phibbs, R.H. (1981). Aortic blood pressure during the first 12 hours of life in infants with birthweights from 610 to 4220 grams. *Pediatrics, 67,* 607.

Weaver, R.H. & Cranley, M.S. (1983). An exploration of maternal-fetal attachment behavior, *Nursing Research, 32,* 68-72.

Chapter 11 *Developmental Assessment*

Margaret A. McCabe

Purpose

The early detection of a deviation in a child's pattern of development is critical to the implementation of appropriate intervention and future outcome. Therefore it is essential that primary care practitioners (PCPs) include developmental screening as a routine part of their practice. Developmental screening is easily integrated into the well-child visit and is a necessary component of providing comprehensive health care to children. The goal is to accurately assess the true state of a child's development. Systematic interview of parents and older children along with routine use of screening instruments and direct observation should provide the practitioner with appropriate information. The actions taken or not taken, based on those results, can have a significant effect on a child's future. It is important that practitioners do their best to ensure that an adequate amount of screening occurs in their practice.

A formal *developmental assessment* is an involved process requiring the input of developmental specialists. The instruments used often require formal training and reliability checks to ensure an adequate level of expertise in the use of the instrument. However, for the PCP, routine developmental screening does not need to be so complicated. *Developmental screening* in primary care practice is a simple and time-efficient mechanism to ensure adequate surveillance of a child's developmental progress. It is important to clarify the differences between developmental assessment and developmental screening, which are summarized in Table 11-1.

Instruments

Many screening instruments are available for professionals to use in clinical practice. Review of the available resources should occur with the following issues in mind: the quality of the tool, the purpose of the tool, clinical practice style, the clinical setting, and the population served. Box 11-1 summarizes the characteristics to consider when one is selecting a screening instrument.

When a screening instrument for a patient is being selected, practitioners should consider their own educational background and physical practice setting (that is, space, equipment, and financial resources). Characteristics of the patient to con-

sider include age and culture. Table 11-2 includes purchasing information for several instruments.

The domains of development a practitioner needs to assess are cognitive, motor, language, social and behavioral, and adaptive. Cognitive development begins in infancy. Examples of areas screened for cognitive development includes language skills in young children and school performance in older children. Motor development occurs at the greatest rate between birth and school age. Assessment focuses on the categories of fine motor and gross motor skills. Language development is tied to cognitive development at all ages. The theoretic foundation of language development continues to evolve. Language assessment is often broken into two categories, receptive (un-

---

Box 11-1 Characteristics to Consider When Selecting a Screening Instrument

Instrument Quality

Sensitivity—Characteristic truly present; probability that a child fails a screening when a difference in development is present

Specificity—Characteristic truly absent; probability that a child passes a screening when a difference in development in not present

Predictive value of a positive test—Probability that a child has a difference in development, given a positive test

Predictive value of a negative test—Probability that a child is developmentally appropriate, given a negative test

Clinical Utility

Child's age
Stated purpose of the screening tool according to the author's original work
Domains of development screened
Length of time to administer
Equipment necessary to administer the instrument
Cost

Table 11-1 Basic Characteristics of Developmental Screening Versus Developmental Assessment

DEVELOPMENTAL SCREENING	DEVELOPMENTAL ASSESSMENT
Detects differences or deviance in the pattern of development	Detects strengths and weaknesses in the pattern of development
Not diagnostic	Diagnostic of delay
Brief in length	Longer, focused items
Does not require formal training	Often requires formal training

Table 11-2 Purchasing Information for Frequently Used Screening Instruments

INSTRUMENT	CHILD'S AGE	TIME TO ADMINISTER	DOMAINS SCREENED	PUBLICATION INFORMATION
Battelle Developmental Inventory Screening Testz	6 months to 8 years	30+ minutes	Gross/fine motor, personal, adaptive, expressive/ receptive language, cognitive	Riverside Publishing 8420 Bryn Mawr Avenue Chicago, IL 60631 800-767-8378
Denver Articulation Exam (DASE)*	2.5 years to 6 years	5 minutes	Language	DDM Inc. PO Box 6919 Denver, CO 80206-0919
Denver II*	Birth to 6 years	15-30 minutes to administer, 5-7 minutes to score	Personal/social, fine motor/adaptive, language, gross motor	DDM Inc. PO Box 6919 Denver, CO 80206-0919
Developmental Profile II	Birth to 9.5 years	20-40 minutes	Physical, self-help, social, academic, communication	Western Psychological Services 12031 Wilshire Boulevard Los Angeles, CA 90025
Early Language Milestone (ELM)*	Birth to 36 months	5-10 minutes	Auditory expressive, auditory receptive, visual	PRO-ED, Inc. 8700 Shoel Creek Boulevard Austin, TX 78758-9867
Miller Assessment for Preschoolers	2.9 years, 9 months to 5.8 years	20-30 minutes	Sensory, motor, cognitive	Foundation for Knowledge in Development 1855 West Union Avenue Suite B-8 Englewood, CO 80110
Peabody Picture Vocabulary Test (PPVT-R)	2.5 years to 40 years	10-20 minutes	Receptive vocabulary	American Guidance Service Circle Pines, MN 55015

Copy of instrument included in Appendix A.

derstanding input) and expressive (formulating and producing output). Surveillance of language skills should begin in infancy. Behavioral assessment should combine a discussion of the child's social relationships and developmental level. Parent-child interaction directly affects socialization of young children. For older children, discerning patterns of a child's performance and participation in school and organized group activities yields useful behavioral information. A combination of screening instruments, parent and child interview, and direct observation best meet social and behavioral screening needs. Developmental milestones and warning signs are discussed in Table 11-3.

Developmental Screening Process

The screening and assessment process is based on evidence that development occurs in an orderly fashion at a predictable rate. To achieve the goal of early identification of delays, developmental screening needs to be a continuous process occurring at each well-child visit. Generally a well-child care schedule provides for approximately 12 visits by 3 years of age and then yearly through adolescence. Normal stages of human development are outlined in Table 11-4. During school age and adolescence cognitive, motor, and language milestones are occurring at a decreased rate. (Table 11-5 outlines typical milestones in language development.) During this time, behavioral and psychosocial concerns also become prominent. Table 11-6 outlines the stages of intellectual development in children and adolescents. Children who have borderline delay, produce questionable findings, or are at increased risk need to be monitored more frequently than those who do not have such conditions.

Risk Factors
Biologic
- High-risk pregnancy:
  - Prematurity
  - Postmaturity
  - Congenital disorder
  - Intrauterine substance exposure
  - Intrauterine growth delay
  - Maternal chronic illness
- Decreased Apgar scores
- Maternal age (teenage or advanced)
- Failure to thrive (FTT)
- Chronic illness
- Central nervous system (CNS) insult
- Recurrent infection

Environmental
- Family history of noncompliance with health care:
  - Poor prenatal care
  - Delayed well-child care and immunizations
- Lack of adequate supports (social and financial)
- Parental substance abuse
- Maternal depression
- Inadequate parenting skills
- Level of parent education
- Family history of child abuse or neglect
- Impaired parent-child interaction:
  - Child temperament
  - Impaired attachment
- Prolonged hospitalization

Interviewing parents to identify parental concern is an important first component in the process of developmental

Table 11-3 Developmental Milestones and Warning Signs

AGE	HIGHLIGHTS OF DEVELOPMENTAL MILESTONES (NORMAL AGE RANGE IN MONTHS)	DEVELOPMENTAL WARNING SIGNS
2 weeks	Lifts chin when prone, lies in flexed position, fixates to close objects and light	Femoral click or hip instability (through age 12 months), undue maternal anxiety (true for all ages)
2 months	Smiles, squeals, coos, follows objects with eyes past midline, regards face in direct line of vision	Persistent heart murmur, absent response to noise, failure to fix gaze on face or poor eye contact, lack of responsive smiling
4 months	Lifts head and chest from prone, smiles at others (1½-4 months), rolls over front to back, follows objects with eyes 180 degrees, grasps rattle, coos and says, "ah," plays with hands	Lack of bonding (a concern at any age), head drag, continued grasp reflex, scissoring of legs when supported under arms
6 months	Sits without support (5-8 months), transfers objects hand to hand (4½-7 months), babbles ("bababababa"), laughs, rolls both ways, bears weight, displays raking hand pattern	Failure to follow objects 180 degrees, persistent fisting, strabismus, failure to reach for objects
9 months	Bears weight, crawls, demonstrates pincer grasp (8½-12 months), uncovers hidden toy, says nonspecific "mama" or "dada," cruises holding furniture, understands "no"	Nystagmus, absence of babble, unable to sit alone
12 months	Stands alone (10-14 months), says "mama" or "dada" (9-13 months), walks well (11-15 months), says three words in addition to "mama"	Unable to transfer objects hand to hand, absence of weight bearing while held
15 months	Walks backward (12½-21½ months), self-feeds with fingers, eats with spoon, says 4 to 6 words, walks alone	Unable to pull self to stand, abnormal grasp or pincer grip
18 months	Walks up steps (14-22 months), finds hidden object (14-20 months), stacks four cubes (15-20 months), puts three words together, says 7 to 20 words	Open anterior fontanel, inability to walk alone, absence of constructive play, lack of spontaneous vocalization
24 months	Pedals tricycle (21-28 months), combines 2 words (14-24 months), says 50 words, kicks a ball forward on request	Absence of recognizable words
3 years	Uses plurals (21-36 months); balances on one foot (30-44 months); goes up stairs; knows age, name, sex; counts three objects; pedals tricycle; speaks well enough for stranger to understand	Speech unintelligible to strangers
3-6 years (preschool)	Stands 10 seconds on one foot by 5 years; by school age, knows colors, counts to 10, hops on one foot, can heel-toe walk, speaks sentences of at least 10 syllables	Inability to perform self-care tasks: handwashing, simple dressing, daytime toileting
6-12 years (school age)	Can take formal tests to assess developmental level of achievement; sexual maturation begins around 10 years in girls and 12 years in boys	School failure, aggressive behavior such as firesetting
13-18 years (adolescence)	Can use formal assessment tools to quantitate level of functioning	School absenteeism or school failure

Modified from Puls, J.E. & Osburn, A.E. (Eds.). (1996). *Oklahoma notes pediatrics (2nd ed.).* New York: Springer.

screening. Parents are often the first to identify areas of deviation in their child's growth and development. It is important to acknowledge this and weigh parental concern while one is assessing a child. As a child gets older, it becomes important to consider information from teachers and the child.

During the actual screening it is optimal to observe the child in a quiet, calm environment. This is often difficult to achieve in a clinical environment. Nonetheless, it remains a goal. The child should feel as comfortable as possible in the environment to encourage cooperation and promote optimal performance of the screening items.

If the screening leads to *normal results,* it is important to reassure the child and family, offer age-appropriate anticipatory guidance, and provide parental education. A follow-up interview on the next scheduled visit is necessary to monitor the child's progress.

If the screening leads to *abnormal results,* the next step should include educating the parents regarding the meaning of the results, scheduling a follow-up interview for rescreening as a monitoring mechanism, and possible referral for diagnostic evaluation or early intervention services. The extent of monitoring that is appropriate before referral varies and depends on the screening instrument being used, the level of expertise of the practitioner, and the level of expert support available within the ambulatory care setting. Timely and appropriate referral is vital because it may significantly affect a child's future.

Guidelines for Counseling Parents to Promote Optimal Development

Parent education focused on age-appropriate behaviors and what to expect as a child progresses to the next stage of development is known as *anticipatory guidance.* As part of anticipatory guidance, practitioners should provide parents with suggestions for parent-child activities that promote optimal development. The time parents spend interacting with their child is important. Activities can be inexpensive and convenient. Many web-based resources provide information about normal growth and development as well as recommended developmentally appropriate activities. Advise parents to follow age-appropriate recommendations when purchasing toys. Table 11-7 contains guidelines for activities to promote optimal development.

Table 11-4 Normal Stages of Human Development (Birth to 5 Years)

This table presents an overview of child development from birth to 5 years of age. It is important to keep in mind that the time frames presented are averages and that some children may achieve various developmental milestones earlier or later than the average but still be within the normal range. This information is presented to help parents understand what to expect from their child. Any questions you may have about your child's development should be shared with a physician.

PHYSICAL AND LANGUAGE	EMOTIONAL	SOCIAL
Birth to 1 Month		
Feedings: 5-8 per day	Generalized tension	Is helpless, asocial, and fed by mother
Sleep: 20 hours per day		
Sensory capacities: makes basic distinctions in vision, hearing, smelling, tasting, touch, temperature, and perception of pain		
2 to 3 Months		
Sensory capacities: color perception, visual exploration, oral exploration	Delight	Visually fixates at a face, smiles at a face, may be soothed by rocking
Sounds: cries, coos, grunts	Distress	
Motor ability: control of eye muscles, lifts head when on stomach	Smiles at a face	
4 to 6 Months		
Sensory capacities: localizes sounds	Enjoys being cuddled	Recognizes mother, distinguishes between familiar persons and strangers, no longer smiles indiscriminately
Sounds: babbling, makes most vowels and about half of the consonants		
Feedings: 3-5 per day		Expects feeding, dressing, bathing
Motor ability: control of head and arm movements, purposive grasping, rolls over		
7 to 9 Months		
Motor ability: control of trunk and hands, sits without support, crawls about	Specific emotional attachment to mother (protests separation from mother)	Enjoys "peek-a-boo"
10 to 12 Months		
Motor ability: control of legs and feet, stands, creeps, apposition of thumb and forefinger	Anger	Responsive to own name, waves bye-bye, plays pat-a-cake, understands "no-no!", gives and takes objects
Language: says one or two words, imitates sounds, responds to simple commands	Affection	
Feedings: 3 meals, 2 snacks	Fear of strangers	
Sleep: 12 hours, 2 naps	Curiosity, exploration	

From Child Development Institute. (2001, January 22). Normal stages of human development (birth to 5 years). Child Development Institute. Available online at childdevelopmentinfo.com/development/normaldevelopment.shtml.

Table 11-4 Normal Stages of Human Development (Birth to 5 Years)—cont'd

PHYSICAL AND LANGUAGE	EMOTIONAL	SOCIAL
1 to 1½ Years Motor ability: creeps up stairs, walks (10-20 minutes), makes lines on paper with crayon	Dependent behavior Very upset when separated from mother Fear of bath	Obeys limited commands, repeats a few words, interested in mirror image, feeds self
1½ to 2 Years Motor ability: runs, kicks a ball, builds 6-cube tower (2 yrs), capable of bowel and bladder control Language: vocabulary of more than 200 words Sleep: 12 hours at night, 1-2 hour nap	Temper tantrums (1-3 years) Resentment of new baby	Does opposite of what he or she is told (18 months)
2 to 3 Years Motor ability: jumps off a step, rides a tricycle, uses crayons, builds a 9- to 10-block tower Language: starts to use short sentences, controls and explores world with language, stuttering may appear briefly	Fear of separation Negativism (2½ years) Violent emotions, anger Differentiates facial expressions of anger, sorrow, and joy Sense of humor (plays tricks)	Talks, uses "I", "me", and "you", copies parents' actions, is dependent, clinging, and possessive about toys, enjoys playing alongside another child, displays negativism (2½ years), resists parental demands, gives orders, has rigid insistence on sameness of routine, inability to make own decisions
3 to 4 Years Motor ability: stands on one leg, jumps up and down, draws a circle and a cross (4 years), self-sufficient in many routines of home life.	Affectionate toward parents Pleasure in genital manipulation Romantic attachment to parent of opposite sex (3 to 5 years) Jealousy of same-sex parent Imaginary fears of dark or injury (3 to 5 years)	Likes to share, uses "we," cooperative play with other children in nursery school, imitates parents, begins identification with same-sex parent, practices sex-role activities, develops intense curiosity and interest in other children's bodies, has an imaginary friend
4 to 5 Years Motor ability: mature motor control, skips, broad-jumps, dresses self, copies a square and a triangle Language: talks clearly, uses adult speech sounds, has mastered basic grammar, relates a story, knows over 2000 words (5 years)	Responsibility and guilt Feels pride in accomplishment	Prefers to play with other children, becomes competitive, prefers sex-appropriate activities

Table 11-5 Language Development in Children

This table presents information on the typical development of language in children. There is a wide range of normal development. Most children will not follow the table to the letter. It is presented so you will know what to expect for your child. If your child seems significantly behind in language development, you should talk with your child's physician regarding your questions and concerns.

AGE OF CHILD	TYPICAL LANGUAGE DEVELOPMENT
6 months	Vocalizes with intonation
	Responds to name
	Responds to human voices without visual cues by turning head and eyes
	Responds appropriately to friendly and angry tones
12 months	Uses one or more words with meaning (may be a fragment of a word)
	Understands simple instructions, especially if vocal or physical cues are given
	Practices inflection
	Is aware of the social value of speech
18 months	Has vocabulary of approximately 5-20 words
	Vocabulary made up chiefly of nouns
	Some echolalia (repeating a word or phrase over and over)
	Much jargon with emotional content
	Is able to follow simple commands
24 months	Can name a number of objects common to surroundings
	Is able to to use at least two prepositions, usually chosen from the following: "in", "on", "under"
	Combines words into a short sentence with largely noun-verb combinations; (mean) length of sentences is given as 1.2 words
	Approximately two thirds of what child says should be intelligible
	Vocabulary of approximately 150-300 words
	Rhythm and fluency often poor
	Volume and pitch of voice not yet well-controlled
	Can use two pronouns correctly: usually "I", "me", or "you", although "me" and "I" are often confused
	"My" and "mine" are beginning to emerge
	Responds to such commands as "Show me your eyes/nose/mouth/hair"
36 months	Use pronouns "I", "you", and "me" correctly
	Is using some plurals and past tenses
	Knows at least three prepositions, usually "in", "on", "under"
	Knows chief parts of body and should be able to indicate these, if not name them
	Handles three-word sentences easily
	Uses approximately 900-1000 words
	About 90% of what child says should be intelligible
	Verbs begin to predominate
	Understands most simple questions dealing with environment and activities
	Relates experiences so that they can be followed with reason
	Able to reason out such questions as "What must you do when you are sleepy, hungry, cool, or thirsty?"
	Should be able to give sex, name, and age
	Should not be expected to answer all questions, even though child understands what is expected
48 months	Knows names of familiar animals
	Can use at least four prepositions or can demonstrate understanding of their meaning when given commands
	Names common objects in picture books or magazines

From Child Development Institute. (2001, May 20). Language development in children. *Child Development Institute. Available online at* childdevelopmentinfo.com/development/language_development.shtml.

Table 11-5 Language Development in Children—cont'd

AGE OF CHILD	TYPICAL LANGUAGE DEVELOPMENT
48 months— cont'd	Knows one or more colors Can repeat four digits when they are given slowly Can usually repeat words of four syllables Demonstrates understanding of "over" and "under" Has most vowels and dipthongs and the consonants *p, b, m, w, n* well established Often indulges in make-believe Extensive verbalization as child carries out activities Understands such concepts as "longer" and "larger", when a contrast is presented Readily follows simple commands even though the stimulus objects are not in sight Much repetition of words, phrases, syllables, and even sounds
60 months	Can use many descriptive words spontaneously (both adjectives and adverbs) Knows common opposites: big/little, hard/soft, heavy/light Has number concepts of 4 or more Can count to 10 Speech should be completely intelligible in spite of articulation problems Should have all vowels and the consonants *m, p, b, h, w, k, g, t, d, n, ng,* and *y* Should be able to repeat sentences as long as nine words Should be able to define common objects in terms of use (hat, shoe, chair) Should be able to follow three commands given without interruptions Should know his or her age Should have simple time concepts: morning, afternoon, night, day, later, after, while Should know tomorrow, yesterday, and today Should be using fairly long sentences and some compound and some complex sentences Speech on the whole should be grammatically correct
6 years	In addition to the above consonants, these should be mastered: *f, v, sh, zh, th, l* Should have concepts of 7 Speech should be completely intelligible and socially useful Should be able to tell a rather connected story about a picture while seeing relationships between objects and happenings
7 years	Should have mastered the consonants *s-z, r,* voiceless *th, ch, wh,* and the soft *g,* as in "George" Should handle opposite analogies easily: girl/boy, man/woman, flies/swims, blunt/sharp, short/long, sweet/sour Understands such terms as: alike, different, beginning, end Should be able to tell time to the quarter hour Should be able to read simple text and write or print many words
8 years	Can relate rather involved accounts of events, many of which occurred at some time in the past Complex and compound sentences should be used easily Should be few lapses in grammatical constructions, including tense, pronouns, plurals All speech sounds, including consonant blends, should be established Should be reading with considerable ease and now writing simple compositions Social amenities should be present in speech in appropriate situations Control of rate, pitch, and volume are generally well- and appropriately established Can carry on conversation at rather adult level Follows fairly complex directions with little repetition Has well-developed time and number concepts

Table 11-6 Piaget's Stages of Cognitive Development

DEVELOPMENTAL STAGE (APPROXIMATE AGE)	CHARACTERISTIC BEHAVIOR
Sensory motor period (0-24 months)	None
Reflexive stage (0-2 months)	Simple reflex activity (e.g., grasping, sucking)
Primary circular reactions (2-4 months)	Reflexive behaviors occur in stereotyped repetition (e.g., opening and closing fingers repetitively)
Secondary circular reactions (4-8 months)	Repetition of actions to reproduce interesting consequences (e.g., kicking one's feet to move a mobile suspended over the crib)
Coordination of secondary reactions (8-12 months)	Responses coordinated into more complex sequences; actions take on an "intentional" character (e.g., infant reaches behind a screen to obtain a hidden object)
Tertiary circular reactions (12-18 months)	Discovery of new ways to produce the same consequence or obtain the same goal (e.g., infant may pull a pillow toward him in an attempt to get a toy resting on it)
Invention of new means through mental combination (18-24 months)	Evidence of an internal representation system; symbolizes the problem-solving sequence before actually responding; deferred imitation
Preoperational period (2-7 years)	
Preoperational phase (2-4 years)	Increased use of verbal representation, but speech is egocentric; beginnings of symbolic rather than simple motor play, transductive reasoning; can think about something without the object being present through use of language
Intuitive phase (4-7 years)	Speech becomes more social, less egocentric; has an intuitive grasp of logical concepts in some areas; still a tendency to focus attention on one aspect of an object while ignoring others; concepts formed are crude and irreversible; easy to believe in magical increase, decrease, disappearance; reality not firm; perceptions dominate judgment
	In moral-ethical realm, not able to show principles underlying best behavior; rules of a game not developed; only uses simple *dos* and *don'ts* imposed by authority
Period of concrete operations (7-11 years)	Evidence of organized, logical thought; ability to perform multiple classification tasks, order objects in a logical sequence, and comprehend the principle of conservation; thinking becomes less transductive and less egocentric; capable of concrete problem-solving
	Some reversibility now possible (quantities moved can be restored, such as in arithmetic: $3 + 4 = 7$ and $7 - 4 = 3$)
	Can class logic-finding bases to sort unlike objects into logical groups; previously sorting was on superficial perceived attributes such as color; categoric labels such as "number" or "animal" now available
Period of formal operations (11-15 years)	Thought becomes more abstract, incorporating the principles of formal logic; ability to generate abstract propositions, multiple hypotheses, and their possible outcomes evident; thinking becomes less tied to concrete reality
	Formal logical systems can be acquired; can handle proportions, algebraic manipulation, other purely abstract processes (e.g., if $a + b = x$ then $x = a - b$)
	Prepositional logic; as-if and if-then steps; can use aids such as axioms to transcend human limits on comprehension

From Child Development Institute. (2001, May 20). *Stages of intellectual development in children and teenagers. Child Development Institute.* Available online at childdevelopmentinfo.com/development/piaget.shtml.

Table 11-7 Guidelines for Counseling Parents to Promote Optimal Development

AGE OF CHILD	ACTIVITY
Birth to 3 months	Play soft music.
	Read books, tell stories, talk to baby.
	Use soft touch and infant massage.
	Pictures with bold black or red on white background are easy for infants to focus on and provide visual stimulation.
3-12 months	Brightly colored toys that are easy for child to handle should be kept within reach of child.
	Toys should be large enough so that they can be mouthed without danger of swallowing or small parts breaking off.
	Change child's position throughout the day to encourage a variety of experiences while interacting with the environment.
	Continue talking and reading to child and providing auditory stimulation with music.
12-18 months	Encourage activities that provide a variety of sensory motor experiences; characteristics to consider include visual stimulation, auditory/verbal stimulation, and tactile stimulation; these experiences can be provided in activites related to eating, play, dressing, and household activities.
	Provide activities that encourage the use of evolving gross motor skills; at this stage, providing a safe environment for child becomes much more challenging than in the previous months.
	Continue talking and reading to child and providing auditory stimulation with music.
18-24 months	Encourage activities that promote a sense of independence.
	Provide opportunities for continued motor development; focus on both gross motor and fine motor skills.
	Encourage appropriate behaviors by paying attention to child and praising child when the child engages in acceptable behaviors.
24-36 months	Begin activities that provide contact and interaction with other children.
	Encourage activities that promote language development: reading and telling stories, vocalization in play.
	Provide activities that promote a sense of autonomy.
	Encourage activities that allow child to imitate a parent and be involved in carrying out a task.
	Encourage activities that promote fine motor skills and increasing manual dexterity: drawing, coloring, simple puzzles, large blocks.
3-5 years	Provide opportunities to begin using imagination in play: dress up, stories, group play, puppets.
	Encourage use of curiosity, creativity, and memory through memory games, storytelling, exposure to environment (animals, nature, people).
	Encourage social and structured interactions with other children.
	Provide child opportunities to make choices related to activities.
	Give opportunity for motor activity and free play.
	At this age children find task-oriented activities enjoyable.
	Monitor information and experiences child is exposed to through television, other children, and group activities.
6-10 years	Peer group experiences become important, including structured group activities with a common group goal: team sports, social groups, boys' club, girls' club, community organizations.
	Provide structured, systematic support for skill development: supervised time to complete homework, participation in activities in the home (e.g., baking, grocery shopping, planning special events).
	Encourage recreational reading.
	Provide opportunities for active gross motor experiences to improve muscle coordination.
11-14 years	Encourage activities to promote sense of self (self-confidence, self-esteem) and increased independence.
	Promote activities that build on individual strengths: music, writing, arts and crafts, sports, dance.
	Engage child in abstract conversation.
	Give firm, direct support encouraging responsible social behaviors; give simple concrete choices.

Resources

Websites
For Parents
Brilliant Beginnings (www.brilliantbeginnings.com)
The National Academy for Child Development (www.nacd.org/resources)
For Parents and Professionals
American Academy of Pediatrics (www.aap.org)
Bright Futures (www.brightfutures.com)
Child Development Institute (www.cdipage.com)
Zero to Three (www.zerothree.org)

Bibliography

Dworkin, P. (1989). British and American recommendations for developmental monitoring: The role of surveillance. *Pediatrics*, *84*(5), 1000-1010.

King-Thomas, L. & Hacker, B. (1987). *A therapist's guide to pediatric assessment.*, Boston: Little, Brown & Co.

Parker, S. & Zuckerman, B. (2001). *Behavioral and developmental pediatrics* (2nd ed.). Boston: Little, Brown & Co.

Chapter 12 *Screening Tests*

Barbara Jones Deloian

Purpose of Screening Tests

Screening is a first level of testing that identifies individuals at risk for specific problems in a broad range of health and development. As a result of screening, further specific assessment can be completed to verify the screening results and determine the need for further treatment. Screening tests usually can be done by paraprofessionals with less training than is needed for diagnostic testing. The use of screening tests has come under increasing scrutiny as the cost effectiveness of health care services and procedures is evaluated. In the past, practitioners have recognized that the history provides approximately 80% to 85% and the physical examination 10% to 15% of important data used in making a diagnosis. Thus screening tests may supply only 5% of the information used in making a diagnosis. Screening tests are valuable, however, in providing a rapid and inexpensive measure to determine who is at risk for a specific problem. Those who are identified with a "positive" screening test may then undergo the more expensive and time-consuming diagnostic testing.

Usefulness of Screening Tests

Frame and Carlson (1975) have identified the following circumstances that must exist for screening tests to be useful:
- The condition must have a significant effect on the quality and quantity of life.
- Acceptable methods of treatment must be available.
- The condition must have an asymptomatic period during which detection and treatment significantly reduce morbidity and mortality.
- Treatment in the asymptomatic phase must yield a therapeutic result superior to that obtained by delaying treatment until symptoms appear.
- Tests that are acceptable to patients must be available, at a reasonable cost, to detect the condition in the asymptomatic period.
- The incidence of the condition must be sufficient to justify the cost of screening.

Sensitivity, Specificity, and Positive Predictive Value

When determining how and when different screening tests should be performed, one should use the concepts of sensitivity, specificity, and positive predictive value. The U.S. Preventive Services Task Force (1996) describes the terms as follows:
- *Sensitivity*—The proportion of persons *with a condition* who test positive when screened. A test with poor sensitivity may miss many individuals who have the condition by showing a large number of false-negative results.
- *Specificity*—The proportion of persons *without a condition* who correctly test negative when screened. A test with poor specificity reports that healthy individuals actually have disease. These are false-positive results.

- *Positive predictive value* (PPV)—The proportion of individuals with a positive test who actually have the condition confirmed. This is related to the prevalence of the disease in the population and the specificity of the test. Because most target conditions for screening are uncommon and most screening tests do not have perfect specificity, the PPV of most screening tests is between 10% and 30%.

Thus many patients with positive screening tests *do not have the disease.* This explains why it is very important to carefully consider the selection of the tests and counseling of parents and children to avoid unnecessary, potentially harmful testing and anxiety.

Principles of Screening

In addition to the circumstances under which screening tests should be used and the concepts of sensitivity, specificity, and PPV, other basic principles must be considered in performing screening tests. These include:
- There is no purpose in performing screening tests without close, consistent tracking and needed follow-up testing. This involves a concerted team effort to track the results, making sure that current patient and family addresses, phone numbers, and message numbers are in the file and providing necessary follow-up.
- Any testing that is done must adhere to the specified standards of training, quality control, testing, and reporting results. The sensitivity and specificity of the tests are only as reliable as the individuals who are conducting the tests.
- Parents and children must be clearly informed of the potential cost and morbidity of the necessary follow-up testing and treatment. Some clinics and centers require informed consent before administering screening tests.
- Consideration should be made for the cultural context of care and the standards of practice in different geographic areas and ethnic backgrounds (e.g., the use of the bacille Calmette-Guérin [BCG] in Mexico and its effect on tuberculin skin testing, the increase in early discharge, the need to repeat phenylketonuria [PKU] screening tests).

Types of Screening Tests
Measurements

Purpose. Routine weight and height measurements are necessary for monitoring a child's rate of growth, failure in growth, or acceleration in growth. A series of accurate measurements, rather than a single measurement, is needed to determine growth trends. Changes in growth are often the first indication of other health problems.

Technique. Measurements must be taken carefully and accurately. Equipment must be in good working order (such as scales being calibrated) and checked regularly against standard measures. All staff should understand the significance of accurate measurements. Measurement should be recorded on a growth chart and rechecked if there is any discrepancy with previous measurements. The percentiles also should be tracked for consistency. Refer to the Centers for Disease Control (CDC), National Center for Health Statistics for updated growth charts, education and training materials, and instructions for calculating body mass index (BMI).

Length and height. Infants and toddlers up to 2 years of age should have their length measured using a fixed measurement board. Marks made on the examination table paper do not provide accurate, consistent results. Children over 2 years of age should always have their height measured with their shoes off.

Weight. Infant weights should be obtained without clothing or a diaper. Children should have consistent clothing when weighed.

Head circumference. A metal or firm tape should be used to measure the broadest part of the head, over the forehead and occipital protuberance. For the greater accuracy, at least two measurements should be taken and three measurements if different.

Body mass index. BMI is another screening tool that is age and gender specific for children. The advantages are that it tracks childhood weight into adulthood, provides a reference for adolescents, and is consistent with adult standards so that it can be used continuously through adulthood. BMI for age is the recommended method for screening overweight and underweight. The formula is: Weight (lb) / [Height (in)]^2 x 703.

Interpretation. During the first 6 months, infants usually follow a fairly standard growth curve. After 6 months changes in growth patterns begin to occur as children assume their own curve based on their parents' stature and nutritional or health conditions. Any changes of two percentiles above the 90th percentile or below the 5th percentile should be followed closely. The stature or hat size (head circumference) of both biologic parents should be determined when concerns arise about the growth curve or head circumference. Follow-up findings for other health problems should be investigated.

Vital Signs

Purpose. Vital signs provide an important indication of the health of the child. Usually the pulse and respirations are measured at each routine visit to establish a baseline value. After 3 years of age the blood pressure (BP) is measured at each well-child visit to screen for hypertension. Premature infants should have their BP measured earlier at their routine visits. Temperatures are usually not taken at each visit but should be considered when immunizations are being given or for each illness visit.

Technique. Because of the routine nature of vital signs, accuracy can become compromised as a result of careless technique. Standardization is important for accurate results. Equipment also should be monitored for infection control and accuracy. Stethoscopes should be cleaned regularly with alcohol.

Interpretation. Vital signs readings should be interpreted along with the child's history, physical examination, and other diagnostic tests.

Laboratory Tests

Blood tests

Newborn screening. In 1962 Dr. Robert Guthrie introduced a technique to screen for PKU using three or four drops of blood on filter paper. This allowed for the collection of blood from newborns on a large-scale basis. Since then it has be-

come possible to screen for many other serious and lethal disorders; newborn screening is no longer just "the PKU test." Currently all states require or offer voluntary initial screening for PKU and congenital hypothyroidism. Some states also require repeat PKU testing because of problems of accuracy with early discharge of newborns after delivery. The requirements for other newborn screening tests vary according to state law. Newborn screening tests are outlined in Table 12-1.

Other newborn screening tests that have been developed include those for tyrosinemia, cystic fibrosis, and toxoplasmosis.

Coombs test

Purpose. A Coombs test is done on the newborn when there is concern about ABO or Rh incompatibility. It measures Rh and other blood type factors.

Interpretation. The Coombs test is read on a scale of 1 to 4. A negative, or normal, reading indicates a complete lack of agglutination or incompatibility. A positive, or abnormal, reading is seen in erythroblastosis fetalis. The higher reading indicates a greater chance of incompatibility and subsequent problems.

Glucose

Purpose. The test measures glucose levels in infants or children.

Hypoglycemia. The incidence varies from 4% to 11.4% depending on the criteria used. Generally criteria include less than 30 mg/dL in low-birth–weight infants and 40 mg/dL in full-term infants. Hypoglycemia is associated with irritability, lethargy, limpness, high-pitched cry, difficulty feeding, sweating, apnea, cyanosis, tremors, and convulsions. It may also be associated with hypocalcemia or polycythemia. Infants of diabetic mothers who are usually large for gestational age may require glucose testing because of symptoms associated with hypoglycemia.

Bilirubin

Purpose. Bilirubin is the byproduct of the hemoglobin destroyed in the liver. Hyperbilirubinemia is one of the most common conditions in full-term infants, with 60% of newborns clinically jaundiced. Total serum bilirubin (TSB) levels include both the direct (conjugated) and indirect (unconjugated) bilirubin fractions. The specific levels of each help determine the possible cause of the hyperbilirubinemia. Serum bilirubin is monitored to prevent kernicterus, which occurs when unconjugated bilirubin enters the nerve cells and produces cell death. The clinical assessment of jaundice should be done in a well-lighted room by blanching the skin with finger pressure. The underlying color of the skin and subcutaneous tissue will be seen. Dermal icterus is observed first in the face (sclerae, nose, and gums), progressing to the chest, trunk, and extremities. All neonates discharged from the hospital within 48 hours of birth should be seen by their health care provider within 2 to 3 days of discharge to be evaluated for jaundice. Infants who experience abnormal difficulty in awakening, feeding difficulty, behavior changes, apnea, or temperature instability should be closely monitored and evaluated. Approximately one-third healthy breast-fed infants may have jaundice that persists after 2 weeks. Dark urine or light stools should prompt evaluation of the TSB. An infant's risk factors (ABO incompatibility), prematurity, weight, age, clinical assessment, and behavior provide guidance for obtaining the TSB (Table 12-2).

Interpretation. High levels of direct (conjugated) bilirubin require further evaluation for more pathologic causes of the jaundice. Indirect (unconjugated) bilirubin levels greater than or equal to 20 mg/dL have the potential to cause neurotoxic effects on an infant's brain development.

Table 12-1 Disorders Commonly Screened for in Newborns

DISORDER	DESCRIPTION	INCIDENCE	SYMPTOMS	TREATMENT
Phenylketonuria (PKU)	Enzyme that converts phenylaline to tyrosine is missing. This is an autosomal recessive aminoacidopathy.	1:10,000 to 1:25,000 live births	Severe, irreversible mental retardation.	With optimal dietary restriction of phenylalanine, most children achieve a normal range of intelligence. Female patients must be followed and require dietary considerations and close monitoring when they become pregnant.
Hypothyroidism	Hypoplastic or dysfunctional thyroid gland.	1:3600 to 1:5000 live births	Leads to irreversible mental retardation, differing levels of growth failure, deafness, and certain neurologic problems that make up the syndrome of cretinism.	Infants who are adequately treated with thyroxine within the first weeks of life are reported to have normal or near-normal IQ when tested at 4 to 7 years of age.
Galactosemia	Lack of or low level of enzyme that converts galactose into glucose.	1:60,000 to 1:80,000 live births	Failure to thrive, vomiting, liver disease, cataracts, and irreversible mental retardation.	Dietary restrictions of galactose-containing foods (e.g., milk) leads to significant improvement, and all clinical features may improve, including intelligence.
Hemoglobinopathies	Carriers are genetic heterozygotes and do not have significant symptoms.	Screening for these diseases includes such conditions as sickle cell anemia, thalassemia, and hemoglobin E. Often the screening is targeted to those individuals of African, Mediterranean, Asian, Caribbean, and South and Central American background.	Problems that may be seen when not identified early include overwhelming sepsis, chronic hemolytic anemia, spasmodic vascular occlusive crises, hyposplenism, periodic splenic sequestration, and bone marrow aplasia.	When identified early, infants with sickle cell disease benefit from prompt intervention for infections and prevention of sequestration crises.

Condition	Description	Incidence	Clinical features	Treatment
Maple syrup urine disease (MSUD)	Enzyme needed to metabolize leucine, isoleucine, and valine is low or absent.	1:250,000 to 1:400,000 live births	Acidosis may occur, causing hypertonicity, vomiting, drowsiness, apnea, and coma. Infant death or severe mental retardation and neurologic and behavioral problems may occur without treatment.	Treatment includes a diet low in leucine, isoleucine, and valine.
Homocystinuria	Deficiency of the enzyme cystothionine synthase, which is needed for cystothionine metabolism.	1:50,000 to 1:150,000 live births	Problems of mental retardation, seizures, behavior disorders, early onset thromboses, dislocated lenses, and tall lanky body are the recognized associated symptoms.	Treatment includes a methionine-restricted diet, cystine supplement, and vitamin B_6 supplement if responsive.
Congenital adrenal hyperplasia (CAH)	21-Hydroxylase enzyme defect.	1:12,000 to 1:20,000 live births	This illness is characterized by hyponatremia, hypokalemia, hypoglycemia, dehydration, and early death because of a defect in the 21-hydroxylase enzyme. Females may have ambiguous genitalia, and progressive virilization may be seen in both males and females.	Corticosteroid replacement and corrective surgery is the treatment when identified early.
Biotinidase deficiency	Low activity of the biotinidase enzyme causes biotin deficiency.	1:72,000 to 1:126,000 live births	Mental retardation, seizures, ataxia, skin rashes, hearing loss, alopecia, optic nerve atrophy, coma, and death.	Treatment is daily administration of biotin.
Cystic fibrosis (CF)	An autosomal recessive disorder characterized by generalized disturbance in exocrine function related to a abnormal transmembrane regulator protein that has properties of a chloride channel.	1:2000 Northern European live births 1:17,000 African-American live births 1:9000 Hispanic live births	Poor growth, with chronic respiratory infections, malabsorption, and gastrointestinal abnormalities.	Improved parenteral and oral nutrition, fat-soluble vitamin supplements, predigested formula, and pancreatic enzyme replacement enable more normal growth. Pulmonary treatments may also be done.
Tyrosinemia	Elevated levels of tyrosine.	Higher in preterm infants but not established	Mild retardation and linguistic delays to acute failure to thrive (FTT), vomiting, diarrhea, hepatomegaly, and ensuing liver disease with death.	Dietary restrictions, liver transplantation, and close follow-up observations are needed.
Toxoplasmosis	Protozoan infection that causes no symptoms in the newborn.	1:1000 to 1:8000 live births	Blindness and mental retardation.	Early treatment may be effective in interrupting the acute disease that progresses to damaging vital organs.

Updated from American Academy of Pediatrics Committee on Genetics. (1996). Newborn screening fact sheets. Pediatrics, 98(3), 473-501.

Table 12-2 Management of the Healthy Newborn with Hyperbilirubinemia

HOURS OF AGE	TOTAL SERUM BILIRUBIN LEVELS, MG/DL (PMOL/L)			
	PHOTOTHERAPY CONSIDERED	PHOTOTHERAPY	EXCHANGE TRANSFUSION IF PHOTOTHERAPY FAILS	EXCHANGE TRANSFUSION AND PHOTOTHERAPY
< 24	—	—	—	—
25–48	> 12 (170)	> 15 (260)	> 20 (340)	> 25 (430)
49–72	> 15 (260)	> 18 (310)	> 25 (430)	> 30 (510)
> 72	> 17 (290)	> 20 (340)	> 25 (430)	> 30 (510)

Adapted from American Academy of Pediatrics, Provisional Committee for Quality Improvement Subcommittee on Hyperbilirubinemia. (1994). Management of hyperbilirubinemia in the healthy term newborn. Pediatrics, 94(4), 558-565.

Table 12-3 Blood Lead Levels in Children

BOOD LEAD LEVELS (μg/dl)	TYPE	CONFIRMATION OF BLOOD LEAD LEVEL TEST	INTERPRETATION OF BLOOD LEAD LEVELS
< 9	I	Screen only	No lead poisoning. No action needed
10–14	IIA	1 month	If still elevated, provide education to decrease lead exposure. Repeat the test in 3 months. Communities with a large proportion of children in this range should undergo community screening.
15–19	IIB	1 month	If still elevated, assess the environment carefully. Provide education to decrease lead exposure. Repeat the test in 2 months.
20–44	III	1 week	If still in this range, the child needs complete medical evaluation (e.g., detailed environmental history, nutritional assessment, physical examination) and follow-up observation. Provide education to decrease lead exposure and lead absorption. Either refer patient to health department (local) or provide case management services (includes detailed environmental investigation with lead hazard reduction and appropriate referrals for support services). If the level is > 25 μg/dl, consider chelation after consultation with clinicians experienced in lead toxicity treatment; chelation therapy is not currently recommended for levels < 45 μg/dl.
45–69	IV	2 days	If still in this range, the child needs complete medical evaluation (e.g., detailed environmental history, nutritional assessment, physical examination) and follow-up observation. Provide education to decrease lead exposure and lead absorption. Either refer patient to health department (local) or provide case management services (includes detailed environmental investigation with lead hazard reduction and appropriate referrals for support services). Begin chelation therapy in consultation with clinicians experienced in lead toxicity therapy.
> 70	V	Immediate	Child should be admitted to the hospital and begin immediate treatment in consultation with clinicians experienced in lead toxicity therapy. The rest of the care should be as noted for management of children with levels between 45 and 69 μg/dl.

Adapted from American Academy of Pediatrics, Committee on Environmental Health. (1998). Screening for elevated blood lead levels. Pediatrics, 101(6), 1072-1078.

Hemoglobin and hematocrit

Purpose. The purpose is to evaluate for anemia or polycythemia. Hemoglobin refers to the amount of hemoglobin (protein) within each red blood cell (RBC). The hematocrit compares the packed RBC volume and the volume of the whole blood. It does not provide information about the quality of the RBCs.

Interpretation. Some children with anemia have enough RBCs but not enough hemoglobin in each cell. Therefore it is often important to know both the hemoglobin and the hematocrit. It is important to consider birth weight or prematurity and the age of the child when one is interpreting normal ranges. The practitioner needs to know the norms for the state and laboratory or equipment used to test the blood. High altitudes and smoking may affect the norms as well.

Polycythemia is defined for term infants as a venous hematocrit level greater than 65%. This level may spontaneously drop within 6 to 18 hours of age. Anemia is defined as a venous hematocrit value greater than 2 standard deviations below the mean, or a value below 46%.

Technique. The first drop of blood should be wiped off and not used. Also, the site should be allowed to dry after an antiseptic was used. The finger or leg should not be "milked" to obtain the blood sample. Proper technique is required to avoid altering the test results.

Lead screening

Purpose. The screening identifies children at risk for lead poisoning, which is a common, yet preventable, childhood environmental health problem.

Interpretation. Refer to Table 12-3, and also note the following ranges:

- *Greater than 10 mg/dl*—About 2.2 % of all children under 6 years of age may have blood lead levels greater than 10 mg/dl. A decrease attributed to removal of lead from gasoline, paint, and food cans has been noted.

Table 12-4 Questions for Evaluating Lead Risk Exposure

SCREENING QUESTIONS	YES/NO
1. Does your child live in or regularly visit a house (perhaps of a friend or relative), day care center, or preschool built before 1950 that contains peeling or chipping paint?	
2. Does your child live in or regularly visit a house built before 1978 that is being renovated or remodeled or has been renovated or remodeled within the last 6 months?	
3. Does your child have a sibling or playmate who has or did have lead poisoning?	
4. Does your child live with an adult whose job or hobby involves exposure to lead? (Examples include those who work with ceramics, furniture refinishing, and stained glass.)	
5. Does your child live near an active lead smelter, battery recycling plant, or other industry likely to release lead?	
6. Has your child used any home or folk remedies in the past year? (Examples include Azarcon, Greta, Pay-loo-ah, Coral, Bali Goli, Rueda, and Alarcon.)	
7. Do you cook or serve food in clay pots or dishes made outside the United States?	
8. Do you live close to a heavily traveled highway or truck route?	
9. Do you live in an area where there is lead in the water supply (e.g., in well water)?	

Based on information from American Academy of Pediatrics, Committee on Environmental Health. (1998). Screening for elevated blood lead levels. Pediatrics, 101(6), 1072-1078; Centers for Disease Control and Prevention. (1997). Screening young children for lead poisoning. Guidance for state and local public health officials. Atlanta: U.S. Department of Health and Human Services, Public Health Service.

- *10 to 14 mg/dl*—This level is associated with impaired neurobehavioral development, diminished intelligence, decreased hearing acuity, and growth inhibition. Higher rates may be found in low-income, inner-city children. No racial, ethnic, socioeconomic, or geographic area can be excluded from screening.
- *Above 20 mg/dl*—This level is associated with severe damage to the central nervous, renal, and hematopoietic systems.

Technique. Universal screening is recommended in areas where 27% or more of the housing was built before 1950 and in populations where the percentage of 1- and 2-year-olds with elevated blood lead levels is 12% or more. For all other children, screening should be targeted based on risk-assessment during specified pediatric visits. When one is using a risk assessment (Table 12-4), any child who answers *yes* to any of the questions is considered at risk and should receive lead screening and monitoring on a regular basis. Screening usually begins at 12 months of age.

Cholesterol

Purpose. Universal cholesterol screening of children is not generally recommended. Screening is recommended for children with a family history of premature cardiovascular disease or if the family history is unknown and risk factors for coronary artery disease are present (Box 12-1).

Interpretation. There are no long-term studies of the correlation of blood cholesterol levels measured in childhood to coronary heart disease in later life. Therefore the relationship has been inferred. Dietary interventions are the treatment of choice for children. No definitive research is available regarding the safety and effectiveness of treating high cholesterol levels in childhood to prevent coronary artery disease in adulthood. (Refer also to Table 12-5.)

Hemoglobinopathies

Purpose. Hemoglobinopathy tests are used to identify individuals who have genetic disorders that may affect the production and function of hemoglobin. Sickle cell disease, sickle cell trait, and thalassemias are included. Universal screening of all newborns for sickle cell disease is now recommended.

Box 12-1 Selective Screening Criteria for Cholesterol

Children whose parents or grandparents, at less than 55 years of age, underwent diagnostic coronary arteriography and were found to have coronary atherosclerosis (includes those who have undergone balloon angioplasty or coronary artery bypass surgery)

Children whose parents or grandparents, at less than 55 years of age, had documented myocardial infarction, angina pectoris, peripheral vascular disease, cerebrovascular disease, or sudden cardiac death

Children of parents with an elevated blood cholesterol level (240 mg/dl or higher)

Children whose parental history is unobtainable, particularly for those with other risk factors.

Optional cholesterol screening may be appropriate for children at a higher risk independent of their family histories (e.g., teens who smoke, are overweight, consume large amounts of saturated fats and cholesterol).

Adapted from American Academy of Pediatrics, Committee on Nutrition. (1998). Cholesterol in childhood. Pediatrics, 101(1), 141-147.

Hemoglobin electrophoresis. Electophoresis identifies both affected individuals and carriers.

Technique. Hemoglobinopathies are identified by electrophoresis, which is considered very accurate in differentiating among hemoglobin disorders.

Urine tests

Urinalysis

Purpose. Urinalysis identifies abnormalities in the urine, including glucose, ketones, protein, red and white blood cells, nitrites, and leukocyte esterase. Positive results may indicate metabolic problems, dehydration, renal disease, infection, trauma, or secondary response to chemicals or drugs. The value of a urinalysis in nonsymptomatic children remains controversial but is warranted in symptomatic children for the diagnosis

Table 12-5   Classification of Total and Low-Density Lipoprotein Cholesterol Levels in Children

CATEGORY	TOTAL CHOLESTEROL (MG/DL)	LDL CHOLESTEROL (MG/DL)	REEVALUATION	INTERVENTION
Acceptable	< 170	< 110	5 years	Provide education on eating patterns recommended for all children and adolescents and on other risk factors.
Borderline	170-199	110-129	1 year	Provide advice about risk factors for cardiovascular disease. Start the American Heart Association (AHA) Step-One diet and other risk factor interventions.
High	> 200	> 130	Examination for secondary causes, including thyroid, liver, or renal disorders	Screen all family members. Start the AHA One Step diet, followed by the Two-Step diet if needed.

Adapted from American Academy of Pediatrics, Committee on Nutrition. (1998). Cholesterol in childhood. Pediatrics, 101(1), 141-147.

Box 12-2 Risk Factors for Tuberculosis in Children in the United States

TB is prevalent in children who:
- Are from families with a suspected or confirmed case of TB or a history of TB
- Have radiographic findings or clinical findings suggestive of TB
- Have present or past contact with adults who are or were residents of countries where there is or was a high prevalence of TB
- Have present or past contact with adults who are or have been residents of correctional facilities or long-term care facilities
- Were born or resided in countries with a high prevalence of TB
- Live in areas considered to be high-risk communities or neighborhoods
- Are in foster care
- Are homeless
- Are children of migrant farm workers
- Who are institutionalized or incarcerated
- Are children of parents or families with a history of intravenous or other drug abuse
- Are users of intravenous or other drugs
- Have HIV
- Live in a household with an HIV-infected person

TB screening may be used as a baseline before any child begins immunosuppressive therapy. Children with other medical conditions, including malnutrition, failure to thrive (FTT), diabetes, chronic renal failure, congenital or acquired immunodeficiencies do not need routine TB screening *unless* they have had recent exposure to infected family members or other individuals or come into contact with such individuals

Adapted from American Academy of Pediatric, Committee on Infectious Disease. (1996). Update on tuberculosis skin testing of children. Pediatrics, 97(2), 282-284; Hoekelman, R.A., Adam, H.M., Nelson, N.M., Weitzman, M.L., & Willson, M.H. (Eds.). (2001). Primary care pediatrics (4th ed.). St Louis: Mosby; Pickering, L.K. (Ed.). (2000). 2000 Red book: Report of the Committee on Infectious Diseases (25th ed.). Elk Grove Village, IL: American Academy of Pediatrics.

and management of pathologic conditions. Currently the recommendations for healthy children include a single urinalysis before school entry and again during adolescence. If the results are positive, the urinalysis should be repeated once or twice more before an extensive evaluation is completed. Microscopic evaluation should then be considered for confirmation.

Screening for evidence of infection, such as white blood cells and bacteria, may result in the most effective screening for treatment. Screening for RBCs and protein is usually not so useful because of the transiency of the conditions that cause them. Glucosuria is also of questionable usefulness because of the variation of the renal thresholds and the rapid onset of the symptoms of diabetes mellitus after glucosuria.

Interpretation. The leukocyte esterase dipstick test has good sensitivity and specificity for bacteremia. The nitrate test is inadequate for screening purposes because of low sensitivity (30%), but it does have high specificity (99%) for significant bacteriuria. The current goal of screening is identification of bacteriuria or renal disease in infants and young children (infants: males, 2.8%, females, 0.9%; toddlers and preschoolers: males, 0.1%, females, 1% to 2%). It is also recommended to identify asymptomatic sexually transmitted diseases (STDs), such as that caused by *Chlamydia trachomatis,* in adolescents and young adults (males, 6% to 11%).

Technique. The method of obtaining the urine determines the accuracy of the screening urinalysis. Usually the first voided specimen of the day, which is more concentrated, contains higher amounts of bacteria and bacterial breakdown material. Later voids may be more practical and are acceptable. Midstream urine specimens are generally the most desirable, except when males for STDs are being screened. The first 15 to 20 ml of a void should be used. Cleansing with a mild soap solution is very important to avoid contamination. Antiseptic solutions should not be used because of the possibility of suppressing bacterial growth. Male cultures for *Chlamydia* or *Gonococcus* organisms should be completed before voiding or done at least 1 hour after voiding. The technique for obtaining a urine specimen from infants and toddlers requires bagged urine collection after the area is cleaned well. After the area is allowed to dry thoroughly, the bag is secured in place. The urine should be tested as soon as collected.

Skin tests
Tuberculin skin testing

Purpose. Tuberculin skin testing is now focused on children who are at increased risk for acquiring tuberculosis (TB). Routine testing of low-risk populations has not been considered an efficient use of health care resources. Those children who have no risk factors and live in areas of low prevalence do not need routine tuberculin screening. The current criteria for identifying children at risk is identified in Box 12-2. The Mantoux test,

Table 12-6 Definition of Positive Mantoux Skin Test (Purified Protein Derivative)

PPD RESULTS	RECOMMENDED INTERPRETATION FOR POSITIVE RESULTS*
5-10 mm	Children in close contact with persons who have known or suspected infectious cases of TB: • Households with active or previously active cases if: (1) treatment cannot be verified as adequate before exposure, (2) treatment was initiated after period of child's contact, or (3) reactivation is suspected Children suspected to have TB disease: • Chest roentgenogram consistent with active or previously active TB • Clinical evidence of TB[†] Children with immunosuppressive conditions or HIV infection[‡]
10-15 mm	Children younger than 4 years of age Children with increased environmental exposure (e.g., those born in [or to parents who come from or were born in] regions of the world where TB is highly prevalent Children in close contact with high-risk adults (adults who are infected with HIV, homeless people, users of intravenous and other street drugs, poor and medically indigent city dwellers, residents of nursing homes, incarcerated or institutionalized persons, and migrant farm workers) Children or adults who are residents of institutions, prisons, or nursing homes in which many persons are living Children with medical risk factors, including Hodgkin's disease, lymphoma, diabetes mellitus, chronic renal failure, and malnutrition
> 15 mm	Children 4 years of age and older without *any* risk factors

*These recommendations should apply regardless of whether BCG has previously been administered.
†Physical examination, lab, or radiographic examinations that include TB in the working diagnosis.
‡Including immunosuppressive doses of corticosteroids.
From American Academy of Pediatrics, Committee on Infectious Disease. (1996). Update on tuberculosis skin testing of children. Pediatrics, 97(2), 282-284; Hoekelman, R.A., Adam, H.M., Nelson, N.M., Weitzman, M.L., & Willson, M.H. (Eds.). (2001). Primary care pediatrics (4th ed.). St Louis: Mosby; Pickering, L.K. (Ed.). (2000). 2000 Red book: Report of the Committee on Infectious Diseases (25th ed.). Elk Grove Village, IL: American Academy of Pediatrics.

0.1 ml of purified protein derivative (PPD), is the accepted standard of skin testing.

Interpretation. Refer to Table 12-6.

Technique

- *Mantoux test with tuberculin PPD*—The Mantoux test is recommended because of its specificity and sensitivity. Care should be taken with the technique of administering the PPD. It is necessary to read the test 48 to 72 hours after the injection.
- *Multiple-puncture device (MPD) tine test*—The MPD is no longer recommended because of its inaccuracies and limitations.

Sensory Tests

Hearing screening

Purpose. Early identification of children with hearing problems is necessary to intervene and support normal development of speech, language, and psychosocial skills. Most speech and language development occurs before 3 years of age. Problems are identified early by means of history taking, a physical examination, and developmental screening. Approximately 1 of 1000 children have profound sensorineural hearing loss at birth, and when mild to severe hearing loss is considered, the prevalence increases to 7 of 1000. Because the first 18 to 24 months of life are critical for the development of language, early identification and intervention for hearing problems is crucial.

High-risk criteria are identified in Table 12-7. Infants at high risk should be screened before hospital discharge but no later than at 3 months of age. Children under 2 years of age should be screened within 3 months after being identified as high risk. Screening for the school-age child is focused on the maintenance of optimal educational hearing and the detection of an otopathologic condition. The same screening procedures used for younger children should be continued for school-age children.

Technique

Pure-tone audiometry. The audiometer should be calibrated. The ideal screening protocol comprises pure-tone hearing screening, acoustic immittance testing (tympanometry), otoscopic inspection of the ear canal, and parental reports of concerns that include obtaining a family medical history and assessing the child's auditory responsiveness and speech and language development annually, and the individual administering the testing should be trained in the correct technique and should know when repeat testing is necessary. Pure-tone audiometry can be started with children as young as 3 years of age, depending on their cooperation. It must be done in a quiet environment using earphones. It is important that children's performance not be affected by their ability to understand instructions or cooperate. Starting at a 50 dB tone at 1000 Hz and then decreasing to 20 dB at 4000, 2000, and 1000 Hz respectively is the current recommendation for testing 3 to 4 year olds. For the school-age child, one should begin pure-tone stimuli at 20 dB and evaluate frequencies of 1000, 2000, and 4000 Hz. Follow-up on any failures should be with rescreening and then a more thorough evaluation.

Tympanometry. Tympanometry can reliably detect the presence of eustachian tube dysfunction and middle ear effusion. It is also especially helpful in identifying those children who have a slight hearing loss but still "pass" the auditory screening tests. It provides an estimate of middle ear air pressure and an indirect measure of tympanic membrane compliance. The majority of middle ears with normal tympanograms are in fact normal and typically show a negative predictive value, while half the ears with abnormal tympanograms (showing a positive predictive value) may have otitis media with effusion. Used with pneumatic otoscopy, the weaknesses of each can be overcome.

Pneumatic otoscopy. During the physical examination, attention should be paid to structural defects of the ear, the head,

Table 12-7 Screening Criteria for Sensorineural or Conductive Hearing Loss Testing

RISK CRITERIA (NEONATAL)*	RISK CRITERIA (29 DAYS TO 3 YEARS OF AGE)
Family history of congenital early onset or delayed onset childhood sensorineural or conductive hearing loss, or both.	Parent or other caregiver with concerns regarding speech, hearing, language, or developmental delay
Birth weight of less than 1500 g	Infection with bacterial meningitis
Presence of craniofacial abnormalities	Family history of hereditary childhood hearing loss
Presence of congenital infection with toxoplasmosis, syphilis, rubella, cytomegalovirus (CMV), or herpes	Head trauma associated with loss of consciousness or with skull fracture
Bacterial meningitis	Stigmata or other findings associated with a syndrome know to include sensorineural or conductive hearing loss
Hyperbilirubinemia requiring exchange transfusion	Ototoxic medications including but not limited to chemotherapeutic agents, aminoglycosides used in multiple courses or in combination with loop diuretics
Ototoxic medications used for more than 5 days	Recurrent or persistent otitis media with effusion for at least 3 months
Loop diuretics used with aminoglycosides	Neonatal risk factors that may be associated with delayed onset or progressive sensorineural hearing loss such as persistent pulmonary hypertension
Severe depression at birth, including Apgar scores of 0 to 4 at 1 minute or 0 to 6 at 5 minutes	History of uterine infections (e.g., CMV, toxoplasmosis, syphilis, rubella, herpes)
Prolonged mechanical ventilation lasting 5 days or longer (e.g., persistent pulmonary hypertension)	Infectious disease known to be associated with sensorineural hearing loss (e.g., mumps, measles)
Problems or other findings associated with syndromes that may include sensorineural or conductive hearing loss	Neurodegenerative disorder associated with hearing loss (e.g., neurofibromatosis type II, neurodegenerative disorders)
Neonatal intracranial hemorrhage	Anatomic deformity and other disorders that affect eustachian tube function

For use when Universal Hearing Screening is not available.

From American Academy of Pediatrics, Task Force on Newborn and Infant Hearing. (1999). Newborn and infant hearing loss: Detection and intervention. Pediatrics, 103(2), 527-530; Hoekelman, R.A., Adam, H.M., Nelson, N.M., Weitzman, M.L., & Willson, M.H. (Eds.). (2001). Primary care pediatrics (4th ed.). St Louis: Mosby.

or the neck, and abnormalities of the ear canal (inflammation, cerumen, impactions, tumors, or foreign bodies) and eardrum (perforations, retractions, or effusion) should be noted. Otoscopy and pneumoscopy are recommended for assessment of the middle ear because, with an experienced examiner, they provide an accurate diagnosis of otitis media with effusion at 70% to 79% reliability.

Vision screening

Purpose. Vision screening is intended to identify (as early as possible) children with vision problems, such as refractive errors (e.g., myopia, hyperopia, astigmatism, anisometropia), functional visual loss, amblyopia (e.g., strabismus, anisometropic, occlusion, bilateral ametropic, deprivation), disorders causing visual loss, and ocular and neurologic disorders. Amblyopia can occur until 9 years of age, when visual development is complete, but the risk is greatest between 2 and 3 years of age. Other visual problems that must be identified include cataracts (1 per 1000 live births), congenital glaucoma (1 per 10,000 live births), retinoblastoma (1 per 20,000 live births), and retinopathy of prematurity (ROP) (16% to 34% in infants weighing less than 1500 g). Eye injury also should be evaluated carefully and treated appropriately. Vision screening comprises three components: (1) assessment of ocular alignment and movement, (2) assessment of the red light reflex and fundus, and (3) measurement of visual acuity in each eye.

Technique. Visual screening for infants and toddlers is focused within the physical examination. Vision testing for acuity in preschool children, school-age children, and adolescents includes the physical examination and measurements for visual acuity. Table 12-8 provides those areas of the physical examination and visual acuity testing that should be considered at various ages and the indications for follow-up and referral.

Interpretation. Refer to Table 12-8.

Developmental Screening and Testing

Refer to Chapter 11 for more information.

Purpose. Developmental screening provides a mechanism to evaluate a child's ongoing development and a basis for providing parent education about age-appropriate expectations and activities. Although developmental screening has been a standard for well-child care, developmental surveillance is needed to ensure the overall physical and emotional health of a child. The focus of current approaches to development recognizes the family's primary influence on the child's development. Therefore developmental screening and approaches to care now include assessment of a child's world beyond just the child's developmental tasks. Including the parents and child in the clinical interview provides information about the family's strengths and stressors, along with information about the child's place in the family, school, and community. A family-directed interview model is suggested so that there is recognition of the developmental potential for the child as affected most by his or her environment.

Implementation. Because of time constraints, developmental testing or screening has decreased. Many offices have begun to use a "development-based office" to overcome some of these constraints. The use of prenatal visits, questionnaires, children's picture drawings, and in-office parent education classes are just some of the strategies being used.

Technique. All developmental tests have limitations in their use in clinical practice. Often the time needed for testing and training of staff is difficult to maintain. Screening tests include parent questionnaires (e.g., Ages and Stages), history, components of the physical examination, and specific tests (e.g., Denver II). (A list of different developmental screening tests can be found in Chapter 11.)

Table 12-8 Visual Screening and Testing for Children

AGE	VISION SCREENING AND TESTING	RESULTS REQUIRING FOLLOW-UP OR REFERRAL
Birth-3 months	History: • Family: vision problems • Prenatal: infection • Birth: prematurity, oxygen Physical examination (PE): • Anatomy • Red light reflex • Corneal light reflex • Fixes and follows examiner's face (3 to 6 months)	Family history of congenital vision problems, genetic problems, metabolic disease, VD, or HIV Prenatal history of infection (e.g., rubella, CMV) Neonatal problems of prematurity (< 28 weeks), oxygen, or low birth weight (< 1500 g) Asymmetric findings Structural abnormalities Absence of red light reflex or opacity, dimness, or asymmetry Inability to fix and follow
6 months-1 year	History: • Parental concerns and observation regarding child's visual ability PE: • Anatomy • Fixes and follows toy (6 to 12 months) • Red light reflex • Corneal light reflex • Cover/uncover test	ROP or other family or birth problems (follow-up by ophthalmologist) Asymmetric findings Structural abnormalities Absence of red light reflex or opacity, dimness, or asymmetry Asymmetric or ocular fixation movements
1-3 years	History and PE: • As above • Localizes small object in hand (12-30 months) Visual acuity: • Picture chart (30-60 months) Color perception: • Ishihara test	As above 20/50 Vision or worse (3-year-olds) Difference of two lines between eyes
4-5 years and up	History and PE: • As above • School performance, including worsening grades Visual acuity: • Tumbling E (5-6 years) • Snellen (6 or more years) Color perception: • Ishihara test	As above Visual screening Children 4 years and older who cannot be screened successfully after repeated attempts 20/40 Vision or worse (5-year-olds) Difference of two lines between eyes 20/30 Vision or worse (school-age children or adolescents) Children who fail binocular vision

Adapted from American Academy of Pediatrics, Committee on Practice and Ambulatory Medicine, Section on Ophthalmology. (1996). Eye examination and vision screening in infants, children, and young adults. Pediatrics, 98*(1), 153-157; Hoekelman, R.A., Adam, H.M., Nelson, N.M., Weitzman, M.L., & Willson, M.H. (Eds.). (2001).* Primary care pediatrics *(4th ed.). St Louis: Mosby.*

Interpretation. Each developmental screening test has a manual that provides an explanation of the techniques for testing and the standards for retesting and referral. If there are any questions about the results of a particular screening test or if the child was uncooperative, the child should be retested or referred to a specific developmental screening program such as Child Find. Child Find programs are the result of federal legislation (Public Law 99-457) and are intended to provide early identification of developmental problems.

Integration of Screening into Practice

Pediatric screening has come under considerable debate and evaluation of cost effectiveness. Greater emphasis is being placed on individual monitoring and surveillance rather than mass screening. Surveillance encompasses all primary care activities related to the monitoring of development of children; it includes preparing a relevant developmental history, making accurate and informative observations of children, and eliciting and attending to parental concerns. Establishing a primary care "home" where each child is evaluated on an ongoing basis is essential for health care surveillance. Through the primary care practitioner (PCP), parents develop an appreciation of the importance of continuity of care and are involved in their child's health care plan.

Follow-Up of Screening Tests

Establishment of follow-up program standards for screening tests (and other tests) should include the person who has the primary responsibility for the follow-up, the type of follow-up evaluation that is appropriate for each test, and the follow-up documentation procedure. Practitioners' participation in follow-up varies, but the practitioner needs to ensure that it is being completed. A benefit of tracking test results is that it provides an internal system for monitoring the effectiveness of certain tests. If *no* positive results are found or if an *increase* in positive tests are noted, follow-up examination can be completed to determine why this is happening. Staff education is needed to resolve the problem.

Systems for follow-up of newborn screening tests are often not in place in pediatric practices. This is based on an assumption that the state or agency completing the test will complete the follow-up process. Some families move, leaving no forwarding address, and contact is lost. Others have not established ongoing pediatric care at the time of delivery or change providers within the first or second month of the child's life. It is important for all pediatric practitioners to know the actual newborn screening results for newborns and infants in their practices.

Education of parents as to why the screening tests are being done, when they will be notified about positive results, and what follow-up evaluation might be needed is important. Parental expectations must be included in the plans for performing screening tests. If parents are not committed to follow up or have no means of paying for follow-up testing, community resources need to be used.

Follow-up on test results usually includes a phone call or letter to the patient or parents. Care needs to be taken that current phone numbers and message numbers are obtained with each visit. Follow-up contact with adolescents needs to be made in a form that does not breach confidentiality. Follow-up plans should be made *before* the tests are completed.

Resources

Websites
American Academy of Pediatric (www.aap.org)

National Center for Health Statistics (www.cdc.gov/nchs/growthcharts)

National Guideline Clearinghouse, including *Pediatric preventive care: health assessments and anticipatory guidance* (www.guidelines.gov)

Centers for Disease Control and Prevention, *Immunization schedule* (www.cdc.gov/nip/recs/child-schedule.pdf)

Bibliography

American Academy of Pediatrics, Committee on Environmental Health. (1998). Screening for elevated blood lead levels. *Pediatrics, 101*(6), 1072-1078.

American Academy of Pediatrics, Committee on Fetus and Newborn. (1993). Routine evaluations of blood pressure, hematocrit, and glucose in newborns. *Pediatrics, 92*(3), 474-476.

American Academy of Pediatrics, Committee on Genetics. (1996). Health supervision for children with sickle cell diseases and their families. *Pediatrics, 98*(3), 467-472.

American Academy of Pediatrics, Committee on Genetics. (1996). Newborn screening fact sheets. *Pediatrics, 98*(3), 473-501.

American Academy of Pediatrics, Committee on Infectious Disease. (1996). Update on tuberculosis skin testing of children. *Pediatrics, 97*(2), 282-284.

American Academy of Pediatrics, Committee on Nutrition. (1998). Cholesterol in childhood. *Pediatrics, 101*(1), 141-147.

American Academy of Pediatrics, Committee on Practice and Ambulatory Medicine. (2000). *Recommendations for preventive pediatric health care: Policy statement.* Elk Grove Village, IL: American Academy of Pediatrics.

American Academy of Pediatrics, Committee on Practice and Ambulatory Medicine, Section on Ophthalmology. (1996). Eye examination and vision screening in infants, children, and young adults. *Pediatrics, 98*(1), 153-157.

American Academy of Pediatrics, Provisional Committee for Quality Improvement Subcommittee on Hyperbilirubinemia. (1994). Management of hyperbilirubinemia in the healthy term newborn. *Pediatrics, 94*(4), 558-565.

American Academy of Pediatrics, Task Force on Newborn and Infant Hearing. (1999). Newborn and infant hearing loss: Detection and intervention. *Pediatrics, 103*(2), 527-530.

Dixon, S. & Stein, M. (2000). *Encounters with children.* St Louis: Mosby.

Frame, P.S. & Carlson, S.J. (1975). A clinical review of periodic health screening using specific criteria. *Journal of Family Practice, 2,* 29-36.

Hoekelman, R.A., Adam, H.M., Nelson, N.M., Weitzman, M.L., & Willson, M.H. (Eds.). (2001). *Primary care pediatrics* (4th ed.). St Louis: Mosby.

Pickering, L.K. (Ed.). (2000). *2000 Red book: Report of the Committee on Infectious Diseases* (25th ed.). Elk Grove Village, IL: American Academy of Pediatrics.

U.S. Preventive Services Task Force. (1996). *Guide to clinical preventive services* (2nd ed.). Baltimore: Williams & Wilkins.

Chapter 13 *Immunizations*

Mary Koslap-Petraco

Immunizations are agents that provide protection from infectious disease by stimulating production of cellular or hormonal responses. These agents are a most important and cost-effective element of preventive health care for children. Before the advent of routine immunization, millions of lives were lost and permanent disabilities sustained as a result of infectious diseases. Many parents have not witnessed the ravages of polio, rubella, rubeola, mumps, and pertussis. These diseases, which are still occurring, cost millions of dollars because of loss of function from permanent disabilities and loss of time for parents at work and children in school.

Benefits

By conferring protection against communicable disease, immunizations prevent the sequelae associated with the naturally occurring disease. Communicable diseases can cause brain damage as a result of meningitis, paralysis, deafness, birth defects, blindness, lung damage, cancer of the liver, and death.

Contraindications

Table 13-1 describes the true contraindications for all vaccines. Many practitioners withhold immunizations based on personal opinion rather than true contraindications. Missed opportunities for immunization often result when personal opinion is followed rather than the guide to contraindications and precautions issued by the Centers for Disease Control and Prevention (CDC).

Practitioners need to be prepared to deal with caregivers who fear the consequences of immunization. Risk and benefits have to be assessed. There is a far greater chance for permanent damage to a child as a result of disease than from a vaccine. Often a vaccine such as diphtheria-tetanus-acellular pertussis (DTaP) is blamed for the development of seizures. Administration of pertussis may hasten the recognition of febrile seizures or epilepsy but does not cause them. Refer the child who has a seizure disorder or experiences febrile seizures to a pediatric neurologist to determine the feasibility of future doses of pertussis.

Indications for delaying immunizations are described in Table 13-1 and include moderate or severe illnesses with or without a fever and known altered immunodeficiency (for measles-mumps-rubella [MMR] and varicella [VAR] vaccines only).

Terms

- *Vaccine* is a suspension of live attenuated (live but modified) or inactivated (consisting of either whole or parts of bacteria or viruses that have been killed) microorganisms administered to produce immunity to prevent disease.
- *Toxin* is a poisonous substance secreted by an organism that causes illness.
- *Antigen* is a live or inactivated substance (such as protein, polysaccharide) coproducing an immune response.
- *Antibody* is a protein molecule (immunoglobulin) produced by B lymphocytes to help eliminate an antigen. Antibodies are produced in response to an antigen.
- *Toxoid* is a modified bacterial toxin that has been rendered nontoxic but still has the ability to stimulate the formation of antitoxin.
- *Antitoxin* is a solution of antibodies obtained from serum of animals immunized with specific antigens used to achieve passive immunity for treatment.
- *Active immunization* is the production of antibodies or other immune response to the administration of vaccine or toxoid.
- *Passive immunization* is the provision of temporary immunity by the administration of preformed antibodies or the acquisition of those antibodies from the mother before birth.
- *Adjuvant* is a substance added to a vaccine that can be the vehicle for the active components of the vaccine or the preservative.
- *Live virus vaccine* is derived from a wild agent (found naturally) that has been attenuated (weakened). The virus must replicate to be effective. The immune response is similar to the natural effect of the disease. Examples are VAR and MMR vaccines.
- *Killed virus vaccine* is composed of either whole or partial bacteria or viruses. The virus does not replicate, and the antibody level falls over time. Little or no cellular immunity results. Examples are diphtheria-tetanus-pertussis (DTP) vaccine and inactivated poliovirus vaccine (IPV).
- *Polysaccharide vaccine* is a unique type of inactivated fraction (part of virus or bacteria) composed of long chains of sugar molecules that make up the surface capsule of certain bacteria. Examples are *Haemophilus influenzae* type B (Hib) vaccine and pneumococcal vaccine.

Vaccines

Diphtheria-Tetanus-Acellular Pertussis Vaccine

DtaP vaccine is used for the basic series of four immunizations for all children up to 7 years of age. Because of the increased likelihood of untoward effects, the use of whole-cell DTP has been phased out. The only acceptable vaccine to be used is the acellular product, DTaP. This vaccine greatly decreases the likelihood of reactions such as fever, irritability, listlessness, redness, and swelling at the site of the injection. In DTaP the piece of the bacteria that invokes the immune response has been isolated. The extraneous part of the cell wall that causes the side effects has been eliminated.

Table 13-1 Guide to Contraindications and Precautions to Immunizations

VACCINE	TRUE CONTRAINDICATIONS AND PRECAUTIONS	NOT TRUE (VACCINES MAY BE GIVEN)
General for all vaccines	Anaphylactic reaction to a vaccine contraindicates further doses of that vaccine	Mild to moderate local reaction (soreness, redness, swelling) after dose of an injectable antigen
(DTP, DTaP, OPV, IPV, MMR, Hib, HBV, Var)	Anaphylactic reaction to a vaccine constituent contraindicates the use of vaccines containing that substance Moderate or severe illnesses with or without a fever	Low-grade or moderate fever after a prior vaccine dose Mild acute illness with or without low-grade fever Current antimicrobial therapy Convalescent phase of illnesses Prematurity (same dosage and indications as for normal, full-term infants) Recent exposure to an infectious disease History of penicillin or other nonspecific allergies or fact that relatives have such allergies Pregnancy of mother or household contact Unvaccinated household contact

DTP/DTaP	Encephalopathy within 7 days of administration of previous dose of DTP/DTaP
	Precautions[1]
	   Fever of 105° F (40.5° C) within 48 hours after vaccination with a prior dose of DTP/DTaP and not attributable to another identifiable cause
	   Collapse or shocklike state (hypotonic-hyporesponsive episode) within 48 hours of receiving a prior dose of DTP/DTaP
	   Seizures with 3 days of receiving a prior dose of DTP/DTaP (see footnote 2 regarding management of children with a personal history of seizures at any time)
	   Persistent, inconsolable crying lasting 3 hours, within 48 hours of receiving a prior dose of DTP/DTaP
	   Guillain-Barré syndrome (GBS) within 6 weeks after a dose[3]
		Temperature of < 105° F (40.5° C) after a previous dose of DTP/DTaP
		
		Family history of convulsions[2]
		
		Family history of sudden infant death syndrome (SIDS)
		Family history of an adverse event after DTP/DTaP administration

OPV	Infection with HIV or a household contact with HIV infection Known immunodeficiency (hematologic and solid tumors, congenital immunodeficiency, and long-term immunosuppressive therapy) Immunodeficient household contact Precaution[1] Pregnancy	Breastfeeding Current antimicrobial therapy Mild diarrhea

From Centers for Disease Control and Prevention. Atlanta.
[1]*The events of conditions listed as precautions, although not contraindications, should be carefully reviewed. The benefits and risks of administering a specific vaccine to an individual under the circumstances should be considered. If the risks are believed to outweigh the benefits, the immunization should be withheld; if the benefits are believed to outweigh the risks (e.g., during an outbreak of foreign travel), the immunization should be given. Whether and when to administer DTP/DTaP to children with proven or suspected underlying neurologic disorders should be decided on an individual basis. Avoiding administration of certain vaccines to pregnant women is prudent on theoretic grounds. If immediate protection against poliomyelitis is needed, either OPV or IPV is recommended.*
[2]*Acetaminophen given before administration of DTP/DTaP and thereafter every 4 hours for 24 hours should be considered for children with a personal or with a family history of convulsions in siblings or parents*
[3]*The decision to give additional doses of DTP/DTaP should be based on consideration of the benefit of further vaccination vs. the risk of recurrence of GBS. For example, completion of the primary series in children is justified.*

Table 13-2 is a summary of the rules of childhood immunizations, and Table 13-3 describes the dosage, route, side effects, and teaching for each vaccine.

Pediatric Diphtheria Tetanus Vaccine

Pediatric diphtheria tetanus vaccine, or diphtheria and tetanus toxoids (DT), is used when there has been a reaction to a previous dose of DTaP. In this vaccine the pertussis component has been removed. A true contraindication to DTaP should exist before the child is given DT. Tables 13-1 and 13-4 provide additional information. Invalid contraindi-

cations account for far too many children being given DT. As a result communities are seeing a resurgence of pertussis disease.

Adult Diphtheria Tetanus Vaccine

Adult diphtheria tetanus vaccine, or tetanus and diphtheria toxoids absorbed for adult use (Td), is used for children 7 years of age and older. It contains no pertussis vaccine because the pertussis component would cause a severe local reaction in this age group. This vaccine contains a lower dose of the diphtheria component than the pediatric formulation. Im-

Table 13-1 Guide to Contraindications and Precautions to Immunizations—cont'd

VACCINE	TRUE CONTRAINDICATIONS AND PRECAUTIONS	NOT TRUE (VACCINES MAY BE GIVEN)
IPV	Anaphylactic reaction to neomycin, streptomycin, or polymyxin B Precaution[1] Pregnancy	
MMR	Anaphylactic reaction to neomycin or gelatin Pregnancy Known immunodeficiency (hematologic and solid tumors; congenital immunodeficiency; long-term immunosuppressive therapy; HIV infection with evidence of severe immunosuppression) Precaution[1] Recent (within 3 to 11 months, depending on product and dose) administration of a blood product or immune globulin preparation Thrombocytopenia[5] History of thrombocytopenic purpura[5]	Tuberculosis or positive PPD Simultaneous tuberculin skin testing[4] Breastfeeding Pregnancy of mother or household contact of vaccine recipient Immunodeficient family member or household contact HIV infection without evidence of severe immunosuppression Allergic reaction to eggs[6] Nonanaphylactic reactions to neomycin
Hib	None	
Hepatitis B (HBV)	Anaphylactic reaction to baker's yeast	Pregnancy
Var[7]	Anaphylactic reaction to neomycin or gelatin Pregnancy Known immunodeficiency (e.g., hematologic and solid tumors, congenital immunodeficiency, long-term immunosuppressive therapy) Precaution[1] Recent (within 5 months) administration of an immune globulin preparation[8] Family history of immunodeficiency[9]	Immunodeficiency of a household contact HIV infection in a household contact Pregnancy in the mother or other household contact of the recipient

[4]*Measles vaccination may temporarily suppress tuberculin reactivity. MMR vaccine may be given after or on the same day as TB testing. If MMR has been given recently, postpone the TB test until 4 to 6 weeks after administration of MMR. If giving MMR simultaneously with tuberculin skin test, use the Mantoux test and not multiple puncture tests, because the latter require confirmation if positive, which would have to be postponed 4 to 6 weeks.*

[5]*The decision to vaccinate should be based on consideration of the benefits of immunity to measles, mumps, and rubella versus the risk of recurrence or exacerbation of thrombocytopenia after vaccination, or from natural infections of measles or rubella. In most instances, the benefits of vaccination will be much greater than the potential risk and justify giving MMR, particularly in view of the even greater risk and justify giving MMR, particularly in view of the even greater risk of thrombocytopenia after measles or rubella disease. However, if a prior episode of thrombocytopenia occurred in close temporal proximity to vaccination, it might be prudent to avoid a subsequent dose.*

[6]*Recent data suggest that most anaphylactic reactions to measles- and mumps-containing vaccines are associated with hypersensitivity not to egg antigens but to other components of the vaccines. Because the risk of anaphylactic reactions after administration of measles- or mumps-containing vaccines in persons who are allergic to eggs is extremely low and skin testing with vaccine is not predictive of allergic reactions to these vaccines, skin testing and desensitization are no longer required before administration of MMR vaccine to persons who are allergic to eggs.*

[7]*Varicella virus vaccine preferably should be administered routinely to children at the same time as MMR vaccine. Varicella virus vaccine is safe and effective in healthy children 12 months of age when administered at the same time as MMR vaccine at separate sites and with separate syringes or when administered separately 30 days apart.*

[8]*Varicella vaccine should not be given for at least 5 months after administration of blood (except washed red blood cells), plasma transfusions, immune globulin, or Varicella zoster immunoglobin (VZIG). Immune globulin or VZIG should not be given for 3 weeks after vaccination unless the benefits exceed those of the vaccination. In such cases, the vaccinee should either be revaccinated 5 months later or tested for immunity 6 months later and revaccinated if seronegative.*

[9]*Varicella vaccine should not be given to a member of a household with a family history of immunodeficiency until the immune status of the recipient and other children in the family is documented.*

Note: This information is based on the recommendations of the Advisory Committee on Immunization Practices (ACIP) and those of the Committee on Infectious Diseases (Red Book Committee) of the American Academy of Pediatrics (AAP). Sometimes these recommendations vary from those contained in the manufacturers' package inserts. For more detailed information, providers should consult the published recommendations of the ACIP, AAP, the AAFP, and the manufacturers' package inserts.

munity to pertussis acquired by vaccination in childhood wanes by approximately 12 years of age. Older children and adults can develop pertussis, but it is not so devastating an illness in the older age groups. (For additional information, see Tables 13-2 and 13-3.)

Haemophilus Influenzae Type B Vaccine

Hib vaccine prevents Hib meningitis and other invasive bacterial diseases in children. Since most fatalities occur from this organism before 18 months of age, it is essential to adequately immunize infants. Hib vaccine is a polysaccharide conjugate vaccine. A polysaccharide (a poor antigen) is chemically bonded to a protein carrier in a process called "conjugation. The process greatly improves immunogenicity, particularly in young children." Three products are licensed for use in infants. Limited data indicate that three doses of any of these vaccines may confer immunity (see Tables 13-2 and 13-3). A combined DTaP/Hib vaccine is available for the fourth dose but may be used only if three separate doses of DTaP and three separate doses of Hib vaccine have been given previously. This combination vaccine cannot be given before the 15-month birthday.

Table 13-2 Summary of Rules for Childhood Immunization*

VACCINE	AGES USUALLY GIVEN AND OTHER GUIDELINES	IF CHILD FALLS BEHIND (MINIMUM INTERVALS)	CONTRAINDICATIONS (REMEMBER: MILD ILLNESS NOT A CONTRAINDICATION)
DTaP (Diphtheria, tetanus, acellular pertussis) Give IM	• DTaP (not DTP) is recommended for all doses in the series. • Give at 2 months, 4 months, 6 months, 15–18 months, 4–6 years of age. • May give #1 as early as 6 weeks of age. • May give #4 as early as 12 months of age if 6 months have elapsed since #3 and the child is unlikely to return at age 15–18 months. • If started with DTP, complete the series with DTaP. • Do not give DTaP to children ≥ 7 years of age (give Td). • May give all other vaccines but as a separate injection. • It is preferable but not mandatory to use the same DTaP product for all doses.	• #2 and #3 may be given 4 weeks after previous dose. • #4 may be given 6 months after #3. • If #4 is given before fourth birthday, wait at least 6 months for #5 (4–6 years of age). • If #4 is given after fourth birthday, #5 is not needed. • DO NOT restart series, no matter how long since previous dose.	• Anaphylactic reaction to a prior dose or to any vaccine component. • Moderate or severe acute illness. Don't postpone for mild illness. • Previous encephalopathy within 7 days after DTP/DTaP. Precautions for DTP/DTaP: The following are precautions, not contraindications. Generally when these conditions are present, the vaccine shouldn't be given. But in situations when the benefit outweighs the risk (e.g., community pertussis outbreak), vaccination should be considered. • T ≥ 105° F (40.5° C) within 48 hours after previous dose. • Continuous crying lasting ≥ 3 hours within 48 hours after previous dose. • Previous convulsion within 3 days after immunization. • Pale or limp episode or collapse within 48 hours after previous dose. • Unstable progressive neurologic problem (defer until stable).
DT Give IM	• Give to children < 7 years of age if child had a serious reaction to "P" in DTaP/DTP or if parents refuse the pertussis component. • May give with all other vaccines but as a separate injection.		• Anaphylactic reaction to a previous dose or to any vaccine component. • Moderate or severe acute illness. Do not postpone for minor illness.
Td Give IM	• Use for persons ≥ 7 years of age. • A booster dose is recommended for children 11–12 years of age if 5 years have elapsed since last dose. Then boost every 10 years. • May give with all other vaccines but as a separate injection.	For those never vaccinated or with an unknown vaccination history: dose #1 is given now, dose #2 is given 4 weeks later, dose #3 is given 6 months after #2, then give booster dose every 10 years. If the series is incomplete, continue from where you left off. DO NOT restart the series.	
MMR (Measles, mumps, rubella) Give SC	• Give #1 at 12–15 months of age. Give #3 at 4–6 years of age. • Make sure that all children (and teens) over 4–6 years of age have received both doses of MMR. • If a dose was given before 12 months of age it doesn't count as the first dose, so give #1 at 12–15 months of age with a minimum interval of 4 weeks between these doses. • If MMR and Var (and/or yellow fever vaccine) are not given on the same day, space them ≥ 28 days apart. • May give with all other vaccines, but as a separate injection.	• Two doses of MMR are recommended for all children ≤ 18 years of age. • Dose should be given whenever it is noted that a child is behind. Exception: If MMR and Var (and/or yellow fever vaccine) are not given on the same day, space them ≥ 28 days apart. • There should be a minimum interval of 28 days between MMR #1 and MMR #2. • Dose #2 can be given at any time if at least 28 days have elapsed since dose #1 and both doses are administered after 1 year of age. • DO NOT restart the series, no matter how long since previous dose.	• Anaphylactic reaction to a prior dose or to any vaccine component. • Pregnancy or possible pregnancy within next 3 months (use contraception). • Moderate or severe acute illness. Don't postpone for minor illness. • If blood, plasma, or immune globulin were given in past 11 months, see ACIP recommendations or 2000 Red Book regarding the time to wait before vaccinating. • HIV is NOT a contraindication unless severely immunocompromised. • Immunocompromised persons (e.g., because of cancer, leukemia, lymphoma). Note: For patients on high-dose immunosuppressive therapy, consult ACIP recommendations regarding delay time. Note: MMR is not contraindicated if a PPD test was recently applied. If PPD and MMR weren't given on same day, delay PPD for 4–6 weeks after MMR.

Vaccine		Contraindications/Precautions
Varicella (Var) (Chickenpox) Give SC	• Routinely give at 12-18 months of age. • Vaccinate all children ≥ 12 months of age including all adolescents who have not had chickenpox. • May use a postexposure prophylaxis if given within 3-5 days. • If Var and MMR (and/or yellow fever vaccine) are not given on the same day, space them ≥ 28 days apart. • May give with all other vaccines but as a separate injection.	• Do not give children <12 months of age. • Susceptible children <13 years of age receive one dose. • Susceptible persons ≥ 13 years of age receive two doses 4-8 week apart. • DO NOT restart series, no matter how long since previous dose.	• Anaphylactic reaction to a prior dose or to any vaccine component. • Moderate or severe acute illness. Don't postpone for minor illness. • Pregnancy or possibility of pregnancy within 1 month. • If blood, plasma, or immune globulin (IG or VZIG) were given in past 5 months, see ACIP recommendations or AAP's 2000 Red Book regarding the time to wait before vaccinating. • Persons immunocompromised due to high doses of systemic steroids, cancer, leukemia, lymphoma, or immunodeficiency. **Note:** For patients with humoral immunodeficiency, HIV infection, or leukemia, or for patients on high doses of systemic steroids, consult ACIP recommendations. • For use in children taking salicylates, consult ACIP recommendations.
Polio (IPV) Give SC or IM	• Give at 2 months, 4 months, 6-18 months, and 4-6 years of age. • May give #1 as early as 6 weeks of age. • Not routinely recommended for those 18 years of age (except certain travelers). • May give with all other vaccines but as a separate injection.	• All doses should be separated by at least 4 weeks. #4 is given at 4-6 years of age. • If #3 of an all-IPV or all-OPV series is given at ≥ 4 years of age, dose #4 is not needed. • Those who receive a combination of IPV and OPV doses must receive all four doses. • DO NOT restart series, no matter how long since previous dose.	• Anaphylactic reaction to a previous dose or to any vaccine component. • Moderate or severe acute illness. Do not postpone for mild illness.
Hib Give IM	• HibTITER (HbOC) and ActHib or OmniHib (PRP-T): give at 2 months, 4 months, 6 months, 12-15 months. • PedvaxHIB (PRP-OMP): give at 2 months, 4 months, 12-15 months. • Dose #1 of Hib vaccine may be given as early as 6 weeks of age but no earlier. • May give with all other vaccines but as a separate injection. • Hib vaccines are interchangeable. • Any Hib vaccine may be used for the booster dose. • Hib is not routinely given to children ≥ 5 years of age.	**Rules for all Hib vaccines:** • The last dose (booster dose) is given no earlier than 12 months of age and minimum of 2 months after the previous dose. • For children ≥ 15 months and <5 years of age who have never received Hib vaccine, give only one dose. • DO NOT restart series, no matter how long since previous dose. **Rules for HbOC (HibTITER) and PRP-T (ActHib, OmniHib) only:** • #2 and #3 may be given 4 weeks after previous dose. • If #1 was given at 7-11 months, only three doses are needed; #2 is given 4-8 weeks after #1, then boost at 12-15 months. • If #1 was given at 12-14 months, give a booster dose in 2 months. **Rules for PRP-OMP (PedvaxHiB) only:** • #2 may be given 4 weeks after dose #1. • If #1 was given at 12-14 months, boost 8 weeks later.	• Anaphylactic reaction to a prior dose or to any vaccine component. • Moderate or severe acute illness. Don't postpone for mild illness. • Anaphylactic reaction to a previous dose or to any vaccine component. • Moderate or severe acute illness. Do not postpone for mild illness.

The newer combination vaccines are not listed on this table but may be used whenever administration of any component is indicated and none is contraindicated. Read package inserts. For detailed information, see the ACIP... ments which are published in the MMWR. To obtain visit www.cdcgov/nip/publications/ACIP-list.htm or visit the Immunization Action Coalition's (IAC) website at www.immunize.org/acip. For recommendations of American Ac... Pediatrics (AAP), consult AAP's 2000 Red Book and the journal Pediatrics at www.aap.org.

This table is published annually by the Immunization Action Coalition, 1573 Selby Ave, St. Paul, MN 55104, (651) 647-9009. The most recent edition is found on IAC's website at www.immunize.org/childrules.

Table 13-2 Summary of Rules for Childhood Immunization—cont'd

VACCINE	AGES USUALLY GIVEN AND OTHER GUIDELINES	IF CHILD FALLS BEHIND (MINIMUM INTERVALS)	CONTRAINDICATIONS (REMEMBER: MILD ILLNESS NOT A CONTRAINDICATION)
Hep B Give IM	• Vaccinate all infants at 0-2 months, 1-4 months, 6-18 months of age. • Vaccinate all children 0 through 18 years of age. • For older children/teens, spacing options include: 0, 1, 6 months; 0, 2, 4 months; or 0, 1, 4 months. • Children born (or whose parents were born) in countries of high HBV endemicity or who have other risk factors should be vaccinated ASAP. • If mother is HBsAg positive: Give HBIG and hep B #1 within 12 hours of birth, #2 at 1-2 months, and #3 at 6 months of age. • If mother's HBsAg status is unknown: Give hep B #1 within 12 hours of birth, #2 at 1-2 months, #3 at 6 months of age. If mother is later found to be HBsAg positive, her infant should receive HBIG within 7 days of birth. • May give with all other vaccines but as a separate injection.	• DO NOT restart series, no matter how long since previous dose. • Three-dose series can be started at any age. • Minimum spacing for children and teens: 4 weeks between #1 and #2, and 8 weeks between #2 and #3. Overall there must be ≥ 16 weeks between #1 and #3. • Dose #3 should not be given earlier than 6 months of age. **Dosing of hepatitis B vaccines:** Vaccine brands are interchangeable for three-dose schedule. For Engerix-B, use 10 μg for 0 through 19 years of age. For Recombivax HB, use 5 μg for 0 through 19 years of age. **Alternative dosing schedule for adolescents aged 11 through 15 years:** For Recombivax HB *only*, use 10 μg (adult dose) in two doses spaced 4-6 months apart. May only be given to adolescents 11 through 15 years of age.	• Anaphylactic reaction to a previous dose or to any vaccine component. • Moderate or severe acute illness. DO NOT postpone for mild illness.
Hep A Give IM	• Vaccinate children ≥ 2 years old who live in areas with consistently elevated rates of hepatitis A, as well as children who have specific risk factors. (See ACIP statement and column 2 of this table for details.) • Children who travel outside of the U.S. (except Western Europe, new Zealand, Australia, Canada, or Japan). • Give dose #2 a minimum of 6 months after dose #1. • Dose #1 may not be given earlier than 2 years of age. • May give with all other vaccines, but as a separate injection.	• DO NOT restart series, no matter how long since previous dose. • The minimum interval between dose #1 and #2 is 6 months. • Hepatitis A vaccine brands are interchangeable. • Consult your local or state public health authority for information regarding your city, county, or state hepatitis A rates. States with consistently elevated rates (average ≥ 10 cases per 100,000 population from 1987-1997) include the following: AL, AZ, AK, CA, CO, ID, MO, MT, NV, NM, OK, OR, SD, TX, UT, WA, and WY.	• Anaphylactic reaction to a previous dose or to any vaccine component. • Moderate or severe acute illness. DO NOT postpone for mild illness.

Pneumococcal conjugate (PCV7) Give IM	• Give at 2 months, 4 months, 6 months and 12-15 months of age. • For children age 24-59 months of age, give two doses to high-risk children, and consider one dose for moderate-risk children. (See below for list of high- and moderate-risk children.) • If both PCV7 and PPV23 are indicated, PPV23 is given ≥ 8 weeks after PCV7. • May give one dose to unvaccinated healthy children 24-59 months. • PCV7 not routinely given to children ≥ 5 years of age. • May give with all other vaccines but as a separate injection. **High-risk children:** Those with sickle cell disease; anatomic or functional asplenia; chronic cardiac, pulmonary, or renal disease; diabetes mellitus, CSF leak; HIV infection; or immunosuppression. **Moderate-risk children:** Children aged 24-35 months; children aged 24-59 months who attend group day care centers or are of Alaska Native, Native American, or African-American descent.	• Minimum interval for infants ≤ 12 months of age is 4 weeks, for >12 months of age is 8 weeks. • For infants 7-11 months of age: If unvaccinated, give dose #1 now, give dose #2 4-8 weeks later, and boost at 12-15 months. If infant has had one or two previous doses, give next dose now, and boost at 12-15 months. • For infants 12-23 months: If not previously vaccinated or only one previous dose before 12 months, give two doses ≥ 8 weeks apart. If infant previously had two doses, give booster dose ≥ 8 weeks after previous dose. • DO NOT restart series, no matter how long since previous dose.	• Anaphylactic reaction to a prior dose or to any vaccine component. • Moderate or severe acute illness. DO NOT postpone for mild illness.
PPV23	There are children ≥ 2 years of age for whom pneumococcal polysaccharide vaccine (PPV23) is recommended. Give IM or SC. Consult the ACIP statement *Prevention of Pneumococcal Disease* (4/4/97) for details.		
Influenza	There are children ≥ 6 months of age for whom influenza vaccine is recommended. Give IM. Consult the current year's ACIP statement *Prevention and Control of Influenza* for details.		
Lyme	There are teenagers (≥ 15 years of age) for whom Lyme disease vaccine is recommended. Give IM. Consult the ACIP statement *Recommendations for the Use of Lyme Disease Vaccine* (6/4/99) for details.		
Mening	Meningococcal disease risk and vaccine availability should be discussed with college students. Give SC. Consult the ACIP statement *Meningococcal Disease and College Students* (6/30/00) for details.		

This table is published annually by the Immunization Action Coalition, 1573 Selby Ave., St. Paul, MN 55104, (651) 647-9009. The most recent edition is found on IAC's website at www.immunize.org/childrules.

Table 13-3 Summary of Vaccine Administration, Side Effects, and Teaching

VACCINE	DOSE AND ROUTE	SIDE EFFECTS	TEACHING
DTaP Diphtheria-tetanus-acellular pertussis	0.5 ml IM	*Occasional* Redness and/or swelling at site, fever < 105° F, irritability, restlessness, listlessness; at least one of these in 80% of children *Unusual* Fever of 105° F or higher Collapse, shocklike state within 48 hours of receiving DTP Seizures within 3 days of receiving DTP Persistent, inconsolable crying lasting 3 hours or more within 48 hours of receiving DTP *Very unusual* Encephalopathy within 7 days of receiving DTP	Ice pack to site as long as warm and red swelling as needed Warm soaks to site for head lump Acetaminophen as needed for temperature > 101° F or for discomfort Go to emergency department if unable to reduce fever with acetaminophen, fever is 105° F, develops seizures, encephalopathy, continuous crying for more than 3 hours
DT Diphtheria and tetanus toxoids	0.5 ml IM Used only if child has had serious reaction to "P" in DTP or has unstable neurologic disorder	Does not cause fever usually associated with DTaP	Same as DTaP; does not need acetaminophen prophylactically
Td Tetanus and diphtheria toxoids (adsorbed for adult use) Children > 7 years of age	0.5 ml IM Contains less diphtheria vaccine than children's strength	Redness, swelling, or lump that can last from several days to weeks	Ice pack to site as long as warm and red Warm soaks to site thereafter
Polio vaccine	0.5 ml PO		
IPV Inactivated poliovirus vaccine	0.5 ml SC	Redness, swelling, or lump that can last from several days to several weeks	Ice pack to site for first 24 hours for discomfort Warm soaks to site thereafter
MMR Measles-mumps-rubella	0.5 ml SC	7-10 days after immunization can develop generalized rash and fever Occasional transient myalgia, which can last from several days to several months in adolescents and adults Statistical chance of teratogenic damage to developing fetus	Ice to site as long as warm and red Warm soaks to the site thereafter Ask if female is pregnant; document last menstrual period Advise avoiding pregnancy for 3 months following immunization Acetaminophen every 4 hours as needed for transient myalgia
Hib *H. influenzae* type B conjugate Consider DTaP/Hib for fourth dose of both vaccines	0.5 ml IM	Occasional fever (100° F), redness, swelling If using DTaP/Hib, same as DTaP	Acetaminophen every 4 hours for fever Ice pack to site as long as warm and red Warm soaks to site thereafter

Polio Vaccine

The use of polio vaccine has eliminated wild polio from the United States. Oral polio vaccine (OPV), though largely responsible for the demise of wild polio, also carries the risk of causing vaccine-associated paralytic polio (VAPP). To eliminate VAPP, an all IPV schedule has gradually been introduced. This change will be the last to the polio schedule until polio vaccination is most likely eliminated some-time within the next 10 years. OPV is no longer available for general distribution. The use of OPV is restricted to those children traveling to a polio endemic area in less than 4 weeks or in the event of a polio outbreak. Use of IPV will ultimately eliminate VAPP. The use of IPV eliminates any risk to either the immune-suppressed child or a family member (see Tables 13-2 and 13-3).

Table 13-3 Summary of Vaccine Administration, Side Effects, and Teaching—cont'd

VACCINE	DOSE AND ROUTE	SIDE EFFECTS	TEACHING
Hib *H. influenzae* type B conjugate Consider DTaP/Hib for fourth dose of both vaccines	0.5 ml IM	Occasional fever (100° F), redness, and swelling If using DTaP/Hib same as DTaP	Acetaminophen every 4 hours for fever Ice pack to site as long as warm and red Warm soaks to site thereafter
Hep B Hepatitis B	Recombivax-HB 5 μg for 0-19 years of age, including infants and infants born of HbsAG 6 positive mothers Engerix 10 μg for 0-19 years of age, including infants born of HBsAG-positive mothers Recombivax-HB 10 μg for adolescents 11-19 years of age two doses separated by 4 months	Occasional fever (100° F), redness, and swelling at site	Acetaminophen every 4 hours as needed for fever Ice pack to site as long as warm and red Warm soaks to site thereafter
VAR Varicella	0.5 ml SC 0.5 ml < 3 years of age	Redness, swelling at site, and fever Injection site rash and/or generalized varicelliform rash	Acetaminophen every 4 hours for fever Ice pack to site as long as warm and red Warm soaks to site thereafter
Influenza vaccine Recommended for children 6 months of age with chronic metabolic diseases, HIV, some drug therapies, renal dysfunction, hemoglobinopathies	0.5 ml IM ages 3 and above If receiving influenza vaccine for first time children < 8 years of age need two doses spaced 28 days apart Split virus only until age 8	Redness, swelling, and discomfort at site Occasional mild influenza-like symptoms	Acetaminophen for fever every 4 hours as needed Ice pack to site as long as warm and red Warm soaks to site thereafter
Pneumococcal vaccine Recommend for children > 2 years of age, same as for influenza indications	0.5 ml IM	Redness, swelling, and discomfort at site	Ice pack to site as long as warm and red Warm soaks to site thereafter

Hepatitis B Vaccine

Hepatitis B vaccine (Hep B) is a recombinant DNA vaccine. It provides excellent protection against the hepatitis B virus. The vaccine is known to confer immunity for 13 years or more. It is one of the safest vaccines ever manufactured and produces minimal side effects. Infants born of hepatitis B surface antigen (HbsAg)–positive mothers are to be immunized at birth (see Tables 13-2 and 13-3). Infants born to HbsAg-positive mothers have up to a 90% chance of becoming chronic hepatitis B carriers if not immunized at birth. A two-dose Hep B schedule has been approved for adolescents 11 to 19 years of age. This schedule is limited to Recombivax HB adult formulation only (see Tables 13-2 and 13-3). Only this vaccine has been approved for the two-dose series. Because of the limitations

Text continued on p. 170

Table 13-4 National Childhood Vaccine Injury Act: Reporting and Compensation Tables[a]

VACCINE	ADVERSE EVENT	INTERVAL FROM VACCINATION TO ONSET OF EVENT	
		FOR REPORTING[b]	FOR COMPENSATION[c]
I. Tetanus toxoid–containing vaccines (e.g., DTaP, DTP, DT; Td, or TT)	A. Anaphylaxis or anaphylactic shock	0-7 days	0-4 hours
	B. Brachial neuritis	0-28 days	2-28 days
	C. Any acute complication or sequela (including death) of above events	No limit	No limit
	D. Events described in manufacturer's package insert as contraindications to additional doses of vaccine	No limit	Not applicable
II. Pertussis antigen–containing vaccines (e.g., DTaP, DTP, P, DTP-Hib)	A. Anaphylaxis or anaphylactic shock	0-7 days	0-4 hours
	B. Encephalopathy (or encephalitis)	0-7 days	0-72 hours
	C. Any acute complication or sequela (including death) of above events	No limit	No limit
	D. Events described in manufacturer's package insert as contraindications to additional doses of vaccine	No limit	Not applicable
III. Measles, mumps, and rubella virus–containing vaccines in any combination (e.g., MMR, MR, M, R)	A. Anaphylaxis or anaphylactic shock	0-7 days	0-4 hours
	B. Encephalopathy (or encephalitis)	0-15 days	5-15 days
	C. Any acute complication or sequela (including death) of above events	No limit	No limit
	D. Events described in manufacturer's package insert at contraindications to additional doses of vaccine	No limit	Not applicable
IV. Rubella virus–containing vaccines (e.g., MMR, MR, R)	A. Chronic arthritis	0-42 days	7-42 days
	B. Any acute complication or sequela (including death) of above event	No limit	No limit
	C. Events described in manufacturer's package insert as contraindications to additional doses of vaccine	No limit	Not applicable
V. Measles virus–containing vaccines (e.g., MMR, MR, M)	A. Thrombocytopenic purpura	0-30 days	7-30 days
	B. Vaccine-strain measles viral infection in an immunodeficient recipient	0-6 months	0-6 months
	C. Any acute complication or sequela (including death) of above events	No limit	No limit
	D. Events described in manufacturer's package insert as contraindications to additional doses of vaccine	No limit	Not applicable
VI. Polio live virus–containing vaccines (OPV)	A. Paralytic polio:		
	• In a non-immunodeficient recipient	0-30 days	0-30 days
	• In an immunodeficient recipient	0-6 months	0-6 months
	• In a vaccine-associated community case	No limit	No limit 30 days

From the Centers for Disease Control and Prevention. Atlanta.
[a]*Effective date: October 22, 1998.*
[b]*Taken from the Reportable Events Table (RET), which lists conditions reportable by law (42 USC 300aa-25) to the Vaccine Adverse Event Reporting System (VAERS), including conditions found in the manufacturer's package insert. In addition, individuals are encouraged to report ANY clinically significant or unexpected events (even if you are not certain the vaccine caused the event) for ANY vaccine, whether or not it is listed on the RET. Manufacturers are also required by regulation (21 CFR 600.80) to report to the VAERS program all adverse events made known to them for any vaccine. VAERS reporting forms and information can be obtained by calling (800) 822-7967 or from their website at www.fda.gov/cber/vaers/report.htm.*
[c]*Taken from the Vaccine Injury Table (VIT) used in adjudication of claims filed with the National Vaccine Injury Compensation Program. Claims may also be filed for a condition with onset outside the designated time intervals or a condition not included in the Table. The Qualifications and Aids to Interpretation below define conditions or injuries listed on the VIT. Information on filing a claim can be obtained by calling (800) 338-2382 or through the Vaccine Injury Compensation Program's website at www.hrsa.gov/bhpr/vicp.*

Table 13-4 National Childhood Vaccine Injury Act: Reporting and Compensation Tables*ᵃ*—cont'd

VACCINE	ADVERSE EVENT	INTERVAL FROM VACCINATION TO ONSET OF EVENT	
		FOR REPORTING*ᵇ*	FOR COMPENSATION*ᶜ*
VI. Polio live virus–containing vaccines (OPV)–cont'd	B. Vaccine-strain polio viral infection		
	in a non-immunodeficient recipient	0–30 days	0–6 months
	in an immunodeficient recipient	0–6 months	No limit
	in a vaccine-associated community case	No limit	No limit
	C. Any acute complication or sequela (including death) of above events	No limit	Not applicable
	D. Events described in manufacturer's package insert as contraindications to additional doses of vaccine	No limit	No limit
VII. Polio inactivated–virus containing vaccines (e.g., IPV)	A. Anaphylaxis or anaphylactic shock	0–7 days	0–4 hours
	B. Any acute complication or sequela (including death) of above event	No limit	No limit
	C. Events described in manufacturer's package insert as contraindications to additional doses of vaccine	No limit	Not applicable
VIII. Hepatitis B antigen–containing vaccines	A. Anaphylaxis or anaphylactic shock	0–7 days	0–4 hours
	B. Any acute complication or sequela (including death) of above event	No limit	No limit
	C. Events described in manufacturer's package insert as contraindications to additional doses of vaccine	No limit	Not applicable
IX. *Haemophilus influenzae* type B polysaccharide vaccines (unconjugated PRP vaccines)	A. Early-onset Hib disease	0–7 days	0–7 days
	B. Any acute complication or sequela (including death) of above event	No limit	No limit
	C. Events described in manufacturer's package insert as contraindications to additional doses of vaccine	No limit	Not applicable
X. *Haemophilus influenzae* type B polysaccharide conjugate vaccines	A. No condition specified for compensation	Not applicable	Not applicable
	B. Events described in manufacturer's package insert as contraindications to additional doses of vaccine	No limit	Not applicable
XI. Varicella virus–containing vaccine	A. No condition specified for compensation	Not applicable	Not applicable
	B. Events described in manufacturer's package insert as contraindications to additional doses of vaccine	No limit	Not applicable
XII. Rotavirus live virus–containing vaccine	A. No condition specified for compensation	Not applicable	Not applicable
	B. Events described in manufacturer's package insert as contraindications to additional doses of vaccine	No limit	Not applicable
XIII. Any new vaccine recommended by the CDC for routine administration to children, after publication by Secretary HHS of a notice of coverage	A. No condition specified for compensation	Not applicable	Not applicable
	B. Events described in manufacturer's package insert as contraindications to additional doses of vaccine	No limit	Not applicable

Continued

Qualifications and Aids to Interpretation of Table 13-4

(1) *Anaphylaxis and anaphylactic shock* mean an acute, severe, and potentially lethal systemic allergic reaction. Most cases resolve without sequelae. Signs and symptoms begin minutes to a few hours after exposure. Death, if it occurs, usually results from airway obstruction caused by laryngeal edema or bronchospasm and may be associated with cardiovascular collapse. Other significant clinical signs and symptoms may include the following: cyanosis, hypotension, bradycardia, tachycardia, arrhythmia, edema of the pharynx and/or trachea, and/or larynx with stridor and dyspnea. Autopsy findings may include acute emphysema resulting from lower respiratory tract obstruction; edema of the hypopharynx, epiglottis, larynx or trachea; and minimal findings of eosinophilia in the liver, spleen and lungs. When death occurs within minutes of exposure and without signs of respiratory distress, there may not be significant pathologic findings.

(2) For purposes of the Vaccine Injury Table (VIT), a vaccine recipient shall be considered to have suffered an *encephalopathy* only if such recipient manifests, within the applicable period, an injury meeting the description below of an acute encephalopathy, and then a chronic encephalopathy persists in such person for more than 6 months beyond the date of vaccination.

(i) An *acute encephalopathy* is one that is sufficiently severe so as to require hospitalization (whether or not hospitalization occurred).

  (A) *For children less than 18 months of age* who present without an associated seizure event, an acute encephalopathy is indicated by a "significantly decreased level of consciousness" (see "D" below) lasting for at least 24 hours. Those children less than 18 months of age who present following a seizure shall be viewed as having an acute encephalopathy if their significantly decreased level of consciousness persists beyond 24 hours and cannot be attributed to a postictal state (seizure) or medication.

  (B) *For adults and children 18 months of age or older*, an acute encephalopathy is one that persists for at least 24 hours and characterized by at least two of the following:

    (1) A significant change in mental status that is not medication related; specifically a confusional state, a delirium, or a psychosis

    (2) A significantly decreased level of consciousness, which is independent of a seizure and cannot be attributed to the effects of medication

    (3) A seizure associated with loss of consciousness

  (C) Increased intracranial pressure may be a clinical feature of acute encephalopathy in any age group.

  (D) A "significantly decreased level of consciousness" is indicated by the presence of at least one of the following clinical signs for at least 24 hours or greater (see paragraphs (2)(I)(A) and (2)(I)(B) of this section for applicable timeframes):

    (1) Decreased or absent response to environment (responds, if at all, only to loud voice or painful stimuli)

    (2) Decreased or absent eye contact (does not fix gaze upon family members or other individuals)

    (3) Inconsistent or absent responses to external stimuli (does not recognize familiar people or things)

  (E) The following clinical features alone or in combination do not demonstrate an acute encephalopathy or a significant change in either mental status or level of consciousness as described above: sleepiness, irritability (fussiness), high-pitched and unusual screaming, persistent inconsolable crying, and bulging fontanelle. Seizures in themselves are not sufficient to constitute a diagnosis of encephalopathy. In the absence of other evidence of an acute encephalopathy, seizures shall not be viewed as the first symptom or manifestation of the onset of an acute encephalopathy.

(ii) *Chronic encephalopathy* occurs when a change in mental or neurologic status, first manifested during the applicable time period, persists for a period of at least 6 months from the date of vaccination. Individuals who return to a normal neurologic state after the acute encephalopathy shall not be presumed to have suffered residual neurologic damage from that event; any subsequent chronic encephalopathy shall not be presumed to be a sequela of the acute encephalopathy. If a preponderance of the evidence indicates that a child's chronic encephalopathy is secondary to genetic, prenatal or perinatal factors, that chronic encephalopathy shall not be considered to be a condition set forth in the Table.

(iii) An encephalopathy shall not be considered to be a condition set forth in the Table if in a proceeding on a petition, it is shown by a preponderance of the evidence that the encephalopathy was caused by an infection, a toxin, a metabolic disturbance, a structural lesion, a genetic disorder or trauma (without regard to whether the cause of the infection, toxin, trauma, metabolic disturbance, structural lesion or genetic disorder is known). If at the time a decision is made on a petition filed under section 211(b) of the Act for a vaccine-related injury or death, it is not possible to determine the cause by preponderance of the evidence of an encephalopathy, the encephalopathy shall be considered to be a condition set forth in the Table.

(iv) In determining whether or not an encephalopathy is a condition set forth in the Table, the court shall consider the entire medical record.

(3) A petitioner may be considered to have suffered a *residual seizure disorder* for purposes of the Vaccine Injury Table, if the first seizure or convulsion occurred 5-15 days (not less than 5 days and not more than 15 days) after administration of the vaccine and two or more additional distinct seizure or convulsion episodes occurred within 1 year after the administration of the vaccine which were unaccompanied by fever (defined as a rectal temperature equal to or greater than 101° F or an oral temperature equal to or greater than 100° F. A distinct seizure or convulsion episode is ordinarily defined as including all seizure or convulsive activity occurring within a 24-hour period, unless competent and qualified expert neurologic testimony is presented to the contrary in a particular case.

  For purposes of the VIT, a petitioner shall not be considered to have suffered a residual seizure disorder, if the petitioner suffered a seizure or convulsion unaccompanied by fever (as defined above) before the fifth day after the administration of the vaccine involved.

Qualifications and Aids to Interpretation of Table 13-4—cont'd

(4) For purposes of paragraphs (2) and (3) of this section, the terms *seizure* and *convulsion* include myoclonic, generalized tonic-clonic (grand mal), and simple and complex partial seizures. Absence (petit mal) seizures shall not be considered to be a condition set forth in the Table. Jerking movements or staring episodes alone are not necessarily an indication of seizure activity.

(5) The term *sequela* means a condition or event which was actually caused by a condition listed in the VIT.

(6) For purposes of the VIT, *chronic arthritis* may be found in a person with no history in the 3 years before vaccination of arthropathy (joint disease) on the basis of:

    (A) Medical documentation, recorded within 30 days after the onset, of objective signs of acute arthritis (joint swelling) that occurred between 7 and 42 days after a rubella vaccination

    (B) Medical documentation (recorded within 3 years after the onset of acute arthritis) of the persistence of objective signs of intermittent or continuous arthritis for more than 6 months following vaccination

    (C) Medical documentation of an antibody response to the rubella virus

    For purposes of the VIT, the following shall not be considered as chronic arthritis: musculoskeletal disorders such as diffuse connective tissue diseases (including but not limited to rheumatoid arthritis, juvenile rheumatoid arthritis, systemic lupus erythematosus, systemic sclerosis, mixed connective tissue disease, polymyositis/dermatomyositis, fibromyalgia, necrotizing vasculitis and vasculopathies, and Sjögren syndrome), degenerative joint disease, infectious agents other than rubella (whether by direct invasion or as an immune reaction), metabolic and endocrine diseases, trauma, neoplasms, neuropathic disorders, bone and cartilage disorders and arthritis associated with ankylosing spondylitis, psoriasis, inflammatory bowel disease, Reiter syndrome, or blood disorders. Arthralgia (joint pain) or stiffness without joint swelling shall not be viewed as chronic arthritis for purposes of the VIT.

(7) *Brachial neuritis* is defined as dysfunction limited to the upper extremity nerve plexus (i.e., its trunks, divisions, or cords) without involvement of other peripheral (e.g., nerve roots or a single peripheral nerve) or central (e.g., spinal cord) nervous system structures. A deep, steady, often severe aching pain in the shoulder and upper arm usually heralds onset of the condition. The pain is followed in days or weeks by weakness and atrophy in upper extremity muscle groups. Sensory loss may accompany the motor deficits, but is generally a less notable clinical feature. The neuritis, or plexopathy, may be present on the same side as or the opposite side of the injection; it is sometimes bilateral, affecting both upper extremities. Weakness is required before the diagnosis can be made. Motor, sensory, and reflex findings on physical examination and the results of nerve conduction and electromyographic studies must be consistent in confirming that dysfunction is attributable to the brachial plexus. The condition should thereby be distinguishable from conditions that may give rise to dysfunction of nerve roots (i.e., radiculopathies) and peripheral nerves (including multiple mononeuropathies), as well as other peripheral and central nervous system structures (e.g., cranial neuropathies, myelopathies).

(8) *Thrombocytopenic purpura* is defined by a serum platelet count less than 50,000/mm^3. Thrombocytopenic purpura does not include cases of thrombocytopenia associated with other causes such as hypersplenism, autoimmune disorders (including alloantibodies from previous transfusions) myelodysplasias, lymphoproliferative disorders, congenital thrombocytopenia or hemolytic uremic syndrome. This does not include cases of immune (formerly called idiopathic) thrombocytopenic purpura (ITP) that are mediated, for example, by viral or fungal infections, toxins or drugs. Thrombocytopenic purpura does not include cases of thyombocytepenia associated with disseminated intravascular coagulation, as observed with bacterial and viral infections. Viral infections include, for example, those infections secondary to Epstein Barr virus, cytomegalovirus, hepatitis A and B, rhinovirus human immunodeficiency virus (HIV), adenovirus, and dengue virus. An antecedent viral infection may be demonstrated by clinical signs and symptoms and need not be confirmed by culture or serologic testing. Bone marrow examination, if performed, must reveal a normal or an increased number of megakaryocytes in an otherwise normal marrow.

(9) *Vaccine-strain measles viral infection* is defined as a disease caused by the vaccine strain that should be determined by vaccine-specific monoclonal antibody or polymerase chain reaction tests.

(10) *Vaccine-strain polio viral infection* is defined as a disease caused by poliovirus that is isolated from the affected tissue and should be determined to be the vaccine-strain by oligonucleotide or polymerase chain reaction. Isolation of poliovirus from the stool is not sufficient to establish a tissue specific infection or disease caused by vaccine-strain poliovirus.

(11) *Early-onset Hib disease* is defined as invasive bacterial illness associated with the presence of Hib organism on culture of normally sterile body fluids or tissue, or clinical findings consistent with the diagnosis of epiglottitis. Hib pneumonia qualifies as invasive Hib disease when radiographic findings consistent with the diagnosis of pneumonitis are accompanied by a blood culture positive for the Hib organism. Otitis media, in the absence of the above findings, dose not qualify as invasive bacterial disease. A child is considered to have suffered this injury only if the vaccine was the first Hib immunization received by the child.

imposed upon this particular vaccine regimen, vaccine brands and doses may not be interchanged.

Measles-Mumps-Rubella Vaccine

MMR is a live virus vaccine. One dose usually confers life-long immunity in 95% of recipients. The second dose of measles vaccine was added to the schedule to cover the 5% of the population, which does not seroconvert after one dose. Leaving 5% of the population unimmunized had continued to lead to periodic measles outbreaks. Single-antigen measles, mumps, or rubella vaccine is rarely given, which has led to the more common use of MMR for the second dose.

Antibodies begin to rise approximately 5 to 12 days after immunization. MMR is contraindicated during pregnancy because of the statistical chance of teratogenesis. Menstrual history must be assessed, and the female of childbearing age advised to avoid pregnancy for 3 months after MMR immunization. It may be safely given to the human immunodeficiency virus (HIV)–positive person if the CD4T cell count is 25% or higher. (For additional information, refer to Tables 13-2, 13-3, 13-5, and 13-6.) Issues have been raised about a possible connection between MMR vaccine and autism. Recently the National Academy of Medicine has published findings that disprove this theory.

Varicella Vaccine

Varicella-zoster virus (VAR) vaccine, a live virus vaccine, is highly effective. As with MMR, it should not be given to pregnant women. The same precautions for MMR are in effect for VAR. Asymptomatic HIV-positive individuals and those with impaired humoral immunodeficiency may be given VAR if the CD4T cell count is 25% or higher. (For more information, refer to Tables 13-2, 13-3, and 13-6.)

VAR may also be used for prophylaxis. The vaccine prevents infection in 70% to 100% of individuals if given within 3 days of exposure and could possibly offer protection after as much as 5 days. Giving VAR after 5 days will not prevent infection but will confer immunity should the disease not develop.

Influenza Vaccine

Influenza vaccine is not routinely given to children unless they suffer from a chronic illness such as asthma or diabetes mellitus or are immunocompromised. The child must be at least 6 months of age before influenza vaccine can be given (see Tables 13-3 and 13-6).

Pneumococcal Vaccine

Until recently, only polysaccharide-chain pneumococcal vaccine was available. This vaccine did not invoke immunity in children less than 2 years of age. A protein conjugate pneumococcal vaccine (PCV7, or Prevnar) that confers excellent immunity is now recommended for use in children less than 2 years of age. Pneumococcal conjugate vaccine 7 valent (PCV7) is recommended for all children 24 to 59 months of age who are at high risk for invasive pneumococcal infection, such as those with sickle cell disease, HIV, asplenia, congenital immune deficiency, chronic cardiac disease, chronic pulmonary disease, cerebrospinal fluid leads, chronic renal insufficiency, malignancies, solid organ transplantation, and diabetes mellitus. The next highest priority groups for the vaccine are children 24 to 35 months of age, followed by children 36 to 59 months of age who attend out-of-home day care. Children 36 to 59 months of age who are of Native American or African-American descent are also a priority (see Tables 13-3 and 13-6). Polysaccharide-chain pneumococcal vaccine is recommended for children over 2 years of age even if they have received conjugated vaccine, should they be in the high-risk group for invasive pneumococcal infection. The polysaccharide-chain vaccine covers the seven most virulent serotypes of the organism found in this age group in the United States, more than the conjugate vaccine does.

Meningococcal Vaccine

Meningococcal disease generally occurs in small settings. First-year college students living in campus housing have been found to be at slightly higher risk for this disease than the general public. It is now recommended that health care providers counsel parents and guardians regarding the risk of this disease to their adolescent children. Pneumococcal vaccine should be offered as an option. The currently licensed vaccine covers about 50% of the most virulent serotypes of the organism. Meningococcal vaccine is safe and effective, but immunity generally lasts only from 3 to 5 years.

Hepatitis A Vaccine

Hepatitis A is the most commonly reported type of hepatitis in the United States and is generally asymptomatic in children. Children are the usual source of infection. Hepatitis A vaccine (Hep A) is recommended for all children 2 years of age and older in communities identified as high risk for hepatitis A, international travelers, and homosexual men. This vaccine has an excellent rate of seroconversion and confers lifelong immunity.

Table 13-5 Guidelines for Spacing Live and Killed Antigen Administration

ANTIGEN COMBINATION	RECOMMENDED MINIMUM INTERVAL BETWEEN DOSES
≥ two killed antigens	None. May be given simultaneously or at any interval between doses*
Killed and live antigens	None. May be given simultaneously or at any interval between doses†
≥ two live antigens	4-week minimum interval if not administered simultaneously

From the Centers for Disease Control and Prevention. Atlanta.

If possible, vaccines associated with local or systemic side effects (e.g., cholera, typhoid, plague vaccines) should be given on separate occasions to avoid accentuated reactions.

†*Cholera vaccines with yellow fever vaccine are the exception. If time permits, the antigens should not be administered simultaneously, and at least 3 weeks should elapse between administration of yellow fever vaccine and cholera vaccine. If the vaccine must be given simultaneously or within 3 weeks of each other, the antibody response may not be optimal.*

Table 13-6 Summary of the Advisory Committee on Immunization Practices of the American Academy of Pediatrics' Recommendations on Immunization of Immunocompromised Infants and Children

VACCINE	ROUTINE (NOT IMMUNOCOMPROMISED)	HIV INFECTION/AIDS	SEVERELY IMMUNOCOMPROMISED (NON–HIV RELATED)*	ASPLENIA	RENAL FAILURE	DIABETES
Routine Infant Immunizations						
DTaP (DT/T/Td)†	Use if indicated	Recommended	Recommended	Recommended	Recommended	Recommended
eIPV	Use if indicated	Recommended	Recommended	Use if indicated	Use if indicated	Use if indicated
MMR (MR/M/R)	Recommended	Recommended/considered	Contraindicated	Recommended	Recommended	Recommended
Hib	Recommended	Recommended	Recommended	Recommended	Recommended	Recommended
Hepatitis B‡	Recommended	Recommended	Recommended	Recommended	Recommended	Recommended
Other Childhood Immunizations						
Pneumococcal§	Use if indicated	Recommended	Recommended	Recommended	Recommended	Recommended
Influenza||	Use if indicated	Recommended	Recommended	Recommended	Recommended	Recommended
Varicella	Recommended	Recommended/considered	Not recommended	Not recommended	Not recommended	Recommended

From Centers for Disease Control and Prevention. Atlanta.
*Severe immunosuppression can be the result of congenital immunodeficiency, HIV infection, leukemia, lymphoma, aplastic anemia, generalized malignancy or therapy with alkylating agents, antimetabolites, radiation, or large amounts of corticosteroids.
†Including DTaP boosters.
‡Hep B vaccine is now recommended for all infants.
§Recommended for persons ≥ 2 years of age.
||Not recommended for infants <6 months of age.
For further information refer to the latest MMWR publication on immunizations.*

Recommended Childhood Immunization Schedule
United States, January-December 2001

Vaccines[1] are listed under routinely recommended ages. [Bars] indicate range of recommended ages for immunization. Any dose not given at the recommended age should be given as a "catch-up" immunization at any subsequent visit when indicated and feasible. (Ovals) indicate vaccines to be given if previously recommended doses were missed or given earlier than the recommended minimum age.

Updates to this schedule may be found at the American Academy of Pediatrics' Website (www.aap.org/family/parents/immunize.htm).

Age ▶ Vaccines ▼	Birth	1 mo	2 mos	4 mos	6 mos	12 mos	15 mos	18 mos	24 mos	4-6 yrs	11-12 yrs	14-16 yrs
Hepatitis B[2]		Hep B #1	Hep B #2		Hep B #3						Hep B[2]	
Diphtheria, Tetanus, Pertussis[3]			DTaP	DTaP	DTaP		DTaP[3]			DTaP	Td	
H. influenzae type B[4]			Hib	Hib	Hib	Hib						
Inactivated Polio[5]			IPV	IPV	IPV[5]					IPV[5]		
Pneumococcal Conjugate[6]			PCV	PCV	PCV	PCV						
Measles, Mumps, Rubella[7]						MMR				MMR[7]	MMR[7]	
Varicella[8]						Var					Var[8]	
Hepatitis A[9]									Hep A (in selected areas)[9]			

Approved by the Advisory Committee on Immunization Practices (ACIP), the American Academy of Pediatrics (AAP), and the American Academy of Family Physicians (AAFP).

1. This schedule indicates the recommended ages for routine administration of currently licensed childhood vaccines, as of 11/1/00, for children through 18 years of age. Additional vaccines may be licensed and recommended during the year. Licensed combination vaccines may be used whenever any components of the combination are indicated and its other components are not contraindicated. Providers should consult the manufacturers' package inserts for detailed recommendations.

2. **Infants born to HBsAg-negative mothers** should receive the first dose of hepatitis B (Hep B) vaccine by age 2 months. The second dose should be at least one month after the first dose. The third dose should be administered at least 4 months after the first dose and at least 2 months after the second dose, but not before 6 months of age for infants.

Infants born to HBsAg-positive mothers should receive hepatitis B vaccine and 0.5 ml hepatitis B immune globulin (HBIG) within 12 hours of birth at separate sites. The second dose is recommended at 1-2 months of age and the third dose at 6 months of age.

Infants born to mothers whose HBsAg status is unknown should receive Hep B vaccine within 12 hours of birth. Maternal blood should be drawn at the time of delivery to determine the mother's HBsAg status; if the HBsAg test is positive, the infant should receive HBIG as soon as possible (no later than 1 week of age).

All children and adolescents who have not been immunized against hepatitis B should begin the series during any visit. Special efforts should be made to immunize children who were born in or whose parents were born in areas of the world with moderate or high endemicity of hepatitis B virus infection.

3. The fourth dose of DTaP (diphtheria and tetanus toxoids and acellular pertussis vaccine) may be administered as early as 12 months of age, provided 6 months have elapsed since the third dose and the child is unlikely to return at age 15-18 months. Td (tetanus and diphtheria toxoids) is recommended at 11-12 years of age at least 5 years have elapsed since the last dose of DTP, DTaP or DT. Subsequent routine Td boosters are recommended every 10 years.

4. Three *Haemophilus influenzae* type B (Hib) conjugate vaccines are licensed for infant use. If PRP-OMP (PedvaxHIB or ComVax [Merck]) is administered at 2 and 4 months of age, a dose at 6 months is not required. Because clinical studies in infants have demonstrated that using some combination products may induce a lower immune response to the Hib vaccine component, DTaP/Hib combination products should not be used for primary immunization in infants at 2, 4, or 6 months of age, unless FDA-approved for these ages.

5. An all-IPV schedule is recommended for routine childhood polio vaccination in the United States. All children should receive four doses of IPV at 2 months, 4 months, 6-18 months, and 4-6 years of age. Oral polio vaccine (OPV) should be used only in selected circumstances. (See *MMWR* May 19, 2000/49(RR-5);1-22).

6. The heptavalent conjugate pneumococcal vaccine (PCV) is recommended for all children 2-23 months of age. It also is recommended for certain children 24-59 months of age. (See *MMWR* Oct. 6, 2000/49(RR-9);1-35).

7. The second dose of measles, mumps, and rubella (MMR) vaccine is recommended routinely at 4-6 years of age but may be administered during any visit, provided at least 4 weeks have elapsed since receipt of the first dose and that both doses are administered beginning at or after 12 months of age. Those who have not previously
received the second dose should complete the schedule by the 11-12 year old visit.

8. Varicella (Var) vaccine is recommended at any visit on or after the first birthday for susceptible children, (i.e., those who lack a reliable history of chickenpox [as judged by a health care provider] and who have not been immunized). Susceptible persons 13 years of age or older should receive two doses, given at least 4 weeks apart

9. Hepatitis A (Hep A) is shaded to indicate its recommended use in selected states and/or regions, and for certain high risk groups; consult the local public health authority. (See *MMWR* Oct. 1, 1999/48(RR-12); 1-37).

For additional information about the vaccines listed above, please visit the National Immunization Program Home Page at www.cdc.gov/nip or call the National Immunization Hotline at (800) 232-2522 (English) or (800) 232-0233 (Spanish).

Fig. 13-1 Recommended Childhood Vaccination Schedule. (From Centers for Disease Control and Prevention. [2000]. Atlanta.)

Thimerosal Issues

Thimerosal is a preservative used in vaccines since vaccines were introduced in the 1930s. Because thimerosal contains trace amounts of mercury, a heavy metal, efforts have been made to eliminate thimerosal from all vaccines. Several vaccines in use in the United States are already thimerosal free. This measure was taken to eliminate any theoretical risk to a small infant from mercury and was not triggered by any adverse events. Any newly licensed vaccines in the United States will no longer contain thimerosal.

Scheduling of Immunizations

Fig. 13-1 includes the Recommended Childhood Vaccination Schedule for the United States (January-December 2001; updates at www.aap.org/family/parents/immunize.htm). Table 13-7 includes the accelerated immunization schedule for infants and children under 7 years of age, and Table 13-8 describes the recommended schedule for children 7 years of age and older.

- Intervals between doses that are longer than recommended do not lead to a decrease in final antibody levels. It is not necessary to restart an interrupted series or give extra doses.
- Giving doses of vaccine or toxoid closer than recommended intervals may lessen the antibody response and therefore should be avoided. If a subsequent dose of vaccine is given at less than the recommended interval, the previous dose does not count as part of the series. The appropriate time must elapse before the next dose is administered (see Tables 13-5 and 13-9).
- Live virus vaccines (e.g., MMR) must be separated by a minimum of 28 days, but more than one live virus vaccine (e.g., VAR) can be given on the same day. Shorter intervals limit the antibody response and render the second dose ineffective (see Tables 13-5 and 13-9).

- MMR should *not* be given if the individual has received gamma globulin within the last 5 months. There is a 6-month interval between the administration of blood and MMR, and 7 months must pass after the administration of plasma or platelets. Blood products decrease immune response.
- Historically, immunization providers gave half doses of vaccines such as DTP in an effort to decrease the reaction to the vaccine. However, these half doses do not stimulate an adequate immune response. Therefore any half-dose vaccine is to be discounted as part of a series. A full dose must be repeated to confer adequate protection.

Special Considerations

Immunocompromised Children

Immunizations present special challenges for immunocompromised children. These children still need to be immunized, even considering their inadequate antibody response to vaccines. It is believed that for the HIV-positive child limited protection from immunizations is better than no protection at all. The routinely given live virus vaccines MMR and VAR may be administered to asymptomatic HIV-positive children and those with impaired humoral immunodeficiency. The indications for these vaccines are discussed in the previous sections on MMR and VAR vaccines. Since the virus replicates in the blood, it does not pose the danger of reinfecting the child. Limited studies of MMR vaccine in HIV-positive patients have not documented serious or unusual adverse effects. Because measles and varicella may cause severe illness in children with HIV infection, MMR and VAR vaccines are recommended for all children without overt symptoms of infection and adequate CD4T cell counts at the time of immunization. All other immunizations are given as scheduled to the HIV-positive child. Additionally, immunocompromised children should receive PCV7

Table 13-7 Recommended Immunization Schedule for Children Who Are Older than or at 7 Years of Age Who Were Not Vaccinated at the Recommended Time in Early Infancy

TIMING	VACCINE(S)	COMMENTS
First visit	Td*, OPV†, MMR‡, hepatitis B§	Primary poliovirus vaccination is not routinely recommended to persons ≥ 18 years of age
Second visit (6-8 weeks after first visit)	Td, OPV, MMR‖‡, hepatitis B§	
Third visit (6 months after second visit)	Td, OPV, hepatitis B§	
Additional visits	Td	Repeat every 10 years throughout life

From the Centers for Disease Control and Prevention. Atlanta.

*The DTP and DTaP doses administered to children < 7 years of age who remain incompletely vaccinated at age ≥ 7 years should be counted as previous exposure to tetanus and diphtheria toxoids (e.g., a child who previously received two doses of DTP needs only one dose of Td to complete a primary series for tetanus and diphtheria).

†Inactivated polio virus is recommended for all doses except in limited circumstances. For the immunization schedule for IPV, see the specific ACIP statement on the use of polio vaccine.

‡Persons born before 1957 can generally be considered immune to measles and mumps and need not be vaccinated. Rubella (or MMR) vaccine can be administered to persons of any age, particularly to nonpregnant women of childbearing age.

§Hepatitis B vaccine, recombinant. Selected high-risk groups for whom vaccination is recommended include persons with occupational risk, such as health care and public safety workers who have occupational exposure to blood, patients, and staff of institutions for the developmentally disabled, hemodialysis patient, recipients of certain blood products (e.g., clotting factor concentrates), household contacts and sex partners of hepatitis B virus carriers, injecting drug users, sexually active homosexual and bisexual men, certain sexually active heterosexual men and women, inmates of long-term correctional facilities, certain international travelers, and families of HBsAg-positive adoptees from countries where HBV infection is endemic. Because risk factors are often not identified directly among adolescents, universal hepatitis B vaccination of teenagers should be implemented in communities where injection of drugs, pregnancy among teenagers, and sexually transmitted diseases are common.

‖The ACIP recommends a second dose of measles-containing vaccine (preferably MMR to ensure immunity to mumps and rubella) for certain groups. Children with no documentation of live measles vaccination after the first birthday should receive two doses of live measles-containing vaccine not less than 1 month apart. In addition, the following persons born in 1957 or later should have documentation of measles immunity (i.e., two doses of measles-containing vaccine [at least one being MMR], physician-diagnosed measles, or laboratory evidence of measles immunity): (a) those entering post-high school educational setting; (b) those beginning employment in health care settings who will have direct patient contact (New York State requires all employees in health care settings); and (c) travelers to areas with endemic measles.

Table 13-8 Recommended Accelerated Immunization Schedule for Infants and Children Who Are Younger than 7 Years of Age Who Start the Series Late* or Who Are More than 1 Month Behind in the Immunization Schedule‡ (i.e., Children for Whom Compliance with Scheduled Return Visits Cannot Be Ensured)

TIMING	VACCINE(S)	COMMENTS
First visit (≥ 4 months of age)	DTP⁺, IPV, Hib§⁺, hepatitis B, MMR (should be given as soon as child is age: 12-15 months)	All vaccines should be administered simultaneously at the appropriate visit
Second visit (1 month after first visit)	DTP⁺, Hib§⁺, hepatitis B	
Third visit (1 month after second visit)	DTP⁺, IPV, Hib§⁺	
Fourth visit (6 weeks after third visit)	IPV	
Fifth visit (≥ 6 months after third visit)	DTaP⁺ or DTP, Hib§⁺, hepatitis B	
Additional visits (age 4-6 years)	DTaP⁺ or DTP, IPV, MMR	Preferably at or before school entry
(Age 14-16 years)	Td	Repeat every 10 years throughout life

From the Centers for Disease Control and Prevention. Atlanta.
*If initiated in the first year of life, administer DTP doses 1, 2, and 3 and OPV doses 1, 2, and 3 according to this schedule; administer MMR when the child reaches 12-15 months of age.
†See individual ACIP recommendations for detailed information on specific vaccines.
‡Two DTP and Hib combination vaccines are available (DTP/HbOC [TETRAMUNE] and PRP-T [ActHIB, OmniHIB], which can be reconstituted with DTP vaccine produced by Connaught). DTaP preparations are currently recommended only for use as the fourth and/or fifth doses of the DTP series among children 15 months through 6 years of age (before the seventh birthday). DTP and DTaP should not be used on or after the seventh birthday.
§The recommended schedule varies by vaccine manufacturer. For information specific to the vaccine being used, consult the package insert and ACIP recommendations. Children beginning the Hib vaccine series at age 2-6 months should receive a primary series of three doses of HbOC [Hib TITER] (Lederle-Praxis), PRP-T [ActHIB, OmniHIB] (Pasteur Merieux; SmithKline Beecham; Connaught), or a licensed DTP-Hib combination vaccine; or two doses of PRP-OMP [PedvaxHIB]; (Merck, Sharp, and Dohme). An additional booster dose of any licensed Hib conjugate vaccine should be administered at 12-15 months of age and at least 2 months after the previous dose. Children beginning the Hib vaccine series at 7-11 months of age should receive a primary series of two doses of an HbOC, PRP-T, or PRP-OMP-containing vaccine. An additional booster dose of any licensed Hib conjugate vaccine should be administered at 12-18 months of age and at least 2 months after the previous dose. Children beginning the Hib vaccine series at ages 12-14 months should receive a primary series of one dose of an HbOC, PRP-T, or PRP-OMP-containing vaccine. An additional booster dose of any licensed Hib conjugate vaccine should be administered 2 months after the previous dose. Children beginning the Hib vaccine series at age 15-59 months should receive one dose of any licensed Hib vaccine. Hib vaccine should not be administered after the fifth birthday except for special circumstances as noted in the specific ACIP recommendations for the use of Hib vaccine.

Table 13-9 Minimum Age for Initial Vaccination and Minimum Interval between Vaccine Doses, by Type of Vaccine

VACCINE	MINIMUM AGE FOR FIRST DOSE	MINIMUM INTERVAL FROM DOSE 1 TO 2*	MINIMUM INTERVAL FROM DOSE 2 TO 3*	MINIMUM INTERVAL FROM DOSE 3 TO 4*
DTP/DTaP (DT)⁺	6 weeks	4 weeks	4 weeks	6 months
Hib (primary series)				
HbOC	6 weeks	4 weeks	4 weeks	§
PRP-T	6 weeks	4 weeks	4 weeks	§
PRP-OMP	6 weeks	4 weeks	§	
Polio¶	6 weeks	4 weeks	4 weeks**	⁺⁺
MMR	12 months	4 weeks		
Hepatitis B	Birth	4 weeks	8 weeks§§	
VAR	12 months	4 weeks		
Hepatitis A	2 years	6 months		

From the Centers for Disease Control & Prevention. Atlanta.
*These minimum acceptable ages and intervals may not correspond with the optimal recommended ages and intervals for vaccination. See the ACIP's General Recommendations on Immunization and the current ACIP Recommended Childhood Immunization Schedule, United States for the current recommended routine and accelerated vaccination schedules. This table contains some information that has not yet been published in the ACIP's recommendations.
†The total number of doses of diphtheria and tetanus toxoids should not exceed six each before the seventh birthday.
§The booster dose of Hib vaccine that is recommended following the primary vaccination series should be administered no earlier than 12 months of age and at least 8 weeks after the previous dose of Hib vaccine (Tables 3 and 4 of ACIP's General Recommendations on Immunization).
¶IPV is recommended for all doses except in limited circumstances. Intervals also apply to any combination of IPV and OPV or all OPV.
**For unvaccinated adults at increased risk of exposure to poliovirus with < 3 months but > 2 months available before protection is needed, three doses of IPV should be administered at least 28 days apart.
⁺⁺If the third dose is given after the fourth birthday, the fourth (booster) dose is not needed.
§§This final dose is recommended at least 16 weeks after the first dose and no earlier than 6 months of age.

vaccine as discussed previously. Annual influenza immunization should begin after 6 months of age.

Immunization during chemotherapy or radiation should be avoided because of poor antibody response. Immunization in these children should be delayed until at least 3 months after their treatments have been completed and adequate immune response is demonstrated.

Preterm Infants

Preterm infants are immunized with full doses of DTaP, IPV, Hib, PCV7, MMR, and VAR vaccines at the appropriate chronologic ages regardless of their present weights. Hep B vaccine is not administered until the child weighs 4000 g (4.4 pounds). Seroprotection rates in very low birth weight infants (1 kg) vaccinated soon after birth are lower than in term infants. If the infant does not weigh 2 kg at discharge from the hospital, vaccination should be given at 2 months of age regardless of weight. If there is concern that the infant may not begin vaccination as an outpatient, the first dose should be administered before hospital discharge.

Preterm infants born to HBsAG-positive mothers should receive hepatitis B immune globulin (HBIG) and vaccine within 12 hours of birth regardless of their weight.

Tuberculosis Skin Testing

Live virus vaccines such as MMR and VAR suppress the reactivity of tuberculosis (TB) skin testing. If a child receives MMR or VAR vaccine, TB skin testing must be postponed for 6 weeks. Additionally a child with active TB will have a less-than-adequate immune response to MMR or VAR vaccine. TB testing is currently indicated only for children who have increased risk of exposure. Children who have no risk factors but who reside in high-prevalence regions and children whose histories for risk factors are incomplete or unreliable should be considered for TB testing. An acceptable schedule for testing of these children is 4 to 6 years of age and 11 to 16 years of age (see the section on tuberculosis in Chapter 44).

The Mantoux test, also referred to as purified protein derivative (PPD) skin testing, is the only acceptable testing method. Previously tine testing was considered adequate for mass screening, but it is no longer considered reliable. Ideally the PPD should be administered first, followed by the MMR or VAR on the day the child returns for the PPD reading. Often this is not feasible, and it is acceptable practice to administer these vaccines along with the PPD at the same visit.

Records

Adequate record-keeping is essential; an immunization history must follow a child throughout life. If a record is unobtainable, it results in the child having to repeat all immunizations. Reimmunization is costly, time consuming, and uncomfortable for both the child and parent or guardian. The most recent development in record keeping is the creation of an immunization database. The CDC is presently funding the creation of such a database in individual states. This system eliminates the problem of missing records. Presently the CDC mandates storing immunization records for 25 years.

A well-documented history must be completed before immunization to minimize reactions and to determine which vaccines are to be given. Several questionnaires exist, though the one chosen must include all pertinent information (Fig. 13-2). Parents do not always accompany children for immunizations.

The CDC states that any blood relative who is at least 18 years of age may consent. The parent or guardian must be provided with a record of each immunization and reminded to bring the immunization record to each health care visit.

In addition, all health care providers (defined as any licensed health care professional, organization, or institution, whether private or public, under whose authority a specified vaccine is administered) are required to ensure that the following are recorded on the vaccine recipient's permanent record or office log or file:

- Date the vaccine was administered
- Manufacturer and lot number of vaccine
- Name, address, and title of person administering the vaccine

These records must be accessible to a legal representative or parent or guardian upon request.

Parent Education

One of the most important aspects of immunization administration is adequate parent teaching. It is essential to give the parents all the information available so that they can make informed decisions for their children (see Table 13-3). Parents should be given every opportunity to ask questions and to have those questions answered to their satisfaction. Current vaccine information sheets are supplied by the CDC, and they must be given to parents before vaccines are administered.

Remind parents and caregivers that an immunization can cause a lump at the site of the injection that can last from several days to several weeks. An ice pack applied to the site as long as it is warm and red followed by warm soaks thereafter can be very soothing. If the child is still uncomfortable, the parent can give acetaminophen. Give the parent a copy of an acetaminophen dosing sheet and advise that the dose is based on weight, not age. Encourage the parent to offer extra fluids as an additional precaution should the child develop a fever. Inform parents which potential side effects necessitate calling the practitioner or going to an emergency department.

Immunization Techniques

- For children under 2 years of age, intramuscular injections should be limited to the anterolateral aspect of the upper thigh. The buttock should never be used to prevent injury to the sciatic nerve.
- Reports of decreased immune response to hepatitis B vaccine presumably are attributable to inadvertent subcutaneous injection or injection into deep fat when the vaccine is injected into the buttock.
- Toddlers (not preferred) and older children: the deltoid is an acceptable injection site for both intramuscular and subcutaneous injections.
- It is best to use a separate site for each immunization.
- When multiple injections are required, it is acceptable to use the same limb, but the sites should be separated by at least 1 inch.
- Needle size for intramuscular injections: infants $7/8$ to 1 inch, 22- to 25-gauge needle; toddlers and older children 1 to $1\frac{1}{4}$ inch, 22- to 25-gauge needle.
- The Minnesota State Health Department immunization website provides excellent diagrams on immunization administration sites for children and adults.

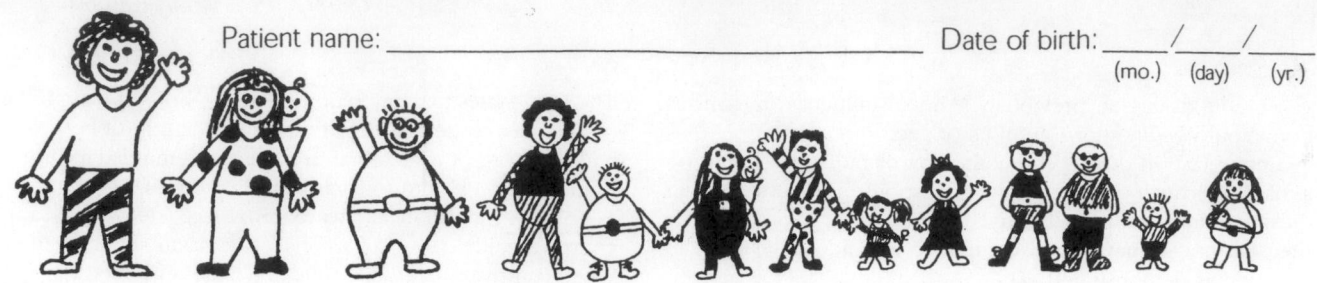

Patient name: _____ Date of birth: ____/____/____
                                                                (mo.) (day) (yr.)

Screening Questionnaire
for Child and Teen Immunization

For parents/guardians: The following questions will help us determine which vaccines may be given today. If a question is not clear, please ask the nurse or doctor to explain it.

	Yes	No	Don't Know
1. Is the child sick today?	☐	☐	☐
2. Does the child have allergies to medications, food, or any vaccine?	☐	☐	☐
3. Has the child had a serious reaction to a vaccine in the past?	☐	☐	☐
4. Has the child had a seizure or a brain problem?	☐	☐	☐
5. Does the child have cancer, leukemia, AIDS, or any other immune system problem?	☐	☐	☐
6. Has the child taken cortisone, prednisone, other steroids, or anticancer drugs, or had x-ray treatments in the past 3 months?	☐	☐	☐
7. Has the child received a transfusion of blood or blood products, or been given a medicine called immune (gamma) globulin in the past year?	☐	☐	☐
8. Is the child/teen pregnant or is there a chance she could become pregnant in the next 3 months?	☐	☐	☐
9. Has the child received any vaccinations in the past 4 weeks?	☐	☐	☐

Form completed by: _____ Date: _____

Did you bring your child's immunization record card with you?   yes ☐   no ☐

It is important to have a personal record of your child's vaccinations. If you don't have a record card, ask the child's health care provider to give you one! Bring this record with you every time you seek medical care for your child. Make sure your health care provider records all your child's vaccinations on it. Your child will need this card to enter daycare, kindergarten, junior high, etc.

Item #P4060 (3/01)

Immunization Action Coalition • 1573 Selby Avenue • St. Paul, MN 55104 • (651) 647-9009 • www.immunize.org

Fig. 13-2 Screening Questionnaire for Child and Teen Immunization. (From Immunization Action Coalition. [2001, March]. St. Paul, MN, and Chicago.)

Standards for Pediatric Immunizations

The CDC has developed standards for pediatric immunization practices (Box 13-1) to maintain consistent quality assurance in the administration of immunizations. All providers using federally supplied vaccine are expected to conform to these standards to ensure the safe, efficient, and cost-effective administration of immunizations.

Handling and Storage of Vaccines

Vaccines, also referred to as "biologicals," are very fragile and must be handled carefully to maintain potency. Table 13-10 discusses the proper storage and handling of vaccines.

National Childhood Vaccine Injury Act

The National Childhood Vaccine Injury Act of 1986, which became effective in 1988, includes requirements for detailed notification of parents and patients about vaccine benefits and risks in both the private and public sectors. This legislation requires the development and distribution of standardized benefit-risk statements when one is administering vaccines for which vaccine injury compensation is available. Table 13-4 lists reportable events after vaccination.

Currently these requirements apply to DTaP, single-antigen measles, mumps, rubella, MMR, VAR, Td, TOPV, IPV, Hep B, Hib, Hep A, and PCV7. The withdrawal of rotavirus vaccine was the result of diligent monitoring for vaccine side effects by the VAERS system.

Adverse events after vaccination purchased with public funds must be reported on the Vaccine Adverse Event Reporting System (VAERS) form (Fig. 13-3) and sent to VAERS, c/o ERC BioServices Corporation, 1055 First Street, Suite 130, Rockville, MD 20850-9788.

Vaccine Reactions

Tables 13-2 to 13-4 describe contraindications, side effects of vaccines, and reportable events after vaccination.

- Shock-collapse or hypotonic-hyporesponsive collapse may be evidenced by signs or symptoms such as decrease in or loss of muscle tone, paralysis (partial or complete), hemiplegia, loss of color or turning pale white or blue, unresponsiveness to environmental stimuli, depression of or loss of consciousness, prolonged sleeping with difficulty arousing, or cardiovascular or respiratory arrest.
- Residual seizure disorder may be considered to have occurred if: (1) *before* the vaccination the child had no seizure or convulsion either unaccompanied by fever or accompanied by fever of less than 102° F, and (2) two or more seizures or convulsions occur within 1 year after the vaccination either unaccompanied by fever or accompanied by fever of less than 102° F.
- The terms *seizure* and *convulsion* include grand mal, petit mal, myoclonic, tonic-clonic, and focal motor

Box 13-1 Standards for Pediatric Immunization Practices

1. Immunization services are readily available.
2. There are no barriers or unnecessary prerequisites to the receipt of vaccines.
3. Immunization services are available free or for a minimal fee.
4. Providers utilize all clinical encounters to screen and, when indicated, vaccinate children.
5. Providers educate parents and guardians about immunization in general terms.
6. Providers question parents and guardians about contraindications and, before vaccinating a child, inform them in specific terms about the risks and benefits of the vaccinations their child is to receive.
7. Providers follow only true contraindications.
8. Providers administer simultaneously all vaccine doses for which a child is eligible at the time of each visit.
9. Providers use accurate and complete recording procedures.
10. Providers co-schedule immunization appointments in conjunction with appointments in conjunction with appointments for other child health services.
11. Providers report adverse events following vaccination promptly, accurately, and completely.
12. Providers operate a tracking system.
13. Providers adhere to appropriate procedures for vaccine management.
14. Providers conduct semiannual audits to assess immunization coverage levels and to review immunization records in the patient populations they serve.
15. Providers maintain up-to-date, easily retrievable medical protocols at all locations where vaccines are administered.
16. Providers practice patient-oriented and community-based approaches.
17. Vaccines are administered by properly trained persons.
18. Providers receive ongoing education and training regarding current immunization recommendations.

From the Centers for Disease Control and Prevention. Atlanta.

seizures and signs. Encephalopathy means any significant acquired abnormality of, injury to, or impairment of function of the brain. Among the frequent manifestations of encephalopathy are focal and diffuse neurologic signs, increased intracranial pressure, or changes lasting at least 6 hours in levels of consciousness, with or without convulsions. The neurologic signs and symptoms of encephalopathy may be temporary with complete recovery, or they may result in various degrees of permanent impairment. Signs and symptoms such as high-pitched and unusual screaming, persistent inconsolable crying, and bulging fontanels are compatible with a diagnosis of encephalopathy but in and of themselves are not conclusive evidence of encephalopathy. Encephalopathy usually can be documented by slow-wave activity on an electroencephalogram.

Table 13-10 Vaccine Management: Recommendations for Handling and Storage of Selected Biologicals

BIOLOGICAL	SHIPPING REQUIREMENTS	CONDITION ON ARRIVAL*	STORAGE REQUIREMENTS
DTaP: Diphtheria toxoid, tetanus toxoid, acellular pertussis vaccine DTaP/ACTHIB: Diphtheria toxoid, tetanus toxoid, acellular pertussis vaccine combined with *Haemophilus* conjugate vaccine DTP: Diphtheria toxoid, tetanus toxoid, whole cell pertussis vaccine DTP/HIB: Diphtheria toxoid, tetanus toxoid, whole cell pertussis vaccine combined with *Haemophilus* conjugate vaccine†	Should be shipped in insulated container. Maintain temperature at 35° to 46° F (2° to 8° C). **Do not freeze** or store vaccine in direct contact with refrigerant.	Should not have been frozen. Refrigerate on arrival.	Refrigerate immediately on arrival. Store at 35° to 46° F (2° to 8° C). **Do not freeze.**
HBIG: Hepatitis B immune globulin	Should be shipped in insulated container.	Should not have been frozen. Refrigerate on arrival.	Refrigerate immediately on arrival. Store at 35° to 46° F (2° to 8° C). **Do not freeze.**
Hepatitis vaccine: Hepatitis A and hepatitis B	Use insulated container. Must be shipped with refrigerant.†	Should not have been frozen. Refrigerate on arrival.	Refrigerate immediately on arrival. Store at 35° to 46° F (2° to 8° C). **Do not freeze.**
Hib or HBCV: *Haemophilus* conjugate vaccine	Should be shipped in insulated container to help prevent freezing.	Should not have been frozen. Refrigerate on arrival.	Refrigerate immediately on arrival. Store at 35° to 46° F (2° to 8° C). **Do not freeze**—this reduces potency.
Influenza vaccine	Should be delivered in the shortest possible time. Should not be exposed to excessive temperatures.	Should not have been frozen. Refrigerate on arrival.	Refrigerate immediately on arrival. Store at 35° to 46° F (2° to 8° C). **Do not freeze.**
IPV: Inactivated poliovirus vaccine	Should be shipped in insulated container with refrigerant.	Should not have been frozen. Refrigerate on arrival.	Refrigerate immediately on arrival. Store at 35° to 46° F (2° to 8° C). **Do not freeze.**

If you have questions about the condition of the material at the time of delivery, you should: (1) Immediately place material in recommended storage, and (2) notify the Quality Control office of the vaccine manufacturer, or (3) notify the National Immunization Program, CDC, Atlanta, Georgia.

†*ACTHIB (Connaught) should be used within 24 hours of reconstitution if used alone or when reconstituted with Connaught DTP. If Connaught DTaP is used to reconstitute ACTHIB, the TriHibit vaccine must be used within 30 minutes. Only Connaught DTP, DTaP, or the diluent shipped with the product may be used to reconstitute the Connaught ACTHIB product. Pedvax Hib-Merck-available in liquid and lyophilized one-dose vials good for 24 hours after reconstitution if kept at 35° to 46° F (2° to 8° C).*

†*Engerix by SmithKline Beecham may be shipped without refrigerant for up to 96 hours as long as the vaccine does not exceed 86° F.*

SHELF-LIFE EXPIRATION	INSTRUCTION ON RECONSTITUTION OR USE	SHELF-LIFE AFTER RECONSTITUTION, THAWING, OR OPENING	SPECIAL INSTRUCTIONS
Up to 18 months. Check date on vial or container.	Shake vial vigorously before withdrawing each dose.	Until outdated, if not contaminated.	Rotate stock so that the shortest dated material is used first.
Up to 1 year. Check date on vial or container.	Shake vial vigorously before withdrawing each dose.	Until outdated, if not contaminated.	Rotate stock so that the shortest dated material is used first.
Up to 3 years. Check date on vial or container.	Shake vial vigorously before withdrawing each dose.	Until outdated, if not contaminated.	Rotate stock so that the shortest dated material is used first.
Up to 2 years. Check date on vial or container.	If the product requires reconstitution, record date of reconstitution on vial. Use only diluent supplied.	*Multidose vials*—Stable until date of expiration, if stored at 35° to 46° F (2° to 8° C) when not in use. *Single-dose vials*[†]— Discard unused reconstituted vials after 24 hours.	Rotate stock so that the shortest dated material is used first.
Formulated for use within current influenza season.	Shake vial vigorously before withdrawing each dose.	Until outdated, if not contaminated.	Rotate stock so that the shortest dated vaccine is used first.
Up to 18 months. Check date on package.	*Ampule (1 dose)*—Tap the ampule to ensure that the solution is in the lower portion rather than in the neck of the ampule. With sterile needle and syringe, withdraw the contents of the ampule into syringe, holding the ampule in such a way that the point of the needle is kept immersed throughout the withdrawal.	*Ampule*—Discard if not used immediately.	Rotate stock so that the shortest dated vaccine is used first. The vaccine should be perfectly clear. Any vaccine showing particulate matter, turbidity, or change of color should be discarded.
	Vial (10 doses)—Withdraw 0.5 ml of vaccine into separate sterile needle and syringe for each immunization.	*Vial*—Until outdated if not contaminated.	

Continued

Table 13-10 Vaccine Management: Recommendations for Handling and Storage of Selected Biologicals—cont'd

BIOLOGICAL	SHIPPING REQUIREMENTS	CONDITION ON ARRIVAL*	STORAGE REQUIREMENTS
Measles virus vaccine, mumps virus vaccine, rubella virus vaccine measles/mumps/rubella-MMR vaccine, measles/rubella-MR vaccine Note: All materials used for administering live virus vaccines should be burned, boiled, or autoclaved before disposal.	*Vaccine*—Use insulated container. Must be shipped with refrigerant. Maintain at 50° F (10° C) or less. If shipped with dry ice, diluent must be shipped separately. *Diluent*—May be shipped with vaccine but **do not freeze.**	Should be below 50° F (10° C). If above this temperature, see footnote. **Do not use warm vaccine.** Refrigerate on arrival.	Vaccine may be stored separately from diluent. Store as follows: Vaccine—refrigerate immediately on arrival. Store at 35° to 46° F (2° to 8° C). **Protect from light at all times,** since such exposure may inactivate the virus. Diluent may be stored at 59° to 86° F (15° to 30° C) room temperature. **Do not freeze.** Note: Freeze dried (lyophilized) vaccines may be maintained at freezer temperatures.
TD (adult): Tetanus-diphtheria toxoids DT (pediatric): Diphtheria-tetanus toxoids	Should be shipped in insulated container. Maintain temperature at 35° to 46° F (2° to 8° C). **Do not freeze** or store vaccine in direct contact with refrigerant.	Should not have been **frozen.** Refrigerate on arrival.	Refrigerate immediately on arrival. Store at 35° to 46° F (2° to 8° C). **Do not freeze.**
Pneumococcal polysaccharide vaccine (polyvalent)	Should be shipped in insulated container with refrigerant. **Do not freeze.**	Should not have been frozen. Refrigerate on arrival.	Refrigerate immediately on arrival. Store at 35° to 46° F (2° to 8° C). **Do not freeze.**
Varicella (chickenpox) vaccine	Ship with dry ice only. Should be delivered within 2 days.	Should be frozen. Vaccine should remain at −5° F (−20° C) until arrival at health care facility. Dry ice should still be present in the shipping container when vaccine is delivered.	Maintain in a continuously frozen state at 5° F (−15° C) or colder. **No freeze thaw cycles are allowed with this vaccine.** Vaccine should only be stored in freezers or refrigerator/freezers with separate doors and compartments. Acceptable storage may be achieved in standard household freezers purchased in the last 10 years, and standard household refrigerator/freezers with a separate, sealed freezer compartment. In order to maintain this temperature it will be necessary in most refrigerator/freezer models to turn the temperature dial down to the coldest setting. This may result in the refrigerator compartment temperature being lowered as well. Careful monitoring of the refrigerator temperature to avoid freezing killed or inactivated vaccines will be necessary.

*If you have questions about the condition of the material at the time of delivery, you should: (1) Immediately place material in recommended storage, and (2) notify the Quality Control office of the vaccine manufacturer, or (3) notify the National Immunization Program, CDC, Atlanta, Georgia.
†ACTHIB (Connaught) should be used within 24 hours of reconstitution if used alone or when reconstituted with Connaught DTP. If Connaught DTaP is used to reconstitute ACTHIB, the TriHibit vaccine must be used within 30 minutes. Only Connaught DTP, DTaP, or the diluent shipped with the product may be used to reconstitute the Connaught ACTHIB product. Pedvax Hib-Merck-available in liquid and lyophilized one-dose vials good for 24 hours after reconstitution if kept at 35° to 46° F (2° to 8° C).
‡Engerix by SmithKline Beecham may be shipped without refrigerant for up to 96 hours as long as the vaccine does not exceed 86° F.

SHELF-LIFE EXPIRATION	INSTRUCTION ON RECONSTITUTION OR USE	SHELF-LIFE AFTER RECONSTITUTION, THAWING, OR OPENING	SPECIAL INSTRUCTIONS
Vaccine—Up to 2 years. Check date on container or vial. *Diluent*—Check date on container or vial.	Use **only** the diluent supplied to reconstitute the vaccine. *Single-dose vials*—Inject diluent into the vial of lyophilized vaccine and agitate to ensure thorough mixing. Withdraw entire contents into syringe and inject total volume of vaccine subcutaneously. *Multidose vials*—Withdraw **all** diluent from vial into syringe. Inject into vial of lyophilized vaccine and agitate to ensure thorough mixing. *10-Dose vials*—Withdraw 0.5 ml of reconstituted vaccine into separate sterile needle and syringe for each immunization. Licensed for jet injector use. *50-Dose vials*—Use on jet injector only, with dosage set at 0.5 ml.	After reconstitution, use immediately or store in a dark place at 35° to 46° F (2° to 8° C). **Discard if not used within 8 hours.**	Rotate stock so that the shortest dated vaccine is used first. *10-Dose vials*—May be used for both jet injector and needle and syringe methods of immunization.
Up to 2 years. Check date on vial or container.	Shake vial vigorously before withdrawing each dose.	Until outdated, if not contaminated.	Rotate stock so that the shortest dated vaccine is used first.
Up to 2 years. Check date on container or vial.	*Vials*—Shake vial vigorously before withdrawing each dose. *Prefilled syringes*—Follow manufacturer's directions.	Until outdated, if not contaminated.	Rotate stock so that the shortest dated vaccine is used first. **Do not inject intravenously.** Intradermal administration may cause severe local reactions and should be avoided.
Up to 18 months. Check date on package and use the earliest expiration date first.	This product is a lyophilized (freeze-dried) product and should only be reconstituted with the diluent provided with the vaccine. This vaccine must be used within 30 minutes of reconstitution or should be discarded.		If this vaccine is stored at a temperature warmer than −15° C, it will result in a loss of potency and a reduced shelf life. If a power outage or some other situation occurs that results in the vaccine storage temperature rising above the recommended storage, the health care provider should contact Merck, the manufacturer, at (800) 827-4829 for a reevaluation of the products potency before using the vaccine.

VAERS

VACCINE ADVERSE EVENT REPORTING SYSTEM
24 Hour Toll-free information line 1-800-822-7967
P.O. Box 1100, Rockville, MD 20849-1100
PATIENT IDENTITY KEPT CONFIDENTIAL

For CDC/FDA Use Only

VAERS Number _____

Date Received _____

Patient Name:	Vaccine administered by (Name):	Form completed by (Name):
Last　　First　　M.I.	Responsible Physician _____	Relation ☐ Vaccine Provider ☐ Patient/Parent to Patient ☐ Manufacturer ☐ Other
Address	Facility Name/Address	Address *(if different from patient or provider)*
City　State　Zip	City　State　Zip	City　State　Zip
Telephone no. (____)____	Telephone no. (____)____	Telephone no. (____)____

1. State	2. County where administered	3. Date of birth ___/___/___ mm dd yy	4. Patient age	5. Sex ☐ M ☐ F	6. Date form completed ___/___/___ mm dd yy

7. Describe adverse event(s) (symptoms, signs, time course) and treatment, if any	8. Check all appropriate:
	☐ Patient died　(date ___/___/___) mm dd yy
	☐ Life threatening illness
	☐ Required emergency room/doctor visit
	☐ Required hospitalization (_____days)
	☐ Resulted in prolongation of hospitalization
	☐ Resulted in permanent disability
	☐ None of the above

9. Patient recovered ☐ YES ☐ NO ☐ UNKNOWN	10. Date of vaccination	11. Adverse event onset
12. Relevant diagnostic tests/laboratory data	___/___/___ mm dd yy Time_____ AM PM	___/___/___ mm dd yy Time_____ AM PM

13. Enter all vaccines given on date listed in no. 10

	Vaccine (type)	Manufacturer	Lot number	Route/Site	No. Previous doses
a.	_____	_____	_____	_____	_____
b.	_____	_____	_____	_____	_____
c.	_____	_____	_____	_____	_____
d.	_____	_____	_____	_____	_____

14. Any other vaccinations within 4 weeks of date listed in no. 10

	Vaccine (type)	Manufacturer	Lot number	Route/Site	No. Previous doses	Date given
a.	_____	_____	_____	_____	_____	_____
b.	_____	_____	_____	_____	_____	_____

15. Vaccinated at: ☐ Private doctor's office/hospital ☐ Military clinic/hospital ☐ Public health clinic/hospital ☐ Other/unknown	16. Vaccine purchased with: ☐ Private funds ☐ Military funds ☐ Public funds ☐ Other /unknown	17. Other medications

18. Illness at time of vaccination (specify)	19. Pre-existing physician-diagnosed allergies, birth defects, medical conditions (specify)

20. Have you reported this adverse event previously? ☐ No ☐ To health department ☐ To doctor ☐ To manufacturer	*Only for children 5 and under*
	22. Birth weight ____ lb. ____ oz.	23. No. of brothers and sisters

21. Adverse event following prior vaccination (check all applicable, specify)	*Only for reports submitted by manufacturer/immunization project*	
Adverse Event / Onset Age / Type Vaccine / Dose no. in series	24. Mfr. / imm. proj. report no.	25. Date received by mfr. / imm. proj.
☐ In patient _____ _____ _____ _____		
☐ In brother or sister _____ _____ _____ _____	26. 15 day report? ☐ Yes ☐ No	27. Report type ☐ Initial ☐ Follow-Up

Health care providers and manufacturers are required by law (42 USC 300aa-25) to report reactions to vaccines listed in the Vaccine Injury Table. Reports for reactions to other vaccines are voluntary except when required as a condition of immunization grant awards.

Form VAERS -1

Fig. 13-3 Vaccine Adverse Event Reporting System form. (From VAERS. Rockville, MD.)

DIRECTIONS FOR COMPLETING FORM
(Additional pages may be attached if more space is needed.)

GENERAL

- Use a separate form for each patient. Complete the form to the best of your abilities. Items 3, 4, 7, 8, 10, 11, and 13 are considered essential and should be completed whenever possible. Parents/Guardians may need to consult the facility where the vaccine was administered for some of the information (such as manufacturer, lot number or laboratory data.)
- Refer to the Vaccine Injury Table (VIT) for events mandated for reporting by law. Reporting for other serious events felt to be related but not on the VIT is encouraged.
- Health care providers other than the vaccine administrator (VA) treating a patient for a suspected adverse event should notify the VA and provide the information about the adverse event to allow the VA to complete the form to meet the VA's legal responsibility.
- These data will be used to increase understanding of adverse events following vaccination and will become part of CDC Privacy Act System 09-20-0136, "Epidemiologic Studies and Surveillance of Disease Problems". Information identifying the person who received the vaccine or that person's legal representative will not be made available to the public, but may be available to the vaccinee or legal representative.
- Postage will be paid by addressee. Forms may be photocopied (must be front & back on same sheet).

SPECIFIC INSTRUCTIONS

Form Completed By: To be used by parents/guardians, vaccine manufacturers/distributors, vaccine administrators, and/or the person completing the form on behalf of the patient or the health professional who administered the vaccine.

Item 7: Describe the suspected adverse event. Such things as temperature, local and general signs and symptoms, time course, duration of symptoms diagnosis, treatment and recovery should be noted.

Item 9: Check "YES" if the patient's health condition is the same as it was prior to the vaccine, "NO" if the patient has not returned to the pre-vaccination state of health, or "UNKNOWN" if the patient's condition is not known.

Item 10: Give dates and times as specifically as you can remember. If you do not know the exact time, please
and 11: indicate "AM" or "PM" when possible if this information is known. If more than one adverse event, give the onset date and time for the most serious event.

Item 12: Include "negative" or "normal" results of any relevant tests performed as well as abnormal findings.

Item 13: List ONLY those vaccines given on the day listed in Item 10.

Item 14: List ANY OTHER vaccines the patient received within four weeks of the date listed in Item 10.

Item 16: This section refers to how the person who gave the vaccine purchased it, not to the patient's insurance.

Item 17: List any prescription or non-prescription medications the patient was taking when the vaccine(s) was given.

Item 18: List any short term illnesses the patient had on the date the vaccine(s) was given (i.e., cold, flu, ear infection).

Item 19: List any pre-existing physician-diagnosed allergies, birth defects, medical conditions (including developmental and/or neurologic disorders) the patient has.

Item 21: List any suspected adverse events the patient, or the patient's brothers or sisters, may have had to previous vaccinations. If more than one brother or sister, or if the patient has reacted to more than one prior vaccine, use additional pages to explain completely. For the onset age of a patient, provide the age in months if less than two years old.

Item 26: This space is for manufacturers' use only.

Fig. 13-3, cont'd

Resources

Immunization practices are changing continuously and are constantly being updated. It is essential that the practitioner check with the local health department to determine the most up-to-date information regarding the administration of immunizations. Another resource is the *Morbidity and Mortality Weekly Report* (MMWR) published by the CDC. The CDC also maintains an information services directory to provide the latest information. The directory is divided into sections for the general public, health care workers, and the Advisory Committee on Immunization Practices (ACIP) of the American Academy of Pediatrics (AAP). The following documents are available from the CDC Fax Information Service Immunizations Directory and are updated as necessary. To receive a document, call (404) 332-4565 and follow the prompts. To enter document numbers, choose option 1, and, when asked, enter the six-digit document number and then press the # key. You may then request additional documents or enter your fax number. Your fax number should include your area code plus telephone number (10 digits), followed by the # key. You may enter up to five documents. If you do not receive your fax in a reasonable amount of time, check to see if your fax machine is on and available for transmission. The fax system will make five attempts to deliver the document. After each attempt the fax system waits 5 minutes and then inserts the request at the bottom of the queue. Please retry your call if your fax does not arrive within an hour.

For the General Public

000004	Other diseases directory
000005	International travelers' health information

General Information Documents

240000	Overall immunization schedule
240001	How to report vaccine adverse reactions
240002	Theory of immunizations

General Vaccine Information Pamphlets

246084	Measles, mumps, and rubella
246085	Diphtheria, tetanus, and pertussis
246059	Polio

Measles Information

241001	Disease and immunity information
241002	Vaccine
241003	Vaccine side effects
241004	Recommendations for immune suppressed
241005	Statistics

Mumps Information

242001	Disease and immunity information
242002	Pregnancy
242003	Vaccine information
242004	Statistics

Rubella Information

243001	Disease and immunity information
243002	Congenital rubella syndrome
243003	Postexposure treatment
243004	Rubella vaccine
243005	Pregnancy
243006	Statistics and goals for rubella vaccine program

Diphtheria Information

244001	Disease information
244002	Pregnancy
244003	Vaccine information
244004	Statistics

Tetanus Information

245001	Disease information
245002	Pregnancy
245003	Wounds
245004	Vaccine information
245005	Statistics menu

Pertussis Information

246001   Disease information
246002   Vaccine information (new and old)
246003   Pregnancy
246004   Pertussis vaccine controversy
246005   Statistics menu

H. Influenzae Type B Information

247001   Disease information
247002   Exposure and transmission
247003   Vaccine information

Chickenpox, Varicella, and Shingles Information

248001   Disease information
248002   Pregnancy and infants
248003   Exposed
248004   Varicella-zoster immune globulin (VZIG)
248005   Prevention and treatment
248006   Statistics
248007   Shingle and zoster disease information transmission and treatment

Polio Information

249001   Disease information
249002   Travel recommendations
249003   Pregnancy and polio
249004   Vaccine information
249005   Adult immunizations with polio vaccine
249006   Recommendations for immune suppressed
249007   Statistics for polio

For Health Care Workers

General Information Documents

000002   Childhood immunization directory
000004   Other diseases directory
000005   International travel
000103   ACIP recommendations for MMR, DTP, Hib, and VAR

Measles Information

241101   Postexposure information
241102   Vaccine information
241003   Side effects
241104   Recommendations for the immune suppressed
241105   Diagnosis
241106   Outbreak control
241107   Pregnancy

Mumps Information

242101   Vaccine information, diagnosis, and outbreak information

Rubella Information

243101   Vaccine
243102   Inadvertent use of rubella vaccine during pregnancy
243103   Outbreak control
243104   Congenital rubella syndrome (CRS)
243105   Testing and diagnostic information

Diphtheria Information

244101   Prevention among close contacts
244102   Vaccine information
244103   Diagnosis and treatment

Tetanus Information

245101   Vaccine information
245102   Pregnancy
245103   Wounds

Pertussis Information

246101   Diagnosis and treatment of cases and contacts
246102   Vaccine information
246103   Pertussis vaccine controversy

H. Influenzae Type B Information

247101   Vaccine information
247102   Outbreaks
247103   Diagnosis and treatment

Varicella Information

248101   VZIG
248102   Postexposure situations
248103   Treatment and diagnosis

Poliomyelitis

249101   eIPV vaccine information
249102   Travel recommendations and polio vaccine
249103   Adult immunization information
249104   OPV or eIPV: advantages and disadvantages
249105   Recommendations for the immune suppressed

ACIP Recommendations

000002   Childhood immunization directory
000004   Other diseases directory
000005   International travel
000102   Health-care workers' immunization directory

Measles ACIP Information

241151   Introduction and background
241152   Vaccine indications
241153   Side effects and adverse reactions
241154   Precautions and contraindications
241155   Outbreak control
241156   Surveillance and reporting adverse events
241157   References

Mumps ACIP Information

242151   Introduction and background
242152   Mumps virus vaccine
242153   Mumps outbreak control
242154   Surveillance and reporting adverse events
242155   Recommendations for travelers
242156   References

Rubella ACIP Information

243151   Introduction
243152   Live rubella virus vaccine
243153   Adverse events, precautions, and contraindications
243154   Simultaneous administration of certain live virus vaccines
243155   Strategies for eliminating CRS
243156   International travel
243157   Laboratory diagnosis
243158   References

DTP ACIP Information

244151   Introduction, background, and statistics
244152   Vaccine information
244153   Vaccine side effects and adverse reactions
244154   Reduced dosage and simultaneous administration
244155   Precautions and contraindications
244156   Prevention of diphtheria among contacts of a diphtheria patient
244157   Tetanus prophylaxis in wound management
244158   Prophylaxis for contacts of pertussis patients
244159   Bibliography
244160   References

Haemophilus Influenzae Type B ACIP Information

247151   Conjugate vaccines—1990
247152   Conjugate vaccines—background
247153   Conjugate vaccines—use
247154   Conjugate vaccines—references

Organizations

American Liver Foundation: (800) 223-0179

Center for Disease Control and Prevention National Immunization Program: (800) CDC-SHOT

Every Child by Two: (202) 544-0808

Hepatitis Branch of the Centers for Disease Control and Prevention: (404) 639-2327

Hepatitis Foundation International: (800) 891-0707

Immunization Education and Action Committee: (202) 863-2414

Merck & Co, Inc.: (800) 672-6372

National Coalition for Adult Immunization: (301) 656-0003

National Coalition of Hispanic Health Organizations (COSSHMO): (202) 387-5000

National Council of La Raza: (202) 785-1670

National Digestive Diseases Information Clearinghouse: (301) 654-3810

National Hepatitis Detection, Treatment, and Prevention: (800) 822-4633

Pan American Health Organization: (202) 861-3279

Parke-Davis: (800) 223-0432

SmithKline Beecham Pharmaceuticals: (800) 366-8900; ex. 5231, product info; ex. 3670, patient education materials

Task Force for Childhood Survival and Development: (404) 872-4122

Wyeth-Lederle Vaccines: (800) 820-2815

Websites

Centers for Disease Control and Prevention (www.cdc.gov)

Centers for Disease Control and Prevention Immunization Website (www.cdc.gov/nip)

Immunization Action Coalition (www.immunize.org)

Minnesota State Health Department Immunization Website (www.heath.state.mn.us/divs/dpc/adps/news/tr/admin.pdf/)

National Coalition for Adult Immunization (www.medscape.com/ncai)

Pan American Health Organization (www.paho.org)

Immunization questions for the CDC (e-mail inquiry) (Nipinfo@cdc.gov)

National discussion about immunization tracking systems (to subscribe, send e-mail to Listserv@listserv.dartmouth.edu)

Bibliography

American Academy of Pediatrics. (2000). *2000 Red book: Report of the Committee on Infectious Diseases* (25th ed.). Elk Grove Village, IL: American Academy of Pediatrics.

Atkinson, W., Wolf, C., Humiston, S., & Nelson, R. (Eds.). (2000). *Epidemiology and prevention of vaccine-preventable diseases: The pink book* (6th ed.). Atlanta: Centers for Disease Control and Prevention.

Centers for Disease Control and Prevention. (1994). General recommendations on immunizations: United States. *Morbidity and Mortality Weekly Report, 43*(RR-1), 1-38.

Rennels, M., Edwards, K., Deyserling, H., et al. (1998). Safety and immunogenicity of heptavalent pneumococcal vaccine conjugated to CRM197 in United States infants. *Pediatrics, 101,* 604-611.

Shinefield, H., Black, S., Ray, P., et al. (1999). Safety and immunogenicity of heptavalent pneumococcal CRM197 conjugate vaccine in infants and toddlers. *Pediatric Infectious Diseases Journal, 18,* 757-763.

Chapter 14 *Injury Prevention*

Theresa M. Eldridge

Accidents are the leading cause of death and disability in children 1 to 19 years of age, and injuries kill more children than all diseases combined. Studies have shown that one fourth of children in the United States have a medically attended injury each year, and one third of these are severe enough to require surgery, bed restriction, and loss of school or normal activity for 1 day or more. Additional studies reveal that on average a child will have eight or more accidents per year.

In the past decade the term *accident* has been replaced with the term *injury*. *Accident* is defined as a happening or an event that is not expected and thus not controllable. *Injury* is defined as a wrongful or unjust happening that causes physical harm or damage and is describable, preventable, and controllable. Injuries are either unintentional (accidental) or intentional (deliberate). Unintentional injuries include motor vehicle injuries, burns, falls, drownings, and poisonings. Homicide, suicide, and child abuse are considered intentional injuries. This change in perspective is a result of using an epidemiologic groundwork of host, environment, and agent. Haddon (1980) proposed a model that identified injury events as attributable to only five agents: the five forms of physical energy (*kinetic, chemical, thermal, electrical,* and *radiation*). Haddon also divided injury events into the following phases: (1) a preinjury phase during which control of the energy source is lost, (2) a brief injury phase during which the energy is transferred to people and causes damage, and (3) a postinjury phase during which attempts are made to repair the damage. For example, hot tap water is a vehicle of thermal energy (and may result in burns);

a frayed extension cord is the conduit for electrical energy; and medical containers contain chemical energy. Injuries do not necessarily occur after all events: the use of car seats may prevent injury even though a collision does occur.

Injury death rates vary greatly with age. The leading cause of mortality in children under 1 year of age is congenital anomalies; injury is seventh in the ten leading causes of death. One fourth to one fifth of children and adolescents in the United States experience an injury serious enough to require medical attention. In children over 1 year of age, motor vehicle–related injury is the leading cause of death; homicide and suicide rank second and third respectively for the child over 14 years of age (Tables 14-1 to 14-3). Of all fatal injuries from birth to 19 years of age, 47% are attributable to motor vehicle–related injuries.

Child (Host) Characteristics

The type and severity of injury are closely related to a child's developmental stage and physical, cognitive, and psychosocial needs and skills. At each stage, a child may have unintentional injuries when the demands of a particular task exceed the ability to complete the task. A preschool-age child can safely negotiate stairs that represent a danger to a toddler. However, the preschool-age child cannot safely cross streets alone. The more physically competent and inquisitive a child becomes, the more risks are involved in the environment. At this stage the environment must be modified to protect the child.

Table 14-1 Leading Causes Of Death According To Age: United States (1998)

RANK ORDER	UNDER 1 YEAR	1-4 YEARS	5-14 YEARS	15-24 YEARS
1	Congenital anomalies	Unintentional injuries	Unintentional injuries	Unintentional injuries
2	Disorders relating to short gestation and unspecified low birth weight	Congenital anomalies	Malignant neoplasms	Homicide and legal intervention
3	Sudden infant death syndrome	Homicide and legal intervention	Homicide and legal intervention	Suicide
4	Newborn affected by maternal complications of pregnancy	Malignant neoplasms	Congenital anomalies	Malignant neoplasms
5	Respiratory distress syndrome	Diseases of the heart	Diseases of the heart	Diseases of the heart
6	Newborn affected by complications of placenta, cord, and membranes	Pneumonia and influenza	Suicide	Congenital anomalies
7	Infections specific to the perinatal period	Septicemia	Chronic obstructive pulmonary diseases	Chronic obstructive pulmonary diseases
8	Unintentional injuries	Certain conditions originating in the perinatal period	Pneumonia and influenza	Pneumonia and influenza
9	Intrauterine hypoxia and birth asphyxia	Cerebrovascular diseases	Benign neoplasms	Human immunodeficiency virus infection
10	Pneumonia and influenza	Benign neoplasms	Cerebrovascular diseases	Cerebrovascular diseases

From Centers for Disease Control and Prevention, National Center for Health Statistics, National Vital Statistics. (2000, July 24). National vital statistics system (Vol. 48).

As a child grows and learns, parental supervision is lessened. During the school years children are involved in new activities away from home, such as crossing the street, playing in playgrounds, and riding bicycles. As adolescence approaches, there is increased independence and mobility, resulting in more sources of injury, including motor vehicles.

Injury prevention combines the physiologic and psychologic factors of the host that influence the potential for injury at the various developmental stages. For example, a child's skin is less mature and a less effective barrier to damage than an adult's. When this is combined with cognitive immaturity, increased mobility, and curiosity, a toddler is predisposed to more severe scalding burns from hot tap water than an adult. Table 14-4 lists approximate ages for certain developmental behaviors, potential injuries, and intervention strategies. However, children vary greatly in their accomplishment of various developmental milestones, and the ages listed for various interventions may vary. Some children walk as early as 9 months of age, and others, not until 14 months. The key to injury control is to implement injury-prevention strategies before the child is at risk.

The concept of accident proneness has been discounted by scientific studies; however, certain other factors that influence injury rates have been identified. Boys are well known to have a higher risk of injuries, in most cases beginning after their first birthday. The increased injury rate in boys is even more pronounced during the teenage years. Certain behavioral characteristics such as aggressive behavior, risk-taking behavior, higher impulsivity, overactivity, and poor self-esteem have also been associated with higher injury rates. Furthermore, children with cognitive and motor delays are at increased risk.

Parental behaviors may also contribute to injury rates in children. Some parents may demand certain behaviors and tasks that are not accomplishable or appropriate for the developmental age of the child. Placing an infant in an infant walker converts a premobile infant to a mobile toddler who does not have the necessary judgment or skills to prevent injury. In a survey of 2400 parents of children in kindergarten through fourth grade, most parents stated that 5- and 6-year-old children were not able to reliably and safely cross streets alone. Yet, one third of those parents allowed their first grader to walk to school alone.

Agent (Vector) Characteristics

The vehicle causing injury is the *agent*, or *vector*. As previously mentioned, Haddon (1980) identified five forms of physical energy that make up injury agents. The characteristics of the agent determine the degree of potential injury for the child. Tap water hotter than 120° F causes 24% of the scald burns of children under 4 years of age. The major cause of burn deaths in children is smoke asphyxiation. One can cut these risks in half by using operable smoke alarms and turning hot water heaters to 120° F. Poisonings have decreased greatly in the last 12 years, probably as a result of the packaging of drugs in child-resistant containers and the reduction of medication

Text continued on p. 192

Table 14-2 Death Rates For Motor Vehicle Traffic Accidents According To Age: United States (1995)

AGE (YEARS)	DEATHS PER 100,000 RESIDENT POPULATION
Under 1	4.5
1-4	4.5
5-9	4.4
10-14	5.8
15-19	28.3

From American Academy of Pediatrics. (1997). Injury prevention and control for children and youth, Elk Grove Village, IL: American Academy of Pediatrics.

Table 14-3 Rank Order of Fatal and Nonfatal Injuries by Age-Group: United States

	AGE (YEARS)			
	1 TO 4	5 TO 9	10 TO 13	14 TO 17
Fatal	Burns	Pedestrian accidents	Motor vehicle	Motor vehicle
	Drowning	Motor vehicle	Pedestrian	Suicide
	Motor vehicle	Burns	Drowning	Assault/abuse
	Pedestrian	Drowning	Assault/abuse	Pedestrian
	Assault/abuse	Assault/abuse	Other accidents	Drowning
	Suffocation	Bikes/skates	Burns	Other accidents
	Other accidents	Suffocation	Bikes/skates	Bikes/skates
	Poisoning	Other accidents	Suicide	Poisoning
	Falls	Falls/lacerations	Suffocation	Burns
Nonfatal	Falls/lacerations	Falls/lacerations	Falls/lacerations	Sports
	Other accidents	Bikes/skates	Sports	Falls/lacerations
	Poisoning	Other accidents	Bikes/skates	Other accidents
	Burns	Motor vehicle	Other accidents	Motor vehicle
	Animal bites/stings	Animal bites/stings	Motor vehicle	Bikes/skates
	Suffocation	Sports	Animal bites/stings	Animal bites/stings
	Motor vehicle	Suffocation	Assault/abuse	Assault/abuse
	Bikes/skates	Burns	Poisoning	Poisoning
	Sports	Poisoning	Burns	Burns
		Pedestrian		

From Schneidt, P.C. (1995). The epidemiology of nonfatal injuries among U.S. children and youth. American Journal of Public Health, 85, 932-938.

Table 14-4 Injury Prevention and Normal Developmental Behavior in Childhood

Birth Through 5 Months of Age
Developmental behavior

Newborn

Newborn sleeps a great deal and does little else except eat and cry.

Head flops and needs support.

Infant wiggles a lot.

4 Months

Infant begins to hold rattle and puts hands in mouth.

Infant sucks on everything.

Some children able to roll over before 4 months.

Average infant can roll from side to back or back to side, hold head erect, and reach for objects; retains grasped rattle.

Moves self by pushing with feet and may flip over.

Injury	*Prevention*
Falls/trauma	Never leave child unattended at any time.
	Do not shake baby.
	Carry baby firmly and support the head and neck.
	Use car restraint device.
	Keep crib rails up when infant is in crib.
	Keep one hand on baby while changing or reaching for supplies.
	Do not sit a child infant seat on the table or counter.
	Avoid infant walkers at any age.
Burns	Keep child's exposure to sun brief.
	Install smoke alarms.
	Keep child away from stove and work counters.
	Do not smoke or drink hot liquids while holding a baby.
	Use nonflammable rattles and toys.
	Use flame-retardant clothes.
	Set hot water heater at 120° F; use special scald-prevention fixtures.
	Check bath water temperature carefully before bathing baby.
	Avoid microwave use for heating bottles.
	Check bottles and foods for temperature.
Suffocation or strangulation	Do not prop the baby bottle.
Foreign body aspiration	Keep baby on back or side when asleep.
Inhalation or ingestion of toxic substances	Make sure furniture and toys are finished with lead-free paint.
	Keep dangerous objects out of reach (e.g, buttons, pins, beads, sharp objects, razor blades, knives, hairpins).
	Avoid jewelry and pacifiers around the neck.
	Avoid waterbeds, bean bags, and overly padded bedding (suffocation).
	Crib and playpen slats should be no more than $2^3/_4$ inch apart and mattress should fit crib snugly.
	Keep baby powder out of reach and use carefully to avoid inhalation.
	Toys should be too big to fit in the mouth, with parts that cannot be removed.
	Toys should be tough, with no sharp edges or points.
	Educate siblings regarding food, toys, and handling baby.
	Turn head to side and down when vomiting.
	Avoid easily aspirated foods or toys.
Drowning	Never leave child alone in tub or sink.

6 Through 11 Months of Age
Developmental behavior

6 Months

Sits with support.

Rolls back to stomach and vice versa.

Reaches for and grasps objects.

Imitates.

7 Months

Sits alone.

Pushes self to hand-knee creeping position; may crawl.

May be teething and chewing on everything.

Oral exploration of all objects.

8 Months

Looks for toys that have fallen from sight.

9 Months

Pulls self to knees, then to standing position.

Stands fairly steadily while holding onto support.

10 Months

Is able to stand without support, occasionally walks fairly well holding onto support.

11 Months

Stands alone but only for short periods.

General

Perfects crawling and begins standing and walking.

Child scares quickly.

Begins to climb, pulls self up and everything else down.

Opens drawers, cupboards, bottles, and packages.

Chews on everything.

Table 14-4 Injury Prevention and Normal Developmental Behavior in Childhood—cont'd

6 Through 11 Months of Age—cont'd

Injury	*Prevention*
Falls/trauma	See Birth through 5 Months of Age.
	Child still requires full-time protection.
	Accidents are more frequent because baby can move and grasp more.
	Put gate across bottom and top of stairs.
	Keep dangling electric cords, drapery cords, and mobiles out of reach.
	Lower crib mattress.
	Install safety devices on windows.
Burns	See Birth through 5 Months of Age.
	Keep high chair and playpen away from cords, appliances, and stoves.
	Teach meaning of "hot"; set limits.
	Limit sun exposure, use sunscreen.
	Place guards around fireplaces, registers, floor furnaces, and open hearths.
	Put safety caps over electric outlets.
	Keep electric cords out of reach.
	Keep faucets out of reach.
	Turn pot handles inward.
	Do not let child play in kitchen during meal preparation.
	Do not leave heavy objects or containers of hot liquid on tablecloths, or table scarves; infant may pull them down.
Suffocation or strangulation	See Birth through 5 Months of Age.
Foreign body aspiration	Lock up all poisonous materials and medicines.
Inhalation or ingestion of toxic substances	Keep foods that may choke baby out of reach (popcorn, nuts, seeds, hard candy, raw carrots and celery, hot dogs, raisins, grapes, raw apples, chewing gum).
	Have syrup of ipecac in the home.
	Install safety latches on cupboards and drawers.
	Have poison control center and emergency medical numbers by phone.
Drowning	Do not leave child alone in or near a tub, pail of water, toilet, or swimming pool.

12 Through 35 Months of Age

Developmental behavior

12 Months
  Cruises.
  Holds cup and uses spoon.
  May begin to walk alone.
15 Months
  Walks alone.
  Stoops to pick up objects.
  Drinks from cup with little spilling.
  Rolls or tosses ball.
18 Months
  Walks well alone.
  Runs.
  Climbs down stairs.
  Uses spoon, spilling little.
  Can turn doorknob.

General
  Continual exploration of environment, both inside and outside.
  Imitates household tasks.
  Has basic language development.
  Insists on doing everything for self.
  Often tests parent to see if limits are set and kept.

Critical period
  Time for complete protection is past, and teaching begins.

Injury	*Prevention*
Falls/trauma	See 6 through 11 Months of Age.
Cuts and lacerations	Sharp objects are an increased danger.
	Teach child not to approach strange animals.
	Keep screens on windows and doors locked and latched, and use window guards.
	Keep garage locked and tools out of reach.
	Never leave child alone in car or house.
	Pad sharp corners on furniture or remove from play area.
	Keep child in fenced yard.
Burns	See 6 through 11 Months of Age.
	Keep child away from fireplace, curling irons, stove, space heaters, and irons.
	Teach child not to play with matches.
	Keep cigarettes, lighters, and matches locked up.

Continued

Table 14-4 Injury Prevention and Normal Developmental Behavior in Childhood—cont'd

12 Through 35 Months of Age
Injury—cont'd

Suffocation or strangulation	See 6 through 11 Months of Age.
Foreign body aspiration	Keep houseplants and outdoor plants out of reach; many are poisonous (see Box 14-1).
Inhalation or ingestion of toxic substances	No area is safe from the climbing toddler; lock up all poisons and hazardous substances.
	Teach child not to run or walk with mouth full of food.
Motor vehicle	Keep child away from street and driveway.
Drowning	See 6 through 11 Months of Age.
	Supervise child when around toilets, buckets of water, and so forth.
	Never leave child alone during bathing or swimming.
	Be sure to empty wading pool.
	Child should be taught basic swimming and survival techniques.
	All swimming pools should be enclosed by a fence that locks.

3 Through 5 Years of Age
Developmental behavior

3 Years
  Jumps.
  Pedals a tricycle.
  Washes and dries hands.
  Helps dress and undress self.
  Able to understand 90% of speech.
  Is toilet-trained.

4 Years
  Can throw a ball overhand.
  Buttons clothes.
  Broad jumps.
  Plays games with other children.
  Runs, skips.

5 Years
  Can dress and undress self.
  Hops.
  Can catch a ball.

Injury	*Prevention*
Falls/trauma	See 12 through 35 Months of Age.
	Use safety glass on house, doors, and shower doors.
	Teach about "good" and "bad" touching.
Cuts and lacerations	Use adhesive strips on bathtub.
	Keep stairways and play areas well lighted.
	Teach child how to handle scissors and knives.
	Teach playground and pedestrian safety.
Burns	See 12 through 35 Months of Age.
	Teach child not to run if clothes catch fire, but to drop and roll until fire is out.
	Conduct fire drills at home.
Suffocation or strangulation	See 12 through 35 Months of Age.
Foreign body aspiration	Child still needs supervision regarding poisons but is past oral stage and is learning limits of what can
Inhalation or ingestion of toxic substances	and cannot be played with.
	Never allow child to run or walk while eating.
	Continue to keep nuts, popcorn, and hard candy out of reach until child is 4 or 5 years old.
	Check neighborhood for ditches, abandoned refrigerators, and ice chests.
	Teach about cosmetics and other items used for "playing house."
Motor vehicle or bicycle	Instruct child in traffic and pedestrian safety; wear white at night.
	Never allow playing near garage, driveway, or street.
	Teach child to refuse rides from strangers.
	Child should lean his or her full name, address, and phone number.
	Child should wear bike helmet when riding on bicycle, or as a passenger on an adult's bicycle.
Firearms	Keep firearms locked up.
	Store weapons and ammunition separately.
	Teach child the danger of weapons and instruct never to play with them.
	Never keep a loaded weapon in car or at home.
Drowning	See 12 through 35 Months of Age.
	Continue close supervision of bathing and swimming.
	Teach safety rules for swimming.

Table 14-4 Injury Prevention and Normal Developmental Behavior in Childhood—cont'd

6 Through 11 Years of Age
Developmental behavior
General

Most children have basic motor skills for running, jumping, throwing, catching, and balancing.
Physical growth is slowed down.
Plays games such as tag, hide-and-seek.
Balancing and coordination important for hopscotch, gymnastics, jump rope, bicycling, and skating.
Cooperative play; baseball, tag.
Involved outside of home, such as time spent in school.

Increased independence.
Young school-age child may be clumsy.
Increased interest in sports, groups.
Children continuing to imitate parents and other adults.
Daring, adventurous, wanders away from home.
Likes to climb fences and trees.
Impulsive.
Full of energy.

Injury	*Prevention*
Motor vehicle	See 3 through 5 Years of Age. Teach bike safety, emphasize avoidance of street play. Teach rules of road, traffic signals, and respect for traffic officers.
Drowning	See 3 through 5 Years of Age Teach child rules of water safety. Do not play in drainage ditch. Do not swim alone. Teach boating safety rules. Supervise ice skating and other water sports.
Injuries or fractures	See 3 through 5 Years of Age.
Suffocation	Teach sport safety and playground safety (wearing appropriate safety gear). Use appropriate protective gear (knee and elbow pads, helmets with skateboards). Teach safety for skateboard and trampoline. Teach safety related to hobbies, sports, handicrafts, mechanical equipment. Check yard for rusty nails and glass. Encourage children to wear shoes when playing outside. Advise parents of hazards for school-age children associated with sports. Teach child safety precautions, not to take chances. Give child sense of confidence and responsibility. Teach child to use kitchen implements, machines (e.g., sewing machines) correctly. Teach safe use of tools. Teach rules of sports and proper use and maintenance of equipment. Teach hazards of playing in excavations, old refrigerators, and deserted buildings.
Burns	See 3 through 5 Years of Age. Use approved electric toys (Underwriters' Laboratory [UL]). Use electric toys under supervision. Avoid conductive kites. Supervise and teach appropriate use of matches, fires, and flammable chemicals.
Firearms	See 3 through 5 Years of Age. Teach child respect for weapons. Never keep loaded weapons in the house. Do not buy firearms as a gift unless child is responsible enough to handle under close supervision.
Inhalation or ingestion	Infrequent in this age group, but continue supervision. Child still needs reinforcement and teaching—needs to know "why." Ask questions about glue sniffing, smoking, drinking, and drug use.
Trauma	See 3 through 5 Years of Age Teach how to prevent injury from cold and heat. Avoid high noise levels, especially in headsets and at concerts.

Continued

Table 14-4 Injury Prevention and Normal Developmental Behavior in Childhood—cont'd

12 To 18 Years of Age
Developmental behavior
General

Many physical changes and rapid growth.

Large muscles develop faster than small muscles; poor posture, increased clumsiness, decreased coordination.

Development of secondary sex characteristics.

Increased interest in extracurricular activities.

Varying degree of physical activities.

Increased mobility.

High level of imaginative and creative thinking.

Adolescent's mind at point of greatest ability to acquire and use knowledge.

Able to problem solve.

Activities include sports, dating, hobbies, dancing, and day-dreaming.

Mood swings.

Increased freedom and independence.

May get a job.

Learns to drive.

Develops adult characteristics.

Injury	*Prevention*
Motor vehicle	See 6 through 11 Years of Age
	Always wear a seat belt and be sure passengers wear seat belts.
	Have adolescent take driver's education.
	Drive at speed limit.
	Involve adolescent in decision-making regarding rules of car use.
	Do not drink and drive.
	Encourage adolescent to use responsibilities and freedom wisely.
	Instruct adolescent in safety for motor scooters, motorcycles, and minibikes and the use of helmets.
Injuries or fractures	See 6 through 11 Years of Age
	Encourage proper use of equipment and safety regulations for sports.
	Advise about consequences of sports injuries.
Drowning	Instruct in emergency care procedures.
	Instruct in water safety, routine safety practices.
Firearms	See 6 through 11 Years of Age.
Inhalation or ingestion	Drug abuse prevention: give adolescent freedom to make decisions while providing information for an adequate knowledge base.
	Provide healthy influence for adolescent.
	Provide appropriate role model.
Trauma	See 6 through 11 Years of Age.
	Date-rape prevention.
	Teach cardiopulmonary resuscitation and first aid.

Box 14-1 Plant Exposures* by Plant Type

BOTANIC NAME	COMMON NAME	BOTANIC NAME	COMMON NAME
Philodendron species	Philodendron	*Brassaia actinophylla*	Umbrella tree
Capsicum annuum	Pepper	*Saintpaulia ionantha*	African violet
Dieffenbachia species	Dumbcane	*Rhododendron* species	Rhododendron, azalea
Euphorbia pulcherrima	Poinsettia	*Taxus* species	Yew
Ilex species	Holly	*Eucalyptus globulus*	Eucalyptus
Phytolacca americana	Pokeweed, inkberry	*Pyracantha* species	Pyrancantha
Spathiphyllum species	Peace lily	*Chlorophytum comosum*	Spider plant
Crassula species	Jade plant	*Schlumbergera bridgesii*	Christmas cactus
Epipremnum aureum	Pothos, devil's ivy	*Hedera helix*	English ivy
Toxicodendron, or *Rhus radicans*	Poison ivy	*Solanum dulcamara*	Climbing nightshade

From Litovitz T., Clark, L.R., & Soloway, R.A. (1994). *1993 Annual Report of the American Association of Poison Control Centers Toxic Exposure Systems.* American Journal of Emergency Medicine, 12, 546-599.
*Exposures are in descending order of occurrence.

doses to sublethal doses. Intervention that is directed at agents through packaging drugs in child-safe containers, producing flame-retardant children's clothing, and making cribs with bars no greater than 2⅜ inches apart are examples of *passive* intervention strategies. *Active* strategies require a change in behav-

ior of the host. Using motor-vehicle restraint devices and wearing bicycle helmets involve behavior that may alter the injury agent but not necessarily prevent the event (e.g., wearing a helmet may reduce the extent of a head injury in a bicycle crash).

Environment

Sociocultural and physical environmental factors are key determinants of both intentional and unintentional injuries in childhood and adolescence. Time of day, type of equipment, and physical arrangement of the environment (e.g., crowded neighborhoods) can contribute to injury. Children in urban environments face hazards different from the hazards of those who live in rural areas. Cultural differences also exist; the highest injury death rate occurs in Native Americans, followed by African Americans, Caucasians, and Asian Americans. Socioeconomic factors such as stress, loss of employment, death in the family, substance abuse, single-parent families, and poverty have significant influence on injury rates. Children from lower socioeconomic groups have a twofold increase in injury death rates, a fourfold greater risk of drowning, and a fivefold greater rate of fatal injury from fire and burns.

Modifications of the environment to improve safety are accomplished through organizations such as the Consumer Product Commission and legislative efforts of local and national governments. The Seattle Children's Bicycle Helmet Campaign is a notable example of a community program that had a significant influence on the use of bicycle helmets in school-age children. Other communities have enforced curfews; these curfews have led to a demonstrated decrease in motor vehicle accidents (MVAs) and homicides in teenagers.

Prevention Strategies

The following strategies for injury prevention have been identified by the National Research Council on Injury Prevention:

- Persuade and educate at-risk individuals (and their parents) to change their behavior.
- Require individuals to change their behavior through legislation or regulation.
- Modify the design of products and the environment to protect the public safety.

In a resurgence of interest and effort in injury control, Congress requested the National Academy of Sciences establish a committee on trauma. The committee published *Injury in America* in 1985, which attempted to document the extensive public health problem of intentional and unintentional injuries. The report also noted that no single agency or organization had responsibility for coordination of injury research and endeavors. The Centers for Disease Control and Prevention (CDC) were mandated by Congress to coordinate and supervise injury control activities, and the CDC has developed a comprehensive National Center for Injury Prevention and Control.

Each of the preceding strategies has an important role in the control of injuries to children and adolescents; however, no single method of prevention is effective. Although passive intervention strategies such as modification of a product or the environment are more likely to protect individuals, injuries occur as a result of complex interactions of host, agent, and environment, and to be effective a combination of strategies is often required. Following is a review of common injuries that occur in childhood and adolescence, including prevention and control strategies directed at the host, agent, and environment. Table 14-5 reviews the safety issues and prevention strategies common to all age groups; these safety issues should be addressed at each visit and reflect the developmental progression of the child (e.g., using a car seat for infants and lap and shoulder belts for older children). Box 14-2 contains questions parents can be asked regarding their safety practices.

Table 14-5 Safety Issues and Prevention Strategies

SAFETY ISSUES	PREVENTION STRATEGIES
Motor vehicle (occupant, pedestrian bicycle)	Use child-restraint device that is age appropriate.
	Never leave child alone in car.
	Wear safety helmets appropriate for activity (e.g., bicycling, skateboarding, skating, horseback riding).
	Teach rules of pedestrian safety.
	Be a role model for appropriate behavior (e.g., parents use seat belts, helmets).
Burns	Reduce hot water temperature.
	Purchase, install, and check smoke alarms and fire extinguishers.
	Use nonflammable clothing, toys, and household products.
	Avoid smoking.
Poisoning	Safely store drugs, cleaning agents, chemicals, and corrosives.
	Use child-resistant caps on drug containers.
	Keep syrup of ipecac in the home.
	Post poison control and emergency facility number by the phone.
Drowning	Supervise children around water.
	Lock gates around swimming pools.
	Teach water safety and swimming.
Play	Monitor safety of toys and activities.
Violence	Remove handguns from the home or lock all weapons and ammunition in separate areas.
	Assess family for substance abuse, child abuse, and family violence.
General	Provide education and guidance before child exhibits behaviors or skills that may lead to injury.
	Assess risk factors, environmental factors, and stress-related factors at each clinic visit.

Motor Vehicle–Related Injuries

MVAs are the leading cause of death in children older than 1 year of age. Motor vehicle–related injuries include injuries to vehicle occupants, motorcyclists, bicyclists, and pedestrians and accidents involving all-terrain vehicles. Injuries also result from children being left alone and unsupervised in vehicles.

Special circumstances require various strategies and intervention to prevent injuries. The premature infant needs to be positioned in such a way as to prevent the head from falling forward and causing respiratory compromise. Disabled children also have special needs that must be addressed when they ride in a vehicle.

Use of seat belts and appropriate child-restraint seats has significantly decreased motor vehicle–related injuries. However, children are often improperly restrained, and many older children and adolescents are not restrained at all. Also, misuse of restraint devices and improper positioning continue to be problems. A multidisciplinary approach involving legislation, education, and consumer product safety is needed to reduce morbidity and mortality in children and adolescents.

Box 14-2 Parents' Quiz for Injury Prevention

Most serious accidents can be prevented. Parents should ask themselves these questions and take appropriate preventive measures when necessary to avoid injuries to their child.

Your Habits: Do You . . .

- Always have your child safely buckled in when you are driving with him or her in the car (with an appropriate safety restraint for age)?
- Put medicine away in a childproof place after use?
- Place the baby's high chair or playpen well away from stove and kitchen counters?
- Turn pot and pan handles toward the back of the stove?
- Keep plastic wrappers, bags, and balloons away from children?
- Keep matches and lighters away from small children?
- Keep electric cords out of the reach of infants and toddlers?
- Consider flammability when purchasing clothing and toys?
- Check your child's toys for safety hazards?
- Keep tiny things (e.g., buttons, pins, tacks) away from infants and toddlers?
- Store knives and scissors well out of reach of young children?
- Carry hot liquids when holding your child?
- Smoke?
- Ever leave your child unattended?
- Stay with your child when he or she is in the bathtub or wading pool?
- Use guns?
- Know cardiopulmonary resuscitation (CPR) and the abdominal thrust maneuver?

Your Home: Do You . . .

- Have smoke alarms installed in your home?
- Keep poisons and flammable substances locked away from young children?
- Have gates at stairways to keep baby or toddler from falling?
- Light stairwells?
- Fit stairs with treads and handrails?
- Anchor scatter rugs so they won't slip?
- Have a fire extinguisher?
- Screen or bar high windows to keep children from falling?
- Keep the telephone number of the poison control center next to your phone?
- Have syrup of ipecac?
- Lock or latch doors that lead to danger for a toddler?
- Put dummy plugs into unused electric outlets?
- Keep electric cords in good condition and out of reach?
- Dispose of any combustible litter in your attic and basement?
- Use flame-retardant fabrics for home furnishings?
- Lock up firearms?
- Set the hot water heater thermostat to less than 120° F?

Adapted from American Academy of Pediatrics. (1994). The injury prevention program. *Elk Grove Village, IL: American Academy of Pediatrics; Green, M. (Ed.). (1994).* Bright Futures: Guidelines for health supervision of infants, children and adolescents. *Arlington, VA: National Center for Education in Maternal Child Health.*

Scope of the problem

- Motor vehicle traffic injuries were the leading cause of death in 1995 among children 1 to 14 years of age.
- Among teenagers 15 to 19 years of age, motor vehicle–related injuries and firearm-related injuries were the two leading causes of death in 1995.
- Mortalities for adolescents are 10 times greater than those of younger age groups.
- In MVAs involving teens, approximately 50% of the incidents occur between 9 PM and 6 AM and 58% occur on weekends. Of fatally injured teens, 63% sustain their injuries in cars driven by other teenagers.
- Motor vehicle occupant death rates among Native Americans are double that for any other race.
- Of teenagers 16 to 19 years of age involved in fatal crashes, 31% had elevated blood alcohol levels.
- National statistics show that 80% to 90% of child safety seats are incorrectly used.

Prevention strategies

- Advise parents to position their child and child restraints away from all air bags. Front and side air bags have been shown to severely injure children. Children should not ride on the front passenger side of a vehicle with an air bag until 13 years of age.
- Infants must ride facing the rear in a child restraint until they weigh 20 pounds and 1 year of age. Both of these milestones must be met before the restraint is placed in a forward-facing position. Some safety seats are designed for children up to 30 pounds, and parents should be advised to use the rear-facing position as long as possible.

- It is critical that the parents read the manufacturer's instructions carefully on safety seats that are convertible from rear facing to forward facing and follow those instructions carefully. (Often a kickstand must be used, the path that the seat belt is routed changes, and the shoulder harness is moved.)
- Safety seats must be secure in the vehicle and the child secure in the seat. The child should fit snugly in a 5-point harness with no more than one finger's gap between the harness and the clavicle, and the positioning clip should be at armpit level.
- Booster seats should be used until the child weighs approximately 80 pounds or is 9 years of age, again with a 5-point harness. Booster shields have been shown to be ineffective in preventing injuries.
- Certified safety seat technicians are available in each state to check child-restraint systems. A list of contacts for each state is listed on the National Highway Traffic Safety Administration website.
- Special safety restraint devices are available for children with special needs. Advise parents to use these devices as needed.
- Health care providers should visit websites frequently to keep updated on current information.

Pedestrian Injury

Scope of the problem

- Nearly one sixth of traffic deaths are the result of pedestrian injuries.
- Pedestrian injury is highest in the 5- to 9-year-old age group.

- Poor children have a risk two to three times higher than that of other children.
- "Dart-out" injuries (in which the child darts out into the middle of the street) account for 50% to 70% of pedestrian injuries.
- Of injured children, 75% are boys.
- Peak times for injury are late afternoon and early evening.
- The highest injury rates are in non-Caucasian, low-income, female-headed households with large numbers of children.
- Children who are playing have no perception of potential hazards because of absorption in play and peers.
- Children who exhibit behaviors such as impulsivity, have poor visual acuity and depth perception, show poor auditory discrimination; and have difficulty judging distance and velocity have a higher incidence of injuries.

Prevention strategies

- Provide off-street play areas.
- Provide education programs to teach road safety.
- Adopt "neighborhood traffic control" (i.e., local streets designed as cul-de-sacs with homes having two entrances: a garage entrance in the rear for motor vehicles and a main entrance facing a grassy area with paths for bicyclists and pedestrians).
- Provide pedestrian traffic areas (e.g., walkways separate from motor vehicles).
- Improve and simplify traffic flow in neighborhoods and city streets.

Bicycle, Motorcycle, Rollerblading, Skateboarding, and Recreational Injury

Scope of the problem

- Head injury from cycling is the most common cause of death and the leading cause of disability.
- Helmet use reduces risk of head injury by 85% and brain injury by 88%.
- Less than 5% of children riding bicycles wear helmets.
- Helmet use reduces head injury rates by 75% in motorcycle accident victims.
- Wearing helmets and protective gear while skateboarding and rollerblading significantly reduces injury.

Prevention strategies

- Encourage helmet and protective gear use.
- Wear properly fitted, safety-inspected helmets.
- Formulate programs to provide helmets at a low cost.
- Encourage development of safe areas for biking, rollerblading, and skateboarding.
- Develop programs to promote awareness and availability of helmet use.
- Teach helmet use safety.
- Urge local and municipal governments to enact legislation mandating helmet use for bicyclists, motorcyclists, skateboarders, and rollerbladers.
- Urge the media to show properly helmeted individuals on television, in advertisements, and in promotional materials.

Homicide, Assault, and Abuse

Discussions of injury control would not be complete without including injuries resulting from child abuse, homicide, and assault. The practitioner has both a legal and a moral obligation to report child abuse. All 50 states have child-protection laws, and all practitioners are responsible for knowing their state laws and regulations. In 1994 more than 1 million children under 19 years of age were victims of abuse and neglect. Shaken-baby syndrome (SBS), a previously less-recognized form of child abuse, has received national attention. The practitioner must be alert to signs of neglect or abuse and investigate any suspicious injury. Chapters 31 and 47 discuss abuse in more detail.

Child abuse and assault injury

Scope of the problem

- Over 1 million children were neglected and abused in 1994.
- Approximately 60% of these cases involved physical abuse or neglect, and 55% of the abused were girls.
- Of sexual assaults, 50% involve verbal force, 27% to 40% involve minimal force, and 15% involve beating or the presence of a weapon.

Prevention strategies

- Practice firearm control.
- Teach children self-protection.
- Teach parents child development and parenting skills.
- Provide respite care for stressed parents (e.g., drop-in care centers).
- Mobilize social supports for parents (e.g., housing, health care, food, legal aid, counseling, transportation, community resources).
- Use home health care visitors for support and for educating parents on parenting skills and role modeling.
- Decrease the effects of poverty by using appropriate resources.
- Consider foster care placement.
- Use support and counseling programs for abuse victims.
- Teach children and adolescents parenting and child-rearing skills.
- Identify children and families who are at risk for abuse.
- Evaluate children and adolescents for abuse.
- Refer potential perpetrators to prevention programs.

Homicide

Homicide is now a leading cause of injury death among all children. Homicide rates for African-American males are five times greater than for Caucasian males and twice those of females. According to the CDC (2000), firearms will replace motor vehicles as the leading cause of injury death in the United States by the year 2003. Several states, including California, Nevada, Texas, and New York have already experienced this change. It is estimated that half of American homes contain firearms, and rates of homicide in the United States resulting from firearms are significantly higher than those of other developed countries.

Studies have shown that 20% of adolescents have carried a weapon to school. Homicides of adolescents are often caused by arguments and crime involving peers and gangs, and approximately 62% of pediatric homicide victims were 15 to 19 years of age. Many schools have installed metal detectors in response to the increased handgun use in children and adolescents. A survey of nurse practitioners (NPs) in New York found that only 7% of those surveyed discussed firearms in the home, though homicide is the leading cause of injury death for children and youth in New York City, with 59% of those deaths are attributed to firearms. Information regarding injury assaults is not consistent or reliable, though most violent injuries have been found to involve a family member or an individual from a social relationship rather than being random acts of violence. Ozmar (1994) defines the former as *interpersonal violence,* a term that includes child abuse, sexual assault, spousal abuse, psychologic and physical abuse, elder abuse, and homicide. Data collected from telephone interviews indicate that each year 80% of siblings engage in violent interactions ranging from pushing to threatening with a gun.

Risk-taking behavior in adolescents (e.g., substance abuse, hitchhiking, going to unprotected environments with new acquaintances) has been shown to contribute to adolescent sexual assaults. Approximately 80% of sexual assault offenders are known to their victims. The National Crime Survey (as cited in Baker, O'Neill, Ginsburg, et al, 1997) emphasizes the vulnerability of adolescents to assault and notes that victims and offenders tend to be the same age. Costs of fatal and nonfatal violent injury are difficult to determine, and studies often apply only to adults. Reporting is also inconsistent, and in most cases data are underreported; it is estimated that less than 50% of injuries that are the result of violence are reported to the police.

Although homicide, suicide, abuse, and assault are intentional injuries, firearms also contribute to unintentional fatalities from accidental shootings and self-inflicted injuries. Firearms are believed to be the fourth leading cause of accidental death among children 5 to 14 years of age. Firearm education should now be a routine part of anticipatory guidance for all children. The American Academy of Pediatrics (AAP) has even issued a position statement recommending the removal of firearms from the home and supporting legislation to reduce the availability of handguns in the environment in which children play.

Scope of the problem
- One third of homicides among females are inflicted with firearms.
- Among males, 50% of homicides are inflicted with firearms.
- Approximately 50% of homicides of children 1 to 4 years of age are inflicted with blows and 10% by firearms.
- Homicide rates for African-American children are five times higher than those for Caucasians.
- African-American female homicide rates are two to four times higher than Caucasian female rates.
- Youth-violence risk factors include:
  Past victim of violence
  Low socioeconomic status
  History of family violence (possibly including abandonment by a father or lack of strong family unit)
  African American, Hispanic, or Latino race
  Male gender
  Poor education
  Unemployed
  Involvement with violence-prone peers
  Poor impulse- and anger-control skills
  Depression
  Substance abuse
  History of juvenile detention

Prevention strategies
- Practice firearm control.
- Reduce toy-gun play.
- Offer gun safety education.
- Offer violence prevention education in schools.
- Identify high-risk children and adolescents and refer them for conflict-resolution training, family counseling, and substance-abuse counseling.
- Teach conflict-resolution skills.
- Identify and report domestic violence and refer to appropriate social service agencies and shelters.
- Use metal detectors in schools.
- Use community programs for the following:
  After-school care
  Curfews
  Drug-free communities
  Weapon-free communities
- Decrease the effects of poverty by using appropriate resources.

- Decrease media violence that is seen by children.
- Encourage parents to remove firearms from the home.
- If guns are in the home, advise parents to lock up guns and ammunition and use trigger-locking devices.

Suicide

Although suicide is rare in children younger than 10 years of age, it is the third leading cause of death in children 10 years of age or younger (see Chapter 39). Late adolescence (15 to 19 years of age) is associated with an increase in overall mortality, and 87% of self-inflicted deaths occur in this age group. Native Americans and Caucasian males have the highest suicide rates. Suicide rates for children 10 to 19 years of age have more than doubled in recent years. More than half the suicides among 10- to 14-year-olds resulted from the use of firearms, and 20% of the suicides in 15- to 19-year-olds were caused by the same. Known suicide attempts cost society more than $8 million in direct medical care alone. This is a conservative estimate, since the number of suicide attempts and deaths is generally underrepresented. Strategies such as suicide-prevention curricula and crisis centers have not been adequately evaluated for their effectiveness, but restricting handguns has shown promise as an effective strategy.

In a recent study, comparison of suicide mortalities in Vancouver, British Columbia, and Seattle showed 1.37 times more suicides in Seattle than in Vancouver. This difference was attributed to the finding that handgun suicides were nine times more common in Seattle. A general unavailability of handguns in Vancouver did not show an increase in suicides by other methods, as was evident in older adults. The practitioner can have a significant effect on suicide prevention by identifying risk factors for children and adolescents and inquiring about the availability of firearms. Appropriate counseling and referral can then be implemented for a person who might be contemplating suicide.

Scope of the problem
- The number of suicide deaths has doubled in past 30 years in 10- to 19-year-olds.
- Of those who die, 80% are male.
- Rates are 1.5 to 2.5 times higher in Caucasians (excluding Native Americans)
- Approximately 51% of deaths are by gunshot in 10- to 14-year-olds; about 60% involve firearms in 15- to 19-year-olds.
- Approximately 10% of those who attempt suicide complete suicide.
- There are eight or more suicide attempts for every death.
- Attempt rates are higher for females than for males.
  Risk factors for suicide include:
- History of previous suicide attempts (which makes a person 20 to 50 times more likely to succeed)
- Depression
- Alcohol and substance abuse
- Availability of firearms
- Loss of a friend or family member to suicide
- Acute conflict or disruption of a relationship

Prevention strategies
- Use screening programs to detect at-risk children and adolescents.
- Teach suicide detection and prevention in schools.
- Use suicide-prevention crisis centers and hotlines.
- Restrict available firearms.
- Assess children and adolescents for risk factors and for present and past suicidal behaviors.

- Train teachers, health professionals, parents, and others to recognize high-risk children and adolescents.

Violence, as evident in the overwhelming unintentional-injury death rates in children and adolescents, is a major societal problem with multifactorial causes. Prevention and intervention strategies must address such global issues as poverty, substance abuse, family and gang violence, and the moral and ethical values of today's society. Strategies should reflect an interdisciplinary approach at the individual, family, community, state, and national levels.

Poisoning Injury

A poison is any substance that can be harmful when exposure to that substance occurs. Poisoning can occur through ingestion, inhalation, skin exposure, and eye contact. The highest incidence of poisoning occurs in 1- to 2-year-olds, though poisoning is still a major problem in all children under 6 years of age. Boys have a higher incidence of poisoning under 13 years of age, and girls have a higher incidence over 13 years of age. In girls over 13 years of age, ingestion of poisons is a primary method of suicide attempts.

The incidence of poisoning has decreased in recent years, primarily because of childproof packaging and decreased lethality of medication doses. Iron supplements are the most frequent cause of poisoning deaths in children, followed by antidepressants, cardiovascular medications, and methylsalicylate preparations. Hydrocarbons (including lamp oil) and pesticides are also frequent causes of death in the pediatric age group. Poisonings are categorized by rating the *hazard factor*, which is an attempt to determine the fatal or near-fatal risks of certain substances or exposures. This hazard factor rating is used by many poison control centers to determine areas needing further study.

It is also important to recognize that 10% of poisonings are intentional (suicide attempts) and are probably unreported. Medication errors also account for a small percentage of poisonings. The majority of poisonings occur in the home, including ingestion of lead paint or lead-based products. Boxes 14-3 to 14-6 review information pertinent to poisoning injury prevention.

Scope of the problem
- The number of calls to poison control centers peaks between 4 PM and 10 PM.
- Children under 3 years of age account for 42% of poisonings; children under 6 years of age account for 56%.
- Approximately 86% of poison exposures are unintentional, while 8% are intentional and 5% are caused by therapeutic error).
- Of poisonings, 71.5% are managed in the home (with no hospitalization or emergency room visit).
- Of all poisoning exposures managed by poison control centers, 60% involve children under 6 years of age.
- Of poisoning exposures to children under 6 years, 34% are caused by cosmetics and personal care products, cleaning substances, and plants.
- Of all poisoning cases, 90% occur in the home.
- About 9% of preschool children have a potentially harmful lead level.

Prevention strategies
- Teach parents about potential dangers for each developmental stage (see Table 14-4).
- Modify the environment before a child accomplishes the skill that places him at risk (e.g., crawling, pulling up to stand, climbing).
- Modify the environment from a child's eye level.
- Support and use poison control centers.
- Identify risk factors.
- Conduct widespread screening and early intervention.
- Use childproof packaging.
- Keep syrup of ipecac on hand.
- Poison-proof the home and child care areas (see Box 14-2).
- Follow safety tips (see Box 14-3).
- Use lead-free paint, and do not allow child to chew on items that may contain lead (e.g., paint, toys). Also check bathtubs, which may be leaching lead into the water.
- Teach about drug abuse and prevention.

Box 14-3 Checklist for Poison-Proofing Areas at Home

Kitchen
- No medicines on counters, open areas, refrigerator top, or window sills ☐
- No household products under the sink ☐
- All medicines, cleaners, and household products in original, safety-top containers ☐

Bathroom
- All medicines in original, safety-top containers ☐
- Medicine chest cleaned out routinely ☐
- All old medications flushed down toilet ☐
- All medicines, powders, sprays, cosmetics, hair-care products, and mouthwash locked in medicine chest or out of reach ☐

Bedroom
- No medicines in or on dresser or bedside table ☐
- All perfumes and cosmetics out of reach ☐

Laundry Area
- All products in original containers ☐
- All bleaches, soaps, detergents, and fabric softeners out of reach or locked away ☐

Garage and Basement
- Gasoline and car products locked up ☐
- Paints, turpentine, and paint products locked up ☐
- All products in original containers ☐
- All gardening and workshop tools out of reach or locked up ☐

General
- Plants out of reach ☐

Household
- Alcoholic beverages out of reach ☐
- Paint in good repair ☐
- Ashtrays empty and out of reach ☐
- Purses out of reach ☐
- All household and personal products out of reach ☐

Back Yard
- Poisonous plants fenced off ☐
- All gardening tools, pesticides, seeds, and bulbs locked up ☐
- Charcoal lighter fluid and charcoal briquettes locked up ☐

Box 14-4 Safety Tips to Remember for Prevention of Accidental Poisoning

- Young children will eat and drink almost anything, so keep all liquid and solids that may be poisonous out of their reach.
- The following are the most commonly ingested items:
  Acetaminophen
  Ibuprofen
  Iron
  Aspirin
  Soaps, detergents, and cleaners
  Plants
  Vitamins
  Antihistamines and cold medicines
  Disinfectants and deodorizers
  Miscellaneous medicines
  Perfume and toilet water
- Most accidents (up to 90%) are preventable.
- Keep all medicines and hazardous products locked away when not in use.
- Never call medicine "candy."
- Keep all products in original containers.
- Read labels on all household products and medicines, and follow directions carefully.
- Destroy old products.
- Keep foods and household products separated.

- Always turn on the lights when giving or taking medicine.
- Since children imitate adults, avoid taking medicines in their presence.
- Use safety closures on as many products as possible, but realize that children may still be able to open them.
- Keep a bottle of syrup of ipecac for each child at home. Do not use unless instructed by a physician or poison control center.
- Accidental poisonings often occur when the usual household routine is upset (e.g., holidays, relatives or friends visiting, a new baby at home, a family move).
- Holidays often present special poisoning problems. Christmas ornaments (e.g., lights, bulbs, tinsel, "snow," "angel hair") may cause injury or contain poisonous materials. Christmas plants such as poinsettia, holly, mistletoe, and Christmas greens may be harmful if swallowed.
- Remember that many poisonings occur in the homes of babysitters, relatives, and friends, so help them "poison-proof" their homes.
- Use safety stickers on poisonous items, and teach children to recognize and avoid items with safety stickers. (Stickers can be obtained from local poison control centers.)
- Keep the telephone number of the family health care provider, poison control center, hospital, and police and fire departments near the telephone.

Box 14-5 First Aid for Poisoning

Inhaled Poisons
- If gas, fumes, or smoke have been inhaled, immediately drag or carry child to fresh air.
- Contact the poison control center or emergency medical system.

Poisons on the Skin
- If the poison or chemical has been spilled on the skin or clothing, remove clothing, gently brush off any dry material (wear rubber gloves if possible), and flush the involved skin area with water for 2 to 3 minutes. Then gently wash with soap and water and rinse.
- Contact the poison control center.

Swallowed Poisons
- If *any* poison has been swallowed, contact the poison control center or emergency medical system.
- Antidote labels on products may be incorrect.
- *Do not* give salt, vinegar, or lemon juice.
- If a child is unconscious, becoming drowsy, having convulsions, or having trouble breathing, call 911 or an emergency ambulance.

- Always keep syrup of ipecac at home. Ipecac causes vomiting and is sometimes used when poisons are swallowed. *Do not* use it unless the poison control center or family health care providers has given instructions to do so.

Poisons in the Eyes
- If the poison or chemical is in the eye, flush the eye with lukewarm water from a pitcher. Hold the pitcher 1 to 2 inches from the eye and flush the eye for 15 minutes.
- Contact the poison control center.

Plant Poisons
- If poisonous plants are swallowed or chewed, contact the poison control center or emergency medical service.
- For skin contact with poisonous plants, gently wash the skin with soap and water and rinse thoroughly.
- Contact the poison control center.

Call 911 or an emergency ambulance for any severely injured child.

Box 14-6 Telephone Management for Poisoning and Overdose

Telephone number—Obtain caller's number in case of a disconnection or for follow-up.
Address—Obtain caller's address in case emergency equipment needs to be dispatched.
Evaluation of severity—Identify whether child is in immediate danger, potential danger, or no danger.
Weight and age—Information helps in estimating potential toxicity and lethality.
Time of ingestion—Information helps in interpreting onset of signs and symptoms.

Past medical history—Ask about allergies, chronic medication use, and chronic health conditions.
Type of exposure—Specify product name and ingredients from the label and from toxicology text or poison control center.
Amount of exposure—Determine number of tablets or amount of fluid ingested; caller may need to count remaining tablets or measure remaining fluid.
Route of exposure—Determine whether exposure is ingestion, inhalation, contact with eyes or skin, or parenteral.
Caller's relationship to child—Identify caller (e.g., parent, babysitter, friend).

Suffocation, Aspiration, and Choking Injury

Suffocation is a serious injury threat for infants under 1 year of age because of their ability to move and wiggle but inability to untangle or remove themselves from a constricting object. Bedding should be kept to a minimum, and crib mattresses should fit snugly to prevent suffocation between the mattress and crib sides. Mobiles, hanging drapery cords, strings, pacifiers, and bibs present a strangulation hazard once the baby can sit or reach. Avoid placing infants on pillows or large cushions that could suffocate if the baby rolls over face down and lacks the strength and skills to escape. As the child becomes mobile and walks and climbs, entrapment in abandoned refrigerators and trunks poses an additional concern. Even the school-age child is at risk for entrapment in abandoned equipment, wells, mines, caves, and deserted buildings. (See also the discussion of various emergencies and airway obstruction in Chapter 48.)

Asphyxiation resulting from aspiration of a foreign body poses a significant safety concern. Any small object can be swallowed and aspirated. Table 14-4 reviews prevention strategies for various age groups. Aspiration of food is common in childhood and can be avoided by refraining from giving such foods as nuts, LifeSavers, and raisins to small children (under 4 years of age). Food should be cut into small pieces and chewed thoroughly while the child is sitting. Running and walking while eating predisposes children to aspirate food particles. Also, children should not eat and drink while supine.

The Consumer Product Safety Commission (CPSC) was developed to investigate reports of injury and mortality related to manufactured objects. It has legislative power to ban any toy that presents a risk for injury through normal use. The Federal Hazardous Substances Act provides for a test of object size and the use of the Small Parts Test Fixture (SPTF), a cylinder with a diameter of 3.17 cm and a depth of 2.54 to 5.71 cm. Objects intended for use by young children (less than 3 years of age) must pass the SPTF test (that is, have a diameter greater than 3.17 cm or a length greater than 5.71 cm). A recent study demonstrated that asphyxiation occurred even when spherical parts met the SPTF standards and that one third of the deaths occurred in children older than 3 years of age.

The CPSC recorded 449 deaths from aspirated foreign bodies between 1972 and 1992 in children 14 years of age and younger. Sixty-five percent of the aspiration victims were under 3 years of age. Twenty percent of the deaths were caused by toy products or parts and 19% by balls and marbles. The remaining 32% of deaths were caused by products not intended for young children's use. Balloons and latex gloves caused 29% of the deaths.

Scope of the problem

- Asphyxiation resulting from aspiration of a foreign body into the respiratory tract is a leading cause of death in children under 7 years of age.
- Food items cause 70% of aspirations.
- Of all choking deaths, 77% occur in children under 3 years of age.
- Asphyxiation risk attributable to balloons doubles in the 3-years-and-older age group.
- Spherical objects (e.g., balls, marbles) can cause asphyxiation even if they meet SPTF standards.
- Other objects frequently aspirated include children's toys, hardware (e.g., nails, screws, metal wire), coins, and household products (e.g., pen caps, paper clips, chalk, buttons, beads, staples, string)

Prevention strategies

- Teach parents about hazards and prevention strategies (see Table 14-4).
- Teach parents and caregivers the abdominal thrust maneuver and cardiopulmonary resuscitation (CPR).
- Do not allow children to play with toys with small, removable parts. Check toys for safety hazards.
- Continue testing of toys and objects for safety.
- Report aspiration and choking of manufactured objects to the CPSC.
- Develop standards for toys intended for children between 3 and 6 years of age.
- Conduct additional research to determine whether SPTF standards should be changed for children 3 years of age and younger.

Fire and Burn Injury

Burns cause excruciating pain and rehabilitation. Often, reconstructive surgery for scarring is needed, and the emotional and physical trauma lasts a lifetime. Nonfatal injuries resulting from chemical, electrical, thermal, or radiation energy are considered the most serious injuries to the human body. (See also the discussion of burn injury in Chapter 48.)

Scope of the problem

- Fire and burn injury is the fifth leading cause of death in children from birth to 19 years of age.
- Fire is the second leading cause of death in 1- to 4-year-olds.
- Kitchens and bathrooms are the most hazardous areas.
- Risk of flame burns is increased in children 5 to 13 years of age.
- Scalding burns cause 56% of burns (e.g., from hot water and other liquids, hot foods).
- Home fires cause 84% of deaths from fire and burns, usually because of smoke inhalation.
- Boys have a higher risk for injury.
- Groups at increased risk for house fire deaths include African Americans and Native Americans (who are at greater risk than Caucasians) and poor children.
- Cigarettes are the source of 35% of all fatal fires.
- Playing with matches and lighters causes one third of fires that kill children under 5 years of age.
- Burn injuries involving gasoline resulted in 62% of hospital admissions at one hospital surveyed; gasoline thrown on a fire and gasoline "sniffing" are frequent causes.
- Burns are involved in 10% of child-abuse cases.
- Developmental circumstances for burns include:
  Infants—Hot-water scalding, overheated liquids (e.g., microwave heating of bottles and solids)
  Toddlers—Spilled hot foods and drinks, hot tap water, household electricity, caustic chemicals, hot surfaces (e.g., stoves, irons)
  Preschoolers—Matches, lighters, stoves
  Preadolescents and adolescents—Matches, gasoline, high-voltage electricity

Prevention strategies

- Reduce hot-water temperature to 120° F.
- Place smoke detectors and fire extinguishers on each level of the home.
- Teach children appropriate skills and provide protection (see Table 14-4).
- Modify ignition sources (e.g., develop cigarettes that have reduced propensity to ignite upholstered furniture and mattresses, use childproof lighters).

- Extinguish flames by use of fire sprinkler systems in all residences.
- Install antiscald devices in faucets and showerheads.
- Create a safe environment by:
  Meeting building codes.
  Teaching parents about safety and supervision.
  Using a ground fault circuit interceptor (GFI).
- Protect from the sun.
- Be a role model for appropriate, safe behaviors.
- Clean the fireplace and creosote.
- Keep space heaters 36 inches away from flammable objects; check kerosene heaters.
- Remember the following holiday safety tips:
  Use a fresh, not dry, natural Christmas tree or an artificial, flame-retardant tree.
  Check lights and discard broken, frayed lights.
  Read and follow directions (e.g., do not use indoor lights outdoors).
  Place Christmas trees away from heating vents. Do not block stairs, hallways, or exits.
  Keep candles out of reach of children and away from flammable objects.
  Never leave tree lights on or lighted candles unattended.
- Model healthy behaviors (for example, use sunscreen; provide adequate sun protection for children; avoid tanning booths).
- Use sunscreen with a sun-protection factor (SPF) of 15 or higher on children over 6 months of age as much as possible during their first year of life.
- Use appropriate cover-ups (e.g., hats, long sleeves, pants).
- Wear sunglasses with lenses that absorb 99% to 100% of ultraviolet radiation.
- Limit sunlight exposure. The sunlight is most intense from 10 AM to 2 PM.
- Be aware that even on cloudy days 80% of the sun's radiation reaches the ground, that radiation increases 4% to 5% for every 1000 feet above sea level, and that the sun's radiation is intensified through glass.
- Consult a practitioner or pharmacist to determine whether certain medications cause photosensitivity, and avoid sun exposure if necessary. (See also the discussion of sunburn in Chapter 37.)

Drowning Injury

Childhood drowning is the fourth leading cause of death in children from birth to 19 years of age. The majority of drownings are preventable, and survival depends on early intervention. (See also the discussion of near drowning in Chapter 48.)

Scope of the problem
- Approximately 78% of drowning victims are male.
- Approximately 86% of drowning victims are under 5 years of age.
- Up to 20% of survivors have permanent neurologic disability.
- The risk for African-American children is two times greater than for Caucasian children, except in the 1- to 3-year-old age group, in which the chance is reversed.
- Those of a high socioeconomic status may have greater pool exposure and higher risk.
- Children with a seizure disorder have a four times higher risk than those without seizures.
- Approximately 98% of drownings occur in fresh water.

- For every drowning death, there are 10 nonfatal immersion events.
- About 60% to 90% of drownings in children from birth to 4 years of age occur in swimming pools. About 50% of these occur in the child's own home pool, while 33% occur at a friend's, family member's, or neighbor's pool. Public pool drownings are infrequent.
- At the time of drowning, 69% of children are being supervised by one or more parents, with a lapse in supervision of only a few minutes.
- Drowning occurs in less than 5 minutes.
- Alcohol is involved in 40% to 50% of drownings of adolescent males.
- Drownings in adolescents are generally the result of boating accidents or drownings in rivers and lakes, not in pools.
- Survival depends on prompt resuscitation.
- Children who receive prompt CPR and are spontaneously breathing within 5 minutes after extraction from the water have good outcomes. Children who do not receive prompt CPR or still require CPR in the emergency room have a poor prognosis.
- Survival without impairment is unusual after immersion for longer than 5 minutes. Irreversible brain damage occurs after 4 to 6 minutes.
- Survival after prolonged immersion in cold water is rare in the United States.

Prevention strategies
- Fencing swimming pools with locked gates could prevent 50% to 90% of pool drownings. (The fence should be 4 to 6 feet in height).
- Strict supervision of children around bodies of water is necessary.
- Use only approved life vests for protection, not inflatable arm bands or toys.
- Provide swimming lessons for children over 3 years of age (and do not consider them "safe," even if they are competent swimmers.)
- Provide water safety and lifesaving courses for school-age and older children.
- Teach the proper use of any water equipment (e.g., boogie boards, snorkeling equipment).
- Teach children not to:
  Swim alone
  Swim during electrical storms
  Run in pool areas
  Dive in shallow pools or lakes
  Swim after eating a heavy meal or after taking medication
  Stand in small boats
  Walk, skate, or ride on thin or weak ice
- Pool covers may be helpful, but a child can fall under a pool cover and go undetected.
- Provide CPR training for pool owners, parents, and children over 12 years of age.
- Teach alcohol and drug abuse prevention.
- Limit alcohol use at water recreation sites.
- For high-risk children (e.g., those with a seizure disorder):
  Provide strict supervision with high visibility (e.g., distinctive swimsuits or caps).
  Be sure the child's condition is well controlled with anticonvulsant therapy and that child has been seizure-free for 2 years.
  Supervise high-risk children for bathtub drownings.

Falls, Trauma, and Head Injury

Falls of newborns and infants are a frequent concern. Table 14-4 identifies age-specific prevention strategies, and global prevention strategies are listed shortly. (See also the discussion of head injury in Chapter 48.)

Scope of the problem

- Head injuries result from:
  MVAs
  Falls
  Sports and recreation injuries
  Assaults and abuse
- Head injury is common in injured children and can cause serious disabilities.
- Approximately 30% of all childhood injury deaths are from head trauma.
- Brain injury rates are two times higher in males, highest in males 15 to 19 years of age, and highest in females from birth to 4 years of age.
- With brain injury incidents, 82% cause mild brain injury, 14% cause moderate to severe injury, and 5% cause death.
- Causes of brain injuries are as follows:
  37% of *all* injuries are from MVAs.
  50% are from falls of newborns to 4-year-olds.
  43% are from sports or recreation accidents in 10- to 14-year-olds.
  55% are from motor vehicle crashes in 15- to 19-year-olds.
- Elevated blood alcohol levels are associated with injuries in 15- to 19-year-olds.
- Child abuse is a frequent cause of both body and brain injury in young children.

Prevention strategies

- See Table 14-4 for age-specific prevention strategies.
- Offer parent education programs on normal growth and development and injury prevention.
- Support pediatric-trained emergency medical personnel.
- Develop guidelines for transporting pediatric patients with trauma and performing triage.
- Perform triage on pediatric patients to pediatric trauma centers when possible.
- Develop rehabilitation services for trauma survivors to prevent increased morbidity.
- Develop community programs to increase awareness and support prevention programs (e.g., bike paths).
- Develop trauma-care systems for children:
  Identify community needs.
  Identify resources.
  Determine how to allocate resources.
  Evaluate and monitor trauma systems.

Sports Injury

There is a need for increased awareness of sports injuries and injury prevention. The practitioner can identify children and teenagers at risk for athletic injury through assessment and can stress importance of injury prevention. (See the discussion of athletic injuries in Chapter 38.) Table 14-6 identifies injuries that are most prevalent in common sports. The magnitude of sports injuries and possible global prevention strategies are listed below. Tables 14-7 and 14-8 review accidental and overuse injuries and sport-specific prevention strategies. Accident- and overuse-prone profiles of boys and girls can be found in Table 14-9. Suggestions for overall sports training, strengthening, conditioning, and stretching basics are described in the beginning of Chapter 38.

Injury prevention is the key to enjoyable sports participation. Children, adolescents, parents, and coaches need to acknowledge the risks and contribute to the prevention of injury. The practitioner may also need to help children become more realistic in their expectations of sports participation. Not all teenagers are going to end up playing professional sports, so the practitioner can encourage a realistic view of sports participation that emphasizes enjoyment, physical conditioning, self-discipline, and cooperation.

Scope of the problem

- There are 600,000 high school sports injuries a year.
- Injury is more likely to occur during practices and organized competition than during physical education classes.
- Athletes over 14 years of age have twice the injury risk of elementary school children.
- The risk and incidence of injury increase as a child gets older and bigger.
- Increased sports participation increases the risk of injury.
- Common sports that cause injury (in order of injury incidence) are:
  Football
  Gymnastics
  Wrestling
  Ice hockey
- Approximately 57% of sports injuries are sprains and strains, followed by contusions and fractures.
- Injury types are as follows:
  Accidental injury is trauma from an outside source.
  Overuse injury is repetitive, smaller trauma with an insidious onset and an intrinsic source.
  Overuse injuries lead to more permanent damage than accidental injuries (because they are present long before diagnosed and treated and cause deleterious effects on growing bones).
- Up to 68% of sports injuries occur during sports practices.
- Risk factors include:
  Gender, size, and weight mismatches
  Physical immaturity
  Rapid nonlinear growth (e.g., bone growth greater than muscle growth during rapid-growth phases, causing clumsiness)
  Body type (increased upper-body strength and muscle flexibility contribute to accident-prone injuries; tall stature, decreased muscle strength and flexibility, and increased ligament laxity contribute to overuse injuries)
  Active joint mobility
  Ligamentous laxity
  Muscle tightness
  Excessive risk-taking or anxiety behaviors
  Poor stress-related coping capabilities
  Major life changes

Prevention strategies

- Enforce the use of appropriate protective equipment (e.g., hockey face gear, protective helmets and pads for racquetball.
- Provide medical coverage at practices and competitions (e.g., athletic trainers, physicians, NPs).
- Ensure that coaches have adequate knowledge of growth and development, injury casualties, injury prevention, and appropriate coaching techniques.
- Ensure accurate reporting of injuries and injury data collection so that safety rules can be made and equipment changes can occur.

Table 14-6 Most Prevalent Injuries in Common Sports

	MOST COMMON INJURY	
SPORT	**TYPE**	**LOCATION**
Baseball	Epicondylitis (epiphysitis of the medial epicondyle of humerus) Traumatic (collision with ball or another player)	Elbow and shoulder
Football	Sprain or strain (late adolescence) Fracture (early adolescence) Contusions Spondylolysis of spine (three times that of general population)	Wrist, knee, shoulder, ankle; upper body equals lower body in frequency
Basketball	Sprain or strain	Ankle, knee (females); shoulder (males)
Wrestling	Sprain or strain Contusion Skin infections (friction from mat or contagious opponent)	Knee, back, shoulder, writs
Soccer	Sprain or strain Fracture Multiple overuse injury Contusion (especially shin)	Ankle, knee, foot, head (brain injury is now being suspected from repeated heading of ball)
Skiing	Fracture Sprain or strain Contusion, laceration	Tibia, fibula ("boot-top" fractures increasing), knee (incidence increases with age), hand, thumb
Track	Almost entirely repetitive microtrauma syndromes Acute strains Most common events causing injury are sprinting, distance running, and pole vaulting	Knee, ankle, thigh, tibia, low back
Gymnastics	Sprain or strain Contusion Fracture Dislocation Spondylolysis of spine (four times that of general population) Equal amount of accidental and overuse injuries Most common events causing injury are floor exercises	Lower extremity most common (ankle, knee), elbow, wrist, back
Ice hockey	Contusions, lacerations Sprain or strain Fracture Dislocation Dental injury Eye injury Body contact and illegal plays are the most common causes of injury	Head, neck, knee, groin, shoulder, spine

From Overbaugh, K.A. & Allen, J.G. (1994). Adolescent athlete. Part II: Injury patterns and prevention. Journal of Pediatric Health Care, 8, 208.

- Encourage athletic programs to use certified athletic trainers.
- Ensure that coaches and support personnel are adequately trained in CPR, first aid, and management of acute trauma.
- Group participants by physical maturation, height, size, and skill level. (Chronologic age is not a good indication.)
- Identify factors that might affect performance, such as:
  Academic concerns
  Peer pressure
  Family dysfunction
  Drug abuse
  Major life changes

- Properly maintain equipment, playing grounds, and arenas. Be sure equipment and shoes fit well and are broken in.
- Encourage appropriate role models who model safe training and playing behaviors.
- Guide children and adolescents in appropriate training, strengthening, and conditioning (see Chapter 38).
- Encourage participation in a variety of sports (i.e., cross-training) to increase overall fitness and decrease the risk for injury.
- Teach parents, coaches, peers, children, and adolescents about injury prevention.
- Assess children and adolescents by performing a health history, identifying risk factors, and performing physical examinations.

Table 14-7 Traumatic Injury in Common Sports

INJURY	COMMON SPORT	PREVENTION
Sprains and strains	All sports, especially those with heavy lower extremity involvement: soccer, football, basketball, baseball, skiing	Lengthy strengthening, especially ankles and knees (wobble board very good for this) Taping site of previous injury if its not 100% strength after complete rehabilitation Warm up body temperature before stretching
	Sports with unreliable playing surfaces (outdoor fields, slippery floors)	Improved playing surface condition (all holes repaired, use of mats) Proper footwear Limited practice time Adequate supervision (use of spotters)
Contusions	All sports, especially collision and contact sports	All athletes screened for underlying blood disorders Use of appropriate padding and protective gear Limited-contact programs
Fracture	Horseback riding Football Wrestling Gymnastics In-line skating/roller skating Skiing (downhill)	Strength conditioning Instruction on proper skill technique Safety precautions Properly fitting protective gear
Head	Football Soccer Ice hockey Golf Baseball Horseback riding	Appropriate supervision Strict adherence to and enforcement of rules Appropriate equipment at all times (helmets, face gear) Emphasis on strong neck muscles
Spine	Water sports (e.g., diving, water-skiing, surfing)* Football† Ice hockey	Appropriate supervision Assessment of dangers Increased strengthening of neck muscles Strict adherence to safety rules (e.g., backchecking into boards in hockey is illegal and requires severe enforcement)
Chest	Baseball Softball	New chest shields being studied for all players regardless of position to prevent chest trauma from a hard pitch or hit
Eye	Racquet sports Baseball Ice hockey	Provision of and enforcement in wearing of head gear and protective glasses Conditioning should include hand/eye coordination and decreased reflex time for defensive movement
Dental	Ice hockey Soccer Baseball	Mouth and face protective gear

From Overbaugh, K.A. & Allen J.G. (1994). Adolescent athlete. Part II: Injury patterns and prevention. Journal of Pediatric Health Care, 8, 204.
*75% of all cervical spine injuries.
†Now approximately 10% of all cervical spine injuries.

Farm Injury

There are serious hazards for children and adolescents in rural communities. Farm-related injuries for minors are not within the jurisdiction of the Occupational Safety and Health Administration if they occur on farms operated by the parents. These injuries are often underreported and are not regulated by the National Safety Council. Therefore, practitioners in rural areas have a unique role in the prevention of farm injuries.

Scope of the problem

- The highest rate of injuries in farms are in 10- to 19-year-olds.
- Moving machinery causes 55% of all farm injury deaths.
- Data are not available on children under 14 years of age, so the incidence of farm injuries is underestimated.

- Farm equipment (e.g., tractors, conveyor belts, hay balers, pitchforks, combines) causes the majority of injuries requiring hospitalization.
- Amputation of limbs is a frequent result of farm injury.
- Many injuries are sustained by children playing in vicinity of equipment.

Prevention strategies

- Develop safety programs for children in rural areas.
- Provide parent education programs to increase awareness of risks, injuries, and prevention.
- Support federal and state legislation to report and monitor safety standards.
- Develop regional trauma centers to improve emergency care, assessment, and rehabilitation services for children and adolescents in rural areas.

Table 14-8 Overuse Injury

INJURY	COMMON SPORT	PREVENTION
Result of Microtrauma		
Stress fracture	Sports requiring endurance or high limb repetition:	Soft running, playing surfaces
	Distance running	Proper footwear
	Distance running	Strengthening
	Softball	Avoid sudden surface changes
	Baseball	No activity past point of pain
	Field events	
Anterior leg pain syndrome ("shin splints")	Sports with quick stop-start and jumping action:	Thorough, gradual stretching before and after activity
	Basketball	Purposeful pronation and supination of feet when standing (ankle wobbling)
	Soccer	Soft running, playing surfaces
	Football	Treatment at first hint of discomfort
	Sports with hard playing surfaces	Proper footwear
	Sports of endurance or high repetition:	Limitations of forceful, extensive use of foot flexors
	Ballet	Avoiding sudden increase in activity, especially if inadequately conditioned
	Distance running	
	Gymnastics	
Tendinitis or arthritis	Sports with repetitive single-limb action:	Decreasing friction areas
	Baseball (pitching)	Warming up the target limb well (stretching, light practice throws and hits, and heat)
	Football (quarterbacking)	
	Racquet sports	
	Field events	
Shoulder impingement syndromes (including rotator cuff strains)	Tennis, racquet sports	Lightweight program of strengthening and passive resistance
	Baseball	Range-of-motion exercise
	Volleyball	Breathing to both sides when swimming
	Football	
	Skiing	
	Field events	
	Swimming (freestyle, butterfly)	
	Gymnastics	
Epicondylitis ("tennis elbow," "pitcher's elbow")	Sports with repeated forearm pronation and supination movement:	Use of proper technique
		Thorough conditioning and strengthening
	Racquet sports	Slow warm-up and cool-down
	Javelin throw	Limiting curveballs and pitching time
	Fencing	Large-headed racket
	Golf	Hitting ball close to center of racket
	Baseball (pitching)	
Chronic bursitis	Baseball (catching)	Longer preseason conditioning of gastrocnemius muscle
		Strengthening muscles
		Taking breaks; six to seven innings maximum catching time per game

From Overbaugh, K.A. & Allen, J.G. (1994). Adolescent athlete. Part II: Injury patterns and prevention. Journal of Pediatric Health Care, 8, *206-207.*

Table 14-8 Overuse Injury—cont'd

INJURY	COMMON SPORT	PREVENTION
Result of Microtrauma—cont'd		
Chronic spondylolysis	Football (blocking) Gymnastics	Stretching and strengthening back and hip muscles (with assistance of a second person)
	Wrestling	Avoiding hyperextension by proper technique
	Diving	Soft landing pads
Plantar fasciitis	Running (both sprint and distance) Also common in all athletes who have feet that pronate (roll inward or flatten) or wear stiff shoes	Proper footwear (cushioned with fitted heel counters) Heel lifts (if needed) Thorough stretching, especially calf and Achilles tendon Ice massage before event or practice Correct biomechanical or technique errors Limiting hills and speed work; increase soft-surface running
Blisters	Almost all sports!	Always wearing socks (one or two pairs) with shoes Properly fitting shoes that are broken in Lightly lubricating "hot spots" with petroleum jelly or powder (base of Achilles heel tendon, ball of foot, ends of toes, outer edges of foot)
Ingrown toenails	All sports	Properly fitting shoes with socks Toenails trimmed straight across, weekly
Heel-pad contusion	Jumping sports: Long jump High jump Hurdles	Cushioned heel cup, pad Full-length insole Rest
Result of Microtrauma, Especially to Growing Skeletal System		
Osgood-Schlatter disease (apophysitis of the tibial tubercle)	Not very sport specific, but usually sports needing more lower body strength; higher incidence in males than in females	Stretching slowly and thoroughly Heating tibial tubercle before activity Recognizing and beginning treatment early to prevent worsening (difficult to prevent) Limiting activities that require repeated extension and flexion directly at knee
Achilles tendinitis (Sever disease)	Distance running Basketball (landing foot) Soccer (stabilizing foot)	Slow stretching, especially legs, feet, and back muscles Soaking lower legs in warm whirlpool before stretching Avoiding uneven running surfaces and unstable shoes Heel cup Rest between activities
Patellar-femoral arthralgia or pain syndrome (chondromalacia is one type)	Sports with twisting or jumping: Football Basketball Volleyball Baseball (catching) Skiing	Good preseason stretching and strengthening program to decrease muscle imbalance and decrease forces exerted across knee joint Avoiding deep squatting and stair-climbing routines Pain-free isometric exercises Proper footwear Screening for anatomic abnormalities (e.g., excessive internal hip rotation, tibial torsion, foot pronation, quadriceps weakness, tight heel cords, patellar weakness)

Table 14-9 Accident- and Overuse-Prone Profiles

	MALE	FEMALE
Accident prone	Short stature Increased upper body strength Increased limb speed Increased muscle flexibility	Increased upper body strength Increased body weight
Overuse prone	Tall stature Endomorphic body structure Decreased muscle strength Decreased muscle flexibility Increased ligament laxity	Tall stature Decreased upper body strength Decreased static strength Increased limb speed Increased muscle tightness Increased ligament laxity

From Overbaugh, K.A. & Allen, J.G. (1994). Adolescent athlete. Part II: Injury patterns and prevention. Journal of Pediatric Health Care, 8, 209.

Conclusion

Childhood injuries present a serious health problem for children and adolescents. The majority of injury deaths can be prevented through active and passive prevention strategies. Unintentional injuries cost the nation more than $8 billion annually in direct health care costs, and this does not address the economic repercussions of lost future earnings of the child or the parents who miss work as a result of the child's injury (i.e., the indirect costs). Pain, suffering, and lost quality of life are also significant for children and families. Studies have shown a clearly positive effect from injury prevention counseling. One study estimated that use of The Injury Prevention Program (TIPP) with children from birth to 4 years of age would save $230 million in medical costs annually. Practitioners can help children keep healthier by counseling parents and children in injury prevention.

Barriers to Injury Prevention Counseling

- Children and parents have a low level of perceived vulnerability. (One third of parents perceived kidnapping of their child as more likely to occur than injury from an MVA.)
- Parents have a poor knowledge of many childhood safety issues (i.e., underestimating dangers of burns, pedestrian injury, drowning, and the like).
- Parents have erroneous beliefs that caution (e.g., the use of "Be careful" and vigilance) is an effective means of preventing injuries.
- Families of lower socioeconomic status are more likely to underestimate risks for injury.
- Parents often believe they already know how to prevent childhood injuries.
- Parents find safety to be a boring subject.
- Parents often expect accidents as part of growing up (i.e., "Children will be children").

Strategies for Promoting Injury Prevention

- Promote passive intervention strategies (e.g., flameproof sleepwear, child-resistant safety caps).
- Support and promote product regulation, government legislation, and community interventions.
- Find out what a parent or child knows and wants to know about injury prevention.
- Identify high-risk children and situations.
- Assess for attitudinal barriers.
- Correct misinformation.
- Increase awareness of the magnitude of injury morbidity and mortality.
- Promote teaching of children by parents and in the schools, and teach children and parents during health supervision visits.
- Provide readable written instructions to parents and children in their primary language and at a reading level they can understand.
- Encourage parents to be role models for appropriate safe behaviors. (Older siblings can also be encouraged to model safe behaviors for younger children in the family.)
- Maintain a nonjudgmental attitude.
- Employ multiple education strategies (e.g., magazines, printed materials, videos, national programs such as the National SAFE KIDS Campaign).
- Serve as an advocate for child safety and injury prevention.

Resources

Organizations

American Academy of Pediatrics, Committee on Injury and Poison Prevention, The Injury Prevention Program (TIPP), PO Box 747, Elk Grove Village, IL 60009; (888) 227-1770; www.aap.org

Centers for Disease Control and Prevention (CDC) Injury Prevention, 6 Executive Park, Mailstop E 19, Atlanta, GA 30329; (404) 639-2500; www.cdc.gov

Consumer Product Safety Commission, Office of Information, Washington, DC 20207; (800) 638-2772 or (800) 638-2772 (for the hotline); www.cpsc.gov/talk.html

National Child Safety Council (NCSC), 4065 Page Avenue, PO Box 1368, Jackson, MI 49204-1368; (800) 222-1464

National Injury Information Clearinghouse; (800) 638-2772; www.cpsc.gov

National SAFE KIDS Campaign, 111 Michigan Avenue NW, Washington, DC 20010-2970; (202) 662-0600

National Safety Council, 1121 Spring Lake Drive, Itasca, IL 60143-3201; (630) 285-1121; www.wwnsc.org

U.S. Department of Transportation, National Highway Traffic Safety Administration, Traffic Safety Programs, 400 7th Street SW, Washington, DC 20590; (202) 366-0123

Publications

A variety of safety pamphlets (often published in different languages) are available from the following sources:

Gerber Products Company, 445 State Street, Fremont, MI 49413; (800) 595-0324

Johnson & Johnson, Skillman, NJ 08558-9418; (800) 526-3967; www.jnj.com/home.html; www.johnsonsbaby.com

Mead Johnson & Co., Evansville, IN 47721; (800) 222-9123

Ross Laboratories (a division of Abbott Laboratories), 625 Cleveland Avenue, Columbus, OH 43215-1724; (800) 624-7677; www.ross.com

Websites

(See also Chapter 3)

Babycenter (www.babycenter.com)

Center for Disease Control and Prevention General Information (www.cdc.gov/ncipc/ncipchm.htm)

Center for Disease Control and Prevention National Center for Health Statistics' FASTSTATS (www.cdc.gov/nchs/fastats/acc-inj.htm)

Injury Mortality Reports (webapp.cdc.gov/sasweb/ncipc/mortrate.html)

National Center for Injury Prevention and Control (www.cdc.gov/ncipc/osp/othrdata.htm)

Parent Center (www.parentcenter.com)

Bibliography

American Academy of Pediatrics, Committee on Injury and Poison and Prevention. (2000). Reducing the number of deaths and injuries from residential fires. *Pediatrics, 105,* 1355-1357.

American Academy of Pediatrics. (1999). Safe transportation of newborns at hospital discharge. *Pediatrics, 104,* 986-987.

American Academy of Pediatrics. (1999). Transporting children with special health care needs. *Pediatrics, 104,* 988-992.

American Academy of Pediatrics. (1997). *Injury Prevention and Control for Children and Youth.* Elk Grove Village, IL: American Academy of Pediatrics.

American Academy of Pediatrics. (1994). *The injury prevention program (TIPP).* Elk Grove Village, IL: American Academy of Pediatrics.

American Academy of Pediatrics, Committee on Injury and Poison Prevention. (1995). Bicycle helmets. *Pediatrics, 95,* 609-610.

American Academy of Pediatrics, Committee on Injury and Poison Prevention. (1995). Skateboard injuries. *Pediatrics, 95,* 611-612.

Baker, S.P., O'Neill, B., Ginsburg, M.J., et al. (1997). *The injury fact book.* New York: Oxford University Press.

Bergman, A.B., Rivara, F.P., Richards, D.D., et al. (1995). Seattle Children's Bicycle Helmet Campaign. *American Journal of Diseases of Children, 144,* 727-731.

Bull, M.J. & Sheese, J. (2000). Update for the pediatrician on child passenger safety: Five principles for safer travel. *Pediatrics, 106,* 1113-1144.

Centers for Disease Control and Prevention, National Center for Health Statistics, National Vital Statistics. (2000, July 24). *National vital statistics system.* Vol. 48.

Coody, D., Brown, M., Montgomery, D., et al. (1994). Shaken baby syndrome: Identification and prevention for nurse practitioners. *Journal of Pediatric Health Care, 8,* 50-56.

Department of Health and Human Services, Centers for Disease Control and Prevention, National Center for Health Statistics. (1997, July). *Health United States 1996-97 and injury chart book,* DHHS No. (PHS) 97-1232. Atlanta: Centers for Disease Control and Prevention.

Green, M., (Ed.). (2001). *Bright futures: Guidelines for health supervision of infants, children and adolescents* (2nd ed.). Arlington, VA: National Center for Education in Maternal Child Health.

Grossman, D.C., Cummings, P., Koepsell, T.D., et al. (2000). Firearm safety counseling in primary care pediatrics: A randomized, controlled trial. *Pediatrics, 106,* 22-26.

Grossman, D.C., & Rivara, F.P. (1992). Injury control in childhood. *Pediatric Clinics of North America, 39,* 471-485.

Haddon, W. (1980). Advances in the epidemiology of injuries as a basis for public policy. *Public Health Reports, 95,* 411-421.

Holinger, P.C. (1990). The causes, impact, and eventability of childhood injuries in the United States. *American Journal of Diseases of Children, 144,* 670-676.

Jones, N.E. (1992). Child injuries: An epidemiologic approach. *Pediatric Nursing, 18,* 30-35.

Jones, N.E. (1992). Injury prevention: A survey of clinical practice. *Journal of Pediatric Health Care, 6,* 182-186.

Kraus, J.F., Rock, A., & Hemyari, P. (1990). Brain injuries among infants, children, adolescents and young adults. *American Journal of Diseases of Children, 144,* 684-691.

Kunkel, N.C., Nelson, D.S., & Schunk, J.E. (2001). Do parents choose appropriate automotive restraint devices for their children? *Clinical Pediatrics, 40,* 35-40.

Litovitz, T.L., Klein-Schwartz, W., White, S., et al. (2000). 1999 Annual report of the American Association of Poison Control Centers Toxic Exposure Surveillance System. *The American Journal of Emergency Medicine, 18,* 517-574.

Overbaugh, K.A. & Allen, J.G. (1994). The adolescent athlete. II. Injury patterns and prevention. *Journal of Pediatric Health Care, 8,* 203-211.

Ozmar, B. (1994). Encountering victims of interpersonal violence. *Critical Care Nursing Clinics of North America, 6,* 515-522.

Rimell, F., Thome, A., Stool, S., et al. (1995). Characteristics of objects that cause choking in children. *Journal of the American Medical Association, 274,* 1763-1766.

Scheidt, P., Hareb, Y., Trumble, A.C., et al. (1995). The epidemiology of nonfatal injuries among U.S. children and youth. *American Journal of Public Health, 85,* 932-936.

Waller, J.A. (1994). Reflections on half a century of injury control. *American Journal of Public Health, 84,* 664-670.

Winston, F.K., Durbin, D.R., Kallan, M.J., et al. (2000). The danger of premature graduation to seat belts for young children. *Pediatrics, 105,* 1179-1354.

Wittenberg, E., Nelson, T.F., & Graham, J.D. (1990). The effect of passenger airbags on child seating behavior in motor vehicles. *Pediatrics, 104,* 1247-1250.

Zavoski, R.W., Lapidus, G.D., Lerer, T.J., et al. (1995). A population-based study of severe firearm injury among children and youth. *Pediatrics, 96,* 278-282.

Chapter 15 *Nutritional Assessment and Guidelines for Infancy through Adolescence*

Clare McLaughlin

There are several tools available to complete the dynamic process of nutritional assessment in children. Gaining skill and experience help the professional complete the best nutritional assessment possible. The most important process is learning to observe normal, healthy children throughout the life cycle for physical appearance in relationship to age and genetic potentials. Observation of the act of eating (what, how, and when) and listening to the child and his or her caregivers can provide the best information. Children are at highest risk for nutritional issues related to excess and inadequate or imbalanced nutrient intake and output. Children have increased nutrient needs related to their size and activity levels and fewer nutrient stores. They often depend on others for their nutrient sources and opportunities for activity.

Normal growth and development through adequate but not excessive intake can maximize quality and quantity of life. A nutrition assessment can help identify problem areas, so that appropriate recommendations and education and therapies can be implemented. Undernutrition is the most significant cause of growth retardation. The incidence of overnutrition has increased in the United States over the past three National Health and Nutrition Examination Surveys (NHANES) (a nationally representative health reference) and has been associated with chronic diseases in adults. Iron deficiency is the number one nutrient deficiency in this country, affecting children. Nutrition assessment should be an ongoing process for all children to identify and prevent nutritional issues such as these that prevent achievement of optimal health and wellness.

Nutritional Assessment

Assessment of a child's nutritional status is completed through careful *clinical assessment,* including a health and dietary history; *physical assessment,* including use of accurately obtained anthropometric measurements; and careful assessment of appropriate *biochemical indices.* Physical, family, and socioeconomic status along with cultural beliefs need to be considered. Nutritional assessment requires various methods and tests with no single component able to make a complete assessment. The use of the tools may require selection of the best tool for the individuals and should always be an ongoing process.

Clinical Assessment
History
- Age
- Birth weight, gestational age at birth, weight-gain history, and deviation from previously established growth curve
- Concern of parents and patient

- Past medical history (especially associated with malabsorption or altered nutrient metabolism) and family medical history requiring diet modification (e.g., diabetes, cardiac disease, vegetarianism)
- Diet recall (e.g., breastfed or formula fed [what formula, how prepared, how tolerated, volume taken], introduction of solid foods and progression to age-appropriate feeding skills)
- History of acute or chronic illnesses
- Surgical history
- Developmental history
- Feeding behavior
- Feeding difficulty (e.g., anorexia, vomiting, use of nutritional support systems)
- Medication or supplement use history by child or family (e.g., of vitamins, minerals, herbal supplements, recreational drugs, alcohol)
- Allergies
- Elimination pattern
- Family history (e.g., of high blood pressure, stroke, heart condition, diabetes, obesity, hyperlipidemia, hypercholesterolemia, eating disorders)
- Participation in food programs (e.g., Women, Infants, and Children [WIC], school lunch programs)

Diet history. A caregiver or older child or adolescent can provide information about typical dietary patterns followed by the child or family. Sample tools such as food frequency questionnaires, diet recalls from families, or 3- to 5-day diet records (if obtained and reviewed by a skilled practitioner) can be compared to normal intakes recommended for age. The U.S. Department of Agriculture (USDA) food guide pyramid (Fig. 15-1) provides foods in groups based on their important nutrient content, along with recommended portion sizes for different age groups to meet nutrient needs over time. The diet recall and activity history or food frequency review can be compared with these age-appropriate guidelines to identify if there are possible nutrition risks. The diet record can be analyzed in more detail based on nutrient content for food references (Pennington, 1998) and compared with the recommended dietary allowances (RDAs) for nutrients for various life stage groups. Knowledge and experience with age-appropriate and culturally acceptable foods helps with obtaining an accurate history (Table 15-1 and Box 15-1). It is important to check the infant formula, baby food, or pediatric vitamin or mineral supplement label for the most accurate and up-to-date nutrient information and the preparation or dosage recommendations, as they change periodically. (Notice the website addresses and phone numbers provided in Table 15-1 for more detailed and current information.)

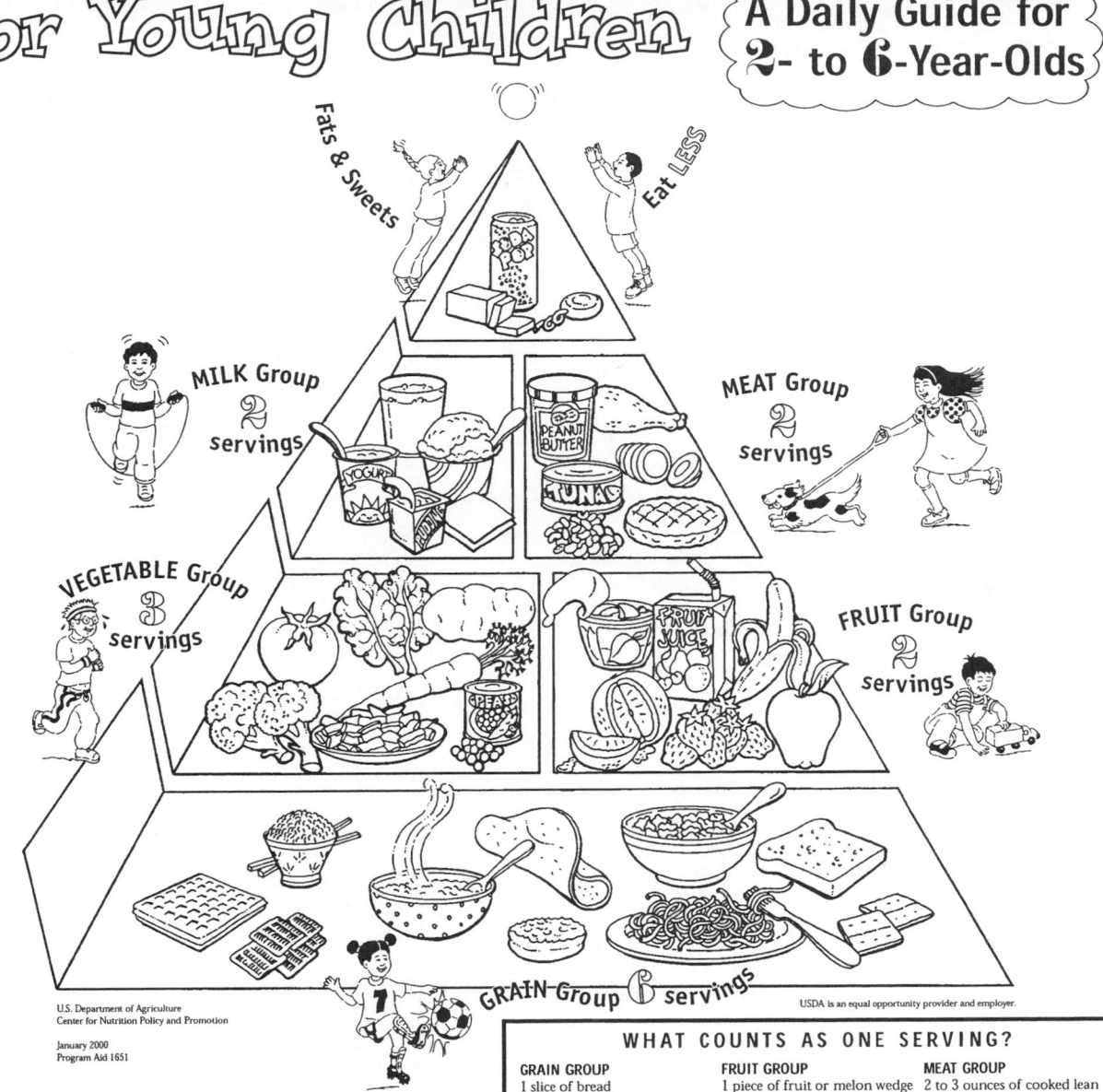

FOOD IS FUN and learning about food is fun, too. Eating foods from the Food Guide Pyramid and being physically active will help you grow healthy and strong.

WHAT COUNTS AS ONE SERVING?

GRAIN GROUP
1 slice of bread
½ cup of cooked rice or pasta
½ cup of cooked cereal
1 ounce of ready-to-eat cereal

VEGETABLE GROUP
½ cup of chopped raw
or cooked vegetables
1 cup of raw leafy vegetables

FRUIT GROUP
1 piece of fruit or melon wedge
¾ cup of juice
½ cup of canned fruit
¼ cup of dried fruit

MILK GROUP
1 cup of milk or yogurt
2 ounces of cheese

MEAT GROUP
2 to 3 ounces of cooked lean meat, poultry, or fish.

½ cup of cooked dry beans, or 1 egg counts as 1 ounce of lean meat. 2 tablespoons of peanut butter count as 1 ounce of meat.

FATS AND SWEETS
Limit calories from these.

Four- to 6-year-olds can eat these serving sizes. Offer 2- to 3-year-olds less, except for milk. Two- to 6-year-old children need a total of 2 servings from the milk group each day.

Fig. 15–1 Food guide pyramid for young children. (From the U.S. Department of Agriculture).

Table 15-1 Formula Information

	MANUFACTURER	FORM	MACRONUTRIENT STANDARD CALORIES PER OUNCE (PER ML)	PROTEIN SOURCE (GRAMS PER 100 CALORIES/ % OF CALORIES) (WHEY:CASEIN)*
Breast milk (mature)	Mom	RTF	20 (0.67)	Human (1.54/6) (70:30)
Infant Formulas				
Enfamil with Iron	MJ	RTF, C, P	20 (0.67)	W, NFM (2.1/9) (60:40)
Similac with Iron	R	RTF, C, P	20 (0.67)	NFM, WPC (2.07/8) (48:52)
Carnation Good Start	C/N	RTF, C, P	20 (0.67)	DWPC (2.4/10) (100:0)
Generic	W	RTF, C, P	20 (0.67)	FM, DW (2.2/9) (60:40)
Similac PM 60:40	R	P	20 (0.67)	WPC, NaC (2.22/9) (60:40)
Enfamil Lacto Free	MJ	RTF	20 (0.67)	NFM, PI (2.07/8) (18:82)
Similac Lactose Free	R	RTF	20 (0.67)	MPI (2.14/9) (18:82)
Enfamil AR	MJ	RTF, P	20 (0.67)	NFM (2.5/10) (18:82)
Similac Neosure	R	P, RTF	22 (0.73)	NFM, WPC (2.6/10) (50:50)
Enfamil Enfacare	MJ	P, RTF	22 (0.73)	NFM, WPC (2.8/10) (60:40)
Special Infant Formulas				
Similac Special Care	R	RTF	24 (0.8)	NFM, WPC (2.7/11)
Enfamil Premature	MJ	RTF	24 (0.8)	NFM, WPC (3/12)
Modified				
Alimentum	R	RTF	20 (0.67)	CH, LC, LTRY, LTYR (2.75/11)
Nutramigen	MJ	RTF, C, P	20 (0.67)	CH (2.8/11)
Pregestimil	MJ	P	20 (0.67)	CH, LC, LTYR (2.8/11)
Neocate	SHS	P	20 (0.67)	LAA (3.1/13)
Portagen	MJ	P	20 (0.67)	C (3.5/14)
Soy				
Isomil	R	RTF, C, P	20 (0.67)	SPI, LM (2.45/10)
Isomil DF	R	RTF	20 (0.67)	SPI, LM (2.66/11)
Prosobee	MJ	RTF, C, P	20 (0.67)	SPI, LM (2.54/12)
Alsoy	C/N	RTF, C, P	20 (0.67)	SPI, LM, T (2.8/11)
Generic	W	RTF, C, P	20 (0.67)	SPI, LM, T (3.15/12)
Toddler and Pediatric Formulas				
Similac 2	R	P	20 (0.67)	NFM, WPC (2.07/8)
Enfamil Next Step	MJ	P	20 (0.67)	NFM (2.6/10)
Carnation F/U	C/N	P	20 (0.67)	NFDM (18:82) (2.6/11)
Isomil 2	R	P	20 (0.67)	SPI, LM (2.45/10)
Enfamil Next Step Soy	MJ	P	20 (0.67)	SPI (2.7/10)
Carnation Soy F/U	C/N	P	20 (0.67)	SPI (3.1/12)
Pediasure	R	RTF	30 (1.0)	NAC, WPC (3/12)
Kindercal	MJ	RTF	30 (1.06)	MPC, NAC, CAC (2.8/11)
Nutren Jr	C/N	RTF	30 (1.0)	W (50%), MPC (3/12)
Resource Just for Kids	N	RTF	30 (1.0)	NAC, WP (3/123)
Complete Pediatric	N	RTF	30 (1.0)	BF, NAC, CAC (3.8/15)
Peptamen Jr	C/N	RTF	30 (1.0)	EHW (3/12)
Ped Vivonex	N	P	24 (0.8)	AA (3/12)
Neocate Jr	SHS	P	30 (1.0)	AA (3/12)
Ele Care	R	P	30 (1.0)	AA (3/15)

Major Infant and Pediatric Formula Food Companies in the United States (Including Chart Abbreviations):
Beechnut (B): (800) 622-4726; www.beechnut.com
Carnation/Nestle (C/N): (800) 782-7766
Gerber (G): (800) 443-7237; www.gerber.com
Heinz (H): (800) 872-2229; www.heinzbaby.com
Mead Johnson (MJ): (800) 457-3550; www.meadjohnson.com
Novartis (N): (800) 333-3785; www.resourceathome.com
Ross (R): (800) 515-7617 or (800) 227-5767; www.similac.com
Scientific Hospital Supply of North America (SHS): (800) NEOCATE; www.shsna.com
Wyeth (W): (800) 272-5095; www.storebrandformulas.com

Other Chart Notations:
Forms: *C, Concentrate; P, powder; RTF, ready-to-feed.*
Protein Sources: *BF, Beef; C, caseinate; CaC, calcium caseinate; CH, casein hydrolysate; DW, demineralized whey; DWPC, demineralized whey protein concentrate; EHW, enzymatically hydrolyzed whey; LAA, L-amino acids; LC, L-cystine; LM, L-methionine; LTRY, L-tryptophan; LTYR, L-tyrosine; MPC, milk protein concentrate; MPI, milk protein isolate; NaC, sodium caseinate; NFM, nonfat milk; PH, protein hydrolysate; PI, protein isolate; SPI, soy protein isolate; T, taurine; W, whey; WP, whey protein; WPC, whey protein concentrate; WPH, whey protein hydrosylate.*
Fat Sources: *C, Corn; CA, canola; CO, coconut; HOSF, high-oleic safflower; HOSUN, high-oleic sunflower; LCAR, L-carnitine; MCT, medium-chain triglyceride; O, oleic; PO, palm olein; S, soy; SAF, safflower; SUN, sunflower.*
Carbohydrate Sources: *AJ, Apple juice; CSS, corn syrup solid; CS, corn starch; FRT, fruit; HCS, hydrolyzed corn starch; L, lactose; MCS, modified corn starch; MD, maltodextrine; MTS, modified tapioca starch; RS, rice starch; S, sugar; SU, sucrose; V, vegetable.*
*Only applies to breast milk and cow's milk products.

FAT SOURCE (GRAMS PER 100 CALORIES/ % OF CALORIES)	CARBOHYDRATE SOURCE (GRAMS PER 100 CALORIES/ % OF CALORIES)	OSMOLALITY (mOsm)	RECOMMENDED USES AND INDICATIONS
Human (5.74/52)	L (10.5/42)	280-300	None
PO, CO, HOSUN, S (5.3/50)	L (10.9/41)	300	All non-breastfed healthy infants
HOSF, CO, S (5.4/49)	L (10.8/43)	300	All non-breastfed healthy infants
PO, HOSF, CO, S (5.1/46)	L (70%, MD (30%) (11/44)	260	All non-breastfed healthy infants; may be useful for some protein intolerances; slow gastric emptying on standard formula
O, CO, SAF, S (5.3/48)	L (10.6/43)	280	All non-breastfed healthy infants; generally less expensive than standard formulas
C, CO, S (5.59/50)	L (10.2/41)	280	Renal, cardiac, or electrolyte imbalances
PO, CO, HOS, UN, S (5.3/48)	CSS (10.9/44)	200	Lactose intolerance
S, CO (5.4/49)	CSS, SU (10.7/43)	200	Lactose intolerance
PO, S, CO, HOSUN (5.1/46)	RS (30%, L, MD (11/44)	240	Reflux in term infants
S, CO, MCT (25%) (5.5/49)	MD (50%), L (50%) (10.3/41)	250	Premature infants at discharge
HOSUN, S, MCT (20%) (5.3/47)	MD, L (10.9/43)	230	Premature infants at discharge
MCT (50%), S, CO (5.43/49)	CSS, L (10.6/42)	280	Premature infants
MCT (40%), S, CO (5.1/44)	CSS, L (11.1/44)	300	Premature infants
SAF, MCT (33%), S (5.54/48)	SU, MTS (10.2/41)	370	Milk protein intolerance; malabsorption
PO, S, CO, HOSUN (5/45)	CSS, MCS (11/44)	320	Milk protein intolerance
MCT (55%), S, C, HOSF (5.6/58)	CSS, D, CS (10.2/41)	320	Milk protein intolerance; malabsorption
HSAF, C, O, S (4.5/41)	CSS (11.7/45)	342	Protein allergy
MCT (85%), C (4.8/41)	CSS, SU (11.5/45)	320	Long-chain fat intolerance
HOSF, CO, S (5.46/49)	CSS, SU (10.3/41)	200	Milk protein or lactose intolerance
S, CO (5.46/49)	CSS, SU (10.1/40)	240	Diarrhea; use for less than 2 weeks; contains 6 g of fiber
PO, S, CO, HOSUN, LCAR (5.3/48)	CSS (10.6/40)	200	Milk protein or lactose intolerance
S, HOSUN, LCAR (4.95/45)	SU, MD (11.1/44)	270	Milk protein or lactose intolerance
CO, SAF, O, S, LCAR (5.4/47)	SU, CSS (10.35/41)	296	Milk protein or lactose intolerance
HOSF, CO, S (5.49/49)	L (10.6/43)	300	Toddlers 8 to 18 months with poor solid food intake
PO, S, CO, HOSUN (5/45)	CSS, L (11.1/45)	260	Toddlers 8 to 18 months with poor solid food intake
PO, S, CO, HOSF (4.1/35)	CSS, L (13.2/54)	326	Toddlers 8 to 18 months with poor solid food intake
HOSF, CO, S (5.46/49)	CSS, SU (10.3/41)	200	Toddlers 8 to 18 months with poor solid food intake
PO, S, CO, HOSF (5.1/45)	CSS, L (11.1/45)	270	Toddlers 8 to 18 months with poor solid food intake
S (4.4/40)	MD, S (12/48)	270	Toddlers 8 to 18 months with poor solid food intake
HOSF, S, MCT (20%) (5/44)	MD, S (11/44)	345-440, (tube feeding), 430-520 (oral)	1- to 10-year-olds as a sole source of nutrition or as an oral supplement
CA, HOSF, MCT (20%), C (4.2/37)	S, MD (12.7/52)	345-440, (tube feeding), 430-520 (oral)	1- to 10-year-olds as a sole source of nutrition or as an oral supplement
S, CA, MCT (25%) (4.2/37)	MD, S (12.7/51)	350	1- to 10-year-olds as a sole source of nutrition or as an oral supplement
HOSUN, S, MCT (20%) (5/44)	CST, S (11/44)	390	1- to 10-year-olds as a sole source of nutrition or as an oral supplement
HOSF, S, MCT (20%) (3.9/35)	HCS, AJ, FRT, VEG (13/50)	380	1- to 10-year-olds as a sole source of nutrition or as an oral supplement
S, CO, MCT (60%) (3.9/33)	MD, CS (13.8/55)	260	1- to 10-year-olds as a sole source of nutrition or as an oral supplement
S, MCT (68%) (3/25)	D, MS (16/63)	360-490	1- to 10-year-olds as a sole source of nutrition or as an oral supplement
MCT, CA, SAF (5/46)	CSS (10.4/42)	607	1- to 10-year-olds as a sole source of nutrition or as an oral supplement
HOSF, MCT (33%), S (4.8/42)	CSS (10.7/43)	596	1- to 10-year-olds as a sole source of nutrition or as an oral supplement

Box 15-1 Baby Foods

Is the food commercial or homemade?

If commercial baby food is used, what stage/jar size is used?

If the food is home made, was anything added to it (e.g., water, sugar, salt)?

Generally, commercial baby foods come in stages:

Stage 1: $2\frac{1}{2}$ oz jar

Stage 2: $4\frac{1}{2}$ oz jar

Stage 3: $6\frac{1}{2}$ oz jar

Commercial food for graduates or toddlers, as well as table foods, can be measured in ounces or tablespoons.

Are the baby foods single or combination foods?

For specific nutrition information, one may check the baby food companies' websites.

Box 15-2 Pediatric Vitamin and Mineral Supplement Recommendations

Routine supplements not needed in healthy, growing children
At-risk populations include:

- Deprived families; victims of parental neglect or abuse
- Those with anorexia or decreased appetite; those on fad diets
- Those with chronic disease (e.g., cystic fibrosis (CF), inflammatory bowel disease (IBD), liver disease)
- Those in obesity management programs
- Those on vegetarian diets without a dairy group
  Keep supplements out of the reach of children.
  If an infant is breastfed, consider supplementing with:
- *Vitamin D*—Especially if the infant receives limited sunlight exposure. If an infant spends less than 30 minutes per week (in a diaper) or less than 2 hours per week (in full clothes) in the sun (with no sunscreen for this period), supplement with 300 international units (IU) (0 to 6 months of age) or 400 IU (6 to 12 months) of vitamin D. (Controversy exists regarding if all breastfed infants should receive a vitamin D supplement.)
- *Iron*—After the age of 4 to 6 months if there is a minimum of iron intake from solids containing iron. Supplement with 1 mg/kg per day to a maximum of 10 to 15 mg/day (for a term infant) or 2 mg/kg per day to a maximum of 10 to 15 mg/day (for a preterm infant). Iron is available in multivitamin-with-iron infant drops (10 mg/ml) and separate iron supplements (Fer-In-Sol drops at 0.6 ml, providing 15 mg of elemental iron)
- *Fluoride*—See Chapter 16.
- B_{12}—Infants of vegan mothers who breastfeed may be at risk. Encourage B_{12}-fortified foods or supplementation (0.3 to 2 μg per day is the RDA from birth 50 years of age)
- *Folic acid*—All women of childbearing age should receive 400 μg per day. (Information obtained from www.cdc.gov/nceh/prevent/birthdef.)
  Further information regarding the use of other nutritional supplements in children may be helpful. See the article by Buck, M. & Michel, R. (2000). Talking with families about herbal therapies. *Journal of Pediatrics, 136*(5), 673-78, or the following websites:
- www.ftc.gov/bcp/conline/features/kidsupp.htm
- www.supplementwatch.com/sup-atoz/index.html
- www.cc.nih.gov/ccc/suplements/intro.html

Data adapted from American Academy of Pediatrics. (1998). Pediatric nutrition handbook. Elk Grove, IL: American Academy of Pediatrics.

The American Academy of Pediatrics (AAP) recommends that all infants be breastfed if possible for at least the first year of life, with solid foods being introduced at 4 to 6 months adjusted or corrected age (chronologic age minus the number of weeks a child was born prematurely, if any), one at a time over a 3- to 5-day period so that the infant can be observed for food allergies or intolerances. The most common food allergies are to cow's milk, eggs, soybeans, wheat, peanuts, tree nuts, fish, and shellfish. If the infant cannot be breastfed, an iron-fortified infant formula should be provided until the child turns 1 year of corrected age (see Table 15-1) (Shandler, 2001).

Topics the practitioner may cover while gathering a child's diet history include:

- Introduction of solid foods, including:
  Timing
  Method
  Frequency and quantity offered (frequency and quantity of specific foods and food groups; who is the primary feeder)
- Nighttime nutrition
- Satisfaction with feeding method
- Use of pacifier or thumbsucking

The primary caregiver may be asked the following questions related to an infant (taken from the Bright Futures website):

- How do you think feeding and meal times are going? Do you have any questions about breastfeeding?
- How does the baby let you know when he or she is hungry or full?
- How often is the baby eating?
- Have you noticed any changes in how the baby eats?
- How do you feel about how your child is growing?
- What is the longest time your child has slept at one time?
- How much rest are you getting?
- How many wet diapers do you change per day?
- Do you burp the baby during or after feeding?
- Is anyone helping you feed your child?
  If an infant is breastfeeding, questions may include:
- Do you have any questions or concerns?
- Do you need help?
- How often do you feed?
- Any problems with the breast?
- Do you restrict any foods?
- What vitamin or mineral supplements do you take or plan to take or plan to give to your infant?
  If an infant is being fed formula, the following questions apply:
- What are you feeding your infant? Is it iron fortified?
- How do you prepare the infant formula?
- How do you store the infant formula after you make it?
- How do you clean the equipment?
- What do you do with the formula in the bottle after the feeding?
- How does your baby take the formula (i.e., how do you hold your baby during feedings)?
- Do you think that the bottles, nipples, and formula are appropriate for your baby?

For toddlers, preschoolers, school-age children, and adolescents, questions may relate to the following topics:

- Daily frequency of meals and snacks
- Daily and weekly consumption of proteins, vegetables, fruits, carbohydrates, fats and oils, sugar, and salt
- Food preferences

- Person primarily responsible for planning, shopping, and preparing meals
- Family food budget
- Dental history (e.g., hygiene, dental care regimen, visits to the dentist)
- Participation in athletics
- Prescribed and self-imposed diets

Vitamin and mineral supplementation recommended by the AAP is discussed in Box 15-2.

If the infant or child's history and physical examination indicate that there are nutritional concerns, further investigation is necessary. Specific biochemical measures might be useful if the diet history reveals data indicating a nutritional problem. An example might be an infant with the following history: breastfed until 14 months of age, no vitamin or mineral supplements, now 24 months of age, described as a picky eater, does drink five to seven 8-ounce glasses of whole milk a day. This child might need a screen for iron deficiency and then might require a supplement and recommendations regarding limiting whole milk, with the goal of increasing iron-containing solid food intake.

Physical Assessment

Physical examination. A complete physical examination should be performed with an emphasis on the following actions most pertinent to nutritional status:

- Observe general appearance.
- Assess hydration status. (Signs and symptoms of dehydration include poor skin turgor, dry mucous membranes, sunken eyes, sunken fontanel, tachycardia, and tachypnea).
- Assess skin color, turgor, and presence of subcutaneous fat.
- Inspect scalp and hair luster.
- Inspect and palpate fontanels (for children up to 2 years of age).
- Notice color of conjunctiva.
- Palpate thyroid.
- Inspect oral cavity.
- Palpate gums, palate, and tongue.
- Make digital assessment of oral tone, tongue placement, and coordination of infant's suck.
- Inspect, auscultate, percuss, and palpate abdomen.
- Perform a neurologic and developmental examination (using the Denver II test).
- Inspect stool, if possible.

Table 15-2 lists clinical signs associated with nutrient deficiencies and specific laboratory findings required to substantiate the diagnosis.

Anthropometrics. Anthropometric data (body measurements) are a major tool for the physical assessment and are often used as an initial step in a nutritional assessment. Height, weight, and head circumference as compared with gender and age averages serve as a nutritional screen or part of a nutritional assessment. Newly revised growth charts have been released by the Centers for Disease Control and Prevention (CDC) and the National Center for Health Statistics (NCHS) that now provide for assessing children's growth compared to others of similar age and sex for up to 20 years of age. These charts include a chart to plot and compare a 2- to 20-year-old's body mass index (BMI) with others their age. The BMI can be used to help assess children for development of overweight or obesity (see Appendix A). BMI is defined as the person's weight in kilograms (pounds divided by 2.2) divided by the height in meters (inches times 2.54) squared. Special growth charts for premature infants or children with specific medical

diagnoses such as Down syndrome, cerebral palsy, and Turner syndrome are available (Feucht, 2000; Trahms & Feucht, 2000).

Obtaining accurate measurements is important. Appropriate tools for obtaining weights, lengths or heights, head circumferences, and skinfold measurements should be used, and the person obtaining these measurements should be trained on obtaining and interpreting the data accurately. The NHANES III survey group provides a training tape on the methods and equipment used to gather anthropometric data. If the individual child's growth data are gathered in the same way as the standard data was measured, the comparison will be more meaningful. The CDC has a website for professionals to use to learn and to teach about the use of the new growth charts. The site includes training programs with case studies that can be downloaded or viewed for refreshers or training for new practitioners completing nutritional assessments. Instructions include measuring the length (0 to 36 months) or height and weight (2 to 20 years) without clothes for children less than 36 months old or in light dress for children 2 to 20 years of age, as well as the head circumference for children 0 to 36 months, then plotting the results on standard growth charts. (The year 2000 charts are available at www.cdc.gov/growthcharts.) A practitioner should check for any deviations from the expected growth pattern. (The deviations may turn out to be normal or may indicate a possible difficulty with nutrition or a medical problem.)

Biochemical Assessment

Laboratory measures of blood, urine, or other body tissue are available to assess nutrient levels or serve as markers of nutritional status. Specific tests can be used to identify excesses or deficiencies of nutrients or nutrient-related disease states. Some lab tests may be recommended as a screening for common nutrition-related issues noticed in children (e.g., checking hemoglobin or hematocrit as a screen for anemias, checking cholesterol levels for those with family history of heart disease). Screening recommendations are based on the risk of deficiencies and excesses and the effect on long-term health. There need to be accurate, effective tests that have age-specific and population-specific norms to go along with the physical and medical history to help with nutritional assessment. Normal values for lab tests vary with the specific labs, and so it is important to note normal values at the institution where the level is drawn. A practitioner should always double check the units in which the levels are reported, and laboratory data should be patient specific. There are useful references for determining specific laboratory tests to help with assessment for specific vitamin and mineral status for different ages, or one may consult with laboratory managers regarding specific age-appropriate tests that might be best for a particular child based on his or her diet and medical history and current medical status. (Appendix C lists some normal laboratory values.)

Promotion of Nutritional Well-Being

Nutrition is important throughout life. It is especially important during the gestational and neonatal periods. Many health practitioners believe that the foundation for health is established during childhood. Educating an expectant or new mother to make appropriate nutritional choices can potentially also benefit a child. Counseling and education, intervention, follow-up evaluation, and appropriate referrals are important components in helping families establish healthful eating patterns.

Table 15-2 Clinical Signs and Laboratory Findings in Malnourished Children and Adults

CLINICAL SIGN	SUSPECT NUTRIENT	SUPPORTIVE OBJECTIVE FINDINGS
External Systems		
Epithelial		
Skin		
Xerosis, dry, scaling	Essential fatty acids	Triene/tetraene radio > 0.4
Hyperkeratosis, plaques around hair follicles	Vitamin A	↓ Plasma retinol
Ecchymoses, petechiae	Vitamin K; vitamin C	Prolonged prothrombin time; ↓ serum ascorbic acid
Hair		
Easily plucked, dyspigmented, lackluster	Protein-calorie	↓ Total protein; ↓ albumin; ↓ transferrin
Nails		
Thin, spoon-shaped	Iron	↓ Serum Fe; ↓ TIBC
Mucosal		
Mouth, lips, and tongue	B vitamins	
Angular stomatitis (inflammation at corners of mouth)	B_2 (riboflavin)	↓ RBC glutahione reductase
Cheilosis (reddened lips with fissures at angles)	B_2; B_6 (pyridoxine)	See above ↓ Plasma pyridoxal phosphate
Glossitis (inflammation of tongue)	B_6; B_2; B_3 (niacin)	See above ↓ Plasma tryptophan; ↓ urinary N-methyl nicotinamide
Magenta tongue	B_2	See above
Edema of tongue, tongue fissures	B_3	See above
Gums		
Spongy, bleeding	Vitamin C	↓ Plasma ascorbic acid
Ocular		
Pale conjunctivae secondary to anemia	Iron; folic acid; vitamin B_{12} (thiamine); copper	↓ Serum iron, ↑ TIBC, ↓ serum folic acid or ↓ RBC folic acid; ↓ serum B_{12}; ↓ serum copper
Bitot's spots (grayish, yellow, or white foamy spots on the whites of the eye)	Vitamin A	↓ Plasma retinol
Conjunctival or corneal xerosis, keratomalacia (softening of part or all of cornea)	Vitamin A	↓ Plasma retinol
Musculoskeletal		
Craniotabes (thinning of the inner table of the skull); palpable enlargement of costochondral junctions ("rachitic rosary"); thickening of wrists and ankles	Vitamin D	↓ 25-OH-vitamin D; ↑ alkaline phosphatase ↓ Calcium, ↓ phosphorus; long-bone films

From Kerner A. (Ed.). (1983). Manual of pediatric parenteral nutrition. *New York: Churchill Livingstone.*
Fe, *Iron;* PBI, *protein-bound iodine;* RBC, *red blood cell;* TIBC, *total iron-binding capacity.*

Infants

During the first few days of life, infants lose weight, but their birth weight is usually regained by the seventh to tenth day of life. Infants usually double their birth weight by the age of 4 months and triple it by 1 year old. Infants increase their length by 50% during the first year of life.

Parent education and counseling tips

- Breastfeeding or feeding of iron-fortified infant formula should be done for the first 12 months of life (see Table 15-1).
- Evaporated milk is not recommended but may have to be acceptable in some cases (e.g., breastfeeding is unsuccessful, cost of commercial formulas is prohibitive). The usual recipe for a 1-day supply is as follows: 1 can of evaporated milk (13 ounces), 19½ ounces of water, and 3 tablespoons of sugar or corn syrup. A vitamin A and vitamin D supplement is needed unless the evaporated milk is fortified. Additional vitamin C and iron are required unless the

infant eats sufficient quantities of solid foods. Unless the water used in the preparation is fluoridated, supplementary fluoride is also needed.

- Goat milk contains inadequate folic acid and excessive protein and electrolytes and is not appropriate for infants.
- Solid foods (Table 15-3) can be introduced when the infant shows developmental readiness, including head control and loss of extrusion reflex, which indicate developmental skills to show hunger or fullness; generally this occurs around 4 to 6 months of age. It may take 15 to 20 attempts before an infant accepts a new food. Solid foods should be introduced in small amounts, one at a time over a 3- to 5-day period so that the caregiver can watch for food allergies or intolerances.
- No solids should be given in a bottle unless it is recommended for reflux. Solid foods change the nutrient distribution of the feeding and, if given in the bottle, change sensory motor development.

Table 15-2 Clinical Signs and Laboratory Findings in Malnourished Children and Adults—cont'd

CLINICAL SIGN	SUSPECT NUTRIENT	SUPPORTIVE OBJECTIVE FINDINGS
External Systems—cont'd		
Musculoskeletal—cont'd		
Scurvy (tenderness of extremities, hemorrhages under periosteum of long bones; enlargement of costochondral junction; cessation of osteogenesis of long bones)	Vitamin C	↓ Serum ascorbic acid; long-bone films
Skeletal lesions	Copper	↓ Serum copper; x-ray film changes similar to scurvy, since copper is also essential for normal collagen formation
Muscle wasting, prominence of body skeleton, poor muscle tone	Protein-calorie	↓ Serum proteins; ↓ arm muscle circumference
General		
Edema	Protein	↓ Serum proteins
Pallor resulting from anemia	Vitamin E (in premature infants)	↓ Serum vitamin E; ↑ peroxide hemolysis; evidence of hemolysis on blood smear
	Iron	↓ Serum iron, ↑ TIBC
	Folic acid	↓ Serum folic acid; macrocytosis on RBC smear
	Vitamin B$_{12}$	↓ Serum B$_{12}$; macrocytosis on RBC smear
	Copper	↓ Serum copper
Internal Systems		
Nervous		
Mental confusion	Protein	↓ Total protein; ↓ albumin; ↓ transferrin
	Vitamin B$_{12}$	↓ RBC transketolase
Cardiovascular		
Beriberi (enlarged) heart, congestive heart failure, tachycardia)	Vitamin B$_1$	Same as above
Tachycardia resulting from anemia	Iron	See above
	Folic acid	
	Vitamin B$_{12}$	
	Copper	
	Vitamin E (in premature infants)	
Gastrointestinal		
Hepatomegaly	Protein-calorie	↓ Total protein, ↓ albumin, ↓ transferrin
Glandular		
Thyroid enlargement	Iodine	↓ Total serum iodine; ↑ inorganic, protein-bound iodine

- The family history should be reviewed for food allergies. The Food Allergy Network (www.foodallergy.org) is a resource for families of children with common food allergies.
- No honey can be given during the first year of life because of the risk of botulism from botulism spores.
- Choking may be a problem for infants and young children because of limited muscle control to chew and swallow. Foods that are small or slippery (e.g., hard candy, whole grapes, hot dogs), are dry or difficult to chew (e.g., popcorn, raw carrots, nuts), or are sticky or tough to break apart (e.g., peanut butter, large chunks of meat) should be modified or avoided.
- To prevent baby bottle tooth decay, caregivers should be warned about prolonged bottle feedings or allowing snacking on sugary or carbohydrate-rich foods, which can increase the risk of tooth decay. Nothing but water should be given in a bottle to encourage sleep or quiet the

infant before sleep. Introduction of the cup for drinking at 6 months of age and weaning of the infant from the bottle by 12 to 14 months of age may help with prevention. Juice should be limited to around 4 ounces of pasteurized juice per day from a cup to prevent excess intake of juice from diluting more nutrient-dense foods like formula or solid foods and to prevent diarrhea caused by excessive juice intake.

Vitamin and mineral supplementation. Nutrient goals are RDA 108 kcal/kg and 2.2 g protein/kg or 13 g/day (National Research Council, Food and Nutrition Board, 1989 (for infants up to 6 months of age) and RDA 98 kcal/kg and 14 g protein/day (27) (for infants 6 to 12 months of age). (See also Box 15-2). To calculate the amount of formula per day, divide the total calories by 0.67 calories/ml, or 20 calories per ounce of standard concentrated formula to find milliliters (cubic centimeters) or ounces of formula per day; then divide that number into the number of feedings per day, depending on whether

Table 15-3 Progression of Solid Foods in the First Year

AGE	TYPES OF FOOD	SUGGESTED ACTIVITIES
Birth to 4 months	Breast milk or infant formula	Breastfeed or bottle-feed.
5 months		Possibly introduce cereal.
6 months	Infant cereal, strained fruit or vegetables, finger foods (if ready)	Prepare cereal with formula or breast milk to a semiliquid texture; use spoon; feed from a dish; advance to $1/_3$ to $1/_2$ cup of cereal with added fruits or vegetables. Start cup introduction; if juice is offered, offer from a cup.
7 months	Infant cereal, plus continue as above	Provide thicker to lumpier texture for foods; seat in high chair with feet supported; introduce cup.
8 to 10 months	Juices; soft, mashed, or minced table foods	Do not add salt, sugar, or fats to food. Offer soft chunks ready for finger-feeding.
10 to 12 months	Soft, chopped table foods	Provide meals in pattern similar to rest of family. Use a cup with meals.

the infant sleeps through the night. These are estimates of goals for feedings; it is best to pay attention to an infant's hunger and satiety cues for the volume of formula needed.

Preparation of infant formulas. Formulas usually come packaged in three forms: (1) ready to feed (32-ounce cans), (2) concentrated liquid (13-ounce cans), and (3) powder (12- to 16-ounce cans).

Concentrated liquid is cheaper than ready-to-feed formula and readily available. It is easily mixed, though this process should be reviewed with families. It can be a source for fluoridated water after 6 months of age. Once prepared, this formula can be kept in the refrigerator for 24 to 48 hours after opening.

Powdered formula is generally the cheapest formula available. General guidelines to mix are for 1 scoop (specific to the formula can) to be added to 2 ounces of water to make the standard dilution of 20 calories per ounce of formula. It is important to check the specific formula can for preparation directions. For example, the standard preparation guidelines for Neocate Powder (made by the Scientific Hospital Suppliers of North America) are 1 scoop to 1 ounce of water. Some powdered formulas specify that unpacked-level or packed-level scoops should be used in preparation, so again, the specific label should be checked. Powdered formulas are generally available in 12- to 16-ounce cans (making 87 to 130 ounces of reconstituted 20-calorie-per-ounce standard dilution formula).

Sterilization of mixing equipment is unnecessary if:
- The formula source is a sterile, commercially prepared formula.
- The water source is from a supervised city filtration plant.
- Hands are washed during preparation and before feeding.
- Equipment is washed well in warm, soapy water and rinsed thoroughly.
- Formula is promptly refrigerated after preparation and must be kept in refrigerator until used.

The practitioner should teach parents to:
- Warm bottles in a pan of hot water, not in a microwave.
- Discard partially used bottles after a feeding.
- Keep bottles cold until used (when transported with a baby).

Toddlers and Preschoolers

Physical growth rate decreases, motor development matures, cognitive ability increases, and the personality continues to evolve during this period. The child develops self-feeding skills, food preferences, and individual patterns of food intake. By the end of the second year of life, birth weight is quadrupled. Birth length is doubled at approximately 4 years of age. Energy and protein goals are approximately 1300 to 1800 calories and 16 to 24 g of protein per day.

Parent education and counseling tips

- Between approximately 1 and 3 years of age, a child may become disinterested in food, with a decrease in appetite.
- Milk intake usually decreases.
- Food preferences are common, and the child's tastes and behaviors become unpredictable.
- Between-meal snacks should be carefully selected (e.g., dry cereal, fruit, juice, skim milk, raw fruit, cheese, crackers).
- Often the child demands that milk be served in the same glass or that a sandwich be served on the same plate.
- Parents should prepare small portions of foods that are simple; have a variety of colors; have a combination of textures; are easy to eat; are cut large enough for the fork, yet small enough to be eaten; and are served at room temperature.
- The child should be situated in a sturdy, well-balanced chair with the feet supported. Food should be kept within reach, and unbreakable dishes and glasses should be used.
- Parents should have the child use a spoon with a handle that is blunt, short, and held easily. A child's fork should have short, blunt tines that adapt easily to the child's palm.
- Parents must be patient and understanding with each new stage of development in the feeding process.
- New tastes and textures must be introduced slowly.
- An emotionally and physically comfortable eating environment should be provided.
- When children get hungry enough, they will eat. Parents need to remain flexible to avoid potential feeding problems.
- A preschooler should have at least 16 ounces of milk or milk substitute daily; 24 ounces is better. Some children refuse to drink milk, so parents should be given a list of foods that are rich in calcium.
- A creative way to encourage milk intake is to add milk to cereal or to serve creamed soups, yogurt, pudding, or ice cream desserts.
- A preschooler should be offered six small meals. Intake of fried or salted snacks and high-calorie, low-nutrient baked goods should be limited.

- Eating with other children or adults provides a child with a pleasurable social experience and an opportunity to learn by imitating others. At such times, a good nutritional role model should be provided.
- The National Cholesterol Education Program recommends that children older than 2 years of age consume a diet that provides no more than 30% of calories from fat (10% to 15% from monounsaturated fats, 10% or less from saturated fats, and up to 10% from polyunsaturated fat) and no more than 300 mg of cholesterol per day. The panel also recommends cholesterol screening for children at risk, children with parents or grandparents who have been diagnosed with coronary heart disease or have had a myocardial infarction before 55 years of age, and children with one or both parents having a serum cholesterol of 240 mg or higher.
- For overall health promotion, moderation is the best policy. For healthy, growing children, the use of low-fat dairy products and a reduced number of high-fat foods is appropriate for children older than 2 years of age.
- Parents and children, when it is age appropriate, should be instructed how to read food labels.
- Parents and caregivers should be encouraged that their job is to provide nutritious foods at regular intervals in a safely prepared, age-appropriate form. The job of the infant, toddler, or child is to decide if and how much to eat.

School-Age Children

The healthy school-age child usually presents few nutritional problems and adapts to family eating patterns. Snacks continue to be a primary source of nutrients, and an increasing amount of nutrition is obtained outside the home. Growth is steady during the school-age years, but it may be erratic in individual children. Weight increases an average of 4½ to 6½ pounds a year until 9 or 10 years of age. Height increases 2⅓ to 3⅓ inches per year until the pubertal acceleration. Calorie and protein goals vary with age and sex to a range of 1800 to 2000 kcal and 24 to 28g of protein per day.

Parent and child education and counseling tips
- Children can begin to select some of their own foods.
- Fluctuations in appetite are caused by growth patterns and activity levels.
- Because growth is slow, the caloric needs, when compared with the stomach size, are not so great as when the child was younger.
- The child should eat foods high in protein, minerals, and vitamins.
- Parents should be cautioned about allowing the child excessive soft drinks and candy.
- Breakfast is an important meal. Many studies have linked breakfast consumption with improved school performance.
- Participation in sports requires a greater caloric intake. Food intake should be increased without changing the proportions of nutrients.
- Intervention for childhood obesity should be directed toward increasing the child's physical activity and reducing dietary fat intake to 30% of total calories.

Adolescents

Nutritional needs are influenced by the physical and emotional adjustment of this period. Caloric needs increase as a result of the adolescent growth spurt; growth during adolescence is as rapid as in early infancy. The adolescent gains about 20% of adult height and 50% of adult weight during this period, and growth continues throughout pubertal development (occurring earlier in girls than in boys). Energy and protein goals vary with sex, age, and activity level but run around 2200 to 3000 calories and 45 to 59 g of protein per day.

This is a common time for rebellion against previously acquired family eating habits. Activities outside the home increase, and snacking becomes a major source of nutrients. Adolescents become concerned about body image and are striving for self-identity. Cultural and familial importance placed on food also plays an important role in adolescent eating behaviors.

Parent and adolescent education and counseling tips
- Over one quarter of calories in teenagers are typically derived from snacks.
- Snacks such as fresh fruits, fruit juices, dried fruits, cheese, milk beverages, peanut butter and crackers, raw vegetables, and nuts should be suggested.
- Do the adolescent or their friends or family skip meals?
- A pregnant adolescent should take a prenatal multivitamin pill if her diet history indicates inadequate intake to meet nutritional needs during pregnancy.
- A minimum of 2300 calories may be required for those involved in very strenuous exercise. Adolescents should be asked if any type of special diet or dietary supplements have been used by them or their friends or recommended by coaches or caregivers.
- Protein should be 10% to 15% of the diet; fat, 25% to 35%; and carbohydrates, 50% to 65%.
- Both adolescent girls and boys need 8 to 15 mg of iron daily.
- Girls frequently lack adequate iron and calcium.
- Fast foods are typically low in iron and vitamin C, calcium, folic acid, vitamin A, and riboflavin and high in fat, cholesterol, and sodium.
- Do any family members or friends follow any type of special dietary practices, including fad diets and herbal or amino acid supplements? (Box 15-3)

Box 15-3 Special Nutritional Considerations and Management: Pediatric Populations

Obesity—See Chapter 43.

Vegetarian—Counseling depends on the classification. *Vegans* consume no animal products. *Lactovegetarians* eat plant foods and dairy products but exclude all meat, fish, poultry, and eggs. *Semivegetarians* eat plant foods and dairy products, eggs, and some fish and poultry. Red meat is avoided or eaten only occasionally. Vitamin B$_{12}$ and a vitamin D supplement may be needed. Consult or refer to a nutritionist if needed.

Food faddism—Discuss the implications of the food fad. Advise that food faddism is normal behavior at certain ages. Help parents explore ways to balance a diet over a week rather than from meal to meal or day to day. Assist parents to understand natural food faddism and how to avoid calling undue attention to diet and behavior. *Nutrition should not be a focus of family conflict.*

Specific disease states—If a child requires a modified diet for a specific condition, he or she should be carefully followed through scheduled health care visits.

- If an adolescent follows a self- or medically imposed diet modification, he or she should be evaluated for nutritional adequacy and followed closely for nutritional, medical, and emotional issues that might require special referrals for further evaluation and treatment.
- Knowledge of the appropriate use of nutrition assessment tools and age and developmental nutrition goals provides adequate information to help maintain or improve an individual's health status. Nutrition assessment should be ongoing for all children.

Resources

Websites

Eat 5 a Day (www.5aday.com)

American Dietetic Association, Pediatric Practice Group; (800) 877-1600; (800) 366-1655; www.eatright.org

American Heart Association (www.americanheart.org)

American School Food Service Association (www.asfsa.org)

American Society of Parenteral and Enteral Nutrition (ASPEN) (www.nutritioncare.org)

Centers for Disease Control and Prevention (CDC) (www.cdc.gov; www.cdc.gov/nchs/about/major/nhanes/growthcharts/charts.htm; www.cdc.gov/growthcharts)

Food Allergy Network; (800) 929-4040; www.foodallergy.org

Food and Drug Administration (www.fda.gov)

Food and Nutrition Board, Institute of Medicine, National Academy Press; (800) 624-6242; www.nap.edu

Food and Nutrition Information Center (www.nal.usda.gov/fnic)

International Food Information Council (www.ific.org)

National Heart, Lung, and Blood Institute (NHLBI) (www.nhlbi.nih.gov)

Nutrition Focus (depts.washington.edu/chdd/uap/co/co29.html)

Quack Watch (www.quackwatch.com)

U.S. Department of Agriculture Food and Nutrition Services (www.fns.usda.gov/fns; www.usda.gov/news/usdakids/food_pyrhtml)

U.S. Department of Health and Human Services, Maternal and Child Health Bureau (www.ncemch.org; www.brightfutures.org)

Using the Food Guide Pyramid (www.nutrition.gov)

Bibliography

American Academy of Pediatrics. (1999). *The official, complete home reference guide to your child's nutrition*. New York: Villard Books.

American Academy of Pediatrics. (1998). *Pediatric nutrition handbook* (4th ed.). Elk Grove village, IL: American Academy of Pediatrics.

American Academy of Pediatrics, Committee on Nutrition. (2001). The use and misuse of fruit juice. *Pediatrics, 107*(5), 1210-1213.

American Academy of Pediatrics, Committee on Nutrition. (2000). Hypoallergenic infant formulas. *Pediatrics, 106*(2), 346-349.

American Academy of Pediatrics, Committee on Nutrition. (1999). Iron fortification of infant formulas. *Pediatrics, 104*(1), 119-123.

American Academy of Pediatrics, Committee on Nutrition. (1998). Atherosclerosis: Cholesterol in childhood. *Pediatrics, 101*(1), 141-147.

American Academy of Pediatrics, Committee on Nutrition. (1998). Soy protein-based formulas: Recommendations for use in infant feeding. *Pediatrics, 101*(1), 148-153.

American Academy of Pediatrics, Committee on Nutrition. (1995). The role of dietary fiber in children. *Pediatrics, 96*(5).

Aldous, M. (1999). Nutrition issues for infants and toddlers. *Pediatric Annals, 28*(2), 101-105.

Baer, M. & Bradford Harris, A. (1997). Pediatric nutrition assessment: Identifying children at risk. *Journal of the American Dietetic Association, 97*(10, Suppl 2), S107-S115.

Barlow, S. & Dietz, W. (1998). Obesity: Obesity evaluation and treatment: expert committee recommendation. *Pediatrics, 102*(3).

Behrman, R.D., Kliegman, R.M., & Jensen, H.B. (2000). *Nelson's textbook of pediatrics* (16th ed.). Philadelphia: W.B. Saunders.

Buck, M. & Michel, R. (2000). Talking with families about herbal therapy. *Journal of Pediatrics, 136*(5), 673-678.

Centers for Disease Control and Prevention. *NHANES III training video: Anthropometric (body measurement) procedures*. CDC 301-436-8500. Hyattsville, MD: National Center for Health Statistics, National Health and Nutrition Examination Survey.

Feucht, S. (2000). Assessment of growth. Part 1: Equipment, technique and growth charts. *Nutrition Focus, 15*(2).

Fleisher, D. (1995). Comprehensive management of infants with GER and FTT. *Current Problems in Pediatrics, 25*, 247-253.

Gidding, S. (2001). Controlling cholesterol in children. *Contemporary Pediatrics, 18*(3), 77-100.

Hall, R. & Carrol, R. (2000). Infant feeding. *Pediatrics in Review, 21*(6). Available online at www.ftc.gov/bcp/conline/features/kidsupp.htm.

Institute of Medicine. (2001). *DRI, Dietary reference intakes, applications in dietary assessment*. Washington, DC: National Academy Press.

International Paediatric Association (IPA) and the Committee on Nutrition of the European Society of Paediatric Gastroenterology, Hepatology, and Nutrition (ESPGHAN) Workshop. (2000). Research priorities in complementary feeding. *Pediatrics, 106*(5), Supplement.

Johnson, T.S., Engstrom, J.L., Haney, S.L., et al. (1999). Reliability of three length measurement techniques in term infants. *Journal of Pediatric Nursing, 25*(1), 13-17.

Kanakoudi, F., Drossou, V., Tzimouli, V., et al. (1995). Serum concentrations of 10 acute-phase proteins in healthy term and preterm infants from birth to age 6 months. *Clinical Chemistry, 41*(4), 605-608.

Queen Samour, P., King Helm, K., & Lang, C.E. (1999). *Handbook of Pediatric Nutrition*. (2nd ed.). Gaithersburg, MD: Aspen.

Klotz, K., et al. (1998). *Goals of pediatric nutrition support and assessment: The ASPEN nutrition support manual*. Gaithersburg, MD: Aspen.

Lipman, T.H., Hench, K., Logan, J.D., et al. (2000). Assessment of growth by primary health care providers. *Journal of Pediatric Health Care, 14*(4), 166-171.

Lohman, T.G., Roche, A.F., & Martorell, R. (Eds.). (1988). *Anthropometric standardization reference manual*. Champaign, IL: Human Kinetics.

Miller, E. & Maropis, C. (1998). Nutrition and diet related problems. Primary care. *Adolescent Medicine, 25*(1), 193-210.

National Research Council, Food and Nutrition Board. (1989). *Recommended dietary allowances* (10th ed.). Washington, DC: National Academy Press.

Parkman-Williams, C. (1998). *Pediatric manual of clinical dietetics*. Chicago: American Dietetic Association.

Pennington, J. (Ed.). (1998). *Bowes and Church's food values, portions commonly used* (17th ed.). Philadelphia: J.B. Lippincott.

Picciano, M. (2001). Nutrient composition of human milk. *Pediatric Clinics of North America, 48*(1), 53-67.

Picciano, M.F., Smiciklas-Wright, H., Birch, L.L., et al. (2000). Nutrition guidance is needed during dietary transition in early childhood. *Pediatrics, 106*(1), 109-114.

Satter, E. (2000). *Child of mine* (Revised and updated edition). Menlo Park, CA: Bull Publishing.

Sauberlich, H. (1999). *Laboratory tests for assessment of nutritional status* (2nd ed.). Washington, DC: CRC Press.

Shandler, R. (Ed.). (2001). Breastfeeding, Parts 1 & 2. *Pediatric Clinics of North America, 48*(1 & 2), 1-539.

Story, M., et al. (Ed.). (2000). *Bright futures in practice: Nutrition.* Arlington, VA: National Center for Education in Maternal/Child Health, Georgetown University, Health Resources and Services Administration. Available online at www.brightfutures.org.

Summer, B. (2000) *Eating expectantly* (2nd ed.). New York: Simon & Schuster.

Trahms, C. & Feucht, S. (2000). Assessment of growth. Part 2: Interpretation of growth. *Nutrition Focus, 15*(3 & 4).

Trumbo, P., Yates, A.A., Schlicker, S., et al. (2001). Dietary reference intakes: Vitamin A, vitamin K, arsenic, boron, chromium, copper, iodine, iron, manganese, molybdenum, nickel, silicon, vanadium, and zinc. *Journal of the American Dietetic Association, 101*(3), 294-301.

U.S. Department of Agriculture, Agricultural Research Service. (1998). *Food and nutrient intakes by individuals in the United States by sex and age 1994-1996.* Washington, DC: U.S. Department of Agriculture, Nationwide Food Surveys Report 96-2, 197.0.

Walker, W. & Watkins, J. (1997). *Pediatric nutrition* (2nd ed.). Boston: Little, Brown & Co.

Yates, A.A., Schlicker, S.A., & Suitor, C.W. (1998). Dietary reference intakes: The new basis for recommendations for calcium and related nutrients, B vitamins, and choline. *Journal of the American Dietetic Association, 98*(6), 699-706.

Chapter 16 *Dental Health*

Linda Gilman

An important component of health promotion is that of educating parents in their role in ensuring their child's oral health now and into adulthood. Good oral health practices begin in infancy, are provided by the parent in the child's early years, and are maintained into adulthood by instructing, monitoring, and motivating the child and by modeling good oral habits as the parent. The primary care practitioner (PCP) is in a crucial position to assess oral health because dental disease continues to be a significant health problem in many segments of the pediatric and general population. Practitioners are in the unique position to reinforce healthful oral habits and successfully guide the parent through the growth and developmental years, free of dental disease in a pediatric dental home.

Prenatal Factors Influencing Dental Health

- Nutrition of the mother is a primary factor in the healthful development of the infant's teeth.
- Severe maternal and neonatal vitamins A and D, phosphorus, and calcium deficiencies can cause enamel hypoplasia (chalky, chipping enamel) and hypocalcification (discoloration). A maternal diet of fresh vegetables, protein, and vitamin D–fortified milk can prevent this.
- Maternal rubella and syphilis can have adverse effects on the neonate's dental health.
- Tetracycline and phenytoin sodium (Dilantin) ingested during gestation can cause abnormal staining of infant's teeth.
- Calcium needs of the infant are provided by the mother's diet. If the diet is inadequate, calcium comes from the mother's bones.
- Increased hormone levels of estrogen and the tendency of gingival tissue to undergo hypertrophy during pregnancy may exaggerate the mother's reaction to toxins produced by bacteria in plaque, causing the gums to become red and tender and to bleed more easily. Brushing, flossing, and regular dental visits during pregnancy should be encouraged.

Stages of Tooth Development and Eruption

Enamel formation of the primary dentition occurs from 6 weeks in utero through the first 6 years of life, to a varying degree. At the same time, calcification of the crowns of the permanent dentition starts at birth and continues until 16 years of age with the formation of the occlusal surfaces of the wisdom teeth. Tooth eruption begins at about 6 months with the primary mandibular central incisors and concludes with the eruption or extraction of the permanent third molars (wisdom teeth) between 17 and 21 years of age (Table 16-1).

Table 16-1 Chronologic Development of Normal Dentition

PRIMARY TEETH	ERUPTION (MONTHS)	SHEDDING (YEARS)
Central incisor	6-9	7-8
Lateral incisor	7-10	7-9
Canine	16-20	10-12
First molar	12-16	9-11
Second molar	20-30	11-12

SECONDARY TEETH	ERUPTION (YEARS)	
	LOWER	UPPER
Central incisor	6-7	7-8
Lateral incisor	7-8	8-9
Canine	9-11	11-12
First premolar	10-12	10-11
Second premolar	11-12	10-12
First molar	6-7	6-7
Second molar	11-13	12-13
Third molar	17-25	17-25

Current Concepts of the Caries Process

Dental caries is a disease of the dental hard tissues characterized by the decalcification of the enamel and eventual breakdown of the organic portions of the tooth. Bacteria in the mouth, mainly *Streptococcus mutans* and *Lactobacillus acidophilus,* use dietary carbohydrates (i.e., sucrose, glucose, lactose, fructose) as a substrate for acid production. It is this acid produced by the bacteria that begins the process of demineralization. The lactic acid produced by carbohydrate metabolism lowers the pH in the plaque from 6 to 4 within minutes. The organisms proliferate in the acid environment, adhere to the enamel surface growing in the small pits and fissures of the occlusal (chewing) surfaces, and form plaque on the smooth surfaces. Mastication stimulates salivation, which buffers the acid and washes the sugars from the oral cavity. But the sugars also affect the rate at which saliva can enter the plaque to buffer the acid and reverse the demineralization. During sleep, when salivary gland secretion stops, the teeth are more susceptible to the acid attack of residual sugars in the mouth, which causes nursing syndrome (i.e., baby bottle disease).

The earliest sign of caries on smooth enamel is a white spot of chalky, opaque enamel, typically seen at the gingival (gum) margin. The white spot is an indication that the underlying enamel has become decalcified. Acids produced by plaque bacteria diffuse into the enamel matrix and begin the process of demineralization below the surface layer. Once demineralization has begun, remineralization takes place in a simultaneous process as long as calcium and phosphate ions are available in the saliva. The presence of fluoride ions accelerates the remineralization process and slows demineralization and caries formation.

Periodontal diseases afflict the gums and bones that support the teeth. Although these diseases are most common among adults, some form of periodontal disease affects 39% of children and 68% of youths in the United States. Studies show that many periodontal problems that occur later in life could be caused by the neglect of oral care during childhood and adolescence. An early sign of periodontal disease is swollen gums that bleed easily, especially when teeth are brushed. If bacteria-laden plaque is not removed by daily brushing and flossing, toxins created by these bacteria can irritate the gums, making them tender and likely to bleed. The progressive irritation can eventually lead to bone deterioration and tooth loss.

Caries Prevention and Preventive Dentistry

Prevention of Small Surface Lesions

- Use of fluoride in its various forms
- Good oral hygiene
- Nutritious diet

Prevention of Pit-and-Fissure Lesions on Occlusal Surfaces

Sealants. A dental sealant is a thin plastic film painted on the chewing surface of teeth. Scientific studies have proved that sealants are effective in protecting the tooth surface from caries. Sealant act as a physical barrier to decay, and as long as the sealant remains intact, small food particles and bacteria that cause cavities cannot penetrate through or around a sealant. Sealants provide a smoother tooth surface, one that is less likely to trap food and plaque. Molars are especially difficult to clean because of the deep and narrow grooves in the chewing part of the tooth. Sealants make it easier to effectively clean with a toothbrush, cutting off the supply of nutrients to the bacteria that cause cavities.

Preventive resin restoration techniques. Resin restorative techniques are used to treat dental caries. The resin is a paste that is applied in layers once the decay has been removed from the tooth. The final layer of resin is hardened with use of a special curing light. Resins are tooth colored and tend to have an esthetic advantage.

Fluoride

There has been a significant reduction since the early 1940s in the prevalence of dental caries, which is attributable to the use of fluoride. Studies have documented caries reduction of 40% to 50% in the primary dentition and 50% to 65% in the permanent dentition of children drinking fluoridated water from birth.

Fluoride is believed to prevent caries by: (1) increasing the resistance of the tooth structure to acid dissolution, (2) enhancing the process of remineralization, and (3) reducing the cariogenic potential of dental plaque.

Fluoride is administered either systemically or topically. Systemic fluoride is ingested via foods or water that contain naturally occurring fluoride, fluoride-adjusted water supplies, and dietary fluoride supplements. Topical fluoride is administered in the form of fluoridated toothpastes, professionally applied treatments, fluoride rinses, and the ingestible fluorides as they pass through the mouth and contact the teeth.

Water fluoridation remains the most effective, reliable, convenient, and cost-effective method of providing fluoride to the population, since it does not depend on individual compliance. The "optimal level" is related to a geographic area's average temperature. This is usually 1 part per million (ppm), which is equivalent to 1 mg of fluoride in 1 liter of water. Many areas of the country have naturally occurring fluoride in the water supply, especially in the Midwest and Southwest. This has led to a higher incidence of fluorosis, or mottled teeth, because of the overingestion of fluoride. Therefore it is imperative to have private well water tested for fluoride levels before fluoride supplementation.

It is also important to assess the ingestion of fluoride from other sources including food, beverages, vitamin supplements, toothpaste, and mouth rinses. Breast milk, cow milk, and ready-to-feed formula have negligible amounts of fluoride, though the fluoride in breast milk is most completely absorbed and used by the infant. If concentrated or powdered formula is reconstituted with fluoridated water, the infant receives adequate amounts of fluoride. If bottled or distilled water is used, fluoride is negligible. Reverse-osmosis filtering systems effectively remove fluoride from the water; charcoal filters do not. Carbonated beverages have varying amounts of fluoride, depending on the supply at the bottling plant. Parents should have well water tested for fluoride content before a child is given supplements. It is also important to know the fluoride exposure from other settings such as day-care centers and schools. Optimum fluoride ingestion provides maximum anticaries protection with minimal fluorosis effects to the teeth. Concern about fluorosis has led to the adoption of revised fluoride supplementation guidelines by the American Dental Association's Council on Dental Therapeutics (ADA), the American Academy of Pediatric Dentistry, and the American Academy of Pediatrics (AAP) (Table 16-2).

To produce both topical and systemic effects, fluoride supplements should be allowed to contact the teeth before being swallowed. Liquid drops can be placed directly on the child's teeth or in a small amount of water. Because fluoride absorption is reduced to 60% or 70% when given with milk or formula, it is recommended that it be given 20 minutes before a feeding. Older children should chew and swish the tablets or allow them to dissolve in the mouth before swallowing, to prolong the contact of the fluoride with the teeth. Supplements should be continued until 14 to 16 years of age, when the third-molar crowns are completely calcified.

Table 16-2 Fluoride Supplementation Schedule of the American Dental Association

AGE	CONCENTRATION OF FLUORIDE IN THE DRINKING WATER (ppm)		
	< 0.3	0.3 TO 0.6	> 0.6
Birth to 6 months	0*	0	0
6 months to 3 years	0.25	0	0
3 to 6 years	0.50	0.25	0
6 to 16 years	1.00	0.50	0.25

*Mg of fluoride per day.

In most instances the regular use of a fluoride-containing toothpaste is the only topical application that children need up to 3 years of age. Because children under 4 years of age cannot effectively expectorate, care must be taken to minimize the amount of toothpaste that is used and swallowed. Generally children under 2 years of age should not use toothpaste or use only a scant smear on the brush. Children over 2 years of age should have a pea-size amount placed on the brush, and parents should supervise the brushing session so that the dentifrice and saliva are expectorated. Preschoolers should not use fluoride rinses. Topical applications of fluoride in a concentrated solution or gel may be applied to the permanent teeth by the dentist or hygienist at regular 6-month intervals. There is a cumulative, enhanced effect on the teeth by the use of both topical and systemic fluoride. Look for the ADA seal of approval on dentifrice and topical products to ensure quality.

Acute toxic effects can result from the accidental ingestion of excessive amounts of fluoride. Although nausea and vomiting are the most common manifestations, on at least one occasion death of a child resulted. The lethal dose of fluoride for a typical 3-year-old is approximately 500 mg. If excessive fluoride is ingested, vomiting should be induced with ipecac syrup. If syrup of ipecac is not readily available, absorption of fluoride can be delayed by administration of milk or milk of magnesia. The patient should be referred to a poison control center.

Dietary Control

It is important that, early in an infant's life, dietary habits be established that promote not only physical growth and development but also an environment conducive to optimal oral health. Although not eating between meals is recognized as one way to decrease caries development, because of a child's small size and developmental level, snacks between meals are recommended. Of more importance are the frequency, duration, retentiveness, and cleaning properties of the foods consumed. Frequency refers to how often foods are in the mouth. Nursing on demand is recommended through 6 months of age, but once the teeth begin erupting the infant is able to have regularly spaced feedings with appropriate care of the teeth. Likewise, babies should not use a bottle as a pacifier because of the frequency with which the teeth will be milk coated. Babies should never hold their own bottles to feed, especially while lying down, because of the increased risk of the nursing syndrome and the increased frequency of otitis media. Although the sugar content of a food is a factor, if it is eaten with other foods, it will not be as detrimental. Retentiveness, or "stickiness," of foods such as dry sugared cereal, caramel, or raisins keeps the sugars in contact with the enamel for longer periods. Suggest that cereal be eaten with milk to rinse the sugars and that sticky foods be eaten at mealtime with other foods. Raw fruits and vegetables, though having natural sugars in them, also provide a mechanical cleansing action to the tooth surface as well as stimulating salivation, which reduces the acidity in plaque. Of utmost importance is brushing the teeth within 20 minutes of eating to cleanse sugars and bacteria from the tooth surfaces.

Oral Care

Oral care should begin in infancy with the gentle cleaning of the baby's gums and teeth with a damp washcloth after each feeding. This is especially important if the infant falls asleep while being fed. If milk, formula, or juice pool around the child's teeth during sleep, the teeth will be attacked by acids for long periods, and serious decay can result. When putting the young child to bed, use only water in the bottle, or give the baby a pacifier. Weaning from the bottle should begin at 9 months of age, when the child is able to drink from a "sippy" cup or glass, and be completed by 12 months of age. If a bottle continues to be used at night, it should contain water only, which may be accomplished by diluting feedings over several nights. Parents should be prepared for several sleepless nights while the child is weaning.

Teething discomfort often occurs when an infant's teeth begin to erupt. Many symptoms have been associated with teething, such as increased fussiness, drooling, interrupted sleep, changes in bowel habits, and decreased feeding. Fever is not a symptom of teething, and the child should be further evaluated if symptoms of illness develop. The coincidental illness may occur because the infant's level of immunity lowers at about the same time that teething begins, at 6 months of age. Symptomatic treatment consists in offering cold-gel teething rings or a wet washcloth on which to chew. Over-the-counter, topical teething anesthetic products (e.g., Orajel) or the judicious use of acetaminophen may provide relief.

As soon as primary teeth begin to erupt, regular brushing with a child-size, soft-bristled brush should begin. It is preferable to place the child on a changing table or bed so that there is good visibility of the oral cavity. Having the child's head in the parent's lap is a comfortable position for both parent and child. At 12 months of age the child should be taken to a dentist, preferably pediatric, for the first dental examination. This not only ensures that dental abnormalities will be identified but also prevents fear of dental care from developing. During the developmental stage of independence in the 2-year-old, advise the parents to make a game of brushing by allowing the child to help brush the parent's teeth. As soon as tooth surfaces touch, flossing should be initiated by the parent to ensure removal of plaque from between the teeth. Parents are responsible for the child's oral care until 7 or 8 years of age, when there is manual dexterity to brush and floss adequately. Even then, supervision on a regular basis is advised. Children are generally seen by a dentist or hygienist at 6-month intervals. Topical fluoride treatments may be applied to the smooth surfaces of the teeth starting at 3 years of age, and sealants may be applied to the occlusal surfaces of the sixth-year molars to protect the pits and fissures from bacterial attack. As the primary dentition is shed, the permanent teeth are observed for malocclusions, and orthodontic treatment is initiated when indicated.

The key to healthy teeth for teenagers is helping them find a motivation that is significant. Peer pressure and their natural developmental focus on appearance often provide the key. There is a strong desire to look attractive, and the mouth, being the center of the face, takes on significant importance to the teenager. Another motivator is the adolescents' desire to be viewed as autonomous and able to take care of themselves. Overall balance of the diet with reduction of frequency of snacking and selection of nonretentive foods should be advised. Adolescent girls should be encouraged to have adequate intake of calcium and iron, if not from foods then from supplements. It is noted that carbonated colas reduce the acidity of the mouth to 2.5 pH, an environment conducive to tooth decay. Teenagers may consume these frequently throughout the day. Because of hormonal changes, dietary habits, decreased oral hygiene, and developmental rebellion and independence, adolescents are at higher risk for dental caries and periodontal disease. The goal should be one thorough cleaning each day before bedtime, which includes routine brushing and flossing. A vigorous rinsing of the mouth with water after meals and snacks should be encouraged, to reduce the risk of decay from the frequent-eating pattern known as "grazing." Because most of the permanent dentition has erupted by adolescence, topical fluorides, along with occlusal sealants, become the primary preventive agents. The presence of orthodontic appliances may make flossing more difficult, but thorough cleaning should be encouraged to prevent caries and periodontal disease. A suggested schedule for anticipatory guidance and preventive dental education is contained in Table 16-3.

Children with Disabilities

Children who have serious physical or intellectual problems are often at higher risk of having dental caries and periodontal disease. With good home and professional care these problems can be avoided. Only a few disabling conditions directly cause dental problems. Children with some genetic disorders have teeth with defective, pitted enamel that decays easily. Missing teeth and malocclusion are common in children with cleft palates. Children with Down syndrome often have gum problems.

Children with disabilities often have additional risk factors. Sometimes they have special diets and eating patterns that can affect the amount of dental caries they have. Children with metabolic conditions must eat diets rich in carbohydrates to get adequate energy. Those with cerebral palsy often need their food blenderized, which tends to increase the stickiness of the carbohydrates. It also prevents the normal mechanical cleansing of the teeth that chewing provides. Many disabled children need to drink from a bottle longer, and such a need may increase the risk of nursing syndrome. Children who cannot drink independently often drink less fluid than other children do. Fluids wash food particles from around the teeth, and fluoridated water helps prevent demineralization. Medications in sugar-based syrup also contribute to caries. Phenytoin, which is used to control seizures, may cause abnormal growth of gingival tissue, and tetracycline stains the teeth. High fevers can also discolor the dentition. Sedatives, barbiturates, and drugs used for muscle control may reduce the flow of saliva, preventing dilution of the acids in the mouth. Some disabled children are unable to chew and swallow properly; others bite or gag when their teeth are brushed. Some are mouth breathers or tongue thrusters, which also makes good dental hygiene difficult.

Preventing dental disease for disabled children involves the same principles as for all children: eating a nutritious diet, cleaning the teeth daily, using fluorides, and visiting a dentist regularly. Children without food restrictions should eat limited

Table 16-3 Suggested Schedule for Anticipatory Guidance and Preventive Dental Education

AGE	ANTICIPATORY GUIDANCE AND PREVENTIVE DENTAL EDUCATION	AGE	ANTICIPATORY GUIDANCE AND PREVENTIVE DENTAL EDUCATION
Prenatal	Nutrition and dental health of the mother	15 months	Oral care and feeding
2 weeks	Nonnutritive sucking needs (e.g., pacifiers)		Symptomatic treatment for teething
	Holding of infant for all feedings		Increased independence
	Nonoral comfort measures		Fluoride need, use, and compliance
2 months	Cleaning of gums after feeding		Injury prevention during climbing stage
	Hazards of bottle-propping	18 months	Nutritious snacks
4 months	Salivation (drooling)		16 ounces of milk per day
	Nutrition; introduction of solids and juice at 5 to 6 months	2 years and annually	Toothpaste use: pea-size amount
	Cleaning of gums and teeth		Oral care: brushing, flossing done by parent
	Private well water treated for fluoride level		Nutritious meals and snacks
6 months	Teething, with symptomatic treatment		Fluoride need, use, and compliance
	Nutritious snacks for dental health		Dental examination every 6 to 12 months
	Brushing and cleaning of teeth	3 years	As above
	Introduction cup feedings		Discontinue pacifier
	Fluoride assessment, supplementation, and safety	4 to 6 years	As above
9 months	Encouragement of liquids by cup or glass		Prevention and treatment of dental trauma
	Only water in bottle at nap and night		Effects of digit-sucking
	Weaning from bottle		Shedding of primary dentition
	Fluoride use and compliance	School-age child	As above
12 months	First visit to dentist		Occlusal sealants by dentist
	Fluoride need, use, and compliance		Child assumes oral care with parental supervision
	Complete weaning from bottle		Three to four dairy servings daily
	Oral care	Preteen and adolescent	As above
	Healthy snacks and fluid intake		Malocclusion and orthodontia
	Assessment for pica		Injury prevention during sports
	Eruption of molars, with symptomatic treatment		Risk behaviors: smokeless tobacco
			Eating disorders
			Extraction of wisdom teeth at ages 17 to 21 years if indicated
			Higher risk of periodontal disease

amounts of foods containing simple sugars, eat them only with meals, and eat nutritious snacks between meals, such as cheese, hard-boiled eggs, vegetables, pizza, nuts, and popcorn. Milk, vegetable juices, or water should be offered instead of carbonated beverages or fruit juices.

Gingivitis is a chronic inflammatory condition around the gingivae that surround the teeth, and this inflammation is related to bacteria in the mouth. The gingival tissue becomes red and swollen in adjacent areas where plaque formation has occurred on the teeth. Bleeding while teeth are being brushed may be an early feature of gingivitis. Prevention is through regular plaque removal with flossing and brushing with a soft toothbrush. Gingivitis is preventable and reversible; however, the need for early prevention care is necessary. Gingivitis is seen in children with disabilities and may harbor a chronic low-grade infection.

Brushing and flossing daily should be done by the child, if at all possible, or by an adult if the child is physically unable to perform adequately. The teeth may be cleaned in any room that is convenient, which may be the kitchen or bedroom. The child can be given water from a straw or squeeze bottle and can spit into a basin. A child's toothbrush that has soft bristles with rounded ends should be used. The toothbrush handle can be adapted for the child with hand, arm, or shoulder problems by the following methods: attach the brush to the hand with a wide elastic band; enlarge the brush handle with a sponge, rubber ball, or bicycle handle grip; lengthen the handle by adding a ruler or tongue blade; bend the toothbrush handle after running hot water over the handle; or use an electric toothbrush. Flossing can be aided by use of a floss holder. When a child cannot or will not keep the mouth open, you can make a mouth prop by taping together several tongue blades or by using a rubber stopper. Parents should consult a dentist about proper insertion of a prop to prevent injury to the teeth and gums. Fluoride, sealant, and professional dental care should be provided as it is to other children.

Cosmetic Dentistry

Tooth discoloration may be caused by staining, as with the administration of antibiotics, aging, or chemical damage to the teeth. Dental bleaching may be 80% to 100% effective and may be instituted before the use of crowns or veneers. Bleaching treatment is a low-cost treatment for tooth discoloration. The disadvantage in using the bleaching process is the sore gums or teeth from the bleach.

Dental Risk Factors

Refer to Table 16-4.

Nursing Syndrome (Baby Bottle Disease)

Nursing syndrome is a serious form of decay that is estimated to occur in 5% of children in the United States. This condition can occur when an infant is allowed to nurse continuously

Table 16-4 Identification and Disposition of Dental Conditions

CONDITION	AGE/RISK FACTORS	SYMPTOMS	CAUSE	TREATMENT
Nursing caries	6 to 18 months	Discolored or chalky maxillary incisors, first apparent on lingual surfaces	Prolonged bottlefeeding or breastfeeding	Refer to pediatric dentist (DDS)
Fluorosis	All ages	Hypoplasia, pitting, hypocalcification	Excess fluoride ingestion	Refer to DDS and assess and modify fluoride intake
Nonnutritive sucking	Past 6 years	Malocclusion	Pressure of digits on palate and teeth	Refer to DDS for evaluation and support efforts to stop
Trauma	All ages/sports involvement	Avulsion, intrusion, subluxation	Injury	Reinsert permanent teeth with immediate referral to DDS
Eating disorders: bulimia and anorexia	Puberty to adulthood/involvement in dance, gymnastics, modeling, and wrestling	Transparent or shortened maxillary incisors, caries on lingual incisors and maxillary molars, periodontal disease	Gastric acid effects during self-induced emesis, starvation	Refer to DDS and mental health professional
Periodontal disease	All ages/smokeless tobacco use	Gingivitis, loose teeth, halitosis	Poor oral hygiene, heredity	Refer to DDS or periodontist
Bacterial endocarditis	History of rheumatic heart disease or congenital heart defect	Acutely ill	Oral bacterial infection during dental treatment	Provide prophylactic antibiotics and refer to physician
Malocclusion	8 to 16 years/eruption of permanent teeth	Crowded, misaligned teeth, periodontal disease	Inadequate space in dental arch	Refer to DDS or orthodontist
Lip habits and bruxism	6 to 12 years	Red, inflamed lips; wear of canines, molars, temporomandibular joint	Occlusal interference, nutritional factors, allergies, stress	As this is common in children, refer to DDS for adjustment or splint
Ankyloglossia	Newborn	Unable to suckle or swallow, speech affected, gingival stripping	Shortened frenum	Refer to speech therapist; if speech is affected, refer to DDS for gingival stripping, or to physician

from the breast or from a bottle of milk, formula, sugar water, or fruit juice during naps or at night. The second predisposing factor is infection with *S. mutans,* the primary pathogen in nursing syndrome. It is believed that *S. mutans* is transmitted from an infant's caregiver to the infant, possibly through blowing on the baby's food, kissing the infant on the lips when the provider has a high level of *S. mutans* in his or her mouth, or tasting the food to determine temperature. The prolonged attack on the teeth by acids causes demineralization of the primary dentition. The teeth most frequently affected are the maxillary incisors and then the occlusal surfaces of the first primary molars (Fig. 16-1). The carious lesions first appear as a white band or spots on the lingual surfaces of the incisors and then progress to discolored and pitted lesions. The mandibular incisors are usually not damaged because the tongue protects them during nursing.

Prevention involves the encouragement of regular feeding schedules once primary teeth start erupting. Long-term dental effects of nighttime and on-demand feeding should be explained to the parents. It is important to use visual aids to demonstrate the effects of nursing syndrome when educating parents. At night, only water should be allowed in the bottle. For breastfed infants, sleeping with the mother should be discouraged because of the frequency and duration of nursing. Rather, the child should be held for all feedings, and the teeth wiped with moist gauze at the end of each feeding. Bottles should never be propped because of the likelihood of the child's falling to sleep with milk in the mouth, the risk of choking, and the higher risk of ear infections and eustachian tube dysfunction. For serious decay, restoration may involve general anesthesia, or extraction may be the only option.

A strategy to reduce high-level transmission of cariogenic microorganisms such as *S. mutans* to the infant from the mother or caregiver is the use of chlorhexidine. The use of chlorhexidine and sodium fluoride to reduce level of *S. mutans* infection in the mother or caregiver has proved to be an important intervention.

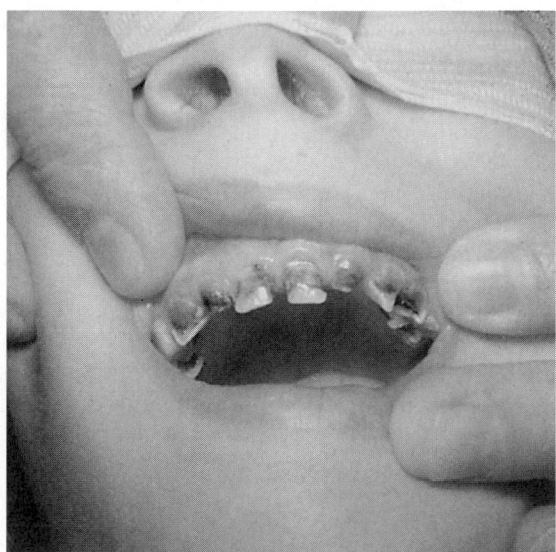

Fig. 16-1 Nursing bottle caries. (Reproduced with permission from Martof, A. [2001]. *Pediatrics in Review, 22,*13-15, Figure 14.)

Trauma

Almost half of all children will incur an accidental dental injury by the time they reach adolescence. Injuries to primary teeth usually involve intrusion (being pushed into the gum) or subluxation (loosening), though avulsion (being knocked out) or fractures may also occur. All dental injuries require referral to a dentist (preferably pediatric) for evaluation, radiographs, and management because, although the teeth may appear intact, root fractures may have occurred, an intruded tooth position may affect the permanent dentition, or an avulsed tooth may be elsewhere in the oral cavity. Other structures such as facial bones may have been damaged. In addition, the possibility that child abuse may have caused the injury must be evaluated. Ideally all children who have orofacial trauma should be seen by a pediatric dentist who will examine dental radiographs for subtle injuries that may not be apparent to the health care provider. Oral facial trauma of a young child may result from the child's learning to walk, whereas older children may experience dental trauma related to contact sports and activities such as bicycling and skate boarding. More serious trauma occurs as a result of automobile or other terrain vehicles and is seen in the early to late adolescent years.

In general, intruded primary teeth sometimes may re-erupt. Loose primary teeth are removed if they interfere with closing or are loose enough to threaten aspiration. Fractured teeth are smoothed or restored as needed. Avulsed primary teeth are not replaced into the socket because of possible damage to the permanent tooth and eruption process. With the traumatic loss of any primary teeth, the need for spacers must be evaluated to ensure proper placement of permanent teeth.

Injuries to permanent teeth are most commonly fractures of the dental crown, subluxation, and avulsion. Fractured permanent teeth are restored; splints are placed on those loosened and can be placed within a day after the accident. Avulsed teeth should be reinserted into the socket immediately. The tooth may be rinsed in water but should not be scrubbed. It can be transported in the cheek of an older child or should be kept moist by being placed into any liquid, including milk, saliva, blood, or the parent's mouth. Teeth reimplanted within 30 minutes of avulsion are much more likely to be saved. When dental trauma occurs, make sure the injured child's tetanus immunizations are up to date.

The importance of mouthguards while children are engaged in sports should be emphasized to parents. Children are "learning" the sport and therefore are at more risk of injury because their coordination and skills are still being developed. Because most dental injuries happen during sport practices, children need to wear protective mouthguards at those times, in addition to game times. The child should wear a mouthguard whenever participating in any activity that may involve falls, head contact, tooth clenching, or flying equipment. Particularly dangerous are hockey, basketball (being hit with elbows), and in-line skating. Of the three types of mouth protectors—ready made, mouth formed, and custom made—the custom-made protectors are usually the most comfortable because of the fit and therefore will improve compliance. The practitioner in evaluating an injured child from a sports injury should include in the oral examination any notation of contusion, laceration, bruising, and palpation of orofacial structures with observance of jaw movement. In a chin wound, the practitioner should consider a jaw fracture. If there is asymmetry observed during palpation or opening or closing of the mouth, a jaw fracture may be present. You should begin an oral examination of the mouth with the soft tissue and then move to the mucosal gingivae, checking the tongue for lacerations, hemorrhage, or swelling. Dentition injury will have pain when the patient is biting down and may indicated displacement or fracture of teeth. Abnormal tooth mobility or tenderness to gentle percussion may be evaluated with a tongue blade. Appropriate referral to a pediatric dentist is indicated. A child who has lost teeth and lost consciousness at the time of the injury should have a radiograph to eliminate the possibility of aspiration of a tooth.

Smokeless Tobacco

Smokeless tobacco is an increasing risk for teenagers. The use of snuff and chewing tobacco for as little as 3 to 4 months can cause precancerous lesions and serious periodontal disease. Because of the abrasives and sugars in smokeless tobacco, teeth are at greater risk for abrasion and decay. The use of tobacco in any form should be discouraged.

Eating Disorders

Preteen and adolescent girls are increasingly developing eating disorders, which adversely affect dentition. These girls often engage in activities that emphasize a small body such as gymnastics, dance, or modeling. However, eating disorders are increasingly found across all body types. Also at increased risk are boys who engage in strenuous exercise and dieting in sports such as wrestling and gymnastics. A careful examination of the lingual surfaces of the maxillary incisors for decay may be a clue to bingeing or purging behaviors, even though the patient is in denial. The front teeth may appear translucent or shortened from the acid demineralization. The starvation of anorexia affects the gums, causing periodontal disease. These patients should be referred to a dentist and mental health professional for further evaluation.

Nonnutritive Sucking

Nonnutritive sucking, or the sucking of digits, pacifiers, and other objects not related to the ingestion of nutrients, is considered a normal part of fetal and neonatal development. Often it is apparent in utero and is related to the rooting and sucking reflexes. Although the rooting reflex disappears around 7 months of age, the sucking reflex remains intact until 12 months of age. The prevalence of nonnutritive sucking is 50% to 70% in the first year of life and decreases as the child matures, with most children stopping by 4 years of age. Newborns have an infantile swallow that gradually changes to an adult swallow as the infant's diet changes from liquid to solid foods. For most children this is accomplished between 3 and 10 years of age. Chronic sucking is simply a learned habit of prolonged infant sucking that has never been stopped. It is not an indication of emotional problems. Sucking on fingers, thumbs, toes, and toys is healthy and normal in infancy and should not be a cause of parental alarm. Although toddler sucking is essentially harmless and generally socially acceptable, setting thoughtful limits on how often and where sucking occurs can be helpful. Assessing the reason for crying by a toddler and offering a reassuring hug instead of food or a pacifier can teach a child alternative ways of dealing with the distresses of fear, boredom, hunger, fatigue, and hurt.

The most common form of digit-sucking is thumbsucking, though finger-sucking is also frequently seen. Use of a pacifier is also common, and because parents control its availability, its use is discontinued at a younger age. Malocclusion of the teeth and arches is the primary concern expressed by parents in regard to digit-sucking. Three modifying factors influence the occurrence and degree of malocclusion: duration, frequency, and intensity of the sucking. When pressure is exerted by the thumb against the hard palate and lingual aspect of the maxillary incisors, overbite and overjut can occur. At the same time, pressure on the mandibular incisors pushes them inward toward the tongue. The upward pressure on the palate alters the shape of the arch and causes cross-bite, in which the upper molars sit inside the lower molars. Although a pacifier may exert less pressure against the teeth and palate than a digit, the intensive sucking can still affect the arch. Although many pacifier styles and shapes exist, there are no long-term, controlled studies that support the claims that physiologically designed pacifiers are best for an infant's growth and development.

The disadvantage of pacifiers over digits is that a young infant cannot put a pacifier into the mouth unaided and requires repeated reinsertion by the parent, whereas fingers and thumbs are readily available. Research about the effects of thumbs versus pacifiers in infancy is inconclusive. If parents choose to have their infant use a pacifier, it should never be attached to a ribbon or string around the child's neck because of the risk of strangulation. Parents should look for a pacifier that has the approval of the U.S. Consumer Products Safety Commission, which requires that the pacifier:

- Be a sturdy, one-piece construction of nontoxic, flexible, and firm but not brittle material
- Possess easily grasped handles
- Possess inseparable nipples and mouthguards
- Possess two ventilation holes and a mouthguard large enough to prevent aspiration
- Bear a warning label against being tied around the infant's neck

In the infancy stage, active intervention to discourage nonnutritive sucking is contraindicated. Most children spontaneously stop the habit between 2 and 4 years of age without ill effects on the permanent dentition. One third to one half of 3- to 5-year-olds continue to suck digits, especially when they are tired, bored, or watching TV. The activity and stimulation of toys, games, friends, or outdoor playtime are preferable alternatives to sucking. Occasional or weak sucking is unlikely to harm teeth or mouth shape. Shy children who suck their thumbs may be ignored or ostracized and are more likely to be left on the social outskirts. Past 6 years of age and the arrival of permanent teeth, the child is at more risk for malocclusion of the permanent teeth. Peer pressure may influence the child to not suck in public, but he or she may continue at home, as an estimated 13% of adults do, leading one to question whether there is a genetic aspect to the behavior.

Effective methods to break the habit include self-motivation, behavior modification with rewards, and the use of "reminders" such as a Band-Aid on the digit, a sock on the hand at night, or a dental device. The last sucking time to persist is that at bedtime because of the separation, darkness, and perhaps fear of the night. It is important for parents to sit down and talk with the child at bedtime to give positive reinforcement for the events of the day. Asking "What was fun today?" puts the child in a space of warmth, comfort, and relaxation. Between 3 and 5 years of age, the habit can be talked about using personification of the digit (e.g., "Mr. Thumb") It can be explained that when Mr. Thumb jumps into the child's mouth, even when the child does not want him to, he can bend the teeth and make them not fit right. The child can be empowered to "tuck Mr. Thumb under the pillow or blanket and make him stay there all night." For a 5- to 6-year-old, it will take 3 weeks to 3 months to stop the habit. The child should never be punished for the behavior. In more severe cases a "reminder appliance" may be devised by the dentist to help stop the habit. This should not be thought of as a punishment but rather as an aid to helping the child reach a goal. An excellent resource for parent and child is *David Decides About Thumbsucking,* by Susan Heitler (Heitler, 1985).

Lip Habits and Bruxism

Lip habits include such behaviors as lip-licking and lip-pulling have little effect on the dentition. The resulting red, inflamed, and chapped lips and perioral tissues can be treated symptomatically with moisturizers. Lip-sucking and lip-biting can maintain an existing malocclusion, and referral to a dentist for further evaluation is recommended. Bruxism is a grinding of the teeth and usually happens at night. It is very common in children between 6 and 12 years of age as the permanent dentition erupts and may be attributed to various causes including occlusal interference, parasites, nutritional deficiencies, allergies, endocrine disorders, and increased stress. For most children engaged in bruxism, it results in moderate wear of the primary canines and molars, occasionally with temporomandibular joint pain. The patient should be referred to a dentist for adjustment of the occlusal surfaces and a mouthguard in severe cases.

Ankyloglossia (Tongue-Tie)

Tongue-tie is evident at birth at the ventral surface of the tongue and is caused by a short lingual frenum or an anterior attachment of the frenum to the tip of the tongue. It is rarely a problem with movement of the tongue for sucking, swallowing, or speaking. Occasionally it results in gingival recession of the mandibular incisors, the stripping of gum tissue behind the front teeth. Only the most severe conditions significantly affect speech; therefore frenectomies are seldom performed. Referral to a speech therapist for further evaluation is recommended where warranted.

Standard Prophylaxis

Rheumatic heart disease, pathologic murmurs, and congenital heart defects are common cardiac anomalies in children and require antibiotic prophylaxis of all bacteremia-inducing dental procedures. These encompass any dental procedure known to cause gingival or mucosal bleeding, including professional cleaning. Recommended prophylactic treatment is included in Fig. 16-2.

This wallet card is to be given to patients by their physician.

Name:

_____

needs protection from
BACTERIAL ENDOCARDITIS
because of an existing
HEART CONDITION

Diagnosis:

_____

Prescribed by:

_____

Date:

_____

Prophylactic Regimens for Dental, Oral, Respiratory Tract, or Esophageal Procedures. (Follow-up dose no longer recommended. Total children's dose should not exceed adult dose.)

I. Standard general prophylaxis for patients at risk:
Amoxicillin: Adults, 2.0 g (children, 50 mg/kg) given orally 1 hour before procedure.

II. Unable to take oral medications:
Ampicillin: Adults, 2.0 g (children, 50 mg/kg) given IM or IV within 30 minutes before procedure.

III. Amoxicillin/ampicillin/penicillin-allergic patients:
Clindamycin: Adults, 600 mg (children, 20 mg/kg) given orally 1 hour before procedure.
-OR-
Cephalexin* or Cefadroxil*: Adults, 2.0 g (children, 50 mg/kg) orally 1 hour before procedure.
-OR-
Azithromycin or Clarithromycin: Adults, 500 mg (children, 15 mg/kg) orally 1 hour before procedure.

*Cephalosporins should not be used in patients with immediate-type hypersensitivity reaction to penicillins .

IV. Amoxicillin/ampicillin/penicillin-allergic patients unable to take oral medications:
Clindamycin: Adults, 600 mg (children, 20 mg/kg) IV within 30 minutes before procedure.
-OR-
Cefazolin: Adults, 1.0 g (children, 25 mg/kg) IM or IV within 30 minutes before procedure.

Prophylactic Regimens for Genitourninary and Gastrointestinal Procedures. (Total children's dose should not exceed adult dose.)

I. High-risk patients:
Ampicillin plus gentamicin: Ampicillin (adults, 2.0 g; children, 50 mg/kg) plus gentamicin 1.5 mg/kg (for both adults and children, not to exceed 120 mg) IM or IV within 30 minutes before starting procedure. 6 hours later, ampicillin (adults, 1 g; children, 25 mg/kg) IM or IV, or amoxicillin (adults, 1.0 g; children, 25 mg/kg) orally.

II. High-risk patients allergic to ampicillin/amoxicillin:
Vancomycin plus gentamicin: Vancomycin (adults, 1.0 g; children, 20 mg/kg) IV over 1-2 hours plus gentamicin 1.5 mg/kg (for both adults and children, not to exceed 120 mg) IM or IV. Complete infection/infusion within 30 minutes before starting procedure.

III. Moderate-risk patients:
Amoxicillin: Adults, 2.0 g (children, 50 mg/kg) orally 1 hour before procedure.
-OR-
Ampicillin: Adults, 2.0 g (children, 50 mg/kg) IM or IV within 30 minutes before starting procedure.

IV. Moderate-risk patients allergic to ampicillin/amoxicillin:
Vancomycin: Adults, 1.0 g (children, 20 mg/kg) over 1-2 hours. Complete infusion within 30 minutes of starting the procedure.

Fig. 16-2 Wallet card for patients at risk for bacterial endocarditis. (Reproduced with permission from American Heart Association. [2000]. *Heart and stroke guide.* Available online at www.americanheart.com.)

Resources

Organizations

American Academy of Pediatric Dentistry, 211 East Chicago
Avenue, Chicago, IL 60611; (800) 544-2174; (312) 337-2169;
(312) 337-6329 (fax); www.aapd.org

American Dental Association, 211 East Chicago Avenue, Chicago, IL
60611; (312) 440-2500; www.ada.org

American Society of Dentistry for Children, 211 East Chicago
Avenue, Suite 1430, Chicago, IL 60611; (312) 440-2500;
asdckids@aol.com

Websites

Alberta Dental Association (www.abda.ab.ca/u9712-7.html)

Bright Futures (www.brightfutures.org)

Centers for Disease Control and Prevention (CDC)
(www.cdc.gov/nccdphp/oh)

National Library of Medicine (www.nlm.nih.gov)

Sports and Mouthguards (www.umanitoba.ca/outreach/
wisdomtooth/sports.htm)

University of Southern California (USC) School of Dentistry
(www.usc.edu/hcs/dental)

Bibliography

American Academy of Pediatric Dentistry. (2000). *Reference manual
2000-2001.* Chicago: American Academy of Pediatric Dentistry.

American Dental Association. (1982). *Caring for the disabled
child's dental health.* Chicago: Bureau of Health Education and
Audiovisual Services.

Anderson, K. (2000). Are sealants doing more than preventing
caries? *California Dental Services Review, 93*(6), 10-14.

Benn, D., Clark T., Dankel, D., & Kostewicz, S. (1999). Practical approach to evidence based management of caries. *Journal of the
American College of Dentists, 66*(1), 27-35.

Caufield, P. & Griffen, A. (2000). Dental caries and infection and
transmissible disease. *Pediatric Clinics of North America,
47*(5), 1001-1019.

Frazier, J., Countie, D., & Elerian, L. (1998). Parental barriers to
weaning infants from the bottle. *Archives of Pediatric and Adolescent Medicine, 152*(9), 889-892.

Harris, J. & Coley-Smith, A. (1998). An overview of dental care for the
young patient: Early diagnosis. *Dental Update, 24*(3), 116-123.

Heitler, S. (1985). *David decides about thumbsucking.* Denver:
Reading Matters.

Martof, A. (2001). Dental care. *Pediatrics in Review, 22,* 13-15.

Mascarenhas, A. (2000). Risk factors for dental fluorosis: A review
of the recent literature. *Pediatric Dentistry, 22,* 4.

Nowak, A. (1978). Early intervention: prenatal and postnatal counseling and infant dental care. In *Pediatric dental care.* New
York: Medcom.

Padilla, O. & Davis, M. (2001). Fluorides in the new millennium.
New York State Dental Journal, 67(2) 34-38.

von Burg, M., Sanders, B., & Weddell, J. (1995). Baby bottle tooth decay: A concern for all mothers. *Pediatric Nursing, 21*(6), 515-519.

Chapter 17 *Issues of Sexuality*

Susan Hagedorn

Role of Sexuality Education in Primary Care

Sexuality education is often not addressed in nursing or medical education. Adults, including parents and health care professionals, though primarily responsible for growth education, are often ignorant or inhibited about discussing sexual issues. Practitioners have the opportunity to be role models by being approachable and can provide support to children and families by facilitating family involvement in children's sexuality education. The role of the practitioner in primary health care is one of promoting healthful sexual development.

Definition of Sexuality

Sexuality is a natural and positive aspect of human experience. Sexuality is *not* just sexual intercourse; it is feeling good physically, having positive self-esteem, and touching and giving pleasure to one's self and others. Sexuality education provides the information and tools with which to process information about different kinds of social relationships, differences in families, and sexual orientation. Sexuality education refers to comprehensive growth education about life cycles, birth, abuse, self-care, wellness, human reproduction, hygiene, safety, sexual orientation, relationships, acquired immune deficiency syndrome (AIDS) and other sexually transmitted diseases (STDs), and decision-making. Sexuality education provides information and tools with which each child can develop self-respect and community respect.

Why Children Need to Know about Sexuality

Children are faced with a myriad of choices related to sexuality and relationships as well as issues related to reproduction, life cycles, and wellness. To make informed life decisions in the context of positive self-esteem, family-centered sexuality education is vital.

Responsibility for Sexuality Education

A partnership between families, health care professionals, and schools is required to offer a balanced perspective. Family- and community-based sexuality education allows the sharing of family and community values and encourages effective decision-making skills. It is imperative that the primary care practitioner work cooperatively with children, schools, *and* parents in sexuality education programs. Practitioners are urged to prepare and make available to families an age-appropriate resource list of books, videos, activities, and games that facilitate family-based sexuality education and discussion.

Child Issues

Children, as they grow into adolescence, have the right to confidentiality within the primary care relationship. As long as a child's behavior is not threatening to self or others, it is the primary care practitioner's responsibility to facilitate the child's independent ability to make healthy choices. The practitioner, while establishing a trusting relationship with the child, must remain cognizant of the child's need for parental involvement and support. Therefore, whenever possible and with the help of the practitioner, the child must be encouraged to share decision-making with the family.

Parental Issues

Parents are the first and primary sexuality educators of their children. Families provide children with their first ideas of gender roles, relationships, values, self-esteem, and caring. Eighty percent of parents desire a role in the sexuality education of their children, though only 25% of adults in the United States report that they learned about sexuality from their parents. Parents often are uncomfortable discussing sexuality with their children, believing that they are ignorant of adequate information about sexuality. Although parents report that they believe their children do not want to discuss sexuality with them, the majority of children do want to discuss sexuality with their parents. In focus groups facilitated by the Children's Defense Fund, young adolescents placed parents at the top of the list of influences on their sexual attitudes and behaviors.

Media Influences

The media, particularly television, videos, and movies, have an ever-increasing influence on what children believe is the norm, whether related to sexuality, violence, gender roles, or other social forces. Because of the enormity of their influence, the media need to be monitored by parents and health care practitioners. If children cannot be protected from media influences, parents and health practitioners can base their discussions about wellness and decision making on examples provided by the media.

Cultural Issues

Cultural issues affect the sexual attitudes, mores, and expression of sexuality. Therefore sexual education must be culturally appropriate and sensitive. It is helpful to involve culturally diverse community groups and parents in the planning and implementation of sexuality education programs to ensure cultural sensitivity.

Developmental Issues

Table 17-1 illustrates the developmental stages pertaining to various ages of the child and adolescent.

Table 17-1 Developmental Issues

AGE	OVERVIEW	ASSESSMENT OF	ANTICIPATORY GUIDELINES	COMMUNITY EDUCATION
Infant	Newborns base their self-image on the safe cuddling, sucking, and loving touch they receive. Body-to-body safe touch establishes the foundation for life-long trust and affection.	Parents' attitudes toward sexuality Parent's degree and style of safe touching	Teach importance of skin-to-skin contact. Teach importance of breastfeeding or breastfeeding-like bottle-feeding techniques.	Family support groups
6 months	Infants explore their own bodies and learn about their bodies through the ways they are held, touched, and gazed at by adults. Infant boys have erections; infant girls' vaginas lubricate themselves.	Parents' ability to distinguish infant's needs Parents' understanding of developmental stages	Reassure parents about normal development of self-stimulation. Teach parents about anatomy, using correct terminology. Encourage parental questions about sexually related subjects.	Parent groups that encourage responsiveness to infants
1 year	Curious, active, and beginning to distinguish gender differences and initiate individuation.	Names used by parents for genitalia Parents' experience and attitudes regarding discipline	Help parents explore their own attitudes about sex and nudity. Encourage parents to take care with gender-based expectations of their child.	Parent groups that encourage parental enjoyment of children and communication skills
Toddler	Imitates parents and significant adults. Will imitate observed sexuality on media without understanding implications. Toilet training heightens attention to genitalia, requires vocabulary for sex language. Effectiveness of toddler discipline determines later ability to handle frustration and impulse control. A sense of privacy develops.	Parents' information and attitudes regarding toilet training Parents' attitudes and knowledge about sexuality Toilet training by observation, if possible	Encourage parents to use correct vocabulary for genitalia. Encourage positive toilet training, including using rewards and reinforcing positive attitudes about genitals. Discuss the development of self-esteem. Encourage parents to use positive feedback, praise, and timeouts in discipline.	Support groups related to discipline and toilet training; education groups about sexuality education and discipline
Preschool-age child	Preschoolers "play doctor," often to identify gender differences. Children from about 3 years of age are curious about reproduction. Preschoolers commonly masturbate, particularly when upset. Children at ages 4 to 5 years often become particularly attached to an adult or parent of the opposite sex, which appears to be sexually seductive. Preschoolers need answers to their sexual questions that are cognitively appropriate to their developmental level.	Child's sexuality knowledge Child's gender-role flexibility	Encourage parental discussion of sexuality in the primary care relationship. Preschoolers *will* ask parents questions about reproduction. Parents want to know how to answer.	Education groups for parents about answering child's questions regarding reproduction

Age	Characteristics	Assessment	Interventions	Community Resources
		Parents' openness to child's questions about sexuality	Encourage parents to determine their child's level of understanding by beginning to answer questions by asking the child what *he* or *she* believes is the answer. For example, when a child asks where babies come from, a parent can begin the discussion by asking, "Where do *you* think they come from?" Prepare parents for preschooler's normal seductive behavior. Remind parents that their child will model the parents' relationships. It is vital that parents attend to their own relationships. Teach parents and children sexual abuse preventions.	Educational groups for parents about child development
5 to 7 years	Early school-age children often reattach to a same-sex adult or parent. Often early school-age children isolate themselves from different-gender children. Elementary school-age children often become exquisitely shy about sharing their growth-related questions with adults. Dirty jokes are common among peers, offering peer-provided sexuality education. Four-letter words are sometimes used to test limits. Often children harbor sexual fantasies about adults. Masturbation is common. Children are in the process of moving away from the family; therefore stranger awareness is important.	Parents' attitudes and knowledge about sex; Child's sexuality knowledge; Cultural perspectives of sexuality	Encourage parents to use everyday events as "teachable moments" (e.g., watching television with their child and discussing issues raised). Discuss parental experiences with sexuality during this age, particularly the common "playing doctor" sexuality exploration game. Discuss sexual abuse and its prevention and warning signs with parents and child. Reinforce that parents may not know all the answers to sexuality-related questions that children ask. Encourage them to bring those questions to their primary practitioner.	
7 to 9 years	Some 7- to 9-year-olds are beginning to develop pubertal changes. Children need a preview of pubertal development. Children need more sophisticated answers to reproductive and other sexual questions. Social values such as kindness and self-responsibility develop.	Child's exposure and response to sexually explicit media; Child's knowledge of pubertal development; Tanner staging as needed*	Teach parents and children the wide range of pubertal development. Dispel the myth that discussing sexuality encourages sexual acting-out. Discuss family values.	Human immunodeficiency virus (HIV) prevention education programs to decrease fear of HIV-positive individuals; teaching in context of respect of differences. Parent education groups and seminars: how to talk about sexuality and pubertal changes with a child

Tanner stages are used to characterize maturation of external genitalia. See Box 42-1.

Continued

Table 17-1 Developmental Issues—cont'd

AGE	OVERVIEW	ASSESSMENT OF	ANTICIPATORY GUIDELINES	COMMUNITY EDUCATION
10 to 12 years	Pubertal changes are of great importance. Both sexes need to know about pubertal changes of both genders (e.g. menarche, wet dreams, sexual fantasies, body changes). Preadolescents are concerned with social development and anxious to "fit in" with their peers. Children are concerned about being "normal." Height is an issue for both girls and boys, with breast and penile development of concern for girls and boys. Peers become a major source of sexuality education. Same-sex crushes and sexual activity are not uncommon. Questions about sexual orientation arise. Concrete thinking persists. Exposure to sexually explicit and violent media, with little parental involvement, is common. Children are curious about sexuality, viewing sex magazines and videos, if available. Sex games (e.g., spin the bottle, "do or dare") are commonly played. The need for privacy intensifies, and self-esteem may be fragile.	Child's sexuality knowledge Child's sexual behaviors Child's resistance to peer pressure How parents have discussed their values about adolescent sexuality with their teens Cultural perspectives of sexuality Cognitive development to determine level of concreteness needed in education strategies Child alone for part of the health visit to encourage the child to discuss sensitive issues Tanner staging*	Provide anticipatory guidance directly to the prepubescent child, as well as the parents. Encourage parents to provide ample encouragement to their prepubescent child. Self-esteem is directly related to the adoption of healthy sexual attitudes and behaviors. Introduce a discussion of sexuality, decision making, substance use, and delinquent behaviors in generalities to children (e.g., "A lot of kids your age do . . . " "What do you think about . . . ?") Provide a chart in the primary care office describing the stages of pubertal development. Discuss future planning with prepubescent children. A sense of future is the best teen pregnancy prevention strategy.	Parent education groups and seminars on adolescent health issues: Confidential adolescent health care: Decision-making education: abstinence education; make decision-making education contextual and relational; practice and discuss situations that children may eventually confront; sexual coercion prevention education HIV and sexually transmitted disease (STD) prevention education: epidemiology, prevention strategies Contraception education: concept of contraception; discussion group format, with more emphasis on interpersonal skills and value clarification Substance use prevention education: relationship between substance use and decision-making
12 to 15 years	Peer pressure and the desire to be popular are major issues for young teens. Peers remain a primary source of sexuality education. Early adolescents may be obsessed with their physical appearance. Experimentation in sexuality, substance use, and other risky behaviors puts young adolescents at high risk.	How parents have prepared their teen to use contraception and safer sex Parents' attitudes and knowledge about sexuality Child's sexuality knowledge	Encourage parental reflective listening. Remember that parents need considerable support. Encourage parents to affirm wholesomeness of sexual feelings, while conveying their own opinions.	Parent education and support groups: How to be supportive of your child in his or her sexual decision-making

Age				
	The need for assertiveness skills (i.e., the right to say no) is important. One quarter to one half of young teens have become sexually active. Exposure to sexually explicit and violent media is common. Young teens are emotionally labile. Still often concrete in their thinking, it is difficult for young teens to assess the potential for danger in their experimentation. Education about STDs, HIV, and contraception is a priority. Many teens, particularly boys, are still developing and continue to question their "normality." The highest proportion of sexual abuse occurs in early adolescence. Children who have been sexually abused are at the highest risk for teen pregnancy.	Child's resistance to peer pressure Teen's attitudes and knowledge about substance use, contraception, safe sex, and abstinence Cognitive development to determine level of concreteness needed in educational strategies Tanner staging as needed*	Remember that parents and teens need education about contraception and safer sex. Encourage parents to become comfortable with sexuality issues in order to discuss issues with their teen. Even if parents disapprove of teen sex, adolescents need to know that they can ask them for assistance. Encourage parents to continue to reinforce positive self-esteem and to discuss personal values. Encourage the discussion of the risks of premature pregnancy, HIV, and STDs. Teens need help planning for self-protection (e.g., abstinence, monogamy, condoms).	How to help your child stay sexually safe Parent support groups: support abstinence education in the context of contraceptive and safer-sex education programs
15 to 20 years	Older adolescents are commonly sexually active, often without contraception or safe sex practices during the first year. Intimate relationships inspire questions about the meaning of commitment and love. Life planning becomes more serious. Sexual orientation becomes apparent to teens, putting the gay or lesbian teen at higher risk for depression and suicide, if not supported. Substance (alcohol and other drugs) use is common. Social affiliation tends toward romantic relationships, whether other sex or same sex. Older teens desire inclusion in the development and implementation of sexuality education programs.	Teen's need for an practice of contraception Teen's need for and practice of safe sexual practices Teen's sense of future and role of parenting in achievement of future goals	Remember that teens need confidentiality and independence in their health care. Discuss sexual assault prevention strategies. Keep in mind that sexual orientation may be an issue for middle to late adolescents. Encourage discussion within the family and in the primary care relationship about sexual orientation.	HIV/STD prevention education: Scientific data Prevention strategies in context of healthy choices Contraception education: Clinic-based contraception education to teens and parents School-based contraceptive education to teens Encouragement of teens to develop peer leadership programs to teach younger peers Substance abuse: Reinforce the relationship between substance abuse and faulty decision-making HIV/STD education: Support organization of health education peer leaders Continue to discuss prevention strategies

*Tanner stages are used to characterize maturation of external genitalia. See Box 42-1.

Special Needs

- Inappropriate exposure to sexually explicit situations
- Delayed sexuality education
- Children with special needs, including cases of:
  Sexual abuse (see Chapter 47)
  Developmental delays (see Chapter 46)
  Learning disabilities (see Chapter 46)
  Deafness (see Chapter 34)
  Blindness (see Chapter 34)
- Parents with histories of being abused as children

Consultations and Referrals

The practitioner should consult or refer to a physician or mental health professional if there is suspicion of sexual abuse, family violence, or depression, or if a child victimizes other children.

Resources

Publications

Adolescents

Bell, R. (1998). *Changing bodies, changing lives: A book for teens on sex and relationships* (3rd ed.). New York: Simon & Schuster.

Bourgeois, P. & Wolfish, M. (1994). *Changes in you and me: A book about puberty mostly for boy*s. Kansas City, MO: Andrews & McMeel.

Bourgeois, P. & Wolfish, M. (1994). *Changes in you and me: A book about puberty mostly for girl*s. Kansas City, MO: Andrews & McMeel.

Loulan, J., & Worthen, B. (2001). *Period. A girl's guide.* Minnetonka, MN: Book Peddlers.

Terkel, S.N. (1995). *Finding your way: A book about sexual ethics.* Danbury, CT: Franklin Watts.

Children

Cole, J. (1993). *How you were born.* Scranton, PA: HarperCollins.

Gordon, S. & Gordon, J. (1992). *Did the sun shine before you were born? A sexuality education primer.* Amherst, NY: Prometheus.

Harris, R. H. (1999). *It's so amazing: A book about eggs, sperm, birth, babies and families.* East Rutherford, NJ: Penguin Putnam.

Families

Family Health Council, Inc., Center for Adolescent Pregnancy Prevention. (1996). *Family connections: A guidebook for parents of children.* Pittsburgh: Family Health Council. Available from www.fhcinc.org.

Haffner, D.W. (1999*). From diapers to dating: A parent's guide to raising sexually healthy children.* New York: Sexuality Information and Education Council of the United States. Available from www.siecus.org.

Moglia, R.F. & Knowles, J. (1997). *All about sex: A family resource on sex and sexuality.* New York: Planned Parenthood Federation of America. Available from www.plannedparenthood.org/store.

Planned Parenthood Federation of America. (1996). *Talking About sex: A guide for families* (multimedia package, including video). New York: Planned Parenthood Federation of America. Available from www.plannedparenthood.org/store.

Websites

Planned Parenthood Federation of America (www.plannedparenthood.org)

Sexuality Information and Education Council of the United States (www.siecus.org)

Chapter 18 *Assessing School Readiness*

Joyce Pulcini

The assessment of readiness for school has taken on increasing importance over the past 15 years as kindergarten curricula have accelerated into higher-level concepts. Also, legislation such as PL 94.142, the Education for All Handicapped Children Act of 1975, and PL 99.457, the Education of the Handicapped Amendments of 1986, promoted the integration into the public school system of children with special health care needs, including very-low-birth-weight children, children with low-level lead exposure, or those influenced by adverse social factors such as poverty and prenatal drug exposure.

Pediatric health care practitioners have always monitored children's development during routine health supervision. The goal of this monitoring process is to "identify, as early as possible, developmental disabilities and signs of future disabilities in children at high risk to ensure the provision of appropriate services and support." In addition, the opportunity to identify potential school problems increased as more and more children enrolled in preschool programs such as Head Start. Today health care practitioners are much more likely to identify potential school problems and to collaborate effectively with schools in managing these problems. But in today's managed care environment, the practitioner must identify ways to perform this screening in the most efficient manner increasing the chance for correct early identification and minimizing the time to perform the assessment. Evidence-based practice research indicates that parental report may be an important component of surveillance and an efficient and effective surveillance technique.

Preschool screening, then, is one avenue for health care practitioners to identify children at risk for school problems. This chapter particularly focuses on screening before entry of a child into prekindergarten and kindergarten, but this screening process has its foundation in the developmental surveillance that has occurred since birth.

Key Concepts

School Readiness

School readiness indicates that a child has the psychoneurologic processes necessary for academic learning to proceed (Shapiro, 1999).

Preschool Screening

Preschool screening includes the identification of children at risk for subtle learning or developmental disabilities, speech and language delays, mild or borderline mental retardation, motor deficits, or social or emotional problems that otherwise might not be detected and that may affect school performance. Children who are identified to be at risk by screening tools or parental report should have further testing using full-scale tests.

Surveillance

Surveillance is a flexible, continuous process of skilled observations that occur throughout all health care encounters. Once a

child is suspected of having a potential school problem, a more comprehensive, interdisciplinary assessment is applicable.

Risk Factors for School Problems

Both biologic and environmental factors have been implicated in failure to perform well in school. Box 18-1 includes a list of biologic and environmental risk factors that should be considered in identifying high-risk children. An important high-risk group is the increasing numbers of children born with a very low birth weight. Other high-risk groups include children exposed to drugs (e.g., cigarettes, alcohol, cocaine) during pregnancy and children who fail to thrive. Full-term low–birth weight children in low- or moderate-risk environments have been found to have no greater risk for school problems than normal–birth-weight children.

Box 18-1 Risk Factors

Biologic Factors

Maternal age less than 15 years or more than 35 years
Congenitally acquired infections
Maternal drug or alcohol use during pregnancy
Complicated pregnancy
Genetic or metabolic disorders
Brain malformations
Prematurity or very low birth weight
Postmaturity
Central nervous system infections, especially bacterial meningitis and viral encephalitis
Intrauterine growth retardation
Complicated perinatal course
Head injuries
Lead poisoning
Failure to thrive or malnutrition
Early recurrent otitis
Chronic illness

Environmental Factors

Poor prenatal care
Parents with disabilities
Parental drug or alcohol use or smoking
Lack of adequate social supports
Maternal depression
Parent/child temperament (i.e., "goodness of fit")
Parent/child interaction and attachment
"Vulnerable child syndrome"
Prolonged hospitalization
Educational background of parents
Financial status
Child abuse or neglect

Modified from Curry, D.M. & Duby, J. (1994). Developmental surveillance by pediatric nurses. Pediatric Nursing, 20*(1), 41.*

Comprehensive Assessment for School Readiness

Comprehensive assessment involves:

- A comprehensive history and physical examination, including at least a screening neurologic examination (see Chapter 39)
- Familiarity with a few preschool readiness tests that can be used routinely in practice
- Practitioner openness to changing to a new test that demonstrates improved effectiveness in the clinical setting, since so many preschool readiness tests are in use today
- Continued use of a test, which not only increases the ease with which it is administered but also gives the practitioner experience with which to evaluate results
- A practitioner having a standard history and physical examination that is used for all preschool children who are about to enter school

Most school systems perform some type of preschool screening on their own, be it in the spring before kindergarten begins, just before school entry, or in the first weeks of school. This screening usually focuses on social, cognitive, or language problems. For example, the *Developmental Indicators for Assessment of Learning, third edition* (DIAL-3) is commonly used. A practitioner may want to survey local school districts to get a sense of what screening instruments they use and how their screening procedure works. This information may be beneficial when selecting screening materials and counseling parents. Parental reports have also been found to be an important predictor of early school problems and must be incorporated into appropriate developmental surveillance for children. If abnormalities are found or problems are suspected on a preschool screening, a practitioner needs to have additional tools available to assess the child and should:

- Perform additional tests on another day when the child is functioning optimally.
- Supplement direct testing with parent checklists.
- Inform parents of the suspected problem.
- Prepare parents to become advocates for their child.
- Work closely as a member of the interdisciplinary team (e.g., of nurse, psychologist, social worker, educator) and provide information about the child.
- Foster optimal collaboration between the health care practitioner, the school, and the family.
- Refer appropriately for diagnosis and intervention.

The following section expands on the assessment process for screening a child who is about to enter school. Subjective information (history), objective information (physical examination, observations, and testing), assessment (factors influencing the assessment), and planning (counseling and prevention, referral, and follow-up evaluation) are included.

Subjective Data

- Parents or caregiver suspicions or concerns. Parents can provide important clues that could lead to a suspicion of potential school problems. Parents may notice a difference in a child's development compared with other children, particularly in the areas of gross motor milestone acquisition and speech and language development. An important clue is a parent's concern about the child's behavior, level of activity, or temperament. Parents may not make the connection between behavior problems and potential

school problems but often have the sense that something is not quite right with their child.

- Identification of biologic and environmental risk factors (as described in Box 18-1).
- Careful developmental surveillance throughout life now comes to fruition as the child enters school. The history-taking process remains the same, but certain aspects of the history are expanded at the time of school entry.

Parental concerns

- Do the parents suspect that this child is not progressing as well as other children in one or more areas?
- Is this child difficult to handle at home?
- Are there any concerns about the child's ability to perform well in school?

Growth and development

- Did this child develop milestones later than other children or siblings in one or more areas?
- Have there been any recent changes in the child's development?
- Has the child shown any evidence of problems with vision or hearing (e.g., sitting close to the television, holding books close to the eyes, squinting, not listening or responding to commands)?
- Can the child speak clearly, with a large vocabulary of words? Follow and recount stories?
- Is the child easily frustrated with tasks or with failure?
- Does the child use a pencil or crayon to draw? How does he or she hold the pencil or crayon? Does the child use scissors?
- Can the child tie his or her shoes?
- Does the child know his or her first and last name, address, or phone number?
- Is the child toilet trained?
- Can the child dress himself or herself? Wash and dry his or her hands?
- Does the child have any difficulty with separation from parents or with transitions between activities?
- Does the child have any signs of depression (e.g., sleep problems, change in affect, loneliness or separation from normal activities, change in eating habits)?
- Is the child clumsy or uncoordinated, having frequent accidents or falls?
- Does the child have any unusual fears or magical friends?
- Can the child follow directions when spoken to?
- Can the child play and work independently?
- Can the child recite the alphabet, write his or her own name, count to 10, and draw a person and a square?
- How is the child's attention span? Is the child easily distracted from activities?
- Does the child interact well with other children?
- Does the child know the basic colors?

Environment

- How much television is watched at home (in hours per day)?
- What is the child's normal routine when home?
- What kinds of activities are encouraged at home?
- Do the parents read to the child? Does the child have access to books to read or look at?
- What kind of toys does the child have access to?
- What opportunities does the child have to exercise gross motor activities (e.g., going to the park, riding a bike)?
- Any exposure to lead paint at home? Recent construction in the home?

- What is the child's experience in preschool or day care or in group activities with other children? What feedback did the parents receive from those working with the child?

Habits

- What are the child's favorite activities?
- Does the child have opportunities to play with other children? How does he or she play or interact with them?
- Does the child have a regular playmate?
- Does the child know how to share and take turns?
- Does the child become aggressive or overly passive with other children?

Family

- What do the parents and child child enjoy doing together?
- Have there been any stressful events or changes in the family recently?
- Any changes in the family routine (e.g., moves, work changes for parents, changes in caregivers for the child)?
- Have there been any losses, deaths, or divorce in the family or among close friends?
- Are there any siblings or family members with learning problems, developmental delays, or school adjustment problems?
- Has the child been a victim of or exposed to violence in the home?

A small sample of additional questions to be asked of the child are included in Table 18-1.

Objective Data: Physical Examination, Observations, and Testing

Carefully observe and evaluate the preschool child. Direct observation is essential. Children should be observed informally in free or unstructured play if possible (ideally for 10 to 20 minutes while history-taking is going on). If the child refuses to cooperate, this may indicate problems, especially in high-risk children.

Complete a physical examination, including the following:

- Administration of an appropriate developmental or screening test (see Table 18-1 for items to supplement the developmental testing)
- Speech and language assessment
- Complete vision and hearing screen to rule out any sensory loss

The practitioner should also perform a screening neurologic examination (including the tasks shown in Table 18-2). If any abnormalities are present, a complete neurologic examination is warranted. Findings should be evaluated in an age-specific manner, allowing for neuromaturational changes in the child over time. Observe for signs of neuromotor dysfunction, including asymmetry of muscle tone or function, hypertonia, hypotonia, and persistence of primitive reflexes interfering with the acquisition of motor milestones.

Assessment

The determination of a potential school problem requires not only skillful assessment but also appropriate interpretation of results, including parent reports and factors intrinsic to the child or test situation. Factors to consider when you are interpreting parent reports or descriptions are:

- Some parents tend to lack objectivity or overestimate their child's ability.
- Parents may not have any basis for developmental comparison except with siblings or friends, but most have a sense that their child is not performing as well as expected.

- Parents usually know when a serious problem exists but may not identify subtle or mild problems.

Factors intrinsic to the child or test situation are:

- Timing (e.g., child may not be ready to begin school or associate testing with invasive or disturbing procedures, and other concurrent illness)
- Child's experience with formal testing or testing materials (e.g., scissors, blocks)
- Level of stimulation in the family environment
- Temperament of the child
- Fatigue or hunger
- Typical or atypical level of functioning (according to the parents)

If the practitioner doubts the reliability of the results or if the child refuses to cooperate, testing should be repeated at a separate time and place from any invasive procedures or examinations.

Management

Counseling and Prevention

- Reassure parents that children grow and develop at different rates and that neuromaturation is an ongoing process for children in the early school-age years.
- Encourage developmentally appropriate activities for preschool children before school entry, as well as while the children are in school.
- Teach parents how to provide educational stimulation for children. Several tools have been developed for home instruction of preschool children.
- Encourage parents to read to their children (see Chapter 11).
- Emphasize the importance of maintenance and building of self-esteem in children, whatever the school problem. Teach children what their strengths are and emphasize these rather than their weaknesses.
- If parents are having significant difficulty accepting a problem with their child, recommend that counseling to help them cope with the problem and to help them be open to further education so that they may better assist and advocate for the child. Provide a list of local support groups and therapists.
- Provide a list of books and references on parenting and specific problems that commonly affect school performance.

Follow-Up

- Keep involved with the interdisciplinary team following the child.
- Assist parents in interpreting any further testing that is done.
- Assist parents in acting as advocates for the child in the educational system by teaching them their rights within the law and how to manipulate the system to maximize services for their child.
- Continue developmental surveillance, particularly focusing on maturational changes that may positively affect performance.

Consultations and Referrals

- If the findings indicate a potential school problem in a preschooler, refer the child for more specific testing by an appropriate psychologist or developmental specialist. Even if the child is of preschool age (above 3 years old), the school district is responsible for evaluating this problem.

Table 18-1 Gathering Data

COGNITIVE DEVELOPMENT

QUESTIONS FOR CHILDREN	OBJECTIVE
Where do you go to school? What grade are you in? What are you learning in school? Are there some things you do at school that you really like? Are there things about school that you don't like?	To assess whether the 6-year-old can provide acceptable answers to nearly all of these questions. Answers may indicate that the child is having difficulty in particular areas. When the child is reluctant to talk about school or provides very little information, the health care practitioner should then invite the parent to enter the discussion.
What town do you live in? On what street? Do you know your address? Do you know your telephone number?	To assess the child's attention to basic information important to his or her well-being as he or she spends increasing amounts of time away from his family; to assess visual or auditory memory skills.
Ask the child to copy a cross (4-year-old), a square (5-year-old), a triangle (6-year-old), or a diamond (7-year-old).	To observe the child's handedness, ability to grasp and control a writing instrument, and competence in increasingly difficult fine-motor and visual-perceptual tasks.
Ask the child to draw a person while you are interviewing the parent.	An estimated mental age may be obtained by using Goodenough's scoring criteria. In addition, information may be obtained about the child's attentiveness, tendency to cooperate, compulsivity, and even emotional health if the drawing is atypical.
What makes the sun come up in the morning? What makes the clouds move in the sky? How can you tell if something is alive?	To assess the child's beliefs regarding causality and to help parents understand that the child remains in a transitional period relative to his or her cognitive abilities. Most 6-year-olds, regardless of intelligence, will respond to these questions with magical thinking characterized by animism and egocentricity (e.g., "The sun comes up in the morning so that I can play").
How do you get to your house from school?	Children at this age continue to be highly egocentric in their ability to give directions and will often leave out important details. This should be interpreted to parents as a normal developmental stage and will help parents understand why it is difficult for children to reverse directions or see the world from another person's perspective.
Have you seen a recent movie or video? Tell me about the story.	To assess child's capacity for sequencing events, memory, and content of story.
Do you ever have dreams? Do the dreams ever really happen? Where do the dreams take place? What really happens to the people on television who fly or get hurt?	To assess the child's capacity for distinguishing between reality and fantasy, which should be well developed at this age.

COGNITIVE DEVELOPMENT

QUESTIONS FOR PARENTS	OBJECTIVE
Does (name) have a problem concentrating or paying attention? Do you think that (name) is more active, less attentive than other children his age?	To assess the parent's perception of the child's ability to attend to a classroom learning environment.
How is school going? Have you had a conference with the teacher? How does (name) fit in with the classroom? What are the teacher's expectations for (name)?	To assess the parent's understanding and involvement with the school; to model the expected close interaction between parent and school personnel.
Do you frequently find yourself repeating directions or instructions?	To assess auditory processing maturation.

SOCIAL AND EMOTIONAL DEVELOPMENT

QUESTIONS FOR CHILDREN	OBJECTIVE
Do you know the name of the team that plays baseball or football for your city? What is your favorite movie? What is your favorite television show? Where did you go on your vacation?	To assess the child's general fund of information and the child's interest in and retention of information about events that occur outside the home.
Who are your good friends?	To assess the child's relationships outside the home. By this time a child should have formed several close relationships outside the home. The child should name one and preferably more friends close to his or her age. A child who does not name anybody or who names an adult, a family member, or a much younger child requires further evaluation. The parent may be asked to comment on the child's response.

From Dixon, S. & Stein, M. (2000). Encounters with children: Pediatric behavior and development (3rd ed.). St. Louis: Mosby.

Table 18-1 Gathering Data—cont'd

SOCIAL AND EMOTIONAL DEVELOPMENT—cont'd

QUESTIONS FOR CHILDREN	OBJECTIVE
What games do you like to play?	To assess the child's preferences for solitary versus peer activities. Is he or she comfortable with the give and take of peer group activities? Does he or she understand the necessity for and the nature of rules? Is he or she involved in organized communitywide activities, such as team sports or a religion-based peer group?
Who lives at your house? What do you think about your brother/sister/the new baby?	To assess the child's capacity to express both positive and negative affects relating to family members and the degree of sibling rivalry that may be present.

SOCIAL AND EMOTIONAL DEVELOPMENT

QUESTIONS FOR PARENTS	OBJECTIVE
How long is (name) in school? What does (name) do after school? What jobs does (name) do around the house? How much television does (name) watch each day? What programs?	To assess the demands on the child's and family's circumstances and arrangements; to assess family responsibilities that the child shares.

Table 18-2 Neurologic Tasks with Scoring Criteria to Determine Readiness for School

TASK	DESCRIPTION	PASSING PERFORMANCE
Walk on toes ↑ ↕	Walk across room on toes after task is demonstrated by tester.	Walks on toes with both feet.
Walk on heels ↑ ↕	Walk across room on heels after task is demonstrated by tester.	Walks on heels with both feet.
Tandem gait forward ↑	Walk heel to toe on a line marked by tape after demonstration by tester.	Walks with sufficient balance to avoid stepping off line.
Tandem gait backward ↕	Walk heel to toe on tape line after demonstration by tester.	Walks with sufficient balance to avoid stepping off line.
Touch localization ↕	Child is asked to close eyes and to point to or report where he or she is touched. The examiner touches, in turn, the dorsum of one hand, the other hand, and both hands.	Reports all stimuli correctly.
Restless movements ↑ ↕	Child sits on a chair with feet off the floor, hands in lap; he or she is asked to sit completely still for 1 minute (timed).	Child remains seated throughout the 1-minute test and is motionless for at least half the test period.
Downward drift ↕	Child stands with outstretched pronated hands for 20 seconds, eyes closed.	No downward drift of either arm.
Hand coordination ↑ ↕	Child is asked to initiate rapid alternating supination and pronation of one hand at a time.	Smooth supination-pronation for at least 3 cycles with each hand.
Hopping (2 tasks) ↕	Child is asked (or shown) to hop on one foot 10 times, twice.	Able to hop on each foot.
Alternate tapping ↕	Child is asked to imitate 3 tapping tasks: (1) tap 5 times with right index finger (at a rate of about 2 taps per second), (2) tap 5 times with left index finger, and (3) tap alternately with left and right index finger for 4 cycles.	Performs all 3 tasks.
Complex tapping ↕	Child is asked to imitate 2 tapping tasks: (1) tap twice with left index finger and then twice with right index finger, repeating the pattern 5 times at a rate of about 2 taps per second; (2) tap once with left index finger and twice with right index finger, repeating the pattern 5 times.	Performs either task correctly.

From Huttenlocher, P.R., Levine, S.C., Huttenlocher, J., et al. (1990). Discrimination of normal and at risk preschool children on the basis of neurological tests. Developmental Medicine Child Neurology, 32, *394-402.*
↑, *3-year-old task;* ↕, *5-year-old task.*

Evaluations, specific therapy, and special schools and programs may be available if the need is found.

- Refer to a pediatric neurologist if a neurologic problem is suspected.
- If the child is in school, refer him or her to the school psychologist or school interdisciplinary team.

Common Parental Concerns Regarding School Readiness

Children Having Problems that Might Interfere with School Function

Currently about 2% of children have severe developmental disabilities, and at least 17% of children have learning disabilities, mild mental retardation, speech and language impairment, and attention deficit disorders.

Children with Different Learning Styles

Some children have different learning styles and need to be approached individually within integrated classrooms, rather than labeled early with school problems. Health care practitioners should be prepared to work collaboratively with schools to identify appropriate strategies for such children.

Best Time for Preschool Screening

Testing should be done as close as possible to entry to school. Many school districts require a physical examination in the spring or summer before school entry, facilitating a preschool screening for potential school problems. Testing that is conducted too early may reflect behavioral or maturational problems that will not be present when the child enters school.

Cutoff Age for Kindergarten

The age of 5 years is generally accepted as the optimal age for kindergarten entry. Parents of the youngest children entering school often ask health care practitioners about their views on holding a child back for later school entry. Parents should be advised that school screening tests are often beneficial in identifying immature children. Each child is individual in his or her needs, but holding back a young child may be an option for some immature children with birth dates near the cutoff date.

Children Kept Back in School

Grade retention has been in favor during various periods in the United States, especially among minority populations who have limited English proficiency and other educationally high-risk students (see Box 18-1). However, it is known that positive environmental factors appear to "wash out" all but the most severe perinatal complications by 10 years of age, and early intervention services improve both short- and long-term outcomes for environmentally and biologically high-risk children. Research has shown that children retained or placed in transition classrooms during their early school years do not demonstrate any academic benefits compared to those in their normal age group and that such retained children demonstrate more social adjustment and self-esteem problems (Casey & Evans, 1993).

Choosing a Developmental Test

Choosing a developmental tool for use in primary care practice should involve several important parameters. Glascoe and others (1990) evaluated 19 developmental tests that were con-

sidered useful as developmental screening tests for young children. For primary care providers (PCPs), the best approach may be to choose several tools, including a parent checklist, and use these consistently in practice while keeping in mind the importance of referring to developmental or educational specialists when questions arise.

The Denver II may be the most commonly used developmental screening tool in primary care pediatrics. It includes 125 items that are easy to administer and score, has items that appeal to the child and examiner, and has improved test/retest and interrater reliability. Compared to previous versions, the Denver II also has more language and articulation items, an age scale that coincides with the American Academy of Pediatrics' (AAP's) recommendations for well-child visits, fewer parent report items, a category of item interpretation to identify milder delays, and extensive training materials. In addition, a rating scale that indicates the child's behavior on the day of testing compared with what is perceived to be normal by the parent or guardian is included. Although the Denver II now has a high sensitivity compared with the Denver Developmental Screening Test (DDST), it has a limited specificity and a potentially high overreferral rate. This test is best used as a tool to monitor the child's overall development rather than the child's development in isolation. The criteria for choosing a developmental test can be found in Chapter 11.

Preschool Screening Tools: What to Look For

Domains. The domains included in a tool are critical when choosing a developmental test. The inclusion of the cognitive domain can be very helpful in assessing the ability of a child to problem-solve or process thought at an age-appropriate level. Assessment of adaptive or self-help skills can also be helpful in terms of ability to perform activities of daily living (e.g., dressing).

Examples from selected tests include the following (see also Table 18-3):

- The *Battelle Developmental Inventory Screening Test* separates both the cognitive area and the adaptive skills or self-help area.
- The *DIAL-3*, which is often used in Head Start programs and public schools as a screening tool, focuses more specifically on cognitive skills but does not include self-help skills.
- The *Denver II*, which is commonly used in pediatric practices, includes personal-social, fine motor/adaptive, gross motor, and language domains. Self-help skills such as dressing and eating are included in the personal-social domain, but problem-solving and cognitive skills are not specifically separated.

Behavior. Inclusion of items that measure behavior, self-control, and emotional functioning is important. Few developmental tests or screening tools actually include this important area, and other tools may be added to complete the assessment. Examples from selected tests and inventories include:

- Parent checklists such as the *Child Behavior Checklist, Child Development Inventory, Parents' Evaluations of Developmental Status* (PEDS), and *Pediatric Symptom Checklist* include parent ratings of child behavior.
- The *Conners Parent and Teacher Rating Scales* and the *McCarney Attention Deficit Disorder Evaluation Scales* elicit information on children's behavioral functioning both at home and at school. To assess emotional functioning, the practitioner must be alert to signs of childhood depression or mental illness (see Chapter 39).

Table 18-3 Selected Instruments Used in Preschool Screening

TYPES OF SCREENING TOOLS	TEST/SOURCE	AGE LEVEL	METHOD	COMMENTS
General development	Battelle Developmental Inventory (BDI) (1984) Author: J Newborg, J Stock, L Wnek, J Guidubaldi, J Svinicki Source: Riverside Publishing 425 Springlake Dr. Itasca, IL 60143-9921	Birth to 8 years	Structured test format Parent and teacher interview Observation	Includes a screening test that can be used to identify areas of development in need of a complete, comprehensive BDI. Full BDI consists of 341 test items in 5 domains: personal-social, adaptive, motor, communication, and cognitive. Administration time: 1 to 1½ hours. Screening test consists of 96% of these items, taking 20 to 35 minutes to administer.
	Brigance Diagnostic Inventory of Early Development (Revised) (1991) Author: A Brigance Source: Curriculum Associates, Inc. 5 Esquire Road North Billerica, MA 01862-2589	1 month to 7 years	Performance task by child	Assesses skills in all areas required for PL 101–476 eligibility. Criterion and normative referenced; curriculum based. May be administered by paraprofessional with supervision. Does not require special equipment for testing.
	Denver II (1990) Author: WK Frankenburg, JB Dodds Source: Denver Developmental Materials, Inc. PO Box 371075 Denver, CO 80237-5075	Birth to 6 years	Structured test format Parent report Observation	Revised version of DDST (1978). 125 items. Increased language/articulation items. A behavioral rating scale. Administration time: 7 to 10 minutes.
	Early Screening Inventory (Revised) (1997) Author: SJ Meisels, D Mardsen, MS Wiske, L Henderson Source: Psychological Corp. Harcourt Health Sciences 555 Academic Ct. San Antonio, TX 78204-2498	3 to 6 years	Observation	Quick inventory to assess children who need further testing. Excellent psychometric properties. Tests perceptual motor and language functioning. Administration time: 15 to 20 minutes.
	Minnesota Preschool Development Inventory (1984) Author: H Ireton, E Thwing Source: Behavior Science Systems PO Box 580274 Minneapolis, MN 55458	3 to 6 years	Observation/interview Parent report True/false	Provides a profile of the child's strengths and weaknesses. 60 items. Administration time: 10 minutes.

Continued

Modified from Jackson, PL & Vessey, JA. (2000). Primary care of the child with a chronic condition (3rd ed.). St Louis: Mosby.
ADHD, Attention deficit-hyperactivity disorder; DDST, Denver Developmental Screening Test.

Table 18-3 Selected Instruments Used in Preschool Screening—cont'd

TYPES OF SCREENING TOOLS	TEST/SOURCE	AGE LEVEL	METHOD	COMMENTS
	Mullen Scales of Early Learning (1997) Author: E Mullen Source: American Guidance Service 4201 Woodland Rd. Circle Pines, MN 55014	Birth to 68 months	Structured test format	IConsists of 4 subscales, including visual and language, expressive and receptive organization. Administration time: 15 to 45 minutes, depending on age. Useful for very-low–birth weight children to detect academic risk.
	Temperament Assessment Battery for Children (TABC) (1988) Author: RP Martin Source: Clinical Psychology Publishing Co., Inc. No. 4 Conant Square Brandon, VT 05733	3 to 7 years	Structured test format	Measures basic personality and behavioral dimensions in the areas of activity, adaptability, approach/withdrawal, intensity, distractibility, persistence. Administration time: 10 to 20 minutes.
	Carey and McDevitt Revised Temperament Questionnaire: Behavior Style Questionnaire Author: SC McDevitt, WB Carey Source: SC McDevitt Dev Profile II Devereaux Center 6436 E. Sweetwater Scottsdale, AZ 85254	3 to 7 years	Interview	Provides an objective measure of the child's temperament profile. Fosters more effective interactions between parent and child. Intelligence quotient used to assess receptive vocabulary, not a measure of speech and language skills.
Speech and language	Peabody Picture Vocabulary Test, Revised (PPVT–R) (1981) Author: LM Dunn, LM Dunn Source: American Guidance Service 4201 Woodland Road Circle Plains, MN 55014-1796	2$\frac{1}{2}$ to 10 years	Interview Individual "point to" response test	Measures hearing vocabulary for standard American English. Used with non-English speaking students to screen for mental retardation of giftedness. Requires a qualified practitioner to administer. Intelligence quotient (IQ) used to measure a person's receptive vocabulary, not used as a measure of speech and language skills. Administration time: 10 to 20 minutes.
	Denver Articulation Screening Exam (DASE) (1971-1973) Author: AF Drumwright, WK Frankenburg Source: Denver Developmental Materials, Inc. PO Box 6919 Denver, CO 80206-0919	2$\frac{1}{2}$ to 7 years	Observation	Designed to identify significant developmental delay in the acquisition of speech sounds. Good for screening children who may be economically disadvantaged and have a potential with a speech problem (articulation) or pronunciation. Administered by a qualified professional; special training required for the nonprofessional. Administration time: 10 to 15 minutes.

Category	Instrument / Author / Source	Age range	Type	Description
Child behavior and cognition	**Attention Deficit Disorders Evaluation Scale (1995)** Author: S McCarney Source: Hawthorne Educational Services 800 Gray Oak Dr. Columbia, MO 65201	4½ to 21 years	Checklist	Three scales available: prereferral behavior checklist, school version, and home version. Profile of symptoms of ADHD. Administration time: 15 to 20 minutes.
	Conners' ADHD/DSM-IV Scales	6 to 17 years	Checklist	Scales to assess for ADHD.
	Conners' Rating Scales (Revised) (1997) Author: CK Conners Source: Multi-Health Systems 908 Niagara Falls Blvd. N Tonawanda, NY 14120–2060	3 to 17 years	Checklist	Comprehensive assessment of psychopathology and problematic behavior patterns. Parent and teacher rating scales.
	Child Behavior Checklist Author: TM Achenbach Source: Center for Children, Youth, and Families University of Vermont 1 S. Prospect St. Burlington, VT 05401	2 to 30 years	Observation/ interview	Provides an overview of the child's behavior. Parent and teacher forms available. Administration time: 15 to 20 minutes.
Parent checklists for developmental behavior problems	**Child Development Inventories** Source: Behavior Science Systems PO Box 580274 Minneapolis, MN 55458	3 to 72 months	Checklist	Three separate instruments each with 60 yes/no descriptions geared to parents and caregivers. Administration time: 10 minutes.
	Parents' Evaluations of Developmental Status (PEDS) Source: Ellsworth & Vandermeer Press, Ltd. PO Box 68164 Nashville, TN 37206	Birth to 8 years	Checklist	A guidance system and triage tool involving 10 questions to elicit parents' concerns. In English and Spanish. Administration time: 2 minutes.
	Pediatric Symptom Checklist Source: Jellineck, M.S., Murphy, J.M., Robinson, J., et al. (1988). Pediatric symptom checklist: Screening school-age children for psychosocial dysfunction. *Journal of Pediatrics, 112,* 201-209.	4 to 16 years	Checklist	Contains 35 short statements of problem behaviors, including both externalizing (conduct) and internalizing (depression, anxiety, adjustment). Administration time: 7 minutes.

Modified from Jackson, P.L. & Vessey, J.A. (2000). Primary care of the child with a chronic condition (3rd ed.). St Louis: Mosby.
ADHD, Attention deficit-hyperactivity disorder; DDST, Denver Developmental Screening Test.

Age intervals. The smaller the age intervals on a test, the more likely it is to take into account the developmental level of a child.

Cultural sensitivity. The practitioner must be aware of the population on which the specific test was standardized and compare this with the background of the child being assessed. Children who have recently moved to this country, those from different cultural environments, or those who have English as a second language are particularly vulnerable to having test results inappropriately applied or interpreted.

Table 18-3 lists selected instruments for assessment of school readiness and potential behavior problems.

Resources

Publications

American Academy of Pediatrics. (1995). *The inappropriate use of school "readiness" tests* (RE9512). Available online at www.aap.org.

Freighter, J.W. (1994). Preschool screening for developmental problems. In Canadian Task Force on the Periodic Health Examination. *Canadian guide to clinical preventive health care*. Ottawa: Health Canada. Available online at www.ctfphc.org.

Vacc, N.A. & Ritter, S.H. (1995). Assessment of preschool children. *Eric Digest*.

Available online at ericae.net/edo/ED389994.htm.

Websites

Pediatric Development and Behavior Homepage (www.dbpeds.org)

Bibliography

Achenbach, T.M. (1991). *Child behavior checklist and revised child behavior profile.* Burlington, VT: University of Vermont Department of Psychiatry.

Adams, E., Shannon, A., & Dworkin, P. (1996). The ready to learn program: A school-based model of nurse practitioner participation in evaluating school failure. *Journal of School Health, 66* (7), 242-246.

American Academy of Pediatrics. (1995). The inappropriate use of school "readiness" tests. *Pediatrics, 95*(3), 437-438.

Baker, A., Piotrkowski, C., & Brooks-Gunn, J. (1999). The home instruction program for preschool youngsters (HIPPY). *The Future of Children, 9*(1), 116-133.

Casey, P., & Evans, L. (1993). School readiness: An overview for pediatricians. *Pediatrics in Review, 14*(1), 4-10.

Conners, K.C. (1997). *Conners parent and teacher rating scales.* N. Tonawanda, NY: MultiHealth Systems.

Curry, D.M. & Duby, J. (1994). Developmental surveillance by pediatric nurses. *Pediatric Nursing, 20*(1), 41.

Dixon, S.D., & Stein, M.T. (2000). *Encounters with children: Pediatric behavior and development* (3rd ed.). St. Louis: Mosby.

Dworkin, P. (1993). Detection of behavioral, developmental, and psychosocial problems in pediatric practice. *Current Opinon in Pediatrics, 5*, 531-526.

Farran, D. & Shonkoff, J. (1994). Developmental disabilities and the concept of school readiness. *Early Education and Development, 5*(2), 141-151.

Frankenburg, W., Dodds, J., Archer, P., et al. (1992). The Denver II: A major revision and restandardization of the DDST. *Pediatrics, 89*(1), 91-97.

Glascoe, F.P. (2000). Evidence-based approach to developmental and behavioral surveillance using parents' concerns. *Child care, health and development, 26*(2), 137-149.

Glascoe, F.P. (1999). Using parents' concerns to detect and address developmental and behavioral problems. *Journal of the Society of Pediatric Nurses, 4*(1), 24-35.

Glascoe, F. P. (1997). Parents concerns about children's development: Prescreening technique or screening test. *Pediatrics, 99*(4), 522-528.

Glascoe, F., Foster, M., & Wolraich, M. (1996). An economic analysis of developmental detection methods. *Pediatrics, 99*(6), 830-837.

Glascoe, F., Martin, E., & Humphrey, S. (1990). A comparative review of developmental screening tests. *Pediatrics, 86*(4), 547-554.

Huttenlocher, P.R., Levine, S.C., Huttenlocher, J., et al. (1990). Discrimination of normal and at risk preschool children on the basis of developmental tests. *Developmental Medicine Child Neurology, 32*, 394-402.

Ireton, H. & Glascoe, F.P. (1995). Assessing children's development using parents' reports. *Clinical Pediatrics, 34*(5), 248-255.

Jackson, P.L. & Vessey, J.A. (2000). *Primary care of the child with a chronic condition* (3rd ed.). St. Louis: Mosby.

Jellinek, M.S., Murphy, J.M., Pagano, M.E., Comer, D., & Kelleher, K. (1999). Use of the pediatric symptom checklist to screen for psychological problems in pediatric primary care: A national feasibility study. *Archives of Pediatrics and Adolescent Medicine, 153*, 254-260.

Langkamp, D. & Brazy, J. (1999). Risk for later school problems in preterm children who do not cooperate for preschool developmental testing. *The Journal of Pediatrics, 135*(6), 756-760.

McCarney, S. (1995). *The attention deficit disorders evaluation scale.* Columbia, MO: Hawthorne Educational Services.

Shapiro, B. (1999). School readiness. In Dershewitz, R. (Ed.). *Ambulatory pediatric care* (3rd ed.). Philadelphia: Lippincott-Raven.

Chapter 19 *Common Parenting Concerns*

Jane A. Fox

Breath-Holding, p. 245
Bullies and Victims, p. 247
Child Care, p. 249
Circumcision, p. 251
Discipline, p. 252
Fears, p. 253
Fighting, p. 254
Latchkey Children, p. 255
Lying, Stealing, and Cheating, p. 256
Masturbation, p. 257
Separation Anxiety, p. 258
Sleep Problems, p. 260
Sibling Rivalry, p. 262
Stranger Anxiety, p. 263
Temper Tantrums, p. 264
Thumbsucking and Digit-Sucking, p. 265
Toilet Training, p. 266

Breath-Holding

Alert

Consult with or refer to a physician when parents require assistance managing pallid or cyanotic breath-holding episodes in their child.

Etiology

The exact physiologic mechanism of breath-holding spells is not well understood. Children who have breath-holding spells react differently to negative stimuli than other children. These spells represent an interaction among the respiratory control center of the central nervous system (CNS), the autonomic nervous system, and cardiopulmonary mechanics. Although the belief is controversial, iron deficiency anemia may also contribute to breath-holding spells.

Incidence

- About 5% of all children have breath-holding spells.
- Children from 6 months to 6 years of age hold their breath, with peak incidence from 1 to 3 years of age.
- A family history of breath-holding is present in almost 25% of all cases.
- Approximately 62% of children have the cyanotic type of spells, 19% have the pallid type, and 19% have spells with features from both types.

Risk Factors

- Previous history of a breath-holding episode(s)
- Family history of breath-holding
- Presence of a known "trigger" for a susceptible child
- Presence of iron-deficiency anemia

Differential Diagnosis

There are two types of breath-holding spells. *Cyanotic,* or *type 1, spells* are the most common form of breath-holding in children and mostly affect toddlers. Any situation that precipitates fear, anger, pain, surprise, or frustration (i.e., any situation that could result in a temper tantrum) could cause cyanotic breath-holding. The child's crying is interrupted, and a sudden gasp is followed by apnea, cyanosis, stiffness, and frequently brief unconsciousness. The episode lasts less than 1 minute, and recovery is spontaneous. These spells are self-limited and harmless.

Pallid, or *type 2, spells* are rare. After a sudden shock, the child becomes pale, white, and limp and is unconscious for several minutes. Trauma to and immunization of an unprepared child are two known triggers for this type of episode. Opisthotonos and seizures with incontinence may or may not occur. Recovery is spontaneous and fast. The neurologic examination is normal in most of these children.

The most common differential diagnosis of both types of breath-holding spells is epilepsy. Table 19-1 discusses how to differentiate breath-holding spells from epilepsy (see also Chapter 39).

Several distinguishing factors should be considered when evaluating a child:

- Breath-holding spells are common during infancy. Grand mal seizures are rare.
- There is usually no precipitating factor before a seizure, as there is before an anoxic convulsion.
- Perspiration is warm with a seizure but cold with a breath-holding spell.
- Breath-holding spells usually last less than 1 minute. Seizures last longer.
- There normally is not any confusion accompanying a breath-holding spell.
- During a breath-holding spell, the heart rate is usually decreased, in asystole, or slightly increased, not markedly increased, as with a seizure.
- No permanent electroencephalographic changes are associated with a breath-holding spell.

Other conditions to consider in the differential diagnosis are discussed in Box 19-1 and can be easily dismissed with a thorough history and physical examination.

Management

Treatments and medications. Treatment with anticonvulsant medications is not indicated for breath-holding episodes. A therapeutic trial of iron is appropriate (6 mg/kg/day for 3 months).

Counseling and prevention

- Inform parents that by the age of 6 years, 90% of children no longer have breath-holding spells.
- Be sympathetic to parents. This is terrifying for them, and frequently parents become overprotective or overindulgent to prevent these attacks. Reassure parents, family, and caregivers that the episodes are harmless.

Table 19-1 Differentiating Breath-Holding Spells from Epilepsy

CHARACTERISTIC	BREATH-HOLDING SPELLS	SEIZURE DISORDER
Age of onset	6-18 months	Rare in infants with normal neurologic examinations
		Onset usually 3-18 months
Precipitated by event	Usually	Rarely
Crying at onset of episode	Always in cyanotic spell; usually in pallid spell	Rarely
Cyanosis	Nearly always at onset of cyanotic spell	Rare at onset of episode; may occur later
Heart rate	Asystole or bradycardia	Rapid
Seizure activity visible	In 20% to 25% of episodes	Almost always
Incontinence	Never	Sometimes
Postictal confusion	Occasionally of short duration	Common; sleepiness
Family history of breath-holding spells	In 30% of children	In 11% of children

From Anderson, J.E. & Bluestone, D. (2000). Breath-holding spells: Scary but not serious. Contemporary Pediatrics, 17(1), 68. Copyright 2000 by Medical Economics Company. Reprinted with permission.

Box 19-1 Differential Diagnosis of Cyanotic Spells

Central Nervous System

Seizures (epilepsy)
- Idiopathic infection (e.g., meningitis)
- Congenital malformation
- Hypoxia
- Trauma; shaken baby syndrome
- Metabolic disorder (e.g., hypoglycemia, electrolyte imbalance)
  Ingestion of drugs (e.g., phencyclidine [PCP], cocaine, isoniazid, aminophyline, antihistamine)
  Tumor (accult) of the brain stem

Respiratory System

Infection
- Bronchiolitis
- Laryngotracheobronchitis
- Pneumonia (e.g., from pertussis, Group B streptococcus, diphtheria, botulism)
  Congenital malformation
- Laryngomalacia
- Tracheomalacia
- Laryngeal web
- Vascular ring
- Tracheostenosis
- Tracheoesophageal fistula
  Bronchospasm
  Emboli
  Pulmonary edema

Nasal Obstruction

Bacterial infection (e.g., syphilis, diphtheria, chlamydia)
Viral infection (e.g., respiratory syncytial virus)
Congenital malformation (e.g., unilateral choanal atresia)

Mass
- Encephalocoele
- Polyps; hemagiomas; lymphangiomas
- Glossoptosis (i.e., large tongue)
- Foreign body
  Medication reaction (e.g., rebound phenomenon)

Cardiovascular System

Polycythemia
Constrictive pericarditis
Orthostatic syncope
Arrhythmias; heart block
Atrial myxoma
Congenital heart disease (e.g., Tetralogy of Fallot)
Prolonged QT syndrome

Gastrointestinal System

Gastroesophageal reflux; Sandifor syndrome
Hiatal hernia

Neuromuscular System

Myasthenia gravis
Poliomyelitis
Familial dysautonomia

Miscellaneous

Methemoglobinemia
Hypoglycemia
Rett syndrome
Munchausen syndrome by proxy

From Anderson, J.E. & Bluestone, D. (2000). Breath-holding spells: Scary but not serious. Contemporary Pediatrics, 17(1), 66. Copyright 2000 by Medical Economics Company. Reprinted with permission.

- Advise parents that if the child is having an episode to be sure he or she is in a safe place and position. They should lay child on the back on a padded surface and can then leave the room.
- Educate parents that unconsciousness is the result of oxygen deprivation, not neurologic damage.

- Inform parents the episodes are involuntary and that the child will begin breathing without parental action.
- Reassure parents that the child cannot and will not hold the breath long enough to cause permanent damage. Isolated breath-holding incidents are not fatal.

- Remind parents that children do not have breath-holding spells when there is no one to witness them, so they need not worry what will happen in their absence.
- Instruct parents to watch the child closely if an obvious trigger is impending.
- Do not shake, smack, or throw water on the child!

Follow-up. Schedule a short follow-up visit or make a telephone call to ensure that parents are managing these episodes effectively.

Consultations and referrals

- Advise parents to always consult their health care practitioner immediately in the event of an unconscious episode.
- Advise parents to telephone the practitioner's office if the breath-holding episode lasts for longer than 1 minute (by the clock).
- Refer the child to a physician if true seizure activity is suspected.

Bullies and Victims

Alert

Consult with or refer to a mental health professional for the following:
- Child who describes self as a victim of bullying and presents with somatic complaints
- Child who exhibits violence against others, including family members (e.g., threatens with a weapon, inflicts bodily harm)
- School avoidance
- Dysfunctional family
- Family with impulse control problems or difficulty managing anger

Etiology

Many school-age children avoid school activities because they fear continual harassment by another more powerful child—a bully. These children, the victims, are unable to defend themselves. Many factors contribute to aggressive or violent behaviors in children, including cold, inconsistent child-rearing; child abuse; excessive corporal punishment; witnessing violence in the home and community and on television; socioeconomic disadvantage; substance abuse; difficult or intense temperament; failure to learn self-control; difficult situation at home (e.g., divorce); and stress. Bullying behavior can include physical (the most obvious form), verbal, emotional, racist, or sexual bullying.

Incidence

- According to the National Education Association, every hour of every school day 2000 students are physically attacked on school grounds, 1 in 5 children regularly carries a weapon to school, more than 6000 teachers are threatened with injury, and 260 teachers are assaulted.
- About 10% of all children attending school are frightened and afraid most of the day.
- Most bullying takes place at school.
- Both girls and boys are equally likely to be victims of bullies; however, they are bullied differently. Boys are more likely to be bullied by other boys, and physical aggression is used more often. Girls are bullied by both sexes and by social alienation and intimidation.
- Boys and girls both bully. In grades one through three, girls are more often the bullies. From the fourth grade on, boys do most of the bullying.
- In one survey, 10% of youth in grades six through ten reported they bullied other children sometimes, and over 8% of the youth reported bullying others more than once a week.
- Almost 30% of children in one study said they were involved in bullying, whether they bullied, were targeted by bullies, or both.
- Of children identified as bullies in the second grade, 60% had at least one felony conviction by the age of 24 years.
- In one study, 33% of special needs children who were mainstreamed were the targets of bullies, compared with 8% of their other classmates.

Risk Factors

Children with the following characteristics are at risk of becoming victims:

- Physical attributes that set them apart from others (e.g., being overweight, having an accent, being very tall or short, having a physical handicap)
- Learning disabilities
- Attention deficit hyperactivity disorder (ADHD)
- Shyness
- Special needs children who are mainstreamed

A victim is at risk for the following:

- Low self-esteem
- Depression
- Anxiety disorders
- Academic difficulties
- Having no or few friends
- Entering abusive relationships (as female victims grow older)
- Attempting suicide out of desperation, believing no one will help

Several causes put a child at risk for becoming a bully:

- Family discord
- Family who has difficulty with impulse control and anger management
- Sibling aggression (see the sections on fighting and sibling rivalry later in this chapter)
- Violence in the home
- Male student in the sixth to eighth grades
- Substance use

A bully is at risk for the following:

- Dropping out of school
- Difficulty holding jobs
- Inability to have long-lasting intimate relationships
- Behavior disorders
- Delinquency

Differential Diagnosis

In primary care pediatrics it is important to identify those children who are victims and those who are bullies and address the issue immediately. (See also the sections on fighting and sibling rivalry later in this chapter.) Garrity and Baris (1996) have developed a brief screen for identifying bully and victim problems (Fig. 19-1). Specific bullying behaviors are described in Table 19-2.

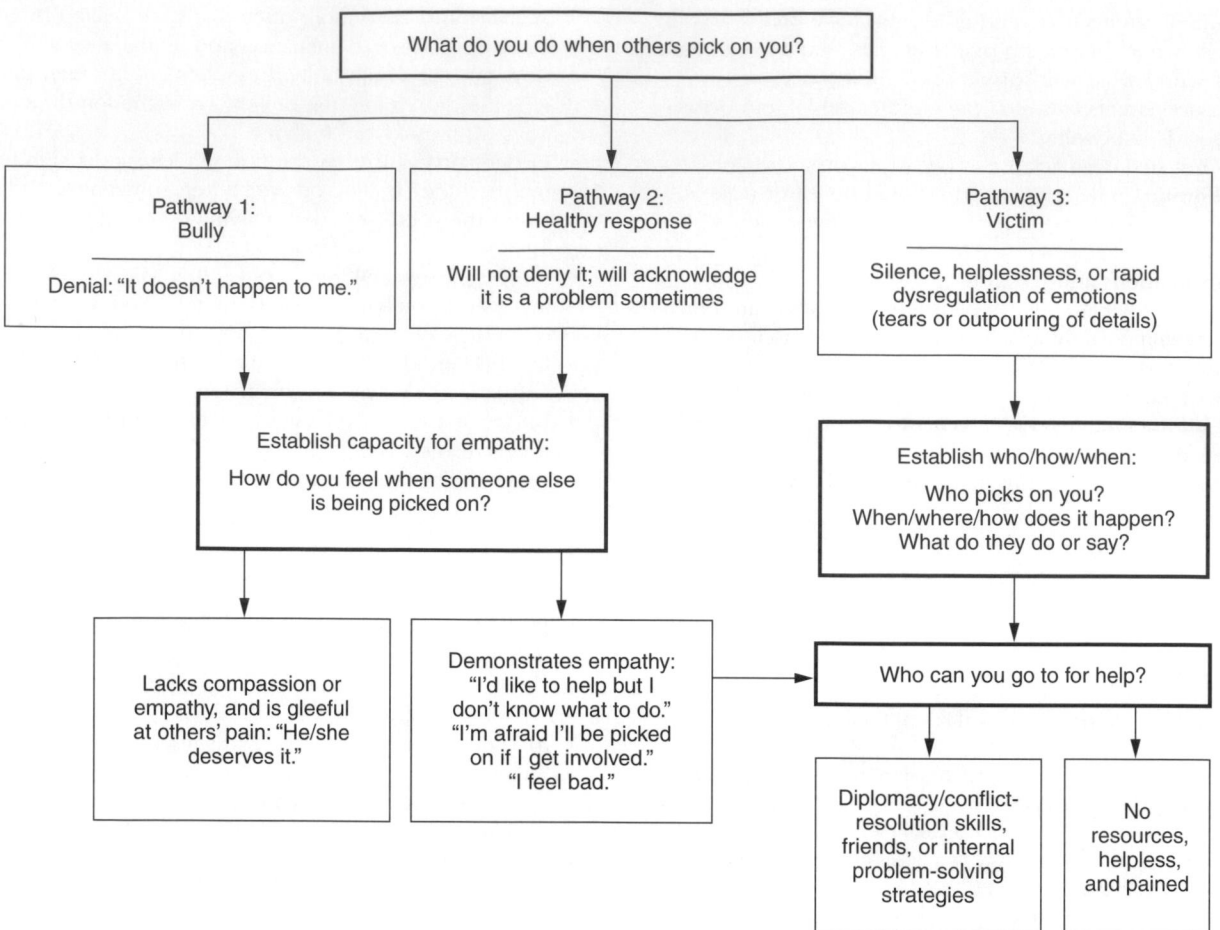

Fig. 19-1 Brief screen for bully-victim problems. (From Garrity, C. & Varis, M. [1996]. Bullies and victims: A guide for pediatricians. *Contemporary Pediatrics, 13*[2]: 105.)

Table 19-2 Bullying Behaviors

MILD		MODERATE		SEVERE	
Physical Aggression					
Pushing	Kicking	Defacing	Demeaning act	Violence against family or	Threatening with a
Shoving	Hitting	property	Locking in closed	friends	weapon
Spitting		Stealing	space		Inflicting bodily harm
Social Alienation					
Gossiping	Setting up to	Ethnic slurs	Public humiliation	Malicious excluding	Threatening total isola-
Embarrassing	look foolish	Setting up	Excluding from	Manipulating rejection	tion from peers
Dirty looks	Spreading	for blame	group	Malicious rumor-mongering	
	rumors		Social rejection		
Verbal Aggression					
Mocking	Teasing about	Teasing about	Intimidating	Threats against property	Threatening bodily
Name-calling	clothes	appearance	phone calls		harm
Taunting					
Intimidation					
Threatening to reveal	Defacing	Taking	Extorting	Threats against family or	Coercion
information	property	possessions		friends	Threatening with a
Graffiti	Dirty tricks	(lunch,			weapon
Daring		toys)			

From Garrity, C. & Baris, M. (1996). Bullies and victims: a guide for pediatricians. Contemporary Pediatrics, 13(2), 91.

Management

Counseling and prevention

For the victim

- Reassure children that no one deserves to be treated the way they are being treated at this time and that their parents and the practitioner can help them. Let children know they are not alone. The bullying can be stopped if everyone works together.
- Offer suggestions to the child on how to respond to being bullied (e.g., try not to react to the bully, do not give in to their demands). A bully likes to feel in control and to intimidate others, so recommend the child walk away. If this does not work, help the child to react assertively to the bully. This action may cause the bully to move on to another, weaker victim. Have the child practice responses to various scenarios involving the bully. Suggest the child avoid places where the bully goes. Encourage the child to tell a teacher. Encourage the child to form close friendships.
- If the situation persists, encourage the parents to stay calm. Suggest the parents first approach the child's classroom teacher. Next, discuss their concerns with the principal and a school counselor. Reassure the parents that they are not alone. Other children in the class are probably also being bullied.
- Suggest the parents promote and rebuild the child's self-esteem at home. Praise special talents and accomplishments.
- Remind the parents that children model their parents' behavior.
- Discuss how anger is controlled and conflicts are resolved in the family. Offer suggestions for change, if indicated.

For the bully

- Discuss the problem of bullying with the parents. This is often difficult for parents, but it is critical. The bully must learn compassion and empathy for others and that relationships should not be based on power, fear, and intimidation.
- Inform the parents and child of the likely consequences of the behavior as the child grows older. No one likes a bully, and the child will have few friends. Once a child develops a reputation as a bully, it is difficult to change.
- Help the family examine how they express anger and resolve conflict. If the family exhibits an aggressive style, it is important for them to change this pattern.
- Advise parents to express to the child their disappointment in the specific aggressive behavior, being careful not to imply the child is bad. Suggest that they review the situation that occurred and offer other options the child might have taken. Respond to bullying behavior with negative consequences, such as having the child spend time alone. A bullying child does not like to be alone.
- Have the parents help the child feel what it might feel like to be bullied by someone. Books are often helpful. (See Resources at the end of this chapter.)
- Do not allow fighting at home. Encourage the child to use words, not fists, in settling conflicts. Have the child put feelings into words rather than acting them out. Reward the child (e.g., with praise, stickers, stars) for settling conflicts without fighting and expressing anger in more acceptable ways.
- Encourage the child to get involved in sports. This sometimes can be an outlet for aggression.
- Help the child develop self-control. At home this can be done with timeouts. Children should remain in their room until they get themselves back under control.

- Stress to parents that they must not be intimidated by their child or avoid situations that might cause conflict. In these situations the parents must take charge, be consistent, and help the child control aggression.
- Enroll the child in conflict resolution classes at school or in the community.

Follow-up

- Remember that telephone contact is important to assess for resolution and offer support.
- Assess social development at each well-child visit.
- Schedule a return visit as needed.

Consultations and referrals

- See the Alert Box at the beginning of this section on bullies and victims.
- Refer the child to a mental health professional if the recommended interventions are unsuccessful or the family believes they will not help.
- Remember that the legal and justice systems are possible resources for children and families when aggressive behavior is not responsive to mental health interventions.

Resources

Publications

Early Elementary Grades

Alexander, M. (1981). *Move over twerp*. New York: Dial.

Carlson, N. (1983). *Loudmouth George and the sixth grade bully*. New York: Puffin.

Henkes, K. (1991). *Chrysanthemum*. New York: Greenwillow.

Middle Elementary Grades

Bosch, C. (1988). *Bully on the bus*. Seattle, WA: Parenting Press.

Carrick, C. (1983). *What a wimp*. New York: Clarion.

Millman, D. (1991). *Secret of the peaceful warrior*. Tiburon, CA: H.J. Kramer.

Parents, Teachers, and Mental Health Professionals

Collins, C. (1995, August). Bully proof your child. *Working Mother*, 43.

Eyre, L. & Eyre, R. (1993). *Teaching your children values*. New York: Simon & Schuster.

Kneidler, W.J. (1984). *Creative conflict resolution*. Glenview, IL: Scott, Foresman & Co.

Shure, M.B. (1994). *Raising a thinking child: Help your child learn to resolve conflicts and get along with others*. New York: Holt.

Websites

Bullying.org (www.bullying.org)

Child Abuse Prevention Services (www.kidsafe-caps.org/bullies.html)

Stop Bullying Now (www.stopbullyingnow.net)

Child Care

Alert

Consult with or refer to a mental health professional for separation or adjustment problems that are prolonged or severe.

Etiology

Over the past 30 years, a significant change in the traditional patterns of raising and caring for children has evolved as more women work outside the home. The genesis of this trend is multidimensional, including the economic needs of modern families and the need for two-income families; more varied and numerous employment opportunities for women in today's

Table 19-3 Child Care Options: Advantages and Disadvantages

TYPE	DESCRIPTION	ADVANTAGES	DISADVANTAGES
Child or day care centers	Range from small privately owned or parent-run facilities to large corporate-based or franchise operations. Center should be licensed. Programs may be accredited by the National Academy of Early Childhood Programs or the National Association for the Education of Young Children, which usually uphold stricter standards than state or local agencies.	Continuity of care is provided. If an individual caregiver is sick, the center will most likely remain open and parents will not be stranded. Contact with other children fosters a child's social skills. Programs provide the widest variety of activities and toys (especially in high-quality centers). Programs subject to state and local oversight and health and safety regulations.	There is the possibility of exposure to infection from other children. A caregiver's attention is divided, especially if there's a high ratio of children to teachers. Schedule may be less flexible than in other options.
Family day care	A child goes to a caregivers' home with a number (ideally, a small number) of other children. A provider may be licensed, but many are not. It is important to ask. Even in states that do require licensing, enforcement of regulations may be lax.	Schedules are usually more flexible than at formal child care centers. Contact with other children fosters a child's social skills. This is usually the least expensive option. A child may receive a good amount of one-on-one attention if the group is small.	It may be hard to find backup if the caregiver is sick. There is a possibility of exposure to infection from other children. Programs may be subject to less oversight and have fewer health and safety regulations than formal centers.
In-home care	A babysitter or nanny comes to the home, either as live-in help or on a daily basis. It is important to choose a person who can be trusted to provide the best possible physical and emotional care for a child. As with any option, references should be checked thoroughly, even if the caregiver is found through an agency. Filing taxes and providing other compensation, such as paid sick leave and vacation is the parents' responsibility.	It is convenient, with no pick-ups or drop-offs. There is less exposure to infection from other children. A child gets the undivided attention of one adult in familiar surroundings.	This is usually the most expensive option. It may be hard to find backup if a caregiver is sick. There are fewer opportunities for socializing with other children.

Data from Immerman, R. (2001, July 31). Finding great childcare. Available online at www.parents.com.

work force; and—not isolated from the other two reasons—an ever-increasing number of single-parent families.

Incidence

- Over 54% of the mothers of infants younger than 1 year of age work outside the home. This percentage is expected to increase.
- Approximately 60% of American women with children less than 3 years of age are working outside the home.
- It has been reported that 50% of all parents obtain day care that they do not deem optimal. This statistic speaks to the inadequate availability of affordable child care in the United States today.
- It is estimated only one in seven child care centers and one in ten child care homes enhance child development.

Risk Factors

- Parental concerns and anxiety concerning child care arrangements
- Child's exhibition of negative behavior responses from being in child care

- Questions about whether the long-term effects of child care will be beneficial or detrimental to a child's overall development and behavior

Management

Counseling and prevention. Choosing the appropriate child care situation is one of the most anxiety-producing tasks for parents. It always requires thought and investigation, regardless of the age of the child. Therefore procuring child care arrangements ahead of time is far more desirable than doing so at the last minute. Encourage new parents to explore possibilities before the birth of their child, especially if both parents are returning to work within 4 to 8 weeks after the baby is born. Help parents decide which type of child care best meets their needs. Explain each type and discuss the advantages and disadvantages of each (Table 19-3).

Some general tips for parents seeking child care include:

- Remember that the ideal situation for a young infant is one-on-one care. If there is more than one baby in care, the children preferably should be close in age. This allows the caregiver to establish feeding, diapering, and cuddling

Table 19-4 American Public Health Association and American Academy of Pediatrics Recommendations for Child-to-Adult Ratios and Group Size (1992)

AGE	CHILD:STAFF RATIO	MAXIMUM GROUP SIZE
Birth–24 months	3:1	6
25–30 months	4:1	8
31–35 months	5:1	10
3 years old	7:1	14
4–5 years old	8:1	16
6–8 years old	10:1	20
9–12 years old	12:1	24

time without the joyous distractions a toddler tends to provide. In addition, toddlers tend to be infected with more contagious illnesses that could pose significant risk to infants.

- Seek out parents in prenatal classes who may have similar needs and form a group to hire a mutually satisfactory caregiver for all their babies. (At this age, the ratio should not exceed three babies to one adult.) Table 19-4 gives further child-to-staff ratio guidelines.
- Investigate the possibility of grandparents, from the parents' own family and of friends who may wish to participate. Grandparents, if not full-time sitters, can be invaluable as backup for sick children or sick or absent sitters.
- Share with parents a copy of Box 19-2.
- Encourage parents to spend a minimum of 1 to 2 hours when observing a facility.
- Keep in mind that family-centered day care provided in the home and center-based care both require licensure.
- Remember that children who play together and share toys in day care tend to share infections (both viral and bacterial).
- Reassure parents that a child in an organized day care situation with other children will probably become ill more frequently than a child who is not. Program caregivers who follow good hygiene and specific infection-control guidelines can significantly reduce the incidence.
- Once a decision regarding care is made and a child is placed, parents should continue to monitor the program, observing it at the beginning or end of the day. Good day care programs do not restrict parents' access to their child.

Circumcision

Alert

Consult with or refer to a physician for the following:
- Multiple urinary tract infections (UTIs)
- Severe infection after circumcision
- Unusually long or redundant foreskin that interferes with normal urination

Box 19-2 Checklist for Parents Considering Day Care

Is the caregiver attentive to the children's safety?

Is the home or center licensed?

Are emergencies planned for and well handled?

Is good nutrition promoted? Is food prepared in a clean, separate area?

Is the atmosphere bright, pleasant, and fun, or is it tense and glum?

If it is a home, are there smoke detectors, carbon monoxide detectors, and multiple exits?

What is the schedule of feeding, sleeping, and diapering? Is the schedule based on the children's needs or on a rigid schedule? What are the procedures for diaper changing (e.g., clean, separate area; use of bleach and gloves)?

How often does the caregiver leave several children to tend to one?

Are there signs of individual attention for each child?

Does the caregiver accept your philosophy on safety, hygiene, and schedules?

Would you want to stay in this place?

How does the caregiver handle separation?

Can you visit anytime, including unannounced?

Does the center or home require that children be immunized and that immunizations are up to date?

Can you voice needs in the morning and receive a report at the end of the day?

What is the policy for sick children?

Is there an emphasis on early teaching, or is teaching dictated by a child's emotional development?

What are the facilities, philosophy, and procedures for discipline? Will the caregiver accept your philosophy, if it is different?

Etiology

Circumcision is the surgical removal of the foreskin from the glans of the penis, exposing the tip of the penis. Normally a loose cuff, at birth the foreskin is very tightly adhered and not easily retractable. The foreskin usually becomes retractable over the first 2 years of life. In 90% of uncircumcised males the foreskin is retractable by the age of 5 years.

The decision about circumcision is usually made before or immediately after birth. Parents should be supported in whatever decision they make and be reassured there is literature that supports whatever they choose. Parental points of view can be dictated by personal or religious beliefs.

Incidence

- Circumcision is medically indicated in about 1% of the male infant population.
- The vast majority of elective circumcisions are performed during the first 2 weeks of life.
- Approximately 1.2 million newborn males are circumcised in the United States each year at a cost of about $200 million.

Risk Factors

Complications (occurring in between 0.2% and 0.6% of cases and mostly minimal) associated with the procedure include:
- Bleeding (the most common complication)
- Infection (local redness and purulence)
- Phimosis

- Adhesions
- Urinary retention
- Penile lymphedema
- Penile cyanosis

Benefits

- Several studies show there is a lower risk of getting cancer of the penis after circumcision. However, this type of cancer is very rare in all males.
- Cancer of the cervix may be less common in the partners of circumcised males.
- Many sexually transmitted diseases (STDs) are less easily acquired by circumcised males.
- There is a slightly lower risk of UTIs in uncircumcised males.
- With circumcision, foreskin infections and phimosis are prevented.

Management

Counseling and prevention

- Review with parents the potential benefits and risks of circumcision (Box 19-3). If the procedure is not essential to the child's current well-being, the parents should determine what is in the best interest of the child.
- Provide parents with an opportunity to discuss their decision.
- If circumcision is chosen, advise parents that after circumcision the area may develop a yellowish crust of healing tissue. Infection is indicated by the presence of yellow pus accompanied by a swollen, red penis shaft.
- Instruct parents to call if they observe signs of infection.
- After circumcision, instruct parents to gently wash the area with mild soap and water and pat dry, then apply petroleum jelly to the tip of the penis or to the diaper in front of the circumcised area to avoid irritation caused by rubbing.
- Avoid the use of powder, because adhesions can develop around the area where the glans meets the shaft of the penis.

Box 19-3 Issues Concerning the Decision to Circumcise

Analgesics should be provided.

Studies show that babies who receive local anesthesia or suck on a sugar-dipped pacifier cry less during a circumcision. Topical enteric mixture of local anesthetics (EMLA) lidocaine and prilocaine applied before the procedure seems to make it painless. However, it is possible that an infant will feel pain despite a physician's best attempts at local anesthesia.

When an older child has a circumcision, it must be done under general anesthesia, which in and of itself poses significant risk to the patient.

Despite the circumcised area being exposed to a dirty field, documented infections are rare. The procedure itself is performed under sterile conditions.

Studies indicate that cancer and STD rates are lower in circumcised males.

UTIs occur less frequently in circumcised males, although this benefit can be replicated in uncircumcised males by using careful hygiene.

Many insurance companies will not pay for circumcision if it is considered an elective procedure.

Follow-up

- The parents should telephone at the first sign of infection.
- In a normally healing circumcision, the site can be checked at the 2-week visit.

Consultations and referrals

- Refer to a physician any child with severe infection after circumcision.
- Refer older children to a surgeon if conditions warrant it (e.g., repeated UTIs, unusually long or redundant foreskin that interferes with normal urination, personal requests by the family).

Discipline

Alert

Consult with or refer to a mental health professional for the following:
- Underlying family dynamics or psychologic problems that prohibit parents from actualizing effective discipline techniques
- Signs and symptoms of abuse, either physical or psychologic (see Chapter 47)

Etiology

Discipline is not only an attempt to control a child's behavior but also a means to direct and shape it. Discipline is driven by the relationship a parent has with a child, not solely by the behavior-controlling techniques a parent chooses to employ. Discipline methods can be classified into three categories: (1) the authoritarian style, (2) the communication approach, and (3) the behavior-modification approach. Guidance for parents should include a discussion of all three, as a combination of all of them may be necessary at various times. (See also Chapter 3.)

The authoritarian style is the traditional way of disciplining children, which focuses on the parents as firm authority figures whom the child must obey or face an undesired set of consequences. Many parents who use this style tend to focus solely on eliminating bad behavior and ignore anything good. The emphasis on punishment tends to preclude the opportunity for education and problem-solving, which would prevent the need for future punishment. The authoritarian style does not allow children to go through the learning process necessary to develop inner controls; they merely react out of fear.

The communication approach focuses on communication rather than punishment. This philosophy is based on the premise that children are fundamentally good, and problems arise when communication is bad. Parents need to listen so children will talk to them and talk to children in a fashion that promotes listening. This style encourages parents to explore the feelings behind their children's behavior.

The behavior-modification approach proposes that children's behavior can be influenced positively or negatively according to the manner in which a child's environment is structured. Behavior modification gives parents techniques (e.g., timeouts, positive reinforcements, allowing natural consequences) that can be called on when all else fails. Behavior modification is especially useful for children with difficult temperaments or emotional disturbances.

Risk Factors

- "Disconnected" parent-child relationships
- Insensitivity of parents to a child's needs
- Parents' lack of understanding of age-appropriate behavior
- Inappropriate concept of punishment experienced by parents as children
- Parental history of abuse

Management

Counseling and prevention

- Share with parents general guidelines regarding discipline (e.g., be consistent, never belittle, discipline with praise, teach consequences, convey values).
- Encourage parents to be sensitive to their child and spend the majority of their time promoting desirable behavior, rather than disciplining.
- Educate parents to have a good understanding of their child's temperament and age-appropriate behavior. Discuss the relationship between the parents' temperament and the child's temperament.
- Suggest to parents that the homes of younger children and toddlers should be made childproof, making it less necessary to say *no* all the time.
- Offer redirection, distraction, and diversion to younger children and toddlers.
- Set limits and secure boundaries; the younger the child, the more secure the boundaries and limits should be.
- Encourage parents to be realistic when planning activities for younger children and toddlers and remember that family schedules should be planned as much as possible to fit the children. Encourage parents to plan ahead and provide regular routines for children.
- Advise parents to say no only when they really mean it and try to create alternatives whenever possible (e.g., "danger," "stop," "not for Suzie").
- Encourage parents to allow children to express their feelings and help construct alternatives.
- Caution parents to avoid hitting the child, which ultimately devalues the child and the parent, can lead to abuse, and does not improve the behavior.
- When offering praise or criticism, encourage parents to be sure the focus is always on the behavior, never on the child.
- Encourage parents to explain their directives, offer choices (all of which would be acceptable to parents), and offer likable alternatives if possible.
- Counsel parents in the art of selective ignoring and in prioritizing what is really important for them to focus on.
- Remember that a timeout should be viewed not as a punishment, but rather a break in the undesired action. It provides everyone time to regroup and reflect and is ineffective when used as a punishment. Timeouts should be kept brief, quiet, and in the right place, which preferably should not be the child's crib or bed or a place with built-in rewards, such as in front of the television.
- Keep in mind that experiencing the consequences of various behaviors can be one of the best ways children learn self-discipline.
- Recommend that parents guide children to consider logical consequences.
- Help parents consider rewards that work. Keep the reward simple, keep it fun, and allow it to involve the child. An example is a reward chart made by the child, with stars or stickers placed by the child daily or at the appropriate time; such charts should be visible and easily accessible to the child.
- Keep in mind that reminders can be helpful. They will meet less resistance if they are not postured as outright commands.
- Remember that loss of privileges can work if it is part of a management strategy agreed on in advance. Parents can work a strategy out ahead of time at family meetings.
- Offer parents support and encouragement. Reassure them there is plenty of time to learn; the discipline process is ongoing!

Follow-up. Remember that a brief visit or telephone follow-up may be necessary to offer parents support and ongoing advice.

Consultations and referrals

- Referral to a mental health professional may be indicated if excessive corporal punishment is used. Each state has its own reporting procedures to protect children, and it is the practitioner's responsibility to be familiar with them.
- Parenting classes are helpful. Encourage parents to join them if appropriate. These classes also provide parents with the support of other parents with similar experiences.

Resources

Publications

(See also Chapter 3.)

Sears, W. & Sears, M. (1995). *The discipline book*. New York: Little, Brown & Co.

Fears

Alert

Consult with or refer to a mental health professional for the following:
- Fears that begin to generalize from a specific origin
- Fears that significantly alter the child's everyday functioning
- Fears that are felt to be justified in response to a legitimately threatening environment

Etiology

Fears are normal. All children have fearful responses to something. Fears have cognitive, behavioral, and physiologic components and occur in response to a perceived source of danger to the child. This threat could be real or imagined. Fears help children solve developmental issues and help make parents aware of these struggles. Being afraid produces an adrenalin surge and subsequent rapid learning on how to control the fear. If the child's reaction is overwhelming, constructive learning is not possible.

Parents cannot eradicate a child's fear, but they can help the child learn from and overcome it. Fearfulness occurs at predictable times during childhood. Table 19-5 delineates common fears throughout the child's development; the objects of fears are consistent across all children.

Incidence

- Fears are universal in childhood.
- Studies of identical twins suggest a genetic predisposition to fearfulness in some children.
- Females report fears more often than males.

Table 19-5 Fears in Childhood

AGE	FEARS
0-7 months	Change in stimulus level; loss of support; loud, sudden noises
8-18 months	Separation, strangers, loud events, sudden movements, touching, physical restraints, large crowds, water, being bathed
2 years	Loud sounds, dark colors, large objects, large moving things, hats, mittens, changes in location of physical things, going down the drain or toilet, wind and rain, animals
2½ years	Movement, familiar objects moved, moving objects, unexpected events linked (e.g., Grandma in Mom's hat)
3 years	Visual fears, masks, old people, people with scars, deformities, the dark, parents going out at night, animals, burglars
4 years	Auditory fears, the dark, wild animals, mother's departure, imaginary creatures, recalled past events, aggressive actions, threats
5 years	Decrease in fears; injury; falls; dogs
6 years	Supernatural events, hidden people, being left or lost, small bodily injuries (e.g., splinters, small cuts), being left alone, death of loved ones, the elements, fire, thunder
7 years	Spaces (e.g., cellars); shadows; ideas suggested by television or movies; being late for school; missing answers in school
8-9 years	School failure, personal failure, ridicule by peers, disease, unanticipated events
10-11 years	Wild animals, high places, criminals, older kids, loss of possessions, parental anger, remote possibilities of catastrophe (e.g., earthquake), school failure, pollution
12-17 years	Physical changes in own body, isolation, sexual fears, loss of face, world events

Modified from Jersild, A.T. & Holmes, F.B. (1935). Child Development Monograph, 20, 358; and Ilg, F.L., Ames L. & Baker SM. (1981). Child behavior. New York: Harper & Row.

Risk Factors

- Fearful, anxious parents tend to have fearful, anxious children.
- The onset of a fear is often related to a triggering event. Fears may be the result of a genuine threat or displaced feelings from another stressor.
- Extremely shy children are at higher risk.

Management

Counseling and prevention

- Assure parents that fears are normal for all children and cannot be avoided. It is the role of parents not to banish the fear but to help the child understand, learn from, and eventually overcome it.
- Advise parents to listen closely and respect what the child tells them about the fear. The fear is real even if the object of fear is not.
- Explain that fears serve an important purpose. They help to keep the child safe, inhibit behavior, and help the child get what is needed from the environment.
- Suggest parents allow the child to withdraw from what is feared and to temporarily regress while struggling to find ways to handle fears.
- Suggest that parents should not belittle the fear or overreact to or dismiss a child's fear.
- Remember that parents should attempt to help the child understand the reasons for the fears. Support the child who is trying to learn about new and scary situations.
- Remember that teaching a child how to rate the fear on a scale of 1 to 10 (highest) may be helpful.
- Advise parents to plan discussions about the fear and attempt to correct any misconceptions, which might include a gradual reintroduction to the feared stimulus. Keep in mind that being able to talk about the fear does help.
- Teach the child various coping strategies. For example, drawings and pretend play with dolls and others may be helpful in coping with the fear.
- Have parents reassure the child that all children have fears and discuss the history of their own childhood fears and how they transcended them.

- Once the fear is overcome, have parents praise the child and use the example of the resolved issue when new fears arise.

Follow-up. A short visit or telephone follow-up may be necessary to ascertain if resolution is forthcoming and the problem is not becoming worse. Shy and fearful children require close follow-up as they are at high risk for emotional disorders.

Consultations and referrals. Referral to a mental health professional may be necessary if the fear becomes a phobia, if the problem lasts longer than 6 months, or if the fear affects social and developmental growth.

Fighting

Alert

Consult with or refer to a mental health professional for the following:
- Failure of normal management strategies instituted by the parents, with the behavior being prolonged or placing the child in excessive or repeated physical danger
- Parents concerned over excessive aggressive behavior of their children and lacking the intervention skills necessary to provide proper supervision and guidance
- Overly aggressive behavior reported by a preschool teacher, or a child being thrown out of preschool
- A child who appears chronically angry or anxious
- Biting behavior after the age of 2½ years

Etiology

One of the most commonly voiced parental concerns is how to deal with fighting. Children often demonstrate hostile and aggressive behavior. Children who are closest in age tend to demonstrate this behavior more often, and it tends to be more extreme. Also, younger children who cannot yet cope with principles such as sharing tend to engage in physical fighting.

It is a well-documented fact that children mimic the behavior of their parents. If conflict resolution is of a hostile or ag-

Box 19-4 Fighting Levels and Prescribed Parent Interventions

Level I fighting: **Normal bickering**

This may be ignored to allow those involved the opportunity for their own conflict resolution.

Level II fighting: **Situation heats up**

Adult supervision may be helpful.

Level III fighting: **Possibly dangerous**

Parents should inquire whether the fighting is real or play-fighting by mutual consent

Level IV fighting: **Definitely dangerous**

This requires adult intervention. Parents should describe what they see and separate the children.

According to Faber and Mazlish (1987), if parent-mediated intervention is necessary, the following steps should be followed:
1. Start by acknowledging the children's anger toward each other. That alone should help calm them.
2. Listen to each child's side with respect.
3. Show appreciation for the difficulty of the problem.
4. Express faith in their ability to work out a mutually agreeable solution.
5. Leave the room.

If children require assistance to resolve a difficult conflict, the following should be suggested:
1. Call a meeting of the concerned parties and explain the purpose of the meeting.
2. Explain the ground rules to everyone.
3. Write down each child's feelings and concerns. Read them aloud to all the children involved to confirm that all the issues are correctly understood.
4. Allow each child time for rebuttal.
5. Invite everyone to suggest as many solutions as possible. Write everything down without evaluating. Allow the children to go first.
6. Decide on all the solutions you can live with.
7. Provide follow-up care.

Modified with permission from Faber, A. & Mazlish, E. (1987). Siblings without rivalry. New York: W.W. Norton.

gressive nature between two parents, similar behavior is likely to be patterned among the children.

Incidence

- The prevalence of conflicts involving older children is not available.
- As reported by their parents, 30% to 45% of school-age children engage in physical fighting at home.
- Physical fighting among siblings that results in significant injury is rare.

Risk Factors

- Children who are close in age; such children tend to fight more aggressively, more hostilely, and more physically.
- Younger children, who are not cognitively ready to share tend to physically fight more frequently; this is also the group that lacks the capacity for employing other resolution strategies.
- Violence in the home.
- Children who are exposed to aggressive and hostile conflict resolution by their parents; these children tend to use the same behaviors.
- Children labeled by other children as bullies.

Management

Counseling and prevention

- Instruct parents to give children clear messages regarding the behavior they expect them to demonstrate.
- Advise parents to state their expectations early, frequently, and before arguing and fighting have become institutionalized in the home.
- Remind parents that they must be consistent, fair, and conscious of various "triggers" that generally set children off.
- Recommend that parents carefully decide which quarrels they want to referee and which ones might be settled through appropriate children-mediated resolution (Box 19-4). Refer to the section on discipline earlier in this chapter.

Follow-up. Following the initial consultation, phone calls or short visits may be necessary. Inform parents that the frequency of conflicts may actually increase for a brief period until the children are more adept at settling their own disputes. The follow-ups may be viewed primarily as a mechanism to provide much-needed moral support to frazzled parents.

Consultations and referrals. If problems persist or the family dynamics are overly stressed by this persistent behavior, refer for family therapy or counseling as needed. (See also the Alert box at the beginning of this section.)

Latchkey Children

Alert

Consult with or refer to a mental health professional or appropriate authorities for the following:
- Safety or health issues are compromised by a lack of adequate supervision after school
- A school-aged child is experiencing emotional stress or other problems related to being left alone after school
- Undesirable social issues present as a result of improper supervision

Etiology

School-aged children of working parents may require care before school begins and after it ends. Many families in this situation utilize school-based programs that are well supervised, safe, and provide ample activity and peer companionship. However, for many families such programs are not available. Those children who do not participate in school-based or other child care programs fall into the category of self-care children (latchkey children).

Risk Factors

- School-aged children of families for which the cost of after-school care is prohibitive
- Older children who, for independent reasons, object to being in organized after-school care
- Children who are at social risk as a result of self-care

Management

Counseling and prevention

- Recommend to parents that children under the age of 12 years not be left alone.
- Remind parents that they should always take into account the emotional and behavioral maturity of their child before making the decision to pursue self-care.
- Remember that, after school, children require time to relax and play with their peers. If a full-week program is prohibitive financially, suggest that parents pursue other after-school activities (e.g., Boy or Girl Scouts, sports, recreation activities) that tend to be less expensive.
- Suggest to parents that they encourage school-aged children to actively participate in extracurricular activities. If self-care is the choice for a child, activities once or twice a week provide social integration and physical activity.
- Advise parents that during periods when children are home by themselves, the parents should still make provisions for contact with the children. Telephone calls serve to reassure a child and provide a method of monitoring to some degree the activities of the afternoon.
- Review emergency procedures and resources with the child. Perhaps a neighbor could be a "standby adult" for the child.
- Suggest that parents set limits regarding acceptable activities during periods when they are absent.
- Counsel parents that self-care is probably not the best child care alternative for social, emotional, and safety reasons.
  Follow-up. See the child for well-child visits and as needed.
  Consultations and referrals. Report to appropriate authorities if the child's safety is compromised. Refer to a mental health professional children with severe emotional stress or families experiencing undesirable social issues as a result of improper supervision of the children.

Lying, Stealing, and Cheating

Alert

Consult with or refer to a mental health professional for the following:
- A child (by 8 or 9 years of age) not achieving developmental mastery sufficient to consistently comply with basic social rules, with disruptive behavior persisting on a routine basis
- Acting-out behavior as a result of low self-esteem, group pressure, or a disruptive life event (e.g., divorce, death of a parent, other family dysfunction)

Etiology

Lying, stealing, and cheating can all fall into the category of disruptive behavior disorders (DBDs) and be symptomatic of diverse underlying problems. While a DBD is classified as pathologic, many described behaviors are developmentally predictable, especially for children under 6 to 7 years of age.

Preschoolers lie for a variety of reasons. It can be to avoid punishment or because they are imitating behavior they have observed in adults (commonly referred to as "little white lies"). More often than not, in this age group children become carried away with their fantasies. Telling tall tales is quite different from lying, being just an expression of imagination and becoming harmful only when a child has difficulty differentiating fantasy from reality.

Similar to the concept of lying, young children do not equate the activity of stealing with the socially unacceptable behavior it is. To young children (under 4 or 5 years of age), possession is ownership. For children under 4 years of age, it is difficult to differentiate "mine" from "yours"; as a result, everything often becomes "theirs." In the children's minds, they have done nothing wrong until they meet with the disapproving response of their parents. Preschool children typically have trouble controlling their impulses, and rather than feel guilt over taking something that does not belong to them, they are merely satisfied to have what they want. Between 5 and 7 years of age, children develop the ideas of ownership and respect for the property rights of others. They also establish the principles of honesty and the wrongness of stealing.

In the same vein, the adult concept of cheating is not well understood by children until the age of 7 years. Young children tend to fabricate their own rules as they progress on and find rigid rules hard to comprehend. By 6 years of age, all children understand the concept of "play fair" as a method of ensuring parity for all involved in the game. If children older than age 7 years cheat in school, there may be several causes. Children can be motivated to cheat in school because of peer competitiveness, strong parental pressure to excel, or a lack of self-esteem in a child who equates self-worth with accomplishments.

Incidence

- DBDs are four times more common in boys than girls.
- Significant stealing is done by approximately 5% of all children.
- Up to 9% of all boys and 2% of all girls have the most severe form of DBDs.
- DBDs are associated with family psychosocial dysfunction and poverty.
- There is no known correlation of DBDs to race or ethnicity.

Risk Factors

- Poor self-esteem
- Poor role models
- Impulsive and strong desire, but weak control
- Insensitivity to others
- Family dysfunction
- Poverty
- Not being connected to others
- Anger
- Changes in the family situation
- Being bored or lonely

Management

Counseling and prevention

Lying

- Encourage parents to strengthen their attachment to their child. Encourage a strong sense of self in children, eliminating the need to lie. If a young child does lie, encourage parents to matter-of-factly confront the child, saying they are disappointed and explaining that lying is not an acceptable behavior.

- Before any intervention, assist parents in attempting to understand the circumstances that prompted the lie.
- Advise parents that punishments that are too rigid or severe could undermine a child's sense of self.
- Suggest that parents model their own behavior according to what they teach and expect from their child.
- Remember that parents should not label a child who has lied.
- Instruct parents to avoid setups for lies and putting children in a position where lying is an easy out.

Stealing

- Have parents try to prevent stealing before it happens. Encourage children to be careful with their money and belongings and try not to make them too tempting for people on the prowl.
- Remember that if parents know their child has stolen something, the first thing they should do is avoid making a scene; this would probably frighten the child and might label the child as well.
- Remind parents that they should confront the child with words like, "I'm sorry you took something that is not yours," then ask the child to produce it.
- Advise parents to help the child return the object to its owner and then apologize. If the object is from a store, it should be paid for, if possible, by the child. Parents must be consistent each time this happens.
- Advise parents to use the opportunity to try to educate the child about ownership and the rights of others. Also, attempt to identify why a child steals if it is a recurrent activity.
- When the child succeeds in not stealing, encourage parents to offer praise and positive reinforcement for honesty.

Cheating

- Counsel parents that to truly understand cheating, the child must be mature enough to understand the concept of rules, both at home and at school.
- Instruct parents that around age 5 to 6 years of age, children can learn the concept of open bargaining rather than subversive cheating.
- Encourage parents to handle cheating gently and openly. Harsh or inappropriate punishments could undermine the child.
- Encourage parents to express their disappointment to the child and then proceed to explain the consequences of cheating in a nonjudgmental way.
- Help parents to understand the cause for the behavior, and if possible, modify the trigger. For example, if a parent is putting too much pressure on a child to succeed academically and this is causing the child to cheat in school, significant behavior modification by the parent is necessary.

Follow-up. See the child as needed for parent and child support and counseling and well-child visits.

Consultations and referrals. If a DBD is demonstrated in an older child for a prolonged period, a psychiatric referral should be considered. While this behavior is diagnosed primarily through history and observation, further psychologic testing may be indicated to assess cognitive function and evaluate emotional or behavioral disturbances.

Masturbation

Alert

Consult with or refer to a physician or a mental health professional for the following:
- Family or interpersonal pathology
- Impeded adaptive or social functioning
- Suspected sexual abuse (see Chapter 47)

Etiology

Masturbation is defined as deliberate self-manipulation of the genitals that results in sexual arousal. It is a normal activity at any age. Masturbation-like activity has been observed in the male fetus in utero and during the first few months of life. Childhood sexuality is very much a part of a child's development and maturation. Parental responses to a child's sexual behavior are greatly influenced by their cultural patterns and orientation.

Most children masturbate because it feels good and do it as much as several times a day or as infrequently as once a week. Children generally engage in masturbation when they are sleepy, bored, watching television, unhappy, or under stress. The most common masturbatory activity in infants and toddlers involves a particular posturing, tightening of the thighs, and handling of the genitalia. It may also involve less obvious behavior, such as leaning on a firm edge or posturing the lower body with various rocking movements. These behaviors may be followed by symptoms of sexual arousal.

Incidence

- Masturbation is deliberate in all children of both sexes by the age of 5 to 6 years.
- Almost all boys and 25% of all girls have masturbated to the point of orgasm by the age of 15 years.
- Up to one third of children discover masturbation while exploring their bodies at 1 to 2 years of age.

Risk Factors

Children who demonstrate persistent, compulsive, and excessive masturbatory behavior should be closely investigated to rule out sexual abuse. A child in psychologic distress may also demonstrate compulsive and excessive masturbatory behaviors.

Differential Diagnosis

Masturbatory activities that include tonic posturing and irregular breathing, with or without facial flushing, can be mistaken for seizure activity. Symptoms of masturbation can be confused with abdominal pain or constipation, although this is rare.

Management

Counseling and prevention

- As a practitioner, be open to and comfortable with discussions of sexuality with parents.
- Educate parents that masturbation is universal, normal, and a necessary part of their child's development. Such guidance should be offered early in the child's life to avoid confused or scornful responses from parents after the behavior is noticed.

- If parents view masturbation as a problem, explore further with them to determine the level and the cause of their concern and discomfort.
- Initiate intervention with the intention of alleviating parental anxiety, thereby reducing or eliminating any fear, anxiety, or shame the child may feel.
- Advise parents not to overreact to their child's behavior. Encourage them to adopt a realistic approach. Suggest that parents encourage limit-setting, if necessary, and include discussions of privacy.
- Keep in mind that a child will masturbate but the parents can control where it is done (e.g., bedroom, bathroom).
- Instruct parents to avoid punitive actions of any kind, as these could have long-term negative effects on the child's self-esteem and sexual development.
- Recommend that if a child masturbates in public places and this is of concern to parents they should distract the child, offering him or her things to carry or something to eat.
- Recommend the parents increase physical contact with the child (i.e., more hugs and kisses). This may help to decrease the frequency of masturbation.
- Instruct parents that positive reinforcement and other behavior modification techniques may be useful to control excessive masturbatory behaviors.

Consultations and referrals. Refer to a mental health professional for evaluation when the following occur:

- Parents report that the child is in psychologic distress
- Unusual manifestations or excessive masturbation undermine the self-esteem and social and adaptive functioning of the child.
- A behavioral or developmental problem is observed in the child.

Separation Anxiety

Alert

Consult with or refer to a mental health professional for the following:

- Behavior lasting longer than 4 weeks in older children
- Behavior interfering with attainment of social and developmental milestones
- A child refusing to go to school
- Parents voicing resentment over a perceived lack of privacy

Etiology

Separation anxiety is the conflicting feelings children have when they are separated from the person or people to whom they are most attached. It is a sign the child has reached an important developmental milestone. During infancy, wariness and apprehension with unknown people begins around the age of 3 to 9 months; this is one of the first affective and cognitive milestones infants reach. The degree and duration of separation anxiety is determined by the infant's developmental age, health, fatigue, and hunger. Temperament also plays a large part in contributing to the infant's level of separation anxiety. Some babies experience mild behavior changes lasting only a brief period. For others, a much stronger response can last throughout the second year of life. The basis for most infant separation anxiety was described by Piaget in 1952. It is postulated that infants begin to remember their parents dur-

---

Box 19-5   Factors Contributing to Separation Anxiety

Biologic—Autonomic/central nervous system tone and responsiveness

Genetic—Family history of anxiety, depression, and other comorbid disorders

Temperamental—Threshold, behavioral inhibition, and so on

Psychodynamic—Attachment, identification with parent, and inhibited autonomy

Cognitive—Stability of object permanence

Cultural—Expectations concerning child care

Situational—Changing schools, moving, or experiencing a loss in the family; parental divorce; tension in school; or family violence

Behavioral—Operant and modeling of parental behavior

Reproduced with permission from Jellinek, M.S. & Kearns, M.E. (1995). Separation anxiety. Pediatrics in Review, 16(2), 57-61, Tables 1 and 2.

---

ing absent periods concurrently with the infants' development of object permanence, which is the ability to remember an object even when it is not physically present. During the first year of life, children lack the coping skills necessary to know their absent parents will return, but refined cognitive capacities allow for more successful resolution during the child's second year.

Another peak of separation anxiety may occur during toddlerhood (at age 18 to 20 months). This diminishes gradually as the toddler's language skills increase and a child can communicate more effectively and independently.

Separation anxiety can continue beyond the expected age and interfere with the child's social and cognitive development. Factors contributing to separation anxiety are categorized in Box 19-5.

Incidence

- Separation anxiety normally begins at 3 to 9 months of age, with reactions lessening during the second year of life.
- A peak can occur at 18 to 20 months of age.
- Children with separation anxiety disorder have higher baseline heart rates and blood pressure levels, leading to a questionable association of anxiety with increased noradrenergic and endocrine function.

Risk Factors

- Previous history of depression
- Shy temperament or behavioral inhibition
- Family history of psychiatric disorders (e.g., parental anxiety disorder, parental depression)
- History of numerous environmental stressors

Differential Diagnosis

The *Diagnostic and Statistical Manual of Mental Disorders, fourth edition* (DSM-IV) criteria for separation anxiety disorder are provided in Box 19-6.

Management

Management must include the cooperation of the parents, the teacher and school, and the child's caregiver (if applicable).

Box 19-6 DSM-IV Diagnostic Criteria for Separation Anxiety Disorder

A. Developmentally inappropriate and excessive anxiety concerning separation from home or from those to whom the individual is attached, as evidenced by three or more of the following:

   1. Recurrent excessive distress when separation from major attachment figures occurs or is anticipated
   2. Persistent and excessive worries about losing, or about harm befalling, major attachment figures
   3. Persistent and excessive worry that an untoward event will lead to separation from a major attachment figure (e.g., getting lost, being kidnapped)
   4. Persistent reluctance or refusal to go to school or elsewhere because of a fear of separation
   5. Persistent and excessively fearful or reluctant to be alone without a major attachment figure at home or without significant adults in other settings
   6. Persistent reluctance or refusal to go to sleep without being near a major attachment figure or to sleep away from home
   7. Repeated nightmares involving the theme of separation
   8. Repeated complaints of physical symptoms (e.g., headaches, stomachaches, nausea, vomiting) when separation from major attachment figures occurs or is anticipated

B. The duration of the disturbance is at least 4 weeks.

C. The onset is before 18 years.

D. The disturbance causes clinically significant distress or impairment in social, academic (occupational), or other important areas of functioning.

E. The disturbance does not occur exclusively during a pervasive developmental disorder, schizophrenia, or other psychotic disorder, and in adolescents and adults is not better accounted for by panic disorder with agoraphobia.

Reproduced with permission from Jellinek, M.S. & Kearns, M.E. (1995). Separation anxiety. Pediatrics in Review, 16(2), 57-61, Tables 1 and 2.

Counseling and prevention. The following are general guidelines for aiding parents of infants and toddlers:

- Explain to parents the developmental and cognitive basis for stranger anxiety. Give them a time frame that will put separation in a more normative context.
- Assure parents that it is all right if their child does not want to show affection to a new person. Such guarded behavior is developmentally normal.
- Advise parents that leave-taking and sleep rituals should be as routine as possible. The repeated familiarity of a routine helps children cope with separation.
- Keep in mind that scheduling departures after naps, when the child is less susceptible to stress and not as tired, may be helpful.

The practitioner may also suggest parents use the following techniques:

- Practice short-term separations around the house. Keep in voice contact with the child when moving from room to room and try to reappear regularly.
- Never sneak out or leave after children have fallen asleep; this violates their trust. Expect and tolerate their protest over such an action.
- Prepare the child when they leave that they will return. Use timeframes they understand (e.g., "I will be back after you eat lunch"). Stick to the timeframe or call if delayed.

- Prepare in advance for extended separations (e.g., business trips, vacations that do not include the child). Discuss what can be done to support the child during this period (e.g., regularly scheduled phone calls).
- Avoid changes in custody, babysitters, and so on when the child is 6 to 18 months if this is at all possible.
- Always remain with children during medical procedures (if possible).
- Introduce the child to friendly adults and children; this is an opportunity for growth.
- Establish bedtime routines with the child and plan them so the pattern can be utilized again should the child awaken during the night.
- Use transitional objects, which may be helpful for a child having trouble separating.
- Remember that separation anxiety is a part of normal development and usually resolves on its own with little or no intervention.
- Anticipate exacerbations during periods of stress (e.g., when the child faces a loss or move, experiences the birth of a sibling).
- Remember the importance of being supportive and patient with the child. When the child is showing signs of distress, parents should stay calm, matter of fact, and sympathetic.

The following are general guidelines for aiding parents of children attending day care or school:

- Advise parents that the initial intervention phase can take up to 2 weeks. The child should attend school regularly during this period.
- Stress to parents that consistency is important; whatever specific interventions are initiated must be faithfully followed.
- Encourage parents to develop graduated expectations for their child.
- Counsel parents that if a child is having difficulty going to school, one of them may need to remain at school with the child for a limited period, either in the hall or in the car parked in front of the school. Gradually the child can be left for the duration of the day.
- Remind parents to support their child's positive progression.

Follow-up. Telephone contact with the parents may be necessary to evaluate the success or needed modifications of intervention strategies.

Consultations and referrals. Consider a referral to a mental health professional in the following situations:

- The child does not improve or worsens, or there is a history of environmental stressors or family history of psychiatric illness.
- Medications such as alprazolam, imipramine, clonazepam, and monoamine oxidase inhibitors are needed. (These are not first-line solutions, and their use should be reserved for experienced child psychiatrists.)
- Psychotherapy and play therapy treatments are indicated.

Resources

Publications

Bailey, B. (1992). "Mommy, don't leave me!" Helping toddlers and parents deal with separation. *Dimensions of Early Childhood, 20*(3), 25-27, 39.

Piaget, J. (1952). *The origin of intelligence in children.* New York: International University Press.

Websites

Coping with Separation Anxiety (from the National Parent Information Network) (npin.org/library/pre1998/n00205/n00205.html)

Easing Separation Anxiety (from the National Network for Child Care) (www.nncc.org/Guidance/dc11_ease.transit.html)

Sleep Problems

Sleep Difficulty

Alert

> Consult with or refer to a physician when an underlying pathology is suspected to be the cause of the sleep disturbance

Etiology. Sleep problems are typically classified as developmental or situational. Most sleep problems begin during infancy and occur through 2 to 3 years of age, which is typically when separation anxiety peaks. Illness, changes in routine, or stressful events for a child may also exacerbate sleep problems.

What is defined as normal varies even for infants. Infants sleep in short spurts and can not differentiate between day and night. During normal sleep a child typically cycles between rapid eye movement (REM) and non–rapid eye movement (NREM) sleep. Each REM/NREM cycle lasts 50 to 60 minutes during infancy and increases to 90 minutes at school age. REM sleep is characterized by jerky, rapid eye movements, absence of motor movements, and irregular pulse and respiratory rate. Dreaming occurs during REM cycles; it is the lightest stage of sleep and the one in which the child most often awakens. The four stages of NREM sleep constitute much deeper sleep.

Generally a newborn sleeps about 16 hours daily, and this amount decreases as a child gets older. At 6 months of age a child sleeps approximately 14.5 hours, and at 12 months about 13.5 hours. Between 1 and 5 years of age, a child generally sleeps 8 to 12 hours nightly. Most children nap until between 2 and 4 years of age. By the age of 4 months, an infant can sleep 6 to 8 hours without waking; by 6 months of age an infant can sleep uninterrupted for 10 to 12 hours. Though it is a common misconception, neither the introduction of solid food nor the baby's weight is associated with uninterrupted night sleep.

Several factors associated with problems of night waking include the following:

- Perinatal problems such as prematurity and perinatal asphyxia
- Children with a difficult temperament and lower sensory thresholds
- Night feedings (typically less necessary by the age of 4 to 6 months)
- Family stress, maternal depression, and maternal employment (all possible but unconfirmed factors)

How parents put a child to sleep greatly influences the child's ability to go back to sleep after awakening. If a child falls asleep while being held or fed, this procedure will need to be repeated after nocturnal awakenings. A child may also call out to his or her parents before falling asleep or during an REM awakening; if parents do not allow the child to go back to sleep independently, the immediate response of the parents can perpetuate night-waking problems.

Incidence

- By the age of 9 months, 84% of all infants awaken only once nightly, and the majority of these infants put themselves back to sleep without parental intervention.
- Sleep problems, which include night-waking and difficulty going to sleep, are present in 20% to 30% of all infants and children.

- About 70% of parents of 3-month-olds report that their infants sleep unaided from midnight to 5 AM.

Risk factors

- Perinatal problems
- Difficult temperament
- Breastfeeding
- Night feeding
- Co-sleeping with parents
- Family stress
- Resistance to sleep based on autonomy of child an inappropriate expectations of parents

Differential diagnosis. The practitioner needs to identify other problems that may be causing a child to have sleep problems. A careful history and physical examination should reveal sources of stress (e.g., family dysfunction, maternal depression, maternal isolation) and occult medical problems (e.g., otitis media) that could be causing the sleep disturbance, as well as normal variations in developmentally appropriate sleep patterns.

Management

Counseling and prevention

- Discuss sleep patterns during well-child visits. Offer suggestions for developing good sleep patterns in infancy (Box 19-7).
- Encourage parents and remind them that patience and consistency are essential.
- Remember that parents can still hold or feed a child as part of a bedtime routine, but the child must be put into bed while awake and fall asleep without parental assistance. This way, if the child wakes during the night, the child can put himself or herself back to sleep. Transition objects may be helpful to diminish separation issues.
- For older infants, suggest parents gradually decrease the amount and/or concentration of formula over a 10-day period so that it eventually contains only water.
- Recommend that parents establish a firm bedtime routine and let an older child participate in deciding what activities should be included. Keep it simple and consistent.

Box 19-7 Developing Good Sleep Habits in Infancy

Be as consistent as possible in *times* of sleep.

Be as consistent as possible in the *place* where the baby sleeps.

Develop a simple *pattern* of putting the baby to sleep.

Put the baby down while he or she is *drowsy,* not asleep, unless you want ot put the child back to sleep all night long through rocking.

Don't give the baby a bottle with which to fall asleep.

Don't respond instantly to every whimper during the night. Give the baby a chance to settle back down.

When you do respond at night, do it *quietly and calmly.* Avoid vigorous play, lots of talk, jiggling, and vigorous diaper changes.

Respond to real crying with calm reassurance, patting, or nursing.

Remember that small infants shouldn't be allowed to "cry it out."

As parents, talk to each other about how to handle sleep issues. Remember that underlying assumptions, ghosts from your past, and perceptions of the child's needs may vary wildly, so now is the time to discuss the subject.

Modified from Dixon, S.D. & Stein, M. (2000). Encounters with children: Pediatric behavior and development (3rd ed.). St. Louis: Mosby.

If parents wish to modify night-waking patterns in an infant, instruct them in the following ways:

1. Over a period of 1 to 2 weeks, a gradual program of reducing contact with the child while he or she is falling asleep can be started. Parents must be assured that crying is to be expected and that it is important they not "cave in."
2. For the first few nights, a parent can stand next to the bed and comfort the child, placing a hand on the child but not picking him or her up.
3. For the next few nights, the parent can stay next to the bed, talking to the child but not touching him or her in any way.
4. For the next few nights, the parent cannot talk or make eye contact with the child in any way and should gradually move farther and farther away from the child until out of the room.
5. This procedure may need to be repeated if the child relapses secondary to illness or a change in routine.

If parents wish to modify night-waking patterns in an older child, they should discuss the plan with the child during the day. A sleeping bag may be placed next to the parents' bed and, over a period of 2 to 3 weeks, moved closer and closer to the child's room and bed until gradually the child is sleeping in his or her own bed.

If parents are experiencing trouble getting the child to bed, they should set firm, clear, consistent rules. It may necessitate eliminating an afternoon nap or waking the child up earlier in the morning if the child is not becoming tired at the predetermined bedtime. This should make the child more fatigued at night.

Co-sleeping with a child is an independent choice. Parents should be assured that it is probably not harmful as long as they are comfortable with the decision.

Follow-up. A few planned follow-up visits or phone calls might be in order to measure the results of the management plan and advise and support parents in their often sleep-deprived endeavor. It may be helpful for the parents to keep a log to really enable them and the practitioner to review the dynamics of the problem.

Consultations and referrals. Refer the child to a physician if an underlying pathology is suspected or identified.

Nightmares

Alert

> Consult with or refer to a mental health professional for any independent problem suspected to be the cause of recurrent nightmares

Etiology. Nightmares are bad dreams that affect all children. They are a normal part of a child's development. Nightmares can be related to many things (e.g., separation anxiety, toilet training) but are usually not attributed to any significant definable environmental problem. Nightmares occur in the REM stage of sleep, and children do remember them. Children are easily consoled after an episode but may experience some difficulty returning to sleep after it ends.

Incidence. Nightmares are a universal occurrence in childhood.

Risk factors

- Fear of sleeping alone
- Family upsets (e.g., moving, divorce, illness, death)
- Change of school
- One parent being away
- Emotional disturbance in a family member
- Scary costumes, television shows, movies, or stories
- Problems with parents, siblings, peers, or teachers

Differential diagnosis. Nightmares can be confused with night terrors (see the discussion of night terrors later in this chapter).

Management

Counseling and prevention

- Advise parents that nightmares are very frightening for children, even though they may understand they are not real. Parents should not trivialize the nightmare, but they should not overreact either.
- Remind parents to never dismiss a nightmare. They should accept the child's fear.
- Have parents console and physically comfort the child until the child is comfortable. Take a few moments to reassure the child and then leave the room.
- Suggest that parents reassure the child that even though they cannot make the nightmare go away, they will always try to be there if the child is frightened.
- Advise parents to gently remind the child that as real as the nightmare seemed, the child is not in any physical danger.
- Suggest transitional objects that may offer additional security to the child experiencing the nightmare. Nightlights are also useful.
- Recommend that parents turn on the light, look out the window, open the closet door, and check under the bed if necessary to allay the child's concern. They should allow the child to participate if he or she chooses.
- Instruct parents to discuss the nightmare the next day (in broad daylight) and utilize storybooks about fictitious children and their bad dreams to help the child work through trepidations. (Note that some experts recommend the parents not ask the child about the dream and recommend only discussing the dream if the child initiates the discussion.)

Follow-up. Schedule a short visit or telephone call to evaluate the parents' effectiveness in dealing with these episodes.

Consultations and referrals. Refer to a mental health professional if an independent problem is suspected as the cause of prolonged and recurrent nightmares.

Night Terrors

Alert

> Consult with or refer to a physician for cases when traditional intervention methods have failed and medication is being considered.

Etiology. Night terrors are actually more terrifying for parents than for a child. They are common in preschool and elementary school children. Night terrors cause children to bolt upright from their sleep, rage, yell incoherently, and cry inconsolably for an average of 5 to 20 minutes. They are associated with autonomic signs, including a rapid pulse, increased respiratory rate, and sweating. The child tends to have a glassy-eyed stare due to the fact that the child is in REM sleep and actually not awake. Night terrors are a disorder of arousal that occurs during an abrupt transition from stage 4 NREM sleep to REM sleep. A child experiencing a night terror is not consolable and does not remember the event. It is unclear what causes night terrors.

Incidence
- Night terrors can start in children as young as 9 months of age and occur most often between the ages of 5 and 7 years.
- Night terrors occur in approximately 5% of children.
- About 96% of children with night terrors have another family member who has night terrors or who walks in his or her sleep.

Risk factors
- Sleep deprivation in general.
- Triggers such as a car horn, an explosion, or a jolted or bumped bed.
- Fever, illness, or sudden pain, possibly from otitis media or abdominal pain caused by gas, constipation, or parasite infections.
- Stressful times
- Family history of night terrors or sleepwalking
- Strange places

Differential diagnosis. Night terrors can sometimes be confused with nightmares (see the preceding discussion of nightmares). Night terrors occur 1 to 2 hours after falling asleep. The child will later have no memory of the event, as he or she is between being asleep and being awake. During the event, the child avoids being comforted.

Management
Treatments and medications. No medications are usually given. Diazepam stops attacks by suppressing REM sleep and providing temporary relief. However, this should be used rarely, as a last measure, and with extreme caution.

Counseling and prevention
- Reassure parents as to the benign nature of these episodes. Explain the physiologic basis of the behavior. Reassure parents that night terrors are not caused by psychopathology or a single life event; this helps parents better tolerate the behavior.
- Inform parents most children outgrow night terrors by puberty.
- Instruct parents not to attempt to wake the child. Waking only causes the child to become confused and distraught. Parents must be encouraged to pull back and observe (as hard as it may seem). Within 15 to 20 minutes the child will stop screaming, curl up, and resume normal sleep. Parents may try to guide the child back to bed, but if the child resists the parents should leave the child alone.
- Discuss how to keep the child safe.
- Suggest increasing sleep time, as sleep deprivation may contribute to night terrors.
- Stress the importance of maintaining a regular sleep schedule.
- Allay the child's fears.
- Advise parents that if the night terrors are recurrent or if they disturb other family members, the child can be awakened before the time the episode normally occurs. This may alter the sleep-cycle pattern and prevent the episode.

Follow-up. Schedule a short office visit or telephone contact to measure the success of the intervention.

Consultations and referrals. Consult a physician if intervention is unsuccessful and medication is being considered.

Resources

Publications
Cohen, G.J. (Ed.). (1999). *1999 Guide to your child's sleep: Birth through adolescence.*

Elk Grove Village, IL: American Academy of Pediatrics

Ferber, R. (1986). *Solve your child's sleep problems.* New York, Simon & Schuster.

Huntley, R. (1991). *The sleep book for tired parents: Help for solving children's sleep problems.* Seattle, WA: Parenting Press.

Sadeh, A. (2001). *Sleeping like a baby: A sensitive and sensible approach to solving your child's sleep problems.* New Haven, CT: Yale University Press.

Symon, B. & Symm, B. (1998). *Silent nights: Overcoming sleep problems in babies and children.* Oxford: Oxford University Press.

Sibling Rivalry

Alert
Consult with or refer to a mental health professional for the following:
- Aggressive and hostile behavior posing a physical danger.
- Behaviors that are prolonged despite the attempts of parents to manage the conflict
- Behavior that places adverse and severe stress on the dynamics of the entire family

Etiology
Parental concerns about sibling rivalry often begin after the birth of a second child. Older children frequently demonstrate aggressive behaviors toward the baby or manifest regressive behaviors themselves. Sibling rivalry takes a different shape with school-age children. Children who independently are easygoing and nonaggressive regularly engage in physical and psychologic warfare with their brothers and sisters at home. Parents often do not have the energy to deal with this ongoing, seemingly neverending confrontational activity. However, as children get older, they do tend to become closer, and valuable lessons (e.g., sharing, independent conflict resolution) can be learned early in life.

Incidence
- The peak period for sibling rivalry usually occurs between the ages of 1 and 3 years, although in some cases it can be prolonged indefinitely.
- Sibling rivalry is usually more intense if the siblings are close in age and the same sex. Twins and children born 3 or more years apart tend to demonstrate less sibling rivalry.
- One third of older siblings show developmental gains after a sibling's birth. However, many exhibit transient regression, and often children experience a combination of both.
- Reportedly, 60% of all parents become regularly involved in sibling conflicts. In these cases the frequency and number of conflicts tend to increase, and the resolution is generally of a more verbal, less physical nature.

Risk Factors
- Siblings spaced about 2 years apart tend to experience the most intense sibling rivalry.
- Parental favoritism tends to exacerbate conflicts.
- Labeling and typecasting children into roles (positive and negative) can enhance sibling rivalry.
- Comparing siblings can increase sibling rivalry.

Management

Counseling and prevention

- Increase parental understanding. Parents must have reasonable expectations. They cannot totally prevent all sibling rivalry, but they can enforce a minimum standard of behavior and model their own parenting practices to minimize the amount of competition and rivalry between their children.
- Advise parents to prepare a young child for the birth of a sibling. A child who is 4 years of age or older should be told of the expected birth of a sibling as soon as parents begin telling family and friends. Depending on the child's developmental level and cognitive abilities, basic facts about conception, pregnancy, and birth should be explained. Children's books are available in local bookstores to help parents with this (see the Resources at the end of this chapter). If a child is younger than 4 years of age, parents can wait until further along in the pregnancy before telling him or her; children are self-centered at this age, and the concept of pregnancy is too abstract.
- As the pregnancy progresses, suggest that parents answer questions and explain as much as an older child is capable of understanding. Again, storybooks are very helpful.
- Remind parents to include the child in as many of the preparatory activities as possible.
- Advise parents to try to complete any major changes for the child before the birth of the baby, if at all possible. These include toilet training, switching from a crib to a bed, starting preschool, and so on.
- Counsel parents that it is not unusual to expect some regression from a child after the birth of the baby. Parents should be supportive of this.
- Help parents recognize that the actual birth of the baby may be confusing and threatening to a child, depending on the child's developmental level. The birth experience includes the disappearance of the mother for a time and possibly the first visit to the hospital, which could be overwhelming and frightening.
- Remind parents to recognize the sibling's jealousy, give that child extra and special time, and again try to involve the child in caring for the infant whenever appropriate.
- Remember that toddlers may benefit from having a doll of their own to take care of.
- As an infant grows and begins to become independently mobile, keep in mind that new problems may arise as sharing and private space become issues. Remind parents to respect the rights of the older child.
- For older children, advise parents to simply and concretely explain the rules of the house and the general code of behavior to be followed by all. For a variety of reasons, specific responsibilities and privileges may not be equal for each child. The reasons for this should be carefully explained to avoid jealousy and resentment.
- Encourage parents not to overreact unless there is danger of physical harm. Many experts believe that children should be given the opportunity to work out their differences without parents becoming involved or acting as referees. However, if children are in danger of physical harm, they should be separated and a timeout initiated. Parents should resolve the crisis with their children, not for them.
- Remind parents that children commonly pattern their behavior on, and learn coping strategies from, their parents. Adults who address differences in a confrontational manner can expect the same behavior from their children.

Follow-up. Several brief monthly follow-up visits or telephone calls may be necessary. These contacts may be more important for the parents, who may feel frustrated or concerned that progress is not as forthcoming or rapid as they may wish.

Consultations and referrals. A referral for family therapy may be indicated if:

- Prolonged and extreme sibling rivalry undermines the family's dynamics.
- The parents are unable to actualize the management strategies suggested.
- Sibling rivalry is severe enough that it leads to marital problems.
- It is damaging to the self-esteem or psychologic well-being of one or more family members.
- The sibling rivalry is related to another psychologic disorder (e.g., depression, drug abuse).

Stranger Anxiety

Alert

Consult with or refer to a mental health professional for the following:
- Stranger anxiety continuing beyond the normally anticipated ages
- Stranger anxiety interfering with the child's normal, social, and developmental achievements

Etiology

As with separation anxiety, the basis for stranger anxiety is rooted in Piaget's concept of object permanence, or the child's ability to remember an object once it is removed. Stranger anxiety is normal and should be anticipated as an emergent stage of an infant's cognitive growth. The quality of an infant's stranger anxiety is a function of developmental age, temperament, presence of illness or fatigue, the way a stranger appears, and the presence or absence of a familiar figure. The baby's stranger anxiety may be intensified by being in unknown surroundings, the appearance and speed of approach by the stranger, and the physical proximity of a parent or familiar person during the new encounter.

A child's temperament dictates to a large extent the magnitude of stranger anxiety experienced and the length of time it lasts. Children who are exposed to many different adults during infancy tend to experience less stranger anxiety than those who are not, and strange children tend to elicit less anxiety in infants and toddlers than strange adults. Infants who have extreme and prolonged stranger reactions tend to be shy and more sensitive, so it sometimes takes them longer to warm up.

Incidence

Stranger anxiety, in the vast majority of children, has the following peaks during early childhood:

- Stranger awareness begins to appear around 3 to 9 months of age.
- Crosscultural studies show that the first peak in stranger anxiety is generally uniform, occurring at about 8 months of age.
- A second peak in stranger anxiety occurs around 18 to 20 months of age, or before the time when the toddler's language skills are secure.

- Most developmentally based stranger anxiety lessens or gradually dissipates by 2½ to 3 years of age.

Risk Factors

Children tend to experience greater stranger anxiety if they undergo stressful events during peak ages. These events include, but are not limited to, the following:

- The parent who has been a primary caregiver returns to work.
- A change in a babysitter or caregiver is necessary.
- The family moves to a new home.
- The family constellation changes (e.g., birth of a new sibling, separation of parents).
- The child requires hospitalization.

Management

Counseling and prevention

- Advise parents that major changes (if possible) should be minimized during peak stranger anxiety ages. If changes are unavoidable, they should be made gradually and with as much support to the child as possible. Parents should expect a heightened or prolonged response or some regression during these times.
- Remind parents that stranger anxiety is normal.
- Suggest strangers be introduced in the presence of a parent or familiar adult, with the stranger's approach being gradual.
- Advise parents never to force a child who is reluctant to sit with or be held by a new person or unfamiliar face until the child has had time to "warm up."
- Keep in mind that transitional objects may be helpful for the child to carry (e.g., cuddly toy or animal, favorite blanket) and provide the child with security. The need for a special object is most prevalent in 1- to 2-year-olds.
- Remember that parents should never sneak away from children.
- Recommend parents try to familiarize the child with a new setting before introducing strangers. Encourage strangers to respect the child's reluctance and give them adequate time to adjust.
- Inform parents that most children resolve the issue of stranger anxiety on their own as they mature.
- Encourage parents to be supportive and patient.

Follow-up. Schedule follow-up visits or telephone calls as needed.

Consultations and referrals. Refer to a mental health professional if the response to strangers is prolonged, if there is a possible separate underlying cause of the behavior, or if the behavior interferes with the attainment of the child's social and developmental milestones.

Temper Tantrums

Alert

Consult with or refer to a mental health professional for the following:
- Temper tantrums occurring regularly before the age of 1 year or after the age of 4 years
- Temper tantrums caused by underlying family dysfunction or pathology in the child

Etiology

Temper tantrums occur during childhood when children's emotions exceed their ability to control them. Tantrums can be frustrating and embarrassing for parents, especially when they occur in public places. Tantrums are often an expression of frustration for the children. Preschoolers, in their eagerness to control the world around them, may want to be more independent than their skills or safety allow. They may also have trouble expressing their feelings in words, resulting in a temper tantrum. Tantrums typically manifest themselves as bouts of screaming, crying, kicking, foot-stomping, and excessive frustration. During toddlerhood, a likely cause of tantrums is the need for autonomy, which is restricted by dependence. The tantrum is the result of a child's overwhelming frustration and compounded by the lack of verbal skills normally possessed at this often immature age.

Temperament plays an important part in determining the intensity, duration, and frequency of tantrums. Intense children tend to have more exaggerated outbursts, while the tantrums of persistent children tend to last longer. Irregular sleeping and eating patterns make it harder to anticipate when a child will reach the point of maximum frustration, thereby making it difficult to prevent the incident.

Environmental factors associated with causing tantrums include overcrowded or confined personal or living space (especially for active children), domestic violence or stress, parental depression or substance abuse, frequent corporal punishment, and parental inability to set firm limits.

Incidence

- Temper tantrums occur at least weekly in 50% to 80% of all children between the ages of 2 and 3 years.
- Daily temper tantrums occur in 20% of all children between the ages of 2 and 3 years.
- Of 2-year-olds with frequent temper tantrums, 60% continue to have them at the age of 3 years; of these, 60% also have them at the age of 4 years.
- Temper tantrums are not related to gender or social class.
- There is no known genetic or familial predisposition for temper tantrums.

Risk Factors

- Recurrent upper respiratory tract infections
- Respiratory allergies
- Inadequate or disturbed sleep
- Hearing loss
- Speech and language delay
- Autism, traumatic brain injury, and severe mental retardation

Management

Counseling and prevention. The practitioner should take a careful history before counseling. This enables priorities to be set during the intervention. The following should be included in the parental interview:

- When, where, why, and how do the child's temper tantrums usually occur?
- How do the parents feel, respond, and intervene when the child has a temper tantrum?
- Is there any specific time, place, or person more likely to provoke a temper tantrum from the child?

Once a thorough history has been obtained, the practitioner should:

- Help parents identify possible triggers and determine ways to alleviate or remedy them, if possible.

- Help parents understand their child's temperament and set realistic goals based on it.
- Instruct parents to organize or childproof their home, making it less necessary to say "no" to a child.
- Advise parents to make sure they really mean it when they do say "no." There is no better way to reinforce negative behavior than to give in to it. Children become aware of this very quickly.
- Assist parents to empower their young children to participate in decision-making. Offer only choices for which any outcome is acceptable (e.g., "Do you want to wear the pink hat or the white hat today?", "Should we have string beans or corn for dinner?")
- Help parents try to limit the frustrations their children feel by respecting their individual needs for activity, sleep, and food. Help parents recognize when their child is fatigued and in need of assistance to reduce frustration.
- Have parents attempt to ignore tantrums as much as possible, or at the very least minimize their attention and response to them. Children should be watched to ensure they are out of physical danger, but parents remaining calm and indifferent is crucial to avoiding reinforcing the behavior.
- Instruct parents to avoid punitive actions as a method of remedying tantrums. Any discussion of tantrums should be focused on the behavior, not on labeling the child as a "bad" boy or girl; such labeling could seriously threaten a child's self-esteem.

Follow-up. Encourage a telephone call from the parents to report if interventions are effective, and discuss the situation at well-child visits. Schedule a return visit if tantrums worsen or parents are concerned.

Consultations and referrals. Further evaluation of tantrums, to be performed by a mental health professional, may be indicated in the following situations:
- Traditional intervention recommendations failing repeatedly over time
- Underlying etiologies found to be causing the behavior, which require separate intervention (e.g., parental depression, substance abuse, family dysfunction)

Resources

Publications
Turecki, S. & Tonner, L. (2000). *The difficult child*. New York: Bantam Doubleday.

Thumbsucking and Digit-Sucking

Alert

Consult with or refer to a mental health professional or pediatric dentist for the following:
- Thumbsucking persisting past early childhood
- Child becoming affected by negative comments or ridicule by playmates, siblings, or relatives
- Parents overly criticizing or punishing the child for the behavior, with it adversely affecting their relationship
- Changes in the oral cavity and dentition (primary and permanent)
- Development of related digital abnormalities
- Thumbsucking or pacifier-sucking interfering in any way with a child's normal developmental achievements

Etiology
Thumbsucking is very common. It has calming, soothing, and stress-relieving effects and is often employed by children when they are falling asleep, tired, bored, or unhappy. Many think thumbsucking is a learned behavior, but recent evidence shows that many infants suck their thumb or fingers in utero and continue this behavior immediately after birth. Many psychoanalysts postulate that it is an expression of infantile sexuality. However, prolonged thumbsucking could be indicative of an emotional disturbance.

Incidence
- Estimates of nonnutritive sucking (i.e., of thumbs, fingers, pacifiers) range from 75 to 95% of infants in Western cultures.
- Some studies estimate 30% of those 4 to 6 years old and 26% of those 6 to 9 years old persist in digit-sucking.

Risk Factors
- Severe emotional problems
- Stress-related problems
- Poor parent-child interaction or relationship
- Regressive behavior

Differential Diagnosis
Subjective data. There may be a history of concern by the parents or child because of thumb or digit-sucking. The history may reveal the following about the digit-sucking:
- It is viewed as immature or socially unacceptable.
- It is indicative of an emotional disturbance.
- It is indicative of parent-child discord.
- It has continued despite parents' attempts to alter the behavior. (The parents should describe what steps they have employed thus far.)

Objective data. A physical examination may indicate the following:
- Possible wrinkled, red digit
- Digital callus formation, irritant eczema, paronychia, or herpetic whitlow
- Possible hyperextension finger deformity
- Malocclusion of primary and permanent teeth (common with chronic thumbsuckers)
- Possible anterior overbite and/or posterior crossbite
- Narrowing of maxillary arch secondary to buccal wall contraction

Management
Treatment and medications
- Over-the-counter, unpleasant, bitter substances are available to coat the finger. Apply in the morning, at night, and whenever the behavior occurs. As thumbsucking stops, cut back treatments. Discontinue the nighttime application last. Counsel children that the liquid is a reminder for them, not a punishment.
- The finger may be covered with a bandage or thumb guard (an adjustable plastic cylinder that can be taped on). Socks or gloves also can be used at night.
- Elbow immobilizers prevent the arm from bending, thus keeping the fingers away from the mouth.
- Severe emotional or stress-related problems should be ruled out before behavior modification is attempted.

Counseling and prevention
- Advise parents that intervention should not be required until about 4 to 5 years of age, because most children

spontaneously stop and develop more socially acceptable coping strategies. It is important to consider a child's emotional and intellectual stage of development. The child should be involved in the decision, because the child must want to stop.

- Carefully explain the management strategies and their goals to children. The techniques are not intended to cause excessive anxiety, stress, or tension. If they do, they should be stopped immediately.
- Advise parents that interventions are most successful when they empower the child and offer options, not when they are punitive.
- Encourage parents to give support and remember that patience is essential in this endeavor, as it may take time and the child can relapse.
Counsel parents with children younger than 5 years old to:
- Try to ignore the behavior and do not give it unnecessary negative attention.
- Offer the child alternatives or provide desirable distractions, especially if the behavior is demonstrated at predictable times (e.g., when bored, hungry, tired). This may help the child to avoid the behavior. (Pacifiers are not effective alternatives. They only substitute one sucking behavior for another.)
- Provide praise when the behavior is successfully averted.
- Do not punish or ridicule the child.
Counsel parents with children older than 5 years to:
- Try positive reinforcement as much as possible, with visible tools (e.g., stickers, stars, calendars).
- Provide praise when the behavior is averted.
- Encourage verbalization to validate underlying feelings.
- Designate an assigned time for thumbsucking and allow the child to participate in this decision. Mandatory thumbsucking may cause the child to lose interest.
If the child is told to suck the thumb for several minutes every day under designated conditions, it may not be as appealing.
Follow-up. See the child for well-child care and as needed.
Consultations and referrals. If behavior modification fails, consider referring the child to a pediatric dentist for an orthodontic device such as an intraoral plate bar or crib that blocks the thumb.

Toilet Training

Alert

Consult with or refer to a mental health professional or physician for the following:
- Family dysfunction or other problems that undermine the child's ability to toilet train
- Children 5 years or older who are not toilet trained

Etiology

All normal children will, at one point or another, toilet train themselves. Most parents, however, have difficulty waiting for this to happen. The current unanimous consensus among practicing pediatric providers is that when a child is ready to toilet train, there is little anyone can do to stop the process. However, if parents intervene prematurely, there is much they can do to delay it.

Incidence

- In the United States 26% of all children achieve daytime continence by the age of 2 years, 85% by 2½ years, and 98% by 3 years.
- Toilet training usually can be accomplished within 3 months, and nighttime continence is generally achieved several months after that.
- Girls tend to toilet train earlier than boys.

Signs of Readiness

The following characteristics of a child suggest a developmental readiness for toilet training:
- Understands simple questions and directions
- Has cognitive skills (i.e., the ability to understand cause and effect)
- Is eager to please and imitates parents
- Shows interest in the potty or toilet
- Has the necessary motor skills required to manipulate pants and sit for extended periods
- Has the body awareness needed to differentiate between a wet and a soiled diaper or to recognize the urge to void or defecate before it actually happens

Management

Parents should begin with bowel training; this is easier than bladder training. Bowel movements happen less frequently and the child usually has a longer warning time. Warning of the need to urinate may be only a few seconds.

Brazelton (1992) advocates eight steps to successful toilet training, which probably happen sometime during the third year. These are listed in Box 19-8.

Box 19-8 Eight Steps to Successful Toilet Training by Parents

1. Place a potty chair on the floor that the child knows is his or hers, and allow the child to take it wherever he or she chooses.
2. After a week or so, allow the child to sit on the potty, wearing clothes if the child prefers. The goal here is to establish the routine of sitting on the potty.
3. Next, ask the child's permission to remove the diaper while sitting on the potty. Allow the child to see you sitting on the toilet; he or she will try to imitate you.
4. Place the contents of dirty diapers in the toilet. The child can then learn where excreta go. If flushing frightens the child, it is better to flush after the child loses interest and leaves the bathroom.
5. Allow the child a period to keep the pants off. If the child is ready to use the potty, this is great. If the child soils on the floor, put the diaper back on and hold off for a while.
6. If the child displays temper tantrums or episodes of stool-holding, delay the process for a while. *Parents should never be demeaning or punitive to the child who fails!*
7. When learning to urinate, boys should sit down. When mastering this, the boy can watch a male family member use the toilet and at that point begin to stand up.
8. Nighttime training should not begin until the child is dry during a nap and until the child gives some signal of wanting to stay dry at night. Many children are not ready to stay dry at night until they are 4 to 5 years of age.

Some children resist toilet training despite appropriate, secure, and consistent efforts of their parents. In these cases the following suggestions to parents may be useful:

- Be sympathetic and understanding to the child. *Never* fight, argue, insult, or shame the child.
- Rather than engage in a power struggle that a parent is sure to lose, hold off toilet training for several weeks, then begin fresh.
- Continue toilet training discussions with the child (or read toilet training children's stories) in a nonstressful, empathic, and nondemanding manner.
- Encourage the child to imitate siblings or parents.
- Encourage the child to try to change his or her own diapers.
- At the first sign of defecation, ask the child if he or she would like to use the potty.
- Institute a reward system (e.g., sticker or star chart) for successful attempts.
- Address the issue of constipation through diet modification if this is an impeding factor.
- If the child is emphatically resistant but clearly able emotionally and developmentally to master the task and is more than 3 years old, have a ceremony to throw away the diapers.
- Announce that the child is a "big boy" or "big girl" now and give the child encouragement to do his or her best.

Follow-up. See the child for well-child visits and as needed.

Consultations and referrals. Refer to a mental health professional if there is underlying family dysfunction that is undermining the child's natural toilet training progress.

Resources

Websites

(See also Chapter 3.)
About Our Kids (aboutourkids.med.nyu.edu)
Family.com (www.family.go.com)
Kids Health (www.kidshealth.com)
Knowledge Exchange Network (www.mentalhealth.org)
National Child Care Information Center (www.nccic.org)
National Parent Information Network (www.npin.org)
Tufts University Child and Family Webguide (www.cfw.tufts.edu)

Bibliography

American Academy of Pediatrics Committee on Psychosocial Aspects of Child and Family Health. (1998). Guidance for effective discipline. *Pediatrics, 101*(4) 723-728.

American Academy of Pediatrics Task Force on Circumcision. (1999). Circumcision policy statement. *Pediatrics, 103*(3), 686-693.

Anderson, J.E. & Bluestone, D. (2000). Breath-holding spells: Scary but not serious. *Contemporary Pediatrics, 17*(1), 61-72.

Berezin, J. (1990). *The complete guide to choosing childcare*. New York: Random House.

Brazelton, T.B. (1992). *Touchpoints*. New York: Merloyd-Lawrence.

Christophersen, E.R. (1991). Toileting problems in children. *Pediatric Annals, 20*(5):240-244.

Dixon, S.D. & Stein, M. (2000). *Encounters with children: Pediatric behavior and development* (3rd ed.). St. Louis: Mosby.

Faber, A. & Maslish, E. (1987). *Siblings without rivalry*. New York: W.W. Norton.

Frailberg, S. (1959). *The magic years*. New York: Charles Scribner & Sons.

Garrity, C. & Baris, M. (1996). Bullies and victims: a guide for pediatricians. *Contemporary Pediatrics, 13*(2):90-116.

Glew, G., Rivara, F., & Feudtner, C. (2000). Bullying: Children hurting children. *Pediatric Reviews 21,* 183-190.

Howe, A.C. & Walker, C.E. (1992). Behavioral management of toilet training, enuresis, and encopresis. *Pediatric Clinics of North America, 39,* 413-432.

Jellinek, M.S. & Kearns, M.E. (1995). Separation anxiety. *Pediatrics in Review, 16*(2):57-61.

Leach, P. (1995). *Your growing child*. New York: Alfred A. Knopf.

Nansel, T.R., Overpeck, M., Pilla, R.S., Ruan, W.J., Simons-Morton, B, & Scheidt, P. (2001). Bullying behaviors among U.S. youth: Prevalence and association with psychosocial adjustment. *Journal of the American Medical Association, 285*(16), 2094-2100.

Parker, S. & Zuckerman, B. (2001). *Behavioral and developmental pediatrics* (2nd ed). New York: Little, Brown & Co.

Preiser, G., et.al. (2000). Circumcision: The debate goes on. *Pediatrics 105,* 681-684.

Schachter, R. & McCauley, C.S. (1988). *When your child is afraid*. New York: Simon & Schuster.

Schmitt, B.D. (1992). How to help the training night crier. *Contemporary Pediatrics, 9*(12), 45-49.

Schor, E.L. (Ed.). (1999). *Caring for your school-age child: Ages 5 to 12* (2nd ed.). Elk Grove Village, IL: American Academy of Pediatrics.

Sears, W. & Sears, M. (1995). *The discipline book*. New York: Little, Brown & Co.

Shelov S. & Hannemann, R.E. (2001). Caring for your baby and child, birth to age five (2nd ed.). Elk Grove Village, IL: American Academy of Pediatrics.

Van Norman, R.A. (2001). Why we can't afford to ignore prolonged digit sucking. *Contemporary Pediatrics, 18*(6), 61-81.

Wiswell, T.E. (1997). Circumcision circumspection. *New England Journal of Medicine 336,* 1244-1245.

Chapter 20 *Common Adolescent Concerns*

Linda M. Kollar

Adolescent Office Visits

Adolescence represents a transitional period in the patient–health care provider relationship. The pediatric office visit traditionally focuses on parental concerns about the child's health. During adolescence, the focus begins to shift from the concerns of the parents to the concerns of the adolescent patient. The adolescent and parents require an explanation of this process to decrease discomfort and increase trust between the health care provider and the adolescent. Adolescent health care requires a careful balancing act to gain the trust of the adolescent while the provider maintains a relationship with the parent.

The first impression begins when the teen enters the office. An adolescent-friendly environment includes support staff interested in teens and a waiting room with posters, magazines, and health education pamphlets relevant to teens. The provider must demonstrate genuine interest in the adolescent, perhaps by greeting the adolescent first and then the parent. Adolescents prefer a brief period of small talk before beginning the health history. The visit should be sensitive to the sociocultural norms of the individual adolescent.

Adolescents favor providers who are comfortable with risk-assessment subject matter, and they prefer a direct approach to sensitive topics. Providers need to be cognizant of language, avoiding the use of both adolescent jargon and high-level medical terminology. A nonjudgmental approach with attention to biases increases trust and acceptance. Above all, the practitioner should listen to the teen (rather than lecture) and take the concerns of the adolescent seriously. The goal of the interaction is not to change risk behaviors but to assist with the resources necessary to enable teens to make the choices that are best for them.

Each visit should include some time alone with the adolescent. The amount of time should appropriate to the adolescent's age and developmental level and be guided by the comfort level of the teen and the parents. After a review of confidentiality, the conversation should move from less-sensitive to more-sensitive topics and include an explanation of the context for the questioning.

The health care provider must review the parameters of confidentiality at the beginning of the provider-patient relationship and again at each visit. When a guardian is participating in the care of the adolescent, the guardian should be included in this discussion. The traditional parameters of confidentiality include holding all information confidential except in circumstances of abuse, suicide, or homicidal ideation. Some providers frame confidentiality in a broader context, assuring the adolescent that all information will be held confidential unless the provider believes the adolescent or someone else is at risk and that another adult needs to be involved. If the provider deems that confidentiality should be breached, the adolescent must be informed of this first and given an opportunity to participate in the disclosure; the adolescent can

then have the choice to tell the guardian alone, tell the guardian with the provider present, or have the provider tell the guardian alone or with the adolescent present.

Consent and confidentiality in adolescent health care can be divided into two basic questions: (1) When can adolescents approve their own treatment? and (2) When should parents be informed of their child's health care decision? The regulations governing the answers to these questions are formed by federal and state law as well as institutional policy and guidelines. State laws determine the parameters of minor consent for medical treatment, and specific state statutes fall into two categories: (1) a minor's right to give consent for specific services (e.g., mental health assessment, sexually transmitted disease [STD] testing), and (2) specific groups of minors having the right to give consent (e.g., married minors, minors in the military). All providers working with adolescents must become familiar with their state statutes for consent and confidentiality, and prudent providers will review changes to minor consent statutes after each legislative session.

The American Medical Association (AMA), the Society of Adolescent Medicine (SAM), the American Academy of Pediatrics (AAP), and the American College of Obstetrics and Gynecology (ACOG) have written policy statements in support of a minor's right to confidential health care. All agree that although parental involvement is desirable, confidentiality may be central to encouraging teens to access needed health advice and treatment.

Preventive services are the mainstay of health care to adolescents. The primary and secondary prevention of health risks and threats are the main components of clinical practice. The AMA has developed and published the *Guidelines for Adolescent Preventive Services* (GAPS) (1997), which serve as the framework for the organization and content of preventive health services. Table 20-1 is an adaptation of the guidelines for preventive counseling, with the goal being to address each of the issues at least once during each age period from early to late adolescence. GAPS also outlines recommendations for health screening for adolescents; an adaptation of these guidelines is provided in Table 20-2.

Vaccinations remain an important part of disease prevention for adolescents, and the current immunization status of an adolescent needs to be determined. If the pediatric immunizations are up to date, most of the immunizations required during adolescence are ideally given during the visit at 11 to 12 years of age. The bivalent tetanus-diphtheria toxoid (Td) vaccine booster should be administered if the adolescent has not been vaccinated in the past 5 years and then readministered every 10 years. The second dose of measles-mumps-rubella (MMR) vaccine should be given unless there is documentation of two vaccines in earlier childhood. Pregnancy must be ruled before administration of the MMR. If there is no history of chickenpox or previous immunization, the varicella vaccine should be offered; if started after 13 years of age, a two-dose regimen

Table 20-1 Primary Health Care Services for Adolescent Patients: Recommendations for Health Education

RECOMMENDED COUNSELING	EARLY ADOLESCENCE (11-14 YEARS OLD)	MIDDLE ADOLESCENCE (15-17 YEARS OLD)	LATE ADOLESCENCE (18-21 YEARS OLD)
Preventive visit	Annually	Annually	Annually
Adolescent health guidance related to:	Annually	Annually	Annually
• Physical growth			
• Psychosocial development			
• Active involvement in health care decisions			
• Dietary habits			
• Healthy diet and safe weight management			
• Exercise			
• Abstinence			
• Responsible sexual behaviors			
• STD prevention			
• Condom use			
• Availability of contraception			
• Avoidance of tobacco, alcohol, and other abusable substances			
• Avoidance of steroids			
Parental health guidance	Once	Once	Once
	Related to:	Related to:	Related to:
	• Normative adolescent development	• Normative adolescent development	• Normative adolescent development
	• Signs and symptoms of disease and emotional distress	• Signs and symptoms of disease and emotional distress	• Signs and symptoms of disease and emotional distress
	• Parenting behaviors to promote healthy adjustment	• Parenting behaviors to promote healthy adjustment	• Parenting behaviors to promote healthy adjustment
	• Role modeling of health-related behaviors	• Role modeling of health-related behaviors	• Role modeling of health-related behaviors
	• Weapons	• Driving behaviors	• Driving behaviors
	• Monitoring social and recreational activities	• Weapons	• Weapons
		• Monitoring social and recreational activities	• Monitoring social and recreational activities

Data adapted from American Medical Association (1997). Guidelines for adolescent preventive services. *Chicago: American Medical Association.*

is required because adolescents have a diminished response to the vaccine as compared to children. If the adolescent has not been previously vaccinated, the hepatitis B immunization series should also be initiated. College freshman who will be living in a dormitory setting are at increased risk of acquiring meningococcal disease and should be offered the quadrivalent meningococcal polysaccharide vaccine to decrease this risk (Centers for Disease Control and Prevention [CDC], 2000).

Pubertal Growth and Maturation

Pubertal changes follow a predictable sequence and tempo, and deviations from the predicted timing or in the rate of change require further investigation for factors influencing pubertal maturation. The most prominent biologic changes of puberty are growth and the development of secondary sexual characteristics. The sequence and timing of pubertal events can be seen in Fig. 20-1, and the specific pubertal stages for both males and females have been systematized into Tanner stages (as illustrated in Chapter 40). The provider should assess and document the stage of pubertal development annually.

Nutritional Assessment

In addition to the growth of the reproductive system, pubertal development includes growth of the skeletal, endocrine, and neurologic systems. By the end of puberty the adolescent is 20% taller and 50% heavier than before puberty started. These biologic changes require support with adequate nutrition.

Growth occurs in spurts, with more rapid growth in the spring and summer seasons. Height and weight should be documented annually to adequately follow trends; the body mass index (BMI) is an objective method for evaluating the appropriate range of body weight for a given height, age, sex,

Table 20-2 Primary Health Care Services for Adolescents: Recommendations for Screening

RECOMMENDED SCREENING	EARLY ADOLESCENCE (11-14 YEARS OLD)	MIDDLE ADOLESCENCE (15-17 YEARS OLD)	LATE ADOLESCENCE (18-21 YEARS OLD)
Complete physical examination	Once, unless more frequency warranted by signs and symptoms	Once, unless more frequency warranted by signs and symptoms	Once, unless more frequency warranted by signs and symptoms
Blood pressure	Annually	Annually	Annually
Total blood cholesterol	Once if : • Parents have serum cholesterol > 240 • Unknown family history or multiple risk factors for heart disease (e.g., smoking, obesity, diabetes, high-fat, cholesterol diet) • Parent or grandparent with coronary artery disease, peripheral vascular disease, cerebrovascular disease, or sudden cardiac death at ≤ 55 years of age	Once if meeting the guidelines and not screened in early adolescence	Once when over age 19
Weight and stature; body image and dieting patterns to screen for eating disorders and obesity	Annually	Annually	Annually
Assessment for use of tobacco products; cessation counseling for positive findings	Annually	Annually	Annually
Assessment for use of alcohol or other drugs, including circumstances of use; amount and frequency of use; attitudes and motivation; and physical, psychosocial, and school functioning; also appropriate counseling and treatment for positive findings	Annually	Annually	Annually
Assessment of sexual activity; use and motivation to use condoms; use and motivation to use other contraception; number of partners; any exchanges of sex for money or drugs; pregnancy history; and STD history; also counseling to reduce risk	Annually	Annually	Annually
Screening of sexually active teens for STDs: • Females: cervical culture for gonorrhea, immunologic test for chlamydia, Pap smear • Males: urine leukocyte esterase analysis for gonorrhea and chlamydia • Visual inspection for HPV	Frequency dependent on sexual practices and history of previous STDs	Frequency dependent on sexual practices and history of previous STDs	Frequency dependent on sexual practices and history of previous STDs Annual Pap smear
HIV screening with pre-and post-test counseling for teens at risk of acquiring HIV; screening includes: • Intravenous drug use or partner who uses • More than one sexual partner in the last 6 months • Exchange of sex for drugs or money • Male having sex with other males • Sexual partner at risk for HIV	Frequency determined by the risk factors of the individual	Frequency determined by the risk factors of the individual	Frequency determined by the risk factors of the individual
Assessment for behaviors that indicate recurrent or severe depression or risk of suicide	Annually	Annually	Annually
Assessment for emotional, physical and sexual abuse	Annually	Annually	Annually
Assessment for learning or school problems	Annually	Annually	Annually

Data adapted from American Medical Association (1997). Guidelines for adolescent preventive services. *Chicago: American Medical Association.*

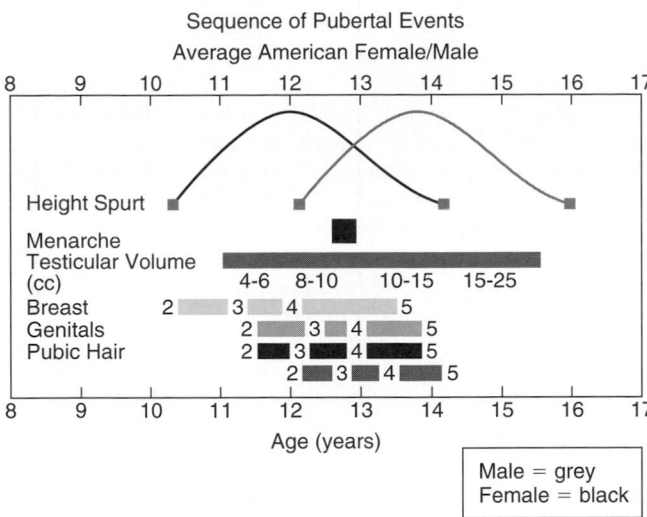

Sequence of Pubertal Events
Average American Female/Male

Age (years)

Male = grey
Female = black

Fig. 20-1 Sequence of pubertal events. (From Tanner, J.M. [1962]. *Growth at adolescence* [2nd ed.]. Blackstone Scientific Publications.)

Table 20-3 Percentile Ranking of Calculated Body Mass Index

UNDERWEIGHT	< 5TH PERCENTILE
At risk for being underweight	≤ 15th percentile
Acceptable weight range	> 15th and < 85th percentiles
At risk for being overweight	≥ 85th and < 95th percentiles
Overweight	≥ 95th percentile

and race. The BMI provides a percentile ranking that a provider should use, rather than the provider relying on traditional growth charts when evaluating body size. (Clinical classifications for interpreting BMI percentile ranking are listed in Table 20-3.)

The food guide pyramid is an excellent tool for counseling adolescents about healthy eating, and most adolescents are familiar with the pyramid from school and on food packaging. The traditional food guide pyramid is modified for adolescents by increasing the milk, yogurt, and cheese group from two or three servings per day to four servings per day; this satisfies the increased calcium needs for growth and bone density. The bread and starch group at the base of the pyramid is increased for adolescents to nine to eleven servings to meet higher energy demands.

Obesity (see Chapter 43) is increasing in all populations in the United States, and currently about 11% of children and adolescents are overweight. Obesity with an onset during adolescence is likely to persist into adulthood, and the physiologic and emotional ramifications of obesity make this an important clinical issue. The stage of growth and development of the adolescent must be considered when one is treating obesity. For those teens still experiencing growth, yet falling between the 85th and 95th percentiles for BMI with no accompanying medical complications, the goal of treatment is weight maintenance.

Before nutritional interventions are considered in any situation, the provider must seek to understand how satisfied the adolescent is with his or her own body size. Is the adolescent concerned about weight? Interested in losing or gaining weight? Is there a family health history of diabetes, heart disease, or elevated cholesterol? What methods has the adolescent tried in the past to gain or lose weight? Nutritional education will not succeed unless an adolescent feels positive about the goals. Changes that are introduced slowly and in small increments are more likely to be adapted and maintained. Parents need to be involved in the education and should be encouraged to be supportive rather than intrusive about nutritional issues.

For adequate strength and fitness, adolescents must have some form of regular exercise. Fortunately, many adolescents are involved in organized athletics. Assessment of activity level should include the amount of time spent watching television and playing computer and video games. Fitness goals should aim toward 30 minutes of physical activity daily. Helping teens discover a variety of activities that they enjoy aids in making physical fitness a lifetime habit.

Family Planning

Counseling about pregnancy prevention is an essential part of primary health care for adolescents. The messages for pregnancy prevention should be reviewed with all male and female patients at least annually. Providers should encourage postponing sexual involvement and review the risks of sexual activity, including pregnancy, STDs, and the psychologic sequelae.

The decision for an adolescent to abstain from sexual activity is supported by various factors. Individual protective factors include orientation toward the future and goals, higher intellectual attainment, and minimal engagement in other risk behaviors. One of the most important protective factors in the peer group is the perception that peers are abstaining from sexual intercourse. Pro-social norms among the peer group and the delay of nongroup dating also delay the age of onset of sexual activity. Family characteristics that increase the likelihood that the adolescent will postpone sexual involvement include monitoring by parents and higher socioeconomic status. Adolescents with a sense of connectedness to their school, separate from academic achievement, are also more likely to postpone sexual involvement. The care provider should conduct a careful assessment of the adolescent's protective factors, intentions for engaging in sexual activity, and sexual experience. This knowledge allows the provider to tailor interventions and educational messages appropriately.

Improved access to contraceptive methods could have an effect on decreasing the more than 1 million pregnancies in the 15- to 19-year age group. Professionals providing primary health care to teens must be familiar with the methods of contraception available. Teens require time and targeted health information counseling to choose the appropriate method for themselves. Frequent follow-up and continued education also helps teens become effective users of contraception.

Discussions about sexuality need to take place in a confidential setting, and there are currently no states with statutes prohibiting the dispensing of contraceptive methods to teens without parental notification. However, this is not meant to preclude the inclusion of parents in discussions of contraceptive choice and compliance with a method. Adolescents are more likely to use a method consistently when parental support of the decision to use contraception is present. Encouraging the teen to involve parents in this decision can facilitate open communication within the family.

A thorough understanding of the adolescent's medical, sexual, and social history is necessary to assist the adolescent in choosing a contraceptive method that is right for her. Box 20-1 provides an outline of the information to obtain at the contraceptive-counseling appointment. A discussion of the adolescent's opinion of the pros and cons of each method assists in dispelling myths and helps determine the right method for the current situation. The clinician should provide accurate unbiased information about the benefits and risks, effectiveness, and return to fertility for each contraceptive method (Table 20-4).

After a method is chosen, careful education about the use, expected side effects, and noncontraceptive benefits of the method must be reviewed. Whenever possible, parents should be included in the teaching. Clear oral instructions with a demonstration with the actual methods enhances learning; written instructions and a contact phone number should be given for future questions. When hormonal methods are chosen, condom use is always included for STD prevention. Frequent follow-up evaluation with a review of any side effects,

a review of usage patterns, and an opportunity to voice concerns increases the likelihood an adolescent will continue to use effective contraception.

The physical examination should include a general examination with measurement of blood pressure, as well as a pelvic examination. Ideally the pelvic examination is a part of preventive health care and does not present a barrier to obtaining contraception. Care providers should make every effort to decrease the anxiety associated with the pelvic examination. A careful explanation of the procedure, the presence of a supportive person, and the use of relaxation techniques can help. Every effort should be made to give the adolescent as much control as possible, including postponing the examination until another visit without withholding administration of a contraceptive method.

Sexually Transmitted Diseases

STDs are prevalent among sexually active adolescents, and there are many explanations for these high rates of occurrence. Behavioral causes include early age of onset of sexual intercourse, low rates of condom use, and multiple lifetime partners. Physiologic causes include the fact that adolescent females have an extension of the columnar epithelium to the exocervix, resulting in a large cervical ectropion. Adolescents also lack knowledge of symptoms and transmission routes of diseases and underestimate their own degree of risk.

Asymptomatic infections are common among adolescents, with as many as one third of affected patients having no symptoms. Screening should begin with a review of symptoms including dysuria, vaginal or penile discharge, genital lesions, odor, and change in menstrual bleeding. STD assessment should be conducted with each change in sexual partners or at least annually. Treatment for each of STD is summarized in Table 20-5.

Chlamydiosis is the most common bacterial STD in the United States. The sequelae of untreated chlamydial infections include pelvic inflammatory disease (PID), ectopic pregnancy, epididymitis, and infertility. Infants born to infected mothers may be born prematurely and develop conjunctivitis and pneumonia. The incidence of asymptomatic chlamydial infections is as high as 50% in men and 75% in women. The diagnosis is confirmed in females by endocervical cultures, rapid antigen tests, or polymerase chain reaction (PCR) or ligase chain reaction (LCR) tests. Table 20-6 provides specificity and sensitivity data on available tests for chlamydia. Diagnosis of urethritis in males can be made with the use of leukocyte esterase activity in a urine specimen. Identification of the pathogen is made with a cell culture or a PCR or LCR test from urethral or urine specimens. Sexual partners should be treated, and affected teens should abstain from sexual intercourse for 7 days after treatment.

Gonorrhea may also have a wide range of presentations and is often asymptomatic. Gonorrhea often appears simultaneously with chlamydiosis. Urethritis is the most common finding in males and occurs about 1 week after exposure, beginning with dysuria and a mucoid discharge. Gonococcal cervicitis is often asymptomatic in females, but a patient may have vaginal discharge, dysuria, urinary frequency, or pain with sexual intercourse. Diagnosis is made by culture from the urethra (in males) or the cervix (in females). Urine leukocyte esterase analysis (for males) and PCR and LCR techniques as outlined for chlamydiosis may also be used. Sexual

---

Box 20-1   Contraception Assessment

Health History

Current health status and any chronic illness
History of venous thromboembolism
History of migraines
Current medications
Age at menarche
Menstrual history, including date of last menstrual period
Dysmenorrhea
Pregnancy history
Family history of stroke, venous thromboembolism, and bleeding disorders

Contraception History

Previous methods, including satisfaction and reason for discontinuation
Concerns and beliefs about the risks and effectiveness of various methods

Sexual History

Range of sexual activity, including frequency
Current condom usage
Partner involvement in contraceptive choice
Motivation to prevent pregnancy
Parental awareness and involvement in contraception decision-making

Other Factors

Financial prohibition
Accessibility to care provider
Future childbearing plans
Need for contraceptive privacy

Table 20-4 Contraceptive Methods

METHOD	MECHANISM OF ACTION	ADVANTAGES	DISADVANTAGES	ANTICIPATORY GUIDANCE
Abstinence	No vaginal penetration with penis. Completely (100%) effective	Increased popularity among adolescents. No risk for pregnancy or STDs	Perceptions of peer sexual activity may stigmatize	Discuss at all visits. Promote refusal skills. Encourage parental discussion and reinforcement.
Withdrawal (coitus interruptus)	Withdrawal of penis from vagina before ejaculation. Pregnancy rate among typical users: 19%	No monetary cost. No devices or chemicals. Available in any situation. No medical side effects	No protection from STDs. Unforgiving with incorrect use. Requires self-control and self-awareness on the part of the male	Support attempts to avoid pregnancy. Advise on more effective methods. Review the availability of emergency contraception if ejaculation in the vagina occurs.
Fertility awareness	Identification of days each menstrual cycle when intercourse is most likely to result in pregnancy. Couples either abstain or use withdrawal or barrier methods during fertile times. Pregnancy rate among typical users: 25%	Increases user's knowledge of reproductive potential. Minimal cost	Risk for STD transmission. Adolescent females often have irregular cycles. Complicated. Limits spontaneity	Teach how to observe, chart, and interpret fertility signs in the female. Review barrier methods.
Condoms	Male—A thin sheath placed over the penis to act as a physical barrier to block the passage of semen. Female—A polyurethane sheath that lines the vagina to block the passage of semen. Pregnancy rate among typical users: 14% male condom, 21% female	Inexpensive (female condom more expensive). No hormonal influence. Rare side effects. Easily available. STD protection	Reduced sensitivity. Limits spontaneity. May be embarrassing to buy. Female condom noisy and may be complicated to insert	Demonstrate condom application. Do not recommend oil-based lubricants. Roleplay techniques for negotiation. Review emergency contraception. Encourage use with all methods. Advise that male and female condom should not be used together.
Spermicides	A chemical barrier inserted into the vagina before sexual intercourse. Pregnancy rate among typical users: 5% to 50%	Readily available. Some STD protection. Rare side effects. Provide lubrication during intercourse	Limits spontaneity. Skin irritation may develop. Messy	Advise use as a backup with condoms. Demonstrate the different products available.
Diaphragm	A dome-shaped rubber cup with a flexible rim that is coated with spermicide and inserted into the vagina to provide a protective barrier over the cervix. Pregnancy rate among typical users: 20%	No systemic side effects. Decreased rates of cervical cancer	Increased rates of urinary tract infections. Requires a health visit for fitting. Female must be comfortable with touching herself. Limits spontaneity	Practice insertion and removal in the office. Advise the female return for a new fitting if weight fluctuates by 10 pounds and postpartum. Advise to check the diaphragm for holes before each use. Advise the female to leave the diaphragm in place for at least 6 hours after intercourse and apply more spermicide if having intercourse more than once during that time.
Combination oral contraceptive pills (OCPs)	Prevents pregnancy by suppressing ovulation, thickening cervical mucus, and thinning the endometrial lining. Pregnancy rate among typical users: 5%	Very effective when taken correctly. Well-studied method with minimal risk in the adolescent age group. Noncontraceptive benefits include decreased acne, menstrual regulation, and decreased dysmenorrhea. Decreased risk of PID	Hormonal changes. Expensive. Require office visit and prescription. Nausea. Daily involvement	Review use with the pill pack present, including how to make up missed pills. Review potential side effects. Provide reassurance regarding the cancer risk. Help an adolescent develop daily pill routine. Recommend frequent visits. Encourage taking with food to decrease nausea. Encourage condom use.

Continued

Table 20-4 Contraceptive Methods—cont'd

METHOD	MECHANISM OF ACTION	ADVANTAGES	DISADVANTAGES	ANTICIPATORY GUIDANCE
Progestin-only OCPs	Prevent pregnancy by thickening cervical mucus and inhibiting ovulation. Pregnancy rate among typical users: 5%	No estrogen complications. Immediately reversible. Noncontraceptive benefits include menstrual regulation, less heavy bleeding, and decreased dysmenorrhea	No STD protection. No STD protection. Hormonal changes. Expensive. Require office visit and prescription	Review use with the pill pack present, including how to make up missed pills. Remember to consider for estrogen-sensitive adolescents. Reinforce strict compliance for maximum effectiveness. Encourage condom use. Recommend frequent visits.
Emergency contraceptive pills (ECPs)	Regimen of combined or progestin-only OCPs administered within 72 hours of sexual intercourse to prevent implantation if fertilization were to occur. Pregnancy rate among typical users: 20% to 25%	May be used as a backup method for condom breakage or slippage of the diaphragm, or for unprotected intercourse. Easy to use	Requires prescription. No STD protection. Nausea with some regimens. Change in next menses	Review availability as part of routine contraceptive counseling. Recommend a return for pregnancy testing if menses does not resume. Explain mechanism of action.
Depo-Provera	Injectable progestin-only contraceptive method that inhibits ovulation, thins endometrial lining and thickens cervical mucus. Injection given every 12 to 14 weeks. Pregnancy rate among typical users: 0.3%	Use is separate from act of intercourse. No estrogen complications. Scanty or no menses. Effective long-term contraceptive method	No STD protection. Requires visit and injection every 12 weeks. Expensive. Change in menstrual pattern. Weight gain. Decreased libido. Bone density decrease	Carefully review side effects and prolonged effects after discontinuation. Encourage condom use. Review the possibility of fertility delay after discontinuation.
Combination contraceptive injection Lunelle	Monthly injectable combination hormonal contraceptive that prevents ovulation, thins endometrial lining and thickens cervical mucus. Pregnancy rate among typical users: 0.2%	Rapid return to ovulation after discontinuation. Use is separate from act of intercourse. Regular menstrual patterns and decreased menstrual cramping	Monthly injection. No STD protection	Review the importance of keeping follow-up appointments on time. Encourage condom use.
Norplant	Levonorgesterol implants inserted beneath the skin in the upper arm, preventing ovulation in at least half the cycles, thickening cervical mucus, and thinning the endometrial lining. Pregnancy rate among typical users: 0.05%	No estrogen effects. Use is separate from act of intercourse. Immediate return to fertility at removal. Provides 5 years of pregnancy protection	Expensive. Nausea. Breast tenderness. Expensive. Requires clinician insertion and removal. Bleeding pattern changes. Weight gain. No STD protection. Removal may be difficult	Careful counseling before insertion. Encourage condom use.
Intrauterine device (IUD)	Copper IUDs prevents sperm from meeting ovum and prevents implantation. Progestin IUDs have a hormonal action that thickening cervical mucus, thinning the endometrial lining. Pregnancy rate among typical users: copper 0.8%; progestin 2.0%	Progestin IUDs decrease menstrual blood loss. Easy to use after insertion. Use is separate from act of intercourse. No systemic side effects	Risk of spontaneous expulsion. Requires office visit for insertion and removal. Risk of infection at time of insertion. Change in menstrual patterns. Dysmenorrhea with copper IUD. No STD protection	Careful selection of candidates for the method, including being in a monogamous relationship. Teach an adolescent to check for the presence of the strings. Encourage condom use. See patients with complaints of abdominal pain immediately.

Table 20-5 Treatment Guidelines for Sexually Transmitted Diseases

DIAGNOSIS	PRIMARY TREATMENT	ALTERNATIVE TREATMENTS
Chlamydiosis	Azithromycin 1 g PO as single dose OR doxycycline 100 mg PO bid for 7 days	Erythromycin base 500 mg PO qid for 7 days OR erythromycin ethylsuccinate 800 mg PO qid for 7 days OR ofloxacin 300 mg bid for 7 days
Gonorrhea	Cefixime 400 mg PO single dose Ceftriaxone 125 mg IM single dose OR ciprofloxacin 500 mg PO single dose (at > 18 years old) OR ofloxacin 400 mg PO single dose (at > 18 years old) PLUS azithromycin 1 g PO as single dose OR doxycycline 100 mg PO bid for 7 days	Spectinomycin 2 g IM single dose Ceftizoxime 500 mg IM single dose Lomefloxacin 400 mg PO single dose (at > 18 years old) PLUS azithromycin 1 g PO as single dose OR doxycycline 100 mg PO bid for 7 days
Trichomoniasis	Metronidazole 2 g PO in single dose	Metronidazole 500 mg PO bid for 7 days
Human papilloma virus	Patient applied: • Podofilox 0.5% solution bid for 3 days, then repeat after 4 days • Imiquimod 5% cream for 3 days a week for 16 weeks Provider applied: • Cryotherapy with liquid nitrogen every 1 to 2 weeks • Podophyllin resin 10% to 25% in benzoin weekly • TCA or BCA 80% to 90% weekly	Intralesional interferon Laser surgery
Herpes	First outbreak—Acyclovir 400 mg PO tid for 7 to 10 days OR acyclovir 200 mg PO five times daily for 7 to 10 days OR famciclovir 250 mg PO tid for 7 to 10 days OR valacyclovir 1 g bid for 7 to 10 days Recurrent—Acyclovir 400 mg PO tid for 5 days OR acyclovir 200 mg PO five times a day for 5 days OR acyclovir 800 mg PO bid for 5 days OR famciclovir 125 mg PO bid for 5 days OR valacyclovir 500 mg PO bid for 5 days Daily suppression—Treat for 1 year, then discontinue, with acyclovir 400 mg PO bid OR famciclovir 250 mg PO bid OR valacyclovir 250 mg PO bid OR valacyclovir 500 mg PO daily OR valacyclovir 1000 mg PO daily	None
Syphilis	Benzathine penicillin G at 2.4 million units IM single dose Latent and tertiary syphilis—Benzathine penicillin G at 7.2 million units IM in three 2.4 million unit doses IM at 1-week intervals	For patients with penicillin allergies— Doxycycline 100 mg PO bid for 2 weeks OR Tetracycline 500 mg PO qid for 2 weeks

From *Centers for Disease Control and Prevention. (1997). 1998 Guidelines for treatment of sexually transmitted diseases.* Morbidity and Mortality Weekly Report, 47 (RR-1), 1-118.
BCA, *Bichloroacetic acid;* Bid, *twice a day;* IM, *intramuscular;* PO, *by mouth;* qid, *four times a day;* TCA, *trichloroacetic acid;* tid, *three times a day.*

partners must be treated for both gonorrhea and chlamydiosis, with abstinence from sexual intercourse for 7 days after treatment.

Trichomoniasis is caused by a protozoon and often accompanies other infections. Symptoms include a malodorous frothy vaginal discharge, pruritus, dysuria, painful sexual intercourse, and menstrual bleeding changes. The diagnosis is made in females by visualization of the flagellated protozoa from saline wet prep examinations. Sexual partners are treated, with abstinence from sexual intercourse for 48 hours after treatment.

Human papillomavirus (HPV) is the most common sexually transmitted infection in the female genital tract. HPV may remain asymptomatic, or it may show an exophytic condyloma on the genitals or cervical dysplasia and carcinoma. The HPV that infects the genital tract has been divided into low– and

Table 20-6 Sensitivity and Specificity for Chlamydiosis Tests

TEST	SENSITIVITY	SPECIFICITY
Culture	70% to 85%	100%
LCR/PCR	99%	90%
DNA Probe	65% to 72%	97%

high–oncogenic risk categories. Types 6 and 11 are categorized as low risk. Types 16, 18, 31, 45, and 56 are classified as high risk and are associated with high-grade cervical changes and invasive carcinomas of the anus, cervix, and penis. Annual Papanicolaou (Pap) smear screening is essential for sexually active adolescent females to detect the presence of cervical cell changes. Deoxyribonucleic acid (DNA) testing for HPV is becoming more widely used to assist with identification of high-risk categories. Patients with warts or cervical dysplasia should be counseled that they may infect sexual partners. Female partners should receive a Pap smear if she is sexually active with a male partner with warts.

The incidence of genital herpes infections has increased in the United States. Symptomatic patients are the most infectious, but asymptomatic people also shed the virus and transmit the herpes virus. The ulcers are painful and occur at the site of infection. There may be burning, dysuria, inguinal lymphadenopathy, and urinary retention. Rectal infections may cause anal discharge, pain, and tenesmus. Systemic symptoms of headache, fever, myalgia, and malaise often accompany the primary herpes simplex virus (HSV) outbreak; the symptoms with recurrent HSV are usually less severe and of shorter duration. A clinical diagnosis is made based on the appearance of tender vesicles, pustules, or ulcers, and HSV can be cultured from the lesions.

Syphilis has variable incidence rates from nearly none to high rates in certain geographic areas of the United States. Screening protocols are based on the incidence in the area. Syphilis causes painless genital ulcers, which increases the risk of acquiring HIV infection. Dark-field examination of exudates from the lesion give a definitive diagnosis in early syphilis. The lesion will spontaneously resolve, and the second stage of syphilis is a generalized maculopapular rash. A serum rapid plasma reagin (RPR) test will show a positive result at this stage. Latent syphilis occurs when the disease is hidden but still sexually transmissible. The late stage of syphilis results in neurologic and cardiovascular changes from vasculitis. Treatment is effective in eradicating the bacteria at any stage of syphilis. The state health department performs careful notification of contacts.

Human immunodeficiency virus (HIV) is discussed in detail in Chapter 45. Adolescents account for a small number of acquired immune deficiency syndrome (AIDS) cases in the United States, but many of the adult infections are acquired during the adolescent period. HIV testing should be considered for all sexually active adolescents, especially those who have other STDs, are pregnant, express concern about HIV infection, and use or have partners who use intravenous drugs.

Issues for Parents

Fortunately, most teens pass through adolescence without great conflict and turmoil within the family. However, parenting a teenager does present new challenges as the teen begins to develop identity and autonomy. The period of adolescence is much harder on parents than it is on teens. As adolescents develop the ability for abstract thought, they begin to question and challenge their parents, and parents and teens interpret these discussions very differently. Parents often view the discussion as a matter of moral codes of right and wrong. Teens walk away from the same argument viewing the issue as a matter of personal choice. Parents feel that the basic values they have tried to instill in the adolescent have been violated; the adolescent leaves the discussion with far less meaning and turmoil related to the outcome. Health care providers play an important role in supporting parents through this exciting and daunting period of family development.

Setting Limits

Parents are responsible for trying to build their child's sense of confidence and security. Without trust, an adolescent cannot build confidence. When a family gets into a cycle of not trusting, the result is distance between the parents and child. A wide gap between children and their parents allows opportunities for outside forces to fill these spaces, and these outside forces may be a harmful peer group or experimentation with drugs or alcohol. To maintain trust, teens need clear boundaries and limits. The consequences for breaking the rules must be realistic and consistently applied. Health care providers should encourage and support parents' efforts to monitor their child's activities and set reasonable limits.

Driving

Adolescents see the driver's license as an important rite of passage into adulthood, but the inexperience of young drivers puts them at incredible risk. Motor vehicle crashes (MVCs) are the leading cause of death among those 15 to 20 years old in the United States. Even more frightening is that the injury rate is nine times the death rate. Nighttime driving, transporting passengers, and drinking and driving are high-risk driving circumstances. Adolescents 16 and 17 years old are more likely to have a fatal crash when transporting male passengers, teen passengers, and passengers 20 to 29 years of age.

Driving is a complex skill that takes time and practice to master, and some states have instituted graduated licensing procedures to allow for time and supervision to learn these skills. Parents can be encouraged to limit teen access to these driving conditions. Parents should also be advised to place limits on adolescent opportunities to ride with other teen drivers. Parents are encouraged to discuss calling for a ride when an adolescent is intoxicated or scheduled to ride with a friend who becomes intoxicated, and some advocate a "no questions asked" policy for rides in such situations.

Sexuality

Effective sexuality counseling is tailored to the developmental level of the adolescent. Parents have varying levels of comfort and skill at discussing sexuality with their children. Strengthening family function and communication serves to protect the adolescent from harm. Ideally, developmentally appropriate discussions of sexuality issues at home have started before the adolescent years, but parents may need encouragement to move past their own uneasiness and start talking about uncomfortable subjects.

During the pubertal changes, preteens (9 to 12 years of age) are interested in the physical changes happening to their bodies. They are keenly concerned with the variability of penis, testicle, and breast size as they seek the answer to the question, "Am I normal?" Preteens seek information about menstruation, nocturnal emissions, birth, and pregnancy. In terms of interpersonal relationships, early adolescents are concerned with their changing role and relationships within the family, their changing feelings toward others, and heterosexual and homosexual feelings.

Early adolescents (11 to 14 years of age) have more complex questions about physical changes, emotional issues, and sexual behavior. Parental discussion of sexual activity should not be limited to values related to engaging in sexual intercourse but should include the range of noncoital behavior and intentions to engage in sexual activity. Young teens benefit from clarification of misconceptions about sexuality, contraception, and STDs. Discussion topics include tolerance, individual respect, and dealing with coercion.

Middle adolescents (15 to17 years of age) benefit from more detailed and deeper discussion of sexual topics. This is a time of significant symbolic movement away from the home environment and strong reliance on peers. The adolescents' perception of their peer group's sexual activity and condom use influences their behavior. Parents and health care providers can provide support for decisions to postpone sexual involvement and provide factual information about pregnancy and STD prevention; adolescents lack information about prevalence, signs and symptoms of STDs, and the incidence of asymptomatic infections.

Late adolescents (18 to 21 years of age) have essentially resolved the issues of emancipation from parents. Interpersonal relationships are based on mutual interests and traits versus peer norms and acceptance. Gay and lesbian teens have often clarified and identified their sexual orientation and begun to incorporate their sexual identity into a positive self-image. Discussion topics include issues of trust and commitment within relationships, satisfaction with sexual activity, dating violence, and the social and psychologic context in which sex occurs.

Special Circumstances

Piercing and Tattooing

The skin is providing another battleground for tensions between adolescents and their parents. Adolescents often view adornment with tattoos and piercings as beautification, whereas parents see opposition and confrontation of authority. The battle is really another struggle for separation from the family. Body art can fill the need for autonomy by singling out an adolescent as unique. Some adolescents also use the negative reaction from adults as a means to keep people at bay, serving as a "keep out" sign. The permanence of a tattoo can allow grounding and a sense of control over an adolescent's rapidly changing body and life.

States are responsible for regulations about tattoos; most states require parental consent for anyone less than 18 years of age to receive one. The health risks for tattooing are minimal if performed under sterile conditions, and no association has been found between viral hepatitis transmission and tattooing. However, the risk for any infection is increased with amateur artists, the source of nearly half of adolescent tattoos. The dyes used pose a risk for allergic reaction, with red and yellow dye being the most allergenic.

Anticipatory guidance for an adolescent considering a tattoo should include considerations about the permanence of the decision, finding a reliable tattoo artist, and aftercare to prevent infection. The new tattoo is cared for as a skin abrasion, with maintenance of a moist protective barrier with antibiotic ointment until healed.

The advent of laser technology has aided in the effective removal of unwanted tattoos. Amateur tattoos generally contain less ink and are therefore easier to remove than those placed by professionals. Multiple treatments are generally needed for complete removal. Scar tissue is often formed when a tattoo is applied and may be more noticeable after the tattoo is removed.

Infection is also a risk with body piercings; infectious agents include *Staphylococcus* and hepatitis B virus, and there have been documented cases of HIV with multiple piercings. The American Red Cross prohibits the donation of blood products for 1 year after a body piercing. Autoclaving has decreased spore formation and the risk for tetanus transmission, and the use of sterile instruments and technique reduces the risk of infection.

Other adverse effects after body piercing include the potential for migration and rejection of the jewelry, especially with naval piercings and those on flat areas such as the chest. If not positioned deeply enough, the jewelry is rejected similar to a splinter. Keloid scar formation and torn tissue are other piercing risks. Allergies to the metals in the jewelry can result in allergic reactions at the piercing site.

Postpiercing care must begin immediately, with twice-a-day cleaning using a mild antibacterial soap until healed. If an infection occurs, the removal of jewelry poses the risk for abscess formation. The infected piercing is treated as a puncture wound, with application of topical antibacterial medications.

Healing times vary with the site of the piercing. Cartilage piercings (e.g., of upper ear, nose cartilage) heal slowly and are prone to infection and scarring. Genital piercings require the use of barrier methods until healed to prevent contact with body fluids. Extra care is needed with condoms to prevent puncture.

A nonjudgmental approach to adolescents with body piercing or tattooing allows more reasonable clinical judgments. Taking the opportunity to explore the thought process behind the decision for body art opens the door to understanding an adolescent and enhancing the provider-patient relationship.

Teen Pregnancy

Incidence

- Nearly 1 million teenage women become pregnant each year, including 10% of all women who are 15 to 19 years of age and 19% of those who have had sexual intercourse.
- Approximately 6 in 10 teen pregnancies occur among those 18 and 19 years of age.
- Approximately 56% of teen pregnancies end in births, 30% in induced abortion, and 14% spontaneous abortion.
- Approximately 1 in 5 infants born to unmarried minors are fathered by men 5 or more years older than the mother.
- Teens account for 31% of all nonmarital births, and 78% of teen mothers are unmarried.
- The United States has the highest rate of teen pregnancy in the industrialized world.
- Teenage women's contraceptive use at first intercourse is 78%; two thirds of these uses are of condoms.
- Approximately 78% of teen pregnancies are unplanned, accounting for one fourth of all accidental pregnancies annually.
- Pregnancy rates are increasing among teens 13 and 14 years of age.
- Approximately 25% of teenage mothers have a second child within 2 years of their first.
- Teens who give birth are more likely to come from poor or low-income families (83%) than teens who have abortions (61%) or teens in general (38%).
- Inadequate prenatal care is received by one third of pregnant teens.

Assessment. The initial evaluation of an adolescent presenting with amenorrhea, a missed menstrual period, or a change in her menstrual pattern must include a urine pregnancy test, even when the adolescent denies sexual intercourse. A low threshold for performing pregnancy testing allows for early identification, timely management, and referral of pregnant adolescents. Ideally, before the test is obtained, the adolescent will have a private discussion with the health care provider to discuss the possibilities of the pregnancy test. The provider should assess whom the adolescent has discussed the possibility of pregnancy with and what she would do if the pregnancy test is positive. A pregnancy test should never be done without the adolescent's knowledge, even when done for "routine" screening (e.g., before initiating contraception, before a surgical procedure).

Reliable urine pregnancy testing is readily available and can be used in the office following clinical laboratory guidelines. The availability of monoclonal antibody testing techniques have made highly sensitive and reliable tests readily available. Qualitative blood pregnancy tests do not have any advantage over immunometric urine tests. Clinical management should not be based on the results of a home pregnancy test.

If the pregnancy test is positive, the adolescent should be told privately. After informing her of the result, the practitioner should elicit a reaction and allow her time to process the results. An unbiased discussion of all available options should be outlined for each adolescent. Options counseling includes discussion of the adolescent's choice to continue the pregnancy and parent the child, to continue the pregnancy and put the child up for adoption, or to have a medical or surgical abortion. The adolescent needs information regarding state laws for parental notification and consent for abortion. This is often the first time an adolescent is faced with such an important deci-

sion; she will need time and support to make the best decision for her situation. The provider should voice unconditional support of the adolescent no matter what choice she makes. The adolescent should be encouraged to discuss the options with her support system and not be encouraged to make a decision at the initial visit. Assistance in notifying a parent or guardian should also be offered at the time of diagnosis but rarely is required at the initial assessment. Box 20-2 provides an outline of assessment questions at the time of a pregnancy diagnosis.

Physical examination begins with palpation of the abdomen. At 11 or 12 weeks of gestation, the uterus is palpable at the pubic symphysis. A pelvic examination is performed to confirm that the pregnancy is in the uterus and to correlate the uterine size with the date of the last menstrual period. Experienced clinicians can recognize enlargement of the uterus by 8 weeks of gestation. Screening tests for STDs are obtained. No matter what choice the adolescent ultimately will make, prenatal vitamins should be started at this time. Nutritional deficits for pregnant adolescents can have consequences for both the adolescent and the developing fetus; there is competition for nutrients between the fetus and the adolescent, especially when pregnancy occurs near the time of menarche. Abstinence from drugs, alcohol, and tobacco should be encouraged.

Unless emergent care is needed for abnormal bleeding or abdominal pain, phone or office follow-up evaluation within 5 to 7 days is necessary to further discuss options and assist with referral for the appropriate care. Follow-up should continue until there is successful referral and appropriate social support is in place. Adolescents seeking prenatal care should be referred to comprehensive adolescent pregnancy programs whenever possible. Teens with prenatal care in comprehensive adolescent programs have better outcomes than those in more traditional prenatal care programs.

Parenting Adolescents

Parenting adolescents and their children are at high risk for poor social and educational attainment. A young mother is at especially high risk to drop out of high school and to live as an impoverished single parent. However, recent longitudinal studies do offer hope, with demonstration of gradual improvement in the mother's educational and economic achievement over time.

Adolescents who postpone the birth of a second child have improved outcomes for themselves and the child. Adolescent mothers require continuous monitoring of contraceptive use, and those who use long-acting contraceptives have much lower rates of repeat pregnancy within 2 years than those who use short-acting contraceptives. Younger adolescent mothers are at particular risk for repeat pregnancy and require close health supervision and fortification of their social supports.

Children of teen parents are at increased risk of low birth weight, neurodevelopmental delay, and death before 1 year of age. As they grow older, they have higher rates of educational underachievement, inadequate health care, behavioral problems, and a greater likelihood of becoming teen parents themselves. The health care provider can assist teen parents by encouraging increased verbal stimulation of the child, teaching methods to handle aggressive behavior and avoid abuse, promoting normal developmental growth and developmental milestones of the infant or child, and reinforcing the social support network of the parents.

Box 20-2 Assessment of the Pregnant Teenager

Social History

Who do you live with currently?

Have you considered the possibility of pregnancy?

Have you thought about what you would do if you were pregnant?

With whom have you discussed the possibility of pregnancy?

How do you think your parent or guardian will react to the news that you are pregnant?

Who do you normally talk to about personal things?

What is your relationship with the father of this baby?

What is your history of substance use, including tobacco?

What is your history of physical and sexual abuse?

Medical and Gynecologic History

What is your current health status, including any chronic illnesses or infectious disease exposures?

When was your last normal menstrual period?

Have you had any breakthrough bleeding?

Have you had any symptoms of pregnancy, including breast tenderness, fatigue, nausea, and frequent urination?

Have you had any abdominal pain?

Are there any symptoms of a urinary tract infection?

Are you taking any medication?

Were you using a method to prevent pregnancy?

Have you ever been pregnant before? What was the outcome?

Have you ever had a sexually transmitted disease?

Have you ever had a pelvic inflammatory disease?

Have you had abdominal or pelvic surgery?

Gay, Lesbian, Bisexual, and Transgender Youths

The way in which sexual identity is developed is not clearly understood; it is most likely a combination of multiple intrinsic and extrinsic factors. Most gay, lesbian, bisexual, and transgender youths become aware of their sexual orientation during early adolescence; however, they often deny this discovery for a variety of internal and external reasons. For most teens, adolescence is a time of clarification of sexual identity and roles. However, homosexual youths often spend their adolescence concealing large areas of their sexual identity from themselves and others. This struggle can result in lower self-esteem and a sense of worthlessness. The fear of discovery can lead to social isolation and a profound sense of loneliness.

Gay, lesbian, bisexual, and transgender youths are at high risk in multiple areas. Suicide is the number-one cause of death among gay youths, with attempt rates much higher than completion rates. Gay youths are also at risk as victims of violence within both their family and within their society. Homosexual and bisexual youths are at higher risk for substance abuse, sexual risk-taking (leading to unplanned pregnancy and STD acquisition), school failure, and running away than their heterosexual peers.

The issues for transgender youths have not been well studied, but these young people are probably at even higher risk. Youths who live outside the societal gender norms are identified as *transgender*. This may include wearing clothes not traditionally associated with one's own gender, displaying an outward appearance that is androgynous, or surgically altering the body to change gender. Transgender youths may self-identify as gay, lesbian, or bisexual.

Health care providers often avoid the subject of sexual orientation because of a lack of comfort and training. Assurances of confidentiality and inclusive language are vital for open discussions about sexuality. When discussing sexual identity, the conversation should not be limited to sexual experience but include sexual desires and self-perception. Homosexual youths may have never had a same-sex sexual encounter but may still recognize that their sexual attractions and fantasies are toward persons of the same gender.

Confidentiality is an important issue for homosexual youths, and coming out to parents is a huge concern. It is not always advisable for youths to disclose their sexual orientation. The official stance of Parents, Friends, and Families of Lesbians and Gays (P-Flag) is that youths should not come out to parents until they are financially independent or unless they are absolutely sure that their family will be accepting.

The ability of health care providers to recognize gay, lesbian, bisexual, and transgender youths as a minority group at high risk and with special health concerns will help in meeting their needs. An accepting health care provider can provide a safe haven for discussions about the realities of dealing with a secret life and about safety issues in today's homophobic society. Information should be shared about how to foster a positive gay relationship for youths who lack positive role models in their lives. Health education for gay and lesbian youths includes STD and HIV prevention, pregnancy prevention, the risk factors of substance use, and the availability of local peer support groups.

Runaway and Homeless Youths

The exact number of runaway and homeless youths in the United States is unknown, with estimates ranging anywhere from 500,000 to 2 million young people. Homeless youths include those abandoned by their parents, as well as others who have left home with parental knowledge. Homeless and runaway youths often live with little or no connection with family or caregivers. Approximately 1 in 12 come into contact with the shelter systems for homeless and runaway youths; others remain on the streets and are referred to as "street youths."

Family problems forcing an adolescent to leave home are long standing. Causes of adolescent homelessness include parental neglect, physical and sexual abuse, family substance abuse, and family violence. This long-standing family dysfunction results in youths without a sense of connectedness to adults and society in general. School failure often predates the departure from home and can usually be traced to the early school years.

Homeless youths often live in high-risk environments both before and after leaving their family. Health problems of homeless youths include high rates of hepatitis, respiratory problems (e.g., asthma, pneumonia), scabies, STDs, injury, depression, and suicidal tendencies and attempts. Homeless youths who are homosexual have much higher rates of depression and suicide.

Sexual risk-taking is high among homeless and runaway youths. High-risk sexual behaviors include multiple partners, casual partners, infrequent condom use, and early age of sexual initiation. A nationally representative sample of homeless youths reports high rates of survival sex (the exchange of sex for shelter, food, drugs, or money). One study found rates of survival sex at 27.5% for street youths and 9.5% for shelter youths. The HIV rate among homeless and runaway youths in the United States is estimated to be 2.3%.

Pregnancy rates are also high for homeless youths. National samples find self-reported pregnancy rates of 50% for street youths and 30% for shelter youths. The pregnancy rates are high no matter how long a young woman has been out of the home, and pregnancy may be what keeps the youth from returning to her home or may be the reason she left.

There are many barriers to health care for homeless youths, including consent and confidentiality, distrust of adults and community systems, lack of knowledge of available services, denial of the need for care, payment issues, transportation issues, and fears related to immigration status. Most homeless youths receive sick care only in area emergency departments.

When providing health care to homeless youths, confidentiality is crucial. Establishing trust is particularly challenging and vital for optimal care. The health care provider must be cognizant of the youth's perception of health problems and prioritize care in concurrence with the youth. An adolescent must have basic survival issues addressed before education regarding long-term health risk reduction begins. For example, safety and violence must be taken into consideration when one is discussing condom use, because adolescents having survival sex may put themselves at risk of injury if a condom is required.

Resources

Publications

Emans, S.J., Laufer, M.R., & Goldstein, D. (1998). *Pediatric and adolescent gynecology* (4th ed.). New York: Lippincott-Raven.

Friedman, S.B., Fisher, M.M., Schonberg, S.K., & Alderman, E.M. (1998). *Comprehensive adolescent health care* (2nd ed.). St. Louis: Mosby.

Hatcher, R.A., Trussell, J., Cates, W., Stewart, G.K., Guest, F., & Kowal, D. (1998). *Contraceptive technology* (17th ed.). New York: Ardent Media.

Lieberman, J.M. (2001). Varicella vaccine: What have we learned? *Contemporary Pediatrics, 18*(1), 50-60.

Lowinson, J.H., Ruis, P., & Millman, R.B. (1992) Substance abuse: A comprehensive textbook (2nd ed.). Baltimore: Williams & Wilkins.

McAnarney, E.R., Kriepe, R.E., Orr, D.P., & Comerci, G.D. (1992). *Textbook of Adolescent Medicine.* Philadelphia: W.B. Saunders.

Neinstein, L.S. (1996). *Adolescent health care: A practical guide* (3rd ed.). Baltimore: Williams & Wilkins.

Rikert, V.I. (1996). *Adolescent Nutrition Assessment and Management.* New York: Chapman & Hall.

Slap, G.S., Jablow, M.M., Spock, B., & McCarthy, P. (1994). *Teenage health care: The first comprehensive guide for the pre teen to young adult years.* New York: Pocket Books.

Speroff, L., Glass, R.H., & Kase, N.G. (1999). *Clinical gynecology, endocrinology and infertility* (6th ed.). Baltimore: Williams & Wilkins.

Websites

Adolescent Pregnancy

Alan Guttmacher Institute (www.agi.usa.org)

Association of Reproductive Health Professionals (www.arhp.org)

Directory of Emergency Contraception Providers (www.not-2-late.com)

Gay/Lesbian/Straight Education Network (www.glsen.org)

National Campaign to Prevent Teen Pregnancy (www.teenpregnancy.org)

Parents, Families and Friends of Lesbians and Gays (www.pflag.org)

Drugs/Alcohol

Campaign for Tobacco-Free Kids (www.tobaccofreekids.org)

Legal Issues

Advocates for Youth (www.advocatesforyouth.org)

American Bar Association Center on Children and the Law (www.abanet.org/child/childhl.html)

Statistics

National Center for Health Statistics (www.cdc.gov/nchs)

Bibliography

Allen, D.M., Lehman, J.S., Green, T.L., et al. (1994). HIV infection among homeless adults and runaway youth. US 1989-92. *AIDS,* (8), 1593-1598.

American Academy of Pediatrics. (1998). Counseling the adolescent about pregnancy options. *Pediatrics, 101*(5), 938-940.

American Medical Association. (1977). *Guidelines for adolescent preventive services.* Chicago: American Medical Association.

Bonny, A.E. & Biro, F.M. (1998). Recognizing and treating STDs in the adolescent. *Contemporary Nurse Practitioner, Spring,* 15-24.

Brill, S.R. & Rosenfeld, W.D. (2000). Contraception. *Medical Clinics of North America, 84*(4), 907-925.

Centers for Disease Control and Prevention. (2000). Meningococcal disease and college students: Recommendations of the advisory committee on immunization practices. *Morbidity and Mortality Weekly Report, 49*(RR-7), 11-20.

Centers for Disease Control and Prevention. (1997). 1998 guidelines for treatment of sexually transmitted diseases. *Morbidity and Mortality Weekly Report, 49*(RR-1), 1-118.

Chen, L., Baker, S.P., Braver, E.R., & Li, G. (2000). Carrying passengers as a risk factor for crashes fatal to 16- and 17-year-old drivers. *Journal of the American Medical Association, 283*(12), 1578-1582.

Coard, S.I., Nitz, K., & Felice, M.E. (2000). Repeat pregnancy among urban adolescents: sociodemographic, family, and health factors. *Adolescence, 35*(137), 193-200.

East, J.A., & Rayess, F. E. (1998). Pediatricians' approach to the health care of lesbian, gay and bisexual youth. *Journal of Adolescent Health, 23,* 191-193.

Elster, A.B. & Kuznets, N. J. (1994). *Guidelines for adolescent preventive services.* Baltimore: Williams & Wilkins.

English, A. & Simmons, P.S. (1999). Legal issues in reproductive health care for adolescents. *Adolescence: Medical State of the Art Review, 10*(2), 181-194.

Greene, J.M., Ennett, S.T., & Ringwalt, C.L. (1999). Prevalence and correlates of survival sex among runaway and homeless youth. *American Journal of Public Health, 89*(9), 1406-1409.

Greene, J.M. & Ringwalt, C.L. (1998). Pregnancy among three national samples of runaway and homeless youth. *Journal of Adolescent Health, 23*(6), 370-377.

Grimes, D.A. (2000). STD update: Incidence trends and new screening test. *The Contraception Report, 11*(3), 4-10.

Hennigen, L , Kollar, L.M., & Rosenthal, S.L. (2000). Methods for managing pelvic examination anxiety: Individual differences and relaxation techniques. *Journal of Pediatric Health Care, 14*(1), 9-12.

Koenig, L.M. & Carnes, M. (1999). Body piercing medical concerns with cutting edge fashions. *Journal of General Internal Medicine, 14,* 379-385.

Lenders, C.M., McElrath, T.F., & Scholl, T.O. (2000). Nutrition in adolescent pregnancy. *Current Opinion in Pediatrics, 12*(3), 291-296.

Montgomery, D.F. & Parks, D. (2001). Tattoos: Counseling the adolescent. *Journal of Pediatric Health Care, 15*(1), 14-19.

Nelson, J.A. (1997). Gay, lesbian, and bisexual adolescents: Providing esteem-enhancing care to a battered population. *The Nurse Practitioner, 22*(2), 94-105.

Patel, D.P., Greydanus, D.E., & Rowlett, J.D. (2000). Romance with the automobile in the 20th century: Implications for adolescents in a new millennium. *Adolescence: Medical State of the Art Review, 11*(1), 127-139.

Perkins, K.C. (1997). Adolescent trends in the late 20th century: Fad or social alienation? *West Virginia Medical Journal, 93,* 313-316.

Polaneczky, M. & O'Connor, K. (1999). Pregnancy in the adolescent patient, screening, diagnosis, and initial management. *Pediatric Clinics of North America, 46*(4), 649-670.

Radkowsky, M. & Siegel, L.J. (1997). The gay adolescent: Stressors, adaptations, and psychosocial interventions. *Clinical Pyschology Review, 17*(2), 191-216.

Rieder, J. & Coupey, S.M. (2000, March). Contraceptive compliance personalizing an adolescents plan for effective birth control. *The Female Patient* (Supplement), 12-19.

Rigsby, D.C., Macones, G.A., & Driscoll, D.A. (1998). Risk factors for rapid repeat pregnancy among adolescent mothers: A review of the literature. *Journal of Pediatric and Adolescent Gynecology, 11,* 115-126.

Seitz, V., Rosenbaum, L.K., & Apfel, N.H. (1985). Effects of family support intervention: a ten year follow-up. *Child Development, 56*(2), 376-391.

Sherwood, N.E. (2000). Epidemiology of obesity. *Healthy Generations, 1*(2), 1-3.

Silverman, A.L., Sekhon, J.S., Saginaw, S.J., Wiedbrauk, D., Balasubramaniam, M., & Gordon, S.C. (2000). Tattoo application is not associated with an increased risk for chronic viral hepatitis. *American Journal of Gastroenterology, 95*(5), 1312-1315.

Smoller, J. (1999). Homeless youth in the United States: Description and developmental issues. In Raeffelli, M. & Larson, R.W. (Eds.). *New Directions for Child and Adolescent Development.* Baltimore: Josey Bass.

Steinberg, L. (2000). The family at adolescence: Transition and transformation. *Journal of Adolescent Health, 27,* 170-178.

Stevens, P.E. & Morgan, S. (2001). Healthcare for lesbian, gay, bisexual, and transgender youth. *Journal of Pediatric Health Care, 15*(1), 24-34.

Williams, A.F. (1999). Graduated licensing comes to the United States. *Injury Prevention, 5,* 133-135.

Section 2
Families with Special Parenting Needs

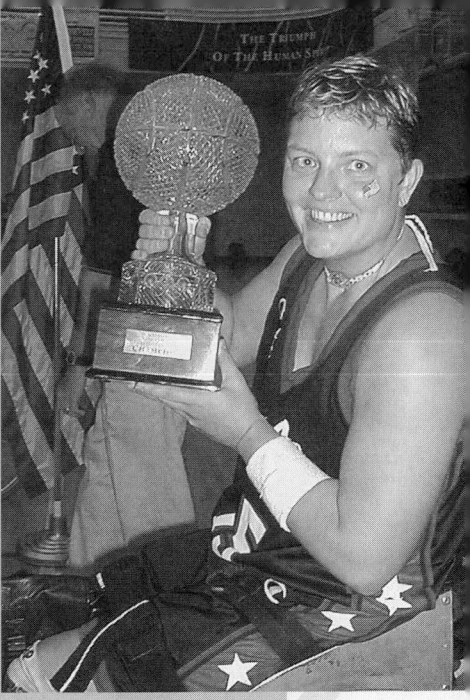

Amy L. Verst, a pediatric nurse practitioner (PNP), exemplifies the "triumph of the human spirit". Amy is a university professor, Olympic athlete, and national presenter. She is known to this readership in particular for her presentations at NAPNAP, Keystone, and other national pediatric symposia and conventions.

Amy's accomplishments are many, but of herself she says only, "I love my job. I love seeing kids, caring for kids, and sharing with students how to care for children and their families. I am also a fierce competitor and enjoy playing all sports, especially basketball."

As Assistant Professor of Pediatric Nursing at Bellarmine University, she serves as a master teacher of pediatric content, and in collaboration with the Louisville Jefferson County Health Department she has developed the role of School Nurse for Southern Middle School. Under Amy's direction, Bellarmine, the Health Department, and the Jefferson County Public School System have supported a program called Fitness Club that has made significant improvement in the physical fitness, attendance, grades, and well-being of its sixth-grade participants.

As a professor, Amy has received University Merit Awards that have recognized her outstanding accomplishments in teaching, scholarship, and service. Her commitment to the Louisville community has resulted in her receiving the esteemed Bell Award for community service, an award given to only 10 Jefferson County and Louisville residents each year. Also, Amy's commitment to the community has gained her recognition from the American Red Cross, the Jefferson County Public School system, and the Coalition for the Homeless.

Besides giving back to her community, which she sees as her civic responsibility, she has participated in numerous summer camps for "special kids." These camps, located all over the United States, have aided children with physical disabilities, cancer, burns, diabetes, and asthma, and their staff have developed sports components at summer camps for girls and boys with physical disabilities.

Another passion for Amy is sports. Amy is certified as an athletic trainer, and she served on the volunteer U.S. Medical Team for the 1996 Olympic Games as an NP and athletic trainer. In addition, she is an elite athlete in her own right. She has rigorously trained for and earned a position on the U.S. Women's Wheelchair Basketball Team. The highlight of her athletic career was the opportunity to represent the United States in Sydney, Australia at the 2000 Paralympic Games. Amy was the co-captain of the team and enjoyed top scorer and top rebounder honors.

Amy's advice for those who ask includes, "When you dream, dream BIG," and "If it is to be, it is up to me."

Jane A. Fox

Chapter 21 *Children with Addicted Parents*

Bonnie Gance-Cleveland

The experience of having a substance-abusing parent has a detrimental effect on children, influencing their physical, psychologic, social, and spiritual development. Furthermore, with the widespread problem of addiction in today's society, significant numbers of children live with substance-abusing parents. Thus nurse practitioners (NPs) are challenged to intervene with this at-risk population.

Besides the devastating effects chemical dependency has on the substance abuser, it is estimated that four to six other lives are also affected by the addiction. The spouse and children of substance abusers are particularly affected by the disease. Black (1982) theorizes (from clinical impressions as a family therapist) that common rules develop in the dysfunctional family that the children learn from an early age. Children are given the message "don't talk," and no one openly discusses the problem of addiction. By the age of 9, the children develop a denial system to cope with the addiction, having learned the rule is not to discuss the real issues. The children also learn "don't trust," discovering very early that they cannot depend on the addictive parent. The children experience many broken promises and disappointments and soon realize that if they don't trust anyone else and rely only on themselves, they will not be disappointed. The denial system is also used to suppress feelings; children learn they can reduce the pain if they "don't feel."

Roles of Children in an Addictive Family

According to Wegscheider-Cruse (1985), the roles of children of addicted parents vary according to their placement within the family.

Oldest Child

An oldest child:
- Is often the hero or "superkid"
- Reverses roles with the parents
- Becomes the caregiver, a role the child is not prepared to perform
- Is a good student and overly responsible
- Is emotionally drained by the role

Second Child

A second child:
- Is often the scapegoat
- Is frequently blamed for all the problems in the family
- Is a poor student and a delinquent
- Is often in trouble at school and with law enforcement

Middle Child

A middle child:
- Is often the lost child
- Avoids the tension in the family by escaping
- Becomes a loner
- Is an average student
- Is quiet, shy, ignored, and careful not to call attention to himself or herself

Youngest Child

A youngest child:
- Often becomes the family mascot
- Uses humor to decrease the tension in the addictive family
- Is a class clown, cheerleader, and "super-cute kid"

Incidence

Substance Abuse in America

- Approximately 105 million Americans (43% of the population) report that they are currently drinkers.
- Binge drinking in the previous 30 days is reported by 45 million people.
- Heavy drinking is reported by 12.4 million people.
- There are 10.5 million adults with symptoms of alcohol dependency.
- About 10% of adult drinkers have problems with substance abuse.
- An illicit drug has been used by 75.5 million adults.

In a 1999 national survey on drug abuse by the Substance Abuse and Mental Health Services Administration:
- Approximately 14.8 million Americans reported current illicit drug use in the previous 30 days.
- Marijuana was the most commonly used illicit drug.
- Approximately 1.5 million Americans reported current cocaine use.
- Current hallucinogen use was reported by 900,000 Americans.
- Current heroin use was reported by 200,000 Americans.

Children of Substance Abusers

- Approximately 76 million Americans have been exposed to alcoholism in their family.
- One out of five Americans report living with an alcoholic parent while growing up.
- It is estimated that 26.8 million children and adults in America have an addicted parent.
- Of the children of alcoholics or addicts, 11 million are under 18 years of age.

- Only 5% of children with addictive parents receive any supportive services.
- It is estimated that there are four to six children with chemically dependent parents in an average classroom of twenty-five students.
- Children with an addicted parent are four to six times more likely to develop a drinking problem.
- A serious drinking problem occurs in one of five adolescents who are children of substance abusers.

Consequences of Addiction

- Approximately 100,000 deaths per year are related to alcohol use.
- In 1995, the economic cost of alcohol or drug abuse was estimated at $276 billion; this includes cost of health care, motor vehicle accidents, crime, and lost productivity.
- Alcohol is a key factor in 68% of manslaughter cases, 62% of assaults, 54% of murders, 48% of robberies, 44% of burglaries, and 41% of motor vehicle fatalities.

Risk Factors

Physical Problems

- Asthma
- Hypertension
- Abdominal pain
- Headaches
- Tics
- Gastrointestinal problems
- Allergies
- Anemia
- Frequent respiratory infections
- Enuresis

Social Problems

- Delinquency
- Rebellion
- Running away
- Social isolation
- Interpersonal problems
- Child abuse
- Child neglect
- Sexual abuse

Emotional Problems

- Chemical dependency
- Eating disorders
- Suicidal behavior
- Depression
- Low self-esteem
- Tension
- Anxiety
- Psychosomatic complaints
- Insomnia
- Nightmares

School Problems

- School difficulties
- Absenteeism
- Tardiness
- Learning disabilities
- Lack of parental support for homework
- Dropping out

Box 21-1 Red Flags: Potential Signs and Consequences of Substance Abuse

Medical Diagnosis of Parents	School Performance
Headaches	Poor student
Back pain	Overachiever
Ulcers	Class clown
Difficulty sleeping	Quiet student

Family Violence	Financial
Spouse abuse	Frequent job changes
Child abuse	Unpaid debts
Child neglect	Bankruptcy
Sexual abuse	Eviction

Adolescence

Running away
Early marriage
Juvenile delinquency
Suicide attempts

Subjective Data

Family History

A genogram (see Chapter 5) is helpful in detecting intergenerational patterns of abuse and dependence. Rarely is only a single family member affected by substance abuse, and beginning with the genogram allows a practitioner to begin learning about potential patterns of abuse before exploring the immediate family member's history of abuse.

The narrative portion of the family history provides a practitioner additional information about possible substance abuse in family members. School-age children can be asked directly, "Does anyone in your family have a problem with drugs or alcohol?" Family assessment tools may also be helpful (see Chapter 1).

The Children of Alcoholics Screening Tool (CAST), developed by John W. Jones (Black, 1982), is a 30-item questionnaire designed for children to identify problems with parental alcohol use. The questionnaire is in a yes/no format, and a score of six or more positive responses indicates the child has an alcoholic parent. The following are examples of questions:

- Have you ever thought that one of your parents had a drinking problem?
- Have you ever lost sleep because of a parent's drinking?
- Did you ever resent a parent's drinking?

Obtaining a psychosocial history can possibly identify a variety of emotional and social problems in the addictive family (Box 21-1).

Objective Data

There are no specific objective data to be collected during the physical examination of children of addictive parents because:

- Individual children may be affected differently.
- The roles the children adopt may affect the physical assessment findings.
- Children and adolescents may have a difficult time talking about issues in the family.
- Children may not make eye contact or may act hesitant in answering questions.

However, the practitioner should be alert for possible signs and symptoms of abuse or neglect.

Primary Care Issues and Implications

Increased public awareness of the economic and social ramifications of addiction, coupled with insurance companies' increased willingness to pay for treatment of addictions, has greatly increased the demand for knowledgeable health care professionals. In response to the growing concern regarding substance abuse, the International Council of Nurses and the World Health Organization (WHO) have jointly produced guidelines that apply to the role of an NP in addressing the problem of addiction (Box 21-2) (Burns & Thompson, 1983).

Management

Treatments and Medications

Individual, peer, or family counseling may be included.

Support groups. Practitioners may refer patient to self-help groups (e.g., Alateen) or support groups offered by professionals, or they may collaborate with colleagues to offer support groups in their practice setting.

Guidelines for support groups. A *self-help support group* is defined as an organized peer support group that typically involves strangers who have united in response to a common need or problem. Aspects include:

- *Pregroup phase*—Contacting appropriate sources of support, obtaining referrals, and screening potential participants (10 to 12 children or adolescents are usually needed to ensure adequate participation on a weekly basis)
- *Early phase*—Establishing trust, clarifying the purpose of the group, and formulating the group's rules, norms, and expectations
- *Working phase*—Sharing of secrets about family situations, gaining information about addictions and their profound effect on the family, supporting one another, engaging in critical self-analysis, identifying goals, making choices, and learning to manage
- *Termination phase*—Evaluating progress of participants, evaluating the group experience, and celebrating the progress participants have made
- *Critical attributes*—Recognition of commonalities, creation of a caring community, establishment of reciprocal relationships, recognition of patterns, and empowerment of patients
- *Individualized outcomes of the support group experience identified by support group participants*—Increased knowledge regarding the profound effect of addictions on families, improvement in relationships, increased coping strategies, increased resiliency, and enhanced school performance

Counseling and Prevention

Substance-abuse education should be offered. Children with a substance-abusing parent need information regarding their risks of developing an addiction and the effects the addiction might have on the various family members. Written information or videos about substance abuse may be provided for later reference (see Resources at the end of this chapter); this is often helpful for families who may not be willing to address the problem during the visit.

Box 21-2 Guidelines for the Role of Nurse Practitioner

Become a political advocate, encouraging a focus on decreasing the demand for, not decreasing the supply of, drugs.

Support the development of a wide range of services related to substance abuse at local and national levels.

Mobilize the community to address substance abuse issues.

Initiate and participate in research to develop interventions.

Support patients and their families.

Develop training courses for all levels of nurses.

Incorporate cultural and ethnic diversity into the care of patients and their families.

Obtain education on substance abuse.

Follow-Up

Children of substance abusers need to have follow-up evaluation based on the other physical and psychosocial issues uncovered during the history and physical examination. Such children should also be informed that the practitioner is available to address problems and questions as they arise, and the issues of parental abuse should be evaluated at each visit.

Consultations and Referrals

Families should be evaluated regarding the need for referral to social services if there is a history of abuse, to counseling for families in crisis, and to support groups for additional support. A parent with a substance-abuse problem should be referred for treatment. The NP should provide a list of resources available in the area and recommend treatment that includes family counseling.

Resources

Organizations

Family

Alateen, Al-Anon Family Group Headquarters, Inc., 1600 Corporate Landing Parkway, Virginia Beach, VA 23454-5617; www.al-anon.alateen.org

Alcoholics Anonymous, Box 459, Grand Central Station, New York, NY 10163; (212) 683-3900; www.aa.org

Children of Alcoholics Foundation, 164 W. 74th Street, New York, NY 10023; (212) 595-5810, x. 7760; www.CoAF.org

National Families in Action, National Drug Information Center, 2296 Henderson Mill Road, Suite 204, Atlanta, GA 30045; www.emory.edu/NFIA

Hazelden Foundation, PO Box 11 CO 3, Center City, MN 55012-0011; (800) 257-7810

National Association for Children of Alcoholics, 31582 Coast Highway, Suite B, South Laguna, CA 92677; (714) 499-3889

National Clearinghouse for Alcohol and Drug Information, PO Box 2345, Rockville, MD 20852; (301) 468-2600

Professional

National Clearinghouse for Alcohol and Drug Information (NCADI), 11426 Rockville Pike, Suite 200, Rockville, MD 20847-2345; (800) 729-6686

National Institute on Alcohol Abuse and Alcoholism, Parklawn Building, Room 14C-20, 5600 Fishers Lane, Rockville, MD 20857; (301) 443-1207

National Institute on Drug Abuse, 5600 Fishers Lane, Rockville, MD 20857; (301) 443-4877

Publications

Family

Alateen. (1987). *Hope for children of alcoholics.* New York: Al-Anon Family Group Headquarters.

Black, C. (1985). *Children of denial: A videotape regarding defenses used by children with addictive parents.* Denver, CO: MAC Publishing.

Black, C. (1985). *My dad loves me, my dad has a disease.* Denver, CO: MAC Publishing.

Black, C. (1985). *Repeat after me.* Denver, CO: MAC Publishing.

Black, C. (1985). *Roles: A videotape describing the roles of children with addictive parents.* Denver, CO: MAC Publishing.

Black, C. (1985). *Sound of silence: A film regarding children of alcoholics.* Denver, CO: MAC Publishing.

Courage to blame: Living with alcoholism. (1996). Virginia Beach, VA: Al-Anon Family Headquarters.

Hyppo, M.H. & Hastings, J.M. (1984) *An elephant in the living room: The children's book.* Minneapolis, MN: CompCare.

Moe, J., Brown, C., & LaPorte, B. (1996). *Kids Power, Too!* Dallas, TX: Imagin Works.

Professional

Burns, E.M. & Thompson, A. (1993). *An addiction curriculum for nursing and other helping professionals.* Vols. I, II. New York: Springer.

Marcus, M.T. (1997). Faculty development and curricular change: A process and outcomes model for substance abuse education. *Journal Professional Nursing, 13*(3), 168-177.

Murphy, S.A., Scott, C.S., & Mandel, L.P. (1996). Clinical knowledge and skill priorities in substance abuse education: A nursing faculty longitudinal survey. *Journal of Nursing Education, 35*(8), 356-360.

Naegle, M.A. (1992). *Substance abuse education in nursing.* Vols. I to III. New York: National League for Nursing Press.

Websites

American Council for Drug Education (www.acde.org)

Center for Substance Abuse Prevention (www.samhsa.gov/centers/csap)

Center for Substance Abuse Treatment (www.samhsa.gov/centers/csat)

National Association for Children of Alcoholics (www.NACOA.org)

National Clearinghouse for Alcohol and Drug Information (www.health.org)

National Institute on Alcoholism and Alcohol Abuse (www.niaaa.nih.gov)

National Institute on Drug Abuse (www.nida.nih.gov)

Substance Abuse and Mental Health Services Administration (www.samhsa.gov)

Bibliography

Black, C. (1982). *It will never happen to me!* Denver, CO: MAC Publishing.

Lynskey, M.T., Fergussen, D.M., & Horwood, L.J. (1994). The effect of parental alcohol problems on rates of adolescents' psychiatric disorders. *Addiction, 89,* 1277-1286.

Burns, E.M. & Thompson, A. (1993). *An addiction curriculum for nursing and other helping professionals.* Vols. I, II. New York: Springer.

National Association for Children of Alcoholics. (1998). *Children of alcoholics: Important facts.* Rockville, MD: National Clearinghouse for Alcohol Information.

Substance Abuse and Mental Health Services Administration. (1999). *National estimates of substance use.* Available online at www.samsha.gov/oas/NHSDA/1999/chapter2.htm.

Substance Abuse and Mental Health Services Administration. (1995). *Annual medical examiner data, 1993: Data from the Drug Abuse Warning Network.* Rockville, MD: Substance Abuse and Mental Health Services Administration.

U.S. Department of Health and Human Services. (2000). *Healthy people 2010.* Washington, DC: Department of Health and Human Services.

Wegscheider-Cruse, S. (1985). *Choicemaking: For co-dependents, adult children, and spirituality seekers.* Deerfield Beach, FL: Health Communications.

Wolin, S. & Wolin, S. (1995). Resilience among youth growing up in substance abusing families. *Pediatric Clinics of North America, 42,* 415-429.

Chapter 22 *Adoptive Families*

Marty Witrak & Arlene E. Johnson

Types of Families

Adoptive families are families not linked by blood but by intended parenting. Adoptive families do have many of the same experiences, joys, and frustrations as other families. These families, however, have one major difference: they are all built on an experience of loss. All adopted children have the circumstance of loss of their biologic parents. Furthermore, the adoptive parent or parents may have encountered the experience of loss in relation to infertility or their inability to be able to have a birth child. For each adoptee, there are adoptive parents, birth parents, and other close family associations. This makes it important for practitioners to be aware of the dynamics in an adoptive family because they will be encountered in practice in one form or another. Understanding the adoptive processes and the dynamics of an adoption is crucial to understanding and working with adoptive individuals and their families.

The common assumption is that adoptive families comprise infertile parents and a newborn; however, many other types of adoptive families are becoming increasingly prevalent. There are several configurations of adoptive families, ranging along a continuum (cited by Feigleman and Silverman [1979]) of traditional families and preferential families. When one looks at these patterns, whether adopting a child is the preferred way to bring a child into the family or adoption is the only choice available for a couple to experience being parents, the basic dynamics are similar, and these two types of patterns are the two ends of the continuum. Most adoptive parents or families fall somewhere in the middle. The concept of *open adoption* has become increasingly more common in recent years. In an open adoption there is contact between the birth parents and the adoptive parents during the adoption process, and the biologic parents may have an ongoing relationship with the adoptive family throughout the child's life. There may also be varying degrees of openness. Couples who choose to adopt through an agency receive preadoptive counseling, while in some private adoptions the adoptive couple may not receive any counseling before the adoptive placement. Some parents may have unresolved feelings related to the adoptive process.

To make the picture even more complex, many families enter into more than one type of adoption. For example, some couples may first adopt a healthy infant and subsequently adopt a child with special needs, or they may first adopt an infant and later adopt one or more older children. Although these configurations are useful theoretically, they may not be useful in practice when working with a family that has multiple configurations in place. Furthermore, it is not the configuration of the family affects the orientation toward adoption. Influencing how these families operate are the reasons why they choose to adopt a particular "type" of child and their expectations of family life and parenting.

What follows is a summary of the basic two types of adoptive families, followed by descriptions of types of children that may be adopted.

Traditional Families

- Have experienced either primary or secondary infertility.
- May already have birth children.
- Are unable to biologically add a child to their family.

Preferential Families

- Choose to adopt as the route to increase their family.
- Include the following:
  Unmarried individuals who choose adoption as a means to become a parent
  Gay or lesbian couples who wish to become parents
  Couples who adopt for ideologic or religious reasons
  Couples who have married late in life
  Foster families who choose to adopt when the child becomes legally available

Types of Children

Infants

- Whether from this country or another country, infants' experience in other families has been minimal.
- In open adoptions, a contract is made between the birth parents and adoptive parents. Both sets of parents retain the right to continuing contact and access to knowledge on behalf of the child.
- Infants may be foreign-born children living in foster care or orphanages.
- There may be few local traditional adoptions.
- Infants may not immediately experience loss. As they grow older (particularly in adolescence), loss issues will surface and the birth parents' decision to relinquish the child may be perceived as rejection.

Sibling Groups

- Sibling groups are children who are primarily from the United States and may have experienced multiple moves in the foster care system and suffered abuse or neglect in their biologic family. These are children who often have had prenatal exposure to cocaine, alcohol, human immunodeficiency virus (HIV), and so on.
- Siblings adopted internationally share a genetic heritage and background.

Older Children

- Older children may have some experience either in a previous family or in an orphanage.
- They may be perceived as "difficult to place" because most couples who adopt desire an infant.
- The experiences that older children have had may make it difficult for them to form relationships with their new family members.
- Children adopted from institutions outside of the United States have often been abandoned by their birth families.

They will experience significant changes in every facet of their existence.

- All children bring with them varying degrees of loss originating from the amount of time they spent with their birth families and the quality of care they experienced in institutions or foster homes. Grief and mourning for their loss may not surface for months or years.
- Children who have lived primarily in institutions may not have a comprehension of what a family is and may have difficulty in adjusting to family life and developing a sense of attachment to parents.

Incidence

- Approximately 1 million children in the United States live with adoptive parents.
- About 2% to 4% of all American families include an adopted child.
- In the 1990s, there were approximately 120,000 adoptions annually in the United States.
- Infants make up less than half of domestic adoptions.
- Nearly half of all adoptions are of children with special needs.

Risk Factors

- School problems
- Signs and symptoms of unresolved grief
- Overweight children
- Secrecy about adoption
- Unknown medical history
- Anger
- Fetal alcohol syndrome/alcohol-related neurologic disorder (FAS/ARND)

Subjective Data

An initial visit with an adopted infant or child requires a comprehensive history with careful attention to the following:

- Is a health history available, including a pregnancy history? If not, can the agency be contacted?
- Many children adopted from outside of the United States do not arrive with a relevant medical history. It is very important to obtain an accurate history of developmental milestones.
- What is the family medical history? The National Committee of Adoption has designed a form to request a complete family medical history for an adopted child. However, in the case of international adoption, many children have been abandoned and a family history is not available.
- What was the child's living arrangement before placement with the adoptive family? What is the placement history of the child? What is the nature and extent of separation and loss experienced by the child? How is the child adjusting to his or her new surroundings?
- What are the legal arrangements and circumstances surrounding the adoption? Is this an open adoption? What is the child's current understanding of the adoption placement?
- What children are in the adoptive family? Birth children? Adopted siblings? Biologic adopted siblings? Were there biologic siblings who were not placed with the same adoptive family?

- What is the adoptive parents' pregnancy history? If there have been infertility issues, to what extent have these been addressed?

Objective Data

Physical Examination

Perform a complete head-to-toe physical examination. A newly arrived foreign-born child should be more thoroughly assessed, and such an examination may include:

Diagnostic Procedures and Laboratory Tests

- Complete blood cell (CBC) count, differential, platelet count, and indices
- Hemoglobin electrophoresis and glucose-6-phosphate dehydrogenase (G6PD) screening
- Hepatitis B panel, HIV test, and rapid plasma reagin (RPR) test
- Urinalysis, tuberculosis skin test, lead level, and a stool test for ova and parasites
- Standard newborn screening (if a young infant)
- Thyroid function test (if not done as part of newborn screening)

Children who have resided in orphanages may have been exposed to a wide range of conditions, and they may suffer from malnutrition, anemia, or a protein deficiency. If a medical history is unavailable, the practitioner should consider screening for congenital conditions, which should be detected early in the child's life. Some children who have been removed from their biologic families because of abuse may have been conceived through an incestuous relationship, resulting in congenital birth defects. Children identified with congenital anomalies should be referred for genetic screening. Other recommended screening tests include:

- Developmental
- Dental
- Hearing
- Vision

Assessment of fetal alcohol syndrome/alcohol-related neurologic disorder. Practitioners should also be particularly aware of screening children in adoptive families for FAS/ARND (see Chapter 47). Many children placed for adoption have unknown prenatal histories and may come from high-risk environments. The practitioner should assess the child for a cluster of symptoms that may indicate FAS/ARND. Not all children will exhibit all these symptoms; it is only a clustering of symptoms that indicates FAS/ARND. The condition is severe and occurs in approximately 1 to 300 (possibly up to 1 in 2000) life births. Characteristics of FAS/ARND include facial dysmorphology with an underdeveloped philtrum, thin upper lip, flat midface, short or upturned nose, low nasal bridge, ear anomalies, short palpebral fissures, epicanthal folds, and growth retardation. Central nervous system (CNS) involvement includes developmental delays, retardation, poor motor control, attention deficits, hyperactivity, and muscle weakness. Brain damage caused by this condition is permanent, and other congenital anomalies may occur (see also Chapter 28).

Attachment disorders. Another specific area for screening is that of attachment disorders (ADs). Situations that frequently produce lack of closeness and can lead to ADs include multiple foster care placements, backgrounds of abuse or neglect, and institutional living. The most common form of institutional living is found in countries that use orphanages extensively (e.g., Romania). Children who do not have consistent caregivers or who are moved from placement to placement are not able to progress through the normal developmental steps. Although the contribution of these experiences to relationship development is self-evident, many other developmental milestones are learned in the context of a relationship. For example, if a baby is hungry and cries, the caregiver responds and satisfies the baby's hunger. This type of reinforcement is the basis of cause-and-effect thinking, but these associations are not developed if the baby's cry elicits no response and hunger is satisfied only on a schedule.

The diagnostic category of AD has recently become better described so that parents and practitioners can make the appropriate diagnosis. The diagnostic criteria for reactive AD in infancy and childhood include the following:

A. The child exhibits greatly disturbed and developmentally inappropriate social relatedness in most social contexts, beginning before 5 years of age, as evidenced by either of the following:
   1. Persistent failure to initiate or respond in a developmentally appropriate fashion to most social interactions, as manifested by excessively inhibited, hypervigilant, or highly ambivalent and contradictory responses (e.g., the child may respond to caregivers with a mixture of approach, avoidance, and resistance to comforting or may exhibit frozen watchfulness)
   2. Diffuse attachments as manifested by indiscriminate sociability with a strong inability to exhibit appropriately selective attachments (e.g., excessive familiarity with relative strangers, lack of selectivity in choice of attachment figures)
B. The disturbance in criterion A is not accounted for solely by developmental delay (as in mental retardation) and does not meet the criteria for pervasive developmental disorder.
C. The child received pathogenic care as evidenced by at least one of the following:
   1. Persistent disregard for the child's basic emotional needs for comfort, stimulation, and affection
   2. Persistent disregard for the child's basic physical needs
   3. Repeated changes of primary caregiver that prevented formation of stable attachments (e.g., frequent changes in foster care)
D. There is a presumption that the care in criterion C is responsible for the disturbed behavior in criterion A (i.e., the disturbances in criterion A began after the pathogenic care in criterion C).

There are two types of AD: (1) inhibited type (if criterion A predominates in the clinical presentation), and (2) disinhibited type (if criterion B predominates in the clinical presentation). Children whose developmental interruptions have resulted in an AD may exhibit many or even all of the symptoms listed in Box 22-1.

Primary Care Issues and Implications

Development

All newly adopted children from birth to 6 years of age should be assessed with the Denver II Developmental Screening Test. School-age children may be evaluated through the local school

---

Box 22-1 Symptoms of Attachment Disorders

Superficial engagement in "charming behavior"
Indiscriminate affection toward strangers
Lack of affection with parents on their terms (i.e., not "cuddly")
Little eye contact with parents on normal terms
Persistent nonsense questions and obsessive chatter
Inappropriate demanding and clinging behavior
Lying about the obvious or lying in a crazy manner
Stealing
Destructive behavior to self, others, and material things (e.g., "accident prone")
Abnormal eating patterns, hoarding of food, or overeating
No impulse controls or frequent hyperactivity
Lags in learning
Abnormal speech patterns
Poor peer relationships
Lack of cause-and-effect thinking
Lack of conscience
Cruelty to animals
Preoccupation with fire

---

system, and children younger than school age who are identified to have developmental or speech delays may receive early childhood special services through their local school district. Language development should be assessed for children who have to acquire a second language, and school-age children may be eligible to receive language services through the local school system. The practitioner should also assess for learning disabilities (see Chapter 46).

Diet and Nutrition

- Assess for hoarding or overeating as symptoms of AD.
- Assess institutionally housed children for proteinemia.
- Support mothers who adopt infants and wish to consider the option of breastfeeding. Refer mothers to a lactation consultant.
- Discuss cultural food preferences if the child is from a foreign country. Advise parents to add new foods to the diet slowly. Refer to a dietitian if there are nutritional concerns.

Discipline

Adoptive parents have often worked very hard to become parents and as such are very committed to their role. However, the negative side of this dynamic is that they may "overvalue" their children. Support for limit-setting and parenting skills may be useful. As adolescents begin to display normal independence and testing behaviors, adoptive parents may personalize conflicts more than necessary, and this is even more likely if these behaviors coincide with the request to search for birth parents. Adoptive children who require constant limit-setting or who are very difficult should be assessed for AD, and the practitioner should not rely on personal interaction with the child because these children are typically better at relating to strangers.

Screening

General areas for screening include:
- Effects of prenatal drug use (e.g., of cocaine, alcohol) (see Chapter 28)

- Mercury for children adopted from some South American countries
- ADs in children who are adopted when they are older, who have been institutionally housed for a length of time, and who have had multiple moves

The International Adoption Clinic at the University of Minnesota Hospital and Clinics has over 20 different sets of informational materials available, including studies on the health of Eastern European, Chinese, and all internationally adopted children; growth charts for Korean, Chinese, and Indian children; materials concerning hepatitis B, cytomegalovirus, and tuberculosis; and other materials for practitioners caring for internationally adopted children. (See also Resources at the end of this chapter.)

Immunizations

All children need careful documentation of immunizations. If immunizations cannot be documented, a child should be considered unimmunized; a full series of immunizations should be given as recommended by the American Academy of Pediatrics (AAP) Committee on Infectious Diseases because there is little risk in repeating immunizations.

Management

Counseling and Prevention

Counseling and assisting parents with the adoption process and parenting issues

Decision to adopt. The first phase that adoptive families routinely go through is reaching the decision to adopt. For infertile couples, this phase is fraught with more loss and pain than for the preferential family. Traditional families need to go through mourning the loss of their own fertility, and for many families this phase can take a very long time as technology becomes more and more sophisticated in assisting infertile couples to have a birth child. As fertility options diminish, the decision for parents becomes a matter of whether they want to parent any child or want to have a birth child. It is important for these families to mourn the loss of their fertility before they engage in trying to nurture and raise an adoptive child, and these processes are usually facilitated by the adoption agency working with a couple. However, infertility is a very difficult and pervasive issue, and many people still experience grief for a long time; this is particularly true if there have been multiple spontaneous abortions or other kinds of pregnancy loss (e.g., stillbirths).

Even for couples not experiencing pregnancy losses, the decision to pursue adoption requires coming to terms with motivations and expectations. Couples who have postponed marriage or who made major commitments to a career and later find themselves wanting a family may have to mourn their earlier decisions or to come to terms with those earlier decisions. Other individuals who are not married but want to pursue single-parent adoption must deal with their single-parent status and the associated social stigma. They must acknowledge that for the immediate future they probably will remain single and will not be part of a marriage. It is important that the motivation of adoptive families be the desire to parent and not the desire to confront society's expectations that couples must parent. Many couples who have issues of infertility choose to pursue a child-free family pattern and do so with no regrets.

Pursuit of adoption. The next major phase that adoptive families go through is the actual pursuit of the adoption. In this phase, families find out what the availability of children is and learn about the process, time frame, cost, and what kinds of children are available to them. Adoptive parents unfortunately find that many adoptions are extremely expensive. Often people who have few resources may be forced to pursue an adoption experience that requires burdensome financial and personal resources, especially if the adoption is a special-needs adoption. In fact, if families are not prepared to cope with all the demands of a special-needs adoption, they may have even more trouble becoming a family and maintaining functional family structure in the future. Another issue in the pursuit of adoption is the profound influence that the new children or child will have on the children already in the family; this may be an area about which families raise questions with the practitioner.

Transition to parenthood. The transition to parenthood for adoptive families is just as intense and in several respects more intense than for birth families. Most families need to reorganize their lives, schedules, and routines when they add a child to the family; in fact, additions to a family change the whole balance of the family system. When a new adoptive child is brought into the family, the family needs to learn the child's personality, be the new child an infant or a 4-year-old, in order to form an attachment. Like birth parents, adoptive parents may not instantly feel love toward their new child. Infertile couples in particular may feel a great sense of mourning or guilt because they have waited for a very long time for a child and now the magic that they were expecting is not there. Practitioner anticipation of these feelings is very useful.

Attachment or claiming of children. Another experience similar to that of biologic families is that of claiming or attaching to the child. Biologic parents may examine their child from head to toe, and the same kind of process happens in adoptive families; they need to get to know and to experience the new addition to their family. A process related to the attachment parents feel is the sense of entitlement to parenting. Society recognizes that biologic parents are entitled to parent their child. Furthermore, this is often taken to extremes when children are kept in neglectful or abusive situations because the members of society believe so strongly in the sense of entitlement of a biologic parent. Therefore, it may be much more difficult for adoptive families to feel that they are now entitled to parent. Adoptive parents need to feel that they are real parents and that these are their real children, as opposed to feeling the children are just in their custodial care. This acceptance of parenting can be even more difficult with special-needs children who have major disabilities and emotional or mental problems.

Entitlement to parent. The entitlement to parent is more difficult to feel for a family who has adopted an older child. Children who are adopted when they are older may come to a family with previous experiences about parenting or previous issues with authority, and they may challenge the new adoptive parents' right to parent. In such cases, the sense of forging a family also may be very difficult. If children have been in multiple foster placements or have been institutionalized, they may not have the same sense of "family" as the family who has adopted them. Furthermore, there may be a large amount of ambivalence or fear about getting close, fear of being moved again and fear of another loss. All these issues are very common in older-child placement. The practitioner needs to be especially alert and ask questions about these issues so that the parents feel it is acceptable to engage in discussions with the practitioner rather than feeling that their problems are very unusual and unique.

Photo listings. One of the most effective methods devised to recruit families for waiting children is the photo listing book. This book shows pictures of waiting children and gives a brief history of each child or, in some cases, each sibling group. Many states maintain these listing books, and there are regional and national books as well. Many families may be unfamiliar with the descriptions or the jargon used and come to a practitioner for help in understanding the terms. Prospective parents may also ask for clarification of the conditions listed for many of the children who have special physical, emotional, or mental health needs.

In general, each photo listing contains the child's name, month and year of birth, a small amount of information about where he or she lives, an identification number, and the date that the child was entered in the book. The photo listing may also explain something about the child's social and medical history, kind of home desired, and likes and dislikes, as well as provide a telephone number to reach the contact person or agency. Practitioners should be aware of several common phrases used in the listings; these include:

- "All boy," "tomboy," "very active," "impulsive," "needs a lot of attention," and "acts out" are phrases that may indicate attention-deficit hyperactivity disorder (ADHD).
- "Requires a lot of structure," "manipulative," "has experienced several losses," "is grieving," "is bossy," and "has had many moves" are phrases indicating that the child may have problems such as AD.
- "Victim of neglect" is a phrase that may indicate a possibility of AD, sexual abuse, or any of the physical repercussions of malnutrition.
- "Developmentally delayed," "small head," "toileting accidents," "difficulty in school," "delayed speech," and "is immature" are phrases that may indicate learning disabilities or emotional or behavioral problems.

Most of these phrases are understated, but the key to helping parents understand the descriptions is to be *aware* that they are understated. Parents should not be discouraged from adopting children with ADs or who are hyperactive, and they should be encouraged to understand exactly what problems children may have. Parents can then decide whether they have the necessary resources and prepare themselves. It can also be very useful for prospective parents to request a conversation with someone who knows the waiting child, which may may provide more information than the listing description.

Addressing adoptive parent and adopted child concerns

Telling of adoption. Another fundamental and distinctive process in adoptive families is that of explaining adoption to the child. This process occurs over time and includes actions and activities surrounding the discussion of adoption with the child and with the public. With children adopted as babies, the parents need to decide at what point to introduce the concept of adoption to the child and in what way. Many contemporary families send out adoptive birth announcements and discuss adoption openly from the very beginning. However, historically this openness was not common, and occasionally individuals still discover much later in life that they were adopted. The process of explaining adoption can be facilitated by a large number of fiction and nonfiction books published to help parents explain to children what it means to be adopted and to normalize the associated feelings. For families who adopt older children who know their adoption status, the issue is not telling a child that he or she is adopted but working with the child to provide a sense of adoption without insecurity. As they begin or continue attending school, it is important for both younger and older children to understand what information related to their adoption status does and does not need to be shared with other people.

Outsiders' questions. In many mixed-race families or mixed-culture families, it is easy for people to observe that the family comprises people who are not biologically related to each other. However, in those situations it is also not unusual to have to deal with intrusive questions such as, "Whose child is this, really?", "Are you the mother of this child?", and "What happened to the child's real family?" How the adoptive family answers these questions conveys a sense of what the family believes about adoption to their adopted child.

Children's questions. As children become older and ask about their own adoptive experience, they may ask questions about issues that are still sensitive to the parents. These questions may include why they were not able to have biologic children. Adoptive parents need to be prepared to answer in a way that the child can understand and that also protects the parents' need for privacy and comfort. In addition, children often ask questions that are uncomfortable for them, such as "Why didn't my parents keep me?" or "Why didn't they like me?" It has often been suggested that when a child asks, "Why didn't they keep me?", an appropriate answer is "They loved you so much that they gave you away so you could have a good family." However, these kinds of answers can be very unsettling for children because they begin to associate love with being sent away, which is very disconcerting to children who lack a sense of permanency. It is also not appropriate to identify birth parents as bad people. One recommended course of action is to tell as much of the truth as a child is capable of understanding or to keep the explanation general while not deviating too far from the truth; elusive or misleading answers become more difficult for a child as he or she grows older and learns the reality of the situation.

What to tell children is very complicated issue and needs to be worked out in a way that is comfortable for both the parents and the future of the child. Often when children ask these questions, feelings of loss are elicited not only from the child but also from the parents, whose infertility issues may once again be brought into focus.

Identity issues. Another common process for adoptive families is supporting an adopted teenager's struggle for identity. In adolescence, many adoptees begin the task of formulating their own identity and their sense of who they are. Furthermore, with this examination of identity come the questions, "Who do I belong to?" and "Where did I come from?" These questions connect the past with the child's future as he or she works to understand their birth and learn more of their biologic family, and this often becomes more of a struggle because aspects of the adoptee's past are often rooted in fantasy. It is not uncommon for children to glorify their birth parents, especially if they are engaged in a struggle for their own independence with their adoptive parents; they may see the issues of limit-setting and discipline as related to being adopted, rather than as an issue of normal parenting and adolescence. Adoptees frequently fantasize that their birth parents could not possibly be like the parents they are living with at the moment.

In addition, parents of transracially or transculturally adopted teenagers need to think about strategies for protecting themselves and their children from social sanctions. When teenagers start dating, many issues around racial prejudice, sexual stereotypes, and social bias can come into focus.

Searching. The developmental influence of adoption continues as a young person moves toward adulthood. Abandonment and separation issues, as well as a sense of belonging, recur throughout the individual's life. However, these issues are usually most poignant in adolescence, when the identity issues are the most acute. It is not unusual that during adolescence or late adolescence a new interest in searching for the birth family surfaces. The practitioner should assist the family and child to have a positive sense of adoption. Over time, the family needs to integrate what it means to be adopted, have a positive sense about how families are constructed through adoption, and ensure that the child has a positive self-concept. If a child comes from another culture, this integration includes their ability to feel positive about both their birth culture and the culture in which they are now living.

Counsel adolescents as they engage in identity issues. The challenge for a practitioner during a child's adolescence is to facilitate reconciliation of the need to search with the need to stay connected with the adoptive family. Talk with both the adolescent and the parents about the child's need to search being a matter of identity, not a desire to be distant from the adoptive parents. Many organizations exist that help adoptees with the search process. Support parents during adolescence because there may be a renewal of grief over the parents' infertility issues.

Follow-Up

Appropriate follow-up should be based on AAP guidelines.

Consultations and Referrals

The practitioner should refer any child with AD (which is frequently misdiagnosed, and for which treatment for related kinds of behavior problems only exacerbates the symptoms), ADHD, or FAS/ARND to a specialized mental health professional.

Resources

Organizations

Adoption Clinic, PO Box 211, 420 Delaware Street SE, University of Minnesota Hospital and Clinics, Minneapolis, MN 55455; (612) 626-6777

Adoptive Families of America (AFA), 3333 Highway 100 North, Minneapolis, MN 55422; (800) 372-3300

The National Committee on Adoption, 2025 M Street NW, Suite 512, Washington, DC

Websites

Adoption Information Services (www.adpotioninfosvcs.com/foreign.htm)

Adopt Vietnam (www.adoptvietnam.org/adoption/health-clinics.htm)

Family Doctor (familydoctor.org/handouts/321.html)

Georgetown University Child Development Center (www.gucdc.georgetown.edu/site.html)

The Joint Council on International Children's Services from North America (JCICS) (www.jcics.org/mission.html)

Medline (www.nlm.nih.gov/medlineplus/adoption.html)

National Adoption Information Clearinghouse (www.calib.com/naic)

Russian Adoption (www.russianadoption.org/specialists.htm)

Bibliography

Albers, L.H., Johnson, D.E., Hosteter, M.K., Iverson, S., & Miller, L.C. (1997, September). Health of children adopted from the former Soviet Union and Eastern Europe: Comparison with preadoptive medical records. *Journal of the American Medical Association, 278*(11), 922-924.

Babb, L.A. & Laws, R. (1997). *Adopting and advocating for the special needs child: A guide for parents and professionals.* Westport, CT: Greenwood Publishing Group.

Bayless, L. & Love, L. (Eds.). (1990). *Assessing attachment, separation and loss.* Atlanta: Child Welfare Institute.

Cermak, S.A. & Daunhauer, L.A. (1997, July/August). Sensory processing in the postinstitutionalized child. *American Journal of Occupational Therapy, 51*(7), 500-507.

Chisholm, K., Carter, M.C., Ames, E., & Morison, S.J. (1995, Spring). Attachment security and indiscriminately friendly behavior in children adopted from Romanian orphanages. *Development and Psychopathology, 7*(2), 283-294.

Evan B. Donaldson Adoption Institute. (1997). *Benchmark adoption survey: Report on the findings.* New York: Evan B. Donaldson Institute.

Feigleman, W. & Silverman, A.R. (1979). Preferential adoption: A new mode of family formation. *Social Casework 60,* 296-305.

Groze, V. & Ileana, D. (1996, December). A follow-up study of adopted children from Romania. *Child and Adolescent Social Work Journal, 13*(6), 541-565.

Hostetter, M. & Johnson, D.E. (1989, March). International adoption: An introduction for physicians. *American Journal of Diseases of Children, 143*(3), 325-332.

Hostetter, M.K., Iverson, S., Dole, K., & Johnson, D. (1989, April). Unsuspected infectious diseases and other medical diagnoses in the evaluation of internationally adopted children. *Pediatrics, 83*(4), 559-563.

Jenista, J.A. (Ed.). (1997, May). Romanian review. *Adoption Medical News, 3*(5), 1-6.

Johnson, D.E. & Hostetter, M. (1997, March/April). Post-arrival evaluations: Identifying medical problems common to internationally adopted children. *Adoptive Families, 30*(2), 14-17.

Keck, G.C. & Kupecky, R.M. (1995). *Adopting the hurt child: Hope for families with special needs kids.* Colorado Springs, CO: Pinon.

Marcovitch, S., Cesaroni, L., Roberts, W., & Swanson, C. (1995, September/October). Romanian adoption: Parents' dreams, nightmares, and realities. *Child Welfare, 74*(5), 993-1017.

Parent Network for the Post-Institutionalized Child. (1995, Spring). Overview of the post-institutionalized child. *The Post, 1,* 1-5.

Rosenberg, E.B. (1992). *The adoption life cycle: The children and their families through the years.* New York: The Free Press.

Rutter, M. (1998). Developmental catch-up and deficit following adoption after severe global early privation. *Child Psychology and Psychiatry, 39* (4), 465-476.

Van Gulden, H. & Rabb, L.B. (1993). *Real parents, real children: Parenting the adopted child.* New York: The Crossroad Publishing.

Chapter 23 *Childhood Loss*

Peggy Vernon

A substantial risk of disruption of the family has always been present for children. Major changes resulting in loss cause insecurity and anxiety. How children deal with the stressful events surrounding loss affects their ability to deal with future stresses in life. Although a child perceives loss in a uniquely individual way, some losses are minimal, whereas others have a great effect. Previously the major cause of disruption was death. Today, however, disruptions are more likely to result from divorce (see Chapter 24). This chapter deals with the major loss of death. Certainly the stages of grief, coping, and defense mechanisms can be applied to other losses as well. In counseling a child and family experiencing loss, it is important to understand the perception of loss and what the loss means to them.

Types of Loss

- Death (e.g., of parent, sibling, grandparent, or other family member; friend; pet)
- Divorce (see Chapter 24)
- Remarriage
- Move (e.g., child's family away from familiar neighborhood or school, child's friend away from neighborhood or school)

Stages of Grief

The stages of grief are the same for children as they are for adults. However, children deal only with as much as they can handle at the time. It is not unusual for them to appear sad at one moment and playful at the next. Therefore the grieving process takes much longer for children, often several years. The mourning process is highly individual, and children have their own timetables. The process of grief resolution for children can be prolonged and is revisited at each new developmental stage. The grief process has the following stages:
- Denial and shock, including emotional numbness
- Anger and confusion
- Resistance
- Depression
- Acceptance

Meaning of Loss to a Child

At a time of loss, a child's greatest need is truth. Explanations should be given according to the child's psychologic and intellectual capabilities. They should be short and factual. Lying and insincerity lead to insecurity and anxiety. Euphemisms such as the following should be avoided:
- "Daddy has gone to sleep."
- "Grandma has passed away."
- "We lost our puppy."
- "He lives with God now."
- "She went to Heaven."

A child's developmental stage should also be considered when explaining the loss and anticipating the reaction.
- When under 3 years of age, children lack the cognitive sophistication to understand the meaning of death. Their reaction is confusion and fear; they often regress to a time in their lives that was comfortable and secure. They may rely on a blanket, suck their thumb, or use other security objects.
- Preschool children understand death as reversible, somewhat like going away but coming back again. Death is a continuation of life in a different form. Their reaction can be egocentric (i.e., "Something I did caused this").
- Children 5 to 9 years of age understand that death is irreversible but believe it will not happen to them. They feel death is caused by an outside source (i.e., "Someone bad caused him to die"). However, because of their greater cognitive maturity, they react to loss with feelings of sadness and depression. They feel personal rejection tied to the loss (i.e., "How could he do this to me?") and place blame for the loss elsewhere, often on a parent who has left or the person who has died.
- Children older than 9 years of age understand that death is irreversible and may involve them and their family or friends. They are able to comprehend the finality and universality of death and to understand that death occurs from within the body, not from an outside source. They respond to loss with increased anger and feelings of helplessness.
- Adolescents understand death realistically. However, since they are less dependent on their family and are more peer oriented, the loss is internalized, and they are concerned with the effect on their own intimate relationships and their ability to maintain long-term relationships.

Grieving Process

When a family experiences a loss, the parents' grieving interrupts the comfort and support normally available to children, causing a change in the family dynamics. Mourning adults give children a model to follow. However, in a child's mind, someone must be in control. Therefore, if the adults are consumed with their grief, children often assume the role of being in charge, seeming unaffected, even becoming the protector while parents grieve. At a later time, when adults are more in control and emotionally available, children will begin their grieving process. In this way children receive permission to grieve from adults. It is important to grant this permission, regardless of the age of the child. Do not assume that the child does not understand or feel the loss.

At the same time, adults tend to project their sense of loss onto the child. Often the child does not feel the loss, or it may not be perceived with the profoundness or sensitivity characteristic of adults.

Children react to loss in a variety of ways, not unlike adults. Reactions include:

- Hurt
- Loneliness
- Sadness
- Fear (i.e., if one parent left or has died, how can the child be sure it will not happen to the remaining parent?)
- Anger (It is natural for children to retaliate against those who have hurt them.)
- Depression (including loss of interest in previously enjoyable activities)
- Guilt (Children tend to feel more guilty than adults and also feel a strong correlation between their behavior and the loss. In addition, they feel guilty that they continue to live.)
- Personal rejection (i.e., "He didn't love me enough to stay.")
- Decreased energy
- Antisocial behavior (e.g., unwillingness to participate in previously pleasurable activities, rowdiness, rudeness)
- Regressive behavior (e.g., bedwetting, thumbsucking, baby talk)
- Academic failure
- Sleep disturbances (e.g., insomnia, nightmares, separation anxiety)
- Appetite disturbances (e.g., weight loss, anorexia, overeating)
- Developmental disruptions
- Suicidal gestures (e.g., giving belongings away, preoccupation with own death, self-destructive behaviors)

A child's response to loss is greatly affected by the response of significant adults, and children resume activities sooner than adults, usually less than 2 weeks after the loss.

Adult Support

- Become comfortable with using correct words with the child (e.g., *dead, divorce*).
- Offer short simple explanations (e.g., "Grandma died because she had cancer. It does not mean that all people die when they get sick").
- Understand what it means for the child (e.g., "Death means a person does not breathe. The body is still and quiet."; "Divorce means that Daddy no longer lives here, but you will still see him.").
- Answer questions honestly. Reassure children that they had no responsibility in the death or divorce and could not have prevented it. Children often ask three questions:
  Did I cause this to happen?
  Will it happen to you?
  Who will take care of me?
- Allow the child to cry and express anger appropriately. Expression of emotions is healthy; suppression is harmful. Ways to help children express their emotions include verbal communication, roleplaying, puppets, painting and art, and books or stories.
- Maintain daily routines as much as possible.
- Maintain discipline and limits. A child's life is disrupted with a loss, but security comes with consistency.
- Understand that a child is not a companion, confidante, or confessor for parents and other adults.
- Be willing to discuss the loss briefly and episodically over a period of months or years. Children need repeated reassurance and will mourn a loss through each developmental phase.

Practitioner's Role

The task of the practitioner is to differentiate between families and children who are experiencing normal grief and those who are exhibiting a pathologic condition requiring referral to a mental health professional. Practitioners must understand their own feelings and experiences with loss and resolve past personal tragedies before being able to help families deal with loss.

Referral to a mental health professional is necessary if, after several months, the child continues to exhibit signs of depression; these include:

- Looking sad
- Appearing tired or having sleep disturbances or insomnia
- Losing interest in personal appearance
- Experiencing appetite changes (including anorexia, bulimia, and purging)
- Experiencing persistent and previously absent health problems and somatic complaints
- Avoiding social situations and choosing to be alone
- Appearing indifferent to school and hobbies
- Experiencing academic failure
- Displaying feelings of worthlessness and poor self-esteem
- Relying on drugs and alcohol
- Experiencing extended guilt
- Displaying regressive or non–age-appropriate behaviors
- Displaying apathy
- Showing hostility

Funerals

Parents may ask the practitioner if a young child should attend the funeral. It is a very sad situation in which adults tend to want to protect children from further hurt and grief. The practitioner can assist and support the family by explaining that funerals are rites of separation, the final stage of life. Grief is resolved by acknowledging it, not by denying or ignoring it. If a preschool or school-age child wants to attend a funeral, it is generally better to assign a familiar adult to accompany the child. This adult should be able to leave the funeral if the child desires to do so. To deny the child the right to attend the funeral is to deny the right to say goodbye. To send children away during this time may be sensed as another rejection or abandonment. Just as children cannot be spared the sadness of death, they should not be excluded from the entire grief process, including the funeral and visits to the cemetery.

In very young and preverbal children, it is important to pay close attention to facial expression, body posture, tone of voice, tempo of language, and level of activity. Cognitive and language skills vary with different age levels, which in turn affect how children interpret questions and their answers. For this reason, when interviewing a very young or preverbal child, questions must be posed simply and concretely.

Conclusion

Helping a child deal with loss can be a painful but rewarding process for a practitioner. The grieving process for children is difficult to observe and therefore often ignored by adults. By approaching the child with kindness, sympathy, and warmth, the practitioner allows the child the opportunity to openly and honestly express emotions and feelings in a safe environment. The course of the grieving process can also be an enlightening experience for the practitioner.

Resources

Organizations

AIDS Support Group, 8119 Holland Avenue, Alexandria, VA 22306

The Compassionate Friends, PO Box 1347, Oak Brook, IL 60521; (312) 323-5010

Good Grief Program, Judge Baker Guidance Center, 295 Longwood Avenue, Boston, MA 02115

Families and Friends of Missing Persons and Violent Crime Victims, PO Box 27529, Seattle, WA 98125; (206) 362-1081

Families and Friends of Murder Victims, PO Box 80181, Chattanooga, TN 80181

Lifeline Institutes, 9108 Lakewood Drive, SW, Tacoma, WA 98499

National SIDS Resource Center, 8201 Greensboro Drive, Suite 600, McLean, VA 22101; (703) 821-8955

Omega, 271 Washington Street, Somerville, MA 02143

Students Against Driving Drunk (SADD), PO Box 800, Marlborough, MA 01752

Survivors of Suicide National Office, Suicide Prevention Center, Inc., 184 Salem Avenue, Dayton, OH 45406

Publications

For Children

Brown, M.W. (1995). *The dead bird.* New York: HarperCollins.

Buscaglia, L. (1982). *The fall of Freddie the leaf.* Thorofare, NJ: Charles B. Slack.

Dodge, N. (1984). *Thumpy's story: A story of love and grief shared by Thumpy the bunny.* Springfield, IL: Prairie Lark.

Fassler, J. (1971). *My grandpa died today.* New York: Behavioral Publications.

Johnson, J. & Johnson, M. (1982). *Where's Jess?* Omaha: Centering Corp.

Mellonie, B. & Ingpen, R. (1983). *Lifetimes: The beautiful way to explain death to children.* New York: Bantam.

Miles, M. (1985). *Annie and the old one.* Boston: Little, Brown & Co.

Viorst, J. (1971). *The tenth good thing about Barney.* New York: MacMillan.

For Parents

Baxter, G. & Stuart, W. (1999). *Death and the adolescent.* Toronto: University of Toronto Press.

Grollman, E. (1976). *Explaining death to children.* Boston: Beacon.

Grollman, E. (1990). *Talking about death: A dialogue between parent and child.* Boston: Beacon.

Kroen, W.C. & Espeland, P. (1996). *Helping children cope with the loss of a loved one.* Minneapolis, MN: Free Spirit.

Kubler-Ross, E. (1993). *On children and death.* New York: Macmillan.

Kubler-Ross, E. (1969). *On death and dying,* New York: Macmillan.

Kushner, H. (1983). *When bad things happen to good people.* New York: First Avon.

Schaefer, D. & Lyons, C. (1993). *How do we tell the children?* New York: Newmarket.

Websites

The Children's Hospital at Westmead (old.nch.edu.au/parents/health/books/booklis8.htm)

GriefNet (www.griefnet.org)

Growth House, Inc. (www.growthhouse.org)

Healing Children's Grief (www.childrensgrief.com)

Three Trees (www.threetrees.org)

Bibliography

Betz, C. Helping children to cope with the death of a sibling. *Child Care Newsletter, 3*(2), 3-5.

The Center for the Future of Children. (1994, Spring). The future of children. *Children and Divorce, 4*(1).

Dershewitz, R. (1988). *Ambulatory pediatric care.* Philadelphia: J.B. Lippincott.

Grollman, E. (1990). *Talking about death.* Boston: Beacon.

Kubler-Ross, E. (1993). *On children and death.* New York: Macmillan.

Serwint, J. (1995). When a child dies. *Contemporary Pediatrics, 12*(3), 55-78.

Shelov, S.P. & Hannemann, R.E. (1991). *Caring for your baby and young child: Birth to age 5.* New York: American Academy of Pediatrics.

Chapter 24 *Divorce*

Jane A. Fox

Divorce is not a single event but a long-term process of transition that changes the family structure, dynamics, and resources. It is stressful for both parents and children and can have devastating effects on children. Divorce is the termination of the family unit and is often characterized by painful losses. The divorce is usually only the first of many major changes in the lives of affected children. Despite increasing trends toward joint legal custody, mothers retain physical custody of most children, and these mothers usually experience a significant reduction in financial resources. The majority of children adjust to their changed family circumstances without significant problems. However, studies indicate up to half of children have a symptomatic response during the first year after their parents divorce. Nurse practitioners (NPs), knowledgeable about child development and acting as child advocates, are in a unique position to help these children and families cope with the effects of divorce. The NP has the responsibility to identify children in these families and the opportunity to work through this increasingly common family transition to promote the best interests of the child. The NP also has the capability to apply developmental considerations to a child's experience of divorce (Table 24-1), health, and illness and to assess and support the child. In addition, the NP can offer anticipatory guidance for the divorcing parents and help them create an environment in which both parents are encouraged to stay involved in their children's lives.

Incidence

- During the 1990s, 15 million children, most under 8 years of age, faced divorce.
- By 2010, over half of school-age children will have spent substantial time living with a single parent or in a stepfamily.
- Over 1 million children every year experience divorce of their parents.
- Half of marriages end in divorce, and 60% of these situations involve children.
- Approximately 32 per 100 children are in families who have experienced divorce.
- Single parenthood can result from divorce, nonmarital childbearing, or death of the other parent. However, divorce is most common. Each of these situations has different implications for adjustment and social support. Out-of-wedlock births and divorce result in 61% of all children living with a single parent.

Table 24-1 Developmental Considerations in a Child's Experience of Divorce

AGE	ERIKSON'S DEVELOPMENTAL TASKS	DIVORCE ISSUES*	REACTIONS TO DIVORCE*
Birth to 1½ years	Trust vs mistrust	Loss of one parent	Regression
		Loss of familiar environment	
1½ to 3 years	Autonomy vs shame/doubt	Abandonment anxiety	Anxiety
		Change in routine	Guilt
		Increased time in child care	
		Upset parent	
3 to 6 years	Initiative vs guilt	Feeling responsible for divorce	Sadness
		Maintaining relationship and	Anger
		contact with noncustodial	Guilt
6 to 11 years	Industry vs inferiority	parent	Loneliness
		Conflicted loyalty	Anxiety
			Somatic symptoms (e.g., headache, stomachache)
			Academic problems
			Aggression (school-age boys)
Adolescent	Identity vs isolation	Concern about own and parents' relationships	Anger
			Depression (early and middle-age adolescent girls)
Young adult	Intimacy vs isolation		Delayed capacity for intimacy and commitment
Adult	Generativity vs stagnation		
Old age	Ego integrity vs despair		

*Some issues and reactions may occur across age groups due to differences in a child's development, situation with respect to parental conflict and resources, changes in environment, and other stress and social support.

Risk Factors

The clinical manifestations of divorce in children are dependent on many variables. Are the parents able, despite their own anger and loss, to focus on their children's feelings and needs during the divorce? What was the predivorce level of psychosocial functioning? What is the child's age.

The major risk factors affecting children's adjustment to parental divorce are as follows:

- Continued interparental conflict.
- Poverty or changes in household resources. (Children in single-parent households are much more likely to be poor than those in two-parent households. Financial resources are often decreased for a postdivorce household, even when the family is well above poverty level.)
- Maternal depression.
- Other psychiatric disorders in either parent.

For each member of the family, divorce involves changes in stress and resources. In addition to the stress caused by one parent leaving the household, divorce is often accompanied by many other changes. One common change for a child is a decrease in the amount of time spent with each parent because one parent moves to a separate residence and the other parent may be less available as a result of increased workload or personal stress. Another common change is moving to a new residence, often necessitating a change of health care provider, school or day care, and friends or other social supports. The changes, chaos, and conflict in divorcing families can also affect exposure, susceptibility, and response to illness. Conflict and resource issues affect a child's level of stress, health, and access to health care, and the outcome for a particular child depends greatly on his or her resilience and circumstances, including environment and social support.

Subjective Data

Because of the prevalence of divorce, it may be helpful to integrate a screening question into all well-child visits (e.g., How are you and your husband getting along? Is there tension that may affect the children?).

A complete history should be obtained at the first encounter with a child. Because of the frequent and multiple changes for children with divorcing parents, it is important to check the current situation at each subsequent visit, including consideration of the age of the child, the source of information, and the information's reliability.

Current Situation

Questions to be asked to remain current on the child's situation include such topics as:

- Where the child spends time and how much time is spent (e.g., longer hours in child care, time unsupervised at home)
- Whether both parents are in contact with the child
- Changes in caregiving
- Changes in residence (e.g., moving, new people in the household)
- Family support systems
- Exposure to conflict
- Financial concerns (e.g., access to health insurance, adequacy of child support)

Age

The current age of a child and the age at the time of parental separation are important factors in assessing the child's adjustment and ability to understand and cope with the stress and changes of divorce. Age is also a factor in expected patterns of illness and injury. The child's gender affects expected behavior, just as the changing composition of the household does (e.g., sons in the mother's custody, remarriage of a parent). It may be difficult to determine if a toddler's irritability is a response to the discomfort of an ear infection or to the anxiety created by parental conflict. (Table 24-1 may be a useful tool in assessing a child's situation.)

Source of Information

Whenever possible, it is important to obtain information from the child in addition to the parent. For all children, this information can help them learn to communicate about their bodies and how they feel. This is especially important for a child of divorced parents because parental perception and assessment may be more reflective of the parent's state or needs than those of the child. Asking children about where and how they are sleeping and eating and how they are currently doing in school may provide clues about their feelings and concerns.

Reliability

Other considerations may affect the reliability of information:

- More time may be spent in the care of someone other than the custodial parent, and so that parent is less aware of details (e.g., symptoms, what medicine has been given).
- Parents may project their own feelings or interparental conflict (e.g., the other parent is not taking good care of the child on weekends).
- The child may minimize symptoms so that the custodial parent will not have to miss work.
- The child may maximize symptoms so that both parents pay more attention.
- Someone less familiar with the child's past medical history may bring the child in for care (e.g., grandparent, parent's new partner).
- Parents may be involved in a child custody dispute.

Health issues may arise in child custody disputes, and the ability to adequately parent may include concerns about the child's health and safety. Parental smoking and alleged sexual abuse are two examples of issues that have been raised as reasons for disputing custody. Unless there is a concern for a child's safety, in general the pediatric practitioner should not side with one parent or the other and should encourage the involvement and cooperation of both parents in the care of the child.

Objective Data

There are a few observations and objective findings that are particular to the child of divorce. The physical examination provides a good opportunity to assess a child's level of stress and to establish rapport and support both the child and the parents. Because of the problems affecting reliability (mentioned previously) and some children's tendencies to somaticize when stressed, the physical examination may be essentially normal despite subjective complaints. However, this should not be assumed.

Acting out and risk-taking behaviors may predispose a child to injury. Careful documentation of findings may be especially important for a child involved in a custody dispute because medical records may be requested as evidence of the provision of adequate care by one of the parents. Any concerns about possible child neglect or abuse should be documented and reported.

Primary Care Issues and Implications

Support of the child within the changing family should be a continuing focus for the practitioner in partnership with the parents. Parents may require assistance in determining what is needed by the child to minimize disruption and maximize safety and support. Helping parents to cooperate "in the best interests of the child" rather than to compete with or condemn each other may remove the biggest obstacle to a child's healthy adjustment to changed circumstances.

Whenever possible, the same practitioner should see the child on subsequent visits to provide continuity, to assess problems and progress, and to create an opportunity for both the parents and child to discuss feelings. This may require juggling of schedules to accommodate visitation or parenting schedules.

The practitioner may be asked for advice in relation to the divorce process. Advocating for the child, encouraging continued involvement of both parents, and providing anticipatory guidance to assist the family with decisions as the child's needs change are appropriate roles for the practitioner; choosing sides and providing legal advice are not. If the child is moving between the parents' two residences, communication, consistency, and continuity of care may become problematic, especially if parental conflict persists. Phone calls or written explanations may be required to keep both parents informed and involved in the child's health care. Supporting both parents in the care of the child should be a goal even in situations of custody or other disputes.

The following potential areas of concern may frequently arise in providing primary care to children in divorcing families:

- *Growth and development*—Interruption of developmental tasks, regression, or early independence
- *Diet and nutrition*—Consistent monitoring of intake and growth, different food rules in different houses, person responsible for meals (e.g., working parent, stepparent), person who can prepare meals and eat with the child, or stress or depression affecting appetite
- *Exercise*—Familiarity with neighborhood resources, availability of friends to play with, or supervision of television time
- *Safety*—Acting out, risk taking, availability of adult supervision (e.g., for latchkey children), different environments, or different sets of rules
- *Immunizations*—Custody of immunization records, different care sites, whose insurance covers what services, or keeping both parents up to date on what services are needed and received
- *Sexuality*—Confusion with parents as social or sexual beings, decreased contact with noncustodial parent for gender role model, increased unsupervised time, acting out, risk taking, or seeking attention and love
- *Specific screening*—Psychosocial (e.g., for stress, depression), or for abuse and neglect

Management
Treatments and Medications

The economic and logistic problems often faced by postdivorce families have important practical implications. If the

---

Box 24-1 Rights of Children of Divorce

Lasting relationships with both parents
Truthful answers to their questions
Relief from feelings of guilt and blame
Freedom from interparental hostility
Attention to children's thoughts and feelings
Input into the visitation schedule
Privacy in communication with family and friends
Recognition of displacement by competing relationships
No requirement to parent the parents
Freedom from the role of messenger
No coercion to keep secrets
Understanding of the divorce agreement

Modified from Sammons, W.A.H. & Lewis, J. (2001). Helping children survive divorce. Contemporary Pediatrics, 18(3), 103-114. Copyright 2001 by Medical Economics Company. Used with permission.

---

child is moving between residences in different areas, communication with other care providers may be required for appropriate treatment, monitoring, and follow-up evaluation or care. As children move from one parent to another, continuity and consistency of treatments may be interrupted, medications may be forgotten or misplaced, monitoring of symptoms may be interrupted, and changes may go unnoticed or unreported. An infection may persist when a course of antibiotics is interrupted or not obtained, or a family activity may be affected by a forgotten inhaler for an asthmatic child.

Counseling and Prevention

Practitioners and parents need to be aware of the effect of stress on child behavior and health. Parents may need help in focusing on their child's needs, especially when their own resources and support systems are changing. Younger children have more frequent contact with practitioners, primarily because of recommended well-child examinations, standard immunizations, and the higher frequency of minor acute illnesses. These opportunities may allow a practitioner to assess the need for additional referrals (e.g., for medication or other counseling, financial or legal assistance).

Older children have fewer medical visits, so it is especially important to create or make use of opportunities for assessing such a child's family situation and to teach about health, stress, and self-care. This is especially important as children begin to make critical decisions that may have long-term implications for their health, such as trying cigarettes, alcohol, or other substances, or beginning sexual intimacy. These issues are difficult enough for two cooperative parents living together to discuss and guide a child through. They may be more difficult or less visible in the chaos of a divorcing family.

The practitioner should advise parents to give truthful, age-appropriate answers when children ask questions about the divorce. Children over 5 years of age usually know what has been going on. False assurances should be avoided. Parents must also understand that their children have both rights and needs (Box 24-1). Written materials can be made available to both parents (Box 24-2), and these guidelines are often applicable to children of all ages.

Follow-Up

Much of the present health care system is better suited to a two-parent situation in which one parent is available to bring a child in for appointments during normal business hours; this

Box 24-2 Helping Your Child Cope with Divorce

1. Reassure your child that both of you love him or her.
2. Keep constant as many aspects of your child's world as you can.
3. Reassure your child that the noncustodial parent will visit (if this is true).
4. If the noncustodial parent is no longer involved, find substitutes.
5. Help your child talk about painful feelings.
6. Make sure that your child understands that he or she is not responsible for the divorce.
7. Clarify that the divorce is final.
8. Try to protect your child's positive feelings about both of you.
9. Maintain normal discipline in both households.
10. Don't argue with each other about your child in the child's presence.
11. Try to avoid custody disputes.

Modified from Schmitt, B. (1992). Instructions for pediatric patients. Philadelphia: W.B. Saunders.

may mean that two working parents cannot bring a child in for recommended follow-up evaluation without taking time off work. Furthermore, if follow-up study is required while the child will be in the care of the other parent, additional communication, coordination, or referral to another health care provider may be required.

Consultations and Referrals

Some common referrals and resources for divorcing families are divorce and child custody mediators; mental health services, including school counselors; single-parent or other support groups; and child-support enforcement agencies. In several states it is now required that divorcing parents attend approved classes on children and divorce before completion of legal proceedings for divorce. Early referral in the divorce process may have the most success.

The practitioner should suggest that parents inform the school. A teacher, principal, or guidance counselor may help identify resources for the child. The practitioner may also recommend that parents request (in writing) that copies of report cards and all announcements be sent to both parents.

Resources

Organizations

Parents without Partners, 401 North Michigan Avenue, Chicago, IL 60611; (312) 644-6610

Single Parent Resource Center, 141 West 28th Street, New York, NY 10001; (212) 947-0221

Publications

Brown, L. & Brown, M. (1986). *Dinosaurs divorce: A guide for changing families.* Boston: Little, Brown & Co.

Christophersen, E.R. (1988). *Little people: Guidelines for common sense child rearing.* (3rd ed.). Chapter 11. Kansas City, MO: Westport Publishers.

Lansky, V. (1991). *Vicki Lansky's divorce book for parents.* New York: Signet.

Lewis, J. & Sammon, W.A.H. (1999). *Don't divorce your children: Parents and children talk about divorce.* Chicago: Contemporary Books.

Smith, G.R. & Abrahams, S. (1998). What every woman should know about divorce and custody. New York: Basic Books.

Thomas, S. (1995). *Parents are forever: A step-by-step guide to becoming successful co-parents after divorce.* Longmont, CO: Springboard.

Wallerstein, J.S. & Blakeslee, S. (1989). *Second chances.* New York: Ticknor & Fields.

Websites

(See also Chapters 3 and 30)

Children and Divorce (www.childrenanddivorce.com)

Divorce Magazine (www.divorcemag.com)

Bibliography

Amato, P. (1993). Children's adjustment to divorce: Theories, hypotheses, and empirical support. *Journal of Marriage and the Family, 55,* 23-38.

Clapp, G. (2000). Divorce and new beginnings: A complete guide to recovery, single parenting, co-parenting and stepfamilies. (2nd ed.). New York: John Wiley & Sons.

Emery, R. & Coiro, M. (1995). Divorce: Consequences for children. *Pediatrics in Review, 16,* 306-310.

Erikson, E.H. (1963). *Childhood and society* (2nd ed.). New York: W.W. Norton.

Furstenberg, F. & Cherlin, A. (1991). *Divided families: What happens to children when parents part.* Cambridge, MA: Harvard University Press.

Hetherington, E.M., Stanley-Hagen, M., & Anderson, E.R. (1989). Marital transitions: A child's perspective. *American Psychologist, 44,* 303-312.

Sammons, W.A.H. & Lewis, J. (2001). Helping children survive divorce. *Contemporary Pediatrics, 18*(3), 103-114.

Visher, J. & Visher, E. (1995). Beyond the nuclear family: Resources and implications for pediatricians. *Pediatric Clinics of North America, 42,* 31-43.

Wallerstein, J.S. (1991). The long-term effects of divorce on children: A review. *Journal of the American Academy of Child and Adolescent Psychiatry, 30,* 349-360.

Wallerstein, J.S., Lewis, J., & Blakeslee, S. (2000). *The unexpected legacy of divorce.* New York: Hyperion.

Chapter 25 *Foster Care*

Susan Nordberg

The foster care system can be very confusing. The current system can be traced back to England of 1590 and the Elizabethan poor laws, but the system has changed just as society's concept of social welfare has changed. President Theodore Roosevelt held the first White House Conference on the Care of Dependent Children in 1909. The report that followed outlined three principles that form the basis of the modern child welfare movement: (1) home is preferable to institutionalized care, (2) poverty alone should not result in separation of children from their family; and (3) there are families who either do not want to provide or cannot provide for their children.

Laws Governing Foster Care

In 1935, Title IV of the Social Security Act provided money for foster care essentials such as shelter, food, and clothing, but Title IV did not address what happened to these children once in the system. This was remedied in 1980 with the passage of Public Law 96-272. Three of that law's most significant provisions are financial incentives to the states to encourage them to make real efforts to reunite children with their birth families or, if that was not possible, to move the children to adoptive homes; federal funds allotted to help with the adoption of children with special needs, including adoption subsidies; and mandated individual case plans and case reviews for children in foster care. The Foster Care Independence Act of 1999 was passed to improve the services and resources available to children in transition from foster care to independence.

In 1991, the National Commission on Family Foster Care, appointed by the Child Welfare League of America and the National Foster Parent Association, published a report entitled *Blueprint for Fostering Infants, Children, and Youth in the 1990s*. This document identifies and discusses fundamental beliefs that collectively define foster care, including the idea that all children, regardless of age, sex, ethnicity, physical and emotional health, intellectual ability, or handicapping condition, are entitled to a family intended to be permanent and the notion that family foster care must fulfill five critical tasks: (1) protecting and nurturing; (2) ameliorating developmental delays and meeting social, emotional, and medical needs; (3) enhancing positive self-esteem, family relationships, and cultural and ethnic identity; (4) developing and implanting a plan for permanence; and (5) educating and socializing children and youth toward successful transitions to young adult life, relationships, and responsibilities.

Types of Foster Placement

There are several types of foster care placements, and some of these placements are specially geared toward therapeutic care for children with severe emotional and behavioral problems. *Group homes* are for children who cannot be maintained in a family environment because of behavioral problems or repeated episodes of running away. *Family foster care* can be divided into *kinship* (or *relative*) *homes* and *nonrelated homes*. The basic premise behind kinship family placements is that children are more comfortable and better cared for by loving relatives. The relatives are usually from the maternal side because many fathers do not claim or are not given the opportunity to claim paternity at birth. If a father has not been legally declared the parent, the paternal family has no legal claim on the infant until after court proceedings. The kinship family may be a grandmother (regardless of age or health) or any other relative willing to care for the child.

Entitlements and requirements vary from state to state and county to county. A kinship family is entitled to a grant to care for the children. However, such families usually receive only some public assistance and Medicaid, and it may take months for the first payment to be received. There may be no specific space requirements. Families may be monitored on an irregular basis, and the health care follow-up evaluation of children in kinship care has been known to be poorer than with family foster care. There may be no requirements for a caregiver to participate in classes or follow specific recommendations for infant/child stimulation. Additionally, when an infant is taken and placed in a particular household, the mother is not to remain in the house, causing many of these women to become homeless.

Nonrelated foster care providers are required to have a home evaluation, participate in classes, and be regularly monitored, and all recommendations must be followed to keep the children. These families receive a monthly payment determined by how much time and medical or psychiatric involvement is required to care for the particular child.

Data contrasting these two systems are inconclusive regarding which type of placement is best for the individual child. In kinship foster care, there seems to be no incentive for returning a child to the natural parent. In nonrelated homes, monitoring is more intense, allowing any abuse to be identified quickly. Furthermore, children are moved out of the system and into permanent homes more quickly.

The newest alternative to foster placement is *family preservation*. In this approach, a parent with an identified problem is allowed to keep the child in the home, but he or she must be involved in intense counseling, monitoring, and community-based services. Individual states must make a commitment of money, resources, and people for this to work.

Incidence

- In 1998, 520,000 children lived in out-of-home care, family foster care, kinship care, or residential care. Of these children, 60% returned to their birth families.
- The average age of the children in foster care was 9.5 years.
- The average time that children remained in foster care was 33 months.
- Children averaged 3.2 different foster home placements.

- Children of color were disproportionately represented, as 45% were African American, 35% were Caucasian, and 13% were Hispanic.
- Providing a family with assistance costs less than placing children in foster care because of a lack of decent housing.
- Compared with the United States population as a whole, children involved in the child welfare system are more likely to be poor and in poor health.
- Adolescents in foster care are among the most at risk for abusing alcohol and drugs, contracting and transmitting of human immunodeficiency virus (HIV), and becoming teen parents.
- Common medical conditions seen in foster care are anemia, asthma, congenital infections, gross dental erosions, dermatologic conditions, enuresis or encopresis, failure to thrive (FTT), hearing and visual problems, neurologic abnormalities, and recurrent otitis media.

Risk Factors

Children may be removed from their parents and placed in foster care for a variety of reasons:
- Family dysfunction or lack of parenting or employment skills in the caregivers
- Drug abuse, mental illness, incarceration, homelessness, alcoholism, illness such as HIV infection (with the mother too ill to care for the child), or intense family conflict
- Physical or sexual abuse (of child or spouse)
- Severe neglect
- Physical, emotional, or behavioral problems of the child
- Abandonment or desertion of the child by the parents

Subjective Data

A comprehensive health history should be obtained whenever possible. This can be a major task for children in the third or fourth placement or in the case of a child removed on an emergency basis. For an infant discharged from the newborn nursery, the foster care agency should receive a discharge summary from the hospital. For an older child, the social worker at the foster care agency can help in obtaining the birth record and any subsequent hospital or health care records. If a sibling group is being placed at the same time, questioning an older sibling about the health of a younger sibling can sometimes yield useful information. By 5 or 6 years of age, a caseworker may obtain general past medical history from the child by asking questions such as, "Do you get sick a lot?", "Do you take any medication or use any machines every day to stay healthy?", and "Have you ever been in the hospital for any reason?" If a biologic parent is available, this can be useful in obtaining the family history and child's past medical history; the caseworker can then relate this information to the agency's medical department. If older children arrive without immunization records, they might be obtained through the last school they attended. In addition to a complete age-appropriate history, the following information should be obtained:
- Reason the child was removed from parents
- Previous number of placements
- Type of placement (e.g., guardianship, kinship, out of family)
- Biologic parents' involvement, such as consent signing for any procedures

- Voluntary or court placement
- Name of foster agency involved or whether the child is being monitored by the child welfare administration
- Name of the caseworker responsible for the child

Gathering and maintaining medical records on children who are in and out of the foster care system is an ongoing challenge for everyone involved in their care. Use of national computerized databases for these children is ideal but not continually used. The use of the "medical passport" for the written documentation of past health care and concerns was first introduced in 1997. Ideally, the passport should travel with the child into and out of placement and be updated as needed whenever the child is seen by any health care professional, with confidentiality issues being kept within the guidelines of the law.

Objective Data

In 1994, the American Academy of Pediatrics (AAP) issued a policy statement regarding the health care of children in foster care. This document proposes four components of health care services:

1. *Initial health screening*—To be done before or shortly after placement. The purpose of this examination is to identify any immediate needs of the child and any additional health conditions that need to be addressed. This examination at the very least should include careful measurement of height, weight, and head circumference; examination of all skin surfaces for any bruises, scars, deformities, or limitation in function of body parts or organ systems; appropriate imaging studies if there is a history of physical abuse or recent trauma; genital and anal inspection of both sexes and testing for sexually transmitted diseases (STDs) if there is a history of sexual abuse or such abuse is indicated by physical findings; observation for signs of infectious and communicable diseases (e.g., pediculosis) and, if noted, prompt treatment; and the status of any known chronic illness to ensure that appropriate medications and treatments are available.

2. *Comprehensive health assessment*—Within 1 month of placement. This examination is not unlike a complete physical given to any child. However, because of the higher incidence of certain medical, developmental, and psychosocial issues inherent in foster children, specific systems need additional consideration:
   - *General appearance*—Assessment areas should include observation of adequate, seasonally appropriate clothing; interaction of child and foster parent, including the ability and willingness of the foster parent to appropriately console the child as needed during any uncomfortable aspects of the examination; and child's general affect.
   - *Growth parameters*—Height, weight, and head circumference (for children younger than 3 years of age) should be plotted carefully on the appropriate growth chart. If past medical records are available, previously recorded measurements should also be plotted to observe for past and current growth rates. Decelerations in height velocity noted before placement with a subsequent return to normal growth velocity can demonstrate that the child is being adequately nurtured in the current placement. If a deceleration is noted during placement, without any other medical cause, this place-

ment may not be ideal for the child to thrive in. Observing a consistent weight gain can allow one to assess adequate nutritional needs. Many children have psychiatric diagnoses requiring the use of a variety of psychotropic medications (e.g., stimulants, antidepressants, antipsychotics) that can increase or decrease their appetites and cause abnormal weight gains or weight losses. There is a higher incidence of microcephaly secondary to prenatal risk factors; therefore monitoring head circumference in infants is also important.

- *Skin*—Complete assessment of all skin surfaces for signs of physical abuse or self-mutilation should be made.
- *Gastrointestinal/genitourinary (GI/GU)*—Any daytime/nighttime urinary incontinence or fecal soiling should be discussed.
- *Status of any chronic illnesses.*
- *Formal dental and visual examinations within the first month of placement*—The practitioner should assess and repair dental caries secondary to nursing bottle syndrome and dental neglect and assess and treat visual problems, especially amblyopia that may not have been previously recognized.
- *Hearing screening.*
- *Laboratory data*—The laboratory tests required at placement are determined by the type of placement, the age of the child, and the agency or state regulations; tests may include:

    Complete blood cell count (CBC) and hemoglobin electrophoresis to rule out sickle cell or other hemoglobinopathies as opposed to iron deficiency anemias

    Lead level (for those 6 years and under or for any child who has a history of excessive mouthing of nonnutritive substances)

    Rapid plasma reagin (RPR) and other screenings for STDs as necessary from the history and physical examination

    Antibodies to the core antigen of the hepatitis B virus (anti-HBc) to screen for current or past hepatitis B infection, with a full hepatitis B panel if positive results

    Screen for hepatitis C antibodies in those children who have been born to a mother with risk factors for hepatitis C

    If HIV infection is suspected in the birth mother (e.g., because of substance abuse, promiscuity, STD, tuberculosis) or in the child, request for HIV testing of the child by the pediatric acquired immune deficiency syndrome (AIDS) unit of the local child welfare administration

    Mantoux test for tuberculosis every 2 or 3 years while in care or more often if the child frequents high-risk areas (e.g., correctional facilities where parents may be incarcerated, extended visits with birth family living in crowded homes or shelters

    Any additional tests deemed necessary by the findings on the physical examination (e.g., liver profile, chromosome analysis, medication levels, bone-age radiographs)

3. *Developmental, mental health, and psychologic assessments*—Use of assessment tools (see Chapter 11) for the child up to 6 years old and the HEADS (Home, Education/Employment, Activity, Drugs/Depression, Sex/Suicide) assessment tool for older children or adolescents.

4. *Monitoring of the child's health while in placement*—Often problems arise during the course of placement that were not apparent at the outset. After the "honeymoon" phase in the new home, distinct behavioral changes may become evident and significant emotional distress may occur after visits from the birth family. Therefore all children in foster care should receive periodic reassessments of their health, development, and emotional status to determine any changes and the need for additional services and interventions.

Primary Care Issues and Implications

Growth and Development

Measure, record, and plot height and weight at each visit to evaluate concerns previously mentioned. Perform developmental assessments at regular intervals. Address and refer to appropriate specialists any consistent failures. Most children in foster care are eligible for Medicaid and are therefore eligible for the Early Periodic Screening, Diagnosis, and Treatment (EPSDT) program. The Omnibus Budget Reconciliation Act of 1989 amendments to EPSDT guarantee access to all federally reimbursed Medicaid services, even those services that are not included in the state's Medicaid plan.

Immunizations

An immunization history is often difficult to obtain, especially if the child has had multiple placements. All attempts should be made to obtain the old records, either through the biologic parents (if feasible) or the last school attended. If the records are unavailable, follow the guidelines for the unimmunized child. For all other children, follow the AAP guidelines (see Chapter 13).

School

Many foster children have school problems such as poor achievement, grade retention, special educational enrollment, and behavior problems. For these children, the school system may be their safe haven, and they may exhibit behavioral problems when removed from the school they knew. Collect past educational and psychologic records and make them available to current schools for appropriate placement and ongoing psychologic or developmental therapies.

Discipline

Discipline is often a major issue for the child and foster parents. Interview both foster parents, as it is often surprising to find out how many couples have different views on discipline. Explore various behavioral interventions (e.g., reward system, timeouts) with the foster parents and encourage them to look for the positive qualities the child exhibits and not dwell on the negative behaviors. Discuss the many and varied reasons why a child may be acting out. Understanding the cause of the behaviors will make it easier for the foster parents to successfully nurture and discipline effectively. Many older children have been placed in foster care because of some type of violence, either verbal or physical, and have never experienced a consistent, positive approach to discipline. Corporal punishment is not acceptable in foster homes and is a major reason for the removal of children from foster parents.

Nutrition

Many children enter foster care malnourished and crave food. It is not unusual for a foster parent to state that the child overeats to the point of vomiting or hoards food under the bed clothing. A foster parent must slowly introduce the major food groups into a child's diet because many young children are reluctant to try unfamiliar foods. Family meals may be a strange concept for the child, but they can be a time for learning communication skills and good eating habits. Cultural differences in food types and preparations can also be a factor. Assist foster parents in referring eligible children to the various federal and state entitlement programs in their community (e.g., Women, Infants, and Children [WIC], Head Start).

Sexuality

Inform foster parents that a sexually abused child may exhibit sexual behaviors far before the expected age. Suggest interventions to handle these behaviors. It is important to counsel such a child about "good touch and bad touch" (not only on how he or she is touched but also on how he or she touches and shows affection to members of the foster family and other acquaintances). Refer for psychotherapy to help children and foster parent work through these concerns. Counsel preadolescents and adolescents on birth control, prevention of STDs, substance abuse, and HIV infection.

Exercise

A formal exercise program, either through the school or in the community, is helpful. It teaches the child to follow rules and helps in "letting off some steam."

Management

Regardless of the type of placement, the foster parents' responsibilities include: (1) helping the foster child maintain or improve relationships with family and friends and adjust at school, (2) nurturing the child's growth and development, (3) maintaining an attitude of respect and understanding toward the child's biologic parents because they are important to the child, (4) helping the agency in the development and implementation of casework plans for the child in the home, and (5) continuing to meet the needs of their own family while the child is in their care.

It is important to remember that people cannot focus on meeting their important individual needs until after their more basic needs of security, nurturance, stimulation, continuity, reciprocity, and value orientation are met. Each child brings a unique set of individual needs into the care situation that are a result of that child's genetic heritage, birth experiences, cultural identity, and past life experiences.

Knowing how the system is supposed to work and being aware of when it does not can help practitioners provide the best possible care for children. Foster care should not be viewed as a detriment to a child's health and emotional development but an opportunity to afford the child a healing environment.

Counseling and Prevention

- Conduct routine well-child counseling.
- Instruct in chronic conditions as indicated.
- Discuss safety and injury prevention. Do a home evaluation when possible.
- Discuss developmentally appropriate counseling for feelings of separation and mourning.

- Educate adolescents about STDs, birth control, and drug, tobacco, and alcohol abuse prevention.
- Teach adolescents how to advocate for their own needs. Depending on the agency or state, foster children usually "age out" by the age of 18 or 21.
- Explore future educational and employment opportunities, emphasizing the individual strengths and interests an adolescent possesses.
- Meet with and update the biologic parents on the child's current health status before the child is discharged back into their care.
- Before adoption, discuss with the foster parents a realistic management plan for chronic illnesses the child might have.

Follow-Up

The practitioner should see the child for well-child care and as needed for any chronic conditions. The periods for these visits vary with agency and state or county policies, AAP guidelines, and the individual provider's recommendations.

Consultations and Referrals

- Care of a foster child is most appropriately handled by an interdisciplinary team consisting of a social worker, the health care practitioner, the parents (biologic and foster), a mental health professional, and an educator.
- Referrals to early intervention programs should be done at the beginning of placement when indicated.
- Support groups, either within the foster care agency or in the community, should be used by both the parents and child.
- Referrals to medical specialists should be made as indicated.

Resources

Organizations

ACTION for Child Protection, 4724 Park Road, Unit C, Charlotte, NC 28203; (704) 529-1080

Child Welfare League of America (CWLA), 440 First Street, NE, Suite 310, Washington, DC 20001; (202) 638-2952

National Children's Advocacy Center, 106 Lincoln Street, Huntsville, AL 35801; (205) 532-3460

National Foster Parent Association, Inc., 226 Kilts Drive, Houston, TX 77024; (713) 467-1850

Publications

American Academy of Child and Adolescent Psychiatry. (1998). *Foster care: AACAP facts for families no. 64.* Online at www.aacap.org/publications/factsfam/64.htm.

American Academy of Pediatrics. (2000). *AAP releases recommendations for young children in foster care.* Online at www.aap.org/advocacy/releases/novfostercare.htm.

Child Welfare League of America. (2000). *Children 2000: Faces of the future national fact sheet.* Online at www.cwla.org/advocacy/nationalfactsheet00.htm.

Child Welfare League of America. (1999). *Foster care independence act of 1999.* Online at www.cwla.org/advocacy/indlivhr3443.htm.

National Clearinghouse on Child Abuse and Neglect Information. (1999). *Blueprint for family foster care in the 1990s.* Online at www.calib.com/nccanch/pubs/usermanuals/subscare/blueprt.htm.

National Clearinghouse on Child Abuse and Neglect Information. (1999). *Children of chemically involved parents: Special risks.* Online at www.calib.com/nccanch/pubs/usermanuals/subabuse/specrisk.htm.

National Clearinghouse on Child Abuse and Neglect Information. (1999). *The needs of abused and neglected children.* Online at www.calib.com/nccanch/pubs/usermanuals/subscare/needs.htm.

National Clearinghouse on Child Abuse and Neglect Information. (1999). *Substitute care and permanency planning.* Online at www.calib.com/nccanch/pubs/usermanuals/subscare/subcare.htm.

Oklahoma Department of Human Service. (1998). *Foster care: Foster parent training manual.* Online at www.homes4kids.org/foster.htm.

Bibliography

American Academy of Pediatrics. (2000). *2000 Red book: Report of the Committee on Infectious Diseases.* (25th ed.). Elk Grove Village, IL: American Academy of Pediatrics.

American Academy of Pediatrics. (2000). Developmental issues for young children in foster care. *Pediatrics, 106*(5), 1145-1150.

American Academy of Pediatrics. (1994). Health care of children in foster care. *Pediatrics, 93*(2), 335-338.

Beall, S. (2000). Addressing the health care needs of children in foster care: An innovative approach. *Advance for Nurse Practitioners, 8*(8), 61-64.

Behrman, R.E., Kliegman, R.M., & Jenson, H.B. (2000). *Nelson textbook of pediatrics.* (16th ed.). Philadelphia: W.B. Saunders.

Gitlitz, B. & Kuehne, E. (1997). Caring for children in foster care. *Journal of Pediatric Health Care, 11*(3), 127-129.

Goldenring, T.M. & Cohen, E. (1988). Getting into adolescent heads. *Contemporary Pediatrics, 5*(7), 75-90.

Hobbie, C. & Braddock, M. (2000). Medical assessment of children going into emergency out-of-home placement. *Journal of Pediatric Health Care, 14*(4), 172-179.

National Commission on Family Foster Care. (1991). *Blueprint for fostering infants, children, and youth in the 1990s.* Available online at www.calib.com/nccanch/pubs/usermanuals/subscare/blueprt.htm.

Roche, T. (2000). The crisis of foster care. *Time, 156*(20), 74-82.

Silver, T.A., Amster, B.J., & Haecher, T. (1999). *Young children in foster care.* Baltimore: Paul H. Brookes.

Simms, M.D., Freundlich, M., Battistelli, E.S., & Kaufman, N.D. (1999). Delivering health and mental health care services to children in family foster care after welfare and health care reform. *Child Welfare, 78*(1), 166-184.

Chapter 26 *Gay and Lesbian Parenting*

Sharon L. Sims

Families with gay or lesbian parents are becoming increasingly visible in the world of primary health care. This may be partly attributable to an increase in the number of such parents coming out about their sexuality after being in a heterosexual relationship, but it is also attributable to the increasing numbers of gay and lesbian partners who are becoming parents through adoption and assisted conception.

Incidence

- It is difficult to estimate numbers of gay and lesbian parents, just as it is difficult to estimate the numbers of gay and lesbian people in the general population.
- It is estimated 2% to 12% of American women are lesbians, and perhaps a third of them are parents.
- It is estimated that there are 2 to 8 million gay- or lesbian-headed families in the United States.

Numbers, however, are not the main issue. If gay and lesbian parents exist in the populations seen by practitioners (and they do), practitioners must be able to help identify and deal with the special concerns of these families. It is important to remember that although health issues for children in gay or lesbian families are often the same as those in other families, the practitioner's problem-solving approach must take the different context into account.

Risk Factors

There are no risk factors applicable to this topic.

Subjective Data

Identification of Gay and Lesbian Families

Gays and lesbians often do not seek health care for themselves because of fears about provider homophobia. These fears may also affect their health care–seeking behavior on behalf of their children. Practitioners should keep the following things in mind:

- Do not assume heterosexuality.
- Remember that one cannot tell who is gay or lesbian by the way a person looks or acts.
- Include questions such as:
  "Do you have a partner?"
  "Who else is responsible for the child's care if you are not available?"
  "Does anyone else share the responsibility of caring for this child with you?"
  "Who else parents this child with you?"
- Assess the level of confidentiality needed. Do the parents want their sexual orientation in the child's record? Are there legal risks to their custody if sexual orientation is revealed?

Objective Data

Normal well-child care is indicated for children in gay and lesbian families. Numerous reported studies have shown that children of gay and lesbian parents function as well as children of heterosexual parents in terms of their behavioral adjustment, sex-role identity, and self-concept (Laird, 1993; Patterson, 1994).

Primary Care Issues and Implications

Coparenting

Many issues related to coparenting in gay and lesbian families may affect the health care of their children. In American culture, the lack of official approval for gay and lesbian relationships makes them appear tentative or temporary, even though they may endure for many years. This lack of legal sanction has some obvious effect on parental status. *Second-parent adoptions* is the term coined by the National Center for Lesbian Rights to describe adoption by nonbiologic and same-sex parents. Many state laws still prohibit adoption of a child by a gay or lesbian coparent. In the year 2000, second-parent adoptions were recognized by statute or court decisions in Connecticut, District of Columbia, Illinois, Massachusetts, New York, New Jersey, and Vermont. Several other states (Alabama, Alaska, California, Hawaii, Indiana, Iowa, Louisiana, Maryland, Michigan, Minnesota, Nevada, New Mexico, Oregon, Rhode Island, Texas, and Washington) report instances of second-parent adoptions granted by judges in some counties. Depending on where they live and what legal actions parents have pursued, a child may have a legal biologic or adoptive parent and an unofficial coparent. Lack of legal parental status may translate into practical problems in the care of the child. For example, if the legal parent is gone, the coparent may not be able to give permission to treat the child. This issue can be brought up as an anticipatory guidance question by a practitioner during routine well-child visits by asking what arrangements have been made for emergency care of the child. If the parents have not considered the question, the practitioner could refer them to an attorney who specializes in alternative family law. Some gay and lesbian couples have obtained a form of unlimited guardianship for the nonadoptive or nonbiologic parent, and this allows the second parent to take legal responsibility for the child's care. However, state laws differ on this issue, and appropriate legal counsel may be the best solution.

Lack of legal status may also interfere with the coparent's ability to fully participate in caring for the child. Some parallels exist in blended families because stepparents must also create a place for themselves as providers of discipline, care, and supervision. Noncustodial parents may find it difficult to determine exactly what authority and responsibility they have in the care of the child, and this can lead to problems in role attainment for them.

Same-sex couples also must negotiate parental roles differently from the way heterosexual couples do, since the traditional male-female division of labor does not apply. This can be an opportunity for creativity in family development, and the practitioner is in the right position to work with gay and lesbian families as they develop their parental and family roles. It is a good practice to ask how parenting has been or is being negotiated between the partners at well-child visits and to offer the opportunity for discussion of this issue.

Gay and lesbian relationships fail sometimes, just as heterosexual marriages do. If a child is involved in the relationship, custody problems may ensue. This is especially problematic if the legal status of one parent is unclear. The legal parent may deny visitation rights to the coparent. The practitioner may need to act as the child's advocate in these cases, as he or she would with any family undergoing change. It may be appropriate to recommend legal or psychologic counseling in such instances.

In summary, the following are the main concerns about coparenting that practitioners should address with gay and lesbian families:

- What are the arrangements for the child's emergency care?
- Do both parents have legal responsibility for the child?
- How have parenting roles been negotiated?
- How comfortable are both partners with their parenting roles?
- If the partners separate, what kind of visitation arrangements will best meet the child's needs?
- If the partners separate, does the child need counseling or therapy support?

Sexuality

In a world where heterosexuality is the "norm," the usual questions about children's sexuality relate to developmental stages, not sexual inclination. Parents may be concerned about whether their adolescent is sexually active, but seldom are they initially concerned that such activity may be with same-sex partners. Gay and lesbian parents and their children cannot avoid either of these issues. It is certainly not a given that children of gays or lesbians will themselves be gay or lesbian, and they may or may not be, but parents must be prepared for either eventuality. What is more important is how parents will, over time, deal with questions of sexuality. A practitioner can assist by helping parents understand how children's developmental level influences what kinds of questions they will ask and how one should give a developmentally appropriate answer. What makes this issue different for gay and lesbian parents is that their children need information about both gay and heterosexual sexuality. It will be evident very early to children of gays and lesbians that their parents are different from most other parents with respect to sexuality, and parents need a plan for educating them appropriately. Jacob (1997) states that children may be more receptive to this information during childhood or late adolescence versus early to middle adolescence.

This increased visibility of gay and lesbian parents' sexuality may present a unique problem for their older children. A well-known joke is that most teenagers believe their parents never have sexual intercourse or had it only once per child. However, children of gays and lesbians do not have this cultural invisibility regarding their parent's sexuality. This may be particularly critical during the adolescent years. These teenagers must strug-

gle with their own sexual identity and behavior as well their awareness of their parent's sexual behavior. The practitioner should be aware of this complicating factor and address it with teenagers when discussing issues of sexual development and sexuality.

- Assess how open the parents are about their own sexuality with their families of origin and with their children.
- Ask if the parents have a plan for their child's sexuality education.
- Assist parents in finding developmentally appropriate answers for their children's questions.
- Be aware that teenagers may have difficulty in dealing with parents' sexuality as they are struggling with their own sexual identity.

Immunizations

Although human immunodeficiency virus (HIV) infection and acquired immunodeficiency syndrome (AIDS) are certainly not limited to the gay community, there may be times in families when issues arise if a parent or close family friends are positive for HIV. For example, a child's immunizations must be managed in a different way. According to the Committee on Infectious Diseases (2000), children in families with immunocompromised members should not receive live attenuated viral immunizations if such viruses are excreted in the stool. Because the Centers for Disease Control and Prevention (CDC) and the American Academy of Pediatrics (AAP) have recommended (since the year 2000) the inactivated polio vaccine for all children, the risks associated with the use of the oral vaccine no longer apply. Other immunizations are made of killed organisms, or they do not have the same viral shedding risk as the Sabin vaccine. There is no reason why a child living in a home with immunocompromised persons should not be fully immunized with DTaP, MMR, HBV, HIB, IPV, VAR, and PCV7 vaccines. Additional consideration should be given to annual influenza immunizations for all healthy contacts of an immunocompromised person. Thus children of parents with HIV or AIDS should receive flu shots yearly.

If a parent is positive for HIV or has AIDS, the practitioner can offer advice about prevention of transmission of common childhood infections from child to parent. This includes information about effective handwashing and perhaps isolating the parent from the child during the early, or most contagious, stage of upper respiratory infections (URIs) and febrile illnesses. This is probably more important than concerns about parent-to-child transmission of HIV infection, which is a much smaller risk.

In summary, the following steps should be considered when immunizing a child living with an immunocompromised person:

- Ask if immunocompromised persons live in the home or are part of the local family network.
- Provide all immunizations as recommended.
- Give influenza vaccine to children and other healthy contacts in the home on an annual basis.
- Provide parent education on decreasing the transmission of common childhood illnesses through effective handwashing and limited isolation of child from immunocompromised person during the early stages of respiratory and febrile illnesses.

Homophobia

The issue of homophobia has relevance for both the practitioner and gay or lesbian parents. The practitioner may experience homophobia as fear, anger, disgust, or confusion about homosexual persons and their way of living, and any of these reactions can prevent the practitioner from working effectively with gay and lesbian families. Often such attitudes are a result of little or no accurate information about gays and lesbians, so the Resources listed at the end of this chapter can provide such information. Talking to a friend or valued colleague who is openly gay or lesbian is another effective way of dealing with homophobia. However, if a practitioner recognizes that homophobia interferes with his or her ability to care for a family with gay or lesbian parents, he or she should suggest another colleague who is better able to provide that care. It is better to admit that an attitude is unlikely to change than to jeopardize the family's care.

Homophobia is often internalized, and gay or lesbian parents are almost always dealing with some degree of this throughout their lives. Their degree of being "out" about their sexual orientation is a direct reflection of internalized homophobia. Of course, this affects their ability to help their children deal with concerns arising from the parents' sexuality. Gays and lesbians with the best chance of success as parents are those who are most comfortable with their own sexuality. Having a high comfort level with their sexuality frees them up to define their families and family boundaries in ways that work best for them and their children and to develop productive ways to talk about issues of sexuality with their children. Of course, any family with appropriate boundaries and good communication skills will have fewer problems with child rearing, whether gay or heterosexual.

In regard to homophobia, the practitioner should:

- Assess himself or herself for problems with homophobia and working with gay and lesbian families.
- Educate himself or herself about gay and lesbian life.
- Assess the parents' comfort level with their sexuality.

Defining Family

How any family defines itself is an important clinical issue for the practitioner. Families with gay or lesbian parents may experience complicating factors as they move through this process. Grandparents, aunts, and uncles may not have an active role in the nuclear gay or lesbian family, depending on their response to the parents' homosexuality. Although it can certainly be a problem and a loss if grandparents or close blood relatives do not participate in the life of children, it can be just as big a problem if their homophobia makes their contribution a negative one. Some gay and lesbian families solve the problem by identifying a "family of choice," which may be a circle of friends who function as a support system to parents and children alike. It may not matter much just what this family structure is; it matters more how well it works.

The practitioner should:

- Assess status of relationships within the family of origin.
- Recognize who makes up the "family of choice."
- Examine how the family boundaries are defined. What information and activities are kept within family boundaries? What information and activities are allowed to cross family boundaries?
- Inquire if parents believe that they have adequate support from their families of origin and choice.

Community Issues

The family-community interface is more permeable in gay or lesbian families with children than it is in heterosexual families. Also, a childless gay or lesbian couple may be able to limit their interactions with the heterosexual community by developing friendships and social networks among only the gay community, but this is simply not possible for families with children. Children attend school, and so parents must interact with school administrators and teachers. Children engage in sports or other activities, and so parents must interact with coaches. Children play with other children, and so parents must interact with other parents. Gay- and lesbian-headed families must have connections in many arenas, including both the heterosexual and homosexual community. They must learn to be boundary dwellers, able to move in and out of communities associated with their children's needs and to be successful in them.

Part of their task is to decide how to present their relationship to these communities. For example, what happens when their child asks another child to stay overnight? Will the parents sleep together or separately? How do they help their children "come out" about their gay or lesbian parents? How will they handle the inevitable problems that arise when other children tease or abuse their children because of their parents' sexuality? How do they interact with a gay or lesbian community that may have problems accepting the presence of children? The practitioner's task is to find out which, if any, of these challenges exist for the family and to help them identify actions they might take or resources they might use in solving the problems.

The practitioner should:

- Assess the parents' comfort level in becoming "boundary dwellers" in multiple communities.
- Inquire how the couple has chosen to present their relationship as parents to their school, church, social network, and neighborhood.

Management

Treatments and Medications

There are none applicable to this topic.

Counseling and Prevention

The practitioner should discuss with parents how they will reveal their sexuality to their children. (See Primary Care Issues and Implications earlier in this chapter.)

Follow-Up

The practitioner should provide follow-up evaluation and care during routine well-child visits.

Consultations and Referrals

The practitioner should:

- Refer to an attorney if parents have not formalized coparenting roles or guardianship or if visitation rights have not been specified after parental separation.
- Refer to a mental health professional if parental separation results in ongoing stress for the child or children.
- Refer to family counseling if parents or children have difficulties dealing with the parents' sexual orientation.
- Refer to a support group for the child or parents if it is desired.

Resources

Organizations

Gay and Lesbian Parents Coalition International, PO Box 50360, Washington, DC 20091; (202) 583-8029

Lambda Legal Defense and Education Fund, 666 Broadway, New York, NY 10012; (212) 995-8585; www.lambda.org

Publications

Arnup, K. (1995). *Lesbian parenting: Living with pride and prejudice.* Charlottetown, PEI, Canada: Gynergy Books.

Burke, P. (1993). *Family values.* New York: Random House.

Curry, H. & Clifford, D. (1991). *A legal guide for lesbian and gay couples.* Berkeley, CA: Nolo Press.

Martin, A. (1993). *The lesbian and gay parenting handbook.* New York: Harper Perennial.

Websites

ACLU Factsheet on Lesbian and Gay Parenting Issues (www.aclu.org/issues/gay/parent.html)

Children of Lesbians and Gays Everywhere (COLAGE) (www.colage.org)

Listing of support groups for gay and lesbian parents (milepost1.com/gaydad/Support.Groups.html)

National Center for Lesbian Rights (www.nclrights.org)

Bibliography

Committee on Infectious Diseases. (2000). *Red book: Report of the Committee on Infectious Diseases.* Elk Grove Village, IL: American Academy of Pediatrics.

Jacob, M.C. (1997). Concerns of single women and lesbian couples considering conception through assisted reproduction. In Leiblum, S. (Ed.), *Infertility. Psychological issues and counseling strategies.* New York: John Wiley & Sons.

Kenney, J.W. & Tash, D.T. (1993). Lesbian childbearing couples' dilemmas and decisions. In Stern, P.N. (Ed.). *Lesbian health.* Bristol, PA: Taylor & Francis Publishers.

Laird, J. (1993). Lesbian and gay families. In Walsh, F. (Ed.). *Normal family processes.* New York: Guilford Press.

Muzio, C. (1999). Lesbian co-parenting: On being/being with the invisible (m)other. In Laird, J. (Ed.). *Lesbians and lesbian families: Reflections on theory and practice.* New York: Columbia University Press.

National Center for Lesbian Rights. (2001). *Second parent adoptions: An information sheet.* Available online at www.nclrights.org/publications.html.

Patterson, C.J. (1995). Lesbian mothers, gay fathers, and their children. In D'Augelli, A.R. & Patterson, C.J. (Eds.). *Lesbian, gay, and bisexual identities over the lifespan.* New York: Oxford University Press.

Patterson, C.J. (1994). Children of the lesbian baby boom: Behavioral adjustment, self-concepts, and sex-role identity. In Greene, B. & Herek, M. (Eds.). *Lesbian and gay psychology: Theory, research, and clinical applications.* Thousand Oaks, CA: Sage Publications.

Patterson, C.J. (1992). Children of lesbian and gay parents. *Child Development, 63,* 1025-1043.

Chapter 27 *The Gifted Child*

Theresa M. Eldridge

Gifted children are developmentally advanced and frequently achieve developmental milestones at an early age. A gifted child has special talents and qualities of character and temperament such as drive, commitment, perseverance, determination, and a high energy level. General characteristics of a gifted child might include superior intelligence (intelligence quotient [IQ] over 120 to 130), insatiable curiosity, retentive memory, insightful, and sensitivity to the environment. The gifted child frequently has a large vocabulary and is intense, compassionate, and able to generalize concepts. A child is often identified as gifted if the child demonstrates above-average ability or potential in one or more of the following categories:

- Academic ability (does well in an academic setting)
- Creativity and productive thinking
- Leadership ability
- Human relationships
- Intellectual ability (e.g., conceptualization, problem-solving)
- Ability in visual and performing arts (e.g., theater, painting)
- Psychomotor and mechanical abilities (e.g., dance, sports)

Giftedness does not appear in pure form because many children have a positive correlation between many abilities and aptitudes. Not all gifted children display the same characteristics, and some traits can mask ability. Gifted children's readiness is far ahead of their peer group. They are ready for challenge, and if the challenge is not met, behavioral problems can occur resulting in underachievement, dropping out of school, and delinquency. Children who are shy or nonverbal or children of color are frequently overlooked. They have become resigned to the boredom and are so emotionally sensitive and fearful of rejection that they do not exhibit their giftedness.

Giftedness is a continuum with different levels of giftedness that need to be addressed differently. Besides levels of giftedness, there are also individual learning styles and cultural differences to consider. Gifted children may learn and process information differently. The auditory learner "gets things" verbally and usually comprehends material in a sequential, step-by-step manner, the way material is ordinarily presented through lecture and textbook. The visual-spatial learner often needs literally to "see the big picture" before the constituent elements make sense. This "global learner" can experience keen frustration in a sequential learning environment. Many gifted children are visual-spatial learners. This variance between the learning style and the usual teaching methods in preschools and schools may lead to the diagnosis of learning disability. In addition, gifted children who have learning disabilities may not be identified as gifted because they have developed coping mechanisms that allow them to compensate for the learning disability.

Gifted and talented students need concerted support and encouragement from parents, the school system, and the community to achieve full development. Contrary to widespread belief, gifted individuals are rarely in positions or environments where they can simply "make it on their own."

Lacking recognition or accommodation for their educational and developmental needs, gifted and talented children and youths are at risk of failing to develop fully and to flourish educationally.

Incidence

There is no specific incidence reported of giftedness, partly because of the difficulty in having specific concrete tests that identify giftedness and partly because giftedness can be missed in many children. There is also no clear cause of giftedness.

- About 2% of the population has an IQ over 130.
- Children from low-income and minority backgrounds are less likely to be identified as gifted, partly as a result of ethnically biased tests.
- African Americans, Hispanics, and Native Americans are underrepresented by 30% to 70% in gifted programs.
- Physically disabled children may be gifted and are often not identified because of the obvious physical disability.
- Giftedness often goes unnoticed in children with learning disabilities. (Up to 16% of the gifted are also learning disabled.)

Risk Factors

Gifted children may be at risk for the following:
- Misdiagnosis
- Underachievement
- School phobia, absence, or failure
- Social and emotional isolation from peers and family
- Lack of appropriate resources and stimulation
- Conforming
- Withdrawal
- Low self-concept
- Rebellion or aggression
- Burnout
- Depression or suicide

Giftedness may also mask other problems and weaknesses, and it should be noted that girls may hide intelligence or be evaluated lower than their male peers.

Subjective Data

Research indicates that parents identify giftedness in their children approximately half the time. Therefore parents can be helpful in identifying gifted children as early as toddlers and preschoolers. In general, children who rapidly progress through the normal developmental milestones such as sitting, smiling, walking, and talking may be exhibiting early signs of giftedness. The preschool age is the best time to identify a gifted child. Preschool children who demonstrate early extensive language development and vocabulary, early ability to read and write, and excellent sense of humor with appreciation of wordplay may benefit from an evaluation for giftedness. Following is a list of questions the practitioner can ask parents to elicit a child's giftedness:

- Does our child readily adapt to new situations?
- Is your child flexible and usually undisturbed when the normal routine is changed?
- Is your child responsible and usually capable of following through on promises?
- Is your child self-confident with peers and adults?
- Is your child verbally expressive and well understood?
- Does your child tend to dominate others and direct others in activities?
- Does your child have strong interpersonal skills?
- Does your child show strong empathy, compassion, and sensitivity to others?
- Does your child express ethical, humanitarian, or global concerns?
- Does your child set and demand high standards for self and others?
- Does your child show good judgment and decision-making capabilities?
- Does your child show independence, nonconformity of thinking, and a willingness to take risks?

- Does your child demonstrate discipline, persistence, and commitment in areas of high interest?
- Does your child demonstrate a longer attention span than that of peers?
- Does your child exhibit an intensity or passion about areas of high interest?

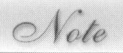

Children often exhibit characteristics of giftedness at a much earlier age than expected (e.g., preschool age).

Initial History

To assess potential giftedness, a history should include the following:

- Age of the child
- Family history:
  Learning disabilities
  Exceptional abilities in any of the specified areas of giftedness (see the overview at the beginning of this chapter)

Box 27-1 Specific Behavioral Characteristics of the Gifted Child

The child may demonstrate characteristics in one or more categories and may also have a combination of qualities from each category or may demonstrate other characteristics not identified here.

Intellectual Ability

- Learns rapidly and easily
- Uses a great deal of common sense and practical knowledge
- Reasons things out; thinks clearly; recognizes relationships; comprehends meanings
- Retains what was heard or read without much rote drill
- Knows about many things of which most students are unaware
- Has a large vocabulary, using it easily and accurately
- Can read books that are 1 to 2 years in advance of the rest of the class
- Performs difficult mental tasks
- Asks many questions; has a wide range of interests
- Does some academic work 1 to 2 years in advance of the class
- Is original in thinking; uses good but unusual methods
- Is alert, keenly observant, and quick to respond

Creative Ability

- Always seems to be full of new ideas pertaining to most subjects
- Invents things or creates original stories, plays, poetry, tunes, sketches, and so on
- Can use materials, words, or ideas in new ways
- Is able to put two or more ideas together to get a new idea
- Sees flaws in things, including own work, and can suggest better ways to do a job or reach an objective
- Is willing to experiment to get answers
- Asks many questions; shows a great deal of intellectual curiosity
- Is flexible and open-minded, willing to try one method after another and to change mind if need be; is not afraid of new ideas and will examine them before rejecting them

Leadership Ability

- Is liked and respected by most class members
- Is able to influence others to work toward desirable goals

- Is able to influence others to work toward undesirable goals
- Can take charge of the group
- Can judge the abilities of other students and find a place for them in the group's activities
- Is able to figure out what is wrong with an activity and show others how to do it better
- Is often asked for ideas and suggestions
- Is looked to by others when something must be decided
- Seems to sense what others want and helps them accomplish it
- Is a leader in several kinds of activities
- Enters into activities with contagious enthusiasm
- Is elected to offices

Scientific Ability

- Expresses self clearly and accurately through either writing or speaking
- Reads 1 to 2 years ahead of the class
- Is 1 to 2 years ahead of class in mathematical ability
- Has greater-than-average ability to grasp abstract concepts and see abstract relationships
- Has good motor coordination, especially eye-hand coordination; can do fine, precise manipulations
- Is willing to spend time beyond the ordinary assignments or schedule on things that are of particular interest
- Is not easily discouraged by failure of experiments or projects
- Wants to know the causes and reasons for things
- Spends much time on own special projects such as making collections, constructing a radio, making a telescope
- Reads a good deal of scientific literature and finds satisfaction in thinking about and discussing scientific affairs

Writing Talent

- Can develop a story from its beginning through the buildup and climax to an interesting conclusion
- Gives a refreshing twist, even to old ideas
- Uses only necessary details in telling a story
- Keeps the idea organized within the story

- Social history:
  Stimulation in the environment
  Freedom for exploration
  Types of activities at home, play, preschool, or school
- Developmental history, including acceleration of milestones (e.g., personal and social, language, fine motor, gross motor)
- Psychosocial history:
  Interrelationships with peers, family, and other adults
  Behavioral characteristics (e.g., determination, drive, high energy [see the questions under the Subjective Data heading])
  Emotional adjustments and behavioral problems
- Parental report of specific behaviors that they perceive to indicate giftedness
- School history (e.g., grades, teacher evaluations)
- Past health history
- Medications (e.g., for hyperactivity)
- History of frequent ear infections; results of hearing testing
- Previous developmental, educational, intellectual, creative, or other testing and results

Objective Data

Objective data also assist in identifying the gifted child. Certain data can be obtained only by educational specialists who are trained in evaluating gifted individuals. Box 27-1 provides a list of specific behavioral characteristics of the gifted child. The gifted child may demonstrate characteristics in one or more categories or may also have a combination of qualities from each category. This is not an all-inclusive list, and gifted children may exhibit other characteristics not identified.

Physical Examination

- Complete physical examination, including vision and hearing screening
- Complete neurologic assessment and evaluation of psychomotor skills
- Language skills

Screening or Testing (Appropriate to Specific Areas of Giftedness and Age)

- Developmental level (e.g., Denver II [see Appendix A], The Developmental Profile)

Box 27-1 Specific Behavioral Characteristics of the Gifted Child—cont'd

Writing Talent—cont'd

- Chooses descriptive words that show perception
- Includes important details that other youngsters miss and still gets across the central idea
- Enjoys writing stories and poems
- Makes the characters seem lifelike; captures the feelings of characters in writing

Dramatic Talent

- Readily shifts into the role of another character
- Shows interest in dramatic activities
- Uses voice to reflect changes of idea and mood
- Understands and portrays the conflict in a situation when given the opportunity to act out a dramatic event
- Communicates feelings by means of facial expression, gestures, and bodily movements
- Enjoys evoking emotional responses from listeners
- Shows unusual ability to dramatize feelings and experiences
- Moves a dramatic situation to a climax and brings it to a well-timed conclusion when telling a story
- Gets a good deal of satisfaction and happiness from play-acting or dramatizing
- Writes original plays or makes up plays from stories
- Can imitate others; mimics people and animals

Artistic Talent

- Covers a variety of subjects in drawings or paintings
- Takes artwork seriously; seems to find much satisfaction in it
- Shows originality in choice of subject, technique, and composition
- Is willing to try out new materials and experiences
- Fills extra time with drawing, painting, and sculpturing activities
- Uses art to express own experiences and feelings
- Is interested in other people's artwork; can appreciate, criticize, and learn four others' work

- Likes to model with clay, carve, or work with other forms of three-dimensional art

Musical Talent

- Responds more than others to rhythm and melody
- Sings well
- Puts verve and vigor into music
- Buys records; goes out of way to listen to music
- Enjoys harmonizing with others or singing in groups
- Uses music to express personal feelings and experiences
- Makes up original tunes
- Plays one or more musical instruments well

Mechanical Skills

- Does good work on craft projects
- Is interested in mechanical gadgets and machines
- Has a hobby involving mechanical devices, such as radios, model trains, construction sets
- Can repair gadgets; can put together mechanical things
- Comprehends mechanical problems, puzzles, and trick questions
- Likes to draw plans and make sketches of mechanical objects
- Reads *Popular Mechanics* and other magazines or books on mechanical subjects

Physical Skills

- Is energetic and seems to need considerable exercise to stay happy
- Enjoys participating in highly competitive physical games
- Is consistently outstanding in many kinds of competitive games
- Is one of the fastest runners in the class
- Is one of the physically best coordinated in the class
- Likes outdoor sports, hiking, and camping
- Is willing to spend much time practicing physical activities (e.g., shooting baskets, playing tennis or baseball, swimming)

- Intellectual ability (done by an educational specialist) (e.g., Stanford-Binet Test, Wechsler Intelligence Scale for Children [WISC])

Observations (by Health Care Provider, Teacher, or Parent)

- *Long attention span*—May work on projects as long as 45 minutes to 2 hours at preschool age (e.g., a 3-year-old who continues a project from one day to the next)
- *Creativity and imagination*—May have unique and innovative ideas for play, toys, and common materials (e.g., a preschooler who designs unusual dramatic play situations such as astronauts landing on the moon)
- *Social relationships*—May be a leader of others, have advanced social skills for age, and prefer to interact with older children and adults (e.g., a preschooler who recognizes that a new child in day care is feeling anxious and fearful and seeks to make that child feel welcome)
- *Number concepts*—Often fascinated with numbers, can tell time at an early age, and demonstrates mathematical abilities at an early age (e.g., a 4-year-old who counts the number of minutes left until snack time)
- *Memory*—Often has an exceptional memory (e.g., a 2-year-old who sits at a window and recites the makes of cars as they drive past)
- *Reasoning ability*—Able to form analogies at a young age and to justify responses; may also be a divergent thinker (e.g., a 4-year-old who is given colored blocks—a yellow triangle, a red triangle, and a yellow circle—and asked to choose a fourth block [a red circle] to complete the analogy, and who is also able to justify the choice)
- *Insight ability*—Has a superior insight from an ability to sift out relevant information, blend the information, and add new information to appropriate information received in the past; can also find solutions to complex problems (e.g., a 3- or 4-year-old who has salient ideas about how to deal with homelessness, nuclear war, or fixing a broken flower pot)
- *Verbal skills*—Shows an early interest in books, has an advanced vocabulary, reads early, or shows interest in foreign languages (e.g., a 3-year-old who can read and has an extensive vocabulary)

- *Attention to detail*—Often notices "insignificant" details (e.g., a 3-year-old who likes to make up elaborate rules for games or roleplaying)
- *High energy level*—Has a very high energy level, often needing little sleep (e.g., a 3-year-year old needing little sleep); may be called hyperactive because of the high energy level

Primary Care Issues and Implications

Growth and Development

Early identification creates opportunities for early intervention. A gifted child may achieve developmental milestones at an early age. Gifted children need time for play and unstructured activities. Parents must decide whether to enroll their gifted child in a private school or a public school. Decisions regarding acceleration (skipping one or more grades) or enrichment (providing classes specifically for gifted and talented children) must be addressed early in the child's life to avoid the negative consequences that can occur when the gifted child is not properly challenged. Issues about acceleration versus enrichment can be found in Table 27-1.

Often a variety of options may not be available to the family; in this instance a practitioner can help parents evaluate the educational program available to see if it is providing an optimal learning environment for their child, one that is difficult enough to increase learning and prevent boredom but not so difficult that it is discouraging. The services provided should also focus on learning experiences that fit the child's specific needs and culture and should be linked to a skill such as problem-solving and organized around issues. Successful gifted and talented programs provide gifted children with imaginative problem-solving, critical-thinking (divergent-thinking) curriculum, and, if possible, the creation of a product.

Immunizations, Exercise, Diet, and Nutrition

The needs of gifted children in these areas are the same as those of other children.

Safety

Gifted children may achieve developmental milestones early, so the biggest issue for parents centers around providing a safe

Table 27-1 Acceleration Versus Enrichment in Gifted Education*

	ADVANTAGES	DISADVANTAGES
Acceleration (starting school early or skipping grades)	Can usually be provided in all schools May provide academic challenge	Difficult to reverse May need to skip more than one grade to provide needed academic challenge Can cause social isolation from peers of same age
Enrichment (staying in same grade but supplementing the regular curriculum)	Classmates same age Provides for learning opportunities that may be lost because of acceleration Appropriate for some gifted children	May be expensive May not be appropriate for highly gifted children May promote an "elite" labeling of gifted children May lead to excessive homework if children have to make up homework for regular classes
Combination (acceleration and enrichment)	May be the best option for gifted children	Need to be sure children are appropriately challenged

*These are options for the child enrolled in a public school. Children can also be enrolled in private schools designed specifically for gifted children. If parents do not have the financial means to enroll their child in a private school, grants and scholarships may be available. Whatever situation is selected, it is important to assess the child and identify specific areas of giftedness that need to be addressed.

environment that provides stimulation and freedom for exploration. Gifted children may be advanced in problem-solving and manual dexterity and therefore can be at higher risk for injuries.

Sexuality

Sexuality issues are the same as for other children. However, a gifted child may be intellectually advanced but emotionally and physically age-inappropriate for dealing with sexuality, potentially causing conflicts.

Discipline

Discipline issues are the same as for other children. A gifted child needs rules and limits and should be treated the same as siblings.

Management

Treatments and Medications

None is needed, though many high-energy gifted children are misdiagnosed as hyperactive and receive Ritalin.

Counseling

Often it is best to work with an education specialist who is knowledgeable about the needs of and resources for gifted children and their families. The practitioner should also:

- Provide for early identification through history, observation, and physical examination.
- Assist parents in identifying unique behaviors and characteristics of the child.
- Provide parents with possible alternatives for maximizing the child's best qualities.
- Reassure and support parents in their recognition and acceptance of their gifted child.
- Provide information and counseling about normal growth and development.
- Educate parents regarding the concept of giftedness and its effect on the child and family.
- Assist the family in developing appropriate coping mechanisms to deal with emotional stresses and adjustment (e.g., experiencing financial stress; having a "different" child; having a child who may not be adjusting and is underachieving, missing school, or acting depressed; making decisions regarding evaluation and placement).
- Assist the family in manipulating environment to meet the needs of the child and in maximizing gifted characteristics (e.g., dance classes, workshops).
- Act as a resource person for the special needs of the family and child.
- Assist parents in evaluating appropriate learning and special programs for the gifted child.
- Encourage parents to participate in support groups for parents of gifted children.
- Encourage parents to provide opportunities for their child to develop peer relationships with other gifted children.
- Help parents identify their expectations of their children and of parenting a gifted child and assist them in reconciling their image with reality.
- Provide parents with resources for parenting a gifted child (see the Resources at the end of this chapter).
- Encourage parents to treat gifted children the same as they do other children.

- Help parents deal with sibling rivalry and encourage self-worth and competence in siblings of the gifted child.
- Help parents be effective and provide support for their gifted child (Box 27-2).
- Encourage parents not to put too much pressure on their gifted children but to provide for unstructured play and activities.
- Provide reassurance if parents are overwhelmed by a gifted child's special talents and intellect.

Follow-Up

The need for follow-up evaluation is the same as that for other children. Check with parents and children on an ongoing basis to see if the child's educational, emotional, and creative needs are being met.

Consultations and Referrals

- Refer the child and family to the state program for exceptional children.

Box 27-2 Nurturing the Gifted Child

- Establish a responsive and expressive climate with the child. Provide emotional support, listen to the child, and allow the child to express feelings.
- Provide encouragement for self-reliance.
- Recognize that a gifted child needs emotional support for being different. Cognitive development may be far ahead of emotional development.
- Respect the individuality and gifted characteristics of the child.
- Expect and allow for comfortable accelerations and regressions in growth patterns.
- Allow and provide for balance between interpersonal and solitary experiences.
- Establish well-defined limits and standards of discipline and conduct.
- Demonstrate an attitude of trust.
- Help the child understand his or her giftedness.
- Let the child act his or her age. An 8-year-old may have the intelligence of an adult but the emotional age of an 8-year-old.
- Do not expect perfection.
- Do not compare the child to other gifted children or to other children in the family.
- Be honest and accepting.
- Do not be overwhelmed by the child's giftedness. Do not be afraid to say you do not know and help the child find the appropriate answers.
- Encourage different areas of interest but also respect the passion that the child may have for one area.
- Nurture self-concept.
- Teach planning and goal setting.
- Teach self-evaluation and distinguish between self and school work. (Many gifted children are perfectionistic and self-critical and need to distinguish between their abilities and themselves as a good person.)
- Include the child in decision-making about acceleration, enrichment, or special placement in a school designed for gifted or talented (e.g., schools specifically for the gifted, schools for the performing arts).

- Refer parents to organizations for gifted children (see the Resources).
- Refer parents and children for testing by educational specialists trained in evaluating gifted children.
- Refer for counseling with a mental health professional such as a psychiatrist who is familiar with gifted children and their issues (if needed).
- Consult with the school principal, teachers, guidance counselors, and school nurse regarding management and psychosocial issues.

Resources

Organizations

Council for Exceptional Children, 348 East 6400 South, Suite 220, Salt Lake City, UT 84107; (703) 620-3660; www.cec.sped.org

Educational Resources Information Center (ERIC), 555 New Jersey Avenue, NW, Washington, DC, 20208-5720; (800) 538-3742; ericec.org

National Information Center for Children and Youth with Disabilities, PO Box 1492, Washington, DC 20013; (800) 695-0285; www.nichcy.org

The National Research Center on the Gifted and Talented, The University of Connecticut, 362 Fairfield Road, U-7, Storrs, CT 06269-2007; (203) 486-4826; www.gifted.uconn.edu/nrcgttxt.html

World Council for Gifted and Talented Children, 18401 Hiawatha Street, Northridge, CA 91326; (818) 368-2163; www.WorldGifted.org

Bibliography

Alvino, J. (Ed.).(1985). *Parents' guide to raising a gifted child: Recognizing your child's potential.* Boston: Little, Brown & Co.

Borland, J.H. & Wright, L. (1994). Identifying young, potentially gifted, economically disadvantaged students. *Gifted Child Quarterly, 38,* 164-171.

Buckley, K.C.P. (1994). Parents' views on education for the gifted. *Roeper Review, 16,* 215-216.

Coleman, M. R., & Gallagher, J.J. (1995). State identification policies: Gifted students from special populations. *Roeper Review, 17,* 268-275.

Frasier, M.M., et al. (1994). *A review of assessment issues in gifted education and their implications for identifying gifted minority students,* Storrs, CT: University of Connecticut, U.S. Department of Education, The National Research Center on the Gifted and Talented.

Stephens, K.R. & Karnes, F.A. (2000). State definitions for the gifted and talented revisited. *Exceptional Children, 66,* 219-238.

Thorkildsen, T.A. (1994). Some ethical implications of communal and competitive approaches to gifted education. *Roeper Review, 17,* 54-57.

Chapter 28 *The Drug-Exposed Infant*

Phyllis K. Marion

An infant exposed prenatally to illegal and legal substances can face a multitude of problems in the struggle for survival. Current estimates indicate 500,000 to 750,000 infants are being born each year who have been exposed in utero to illicit drugs. Adding legal substances such as tobacco and alcohol pushes the number of drug-exposed infants over 1 million. A new group of infants born to mothers being treated with controlled substances for chronic pain has not even been included in these estimates. Addressing the issues for these babies necessitates identifying them as early as possible.

A landmark study done in 1989 in Pinellas County, Florida, and supported by more recent state surveys demonstrates that addicted infants can be of any ethnicity and in all socioeconomic classes and live in any geographic location. The pattern of substance abuse described in this study is one of polysubstance abuse, not the use of a single drug as previously suspected. This polysubstance abuse may place the mother and infant at risk not only from the drugs used but also from the mother's risky lifestyle.

There are several types of legal and illegal substances that may cause problems for infants. Opiates or narcotics have morphine-like pharmacologic actions and can be natural or synthetic substances. Morphine and codeine are two natural opiates, whereas synthetic opiates include heroin, methadone, propoxyphene (Darvon), meperidine, oxycodone (Percodan, Percocet), hydromorphone (Dilaudid), acetaminophen with hydrocodone (Vicodin), and fentanyl. Even when prescribed in therapeutic doses, prolonged use can cause psychologic and physical addiction. Barbiturates used for sedation, insomnia, relief of anxiety, or as an anticonvulsant can also cause physical dependence for the infant with prolonged intrauterine exposure. Cocaine used in several different forms can have a profound effect on the outcome of the pregnancy as well as the neonate. Marijuana is the most widely used illicit drug among American women of childbearing age. Use of hallucinogens has varied over the past 30 years but can affect both the mother and neonate. Three legal and therefore more socially acceptable drugs—alcohol (which is covered in Chapter 47), tobacco, and caffeine—can also affect the fetus and neonate adversely. Table 28-1 details the effects of specific classes of drugs on pregnancy and the newborn.

Incidence

- Of the 4.1 million drug-abusing women of childbearing age, about 3% continued drug use during pregnancy (according to estimates from the 1995 and 1996 National Household Survey on Drug Abuse).
- Approximately 60% of women of childbearing age consume alcoholic beverages (according to the National Institute on Drug Abuse).
- Approximately 119,000 mothers who gave birth in 1992 reported using marijuana during pregnancy, and 820,000 mothers in that same survey reported cigarette smoking during pregnancy.

Risk Factors

The practitioner should be alerted to maternal substance abuse if the following are noted in the mother:

- No or infrequent (less than five visits) prenatal care; care at multiple sites
- History of past or present substance abuse in self or partner; past or present enrollment in drug treatment programs
- History of incarceration
- Current or past involvement in child protective services
- Current or past placement of other children in foster care
- History of placenta previa or precipitous delivery, alone or in combination with extramural delivery; mother's medical history and mental status
- Behavioral indicators, including inconsistent history, difficulty being aroused or falling asleep during visit, refusing to make eye contact, unwarranted hostility, missed appointments for self, and failure to follow up for infant care
- History of asthma without medical documentation (a red flag because "the high" of cocaine is increased with asthma pump use)

Subjective Data

At the first prenatal visit, the issue of substances taken should be addressed, and these questions need to be asked again throughout the pregnancy. It is important to emphasize that the reasons for asking the questions are to ascertain potential problems for mother and baby and to make plans for any necessary care. There may be a reluctance to report the use of illegal substances for fear of the consequences, including the mother's valid concern that her disclosures will mean the infant will be placed in foster care after delivery. The regulations surrounding the reporting of cases of maternal drug use and subsequent fetal exposure to child protective services or law enforcement agencies vary widely from state to state. Each practitioner must be aware of the legal issues in the locality of the practice site.

Social History

The practitioner may begin by asking about family grouping and living arrangements. The medical history and involvement of the father of the baby are also important pieces of information about the expected infant. Previous pregnancies and their outcomes should be discussed. Do the children live with the mother, and what arrangements have been made for their care at the time of delivery? If the mother does not have custody of the children, the circumstances of their placement and whether this was voluntary should be discussed. The mother's past involvement with social services and her reaction to any intervention are important clues. It is also helpful to know what support the mother will have after the baby is born and the availability of supplies for the infant.

315

Table 28-1 Substance Abuse and its Complications and Effects

DRUG OR SUBSTANCE	PRENATAL COMPLICATIONS	EFFECTS ON NEWBORN
Tobacco Used by 25% to 30% of all pregnant women; more than 30 compounds in cigarette smoke are harmful to both mother and infant	Spontaneous abortion Three times increased risk for placenta previa Increased perinatal morbidity fetal hypoxia	Low birthweight, prematurity, tachycardia, poor perfusion, poor feeding, irritability, heightened Moro tremor, greater risk of SIDS
Caffeine Mean caffeine content in foods and beverages vary: Coffee: 66 to 146 mg Nonherbal tea: 20 to 46 mg Colas: 32 to 65 mg	Consumption greater than two caffeine drinks per day increases risks	If used by breastfeeding mother, can cause irritability and poor sleeping patterns in infants
Marijuana Hallucinogen derived from *Cannabis sativa;* active component in THC; used by one of three women in childbearing years	Risk is dose dependent; IUGR with heavier usage; prolonged hypoxia; or prolonged, protracted, or arrested labor	Prematurity, increased meconium passage during delivery, problems of sleep cycling, possible effects on long-term development
Cocaine An alkaloid derivative of the *Erythroxylon coca* plant found in the mountainous regions of South America; Estimated 1% to 5% of neonates are exposed prenatally to one of the many forms by intranasal snorting, smoking, and IV injection	Tachycardia, hypertension, hyperthermia, agitation, anorexia, myocardial infarction/ischemia, CVA placenta previa, premature labor, seizures, abortion	Teratogenetic effects caused by the vasoconstricting effects-intestinal artresia, limb defects, skull defects, congenital heart disease, GU anomalies, small head circumference, SGA, preterm birth, persistent neurobehavioral changes
Hallucinogens LSD and PCP usually used in combination with other drugs	Accidental/self-inflicted trauma, labile mood swings, violent agitation	Severe withdrawal with coarse flapping tremors, facial grimaces with sudden and rapid LOC
Barbiturates Nembutal, Seconal, and Fiorinal are prescription drugs Also used illegally and in combination with other drugs	Sedation	Hyperactivity, excessive crying, restlessness hyperreflexia, seizures caused by sudden withdrawal
Amphetamines Stimulant drugs similar to cocaine and smoked in rock form	Maternal hypertension, tachycardia, proteinuria, placental hemorrhage	Cleft lip, cardiac defects, LBW, growth reduction, small head circumference
Narcotics Heroin and methadone (a synthetic opiate used in the treatment of heroin addiction) are the most commonly used; morphine used for the management of chronic pain	Heroin use, "addict lifestyle", dirty needles, poor nutrition, homelessness, and violence; fetal distress/demise; methadone: larger doses needed near term with increased fetal exposure; morphine: shorter half-life	NAS: high pitched, insistent inconsolable crying, sleep disturbances, irritability; CNS, GI, metabolic, vasomotor and respiratory effects; greater risk for SIDS and long-term developmental issues

GU, *Genitourinary;* LBW, *low birth weight;* LOC, *loss of consciousness;* SGA, *small for gestational age.*

Drug History

In initiating the discussion of substances used, the practitioner may begin with questions about diet and foods eaten. Discuss weight control and ask what methods the patient has used in the past to lose weight. Ask first about prescribed medications and over-the-counter drugs used; these questions are the less threatening. Legal substances should be addressed next, including tobacco and caffeine. Cola drinks, coffee, and tea (both hot and iced) should be included in a count of caffeine consumption. Remember to ask what, if any, stop-smoking aids are being used because there still may be some exposure to nicotine. Ask about alcohol use, remembering to inquire about beer and wine because these may not be considered alcohol by a patient.

Next begin to ask about the illegal substances, emphasizing that the reason for the questions is to help plan for the care of the mother and baby. Marijuana, or "weed" as it may be called, may be considered by some as an acceptable form of tobacco. The final questions should address use of cocaine, crack, heroin, barbiturates, and hallucinogens. A practitioner may use the term "street drugs," but each drug should be mentioned by name to ensure completeness. Some of these drugs will raise the questions of needle use, which has implications for hepatitis B and C and human immunodeficiency virus (HIV) disease.

Questions should be asked in an open-ended manner (e.g., "How many cigarettes or beers do you use in a day or week?"). "When did you start using the particular substance?" and "How often did you use it?" would be helpful questions to ask because those factors are both important in assessing the amount of risk to the mother and the developing fetus. The mother may be more forthcoming with information if she is questioned about the father's use of drugs first. All this information may not be obtained at the first interview, but the mother may become more comfortable over time; then answers may be more truthful. Questions should be repeated at subsequent interviews, even if negatively answered initially, as the situation may change. These questions are all clues to determining possible sequelae because the timing, frequency, and duration of the use of substances is as important as which substances have been used. It is important to remember that these self-reports frequently underestimate drug use.

It may be necessary to obtain this history at different intervals and in multiple settings. The information obtained in the prenatal setting should follow the mother and infant through delivery and the nursery to the primary care setting. The history of maternal drug use has implications for inpatient care, hospital discharge planning, and community health care.

Objective Data

Physical Examination

Since the clinical presentation of the drug-exposed infant in the nursery and the timing of withdrawal vary depending on the drug or drugs used, the timing and amount of maternal use, and both maternal and fetal metabolism and excretion, the maternal history and frequent assessments of the newborn are important. If the period between the last maternal use and the delivery is greater than 1 week or if use was infrequent, the incidence of neonatal withdrawal and complications may be low. On the other hand, prolonged and frequent alcohol use can make the major dysmorphic features of fetal alcohol syndrome (FAS) present at birth and withdrawal begins early, usually during the first 3 to 12 hours after delivery. Depending on the half-life of elimination of the maternal substance used, the appearance of symptoms could also be delayed. Narcotic withdrawal is frequently within the first 48 to 72 hours, but it may take as long as 4 weeks. Even the earlier period may not be long enough for the diagnosis of drug withdrawal to be made in the hospital nursery because many babies are discharged before 48 hours. Sedative withdrawal may also not occur until after the first few days of life and may happen 1 to 3 weeks later. So it is not only in the inpatient newborn nursery but also in the primary care setting that the practitioner must be aware of maternal drug-use history and the signs of neonate withdrawal.

The characteristics of an infant exposed to maternal drug use may include prematurity, unexplained intrauterine growth retardation (IUGR), urogenital anomalies, atypical vascular incidents, and neurobehavioral problems. The presence of anomalies is suggestive of drug use in the first trimester. Poor intrauterine growth may be a result of frequent substance use, while preterm delivery may be the result of use later in pregnancy.

Although initially the newborn may appear normal, there may be some signs occurring as the infant is observed over the first few days of life. Increased tone, an exaggerated Moro reflex, and pulling to a sitting or standing position may be seen. The infant may be irritable and inconsolable. Attempts at feeding are less than successful because of the infant's poorly coordinated suck and swallow. The newborn loses fluid and calories from spitting up and diarrhea that can exceed 10 stools per day. Weight loss also occurs from excessive movement and twitching. Skin excoriation can occur from the frequent stools and the rubbing of bony prominences such as knees, elbows, and noses against fabric. These signs and symptoms may appear during the first 48 hours of life, or they may not appear until the infant is a few weeks old.

Diagnostic Procedures and Laboratory Tests

Although testing of the mother for drugs requires her consent, state and institutional guidelines differ with regard to toxicology screens of an infant. Awareness of these guidelines is necessary before testing of the infant can be ordered. The most frequently reported indicator used to identify mothers whose infants need toxicology screening is no or infrequent prenatal care. It is however, important to consider other secondary indicators to avoid bias in the selection of infants to be tested. Both documentation of the presence of the maternal risk factors previously listed and the infant signs and symptoms that are assessed in the newborn can be used to support the need for testing.

The following are methods of newborn or infant toxicologic screening:

- *Urine*—The urine should be the earliest void possible because urine testing provides confirmation of drugs metabolized quickly and discloses recent use of a substance by the mother. Placement of the urine-collecting bag is difficult; and nursing staff must observe the infant so that the specimen is not lost.
- *Meconium*—Because the infant passes meconium for only the first few stools, this sample needs to be collected promptly. The testing is not available in all laboratories, and the results take longer than the results for urine testing. However, such testing does provide evidence of use throughout pregnancy.
- *Hair*—Testing of the infant's hair is expensive and seldom available and requires clipping strands of hair from the infant; it does however provide evidence of drug use over an extended period.
- *Blood*—Mothers may be tested for hepatitis B and C, syphilis, and HIV disease, while infants may have newborn screening testing for HIV. Positive results on these tests are not conclusive of substance abuse.

Positive results on toxicology screens may be reportable. To whom this information is given, by whom, and what happens as a result vary from state to state. In most states, the social services department is responsible for making the initial report to the state child protective agency. This state agency does the investigation and makes a final decision about the newborn, though the plan does not always require removal of the infant from the mother's custody.

Differential Diagnosis

It may be difficult to differentiate the symptoms of central nervous system (CNS) irritability resulting from infection or metabolic disorders (e.g., hypoglycemia, hypocalcemia) from those resulting from maternal drug use. Clinical signs must be correlated with appropriate diagnostic tests to rule out other causes. The assumption that a positive history of maternal drug use is the sole reason for the infant's symptoms may be an error. Being unaware of the mother's drug history, however, may cause the signs of withdrawal to be mistaken for other common neonatal problems (e.g., colic, formula intolerance).

Primary Care Issues and Implications

Table 28-2 details the primary care issues and suggests necessary assessments and interventions for the post–hospital discharge period.

Management

Management of the drug-exposed infant is dependent on the age of the infant and the drugs to which it has been exposed. The severity of the presentation of neonatal abstinence syndrome (NAS) will determine which infant may need pharmacologic intervention. One common method of assessing a drug-exposed infant is the use of the Neonatal Abstinence Scoring System shown in Fig. 28-1. This scoring system, devised by Finnegan (1986), can be used to assess the onset, progression, and resolution of symptoms, especially in an infant exposed to opioids. If medication is needed, the scoring system will help to monitor its effectiveness. Symptoms are given point values that, when added together, give a total score. Total scores of 1 through 7 will require comfort measures of

swaddling, pacifiers, and so on, as listed in Table 28-3. Scores of 8 or more, especially when measured at three or more consecutive assessments, may require medication. With two consecutive assessments of 12 or higher, appropriate medication therapy should be started within 4 hours.

The infant is assessed 2 hours after birth and then every 4 hours unless the total score rises above 0, at which point the infant should be assessed every 2 hours for a 24-hour period. If scores for that period are 7 or less, assessments may be done every 4 hours. All signs observed during the scoring interval are recorded, not just those seen at a single point in time. A new sheet is begun at the beginning of each day for those infants in the newborn nursery. This scoring sheet can be used at office visits to assess resolution of symptoms by questioning the baby's caregiver.

Treatments and Medications

The decision to use medications to combat the symptoms of withdrawal can be made based on the NAS score. Practitioners should keep in mind that the use of medication delays the infant's discharge, interrupts mother-infant bonding, and increases the mother's feelings of guilt, but it becomes necessary when the infant begins to show signs of distress. The most commonly used medications are phenobarbital and tincture of opium. Paregoric contains additives that themselves have side effects. The dosing of phenobarbital is as follows:

- Loading dose: 5 mg/kg intravenous or intramuscular
- Maintenance dose: 2 to 6 mg/kg/day by mouth, given in divided doses every 6 to 8 hours and increased to a maximum of 10 mg/kg/day
- Weaning: Decrease of 1 mg/kg/day or more depending on the NAS score

The advantages of phenobarbital are that it controls irritability and insomnia and that the infant can be weaned from

Table 28-2 Primary Care for the Infant with Perinatal Drug Exposure

ISSUE	ASSESSMENT/INTERVENTION
Growth and development	Initially see weekly until weight gain is stabilized, then monthly; measure length, weight, and head circumference at each visit; assess developmental milestones; refer to early intervention at 6 months if needed.
Immunizations	Follow American Academy of Pediatrics (AAP) guidelines.
Screening	Consider HIV testing if not part of newborn screening or if history is unknown or questionable.
	Follow AAP guidelines for hearing and vision, hematocrit, lead, tuberculosis, and dental screening.
Neurobehavioral problems	Assess tone and motor skills at each visit.
	Observe interaction between infant and caregiver.
	Observe for signs of depression in both infant and caregiver.
Nutrition	Initially should gain 15 g per day; may need increased calorie formula for several months to achieve that gain.
	Breastfeeding is contraindicated if the mother is still using drugs (with the exception of methadone doses less than 20 mg in 24 hours), is HIV positive, has a history of IV drug use, or has syphilis with drug use
Safety concerns	Home monitoring by child protective agency or public health or visiting nurse.
	Discuss dangers of secondhand smoke.
	Explain increased risks for SIDS; educate about appropriate sleeping position.
	If mother is on methadone—if breastfeeding, should take after a feeding; should be kept in a locked cabinet; question if mother is sleepy or nods off; infant's safety will need to be determined.
Sleep patterns	Has no regular sleep pattern because of irritability and increased sense of sound.
	Needs quiet, dark environment.
	Increasing periods of sleep between feedings promotes growth.
Discipline/parenting skills	Infant may continue to be demanding and irritable, with excessive crying, and is at risk for abuse and neglect.
	Encourage comfort measures.
	Educate regarding appropriate expectations of infant development.

it quickly. Its disadvantages include sedation that can interfere with sucking and no capacity to control the gastrointestinal (GI) symptoms of cramping and frequent stooling. The dosing for tincture of opium (10 mg/ml diluted 25-fold with water to make a solution with a concentration of 0.4 mg/ml) is as follows:

- Loading dose: 0.2 to 0.3 ml dose every 3 to 4 hours, possibly increased by 0.05 ml per dose every 3-4 hours until symptoms abate; maximum dose is 0.7 ml per dose

- Weaning: Decrease of 10% every 2 to 3 days over a 2- to 4-week period, to be started when symptoms have been under control for several days

Tincture of opium works well on the GI system by decreasing bowel motility, affecting cramping and the frequency of stooling. It increases sucking coordination and reduces the incidence of seizures. Its primary disadvantages are that large doses are required and weaning is slow; therefore discharge from the hospital may be delayed.

NEONATAL ABSTINENCE SCORING SYSTEM

	SYSTEM, SIGNS AND SYMPTOMS	SCORE	AM						PM					COMMENTS
CENTRAL NERVOUS SYSTEM DISTURBANCES	Excessive High Pitched (or Other) Cry	2												Daily Weight:
	Continuous High Pitched (or Other) Cry	3												
	Sleeps < 1 Hour after Feeding	3												
	Sleeps < 2 Hours after Feeding	2												
	Sleeps < 3 Hours after Feeding	1												
	Hyperactive Moro Reflex	2												
	Markedly Hyperactive Moro Reflex	3												
	Mild Tremors Disturbed	1												
	Moderate/Severe Tremors Disturbed	2												
	Mild Tremors Undisturbed	3												
	Moderate/Severe Tremors Undisturbed	4												
	Increased Muscle Tone	2												
	Excoriation (Specific Area)	1												
	Myoclonic Jerks	3												
	Generalized Convulsions	5												
METABOLIC/VASOMOTOR/ RESPIRATORY DISTURBANCES	Sweating	1												
	Fever<101 (99-100.8° F/37.2-38.2° C)	1												
	Fever>101 (38.4° C and Higher)	2												
	Frequent Yawning (> 3-4 Times/Interval)	1												
	Mottling	1												
	Nasal Stuffiness	1												
	Sneezing (> 3-4 Times/Interval)	1												
	Nasal Flaring	2												
	Respiratory Rate > 60/min	1												
	Respiratory Rate > 60/min with Retractions	2												
GASTROINTESTINAL DISTURBANCES	Excessive Sucking	1												
	Poor Feeding	2												
	Regurgitation	2												
	Projectile Vomiting	3												
	Loose Stools	2												
	Watery Stools	3												
	TOTAL SCORE:													
	INITIALS OF SCORER													

Fig. 28-1 Neonatal Abstinence Score Sheet. (From Finnegan, L.P. [1986]. Neonatal abstinence syndrome. In Rubatelli, F.F. & Granati, B. [Eds.]. *Neonatal therapy: An update*. New York: Excerpta Medica.)

Table 28-3 Common Symptoms and Interventions for the Drug-Exposed Infant

SYMPTOM	INTERVENTION
High-pitched cry or irritability	Swaddling or wrapping the infant tightly
	Nonnutritive sucking
	Quiet, darkened environment
	Organized care to minimize handling
	Reduced stimuli (e.g., holding but not rocking)
	Vertical rocking more effective than horizontal
	Tepid baths several times a day
Poor feeding	Daily weights
	Frequent feeding
	Slow feeding with frequent burping
	If more than 10% of birth weight is lost, higher-calorie formula until withdrawal symptoms subside and weight gain is consistently improving
	Avoidance of added stimuli of talking to, rocking, or making eye contact while feeding
Gastrointestinal problems	Elevated head of bed
	Tepid bath to relieve cramping once cord is off and healed
	Frequent diaper changes with use of thick cream (e.g., zinc oxide–containing ointments) on buttocks; exposure of buttocks to air
Hypertonicity or tremors	Swaddling
	Cool environment temperature
	Frequent position changes to prevent pressure sores
Skin care	Duoderm for knees, noses, elbows and buttocks that become excoriated from rubbing against linens

The physical care required when symptoms appear can be started in the nursery and will need to be explained to whomever will be taking care of the infant after discharge. The infants can be a challenge to care for while they withdraw from a substance. Table 28-3 provides a summary of care for different symptoms common to the drug-exposed infant.

Once an infant has been medically cleared for discharge, the practitioner's first concern is who will be caring for the infant: the mother, a family member as guardian, or an unrelated foster care family? Each placement has its own special problems. If the infant will be going home with the mother, has monitoring by protective services been put into place?

When the mother and infant return home, it may be to the same setting in which the drug use took place. The home situation may be chaotic, with few support systems and fewer good parenting role models, and drug-exposed infants can be challenging to care for under the best of circumstances. If the mother is the primary caregiver, mother-child interaction and well-being must be assessed frequently and at every contact.

When another family member is caring for the infant, the practitioner may need to assess child-care skills and make suggestions without alienating the caregiver. This person might be older and have long-established parenting skills that now need to be changed, because such a demanding infant will quickly become an active toddler and may tax the older person's physical and emotional energy. Also, family members may not be aware of drug use by the mother and may question why the infant was placed in their care. Secrets can also be revealed if the infant is discharged with a prescription for AZT. This can further isolate the mother from her family and her infant.

Placement in foster care is an additional barrier to mother-infant bonding, but it may be the only choice available. Close medical follow-up study is ensured, but the mother may or may not have access to her child depending on the mother's situation. Instructions for the care of the infant must be given to the foster parent, possibly in writing if he or she is not the one taking the infant from the hospital.

Counseling and Prevention

- Encourage the mother-infant attachment. The infant's primary care provider (PCP) is an important support person for the mother of a drug-exposed baby because the mother may not always be aware of the extent to which her drug use affects her infant and the care required. The mother will also be facing her own drug use issues, as well as those of the infant. If the infant's discharge from the hospital is delayed or the infant is not placed in the mother's care, there may be delayed bonding.

- Explain the treatment plan to the mother. She needs to understand the symptoms her infant is experiencing and the interventions used to ease those symptoms. She may need demonstrations on swaddling. Feeding the infant slowly using jaw-control techniques for infants with a poor suck may need to be demonstrated. Some babies may be very sleepy, hypotonic, and difficult to arouse for feeding; others may move from hyperactive to very quiet.

- Encourage the mother's interaction with her infant, including establishing consistent stable patterns of eating and sleeping. Learning to talk and enjoy her infant are important for the mother. She needs to learn to read the infant's cues and to comfort and quiet the baby. Bathing and massaging the infant can be soothing for both.

- Discuss infant feeding and nutrition. Breast milk is the ideal food source for infants and enhances bonding, which is especially important for drug-exposed infants, who are at increased risk for child abuse and neglect. However, the risks to the infant of exposure to drugs in breast milk must be weighed against the benefits. If the mother has an ongoing problem with the use of illicit drugs, the risks outweigh the benefits, and formula feeding is recommended. Breastfeeding is compatible with moderate use of alcohol, cigarettes, or caffeine and may even encourage the mother to limit her use for the sake of her nursing infant.

Follow-Up

Regular health care for a drug-exposed infant is vital, and prompt follow-up evaluation by the provider of missed appointments is essential. The mother or caregiver must be given emergency contact numbers for after-hours care and clear guidelines on when to seek assistance.

Consultations and Referrals

Consideration of the following referrals should be made:
- Early intervention for developmental delay
- Apnea center, if there is a family history of sudden infant death syndrome (SIDS) or apneic episodes reported by the mother
- Neurologist, if there is persistent hypertonia or hypotonia
- Child protective agency for suspected continued drug use by the mother or abuse and neglect of the child

Resources

Hotlines
Cocaine Helpline: (800) COCAINE
National Institute on Drug Abuse: (800) 662-HELP
Websites
American Academy of Pediatrics (www.aap.org)
CyberZone (www.cyberZone-inc.com)
Parenting: Babies and Toddlers (babyparenting.miningco.com)
University of Washington Medical Center
   (babyparentingabout.com)

Bibliography

Avery, G.B., Fletcher, M.A., & Macdonald, M.G. (Eds.). (1994). *Neonatology, pathophysiology, and management of the newborn.* (4th ed.). Philadelphia: J.B. Lippincott.

Berlin, C.M. (1998). Policy statement: Neonatal drug withdrawal. *Pediatrics, 101*(6), 1079-1088.

Bell, G.L. & Lau, K. (1995). Perinatal and neonatal issues of substance abuse. *Pediatric Clinics of North America, 42*(2), 261-281.

Chasnoff, I., Landress, H., & Barrett, M. (1990). The prevalence of illicit drug or alcohol use during pregnancy and discrepancies in reporting in Pinellas County, Florida. *New England Journal of Medicine, 322,* 1202-1206.

Davidson Ward, S.L. & Keens, T.G. (1992). Prenatal substance abuse. *Clinics in Perinatology, 19*(4), 849-860.

Delaney-Black, V., Covington, C., Templin, T., Ager, J., Martier, S., & Sokol, R. (1998). Prenatal cocaine exposure and child behavior. *Pediatrics, 102*(4), 945-950.

DeVille, K.A. & Kopelman, L.M. (1998). Moral and social issues regarding pregnant women who use and abuse drugs. *Obstetrics and Gynecology Clinics of North America, 25*(1), 237-254.

Finnegan, L. (1986). Neonatal abstinence syndrome. In Rubatelli, F.F. & Granati, B. (Eds.). Neonatal therapy: An update. New York: Excerpta Medica.

Gitlitz, B. (1997). The addicted infant. In Fox, J. (Ed.). *Primary health care of children.* St. Louis: Mosby.

Howard, C.R. & Lawrence, R.A. (1998). Breast-feeding and drug exposure. *Obstetrics and Gynecology Clinics of North America, 25*(1), 195-217.

Johnson, L.M. (1999). *Drug addicted babies.* Available online at babyparenting.miningco.com.

Kuehne, E.A. & Warguska, M. (2000). Prenatal cocaine exposure. In Jackson, P.L. & Vessey, J.A. (Eds.). *Primary care of the child with a chronic condition* (3rd ed.). St. Louis: Mosby.

Kwong, T.C. & Shearer, D. (1998). Detection of drug use during pregnancy. *Obstetrics and Gynecology Clinics of North America, 25*(1), 43-57.

Lee, M. (1998). Marijuana and tobacco use in pregnancy. *Obstetrics and Gynecology Clinics of North America, 25*(1), 65-83.

Novack, A. (1998). Neonatal abstinence syndrome. Available online at babyparenting@about.com.

Plessinger, M.A. (1998). Prenatal exposure to amphetamine: Risks and adverse outcomes in pregnancy. *Obstetrics and Gynecology Clinics of North America, 25*(1), 199-237.

Schydlower, M. (1995). Policy statement: Drug exposed infants. *Pediatrics, 96*(2), 364-367.

Siberry, G.K. & Iannone, R. (Eds.) (2000). *The Harriet Lane handbook: A manual for pediatric house officers* (15th ed.). St. Louis: Mosby.

U.S. Department of Health and Human Services. (1997). *Annual survey of drug abuse in the United States.* Washington, DC: US Department of Health and Human Services.

Wagner, C.L., Kaitikanemi, L.D., Cox, T.H., & Ryan, R.M. (1998). Impact of prenatal drug exposure on the neonate. *Obstetrics and Gynecology Clinics of North America, 25*(1), 169-194.

Chapter 29 *The Premature Infant*

Barbara Jones Deloian

Dramatic decreases in perinatal and infant mortality have been seen in the last couple of decades, and survival rates for preterm infants have improved significantly. Approximately 49% of infants weighing 501 to 750 g, 85% of infants weighing 750 to 1000 g, 93% of infants weighing 1001 to 1250 g, and 96% of infants weighing 1251 to 1500 g survive (Stevenson et al, 1998). The morbidity of these infants, however, is more complicated than mere survival. The morbidities for very-low–birth-weight (VLBW) infants ranges from 40% to 50%, with mild to moderate impairments in 20% to 39% and severe impairments in 20% (Bergman, 1998). Routine well-child care may be inadequate for the needs of these infants and their families because of their early problems. The American Academy of Pediatrics (AAP) Committee on the Fetus and Newborn recommends more frequent appointments for premature infants with medical or weight concerns. This is especially true for VLBW and extremely-low-birth-weight infants (Table 29-1).

The primary care goal for premature infants and their families is normalization. This means helping parents to resume normal daily activities with their newborn infant after an early delivery and long-term hospitalization. Sometimes this early birth has been preceded by a high-risk pregnancy requiring long periods of bed rest, a stressful neonatal course, and a long "roller-coaster" hospitalization. The feedback from early follow-up programs demonstrates the complexity of medical follow-up, high family stress, infant vulnerability, risks of handicaps, and the need for parental reassurance. As a result, premature infant follow-up programs have evolved as an extension of the care provided in neonatal intensive care units (NICUs). These follow-up programs work with the infant's primary care practitioner (PCP) to ensure a healthful outcome.

Incidence

In 1997, 7.4% of all newborns required intensive care (see Table 29-1).

Table 29-1 Incidence of Neonatal Intensive Care Unit Newborn Care

BIRTH WEIGHT	DEFINITION	INCIDENCE
Less than 1000 g	Extremely low birth weight	1% of all NICU admissions
1001–1500 g	Very low birth weight	25% of all NICU admissions
1501–2500 g	Low birth weight	50% of all NICU admissions

Risk Factors

Identifying "at-risk" infants is not straightforward. Prenatal, biologic, and environmental risk factors all contribute to the eventual morbidity of these infants. Infants who have multiple risk factors, including family and environmental factors, and those with more severe neonatal courses are considered to be the most at risk.

Maternal

- Prenatal drug and alcohol abuse
- Teen pregnancy
- Domestic violence
- Limited support systems
- Limited parental contact during hospitalization
- Difficulty with caregiving or technical aspects of infant care
- Uncertain housing, finances, transportation, or primary health care

Neonatal

- VLBW or extremely low birth weight (LBW)
- Central nervous system (CNS) involvement (e.g., infection, seizures, hemorrhage, periventricular leukomalacia)
- Chronic respiratory disease (e.g., bronchopulmonary dysplasia)
- Recurrent infections
- Other chronic medical complications (e.g., cardiac, gastrointestinal [GI] tract problems)
- Feeding problems (e.g., poor suck; suck, swallow, or breathing incoordination; poor endurance)
- Congenital malformations (e.g., cleft lip)
- Genetic syndromes (e.g., Down syndrome)
- Apparent neurologic impairment (e.g., asymmetric tone, poor state control, low tone or high tone)
- Multiple system problems
- Slow progress toward developmental milestones despite adjustments for prematurity

Infant and Child

Nutrition problems
- Growth delay or failure
- Feeding problems
- Gastroesophageal reflux

Frequent infections
- Lower respiratory tract infections and respiratory distress syndrome
- Otitis media or otitis media with effusion
- Gastroenteritis

Neurologic problems
- Movement and strength abnormalities
- Persistent primitive reflexes
- Cerebral palsy (very mild to profound)
- Extra sensitivity to environmental stimulation (e.g., sound, visual stimulus, general activity)
- Epilepsy
- Hydrocephalus

Sensory problems

- Visual problems (e.g., retinopathy of prematurity, amblyopia, strabismus, refractive errors)
- Hearing problems (e.g., sensorineural and conductive loss)

Developmental problems

- Speech and language delay (e.g., speech and articulation disorders, receptive and expressive language problems)
- Motor delays (e.g., hypertonia, hypotonia)
- Cognitive delays (e.g., marginal school readiness, learning disabilities, visual-motor and perceptual problems, low average intelligence or mental retardation)

Behavior disorders

- Excessive crying
- Disturbed sleep-wake pattern
- Impulsiveness or perseveration
- Low frustration threshold
- Short attention span or attention deficit hyperactivity disorder
- Hyperkinesis or inactivity
- Poor neural integration

Social medical problems

- Failure to thrive (FTT)
- Child neglect and abuse
- Vulnerable child syndrome

Subjective Data

A complete history should be obtained on any infant or child with a history of prematurity, with special attention to the following:

Determination of Age

Chronologic age is the age from birth date. *Corrected age* is chronologic age minus the weeks of prematurity (Box 29-1).

Prenatal History

The prenatal history includes information on alcohol or drug exposure; complications of bleeding, pregnancy-induced hypertension, preterm labor, placenta previa, or placental abruption; smoking; poor weight gain; maternal violence or trauma; and TORCH infections (i.e., toxoplasmosis, rubella, cytomegalovirus [CMV], herpes simplex, syphilis).

Birth History

- *Labor and delivery*—Complications of delivery (e.g., asphyxia, very poor Apgar scores [less than 3 at 5 minutes], traumatic delivery, prolonged delivery [greater than 24 hours])

Box 29-1 Adjusting Age for Prematurity

32-week premature infant
  (8 weeks or 2 months early)

Chronologic age:	7 months, 2 weeks
Less:	2 months
Corrected age:	5 months, 2 weeks

29-week premature infant
  (11 weeks or 2 months, 3 weeks early)

Chronologic age:	7 months, 2 weeks
Less:	2 months, 3 weeks
Corrected age:	4 months, 3 weeks

- *Neonatal problems*—Feeding or nippling problems; poor state control (inability to transit any of the six infant states); and medical complications, including apnea and bradycardia, respiratory distress syndrome, bronchopulmonary dysplasia (BPD), extended ventilatory support, patent ductus arteriosus, intraventricular hemorrhage, periventricular leukomalacia, anemia, hyperbilirubinemia, sepsis, and chronic conditions (cardiac, renal, GI tract, prolonged hospitalization [greater than 1 month])

Past History

The past history includes illnesses, emergency room visits, hospitalizations, accidents, operations, age, precipitating factors, frequency, consequences, length of hospitalization, sequelae, follow-up evaluation, and routine well-child care.

Developmental Milestones

- *Rhythmicity and self-regulation*—Early sleep-wake cycle, ability to calm self, requirements for caregiver facilitation, clarity of infant behavioral cues to the caregiver
- *Fine motor skills (feeding, play, and self-care)*—Early feeding experiences (e.g., suckling, swallowing, breathing), progress toward self-feeding, self-care skills (e.g., bathing, dressing)
- *Language skills*—Progress toward expressive and receptive language development
- *Social skills*—Early social skills, smiles and responsiveness to caregiver, behavioral problems
- *Gross motor skills*—Early active and passive muscle tone, head control, sitting, crawling, pulling to stand, walking
- *Adaptive and cognitive skills*—Object permanence; recognizing groups, numbers, time, space, and categories; visual perceptual performance

Immunization Status

Diphtheria, tetanus, and acellular pertussis (DTaP); polio; hepatitis B; and *Haemophilus influenzae* type B (Hib) vaccines should be given in full doses according to chronologic age and the current recommended schedule. Influenza vaccine should be given to infants over 6 months of age with BPD or other chronic illnesses (e.g., cardiac problems). Live virus vaccines (e.g., oral polio vaccine [OPV]) should be omitted until discharged from the NICU. (See also the Management section.)

Allergies

Note should be taken of allergies to medications, foods, and environmental factors. Exposure to secondhand smoke and areas where furniture, carpet, or drapes collect smoke should be minimized or eliminated.

Current Habits

- *Nutrition*—Calories, vitamins, iron, supplements, formula or breastfeeding (including calculation of calories per kilogram per day)
- *Feeding*—Parental satisfaction, location, timing, self-feeding, feeding routines, feeding problems (e.g., gagging, bottle or food refusal, swallowing and chewing problems, vomiting, gastroesophageal reflux [GER], colic, delayed self-feeding)
- *Sleep-wake cycle*—Pattern, endurance, habituation of noise or light, nighttime ritual, problems in sleep pattern or duration

- *Elimination*—Patterns; problems with constipation, retention, or diarrhea; frequency
- *Behavior*—State of transitions and control; irritability; alertness; attention and responsiveness to caregiver

School Performance

This category includes general school problems, language problems, reading problems, and visual motor skills (e.g., writing), as well as likes and dislikes.

Review of Systems

The review of systems includes information on growth problems and delays; sensory defensiveness to oral stimulation, touch (e.g., including water when bathing, clothes textures, brushing teeth, play in sand or grass), noises, or light; inattention, lack of concentration, or transitional problems in activities; persistent clonus; hypotonia or hypertonia; spasticity; tremors; muscle incoordination; and any tripping, falling, or clumsiness.

Family History

The family history may include previous premature births and any history of seizures, learning disorders, school problems, attention deficit disorders (ADDs), hyperactivity, psychiatric disorders, or other children or family members with disabilities or chronic illnesses. The *psychosocial history* includes parental education and learning style, social and financial support systems, problem-solving skills, health insurance benefits, and other family stressors (e.g., divorce, family violence or abuse). A history of the *family environment* includes housing, transportation, community resources, and exposure to passive cigarette, cigar, or pipe smoke.

Objective Data

Physical Examination

A complete physical examination should be done on all infants. When examining a premature infant, the practitioner should especially examine the following areas.

Measurements. Measure weight, height, head circumference, and weight-length ratio at each routine visit. Plot for the corrected age until 2 to 3 years of life. Growth for premature infants may be below the fifth percentile but should parallel standard growth curves for weight and length. Head circumference is usually the first to catch up, then weight, and finally length. The 2000 Centers for Disease Control and Prevention (CDC) growth charts should be used. Infants born at less than 1500 g are excluded from the reference data because they demonstrate a different growth pattern, but growth charts for premature infants 1500 to 2500 g and less than 1500 g are available. Share with parents the growth curve and offer reassurance. The most important aspect of a premature infant's growth is that he or she maintain the growth curve and that weight, length, and head circumference are proportional. If poor growth exists, with or without associated feeding problems, or there is a history of respiratory problems, check the oxygen saturation (O_2 Sat) level.

Vital signs. Observe for temperature instability, poor autonomic control for respiratory rate, and heart rate, and other physical signs (e.g., color, hiccups, gags, flatus). Blood pressure measurements should also be completed for premature infants.

General. Observe overall appearance, state transition, organization, control, amount of caregiver facilitation needed, ability to sustain alert state, attention during examination, endurance, and energy consumption.

Skin. Observe autonomic system control through color, scars, rashes, jaundice, scalp alopecia, contractures, and hypertrophic scarring.

Head, eyes, ears, nose, and throat (including mouth and teeth). Observe for:
- *Head*—Fontanel, sutures, shape
- *Eyes*—Red reflex and corneal light reflex, strabismus, amblyopia, fixing and tracking, refractive errors, glasses
- *Ears*—Infection, fluid level, pneumoscopy, hearing
- *Nose*—Patency, breathing pattern, nasal deformities, scarring, contractures, and stenosis
- *Throat*—Suck-swallow rhythm, tongue thrust, highly arched palate, palatal grooving, oral aversion, uvula movement, hyperactive or hypoactive gag reflex
- *Mouth and teeth*—Dentition, deformities, posterior cross bites, missing teeth, enamel defects

Respiratory tract and chest. Observe for symmetry of chest, movement, respiratory distress, retractions, stridor, and pectus. Monitor closely for respiratory syncytial virus (RSV) with wheezing, accompanied by rhinorrhea, pharyngitis, cough, sneezing, and low-grade fever.

Cardiovascular system. Observe for rhythm, murmurs (e.g., patent ductus arteriosus), radial-femoral pulse equality, and color.

Abdomen and gastrointestinal tract. Observe for umbilical hernia, hepatosplenomegaly, pyloric stenosis, bowel obstructions, and scars indicating previous surgery.

Genitourinary tract. Observe the general anatomy, as well as for hernias, circumcision, hypospadias, and hydrocele.

Extremities and musculoskeletal system. Observe for:
- *Back and spine*—Dimples, cysts
- *Neck and shoulders*—Delayed or poor head control, tight scarf sign, decreased shoulder tone (distress in being placed prone), difficulty bringing hands to midline
- *Trunk*—Arching, decreased range of motion, hypotonia (decreased strength or delayed sitting)
- *Extremities (upper and lower)*—Hypertonia or hypotonia, passive tone (e.g., range of motion [ROM]), active tone (e.g., strength, ease of movement, symmetry of movements).

Neurologic system. Observe for:
- *General (cerebral) functioning*—Poor state control and poor state transition, poor affect, memory, math calculation, Goodenough-Harris Draw-A-Man
- *Cranial nerves*—Presence, symmetry
- *Coordination*—Suck, swallow, breathing, hand-mouth coordination, eye-hand coordination, gait
- *Motor*—See the previous section on Extremities and Musculoskeletal System
- *Sensory*—Aversive behaviors to touch, especially around the mouth; difficulty being held; poor sensory integration.
- *Deep tendon reflexes*—Symmetry, hyperreflexia, clonus.
- *Delayed integration of primitive reflexes*—Moro reflex, asymmetric tonic neck reflex, palmar or plantar grasp, placing, step, Landau reflex.
- *Delayed emergence of protective reflexes*—Lateral prop and parachute reflex

Diagnostic Procedures and Laboratory Tests

Hearing assessment. Infants who are considered at risk for hearing loss require more extensive hearing evaluations. Risk factors include prematurity, family history of hearing loss, TORCH disease, high bilirubin level, severe asphyxia, ototoxic drugs, persistent pulmonary hypertension, diuretics, birth defects, and history of sepsis or meningitis.

Brainstem auditory evoked response. Completed before discharge and at 3 to 4 months of age, this test diagnoses unilateral hearing loss and conductive and sensorineural loss and classifies the loss from mild to profound.

Visual response audiometry. This test is completed on at-risk infants between 6 and 8 months of age (see Chapter 12).

Vision assessment. Infants who are considered at risk for vision problems should be referred to an ophthalmologist; at-risk infants include those with gestational ages less than 32 weeks who received oxygen, as well as all infants with gestational ages less than 28 weeks, whether they received oxygen or not. Standard testing at 6 to 8 weeks of age involves the initial ophthalmology examination, with follow-up depending on findings. At 6 months of age, infants with gestational ages less than 28 weeks should be examined if no problems were noted at discharge. For older children, refractive errors may not be sensitive enough to identify early vision problems; thus an examination by an ophthalmologist is recommended.

Blood tests. Blood tests include a complete blood cell (CBC) and reticulocyte count; this should be checked when a child is between 2 and 4 months of age because of the higher risk for anemia, or sooner if epoetin (Epogen) was used. Hemoglobin and hematocrit should be checked according to chronologic age, or sooner if indicated (e.g., because of tachycardia, tachypnea, pallor, lethargy, apnea with bradycardia, poor feeding, weight loss, elevated lactic acid concentrations).

Respiratory status. O_2 Sat levels should be monitored during alert periods, feeding, and sleep. Decreased O_2 Sat levels frequently occur during feedings and sleep; thus low levels may not be identified if tests are completed for only one activity. Upper respiratory tract illnesses, lower respiratory tract infections, and high altitude may also change an infant's O_2 Sat levels. Even if an infant has not required oxygen in the past, any changes that may influence the infant's respiratory status should cause consideration of the infant's O_2 Sat levels. Heart rate, respiratory rate, and respiratory effort should also be observed. It is recommended that the O_2 Sat level ideally be maintained at or above 95%; for infants with persistent pulmonary hypertension or BPD, the level should also be maintained at or above 95%. For the older child, observe any cough or wheezing with play, any need for the child to stop and rest during exercise or play, and any inability to keep up with peers.

Developmental screening. Developmental screening tools that have been standardized for preterm infants (e.g., Bayley, First Step) should be used because tools that have been standardized for healthy, full-term infants (e.g., Denver II) may not be sensitive enough to identify problems with preterm infants. Table 29-2 provides "red flags" for the first year, whereas most developmental screening tools lack specific items for premature infants. Parent questionnaires (e.g., Ages and Stages Questionnaire) may also be used to monitor development. Many early infant education programs use these tools.

Dental examination. Infants weighing less than 1500 g should have their first examination after their first tooth erupts.

Primary Care Issues and Implications

Facilitating the Parent Role

- Confirm and reinforce parental knowledge regarding their infant. Provide parents with a mechanism to organize information, appointments, resources, and medical information. (Early intervention programs may provide a notebook to assist with this.)
- Support parent caregiving through demonstration, teaching, reading materials, parental support groups, and feedback.
- Facilitate parental decision-making through discussions of different treatment plan options and the timing of referrals.
- Normalize the daily routine for parents through flexible planning, medication schedules, child care resources, integration of family members into caregiving routines, and selective referrals, and provide initial care coordination.
- Ask parents for their input regarding the best timing for appointments.
- Facilitate parent-child interaction by discussing play activities in addition to medical activities. The child's temperament and personality, the child's communication style and cues, and the child's ways of responding to the caregiver are important considerations.
- Encourage parents to connect with parent groups, offer recommendations for reading materials, and support and reinforce the parent's strengths.

Monitoring Growth

- Keep in mind that premature infants should gain at least 1 ounce per day once their feeding routine is established. Infants gaining less than 0.5 to 1 ounce per day should be monitored for their nutritional status, feeding problems, and growth problems. Head growth should be approximately 0.5 cm per week (up to 3 months) and 0.25 cm per week (3 to 6 months). Rapid head circumference growth exceeding 1.25 cm per week should be evaluated for hydrocephalus. Length measurements should be proportional.
- Remember that most healthy low–birth-weight (LBW) and appropriate-for-gestational-age infants achieve catch-up growth in the first 2 years of life. About 16% remain below the normal growth curve beyond 3 years of age. Small-for-gestational-age (SGA) infants or infants with intrauterine growth retardation may have proportional growth asymmetry. Many infants achieve normal catch-up growth by 8 to 12 months of age. Half of these infants finally achieve normal catch-up growth at 3 years of age.
- Remember that premature infants with chronic illnesses often have an altered growth pattern. Chronic lung disease and spastic cerebral palsy are the most common causes of growth retardation. Management of adequate nutrition and oxygen requirements is critical in ensuring adequate weight gain and respiratory status.

Monitoring Development

- Counsel parents regarding their individual child's development according to the adjusted age and individual characteristics.
- Assist parents in understanding the infant's signs of readiness for interaction (e.g., open eyes, relaxed muscles, flexion of extremities, smiling, eye contact) and signs of distress (e.g., yawning, face shielding, hiccups, gas, arching, crying, apnea and bradycardia, gaze aversion). Teach parents how to avoid overstimulation and how to encourage the infant's readiness for interactions through positioning, slow movement, and decreased noise and lights.
- Demonstrate the infant's capabilities and development throughout the examination. Explain the variability in developmental progress for motor skills, visual skills, and language skills.

Table 29-2 Developmental Red Flags

CORRECTED AGE	SLEEP/WAKE CYCLES AND BEHAVIOR	FEEDING SKILLS AND FINE MOTOR SKILLS	REFLEXES AND GROSS MOTOR SKILLS	SOCIAL INTERACTION AND LANGUAGE
2 months	Problems with autonomic responses to stimuli Continued difficulty with establishing regular sleep/wake cycles	Prolonged feedings (over 40 minutes) Food refusal or resistance Problems with choking or gagging Hands fisted and do not open and close	Scissoring or stiffness or low tone Back arching Lack of reflexes, startle reflex or excessive clonus Unable to lift head off mattress or turn side to side when prone Minimal arm and leg movements Asymmetric arm or leg movements	Inability to hold alert state and look at parents face or an object Interaction cues, hunger cues, and satiation cues difficult to understand
4 months	Difficult to console Easily overstimulated Sleeps a lot or very little Tremors or jittery	Back arches and child cries with feeding Difficulty giving appropriate volume Gagging or choking with feedings or at other times Does not enjoy eating	Persistence of primitive reflexes Asymmetric reflexes and asymmetric movements Fisted hands, scissoring, and hypertonia Resists being placed on stomach Hypotonia and difficulty holding head up while supported	No facial interaction or smiling Little interest in surrounding or toys Does not self-control bringing fingers to mouth
6 months	Continues to be overstimulated by caregiving routines Inability to calm self Poor sleep/wake patterns	Coughing, gagging, or food aversions or refusals Refuses to smell, look at, touch, or taste foods Refuses spoon Continued tongue thrust	Asymmetries or hand preference. Delayed or absent protective reflexes Persistent primitive reflexes (e.g., ATNR) Refusal to stand Back arches or rounds when sitting	Unable to reach for objects with open hands, even when lying down Does not explore toys with mouth No babbling or vocalizing Does not respond to social interactions
9 months	Transitions rapidly through states Difficulty transitioning to new environments or experiences	Not yet chewing on toys, chewing or munching foods, or making efforts at finger foods Refuses textures Feeding thrown off in new situations or with new foods	Babinski, hyerreflexia, or clonus Absence of protective reflexes Arching, refusal to sit or roll over, refusal to bear weight on legs when supported Stands on toes with stiff legs	Does not imitate facial expressions, sounds, or games Unable to bring hands together at midline, hold toy in each hand, or transfer toys Poor social interactions
12 months	Inconsistent care because of unpredictable sleep/wake patterns Resists new experiences Does not initiate	Refusal to transition to table foods because of chewing, taste, or texture No effort at self-feeding Inability to swallow or holds food in mouth for a prolonged time Continues to have tongue thrust and spit out food	Lack of integration of primitive reflexes Refuses to sit, crawl, pull to stand, or cruise Unable to move out of sitting without help "W" sitting Poor range of motion in arms or legs	Excessive mouthing of toys Lack of imitation of sounds or expressions Unable to follow simple requests Lack of object permanence Does not respond to reciprocal play or cause-and-effect games

- Encourage consistency in other health care providers in order to monitor development and establish rapport between the parents and practitioners.
- Encourage parents to participate in premature infant follow-up programs or early intervention programs.
- Closely monitor language development, attention, social and behavioral progress, cognitive functioning, academic performance, special education needs, and school retention.
- Refer infants who exhibit development "red flags" (see Table 29-2)

Normalizing Family Life

- Assist parents to normalize the life of their infant or child and family by focusing on normal daily activities (e.g., including "therapy" in play time or bath time rather than setting up a special time for therapy).
- Assist parents in travel plans when needed.
- When infants have multiple medical problems, help parents find respite care and community resources, as well as focus on the strengths of the child.
- Discuss the effect of major milestones (e.g., birthdays, first day of school, transition to junior high or high school) on the family. These may be stressful times for parents.
- Discuss with parents the child's school readiness and the decision concerning when to start school.
- Encourage daily routines that are consistent and predictable.
- Discuss options for parents in handling equipment needs during vacations and travel for children with special needs.

Management

Treatments and Medications

Nutritional needs

Breastfeeding. The mother's breast milk is the first choice for premature infants and is associated with long-term benefits for the infant and mother. It is denser and contains higher concentrations of fat, protein, and sodium. Because of the infant's increased caloric need during the first year of life, he or she may need to have human milk fortifier added to the breast milk. Most mothers of premature infants need assistance with their diet, especially vegetarian mothers; they need to be reminded to get plenty of fluids as well. Unless the infant is nursing well upon discharge, most mothers need to continue to pump to ensure an adequate milk supply until the infant is nursing consistently every 2 to 3 hours for at least 20 to 30 minutes; this usually takes 2 to 4 weeks after discharge. Preterm infants often need a supplement feeding (of breast milk or formula) by bottle at least for one feeding a day for the first 2 to 4 weeks after discharge. In such cases, some mothers may choose to offer 0.5 to 1 ounce after each feeding, but current recommendations show that this may require more energy than offering a bottle once a day.

Vitamin, mineral, and iron requirements

- *Iron*—All formula-fed preterm infants should be given an iron-containing formula by 36 to 40 weeks. Breastfed infants should be given a multivitamin dose with iron or ferrous sulfate drops (4 mg per kg per day of elemental iron).
- *Vitamins A, B, C, and D*—These are provided in most formulas. Breastfed infants and those receiving less than

450 ml (15 ounces) of formula per day should receive appropriate vitamin supplements according to current recommendations.
- *Vitamin E*—This may be given during hospitalization but is usually discontinued at discharge.
- *Folate*—This may be given until the infant weighs 4.5 to 5.5 pounds (2.04 to 2.5 kg). It is not available in standard vitamin preparations and is usually discontinued at discharge.
- *Fluoride*—The same dosage schedule for full-term infants should be maintained based on local geographic standards. Infants on ready-to-feed formula or breastfeeding infants should have fluoride prescribed until they begin taking water, even in geographic areas with fluoride in the water, after 6 months of age.

Caloric requirements. Healthy preterm infants need 110 to 150 kcal per kg per day to achieve adequate growth. Infants with BPD, gastroesophageal reflux (GER), cerebral palsy, cardiac problems, formula intolerance, or other chronic illnesses may need as much as 200 kcal per kg per day.

Increasing calorie intake. If a premature infant's daily intake is inadequate to sustain expected growth, it may be necessary to increase the calories the infant is receiving in the breast milk or formula (Table 29-3). Several options are available to accomplish this. Human milk fortifier can be added to breast milk. Similac Neosure (24 calories per ounce) or Enfamil 22 is most often recommended for the first year of life or until the infant is taking 26 ounces of formula per day to ensure adequate growth. The calorie content of formulas can be increased by adding polycose, vegetable oil, or medium-chain triglyceride (MCT) oils. Because of the hyperosmolarity of the higher calorie formulas, there is a risk of dehydration; therefore it is best to consult with a pediatric dietitian if an infant shows weight loss, poor catch-up growth, or failure to stay at or above the fifth percentile.

Increased feeding volumes with nasogastric tube feedings or gastrostomy feedings with overnight infusions may be needed after all other efforts have failed. Solid foods such as cereal for the older infant (6 to 12 months of age) may be used

Table 29-3 Methods of Increasing Caloric Density

OPTIONS TO INCREASE CALORIES	CALORIES PER OUNCE	FORMULA SCOOPS	OUNCES OF WATER
Regular powder formula (e.g., Similac, Enfamil)	20	1 scoop	2.0 oz
	22	1 scoop	55.0 ml
	24	1 scoop	50.0 ml
Concentrated liquid formula	20	13 ounces	13.0 oz
	22	13 ounces	10.5 oz
	24	13 ounces	8.5 oz
Similac Neosure	20	3 scoops	5.5 oz
	22	3 scoops	5.0 oz
	24	3 scoops	4.5 oz
Enfamil 22	20	2 scoops	4.5 oz
	22	1 scoop	2.0 oz
	24	2 scoops	3.5 oz

Similac Neosure or Enfamil 22 is most often recommended until 6 to 12 months of age to ensure adequate growth in the first year of life.

as a supplement but do not replace high-calorie formulas. Rice cereal is often used for GER. Foods with the highest calorie content include bananas, avocados, sweet potatoes, and meats.

Inappropriate feedings. Whole cow's milk is poorly tolerated by a premature infant's GI tract and is also low in essential nutrients. Once an infant has reached 12 months corrected age, whole cow's milk is appropriate unless the child continues to have growth or feeding problems. After 12 months corrected age, Pediasure may be recommended. Soybean formulas are not generally recommended because of their low phosphorus content (which reduces weight and length growth). Solid foods should not be introduced before appropriate developmental skills develop in the infant and before approximately 4 to 6 months corrected age. Appropriate developmental skills include coordinated swallow without tongue thrust, good head and neck control, sitting with support, and taking more than 26 ounces of formula a day.

Management of feeding problems

- Clarify parental expectations, knowledge, developmental concerns, successes, and challenges.
- Assess feeding status by completing a feeding history that includes patterns, preferences, restrictions, mealtime experiences, and family beliefs.
- Complete a feeding observation of the parent-child interaction (e.g., NCAST Feeding Scale), noting parental sensitivity to the infant and the infant's responsiveness to the parents.
- Interventions include educating the parents about the infant's feeding needs, supporting the infant's developmental skills, making suggestions about environmental modifications, providing behavior-modification recommendations, addressing parent-child interaction needs, and providing early referrals to therapists who specialize in feeding problems.

Immunizations. Preterm infants should receive full-dose immunizations according to their chronologic age or birth age. This includes DTaP; measles, mumps, and rubella (MMR); hepatitis B (Hep B); and Hib vaccines (see Chapter 13 for a complete overview). Because changes occur so frequently, it is recommended that updates be obtained from the CDC website.

- *Diphtheria, tetanus, and acellular pertussis*—The AAP recommends that pertussis be omitted for infants with active seizures or a previous history of a reaction to pertussis.
- *Polio*—*Inactivated* polio vaccine should be given on NICU hospital discharge if the infant is 2 months of chronologic age. Inactivated polio vaccine should also be used in infants who are hospitalized at greater than 2 months of age and in infants with compromised immunity, human immunodeficiency virus (HIV), or an immunodeficient household contact.
- *Influenza*—Infants with chronic lung disease, cardiac and GI tract problems, immunosuppression, or hemoglobinopathies should receive this vaccine after 6 months of age.
- *Palivizumab (synagis)*—Monthly injections are now recommended for RSV prevention for premature infants from the onset of the RSV season (approximately October to December). Those who should receive these injections include infants less than 32 weeks of gestation and children under 2 years of age with chronic lung disease who required mechanical therapy within the previous 6 months. Because of differences by community, consultation with the local health department is recommended.

Developmental surveillance. Assessment of a preterm infant's development should be based on the infant's corrected age until the infant is 2 years old. Parental concerns, symmetry of skills, and overall rate of progress should be taken into consideration. The goal of developmental surveillance should *not* be a prediction of later cognitive functioning. The goal is to provide parental anticipatory guidance, referral to early education programs, appropriate therapies, and further evaluation.

Both formal (developmental screening tests) and informal observations should be included in the primary care of the preterm infant. The formal tools used should be developed for use with preterm infants and have a balance of items measuring gross and fine motor and expressive and receptive language skills. Informal observations should include the quality of the infant's skills, changes in a child's rate of development, understanding as to why the infant or child fails a particular task, identification of behavioral issues, and assessment of the child's environment.

Counseling and Prevention

Assess parental adaptation and parent-child interaction

Monitoring of the parental experience during hospitalization. The PCP may follow the family during initial hospitalization to provide continuity of care during the transition to home. This may involve a phone call or an actual hospital visit. This contact provides information about the infant's status and ensures the parents' understanding of and adjustment to the events surrounding their child's care. A discharge summary should be sent to the PCP and should provide information about the parents' concerns and what the parents have been told about their baby.

Transition to home. The first days and nights at home are extremely stressful for parents. Often the infant's medical condition has stabilized, but feeding patterns, sleep patterns, and behavior may be unsettling to parents who are very anxious. A home visit provides the parents with reassurance and problem-solving support during this time. It also provides the practitioner with insight as to the special needs of the family.

Parental knowledge, understanding, beliefs, and concerns. Parents of premature infants often require more time for questions and concerns. Anticipating these concerns and prioritizing them can be helpful for the parents and save time for the practitioner. Identifying the greatest parental concern to be addressed at each visit and planning for subsequent visits prevents overload for both parents and practitioner. Strategies for assessment include interviewing, questionnaires, and observation; each has different benefits. The important issue is to develop a system to approach the parent and have appropriate resources available.

Observation of the parent-child interaction (attachment). A great deal can be learned through the observation of the parent-child interaction during feeding. Often this occurs in the office during the early months of life. One can make similar observations by asking a parent to teach the older infant or child a task the child has not yet learned. This usually takes less than 5 minutes but provides valuable information about the parent-child interaction, which can then be used in anticipatory guidance, follow-up recommendations, and referrals.

Monitoring of social and emotion development. More recent studies are identifying a greater incidence of behavioral, social, and emotional problems in infants with birth weights less than 1500 g. Hyperactivity, aggressiveness, social and peer conflicts, and problem temperamental characteristics of less adaptability, rhythmicity, activity, attention, and persistence have been seen in school-age children. Families need guidance and recommendations in early management of these issues before school entry.

Facilitation of school readiness and performance. Anticipation of school problems can be accomplished with astute developmental surveillance. VLBW infants are at greater risk for needing special education services for learning difficulties, grade failure, and overall poorer academic achievement. With early intervention services these problems will at least be minimized.

Focusing on the child and family strengths. Families often hear only of the failures and problems. Focusing on the child and the family strengths builds confidence and competence to a greater degree than pointing out problems. Understanding how much and to what degree the family and the child can handle referrals, resource recommendations, and consultations is important in maintaining a strong relationship among the family, child, and practitioner.

Review infection control. Parents should minimize the child's exposure to infection through good handwashing and reduced contacts, especially contacts with other young children. Encourage avoidance of exposure to passive smoke. Early medical evaluation is needed for illnesses, especially respiratory illnesses. Rehospitalization may occur during the first year of life, and parents should not consider this a failure on their part.

Address differences and similarities in full-term and premature infants. Premature infants may be difficult infants when first brought home from the hospital. Preparing parents for some of their behaviors prevents parents from blaming themselves or from thinking there is something wrong with their infant.

Feeding patterns. Premature infants may have poor sucking, swallowing, and breathing coordination, which may lead to them becoming tired during feeding, having shorter feeding times, or needing more frequent feedings.

Sleep patterns. Premature infants spend less time awake than full-term infants do. When they are awake, they may be less alert and responsive than full-term infants; they may also be more fussy and less active when awake. They have shorter sleep-wake cycles, and there is a greater likelihood of their awakening with fussiness during the night.

Behavior patterns. Premature infants give less-clear cues than full-term infants would, and it is more difficult for parents to determine their specific needs.

Motor problems. Because of hypertonia or hypotonia, premature infants may be difficult to hold, may appear to push away from their parents, and may have delays in motor self-help skills (e.g., head control, sitting).

Need for consistency, predictability, and a contingent environment. Premature and term infants and children need an environment that provides consistency and predictability so that they can learn to trust their caregivers and understand the limits of their behavior. They also need caregivers who are sensitive to their needs and respond through paced caregiving based on the child's responses. Further, they need caregivers who respond to their development and abilities in order to support and strengthen their motivation to learn.

Teach about growth and development of premature infants

- Help parents know how to respond to questions about the infant's growth and weight, developmental level, and chronologic age. Allow them to talk about the frustration of having a child that is "different" from the norm.
- Keep parents informed about their child's developmental strengths and struggles. Help them understand how their child may need assistance to overcome difficult tasks and how they can best help their child.
- Help parents understand the importance of therapies, developmental evaluations, and follow-up appointments.
- Assist in identifying barriers and solving problems.
- Assist parents with behavioral and discipline issues early.

Discuss child care. Traditional group day care is generally not recommended for premature infants under 6 months of age because of exposure to viral illnesses, especially GI tract and respiratory illnesses. Discuss options for child care and respite care within the community.

Provide parent education materials. Parents appreciate written and audiovisual materials that are specific to their needs and the needs of their premature infant. Materials used by early infant education programs, occupational therapists, and physical therapists may provide information for the practitioner and parents to assist with parenting concerns. The practitioner should:

- Make sure updated materials are provided to parents because they can become very distressed when they are told one "fact" by their health care provider and then read the opposite in outdated parent information.
- Provide information about smoking-cessation programs for parents and about the risk to the infant of secondhand smoke. Negotiate steps to decrease the risk to the infant if smoking is continued (e.g., avoiding smoking in the car and house). Advise of the risks of oxygen use and smoking.
- Provide information that can be shared with grandparents about the special needs of the premature infant. Encourage the parents to invite the grandparents to a visit if there are questions or conflicts.

Follow-Up

- Despite normal development, parents of premature infants need reassurance and specific examples of social, motor, language, and behavioral milestones that the child achieves. As with all parents, they need assistance with upcoming stages and the need for consistency.
- The child's strengths needs to be emphasized along with how the parents perceive the child's development. The parents should be taught what can be done to strengthen performance in the child's areas of delay. It is best to initiate an early referral to provide the family and child with more intensive support and follow-up care. All preterm infants with questionable development should be evaluated more frequently than routine well-child visits.
- Discussion of abnormal developmental findings with parents requires sensitivity and rapport. Using a positive but realistic approach in a language the parents can understand is very important. Labels can often be emotion laden and should be used with care but not avoided. Parents often feel better when they can place a name on their child's problem. The community agencies that specialize in the evaluation of developmental disabilities are extremely beneficial. These agencies have staff who provide diagnostic evaluations, give explanations to parents that may relieve parental guilt, work with preschool and school programs, and provide recommendations for follow-up care and other community referrals.

- Screening and diagnostic tests that were recommended at the premature infant's discharge or during the first year of life (e.g., recommended vision and hearing tests) must be monitored and followed up by the PCP.

Consultations and Referrals

The PCP often needs to use other specialists and community agencies in the care of a preterm infant. Collaboration and communication are vital in helping a family maximize the care for their child.

It may be necessary for the PCP to make referrals to specialists such as pulmonologists, cardiologists, surgeons, or special clinics. It is important to make sure the family understands the need for the referral and is assisted as needed in arranging an appointment. Parents often need written instruction and information to keep track of appointments.

Special programs may be also available for follow-up care of premature infants. These programs may provide primary care, pulmonary care, developmental care, or follow-up for particular research studies. The PCP must understand the benefits and limitations of these programs to maximize their utilization.

PCPs are not usually able to provide all the support needed for families, though often there is hesitation to refer "their" patients to outside agencies. The availability and timing of referral to community resources must be discussed with parents very early in a child's infancy to allow them the choice of when to use community agencies.

Resources that are available for families include:

- Parent support groups and parents of other premature infants
- Community health or home health nursing
- Early infant intervention programs
- Occupational and physical therapists
- Speech and language therapists
- Regional centers or community center boards for developmental disabilities
- Reading materials (e.g., books, parent journals) and videos

In the initial stages of parenting a child with special needs, the coordination of community services, medical resources, financial resources, medical equipment, and nursing services may be overwhelming to parents. A service coordinator (individual who advocates for the family and child) is frequently needed. The PCP may not be able to do this because of the time involved but should ensure that someone is available from his or her office or the community.

Special funding sources for medical care (e.g., handicapped children's programs, social security disability insurance, medical supply companies, early intervention programs, Women, Infants, and Children [WIC]) are needed by families. PCPs should be aware of these programs or refer to agencies who can assist families with appropriate contacts.

A report from the PCP can be invaluable for a specialist when a child is being seen on a regular basis, just as a report from the specialist can be very important to the PCP.

Resources

Publications

Exceptional Parent; (800) 247-8080

March of Dimes Birth Defects Foundation. (1997). *Breastfeeding the infant with special needs.* White Plains, NY: March of Dimes.

Rosenfeld, L. R. (1994). *Your child and health care: A "dollar and sense" guide for families with special needs.* Baltimore: Paul H. Brookes.

Tracy, A.E., & Maroney, D.I. (1999). *Your premature baby and child: Helpful answers and advice for parents.* New York: Berkley.

Websites

For Parents

American Association for Premature Infants (www.aapi-online.org)

Baby Place (www.baby-place.com)

Coming Home Advice (www.home.earthlink.net/gbangs/advice.html)

March of Dimes (www.modimes.org)

Parents of Premature Infants Support Group (www.home.cicnet.net.au)

Premature Infants (www.snugbuds.com)

Tiny Things, Inc. (www.tinythings.com)

For Professionals

American Academy of Pediatrics (AAP) (www.aap.org)

The Future of Children (www.futureofchildren.org)

Centers for Disease Control and Prevention (CDC) (www.cdc.gov)

National Guideline Clearinghouse (www.guideline.gov)

Respite Care for Children Who Are Medically Fragile (www.chtop.com)

VORT Corporation—Premature Infants (www.vort.com)

Bibliography

Ambalavanan, N., Nelson, K.G., Alexander, G., Johnson, S.E., Biasini, F., & Carlo, W.A. (2000). Prediction of neurologic morbidity in extremely low birth weight infants. *Journal of Perinatology, 20*(8), 496-503.

American Academy of Pediatrics, Committee on Fetus and Newborn. (1998). Hospital discharge of the high-risk neonate-proposed guidelines. *Pediatrics, 102*(2), 411-417.

American Academy of Pediatrics, Committee on Fetus and Newborn. (1998). Prevention of respiratory syncytial virus infections: Indications for the use of palivizumab and update on the use of RSV-IVIG. *Pediatrics, 102*(5), 1211-1216.

American Academy of Pediatrics, Task Force on Newborn and Infant Hearing. (1999). Newborn and infant hearing loss: Detection and intervention. *Pediatrics, 103*(2), 527-530.

Berger, S.P., Holt-Turner, I., Cupoli, J.M., Mass, M., & Hageman, J.R. (1998). Caring for the graduate from the neonatal intensive care unit. *Pediatric Clinics of North America, 45*(3), 701-713.

Bregman, J. (1998). Developmental outcomes in very low birth-weight infants: Current status and future trends. *Pediatric Clinics of North America, 45*(3), 673-690.

Daley, H.K. & Kennedy, C.M. (2000). Meta-Analysis: Effects of interventions on premature infant feeding. *The Journal of Perinatal and Neonatal Nursing, 14*(3), 62-70.

Deloian, B. (1998). *Caring connections: Nursing support transitioning premature infants and their families home from the hospital.* Denver, CO: University of Colorado Health Sciences Center, School of Nursing.

McKinley, L.T. (1997). Optimal nutrition approaches for low birth weight infants. *Infants and Children, 4*, 3-7.

Newton, N.R., Leonard, C.H., Piecuch, R.E., & Phibbs, R.H. (1999). Neurodevelopmental outcome of prematurely born children treated with recombinant human erythropoietin in infancy. *Journal of Perinatology, 19*(6), 403-406.

Stevenson, D.K., Wright, L.L., Lemons, J.A., Oh, W., Korones, S.B., Papile, L., Bauer, C.R., Stoll, F.J., Tyson, J.E., Shankaran, S., Fanaroff, A.A., Donovan, E.F., Ehrenkranz, R.A., & Verter, J. (1998). Very low birth weight outcomes of the National Institute of Child Health and Human Development Neonatal Research Network, January 1993 through December 1994. *American Journal of Obstetrics and Gynecology, 179*, 1632-1639.

Chapter 30 *The Stepfamily*

Marty Witrak

During the past decade, the number of stepfamilies has risen dramatically. As the number of divorces in this country rises or remains stable, so will the number of stepfamilies. Although there is more recognition of stepfamilies, American institutions such as schools and health care systems have not kept pace with many of the needs of these families, and many of the stereotypes of stepfamilies are negative. No one ever had a "fairy stepmother"; all stepmothers were wicked.

Remarriages are often built on unrealistic expectations. Stepparents expect to love the new children immediately. Stepmothers try to be "supermoms," and stepfathers try to immediately assume the parental authority. Children often feel they have no choice in the living arrangements. Further, children often resist the new marriage, since it ends the fantasy that their biologic parents will reunite.

In most new families, spouses have time to adjust to marriage before children enter the picture. The couple is able to work on blending their respective backgrounds and perceptions of family. When children do enter the family, they are infants whose needs allow the parents time to negotiate parenting styles and attitudes. However, even under these circumstances, parenting is frequently a source of conflict.

In stepfamilies, there is no time to blend family styles or negotiate parenting. Further, there has not been time to establish and nurture the marriage. By the time parents and their children become part of a stepfamily, all have been members in two other family forms: (1) the original family and (2) a single-parent family. Although the original family may be a more critical experience, the single-parent family is the most recent experience. Stepfamilies are families in transition; several types of stepfamilies exist, and the issues are different in each.

Types of Stepfamilies

Stepfather Families

These are stepfamilies in which the man is the stepparent. They tend to have less stress than other types of stepfamilies. In particular, the response of boys is more favorable than that of girls to a stepfather.

Stepmother Families

These are stepfamilies in which the woman is the stepparent. In such families, more stress than in stepfather families is reported by both children and stepmother. Because mothers often nurture family relationships and set the emotional tone of the family, stepmother families have more loyalty conflicts. This type of family is less common than the stepfather family.

Complex Stepfamilies

These are stepfamilies in which both adults have children from a previous marriage living with them. The more children present, the greater is the stress. This type of family has the greatest incidence of re-divorce.

Stepfamilies with a Mutual Child

This type of stepfamily encompasses about half of all stepfamilies. The key to success is whether the mutual child is born before or after integration of the new family. Successful integration is impeded if the child is born early in the new marriage. However, if the child is born after the integration of the new stepfamily, he or she may provide a positive influence on the integration.

Incidence

- Approximately 40% of all marriages today are remarriages for at least one of the partners. Approximately 65% of these remarriages involve children from a previous marriage.
- More than 33% of all United States children are expected to live in a stepfamily before 18 years of age.
- Stepfather families are the most common type of stepfamily (65%).
- African-American children are most likely to live in stepfamilies; about 32.3% of African-American children under 18 years of age living in married-couple families live with a stepparent, compared with 16.1% of Hispanic children and 14.6% of Caucasian children.
- The most common problem experienced by stepfamilies is conflict over the relationship between the stepparent and a child.

Risk Factors

Children in stepfamilies may be at risk for the following:
- Depression
- Anxiety
- Fighting at school
- Poor peer relationships
- School-related problems (e.g., absences, expulsion)
- Alcohol use (in teens)
- Increased conflict between stepparent and child

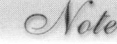

Note

If there is a history of domestic violence for one or both spouses, there is an increased likelihood of abuse occurring in the stepfamily. This is a result of the conflicts inherent in forging a new stepfamily.

Subjective Data

The following information should be included in the history of any child who is a member of a stepfamily and should be updated as needed:
- Loyalty (e.g., Does the child feel loyalty conflicts? If so, do the parents handle the child's concerns?)

- The parents' ability to negotiate child support and visitation, and the ability of parents to resolve these issues positively (because they do affect the child)
- History of domestic abuse
- The child's attitude toward the stepfamily
- Length of time as a stepfamily
- Type of stepfamily household (e.g., stepfather, stepmother)
- Specifics of the custody arrangement
- Legal right to information (i.e., Who is legally entitled to access information? What are their current phone numbers and addresses?)
- Health care decision-making (i.e., Who participates in health care decisions, especially in an emergency?)

Objective Data

Gathering of objective data includes a complete physical examination at the initial visit.

Primary Care Issues and Implications

Many stepfamilies may not identify themselves as stepfamilies to a practitioner because of the negative social stereotype. It is extremely important for practitioners to remain aware of the strengths and rewards in stepfamilies while helping them deal with normative challenges. Stepfamilies go through normal developmental stages. Although these stages are unique to stepfamilies, a stepfamily can take comfort in knowing that these challenges are not unique to their particular family. The result or desired outcome of these developmental stages is to achieve stability as a family group.

Stepfamily Developmental Stages

Stage 1—fantasy: the invisible burden

- Fantasies about the past or the future predominate. Children may be grieving over the fantasy that their biologic parents would remarry.
- Adults may believe that other stepfamilies have troubles but everything will be better for them. The mother may fantasize that her new husband will be more loving and responsible.
- Developmental tasks:
  Family members understand and express fantasies about the past and present family.
  Family members let go of their fantasies and are allowed to grieve their loss.
- Dangers and dilemmas include situations in which the fantasies are not understood or acknowledged, making the requirements for the family or spouse to succeed impossible to meet.

Stage 2—immersion: sinking versus swimming

- Stepfamily members are intensely aware of feelings of jealousy, resentment, and confusion as boundaries become clearer. These boundaries include insider-outsider, adult-child, and stepparent–biologic parent differences.
- Feeling isolated, overrun, torn, or disloyal to the absent parent is common at this stage.
- Developmental tasks:
  Each family member needs to "keep swimming."
  Family members need to get comfortable with the discomfort they feel.

Family members need to identify feelings and listen to each other's stories.
- Dangers and dilemmas include unrealistic expectations of the new family, stepparent, or spouse resulting in shaming and blaming.

Stage 3—awareness: mapping the territory

- The mapping stage is the most important. Stepfamily members develop more realistic expectations of the family.
- Explicitness and acceptance supplant confusion and self-doubt.
- Empathetic responses provide the groundwork for understanding, which in turn leads to mutual decision-making.
- Developmental tasks:
  Family members identify the feelings and needs of the stepfamily.
  Family members should be "curiously empathetic."
- Dangers and dilemmas include not being able to move beyond emotions of shaming and blaming.

Stage 4—mobilization: exposing the gaps

- Increased willingness exists as family members are able to discuss stepfamily issues.
- The stepparent takes a stand on an issue or a conflict, thus initiating the middle stage.
- Conflict can be emotionally intense.
- Developmental tasks:
  Family members should be able to discuss and actively deal with differences in family culture so that positive changes can take place, rather than such differences creating increased tension.
- Dangers and dilemmas include situations in which the stepparent takes a stand on an issue, at which time the family may either move forward or move backward developmentally.

Stage 5—action: going into business together

- New family traditions, rules, and activities are initiated.
- Clearer boundaries form around the stepfamily as loyalty conflicts with the biologic parent lessen.
- Developmental tasks:
  The original subsystem provides the groundwork on which the new family customs, rituals, and traditions are built.
- Dangers and dilemmas include the fact that if the family has intense difficulty with conflict, they may move too quickly into this phase. If this happens, the trust and understanding resulting from the previous stages will not be there. Too many new rules and regulations may appear in an attempt to find order.

Stage 6—contact: intimacy and authenticity in steprelations

- Open communication can occur.
- Family members allow the stepparent to assume an "intimate outsider" role.
- Developmental tasks:
  The stepparent role is solidified through open communication, awareness, and constructive, authentic conflict resolution.
- Dangers and dilemmas include the original family dysfunction showing up in the adults. Responses may range from discomfort to sabotage of communication.

Stage 7—resolution: holding on and letting go

- Great change has taken place.
- The stepfamily functions effectively as a family, with clear rules, boundaries, and roles.
- All members have a sense of family.

- Members feel secure and are able to get their needs met through multiple family members.
- Developmental tasks:
  Adults can share children with ex-spouses.
  Normal life transitions such as weddings, graduations, and deaths provide opportunities for unresolved grief to emerge. (This can be either a problem or an opportunity.)
- Dangers and dilemmas include the fact that as disputes are resurrected, the family may regress to previous stages. Loyalty conflicts may reemerge in children whose divorced parents are unable to cooperate around these occasions.

Characteristics of Successful Remarried Families

- Expectations are realistic.
- Losses can be mourned.
- Satisfactory steprelationships have formed.
- Satisfying rituals are established.
- The separate households cooperate.

Safety

Stepfathers are more likely than biologic fathers to be sexually abusive. Many studies report that children are more likely to be abused by a stepparent than a biologic parent; however, other reports suggest that biologic parents are more likely to severely abuse or kill their children. The overall rate of violence is substantially lower for stepchildren than for all other children. If a practitioner suspects abuse or neglect, the child should be evaluated and a report given to the appropriate agency.

Growth and Development

An individual child's physical growth and development are not affected directly by being a member of a stepfamily.

Discipline

In the same way that a stepparent should not expect to love a stepchild immediately, the new stepparent should not expect to "parent" immediately. In no area is this more crucial than discipline. The initial focus may be on building a friendship based on mutual appreciation and respect. The development of this relationship takes time and will be tested frequently along the way. Although the stepparent may coparent in terms of upholding family rules and nurturing, discipline may be a source of intense conflict. Further, this conflict is not limited to the stepparent and child; discipline issues are often a source of conflict between the new spouses.

Stepparents may need to be tolerant and attempt to understand the apparently offensive or disrespectful behavior patterns. Immediate attempts to correct a child often escalate the existing tension of creating the new family. Children feel intense loyalty conflicts and may act out to avoid the feelings of guilt.

New spouses in stepfamilies need to support each other in understanding the dynamics of children's behavior and the appropriate style of discipline. The most difficult situations occur with adolescent children. These sources of conflict can be destructive to the new family.

Sexuality

Research is mixed on the effect of divorce and remarriage on adolescent sexual behavior. Some studies show that the pres-ence of a stepparent is predictive of adolescent sexual behavior more like that of teens in intact families.

Management

Counseling and Prevention

A practitioner should help parents address and understand the issues that may confront stepfamilies. Stepfamilies have no uniform profile; some are small, some are large, and some fluctuate in size from weekend to weekend. However, the issues confronting stepfamilies fall into the following several key areas.

Outsiders versus insiders. The goal in a stepfamily is a sense of family unity. Stepfamilies need to help all members find a place in the family, and this is particularly true for the "outsiders." An outsider can be the new stepparent, the child who is visiting each weekend, or the child who is changing residence. Feelings of exclusion, intrusion, rejection, and resultant anger and depression can be common. Insiders may also feel displaced and worry about their importance in the family. Tolerance for ambiguity, understanding, and patience are essential in accommodating the changes in the family structure.

Boundary disputes. Because children in stepfamilies often move between both parents' households, the boundaries may become indistinct as the parents cooperate in activities and arrangements involving the children. However, each household must develop unique boundaries in their quest for cohesion. Parents do not need to have the same responses to events that take place within the family unit. As the two families develop internal cohesion, maintaining these differences becomes important. "Turf" disputes are common as the numbers in the family increase and decrease with weekend or summer migrations of children. Each member of the family needs to have some privacy and some personal space. Children and adults need time to adjust to these household transitions and should not expect to become an "instant family."

Power issues. One of the common arenas for conflict in any marriage is the issue of control and how to make decisions. Power issues can be more intense for stepfamilies for several reasons. First, power may have been a key ingredient in the disintegration of the previous marriage. Further, many wives feel that after they divorced, they took control of their lives for the first time. Therefore, remarriage is usually a difficult transition and one that involves much pride. Wives are often reluctant to share power after they have proved themselves as single parents. Husbands may feel robbed of power through restrictions on access to children, child support payments, and so forth. Financial matters are often highly charged as a result of previous bad experiences. All new couples need to negotiate the balance of power in the relationship. The difference in the negotiation process for stepfamilies is that they must negotiate in the presence of stepchildren, and they must negotiate power issues over children with previous spouses. Further, even children who may be more or less happy with the new family may use the divide-and-conquer technique (e.g., a child may threaten loss of affection or relocation to the other parent's household). Child-centered issues are more difficult if the original parents are not cooperative with each other. Power issues cannot be avoided, but the new stepfamily may need help in getting perspective on the process.

Conflicting loyalties. In a traditional family, children may not feel the same level of closeness toward each parent, but the child seldom has to choose between the two. Further, the marriage bond allows for accommodation between the strengths and talents of the parents. Loyalty conflicts for children and remarried parents are inevitable. This is true whether the stepfamily was established after a divorce or a death. However, adults who have not been able to achieve a satisfying marriage can still parent effectively together. Ideally, all parents (biologic parents and stepparents) can work together for the best interests of the children. If this is not possible, comments about former spouses should not be made in front of children; children tend to personalize attacks on an absent parent. Parents need to understand that the acrimony is more damaging to the children than to the former spouse who is the target of the comments.

Rigid, unproductive triangles. Although triangle relationships are common in all families, triangles in stepfamilies frequently are rigid and unproductive. Unproductive triangles contain three people in a conflict such that clear, dyadic relationships are not workable. Typical triangles in stepfamilies include:

- Remarried parent in the middle, not allowing a direct relationship between a stepparent and a child
- Remarried parent and stepparent standing together against an ex-spouse
- Child caught in the middle between hostile ex-spouses
- Child caught in the middle between a parent and stepparent of the same sex

If these triangles are intense and allowed to go on for a long time, they become difficult to break down. As long as triangles exist, clear relationships between any two of the three persons are not feasible.

Unity versus fragmentation of the new couple relationship. Forming a solid marital relationship is difficult under the best of circumstances, and a new couple has many issues to negotiate. The process of establishing this relationship is hindered by the adjustment difficulties of children, grandparents, and other significant persons in the environment. However, the strength of the new marriage is the foundation for the success of the stepfamily. Partners should be encouraged to preserve time for their relationship, despite pressures from children and their activities.

Follow-Up

Schedule follow-up visits as needed for well-child care or to address parenting concerns.

Consultations and Referrals

- Refer, as needed, to support groups that can be useful in providing information and education (e.g., the Stepfamily Association of America).

- Consult with or refer to a mental health professional with training in stepfamily issues for families who are having difficulty.

Resources

Organizations
Stepfamily Association of America, 212 Lincoln Center, 215 South Centennial Mall, Lincoln, NE 68508; (402) 477-7837; www.stepfam.org

Websites
Parents Place (www.parentsplace.com/readroom/aacap/stepfmly.html)
Center for Law and Social Policy (CLASP) (www.clasp.org/whoweare.htm)
American Psychological Association (helping.apa.org/family/step.html)
Stepping Stones Counseling Center (www.stepfamilies.com)
Stepfamily in Formation (www.sfhelp.org)
Blended Family Resource Guide (www.blendedfamily.com)
My Two Homes (www.mytwohomes.com)

Bibliography

Bumpass, L.L., Raley, R.K., & Sweet, J.A. (1995). The changing character of stepfamilies: Implications of cohabitation and nonmarital childbearing. *Demography, 32,* 425-436.

Glick, P.C. (1989). Remarried families, stepfamilies, and stepchildren: A brief demographic profile. *Family Relations, 38,* 24-28.

Huntley, D.K. (Ed.). (1995). *Understanding stepfamilies: Implications for assessment and treatment.* Alexandria, VA: American Counseling Association Press.

Larson, J. (1992). Understanding stepfamilies. *American Demographics, 14,* 360.

Norton, A.J. & Miller, L.F. (1992). Marriage, divorce, and remarriage in the 1990s. In *Current population reports* (series P23-180). Washington, DC: Government Printing Office

Papernow, P.L. (1993). *Becoming a stepfamily: Patterns of development in remarried families.* San Francisco: Jossey-Bass.

U.S. Bureau of the Census. (1998). Marital status and living arrangements. In *Current population reports* (series P20-514). Washington, DC: Government Printing Office.

Visher, E.B. & Visher, J.S. (1988). *Old loyalties, new ties: Therapeutic strategies with stepfamilies.* New York: Brunner Mazel.

Chapter 31 *The Violent Family*

Jane A. Fox

Family violence is a universal problem. It has no age, race, income, religious, or educational boundaries. Health care practitioners are in the ideal position to address the issue of violence in the family. *Family violence* is defined as any violence against partners, children, or older adult relatives. The American Psychological Association (APA) states that family violence and abuse means the physical, sexual, and emotional maltreatment of one family member by another. Violence is identified more frequently in families of low income because they often use clinics and hospitals for health care rather than a private practitioner who may not recognize an injury or be willing to report to the authorities.

To be able to identify a family at risk, a practitioner needs to be aware of the problems that can occur as a result of violence. The American Medical Association (AMA) has reported that nearly one quarter of the women in the United States will be abused by a current or former partner during their lives. Spousal abuse often occurs in homes where children are present, and these children are at increased risk of also being victims of abuse. Some reports estimate that children are at twice the risk for abuse when the mother is being abused. Notably, children are often exposed to hours of television portraying violence as a way of life, without showing any realistic consequences. It has been reported that television has a negative influence on behavior, resulting in children and adolescents acting more aggressively towards others or passively accepting the role of victim.

The availability of firearms in the home and on the street has increased the risk of children accidentally being shot. Young children now carry guns at alarming rates because they believe they need them for protection. When a practitioner is evaluating a child, it is imperative that the differential diagnosis considers that violence may be the cause of behavioral and physical symptoms. In addition, practitioners are in the ideal setting to incorporate (into anticipatory guidance) various alternatives to physical discipline, the need to limit and monitor watching television programs that contain violence, and the issue of firearms in the home.

An important function of the family is to provide a safe and nurturing environment for its members. Family violence occurs within ongoing relationships that are expected to be protective, nurturing, and supportive, and it has a powerful influence on children. Children begin to believe that violence plays an integral part in any close relationship and may expect violent behavior from others. Children who are exposed to family violence also learn that violence is an acceptable way to solve problems and end disputes.

Incidence

- More than 3 million children are reported for abuse or neglect yearly.
- Of every 1000 children, 47 are victims of abuse.
- It is estimated that nationally more than 3 children die each day as a result of maltreatment.

- Approximately 35% of all child abuse cases involve parental substance abuse.
- About 1 of every 4 parents who grew up in a violent home will seriously injure a child.
- Over 3 million children are at risk of witnessing violence between their parents.
- Approximately 4 million women in the United States suffer some kind of violence each year.
- An act of domestic violence occurs every 15 seconds, more frequently than any other crime in the United States.
- Studies indicate child abuse occurs in 33% to 77% of families in which there is abuse of adults.
- Guns are in 43% of all U.S. homes, and 30% of the time they are loaded. A gun takes the life of a child every 2 hours.
- About 17% of adolescent girls and 37% of adolescent boys will at one time take a weapon to school.
- Approximately 65% of child homicides and 82% of adolescent homicides are the result of firearms.

Risk Factors

- Parental history of violence as a child
- History of mental illness, previous domestic violence, or substance abuse in parents or other family members
- Witnessing domestic violence during childhood and adolescence
- Exposure to violence in the home, school, or community
- Family stresses that could lead to violence (e.g., unemployment, divorce, death, chronic illness)
- Corporal punishment or emotional abuse in the home
- Children with physical and mental disabilities
- Violence on television
- Social isolation
- Victim of physical assault or sexual victimization
- Firearms in the home, or access to firearms at a neighbor's or relative's home or in the community
- Poor self-esteem or depression
- Poverty
- Gang involvement or exposure

Signs and Symptoms of Violence in the Home

Physical Indicators

For possible domestic violence (which may be asked about directly):
- Obvious maternal depression
- A partner who never allows the mother to be alone with health care personnel
- Bruises, welts, lacerations, or unexplained injuries
For abuse toward children:
- Harsh, demeaning parenting style

- Unexplained bruises, welts, and lacerations
- Failure to thrive (FTT)
- Lags in development, including speech disorders
- Secondary enuresis
- Violent tantrums in the office or clinic
- Encopresis
  For adolescents:
- All signs listed for children
- Dress style of a particular gang known to be violent
- Observing a weapon on a patient, or noting injuries that could be caused by violence

Behavioral Indicators

- Cold, inconsistent parenting
- Behavioral extremes
- Cowering at any noise or quick movement
- Apprehensive and fearful to go home
- Low self-esteem
- Conduct disorders
- Habit disorders (e.g., sucking, biting)
- Threatening behavior in the older child and adolescent

Subjective Data

A detailed history is essential when it is suspected that a child has been a victim of abuse (see Chapter 47) or is living in a violent home. It is beneficial to interview the child alone without a parent present; if domestic violence is suspected and the child is verbal (able to speak), interview the victim (usually the mother) alone. Either way, this allows a person the opportunity to respond to questions without the stress of a parental or child knowledge or reaction.

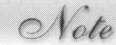

Note

Ask open-ended questions. Never ask leading questions. Any disclosure needs to be documented in "direct quotes" in the medical records.

History

The goal is to assess for the presence of or to identify risk factors for violence.

Parent Interview

In addition to a complete health history of the child, explore the following:

- Has child been exposed to violence at home, at school, in the neighborhood, or at other places?
- What about domestic violence? How do the parents get along? If they're not married, how does the mother get along with the child's father. Do they have yelling or screaming fights? How often? Any pushing or shoving fights?
- Is there a gun in the house or any place where the child spends time. What kind? Is it loaded? What is it used for?
- Are there behavioral problems or school problems, including aggressive behavior?
- Do the parents have concerns about their child?
- What do the parents do if the child "drives them crazy"?
- Is there any support to help with the child?
- How do the parents discipline the child?

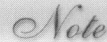

Note

This is an ideal time to observe the child-parent relationship. Parents who are abusive, neglectful, or are themselves victims of violence often sit in the examining room and appear distant, with little or no interaction with the child.

Child Interview

- Ask the child if he or she feels safe in the home, school, and neighborhood. Does the child ever hear gunshots?
- Ask the child with whom he or she lives. Have the child name the people who provide care.
- Inquire as to where the child sleeps, if he or she shares a bed, and with whom.
- Ask if there are any problems with sleep (e.g., nightmares, bedwetting).
- If the child is of school age, ask about school, interest in school, how safe he or she feels in school, and if there are any problems. Inquire how many fights the child has had in the past year and if he or she knows how to avoid a fight.
- If the child is an adolescent, ask about interests, peer relationships, participation in school activities, alcohol and drug use (including tobacco), rape, depression, sexuality, and how safe he or she feels in school. Explore violence (e.g., use of weapons, fighting). Ask if the adolescent has ever had a pushing or shoving fight with a girlfriend or boyfriend. Ask how many times the adolescent has been hit at home in the past year and how it makes him or her feel. Inquire if the adolescent is a member of a gang or if there is a gang in the neighborhood. Ask if the adolescent has ever carried a weapon for self-protection.
- Ask the child how he or she gets to and from school and who is home after school.
- Ask questions to determine the child's level of development.
- Ask the child who the boss is in the house.
- Inquire what happens if the child does something wrong. Ask how he or she is disciplined.
- Ask the child how disagreements are handled at home.
- Inquire about fighting at home. Do people fight at home? In what way? About what?
- Ask the child what he or she does if something is bothersome.
- Ask the child whom he or she talks to about a problem.
- Inquire about guns in the home and if anyone in the child's home has one
- Ask the child if he or she (or any acquaintance) carries a weapon to school.
- Determine what names the child uses for body parts. Use a picture so the child can point to the body part.
- Assess whether the child can define "good," "bad," and "secret" touch.
- Ask the child if anything hurts on his or her body.
- Ask the child if he or she has ever been touched in an uncomfortable way. If the answer if yes, ask if the child will share the event.
- If the child is an adolescent, explore peer relationships (both friends and dating).
- Use age-appropriate questions to determine sexual knowledge, including knowledge gained from movie, television, and video exposure.

- Ask the child if he or she knows the reason for today's visit.
- Ask the child to tell you three wishes he or she has.
- Inquire if the child has any questions.

Objective Data

Physical Examination

A child suspected of living in a home where violence is present requires a comprehensive physical examination. It should include the following:

- Vital signs
- Height and weight (plotted on an appropriate growth chart)
- Complete head-to-toe examination (including any skin lesions)
- Funduscopic eye examination (including any retinal hemorrhages)
- Genital examination (with a speculum *not* to be used in prepubertal girls)

Diagnostic Procedures and Laboratory Tests

- Hemoglobin and lead levels should be assessed. Children who have been victims of violence often have not had routine health care and are at risk for anemia and lead poisoning.
- Blood disorders need to be ruled out.
- Radiographic studies are needed whenever a child has a suspicious injury or trauma.
- Laboratory studies are needed to rule out sexually transmitted diseases (STDs) whenever a child is suspected of being a victim of sexual abuse.
- Color photographs should be taken if a child has visible lesions. On the photo should be included a rule of measurement, the child's name, and the name of the person taking the photo. A detailed written description needs to be documented in the medical records.

Primary Care Issues and Implications

The care of a child who has been a victim of abuse or living in a violent environment is a complex, multifaceted challenge. Not only does the practitioner have to be concerned about the child's safety, the situation is often complicated by a mother's fear of physical retaliation by her partner. With domestic violence, the majority of the time the man is the aggressor; however, there are reports of men who have also been victimized. The practitioner's role is to identify a child's problem and work with the family to resolve the violence. When the child's safety is in question, it is the responsibility of the practitioner to report suspicions to the proper community agency.

Management

Treatments and Medications

See also Chapter 47 and Counseling and Prevention in this chapter.

Domestic violence in the home (when the child is a witness to the violence). Address the parents' needs, including support and safety. Help the child learn coping mechanisms and responses to deal with the violence (e.g., if there is violent fighting, the child should protect himself or herself, go to his or her room, and close the door). Suggest that the child ask for help from a trusted adult (e.g., at school, church). Stress that the child should try to make a difference verbally but not become violent like the other people. Remind parents that their child sees, hears, and understands more than they may realize. Have parents help the child express feelings about violence through play, drawings, or talking.

Corporal punishment used as discipline. Educate the family that using physical discipline to stop a behavior provides a misconception to the child that violence is acceptable. Discuss alternatives to physical discipline and give suggestions (e.g., timeout, natural and logical consequences). Help the family learn nonviolent conflict resolution. (See also Chapters 3 and 19.)

Children watching television unsupervised. Advise parents to monitor and limit the types of television programs being watched and to be aware of the negative influence these programs may have on their child. Suggest that parents watch television with their child and discuss positive strategies for resolving conflict (as opposed to the negative ones often seen on television).

Firearms in the home. Instruct parents that firearms kept in the home must always be locked in a secure cabinet, with the ammunition never kept in the same location. Discuss the risks of gun ownership.

Firearms and violence at school. Advise the child to inform his or her teacher and parents of the violence. Help parents identify creative ways to help their child explore their world in safe, nonthreatening places. Discuss nonviolent ways to prevent fighting (see Chapter 19).

Parents as substance abusers. Inform parents that children can be intoxicated by passive inhalation or by ingesting substances left lying around by parents. A substance-abusing parent often is neglectful or has a disregard for child's needs (see Chapter 29).

Counseling and Prevention

Prevention, early identification, and intervention

- Incorporate prevention into every health care visit, starting when a family enters the health care system. Prevention of aggressive behavior in a child requires the parents or caregiver to be motivated to learn how to respond to his or her child and others in a positive, nonviolent way.
- Implement age-appropriate anticipatory guidance strategies that address violence.
- If a family who is at risk of violence is identified, recommend counseling. Counseling should address child-parent interactions and offer suggestions on how to improve them into a more positive, nurturing relationship; they should include both the child and the parents. Counseling can involve short-term therapy, crisis intervention, family therapy, parent education programs, and/or self-help parenting groups.
- Explain specific concerns and plans to the parents. A woman living with an abusive spouse needs to be reassured that her privacy will not be invaded until she is ready and motivated to make a change in her life. It frequently takes more than one violent incident for a woman to uproot herself and her children.

Age-appropriate interventions. Discuss the following with parents of infants:

- Normal developmental milestones
- Importance of touching, holding, hugging, and talking in a soft voice

- Crying, and how to respond without shaking the baby
- Childproofing the house, including storage of poisons, medicines, cleaning supplies, and firearms
Discuss the following with parents of toddlers:
- The need to play with their children and teach their children how to play
- Toilet training
- Temper tantrums and alternatives to spanking
Discuss the following with parents of preschoolers:
- Importance of social interaction and how to communicate with other children
- How to approach aggressive behavior (e.g., biting, hitting, kicking)
- How to teach conflict resolution
- The need to monitor television viewing
- The safety issue of firearms, and the need to keep all firearms securely locked away
Discuss the following with parents of school-age children:
- Importance of teaching problem-solving without using physical means
- Sibling play, and the need to listen to what a child is communicating
- Limiting and monitoring what is watched on television
- The need for positive reinforcement
Discuss the following with adolescents:
- Peer relationships
- How to handle conflict with siblings, parents, peers, and other adults
- Temper, and how to control it
- Dating and the need to respect each other without violence

Follow-Up

Follow up is as important as the initial visit when violence is a factor. Be aware of local agencies to assist the family and have their numbers readily available in a discreet location in the office (e.g., the ladies' room). If a scheduled follow-up appointment is planned and not kept, place a telephone call or send a letter asking the parents if assistance is needed and at the same time alerting them of concerns. Often the families have many needs and issues, so once the child appears well, the parent may not see follow-up as a priority. It is imperative to be nonjudgmental and provide assistance as needed to the family. However, the child's safety remains the priority, and the practitioner must *always* advocate for the child.

Consultations and Referrals

- Consult with a local multidisciplinary team on child abuse, or refer to a program experienced in working with similar families.
- Collaborate with other agencies working with the family to not duplicate interviews, and at the same time facilitate communications between professionals to ensure a comprehensive, coordinated plan for the child and his or her family.
- Refer to local community services (e.g., parent education classes, parent support groups, other available services).

Resources

Organizations

American Professional Society on the Abuse of Children (APSAC), University of Chicago, School of Social Service Administration, 969 East 60th Street, Chicago, IL 60637; (312) 702-9419; www.apsac.org

Center to Prevent Handgun Violence, 1225 Eye Street NW, Suite 1100, Washington, DC 20005; (202) 289-7319; www.cphv.org

National Center on Child Abuse and Neglect (NCCAN), Administration on Children, Youth and Families, Department of Health and Human Services, PO Box 1182, Washington, DC 20013; (703) 385-7565

National Children's Advocacy Center: Clinical offices, 106 Lincoln Street, Huntsville, AL 35801; (256) 533-5437; www.ncac-hsv.org; administrative offices, 200 Westside Square, Suite 700, Huntsville, AL 35801; (800) 543-7006; www.ncac-hsv.org

National Committee for Prevention of Child Abuse and Family Violence, 332 South Michigan Avenue, Suite 1600, Chicago, IL 60604; (312) 663-3520

National Domestic Violence Hotline; (800) 799-SAFE (7233)

Publications

Muscari, M. (2000). *Not my kid: 21 Steps to raising a nonviolent child* (book and video). Scranton, PA: University of Scranton Press. Available at (800) 941-3081 or www.scrantonpress.com

Websites

American Bar Association on Domestic Violence (www.abanet.org)

Family Violence (www.famvi.com)

National Coalition Against Domestic Violence (www.ncadv.org)

National Council on Child Abuse and Family Violence (www.nccafv.org)

Violence Against Women Online Resources (www.vaw.umn.edu)

Bibliography

American Academy of Pediatrics, Committee on Child Abuse and Neglect. (1998). The role of the pediatrician in recognizing and intervening on behalf of abused women. *Pediatrics, 101*(6), 1091-1092.

American Academy of Pediatrics, Task Force on Violence. (1999). The role of the pediatrician in youth violence prevention in clinical practice and at the community level. *Pediatrics, 103*(1), 173-181.

Beauchesne, M.A., Kelley, B.R., Lawrence, P.R., & Farquharson, P.E. (1997). Violence prevention: A community approach. *Journal of Pediatric Health Care, 1,* 155-164.

Dubwitz Jr., H. & King Jr., H. (1995). Family violence: A child-centered, family-focused approach. *Pediatric Clinics of North America, 42*(1), 153-166.

Margolin, G. (1998). Effects of witnessing violence on children. In P.K. Trickett & C J. Schellenbach (Eds.). Violence against children in the family and the community. Washington, DC: American Psychological Association.

McClosky, L.A., Figueredo, A.J., & Koss, M.P. (1995). The effects of systemic family violence on children's mental health. *Child Development, 66,* 1239-1261.

Pelcovitz, D. & Kaplan, S. (1994). Child witnesses of violence between parents. *Child and Adolescent Psychiatric Clinics of North America, 3*(4), 745-758.

Reece, R.M. (Ed.). (1994). *Child abuse: Medical diagnosis and treatment.* Philadelphia: Lea & Febiger.

Spivak, H. & Harvey, B. (Eds.). (1994, October). The role of the pediatrician in violence prevention (Proceedings of a conference, Chantilly, VA, Mar 4-5, 1994, #4 [Part II]). *Pediatrics, 94*(4; suppl).

Section 3
Common Presenting Symptoms and Problems

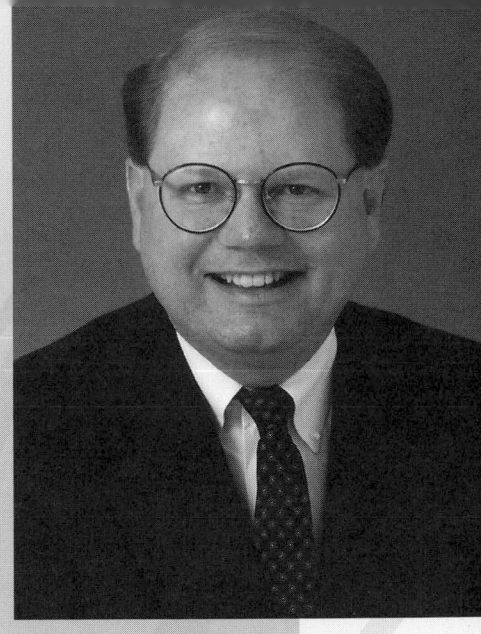

As with many nurse practitioners (NPs), I find myself involved in a practice far different from my original training as a pediatric nurse practitioner (PNP). I began my professional nursing career as a staff nurse on a pediatric oncology inpatient unit at Egelston Children's Hospital in Atlanta, Georgia, but I soon returned to school and completed my Master's education in a dual role as clinical nurse specialist and PNP. Upon graduation, I applied for several positions in primary care pediatrics and ultimately accepted a position with the Division of Urology at Emory University. This practice focused on neurologic urology and included both adults and children.

My practice at Emory primarily involved urodynamic testing (a sophisticated measurement of lower urinary tract function), and I discovered urodynamics to be invaluable for the diagnosis and management of children with paralyzing spinal disorders and multisystem congenital disorders affecting lower urinary tract function. However, while I found these sophisticated evaluations interesting and rewarding, I felt frustrated because treatment modalities seemed limited to pharmacotherapy or surgery. Fortunately, that all changed when I met a 12-year-old boy (I'll call him Jeremy) diagnosed with voiding dysfunction. This young man suffered from daytime urinary incontinence, nocturnal enuresis, recurring urinary tract infections (UTIs), and recurring pyelonephritis. Attempts to teach Jeremy intermittent catheterization were unsuccessful. After urodynamic assessment, I met with his pediatric urologist and psychiatrist (Jeremy had been admitted to an inpatient psychiatry unit for depression and continued voiding problems) who questioned whether "some sort of biofeedback to re-teach him to urinate" might be beneficial. This fascinating case was my introduction to pelvic muscle rehabilitation, a technique that I strongly advocate for children with a variety of bladder and bowel dysfunctions. I soon expanded this aspect of my practice and, working in conjunction with Pediatric Urology and the Department of Psychiatry, demonstrated a remarkably high prevalence of psycho-logic dysfunction and sexual abuse among children with severe voiding dysfunction characterized by pseudo-dyssynergia.

I subsequently completed a doctorate in lower urinary tract physiology. The knowledge gained from my doctoral education only added to my interest in pediatric voiding dysfunction. I moved into a private practice setting and contracted with Egleston Children's Hospital and the Scottish Rite Medical Center in Atlanta, Georgia. My practice focused on urodynamic evaluations, but my work with voiding dysfunction evolved, as did the realization that urodynamic testing plays an invaluable role in diagnosing problems and guiding treatment in these complex cases.

After a long and enjoyable practice in Atlanta, I returned to university-based practice in Charlottesville, Virginia. I continue to evaluate and manage children with a variety of bladder problems related to birth defects, as well as voiding dysfunction in otherwise neurologically intact children. As with many NPs, prescriptive authority has added an important element to my practice. However, the prescription of medications for various conditions remains an adjunct to my primary focus on the reeducation and rehabilitation of the pelvic floor muscles in the management of complex voiding dysfunction.

Voiding problems in children continue to provide many challenges and opportunities for PNPs. From highly prevalent voiding issues such as primary nocturnal enuresis to complex voiding dysfunction associated with encopresis and recurrent UTI, successful management goes beyond selection of a medication or surgical procedure. Instead, practice may center on basic nursing skills involving muscle rehabilitation, alterations in diet and lifestyle, and scheduled or prompted toileting. When combined with advanced practice and evolving prescriptive authority, the PNP is becoming an increasingly critical member of a busy pediatric urology practice and an invaluable resource for children and their families.

Mikel Gray

Chapter 32 *Cardiovascular System*

Kathleen Kenney

Chest Pain, p. 343
Congenital Heart Defects, p. 346
Heart Murmurs, p. 350
Hyperlipidemia, p. 353
Hypertension, p. 356

Risk Factors

- Genetic predisposition for congenital heart defects (CHDs)
- Prenatal exposure to teratogenic agents (e.g., medications, alcohol, tobacco, x-rays)
- Prenatal history of viral illness (coxsackievirus B, cytomegalovirus [CMV], influenza B, mumps, rubella)
- Maternal factors (e.g., age over 40 years, insulin-dependent diabetes, systemic lupus erythematosus [SLE])
- Chromosomal anomalies (e.g., Noonan syndrome; trisomy 13, 18, or 21; Turner syndrome; single-gene abnormality [such as Holt-Oram syndrome])
- Prematurity
- Infection (e.g., rheumatic fever, Kawasaki's disease)
- Autoimmune response (e.g., SLE)
- Tobacco or alcohol use
- Environmental factors (e.g., passive smoke)
- Familial tendencies (e.g., obesity, physical inactivity)
- Myocardial infarction before 55 years of age in family members
- Sudden death (by known or unknown cause) in family members
- Congenital heart disease in siblings or other family members
- Obesity
- Stroke
- Xanthomas
- Family history of rheumatic fever
- Recent history of group A β-hemolytic streptococcal (GABHS) infection
- Medications (e.g., corticosteroids, oral contraceptives, Accutane, anticonvulsants)

Health Promotion

Prenatal

- Genetic counseling for high-risk groups
- Early prenatal care
- Continuation of prenatal care
- Cardiac evaluation for family history of CHDs

Early Childhood

- Prevention of infection through general health maintenance
- Maintenance of immunization schedules into adulthood
- Promotion of breastfeeding

- Anticipatory guidance regarding dietary habits, the food guide pyramid, the benefits of a healthy diet, and safe weight management
- Use of growth charts at each visit to determine patterns of growth
- Instruction to parents on the importance of completing prescribed medication for GABHS infection
- Selected screening of young children to determine the risk of developing adult coronary artery disease (CAD)

Childhood and Adolescence

- Annual health guidance regarding the benefits of safe exercise on a regular basis
- Stressing the importance of a nutritious diet
- Annual health guidance to parents and children regarding avoidance of tobacco, alcohol, and other abusable substances, including anabolic steroids
- Annual hypertension screening beginning at 3 years of age
- Selected screening of children and adolescents to determine the risk of developing adult CAD
- Instruction to parents and child on the importance of completing prescribed medication for GABHS infection

Subjective Data

- *Demographics*—Age, gender, race, socioeconomic status
- *Reason for visit and description of problem*—Perception of parents and child
- *Onset of symptoms*—Sudden, gradual, recurring
- *Precipitating factors*—Feeding, exercise, emotions, stress, infection, trauma
- *Relieving factors*—Medications, rest or sleep, positional change, reassurance
- *Current medications and treatments*—Vasopressors, corticosteroids, contraceptives, antihypertensives, antibiotics, over-the-counter medications, street drugs
- *Prenatal history*—Prenatal exposure to Accutane, alcohol, tobacco, thalidomide, lithium compounds, hydantoin, isotretinoin, trimethadione, x-rays
- *Neonatal history*—Prematurity, respiratory distress syndrome, sepsis, murmur, chronic illnesses, surgeries, procedures
- *Past health history*—Hospitalizations, operations, infectious diseases (e.g., coxsackievirus B, cytomegalovirus [CMV], influenza B, mumps, rubella, GABHS), frequency of upper respiratory infections
- *Chronic illness*—History of recurrent respiratory infections, significant recurrent illnesses
- *Past or recurrent problems related to the cardiovascular system*—Rheumatic fever, heart murmur, congenital heart disease, hypertension, Kawasaki's disease
- *Infections*—Urinary tract infections, acute glomerulonephritis, pyelonephritis

- *Family history*—Congenital heart disease of any kind (surgically or not surgically repaired), sudden unexplained death, SIDS, hypercholesterolemia, early CAD
- *Emotional instability*
- *Allergies*
- *Child's health habits*—Eating or feeding behavior; changes in sleep patterns, personality, school (e.g., performance, number of absences), temperament, medications
- *Immunization history*—Diphtheria, tetanus, acellular pertussis (DPT or DTaP) vaccine; *Haemophilus influenzae* type B (Hib) vaccine; influenza or pneumococcal vaccine
- *Diet history*—Percentage fat intake, poor nutrition, poor feeding, high salt intake
- *Developmental history*—Delayed development
- *Patterns and habits.* Reactions to physical activity and ability to keep up with peers; passive or active smoking; sleep and activity habits
- *Date of last chest radiograph*—Any findings of increased cardiac size or abnormal pulmonary vascular markings
- *Recent history of the following*—Trauma to abdomen or flank, fractures, infections (skin and upper respiratory, especially GABHS), new murmur documented after GABHS
- *Associated symptoms*—Dizziness; headache (especially upon awakening); blurred vision; chest pain, palpitations, or shortness of breath; weakness or easy fatigability; syncope; polyuria; muscle cramps; excessive diaphoresis; recent weight gain or loss; chronic cough; "blue spells," or squatting during play or other activities; digital clubbing; periorbital edema; hemiplegia; intermittent or persistent pallor or cyanosis of the skin, mucous membranes, lips, or nail beds; lethargy or excessive, prolonged napping; paroxysmal tachypnea (hypoxic spells); tiring during feeding; diaphoresis with feeding; failure to thrive (FTT)

Objective Data

Physical Examination

A complete physical examination is generally indicated for all infants and children with significant cardiac signs and symptoms. Most cardiac disorders can be identified with a thorough history and physical examination. All procedures should be explained to the child or parents before the examination is performed. The heart and lungs need to be evaluated early in the examination of infants and young children, before crying and agitation occur.

The physical examination includes the following areas:
- *Measurements*—Height, weight, percentiles
- *Vital signs*
- *Blood pressure (BP) readings*—With the patient quiet and relaxed; using appropriate-sized cuff; in supine position, measurement of all extremities to detect differences; sitting, measurement in right arm; standing (after 3 minutes), measurement for possible postural changes; using mercury manometer placed at the level of the patient; data recorded on percentile charts; flush or Doppler method will be necessary for some infants
- *Heart*—Palpation of point of maximum impulse; palpation for heaves, thrills, increased impulses; auscultation for first and second heart sounds, presence of abnormal heart sounds, rate, pitch, intensity, quality, rhythm, location,

radiation, extra heart sounds, murmurs (including differentiation of innocent versus pathologic murmurs)
- *Pulses*—Radial, brachial, femoral, popliteal, dorsalis pedis, posterior tibial; palpation bilaterally for quality, character, symmetry, rate, rhythm
- *General appearance*—Observation of gait, coordination, speech, physical deformity; observation for congenital anomalies, signs of distress
- *Skin*—Inspection for color, cyanosis (circumoral or peripheral), digital clubbing, edema
- *Neck*—Neck vein prominence or distension
- *Eyes*—Funduscopic examination for vascular changes
- *Chest and lungs*—Chest configuration, size, shape, symmetry, movement; auscultation for crackles, wheezing, adventitious breath sounds
- *Abdomen*—Inspection and palpation for hepatosplenomegaly, liver tenderness, hepatojugular reflex, enlarged kidneys
- *Neurologic examination*—Signs of cerebral vascular disease (e.g., defect in mentation or motor function)

Diagnostic Procedures and Laboratory Tests

A *chest radiograph* provides information regarding cardiac size and contour, size of the cardiac chambers and vessels, and status of the pulmonary blood flow and lungs.

An *electrocardiogram* (ECG) uses the graphic tracing of the electrical activity of the heart from different locations and in different planes, aids in determining size and axis of heart, and identifies potential and present arrhythmias and electrical disturbances.

An *echocardiogram* is a noninvasive procedure that uses reflected sound waves to identify intracardiac structures and their motion. Two-dimensional, M-mode, contrast, and Doppler recordings may be obtained.

Cardiac catheterization provides information regarding oxygen saturation and pressure in the cardiac chambers; cardiac output and function; vascular resistance; and cardiac response to medication and exercise. A catheter is introduced into the heart chambers through the femoral vessel. (In neonates the umbilical vein or artery may be used.) The thin, flexible, radiopaque catheter is observed by means of fluoroscopy.

Magnetic resonance imaging (MRI) is a noninvasive imaging technique that uses low-energy radio waves in combination with a strong magnetic field to visualize heart structures and identify abnormalities.

Arterial blood gas methods reveal arterial levels of oxygen and carbon dioxide. Metabolic acidosis has a higher association with a cardiac cause, and respiratory acidosis has a higher association with a pulmonary cause.

Transcutaneous pulse oximetry is a noninvasive method of assessing arterial oxygen saturation during rapidly changing circulatory states.

A *hyperoxia or oxygen challenge test* involves provision of 100% oxygen, resulting in increased arterial saturation and "pinking" when the origin is primarily respiratory. Minimal or no color improvement or lack of significant increase in oxygen percentile is more indicative of a cardiac problem.

Hemoglobin and hematocrit with indices are diagnostic for anemia or polycythemia and also reflect the degree of desaturation and cyanosis.

Chest Pain

Alert

Consult with or refer to a physician for the following:
- Presence of an obstructive heart lesion
- Murmur of an obstructive heart lesion
- History of chest pain with palpitations
- Family history of sudden death
- Chest pain with syncope
- Chest pain with vigorous activity
- History of Kawasaki's disease
- Chest pain with fever or significant illness
- Heart rate greater than 200 beats per minute
- Signs of respiratory distress or cyanosis
- Clinically significant trauma
- History of drug use or abuse
- History suggestive of myocarditis (e.g., fever, recent viral illness, malaise)
- Chest pain in a young child

Etiology

Chest pain is a frequent complaint encountered in routine pediatric care. The majority of chest pain complaints in the pediatric population are not caused by cardiac disease. The implications of a child having pain in the chest should not be underestimated, and the practitioner must be diligent in the diagnosis and explanation of the cause to both parents and child. Common causes of chest pain include musculoskeletal pain and strain, inflammation, gastroesophageal irritation, and psychogenic origins. Certain chronic conditions (e.g., sickle cell crisis, pulmonary disease, malignancies) may result in chest pain in children. Least common are true cardiac diseases or processes. Congenital heart lesions, arrhythmias, and some acquired cardiac conditions may also manifest as chest pain.

Irritation of the pericardium may also result in complaints of chest pain. Inflammatory processes that result in irritation to the pericardium include viruses, bacterial endocarditis, tuberculosis (TB), pericarditis, and rheumatoid illnesses. Cardiomyopathy of any origin may cause chest pain related to either ischemia or arrhythmias. Supraventricular tachycardia (SVT) is the most common manifesting arrhythmia in children with heart rate irregularities and chest pain. Pain may result from actual ischemia from a sustained fast heart rate or may be expressed in relation to the forcefulness of the rapid heartbeats. Some children may interpret palpitations as chest pain because of a lack of ability to describe what they are feeling.

Noncardiac causes of chest pain include a wide variety of diagnostic categories. Muscle strain or inflammation and costochondritis are among the most common causes of chest discomfort. Various respiratory, thoracic cage, gastrointestinal, and psychogenic diseases may also manifest as chest pain. The emotional origin of chest pain cannot be ignored; stress and anxiety are primary causative factors in many complaints of chest pain within the pediatric and adolescent population.

Incidence

- The most common cause of chest pain in children is costochondritis (20% to 75% of pain).
- Chest pain in children is rarely of cardiac origin.
- The most common arrhythmia with chest pain in children is SVT.
- In 21% to 39% of children and adolescents with chest pain, the cause is found to be idiopathic.
- About 30% of chest pain in children is a result of musculoskeletal causes.
- Anxiety and emotional distress account for as much as 9% to 20% of chest pain in adolescents.
- Gastrointestinal disorders account for 2% to 7% of cases of chest pain.

Risk Factors

- Structural heart defects (e.g., obstructive lesions, mitral valve prolapse, anomalous origin of the left coronary artery)
- Inflammatory processes (e.g., pericarditis, Kawasaki's disease)
- Arrhythmias (e.g., SVT, frequent premature ventricular contractions [PVCs])
- Costochondritis
- Muscle strain
- Trauma to the chest wall
- Abnormalities of the rib cage or spine; pectus excavatum; or scoliosis
- Asthma
- Pneumonia
- Pleural effusion
- Spontaneous pneumothorax
- Viral infections
- Hyperventilation
- Stress and anxiety
- Conversion reaction, somatization, or disorder
- Depression
- Drug use (e.g., of cocaine)
- High caffeine intake
- Exercise

Differential Diagnosis

The ability of a practitioner to differentiate between cardiac and noncardiac causes of chest pain as well as serious, life-threatening, or common diagnoses is crucial. A thorough history and physical examination are essential for determining the appropriate diagnosis and treatment plan. Differential diagnoses of chest pain in children can most easily be divided into two major categories, cardiac and noncardiac (Table 32-1). Cardiac causes of chest pain may be related to structural abnormalities, acquired heart disease, pericardial or myocardial inflammation, or arrhythmias. Myocardial infarction is a rare possibility in healthy children and adolescents. It is imperative that cardiac conditions be ruled out immediately.

Cardiac causes. Structural cardiac abnormalities causing chest pain usually result in an alteration in the myocardial oxygen demands and supply to the heart.

Obstructive lesions are the most common structural causative factors. Aortic stenosis (AS) or subaortic stenosis is the most common obstructive lesion causing pain. Pulmonary stenosis (PS) (valvular and subvalvular) is much less commonly the origin of chest pain. The amount of obstruction is usually severe, resulting in an alteration in oxygen supply and demand. These structural anomalies become evident with an audible stenotic type of murmur. There may be a thrill on palpation and an ECG showing ventricular hypertrophy with or

Table 32-1 Differential Diagnosis: Chest Pain

CRITERIA	NONCARDIAC	CARDIAC*
ICD-9 code	786.59	786.50
Subjective Data		
Age	Any	Any
Onset	Acute, progressive, chronic	Acute, intermittent, progressive, chronic
Associated symptoms	Cough, exercise, shortness of breath, fever, nausea, musculoskeletal pain	Shortness of breath, pain with inspiration, pain with exercise, fever, diaphoresis
Present history	Recent illness, history of asthma, trauma, anxiety, recent increase in physical activity	History of palpitations, congenital heart defect, recent streptococcal infection, syncope
Feeding history	Normal feeding habits	May be history of crying, diaphoresis, tachypnea, or easy fatiguability with feeds
Prenatal history	History of respiratory difficulty	Diagnosis of congenital heart lesion, arrhythmia during prenatal examinations, chromosomal abnormality in utero, maternal drug use, maternal illness during pregnancy
Newborn history	Noncontributory	Diagnosis of obstructive congenital heart lesion, history of cyanosis at rest or with crying or activity; tachypnea, diaphoresis at rest, history of poor weight gain
Family history	Presence of stress disorders, psychiatric illnesses, internal family stress, illness, abuse, neglect, divorce, violence	History of early sudden death, myocardial infarction, elevated serum cholesterol level, hypertension, familial history of congenital heart lesion
Objective Data		
Physical examination		
Vital signs		
Pulse	Normal, slightly elevated (anxiety); sinus arrhythmia	Irregular rapid extrasystole, abnormal beats (premature ventricular contractions)
Blood pressure	Normal for age group	May be normal, low, high, or significant difference between upper and lower extremities
Respiratory rate	May be normal or elevated	May be normal or elevated
Chest examination		
Inspection	May be signs of respiratory distress, retractions, nasal flaring, dyspnea	May be signs of respiratory distress (e.g., retractions, nasal flaring, dyspnea); may be crackles
Auscultation	May be wheezing, crackles, decreased or absent breath sounds	May be crackles
Palpation	May result in reproduction of pain; may be able to produce crepitus	May feel abnormal cardiac heaves in chest, thrill, or abnormal impulses
Percussion	Dullness may be heard over area of consolidation, atelectasis, or pleural effusion; tympany may reflect hyperaeration with asthma; resonance reflects normal lung findings	May be resonance because of normal lung parenchyma
Heart	Normal heart sounds, innocent murmur (less than grade II/VI), normal pulses	Possible murmur present, possible thrill, rapid heart rate, muffled heart sounds, gallop rhythm, pericardial friction rub, altered second heart sound, ejection click
Abdomen	May be able to reproduce chest pain with palpation of epigastric area or right or left upper quadrants	Normal examination; may have hepatosplenomegaly
Musculoskeletal	May reproduce pain with bending or movement of extremities; may see signs of trauma	Normal examination may have long, thin body type and long arm span
Laboratory data	Appropriate tests for suspected underlying cause of chest pain	Electrocardiogram, chest radiograph, echocardiogram, cardiac catheterization

*Refer to a physician.

without strain pattern. An echocardiogram defines the actual lesion and amount of obstruction. Chest radiograph may demonstrate an enlarged cardiac silhouette because of the increased workload of the heart. Severe obstruction resulting in chest pain requires surgical palliation.

Coronary artery anomalies such as the anomalous origin of the left coronary artery may become evident as chest pain that is perceived by the parent in the infant or very young child. Although infants and young children are unable to verbalize pain, they demonstrate common symptoms of chest pain that include crying, irritability with feeding, episodes of paleness, or diaphoresis, and parents may perceive them to be in pain. Once again, physical examination reveals a murmur. Anomalous origin of the left coronary artery may be misdiagnosed within the first few months of life as colic. Attention must be paid to signs of pain with feeding, since sucking is the hardest work the heart must complete during this time. Pain and diaphoresis during feeding are related to actual ischemia. An ECG may show signs of ischemia or an infarction pattern. Obtaining an ECG while an infant is feeding may be most beneficial during the initial evaluation. In contrast to coronary artery anomalies, which result in ischemia and pain during actual physical work (i.e., feeding), colic results in crying and possible abdominal pain after feeding.

Mitral valve prolapse (MVP) causes chest pain more often in adults and adolescents but occasionally may become evident with chest pain in children. The causes of the pain associated with MVP are poorly understood.

Pericarditis, myocarditis, and other inflammatory disorders from a viral, bacterial, or rheumatoid illness may cause diffuse chest pain or sudden, severe midsternal chest discomfort, causing anxiety in both children and parents. Children with acute pericarditis often appear ill and have other associated symptoms of cardiac involvement.

Kawasaki's disease, or *mucocutaneous lymph node syndrome,* is a disease of unknown origin. It is a generalized illness accompanied by fever and significant disease of the heart and may ultimately result in death. A sequela related to Kawasaki's disease is vasculitis of the coronary arteries with possible aneurysm formation. All children with Kawasaki's disease according to the diagnostic criteria require an echocardiogram to confirm cardiac involvement, whether or not they have chest pain.

Arrhythmias, including SVT and extrasystoles (ventricular and junctional), may result in chest pain. Heart rates exceeding 200 beats per minute may cause pain as a result of inadequate myocardial oxygen delivery in response to increased demand. Extrasystoles may be perceived by a child as palpitations or irregularities in the chest, thereby being misinterpreted as chest pain. Isolated PVCs can produce transient chest discomfort or pain that lasts for a few seconds before resolving.

Respiratory causes. Common respiratory illnesses may cause chest pain because of irritation of the chest wall, inflammation, or trauma. Asthmatic children frequently complain of chest pain resulting from prolonged wheezing, cough, or tachycardia related to their medication. Pleural effusions may include symptoms of chest discomfort. Pneumonia incorporating a lobar pattern may become evident as chest, abdominal, or combined pain. Spontaneous pneumothorax should be considered with absent or significantly decreased breath sounds, chest pain, or splinting. Adolescents often have hyperventilation during times of anxiety or crisis; chest pain may be a combined result of the rapid breathing and a stress factor.

Musculoskeletal causes. Inflammation, injury, or irritation to muscles surrounding or connected to the chest wall often result in pain that patients classify as "chest pain." One of the most common musculoskeletal causes is costochondritis. Costochondritis is the result of inflammation over the junction between the anterior ribs and the sternum, which may be the result of vigorous exercise, sneezing, or persistent coughing. The pain of costochondritis often is anterior and is reproducible at the costochondral junction.

Trauma. Direct injury to the chest wall may cause bruising, inflammation, or bleeding into the chest wall or pericardial cavity. History-taking is imperative, especially if some time has passed since the injury occurred. Severe trauma with significant damage to the heart or lungs becomes evident immediately after the initial injury. Auscultation of heart sounds may reveal a rub or decreased crisp heart sounds.

Gastrointestinal causes. Gastroesophageal reflux or irritation may cause pain that is perceived as originating in the chest or is referred to the xiphoid area of the chest.

Idiopathic causes. In a large percentage of children with chest pain a definite diagnosis or origin of the pain is never found. This group of children often has nonspecific, unclear complaints with a normal physical examination.

Psychogenic causes. Emotional causes of chest pain must be considered once other differential diagnoses have been exhausted. The profound effect that stress and psychologic factors have on the body cannot be ignored. Signs of depression (see Chapter 39), severe anxiety, or emotional trauma must be addressed during the history and physical examination.

Miscellaneous causes. Miscellaneous causes may include sickle cell crisis, tumors, lung diseases, and malignant processes.

Management

Treatments and medications

Cardiac causes of chest pain. Any children with strong suspicion of cardiac causes of chest pain should immediately be referred to a specialist or an emergency room. Children with significant respiratory distress resulting in chest pain should be referred to the appropriate physician or emergency room by the emergency services. Patients with suspected infectious or inflammatory origins of chest pain should be referred to a physician for further evaluation and work-up.

Noncardiac causes of chest pain. Children with more common, non–life-threatening causes of chest pain must first be reassured that their heart is normal and that they are in no danger of becoming very ill. Management of chest pain of noncardiac origin includes treatment of the underlying cause of the chest pain. Management of chest pain resulting from idiopathic or psychogenic sources should include emphasizing that the child's heart is not the cause of the pain and that the child is in no danger. Much support and counseling may be required when these diagnoses are under consideration. It may be beneficial to do an ECG and chest radiograph to reassure the child or adolescent and family.

For costochondritis, nonsteroidal medications and treatments include ibuprofen 10 mg per kg per dose every 6 hours as needed for pain; naproxen 10 mg per kg per 24 hours, with one dose every 12 hours; no heavy lifting or excessive activity; and warm, moist heat to chest as needed.

Counseling and prevention

- Reassure the parents and child that the child is in no danger of having a "heart attack" or dying.
- Review with the parents and child management protocols for the specific disease process causing the chest pain (e.g., for asthma, Proventil pump every 4 hours for cough, pain, and wheezing; for costochondritis, ibuprofen 10 mg per kg per dose every 6 hours for pain).
- Educate the patient on the dangers of illicit drug, tobacco, and alcohol use and their effect on the heart.
- Encourage children with musculoskeletal causes to rest, use analgesics, and refrain from strenuous physical activity until pain has resolved.
- Teach children with anxiety or stress that results in chest pain methods of identifying stressors and ways to reduce anxiety.

- Teach children with hyperventilation to concentrate on slowing breathing down and to use a bag to breathe into until breathing returns to normal.

Follow-up

- A return visit should be scheduled in 24 to 48 hours for children with infectious (e.g., pneumonia) respiratory or gastrointestinal causes of chest pain to assess improvement of symptoms and recovery.
- Children with musculoskeletal causes of chest pain may continue with routine pediatric follow-up evaluation unless symptoms do not dissipate within 2 weeks.
- Children with psychogenic causes of chest pain may need frequent telephone calls or visits to identify stressors or help manage acute anxiety attacks.

Consultations and referrals. Refer to a physician those children with signs of acute distress and chest pain; recurring chest pain associated with exercise, palpitations, dizziness, or syncope; known history of cardiac disease; suggestive acute inflammatory process (e.g., pericarditis, myocarditis); or significant respiratory distress, absent breath sounds, hypoxia, or foreign-body aspiration.

Congenital Heart Defects

Alert

Consult with or refer to a physician for the following:
- Infant with new murmur and feeding difficulties
- Infant with murmur, cyanosis, or poor weight gain
- Child with genetic or chromosomal disorder and murmur
- Infant or child with murmur and systemic signs or symptoms of cardiac compromise
- Infant with tachypnea or tachycardia with feeding
- Infant with bounding pulses and tachypnea

Etiology

CHDs are defined as abnormal structural developments of the heart or its vessels that may affect the overall function of the heart. Although the exact causes of the various CHDs are unknown, there are many factors that are believed to contribute to the abnormal development of the structure of a neonate's heart. It has been estimated that up to 10% of CHDs are related to a direct cause (e.g., maternal infection, maternal teratogens) or associated disease (e.g., Down syndrome, Turner syndrome). Inheritance, genetics, and environmental factors are believed to be responsible for up to 90% of CHDs, while certain chromosomal and genetic disorders are associated with specific congenital lesions.

Incidence

- CHDs are relatively common in the pediatric population, occurring in approximately 6 in every 1000 live births.
- CHDs are one of the most common forms of significant congenital defect.
- With recent advances in surgical and medical management of CHDs, up to 85% of children born with a CHD will survive into adulthood.
- The most common CHD seen in children is an isolated ventricular septal defect (VSD).
- Only 40% to 50% of CHDs are diagnosed by 1 week of age.
- Only 50% to 60% of CHDs are diagnosed by 1 month of age.

- The incidence of CHDs increases in families with a history of CHDs in a first-degree relative.
- Certain CHDs may not appear until the pulmonary pressures drop (between 4 and 8 weeks of age).
- Atrial septal defects (ASDs) account for as many as 10% of all CHDs in children.

Risk Factors

- Family history of CHDs
- Maternal illness or use of teratogens during prenatal period
- Maternal chronic illness (e.g., lupus erythematosus)
- Poor feeding
- Prematurity
- Persistent tachypnea
- Easy fatigability
- FTT
- Frequent, recurrent upper respiratory infections
- Diaphoresis with feeding
- Hepatomegaly
- Clubbing
- Central cyanosis
- Bounding pulses
- Presence of a syndrome or chromosomal abnormality

Differential Diagnosis

Many infants with CHDs are asymptomatic at birth and are diagnosed during routine well-child visits (Table 32-2). Early hospital discharge and persistently high pulmonary pressures often delay the presentation of the murmur and the symptoms of certain heart defects. Most of the major defects appear with physical signs and symptoms resulting from the defect, and significant cardiac lesions will affect the infant or child's growth and development. CHDs are divided into two basic categories: acyanotic and cyanotic. Acyanotic defects include those defects that allow for shunting of blood from the left side of the heart to the right side as well as most of the stenotic lesions where there is no actual mixing of oxygenated and deoxygenated blood. The most common defects that are undetected are the acyanotic lesions, which may manifest with only subtle symptoms and take months to a few years to detect. Cyanotic defects allow for shunting of deoxygenated blood from the right side of the heart to the left side. It is important for the practitioner to recognize that cyanosis may be subtle and manifest itself only at times of increased cardiac output, as during crying or feeding. Cyanosis may appear as paleness, a bluish hue, or a gray-appearing child. Clubbing, which can result from chronic cyanosis, may take up to 1 year to develop. Therefore it often does not appear early in the diagnostic period in most infants and children.

Assessment of infants and children with possible CHD should be comprehensive, with a strong focus on respiratory and cardiac function. Feeding problems are a common complaint in infants with CHDs because of the increased workload of the heart required during feeding. Parents often complain of prolonged feeding times and tachypnea or cyanosis with feeding. One can assess exercise tolerance by determining the child's ability to keep up with his or her peers or observing for signs of respiratory difficulty with running or prolonged exercise. Easy fatigability or episodes of shortness of breath, diaphoresis, or squatting during exercise are congruent with a possible CHD. Growth parameters should be measured and plotted at every visit for any child with a CHD, including those

Table 32-2 Common Congenital Heart Defects: Clinical and Radiographic Findings

HEART DEFECT	CLINICAL FINDINGS	RADIOGRAPHIC FINDINGS
Atrial septal defect (ASD)	May be asymptomatic Widely split fixed S2 Systolic ejection murmur at upper left sternal border	May show cardiomegaly with right atrial enlargement, possible right ventricular enlargement, and prominent main pulmonary artery
Ventricular septal defect (VSD)	Grade II to V/VI holosystolic murmur loudest at left lower sternal border May have a thrill	May have with larger defects: cardiomegaly, enlarged left and right ventricles, and increased pulmonary vascular markings
Patent ductus arteriosus (PDA)	May be asymptomatic Grade I to IV/VI continuous murmur (to and fro) at left upper sternal border Bounding pulses	Small PDA: normal Large PDA: cardiomegaly, left atrial enlargement, left ventricular enlargement, and increased pulmonary vascular markings
Partial anomalous pulmonary venous return (PAPVR)	May be asymptomatic Widely split S2	Right atrial and ventricular enlargement Increased pulmonary vascular markings
Pulmonary stenosis (PS)	Systolic ejection murmur II to V/VI along the left sternal border S2 may be widely split Possible thrill present	Heart size normal Main pulmonary artery may be prominent Pulmonary vascular markings can be decreased in severe PS
Aortic stenosis (AS)	Systolic ejection murmur II to V/VI along sternal border; loudest at right and left upper sternal border, sternal notch, and over the carotids Possible thrill	Usually normal
Coarctation of aorta (COA)	Often no murmur present unless with other concurrent defects (e.g., VSD)	May be normal or have cardiomegaly (depends on degree of coarctation) May be signs of pulmonary venous congestion
Transposition of the great arteries (TGA)	No murmur may be present S2 is single If associated with VSD or PS, murmurs may be audible	Cardiomegaly Increased pulmonary vascular marking "Egg-shaped" heart
Tetralogy of Fallot (TOF)	Murmur depends on degree of VSD and RVOT obstruction May have systolic ejection murmur at upper left sternal border May have single S2	May show normal heart size (depends on degree of stenosis and VSD) "Boot-shaped" heart
Total anomalous pulmonary venous return (TAPVR)	S2 is widely split and fixed Grade II to III/VI systolic ejection murmur at upper left sternal border	May see mild to significant cardiomegaly Increased pulmonary vascular markings "Snowman" heart may be seen after the age of 4 months

with acyanotic defects. Often children with even small heart defects (such as atrial septal defect) develop a growth pattern on the lower percentiles (5th to 10th). A history of frequent upper respiratory infections in toddlers and young children may be indicative of certain congenital defects (e.g., ASD, patent ductus arteriosus [PDA]). The presence of a syndrome or chromosomal abnormality should raise suspicion for possible coronary heart disease.

Significant complications and manifestations of CHDs include hypoxemia and congestive heart failure (CHF). These two complications may not appear in the infant or child until a few weeks or months of age because of the increased pulmonary pressure in young infants. As the pulmonary pressures begin to lower, the pressures in the right side of the heart begin to drop to normal levels, thus allowing a greater degree of mixing of oxygenated and deoxygenated blood. This natural process results in the gradual development of symptoms in a previously asymptomatic infant or child. Cyanosis is the bluish discoloration of the skin from an increased amount of deoxygenated blood in the peripheral circulation. Cyanosis is often not easily visible in the extremities and may manifest only at times when the heart is in a hyperdynamic state such as crying, fever, and feeding. The most common sites for assessing for the presence of cyanosis include the mucous membranes, tip of the nose, and the nail beds. This may be more difficult in darkly pigmented skin. Often the onset of cyanosis is gradual; thus many parents may not notice its presentation. Children who are cyanotic have higher hemoglobin concentrations as a result of the body's physiologic response to increase its ability to carry oxygen to the vital organs. Chronic hypoxemia can result in clubbing of the distal area of the digits, with this usually taking up to a year to appear. Infants and children who are cyanotic often show decreased activity levels compared to their peers, tachypnea, and easy fatigability. It is important for the practitioner to identify these signs and symptoms in the history when assessing any child for a CHD.

The three cardinal signs and symptoms of CHF are increasing heart size, tachypnea, and hepatosplenomegaly. Infants and children with CHF often show increased difficulty in feeding, decreased caloric intake, tachypnea, diaphoresis, decreased activity, and possibly lethargy. There may be a complaint of a new-onset cough, periorbital edema, and irritability. CHF may appear early in significant cyanotic heart defects and later in the neonatal period with defects such as VSD, which may not cause increased shunting from left to right until the pulmonary pressures drop between 4 and 8 weeks of age. Those infants or children with CHF usually have a significant defect with numerous findings on both the history and physical examination.

Acyanotic defects

Atrial septal defect. There are three possible types of ASD, all of which have an area along the atrial septum that has not been completely formed. This defect allows for shunting of blood from the left atrium to the right atrium, resulting in an increased workload for the right side of the heart. This increased volume results in an increased amount of pulmonary blood flow, which if significant enough may manifest as CHF. Most infants and children with small to moderate ASDs are asymptomatic, with a grade I to III or grade VI systolic murmur in the upper left sternal border and a widely fixed, split S_2. Children with a large defect may manifest with CHF from the large volume overload on the pulmonary vasculature. Up to 40% of children with ASDs may have spontaneous closure of their defect before 4 years of age. The smaller defects have a much higher rate of spontaneous closure before 18 months of age.

Ventricular septal defect. A VSD results from an incomplete formation of the musculature between the right and left ventricle. Defects range from a small membranous defect, with minimal symptoms, to a large muscular defect, which may result in CHF. The signs and symptoms of VSDs depend on the size of the defect and the pulmonary vascular resistance. Often infants born with VSDs do not demonstrate symptoms of the defect until the pulmonary pressures drop, and such a drop allows for a greater degree of shunting of blood from the left side of the heart to the right. Small VSDs manifest asymptomatically with a holosystolic, grade II to V (possible thrill) murmur at the left lower sternal border. Infants with larger defects demonstrate signs and symptoms of delayed growth and development, tachypnea, diaphoresis with feeding, and possibly CHF. Children with VSDs may have poor exercise tolerance, easy fatigability, frequent upper respiratory tract infections, and delayed growth and development.

Approximately 30% to 40% of VSDs spontaneously close within the first few years of life. Defects that are larger and symptomatic are less likely to close completely or spontaneously. The larger defects may get smaller as the child grows but may not completely close on their own. Infants and children with large VSDs, which cause pulmonary compromise and growth delays, are often surgically repaired within the first few years of life. Those defects not causing significant health problems or growth delays may wait to be repaired until the child is 2 to 4 years of age. Small, insignificant VSDs may go unrepaired.

Patent ductus arteriosus. The defect called PDA represents a persistence in the fetal duct between the aorta and pulmonary artery. It is most common among premature infants but also accounts for up to 10% of all CHD in full-term newborns. The symptoms of PDA are dependent on the width of the lesion. Small lesions often do not demonstrate significant signs beyond a continuous murmur along the upper left sternal border and bounding pulses. Large lesions may manifest as CHF, bounding pulses, and a widened pulse pressure.

Partial anomalous pulmonary venous return. Partial anomalous pulmonary venous return (PAPVR) is differentiated from total anomalous pulmonary venous return (TAPVR) in that not all the pulmonary veins drain into the right atrium. Most infants or children with PAPVR are asymptomatic, with few physical findings. The findings consistent with PAPVR are synonymous with ASDs because many patients with PAPVR have a concurrent ASD. If there is no ASD present, these children may go undetected for many years, with some not being discovered until well into their adult life. In the absence of a murmur or fixed split S_2, these patients with PAPVR are discovered by an ECG that shows right ventricular hypertrophy or a right bundle branch block or by a chest radiograph that demonstrates increased pulmonary vascular markings and right-sided heart enlargement.

Pulmonary stenosis. Mild PS often does not manifest physical symptoms beyond a systolic ejection murmur along the left upper sternal border, a possible thrill, and a widely split S_2. The more severe the PS, the louder is the murmur. Practitioners may be able to assess the progression of the PS by monitoring the intensity of the murmur. Moderate and severe PS may manifest as dyspnea, exercise and activity intolerance, or CHF. Critical PS may produce cyanosis as a result of poor blood flow to the pulmonary bed.

Aortic stenosis. As with PS, AS may be below the aortic valve (subvalvular), at the valve (valvular); or above the valve (supravalvular). Infants and children with mild or moderate AS are often asymptomatic. Those patients with severe AS can experience chest pain and syncope, and infants can have CHF. The murmur of AS is a systolic ejection murmur at the right upper sternal border that is transmitted easily, and there may be a thrill present and a narrow pulse pressure if the AS is severe.

Coarctation of the aorta. Symptomatic presentation of a coarctation of the aorta (COA) depends on the severity of the narrowing of the aorta. Often there are other concurrent defects present in infants (e.g., PDA, VSD). Asymptomatic infants and children may have only a delayed or decreased pulse in the lower extremities with hypertension in the upper extremities. During childhood these children may complain of leg pain or cramps. These patients may have a systolic ejection murmur or no murmur. Physical examination is very important including measurement of the BP along with simultaneous palpation of upper and lower extremity pulses. Symptomatic children manifest in infancy with signs and symptoms of CHF, poor perfusion, and possibly shock early in the newborn period. Hypertension and weak or absent peripheral pulses are among the classic findings in infants with COA.

Cyanotic defects

Tetralogy of Fallot. There are four distinct malformations that occur to create the diagnosis of tetralogy of Fallot (TOF): a large ventricular septal defect, right ventricular hypertrophy, right ventricular outflow tract obstruction (PS or infundibular stenosis), and an overriding aorta. The degree of symptoms for children with TOF depends on the severity of each defect. The VSD associated with most TOFs is often very large, resulting in equal pressure gradients in both ventricles. The degree of right ventricular outflow tract obstruction is the deciding factor in its relationship to the presence or absence of cyanosis. With mild PS, a child will have shunting of blood from the left side of the heart to the right side (not resulting in cyanosis). A child with moderate to severe stenosis has more shunting of blood from the right to the left ventricle (appearing as cyanosis). The presence or absence of cyanosis determines the clinical manifestations of the child with a TOF.

Children with cyanotic TOF are usually symptomatic often having complaints of difficulty feeding, diaphoresis, cyanosis, and hypoxic spells. Hypoxic spells, otherwise known as "tet" spells, most often appear between 2 and 4 months of ages though they can occur at any time before surgical repair. The presence of hypoxic spells is an indicator of the need for surgical or medical intervention.

Transposition of the great arteries. Transposition of the great arteries (TGA) occurs when the pulmonary artery is located off the left ventricle and the aorta originates from the right ventricle, thus producing two completely separate systems within the heart. In order for an infant or child to survive beyond the first few minutes of life there must be an avenue for mixing between these two circuits, which most often occurs by means of an ASD, VSD, or PDA. TGA appears in the early newborn period as increasing cyanosis, poor feeding, and signs and symptoms of CHF.

Total anomalous pulmonary venous return. In the defect TAPVR, the pulmonary veins drain into the right atrium rather than the left atrium. For these infants and children to survive, there must be some mixing of blood between the right and left atrium through an ASD. Clinical symptoms include cyanosis, symptoms of pulmonary overflow (e.g., pneumonia, CHF), and FTT.

Double-outlet right ventricle. In the defect double-outlet right ventricle (DORV), the aorta arises out of the right ventricle alongside the pulmonary artery with a VSD that allows for survival. Clinical manifestation depends on the location of the VSD and the presence or absence of PS. Infants may show signs similar to those for children with a VSD or TOF.

Management
Treatments and medications
- Address primary care issues.
- Follow standard immunization protocols with routine TB screening. Immunizations should not be given for at least 4 weeks before any corrective surgeries and for approximately 6 weeks postoperatively. Additional vaccines such as influenza and pneumococcal vaccines should be considered.
- Reinforce routine dental, vision, and hearing screening with provision of subacute bacterial endocarditis (SBE) prophylaxis before dental and invasive procedures for those lesions requiring it. Infants and children who are cyanotic should have their hemoglobin checked more frequently, because an increase in hemoglobin may be an indicator of worsening cyanosis.

Treatments for specific acyanotic defects include:
ASD
- Assessment for signs or symptoms of CHF.
- Provision of SBE prophylaxis for dental and invasive procedures for significant and symptomatic defects.
- No need for exercise restriction before or after surgical repair.
- ASDs that do not close spontaneously being closed surgically because of the increased risk of cerebrovascular accident from paradoxic embolizations through an ASD. One of the most common complications from surgical repair is the subsequent development of arrhythmias, which occurs in 7% to 20% of patients.
VSD
- Treatment of CHF.
- Optimal nutrition for growth and development.

- SBE prophylaxis, which also needed for up to 6 months postoperatively and can be discontinued if there is no residual shunting after repair.
- Maintenance of good oral hygiene.
- Exercise restriction often not needed. In the presence of CHF, most children restrict their own activities.
PDA
- In infancy, a trial of indomethacin to medically close the defect. Catheterization closure using various devices is another alternative to surgical closure. Beyond the neonatal period and if a device closure in not warranted or unsuccessful, the PDA can be surgically closed by a ligation of the defect.
- Maintenance of SBE prophylaxis on all open lesions and for the first 6 months after closure.
- No exercise restriction needed.
PAPVR
- Surgical repair between ages 2 and 5 years, if diagnosed early.
- No exercise restriction needed.
- Probably no need for SBE prophylaxis. Once surgical closure is complete, with no residual shunting, there is definitely no need for antibiotic SBE coverage.
PS
- Balloon valvuloplasty by cardiac catheterization, which may be performed numerous times during a child's lifetime. After balloon valvuloplasty, the cardiac status of infants and children should be continuously monitored for restenosis through history and physical examination. Surgical repair may also be performed for critical PS or unsuccessful balloon valvuloplasty.
- Exercise restriction not required for mild PS but may be needed for moderate or severe PS, with restriction of children from competitive sports and stressful cardiac exercise.
- Bacterial endocarditis prophylaxis.
AS
- Balloon angioplasty or surgical correction, as with PS.
- Restriction from competitive sports and aerobic exercise of children with moderate or severe AS.
- SBE prophylaxis both before and after repair.
COA
- Management with balloon angioplasty is controversial. Surgical repair is the mainstay of intervention. Infants with critical COA require urgent repair early in the neonatal period incorporating management of CHF.
- Postoperative care, including monitoring for signs of restenosis, SBE prophylaxis, and possible management of residual hypertension.

Treatments for specific cyanotic defects include:
TOF
- Positioning of the child in a knee-chest position or squatting position and provision of morphine sulfate.
- Education of the parents and family on the need to identify hypoxic spells and importance of seeking care when they occur.
- Timing of surgical repair of a child dependent on the degree of cyanosis, presence of hypoxic spells, and stability of the infant or child.
- Ensuring that SBE prophylaxis is implemented, limitation of activity if necessary, and monitoring of the infant or child for possible arrhythmias (which can occur in postoperative children).

TGA

- Surgical correction early in the newborn period.
- Education of the family on the care of a child with a cyanotic lesion, provision of appropriate immunizations and SBE prophylaxis, and monitoring for concurrent arrhythmias.

TAPVR

- Corrective surgery, with no option for palliative procedures to alleviate any symptoms. These children must be followed throughout their lives after surgical repair to assess for the development of pulmonary vein obstruction and arrhythmias. Once surgical repair has been completed there is no need for limitation of activity. If there are no residual defects, SBE prophylaxis is not needed.

DORV

- Management of CHF, provision of SBE prophylaxis, and education of the family related to medical and surgical management. Surgical management most often includes a palliative procedure during infancy and full corrective surgery later in infancy or in early childhood. The timing and type of corrective surgery depends on the degree of the defects associated with the DORV.

Counseling and prevention

- Educate the family about the defect and what to expect; this is of the utmost importance early in the care of these children.
- When the diagnosis is made in the newborn period, provide the parents with a good baseline understanding of the child's defect, his or her baseline data (e.g., normal oxygen saturation), and what changes to look for, and provide any additional training that may be needed (e.g., cardiopulmonary resuscitation [CPR] training).
- Identify support systems for the family.
- Teach the parents and all caregivers how to identify symptoms of CHF, increasing cyanosis, and the need for urgent evaluation.
- Discuss issues related to ensuring adequate caloric intake to ensure adequate weight gain for growth and development. Infants with CHF have a caloric requirement of up to 150 kcal/kg per day and may require high-calorie formulas.
- Remember that sleep patterns of infants with CHDs may be altered. Teach parents the importance of waking the infant for feeding, because such an infant often sleeps more than other infants. Infants with CHF may be unable to satisfy their hunger and may have interrupted sleep, waking up more often.
- Inform parents that children with symptomatic CHDs often have some delay in their growth and development. They are often the "slow-but-sure" growers, making their own curve with a slower rate of weight gain and height increase. Children with significant CHDs or congenital syndromes associated with their heart defect may attain growth and developmental milestones at a later age than their cohorts.
- Provide families with emergency plans of action, including CPR training for all who care for the infant or child, oxygen safety, action plans for power outages, medication safety, and emergency care.
- Discuss issues surrounding contact with sick children and family members.

Follow-up. Follow-up care is determined by the pediatric cardiologist. Schedule visits for routine well-child care.

Consultations and referrals. Initially refer to a pediatric cardiologist.

Heart Murmurs

Alert

Consult with or refer to a physician for the following:
- FTT
- Murmur of intensity greater than grade II or murmur with the presence of a thrill; diastolic murmurs
- Tachypnea, diaphoresis, or tiring with feeding
- Paroxysmal tachypnea (hypoxic spells)
- Chest pain, palpitations, or shortness of breath in the presence of abnormal heart sounds
- New murmur after documented GABHS infection
- New murmur after recent dental procedure
- New murmur after direct trauma
- "Blue spells," or squatting during play or other activities
- Digital clubbing
- Periorbital edema
- Hypertension
- Absent, diminished, or bounding pulses
- Arteriolar changes in funduscopic examination
- Hemiplegia or convulsions
- Cardiac failure (e.g., tachycardia, tachypnea, hepatomegaly, prominent third heart sound, crackles, pitting edema)

Etiology

Heart sounds are described by the following characteristics: frequency (high or low), intensity (loud or soft), duration (short or long), and timing (systole or diastole). Heart murmurs are abnormal sounds heard during the cardiac cycle (affecting one of the above-mentioned characteristics) and caused by turbulent blood flow and collision currents. The origin of the turbulence may be innocent (nonpathologic or physiologic) or pathologic. An innocent or nonpathologic heart murmur occurs in the absence of heart disease or structural abnormality of the heart. Normal blood-flow turbulence may be increased because of a thin chest wall, an increased heart rate from exercise or fever, or altered blood viscosity (e.g., anemia).

Pathologic heart murmurs are caused by significant alteration in cardiovascular structure or function. Most significant alterations in cardiovascular function in the pediatric population are the result of congenital heart disease. Other causative factors of heart murmurs include acquired heart diseases that result in damage to the heart's internal structures (e.g., valves) or function. Acquired heart diseases within the pediatric population include rheumatic fever, bacterial endocarditis, and Kawasaki's disease. This specific set of conditions may become evident as a new murmur in a child who previously had normal heart sounds with specific symptoms relative to the disease process.

Incidence

- During routine health care visits, over 30% of children may have an innocent murmur.
- Approximately 40,000 infants are born with CHD in the United States each year.
- About 8 to 10 infants of every 1000 live births have CHD.
- One third of the children with CHD become critically ill in the first year of life, one third have problems later in childhood or as young adults, and one third never have serious handicaps.

- The incidence of CHD in children of affected mothers or siblings is 15%.
- Acquired cardiac disease (ACD) is less common in the pediatric population.
- ACD results from infection, environmental factors, autoimmune responses, or familial tendencies.

Risk Factors
- Prematurity
- Congenital cardiac disease in siblings or other family members
- Maternal age over 40 years
- Maternal illness, either chronic (e.g., SLE, diabetes) or acute (e.g., viral disease, rubella)
- Chromosomal abnormalities
- Renal abnormalities
- Family history of rheumatic heart disease
- Recent GABHS infection

Differential Diagnosis

The heart rate and rhythm are assessed in each of the auscultatory areas: aortic, pulmonic, Erb's point, tricuspid or right ventricular, and mitral. High-pitched sounds are heard best with a diaphragm; low-pitched sounds are heard best with the lightly applied bell of a stethoscope. Discrepancies between the apical and peripheral pulses are noted. The character and intensity of the heart sounds are analyzed.

It is important to listen selectively to each component of the cardiac cycle. Notice the character and intensity of each heart sound (S_1, S_2, S_3, S_4). Listen for extra sounds, and notice intensity, timing, and pitch. Listen for bruits over the carotids or aorta. Listen for murmurs (turbulent blood flow) and describe intensity (loudness), timing (systolic, diastolic, continuous), quality (musical, blowing, harsh, rumbling), pitch (high, medium, low), location (aortic, pulmonic, tricuspid, mitral), and radiation. It is important to understand that murmurs are intensified by fever, excitement, or exercise.

A systematic technique should be used in auscultation and assessment of the heart sounds. The clinician should listen in all auscultatory areas to assess for radiation of sound to axillae, back, and neck, and observe whether the murmur changes with position from supine to sitting to squatting to standing.

The intensity of the murmur is graded I to VI as follows:
- *Grade I to VI*—Barely audible; heard faintly after a period of attentive listening
- *Grade II to VI*—Soft, medium intensity; easily audible
- *Grade III to VI*—Moderately loud; *not* associated with a thrill (palpable vibration on chest)
- *Grade IV to VI*—Louder; associated with a thrill
- *Grade V and VI*—Loud; associated with a thrill; audible with stethoscope barely on the chest wall
- *Grade VI*—Very loud; audible with stethoscope off the chest; associated with a thrill

The timing of murmurs can help a clinician in the classification of the murmur. Systolic murmurs occur during the contraction of the heart or between heart sounds S_1 and S_2. Diastolic murmurs occur during diastole or between S_2 and S_1 (while no pulse is palpated). A continuous murmur is heard throughout both systole and diastole. Diastolic murmurs are almost always considered pathologic and should immediately alert the practitioner for the need for further diagnostic testing and referral. Combined murmurs have both a systolic and diastolic portion. Combined murmurs should almost always be considered pathologic and require referrals for further evaluation. Murmurs can be further classified as early, middle, or late (systolic or diastolic).

Murmurs may be differentiated into two broad diagnostic categories, innocent (nonpathologic) and pathologic (Table 32-3). The clinician must use the criteria previously listed in assessing the murmur, along with the physical findings to differentiate a nonpathologic murmur from a pathologic one.

Innocent murmurs. The intensity of the murmur may bear no relation to the severity (present or future) of the underlying cardiac defect; however, most innocent murmurs are grades I to II in intensity. Innocent murmurs may be the result of normal, transitional physiologic processes. Table 32-4 lists the types of innocent murmurs. The characteristics of innocent murmurs that help distinguish them from pathologic murmurs include:
- Usually grade I or grades II to VI in intensity and localized
- May change in loudness or intensity with position change
- Variation in loudness and presence from visit to visit
- Systolic in timing except for the venous hum, which is continuous
- Musical or vibratory quality
- Duration usually short (e.g., early systolic)
- Left lower sternal border and the pulmonic area the most common sites
- Rarely transmitted
- Heard best in the supine position, during expiration, and after exercise (except for venous hum)
- Heart sounds S_1 and S_2 normal
- Vital signs normal
- Do not affect growth and development

Pathologic murmurs. Murmurs resulting from a structural abnormality within the heart often can be differentiated from innocent murmurs by means of a thorough history and physical examination. Often there are other complaints or physical findings (including specific characteristics of the murmur) that help identify the specific cardiac lesion causing the murmur. Pathologic heart murmurs may be caused by a variety of different cardiac defects, which can be further differentiated into acyanotic, cyanotic, and acquired. Acyanotic lesions are structural defects in the heart that do not cause significant deoxygenation of the child's blood supply. They include right-to-left shunt lesions and obstructive lesions. Cyanotic lesions include defects that result in significant mixing of oxygenated and deoxygenated blood and lead to blood oxygen desaturation. Acquired lesions are defects within a previously normal heart resulting from another disease process (e.g., rheumatic fever, endocarditis, Kawasaki's disease) or other infectious processes. These murmurs often become evident in combination with an ongoing or previous illness.

Management

Innocent murmurs
Treatments and medications
- Most innocent murmurs need no medical management.
- For murmurs resulting from anemia (see Chapter 36), orally ingested elemental iron at 2 to 6 mg/kg per day in three divided doses for 3 to 6 months may be given.
- For murmurs resulting from fever (see Chapter 43), acetaminophen at 10 to 15 mg/kg per dose every 4 hours as needed for fever may be provided.

Table 32-3 Differential Diagnosis: Murmurs

CRITERIA	INNOCENT MURMUR	PATHOLOGIC MURMUR
ICD-9 code	785.2	785.2
Subjective Data		
Present/past history	May be negative; may report fever, anxiety, recent exercise, loss of blood (anemia), or history of chronic disease (e.g., sickle cell disease)	May have perinatal history of prematurity, chromosomal abnormality, other congenital deformities *Infancy:* may complain of FTT, tachypnea with feeding, diaphoresis with feeding or at rest, fatigability, developmental delays *Older child:* may complain of developmental delays, decreased exercise tolerance, dyspnea, palpitations, tachypnea May be history of "blue spells" during exercise, may be history of frequent respiratory illnesses, may be recent history of documented GABHS infection
Family history	Not significant	May be history of rheumatic fever, congenital heart disease, or genetic syndromes
Objective Data		
Physical examination		
Growth parameters	Normal	May be significant growth delay, FTT
Vital signs		
Temperature	May be normal or elevated (with illness)	Normal or elevated with certain conditions (e.g., rheumatic fever, myocarditis, Kawasaki disease)
Pulse	Normal; may be elevated with fever	Normal; may see bradycardia (heart block), tachycardia, or arrhythmia; may feel bounding pulses (patent ductus arteriosus); diminished or absent peripheral pulses (coarctation of the aorta)
Respiratory rate	Normal	May see tachypnea at rest or with feeding or activity
Blood pressure	Normal	May be elevated (coarctation of the aorta) or low; hypotension (shock)
Head, neck, ears, mouth, throat	Normal; may see signs of active infection if fever is present; may hear murmur in auscultation of neck	May see neck vein distention or cyanosis of mucous membranes and lips
Chest	Normal	May see chest deformities; may hear crackles; may see retractions, tachypnea, precordial bulging
Heart/murmur	Typically grades I to II/VI medium- to high-pitched, musical, early systolic murmur, pulmonic area, does not radiate, supine position only, only present with fever of high output state	May be any grade of loudness; diastolic murmurs are usually pathologic, low- to medium-pitched, harsh; may radiate, may accompany a thrill, does not change with position, present at all times
Abdominal examination	No hepatosplenomegaly	May be hepatosplenomegaly
Extremities	Normal	May see clubbing of fingers; nail beds and extremities may be cyanotic
Laboratory data	Complete blood cell count (for anemia, infection, chronic illness)	Chest radiograph (determine heart size, pulmonary vascular markings) Electrocardiogram (determine rhythm, cardiac enlargement or subtle suggestions of underlying heart disease) Echocardiogram (define cardiac structures, identify cardiac abnormalities) Magnetic resonance imaging (identify cardiac structures and possible abnormalities) Cardiac catheterization (assess cardiac anatomy and physiology, along with cardiac chamber pressures and pulmonary pressures) Arterial blood gas levels (determine oxygenation of blood and assess for deoxygenation)

Table 32-4 Types of Innocent Murmurs

NAME	DESCRIPTION
Still murmur	Soft, medium-pitched, early-systolic to midsystolic, musical or vibratory murmur, heard best at the apex and left lower sternal border, with child in supine position
Physiologic peripheral pulmonic stenosis	Short, systolic murmur, heard best in axillae and back; heard in early postnatal period and infancy; disappears typically by 3 to 4 months of age; also called pulmonary outflow murmur
Venous hum	Continuous, humming murmur heard best in the infraclavicular and supraclavicular areas with child sitting; diminished by having child lie down, by turning the child's head, or by occluding the jugular vessels; intensity may reach grade III/VI

- For fevers greater than 102° F, ibuprofen at 10 mg/kg per dose every 6 hours (for children older than 6 months of age) may be given.
- When the child is afebrile, heart sounds should be reevaluated.
  Counseling and prevention
- Educate the parents and child on the existence of the murmur and the fact that it is innocent and therefore normal for that child at that time, though it may either go away or persist.
- Emphasize to the parents and child that there is no abnormality in the child's heart structure and function and that no treatment or limitations are necessary.
- Encourage the parents and child to ask questions.
- Inform the parents that during times of fever, anxiety, exercise, and other high-cardiac-output, the murmur will sound louder. (This is a normal variant.)
  Follow-up
- Routine pediatric follow-up evaluation for well-child care.
- If a child is presently ill, reevaluate after treatment is completed and the child is afebrile.
- For a child with anemia, reevaluate in 4 to 6 weeks to assess the effectiveness of treatment.
  Consultations and referrals. Usually none are needed.
  Pathologic murmurs
  Treatments and medications. Refer to physician for further evaluation and management.
  Counseling and prevention
- Educate the parents and child on the specific defect, using pictures and models.
- Explain the side effects of defects and possible complications.
- Use a teaching doll and written materials to explain the child's disease and treatment.
- Educate on the prevention of respiratory infections through careful handwashing, good general hygiene, and optimal health maintenance.
- Inform the parents and child of surgical correction (if indicated) and the procedures associated with surgical repair.
- Educate the parents and child on medications to be taken (e.g., dosages, usage, timing, side effects).
- Provide the parents and child an opportunity to express concerns, anxieties, and fears.
- Educate the parents on the need for antibiotic prophylaxis for dental and other surgical procedures.
- Educate the parents and family on the importance of obtaining necessary immunizations and the need for additional precautions during the winter months.

- Encourage the parents to the treat child as normally as possible.
- Promote the child's independence and understanding of the condition.
- Explain to the parents the signs and symptoms of distress or concern.
- Identify important courses of action for the parents to take when or if the child becomes ill.
  Follow-up
- Once child has been referred to a pediatric cardiologist, continue with routine pediatric follow-up.
- Contact the parents by phone to assess the results of the cardiologist's findings, and meet with the parents if necessary to explain the testing or diagnosis.
  Consultations and referrals
- Refer to a cardiologist for diastolic murmurs or any suspected pathologic murmurs.
- Refer the parents to local support groups for parents of children with CHDs.
- Consult a social worker for any identified financial support needs of the family and child.

Hyperlipidemia

Alert

Consult with or refer to a physician for the following:
- Children older than 2 years of age with total cholesterol greater than 175 mg/dl on routine screening
- Family history of premature coronary heart disease or hyperlipidemia
- Genetic disorders for familial hypercholesterolemia, familial hypertriglyceridemia, or hyperlipidemia
- Use of corticosteroids, oral contraceptives, alcohol, or tobacco
- Disease processes (e.g., liver disease, nephrotic syndrome)
- Obesity
- Medications (e.g., isotretinoin [Accutane], anticonvulsants)
- Teenagers with thickening of Achilles' tendon
- Glycogen storage disease
- Congenital biliary atresia

Etiology

Hyperlipidemia is defined as an elevated serum cholesterol level (200 mg/dl). During the past decade major attention has been focused on the control and prevention of CAD. Studies demonstrate that cardiovascular risk factors, most importantly obesity, are present in a significant portion of the pediatric population. It is now recognized that cardiovascular risk factors present in children will track through to there adult years, increasing the potential for CAD. Research indicates a combination of genetic and environmental factors that interact to increase the potential of CAD. Because of the relationship between dietary factors (fat and cholesterol) and atherosclerotic disease, it is important to identify children who are at risk in early childhood. However, it is important that infants and toddlers receive adequate fat intake because of its role in optimal myelinization of the brain. This is exemplified by the fact that 50% of brain growth takes place within the first 2 years of life.

There is no consensus regarding the efficacy of universal cholesterol screening in children. The recommendations of the National Cholesterol Education Program published in 1992 promote an individualized approach to identifying and treating children and adolescents at risk for hyperlipidemia. This includes selectively screening children over 2 years of age for risk factors. These recommendation are based on the unanimity of the expert panel that the incidence of cardiovascular disease would decline with dietary improvements; smoking cessation and prevention; early and sustained management of hypertension, diabetes, and obesity; and a decrease in sedentary lifestyles.

Atherosclerosis begins in childhood and is related to elevated levels of blood cholesterol. Preventing or slowing the atherosclerotic process could prevent early CAD and premature death. Aortic fatty streaks can be seen in children younger than 10 years of age. Children with elevated serum cholesterol levels, particularly low-density-lipoprotein (LDL) cholesterol levels, frequently have a family history of CAD. High blood cholesterol aggregates in families are a result of both common environmental and genetic factors.

Hyperlipidemia is classified according to the plasma lipoprotein pattern on paper electrophoresis or after ultracentrifugation. Total cholesterol values reflect the cholesterol content of several types of lipoproteins, including LDL and high-density lipoprotein (HDL). HDL carries cholesterol away from peripheral tissue for excretion through the liver, whereas LDL is believed to be involved in the generation of the foam cells of the early lesions of atherosclerosis. When classifying hypercholesterolemia in childhood, one must assess the concentrations of HDL and LDL to distinguish the specific type of hypercholesterolemia. High levels of HDL are believed to be protective against atherosclerosis. In contrast, high levels of LDL may be a causative factor in the development of CAD. Therefore it is important to differentiate this form of hyperlipidemia from those forms involving high levels of LDL. Most elevations in cholesterol levels reflect elevations of LDL levels.

Elevated plasma levels of lipids or lipoproteins are divided into two causes or origins, primary and secondary. Primary hyperlipidemia is genetically determined. Secondary hyperlipidemia may result from diets high in saturated fats, disease processes, medications, and other causes. Familial hypercholesterolemia, the best understood of this group of disorders, is an autosomal dominant disease resulting from defective LDL-C receptors.

Secondary causes of hyperlipidemia include diabetes, hypothyroidism, obstructive liver disease, nephrotic syndrome, excessive dietary fat intake, obesity, and high blood pressure, as well as the use of corticosteroids, oral contraceptives, and alcohol. Children, adolescents, and adults in the United States have an increased prevalence of elevated blood cholesterol levels and generally excessive intake of saturated fatty acids

and cholesterol. CAD is a leading cause of morbidity and mortality among adults in the United States, so early identification and management is essential.

Exogenous factors are probably the most prevalent cause of secondary hyperlipidemia in the first 20 years of life. They include oral contraceptives, corticosteroids, cyclosporin A, anticonvulsants, and isotretinoin. The most common causes of secondary hyperlipidemia in the first year of life are glycogen storage disease and congenital biliary atresia. Hypothyroidism, diabetes mellitus, and nephrotic syndrome are the most prevalent of the metabolic causes later in childhood. Table 32-5 presents a summary of clinical features for hyperlipidemia.

Incidence

- Approximately 5% to 25% of children and teens have cholesterol levels in excess of 200 mg/dl.
- There is a higher incidence in children with a familial history of CAD or hyperlipidemia.
- Genetic disorders for familial hypercholesterolemia, familial combined hyperlipidemia, and familial hypertriglyceridemia are found in 0.5% to 1% of the population.
- About 80% of children with CAD have symptoms before 20 years of age.
- Patients with heterozygote familial hypercholesterolemia patients compose 0.2% to 0.5% of the U.S. population.
- Ischemic heart disease develops in 80% of men with CAD by 50 years of age and in 50% of women by 60 years of age.

Risk Factors

- Family history of heart disease or high cholesterol levels
- Lack of exercise
- Obesity
- Diet high in fat content
- Use of certain medications (e.g., oral contraceptives, corticosteroids, cyclosporin A, anticonvulsants, isotretinoin)
- Family history of homozygous familial hypercholesterolemia
- History of glycogen storage disease or congenital biliary atresia within the first year of life
- History of hypothyroidism, diabetes mellitus, or nephrotic syndrome
- Family history of premature death or morbidity from atherosclerotic heart disease in either parent before 50 years of age
- Infants or children with recurrent, unexplained abdominal pain

Differential Diagnosis

Typical findings in individuals with hyperlipidemia are a family history of heart disease and high cholesterol levels, high-fat diet, obesity, and lack of exercise. Hyperlipidemia can be divided into three different categories of causative factors: genetic, environmental, and disease related. Once a child has been identified as having an elevated serum cholesterol level (200 mg/dl), the practitioner must define the category of hyperlipidemia and begin appropriate treatment and counseling to prevent other risk factors. Preventive efforts to aid in lowering cholesterol levels in children may prevent or retard the progress of atherosclerosis, which may cause significant complications by the fourth decade of life. Hyperlipidemia is further divided into five major groups according to plasma lipoprotein patterns on electrophoresis or after ultracentrifugation, regardless of the cause (genetic, environmental, or hereditary). Plasma lipoproteins are lipids and proteins that circulate in the plasma concentration of the blood. The major categories of plasma lipoproteins range from largest and least dense to

Table 32-5 Hyperlipidemia: Summary of Clinical Features

TYPE	LIPOPROTEIN LEVEL ELEVATED	LIPID LEVELS ELEVATED	PREVALENCE IN CHILDHOOD	CLINICAL MANIFESTATIONS	TREATMENT
Type I	Triglyceride (chylomicrons)	Triglyceride (2000–4000 mg/dl)	Rare	Childhood onset (70%); abdominal pain (pancreatitis), eruptive exanthemas, no coronary heart disease	Low-fat diet (10–15 g/day)
Type II-a	LDL	Cholesterol	Common	Childhood or adult onset; xanthomas of eyelids and palms, Achilles' tendinitis, coronary artery disease; common in homozygotes	Diet low in cholesterol and saturated fat, cholestyramine if not responsive to diet alone, weight loss if obese
Type II-b	LDL and VLDL	Triglyceride, cholesterol	Uncommon	Same as type II-a	Same as type II-a
Type III	LDL and VLDL	Cholesterol, triglyceride	Very rare	Xanthomas (palmar and tuberosum); coronary artery disease (+/−)	Low-fat and low cholesterol diet, weight control, clofibrate
Type IV	VLDL	Triglyceride	Relatively uncommon	Obesity, eruptive xanthomas, abdominal pain	Low-fat and low-cholesterol diet, weight control
Type V	VLDL, chylomicron	Triglyceride, cholesterol (+/−)	Very rare	Obesity, eruptive xanthomas, coronary artery disease (not frequent)	Low-fat diet, weight control

Modified from Park, M.K. (1991). Pediatric cardiology handbook. St. Louis: Mosby.

smallest and most dense. The major plasma lipoprotein classes are as follows: chylomicron, very-low–density lipoprotein (VLDL), intermediate-density lipoprotein (IDL), LDL, and HDL. Elevations of specific concentrations of lipoproteins aid in the differential diagnosis in determining the type of hyperlipidemia and the course of treatment.

Hypercholesterolemia. Type II (a or b) occurs as hypercholesterolemia, either without lipoprotein abnormality (type II-a) or with a raised concentration of VLDL (type II-b). In either form the plasma levels of total cholesterol are elevated (250 to 500 mg/100 ml in heterozygotes and 500 to 1000 mg/100 ml in the homozygotes). Homozygous familial hypercholesterolemia is extremely rare. These patients have cutaneous planar xanthomas during the first 6 years of life and atherosclerosis involving the aortic valves and aortic root. About 80% have symptomatic CAD before 20 years of age. Patients with heterozygote familial hypercholesterolemia have thickening of the Achilles' tendon in their teens and xanthomas in their late 30s. Development of ischemic heart disease is quite significant in these patients. Therefore early identification and treatment are imperative to their future.

Hypertriglyceridemia. Type I, IV, and V hypertriglyceridemia is a grouping that comprises elevated plasma levels of triglycerides (200 to 400 mg/dl). Clinical manifestations of this category include eruptive xanthomas, hepatosplenomegaly, lipemia retinalis, and life-threatening pancreatitis. There is no predisposition for CAD in adulthood.

Familial dysbetalipoproteinemia. In type III, plasma levels of both cholesterol and triglycerides are elevated. A hallmark finding is the unusual yellow deposits in the creases of the palms. This form of hyperlipidemia is rare in childhood but when present may cause premature CAD.

Management

Treatments and medications

- Explain that hyperlipidemia screening is recommended with the presence of any risk factors.
- Emphasize physical exercise incorporating aerobic exercise on a regular basis.
- Stress the importance of avoiding or limiting excess calories, alcohol, and smoking.
- Suggest for cholesterol levels of 175 to 200 mg/dl: nutritional counseling, and exercise. Rule out secondary hyperlipidemia.
- For cholesterol levels greater than 200 mg/dl, suggest all of the previously described management in addition to family nutritional counseling and family screening.
- For cholesterol levels greater than 230 mg/dl, suggest all of the previously described management and refer to a lipid specialist.
- Encourage lowering of dietary intake of total fat to less than 30% of total calories and saturated fat to less than 10% of total calories, to less than 300 mg of dietary cholesterol per day (following the American Heart Association's [AHA's] Step I Diet).
- For hyperlipidemia greater than 6 months (following the AHA's Step II Diet and guidelines for management of obesity), use a bile sequestrant as follows: cholestyramine 4 to 16 g of active resin per day or colestipol resin 2 to 12 mg per day (with consultation from a specialist).

Counseling and prevention

- The practitioner should screen for the following risk factors: smoking, hypertension, physical inactivity, obesity, diabetes mellitus.

- Hyperlipidemia screening is recommended with the presence of any risk factors.
- Children and adolescents with risk factors should be screened (per the National Cholesterol Education Program's screening recommendations) after 2 years of age.
- Screening is recommended if the family history cannot be ascertained.
- If the total cholesterol is less than 170 mg/dl or the LDL less than 110, the practitioner should encourage healthful eating, provide education on CAD risk factors, and repeat the analysis in 5 years.
- If the total cholesterol is between 170 and 199 mg/dl and the LDL between 110 and 129, the practitioner should use the previous recommendations, encourage the use of the AHA Step 1 Diet, and reevaluate in 1 year.
- If the total cholesterol between 170 and 199 mg/dL and LDL greater than130, *or* total cholesterol greater than 200 mg/dL and LDL greater than 130, the practitioner should complete the previous recommendations, perform a full clinical evaluation for secondary causes, evaluate for familial disorders, and screen all family members. If the AHA's Step 1 Diet does not work for a compliant patient, the patient may need to go to the Step 2 Diet (with nutritionist consultation and possible consultation with a lipid specialist).
- Patients must be educated on the importance of exercise, weight control, and a prudent diet.

Follow-up. Follow-up should be performed every 3 to 5 years if the cholesterol level is within normal limits. If the cholesterol level is in the moderate-risk category (175 to 200 mg/dl), screening should be done every 6 to 12 months until the level is normal. For cholesterol levels greater than 200 mg/dl, screening should be done every 6 months during treatment until an acceptable level has been achieved.

Consultations and referrals. Refer to a lipid specialist if the cholesterol level is greater than 230 mg/dl, if there is significant family history of premature or sudden death, or if there is persistent hyperlipidemia even with appropriate treatment.

Hypertension

Alert

Consult with or refer to a physician for the following:
- Children with hypertension in conjunction with decreased or absent pulses in lower extremities
- Suspected underlying renal disorders
- Use of certain drugs (e.g., oral contraceptives, cyclosporin A, corticosteroids)
- Suspected drug use or abuse (e.g., of cocaine, anabolic steroids)
- Signs and symptoms of increased intracranial pressure
- Signs and symptoms of hyperthyroidism or hyperparathyroidism
- BP measurement elevation greater than the 95th percentile for age
- Funduscopic changes
- Left ventricular hypertrophy based on electrocardiogram or chest radiograph findings
- Signs of cardiac decomposition
- Left ventricular hypertrophy based on electrocardiogram or chest radiograph findings
- Signs of cardiac decompensation

Etiology

The etiologic factors for hypertension are divided into two categories, primary and secondary. Primary, essential, or idiopathic hypertension refers to an increase in peripheral vascular resistance or cardiac output of unknown origin. Secondary hypertension in children or adolescents is related to an ongoing organic process. The three most common organic causes of hypertension in children are renal parenchymal disease, renal artery disease, and COA. Other causes include endocrine disorders (e.g., hyperthyroidism, adrenal dysfunction, hyperparathyroidism), neurogenic disorders (e.g., increased intracranial pressure, Guillain-Barré syndrome, dysautonomia), drugs, and miscellaneous conditions such as hypovolemia, hypernatremia, or Stevens-Johnson syndrome. Factors that may play an important role in essential hypertension include stress, heredity, obesity, and salt intake or sensitivity.

The role of hypertension in cardiovascular disease is significant. Therefore early intervention to prevent or delay its development may be effective in preventing long-term sequelae or complications. As with CAD, fixed hypertension results from an interplay of genetic and environmental factors with estimates that genetic factors are responsible for 60% of the variance in BP.

Incidence

- Approximately 5% of all children have hypertension; 4% of these cases are significant and 1% are severe.
- About 80% of children with severe hypertension have secondary hypertension with an underlying cause.
- Most children and adolescents with mild hypertension are found to have no discernible cause for their hypertension (i.e., idiopathic).
- Often, the younger the child and the more severe the hypertension, the more likely it is that an underlying cause can be identified.
- There is a higher incidence in African Americans.

Risk Factors

- Neonatal use of umbilical artery catheters
- Congenital heart disease (e.g., COA, conditions requiring cardiac surgery)
- Familial history of hypertension, atherosclerotic heart disease, or cerebrovascular accident
- Familial or hereditary renal disease (e.g., polycystic kidney disease, nephritis)
- History of renal conditions (e.g., obstructive uropathies, urinary tract infections, trauma, glomerulonephritis, hemolytic-uremic syndrome)
- Obesity
- Diet
- Smoking
- Lack of exercise
- Endocrine disorders (e.g., hyperthyroidism, hyperaldosteronism)
- Use of certain medications (e.g., corticosteroids, amphetamines, oral contraceptives, antiasthmatic drugs, cold medications, nephrotoxic antibiotics)
- Use of illicit drugs
- Increased intracranial pressure (e.g., from trauma, infection, congenital malformation, mass)

Differential Diagnosis

Hypertension can be defined as an average systolic or diastolic BP equal to or greater than the 95th percentile for age and sex with measurements obtained on at least three separate occasions (Table 32-6). Hypertension can be further divided into three separate categories: high-normal, significant, and severe. Children with high-normal BP have readings between the 90th and 95th percentiles of systolic or diastolic pressure reading for their specific age and sex. These children should be closely monitored for further development of hypertension. Significant hypertension pertains to BP readings between the 95th and 99th percentiles for age and sex; severe hypertension constitutes BP values greater than the 99th percentiles.

In diagnosing hypertension the practitioner must differentiate between primary and secondary causes of elevations in pressure. Primary hypertension, otherwise known as *essential* or *idiopathic hypertension,* is often identified as the causative factor in a significant amount of children with high-normal and significant hypertension. Secondary hypertension results from an underlying pathologic condition. Renal and cardiac anomalies are the most common underlying diagnoses. Other differential diagnoses consistent with hypertension include central nervous system (CNS) disorders or illnesses, renal trauma, drug-induced causes, and miscellaneous causes such as anxiety, pain, fractures, burns, leukemia, Stevens-Johnson syndrome, hypercalcemia, inappropriate cuff size, and heavy-metal poisoning.

Primary or essential hypertension is believed to incorporate such factors as hereditary, stress, obesity, high salt intake or increased sensitivity to salt, and poor diet. Primary hypertension is diagnosed once secondary causes have been excluded. Most children with primary hypertension can be managed through nonpharmacologic options. Those who may need medical intervention include children whose systolic or diastolic pressure exceeds 95% consistently, with symptoms (e.g., headaches) of hypertension irrespective of the degree of elevation, or with any identified target organ damaged because of the hypertension. These children should be referred to a specialist for evaluation and consultation for management. Treatment for hypertension for children includes beginning with monotherapy and the nonpharmacologic treatment options. Monotherapy most often includes an angiotensin-converting enzyme (ACE) inhibitor, calcium-channel blocker, or beta-adrenergic receptor blocker. Diuretics may be used after a few weeks of treatment with no obvious improvement. Combination therapy consists of using an ACE inhibitor and a calcium-channel blocker.

Management

Treatments and medications. Nonpharmacologic management includes:
- Dietary modification, including a regular, low-fat, low-cholesterol, and restricted-salt diet; minimal caffeine intake; and weight reduction.
- Appropriate exercise
- Stress modification
- Counseling on smoking, weight loss, and lipid reduction

Pharmacologic management includes antihypertensive medications (Table 32-7), which may be prescribed after a thorough examination, diagnostic evaluation, and consultation with a physician.

Counseling and prevention
- Instruct parents about possible causes of hypertension.
- Explain the disease process and reasons for treatment.

Table 32-6 Differential Diagnosis: Hypertension

CRITERIA	ESSENTIAL HYPERTENSION	SECONDARY HYPERTENSION
ICD-9 code	401.9	405.99
Subjective Data		
Prenatal/natal history	Noncontributory	Use of umbilical artery catheters; use of renal-toxic antibiotics and medications; identification of renal abnormalities
Family history	Possible history of stressful events, financial concerns, family dysfunction; history of familial essential hypertension; obesity; poor dietary habits	Familial history of atherosclerotic heart disease, cerebrovascular accident, renal disease
Nutritional history	High salt intake, poorly balanced diet	Noncontributory
Drug history	Use of illicit drugs, smoking	Use of illicit drugs, nephrotoxic drugs, oral contraceptives
Social history	May be identification of stress in social settings, poor interactive abilities, stressful interactions, conflicts, poor school performance	Noncontributory
Objective Data		
Physical examination		
Vital signs		
Pulse	Normal	May be decreased or absent pulses in lower extremities (coarctation of aorta)
Respiratory rate	Normal	Normal
Blood pressure	Above 95th percentile for age on three consecutive occasions	Above 95th percentile for age on three consecutive occasions
Head, eyes, ears, nose, and throat	Noncontributory	Funduscopic changes may be seen
Heart	Noncontributory	May hear murmur, ejection click, altered heart sounds
Abdominal examination	Noncontributory	Noncontributory
Laboratory data		
Urinalysis	Normal	May be positive for protein and/or blood
Blood urea nitrogen and creatinine levels	Normal	May be abnormally elevated
Electrocardiogram	Normal	May show signs of ventricular hypertrophy or strain pattern of ischemia
Chest radiograph	Normal	May show cardiomegaly, abnormal heart silhouette, abnormal pulmonary vascular markings
Fasting serum lipid levels	Normal	May be elevated

- Identify for the parents the predisposing factors of hypertension, including heredity, race, and nutrition. (Saturated fats, cholesterol, and sodium cause increased risk for development of hypertension).
- Explain systolic and diastolic BP.
- Encourage physical exercise, including participation in physical education (with adequate rest).
- Encourage weight reduction in obese patients, and place patients on a moderately salt-restricted diet.
- Demonstrate the technique of BP measurement for monitoring at home, if the parents are able to accept this responsibility.
- Advise the parents to contact the clinic if norms are not achieved or maintained.
- Educate adolescents on reduction of sodium intake through a moderately salt-restricted diet, avoidance of fast foods and sweets, keeping a diet diary, and counting calories.
- Educate regarding avoidance of smoking and secondary smoke.

- Encourage increased, regular aerobic exercise.
- Teach techniques to identify and manage stress, anxiety, and anger.
- Encourage the patient to discontinue the use of oral contraceptives and low-dose estrogen, or discuss other methods of birth control.
- Instruct the parents and child about medications. Emphasize that compliance with treatment and medications is important.
- Educate the parents and child in the importance of following medication schedules and being alert to possible side effects (e.g., lightheadedness, dizziness, urinary frequency, sedation, altered bowel habits, orthostatic hypotension). Advise them to call if side effects are noted.

Follow-up. Arrange return visits at 1- to 4-week intervals to evaluate treatments, adjust medications, and measure BP.

Consultations and referrals. Consult with a physician when hypertension is detected.

Table 32-7 Commonly Prescribed Antihypertensive Medications in Children

CLASSIFICATION/ MEDICATION	INITIAL PEDIATRIC DOSAGE (mg/kg/day)
Angiotensin-Converting Enzyme Inhibitors	
Captopril	
Neonates	0.03-0.15
Children	1.5
Enalapril	0.15
Calcium Channel Blockers	
Nifedipine	0.25
Diuretics	
Hydrochlorothiazide	1
Furosemide	1
Spironolactone	1
β-Adrenergic Blockers	
Propranolol	1
Atenolol	1
Metoprolol	1
Vasodilators	
Hydralazine	0.75
Minoxidil	0.1-0.2

Resources

Websites

American Academy of Family Physicians's *Heart Murmurs in Children: What Every Parent Should Know* (aafp.org/afp/990800ap/990800f.html)

American Family Physician's *Heart Murmurs in Pediatric Patients: When Do You Refer?* (aafp.org/afp/990800ap/558.html)

American Heart Association's *Heart and Stroke A to Z Guide* (www.americanheart.org/Heart_and_Stroke_A_Z_Guide/)

Dr. Koop.com Medical Encyclopedia's *Congenital Heart Defect Corrective Surgery* (highmark.drkoop.com/conditions/ency/article/002948.htm)

Evaluation of Heart Murmurs in Children and Adolescents (www2.kumc.edu/instruction/cardiology/cardiac2/menu.htm)

General Pediatrics.com's *Common Pediatric Health Problems for Patients and Families* (generalpediatrics.com/CommonProbLay.html#19)

Heart Disease and Cardiology (heartdisease.about.com/health/heartdisease/?once=true&)

Journal of Emergency Medicine and Acute Primary Care (www.medical-library.org/j_er.htm)

Karolinska Institutet's *Cardiac Diseases* (www.mic.ki.se/Diseases/c14.html)

The Nephron Information Center's *Hypertension Guidelines* (nephron.com/htnguidelines.html)

New England Journal of Medicine (med.hallym.ac.kr/~medline/public/1996/0335/0026/TOC/1.htm)

Pediheart (Practitioners' Site) (www.pediheart.org/practitioners/)

University of Texas Southwestern Medical Center's *Clinical Guidelines* (irweb.swmed.edu/utshs/CLINICALGUIDELINES/htmls/Hyperlipidemia/HyperlipidemiaTbl.htm)

Bibliography

Ainsworth, S., Wyllie, J.P., & Wren, C. (1999). Prevalence and clinical significance of cardiac murmurs in neonates. *Archives of Disease in Childhood Fetal & Neonatal Edition, 80*(1), F43-45.

Anzai, A.K. & Merkin, T.E. (1999). Adolescent chest pain. *American Family Physician, 53*(5), 1682-1690.

Baum, V. & McDaniel, N. (1999). Cardiac disease in the newborn. In Dershewitz, R.A. (Ed.). *Ambulatory pediatric care.* Philadelphia: Lippincott-Raven.

Chang, R.-K., Chen, A.-Y., & Klitzner, T. S. (2000). Factors associated with age at operation for children with congenital heart disease. *Pediatrics, 105*(5), 1073-1081.

Daberkow-Carson, E. & Smith, P. (1994). Altered cardiovascular function. In Betz, C.L., Hunsberger, M., & Wright, S. (Eds.). *Family-centered nursing care of children.* Philadelphia: W.B. Saunders.

Dershewitz, R.A. (Ed.). (1999). *Ambulatory pediatric care* (3rd ed.). Philadelphia: J.B. Lippincott.

Hohn, A.R. (1997). Diagnosis and management of hypertension in childhood. *Pediatric Annals, 26*(2), 105-110.

Hunter, S. (2000, March-April). Congenital heart disease in adolescence. *Journal of the Royal College of Physicians of London, 34*(2), 150-152.

Kenney, K. (2000). Heart murmurs in children: Pieces of the diagnostic picture. *Advance for Nurse Practitioners, 8*(9).

McCrindle, B.W. (2000). Screening and management of hyperlipidemia in children. *Pediatric Annals, 29*(8), 500-508.

U.S. Preventive Services Task Force. (1996). *Guide to clinical preventive services* (2nd ed.). Baltimore: Williams & Wilkins.

Sapin, S.O. (1997). Recognizing normal heart murmurs: A logic-based mnemonic. *Pediatrics, 99*(4), 616-619.

Chapter 33 *Endocrine System*

Jane A. Fox

Delayed Puberty, p. 363
Precocious Puberty, p. 365
Short Stature, p. 366
Thyroid Disorders, p. 369

Risk Factors

- History of central nervous system (CNS) injury, infection, trauma, or lesions
- Chromosomal abnormalities
- Family history of short stature, delayed puberty, precocious puberty, or thyroid disorder
- Cleft lip or palate
- Spina bifida
- Septo-optic dysplasia
- Cranial-spinal irradiation
- Chronic systemic illness
- Chronic steroid use
- Emotional deprivation
- Neurofibromatosis

Health Promotion

Promoting Optimal Growth and Development and Early Detection of Problems

- Perform newborn screening as required. Do careful follow-up on test results and repeat as needed.
- Review essential components of good nutrition with the parents and child.
- Promote overall good health practices.
- Take routine height and weight measurements. From birth to 3 years of age, take them 3 to 4 times yearly; from 3 years through puberty, take them annually. Plot the results on appropriate growth charts (see Appendix A).
- Assist the parents in providing a nurturing psychosocial and emotional environment.
- Educate the family and child on the signs of puberty and its progression.
- Reinforce with the parents the importance of setting age-appropriate expectations.
- Offer psychosocial intervention to the family if needed.

Assisting the Family and Child in Managing Endocrine Problems

- Assist the family with follow-up visits with a pediatric endocrinologist.
- Assist with administration of medical therapy.
- Educate the parents and family members on the cause of problem (e.g., precocious or delayed puberty), the effects of treatment, and the potential social issues related to sexual precocity or delay.
- Counsel the parents on the potential risk of sexual abuse with precocious puberty.
- Counsel the parents, family members, and teachers to set age-appropriate expectations for the child.
- Assist the child with understanding the presence of secondary sexual characteristics in precocious puberty.
- Assess the family and child for any psychosocial difficulty resulting from precocious puberty and offer counseling if indicated.
- If short stature is an issue, encourage activities in which the child can readily excel despite short stature.

Subjective Data

A complete history should be obtained with special attention to the following:

- Demographics (e.g., age, sex, ethnicity)
- Description of the problem
- Onset (i.e., age) and progression of the problem to date
- Course of the problem and its symptoms (e.g., chronic, acute, recurrent, progressive)
- Precipitating factors (e.g., viral illness, head trauma, medications, cranial-spinal irradiation, CNS infection, emotional stress)
- Current medications and treatments (e.g., dosage, date of onset, side effects)
- Associated signs and symptoms, such as neurologic symptoms (e.g., headaches, visual changes), delayed onset of puberty, poor weight gain, skin changes, lethargy, constipation, loose stooling, hypoglycemia, excessive or rapid weight gain, and unusual pubertal development (e.g., onset, progression)

  Signs and symptoms of Turner syndrome (e.g., cardiac anomalies [such as aortic valve anomalies and aortic stenosis], hypertension, recurrent otitis media, recurrent urinary tract infections [UTIs], phenotypic features [such as webbed neck, cubitus valgus, low hairline, ptosis, high-arched palate, shield chest, hypoplastic nipples, pigmented nevi, low-set ears, spoon-shaped nails])

  Signs and symptoms of Prader-Willi syndrome (e.g., hypotonia in infancy, small hands and feet, obesity, microphallus, cryptorchidism, mental retardation, almond-shaped eyes)

  Signs and symptoms of Russell-Silver syndrome (e.g., intrauterine growth retardation [IUGR], small triangular facies, incurving of fifth finger, asymmetry in extremities)

  Signs and symptoms of Seckel syndrome (e.g., IUGR, premature synostosis, microcephaly, prominent nose, receding forehead, micrognathia, low-set ears, large eyes, mental retardation)

  Signs and symptoms of Noonan syndrome (e.g., webbed neck, pectus excavatum, pigmented nevi, heart disease)

- Child's health habits and nutrition, including a complete eating history (e.g., what, how, where, by whom the child is fed, decreased appetite, decreased intake, fad dieting, anorexia nervosa, bulimia, purposeful weight loss), sleep patterns and activity level (e.g., difficulty sleeping, restlessness, lethargy, increase in napping, low endurance, intensity of exercise), school performance, and medication history (e.g., institution of new therapies, dosage, side effects [certain medications such as glucocorticoids for asthma treatment have been implicated in cases of short stature])

- Past medical history, including hospitalizations (e.g., age, reason, length of stay), surgeries (e.g., surgical procedure, indication, outcome), and chronic illnesses (e.g., onset, progression, medical therapies [including dosage and length of treatment])
- Birth history, including birth length and weight, gestation, pregnancy history to assess for IUGR (e.g., assessment of maternal health, use or abuse of substances, weight gain, nutritional status during pregnancy, infections, illnesses, bleeding), neonatal history (e.g., hypoglycemia and hyperbilirubinemia can be associated with growth hormone deficiency [GHD], peripheral edema can be seen in females with Turner syndrome, seizures can be related to hypoglycemia), history of infections, and feeding history
- Menstrual history
- Sexual activity
- Substance abuse
- Family history, including heights of parents, grandparents, and siblings; the age of pubertal onset and progression in parents, grandparents, aunts, uncles, and siblings, if applicable (i.e., in females, the onset of menses; in males, the age at which final height was achieved); and any history of endocrinopathies (e.g., thyroid disease, infertility, hirsutism, insulin-dependent diabetes mellitus, adrenal disorders)
- Social history, including any family stress, the home environment (e.g., who are the members of the family, level of emotional nurturing, economic status (e.g., related to access to health care, proper nutrition), and parental level of understanding concerning basic health needs
- Description of daily routine
- Child's temperament
- Developmental milestones
- Review of systems

Burgos and Jutte (2000) have also developed a mnemonic, *GROWTH,* to be used when evaluating a child with a potential growth problem:

G–Gather a complete history (as was just described)

R–Remember genetic contribution. Obtain height and weight of the parents and siblings. Familial short stature (FSS) is common. Inquire about parental growth and development as a child and adolescent.

O–Obtain only basic laboratory studies in the initial evaluation

W–Wonder about "zebras (improbable but possible diagnoses)." Consider all possible diagnoses. Continue to explore possibilities.

T–Track growth trends and plot growth over time. A child's growth between the ages of 2 and 9 years generally follows the same percentile. Infants from birth to age 18 months may shift up or down along the height curves.

H–Hospitalize or hormonally treat. If GHD is suspected, refer to an endocrinologist. If failure to thrive (FTT) is suspected, see Chapter 43.

Objective Data

Physical Examination

A complete physical examination is required for all children presenting with endocrine abnormalities. This examination should cover the following areas:

- *Blood pressure and pulse readings*—Measure for both, as hypertension can be seen in Turner syndrome.
- *Height and weight measurements*—Perform all height measurements three times to ensure accuracy, repositioning the patient with each measurement. A wall-mounted stadiometer should be used for all children past the age of 2 years. Proper positioning is essential and includes good posture with heels, buttocks, shoulders, and head against the wall, ankles together, arms by side, head facing forward and level. Shoes must be removed for measurements. Instruct the child to face forward and to relax the shoulders. The examiner should maintain proper positioning by holding the child's mandible while measuring. For children younger than 2 years of age, supine length measurements should be done. This requires at least two examiners to ensure proper measurement technique and positioning. Three measurements should be done to ensure accuracy. The child's head should be held at a 90-degree angle by one examiner while the second examiner extends the legs and measures the lower extremities, with the foot also being held at a 90-degree angle.
- *Upper to lower body (U/L) segment ratio*—Calculate by dividing a patient's upper segment (total height minus the lower segment) by the lower segment (distance from the floor to the upper border of the pubic symphysis). The U/L ration normally declines from about 1.7 at birth to 0.9 in early puberty, then reaches 1.0 at the end of puberty. In delayed puberty, U/L ratios are less than 0.9.
- *Arm span measurements*—Measure arm span if considering a diagnosis of achondroplasia.
- *Head circumference*—Measure head circumference to evaluate the possibility of microcephaly.
- *General appearance*—Note the child's general health, behavior, ability to interact with others, and bonding with family members.
- *Developmental assessment*—Evaluate for signs of developmental delay.
- *Neurologic examination*—Assess the cranial nerves, including funduscopic examination, assessment for hypotonia, and assessment of nerve strength to evaluate possibility of a CNS lesion as the cause of pituitary failure or precocious puberty. Hypotonia is seen in Prader-Willi syndrome, and mental retardation is seen in Seckel, Prader-Willi, and Down syndromes.
- *Skin*—Evaluate for signs of dry skin (seen in hypothyroidism), cafe-au-lait spots (seen in McCune-Albright syndrome as a cause of precocious puberty), unusual birthmarks, pigmented nevi (seen in Turner syndrome), and hyperpigmentation.
- *Neck*—Palpate the thyroid and assess the size, noting any goiter (seen in hypothyroidism. Palpate for any thyroid nodules and note the symmetry of the gland and any evidence of webbed neck (seen in Turner syndrome).
- *Head, eye, ear, nose, and throat (HEENT)*—Remember that low-set, posteriorly rotated ears and scarring in the inner ear related to recurrent otitis media are common findings in Turner syndrome. Note the shape of the eyes and examine for a high-arched palate (seen in Turner

syndrome), cleft lip or palate, triangular facies (seen in Russell-Silver syndrome), and frontal bossing and depressed nasal bridge (seen in GHD).

- *Heart*—Assess for audible murmurs (including aortic valve abnormalities and aortic stenosis in Turner syndrome and pulmonic stenosis in Noonan syndrome), heart rate and rhythm, and abnormal heart sounds, noting location and any change with positioning.
- *Chest and lungs*—Note the quality of breath sounds and the chest shape and configuration.
- *Abdomen*—Assess for evidence of abdominal mass or organomegaly.
- *Bimanual rectal examination*—This examination is indicated only if there is concern about an ovarian mass as the cause of precocious puberty.
- *Extremities*—Evaluate for arm and leg length discrepancies (seen in achondroplasia), shortened fourth metacarpals and spoon-shaped nails (seen in Turner syndrome), and incurving of the fifth finger (seen in Russell-Silver syndrome).
- *Genital and pubertal examination*—Perform Tanner staging for breast development and pubic hair in females and Tanner staging for genital development (e.g., testicular enlargement, penile length, thinning of the scrotum) and pubic hair in males. (Other signs of puberty include axillary hair, facial hair in males, voice changes, and axillary odor).

Diagnostic Procedures and Laboratory Tests

The following is a list of diagnostic tests that may be indicated for children with endocrine abnormalities:

- *Height measurements*—Length and height measurements should be done at each routine visit and at least three to four times a year from birth to 36 months of age. Subsequently, measurements should be done yearly. Growth velocity in the first year of life is 9 to 11 inches. In the second year, a normal growth velocity is 4 to 5 inches, with a decline to 3 to 4 inches between the ages of 2 and 3 years. By 3 years, the growth velocity should be consistent at 2 to 2½ inches per year. Abnormal growth velocity (either a failure to maintain appropriate velocity or excessive growth) requires further evaluation. Increased growth velocity may be a sign of precocious sexual development.
- *Tanner staging*—This is discussed in Chapter 40.
- *Bone age (BA) x-ray*—X-ray examination of the left hand and wrist is used to evaluate the age range of skeletal maturation. The results indicate a delay in maturation, appropriate maturation for one's chronologic age, or advanced skeletal maturation (i.e., advanced for chronologic age). BA is delayed in constitutional delay of growth and puberty (CDGP) but normal in FSS. Precocious puberty results in a BA that is advanced for chronologic age.
- *Magnetic resonance imaging (MRI) and computed tomography (CT) of the head*—This examination allows visualization of the hypothalamic and pituitary region for identification of any anatomic abnormality (e.g., hypoplasia, ectopic gland) or CNS lesions (e.g., craniopharyngiomas, hamartomas, germinomas).
- *Ultrasound*—Ultrasound evaluation may be indicated if an ovarian, adrenal, or testicular tumor is suspected as the cause of sexual precocity. Ovarian tumors may include benign adenomas and malignant carcinomas, while testicular tumors include Leydig cell adenomas. Ovarian neoplasms are rare but include granulosa and theca cell tumors.

- *Skeletal survey*—A skeletal survey is indicated if considering achondroplasia in the differential diagnosis of short stature.
- *Routine laboratory studies*—Complete blood cell (CBC) count, chemistry panel, sedimentation rate measurement, and urinalysis should be performed to evaluate for the possibility of systemic illness (e.g., liver disease, hematologic disorder, renal disease, gastrointestinal disorder) as a cause of growth failure.
- *Thyroid function studies (including triiodothyronine [T$_3$], thyroxine [T$_4$], and thyroid-stimulating hormone [TSH])*—These studies evaluate for the possibility of hypothyroidism as a cause of growth failure. Severe untreated hypothyroidism also can be a cause of precocious puberty. Assessment should also be made for hyperthyroidism (i.e., Graves' disease).
- *Growth factors (including insulin-like growth factor binding protein [IGF-PB3] and IGF-1) measurement*—This measurement is used as a screening test for GHD. IGFs are released by the liver in response to the presence of circulating growth hormone (GH). Levels of growth factors are constant, unlike GH production, which is pulsatile and occurs mainly during deep sleep. If levels of IGF-1 and IGF-BP3 are low, this may indicate pituitary GHD, and further testing may be indicated. Growth factors can also be low in states of malnutrition or malabsorption (e.g., gastrointestinal disease).
- *Luteinizing hormone (LH) and follicle-stimulating hormone (FSH)*—LH and FSH are released by the pituitary gland in response to gonadotropin-releasing hormone (Gn-RH), which is released by the hypothalamus. LH and FSH control puberty through stimulation of the ovaries to produce estrogen in females and of the testes to produce testosterone in males. Low levels indicate either a prepubertal condition or a hypothalamic or pituitary deficiency.
- *Estradiol (estrogen)*—Estradiol is measured to evaluate the estrogen production by the ovaries. Estradiol levels increase at the time of puberty and reach adult levels at the end of puberty. Estrogen is responsible for the development of secondary sexual characteristics in females, which include breast development and increase in growth velocity. Low levels may simply indicate a prepubertal condition or may reflect ovarian failure or pituitary gonadotropin deficiency.
- *Testosterone*—Testosterone is the male hormone released by the testes during puberty. Levels of testosterone begin to rise at the time of puberty and progress throughout puberty until adult male ranges are achieved. Testosterone causes the secondary sexual characteristics in males, including testicular enlargement, pubic hair development, axillary hair and odor, facial hair, acne, voice changes, and pubertal growth spurt. Low levels may reflect a prepubertal condition (e.g., CDGP) or may indicate testicular failure or pituitary deficiency.
- *Prolactin*—Prolactin is a pituitary hormone that stimulates breast development (along with estrogen and progesterone) and is also responsible for lactation during pregnancy. Prolactin can be elevated in the presence of CNS lesions, which may alter pituitary function and result in growth failure, precocious puberty, or delayed puberty.
- *Human chorionic gonadotropin (HCG)*—HCG is a hormone produced during pregnancy after the ovum has

been fertilized. It can however also be released by tumors such as choriocarcinomas of the uterus, testes, and ovary, as well as by hepatoblastomas. Therefore HCG levels are used as a screening test for peripheral tumors as a potential cause of precocious puberty.

- *Adrenocorticotropic hormone (ACTH)–stimulation test—* This test is performed to diagnose primary and secondary adrenal insufficiency when if there is suspicion of central adrenal hyperplasia (CAH).
- *Chromosomal analysis*—Short stature and delayed puberty can be associated with various chromosomal abnormalities or syndromic conditions. These include Turner, Noonan, Prader-Willi, Seckel, Down, and Russell-Silver syndromes. Chromosomal abnormalities have not been identified for all syndromic conditions (see Chapter 5).

Delayed Puberty

Alert

Consult with or refer to a physician for the following:
- Onset of breast development in females by the age of 13 years
- Menses not beginning by the age of 16 years
- Testicular volume in males not increasing by the age of 14 years
- Once initiated, lack of pubertal progression over 1 year
- Pubertal development not completed within 4 to 5 years
- Females with phenotypic features of Turner syndrome

Etiology

The underlying problem causing delayed puberty can be simply described as either *hypergonadotropic hypogonadism* (the gonads not responding to the CNS hormones) or *hypogonadotropic hypogonadism* (the CNS not producing adequate stimulation). Delayed puberty can be a normal variant, referred to as *constitutional delay of growth and puberty* (see Short Stature, later in this chapter.) It can also be associated with a number of endocrine disorders, including isolated gonadotropin deficiency, panhypopituitarism, gonadal agenesis, gonadal failure (either ovarian or testicular), autoimmune destruction of the gonads, and vanishing testes syndrome. A number of syndromic conditions also can be associated with delayed puberty and hypogonadism, including Prader-Willi, Klinefelter, Turner, and Kallmann syndromes. Hypogonadotropic hypogonadism and panhypopituitarism may be idiopathic, or they can result from CNS lesions (e.g., craniopharyngioma, germinoma) or congenital anomalies resulting in the absence of the pituitary.

Incidence

- The incidence of delayed puberty in the United States is less than 1%.
- CDGP is seen in 3% to 5% of the general population.
- Turner syndrome occurs in 1 of 2500 live female births.

Risk Factors

- Family history of CDGD
- CNS tumor, irradiation, or trauma
- Chromosomal abnormalities
- Syndromic conditions

- Congenital anomalies (e.g., absence of the pituitary gland, septo-optic dysplasia)
- Local irradiation of the region of the gonads
- Chemotherapy
- Testicular torsion
- Autoimmune conditions

Differential Diagnosis

The diagnosis of delayed puberty is made if pubertal milestones have not been obtained within two standard deviations of normal (Table 33-1).

For girls, delayed puberty is diagnosed if a girl has:
1. No pubertal development by the age of 13 years
2. Pubertal maturation that is not complete within 4 years of its initiation
3. Failed to menstruate by the age of 16 years

If a girl has had a chronic illness or been engaged in highly competitive athletics, the work-up for delayed puberty can be delayed until the age of 14 years.

For boys, delayed puberty is diagnosed if:
1. Testicular volume has not increased by the age of 14 years
2. Pubertal development has not been completed within 5 years of its initiation

Once the diagnosis is made then a search for the cause begins.

Delayed onset of puberty can occur as a normal variant. In this instance, the child may present with delayed puberty alone or delayed puberty and short stature. With constitutional delay (the most common cause of delayed puberty), there is a positive family history of delay, a delayed BA for chronologic age, normal growth velocity, a negative past medical history, and a negative review of systems. Constitutional delay is more common in boys. Patients with constitutional delay progress normally through puberty once it is initiated and do achieve adult pubertal development, just at a later age. In adolescents with constitutional delay, physical changes of puberty usually begin when the BA is 12 years.

Hypothalamic abnormalities (e.g., hypogonadotropic hypogonadism) can result in Gn-RH deficiency. Gn-RH is responsible for stimulating the pituitary release of LH and FSH, which then stimulate the gonads. Gn-RH deficiency prevents activation of the hypothalamic pituitary gonadal axis, resulting in lack of pubertal development. Gn-RH deficiency can be isolated, or it can be associated with GH-releasing hormone deficiency. Hypothalamic damage from trauma, tumors, cysts, or irradiation can also cause Gn-RH deficiency and subsequent lack of pubertal development. The female athlete triad of disordered eating, amenorrhea, and osteoporosis is most common in gymnasts, ballet dancers, and long-distance runners, and the exercise-induced menstrual changes appears to be secondary to a disturbance of hypothalamic GnRH secretion. Studies have indicated that for every year of premenarchal athletic training, menarche may be delayed by 5 months.

Pituitary failure or *pituitary dysfunction* can result from trauma, autoimmune destruction, congenital malformations in the CNS (e.g., septo-optic dysplasia, absence of pituitary gland), or tumors and cysts (e.g., adenomas, craniopharyngiomas). Pituitary failure results in gonadotropin deficiency with low levels of LH and FSH, resulting in a lack of stimulation of the gonads.

Several congenital anomalies can result in *gonadal failure* or *gonadal dysfunction,* including gonadal dysgenesis as seen with Turner syndrome (45,XO). Patients with

Turner syndrome present with sexual infantilism, although they do have pubic hair development. Elevated gonadotropin levels (both LH and FSH) indicate gonadal failure. A second form of gonadal failure is pure gonadal agenesis without the phenotypic features found in Turner syndrome. The karyotype in such patients can be either 46,XY or 46,XX, although phenotypically they are female. Patients with this condition are at risk for gonadoblastomas, embryonal carcinomas, and dysgerminomas if the karyotype is 46,XY; they also can have renal failure. Premature ovarian failure also can also be idiopathic. In cases of gonadal failure, there is an elevation in serum LH and FSH levels. Although Kallmann syndrome is uncommon, it is associated with underdeveloped genitalia in males, with sexual infantilism and absent olfactory lobes; loss of smell may be partial or complete.

Congenital anorchia is often referred to as *vanishing testes syndrome.* Males with this condition have a male karyotype and a male phenotype; however, they have undescended testes, and upon surgical exploration, no testicular tissue is found. The phallus, scrotum, and wolffian ducts are well formed, indicating that testicular tissue was present until approximately 20 weeks gestation.

Gonadal failure can result from trauma, injury, castration, testicular torsion, and orchitis, which can be seen in mumps.

Management

There are many causes of delayed puberty and almost all are associated with osteoporosis, especially in young women. Girls with pubertal delay should take 1200 to 1500 mg of elemental calcium daily. In some instances hormonal therapy may be considered.

Constitutional delay of growth and puberty. See Short Stature, later in this chapter.

Hypothalamic or pituitary dysfunction

Treatments and medications. Testosterone treatment is used in males to initiate puberty and maintain masculinization. Testosterone is prepared as either testosterone enanthate or testosterone cypionate, then administered as intramuscular injections on a monthly or bimonthly basis depending on the levels achieved. Testosterone is also available in a sublingual form and in a patch worn on scrotal tissue. In females, various forms of estrogen are used. Estrogen therapy is followed by cycling with both estrogen and progesterone to establish regular menstrual cycles. Both therapies must be prescribed and monitored by a pediatric endocrinologist.

Counseling and prevention
- Educate the child and family on the cause of delayed puberty.
- Review the medical therapy, including dosage, schedule of medications, and potential adverse effects.
- Educate the child and family on normal pubertal changes expected from treatment.
- Assess the child and family for emotional distress resulting from the delay in puberty.

Follow-up
- Perform routine follow-up for primary care needs.
- Follow up with the pediatric endocrinologist routinely.
- In cases of constitutional delay, follow up at 6-month intervals to assess for signs of pubertal progression.

Consultations and referrals
- Refer the child to a pediatric endocrinologist if the diagnosis is unclear.
- Refer the child to a mental health professional if indicated.

Table 33-1 Differential Diagnosis: Delayed Puberty (259.0)

CRITERIA	CONSTITUTIONAL DELAY OF GROWTH AND PUBERTY	HYPOTHALAMIC/ PITUITARY FAILURE*	GONADAL FAILURE*
ICD-9 code	259.0	253.	257.2
Subjective Data			
Age/onset	Usually presents by the age of 3 years	Can occur at any age; delayed onset of puberty	Can occur at any age; delayed onset of puberty
Description of problem	Height at less than the 5th percentile; delayed puberty	History of trauma, tumors, cysts, malformation	History indicates gonadal agenesis, radiation induced, trauma, orchitis
Associated symptoms	Delayed dentition	Usually none	None
Family history	Positive	None	None
Objective Data			
Physical examination			
Height	At or below the 5th percentile	Normal unless also has GHD	Normal
Weight	Normal	Normal	Normal
Puberty	Delayed onset	Delayed onset	Delayed onset
BA	Delayed	Can be delayed	Can be delayed
Laboratory data			
LH, FSH	Normal for BA	Low for age	Elevated
Testosterone	Normal for BA	Low for age	Low
Estradiol	Normal for BA	Low for age	Low
IGF-1	Normal	Normal-low	Normal
IGF-BP3	Normal	Normal-low	Normal

*Refer to an endocrinologist.

Precocious Puberty

Alert

Consult with or refer to a physician for the following:
- History of headache or any neurologic changes
- Onset of puberty in girls younger than 8 years
- Onset of puberty in boys younger than 9 years

Etiology

Precocious puberty is defined as the development of secondary sex characteristics in a girl younger than 8 years of age (a new age of 6 to 7 years has been proposed) or a boy younger than 9 years of age. It may be idiopathic (most common) or constitutional in nature or may result from an organic cause (e.g., a tumor in the CNS or gonads). It also can result from an enzymatic defect resulting in overproduction of certain steroids by the adrenal gland; this is known as *congenital adrenal hyperplasia*. Idiopathic sexual precocity can also be hereditary. Trauma to the CNS in addition to CNS irradiation can result in precocious puberty. It can also result from severe cases of long-standing hypothy-roidism or exogenous exposure to either testosterone or estrogen. There are gonadotropin-independent forms of sexual precocity, namely familial male precocious puberty and McCune-Albright syndrome; these are rare causes due to "turned-on" receptors.

Incidence

Sexual precocity is idiopathic in 80% of girls and 50% to 65% of boys.

Risk Factors

- History of CNS damage; cerebral palsy, head trauma, CNS irradiation, seizures, tumor, or infection (e.g., brain abscess, meningitis, encephalitis)
- Exposure or access to estrogen- or testosterone-containing substances
- Severe, untreated, long-standing hypothyroidism
- Congenital malformations (e.g., hydrocephalus, septo-optic dysplasia, craniosynostosis, porencephaly)

Differential Diagnosis

Table 33-2 provides additional information

Benign premature thelarche is breast development, unilateral or bilateral, without other evidence of sexual precocity

Table 33-2 Differential Diagnosis: Precocious Puberty

CRITERIA	BENIGN PREMATURE THELARCHE	BENIGN PREMATURE ADRENARCHE	CENTRAL PRECOCIOUS PUBERTY*	PERIPHERAL PRECOCIOUS PUBERTY*
ICD-9 code	259.1	259.1	259.1	259.1
Subjective Data				
Age/onset	Female typically less than 2 years	Male less than 10 years; female less than 8 years Typically 6 years	Male less than 9 years Female less than 8 years More common in girls	Any age
Description of problem	Premature breast development	Pubic hair development	Secondary sex characteristics	Secondary sex characteristics
Associated symptoms				
Growth velocity	Normal	Normal	Accelerated	May be accelerated
Neurologic symptoms	Negative	Negative	Positive, if tumor	None
Other				Female: vaginal spotting; abdominal discomfort
Family history	None	Positive	Occasionally	Positive
Objective Data				
Physical examination				
Height	Normal	Normal	Advanced	Can be advanced
Weight	Normal	Normal	Normal-advanced	Normal
Pubertal development	Tanner II-III breasts	Tanner I genitals	Tanner II-III genitals, breasts (hyperpigmented areole)	Tanner II-III genitals, breasts
	Tanner I pubic hair	Tanner II-III pubic hair	Tanner I-III pubic hair	Tanner I-III pubic hair
Vaginal mucosa	Red (prepubertal)	Not applicable	Pink (pubertal) with white discharge	Pink (pubertal)
Laboratory data				
BA	BA = chronologic age	BA = chronologic age	Advanced	Normal or advanced
Female: estradiol	Prepubertal	Prepubertal	Nondiagnostic	May be elevated or low
Male: testosterone	Not applicable	Prepubertal	Elevated	Elevated or low
LH	Prepubertal	Prepubertal	Pubertal	Prepubertal
FSH	Prepubertal	Prepubertal	Pubertal	Prepubertal
Beta HCG	Normal	Not applicable	Normal to increased	Can be elevated
Prolactin	Normal	Not applicable	Can be elevated if CNS lesion	Normal

*Refer to a pediatric endocrinologist.

(e.g., increased growth velocity, advanced BA, estrogenization of vaginal mucosa, changes in uterine size). It is an isolated, unsustained phenomenon and is benign. It usually presents in young female infants and can be present at birth, from 6 months to 2 years, and again after age 6 years.

Benign premature adrenarche is the presence of pubic hair in boys or girls without other evidence of sexual development (e.g., increased growth velocity, acne, increased phallic size and testicular size [in boys]). There is often a family history. The most common age of occurrence is 6 to 7 years, but it may occur as early as 4 years of age. The BA is normal to slightly advanced.

Central precocious puberty (CPP) results from the early release of the gonadotropins LH and FSH from the pituitary gland, which lies within the CNS. CPP can be constitutional, resulting from no apparent cause, or it can result from a disruption in the hypothalamus (e.g., trauma, tumor, infection, irradiation, congenital malformations); the latter is often referred to as *organic CPP*. It is more common in girls but an etiology is found more often in boys. CPP also has been reported in cases of severe hypothyroidism that have been long standing and untreated.

Peripheral precocious puberty occurs when there is production of estrogens and androgens from sources in the periphery, unrelated to the CNS. These may include the ovaries, testes, or adrenal gland. Ovarian tumors are quite rare in the pediatric population, but examples of ovarian tumors include granulosa cell tumors, theca cell tumors, teratomas, and chorioepitheliomas. Adrenal tumors can include adenomas and carcinomas. In males, tumors of the testes that cause sexual precocity are usually Leydig cell adenomas. Other tumors such as teratomas, dysgerminomas, hepatoblastomas, and chorioepitheliomas can also produce androgens, resulting in peripheral precocious puberty. Peripheral precocious puberty can also result from exogenous exposure to either estrogen or testosterone (e.g., through facial creams, ingestion of substances that contain either estrogen or testosterone).

There are several genetic disorders that result in peripheral precocious puberty. These include familial male precocious puberty, [testotoxicosis] (a genetically inherited disorder resulting in autonomous function of the testes), and McCune-Albright syndrome, which consists of sexual precocity, cafe-au-lait spots, and polyostotic fibrous dysplasia and autonomous function of the ovaries.

Management

Treatments and medications. No treatment is indicated for benign premature thelarche and premature adrenarche. The treatment for true sexual precocity is dependent on the cause and may include medical treatment, surgery, or radiation. The gold standard of treatment for CPP is GnRH analogues; these are prescribed to decrease the progression of puberty and also to cause the regression of secondary sexual characteristics. GnRH analogues suppress gonadotropins and are given in a monthly depot preparation. There are no significant side effects. Surgical excision is used when possible for tumors in the CNS and peripheral organs. Radiation is also sometimes used for tumors in the CNS. The goal of treatment is to protect against a loss in final height and to minimize the difficulty in management of precocious sexual development.

Medical therapy involves three main categories of drugs: inhibitors of LH and FSH (e.g., Gn-RH agonist, medroxyprogesterone acetate, cyproterone acetate [not available in the United States]; inhibitors of androgen and estrogen production (e.g., ketoconazole, medroxyprogesterone, spironolactone, testolactone), and inhibitors of androgen and estrogen action (e.g., cyproterone acetate [not available in the United States], tamoxifen, flutamide, spironolactone). Most commonly used are the Gn-RH agonists, especially leuprolide acetate (Lupron Depot), which are long-acting medications given on a monthly basis.

Counseling and prevention
- Educate the parents on the risk of sexual abuse in children with sexual precocity.
- Educate the parents on the need for assisting the child with hygienic maintenance (e.g., use of deodorant, menses).
- Assist the parents and child with understanding the development of secondary sexual characteristics.
- If GnRH therapy is initiated, explain the benefits. Breast size and amount of pubic hair should decrease within 6 months of therapy. If menses was present in a female, it should stop. In a male, a decrease in testicular size, amount of pubic hair, acne, and frequency of penile erections; a decrease in aggressive behavior; and an improvement in self esteem should be anticipated.
- Counsel the parents and family members to set age-appropriate expectations based on the child's chronologic age. Inform the parents about the potential emotional lability of children with sexual precocity.
- Assist the parents with answering the child's questions about the presence of secondary sexual characteristics.
- Offer counseling to assist the child and family with coping.

Follow-up. Follow-up should involve routine evaluations for primary care needs. If the diagnosis is benign premature adrenarche or thelarche, follow-up should be provided at 6-month intervals to evaluate for any evidence of progression. If GnRH therapy is initiated, the patient should be evaluated every 3 months, with LH-releasing hormone stimulation testing being performed.

Consultations and referrals. All children with true precocious puberty should be evaluated and followed by a pediatric endocrinologist. If needed, a child may be referred to a mental health professional.

Short Stature

Alert

Consult with or refer to a physician for the following:
- No growth over 6 months to 1 year
- Neurologic symptoms (e.g., headaches, visual changes)
- Females and males below the 3rd percentile in height
- Unusual phenotypic feature
- Persistent hypoglycemia in newborn period
- Suboptimal growth velocity with normal to excess weight gain (for which an endocrine cause should be suspected)

Etiology

Short stature is defined as height below the 3rd percentile for age. It is not a disease but a symptom. There can be many causes for why a child is short, including normal patterns of growth (e.g., FSS, CDGP), primary growth disturbances (e.g., IUGR, genetic disorders, genetic short stature), systemic illnesses, and endocrine disorders (e.g., hypothyroidism, glucocorticoid excess, GHD).

Incidence

- Of the general population, 5% is statistically short (below the 5th percentile in height).
- CDGP occurs in 3% to 5% of the general population.
- Turner syndrome is seen in 1 in 2500 live female births.
- Turner syndrome occurs in 1 in 40 females below the 3rd percentile in height.
- The incidence of classic GHD is 1 in 4000 live births.
- The incidence of achondroplasia is 1 in 10,000 live births.

Risk Factors

- Chronic systemic illness
- Midline defects (e.g., cleft lip or palate, spina bifida, septo-optic dysplasia)
- Chromosomal abnormalities and genetic syndromes (e.g., Turner, Prader-Willi, Noonan, Russell-Silver, Down, Seckel syndrome; neurofibromatosis).
- IUGR (e.g., from placental insufficiency, poor maternal health, prenatal exposure to toxic substances, prenatal infections)
- Low birth weight
- Prematurity
- Medical therapy (e.g., chemotherapy, irradiation, medications [such as Ritalin])
- Emotional deprivation
- Malnutrition
- Family history of short stature
- Family history of constitutional delay

Differential Diagnosis

Table 33-3 provides additional information.

In *familial short stature,* a child's genetics are inclined for short stature and are within the normal range for the family. The pertinent findings for genetic short stature include a negative past medical history, a negative review of systems, a positive family history for short stature, a normal growth velocity for age, a normal BA, and no abnormalities in the laboratory studies. The age for onset of puberty is normal, and final height is consistent for the family genetics.

Constitutional delay of growth and puberty, also considered a variant of normal, refers to delayed maturation resulting in a delayed BA, a delayed onset of puberty, and a stature that is statistically short for a child's chronologic age but normal for the child's BA. The pertinent findings include a positive family history of delayed growth and puberty, a normal growth velocity for BA, a BA that is delayed for chronologic age, and no abnormalities in the laboratory studies. The onset of puberty is delayed, and final height, although achieved at an older age, is appropriate for the family genetics.

Skeletal dysplasia or various forms of *achondroplasia* result in disproportionate short stature. Achondroplasia is caused by an autosomal dominant mutation. Affected children have short stature, shortened limbs, macrocephaly, prominent forehead, and bowing of the legs and can develop lordosis and kyphosis.

Chromosomal abnormalities and *syndromic conditions* can be associated with short stature. Turner syndrome (45,XO) is associated with stature below the 3rd percentile in 99% of affected individuals. The cause of the short stature is unclear, although patients benefit from treatment with GH. Short stature may also be a phenotypic feature in Down, Noonan, Russell-Silver, Prader-Willi, and Seckel syndromes.

Systemic causes can also be the source of growth failure and short stature. Such causes include malnutrition (e.g., fad dieting, poor nutrition, malabsorption, starvation), chronic systemic illness (e.g., diabetes, cardiac disease, hematologic disorders, chronic renal failure, severe respiratory illness and or severe asthma, gastrointestinal disorders, CNS lesions), emotional deprivation, and idiopathic causes.

Endocrine abnormalities that result in short stature include GHD, GH resistance, hypothyroidism (see Thyroid Disorders, later in this chapter), and Cushing disease (rarely). An endocrine cause should be suspected if the child has normal or excess weight gain associated with below normal growth velocity.

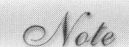

Note

There are continuous and rapid changes in the diagnosis and management of growth anomalies. Any patient needing GH therapy should be referred to a pediatric endocrinologist.

Management

Familial short stature. No treatment is needed.

Constitutional delay of growth and puberty

Treatments and medications. In extreme cases of constitutional delay that are causing psychosocial concern to the child, low-dose hormonal therapy can be used to initiate early pubertal changes and increase growth velocity. This therapy involves low-dose testosterone treatment in males and low-dose estrogen treatment in females and is instituted by a pediatric endocrinologist.

Counseling and prevention

- Reassure the child and family that the genetic potential for size will ultimately be achieved.
- Encourage and direct the child in activities in which he or she can readily excel despite a short stature.
- Educate the child and family on pubertal changes.

Follow-up. Perform routine follow-up for evaluation of growth velocity.

Consultations and referrals

- Refer the child to a pediatric endocrinologist if the diagnosis is unclear or for low-dose treatment if psychosocial implications are manifested.
- Refer the child to a family counselor or mental health professional if needed.

Skeletal dysplasia

Treatments and medications. There is no medical therapy available to augment stature resulting from skeletal dysplasia. Surgical intervention can possibly be offered in extreme cases for patients who are fully grown and who consent to an experimental leg-lengthening surgical procedure.

Counseling and prevention. Offer psychosocial counseling to assist with the implications of extreme short stature. Assistance may be needed in coordinating care from multiple disciplines.

Follow-up. Perform routine follow-up for primary care issues.

Consultations and referrals

- Refer the child to a pediatric endocrinologist if the diagnosis is unclear.
- Refer the child to a mental health professional if needed.

Table 33-3 Differential Diagnosis: Short Stature

CRITERIA	FAMILIAL SHORT STATURE	CONSTITUTIONAL DELAY OF GROWTH AND PUBERTY*	TURNER SYNDROME*	SYSTEMIC ILLNESS*	SKELETAL DYSPLASIA*	GROWTH HORMONE DEFICIENCY*	HYPOTHYROIDISM*
ICD-9 code	783.43	783.40	758.6	783.43	742.9	253.3	244.9
Subjective Data							
Age/onset	Birth to 2 years	Presents usually by age 3 years	Infancy	Any age	Birth	Any age	Any age
Description of problem	Height at or below 5th percentile	Height at or below 5th percentile	Height below 5th percentile	Slow down growth velocity	Short limbs	Lack of growth hormone	Thyroid failure
Associated symptoms	None	Delayed dentition	Associated symptoms of syndrome	Symptoms of illness	Associated symptoms of syndrome	Infant: low glucose	Symptoms of hypothyroidism
Family history	Short stature	Delay in growth and puberty in parents	None	Not applicable	Possible	Possible	Occasionally
Objective Data							
Physical examination							
Height	At or below 5th percentile	At or below 5th percentile Late pubertal growth spurt	Height below 5th percentile	Decline in percentile	Below 5th percentile	Below 5th percentile	Decline in percentile
Weight	Appropriate	Appropriate	Appropriate	May decline	Appropriate	Normal for height	Normal to increased for height
Pubertal development	Normal	Delayed onset	Lack breast development	Can be delayed	Normal	Delayed	Delayed or advanced
Laboratory data							
BA	Normal	Delayed	Normal or delayed	Delayed	Normal	Severely delayed	Delayed
Diagnostic studies	Normal studies	Normal studies	45,X0/variant	Specific for illness	Skeletal survey	Low growth factors	Decreased T4; increased TSH

Refer to an appropriate physician or endocrinologist.

Chromosomal abnormalities. See also Genetic Evaluation and Counseling in Chapter 5 and Down Syndrome in Chapter 46.

Treatments and medications. GH treatment is of benefit in increasing the height of those with Turner and Noonan syndromes. The use of GH in other syndromic conditions is still under investigation.

Counseling and prevention

- Encourage and direct the child in activities in which he or she can readily excel despite stature.
- Remember that counseling by a genetic counselor may benefit the family.

Follow-up. Perform routine follow-up for primary care issues.

Consultations and referrals. Refer the child to a genetics counselor and possibly a pediatric endocrinologist.

Growth hormone deficiency

Treatments and medications. GH therapy is administered by subcutaneous injection. Standard dosing for GH therapy is 0.3 mg/kg per week given as daily injections for 6 to 7 consecutive nights. Potential side effects, although rare, include insulin resistance, increased intracranial hypertension, pseudotumor cerebri, hypothyroidism, slipped capital femoral epiphysis, fluid retention, and a slightly increased risk of leukemia.

New treatment options include GH-releasing hormone, which may be helpful in treating conditions involving hypothalamic dysfunction, and a GH-releasing peptide called hexarelin.

Counseling and prevention

- Encourage and direct the child in activities in which he or she can excel despite a short stature.
- Encourage routine follow-up with a pediatric endocrinologist.
- Instruct the parents on the side effects of medications.

Follow-up. Encourage parents should telephone immediately if side effects develop from the medication. Perform routine follow-up for primary care issues.

Consultations and referrals. Refer the child to a pediatric endocrinologist.

Thyroid Disorders

Alert

Consult with or refer to a pediatric endocrinologist for the following:
- An infant or child suspected of having a thyroid disorder
- A child with a goiter

Etiology

Thyroid disorders can be divided into two categories. *Hypothyroidism* results from an insufficient production of thyroid hormones. It can be congenital, transient, or acquired. Congenital hypothyroidism (CH) may be caused by an embryonic defect in the development or placement of the thyroid gland or inborn errors of thyroid hormone synthesis, secretion, or utilization. Transient primary hypothyroidism is often caused by maternal ingestion of medication during pregnancy (e.g., iodides for asthma, antithyroid drugs, maternal antibodies [if the mother had autoimmune thyroid disease]). Acquired hypothyroidism is most commonly the result of autoimmunity (e.g., from chronic lymphocytic thyroiditis, Hashimoto's disease). Less common causes are treatment with radioactive iodine, thioamide drugs, surgery or thyroidectomy, and infectious agents.

Hyperthyroidism results from an overproduction of thyroid hormones. It is most commonly caused by an autoimmune condition (e.g., Graves' disease). Dysfunction of the hypothalamus or pituitary gland is rare. Hyperthyroidism can be congenital in children whose mother has been diagnosed with Graves' disease.

Incidence

- Congenital hypothyroidism occurs in 1 in 3600 to 5000 live births.
- Of those diagnosed with permanent hypothyroidism, 66% to 75% are female.
- Of those diagnosed with transient hypothyroidism, 65% are male.
- Permanent hypothyroidism occurs in 6% of premature infants.
- Congenital hypothyroidism has a late onset in 10% of the cases.
- There is an increased incidence of congenital hypothyroidism in children with Down syndrome.
- The incidence of hypothyroidism is highest in those areas with an iodine deficiency.
- Hyperthyroidism is more common in females than males.
- Graves' disease has a familial predisposition. About 1% to 10% of women with Graves' disease have children with hyperthyroidism.

Risk Factors

- Family history of thyroid disease
- Autoimmune disease
- Genetic disorders (e.g., Down, Turner, Klinefelter, Noonan syndromes)
- Diabetes mellitus
- Prematurity

Differential Diagnosis

Any infant or child who is suspected of having a thyroid disorder or presents with a goiter (enlarged thyroid gland) requires a comprehensive history and physical examination, including laboratory data to assess thyroid function (Table 33-4).

Congenital hypothyroidism is the most common preventable cause of mental retardation. Usually infants with CH appear normal at birth. Birth weight and head circumference may be slightly above normal, while signs and symptoms are nonspecific and may include feeding difficulty, prolonged jaundice, respiratory problems, hypotonia, constipation, large posterior fontanel, excess sleep, large tongue, rarely cry, umbilical hernia, dry and mottled skin, and slow relaxation of deep tendon reflexes. Early treatment is critical. Neonatal screening is the only means of early diagnosis. All 50 states require newborns to be screened for CH before discharge from the nursery and before day 7 of life. If the screen is done before 24 hours of age, it must be repeated at 1 to 2 weeks of age. T_4 is measured initially. If the T_4 is greater than 6.5, a TSH is done. If the TSH is 20 or higher, the infant should be immediately referred to a pediatric endocrinologist.

Chronic lymphocytic thyroiditis (i.e., Hashimoto's disease, juvenile autoimmune thyroiditis) is the most common cause of acquired hypothyroidism. Symptoms are insidious. The child continues to gain weight despite a reported poor appetite. Associated symptoms may include dry skin, constipation, fatigue, cold intolerance, and anorexia. Puberty is delayed. On palpation the thyroid gland is enlarged with a firm consistency and

Table 33-4 Differential Diagnosis: Thyroid Disorders

| | HYPOTHYROIDISM | | HYPERTHYROIDISM |
CRITERIA	CONGENITAL	ACQUIRED (HASHIMOTO'S DISEASE)	NEONATAL AND GRAVES' DISEASE
ICD-9 code	243.	245.2	242.0/775.3
Subjective Data			
Age	Birth	Any age, most common at 8 to 15 years of age	Birth, if neonatal; others, 12 to 14 years of age
Onset	Several days to weeks after birth	Insidious	Gradual
Prenatal history	Mother may have taken iodides for asthma or antithyroid medication	Unremarkable	Maternal history of Graves' disease
Neonatal history	May include feeding difficulty, constipation, hypotonia, prolonged jaundice, etc.	Unremarkable	Unremarkable
Associated symptoms	See neonatal history above	May be asymptomatic or report weight gain despite reported poor appetite, slow growth velocity, constipation, fatigue, cold intolerance, irregular menses, enlarged thyroid	May report decreased school performance, difficulty concentrating, possible change in stools (diarrhea), hyperactivity, fatigue, weight loss, vision problems, increased perspiration, heat intolerance, sleep problems; may report enlarged thyroid and hoarseness
Past history	Not applicable	Possible past treatment with radioactive iodine, thiomide drugs, surgery, or thyroidectomy; may have history of other autoimmune disease	May have history of autoimmune disease
Family history	Possible	Possible	Possible maternal history of Graves' disease
Objective Data			
Physical examination			
Vital signs		Decreased pulse	Increased pulse
Weight/measurements	Birth weight and head circumference may be slightly increased	Possible weight gain	Weight loss
General appearance	Usually appears normal	May appear sluggish	May appear appear anxious or nervous, have difficulty sitting still for any length of time; eye prominence and exopthalmous
Skin/hair	Skin may appear dry, thick, scaly, coarse with yellowish tinge	Dry skin	Skin: increased perspiration, diffuse hyperpigmentation of skin
	Hair is dry, coarse, brittle	Hair: dry, coarse	Hair: fine, silky, may be some thinning
Musculoskeletal	Infant may have short extremities, hypotonia		
Other findings	May have flat bridge of nose, eyes appear widely spaced, delayed dental eruption, closure of fontanels delayed		Eye or vision changes Hand tremor
Thyroid gland	May be enlarged	Possibly enlarged, nontender, usually symmetric, moderately firm and without nodules; in chronic thyroiditis, cobblestone surface frequently palpated	Diffusely enlarged
Laboratory data			
Total T$_4$	Low	Normal or decreased	Elevated
T$_3$	Low	Normal or decreased	Elevated
TSH	Very elevated	Elevated	Suppressed

a cobblestone surface. Thyroid function tests may be normal, or the TSH may be elevated. As the disease progresses (without treatment) there is a decrease in T_4 and T_3 levels.

Graves' disease is the most common cause of hyperthyroidism in children. The highest incidence is in females age 12 to 14 years. However, it may be present at birth in infants whose mother has been diagnosed with Graves' disease. Older children usually have presenting symptoms of an enlarged thyroid, exophthalmos, decreased school performance, and poor concentration. Other symptoms include irritability, hyperactivity, voracious appetite, weight loss, heat intolerance, tremors, insomnia or restless sleep, poor coordination, excessive sweating, irregular menses, and an increased number of stools. Visual disturbances frequently occur. On palpation the thyroid gland is enlarged. It also has a soft-to-firm consistency, and a bruit is common. Thyroid function tests reveal elevated T_3 and T_4 levels, while TSH is suppressed.

Management

Congenital hypothyroidism

Treatments and medications. Early detection and treatment is critical. Treatment is determined by a pediatric endocrinologist, and levothyroxine is usually the drug of choice. (Practitioners should note that the suggested starting dosage has recently been increased to 10 to 15 g/kg per day.)

Counseling and prevention

- Keep in mind that early identification of infants with congenital hypothyroidism is essential. Newborn screening should be carefully followed and repeated if done before 24 hours of age.
- Remember that a recent study reports that primary TSH screening is more effective for mass screening than the T_4/TSH method. Screening should be performed as close to discharge as possible to avoid false positives.
- Explain the disorder to the parents.
- Instruct the parents about the prescribed medication and the need for lifelong therapy.
- Stress the importance of compliance with the drug therapy. The medication is supplied in pill form and is tasteless. Advise parents to crush the tablet and add it to formula, milk, or food. If a dose is missed, two doses can be given the following day.
- Encourage routine follow-up with a pediatric endocrinologist.
- Educate parents on the signs of drug overdose (e.g., increased pulse, shortness of breath, irritability, restless sleep, fever, sweating, weight loss). Instruct the parents to telephone if any of these symptoms develop. Demonstrate how to take the infant's pulse.
- Instruct the parents on the signs and symptoms of hypothyroidism that may indicate inadequate medication (e.g., decreased appetite, fatigue or increased sleep, constipation). Advise the parents to telephone if any of these signs are observed.

Follow-up. Follow-up care is determined by the pediatric endocrinologist and usually includes a return visit for thyroid function tests 2 weeks after therapy is initiated, every month for the first year of life, every 2 months for the second year of life, every 3 months for ages 3 to 5 years, and every 4 months thereafter. As a child gets older and the levothyroxine dose stabilizes, visits every 6 months are adequate. Repeat thyroid function tests should be performed 6 to 8 weeks after any change in drug dosage. Well-child care follow-up is also needed.

Consultations and referrals

- Refer the child to a pediatric endocrinologist.
- Refer the parents for genetic counseling, if indicated.

Acquired hypothyroidism (chronic lymphocytic thyroiditis or Hashimoto's disease)

Treatments and medications. Treatment is determined by the pediatric endocrinologist. Levothyroxine is usually the drug of choice.

Counseling and prevention

- Educate the parents and child about the disease. Most cases are temporary, and the goiter usually spontaneously regresses in 1 to 2 years.
- Encourage routine follow-up with the pediatric endocrinologist.
- Instruct on medications. Medication is usually very effective in shrinking the goiter. Remember that behavior changes should also be anticipated when the thyroid hormone is restored. If the child was symptomatic, improvement should be expected.

Follow-up. Follow-up as determined by the pediatric endocrinologist. Serum TSH is usually measured at regular intervals to monitor the appropriateness of the drug dosage. Perform follow-up for well-child care.

Consultations and referrals. Refer the child to a pediatric endocrinologist.

Hyperthyroidism (Graves' disease)

Treatments and medications. Neonatal hyperthyroidism requires hospitalization and close monitoring for signs of heart failure. Treatment for hyperthyroidism (Graves' disease) is determined by a pediatric endocrinologist and usually includes medication as initial therapy. Radiation therapy or surgery may be used in a small percentage of patients who do not respond to medical management.

Counseling and prevention

- Educate the parents and child about the disease. Complete remission of the disorder often occurs after 1 to 2 years of therapy, but relapse is possible.
- Instruct the parents and child on the prescribed treatment plan, including the side effects of any medications. Advise the parents to call immediately if side effects are noted. Once treatment is initiated, symptoms should improve in about 2 weeks.
- Discuss possible interventions for the child's physical symptoms before a drug therapy response. Offer frequent rest periods in a quiet environment. Suggest dressing in light cotton clothing at home. Good hydration is also important. Frequent bathing may temporarily help the symptoms of heat intolerance. Careful hygiene is important if increased perspiration is a problem.
- Stress the importance of good nutrition. Recommend six moderate meals a day to help satiate increased appetite.

Follow-up. Follow up in a manner determined by the pediatric endocrinologist. Perform follow-up for well-child care.

Consultations and referrals

- Refer the child to a pediatric endocrinologist.
- Consult with the school nurse and teachers if schoolwork has been affected. Advise them of the medical reason for the problem.

Resources

Organizations

The American Thyroid Association, Inc., Townhouse Office Park, 55 Old Nyack Turnpike, Suite 611, Nanuet, NY 10954; www.thyroid.org

The Endocrine Society, 4350 East West Highway, Suite 500, Bethesda, MD 20814-4410; (301) 941-0200 or (800) ENDO-SOC; www.endo-society.org

Websites

Karolinska Insitutet (www.mic.ki.se/Diseases//c19.html)

Bibliography

Burgos, R. & Jutte, D. (2000). Residents column: "Doctor, is my child growing ok?" *Pediatric Annals, 29*(9), 585-587.

Hopwood, N.J. (2000). The dilemma of the short child without a clear diagnosis. *Pediatric Annals, 29*(9), 542-546.

Kappy M., Steelman, J.S., Travers, S.H., & Zeitler, P.S. (2001). Endocrine disorders. In Hay, W.W., Hayward, A.R., Levin, M.J., & Sondheimer, J.M. (Eds.). *Current pediatric diagnosis and treatment* (ed. 15). New York: McGraw-Hill.

MacGillivray, MH. (2000). The basis for the diagnosis and management of short stature: A pediatric endocrinologist's approach. *Pediatric Annals, 29*(9), 570-575.

Mansbach, J.M. & Gordon, C.M. (2001). Demystifying delayed puberty. *Contemporary Pediatrics, 18*(4), 43-62.

Samuels, R.C. & Cohen, L.E. (2001). Understanding growth patterns in short stature. *Contemporary Pediatrics, 18*(6), 94-122.

Shankar, R.R. & Pescovits, O.H. (1995). Precocious puberty. *Advances in Endocrinology and Metabolism, 6*, 55-89.

Chapter 34 *Eyes and Ears*

Jane A. Fox & Amy Verst

Cerumen: Impacted or Excessive, p. 378
Ear Pain and Discharge, p. 379
Ear Trauma and Foreign Body, p. 386
Hearing Changes or Loss, p. 387
Blindness and Visual Impairment, p. 389
Eye Deviations, p. 393
Eye Injuries, p. 396
Infections of the Eyelid and Orbit, p. 400
Red Eye, p. 402

Risk Factors

- Neonate, infant, or young child (age-related structural differences)
- Inadequate or no prenatal care
- Prenatal or perinatal maternal infection (e.g., toxoplasmosis, cytomegalic inclusion disease, rubella, herpes, syphilis), toxemia, ingestion of medication (e.g., ototoxic, teratogenic substances), exposure to toxins, and substance abuse (e.g., of alcohol, drugs, tobacco)
- Birth trauma
- Low–birth-weight infant, including prematurity
- Hyperbilirubinemia
- Family history of hereditary hearing or vision problems, amblyopia, or "lazy eye"
- Immunization status incomplete
- Parental concerns about vision, hearing, or language
- Failed vision or hearing screen
- Recurrent ear infections
- History of poor compliance with prescribed medication regimen
- Allergies in family or child
- Respiratory conditions (e.g., hypertrophied adenoids, frequent upper respiratory infections [URIs])
- Trauma
- Spectacle therapy (i.e., glasses) or contact lens use
- Exposure to environmental pollutants (e.g., smoke, excessive noise [from urban living, heavy metal or rock music, heavy machinery, airplanes])
- Acute infection (e.g., rubeola, rubella, mumps, encephalitis, meningitis, varicella)
- Exposure to ototoxic drugs (e.g., kanamycin, streptomycin, neomycin, vancomycin, salicylate [aspirin], diuretics, cisplatin [in chemotherapy])
- Developmental delays
- Skeletal defects or anatomic malformations involving the head and neck (e.g., cleft lip, palate)
- Mental retardation, autism, or severe behavioral problems
- Immunosuppressive therapy or chemotherapy
- Chronic diseases (e.g., rheumatoid arthritis, diabetes mellitus)
- Genetic disorders and syndromes associated with deafness (e.g., Down, Alport, Waardenburg, Hurler, Treacher Collins, Klippel-Feil syndrome; Tay-Sachs disease, osteogenesis imperfecta; fetal alcohol syndrome)
- Attendance in day care
- Participation in contact sports without proper protective equipment
- Pacifier use after 6 months of age

Health Promotion

Prevention of Problems during the Prenatal Period

- Provide early prenatal care.
- Screen pregnant women for prenatal infections (e.g., cytomegalic inclusion disease, herpes, sexually transmitted diseases [STDs], rubella, toxoplasmosis).
- Instruct women in safe sex practices, signs and symptoms of STDs, and the importance of treatment.
- Educate women on the dangerous effects of tobacco, alcohol, and other substances on the fetus.
- Perform a rubella titer for women who do not have documented rubella immunizations or immunity and are considering pregnancy. Give rubella vaccination as recommended by the American Academy of Pediatrics (AAP). Do not give the vaccine to pregnant women. For pregnant women with inadequate immunity, provide the vaccine in the immediate postpartum period. Explain the danger of rubella exposure to a fetus and stress the need to use birth control for 3 months after vaccination.
- Instruct pregnant women on the dangerous effects of medications on the fetus. Stress the importance of notifying all health professionals of being pregnant before any medications, radiographic examinations, or other diagnostic tests are performed.

Prevention of Infections

General

- Advise patients to maintain general health through a well-balanced diet, adequate sleep, careful handwashing, and so on.
- Advise patients should avoid exposure to other people with infections.
- Advise parents to keep children's immunization status current.
- Educate parents on age-related structural differences in the eye and ear.

Ears

- Advise parents to avoid exposing children to second-hand smoke. Encourage parents or caregivers not to smoke near the infant or child. Assist parents in smoking cessation.
- Encourage breastfeeding.
- Instruct parents not to prop a bottle.
- Suggest that parents eliminate pacifier use after 6 months of age because it may increase the risk of ear infections.
- Educate school-age children and adolescents in the dangers of tobacco use.

Eyes

- Advise adolescents considering body piercing to avoid the eyelids. Discuss the danger of infection. Recommend piercing be done only by an experienced technician with disposable needles.
- Instruct patients in the proper care of contact lenses, including regular cleaning.

Early Identification of Problems

Vision problems

- Perform routine vision screening (see Chapter 12).
- Identify populations at risk. Screen these children more frequently. The AAP recommends examining newborns and infants for ocular problems and screening for visual acuity and ocular alignment at 3 to 4 years of age and every 1 to 2 years through adolescence.
- Instruct parents on signs and symptoms of vision problems.

Hearing problems

- Perform routine hearing screen (see Chapter 12).
- Identify populations at risk. Screen these children more frequently. The AAP recommends that hearing be assessed and language skills monitored in children with frequent recurring acute otitis media (AOM) or middle ear effusion persisting more than 3 months. These children can be screened at 16 to 24 months of age. the Early Language Milestone Scale (ELMS; see Appendix A) may be used to monitor language skills.
- Advise parents with a child diagnosed with AOM on the importance of taking all medication as prescribed and the need for follow-up evaluation.
- Instruct parents on the signs and symptoms of hearing problems (Box 34-1).

Injury Prevention

General

- See Chapter 14.
- Review age-appropriate safety concerns at well-child visits.
- Discourage substance abuse and stress never drinking and driving.
- Encourage participation in organized sports and the appropriate use of safety equipment.

Eyes

- Advise children to wear sunglasses that block ultraviolet A (UVA) and ultraviolet B (UVB) radiation to protect their eyes when exposed to sun.
- Advise children to wear helmets when riding bikes, skateboarding, rollerblading, motorcycling, or snowmobiling.
- Advise children to wear eye protection when participating in sports where eyes can be injured or if operating dangerous equipment.

Ears

- Advise parents and children to clean ears gently and not to put any objects into the ear canal.
- Advise children to wear ear protection when participating in sports where ears can be injured or if operating dangerous or loud equipment.
- Reduce exposure to loud environmental noises (e.g., loud music). This can cause high-frequency hearing loss.

Box 34-1 Clinical Manifestations of Hearing Impairment

Infants

Lack of startle or blink reflex to a loud sound
Failure to be awakened by loud environmental noises
Failure to localize a source of sound by 6 months of age
Absence of babble or inflections in the voice by 7 months of age
General indifference to sound
Lack of response to the spoken word; failure to follow verbal directions
Response to loud noises as opposed to voices

Children

Use of gestures rather than verbalization to express desires, especially after 15 months of age
Failure to develop intelligible speech by 24 months of age
Monotone quality, unintelligible speech, or lessened laughter
Vocal play, head banging, or foot stamping for vibratory sensation
Yelling or screeching to express pleasure, annoyance (e.g., tantrums), or need
Asking to have statements repeated or answering them incorrectly
Responding more to facial expression and gestures than verbal explanation
Avoidance of social interaction; often puzzled and unhappy in such situations; prefers to play alone
Inquiring, sometimes confused facial expression
Suspicious alertness, sometimes interpreted as paranoia, alternating with cooperation
Frequently stubborn because of a lack of comprehension
Irritable at not making self understood
Shy, timid, and withdrawn
Often appears "dreamy," "in a word of his or her own," or markedly inattentive

From Wong, D. (1999). Nursing care of infants and children (6th ed.). St. Louis: Mosby.

Subjective Data

- Age, sex, and race
- Reason for visit and description of problem
- Onset and surrounding circumstances
- Recent trauma, foreign body, or infection
- Parental concerns about vision or hearing
- Recent use of chemicals (e.g., hair spray, hair dyes)
- Frequent swimming
- Associated symptoms (describe):
  Ear—Pain, tenderness, discharge (including odor), pruritus (itching), pulling or tugging on ears, headache, facial asymmetry, stiff neck, tinnitus (ringing in ears), vertigo (dizziness), URI
  Eye—Pain, discharge, vision changes (e.g., difficulty focusing, blurred vision), unusually large eyes, photophobia (sensitivity to light), excessive tearing, cloudy appearance, inflammation, abnormal movements, constant deviation of one eye
  Other—Fever, headache, irritability, swollen glands, rash
- Past history, including eye or ear injury, infection, or head trauma (with details of the treatment given and results obtained); perforated tympanic membrane; infections or serious illnesses: meningitis, encephalitis, measles, mumps,

frequent URIs, or chronic nasal congestion (with details of the treatment given and results obtained); genetic disorders, chronic diseases, or craniofacial abnormalities; vision or hearing problems (e.g., amblyopia) (with details of testing and results obtained); and exposure to ototoxic drugs (e.g., kanamycin, neomycin)

- Prenatal history, including maternal infection (e.g., rubella, herpes, cytomegalic inclusion disease, toxoplasmosis, syphilis, gonorrhea) and use of ototoxic drugs
- Neonatal history, including birth weight, neonatal problems, and any perinatal infection or asphyxia
- Developmental history, including milestones (e.g., delays in fine motor, gross motor, social, speech or language skills; social or reciprocal smile; social adjustment) and information on the child's hearing, speech, and vision. Ask parents about the following to assess hearing and speech:

  Newborn to 4 months—Quieted by parent's voice; reacts to loud or sudden noises; responds to social gestures with a smile

  4 to 8 months—Turns head in direction of sound; recognizes mother's voice; babbles and coos; responds to environmental sounds

  8 to 12 months—Turns directly to sounds; makes varied noises; imitates simple sounds; responds to "no-no," "bye-bye" and own name

  Toddler (1 to 3 years of age)—Points to familiar objects or body parts; says single words; follows simple commands

  Preschool (3 to 5 years of age)—Uses consonants as well as vowel sounds; speaks intelligibly to parents and others; listens to the radio or television at normal volume levels

  School-age child (5 years and older)—Is attentive in school; follows directions given by the teacher; has good voice quality; uses clear, easily understood speech; shows normal speech pattern for age and developmental level

  To assess vision, ask parents about the following:

  Infant and toddler—Shows responsiveness to parents; shows child's behavior when approached in crib; maintains eye contact and motor excitation versus no eye contact and motor quieting; grasps objects and reaches out for parents; visually searches for sound cues; stumbles or falls easily or knocks into things frequently

  Preschool and school-age child—Holds objects close to the eyes; sits close to the television; has difficulty seeing the blackboard; reads with difficulty

- Medications, especially ototoxic drugs
- Allergies, especially allergic rhinitis or conjunctivitis
- Hospitalizations, including any infections (e.g., meningitis) and surgery
- Immunization history (e.g., of *Haemophilus influenzae* type B [Hib] disease; *Streptococcus pneumoniae* [pneumococcal] pyogenic disorders; measles, mumps, rubella [MMR]), including dates
- Family history, including genetic disorders, chronic diseases, hearing problems, vision problems (e.g., amblyopia, glasses), and allergies
- Social history, including living conditions, pets, emotional or behavioral problems, exposure to smoke, constant exposure to loud noises, attendance in day care or school
- Sports participation, including use of protective equipment
- Alcohol, tobacco, or other substance use

Objective Data

Physical Examination

A complete physical examination should be performed on all infants and young children and include the following general procedures:

- Determine vital signs, including temperature.
- Measure height, weight, and head circumference and plot on an appropriate graph.

  To assess the eyes:
- Perform functional tests first (they are like games to young children), then do the external tests.
- Test visual acuity.
- Inspect extraocular muscle function. Check the corneal light reflex with Hirschberg's method; instruct the child to stare straight ahead while a light is held 12 inches away. Notice the reflection of the light on the corneas; it should be in the same spot in both eyes. Perform the alternative cover test (also known as the *cover-uncover test*) by having the child fixate on an object or stare straight ahead. Cover one eye without touching it and then watch for movement when it is uncovered. Any movement may indicate strabismus. Next, check the child's ability to follow an object in the six cardinal positions of gaze; there should be parallel tracking of the object with both eyes. After each position, return to the center and observe for nystagmus (fine lateral movements).
- Inspect the external structures of the eyes (i.e., the eyebrows, eyelids, eyelashes, eyeballs) for size, shape, and symmetry. Inspect the iris, sclerae, pupils, conjunctivae, and lids. Observe for erythema, discharge, or lid swelling. Notice any pallor near the outer canthus of the lower eyelid, which may be a sign of anemia.
- Palpate the lacrimal sac (punctum) by pressing against the sac just inside the lower orbital ring. This may produce a "pop" of retained secretions from the lacrimal sac, which is diagnostic of an obstructed nasolacrimal duct.
- Test for the pupillary light reflex. Darken the room and have the child look into the distance. This causes the pupils to dilate. Shine a light from the side and observe the pupil response. Normally there will be constriction of the same-sided pupil (a direct light response) and a simultaneous constriction of the other pupil (consensual light reflex) is observed.
- Test for accommodation. Have the child focus on a distant object, which should cause the pupils to dilate. Then have the child shift the gaze to a near object (3 inches away). Observe constriction of the pupils. The normal response is charted as *pupils equal, round, react to light, accommodate* (PERRLA).
- Check for the red reflex.
- Perform a funduscopic examination. This is often difficult with infants and young children. Have the child focus on a distant, fixed object. (A toy can be used for infants and young children.) Focus on the orange-colored retina (following the red reflex) and vessels. Observe for color, hemorrhages, and exudate.
- Inspect the optic disk (observing color, shape, and margins), retinal vessels, and macula.

To assess the cranial nerves (CNs), remember that:

- CN II (the optic nerve) is necessary for vision and transmits visual signals. Test it by assessing visual acuity and visual fields and performing funduscopic examination.
- CNs III, IV, VI (the oculomotor, trochlear, and abducens nerves) innervate all eye muscles and control pupil reaction (constriction and dilatation) and elevation of the eyelids. Test them by assessing the pupils (looking for PERRLA) and extraocular movements and observing for nystagmus.
- CN VIII (the acoustic nerve) controls hearing and balance. Assess by testing hearing acuity.

To assess the ears:

- Inspect the external ears for pinna formation, placement, and patency of the canals. Note pain on movement of the pinna or tragus. Note any swelling, redness, or discharge.
- For otoscopic examination (possibly best if done last for an infant or young child), use an otoscope with a bright light and pneumatic bulb attachment. Choose the largest speculum that fits in the canal without causing pain; this helps to obtain a secure seal. Stabilize the child's head to protect the canal and tympanic membrane from injury with sudden head movement. Gently pull the earlobe straight down on an infant or child under 3 years of age; pull the pinna up and back on older children. Observe any swelling, lesions, redness, foreign bodies, or discharge in the external canal. Observe the color and odor of discharge, if present. Carefully inspect the landmarks of the tympanic membrane. Observe the color and characteristics. The cone-shaped light reflex, a reflection of the otoscope light, should be visualized in the anteroinferior quadrant. Inspect the entire tympanic membrane for perforations.
- Perform pneumoscopy. Ensure a good seal first; then gently blow or squeeze air into the auditory canal through a pneumatic tube attached to the otoscope to determine the mobility of the tympanic membrane. A normal tympanic membrane moves inward with the air puff and outward when the bulb is released.
- Use a tuning fork (512 Hz) to distinguish between conductive and sensorineural hearing loss.
- Perform the Weber test. Place the stem on the midline of the scalp. The sound should be heard equally in both ears. In the presence of conductive loss, the sound is lateralized to the involved side.
- Perform the Rinne test. Place the stem of the tuning fork on the mastoid until sound is no longer heard. Hold the fork 1 to 2 inches in front of the pinna. Air conduction is greater than bone conduction (AC > BC). The child should be able to hear the fork when placed beside the ear, producing a positive Rinne test result. If the sound is heard longer at the mastoid, the Rinne test result is negative.

Other examination procedures should include

- Inspect the nares for patency, color, and condition of mucosa. Note any "allergic salute" if present.
- Inspect the mouth and throat, as the child may have referred pain.
- Palpate and transilluminate the frontal and maxillary sinuses.
- Inspect and palpate the mastoid process and cervical nodes for tenderness and swelling.
- Auscultate the heart for murmurs.
- Auscultate the lungs for wheezes, crackles, or other adventitious sounds.
- Perform a neurologic examination:
- Check Babinski reflex.
- Check for neck rigidity, if indicated (Box 34-2).

Diagnostic Procedures and Laboratory Tests

Ears. *Tympanometry* is used to detect fluid in the middle ear and to determine the mobility of the tympanic membrane. An electroacoustic impedance bridge is used to measure the compliance of the tympanic membrane. A tight seal is necessary. Results are displayed in graphic form (i.e., tympanogram). This test does not measure hearing but the ability of the ossicular complex to reflect or absorb sound. It is most reliable in children over 6 months of age. The basic types of tympanograms can be seen in Fig. 34-1.

Acoustic reflectometry, or *sonar impedance analysis,* is used as an alternative or adjunct to immittance measures to detect middle ear effusion. The tip of an acoustic otoscope is inserted into the ear canal. The device then emits multifrequency sound and measures the incident and reflected sound in the canal. An airtight seal is not required as it is with tympanometry.

Conventional, or *pure tone, audiometry* defines a hearing loss as conductive or sensorineural (see Chapter 12). Each ear is tested separately at the following frequencies: 1000, 2000, and 4000 Hz. Results are interpreted as follows: 0 to 25 dB (normal); 26 to 40 dB (mild loss); 41 to 55 dB (moderate loss); over 55 dB (severe loss). Games may be used to elicit responses in preschool children. Older children should be instructed to raise a hand when a stimulus is heard.

Electrophysiologic audiometry measures the electrophysiologic response of the auditory system to sound. The auditory brainstem response (ABR) test or brainstem auditory evoked response (BAER) audiometry evaluates the hearing threshold and provides an assessment of the integrity of the auditory pathway. This test can be done on any child; it is painless and reliable, and the results are not affected by the child's state of arousal. ABR is currently viewed as the standard for physiologic testing during infancy and the most accurate available method for determining hearing function.

High-risk register (HRR) is another screening test for neonates. This is a specific list of clinical risk factors associated with high rates of impaired hearing in neonates and infants. Those who meet specific criteria then receive more objective testing, usually the ABR.

Evoked otoacoustic emission (EOE) *testing* is a new screening test for neonates and infants. Otoacoustic emissions are

Box 34-2 Suspected Meningeal Inflammation

If meningeal inflammation is suspected, assess for the following:

- *Kernig sign*—Place the child in the supine position. Flex the leg at the hip and knee and then straighten (extend) the knee and note any pain or resistance, which is suggestive of meningeal inflammation and is a positive Kernig sign.
- *Brudzinski sign*—Place the child in the supine position. Rapidly flex the neck. Note any pain or resistance in the neck and flexion of the hips and knees, which is suggestive of meningeal irritation and is a positive Brudzinski sign.

sounds that are generated by the normal cochlear hair cells and are detectable by simple instrumentation. This test has a high rate of false-positive results.

Computed tomography (CT) *scan* defines the bony structures of all parts of the ear and traces the path of the facial nerve through the temporal bone. This test is beneficial in defining congenital anomalies, fractures, and destructive lesions and may be ordered for a child with a newly diagnosed hearing loss.

Tympanocentesis is a diagnostic procedure in which a needle is placed through the tympanic membrane. It is usually performed by an ear, nose, and throat (ENT) surgeon. This test is definitive in identifying fluid in the middle ear and the causative organism (Box 34-3).

Myringotomy is an incision into the tympanic membrane, with a flap left open through which fluid can drain. This is performed by an ENT surgeon (see Box 34-3).

For language screening, the *Denver II* and *ELM* should be administered. (See Appendix A.)

A *TORCH screen* assays immunoglobulin M (IgM) antibody levels in infants and toddlers to toxoplasmosis, other agents, rubella, cytomegalic inclusion disease, and herpes simplex (i.e., TORCH). It may be ordered to determine the cause of sensorineural hearing loss.

Urine dipstick test for blood and protein provides an assessment of kidney function. This is important if there is a family history of deafness or renal problems or suspicion of a syndrome associated with renal problems; further testing may be indicated.

Culture and sensitivity of discharge should be performed to determine the causative organism and appropriate medication.

Eyes. *Vision screening* has no universally accepted screening test or program. An age-appropriate eye screening chart (e.g., illiterate E, tumbling E charts) should be used, and each eye should be tested separately. Allen and Lea individual cards do not always detect amblyopia and should not be used. The AAP standard for passing vision screening is 20/40 at 3 to 4 years of age and 20/30 over 4 years of age; a difference of two lines between eyes requires referral.

Stereopsis is the use of the two eyes for depth perception. Normal stereopsis signifies good vision in each eye and normal alignment. The presence of normal stereopsis alone constitutes sufficient screening; measurement of monocular visual acuity may not be needed. Screening is done using the Random Dot E test.

Photoscreening detects amblyogenic conditions, not amblyopia. Its interpretation is somewhat variable, so it is not endorsed at this time.

Herpesvirus antigen direct fluorescent antibody test identifies herpes simplex virus (HSV) type 1 or 2. Scrapings of a lesion from the conjunctiva or the discharge can be obtained to detect the antigen of HSV. Results are available in 24 hours, much faster than a viral culture.

Viral culture of aspirates should be performed if HSV is suspected. Nasopharyngeal culture is done if chlamydiosis is suspected.

Giemsa stain of the conjunctival scraping or *immunofluorescent monoclonal antibody stains* are needed if chlamydiosis is suspected.

Chest radiographic examination detects pneumonia in infants with neonatal conjunctivitis and respiratory symptoms.

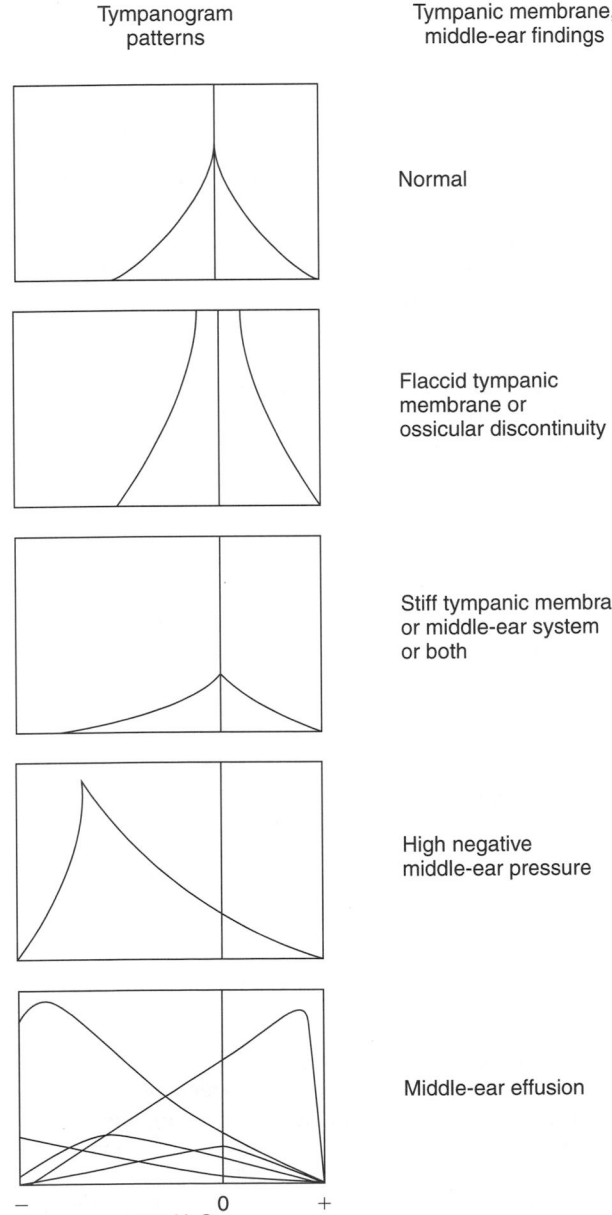

Tympanogram patterns

Tympanic membrane, middle-ear findings

Normal

Flaccid tympanic membrane or ossicular discontinuity

Stiff tympanic membrane or middle-ear system or both

High negative middle-ear pressure

Middle-ear effusion

− 0 +
mm H₂O

Fig. 34-1 Examples of tympanograms related to tympanic membrane compliance and middle-ear pressure (mm H_2O). (From Bluestone, C.D. [1981]. *Pediatric Clinics of North America, 28,* 727.)

Box 34-3 Indications for Tympanocentesis or Myringotomy

Symptomatic infants under 8 weeks of age
OM in a child with severe ear pain or a toxic appearance
Immunocompromised child
Unresponsive to appropriate therapy for OM
Mastoiditis
CNS infection
Facial palsy

Box 34-4 Fluorescein Staining to Assess Corneal Epithelial Integrity

Technique

Instill 1 or 2 drops of a rapid onset and short duration topical anesthetic (e.g., proparacaine Hcl 0.5% [Ophthetic]).

Moisten the fluorescein strip with sterile normal saline (can also touch the trip to the tear film in the lower cul de sac of the affected eye).

Touch the moistened fluorescein strip to the lower conjunctiva of the eye being inspected. (If tear film was used to moisten, this step is unnecessary because dye has already been placed in the eye.)

Ask the patient to blink the eye.

Illuminate the eye with cobalt blue light and inspect for patterns of fluorescence.

Remove excess dye with sterile saline and remind the patient not to rub the eye.

Interpretation

If the corneal epithelium has been disturbed, fluorescein will pool within these areas and stain the hydrophilic stroma. The resultant brighter fluorescence of these pools will delineate the corneal abrasion from surrounding intact epithelium.

The size and pattern of the defect depends on the nature and extent of the injury.

A characteristic pattern that suggests the presence of a foreign body trapped underneath the upper lid is a faint vertically oriented pattern on the cornea.

From Uphold, C. & Graham, M. (1998). Clinical guidelines in family practice (2nd ed.). Gainesville, FL: Barmarrae Books.

Fluorescein staining provides an assessment for corneal abrasion (Box 34-4).

Gram stain and culture of eye discharge are essential for neonates.

Cerumen: Impacted or Excessive

JANE A. FOX

Alert

Consult with or refer to a physician for any child unable to cooperate with a removal procedure or when visualization of the tympanic membrane is essential (e.g., otitis media [OM] suspected)

Etiology

Cerumen, or earwax, has a protective effect on the ear canal. It is produced by the cerumen glands located in the outer portion of the external canal. Overzealous cleaning of the ear canal by parents with a cotton-tipped applicator is the most common cause of impacted cerumen. Narrow ear canals and dermatologic conditions of the preauricular skin and scalp may also cause excessive cerumen.

Incidence

- Common in children with Down syndrome
- May be found in children with ear infections

Risk Factors

- Using cotton-tipped applicators to clean ears
- Down syndrome or other conditions associated with ear problems
- Past history of impacted cerumen
- Otitis externa
- Narrow ear canals

Differential Diagnosis

Excessive cerumen often arises from normal individual variants. The history may reveal overzealous attempts at cleaning the ears. A child may complain of the ears feeling clogged, decreased hearing, or itching. Impacted cerumen may cause otitis externa. Cerumen that impinges on the tympanic membrane may cause a chronic cough that continues until the cerumen is removed. The otoscopic examination usually reveals a large plug of cerumen that prevents visualization of the tympanic membrane. Otitis externa can be ruled out when movement of the tragus does not elicit pain.

Management

Treatments and medications. When visualization of the tympanic membrane is essential (e.g., with a child having a URI, fever, or decreased hearing), the cerumen must be removed. If there is no urgency, recommend instillation of 3 or 4 drops of mineral oil or olive or vegetable oil or instill hydrogen peroxide in the ear for 2 to 3 days to soften the wax. Advise doing this each night for several days followed by insertion of a cotton wick to prevent the oil from dripping out of the ear. If the tympanic membrane must be visualized and there is hard cerumen blocking the canal, place 2 or 3 drops of mineral oil or hydrogen peroxide or docusate disodium (Colace) in the canal to soften the wax. Leave for 20 minutes and then attempt removal.

Earwax can best be removed by two methods: water pressure and curettes. A plastic ear curette can be used to gently remove the wax. Assess progress frequently using the otoscope. Another method for cerumen removal is to gently irrigate the ear canal with tap water at normal body temperature (to avoid vertigo). Never irrigate if a patent tympanostomy tube is in place or if perforation of the tympanic membrane is known or suspected. Explain the procedure and demonstrate all equipment, and instruct the child not to move. Young children may need to be restrained so that the head cannot move. The tubing from a butterfly needle or a dental Water Pik set on low pressure (setting 1 or 2) may be used. Cover the child's shoulder with a towel and place a kidney basin under the ear to collect the draining water. Carefully assess progress with the otoscope. Do not continue if significant pain or bleeding occurs. The cerumen plug may become dislodged intact, but more often the draining water will be yellow tinged. If otitis externa or OM is present, treat appropriately.

Counseling and prevention

- Explain the removal process to the parents and child. Also explain that it is uncomfortable but not painful and that some bleeding is possible. Demonstrate all equipment before use. The child's cooperation is essential.
- Instruct that the outer ear can be cleansed using a washcloth, but no attempt should be made to clean inside the ears. Nothing should be put into the ear canal.
- Demonstrate how to instill mineral oil or peroxide into the canal.

- Advise against using cerumen solvents, and explain that cerumen is normal and protects the canal.
- Recommend instillation of 2 or 3 drops of hydrogen peroxide, mineral oil, or baby oil in the ears twice a week if impaction is a recurring problem.
- Inform the parents and child that if hearing was decreased because of impacted wax, it should return to normal after removal.
- Stress the importance of proper treatment if infection is present.

Follow-up. No follow-up examination is needed except for well-child visits or if pain develops.

Consultations and referrals. No consultations or referrals are necessary.

Ear Pain and Discharge

JANE A. FOX

Alert

Consult with or refer to a physician for the following:
- Signs of meningitis (e.g., full, tense, or bulging fontanel; stiff neck; severe headache; lethargy; irritability; high-pitched cry)
- Head trauma
- Clear or bloody ear drainage
- Infant less than 2 months old
- Severe pain
- Hearing loss or delayed speech
- Child whose condition worsens after 24 hours with treatment or does not improve within 48 hours with treatment
- Three ear infections in 6 months or four episodes in 12 months
- Craniofacial abnormalities (e.g., cleft palate, Down syndrome)
- Mastoid tenderness
- Cholesteatoma
- Chronic perforation of the tympanic membrane
- Child with chronic illness or who is immunosuppressed (e.g., with human immunodeficiency virus [HIV], cancer, chemotherapy, long-term steroid use)

Ear pain and discharge may be caused by many factors. The most common involve the external canal and middle ear. (See also Ear Trauma and Foreign Body and Cerumen: Impacted or Excessive in this chapter.)

Etiology

External canal. *Pseudomonas aeruginosa* is the most common bacterium to cause infection in the external ear canal. Streptococci, *Staphylococcus epidermidis*, protei, and mycoplasmas may also be causative agents. Fungi (aspergilli and *Candida* organisms) and viruses (herpesviruses) may cause pain or discharge in the external ear canal. Trauma caused by digital irritation or foreign body should be suspected, especially if indicated in the history. Other causes include an allergic reaction to chemical or physical agents (e.g., Cerumenex drops, detergents, hair sprays, chemical hair treatments, pigments in clothing); metallic, plastic, or rubber compounds; excessive wetness caused by swimming, bathing, or high humidity; excess cerumen or loss of protective cerumen after exposure of the canal to excessive moisture; stress; or excessive dryness (eczema) if the child or family has a positive history.

Middle ear. *S. pneumoniae* is the most common causative organism of middle ear infections in children and is responsible for about 40% of the cases, or approximately 7 million middle ear infections a year. Nontypeable *Haemophilus influenzae* causes about 27% of the bacterial otitis. Less frequent pathogens include *Moraxella (Branhamella) catarrhalis* and group A β-hemolytic streptococcus. *Staphylococcus aureus* and *P. aeruginosa* are both common in chronic serous OM, especially if a perforation of the tympanic membrane is present. Group A β-hemolytic streptococcus, *Escherichia coli*, and *S. aureus* are more common in neonates. Viruses, particularly respiratory syncytial virus (RSV), influenza virus (types A and B), and adenovirus, put children at risk by possibly impairing eustachian tube function. The increased susceptibility of infants to OM may be caused by the short horizontal position of the eustachian tube. Viruses may be involved in about 40% of cases of AOM, and bacterial resistance is an increasing problem in AOM. Certain strains of *H. influenzae* and most strains of *M. catarrhalis* are resistant to amoxicillin because of β-lactamase production. Another concern is drug-resistant *S. pneumoniae* (DRSP), which has significantly increased in the United States in the past few years. The groups most at risk for DRSP are: (1) children under 24 months of age, (2) those who have recently received β-lactam drugs, were recently treated with antibiotics, or had a recent ear infection, (3) children exposed to large numbers of other children (e.g., those children 2 months to under 5 years of age in day care) or to household crowding after 2 years of age, and (4) those with immune deficiencies (e.g., sickle cell disease, HIV, malignancy). The proportion of penicillin-resistant *S. pneumoniae* strains may be 40% to 50%, and half of these may be highly resistant.

The causes of otitis media with effusions (OME) are multifactorial. They include infection, eustachian tube dysfunction (ETD), and allergies. The most common bacteria found in OME are the same as those for AOM except that the relative frequency of *H. influenzae* is greater in OME than in AOM.

Incidence

- After URI, OM is the most common disease of childhood; its peak prevalence is from 6 to 36 months of age. The incidence declines at about 6 years of age.
- The incidence of OM has dramatically increased during the past 25 years. Most of the increase has been in children younger than 2 years of age.
- OM is the leading reason for the prescription of antibiotics in children.
- By 3 years of age most children have had at least one acute infection, and one third have had three.
- The incidence of OM is highest in winter and spring, which is related to the prevalence of URIs.
- Children who have their first episode of OM early in life are at increased risk for developing chronic ear disease.
- OM is more common in boys than in girls.
- Caucasians, Alaska Natives, and Native Americans have a higher incidence than African Americans.
- OM is more frequent in low-income and large families.
- Those who are immunocompromised, including those with acquired immune deficiency syndrome (AIDS), have a higher incidence of OM.
- Smoking in a household increases the incidence of OM.
- Bottle-fed infants have a higher incidence of OM than breastfed infants.
- The incidence and prevalence of otorrhea increases the longer a child has tympanostomy tubes in place. In one

study, over 83% of children experienced at least one episode of otorrhea if their tubes remained in place for at least 18 months.

Risk Factors

- Under 2 years of age
- Day care attendance
- Male
- Previous history of ear infections
- Native American ancestry
- Conditions that cause ETD or eustachian tube obstruction (ETO) (e.g., allergic rhinitis, URIs, craniofacial abnormalities)
- Bottle-feeding (because breastfeeding for the first 6 to 12 months of life seems to protect against OM, probably because of passive immunity from the mother)
- Inadequate or incomplete immunizations
- Feeding in the supine position
- Bottle-propping
- Secondary smoke
- Use of a pacifier after 6 months of age
- Poor nutrition
- Immunocompromised state
- Iron deficiency anemia
- Children with low birth weights or those born very prematurely
- Tympanostomy tubes in place 18 months or longer
- Crowded living conditions
- Family history of frequent ear infections (i.e., in parents or siblings)
- Winter and early spring
- Recent or existing URI
- Siblings at home
- Low socioeconomic status
- Large family size
- History of allergies: parent or child
- Cleft palate
- Down syndrome

Differential Diagnosis

External ear and canal. Any infant or young child with ear pain or discharge requires a complete history and physical examination (see Table 34-1 and the section on Ear Trauma and Foreign Body and Cerumen: Impacted or Excessive in this chapter.) If discharge or pain is related to the external ear canal, also consider the following:

- *Furuncle*—A furuncle is a localized abscess of a hair follicle in the outer part of the external canal. *S. aureus* is usually the cause. The patient has symptoms of pain and possible ear discharge. The abscess is visualized on otoscopic examination.
- *Foreign body or trauma*—See Ear Trauma or Foreign Body, later in this chapter.
- *Otitis externa*—Otitis externa, or swimmer's ear, is an inflammation or infection of the external ear canal. The child usually experiences a sudden onset of pain, especially when the ear is touched or the earlobe is moved. Hearing loss (caused by debris or edema of the canal) or a feeling of the ear being blocked or clogged are also frequent symptoms. On examination there is pain on movement of the pinna or when pressure is applied to the tragus and when the speculum is inserted into the canal. The external canal is red and swollen, and there may be discharge.

Middle ear. Distinguishing between AOM and OME is critical (Table 34-2). The child with AOM has otalgia and fever,

Table 34-1 Differential Diagnosis: Ear Pain (388.70) or Discharge (388.60)—External

CRITERIA	FURUNCLE OR ABSCESS	OTITIS EXTERNA
ICD-9 code	680.	380.10
Subjective Data		
Age	Any	Any; in infants, may see bottle-in-crib—bacterial growth caused by milk dribbling into ear canal and keeping it moist
Pain	Yes	Yes, especially with movement of earlobe or when ear is touched
Associated symptoms	Possible discharge	Pruritus of ear canal, sensation of fullness in affected ear (early symptoms); hearing loss (often presenting symptom); discharge
Related history	Usually none	May report allergies; frequent swimming (fresh water or pools in winter); frequent showers and shampoos; use of hair sprays, earplugs; ear trauma; excessive cerumen; history of otitis externa or OM with perforation
Systemic symptoms	Usually none	Rare
Objective Data		
Physical examination		
Temperature	Usually normal	Usually normal
External canal	Abscess visualized	Pain on movement of pinna, when pressure applied to tragus, and when speculum inserted into canal (use smaller size); canal may have erythema, edema, or tissue sensitivity
Discharge	Possible	Foul-smelling, bloody, watery, or purulent
Tympanic membrane	Poorly visualized but normal	Often poorly visualized, may appear inflamed with widespread otitis externa; may be perforated if secondary to OM
Lymph nodes	Preauricular or postauricular may be enlarged	Enlarged preauricular or postauricular, or anterior cervical
Laboratory data	Usually none	Culture and sensitivity of discharge if unresponsive to treatment

Table 34-2 Differential Diagnosis: Middle Ear Infections

CRITERIA	ACUTE OTITIS MEDIA (AOM)	CHRONIC OTITIS MEDIA (OTITIS MEDIA WITH EFFUSIONS [OME], SEROUS, NONSUPPURATIVE)
ICD-9 code	382.9	381.01 (381.00)
Subjective Data		
Age/gender	Most common 2 years of age and younger, decreases after 7 years of age; more common in males	Any age, but usually under 15 years; more common in males
Onset	Acute	Gradual, insidious
Presenting complaints	Usually ear pain and fever; pulling, rubbing, or tugging at affected ear in infant or young child; occasionally asymptomatic	Often asymptomatic; may present with hearing loss, clogged ear, crackling sensation in ear, ear feeling plugged
Ear pain	Present in 80% of those with OM	Little or none
Associated symptoms	May report the following: fever (present in 50% of cases); irritability, disturbed sleep; restlessness, rhinorrhea or URI, cough; malaise, sore throat, stiff neck, refusal of bottle by infant, change in eating habits, vomiting or diarrhea	May report turning volume up loud on television, not seeming to hear or pay attention to parents or teachers
Pertinent history	May report the following: recent URI, previous ear infections, allergies, child taking bottle to bed or infant fed supine with bottle propped or flat on mother's lap, sick siblings at home	May report the following: language or speech delays; poor school performance; history of frequent OM; allergies, especially allergic rhinitis; failure of hearing screen at school
Family history	Allergies; frequent OM in siblings	Allergies
Objective Data		
Physical examination		
Fever	Common	Usually none
Irritability	Yes	No
General appearance	May appear toxic	Normal
Nose	May have red and edematous nasal mucosa with thick nasal discharge (URI) or pale and boggy nasal mucosa with clear, watery discharge (allergies)	Possible indicators of allergies: allergic salute; nasal mucosa pale and boggy with clear watery discharge; possible enlarged adenoids
Throat	May be red with enlarged tonsils, pharyngitis	May have enlarged tonsils
Neck	Cervical nodes often enlarged	May have cervical lymphadenopathy
Heart	Normal, heart rate elevated with fever	Normal
Neurologic examination	Normal	Normal
Ear examination (may want to perform last if pain present)		
External canal	If discharge, may have perforation	May have discharge (which must be removed)
Tympanic membrane	Full or bulging (usually regarded as defining AOM with or without systemic symptoms); absent or obscured bony landmarks; erythema of the drum an inconsistent finding; decreased or absent mobility	Usually opaque and retracted or convex; may be translucent with air-fluid level of air bubbles present or amber with blue-gray fluid noted; landmarks blurred; decreased or irregular mobility to both negative and positive pressure; Weber test may show lateralization to involved ear
Hearing impairment	Yes	Usually yes
Laboratory data/ diagnostic tests	Presence of fluid in the middle ear indicated by tympanometry	Presence of fluid in the middle ear indicated by tympanometry

while the child with OME is relatively asymptomatic. The following definitions are useful:

- *Otitis media*—OM is a general term referring to an acute or chronic inflammation or infection of not only the middle ear but also the eustachian tube and mastoid.
- *Acute otitis media*—AOM, acute suppurative or purulent OM, is an acute infection of the middle ear often accompanied by fever and ear pain and precipitated by a URI. On otoscopic examination the tympanic membrane is full or bulging, landmarks are absent or obscured, and mobility is decreased or absent on insufflation. AOM can occur with or without effusion. Children whose middle ear isolates grew *S. pneumoniae* are more likely to have a full or bulging tympanic membrane than children with other middle ear fluid pathogens. Of all the bacterial causes of AOM, *S. pneumoniae* is the least likely to resolve without therapy. Persistent AOM is AOM that persists after initial antimicrobial therapy of 10 to 14 days or recurs soon after the infection has appeared to clear. Recurrent OM is defined as frequent episodes of AOM with complete resolution of the disease between episodes. Persistent middle ear effusion is the presence of fluid in the middle ear after antimicrobial therapy and the resolution of acute symptoms. The fluid usually clears within 3 months.
- *Otitis media with effusion*—OME refers to fluid in the middle ear without signs or symptoms of infection. The child is often asymptomatic or may complain of hearing loss. Chronic OME refers to fluid in the middle ear lasting 3 months or longer. The tympanic membrane appears concave or retracted with decreased or irregular mobility. Middle ear effusion (MEE) is evident on pneumatic otoscopy, but there are no signs of acute inflammation.

Perforations of the tympanic membrane. Perforations of the tympanic membrane may be acute or chronic and result from trauma or chronic OM. The symptom is usually a foul-smelling discharge. There is no pain, and fever is rare. The perforation is visualized on otoscopic examination. Small perforations found on the pars flaccida are often difficult to visualize. Any perforation of the tympanic membrane can be associated with a cholesteatoma (an epidermal inclusion cyst of the middle ear or mastoid). Cholesteatoma should be suspected if the discharge is foul smelling and a pearly white mass is seen within the perforation; this requires an immediate referral to an ENT specialist.

Management

External ear

Furuncle or abscess. See Abscesses in Chapter 37.

Treatments and medications. A broad-spectrum systemic antibiotic such as cephalexin 50 mg/kg per day in four divided doses or dicloxacillin 12.5 to 25 mg/kg per day in four divided doses for 10 days may be prescribed. Referral for incision and drainage may be needed. Acetaminophen and warm soaks may be recommended for discomfort.

Counseling and prevention
- Describe the cause of pain or drainage.
- Explain the treatment plan and review medications.
- Discuss the need for incision and drainage, if indicated.
- Advise parents to telephone if the pain does not improve.

Follow-up. A return visit should be scheduled symptoms worsen or do not improve within 48 hours. Parents should telephone if pain is severe.

Consultations and referrals. Refer the child to an ENT surgeon if incision and drainage are indicated.

Otitis externa
Treatments and medications
- Clean all debris from the canal.
- Gently irrigate the canal with warm water or saline.
- If edema and inflammation of the canal prevent the passage of antibiotic drops, a small gauze wick or absorbent sponge can be inserted into the external canal to carry antibiotic corticosteroid solution into the canal. Have the parent place antibiotic drops on the wick for 2 days. The wick is then removed and drops continued for another 8 days. Ciprofloxacin hydrochloride/hydrocortisone otic suspension (Cipro HC otic) has a broad spectrum for covering resistant organisms. A steroid should be used, especially if the canal is swollen, because it decreases the edema, lessens pain, and may help with compliance. Another choice is combination eardrops of antibiotics, hydrocortisone, and propylene glycol, which help treat the infection and reduce inflammation. The antibiotic-corticosteroid solution may contain neomycin, polymyxin, and hydrocortisone. Neomycin allergy is of concern because it may appear as persistent otitis externa. Another option is ofloxacin solution 0.3% otic drops (Floxin) every 12 hours; this is highly effective for otitis externa caused by *P. aeruginosa* and *S. aureus* in patients 1 year of age and older.
- Prescribe analgesics for pain. Acetaminophen or ibuprofen may be used, but use narcotic preparations sparingly.
- Advise the child and parents to keep the ear dry. No swimming is allowed until the infection is resolved, and showers and shampoos should be limited. The ear must be protected, so the cotton coated with petroleum jelly or lamb's wool should be used to occlude the canal while shampooing, removing it immediately. Earplugs should be avoided.
- Do not use cotton swabs.

Counseling and prevention
- Explain the cause to the parents and child.
- Advise that acute pain should subside within 48 hours.
- Instruct on the treatment plan (e.g., the need to keep ears dry) and medications.
- Instruct on how to instill eardrops. Have the child lie on his or her side with the affected ear up. Pull the tip of the auricle up and back (and demonstrate for the parents). Instill the eardrops without allowing the dropper to touch the ear. Have the child remain in this position for at least 5 minutes.
- Explain the name, dose, frequency, and purpose of the medication.
- Advise the parents and child of the side effects of eardrops (e.g., a local stinging or burning sensation, a rash where the drops have come into contact with the skin).
- Stress the importance of taking medications properly and continuing drops for the prescribed time even though the child feels better.
- Advise that recurrences are common. Prevention is the best treatment:
- Keep foreign objects out of the ears.
- After swimming or showering and during hot humid weather, instill 2 or 3 drops of isopropyl alcohol in both canals as prophylactic treatment. Shake excess water out of the ears.

Follow-up
- Immediately recheck the child if pain worsens or if the child develops sensitivity to the eardrops.

- Schedule a return visit in 2 or 3 days if there is noticeable cellulitis or if the tympanic membrane is not visualized.
- Recheck in 10 days. Continue treatment if the infection is not completely resolved and recheck again in 10 days.
- Schedule a return visit if symptoms recur.
- If otitis externa is not greatly improved at the 10-day recheck, culture and sensitivity are required.

Consultations and referrals. Consult a physician in the following situations:

- The symptoms worsen after 24 hours of treatment.
- There is no response to treatment after 2 to 3 days.
- There is visualization of a foreign body that cannot be easily removed.
- The child has a chronic illness or is immunologically depressed.

Also, send a note to the school nurse or the child's teacher if the child's hearing is decreased.

Middle ear

Acute otitis media (Fig. 34-2)

Treatments and medications. Watchful waiting and symptomatic treatment alone for AOM may be an alternative to antimicrobial therapy for children over 2 years of age whose condition is clinically stable and nontoxic. Suggest warm oil ear drops, Auralgan (antipyrine and benzocaine) otic drops, and acetaminophen or ibuprofen. If the child has not improved or the condition has worsened within 24 to 48 hours, antimicrobial therapy should be started. AOM caused by *M. catarrhalis* or *H. influenzae* or from a viral cause are more likely to respond spontaneously than those caused by *S. pneumoniae*. Antibiotic therapy is indicated for symptomatic AOM, particularly in younger children (less than 2 years of age).

Amoxicillin is the first line therapy in patients with no hypersensitivity and in uncomplicated cases despite the prevalence of DRSP. Increases in the initial dosage of amoxicillin may be justified. Prescribe a dose of 40 to 45 mg/kg per day (which may fail to eradicate DRSP) for 5 to 7 days in uncomplicated cases in children over 2 years of age who do not attend day care and have not taken antibiotics within the past 3 months, except in areas of high resistance. For children who attend day care or those patients who have taken antibiotics recently or have a history of recent AOM prescribe amoxicillin 80 to 90 mg/kg per day in two divided doses for 10 days. (Efficacy against *S. pneumoniae* is most important.) It is important is prescribe an adequate dose for the initial treatment of symptomatic children. Treat children who are allergic to penicillin with azithromycin (for children allergic to β-lactam), orally administered cephalosporins (if not allergic to cephalosporins), macrolides, or trimethoprim-sulfamethoxazole (TMP-SMX) (with rates of resistance to pneumococci being high). Continue treatment for 10 days. In cases of documented amoxicillin failure (e.g., persistent fever, ear pain, irritability, tympanic membrane findings of redness, bulging, or otorrhea after 3 days of therapy), second-line therapy should be initiated. Second-line drug therapy must be active against β-lactamase-producing strains of *H. influenzae* or *M. catarrhalis* as well as DRSP. Initiate a second-line antibiotic such as oral amoxicillin clavulanate (Augmentin) given in higher doses of 80 to 90 mg/kg per day of the amoxicillin component; the clavulanate dose should remain at about 10 mg/kg per day, oral cefuroxime axetil (Ceftin) 30 mg/kg per day, or intramuscular (IM) ceftriaxone (Rocephin) for severe infections. Ceftriaxone has the benefit of being given as one injection or three daily injections, thus eliminating concerns about

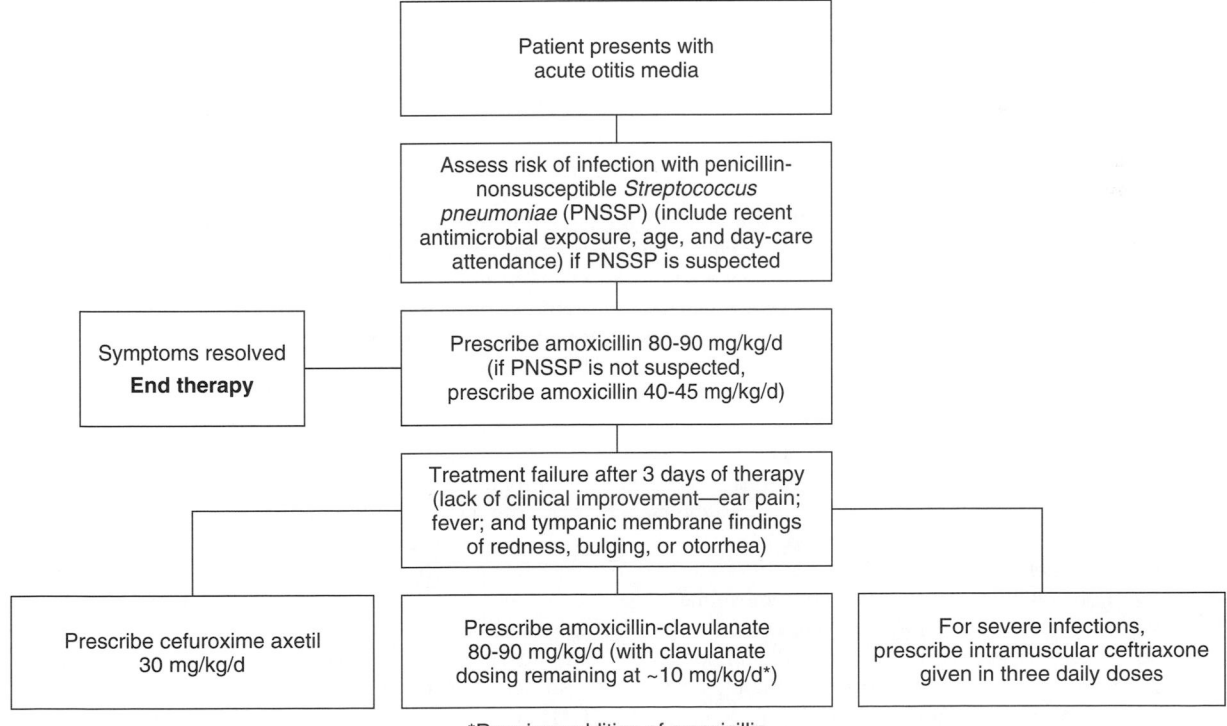

Fig. 34-2 Recommendations from the CDC for the treatment of acute otitis media in an era of pneumococcal resistance. (From Dowell, S.F., Butler, J.C., Giebink, G.S., et al. [1999, January]. *Pediatric Infectious Disease Journal, 18,* 1-9.)

compliance with oral medications. A child who has a recurrence of acute symptoms after a full course of amoxicillin should be retreated with a second-line antibiotic. The first drug of choice is amoxicillin-clavulanate. Oral cephalosporins (except cefuroxime axetil) and macrolides do not provide adequate coverage against resistant strains of *S. pneumoniae*. Administer cephalosporins with caution in those with penicillin allergy because a cross-hypersensitivity among β-lactam antibiotics has been documented in 5% to 10% of children with penicillin allergy. For pain control use warm compresses to the affected ear, an analgesic with antipyretic effects (e.g., acetaminophen, ibuprofen), and eardrops with benzocaine and antipyrine (Auralgan).

Children with frequent AOM should be evaluated for anemia. If iron deficiency is diagnosed (hemoglobin less than 10g/dl), iron supplementation should be started to achieve at least a hemoglobin level of 11g/dl. Persistent AOM is likely to be caused by a pathogen different from the initial infection. Consider treating with an antibiotic other than amoxicillin or ampicillin, such as cefaclor, TMP-SMX, erythromycin-sulfisoxazole, amoxicillin-clavulanate potassium, or cefixime.

With recurrent AOM (because of increasing bacterial resistance), prophylaxis antibiotic therapy should be used carefully and only in select children. The AAP and the Centers for Disease Control and Prevention (CDC) suggest placement of tympanostomy tubes rather than antibiotic prophylaxis. If antibiotics must be prescribed, sulfisoxazole appears to be most effective at preventing recurrences. Administer conjugate pneumococcal vaccine as recommended by the Advisory Committee on Immunization Practices for all infants and children under 2 years of age as well as high-risk children over 2 years of age. Administer *H. influenzae* vaccine in high-risk children. Surgical intervention with insertion of tympanostomy tubes (performed by an ENT surgeon) should be considered in children with chronic middle ear fluid (for 3 months or more) that fails to respond to antimicrobial therapy; children with recurrent AOM; children with suppurative complications; and those with ETD. Adenoidectomy in children over 4 years of age with recurrent AOM is done as a substitute for or in conjunction with insertion of tympanostomy tubes. Adenoid removal helps eliminate obstructing tissue as a source of infection. Tympanocentesis (performed by an ENT specialist) and culture of the exudate should be considered if the diagnosis is uncertain, the child is seriously ill or toxic, the response to antibiotic therapy is unsatisfactory, suppurative complications develop, OM develops in a newborn or in immunologically deficient patients, or AOM develops despite antibiotic therapy.

Counseling and prevention
- Explain to the parents what causes ear infections.
- Identify risk factors and help the parents modify them. Discuss what they can do to prevent ear infections (e.g., breastfeed if at all possible; if bottle-feeding, be sure the infant is not lying flat, and never prop the bottle because this allows milk to get into the eustachian tube; do not smoke in the house with the infant or child; remove the pacifier after 6 months of age; limit exposure to others who are sick; do not allow the child to dive from diving boards or submerge his or her head in water deeper than 2 feet).
- Instruct the parents in the treatment plan.
- Reassure if symptomatic treatment is recommended and stress the importance of a telephone call or return visit if the child's condition does not improve or worsens in the next 24 to 48 hours with antimicrobial therapy.

- If antibiotics are prescribed, emphasize that the antibiotic must be given exactly as prescribed and must not be stopped even if symptoms improve. Review pain relief measures (e.g., acetaminophen or ibuprofen for pain and fever control, antipyrine-benzocaine otic drops [with instructions on how to instill them], propping up the chest and head when the child sleeps, saline nose drops to thin nasal mucus).
- Inform about the need for follow-up care. A return visit is needed after completion of the antibiotics. Instruct on the signs and symptoms that indicate a telephone call or return visit is needed.
- Instruct the breastfeeding mother that the infant may have trouble nursing because of ear pain. Suggest feeding the infant in a semiupright position and expressing milk for a few days.

Follow-up. Infants younger than 3 months of age should routinely be seen in 1 to 2 days because of the increased risk of treatment failure. In children 3 months of age and older, schedule a return visit if there is no improvement in 48 to 72 hours or the child's condition worsens (as this indicates a need to change antibiotics), and schedule a return visit in 4 to 8 weeks to evaluate for OME and reinforce teaching to reduce risk factors. If the infection persists (e.g., persistent AOM), prescribe a second-line antibiotic (as discussed in the Treatments and Medications section) and examine the child every 2 to 4 weeks until the infection clears. If the child has trouble hearing, fevers with or without pain, or signs and symptoms of ear infection, a return visit is indicated.

Consultations and referrals. Consult or refer to a physician in the following situations:
- An infant less than 2 months of age
- Signs and symptoms of meningitis
- Patient unresponsive to appropriate antibiotics in 48 to 72 hours
- More than three episodes of AOM in 6 months or four episodes in 12 months

Also, refer for audiologic testing any child who fails a hearing screen or when hearing loss is suspected. Allow the acute infection to clear before testing.

Otitis media with effusion

Treatments and medications. This is usually not treated unless it becomes chronic. Antibiotic therapy may begin with amoxicillin or ampicillin. However, because of the increasing incidence of β-lactamase–producing strains of causative pathogens, consider beginning with a β-lactamase–resistant antibiotic (Tables 34-3 and 34-4) such as amoxicillin–clavulanate potassium. If the antibiotic trial fails and the child has a 20 dB or greater bilateral hearing loss, he or she should be referred for placement of tympanostomy tubes.

Corticosteroids, antihistamines, or decongestants are not recommended in the treatment of OME. Myringotomy or tympanostomy tubes (bilateral) may be considered in otherwise healthy children 1 to 3 years of age whose OME has lasted 4 to 6 months and who have a hearing deficit of 20 dB or more in the better-hearing ear. Adenoidectomy should be considered only in the presence of an adenoid disorder, and tonsillectomy is not appropriate for treating OME in a child of any age.

Counseling and prevention
- See the discussion of acute OM.
- Explain the diagnosis to the parents and point out that most often OME resolves within 3 months.

Table 34-3 Antibiotics for Acute Otitis Media

DRUG (GENERIC NAME AND TRADE)	DAILY PEDIATRIC DOSAGE
Amoxicillin (Amoxil, Trimox, Wymox)	40-45 mg/kg in three divided doses
Amoxicillin	80-90 mg/kg per day in two or three divided doses
Amoxicillin–clavulanate potassium (Augmentin)	45-90 mg/kg per day of amoxicillin with 6.4 mg/kg per day clavulanate in two divided doses
Ceftriaxone (Rocephin)	50 mg/kg per day, IM once or as three daily doses
Cefuroxime axetil (Ceftin)	125-250 mg twice a day if younger than 13 years; 250-500 mg twice a day if older than 13 years or 30 mg/kg per day
Clindamycin	8-12 mg/kg per day in three divided doses
Erythromycin ethylsuccinate–sulfisoxazole acetyl (Pediazole)	50 mg/kg per day in four divided doses, based on the erythromycin component, every 6 hours

Table 34-4 Antibiotic Susceptibility of Pathogens Common in Persistent AOM*

	PNEUMOCOCCUS			H. INFLUENZAE		M. CATARRHALIS
	PEN^s	PEN^i	PEN^r	β-LAC−	β-LAC+	β-LAC+
High-dose amoxicillin	++++	++++	+++	+++	0	+
High-dose amoxicillin-clavulanate	++++	++++	+++	+++	+++	++++
Ceftriaxone	++++	++++	+++	++++	++++	++++
Cefuroxime	++++	++	0	++++	++++	++++
Cefpodoxime	++++	++	+	++++	++++	++++
Cefprozil	+++	+	0	++	++	+++
Cefaclor	+++	+	0	+++	+++	++++
Loracarbef	+++	0	0	+++	+++	++++
Cefixime or ceftibutin	+++	+	0	++++	++++	++++
Azithromycin	+++	++	+	+++	+++	++++
Trimethoprim-sulfamethoxasole	+++	++	0	+++	+++	+++

Data from Linsk, R, Gilsdorf, J., & Lesperance, M. (1999). When amoxicillin fails. Contemporary Pediatrics, 16(10), 77.

0 = less than 50% effective
+ = 50%-75% effective
++ = 75%-90% effective
+++ = 91%-98% effective
++++ = 98% effective

Pen^s = penicillin-sensitive pneumococcus
Pen^i = penicillin-intermediate pneumococcus
Pen^r = penicillin-resistant pneumococcus
β-lac = β-lactamase

In vitro sensitivity cannot completely predict clinical outcome.

- Instruct in the treatment plan and medications.
- Advise the parents to be aware of the signs of hearing loss.
- Discuss the relationship between speech and language development and hearing.
- Emphasize the importance of follow-up care and testing to evaluate for hearing loss.

Follow-up. Schedule a return visit in 1 month, or sooner if acute symptoms develop. See the child for well-child care.

Consultations and referrals

- Refer for audiologic testing any child who is 1 to 3 years of age with OME for 3 months, fails a hearing screen, or has school or behavior problems related to hearing difficulty.
- Refer the child to an ENT specialist or surgeon if OME does not resolve with appropriate treatment in 3 months or if the child has significant hearing loss on audiometric testing.
- Send a note to the school nurse and the child's teacher explaining that the child has temporary hearing loss.

Perforations of the tympanic membrane and cholesteatoma

Treatments and medications

- For perforations with serous or purulent discharge, prescribe antibiotic-corticosteroid eardrops (because suspensions are less irritating) three times a day for 1 week. Culture the discharge.

- For systemic symptoms, an antibiotic effective against β-lactamase organisms should be prescribed for a 2-week period.

Counseling and prevention

- Explain the condition and carefully review the treatment plan.
- Discuss the relationship between the condition and hearing loss.
- Stress the need for follow-up and the importance of keeping scheduled appointments with specialists.
- Discourage swimming at this time. Diving, jumping into the water, and underwater swimming must be strictly avoided.
- The ears need to be protected before bathing or shampooing. Cotton plugs covered with petrolatum ointment should help keep the ears dry.

Follow-up. Follow-up evaluation may be determined by the specialist; if not, schedule weekly visits until the discharge has cleared. The child should be seen for well-child care.

Consultations and referrals. Refer to an ENT specialist in cases of cholesteatoma (which requires immediate referral) or chronic perforations.

Ear Trauma and Foreign Body

JANE A. FOX

Alert

Consult with or refer to a physician for the following:

- History of significant head trauma
- Clear fluid draining from the ear
- Vertigo
- Ataxia
- Facial paralysis
- Blue or blue-purple tympanic membrane (i.e., Battle sign), raccoon eyes (eyes surrounded by ecchymosis), or bleeding from the ear (which should lead to suspicion of basilar skull fracture)
- Suspected child abuse (i.e., intentional injury)
- Significant hearing loss
- Foreign body that cannot be easily removed, or bleeding or swollen ear canal
- Laceration or hematoma of the pinna
- Alkaline button battery in ear

Etiology

Ear trauma can be divided into external and internal ear trauma. External trauma may be caused by an athletic injury, fall, animal bite, or thermal injury (from heat or cold), resulting in a laceration, hematoma, or burn. Pierced earrings being caught or pulled may lead to tears of the tragus, and infections can result from ear piercing. Internal ear trauma can be further divided into middle and inner ear trauma and frequently results from inquisitive children or their companions placing in the ear objects such as stones, erasers, vegetables (e.g., string beans, peas, beans), paper, pop-apart beads, jelly beans, and small alkaline batteries. Insects may also become lodged in the ear, or chronic irritation or inflammation of the ear (otitis externa) may lead to placement of objects in the ear. Middle ear trauma is often caused by slapping (child abuse), poking, perforations, or barotrauma. Inner ear trauma can be caused by head trauma (concussion) or exposure to loud noise.

Incidence

A foreign body in the ear is most common between 2 and 4 years of age

Risk Factors

- For a foreign body, an age of 2 to 4 years
- Participation in sports without protective head gear
- Neuromuscular disorders (leading to a danger of falling)
- Exposure to loud noises (e.g., being a member of a rock band)

Differential Diagnosis

Trauma. A physical insult to the external ear usually results in injury to the auricle. Athletic injuries, often associated with wrestling and boxing, may cause ecchymosis, hematoma, or seroma of the auricle. The patient's symptom is a painful blue discoloration of the pinna. Hematomas of the external ear appear as smooth masses that distort the contour of the pinna. Animal bites may result in injury to the auricle (see Bites: Animal, Human, Insect and Minor Trauma: Abrasions, Lacerations, Bruises, Puncture Wounds in Chapter 37). Accidental falls may cause abrasions to the external ear. Frostbite and

burns (see Chapter 48) may cause thermal damage to the external ear.

The external ear canal is frequently injured by objects placed in the ear, such as cotton-tipped applicators and bobby pins, to clean the ear (see Cerumen: Impacted or Excessive, in the preceding section). These injuries may cause bleeding and pain. Insects crawling into the ear or foreign bodies placed into the ear by inquisitive children may result in injury to the canal and are visualized on otoscopic examination. Otitis externa and abscess may be present (see Ear Pain and Discharge, earlier in this chapter).

Trauma to the middle ear may cause hemotympanum, or bleeding into the middle ear space, and a conductive hearing loss is noted on physical examination. Barotrauma usually results in a serosanguinous effusion and a moderate to severe conductive hearing loss, and history may indicate recent airline travel or underwater diving. Objects stuck in the ear and blunt trauma may cause perforation of the tympanic membrane. A conductive hearing loss is immediate. Facial nerve paralysis, vertigo, and a sensorineural hearing loss may be noted depending on the structures damaged.

Blunt head insult may cause injury to the inner ear structures, resulting in persistent or transient high-tone sensorineural hearing loss and vertigo. Depending on the structures damaged, the patient may report a sudden onset of vertigo during physical exertion. This indicates a probable perilymph fistula. Fractures of the temporal bone must be considered with bloody or clear (cerebrospinal fluid) otorrhea or facial nerve paralysis. (Immediately refer to a physician.)

Foreign body. The history may reveal that an object was placed in the ear. The child may complain of pain, itching, buzzing (from an insect), a feeling of fullness in the ear, decreased hearing, or discharge from the ear. A foreign object or insect is visualized on otoscopic examination.

Management

Ear trauma

Treatments and medications. Treat minor trauma symptomatically with ice and analgesics (e.g., acetaminophen) for pain.

Counseling and prevention

- Discuss the importance of wearing protective equipment when participating in sports in which ear or other trauma is possible.
- Review age-appropriate injury prevention.
- Explain the treatment plan and need for referral and follow-up care, if indicated.

Follow-up. For minor trauma there is usually no follow-up care. Other care is determined by the consulting physician or specialist.

Consultations and referrals. Refer to an ENT specialist or physician in the following situations:

- History of significant head trauma
- Clear or bloody ear drainage
- Loss of hearing
- Vertigo or ataxia
- Signs of basilar fracture
- Laceration, hematoma, or burn of the pinna

Notify the appropriate local authorities if physical abuse suspected (see Physical Abuse and Neglect in Chapter 47).

Foreign body in the ear canal

Treatments and medications. Extract the foreign object. (If bleeding has occurred, the object must be removed.) Make only one attempt at removal and, if unsuccessful, refer. Have the child lie down and restrain the head if necessary. Do not irrigate if the foreign body is a vegetable or a wood object because it may expand and make removal more difficult, and do not irrigate if perforation of the tympanic membrane is suspected. If an insect is in the ear, it must be killed by filling the ear canal with mineral oil or alcohol before removal. Dislodge ticks by filling the canal with 70% alcohol and then remove. It is best to remove objects using an otoscope with an operating head for visualization. Objects that are soft and unwedged are best removed by irrigation with tepid water (at about body temperature) and a water pik on a low setting or an 18-gauge butterfly catheter with the needle cut off; the pliable tubing can be inserted into the canal behind the foreign body, allowing the pulsating water to help dislodge the object. (See Cerumen: Impacted or Excessive, in the preceding section of this chapter.) If the object does not completely occlude the canal, an ear loop, curette, or forceps can be used.

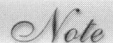

Check all body orifices for foreign objects. After removal of the foreign object, carefully inspect the ear for additional ones.

Counseling and prevention
- Advise parents not to attempt to remove the object.
- Describe the removal process and demonstrate the equipment. Stress that the child must not move his or her head.
- Expect some bleeding.
- Inform the child and parents that any symptoms associated with the foreign object should quickly subside after removal.
- Stress that nothing should ever be put into the ear canal. Advise that cleaning the canal is unnecessary.

Follow-up. Schedule a return visit if symptoms recur, the child complains of ear pain, or there is discharge or other ear symptoms. Follow up for well-child care.

Consultations and referrals. Refer to an ENT specialist or surgeon in the following situations:
- The object is an alkaline button battery. This will cause rapid tissue destruction and ulceration and perforation of the tympanic membrane.
- The object cannot be easily removed, the canal is bleeding or swollen, the object is tightly wedged into canal, or the child is unable to cooperate.

Also, refer to a mental health professional if there is an ongoing history of inserting foreign objects into body orifices.

Hearing Changes or Loss

JANE A. FOX

Alert

Consult with or refer to audiologic evaluation in the following situations:
- Failure in hearing screen
- Infants whose parents suspect a hearing loss
- Delayed speech development
- Lack of response to softer sounds
- Persistent, frequent ear infections
- Infants and children with identified risk factors (e.g., family history of hearing loss during childhood) (see Risk Factors)

Etiology

Hearing deficits can be caused by genetic or hereditary factors, environmental or acquired diseases, or malformations. In almost one third of cases the cause of the hearing impairment is unknown. Congenital cytomegalic inclusion disease and bacterial meningitis cause a significant number of cases. Middle ear effusions and OM and its sequelae frequently cause decreased hearing. Any condition that blocks the ear canal will cause a hearing loss; such conditions include furuncles, cerumen, foreign body, discharge, bony growths, otitis externa, perichondritis, and middle ear anomalies. Congenital causes of hearing impairment include perinatal infections, premature birth, autosomal recessive and dominant inheritance of various deafness syndromes, and meningitis. Continual exposure to high levels of noise can also lead to hearing loss.

Incidence

- Approximately 15% of school-age children have significant conductive hearing losses.
- OM and its sequelae are the most common cause of conductive hearing losses during childhood.
- Profound sensorineural hearing loss occurs in approximately 1 in 1000 children.
- Acquired conductive hearing losses are the most common types of hearing loss in childhood.
- Congenital aural atresia occurs in 1 in 10,000 to 1 in 20,000 live births.
- Hereditary hearing loss occurs in 1 in 4000 live births.
- Hereditary sensorineural hearing loss accounts for 20% to 50% of all cases of severe to profound hearing loss.
- Severe congenital and prelanguage acquired hearing losses occur in 1 in 1000 to 3 in 1000 live births.
- Of children 5 to 8 years of age, 5% to 7% have a 25-dB hearing loss, usually temporary, as a result of OME.
- Deafness occurs in 10% of children diagnosed with meningitis.

Risk Factors

- Family history of hearing loss during childhood or hereditary hearing loss
- Prenatal or perinatal infection (e.g., rubella, cytomegalic inclusion disease, syphilis, toxoplasmosis, herpes)
- Maternal prenatal ingestion of ototoxic or teratogenic drugs
- Malformations involving the head or neck
- Prematurity or birth weight less than 1500 g, or both.
- Birth anoxia as evidenced by an Apgar score of 0 to 5 at 1 minute or less than 6 at 5 minutes, no spontaneous respirations at 10 minutes, or hypotonia persisting longer than 2 hours after birth
- Birth trauma
- Hyperbilirubinemia requiring exchange transfusion (with a bilirubin 20 mg/dl and over)
- More than 24 hours in a neonatal intensive care nursery (NICU)
- Seizures or other neurologic conditions
- History of infection (e.g., sepsis, encephalitis [especially from *H. influenzae*], meningitis, mumps, measles)
- Ototoxic drug exposure (e.g., gentamycin, kanamycin, tobramycin, amikacin, antimalarial drugs [quinine and chloroquine], loop diuretics [ethacrynic acid and furosemide])
- Chronic nasal congestion
- Repeated episodes of OM
- History of head injury

- Incomplete immunization status
- Environmental exposure to continuous loud noise

Differential Diagnosis

A careful history and thorough physical examination, including screening and laboratory data, is essential in identifying those at risk and in the early detection of hearing losses (Box 34-5). Follow screening guidelines at well-child visits. Frequent screening and referral should be initiated for any child with identified risk factors (see Risk Factors). Hearing disorders can be classified into three categories: conductive loss, sensorineural hearing loss, and mixed conductive-sensorineural hearing loss.

Conductive loss, or *middle ear hearing loss,* results from a blockage of the transmission of sound waves from the external ear to the middle ear. It is the most common hearing loss and usually involves an interference with the loudness of the sound. It is characterized by normal bone conduction and reduced air conduction hearing. Causes include middle ear effusions, OM and its sequelae, and blockages of the ear canal (e.g., foreign body, impacted cerumen). These conditions are usually responsive to treatment.

Sensorineural hearing loss, or *perceptive* or *nerve deafness,* comes from a lesion in the cochlear structures of the inner ear or the neural fibers of the acoustic nerve (CN VIII). The most common causes are congenital (e.g., perinatal infections, premature birth, autosomal recessive and dominant inheritance of deafness syndromes) and consequences of acquired conditions (e.g., infection, ototoxic medications, exposure to loud noises). This type of hearing loss results in the distortion of sound and problems in discrimination. Hearing loss often involves high-range frequencies. Children who cannot discriminate high-frequency sounds are unable to perceive consonants. Discrimination and comprehension are severely affected, though the child is able to hear some sounds.

Mixed conductive-sensorineural hearing loss involves a blockage of sound transmission in the middle ear and along neural pathways. This often results from recurrent OME causing damage to the structures of the middle and inner ear. Table 34-5 includes a classification of hearing loss based on symptom severity.

Management

Any child with a suspected hearing loss or identified risk factors should be referred for audiologic testing.

Box 34-5 Assessment of a Child for Suspected Hearing Impairment

History

(See Subjective Data earlier in this chapter.)

Prenatal and perinatal history, including maternal infectious diseases, exposure to ototoxic drugs, other OTC and prescription medications, recreational drug and alcohol use, birth trauma, birth weight, neonatal complications (e.g., jaundice, sepsis, cardiac or respiratory problems, renal disorders, treatments), and NICU stays

Parental concerns about the child's ability to hear, development of language skills, and school or behavior problems

History of ear infections, treatment, and follow-up care

Allergies

History of head or ear trauma

Family history of ear or hearing problems

Physical Examination

(See Objective Data earlier in this chapter.)

Complete examination, with careful attention paid to the following:

- Presence of dysmorphic features
- Size, shape and position of external ear
- Size and shape of external ear canal and any signs of infection or foreign body
- Otoscopic examination, including mobility of the tympanic membrane
- Nares for color and patency
- Sinuses for tenderness
- Oral cavity, noting the number, shape, color, and condition of the teeth, and inspection of the soft and hard palate and pharynx
- Cervical nodes, observing for sinus tracts or embryonic cysts
- Thyroid gland for enlargement or nodules
- Eyes, including visual acuity
- Skin
- Heart for murmurs
- Musculoskeletal and neurologic examination

Laboratory Data

Audiometric testing

Serum TORCH screen (for infants and toddlers)

Serologic test for syphilis (e.g., fluorescent treponemal antibody absorption test) (for older children)

Screening heterophil test (for older children)

Other tests to possibly include:

- CT scan of temporal bones
- Serum chemistry to rule out metabolic disorders
- Electrocardiogram (ECG)
- If renal disease is suspected, complete urinalysis, determination of creatinine level, and abdominal or renal ultrasound examination

---

Table 34-5 Classification of Hearing Loss Based on Symptom Severity

HEARING LEVEL (dB)	EFFECT
Slight; <30 (hard of hearing)	Has difficultly hearing faint or distant speech Usually is unaware of hearing difficulty Likely to achieve in school but may have problems No speech defects
Mild; 30-55 (hard of hearing)	Understands conversational speech at 3 to 5 feet but has difficulty if speech is faint or if not facing speaker May have speech difficulties
Moderate; 55-70 (hard of hearing)	Unable to understand conversational speech unless loud Considerable difficulty with group or classroom discussion Requires special speech training
Profound; 70-90 (deaf)	May hear a loud voice if nearby May be able to identify loud enviornmental noises Can distinguish vowels but not most consonants Requires speech training
Extreme; >90 (deaf)	May hear only loud sounds Requires extensive speech training

From Wong, D. (1999). Nursing care of infants and children, (6th ed.). St Louis: Mosby.

Treatments and medications. Treatment may include medication or surgery for a conductive hearing loss. Amplification (e.g., hearing aids [bilateral is best]) benefits most children. Cochlear implants have shown good results in postlingual children with sensorineural loss if placed within 4 years of hearing loss. Children with identified hearing losses are best managed by an interdisciplinary team. The Food and Drug Administration (FDA) has recently approved the Clarion CII Bionic Ear System for the treatment of deafness. This hardware is able to provide deaf children with more than 10 times more sound than the fastest cochlear implant technology.

Counseling and prevention

- Remember that early detection of hearing loss is imperative. The earlier the hearing impairment occurs, the more serious the consequences can be for language and other development.
- Explain to the parents and child the disease process, type of loss, and causes. Conductive loss is usually reversible, whereas sensorineural loss is often irreversible.
- Discuss with the parents the effect on the child of being hearing impaired, including effects on speech and language development, social development, and the learning process.
- Review the results of the audiogram and explain the technical terminology.
- If the child is prescribed hearing aids, teach about care and function. Inform that hearing aids do not correct the problem or restore normal hearing but amplify remaining hearing.
- Stress to parents the important role they must play in providing stimulation and advocating for their child's education.
- Encourage parents to ventilate and work through their feelings. They need to go through the normal stages of grieving.
- Address the needs of the child:
  Emotional needs—Visual and physical contact is critical. Emphasize to parents that the child is a child first and a child with a hearing impairment second. Stress acceptance of the child and the development of a positive self-image.
  Social needs—The child should have early and continuous contact with hearing children, neighbors, peers, and schoolmates. The child lives in a hearing world and must learn to function within it. Review age-appropriate social expectations and discuss discipline (see Discipline in Chapter 19).
  Educational needs—Early and continuous education and language stimulation are essential for the development of the child's maximum potential. Explain that the child may be taught enhanced methods of communication (e.g., lip reading). The child must learn to watch people's faces. Auditory training may be initiated. Discuss aids in communicating with a deaf child, if indicated. These include attracting the child's attention before speaking; keeping the face visible to the child while one is talking at eye level; using simple, complete phrases with concrete words and specific directions; speaking first and then using a gesture if necessary; using facial expressions; speaking in a clear, distinct voice without exaggerated lip movements; and not shouting at the child. Educate parents and caregivers on the importance of stimulating a deaf child and suggest they use the following techniques: drawing attention to all the sounds in the environment and talking about them; talking more than usual and during all daily activities and explaining everything to the child; talking to the child about what is seen on television or in picture books; and offering positive reinforcement and encouraging the child to talk and make sounds.

- Review the treatment plan, the importance of follow-up care with specialists, and the need to continue with well-child care.
- Address special needs for the hearing-impaired child and interventions to prevent injury (see Chapter 14).
- Instruct the parents that the child should wear a Medic Alert bracelet.
- Recommend that parents attend a support group, offer names of such groups, and so on.

Follow-up. Provide follow up with well-child care and as determined by specialists and interdisciplinary team.

Consultations and referrals

- Refer to an audiologist all children who fail the hearing screen, have frequent or chronic OM, or have facial or external ear deformity.
- Refer to a multidisciplinary team, hearing center, or ENT specialist if hearing impairment is detected.
- Refer for genetic counseling, if indicated.
- Refer to a speech or language therapist.
- Refer to an ophthalmologist for vision testing.
- Remember that infant stimulation programs may be helpful.
- Refer the parents or child to support groups.
- Refer to social services for financial assistance.
- Refer to a mental health professional if counseling is needed.
- Consult with teachers and educational staff if parents desire it.

Resources

Organizations
American Society for Deaf Children (ASDC), PO Box 3355, Gettysburg, PA 17325; (717) 334-7922; www.deafchildren.org

National Association of the Deaf, 814 Thayer Avenue, Silver Spring, MD 20910-4500; (301) 587-1788; www.nad.org

Websites
Agency for Healthcare Research and Quality (ww.ahcpr.gov)

American Academy of Audiology www.audiology.com)

American Academy of Pediatrics (ww.aap.org)

Audiology Net (www.audiologynet.com)

Voice for Hearing Impaired Children (www.voicefordeafkids.com)

Blindness and Visual Impairment

AMY VERST

Alert

Consult with or refer to an ophthalmologist for the following:
- Infant or child who does not have a red reflex
- Sudden loss of vision
- Acute onset of decreased vision
- Sudden onset of diplopia
- Pupils that are not round
- Pupils that do not react to light
- Strabismus
- Pupils that do not accommodate
- Loss of part of the visual field
- Eye pain
- Nystagmus

Etiology

Any interference with an image from the outside to the visual cortex affects the development of vision in a child. It is important to define a child with visual impairments as being blind or having decreased vision. Children with decreased vision have some residual vision to which adaptations or special devices are of assistance, while children who are functionally blind have no residual vision. They can see either nothing or only some light changes and must rely on nonvisual methods to assist them in their activities of daily living. Visual impairment may be caused by congenital defects (e.g., congenital cataract, malignancy), chronic diseases (e.g., diabetes) infections, drugs (e.g., chloramphenicol), trauma, radiation, or enzyme deficiencies.

Incidence

- The incidence of retinoblastoma is 1 in 18,000 infants. There are 200 to 300 new cases per year.

- Retinoblastoma is the most common ocular tumor of childhood.
- The age at diagnosis bilaterally is 12 months and unilaterally is 24 months.
- Of children with congenital cataracts, 60% have other ocular problems. The most common is a lens defect in neonates.
- Glaucoma has an increased occurrence in males, with 75% of cases being bilateral. It is rare in children.
- Gliomas are the second most common intracranial tumor of childhood; they represent in 6% to 10% of all central nervous system (CNS) tumors and 9% of all childhood brain tumors.
- Optic neuritis is more common in adolescence.
- Craniopharyngioma is the third most common brain tumor in children.
- Amblyopia is major public health problem, affecting 2% to 4% of children born in the United States

Table 34-6 Differential Diagnosis: Visual Impairment (369.9)

CRITERIA	AMBLYOPIA*	CONGENITAL CATARACT*	ACQUIRED CATARACT*
ICD-9 code	368.00	743.30	366.9
Subjective Data			
Present history	Frowns, blinks excessively, history of eye surgery or patching; cover/close one eye	May have Down syndrome, Trisomy 21, primary persistent hyperplastic vitreous	May have a history of trauma to the eye or head, radiation, systemic disease
Past history	Hereditary history likely	May have positive history for TORCH	May have a history of long-term steroid use, juvenile onset diabetes
Associated symptoms	Head tilting, strabismus may be present	May have microphthalmos, hypoglycemia, hypoparathyroidism, galactosemia	May have systemic disease
Family history		Maternal infection prenatally; autosomal dominant, recessive, X-linked	May be present
Objective Data			
Physical examination			
Eye examination			
Extraocular movements	Normal—abnormal if associated with strabismus	Abnormal eye movements in one or both eyes; visually inattentive if bilateral; strabismus present	Abnormal eye movements; strabismus present
PERRLA	Normal	Involved eye usually smaller; photophobia	Photophobia
Cover-uncover	Abnormal	Abnormal or poor visual fixation reflexes	Abnormal or poor visual fixation
Fundoscopic	Normal	Abnormal—white fundus reflex (leukocoria); inability to observe retinal details	Abnormal—white fundus reflex (leukocoria)
Red reflex	Normal	Not present or blunted	Not present
Visual acuity	Abnormal—may see differences in two eyes	Abnormal—usually at 20/100 to 20/200 bilateral	Amblyopia

*Refer the child to an ophthalmologist.

- Amblyopia is the leading cause of monocular vision loss
- Amblyopia is treatable especially in infants and young children. The "critical period" is birth to 8 years of age
- Amblyopia is usually passive (suppressed) as the other eye takes over

Risk Factors

- Prematurity (e.g., retrolental fibroplasia)
- Congenital rubella
- Ophthalmia neonatorum
- Congenital syphilis
- Toxoplasmosis
- Anoxic events or birth trauma
- Failure to reach development milestones
- Chromosomal abnormalities
- Cerebral palsy
- Seizure disorder

Differential Diagnosis (Table 34-6)

Congenital cataract is a loss of transparency of the crystalline lens that results from physical or chemical alterations within the lens. Over half the children with congenital cataracts have other ocular problems, most commonly nystagmus, strabismus, and microphthalmia. Opacity is noted on examination of the red reflex when the direct ophthalmoscope is used; excessive tearing may also be seen.

Acquired cataract usually results from a blunt blow to the anterior portion of the eye or a penetrating metal foreign body; it may also result from radiation, long-term use of steroids, enzyme deficiencies, and diabetes. There is slowly progressive visual loss or blurring over months or years and opacification of the normally clear lens.

A solid intraocular malignancy, *retinoblastoma* may appear at any time during the first 4 years of life. The symptoms include leukokoria (white pupil), strabismus (caused by poor vision if the macula is involved), uveitis, or glaucoma.

RETINOBLASTOMA*	GLIOMA*	CRANIOPHARYNGIOMA*	OPTIC NEURITIS*	GLAUCOMA
190.5	191.9	237.0	377.30	
Negative	Negative	Headache	May have concomitant infection (e.g., measles, mumps, chickenpox) meningitis	Photophobia, epiphoria
Negative	May have neurofibromatosis type 1	Negative	History of immunization, ingestion of lead or alcohol, drugs (chloramphenicol)	
Inflammation of eye (e.g., orbital cellulitis) in 10% of cases	Color vision decreased	May have increased intracranial pressure (ICP) or hydrocephalus	Systemic illness	Corneal opacification and enlargement, eye pain
Strong family history	Negative	Eye diseases	Multiple sclerosis, CNS diseases, eye diseases	Primary—can be hereditary; associated with Sturge-Weber syndrome, neurofibromatosis familial hypoplasia
Strabismus present	Central visual field loss, proptosis; may have strabismus and nystagmus	See-saw nystagmus	May be normal	Normal
May have abnormal reaction to light	Afferent pupillary defect	Increased ICP may cause abnormal reaction to light	Sluggish or absent constriction to direct light	
Abnormal	Abnormal	Abnormal	Abnormal	Normal
Abnormal—white pupil	Optic disk swelling	Bilobed papilledema	Swollen optic nerve; may have hemorrhages and exudates on surface of optic disk	Disk-cupping in deep anterior chamber
Abnormal or absent	May be abnormal; abnormal—vision loss in one eye	May be abnormal	May be abnormal	
Abnormal	Abnormal—loss of vision bilaterally	Abnormal—unilateral vision loss	Abnormal—vision loss can be mild to only light perception	Abnormal

Glioma is an intracranial tumor and appears as a gradual, painless proptosis (exophthalmos, or abnormal protrusion of the eyeball) with loss of vision and an afferent pupillary defect. The visual loss is often slow, insidious, and asymptomatic, and the child's symptom may be nystagmus or strabismus.

A brain tumor that originates from the pituitary stalk, *craniopharyngioma* tends to compress the optic chiasm from behind and above. The tumors are slow growing and do not usually appear until the child is 3 or 4 years of age or later. The child's symptom is loss of vision.

Optic neuritis is an inflammation of the optic nerve. It may be caused by CNS tumors, toxins, multiple sclerosis, some drugs (e.g., chloramphenicol), viral infections (e.g., measles, mumps, chickenpox), or immunization. Symptoms include an acute loss of vision, eye pain with movement, light flashes, impaired color vision, afferent pupil defect, and optic disk abnormalities (e.g., swelling, paleness).

Glaucoma is an increase in intraocular pressure. The classic triad of symptoms includes epiphora (tearing), photophobia, and blepharospasm (lid squeezing). Other signs are corneal edema, corneal and ocular enlargement, ocular injection, and visual impairment. Older children have a loss of vision or symptoms of pain and vomiting related to abrupt intraocular pressure elevation.

Amblyopia is a unilateral or bilateral reduction of corrected central visual acuity without a visible organic lesion commensurate with this loss. It is the direct result of failure of the brain to process visual cues accurately. Amblyopia is a disorder of function, not eye structure. It has three main causes: visual deprivation, strabismus, and anisometropia.

Anisometropia, a condition that exists when one eye is more farsighted or nearsighted than the other, is a common cause of amblyopia. The eye with the greater refractive error (blurred image) will be suppressed by the brain. Over time, this suppression will lead to amblyopia.

In strabismic amblyopia the eyes are misaligned. This misalignment causes diplopia, and the brain, which cannot tolerate the diplopia, suppresses vision in one eye.

Management

Amblyopia

Treatments and medications. Refer the child to an ophthalmologist.

Counseling and prevention

- Discuss the cause and course of the condition with the parents and child.
- Explain that the condition has three causes: refractive error, strabismus, and cataract. Treatment is based on the cause of the condition: for refractive error, glasses; for strabismus, patching and surgery; and for cataract, surgery. Parents need to be made aware of how important compliance with the therapy (i.e., glasses, patching) is to the desired outcome.
- Remember that prevention is the best treatment. Amblyopia can and should be prevented. As soon as strabismus or visual impairment is discovered, it should be corrected.

Follow-up. Frequent follow-up examination is necessary based on the reason for the condition and is directed by the ophthalmologist.

Consultations and referrals. Refer all cases to an ophthalmologist as soon as possible.

Blindness

Treatments and medications. Refer the child to an ophthalmologist. Management by a multidisciplinary team is best.

Counseling and prevention

- Keep in mind that parents need to be allowed to grieve (see Chapter 23). If the diagnosis is made at birth, mourning can interfere with normal attachment.
- Teach parents that to assist with attachment a blind baby must be spoken to and held, sung to, and touched to help the baby learn to know the parents and to elicit smiles.
- Remember that acceptance of a child's disability is important for healthful adjustment of both the child and the parents.
- Stress to parents the importance of early intervention. Early intervention can determine to a large degree how independent a blind person will be.
- If the child is older, allow both the child and the parents to grieve over the loss.
- Remember that the younger the child, the more quickly adjustment to the impairment occurs.
- Explain to parents that each blind child has individual needs, just like other children.
- Counsel parents that what the child needs is to have available alternative ways of relating to the environment (i.e., through sound and touch).
- Discuss with parents that motor development and mobility occur much later for a blind child. Explain that developmental delay is secondary to a lack of visual input and not caused by poor parenting or inherent problems (assuming no such problems exist). Sighted babies move to the object, while blind babies need an environment rich in tactile and sounding objects. They react to auditory stimuli, whereas most babies react to visual stimuli.
- Have parents describe as many concrete experiences as possible for the child.
- Stress to parents that handling an object when it is described is extremely important for a blind child.
- Counsel parents that a blind child's ability to learn games is impaired because he or she cannot imitate what cannot be seen (e.g., child cannot follow a rolling ball). However, it can be very helpful to tell a child about the activity. Suggest that parents use physical contact to move a child through the activity to understand it. A high degree of verbal communication must be done with a blind child so that the child understands the objects and the activity.

Follow-up. Schedule follow-up visits as needed for support and well-child care.

Consultations and referrals

- Refer to appropriate agencies such as the National Association for Parents of the Visually Impaired or the American Foundation for the Blind (see Resources).
- Refer to a physical therapist who specializes in visually impaired children.
- Refer to a speech therapist who specializes in visually impaired children.

Congenital cataract

Treatments and medications. Refer the child early to an ophthalmologist for possible surgical intervention.

Counseling and prevention

- Explain to parents the cause and the course of treatment. The condition is caused by congenital cataracts that began to form during the sixth or seventh week of fetal life when the lens was being formed. Explain that the cataract is a clouding of the lens of the eye. The lens normally is transparent and allows light to enter the eye and refract onto the retina; with a cataract, the light cannot be refracted and visual impairment occurs.

- If surgery is suggested, discuss with parents the use of an eye shield postoperatively for about a week.
- Instruct on the administration of eyedrops (as directed by the ophthalmologist) after surgery. Vision does not improve immediately, and a corrective lens is necessary after surgery.

Follow-up. As determined by an ophthalmologist, close follow-up care is important to ensure maximum benefits from the cataract surgery and prescribed lens.

Consultations and referrals. Refer the child to an ophthalmologist.

Acquired cataract

Treatments and medications. Refer the child to an ophthalmologist.

Counseling and prevention

- Explain the cause and course of the condition to the parents and child. Acquired cataracts develop from trauma, foreign body, radiation, long-term use of steroids, and diabetes. The prognosis is fairly good because visual development during the first few months of life is not affected as with congenital cataracts.
- Remember that treatment is the same as for a congenital cataract for children younger than 9 years of age. For children older than 9 years of age, surgery is dependent on the progress of the condition and any physician or patient preferences.

Follow-up. See the section on Congenital Cataract.

Consultations and referrals. Refer the child to an ophthalmologist.

Retinoblastoma. See Neoplastic Disease in Chapter 45.

Treatments and medications. Refer immediately to an ophthalmologist.

Counseling and prevention. Explain the cause and course of the condition to the parents and child. Retinoblastoma is the most common tumor of the eye in infancy and childhood. Surgery to enucleate eye is necessary. The child will be able to have a prosthesis but not until edema from the surgery is gone (in about 3 weeks). Instruction in care of the prosthesis is given at the fitting.

Follow-up. Follow up as directed by the ophthalmologist. Eye examinations of the child's siblings must be done as early as possible.

Consultations and referrals. Refer the parents for genetic counseling, and refer the child to an ophthalmologist.

Gliomas

Treatments and medications. Refer the child to an ophthalmologist.

Counseling and prevention. Explain the cause and course of the condition to the parents and child. Gliomas can be infratentorial or supratentorial. A supratentorial lesion must be surgically excised when one of the optic nerves is involved.

Follow-up. Schedule follow-up care as directed by the ophthalmologist.

Consultations and referrals. Refer the child to an ophthalmologist.

Optic neuritis

Treatments and medications. Refer the child to an ophthalmologist.

Counseling and prevention

- Explain to the parents and child that the condition is an inflammation of the optic nerve caused by CNS tumors, multiple sclerosis, toxins, drugs, or viral infection.

- Inform the parents and child that if the condition is caused by viral infection, the neuritis will run its course and full recovery is usually in 3 weeks.
- Inform the parents and child that if the condition is caused by toxins or drugs, discontinuation of drug or toxin exposure will reverse the condition with full recovery.
- Counsel the parents and child that recurrences are probable if the condition is caused by multiple sclerosis, and a gradual visual deficit should be anticipated.

Follow-up. Schedule follow-up care as directed by the ophthalmologist.

Consultations and referrals. Refer the child to an ophthalmologist.

Resources

Organizations

American Association of University Affiliated Programs, 2033 M Street, Suite 406, Washington, DC 20036

American Foundation for the Blind, 15 West 16th Street, New York, NY 10011; (800) 232-5463

American Printing House for the Blind, Inc, 1839 Frankfort Avenue, Louisville, KY 40200; (800) 223-1839

Association for the Education of the Visually Handicapped, 919 Walnut Street, Philadelphia, PA 19107

Canadian National Institute for the Blind, 1931 Bayview Avenue, Toronto, Ontario M4G 4C8 Canada

Catalog of Optical Aids, Optical Aid Service, New York Association for the Blind, 111 East 59th Street, New York, NY 10022

Catalogue of Large-Type Materials, National Association for Visually Handicapped, 3201 Balboa Street, San Francisco, CA 94121

Council for Exceptional Children, 1920 Association Drive, Reston, VA 22091

Library of Congress, Division for the Blind and Physically Handicapped, Reference Department, 1291 Taylor Street NW, Washington, DC 20542; (202) 707-9275 or (202) 707-5100

National Association for Parents of the Visually Impaired, 2011 Hardy Circle, Austin, TX 78657

National Association for the Visually Handicapped, 305 East 24th Street, New York, NY 10010

National Society for the Prevention of Blindness, Inc., 79 Madison Avenue, New York, NY 10016

Touch, Inc., PO Box 1711, Albany, NY 12201

Vision Center, 1393 North High Street, Columbus, OH 43201

Eye Deviations

AMY VERST

Alert

Consult with or refer to an ophthalmologist for the following:
- Acquired nystagmus
- New-onset diplopia or strabismus
- Absent or abnormal red reflex
- Diminished visual acuity
- Sudden-onset amblyopia
- Unilateral vision loss
- Strabismus that persists beyond 2 months of age

Etiology

Proper alignment of each eye is critical to the development of monocular and binocular vision. If one or both eyes are misaligned, as with stabismus, the light entering the eye falls outside the macula retinae and a blurred image results. The brain does not tolerate blurred images and essentially shuts down nerve impulses to the most affected eye. The result is loss of monocular vision, also known as *amblyopia.*

In pseudostrabismus, the eyes appear to be misaligned because of large epicanthal folds and a flat nose. This condition can be evaluated with the corneal light reflex test.

Nystagmus is another type of eye deviation. Nystagmus is a fine oscillation of the eye in either the horizontal (more common) or vertical plane. It may be idiopathic, familial, or secondary to another systemic condition.

Incidence

- Strabismus is a common condition, affecting up to 3% of children less than 6 years of age.
- Of all children with strabismus, 50% manifest symptoms by 1 year of age and 80% manifest symptoms by 4 years of age.
- Amblyopia occurs in 40% of children with strabismus.
- Amblyopia is the most common cause of visual loss in American children.
- The vision of approximately 80% of children with strabismic conditions can be corrected
- Pseudostrabismus is common in infants with a hereditary flat nasal bridge and broad epicanthal folds.
- Accommodative esotropias are commonly seen between 2 and 4 years of age and are associated with higher degrees of farsightedness.
- The majority of strabismus develops between 18 months and 6 years of age.

- Medial or esodeviations are responsible for 50% of all cases of strabismus.

Risk Factors

- Positive family history of infantile strabismus, accommodative esotropia, exotropia
- Trauma
- Illness
- Large refractive error
- Cataracts
- Lid abnormalities
- Optic nerve hypoplasia
- Glioma
- Different refractory error between the two eyes
- Tumors of the CNS
- Thyroid disease
- Infectious lesion
- Recent viral infection
- Migraine headaches
- Down syndrome
- Cerebral palsy
- Prematurity
- Family history of retinoblastoma

Differential Diagnosis

In *pseudostrabismus,* the infant appears to have esotropia. However, this is a false appearance. Infants commonly have a flat nasal bridge and large nasolabial folds that shield the inner aspect of the eye. The examiner can easily observe the lateral sclera while the medial sclera is hidden, making

Table 34-7 Differential Diagnosis: Eye Deviations (378.87)

CRITERIA	PSEUDOSTRABISMUS	ESOTROPIA*	EXOTROPIA*	NYSTAGMUS*
ICD-9 code	378.9	378.00	378.10	379.50
Subjective Data				
Description of problem	Eyes appear crossed	Eye moves inward	Eye moves outward; complaints of eye strain while reading, eyes may water; needs to close one eye in bright light	May have history of diphenylhydantoin, barbiturates, and other sedative use; may have history of nodding or bobbing of head
Family history	Genetic basis	Hereditary history likely	Hereditary history likely	Familial hereditary history likely
Objective Data				
Physical examination/eye examination				
Extraocular movements	Normal	Constant in medial gaze	Constant in lateral gaze	Movement involuntary from side to side
Cover-uncover test	Normal	Positive with affected eye moving outward	Positive with affected eye moving inward	Eye oscillates in horizontal plane and persists in all fields of gaze
Pupillary reaction	Normal	Normal	Normal	May not be normal depending on cause
Funduscopic examination	Normal	Normal	Normal	May not be normal depending on cause
Corneal light reflex	Normal	Displaced laterally	Displaced medially	Movement causes difficulty in obtaining
Red reflex	Present	Present	Present	May not be present
Visual acuity	Normal	May have amblyopia	May be normal in both eyes	May not be normal depending on cause

*Refer the child to an ophthalmologist.

the eye appear "crossed." A corneal light reflex test will reveal equal reflection of light on each eye ruling out true esotropia.

Strabismus is any condition in which the normal binocular alignment of the eyes to a single point in any and all cardinal fields of gaze is disturbed. Extraocular movements (EOMs) are abnormal. Esotropia (medial deviation) or exotropia (lateral deviation) may be seen. The corneal light reflex test, or Hirschberg test, shows the light reflex to appear off-center in one eye. Eye movement is noted with the cover-uncover test. Vision screening may indicate decreased vision in one eye, and stereopsis screening is abnormal.

Tropia is present when there is constant deviation. *Phoria* is present when there is intermittent deviation expected when binocularity is compromised.

Esotropia (or *esophoria*) is a medial deviation of the eye. It is classified as either accommodative, associated with focusing effort, or nonaccommodative (Table 34-7).

In accommodative esotropia, the eye attempts to correct a refractive error by overaccommodating. The overaccommodation causes a reflexive ocular convergence that forces one eye medially off alignment. Amblyopia develops in the nonfixating eye. Nonaccommodative esotropia is associated with prematurity, trauma, cataracts, or neurodevelopmental problems. The medial malalignment is present at all times.

Exotropia is lateral deviation of the eye; it is classified as intermittent or constant. The majority of lateral deviations are intermittent and worsened by fatigue, illness, visual inattention, and bright sunlight. Exotropia has a more favorable outcome unless the defect becomes constant and amblyopia develops. A child with late-onset, constant exotropia should be evaluated for a CN III palsy.

Vertical deviations occur less frequently than horizontal deviations. They are described as hypertropia (or hyperphoria) if the eye is higher than normal, but hypotropia (or hypophoria) if the eye is lower than normal. The majority of vertical deviations are caused by a paresis of CN IV. This palsy compromises the superior oblique muscle and usually causes a head tilt to the opposite shoulder. It is for this reason that all children with idiopathic torticollis should be evaluated for a CN IV palsy. A palsy of CN III also causes a vertical deviation of the eye.

Because CN III is involved in moving the eye in both horizontal and vertical directions, a palsy of the nerve causes the largest deviation and interruption of motility. Amblyopia is often the result of malalignment caused by CN III.

Nystagmus is spontaneous, rhythmic, back-and-forth movement of one or both eyes. Familial (heredity) nystagmus can appear with back-and-forth movements of the eye that are relatively equal in speed and amplitude. It may also appear as a jerking nystagmus, which has a slow component in one direction and a fast component in the other. Visual acuity is usually decreased. Spasmus nutans is a transient form of nystagmus that is characterized by fine pendular nystagmus and head bobbing or nodding, often asymmetric.

Note

Intracranial tumors or CNS lesions may be associated with nystagmus.

Management

Pseudostrabismus

Treatments and medications. None are necessary.

Counseling and prevention

- Explain the condition to the parents
- Explain the importance of checking with a practitioner to rule out strabismus.
- Reassure and emphasize to the parents that the condition is benign, is caused by anatomic variation, and is a normal variant.

Follow-up. Perform routine vision assessment at each well-child check.

Consultations and referrals. None are necessary.

Esotropia. Refer all eye deviations to an ophthalmologist as soon as possible.

Treatments and medications

Accommodative esotropia. Treatment requires suppression of accommodation. Eyeglasses to correct the refractive error are used to realign the eyes. Bifocal lenses are occasionally required.

Nonaccommodative esotropia. Surgical alignment is needed as soon as possible, especially after 24 months of age for best results. Refractive errors are corrected with eyeglasses, while amblyopia may be treated with patching.

Counseling and prevention. Explain the cause and course of the condition to the parents and child. Esotropia is the most common eye movement disorder in young children. The visual image is focused behind the retina, and the child tries to correct the distorted vision by turning the eye inward, causing double vision. The vision is suppressed in the abnormal eye, also causing reduced vision in that eye. These children are treated with patching and then surgery.

Follow-up. Schedule follow-up care as directed by the ophthalmologist. Assess visual acuity at each well-child visit.

Consultations and referrals. Refer the child to an ophthalmologist.

Exotropia

Treatments and medications

Infants. Surgical alignment may be prescribed because nonsurgical options are limited by the infant's inability to cooperate. Intermittent occlusion may be prescribed.

Children. Nonsurgical approaches such as occlusion, eye glasses, or orthoptic exercises are somewhat successful with older children. Surgical alignment may be necessary in those children with resulting amblyopia.

Counseling and prevention. Explain the cause and course of the condition to the parents and child. The image seen is unclear because the eye does not accommodate, especially when looking at things at a distance. The child uses only the eye with good accommodation and allows the weak eye to deviate. The condition, if not corrected, becomes permanent and vision in the weak eye does not develop normally. Patching and glasses are usually used to correct this condition.

Follow-up. Schedule follow-up care as directed by the ophthalmologist. Assess visual acuity in each well-child visit.

Consultations and referrals. Refer the child to an ophthalmologist.

Vertical deviations

Treatments and medications. Surgical realignment is almost always indicated. Because a CN palsy may signify other neurologic impairment, a thorough neurologic examination is also warranted. The goal of any surgery is to align the eye as normally as possible, but normal motility cannot be restored.

Counseling and prevention. Explain the cause and course of the condition to the parent and the child. Vertical deviations may be the result of many causes. The most common is misalignment with an unknown cause. Head posture is used to achieve binocularity that cannot be obtained when the head is held straight as a result of a nerve palsy of the superior oblique muscle. Surgery and glasses are usually indicated. If this condition is the result of trauma, a "watch and see" approach is usually taken before surgical correction. Stress to the parents that vision testing is to be done frequently to detect developing amblyopia. Also explain to the parents the need for compliance with the treatment plan of the ophthalmologist.

Follow-up. Schedule follow-up care as directed by the ophthalmologist. Assess visual acuity at each well-child visit.

Consultations and referrals. Refer the child to an ophthalmologist.

Nystagmus

Treatments and medications. Refer the child to an ophthalmologist.

Counseling and prevention. Explain the cause and course of condition to the parents and child. Familial nystagmus is the result of an intrinsic defect of the ocular motor control mechanism evident at birth. With familial nystagmus, refractive errors are usually corrected if found. The use of a prism can sometimes diminish nystagmus. Congenital nystagmus may be caused by bilateral visual loss and needs to be ruled out.

Follow-up. Schedule follow-up care as directed by an ophthalmologist.

Consultations and referrals. Refer all cases to an ophthalmologist or a neurologist.

Eye Injuries

AMY VERST

Alert

Consult with or refer to a physician for the following:
- Large laceration of globe
- Prolapse of intraocular lens
- Noticeable asymmetry of limbal configuration
- Suspicion of chemical burn
- Exposure to radiation (ultraviolet or infrared)
- Cloudy or double vision
- Photophobia
- History of blunt trauma or penetrating injury
- Foreign body

Etiology

About one third of all blindness in children results from trauma, usually avoidable. The National Society for the Prevention of Blindness estimates that over 90% of all ocular injuries can be prevented. Boys 11 to 15 years of age are the most vulnerable. Most injuries are related to sports, projectile toys, sticks, and BB guns. BB guns are the single most common cause of significant trauma resulting in visual loss in children. Chemical burns are frequently caused by children using sprays or nozzles on chemicals or cleansers for the garden, garage, or home. Sunlamps, sun reflection off snow, and welding are common causes of ultraviolet burns. Thermal burns tend to damage the eyelid.

Incidence

- Children 11 to 15 years of age have the highest rate of injury to the eye.
- Boys are injured four times more often than girls.
- Superficial corneal abrasions are among the most common injuries.

Risk Factors

- Highest-risk sports (e.g., wrestling, martial arts)
- High-risk sports (e.g., sport with rapidly moving ball or puck, bat, or stick)
- Lowest-risk sports (e.g., swimming, track and field, gymnastics)

Differential Diagnosis (Table 34-8)

Eyelid injury occurs because eyelids are an external surface and exist as a defense mechanism to protect the globe. Lids are very vascular and are capable of a great deal of swelling. Injuries to the globe may be relatively occult and may be overshadowed by obvious lid damage. If injury is from a human bite, consider *Streptococcus viridians* and staphylococci as common organisms. In dog bites, consider *S. aureus, Pasteurella multocida,* and *Bacteroides.* In cat bites, consider *S. aureus* and *P. multocida.*

Corneal abrasion occurs when the superficial corneal epithelium is broken. The patient states that the pain is severe and keeps the lid closed. The eye appears red and irritated. Photophobia and a foreign-body sensation are reported. The critical sign is an epithelial staining defect with fluorescein dye. Conjunctival injection, swollen eyelid, and mild anterior chamber reaction may be seen. It is important to invert the lid to ensure that the foreign body is present.

Ocular irritation or *pain, foreign-body sensation, tearing, red eye,* and *history of trauma to* or *foreign body in the eye* is often reported. If the history indicates ocular penetration (e.g., a moving or flying object hitting the eye), place a patch and shield on the eye. Do not instill any topical medications, and do not manipulate the lids or globe. Refer the child to an ophthalmologist. An irregular pupil is an ominous sign that may indicate penetrating ocular injury.

Black eye is a frequent injury that occurs as a result of a blunt force. The injury itself may not be serious, but sometimes a blow may be severe enough to cause damage to intraocular structures. Palpate the orbit for any interruptions, step-off, or depression, which may indicate orbital fracture.

Orbital fracture results from blunt force that causes injury to one or more of the orbital bones. The usual symptoms are visual loss, diplopia, pain on eye movement, hyperesthesia of the skin on the ipsilateral cheek, displacement of the zygomatic arches, periorbital edema, epistaxis, and, if severe, leakage of cerebrospinal fluid. Periorbital crepitus indicates a possible fracture. Mandibular movement and the CNS should be evaluated.

Chemical burns of the conjunctiva and cornea represent one of the true ocular emergencies. Alkali burns usually result in greater damage to an eye than an acid burn because alkali compounds penetrate ocular tissues more rapidly. All chemical burns require immediate and profuse irrigation and referral to an ophthalmologist.

Table 34-8 Differential Diagnosis: Eye Injuries (921.9)

CRITERIA	EYELID INJURY*	CORNEAL ABRASION*	FOREIGN BODY IN OR ON THE CORNEA*	CHEMICAL BURN†	BLACK EYE— ECCHYMOSIS	ORBITAL FRACTURE*
ICD-9 code	921.1	918.1	930.0	940.0	921.0	802.8
Subjective Data						
Method of injury	Trauma	Trauma	Trauma	Obtain while irrigating	Trauma	Trauma
Associated symptoms	Pain Abrasion/laceration	Pain Foreign body sensation Scratching of eye Photophobia Keeps lid closed Serous, watery discharge	Pain Foreign-body sensation Tearing	Varies Pain	Local tenderness	Pain on vertical eye movement Double vision Local tenderness Eyelid swelling after nose blowing
Objective Data						
Physical examination						
Skin	May be denuded Ecchymosis Laceration Puncture	Swelling possible	Eyelid edema	Immediate referral; periorbital area may appear scalded	Discoloration cycle: black-blue-purple-green-yellow	Ecchymosis Hyperesthesia of ipsilateral cheek and upper lip
Eye						
Conjunctiva	Normal	Injected	Injected		Injected	May have hyphema
Lid movement	Depends on injury	Normal	Normal		Normal	Ptosis
EOM	Intact	Normal	Normal		Normal	Restricted, especially in upward lateral gaze
PERRLA	Normal	Pupil miotic	Pupil miotic		Normal	Normal
Red reflex	Present	Present	Present		Normal	Normal
Funduscopic exam	Normal	Normal	Normal		Normal	May have papilledema
Visual acuity	Normal	Decreased if abrasion is central	Nearly normal		Normal	Double vision
Laboratory data	None	Positive fluorescent stain	None		None	Indicated by radiographic examination (Waters' projection)

*Refer to a physician or opthalmologist.
†Refer immediately to a physician.

Management

Eyelid injury (minor)

Treatments and medications

- Irrigate tissues and débride with saline.
- Apply Polysporin ophthalmic ointment four times a day and a sterile dressing.
- Use cold compresses to decrease swelling.

Counseling and prevention

- Explain the condition and the treatment to the parents and child.
- Demonstrate to the parents or caregiver the application of ointment on the lid. Apply in an even stroke using a cotton-tipped applicator by rolling the applicator across the lid from inside to outside. Use a new applicator each time.
- Instruct the parents or caregiver to inspect the eyelid for swelling, redness, or drainage, and to call if any of these are present.

Follow-up. Schedule a return visit if tissue edema, erythema, or tenderness increase to rule out cellulitis. Also schedule a return visit if the child complains of pain on movement of the eye.

Consultations and referrals. Refer the child to an ophthalmologist or a plastic surgeon if the lid injury is deep and needs to be sutured or if scarring of the lid is possible. (Scarring contracts the skin, and the child may develop exotropia from incomplete closure of the eye.)

Corneal abrasion

Treatments and medications

- Use proparacaine 0.5% as a topical anesthetic for examination of the eye.
- Perform a gross eye examination. Remove the contact lens, if present. Inspect under the upper eyelid for a foreign body.
- Perform a fluorescein stain eye (see Box 34-4).
- If the abrasion is small, apply an antibiotic ointment or drops with gram-positive coverage (e.g., gentamicin ophthalmic drops) into the affected eye every 2 hours for the first day and then every 4 hours for the next 2 days.
- Administer a tetanus booster if the status indicates.
- Remember that patching the injured eye may decrease corneal oxygenation and is not recommended.

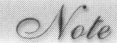

Never use topical steroids, and never discharge a child from the office while he or she is still being affected by a topical anesthesia.

Counseling and prevention

- Explain the condition and the treatment plan to the parents and the child.
- Demonstrate to the parents instillation of the eyedrops.

Follow-up

- Perform an immediate recheck if the pain worsens or if sensitivity to eyedrops occurs.
- Schedule a return visit in 24 hours for reexamination.
- Follow-up daily. If not healed after 3 days, refer to an ophthalmologist

Consultations and referrals. Refer the child to an ophthalmologist if the abrasion is large, or if it is minor and there is no improvement in 24 hours.

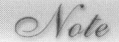

If the history indicates ocular penetration (moving or flying object hitting the eye), place a patch and a shield over the eye. Do not instill any topical medications and *do not* manipulate lids or globe. Refer to an ophthalmologist.

Foreign body in or on the cornea

Treatments and medications

- Refer the child to a physician or ophthalmologist.
- Do not attempt to remove the foreign body or wash it out.
- Lightly patch the eye after estimating visual acuity. Patching lightly or using a shield ensures that no rubbing, wiping, or pressure is applied to the eye.
- If vitreal fluid or an irregular pupil is seen, cover both eyes to decrease eye movements after visual acuity is established and send immediately to the emergency room with the head elevated 30 degrees.
- Administer a tetanus booster if the status indicates.

Counseling and prevention

- Explain the course and the treatment plan to the child and parents.
- If surgery is a possibility, discuss with the parent the necessity of giving the child nothing by mouth (NPO).
- Discuss with the parents that the outcome of the injury varies with each case.
- Remember that some children may take weeks to regain normal vision, whereas others' vision becomes worse with time.
- Keep in mind that prevention is the best treatment. At all well-child examinations, discuss eye safety. Instruct children to use goggles during sports activities. Advise parents to carefully supervise the selection of their child's toys (see Chapter 14).
- Stress to the parents the importance of careful follow-up care by an ophthalmologist.

Follow-up. Follow-up is determined by the physician. If the lens is involved, a cataract often develops. Careful follow-up by an ophthalmologist is very important.

Consultations and referrals. Refer to a physician for removal of the foreign body. Refer to an ophthalmologist if there is loss of vision (e.g., a cataract) or the development of a rust ring on the cornea.

Black eye (ecchymosis)

Treatments and medications

- Refer children with double, blurred, or decreased vision or pain that is continuing or increasing to an ophthalmologist for possible intraocular injury.
- For minor trauma, apply ice to the area for 5 to 10 minutes every hour for the first day.
- Record the child's visual acuity and the type and size of the object that caused the injury.
- Have a radiographic examination performed for possible nasal bone fracture or skull fracture.

Counseling and prevention

- Explain the cause and the course of the injury to the parents and child (i.e., the force of the impact crushes subcutaneous tissue, causing hemorrhage and edema).
- Advise the parents of the discoloration cycle: black to blue to purple to green to yellow.
- Discuss with the parents and child the need for application of ice to the area. Suggest the use of a frozen package of peas or a cold pack on the area for 5 to 10 minutes every hour.
- Alert the parents and child to the possibility of bilateral ecchymosis. Even if only one eye is injured, because of the effects of gravity, fluids cross the nasal bridge during sleep and enter the lower lid and cheeks during wakening.
- Suggest that the parents investigate the use of a helmet and face guard for the child, if appropriate.

Follow-up. Schedule an immediate visit if changes occur or pain increases, and schedule a return visit in 72 hours for follow-up examination.

Consultations and referrals

- Refer the child to a neurologist if radiographs or the physical examination indicates blunt head trauma or a skull fracture.
- Refer to an ENT specialist if radiographs indicate a nasal fracture.
- Refer to a physician and social services if there is suspicion of child abuse.

Orbital fracture

Treatments and medications

- Estimate the child's vision and record it along with the history of injury for referral to a physician.
- Do not allow the child to blow his or her nose until seen by a physician because of possible damage to the sinuses.
- Obtain a Waters' projection radiographic examination or consult with a physician for a CT scan.

Counseling and prevention

- Describe to the parents and child that there are seven bones in the orbital area that protect the eye. The smallest bone is the one lying underneath the eye. When injury occurs in this area, the bone breaks, trapping the inferior rectus and inferior oblique muscles. The resulting movement restriction causes diplopia and prevents the child from looking upward.
- Remember that prevention is the best treatment. Discuss with the parents and child at well-child visits the importance of eye and face protection for sports activities (see Chapter 14).
- Recommend that the child use molded polycarbonate sports goggles secured to the head by an elastic strap for sports that do not require a helmet or face mask. For sports that require helmets and face masks, the child should use polycarbonate face shields and guards.
- Advise children to never wear orthodontic headgear while playing sports because the metallic bow can slip and penetrate the eye.
- Keep in mind that children who have amblyopia are able to participate in most sports. However, boxing, wrestling, martial arts, and any other sport without eye protection should be prohibited.

Follow-up. Schedule follow up as directed by the physician.

Consultations and referrals. All orbital fractures should be referred immediately to a physician.

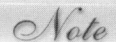

> Chemical burns of the conjunctiva and cornea represent one of the true ocular emergencies. Alkali burns usually result in greater damage to the eye than acid burns because alkali compounds penetrate ocular tissues more rapidly. All chemical burns require immediate and profuse irrigation and referral to an ophthalmologist.

Chemical burns

Treatments and medications

- Immediately irrigate with water or saline for 10 to 30 minutes while consulting with a physician. Flush with intravenous (IV) tubing and a minimum of 2 L of water or saline. Hold the child's head to the side and irrigate from the inner corner of the eye to the side of the head to prevent the chemical from washing into the other eye. Have the child roll the eye around and direct the saline into all corners of the eye and under the lid.
- Use the orbital bones to keep the eye open.
- Do not put pressure on the eye itself.
- Do not apply an eye patch. Continue to irrigate the eye until the emergency room is reached.
- Try to obtain the name of the chemical in the eye, but do not stop irrigating.

Counseling and prevention

- Explain the nature of the emergency situation to the parents and child while irrigating.
- Explain the need for the name of the chemical in the eye to help determine if it was an acid or an alkali. Acid burns tend to affect the cornea and anterior chamber of eye. Alkali chemicals are progressive and can continue causing damage for days.
- Explain to the parents and child that a protective mechanism of the eye is to cause the tissue to coagulate.
- Remember that prevention is the best treatment. At each well-child examination discuss eye safety with the parents and child. Discuss poison ingestion precautions and spray or nozzle precautions. Simple household products sprayed in the eyes can cause a serious emergency and should be locked away. Toilet bowl cleaners, oven cleaners, bleach, and lye are a few examples of such products (see Chapter 14).
- Keep in mind that good role-modeling by parents is important (e.g., using goggles or glasses when spraying products).

Follow-up. Schedule follow up as directed by the ophthalmologist.

Consultations and referrals. Refer immediately because this is a true emergency!

Infections of the Eyelid and Orbit

AMY VERST

Alert

Consult with or refer to a physician for the following:
- Edema and warmth of the eyelid
- Periorbital skin abrasion
- Laceration or other infection site on lid
- Conjunctival chemosis
- Proptosis
- Limited eye movement
- Vision loss

Etiology

Eye and eyelid abnormalities are most likely caused by infection, inflammation, allergy, or trauma. The most common inflammations of the eyelids are those involving the lashes and the lid margins and those that arise within the meibomian glands as an acute lesion or evolve into a chronic lesion. Infections of the orbit itself are life threatening and need to be referred immediately.

Incidence

- Hordeolums (sties) and blepharitis occur frequently.
- Hordeolums tend to recur frequently, especially with itching caused by allergies.
- Blepharitis is relatively uncommon in children.
- Blepharitis is often associated with seborrheic dermatitis.
- Blepharitis is seen more often in adolescents than in children.
- Orbital cellulitis is more common in children over 5 years of age.
- Periorbital cellulitis is more common than orbital cellulitis and occurs more frequently in children under 5 years of age.

Risk Factors

- Immunologic defect
- Not immunized with Hib vaccine
- Diabetes
- Allergies
- Trauma
- Seborrhea
- Recent URI
- Recent trauma to the eyelid
- Impetigo of the eyelid
- History of sinusitis

Differential Diagnosis (Table 34-9)

Hordeolum (sty) is an infection of the gland of Zeis. These infections appear superficially at the margin of the eyelid as red, swollen, tender pustules. *S. aureus* is the most common causative organism.

Erythema, edema, and chemosis are the symptoms of *lid cellulitis*. Fever may be present. Magenta discoloration of the eyelid is distinctive. Proptosis and visual changes are not seen. Hib, *S. pneumoniae,* and *S. aureus* are the most common infecting organisms.

Chalazion is a chronic, noninfectious inflammation of the meibomian gland. This lipogranuloma causes tender, pointed formations of the eyelid but not the lid margins.

Orbital cellulitis usually has an insidious onset with edema of the eyelids and periorbital tissues, proptosis, decreased vision, and limited and painful eye movement. Fever is present, and children often appear toxic. Ninety percent of cases are secondary to sinusitis (especially the ethmoid). In children under 5 years of age the organism most often involved is Hib. Other common organisms are the same as those in acute sinusitis: *S. aureus, S. pneumoniae,* and *Staphylococcus pyogenes.*

Blepharitis is a chronic inflammation of the eyelid margins causing itching and crusting at the eyelash line. It is often bilateral. There are two kinds: (1) seborrheic (oily scales on the lashes, often with seborrhea of the scalp and post-auricular area) and (2) infectious (dry scales with pustules and ulceration of the lid margin, occasionally with loss of lashes). *Staphylococcus* is the most common causative organism.

Management

Hordeolum (sty)

Treatments and medications

- Apply warm moist compresses for 5 to 10 minutes, four or five times per day.
- Scrub lids at bath time with a cotton swab or washcloth and diluted no-tears shampoo.
- Instill trimethoprim sulfate–polymyxin B (Polytrim ophthalmic ointment) (which is just one of many options) four times daily during the acute stage.
- If the child gets repeated infections, rule out possible diabetes mellitus.
- Possibly apply bacitracin ointment to the lid margin.

Counseling and prevention

- Explain the cause and the course of the disease to the parent and child.
- Demonstrate how to instill ointment in the eye. Instruct the parents to wash their hands, warm the ointment in the hands to prevent rolling of ointment ribbon, pull down the child's eyelid, and apply a thin ribbon of ointment. Vision will be blurred temporarily.
- Explain that compresses must be very warm but not burning to the skin, and that they cool down very quickly. It is necessary to change them often.
- Remember that recurrences are very common.

Follow-up. Schedule a return visit if there is no improvement in 48 hours, or sooner if the child's condition worsens (e.g., fever occurs, the child complains of pain with movement of the eye, swelling of the eyelid occurs).

Consultations and referrals. Refer the child to an ophthalmologist if the condition persists.

Lid cellulitis

Treatments and medications. Refer to a physician for a CT scan to rule out orbital cellulitis.

Counseling and prevention. Explain the cause and the course of the disease to the parents and child.

Follow-up. Schedule follow-up as directed by the consulting physician.

Consultations and referrals. Refer to a physician for treatment.

Chalazion

Treatments and medications

- Apply warm compresses to the lid several times a day for as much as 6 weeks.
- Remember that excision may be necessary, and that it may recur even with excision.

Table 34-9 Differential Diagnosis: Eyelid Infections

CRITERIA	HORDEOLUM (STY)	LID CELLULITIS*	CHALAZION	ORBITAL CELLULITIS*	BLEPHARITIS
ICD-9 code	373.11	373.13	373.2	376.01	373.00
Subjective Data					
Onset/description of problem	Recent occurrence of swelling, tenderness of eyelid and margin	Recent occurrence of swelling, tenderness of eyelid	Recent occurrence of swelling, tenderness of eyelid	Sudden onset of swelling and limited movement of eye	History of recurrent inflammation of eyelids that itch
Associated symptoms	None	Recent URI, trauma to lid, lid infection	Lesion fluctuates in size, may have sticky discharge present	Recent URI, toxic-looking child; fever present with pain and restricted eye movement	Has crusting on lids
Objective Data					
Physical examination					
Skin	Localized swelling at lid edge, small abscess on the outside edge	Eyelid swelling, edema of upper lid	Swelling and redness in mideyelid internal to lashes; may have superimposed inflammation	Painful, lid edema	Crusts or scales on lids or lashes; redness present; may experience loss of lashes
EOM	Normal	Normal	Normal	Limited eye movement	Normal
PERRLA	Normal	Normal	Normal	Painful red eye with conjunctival chemosis and infection	Normal
Fundoscopic examination	Normal	Normal	Normal	Normal	Normal
Visual acuity	Normal	Normal	Normal	Visual loss	Normal
Fever	None	May have mild fever	None	Present with acute onset	None

*Refer to a physician.

- Possibly use a combination antibiotic-steroid ointment if there is a lot of inflammation or a superimposed infection is suspected.

  Counseling and prevention

- Explain the cause and the course of the condition to the parents and child.
- Explain to the parents that the condition is chronic.
- Instruct the parents how to apply warm soaks.
- Instruct the child not to pick or squeeze the lesion.
- Discontinue use of the ointment if the child complains of pain or burning.

  Follow-up

- Schedule a return visit in 48 hours if the condition is not better, and sooner if it gets worse.
- Schedule a return visit if the lesion gets larger.
- Schedule a return visit in 2 weeks if not resolved. A chalazion may last up to 6 weeks.

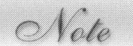

Large chalazion may cause pressure on the globe or astigmatism by obstructing vision.

Consultations and referrals. Refer to an ophthalmologist any child whose lesion obstructs vision or who complains of eye pain. A child with a chronic condition may need an immunologic work-up or an examination for systemic disease.

Orbital cellulitis

Treatments and medications. Refer immediately for hospitalization. This is a life-threatening illness.

Counseling and prevention. Explain the condition and the need for hospitalization to the parents and child.

Follow-up. Schedule follow up as directed by the physician.

Consultations and referral. Refer the child to a physician immediately.

Blepharitis

Treatments and medications

- Scrub the lid at bath time with a cotton swab or washcloth and diluted no-tears shampoo to remove crusts.
- Apply trimethoprim sulfate–polymixin B ophthalmic ointment to the lid at bedtime.
- If concurrent seborrhea of the scalp is present, treat the scalp condition using anti-dandruff shampoos.

  Counseling and prevention

- Explain the condition to the parents and child.
- Discuss with the parents and child that this is a chronic condition and that early institution of soaks can alleviate symptoms.
- Demonstrate the application of ointment. Warm the tube in the hands, pull down the child's lower eyelid, and apply a thin ribbon of ointment along the inner margin of the lower lid.
- Caution the child against rubbing the eyes.
- If eye makeup is usually worn, recommend that it be discontinued for the duration of inflammation. Instruct in the importance of proper eye makeup removal at night, if appropriate.

  Follow-up

- Schedule a return to the clinic in 4 days if no improvement, or sooner if the condition gets worse.

- Discontinue the ointment if the child complains of pain or burning and call the clinic.

  Consultations and referrals. Refer to an ophthalmologist if the condition does not improve.

Red Eye

AMY VERST

Etiology

Red eye is the most common acute disease of the eye seen in children in primary care offices. The most common possible causes can be from trauma (e.g., corneal abrasions, foreign bodies, perforating injuries), congenital anomalies (e.g., nasolacrimal duct obstruction, congenital glaucoma), allergic conjunctivitis (e.g., vernal conjunctivitis), herpes infections, neonatal conjunctivitis (chemical, gonococcal, and chlamydial), and conjunctival infections. The primary causative agents of bacterial conjunctivitis are *H. influenzae* (50% of cases) and *S. pneumoniae* (40% to 50% of cases), while viral conjunctivitis is caused by adenovirus and epidemic keratoconjunctivitis–adenovirus types 3, 8, and 19.

Incidence

- Red eye occurs in 1.6% to 12% of all newborns.
- *Chlamydia trachomatis* infection occurs in 3 in 1000 to 8 in 1000 live births.
- Herpes simplex occurs in 1 in 3000 to 1 in 20,000 live births.
- Nasolacrimal duct stenosis occurs in 2% of newborns.
- Bacterial infection is the cause of conjunctivitis in 50% of cases.
- Adenovirus is the most common cause of viral conjunctivitis.

Risk Factors

- No maternal prenatal care
- Prolonged rupture of membranes
- Prophylactic chemical use
- Maternal history of STD or substance abuse
- No prophylactic chemical use
- Day care setting
- Swimming pools
- Trauma
- History of otitis media
- History of pharyngitis
- History of HSV
- Sexual activity

- Contact lens use
- Makeup use

Differential Diagnosis (Table 34-10)

Neonatal conjunctivitis

Neonatal chemical conjunctivitis. Neonatal conjunctivitis caused by ocular prophylaxis with silver nitrate occurs within 2 days after birth and resolves in a day or so without sequelae. Swelling of lids with serous discharge may be seen in the first 24 to 36 hours of life.

Chlamydia trachomatis. C. trachomatis is the most frequent cause of infectious conjunctivitis in infants. Incubation period is 5 to 12 days after birth. Mucopurulent conjunctivitis starts after the sixth day after birth and becomes copious with obvious lid swelling. The child has a positive immunoassay for C. trachomatis.

Neisseria gonorrhoeae. Gonococcal conjunctivitis is a severe, bilateral purulent conjunctivitis with obvious lid swelling that begins 2 to 4 days after birth. A presumptive diagnosis is made on Gram stain findings of gram-negative diplococci with polymorphonuclear cells.

Herpes simplex. Conjunctivitis caused by herpes infection usually occurs with primary infection by HSV. Most cases are caused by HSV type 1, but type 2 does occur in newborns. The most common manifestation is skin vesicles. In over 70% of affected infants, the disease progresses within days to other sites. Conjunctival involvement usually appears between 3 days to 3 weeks after birth and is characterized by a moderate injection without follicle formation. History of maternal herpetic infection is usually present. Corneal dendrites may be seen.

Bacterial conjunctivitis. Bacterial conjunctivitis manifests with mild to moderate mucopurulent discharge from one or both eyes, beginning within 2 weeks after birth with diffuse conjunctival injection. The most common pathogens are *Haemophilus* organisms, *S. aureus, S. pneumoniae,* and enterococci.

Dacryocystitis. A bacterial infection of the lacrimal sac, dacryocystitis arises in newborns secondary to obstruction of the nasolacrimal duct. Affected infants manifest with a rapid development of erythema and swelling over the lacrimal sac. Systemic signs of illness may occur, and immediate hospitalization is necessary.

Nasolacrimal duct obstruction. Nasolacrimal duct obstruction appears in the first weeks of life with epiphora—tears overflowing onto the cheek without any stimulus. There is frequently an accumulation of mucoid material on the lashes and lower lid margin. The presence of mucopurulent discharge from the puncta on palpation of the lacrimal sac is diagnostic of lacrimal duct obstruction. It may be unilateral or bilateral (though this is less common).

Nonneonatal conjunctivitis

Bacterial conjunctivitis. Symptoms of bacterial conjunctivitis include tearing, mucopurulent discharge, conjunctival injection, and conjunctival swelling, usually seen in both eyes. The child may have concomitant OM without ear pain. The child reports that the eyelids are stuck closed on awakening. Vision is unaffected except for the strands of floating mucus, which can be blinked away to clear the vision.

Viral conjunctivitis. Adenovirus types 3, 7, and 16 are nonepidemic. Types 8 and 19, epidemic keratoconjunctivitis (EKC), are epidemic. Watery discharge starts in one eye, and the eye appears red. Preauricular nodes may be enlarged and tender and the child may complain of a scratchy sensation, swelling of the lower lids, and photophobia. The second eye becomes infected within 10 days. There is no change in visual acuity; otherwise the cornea is most likely involved. It is caused by EKC or HSV.

Acute allergic conjunctivitis. Watery, stringy, milky nonpurulent discharge is present in acute allergic conjunctivitis. Excessive tearing may also be present with mild hyperemia of the conjunctiva, itching, and edema of the lid. The child may have a history of recent exposure to a potential allergen. Acute allergic conjunctivitis is often seen in children with an allergic history (including hay fever and asthma).

Vernal conjunctivitis. Vernal conjunctivitis is an allergic conjunctivitis that is seasonal, recurrent, and bilateral. Itching is intense in the spring and fall. Large papules are observed on the palpebral conjunctivas of the upper lid. The child may complain of photophobia. Vision remains normal.

Primary herpes simplex. Primary HSV appears within 2 days to 2 weeks of contact with a person who has recurrent HSV infection. (Contact is often with a sore on the mouth.) Systemic signs are usually mild. Eye involvement includes obvious eyelid swelling, vesicles on the skin, and ipsilateral preauricular nodes that may be slightly swollen and tender. Acute unilateral redness, irritation, and watery discharge are appear. Dendrites stain with fluorescein.

Management

Neonatal conjunctivitis

Chemical conjunctivitis

Treatments and medications. None are indicated, though the practitioner may use irrigation with saline.

Counseling and prevention. Explain the cause to the parents. Instruct parents that the eye discharge is self-limiting and should resolve in 24 to 36 hours.

Follow-up. Check the neonate in 3 days if the condition does not improve, or sooner if the condition worsens.

Consultations and referrals. None are necessary.

Chlamydia trachomatis

Treatments and medications. Administer oral erythromycin ethylsuccinate 50 mg/kg per day (divided into four doses) for at least 2 weeks.

Counseling and prevention

- Accomplish prevention by early identification and treatment of the infected mother.
- Stress the importance of careful handwashing.
- Explain to parents that the disease is usually transmitted vaginally during delivery.
- Encourage the mother and her sexual partner to seek health care for evaluation and treatment.
- Instruct the parents that eye infection is also associated with neonatal pneumonitis. This pneumonia usually develops during the first 6 weeks of life and is characterized by nasal discharge, cough, and fast breathing. A chest radiograph indicates infiltrates.
- Advise parents that the efficacy of erythromycin therapy is 80%. The child may need a second course of therapy.

Follow-up

- Schedule a return visit in 3 days to monitor the eye infection.
- Schedule a return visit if the infant shows signs of *Chlamydia pneumoniae* or if the parents are concerned about the child's vision.

Table 34-10 Differential Diagnosis: Conjunctivitis (372.30)

CRITERIA	CHEMICAL CONJUNCTIVITIS	N. GONORRHOEAE*	C. TRACHOMATIS*	BACTERIAL CONJUNCTIVITIS (NEONATAL)	HERPES SIMPLEX*
ICD-9 code	372.05	098.40	076.1	771.6	054.43
Subjective Data					
History/description of problem	History of instillation of antimicrobial prophylaxis; serous mucoid discharge	Maternal history of exposure; thick discharge	Exposure from maternal genital tract	Exposure from maternal genital tract or environment	Excessive tearing, usually of one eye; serous discharge
Associated symptoms	None	Systemic infection of blood, CNS, and joints possible	Pneumonia	May be part of other staphylococcal illnesses	May have systemic infection
Onset	24-36 hours of life	2-6 days of life	1-2 weeks of life	First 2 weeks of life	3 days to 3 weeks of life
Objective Data **Physical examination**					
Conjunctiva	Clear	Edematous, hyperemic	Inflammation, hyperemic and edematous	Red, edematous	Corneal dendrites
Exudate	Serous	Purulent and abundant	Mucopurulent	Mucopurulent	Mucopurulent
Tearing	None	None	None	None	Excessive, usually one eye
Preauricular adenopathy	Not present	Not present	Not present	Not present	Not present
Skin	Eyelid edema	Eyelid and conjunctival edema	Edema of eyelid	Eyelid and conjunctival edema	Skin vesicles, herpetic vesicles on eyelid margins
Laboratory findings		Gram stain—gram negative diplococci; culture positive for N. gonorrhoeae	Immunoassay positive for C. trachomatis	Gram stain—white cells and organism; culture to determine organism	Viral cultures positive; Tzanck test of skin scraping—multinucleated giant cells

Refer to a physician/ophthalmologist.

Consultations and referrals
- Refer the child to a physician if the child shows signs of developing a *C. pneumoniae* infection.
- Refer the mother and her sexual partner for treatment.

Neisseria gonorrheae

Treatments and medications. Most pediatricians admit the neonate to the hospital for treatment and to evaluate for signs of disseminated infection. The American Academy of Ophthalmology recommends a single injection of ceftriaxone 25 to 50 mg/kg IM or IV. Frequent eye irrigation with saline are also begun immediately and continued at intervals until purulent discharge is eliminated.

Counseling and prevention

The infection is prevented by an appropriate screening culture of the mother prenatally, and instillation of prophylactic eyedrops is usually mandatory for all newborns at delivery.

NASOLACRIMAL DUCT OBSTRUCTION 375.56	DACRYOCYSTITIS 375.30	BACTERIAL 372.30	VIRAL 077.99	ALLERGIC 372.14	PRIMARY HERPES SIMPLEX* 054.9
Swelling of inner canthus; history of nasolacrimal duct stenosis; mucoid discharge	Redness and swelling over nasolacrimal sac	Eyelids stuck closed upon awakening; close contact with others with same symptoms; mucopurulent or purulent discharge	Scratchy sensation in one eye, then the other, with watery discharge	Watery eyes that itch from a few hours to days; history of other allergic conditions; history of exposure to irritant	Vesicles on skin of lids; reports blurred vision, painful eye; may be associated with varicella
None	Fever common; systemic signs of illness	Recent systemic illness, sore throat, fever, cough, flulike symptoms	May be part of systemic illness (e.g., measles adn rubella or Kawasaki's disease)	Possible signs of allergies (e.g., eczema, asthma)	Fever; no history of trauma to eye
First few weeks of life	First 6 months of life	Within days of exposure	Anytime	Anytime; if seasonal (spring and fall), then vernal conjunctivitis	Anytime
Clear	Nasal conjunctiva may be injected	Hyperemic	Red and edematous; follicular hyperplasia often present	Mild injection	Inflamed—circumcorneal injection
Mucopurulent	Yellowish white mucopurulent	Mucopurulent, yellow discharge in both eyes	Watery, starting in one eye and moving into both	Stringy and milky	Watery
Excessive	May be present	None	Present	Present	Present
Not present Accumulation of mucoid material on the lashes and lower lid margin	Not present Redness, swelling over lacrimal sac	Not present May have small ulcerated areas on lid	Not present Lids are edematous	Not present Lids are edematous; eyelids have cobblestone appearance	May be present Yellow crusts on lid; may or may not have vesicles
Negative	Gram stain and culture to determine organism	None initially, if no improvement, then culture and Gram stain; viral culture if vesicles or superficial corneal ulcerations appear	None initially	None	Fluorescein staining—dendrites seen

Explain to the parents why the child needs to be admitted if *N. gonorrhoeae* is present and why they also need to be treated.

Follow-up. Contact the Public Health Service or health department regarding the child's condition.

Consultations and referrals
- Refer all children with suspected *N. gonorrhoeae* to an experienced physician for hospital admission.

- Refer the mother and her partner for evaluation and treatment of *N. gonorrhoeae* before delivery if it is known, or after delivery if it is unknown.

Herpes simplex virus

Treatments and medications. Refer the child to an ophthalmologist.

Counseling and prevention. The infection is prevented by appropriate cultures of the mother at a prenatal visit. A cesarean section should be scheduled for a mother who has a history of active herpes. Instruct the parents that the child must be treated for the condition, which includes probable hospitalization and treatment for up to 3 weeks. Follow-up visits will also be necessary because of recurrences. Stress the importance of careful handwashing.

Follow-up. Schedule follow up as directed by the physician.

Consultations and referrals. Refer immediately to a physician or ophthalmologist all infants who exhibit signs or symptoms of herpes.

Bacterial conjunctivitis

Treatments and medications. Management of bacterial conjunctivitis is based on Gram stain and culture and sensitivity. If the organism is *Staphylococcus,* erythromycin ophthalmic ointment is instilled in the eyes every 2 to 4 hours. If the organism is not yet identified, prescribe erythromycin ophthalmic ointment until the culture results are received.

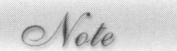

If the infant has fever or signs of systemic toxicity (e.g., poor eating), refer for a septic work-up.

Counseling and prevention. Close monitoring of the mother with prolonged membrane rupture is important. Explain the condition to the parents and instruct on the prevention of spread to others (e.g., washing hands carefully, avoidance of sharing washcloths and towels). Instruct and demonstrate to parents the installation of eyedrops, which can be done in two ways:

- Lay the child down and close his or her eyes, drop 1 drop of solution into the corner of the eye, and have the child open the eye. Repeat with the other eye.
- Put a finger on the bone under the lower eyelid, have the child look up, pull down the lid, and put a drop of solution into the lower lid. Have the child close the eye gently. Repeat with the other eye.

Also, discuss with the parents the signs of an ill infant, and explain to the parents the need to wash hands after diaper changes to prevent spread.

Follow-up. Obtain reports of culture and sensitivities as soon as possible. Schedule a return visit in 2 days to evaluate treatment, or sooner if the child is not improving or is worse.

Consultations and referrals. Usually none are needed.

Dacryocystitis

Treatments and medications. In an afebrile, systemically well, mild case with a reliable parent, prescribe amoxicillin–clavulanate potassium 20 to 40 mg/kg three times daily for 14 days.

In a child with fever or systemic signs of toxicity, refer child for hospitalization.

Counseling and prevention

- Discuss with the parents the cause and the treatment of the condition.
- Instruct on and demonstrate how to measure and give medication to the child.
- State that one of the possible side effects of amoxicillin–clavulanate potassium is an increased number of stools.

Follow-up. Schedule daily visits until the condition improves.

Consultations and referrals. Refer the child to a physician for hospital admission if the child is febrile or seems ill.

Nasolacrimal duct obstruction

Treatments and medications. Treatment requires massage of the nasolacrimal sac region. The parents need to use a firm downward pressure applied to the nasolacrimal sac (from the inner canthus of the eye down along the nose). This pressure allows the residual fluid in the sac to perforate the membrane that is obstructing the flow. This maneuver should be done three or four times a day. If signs of infection appear, treat it as a bacterial infection with erythromycin ophthalmic ointment. Aminoglycosides, gentamicin, or tobramycin should be avoided because of corneal toxicity. Parents may use warm compresses two to four times a day to keep the eyelids clean when discharge is present.

Counseling and prevention

- Explain to the parents that most obstructions are temporary and resolve without surgical probing.
- Demonstrate to the parents the technique used to massage the duct.
- Explain the signs and symptoms of infection.

Follow-up

- Follow up by telephone monthly and check at well-child visits.
- Schedule a return visit if the condition worsens or the parents are unsure.
- Remember that the majority of obstructions resolve spontaneously by 8 months.

Consultations and referrals. Refer the child to an ophthalmologist if the condition worsens or does not improve in 6 months.

Nonneonatal conjunctivitis

Bacterial conjunctivitis

Treatments and medications. Nongonococcal bacterial conjunctivitis can be treated with polymyxin-bacitracin ophthalmic ointment four times a day for 7 days, or erythromycin ophthalmic ointment four times a day for 4 days. An alternative is sulfacetamide sodium 10%, 1 or 2 drops in each eye every 2 hours for first 2 days and then every 4 hours for 3 more days. Do not use soaks or occlude the eyes because it may increase bacterial growth.

Counseling and prevention

- Instruct the parents and child on the cause of the disease.
- Instruct the parents and child on the installation of eyedrops. Have the child lie down and close the eyes, drop a drop of solution into the corner of one eye, and have the child open the eye. Repeat in the other eye. This should be done every 2 hours for the first 2 days and then four times a day until 2 days after all symptoms have disappeared.
- If ointment is prescribed, explain to the parents and child that vision will be blurred because it smears over the cornea.
- Instruct the parents on the installation of ointment. Often the ointment strip curls in upon itself; so hold the tube in the hand to warm it slightly, preventing this curling. Have the child look up and have the parent pull down the lower lid, exposing the cul-de-sac. Place a ½-inch strip of ointment along the cul-de-sac. Then have the child gently close the eye.
- Instruct the parents to immediately discontinue use of the medication if the eye shows a hypersensitivity to the medication.
- Educate the child on finger-to-mouth-to-nose-to-eye behavior.
- Instruct the parents on warm water washes to remove crusts and discharge before installation of medication.

- Teach the parents and child about the prevention of spread to others through good handwashing and no sharing of towels or washcloths.
- Advise the parents there should be no school for the child for 24 hours after the start of antibiotics because of the contagiousness of the condition.

Follow-up. Schedule a return visit in 2 days if no improvement, sooner if worse, for culture and sensitivity.

Consultations and referrals. Parents should notify the school nurse regarding the child's condition. Also, refer the child to a physician if the condition does not improve in 48 hours, or sooner if the condition worsens.

Viral conjunctivitis (epidemic keratoconjunctivitis)
Treatments and medications. None are indicated.
Counseling and prevention

- Instruct the parents on the cause and the course of the disease.
- Stress frequent handwashing to prevent spread to others.
- Advise the child to have a personal towel and bed linen to prevent spread.
- Instruct parents that there should be no school for the child until the virus clears, usually in 1 week.

Follow-up. Schedule a return visit if the symptoms become worse or the child complains of pain. he condition should resolve in 2 weeks, so the parents should call if the condition is not improving.

Consultations and referrals. Refer the child to an ophthalmologist in severe cases.

Acute allergic conjunctivitis
Treatments and medications

- Remove the allergen (e.g., hair spray, shampoo, cosmetics, animals).
- Discontinue any eyedrops or ointments.
- Apply cool compresses to the eyes.
- Use a topical antihistamine, a mast cell stabilizer, or combination eye drops to help relieve symptoms

Counseling and prevention

- Instruct parents on the cause and the course of the illness and the importance of allergen removal in the child's environment.
- Advise the parents and child that the use of over-the-counter (OTC) eyedrops may make the condition worse.
- Suggest washing the child's hair at night to prevent allergens from going on pillows and subsequently into eyes.
- Advise discarding eye makeup applicators when empty. They should not be refilled and reused.
- Recommend not sharing eye makeup applicators with others.

Follow-up. Schedule a return visit if the condition persists or the discharge changes color or consistency.

Consultations and referrals. Refer the child to an ophthalmologist if the condition is chronic.

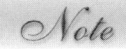

Never give steroids if herpes is present.

Primary herpes simplex virus
Treatments and medications. Refer the child to an ophthalmologist for treatment.

Counseling and prevention

- Instruct the patient on the cause and course of the disease.
- Explain the need for referral.
- Discuss with the parents or others who have "cold sores" on the lips to avoid kissing the child on or near the eyelids.

Follow-up. Schedule follow-up care as directed by the ophthalmologist.

Consultations and referrals. Refer the child to an ophthalmologist.

Herpes zoster
Treatments and medications. Refer the child to an ophthalmologist.

Counseling and prevention. Instruct the parents that the condition is caused by varicella-zoster virus. The virus remains dormant in the trigeminal ganglion until reactivated. It is most commonly encountered in young children and older adults. Explain the need for referral.

Follow-up. Schedule follow-up care as directed by the ophthalmologist.

Consultations and referrals. Refer the child to an ophthalmologist.

Bibliography

Ah-Tye, C., Paradise, J., & Colborn, D.K. (2001). Otorrhea in young children after tympanostomy tube placement for persistent middle ear effusion—prevalence, incidence, and duration. *Pediatrics, 107*(6), 1251-1258.

Alcorn, D.M. (2001, March). Red eye: When to treat and when to refer. *Infectious Diseases in Children* (monograph), 3-8.

Bacal, D.A., Rousta, S.T., & Hertic, R.W. (1999). Why early vision screening matters. *Contemporary Pediatrics, 16*(2), 155-167.

Bluestone, C.D. & Klein, J.O. (2000). *Otitis media in infants and children* (3rd ed.). Philadelphia: W.B. Saunders.

Castiglia, P. (1994). Strabismus. *Journal of Pediatric Health Care, 6*(1), 236-238.

DeRespinis, P.A. (2001). Eyeglasses: Why and when do children need them? *Pediatric Annals, 30*(8), 455-461.

Dowell, S.F., Butler, J.C., Giebink, G.S., et al. (1999). Acute otitis media: Management and surveillance in an era of pneumococcal resistance—a report from the Drug-Resistant *Streptococcus pneumoniae* Therapeutic Working Group. *The Pediatric Infectious Disease Journal, 18*(1), 1-9.

Dowell, S.F., Marcy, S.M., Philips, W.R., et al. (1998). Otitis media: Principles of judicious use of antimicrobial agents. *Pediatrics, 101*(1), 165-171.

Forbes, B.J. (2001). Management of corneal abrasions and ocular trauma in children. *Pediatric Annals, 30*(8), 465-472.

Gegliotti, F. (1995). Acute conjunctivitis, *Pediatrics in Review, 16*(3), 203.

Hoberman, A. & Paradise, J. L. (2000). Acute otitis media: Diagnosis and management in the year 2000. *Pediatric Annals, 29*(10), 609-620.

Kenna, M.A. (2000). Otitis media: The otolaryngologist's perspective. *Pediatric Annals, 29*(10), 630-636.

Kovaliosky, A. (1985). *Nurses' guide to children's eyes.* Orlando, FL: Grune & Stratton.

Leitman, M. (1994). *Manual for eye examination and diagnosis* (4th ed.). Cambridge, MA: Blackwell Scientific Publishers.

Linsk, R., Gilsdorf, J., & Lesperance, M. (1999). When amoxicillin fails. *Contemporary Pediatrics, 16*(10), 67-88.

Magramm, I. (1992). Amblyopia: Etiology, detection and treatment. *Pediatrics in Review, 13*(1), 7-15.

Niemela, M., et al. (1995). A pacifier increases the risk of recurrent acute otitis media in children in daycare centers. *Journal of Pediatrics, 96*(5), 884-888.

Pichichero, M.E. (2000). Recurrent and persistent otitis media. *Pediatric Infectious Disease Journal, 19,* 911-916.

Roddey, O.F. & Hoover, H.A. (2000). Otitis media with effusion in children: A pediatric office perspective. *Pediatric Annals, 29*(10), 623-629.

Rubin, S.E. (2001). Management of strabismus in the 1st year of life. *Pediatric Annals, 30*(8), 474-480.

Simon, J.W. & Kaw, P. (2001). Vision screening performed by the pediatrician. *Pediatric Annals, 30*(8), 446-452.

Stoole, S. (1994). *Otitis media with effusion in young children* (clinical practice guideline no. 12, AHCPR publication no. 94-0622). Rockville, MD: Agency for Health Care Policy and Research, Public Health Service, U.S. Department of Health and Human Services.

Taylor, D. (1990). *Pediatric ophthalmology.* Cambridge, MA: Blackwell Scientific Publishers.

Tigges, B.B. (2000). Acute otitis media and pneumococcal resistance: Making judicious management decisions. *The Nurse Practitioner, 25*(1), 69-80.

Uphold, C.R. & Graham, M.V. (1998). *Clinical guidelines in family practice* (2nd ed.). Gainesville, FL: Barmarrae Books.

Chapter 35 *Gastrointestinal System*

Abdominal Pain, p. 412
Constipation and Fecal Impaction, p. 420
Diarrhea and Loose Stool, p. 425
Hernias: Inguinal, Scrotal, and Umbilical Bulges, p. 434
Infantile Colic, p. 441
Mouth Sores, p. 447
Nausea and Vomiting, p. 452
Perianal Itch and Pain, p. 458
Stool Odor, Color, and Consistency Changes, p. 462

Risk Factors*

- Congenital anomalies of the gastrointestinal (GI) system (e.g., facial, esophageal, intestinal, rectal, anal)
- Failure to pass meconium within the first 24 to 48 hours of life
- Low birth weight (LBW), including prematurity
- Family or child history of GI diseases (e.g., inflammatory bowel disease [IBD], cystic fibrosis)
- Alterations in bowel pattern (e.g., constipation, rectal bleeding)
- Significant weight change
- Alteration in feeding or nutritional intake
- Metabolic disease (e.g., inborn errors of metabolism) or diseases of the liver or pancreas
- Neuromuscular disease (e.g., lesions of the spinal cord)
- Blood dyscrasias
- Immunosuppression
- Systemic disorders (e.g., disorders of liver, biliary system, pancreas, gallbladder)
- Alcohol and drug abuse
- Pharmacologic agents (e.g., antibiotic therapy, iron therapy, antacids)
- Behavioral alterations
- Emotional and physical stress
- Eating disorders (e.g., anorexia nervosa)
- Dysfunctional parenting
- Environmental hazards (e.g., substandard living conditions, contaminated water or food, insufficient toileting or hygiene)
- Sexual abuse
- Anal sex
- Pregnancy
- Immobility and bed rest
- Inadequate or incomplete toilet training or forced training
- Poisoning (e.g., ingestion of caustic agent, overdosage)
- Ingestion of foreign body
- Developmental delay of oral and fine motor development
- Poor suck-and-swallow coordination

*Chapter overview written by Catherine J. Dillon Dolan.

Health Promotion

Prevention of Infection

- Maintenance of general health, including balanced nutrition, adequate fluid intake, adequate rest, exercise, and immunizations
- Handwashing after diapering, toilet use, and before eating
- Enteric precautions, including environmental cleaning (e.g., of surface tops and toys, separation of symptomatic child)
- Proper food preparation, handling, and storage
- Proper laundering of soiled linens and clothing
- Proper disposal of diapers
- Avoidance of exposure to pathogens

General Support Measures

- Recognize early signs of illness (e.g., failure to eat, vomiting, diarrhea, dehydration, weight loss, behavior changes, jaundice).
- Promote a diet that is age appropriate and nutritious.
- Model and encourage good eating habits.
- Use age-appropriate explanations and strategies to teach a child self-care in respect to toileting.
- Discourage substance abuse.
- Introduce toilet training when a child indicates physical and developmental readiness to learn, can communicate his or her needs, and demonstrates a desire to be clean and dry.

Subjective Data

Obtain a comprehensive history with careful attention to the following:

- Description of abdominal pain, including onset, location, pattern, radiation, relieving factors (e.g., medication, position), and precipitating factors (e.g., meal and type of food [greasy, fatty, milk])
- Change in weight in a defined period
- Description of emesis (e.g., nonbilious, bilious, bloody, mucoid, time in relation to meal)
- Description of stool, including frequency, size, color, odor, consistency, presence of blood or mucus, and any change in elimination pattern
- Description of urine, including color, clarity, odor, and any increase or decrease in frequency
- Nutrition history, including eating and feeding behavior, appetite; detailed, 24-hour diet recall, and volume and amount of food
- For a formula-fed infant, the volume and type of formula and how the formula is prepared
- For a breastfed infant, the number of feedings in 24 hours, time on each breast, and mother's diet
- Developmental history
- Immunization history
- Elimination pattern, including number of stools per day and description and the history of toilet training
- Allergy history

- Medication history, including the use of over-the-counter (OTC) or prescribed medication and a list of current medications
- Recent travel
- Recent illness
- Sleeping pattern, including recent changes
- Change in activity level
- Change in personality or temperament
- Birth history, including birth weight and length, passage of meconium, and infant feeding history
- Family health history (with a concentration on any family history of GI disease)
- Level of family stress (both the child's and parents' perceptions), including methods of coping with stress, perception of coping abilities, stability of parental relationship, parent and sibling relationships, any change in job or unemployment, and any recent moves
- Social history, including daily schedule (at school, work, and play), use of alcohol or drugs, and sexual activity (with description)
- Environmental history, including the location and condition of the residence, who lives in the home, number of rooms, sleeping arrangements, cleanliness, occupation of family members (including type of job), any infectious diseases, any chemical or environmental irritants, and the types of pets
- Exposure level, including settings where the child spends time (e.g., day care, preschool, elementary school, high school, camp)
- School, including grade and notable successes or failures
- Economic factors, including a family income sufficient for food, clothing, shelter, and health care treatment (including medications)
- Exposure to smoking (e.g., Does the child smoke or chew tobacco? Do other family members or friends smoke?)
- Child stress level, including friendship patterns, changes in intimate or peer relationships, sports involvement or other competitive outlets, changes in school, or a transition to elementary school, middle school, or high school
- Review of systems (with a concentration on the GI system)

Objective Data

Physical Examination

A complete physical examination is generally performed on all infants and children, with special attention given to the assessment of hydration status and examination of stool. It is recommended that an additional team member be present for a rectal examination. Before proceeding with the examination, explain all procedures to the child and parents. Perform careful examination of the following:

- *Measurements*—Measure height and weight percentiles, weight for height percentile, and head circumference percentile (in a child 3 years of age and under). Plot growth parameters on growth curve and compare with past measurements.
- *Vital signs, including temperature*
- *General appearance*—Inspect body muscle mass, posture or body position, and facial expression, and evaluate interaction between the child and parents and examiner.
- *Skin and lymph*—Inspect for color, edema, rash, and lesions; inspect and assess nails for color, capillary refill, and clubbing; inspect and palpate for lymphadenopathy; and observe the location and size of any findings.
- *Neck*—Palpate for position of trachea, thyroid size, and masses.
- *Eyes*—Inspect sclerae for color, and inspect eyes for position, swelling, tearing, and discharge. Perform funduscopic examination.
- *Ears*—Inspect color, integrity, position, and landmarks of tympanic membrane, and assess mobility by pneumatic otoscopy.
- *Nose*—Inspect for discharge, deformity, swelling, flaring of nostrils, and color and integrity of internal mucosae and turbinates. Assess for patency of nares (palpate over and adjacent to the four paranasal sinuses).
- *Mouth and throat*—Inspect lips, oral mucosa, tonsils, and posterior area of pharynx.
- *Heart*—Auscultate heart sounds.
- *Chest and lungs*—Assess respirations and auscultate breath sounds.
- *Abdomen*—Inspect for skin color, contour, symmetry, peristalsis, and pulsations, and inspect the umbilicus for color, discharge, odor, inflammation, and herniation. Auscultate for bowel sounds in all four quadrants to assess motility and for the presence of any bruits. Percuss over the liver, stomach, and spleen to assess organ size. Liver dullness is present along the right costal margin, and the normal liver span is 6 to 12 cm at the right midclavicular line and 4 to 8 cm along the midsternum line. Stomach tympany may be present in the area of the left lower anterior rib cage (indicating a gastric air bubble), while splenic dullness is percussed near the tenth rib on left side. Palpate over the abdomen to identify the size and shape of the organs and the presence of any masses (e.g., stool) or tumors and to assess for tenderness. The liver edge is normally firm with a sharp, regular ridge with a smooth surface during inspiration. The spleen tip may be palpable 1 to 2 cm below the left costal margin during inspiration. The kidneys are rarely palpable except in neonates. Palpate for inguinal hernia by sliding the little finger into the external inguinal canal, and palpate over the costovertebral angle to check for tenderness.
- *Rectum*—Inspect external anus for presence of fissures, hemorrhoids, skin tags, rash, prolapse, or signs of physical or sexual abuse. Assess anal wink. Perform digital examination to assess tone, identify presence of masses or polyps, and obtain stool for guaiac test.
- *Genitalia*—Inspect external organs, assess development and sexual maturation by Tanner staging (see Chapter 40), and inspect for inguinal and femoral bulges and scrotal masses.
- *Pelvic area*—Examine any sexually active female who has abdominal pain.
- *Neurologic signs*—Assess level of consciousness. Observe any irritability. Examine for meningeal signs.

Diagnostic Procedures and Laboratory Tests

Diagnostic tests are dictated by the history and physical examination findings. The following tests may be ordered.

Stool tests

- *Stool for occult blood*—Screen for the presence of blood.
- *Fecal leukocytes*—Screen for the presence of white blood cells, suggestive of inflammatory enterocolitis.
- *Stool pH*—Screen for carbohydrate malabsorption (pH less than 5.5).

- *Stool for reducing substance (sugar)*—Screen for carbohydrate malabsorption by Clinitest (greater than 0.5%).
- *Stool for fat*—Screen for intestinal malabsorption of fat and pancreatic insufficiency.
  Qualitative—A random stool specimen
  Quantitative—A 72-hour stool collection over 3 consecutive days with a diet recall
- *Stool culture*—Screen for bacterial and viral pathogens.
- *Stool for ova and parasites*—See Parasitic Disease in Chapter 44. Perform microscopic examination of feces to screen for parasites. Often stool samples are collected for 3 consecutive days.
- *Pinworm examination*—Perform transparent tape test or perianal swab to screen for pinworms (see Parasitic Disease in Chapter 44).

Blood tests

- *Blood cell and differential counts*—Order a complete blood cell (CBC) count to evaluate for anemia as in an acute GI tract bleed or chronic inflammation or in response to medication. The total white blood cell count and the total number of neutrophils increase in response to tissue damage related to an infectious process. Eosinophilia can be present in allergic reactions such as milk or soybean allergy or in parasitic infections.
- *Erythrocyte sedimentation rate (ESR)*—Identify the presence of an inflammatory or necrotic process and monitor response to treatment for inflammatory disorders. An elevated ESR can be seen in chronic inflammatory processes such as IBD.
- *Blood chemistries*—Monitor for hydration, electrolyte, and nutritional status. Abnormalities of sodium and potassium are often seen in dehydration. Decreased total protein and albumin indicate poor nutritional state. Disorders causing altered fluid balance affect the blood urea nitrogen level, which is elevated in dehydration and decreased in fluid overload.
- *Liver function tests*—Measure bilirubin levels for indication of known or suspected hemolytic disorders, confirmation of observed jaundice, and determination of the cause of jaundice. Aspartate aminotransferase (AST) (former name was serum glutamate oxaloacetate [SGOT]) and alanine transaminase (former name was serum glutamate pyruvate transaminase [SGPT]) elevations indicate liver disease or liver damage. Alkaline phosphatase elevation indicates disorders associated with the liver, bone, and kidneys; however, levels can be elevated as a result of normal growth in children.
- *Serum amylase*—Evaluate chronic abdominal pain and monitor disease processes of the liver and pancreas.
- *Serum lipase*—Evaluate chronic abdominal pain and monitor disease processes of the liver and pancreas.
- *Hepatitis screening*—Determine the presence of antigen or antibody to a specific type of hepatitis; to determine past exposure, immunity, or carrier status; for screening before donating blood products; and to determine the progression of liver disease (see Chapter 44).
- *Helicobacter pylori*—Remember that the following recommendations for the diagnosis of *H. pylori* infection in children have been endorsed by the North American Society for Pediatric Gastroenterology and Nutrition and the American Academy of Pediatrics.
  Biopsies and histology—Histologic examination of multiple biopsy specimens of the stomach obtained by endoscopy. Currently this is the test of choice for the diagnosis of *H. pylori* in children.
  Rapid urease testing—Rapid urease testing includes pH-sensitive dye tests for urease (such as CLO test) on biopsy specimens. *H. pylori* produces urease, which hydrolyzes urea to ammonia and carbon dioxide (CO_2).
  Serology—This uses the enzyme-linked immunosorbent assay (ELISA) technique; reliable, indirect method to detect presence of serum antibodies; immunoglobulin A (IgA) and immunoglobulin G (IgG) against *Helicobacter* organisms.
  Urea breath test—This measures labeled CO_2 in expired breath after oral administration of radiolabeled urea.
  QuickVue H. pylori gII test—This is a simple one-step 5-minute test that requires as little as two drops of whole blood. It is a lateral-flow immunochromatographic assay intended for the rapid, qualitative detection of IgG antibodies specific to *H. pylori* in human serum, plasma, or whole blood. Results are available in 5 minutes or less. (For additional information, contact Quidel Corp., 10165 McKellar Court, San Diego, CA 92121; [800] 546-8955; www.quidel.com.)

Urine tests. See also Chapter 42.

- *Urinalysis and urine culture*—Detect infection and alteration in kidney and liver function.
- *Urine for specific gravity*—Evaluate hydration status.

Radiographic and ultrasonic procedures. See also Appendix D, Radiologic Tests.

- *Upper gastrointestinal tract series*—Evaluate persistent epigastric pain or heartburn; suspected hiatal hernia; suspected strictures or blood in the lower esophagus; hematemesis or blood in the feces; persistent abdominal pain or diarrhea; unexplained weight loss, anorexia, nausea, or vomiting; inflammatory disorder (e.g., Crohn's disease) or tumor of the stomach or small bowel; congenital anomalies (e.g., pyloric stenosis); malrotation of the bowel causing obstruction; diagnosis of malabsorption syndrome; or suspected foreign body or suspected tumor of the stomach or small bowel.
- *Abdominal radiograph*—Evaluate a palpable abdominal mass or for diagnosis of intestinal obstruction and acute abdominal pain of unknown origin; to evaluate the presence of suspected air, fluid, or foreign objects in the abdomen; to differentiate between genitourinary and GI symptoms; to determine the shape, size, and position of the liver and spleen in evaluating splenomegaly, tumors, and masses.
- *Abdominal ultrasonogram*—Determine the structure or position of organs within the abdomen (e.g., liver, spleen, pancreas, gallbladder, kidneys) and evaluate the patency and function of vessels and ducts of the portal system, renal arteries and veins, splenic vein, superior and mesenteric veins, and biliary and pancreatic ducts.
- *Liver and biliary ultrasonogram*—Evaluate the cause of upper right quadrant pain, diagnose hepatic lesions or cysts, evaluate the patency of the hepatic duct, differentiate between obstructive and nonobstructive jaundice, evaluate potential causes of hepatomegaly (e.g., mass, trauma, abnormal liver function tests), diagnose gallbladder disorders (e.g., cysts, polyps, tumors, stones), and diagnose obstruction of the biliary tree or ducts.

- *Barium swallow*—Diagnose esophageal reflux, esophagitis, or suspected congenital abnormalities (e.g., tracheoesophageal fistula, esophageal atresia), and determine the presence of an ingested foreign object.
- *Barium enema (lower gastrointestinal tract series)*—Determine the cause of rectal bleeding, mucus or blood in the feces, and changes in bowel patterns; use to identify congenital anomalies of the bowel, inflammatory disorders of the colon, Crohn's disease or colitis, polyps or tumors, the cause of weight loss or anemia, persistent abdominal pain or distension of unknown origin (to rule out a suspected foreign body in the colon); and also use as an intervention for the reduction of intussusception in children.
- *Oral cholecystography*—Detect gallstones and use to aid in the diagnosis of inflammatory disease and tumors of the gallbladder.

Nonnuclear medicine scans

- *Computed tomography scan*—Evaluate inflammation or infection (such as abscess of the liver, pancreatitis, appendicitis); diagnose tumors or metastases; identify abdominal aneurysms, obstructions, or congenital anomalies.

Nuclear medicine scans

- *Meckel's scan*—Evaluate unexplained abdominal pain and GI tract bleeding and determine sites of ectopic gastric mucosa by focal increased activity in abnormal structures.
- *Technetium-99m hepatoiminodiacetic acid (HIDA) scan*—Evaluate hepatobiliary function by visualization of the radioisotope taken up by the liver and excreted into the biliary tree, gallbladder, and duodenum.

Manometry procedures

- *Anorectal manometry*—Evaluate the mobility of the internal and external anal sphincter. This test is indicated in suspected Hirschsprung's disease and atypical constipation and useful in biofeedback in bowel training.
- *Esophageal manometry*—Determine whether pyrosis (heartburn) and dysphagia are caused by gastroesophageal reflux (GER) or esophagitis. This test may also be used to diagnose esophagitis and chronic GER, achalasia, or chalasia.

Endoscopic procedures

- *Colonoscopy*—Determine disorders of the lower GI tract, IBD (e.g., Crohn's disease, ulcerative colitis), colitis, polyps, and Hirschsprung's disease and use to remove foreign bodies and polyps from the colon.
- *Endoscopic retrograde cholangiopancreatography (ERCP)*—Differentiate biliary tract obstruction from liver disease in jaundice; diagnose pancreatitis, cholangitis, or carcinoma; and identify anomalies, strictures, stenosis, calculi, or cysts in the ducts, which may cause their obstruction.
- *Esophagogastroduodenoscopy (EGD or upper endoscopy)*—Confirm the diagnosis of reflux esophagitis, esophageal strictures or hiatal hernia, gastric or duodenal ulcer, tumors of the small intestine, anatomic disorders or strictures, and ingested foreign body.

Other tests

- *pH study*—Monitor esophageal pH over a 24-hour period for the evaluation of GER.
- *Human chorionic gonadotropin*—Measure in urine or serum. This test can detect early pregnancy and threatened or incomplete abortion.

- *Sweat test*—Diagnose or confirm cystic fibrosis.
- *Breath hydrogen test*—Evaluate for carbohydrate malabsorption. A rise in expired hydrogen concentration after oral loading with a particular carbohydrate (e.g., lactose) indicates malabsorption.
- *d-Xylose test*—Estimates the functional surface area of the duodenojejunal intestinal mucosa by measuring the absorption of d-xylose taken orally.
- *Rectal biopsy*—Evaluate for Hirschsprung's disease.

Abdominal Pain

MARIE ANN MARINO & SUSAN M. DEVIVIO

Alert

Consult with or refer to a physician for the following:
- Signs of appendicitis (e.g., progressive abdominal pain, localized rebound tenderness at McBurney's point [about 2 inches from the anterosuperior iliac spine on a line to the umbilicus], fever, anorexia, leukocytosis, pain on digital rectal examination)
- Acute abdominal pain lasting more than 6 hours
- Acute abdominal pain in children less than 2 years of age
- Acute abdominal pain associated with bilious emesis
- Sudden onset of acute abdominal pain in a pregnant adolescent
- Rectal bleeding or hematochezia (bloody stools)
- Jaundice
- Sudden onset of severe, paroxysmal, colicky pain, with or without vomiting
- Chronic GI disease
- Persistent abdominal pain without clear cause

Etiology

Table 35-1 identifies some diseases by age that may cause abdominal pain. The diseases, however, may also be seen in patients of other ages. Appendicitis is a significant cause of abdominal pain and the most common disease requiring surgery in childhood. Intestinal obstruction with strangulation, perforated viscus, and ruptured ectopic pregnancy are common surgical emergencies of the abdomen that require immediate identification.

Gastroenteritis (bacterial, viral, or parasitic) often becomes evident with acute abdominal pain, fever, and vomiting, in addition to diarrhea, and must be differentiated from an acute surgical condition. Additionally, gastritis and peptic ulcer disease, both associated with *H. pylori,* may be a significant cause of abdominal pain. Infections of the urinary tract may also become evident with abdominal pain.

Although not commonly encountered in children, peptic ulcer disease, hepatic or biliary tract disease, pancreatitis, IBD, and abdominal tumors should be considered in the etiologic factors of acute abdominal pain. Child abuse and abdominal trauma may insidiously become evident and must also be considered.

Recurrent abdominal pain is defined as acute episodes occurring monthly for at least 3 months in children. In recurrent episodes organic causes are less common, and dysfunctional and psychogenic causes predominate. Common causes include chronic stool retention, reaction to stress and anxiety, hypochondriasis, school phobia, overeating, and depression.

Text continued on p. 417

Table 35-1 Differential Diagnosis: Abdominal Pain (789.0)

CRITERIA	APPENDICITIS*	INTUSSUSCEPTION*	GASTROENTERITIS	URINARY TRACT INFECTION	MECKEL DIVERTICULUM*	CHOLECYSTITIS*	PEPTIC ULCER DISEASE
ICD-9 code	541.	560.0	558.9	599.0	751.0	575.10	533.90
Subjective Data							
Onset/duration	Acute	Variable	Variable	Variable	Insidious	Gradual	Episodic
Fever	Low grade	Common	Variable	Variable	None to low grade	Variable	None
Abdominal symptoms	Vague pain followed by localization to RLQ	Intermittent severe periumbilical abdominal pain with cramping and drawing up of knees	Severe, crampy abdominal pain	Suprapubic pain	RLQ pain	RUQ pain	Intermittent, dull aching abdominal pain
Associated or other symptoms	Anorexia, vomiting, constipation, fever, chills if peritoneal inflammation present	Initially, normal bowel movement followed by bloody, mucoid stools ("currant jelly"); bilious vomiting	Profuse diarrhea, chills, headache, vomiting	Lower back pain, enuresis, foul-smelling urine, dysuria, urgency, frequency, feeding difficulties and irritability in infants	Painless rectal bleeding (pain may be prominent in school-age children)	Pain below right scapula, nausea, vomiting, jaundice, fatty-food intolerance (in older child)	Vomiting, nausea, heartburn, flatulence
Patient and family history	None	None	Attendance at day-care centers, ingestion of contaminated foods	Urinary tract abnormality, sexual activity, poor hygiene, perineal infections (pinworms)	Familial cases have been reported	Usually idiopathic; may be associated with viral illness	Family history in 25% to 50% of patients
Objective Data **Physical examination**							
Vital signs	Low-grade fever	Progression to high fever (106° F); weak, thready pulse–shallow respirations	Variable fever	Variable fever (infants may be hypothermic)	Normal	Variable fever	Normal
Abdominal signs	Abdominal pain with rebound tenderness localized over appendix site (McBurney's point)	Sausage-shaped mass palpable in right side or upper middle of abdomen; increasing abdominal distention	Diffuse and crampy abdominal pain which may be severe	Costovertebral angle tenderness, flank pain, suprapubic pain on palpation	RLQ pain on palpation, palpable mass with ileocolic intussusception, obstruction in 25% of cases	Vague, colicky abdominal pain that gradually localizes to RUQ; may have mass	Periumbilical or epigastric pain that is intermittent (2 to 4 episodes/day), lasting <30 minutes, and is often exacerbated by eating and relieved by vomiting.

*Immediate referral to a physician.
IUD, Intrauterine device; PT/PTT, prothrombin time/partial thromboplastin time; RLQ, right lower quadrant; RUQ, right upper quadrant; WBC, white blood cell.

Continued

Table 35-1 Differential Diagnosis: Abdominal Pain (789.0)—cont'd

CRITERIA	APPENDICITIS*	INTUSSUSCEPTION*	GASTROENTERITIS	URINARY TRACT INFECTION	MECKEL DIVERTICULUM*	CHOLECYSTITIS*	PEPTIC ULCER DISEASE
Associated or other signs	Right-sided tenderness and/or localized mass on digital rectal examination; peritoneal signs: Inability to walk/jump/cough or climb onto examination table without pain	Loud crying and straining with periods of comfort and normal play	Profuse diarrhea which may be bloody, dehydration, vomiting	Turbid urine, irritation of external genitalia, vomiting, hematuria; infants may have jaundice, sepsis, or FTT	Dark maroon or melanotic bloody stools	Jaundice (25% of patients), vomiting	Hematemesis and hemoccult positive stools
Laboratory data	WBC count >15,000 cells/mm³, neutrophil leukocytosis, pyuria, radiopaque fecalith on abdominal radiograph	Barium enema reveals obstruction	Variable serum leukocytosis; evidence of enteric pathogens in stool	Urine culture positive for pathogens, pyuria	Radionuclide scan (Meckel diverticulum scan) may reveal diverticulum lined with gastric mucosa	Ultrasonography may reveal gallstones; radioisotopic scan demonstrates the biliary tree and gallbladder function	Upper GI tract barium series and/or endoscopy

CRITERIA	PANCREATITIS*	ECTOPIC PREGNANCY*	DYSMENORRHEA	PELVIC INFLAMMATORY DISEASE*	PNEUMONIA	TONSILLOPHARYNGITIS (STREPTOCOCCAL)
ICD-9 code	577.0	633.9	625.3	614.9	486.	034.0
Subjective Data						
Onset/duration	Sudden	Variable	Lower abdominal pain, 1 to 2 days before menses through 2 to 4 days of menses	Follows the onset of menses	Bacterial, sudden onset; viral, acute or insidious	Gradual or acute
Fever	Variable	None	None	Variable	Variable	Can be high (to 104° F)
Abdominal symptoms	Steady epigastric pain (often radiates to back)	Lower abdominal tenderness and pain	Crampy spasmodic lower abdominal pain	Lower abdominal pain	Nonspecific abdominal pain	Nonspecific abdominal pain
Associated or other symptoms	Vomiting	Amenorrhea, vaginal bleeding, vomiting, fainting	Nausea, vomiting, diarrhea, lower backache, thigh pain, headache, fatigue, dizziness, syncope, nervousness	Adnexal tenderness, vaginal discharge, chills, menstrual irregularities, dyspareunia, vomiting, constipation, diarrhea, dysuria	Young baby: Tachypnea, nasal flaring, retractions, grunting; Older child: Cough, chest pain, sputum production	Headache, vomiting, sore throat
Patient and family history	May be predisposed by systemic infections, abdominal trauma, diabetes mellitus, cystic fibrosis, systemic lupus erythematosus, drugs (corticosteroids, thiazides, estrogens, L-asparaginase)	May be associated with history of salpingitis, use of IUD, delay in childbearing, prior tubal surgery, use of progestin-only birth control pills	None	May be associated with use of IUDs, acute salpingitis, postpartum or postabortal infection, multiple sexual partners or sexually transmitted endocervical infections	Recent infectious illness in family may be reported	Exposure to streptococcal infection

Objective Data

Physical examination

Vital signs	Variable fever, hypotension in severe cases	Hypotension in ruptured ectopic pregnancy with hemorrhage	Normal	Variable fever	Fever, cough, and tachypnea, especially in a young child	Fever, 102° to 104° F
Abdominal signs	Epigastric or RUQ pain (can progress to severe) that radiates to the back; abdomen is tender, not rigid	Pelvic pain, rebound tenderness, pelvic mass	Lower abdominal cramping	Lower abdominal pain and pelvic tenderness, rebound tenderness if peritonitis is present	Nonspecific abdominal pain without tenderness	Nonspecific abdominal pain without tenderness
Associated or other signs	Vomiting, epigastric tenderness; absent, decreased bowel sounds; in severe cases hypotension and shock may be present	Adnexal tenderness, vomiting, vaginal bleeding, syncope; ruptured: Intraperitoneal hemorrhage and shock	Vomiting and diarrhea	Cervical motion tenderness, adnexal tenderness, vaginal discharge, cervical inflammation, vomiting, diarrhea, breakthrough bleeding	Grunting, nasal flaring, retractions; normal to localized diminished breath sounds to rales	Tonsillar erythema, petechial mottling of soft palate, pharyngeal exudates, anterior cervical lymph nodes
Laboratory data	Elevated serum amylase level, radiograph of abdomen, may show a localized ileus	Serum HCG test, ultrasonography	Menstrual fluid prostaglandin levels, uterine jet washings, endometrial sampling	CBC count and differential, ESR, serologic test for syphilis and HIV, endocervical discharge culture, c-reactive protein, serum HCG test	Chest radiograph, WBC count and differential, blood culture and sensitivity in febrile children, sputum Gram stain and culture	Rapid streptococcal antigen detection tests, pharyngeal culture and sensitivity, monospot (heterophile antibody) test or Epstein-Barr virus serology

CRITERIA	CROHN'S DISEASE	BLUNT ABDOMINAL TRAUMA*	HENOCH-SCHÖNLEIN PURPURA*	PSYCHOGENIC ABDOMINAL PAIN (RECURRENT)
ICD-9 code	555.9	959.1	287.0	789.0
Subjective Data				
Onset/duration	Subtle, often with periods of remissions and exacerbations	Can be sudden and acute or insidious	May be acute	Recurrent (may be acute)
Fever	Variable	None	Low grade	None
Abdominal symptoms	Crampy abdominal pain common	Variable abdominal pain (subtle to acute)	Colicky abdominal pain (may be severe)	Nonspecific abdominal pain
Associated or other symptoms	Diarrhea, anorexia, general malaise, joint complaints, weight loss	Bruising, swelling	Vomiting, rash, malaise, knee or ankle pain	Headache, dizziness, limb pain
Patient and family history	Genetic factors may play a role in increased family incidence	History of recent blunt trauma: Can be accidental or intentional	None	Anxiety, fearfulness, poor self-esteem in children; marital discord, maternal depression/health problems more prevalent in families of these children

*Immediate referral to a physician.

IUD, Intrauterine device; PT/PTT, prothrombin time/partial thromboplastin time; RLQ, right lower quadrant; RUQ, right upper quadrant; WBC, white blood cell.

Continued

Table 35-1 Differential Diagnosis: Abdominal Pain (789.0)—cont'd

CRITERIA	CROHN'S DISEASE	BLUNT ABDOMINAL TRAUMA*	HENOCH-SCHÖNLEIN PURPURA*	PSYCHOGENIC ABDOMINAL PAIN (RECURRENT)
Objective Data				
Physical examination				
Vital signs	Orthostasis	May deteriorate over hours or days	Low-grade fever, moderate hypotension if renal involvement	Normal
Abdominal signs	Periumbilical or RLQ pain	Increasing abdominal tenderness, especially in liver/splenic areas; increasing abdominal girth; absent or decreased bowel sounds	Colicky abdominal pain	Should be considered organic until proven otherwise
Associated or other signs	Growth failure, chronic perianal lesions (skin tags, fissures, abscesses), severe weight loss	Hematuria; severe: Hypotension, tachycardia, tachypnea	Urticarial rash on buttocks and lower extremities progressing to papular purpuric lesions; angioedema of scalp, eyelids, lips, ears, hands, feet, back, scrotum, and perineum; arthritis in large joints; nephritis	Reaction anxiety secondary to stress; depression; school phobia; negative attention gain
Laboratory data	Elevated ESR, leukocytosis, anemia, decreased serum protein and albumin: Radiologic and endoscopic examinations of GI tract; biopsy; granulomas on histologic study	CBC count, PT/PTT, platelet count; abdominal radiograph/computed tomography scan may be helpful	Elevated ESR, WBC count; eosinophilia, gross or occult blood in stools; elevated serum immune globulin A level; hematuria; proteinuria	CBC count, ESR, urinalysis and culture, serum albumin and amylase levels, and stool for occult blood; consider pregnancy test

CRITERIA	GASTRITIS*
ICD-9 code	535.5
Subjective Data	
Onset/duration	Variable
Fever	None
Abdominal symptoms	Epigastric pain
Associated or other symptoms	Postprandial vomiting, irritability, poor feeding, weight loss; rare: chest pain, hematemesis or melena
Patient and family history	Associated with peptic ulcer disease
Objective Data	
Physical examination	
Vital signs	Normal
Abdominal signs	Epigastric pain
Associated or other signs	Vomiting (postprandial), hematemesis (from mild to hemorrhagic)
Laboratory data	CBC count, gross or occult blood in stools; H. pylori antibody, culture of gastric biopsy for H. pylori; upper endoscopy with biopsies.

*Immediate referral to a physician.
IUD, Intrauterine device; PT/PTT, prothrombin time/partial thromboplastin time; RLQ, right lower quadrant; RUQ, right upper quadrant; WBC, white blood cell.

Of the organic causes, urinary tract disease is the most common cause of recurrent abdominal pain and must be considered even in the absence of dysuria and frequency. Other organic causes of recurrent abdominal pain include irritable bowel disease, Henoch-Schönlein purpura (HSP), dysmenorrhea, *mittelschmerz,* and pelvic inflammatory disease, which can mimic a recurrent abdominal syndrome. Organic causes must be ruled out before a diagnosis of dysfunctional or psychogenic pain is considered.

Incidence

- Abdominal pain is a common symptom of many disorders.
- Appendicitis is the most common surgical condition; incidence is greatest in the preadolescent, adolescent, and early adult age groups. It is rare in children less than 2 years of age (less than 1% of all cases of appendicitis). It is estimated that between 7% and 12% of the population will develop appendicitis at one point during their lives. The incidence of perforation is 40% in infants and children.
- Recurrent abdominal pain affects 13% to 17% of middle and high school students; greater than 4% of these students miss more than 6 days of school each year. An organic cause can be identified only in fewer than 10%. Females are affected more often than males.

Risk Factors

Acute abdominal pain
- Dietary factors (e.g., fatty foods, lactose intolerance)
- Medications (e.g., erythromycin, theophylline, amoxicillin with clavulanic acid)
- Sexual activity
- Trauma and child abuse
- Consumption of contaminated food

Recurrent abdominal pain
- Family history of functional GI tract symptoms
- Stressful situations at home or school
- Rigid toilet training practices
- Sexual activity
- School absenteeism
- Dysfunctional coping mechanisms

Differential Diagnosis (see Table 35-1)

Appendicitis is the inflammation of the appendix resulting from obstruction of the appendiceal lumen. Principal diagnostic features include abdominal pain with rebound tenderness localized over the site of the appendix (McBurney's point), pain on digital or rectal examination, and leukocytosis. Untreated appendicitis may lead to appendiceal perforation and peritonitis. Appendicitis requires immediate physician referral.

Intussusception is the invagination, or telescoping, of a proximal portion of the intestine into the distal adjacent intestine, usually in the area of the ileocecal valve. It becomes evident with sudden paroxysmal abdominal pain, palpable sausage-shaped mass, and bloody, mucoid stools ("currant jelly" stools). Intussusception requires immediate physician referral.

Gastroenteritis is a viral, bacterial, or parasitic infection and inflammation of the GI tract. Most common associated symptoms include severe, crampy, abdominal pain; profuse diarrhea; and vomiting.

Urinary tract infection (UTI) is an infection of the urinary tract as evidenced by the presence of bacterial pathogens in the urine. Key diagnostic features include flank pain, dysuria, frequency, and positive urine culture.

Meckel's diverticulum is a persistent remnant of omphalomesenteric duct and is described as the "rule of twos" (i.e., diverticulum is approximately 2 centimeters in length, occurs twice as often in boys, becomes evident before 2 years of age). Painless rectal bleeding and bloody stools are significant findings. Meckel's diverticulum requires immediate physician referral.

Cholecystitis is an acute inflammation of the gallbladder that commonly becomes evident with vague, colicky, abdominal pain localized to the right upper quadrant, nausea, and vomiting. It requires immediate physician referral.

Peptic ulcer disease is an imbalance between gastric acid production and mucosal protective elements resulting in the loss of the tissue lining the stomach, usually in the gastric antrum. It is most often associated with intermittent periumbilical pain that is usually relieved by eating, and it requires immediate physician referral.

Gastritis is an inflammation of the stomach mucosa. *H. pylori* can be a significant cause of severe gastritis. Key diagnostic features include epigastric tenderness, postprandial vomiting, irritability, weight loss, and poor feeding. Gastritis requires immediate physician referral.

Pancreatitis is the inflammation and damage of the pancreas resulting from the autodigestion of the gland by its proteolytic enzymes. Principal diagnostic features include epigastric or right upper quadrant pain that radiates to the back and an elevated serum amylase level. Pancreatitis requires immediate physician referral.

Ectopic pregnancy is a pregnancy located in the fallopian tube. It commonly becomes evident with abdominal tenderness and pain in a female with a positive serum human chorionic gonadotropin (HCG) test result. It requires immediate physician referral.

Dysmenorrhea is painful menses associated with crampy lower abdominal pain. A key diagnostic feature is cervical motion tenderness.

Pelvic inflammatory disease is an infection in the upper genital tract that involves the fallopian tubes. It requires immediate physician referral.

Pneumonia is the acute inflammatory process of the pulmonary parenchyma, small airways, and alveoli. Neonates and young infants require immediate physician referral because these children will likely require hospitalization. In addition, any child who appears acutely ill or has respiratory compromise should be hospitalized.

Streptococcal tonsillopharyngitis is the acute infection of the pharynx with tonsillar edema, pharyngeal erythema, and exudates caused by group A β-hemolytic streptococci.

Crohn's disease is the chronic inflammation of the GI tract, most often affecting the ileum and colon. Common features include crampy abdominal pain, diarrhea, and chronic perianal lesions. It is an immune-mediated inflammation of unknown origin.

Blunt abdominal trauma can be caused by an accidental or intentional insult that results in significant internal abdominal trauma. Immediate surgical intervention may be necessary if internal bleeding is massive or persistent, and in any case it requires referral to a physician or an emergency department to rule out surgical emergency.

Henoch-Schönlein purpura (HSP) is a diffuse vasculitis involving a triad of intestinal symptoms, joint pain, and purpura. The primary manifestations arise from small blood vessel vasculitis. The cause of HSP is unknown. It affects children from

2 to 8 years of age (occurring more often in boys) and requires immediate physician referral.

Psychogenic abdominal pain is recurrent abdominal pain with acute episodes at least monthly for a minimum of 3 months. Multiple causes include school or sleep disturbances and difficulties with family or peers. It is most often seen in school-age children.

Management

Gastroenteritis. See also Diarrhea and Loose Stool and Nausea and Vomiting.

Treatments and medications. Most episodes of acute diarrhea are viral in origin and self-limited, lasting a few days to a week. Antibiotic administration is usually not indicated. Antibiotics are indicated only in cases of salmonellosis in infants younger than 3 months of age; gastroenteritis in infants; immunocompromised patients; sepsis; hemoglobinopathies; infection by *Shigella, Yersinia, Campylobacter, Vibrio cholerae,* or *Aeromonas* organisms; or cases of parasitic disease. Administration of oral rehydration solutions (ORSs) (e.g., Ricelyte, Infalyte, Pedialyte) in small quantities for 4 to 6 hours may be performed. Intravenous rehydration is indicated for patients with severe dehydration (10%) and associated hemodynamic instability, or with diarrhea greater than 10 ml/kg per hour.

After rehydration has been achieved, feeding is started as soon as possible. In formula-fed infants, a lactose-free formula may be better tolerated in the first 48 hours of feeding. Breast milk for nursing infants is usually well tolerated. In older infants and children, a regular diet may be introduced, particularly one with complex carbohydrates (e.g., rice, wheat, potatoes), yogurt, cereals, and meat (chicken). Foods high in fat or simple sugars should be avoided. Antidiarrheal agents are usually not indicated.

Counseling and prevention

- Discuss the benefit of good hygiene practices in reducing the fecal-oral spread of infectious agents.
- Avoid the use of OTC antidiarrheals.
- Explain to the parents the course of the illness and that the symptoms should subside in a few days to a week.
- Ensure adequate understanding of the treatment plan.

Follow-up. Close follow-up study, including daily weights, is indicated for small infants who may rapidly become dehydrated. Schedule a return visit if symptoms do not improve or worsen.

Consultations and referrals. All patients indicating the following should be admitted to the hospital for parenteral fluids and close observation:

- Hemodynamic instability
- Inability to retain orally ingested fluids
- Toxic appearance
- Change in level of consciousness
- Inability to follow treatment regimen

Urinary tract infection. See also Painful Urination in Chapter 42.

Treatments and medications. Many antimicrobials are effective against the bacteria that commonly cause UTIs. The choice of antibiotic should be guided by previous culture and sensitivity. Commonly used antibiotics include amoxicillin, trimethoprim-sulfamethoxazole (TMP-SMX), cephalexin, cefprozil, and nitrofurantoin. The usual duration of therapy is 7 to 10 days.

Counseling and prevention

- Encourage adequate hydration, especially with acidic juices (e.g., apple, cranberry).

- Discuss proper perineal hygiene practices and the avoidance of bubble baths.
- Avoid straining at stool.
- Wear cotton rather than nylon underpants.
- Empty bladder completely with each void.

Follow-up. A culture should be obtained 24 to 48 hours after appropriate antimicrobial therapy has been initiated to confirm therapeutic success.

Consultations and referrals. Infants, especially newborns, and young children should be referred for urologic evaluation to detect any anatomic abnormalities. Children with pyelonephritis require hospitalization and intravenous antibiotics with hydration.

Dysmenorrhea. See also Menstrual Irregularities in Chapter 40.

Treatments and medications. Treatment is directed at symptomatic relief. Mild analgesics such as aspirin, acetaminophen, or ibuprofen usually provide substantial relief. Nonsteroidal anti-inflammatory drugs (NSAIDs) (e.g., naproxen sodium) may also be given. Antiprostaglandin medications are especially effective when started at onset of menses and continued for the first 1 or 2 days of the cycle. If the pain is not responsive to antiprostaglandin drugs, a course of oral contraceptives (e.g., Ortho-Novum 1/35, Ortho-Novum 7/7/7, Tri-Leven/Triphasil, Norinyl 1 and 35) may be tried. If relief is obtained with oral contraceptives, medication is prescribed for 3 to 6 months and then discontinued. If cramps recur, a trial of antiprostaglandins should again be attempted.

Counseling and prevention. Advise that NSAIDs should be taken with food and are contraindicated in pregnant patients, preoperative patients, and patients with ulcer disease, as well as in cases of GI tract bleeding, clotting disorders, renal disease, or allergies to aspirin or NSAIDs.

Follow-up. Patients should be seen initially every 3 or 4 months for evaluation of the effectiveness of the medication therapy.

Consultations and referrals. Refer to a physician if severe dysmenorrhea does not respond to NSAIDs or oral contraceptives, because organic disease (e.g., endometriosis) must be considered and a laparoscopy is indicated.

Pneumonia

Treatments and medications. For older infants and children, appropriate antibiotic therapy for bacterial pneumonia depends on the etiologic agent, child's age, clinical presentation, and time of year. Common bacterial agents include:

- *For neonates—Group B* Streptococcus, Chlamydia trachomatis, Escherichia coli
- *For children 1 month to 5 years of age—Streptococcus pneumoniae, Haemophilus influenzae*
- *For children over 5 years of age—S. pneumoniae, Mycoplasma*

For most children, outpatient antibiotic therapy for mild to moderate severity is appropriate. For young children, amoxicillin for 10 days is sufficient. If there is no improvement in 48 hours, the practitioner may consider changing therapy to a cephalosporin or erythromycin. For patients with penicillin allergy, erythromycin may be considered. If *Mycoplasma* is suspected, erythromycin is the drug of choice.

General supportive care includes rest, fluids, and a cough suppressant at bedtime (if coughing interrupts sleep).

Counseling and prevention

- Inform parents of the name, dose, frequency, and duration of the antibiotic.

- Emphasize the need to finish all medication, even if child is feeling better and fever subsides.
- Advise parents that uncomplicated bacterial pneumonia should improve in 48 hours.

Follow-up

- Provide an immediate recheck if no improvement within 48 hours.
- If improved, recheck at the completion of therapy.
- If there has been no recent tuberculin skin test, place one.

Consultations and referrals

- If tuberculin skin test result is positive and comes with radiographic evidence of infiltrates, refer to a physician.
- Neonates and young infants with clinical symptoms of pneumonia should be referred immediately to a physician.
- Any child with severe symptoms or respiratory compromise should be referred immediately to a physician.

Streptococcal tonsillopharyngitis

Treatments and medications. Penicillin V administered orally for 10 full days is sufficient and produces a prompt clinical response within 24 to 48 hours. If there is a documented history of penicillin allergy, erythromycin ethylsuccinate taken orally for a full 10-day course is a suitable alternative. If noncompliance with a 10-day course of oral antibiotic therapy is suspected, a single intramuscular dose of penicillin G benzathine (Bicillin L-A) is an accepted alternative.

To relieve throat pain, saline gargles, lozenges, and warm compresses to the neck are helpful. Acetaminophen or ibuprofen may be given to reduce fever. Encourage cool, nonacidic liquids (e.g., gelatin water, weak tea, flat ginger ale) progressing to a soft, bland diet as pain resolves.

Counseling and prevention

- Inform the parents of the name, dose, frequency, and duration of the antibiotic.
- Emphasize the importance of finishing all medication, even though the child may feel better and have no fever.
- Instruct that side effects of oral penicillin include nausea, vomiting, diarrhea, and mild epigastric distress; epigastric distress is also a common side effect of erythromycin.

Follow-up

- Recheck immediately if fever continues 48 hours after antibiotic therapy is started or if pain worsens.
- After antibiotic therapy, recheck the child, though a repeated culture is not necessary if symptoms abate.
- Schedule a return visit if symptoms recur.

Consultations and referrals. Consult a physician for the following:

- Signs of rheumatic fever are present (e.g., arthritis, carditis, subcutaneous nodules) (see Chapter 45)
- Development of acute nephrotic syndrome (e.g., edema, hypertension, oliguria)
- Evidence of peritonsillar abscess

Crohn's disease

Treatments and medications. Supportive care is the mainstay of treatment. In severe cases, total parenteral nutrition may be instituted, while in mild to moderate episodes, elemental diets have been shown to induce remissions. Free elemental diets may also relieve diarrhea because they require minimal digestion, thereby reducing the volume of stool. Resting the bowel by these measures also promotes growth. Corticosteroids are used for acute exacerbations for 6 to 8 weeks, with gradual weaning over an additional 8 to 12 weeks.

For ileal Crohn's disease, azathioprine or 6-mercaptopurine used concomitantly with corticosteroids allows for reduced steroid usage. For colonic Crohn's disease, sulfasalazine is given along with corticosteroids. For perianal fistulas, metronidazole is beneficial.

Counseling and prevention. Since the origin of Crohn's disease is unknown, efforts are directed at counseling the child and family in understanding the course of the illness and coping with the effects of this often-debilitating disease. Inform the child and family of name, dose, frequency, side effects, and duration of any pharmacologic therapy, and instruct on the side effects of the most commonly used medications:

- *Corticosteroids*—GI distress may be alleviated when these are taken with meals or antacids. The patient may have an alteration in psyche with associated mood swings and euphoria. He or she may also experience development of a cushingoid state.
- *Azathioprine*—Effects include leukopenia, thrombocytopenia, and GI tract distress. These effects may be less severe if the medication is taken with meals or in divided doses.
- *6-Mercaptopurine*—Effects include leukopenia, thrombocytopenia, and anemia.
- *Sulfasalazine*—Effects include anorexia, headache, and nausea.
- *Metronidazole* (not approved for Crohn's disease by Food and Drug Administration [FDA])—Effects include nausea, headache, anorexia, an unpleasant taste in the mouth, and peripheral neuropathy.

Follow-up. Exacerbations should be monitored frequently to assess for complications, including worsening symptoms, excoriation of anal area, growth status, psychologic adjustment, and medication side effects.

Consultations and referrals

- Provide immediate referral to a physician for extensive perianal or rectal disease, severe growth failure, or failure to respond to treatment modalities.
- Provide immediate referral to a surgeon for signs of intestinal obstruction or perforation.
- Care of the child with Crohn's disease should be in collaboration with a pediatric gastroenterologist.
- Refer to a mental health professional for family and child counseling, if indicated.

Henoch-Schönlein purpura

Treatments and medications. Treatment of HSP is primarily supportive. If the disease followed a bacterial infection, especially streptococcal infection, eradication of the pathogen is essential. Arthritis, edema, rash, fever, and malaise may be alleviated by the use of salicylates or NSAIDs. Corticosteroids (1 to 2 mg/kg every 24 hours) can be used for bowel involvement or arthritis that is unresponsive to salicylates.

Counseling and prevention

- Inform parents of the name, dose, frequency, side effects, and duration of medications.
- Advise that the course of illness runs from a few days (mild illness) to 6 weeks for more severe illness.

Follow-up. Schedule follow-up care as needed.

Consultations and referrals. Refer to a physician if signs of intestinal hemorrhage, obstruction, intussusception, or perforation occur, as well as for cases of renal or central nervous system (CNS) involvement.

Psychogenic abdominal pain

Treatments and medications. Empiric therapy with analgesics (nonopioid anticholinergic or antispasmodic agents) and gastric acid–reducing agents may be tried. Without evidence of organic disease, the primary focus is to lessen abdominal pain by identifying and addressing possible stressors in the child's life.

Counseling and prevention. Explain to the child and family that abdominal pain in children is common and does not necessarily indicate an organic disease.

Follow-up. Children with psychogenic abdominal pain should be seen every 1 to 2 months for evaluation of pain and reassurance.

Consultations and referrals. Consult with a mental health professional when symptoms extend beyond a reasonable period.

Constipation and Fecal Impaction

JANE A. FOX

Alert

Consult with or refer to a physician for the following:
- No meconium passed within first 24 to 36 hours after birth
- History of no stool in 4 days or more in infant less than 1 month old
- Anal or abdominal pain for more than 2 hours
- Soiling in previously toilet-trained child
- Large anal fissure
- No stool for 7 days
- Recurrent constipation
- Rectal bleeding
- Possibility of sexual abuse

Etiology

The most common causes of constipation in children include changes in feeding habits (e.g., dietary mismanagement); environmental, genetic, or constitutional factors; a change in daily habits; toilet-training; pain on defecation; or a degree of dehydration and disease. Medications such as antacids, aluminum hydroxide (Amphojel), iron preparations, narcotics, antidepressants, bismuth compounds, anticonvulsants, barium sulfate, and decongestants and overuse of laxatives and enemas have the side effect of promoting constipation.

Organic causes for constipation are uncommon and include lead poisoning and mechanical obstructions such as Hirschsprung's disease, meconium ileus, intestinal atresia, and stenosis, strictures, or volvulus. Another consideration is psychogenic problems that lead to stool retention. Metabolic disorders such as hypothyroidism, hypercalcemia, cystic fibrosis, hypokalemia, diabetes mellitus, and renal tubular acidosis may also cause constipation. Neuromuscular dystrophy, spinal cord trauma or lesions, and meningomyelocele may lead to constipation. Neurologic disorders, including mental retardation, are often associated with defecation problems.

Incidence

- Constipation is common in children.
- About 3% of all outpatient visits and 25% of visits to gastroenterologists are related to constipation.
- In most children (90% to 95%) no organic cause can be detected.
- Fecal impaction is relatively rare in children.
- Constipation occurs in about 17% of children between 1 and 3 years of age and in 1% of 4-year-old children.

- The ratio of boys to girls is approximately 6:1, but women have a higher incidence of constipation than men.
- There is little or no preference for social class.
- Approximately 85% to 95% of constipation in children is simple or functional.
- About 20% of children have moderate constipation when they are first toilet trained.
- It is estimated that 80% to 90% of all cases of encopresis are the result of chronic constipation.
- Encopresis is rare before 3 years of age with, an increased prevalence in school-age children (1.5% to 3%) and higher incidence in males than females (3:1 to 4:1).
- Hirschsprung's disease is reported in 1 of every 5000 births.

Risk Factors

- Family history of constipation, fecal retention, or encopresis
- Inconsistent toileting habits
- Poor positioning on toilet
- Excessive parental intervention
- Low fiber intake
- Poor dietary habits
- Lack of exercise
- Children with chronic illness
- Depression
- Prolonged bed rest or immobilization
- Neuromuscular impairment impacting feeding and mobility
- Changes in the daily routine
- Stressful situations such as divorce, birth of a sibling, death of a family member
- Uncomfortable lavatory environment
- Traveling
- Constipating drugs (e.g., anticonvulsants, narcotics, OTC cold medications, antihistamines)

Differential Diagnosis

Constipation is a symptom, not a disease. Most important in diagnosing constipation is the history. A clear description of what the parent means by constipation is needed. Often perfectly normal patterns of defecation are misinterpreted as a result of personal, familial, cultural, or social expectations.

Constipation is defined in clinical practice as an alteration in the frequency, size, or consistency of stools (Table 35-2). Numerous studies have shown that frequency of defecation changes with age. Normal stool frequency is variable.

Young infants have an average of five to seven stools a day. This number decreases to one to three during the second half of the first year of life.

Despite patterns of normal stool frequency for age, children still have constipation manifested by hard stools that are difficult to pass. The presenting complaint for the child is most often infrequent bowel movements, but constipation should be clearly defined as hard stools that are difficult to pass, without emphasis on frequency.

Simple constipation or *voluntary withholding* is the most common cause (90% to 95%) of constipation beyond the neonatal period. There is no definite organic cause. It may be influenced by environmental factors or a diet that contains excessive refined carbohydrates and a deficiency in fiber. Functional constipation often first becomes evident during times of dietary transition such as weaning in infancy and in early childhood when the range and composition of what the child eats are changing.

Table 35-2 Differential Diagnosis: Constipation and Fecal Impaction

CRITERIA	SIMPLE CONSTIPATION	FUNCTIONAL/ CHRONIC	FECAL IMPACTION	ENCOPRESIS	ANAL FISSURE	HIRSCHSPRUNG'S DISEASE*
ICD-9 code	564.0	564.0	560.39	787.6	565.0	751.3
Subjective Data						
Age on onset or duration	After 1 year of age	After 2 years of age	More common in children subject to sudden immobility, bed rest, or decreased fluid consumption	About 4 years of age	Any age	At birth
Family history	Can be a family history	Positive family history common	None	Possible	None	Familial patterns in small number of cases
Stools/frequency	Parents report: Dry, hard stools; straining; stool frequency less than five times a week	Parents report very large stools	Regular passage of hard stools at 3–5-day interval; possible continuous soiling that patients describe as diarrhea; straining at stool	Fecal incontinence, large-caliber stools are common	Hard stools; patient suppresses painful defecation; blood on surface of feces, on toilet paper, or in toilet	Parents report small, ribbon-like stools or no stools
Precipitating or aggravating factors	May report excessive intake of refined carbohydrates; low dietary fiber; anal fissure	May report environmental daily habit changes; toilet training; traveling; uncomfortable lavatories; immobilization	ADHD, soiling, prior history of anal fissure	Constipation with maternal overconcern; overaggressive toilet training; extreme family stressors at time of toilet training	Poor dietary habits	None
Associated symptoms	Abdominal pain Acute, self-limiting illness	Encopresis common, pain on defecation, vague abdominal pain	May have vague complaint of abdominal pain associated with vomiting	Increased fecal accumulation; posturing, fecal incontinence; abdominal pain: Periumbilical, dull and crampy	History of painful or hard stools	Diarrhea, vomiting, constipation, and abdominal distention may be present during infancy; abdominal cramps and bloating may be present in older children; occurrence of explosive, watery diarrhea, fever, dehydration may signify the presence of enterocolitis; encopresis uncommon

*Immediate referral to a physician.
ADHD, Attention deficit hyperactivity disorder.

Continued

Table 35-2 Differential Diagnosis: Constipation and Fecal Impaction—cont'd

CRITERIA	SIMPLE CONSTIPATION	FUNCTIONAL/ CHRONIC	FECAL IMPACTION	ENCOPRESIS	ANAL FISSURE	HIRSCHSPRUNG'S DISEASE*
Objective Data						
Physical examination						
Vital signs	Normal	Normal	Normal	Normal	Normal	May have unexplained fever
Growth parameters	Normal growth	Normal growth	Normal	Normal	Normal	Poor growth common
Abdominal examination						
Inspection	Possible abdominal distention	Abdominal distention possible	May be distended	Possible abdominal distention	Normal	Abdominal distention common
Auscultation	Bowel sounds present	Bowel sounds present	Decreased bowel sounds	Bowel sounds present	Normal	Bowel sounds decreased
Palpation	Normal	Moveable fecal masses are often appreciated in the left colon and sigmoid	Palpable feces	Soft, nontender mass midline of left lower quadrant	Normal	Palpable abdominal impaction
Rectal examination	Normal	Cavernous rectum, often filled with feces	Large quantities of hard feces in rectal ampulla	Enlarged stool mass in rectal ampulla	Tear visualized in anal canal at mucocutaneous junction	Ampulla empty, narrowed rectum
Laboratory data	Normal	Abdominal x-ray reveals a large rectal/sigmoid impaction with variable amounts of stool throughout the remainder of the colon	Urine culture may reveal possible urinary tract infection	Abdominal x-ray for new onset (consider); also consider sweat chloride, thyroid, and lead levels	Normal	Abdominal x-ray may be nonspecific during first few days of life; follow-up x-rays may reveal colonic distention with no air in the rectum; barium enema frequently reveals a transitional zone in the colon, accompanied by delayed evacuation of the barium >24 hours
Rectal biopsy	Normal	Normal		Normal		No ganglion cells

*Immediate referral to a physician.
ADHD, Attention deficit hyperactivity disorder.

Chronic constipation usually includes a history of constipation for more than 2 months. There may be soiling and physical symptoms.

Fecal impaction, which some patients actually describe as diarrhea (because it involves liquid passing around hard stools), is most likely to occur in any child subjected to sudden immobility, bed rest, or significant change in diet or fluid consumption. Children with this condition must strain at stooling, do not have normally formed stools, and often have toothpaste-like stool and continuous soiling.

Encopresis is the regular, involuntary fecal soiling after 4 years of age in underpants or other unorthodox places. These children often appear nonchalant about the problem and unaware of the odor and discomfort. Fecal soiling usually occurs at home, not at school.

Anal fissure can occur at any age and may be an acute or a chronic condition. The child may have hard bowel movements with pain on defecation. Blood streaking may be noted on the stool or toilet paper. Constipation results from suppression of defecation because it induces pain. Children with an anal fissure often report blood in the bowel movement. When questioned, they usually recognize that the blood is on the surface of their stool, on the toilet paper, or in the toilet bowl rather than mixed in with the stool.

Hirschsprung's disease results in mechanical obstruction from inadequate motility in part of the intestine. It is characterized by the congenital absence of ganglion cells. Aganglionosis extends no farther than the sigmoid colon in 80% of children, but in 3% it involves the entire colon. It accounts for about one fourth of all cases of neonatal obstruction, though it may not be diagnosed until late in infancy or childhood. It is four times more common in boys than in girls. The typical infant with Hirschsprung's disease is of average weight but fails to pass meconium during the first 24 to 36 hours of life. Progressive abdominal distension develops, and the baby refuses feedings and finally begins vomiting bilious intestinal contents.

The differential diagnosis of constipation in an infant less than 6 months of age should include four conditions:
1. Hirschsprung's disease (discussed previously).
2. Hypothyroidism (see Chapter 33).
3. Imperforate anus. This is a condition that may not be recognized immediately in the newborn period. These infants may have an anteriorly displaced anus that does not allow for the easy passage of stool.
4. Infant botulism. This results in constipation in infants 6 weeks to 6 months of age. History reveals exposure to honey, corn syrup, or homegrown herbal decoctions. These infants are usually breastfed. They are often febrile, hypotonic, and lethargic. A clue to diagnosis is flattened facies and inability to smile or gaze away from a light shined directly into the eye.

Any infant suspected of having one of these disorders should be referred to a physician.

Management

Simple constipation

Treatments and medications. Children with mild constipation may require only dietary changes. Recommend an adequate intake of liquids as well as a high-fiber diet including fruits (whole fruits rather than juices), vegetables, grains, cereals (cereals that have 5 or more g of fiber per serving), breads (whole wheat or whole grain), nuts, seeds, and beans. Skim or low-fat milk may be substituted for whole milk and milk products, which are known to be constipating.

The minimal daily dietary fiber recommended for children 2 years of age and older can be calculated when the chronologic age is taken and 5 is added. For example, a 5-year-old child (5) + 5 equals 10 g of fiber per day. Adolescents require about 20 to 35 grams of fiber a day in their diet. Dietary fiber should be gradually increased over a 2- to 3-week period to minimize the abdominal discomfort sometimes associated with a high-fiber diet.

Recommend limiting the intake of highly processed foods such as white bread, sugared cookies, sugared cereals, and processed meats in children older than 2 years of age. When high-fiber foods are added (Table 35-3), recommend an increase

Table 35-3 Dietary Fiber Content of Selected Foods

FOOD	SERVING SIZE	TOTAL DIETARY FIBER (G)
Fruit		
Apple, unpeeled	1 medium	2.8
Banana	1 medium	1.9
Blueberries	½ cup	2.0
Cantaloupe	¼ of whole	0.9
Grapes	10	0.05
Orange	1 medium	2.5
Orange juice	¾ cup	2.1
Pear, unpeeled	1	4.6
Plum, unpeeled	1	0.8
Raisins	½ cup	3.0
Strawberries	1 cup	2.7
Watermelon	1 cup	0.6
Vegetables (Cooked)		
Broccoli	1 cup	5.4
Carrots	1	1.8
Corn	1 cup	3.5
Potato, with skin	1	5.0
Potato, no skin	1	2.0
Potato, french fries	10	1.2
Spinach	½ cup	2.0
Zucchini	½ cup	1.0
Vegetables (Raw)		
Carrots	1 medium	2.0
Celery	1 stalk	<1.0
Lettuce, romaine	1 cup	1.0
Tomato	1 medium	2.0
Refined Grain Products		
Bagel	1 medium	1.0
Bread	1 slice	0.6
Cereal, corn flakes	1¼ cup	1.2
Cereal, shredded wheat	⅔ cup	3.2
Cookies	2	0.3
Crackers	4	0.4
Macaroni	1 cup	2.8
Legumes/Nuts		
Kidney beans	1 cup	13.3
Peas	1 cup	5.6
Peanut butter	1 tbsp	1.0

in fluid intake to prevent the fiber from having a binding effect. A child weighing less than 10 kg needs 100 ml/kg of fluid per day. Add another 50 ml/kg per day (or approximately 1 pint per day) for a child weighing 10 to 20 kg (a toddler).

For children and adolescents, increasing activity through more outdoor play and walking may also be helpful.

In cases of prolonged constipation a laxative may be required in addition to dietary measures and proper toilet training. Laxatives are prescribed according to age, body weight, and the severity of constipation (Table 35-4).

For infants, add 1 or 2 teaspoons of corn (Karo) syrup to each bottle, or add a bottle of prune juice in a 1:1 ratio with water once or twice daily. If the infant is over 4 months of age, strained fruit may be introduced. Do not change to a low-iron formula. Avoid repeated finger dilatations, enemas, digital disimpactions, and frequent suppositories.

For children over 4 months of age it is possible to modify transit time and stool bulk with a fiber supplement such as Maltsupex, which contains indigestible malt and fermenting dextrins (carbohydrate). The dosage is ½ to 2 teaspoons orally twice a day mixed in water or fruit juice. After 6 months of age, add high-fiber foods to the diet, including pureed fruits and vegetables (e.g., prunes, apricots, plums, peas, beans).

For children over 1 year of age chopped fruits and vegetables can be added to increase fiber in the diet. Senokot may be given. It affects intestinal motility and fluid electrolyte transport and stimulates defecation, and it is available over the counter in syrup, granules, or tablets. Dosages include: for children 1 to 5 years of age, 5 ml at bedtime, with a maximum dosage of 5 ml twice daily; for children and adolescents 5 to

15 years of age, 10 ml at bedtime, with a maximum dosage of 10 ml three times daily. The optimal time to administer Senokot (morning or evening) depends on the parents' and child's schedule. Senokot should be given at the same time each day. A higher single dose is usually more effective than divided smaller doses. The dosage of Senokot requires individual adjustments depending on the child's results.

If diet changes and other measures are not successful, bulk-forming agents may be helpful for adolescents; these include psyllium (Effer-Syllium), methylcellulose (Citrucel), and polycarbophil (FiberCon). Begin with 1 tablespoon a day and increase to 3 tablespoons a day; 16 ounces of water should be taken with each dose. It is important to use such agents on a regular basis for maximum benefit.

Counseling and prevention

- Counsel parents concerning normal bowel function, explain that patterns vary in children as they do in adults, and advise on the early detection of problems. During the first few weeks of life an infant may have a stool after each feeding or less frequently depending if he or she is breastfed or formula-fed. By 3 to 4 months age most infants have one or two stools a day, but less frequent stooling can be normal. By 4 years of age an adult stooling pattern should develop.
- Educate parents about constipation, including the definition, when to be concerned, the practitioner's evaluation, and common interventions.
- Discuss parental attitudes and expectations regarding toilet habits.
- Educate the parents on toilet training.
- Encourage exercise.
- Instruct on diet modifications and medications. Write instructions for parents. Advise parents that Senokot may cause abdominal cramping. If needed, suggest adding foods high in fiber to the diet (see Table 35-4).

Follow-up. Instruct parents to call in 2 days if there is no improvement. Also have them call if the child develops severe abdominal pain or cramping or soils self.

Consultations and referrals. There are usually none.

Chronic constipation and fecal impaction

Treatments and medications. Chronic constipation, often with fecal impaction and encopresis, requires a more aggressive approach after exclusion of organic considerations. The goals of therapy for chronic constipation, fecal impaction, and encopresis are to establish regular bowel habits, restore the urge to defecate, and prevent reimpaction. However, authorities differ greatly on the methods of managing constipation.

The initial therapeutic phase consists of rectal disimpaction by manual removal or by administration of a normal saline enema or pediatric Fleet enema twice daily for no more than 3 days. For a normal saline enema, give 2 oz (60 ml) per year of the child's age to a maximum of 16 ounces (480 ml). For a Fleet hyperphosphate enema, give 1 oz (30 ml) for every 20 pounds (9 kg) of the child's weight. The initial catharsis may be followed by daily laxatives taken orally. The second phase or maintenance schedule is intended to prevent reaccumulation of retained feces. The choice of medication is not so important as the correct dosage and the child's and parents' compliance with the treatment regimen. Treatment failures are the result of laxatives being given either in minimal dosage or for too short a period. The laxative dosage that is required to treat constipation in children is higher than the suggested dosages on the OTC label. The cumulative published data in-

Table 35-4 Suggested Doses of Commonly Used Laxatives

AGENT	PATIENT AGE	DOSAGE
Malt soup extract (Maltsupex)	Breastfed infant	5 to 10 ml in 2 to 4 oz of water or fruit juice twice daily
	Bottle-fed infant	7.5 to 30 ml in day's total formula or 5 to 10 ml in every second feeding
Corn syrup (Karo syrup)	Infant	Same as that for malt soup extract
Milk of magnesia	>6 months	1 to 3 ml per kg of body weight per day, in one to two doses
Mineral oil	>6 months	Same as that of Milk of Magnesia
Lactulose (Cephulac, Chronulac)	>6 months	Concentration 10 g per 15 ml; 1 to 2 ml per kg body weight per day in two doses
Senna syrup (Senokot)	1 to 5 years	5 ml at bedtime; maximum of 5 ml twice daily
	5 to 15 years	10 ml at bedtime; maximum of 10 ml three times daily

Data from Loening-Baucke, V. (1992). In Greydanus, D.E. & Wolraich, M.L. (Eds.). Behavioral pediatrics. New York: Springer-Verlag.

dicate that treatment with multiple modalities may be more successful than a single therapy.

One laxative option is mineral oil. Begin at 1 to 3 ml/kg per day, with a maximum of 5 ml/kg per day in two divided doses to achieve multiple spontaneous, soft bowel movements. The dosage may gradually be increased to a maximum of 300 ml twice a day orally. Continue this therapy for several weeks or up to 3 months. To make mineral oil more palpable, it can be mixed with fruit juices or crushed ice. This medication should be accompanied by vitamin supplements, dietary measures, and a training program on regular defecation habits. The mineral oil dosage should be slowly tapered during a 4- to 6-month period.

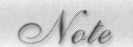

> Reports of lipid pneumonia after aspiration of mineral oil are uncommon but contraindicate its use in infants and children with severe GER or significant neurologic impairment. Mineral oil should *not* be given in combination with antiepileptic drugs or just before bedtime.

Counseling and prevention
- Provide sensitive, careful explanations of the problem to the family.
- Educate the parents and child about the purpose, administration, and side effects of medications.
- Inform the parents and child that treatment failures are most often the result of laxatives being given either in minimal dosage or for too short a time.
- Instruct the parents and child on the importance of stool softeners, laxatives, dietary changes, and exercise in the prevention of stool reaccumulation.
- Instruct the parents and child on the need to develop and maintain a pattern of regular bowel movements that are soft and passed without pain.
- Encourage the child who is toilet trained to sit on the toilet at the same time each day, especially after meals, to take advantage of the gastrocolic reflex.
- Have parents keep a calendar and reward the child for toilet sitting and (later) for bowel movements into the toilet.
- Recommend that parents avoid negative reinforcement.
- Avoid the administration of soap suds, hydrogen peroxide, or tap-water enemas.
- Instruct parents to call immediately if child has abdominal cramps or pain lasting more than 2 hours, or if the child goes 3 days without a bowel movement.

Follow-up
- Remember that it is important to provide support and encouragement during the treatment period through frequent visits or telephone consultation, especially until an appropriate laxative dosage has been established. Follow-up depends on the severity, need for support, compliance, and associated symptoms.
- Review stool records by phone weekly. An abdominal and rectal examination should be repeated to ensure that the constipation is being adequately treated.
- Schedule return visits at 1-month intervals.

Consultations and referrals. If constipation recurs after adequate treatment, refer to a gastroenterologist to rule out an organic disease process.

Anal fissure

Treatments and medications
- Sitz baths in warm salt water for 20 minutes three times a day.
- High intake of fruit, juices, prunes, and bran, which may reduce discomfort when stooling.

Counseling and prevention
- Instruct parents on the treatment regimen, including sitz baths and medications if prescribed.
- Counsel parents in regard to diet and the need to keep the anal area clean and lubricated.

Follow-up. Schedule a return visit in 1 to 2 weeks.

Consultations and referrals. Refer to a physician if the anal fissure is not resolved with the diet change.

Hirschsprung's disease

Treatments and medications. Definitive treatment of Hirschsprung's disease is surgery. Depending on the presentation, it may be an acute, life-threatening condition or a chronic disorder. Delay in the treatment can result in sepsis and death.

Counseling and prevention
- Counsel parents about the disease process.
- Foster infant-parent bonding if the condition is diagnosed during the neonatal period.
- Prepare parents for the medical and surgical intervention.

Follow-up. Follow-up is determined by a physician.

Consultations and referrals. Provide immediate referral to a physician.

Diarrhea and Loose Stool

CATHERINE J. DILLON DOLAN

Alert

> Consult with or refer to a physician for the following:
> - Blood in stool
> - Ill-appearing child with history of large volume of watery diarrhea
> - Signs of moderate to severe dehydration
> - Infants less than 4 months old
> - Febrile infant less than 6 months old
> - Prolonged or persistent diarrhea
> - Immunocompromised child

Etiology

Diarrhea is classified as either acute (an episode lasting less than 2 weeks) or persistent (an episode lasting 2 to 3 weeks or more). Usual stool output is less than 10 g/kg per day in children and 200 g/day in adults. The causes of diarrhea may be infectious (viral, bacterial, parasitic), noninfectious (e.g., food intolerance, food sensitivity, medication induced), or one of many disease processes (e.g., malabsorption syndromes, IBD). The specific origin is not always identified. The possible mechanisms include a decrease in the absorptive capacity of the bowel, a decrease in surface area for absorption, and an alteration of parasympathetic innervation. Proper diagnosis and treatment generally prevents dehydration, malnutrition, and ultimately death.

Incidence

- Diahrrea is most common in those 6 months to 2 years of age.

- Rotavirus is the most common cause of acute infectious gastroenteritis worldwide.
- *Giardia lamblia* is the most common intestinal parasitic organism in the United States.
- Diarrhea-associated illnesses account for 9% of all hospitalizations of children under 5 years of age in the United States.
- Infectious gastroenteritis is second to upper respiratory tract infection as a cause of illness in the pediatric population.
- Crohn's disease is more common in Caucasians.
- IBD is more prevalent among individuals of Jewish descent.

Risk Factors

- Diluted or improper preparation of infant formulas
- Recent travel, especially in late-developing countries such as Africa, Asia, or Latin America
- Contaminated water or food ingestion, especially of fowl, milk, and eggs
- Improper food handling and preparation
- Poor hygiene practices
- Exposure to infectious groups of people (e.g., in hospitalizations, day care)
- Improper handling of soiled infant diapers
- Diet containing an excessive intake of fruit juice or juices
- Family history of IBD
- History of bowel resection or surgery for anal malformation

Differential Diagnosis

Tables 35-5 and 35-6 list and describe the differential diagnoses of acute diarrhea (infectious and noninfectious). Tables 35-7 to 35-9 refer to the differential diagnoses for chronic diarrhea found in specific age groups. These tables represent more common causes. The practitioner is cautioned to consider other conditions leading to chronic diarrhea. Chronic diarrhea may also be associated with malabsorption (see Chapter 45).

Acute infectious diarrhea or *acute gastroenteritis* is one of the most common pediatric illnesses. Viral causes are the most common. Common etiologic agents include rotavirus, enteric adenovirus, Norwalk virus, astrovirus, and calicivirus. The incidence depends on many factors including geographic location, living conditions, climate or season, and daily activities. A bacterial cause is more common in bloody diarrhea. Shigellosis is the most common cause of bacterial dysentery worldwide and is a major cause of diarrhea among children. Enterotoxigenic *E. coli* is the most common cause of traveler's diarrhea. Enteropathogenic *E. coli* can be seen in hospital nurseries and day-care centers. *E. coli* O157:H7 is transmitted by uncooked meat and unpasteurized milk. *Yersinia* infection is rare. Amebiasis, campylobacteriosis, *E. coli* O157:H7 infection, giardiasis, salmonellosis, shigellosis, and yersiniosis must be reported to the local health department where the patient resides. Rotavirus is the most common cause of nosocomially acquired diarrhea in children and is a common cause of acute gastroenteritis in children attending child care.

Antibiotic-associated diarrhea is a commonly seen adverse effect of antimicrobial therapy and is benign in 90% of cases, requiring symptomatic management. It is believed to be related to a change in normal bowel flora, which usually resolves after the discontinuation of antibiotics. Antibiotic-associated colitis caused by toxins produced by *Clostridium difficile* occurs in 0.2% to 10% of patients with antibiotic-associated diarrhea.

Food intolerance includes a variety of problems ranging from simple overfeeding or excessive intake of juices to milk or soybean sensitivity or celiac disease. Cow's milk allergy is a common transient disorder affecting approximately 1% of children, usually in early infancy. There is an intolerance to milk proteins (e.g., whey, casein) found in cow's milk–based infant formulas and breast milk of mothers who ingest cow's milk proteins. There is frequently a sensitivity to soybean-based infant formulas as well. Celiac disease, or gluten-sensitive enteropathy, is a permanent intestinal intolerance to dietary wheat gliadin and related proteins that produces lesions in genetically susceptible individuals.

Lactose intolerance, or *primary acquired lactase deficiency,* is the result of the physiologic decline in lactase production resulting in a subtle, chronic increase in lactose malabsorption after milk ingestion.

Hirschsprung's disease, or *congenital aganglionic megacolon,* is the most common cause of lower intestinal obstruction in neonates. Protracted diarrhea results from enterocolitis or intestinal obstruction.

Munchausen syndrome by proxy or child abuse may be the cause of protracted diarrhea in children, especially infants, if a parent is found or suspected to be giving laxatives surreptitiously.

Chronic nonspecific diarrhea, or *toddler's diarrhea,* is a disorder typically having intermittent, loose, watery stools and believed to be related to altered GI tract motility, a variant of irritable bowel syndrome.

Irritable bowel syndrome or *chronic, recurrent, or functional abdominal pain* in children is believed to be a problem of GI tract motility when histologic, microbiologic, or biochemical abnormalities are absent. It is a diagnosis of exclusion.

IBD is a general term that is used to designate two chronic intestinal disorders: *ulcerative colitis* and *Crohn's disease.* The origin of IBD remains unknown. The child may have abdominal pain, chronic diarrhea, or blood in the stools. GI tract symptoms may not, however, be prominent. The disease may become evident through growth failure or skin lesions or many other extraintestinal signs and symptoms.

Encopresis is the repeated passage of feces into places not appropriate for that purpose (i.e., clothing, floor), whether involuntary or intentional. The pathogenesis is based on retention of stool. It is a complication of constipation.

Management

Acute diarrhea

Treatments and medications. The American Academy of Pediatrics (AAP) no longer advises bowel rest or withholding food and fluids for 24 hours after the onset of diarrhea. Oral rehydration therapy (ORT) is indicated for mild to moderate dehydration. For severe dehydration, intravenous therapy (20 ml/kg boluses) should be used initially until pulse, blood pressure, and level of consciousness return to normal. ORT is contraindicated for shock, intractable vomiting, glucose intolerance, inability to drink, and excessive diarrhea in a short time. ORT is divided into a rehydration, or deficit-replacement, phase and a maintenance phase.

Rehydration phase. For mild to moderate dehydration, give 60 to 80 ml/kg of ORS over the first 4 hours. The type of ORS should contain 60 to 90 mmol of sodium and 111 to 139 mmol of glucose. Such solutions are commercially available (e.g., Pedialyte RS, Rehydralyte, Equalyte, World Health

Table 35-5 Differential Diagnosis: Acute Gastroenteritis (558.9)

CRITERIA	*ESCHERICHIA COLI SPECIES* (BACTERIAL)	*SALMONELLA SPECIES* (BACTERIAL)	*SHIGELLA SPECIES* (BACTERIAL)	*CAMPYLOBACTER SPECIES* (BACTERIAL)	*YERSINIA SPECIES* (BACTERIAL)
ICD-9 code	041.4	003.29	004.9	041.86	027.9
Subjective Data					
Age	Any age; clinically significant in neonates and children <2 years of age	Any age	Any age, peak incidence between 6 months and 5 years of age	Any age	Any age
Onset	Abrupt	Abrupt	Abrupt		
Stool description	Large, watery, explosive bloody stools associated with entero-hemorrhagic *E. coli*	Loose, slimy, green, occasionally bloody or mucoid, spoiled-egg odor	Watery, mucoid, frequently bloody; tenesmus	Mucoid, watery, bloody; tenesmus; foul-smelling	Loose, green, occasionally bloody
Abdominal pain	Crampy	Moderate	Severe	Severe	Crampy in right lower quadrant
Other associated symptoms	Nausea, vomiting, headache, body or joint aches, weaknesses, anorexia	Nausea, vomiting, headache, reports weight loss	Reports weight loss, convulsions, nonsuppurative arthritis	Nausea, malaise, occasionally vomiting	Vomiting, reports weight loss, arthritis
Exposure	Ingestion of contaminated food or water	Ingestion of contaminated food	Ingestion of contaminated food or water, direct contact	Ingestion of contaminated food or water, direct contact	Ingestion of contaminated food or water, or pets
Objective Data					
Physical examination					
Fever	Variable	Variable, possible fever	Common	Common	Variable
Abdominal examination	Hyperactive peristalsis, mild abdominal tenderness	Hyperactive bowel sounds; abdominal tenderness	Hyperactive bowel sounds; abdominal tenderness	Hyperactive bowel sounds; abdominal tenderness	Hyperactive bowel sounds; abdominal tenderness
Laboratory data					
Stool culture	Positive for *E. coli*, specific for strain	Positive for *Salmonella* species	Positive for *Shigella* species	Positive for *Campylobacter* species	Positive for *Yersinia* species

Continued

Table 35-5 Differential Diagnosis: Acute Gastroenteritis (558.9)—cont'd

CRITERIA	*STAPHYLOCOCCUS AUREUS* (BACTERIAL)	*ROTAVIRUS* (VIRAL)	*AMEBIASIS* (PARASITIC)	*CRYPTOSPORIDIUM SPECIES* (PARASITIC INFECTIONS)
ICD-9 code	041.11	008.61	006.9	007.4
Subjective Data				
Age	Any age	Any age, usually <2 years	Any age	Any age
Onset		Abrupt	Gradual	
Stool description	Watery, loose, occasionally bloody or mucoid	Watery, occasionally bloody	Loose, mucoid, blood-tinged, or asymptomatic	Profuse, watery
Abdominal pain	May be present		May be present	Crampy, abdominal pain
Other associated symptoms	Severe nausea, vomiting with retching	Vomiting; concomitant respiratory infection is common; dehydration	Nausea, constipation present between diarrhea	Nausea, vomiting, flulike symptoms; headache, cough, reports weight loss
Exposure	Ingestion of contaminated food	Nosocomial infection; increased incidence in winter months	May report recent travel to foreign region	Person-to-person contact, exposure to farm animals, chronic in immunocompromised
Objective Data				
Physical examination				
Fever	Possible mild fever	Usually present	Low grade	Usually afebrile
Abdominal examination	Normal, probable hyperactive bowel sounds	Normal, probable hyperactive bowel sounds	Normal, probable hyperactive bowel sounds	Normal, probable hyperactive bowel sounds
Laboratory data				
Stool culture	Positive for *S. aureus*	Stool for rotavirus positive by ELISA; stool pH <5.5; stool negative for white blood cells	Positive for ova and parasites; May see guaiac positive stools	Positive for infectious agent

Table 35-6 Differential Diagnosis: Acute Diarrhea (Noninfectious) (787.91)

CRITERIA	FOOD INTOLERANCE	ANTIBIOTIC-ASSOCIATED DIARRHEA/COLITIS	POISONING
ICD-9 code	579.8	960.	973.9
Subjective Data			
Age	Any age	Any age	Any age
Onset	Gradual	Abrupt or gradual	Abrupt
Stool description	Loose, watery	Loose, watery, occasionally mucoid, bloody when associated with *C. difficile*	Large, explosive stools
Abdominal pain	Cramping before bowel movement	Mild abdominal cramping or lower quadrant cramping, generalized abdominal tenderness, hyperactive bowel sounds	Generalized abdominal cramping
Other associated symptoms	Vomiting possible		Nausea, vomiting
Recent diet history, medications, other	Overfeeding or underfeeding; addition of new foods; improper formula or preparation; excessive amount of juices, unripe fruit, or sorbitol	Following administration of cephalosporins, ampicillin, clindamycin, neomycin, or tetracyclines	Ingestion of poison (e.g., iron, food, insecticides, arsenic, other heavy metals)
Objective Data			
Physical examination			
Fever	Usually afebrile	None to low grade	May be present
Abdominal examination	Hyperactive bowel sounds; no localized tenderness	Generalized abdominal tenderness, hyperactive bowel sounds	Appearance of being ill
Laboratory data		Positive toxin assay on stool for *C. difficile* leukocytosis if caused by *C. difficile*	Abnormal and related to the specific poison

Organization [WHO] solution). (Box 35-1 provides the WHO recipe.) Start slowly by offering 5 to 15 ml of ORS by syringe, teaspoon, or cup every 5 to 10 minutes initially, and gradually increase the volume as tolerated. If the child is vomiting, give 2 to 5 ml of ORS every 1 to 2 minutes until the vomiting stops and then gradually return to the regular amount. Rehydration includes the estimated deficit based on the extent of the dehydration, plus any ongoing losses from diarrhea and vomiting. Estimate 4 to 8 ounces for each watery or loose stool and 5 to 10 ml/kg for each episode of vomiting.

Maintenance phase. The goal of the maintenance phase is to provide a usual diet in addition to replacing ongoing losses. Breastfed infants should resume breastfeeding ad libitum. Formula-fed infants should resume their regular formula. If full-strength formula is not initially tolerated, offer half-strength formula (diluted with water). A soybean-based, lactose-free formula with fiber (e.g., Isomil DF) may help to shorten the duration of diarrhea, reduce stool output, and firm stools. Add rice cereal for infants 4 to 6 months of age, or add rice, wheat, or potatoes for infants 6 to 12 months of age if they have had them before. Give an oral maintenance solution (OMS) containing 30 to 60 mmol of sodium and 111 to 139 mmol of glucose (e.g., Pedialyte, Lytren, Infalyte, Resol, Infantile, KaoLectrolyte) as tolerated. Do *not* give beverages such as carbonated drinks, apple or grape juice, sport drinks (e.g., Gatorade), Kool-Aid, tea, chicken broth, or gelatin desserts because they lack the appropriate ratio of ingredients and can cause hyperosmotic diarrhea. Children should continue with their regular diet as tolerated. The BRAT diet (bananas, rice, applesauce, tea) is *not* recommended; instead, a modified BRAT diet (of starchy foods) is encouraged. Such foods include rice, baked potatoes, noodles, soda crackers, toast, and cereals that are not sugar coated. Fresh fruits (especially bananas), yogurt, and clear broths with rice, noodles, or vegetables are also encouraged. Avoid foods that are high in fat (e.g., fried foods) or simple sugars (e.g., juice, soda). Withhold lactose in cases of severe diarrheal illness for at least 1 week after symptoms have resolved because of transient milk protein intolerance. For ongoing losses from diarrhea and emesis, give 4 to 8 oz of OMS for every watery or loose stool and 5 to 10 ml/kg of OMS for each episode of vomiting until the diarrhea stops.

Counseling and prevention
- Educate the parents and child to wash their hands and exposed arms with soap and warm water before eating and after toilet or diaper changes. Fingernails should be kept clean and trimmed.
- Advise the parents to observe the child closely during the initial oral rehydration period.
- Educate the parents or caregiver on how to identify signs of dehydration.
- Describe and demonstrate to parents the amount of ORT to be given using a local measure.
- Instruct the parents to avoid use of antidiarrheal drugs and antiemetics.

Table 35-7 Differential Diagnosis: Chronic Diarrhea in Infants

CRITERIA	MILK AND SOY PROTEIN INTOLERANCE	HIRSCHSPRUNG'S DISEASE	MUNCHAUSEN SYNDROME BY PROXY	OVERFEEDING
ICD-9 code	579.8	751.3	301.51	783.6
Subjective Data				
Age	Most frequently during first 3 months of life	Newborn most common, delay in passage of meconium or if constipation preceded diarrhea		Most frequently during first 6 months of age
Onset	Gradual	Gradual or sudden	Gradual	Gradual
Stool description	Watery, mucoid, sometimes bloody	Foul-smelling		Watery
Abdominal pain	Abdominal pain or cramping			Usually none
Other associated symptoms	May have weight loss, colic, poor feeding	May be present	May be present	Colicky behavior without weight loss
		Vomiting, FTT to hypovolemic shock secondary to obstruction	Vomiting, muscle weakness, lassitude	
Patient and family history	Associated with intake of milk or soy-based formula; may have atopy history	History of constipation; positive family history of trisomy 21	Excessive administration of laxatives, such as lactulose or Milk of Magnesia; overly concerned parent who is usually in constant attendance	Excessive intake of infant formula or food
Objective Data				
Physical examination				
Fever	Possible	Fever in enterocolitis	May be present	Usually normal
Abdominal examination	Hyperactive bowel sounds, generalized abdominal tenderness	Abdominal distention	Varies	Usually normal
Rectal examination	Skin breakdown at rectum	No stool in rectal vault, abnormal rectal examination ("finger in glove feel")	Normal	Normal
Laboratory data	Positive reducing substance; positive stool leukocytes in stool; stool pH <5.5; eosinophilia; guaiac test may be positive or negative	Positive rectal suction biopsy finding for aganglionic cells; abnormal anorectal manometry; barium enema with observed transition zone	Possible hypokalemia	Normal

Table 35-8 Differential Diagnosis: Chronic Diarrhea in Toddlers

CRITERIA	CHRONIC NONSPECIFIC DIARRHEA	GIARDIASIS (PARASITIC INFECTION)	CELIAC DISEASE
ICD-9 code	787.91	007.1	579.0
Subjective Data			
Age	1 to 5 years old	Any age	During first 2 to 3 years of life
Onset	Gradual	Acute or ill-defined in chronic	Gradual
Stool description	About 2 to 3 mushy stools on some days to 6 to 10 loose, watery stools on other days; frequently explosive, foul-smelling; may see whole food particles (e.g., carrots, peas) in stool	Loose, watery, pale, and greasy to asymptomatic carrier; may be foul-smelling	Pale, greasy, bulky, foul-smelling
Abdominal pain	Possible abdominal discomfort	Abdominal cramping	May be present
Other associated symptoms	Normal growth if on regular diet	Self-limiting to vomiting, reports weight loss, anorexia, failure to thrive	Vomiting, failure to thrive, anorexia, irritability, bloating
Patient and family history and exposure	Positive family history of irritable bowel syndrome; may report excessive intake of fluids (e.g., juice and soda)	Transmitted from person-to-person contact, unfiltered water, improperly prepared food, contact with animals	Introduction of solid foods containing gluten, a protein constituent in wheat, oats, barely, rye
Objective Data			
Physical examination			
Abdominal examination	Normal	Abdominal distention	Abdominal distention
Other findings			Muscle wasting, growth delay, delayed dentition, protuberant abdomen, pallor
Laboratory data	Normal	Stool ova and parasite positive for *G. lamblia* by ELISA	Abnormal 72-hour fecal fat collection; abnormal finding on D-xylose test; positive antigliadin antibodies, antireticilin antibodies, and antiendomysial antibodies; abnormal small bowel biopsy showing villous flattening

- Counsel the parents on the need to avoid persistent use of ORS rather than OMS during the maintenance phase because of the risk of hypernatremia.
- Advise parents to avoid using boiled skim milk (because hypernatremia may result from a high-solute load).

Follow-up. Make a telephone call or schedule a return visit immediately if the child refuses to drink, has a high or prolonged fever, has a decrease in urinary output, is unable to retain fluids, has blood in stool, or has ongoing losses greater than intake.

Consultations and referrals. Usually none is needed unless severe dehydration develops that requires hospitalization and intravenous therapy to correct fluid and electrolyte imbalance and acidosis. Refer for intractable vomiting, poor oral intake, high fever, bloody stools, lethargy, irritability, weight loss, and chronic diarrhea.

Infectious diarrhea

Treatments and medications. Provide ORT and correct any fluid and electrolyte imbalances (using selected strategies for mild to moderate diarrhea). Provide antibiotic therapy if indicated. Definitive therapy should be based on culture sensitivities:

- *Enteropathogenic E. coli* (EPEC). If systemic infection is suspected, use TMP-SMX (trimethoprim 5 mg/kg per dose and sulfamethoxazole 25 mg/kg per dose) every 12 hours for 5 days. For mild illness (without inflammatory or bloody diarrhea) in infants less than 3 months of age, use neomycin 100 mg/kg per day orally, divided three times a day for 5 days.
- *Enterotoxigenic E. coli* (ETEC)—Antimicrobials are not recommended for prevention in children; however, empiric treatment with TMP-SMX or ciprofloxacin for 3 days is effective.
- *E. coli 0157:H7*—Treatment is not established.
- *Salmonella.* No treatment is provided for mild illness unless the child is less than 6 months of age or at risk for invasive disease. Cefotaxime or ceftriaxone may be used for 10 to 14 days.
- *Shigellosis*—Treatment is TMP-SMX every 12 hours for 5 days.
- *Campylobacteriosis*—Erythromycin can shorten the duration of the illness and prevent relapse.
- *Yersiniasis*—The efficiency of antibiotic therapy is questionable, but in severe cases TMP-SMX, aminoglycosides, or ceftriaxone are recommended.
- *Amebiasis*—If the patient is asymptomatic, treatment is with paromomycin. For diarrhea, dysentery, or extraintestinal problems, treatment is with metronidazole 35 to 50 mg/kg per day for 10 days, followed by iodoquinol.

Table 35-9 Differential Diagnosis: Chronic Diarrhea in School Aged Children and Adolescents

CRITERIA	IRRITABLE BOWEL SYNDROME	LACTOSE INTOLERANCE	ENCOPRESIS	INFLAMMATORY BOWEL DISEASE	
				ULCERATIVE COLITIS	CROHN'S DISEASE
ICD-9 code	564.1	271.3	787.6	556.9	555.9
Subjective Data					
Age	Any age	Most common at 4 to 8 years of age	Chronologic or mental age of at least 4 years	Adolescence	Adolescence to young adulthood
Onset	Gradual	Gradual	At least one event a month for at least 6 months	Acute	Subtle
Stool description	Child: Loose, foul-smelling, mucus-streaked, three to five times per day; adolescent: Constipation alternating with diarrhea, may be mucoid	Loose, watery	Consistency may vary from normal with intermittent soiling to poorly formed with continuous leakage of liquid stool (soiling)	Often severe, frequently blood and/or mucus, tenesmus	Moderate diarrhea, sometimes bloody or mucoid
Abdominal pain	Crampy or sharp pain (periumbilical or lower), relieved with defecation	Crampy after consumption of lactose	Related to overflow incontinence, secondary to fecal retention, pain may be due to impaction or constipation	Crampy abdominal pain associated with bowel movement	Mild to severe, usually lower abdomen
Other associated symptoms	Pallor, nausea, tiredness, headache, anorexia, sense of incomplete evacuation followed by straining	Flatulence, urgency, bloating	Psychosocial stress, painful defecation, inadequate toilet training, opposition behavior	Anorexia, reports moderate weight loss	Malaise, joint pain, anorexia, reports severe weight loss, arthritis, arthralgia, growth retardation
Family history	Positive	Positive, high prevalence among Asians, Native Americans, and African Americans	More common in boys	High prevalence among Jews	High prevalence among Jews; more common in caucasians
Objective Data **Physical examination**					
Fever	Low grade				Present
Physical findings	Abdominal distention	Abdominal distention, hyperactive bowel sounds	Abdominal distention, palpable mass of stool, retained stool in rectum, anal fissures, excoriated perianal area	Mild growth retardation	Significant growth retardation; right lower quadrant tenderness; anal or perianal lesions
Laboratory data	Normal complete blood cell count, erythrocyte sedimentation rate	Positive result of hydrogen breath test; Stool positive for reducing sugars	Abdomen x-ray shows retained stool or fecal mass; normal rectal manometry; normal rectal biopsy finding	Anemia, ↑ ESR, ↓ Fe, ↓ total protein, ↓ albumin; Small-bowel series shows generalized inflammation, most often in rectum; crypt abscesses on biopsy	Anemia, ↑ ESR, ↓ Fe, ↓ total protein, ↓ albumin; Small-bowel shows narrowing, terminal ileum mostly involved; granulomas on biopsy

Fe, *Total iron.*

- *Cryptosporidium*—Treatment is supportive, and the illness is usually self-limited in immunocompetent patients.
- *Giardiasis*—Treatment is metronidazole 15 mg/kg per day divided three times a day for 5 days, furazolidone 5 mg/kg per day divided four times a day for 7 to 10 days, or quinacrine hydrochloride 6 mg/kg per day divided three times a day after meals for 5 days.
- *Viral gastroenteritis* (e.g., rotavirus, enteric adenovirus, astrovirus, members of the Norwalk agent group)—Treatment is supportive. Lactose intolerance after viral gastroenteritis is common and may persist for months.

Counseling and prevention

- Instruct the patient to avoid exposure to the causative agent.
- Stress the need to follow enteric precautions.
- Emphasize strict handwashing before and after food preparation, feeding, handling of persons and animals, stool elimination, diapering, and laundering.
- Encourage proper storage, preparation, and handling of foods.
- Encourage laundering of contaminated linens, clothes, and other articles.
- Instruct the parents how to collect stool specimens.
- Teach about the cause of diarrhea and any medications, if prescribed.
- Instruct the parents to change diaper frequently, wash area, expose buttocks to air, and apply protective skin ointment.
- Advise the parents that for EPEC, *E. coli* O157:H7, *Shigella*, and *G. lamblia* infections, the child should not reenter school or the day-care center until diarrhea has stopped and stool cultures are negative.

Follow-up. Instruct parents to call if there is no improvement in 72 hours, or earlier if symptoms worsen.

Consultations and referrals. Usually none are needed. Consult with physician for the following:

- Patient under 3 months of age
- Bloody diarrhea or diarrhea persisting over 72 hours
- Moderate to severe dehydration

Report to the local health department as required (e.g., for shigellosis or salmonellosis, yersiniosis, giardiasis, amebiasis, *E. coli* O157:H7 infection, campylobacteriosis, cryptosporidiosis).

Box 35-1 World Health Organization Recipe for Oral Rehydration Therapy

1 L (1.05 qt) clean water
3.5 g sodium chloride
20 g glucose (40 g sucrose) (4 tablespoons sugar)
2.5 g sodium bicarbonate (2.9 g sodium citrate or 1 teaspoon baking soda)
1.5 g potassium chloride (1 cup of orange juice or two bananas)
   Measure ingredients carefully and use within a 24-hour period.
Solution can be made without sodium bicarbonate and potassium chloride, but it is optimal to have them.

Modified from the World Health Organization. (1993). The management and prevention of diarrhea: practical guidelines (3rd ed.). Geneva: World Health Organization.

Antibiotic-associated diarrhea

Treatments and medications. This condition is self-limiting with discontinuation of the implicated antibacterial agent. For *C. difficile*–associated diarrhea or colitis, treatment may be metronidazole 20 mg/kg per day divided every 6 hours for 7 days, or vancomycin 40 mg/kg per day divided four times a day for 7 days in children under 12 years of age (while continuing the antibacterial agent). A second course of treatment is frequently required because of relapse.

Counseling and prevention

- Instruct parent and child in need for strict hand washing.
- Educate the parents and child about the purpose, directions, and side effects of medications.

Follow-up. Make a telephone call if there is no improvement in 72 hours, or earlier if symptoms worsen.

Consultations and referrals. There are usually none.

Food intolerances. See also Allergies in Chapter 43.

Treatments and medications

- Eliminate the offending food from diet.
- For lactose intolerance, use a lactose-restricted diet and use Lactaid caplets or drops as needed (to be taken before a meal containing lactose).

Counseling and prevention

- Stress the need to avoid intestinal irritants (e.g., spices, foods high in roughage) and to eliminate or decrease excessive amounts of fruit juices that contain a large amount of fructose or sorbitol.
- Instruct the parents to maintain a food diary.

Follow-up. Provide follow-up care as needed.

Consultations and referrals. Refer to nutritionist for dietary instructions.

Milk or soybean protein allergy. See also Infantile Colic.

Treatments and medications. Discontinue infant formula containing cow's milk protein and attempt a soybean-based formula. However, approximately 40% of infants are also sensitive to soybean and need a casein hydrolysate formula (e.g., Nutramigen, Alimentum, Pregestimil) for the first year of life. Breastfeeding may be continued; however, the mother must modify her diet and follow a milk-free, soybean-free diet.

Counseling and prevention. Instruct parents to maintain a food diary.

Follow-up. Challenge the infant with milk or a milk-based formula after a prescribed time and check for any recurrence of diarrhea, blood, and reducing substance in stool.

Consultations and referrals

- Refer to gastroenterologist if no improvement is seen with formula or diet change.
- Refer to nutritionist for dietary instructions.

Irritable bowel syndrome

Treatments and medications

- Recommend a high-fiber diet with increased fluids. Limit sorbitol and constipating foods, milk, and milk products.
- Recommend a fiber supplement (e.g., Metamucil, FiberCon). Use half the adult dose in children under 12 years of age.

Counseling and prevention

- Provide appropriate dietary counseling.
- Educate child and parent about symptoms to help promote adherence with treatment.
- Encourage regular toileting habits.
- Offer suggestions to alleviate stressors.

Follow-up. Make a telephone call or schedule a return visit in 1 month for evaluation of the child's response to the treatment plan.

Consultations and referrals. Refer to a gastroenterologist if symptoms persist after 1 month.

Celiac disease

Treatments and medications. Start a gluten-free diet, avoiding wheat, rye, barley, and foods with gluten additives. Rice, corn, and soybeans are allowed.

Counseling and prevention. Educate the child and family about the importance of strict adherence to diet.

Follow-up. Repeat endoscopy with biopsy after 6 to 8 weeks on a gluten-free diet. Schedule periodic visits for growth assessment.

Consultations and referrals

- Refer to a pediatric gastroenterologist for diagnosis and work-up.
- Refer to a nutritionist for dietary instructions and patient education.
- Inform the school's nurse and teachers about the special diet. Refer to national and local support groups, including the Celiac Sprue Association, PO Box 31700, Omaha, NE 68103-0700; (402) 558-0600; e-mail celiacusa@aol.com; members. aol.com/celiacusa/celiac/htm; and the American Celiac Society, 58 Musano Court, West Orange, NJ 07052; (201) 325-8837

Inflammatory bowel disease

Treatments and medications. Treatment is individualized and aimed at reducing or eliminating symptoms, maintaining remission, and promoting a normal lifestyle. Sulfasalazine (Azulfidine) or mesalamine agents (e.g., Asacol, Pentasa) are used in Crohn's disease. Folic acid (1 mg daily) supplementation is the prescribed therapy. Other therapy may include:

- Sulfasalazine or olsalazine (Dipentum) for ulcerative colitis
- Antibiotic therapy (metronidazole) for treatment of refractory perianal lesions in Crohn's disease
- Corticosteroids to induce remission (often used)
- Steroid enemas or mesalamine enemas or suppositories (e.g., mesalamine [Rowasa]) for ulcerative proctitis and severe tenesmus
- High-protein, high-carbohydrate, low-fiber, and normal-fat diet
- Lactose-restricted diet for lactose intolerance
- Vitamin and iron supplements as indicated
- Nasogastric tube feedings to stimulate linear growth and sexual development in the child with Crohn's disease
- Surgical intervention for Crohn's disease (to be used with great caution)

Counseling and prevention

- Educate the child and parents about the cause of symptoms in order to promote adherence with treatment.
- Educate the child and parents about the purpose, directions, and side effects of medications.
- Recommend routine eye and dental visits if the patient is on a long-term regimen of corticosteroids.

Follow-up. Schedule periodic visits every 3 to 6 months if the condition is stable, for the evaluation of the response to the treatment plan, to assess growth, and to promote compliance.

Consultations and referrals

- Refer to a gastroenterologist for diagnostic work-up and ongoing therapy.
- Inform the school nurse if medication is to be given at school, of the need for frequent toilet breaks, and of the need for increased absences as a result of disease exacerbation.
- Refer to national and local support groups, including the Crohn's and Colitis Foundation of America, Inc., 44 Park

Ave. South, New York, NY 10016; (212) 685-3440 or (800) 343-3637.

Hirschsprung's disease

Treatments and medications. Refer to a surgeon for surgical removal of the aganglionic bowel.

Counseling and prevention. See Chapter 49.

Follow-up. Follow-up is determined by a physician. Also, provide well-child care.

Consultations and referrals. Refer to the American Hirschsprung's Disease Association, 22½ Spruce St., Battleboro, VT 05301; (802) 257-0632.

Munchausen syndrome by proxy

Treatments and medications. Separation of the child from the parents or caregiver results in abrupt cessation of symptoms.

Counseling and prevention. None is indicated.

Follow-up. Follow-up is determined by the physician and mental health professional.

Consultations and referrals. Refer to a physician or mental health professional.

Encopresis. See also Constipation and Fecal Impaction.

Treatments and medications. A clean-out regimen is performed for catharsis. This includes normal saline enemas or polyethylene glycol–electrolyte solution (PEG-ES) GoLYTELY oral solution. The maintenance regimen includes oral laxatives (e.g., Senokot, lactulose); scheduled toilet sits after meals for 10 minutes (if toilet trained); a high-fiber diet; increased fluids; and a behavioral modification program.

Counseling and prevention

- Educate parents and child about the problem.
- Review the treatment regimen with the parents and child.
- Instruct and review how to give an enema, if needed.
- Reinforce the need for scheduled toilet sits.

Follow-up. Close telephone contact is needed to determine the success of the clean-out regimen and then a return visit every 6 weeks for at least 6 months. Have the parents call if the child goes 3 days without stool.

Consultations and referrals

- Consult with a pediatric gastroenterologist if needed.
- Refer to a mental health professional if there is an ongoing problem, family dysfunction, or a depressed child.
- Send a note to the school nurse or teacher that the child may require additional toileting breaks.

Hernias: Inguinal, Scrotal, and Umbilical Bulges

ARLEEN NAST STECKEL

Alert

Consult with or refer to pediatric surgeon immediately for the following:

- Sudden onset and severe pain
- Inguinal or scrotal mass that does not reduce
- Hard, firm, tender mass
- Redness or edema over or near bulge or mass
- Cramping abdominal pain
- Vomiting (bilious or feculent)
- Severe irritability
- Empty scrotum

Etiology

Most hernias are the result of congenital defects. Weaknesses in a specific muscle allows abdominal fluid or bowel to escape, causing a bulge. Indirect inguinal hernias are caused by a patent processus vaginalis.

Incidence

- Approximately 80% of all hernias are indirect inguinal, unilateral, and predominantly right-sided.
- Of contralateral hernias, 63% occur at under 2 months of age and 41% at 2 to 16 years of age. Indirect hernias are the most frequent type of inguinal hernia and occur more often in boys than in girls (9:1). Bilateral hernias are 20% to 50% more frequent in females. Direct hernias in children are rare.
- About 10% to 15% of hernias become incarcerated, with an increased incidence in infants less than 2 months of age.
- Greater than one third of all hernias are diagnosed before 6 months of age, and one half are diagnosed before 1 year of age.
- There is an increased incidence of hernias in the following children:
  Premature infants (5% of them)
  Infants weighing 1000 g or less at birth (30%) (more common in girls with LBW)
  Children with cystic fibrosis (15%)
  Children Ehlers-Danlos syndrome and other connective tissue syndromes
  Children with mucopolysaccharidosis (e.g., Hurler and Hunter syndromes)
  Children with myelomeningocele with ventriculoperitoneal shunts
  Children receiving long-term peritoneal dialysis
  Children with developmental dysplasia of the hip (DDH)
- Noncommunicating hydroceles are found in less than 1% of children over 1 year of age.
- Testicular torsion is seen in 1 in 1600 males, with 12% of these occurring in the newborn period.
- Varicoceles are found in 15% to 20% of adolescent boys.
- Spermatocele is most common in the neonatal, late childhood, and early adolescent periods. Incidence peaks at 14 years of age.
- Umbilical hernias can be found in 1 out of every 6 children. It is more common in premature and African-American infants. It is found in 40% of African-American infants less than 1 year of age. It is nine times more common in African Americans than in Caucasians. Umbilical hernias are common in infants with history of congenital thyroid deficiency, Down syndrome, or mucopolysaccharidosis.
- Femoral hernias are rare and are found more frequently in girls.

Risk Factors

- Male gender
- Prematurity
- Bronchopulmonary dysplasia (BPD)
- LBW
- Undescended testes
- Positive family history

- Chronic diseases (e.g., Down syndrome, cystic fibrosis, meningomyelocele, Hunter and Hurler syndromes, Ehlers-Danlos syndrome and other connective tissue disorders)
- Chronic kidney dialysis
- Congenital dislocation of hip

Differential Diagnosis (Table 35-10)

Any child with a suspected hernia requires a thorough history and physical examination including careful attention to documentation of parent- or child-reported symptoms, family history, prenatal history, child's general appearance, vital signs, height and weight, and examination of the abdomen, groin, scrotum, testes, and labia. Document the firmness, tenderness, size, mobility, color, and edema of any masses or bulges and auscultate masses for bowel sounds.

Inguinal hernia is a mass (a protrusion of abdominal structures such as the intestines, ovaries, or testes) in the inguinal area that is caused by the persistence of all or part of the processus vaginalis. If the processus vaginalis fails to obliterate, abdominal fluid or an abdominal structure can be forced into it. This creates a palpable mass or bulge known as an indirect inguinal hernia. The persistent sac may end at any point along the inguinal canal. It may stop at the inguinal ring or extend into the scrotum. Since the inguinal canal is short, the hernia can be present at birth or any time thereafter. The usual age is 2 to 3 months, when the infant has sufficient intraabdominal pressure to open the sac (Fig. 35-1).

Hydrocele is the presence of peritoneal fluid in the scrotum. A communicating hydrocele occurs when the processus vaginalis remains open and fluid is forced into it by intraabdominal pressure and gravity. The length of the hydrocele depends on the length of the processus vaginalis and may extend into the tunica vaginalis in the scrotum. It usually does not extend into the inguinal canal. A communicating hydrocele predisposes a child for a hernia (see Figs. 35-1 and 35-2, *C*).

A *noncommunicating hydrocele* is the presence of fluid in the processus vaginalis. The upper segment of the processus vaginalis has been obliterated, but the tunica vaginalis contains peritoneal fluid. In girls the hydrocele occurs in the Nuck's canal, and fluid cannot be pushed back into the abdomen, which can cause difficulty in distinguishing it from an incarcerated hernia. If a hernia or hydrocele is suspected, palpate over the internal ring with the flat part of the index finger and roll the spermatic cord beneath the fingers as it lies in the inguinal canal. A thin, 1 mm, solid structure going through the ring is palpated.

Testicular torsion (torsion of the spermatic cord) (requiring immediate referral to a physician) usually occurs during puberty and is often associated with sports participation but may also occur in the neonatal period or with undescended testes. Torsion occurs when the normal fixation of the testis is abnormal or absent. Presentation usually includes sudden onset of acute scrotal pain and swelling (Fig. 35-2, *D*).

Adolescent torsion is associated with the bell-clapper deformity (whereby the mesorchium is absent and the tunica vaginalis completely surrounds the testis and epididymis, which hangs dependently and without fixation).

Varicocele is dilated tortuous veins in the venous plexus of the scrotum. It is usually on the left side but can be bilateral. Hormonal deficiency and temperature may be the cause (Fig. 35-2, *A*).

Table 35-10 Differential Diagnosis: Inguinal Bulges and Scrotal Masses

CRITERIA	INGUINAL HERNIA	HYDROCELE	TESTICULAR TORSION*	VARICOCELE	SPERMATOCELE
ICD-9 code	550.90	603.9	608.2	456.4	608.1
Subjective Data					
Age of onset	2-3 months of age	Newborn	Any age; newborn; peaks at 12-14 years	Adolescence	Adolescence
Description of mass	Parent may report: Visible bulge unilaterally or bilaterally; swelling comes and goes, seems to be getting bigger, more persistent, and more difficult to reduce; lump in inguinal area	Parent reports: Scrotal swelling unilateral or lateral swelling that is small in morning but increases with activity (communicating)	Adolescent reports: Scrotal swelling secondary to hydrocele, history of trauma, transient episodes of pain, variability of pain severity	Adolescent reports: Scrotal swelling, prolonged standing leads to engorgement and pain, size decreases when lying down	Adolescent reports: Scrotal swelling
Pain at site of bulge or mass	Yes, if loop of intestine partially obstructed	Usually not	Acute, severe; severity progressively increases within a few hours; can quickly stop if spontaneous detorsion occurs	Usually not	Usually not
Associated symptoms	Parent may report the following: Abdominal distention/pain, fretfulness, irritability, anorexia, nausea/vomiting, difficulty defecating, intermittent or continuous crying, abdominal cramping/pain	Yes, if associated with a hernia	Lower abdominal pain, nausea/vomiting, awakens from sleep because of pain, at times a dull scrotal ache, lower quadrant pain	Usually asymptomatic; noted accidentally by child or examiner	Usually none
History of trauma	Usually not	No	No	May report minor trauma	Usually not
Child and family history	Familial tendency	Usually none	Familial tendency	No	No
Objective Data					
Physical examination					
	Best position for examination: Infants: Legs extended and arms held over head; older child: Supine and erect positions				
Vital signs/temperature	Normal	Normal	Increased temperature and pulse	Normal	Normal
General appearance	Neonate appears ill if hernia is incarcerated	Good	Neonate appears ill	Good	Good
Genitalia (male)	Lump in inguinal and scrotal area (sometimes examiner unable to elicit hernia); go by reliable history plus palpation of the cord or tunica vaginal is rubbing on itself ("silk glove sign") indicative of hernia	No bowel loop felt as pubic ramus and cord structures are palpated at external inguinal ring			

Genitalia (female) Palpation of inguinal area	May see swelling of labia majora Palpate pubic ramus and cord structures at external inguinal ring: If no bowel loop felt, probably hydrocele; bulge in inguinal canal, bulge may or may not be reducible; palpable mass with or without swelling; feels sausage shaped; size changes with crying, coughing, straining, standing; crepitus on palpation and/or during push through external ring			
Scrotum	Bowel sounds in scrotal area; incarcerated: Firm to fluctuant mass in groin and/or scrotum, usually nontender; strangulated: Mass becomes hard, more firm; significant tenderness; skin redness and edema likely	Skin normal; feels ovoid, round and smooth; communicating: Fluid manually compresses into abdomen; painless bulge in scrotal or inguinal area; difficult to palpate other scrotal contents; shine light through mass and fluid in scrotum transilluminates; incarcerated: Bowel in a newborn transilluminates; noncommunicating: Fluid does not shine through mass; mass cannot be reduced	Pubertal period: Acute scrotal pain radiating up to groin, nonreducible mass, no increase in size with crying or increased abdominal pressure, tender to touch, red and swollen, ipsilateral lower abdominal quadrant pain, scrotum elevated on one side; neonatal period: Edema, ecchymosis, does not transilluminate; abdominal examination to rule out incarcerated inguinal hernia, looks ill, little movement, "blue dot" on scrotum indicates testicular appendage torsion	Valsalva maneuver leads to increased size
Testes	Cremasteric reflex present, retractile or undescended testis can be mistaken for hernia, swelling does not transilluminate; incarcerated bowel in newborns: Loop transilluminates; key points: If lump/mass is above inguinal ligament, retractile or undescended testis can be mistaken for a hernia; cold, touch, exercise stimulation tend to make testes ascend higher into pelvic area	Cremasteric reflex present	Pubertal: Testicular pain elevated up toward groin, spermatic cord above testis is thickened and tender, abnormal axis above the testes, elevated testes due to shortened spermatic cord leads to transverse lie; cremasteric reflex usually absent on affected side but may cause ipsilateral hemiscrotum to contract (this is not diagnostic)	Testes may be absent, palpation along spermatic cord feels like "bag of worms" superior to testes; Valsalva's maneuver increases size; usually left side, can be bilateral or on right side
				Cystic nodules above and posterior to testicle; mass varies in size, usually less than 1 cm; size does not change with Valsalva's maneuver; mobile, transilluminates; contains milky, sperm-filled fluid

*Immediate referral to a physician.

Continued

Table 35-10 Differential Diagnosis: Inguinal Bulges and Scrotal Masses—cont'd

CRITERIA	INGUINAL HERNIA	HYDROCELE	TESTICULAR TORSION*	VARICOCELE	SPERMATOCELE
Laboratory data	Ultrasound of inguinal canal and scrotum is study of choice especially if diagnosis of irreducible hernia is in question. Suspected: Ultrasound of inguinal region and scrotum shows bowel loop present in a hernia sac in inguinal region or scrotum, multiple loops, abdominal visceral structures (intestines, ovaries) in inguinal canal, Patent processus vaginalis; Abdominal x-ray shows: Air below inguinal ligament; if incarcerated bowel loop below inguinal ligament is fluid filled, may get a false-negative result	Usually not necessary; ultrasound to rule out other disease (tumor, lymphatic obstruction, infection)	None, unless color-coded duplex Doppler ultrasound available	None	None

Immediate referral to a physician.

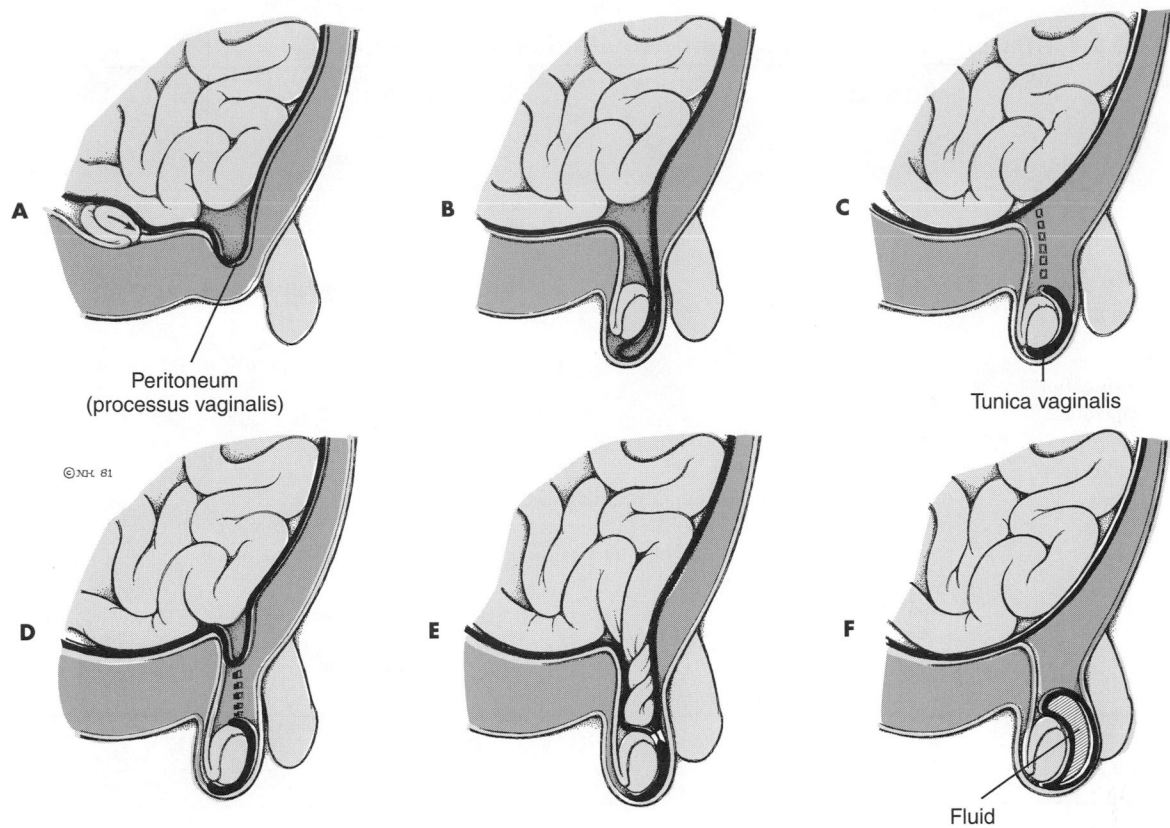

Fig. 35-1 Development of inguinal hernias. **A** and **B,** Prenatal migration of processus vaginalis. **C,** Normal. **D,** Partially obliterated processus vaginalis. **E,** Hernia. **F,** Hydrocele. (From Wong, D. [1995]. *Nursing care of infants and children* [5th ed.]. St. Louis: Mosby.)

Spermatocele is a benign cyst on the head of the epididymis or testicular adnexa. The cysts contain sperm (Fig. 35-2, *B*).

Umbilical hernia (Table 35-11) results from an incomplete closure of the fascia of the umbilical ring. Herniated omentum or bowel is covered by skin.

Femoral hernia (which requires immediate referral to a physician) (see Table 35-11) is seen as a swelling in the groin area. It occurs in the Nuck's canal, which contains the round ligament. The defect is below the inguinal ligament, medial to the femoral artery. The hernia usually contains an ovary or a fallopian tube and may be seen as a mass high in the proximal area of the thigh that increases in size as the intraabdominal pressure increases. Lymph nodes are usually multiple and more discrete and do not increase in size with crying, straining, or other activities. Femoral hernias are associated with severe pain and are rare in children.

Management

Any incarcerated or strangulated hernia or testicular torsion requires immediate referral to a surgeon.

Inguinal hernia

Treatments and medications. Refer for a surgical consult. There is no specific treatment or medication. There is increased risk of incarceration greater than 60% within the first 6 months of life.

Counseling and prevention. Instruct parents about the signs of an incarcerated and obstructed hernia: tenderness or pain; redness in the groin, scrotum, or labia that leads to intermittent or

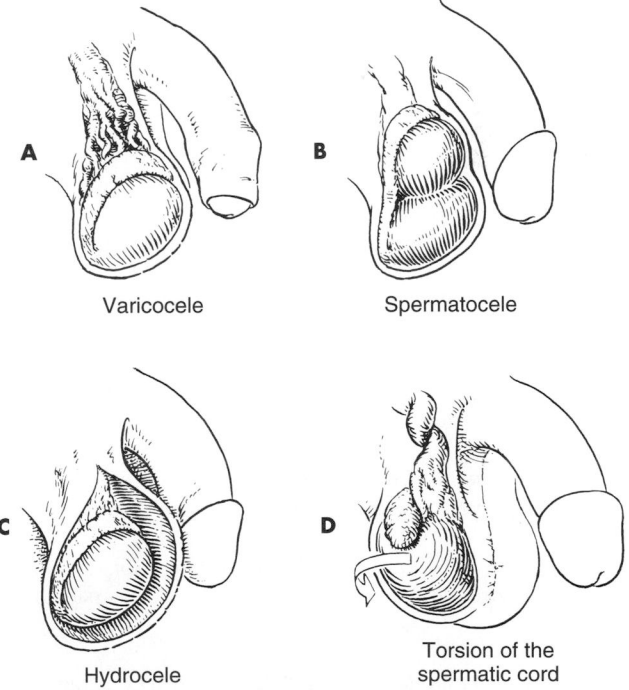

Fig. 35-2 Scrotal abnormalities. **A,** Varicocele. **B,** Spermatocele. **C,** Hydrocele. **D,** Torsion of the spermatic cord. (From Barkauskas, V., Stoltenberg-Allen, K., Baumann, L., et al. [1994]. *Health and physical assessment.* St. Louis: Mosby.)

Table 35-11 Differential Diagnosis: Umbilical and Femoral Hernia

CRITERIA	UMBILICAL HERNIA	FEMORAL HERNIA*
ICD-9 code	553.1	553.00
Subjective Data		
Age of onset	<1 year	Rare in children
Description of mass	Parent reports increased size with crying; straining; coughing, vomiting	Parent reports increased size with crying, straining, coughing
Pain	Yes, if strangulated or incarcerated	Yes, if strangulated or incarcerated
Child and family history	Yes	No
Objective Data		
Physical examination		
Vital signs/temperature	Normal	Normal
General appearance	Good	Good
Examination of abdomen	Protrusion readily seen, feels soft and silky if intestines in sac, gurgling sounds heard as mass reduced incarcerated can be difficult to reduce; strangulated: Nonreducible, painful, redness, abdominal distention, vomiting	Normal
Femoral area	Normal	If hernia present, bulge felt in femoral area, high in proximal thigh; size increases with increased intraabdominal pressure. In males, hernia content is small intestine. In females, content is ovary and fallopian tube.
Laboratory data	None	None

Immediate referral to a physician.

continuous crying; nausea; vomiting; abdominal distension; and lack of flatus and stooling. Advise them to report findings immediately, including any change in mass size.

Follow-up. Assess at well-child visits.

Consultations and referrals. Consult with a physician if changes are observed (e.g., signs and symptoms of strangulation or incarceration, increase in size of bulge).

Hydrocele

Treatments and medications. For a communicating hydrocele, treatment is determined by a urologist or surgeon because surgical repair is often needed. Treatment is not indicated for noncommunicating hydrocele with no other signs or symptoms.

Counseling and prevention

- Instruct parents to monitor for increase and fluctuation in size of scrotum.
- Instruct parents that, with noncommunicating hydrocele, fluid generally reabsorbs within the year.

Follow-up. Carefully monitor noncommunicating hydrocele at each well-child visit for 1 year to assess for a decrease in amount of scrotal fluid.

Consultations and referrals

- Refer to a surgeon if there is a communicating hydrocele or a noncommunicating hydrocele that does not resolve within 1 year.
- Consult with or refer to a pediatric surgeon for communicating hydroceles that fluctuate in size and persist after 1 year.

Testicular torsion

Treatments and medications. Immediately refer to a surgeon.

Counseling and prevention. Advise parents that surgery is generally indicated.

Follow-up. Follow-up is determined by a surgeon and should include visits for well-child care.

Consultations and referrals. Provide immediate referral to a surgeon.

Varicocele

Treatments and medications. Varicoceles in prepubertal boys should be referred to a surgeon.

Counseling and prevention

- Advise the parents and child that varicoceles are generally not problematic.
- Instruct the parents and child to monitor for any increase in discomfort or change in size and shape, and to report noted changes.

Follow-up. Assess at each well-child visit.

Consultations and referrals

- Refer to a surgeon for varicoceles that are painful, have a large testicular volume difference, and show testicular growth retardation over a 6- to 12-month period.
- Refer to a urologist for secondary varicoceles that are usually right-sided and do not disappear in a prone position.

Spermatoceles

Treatments and medications. Spermatoceles that are painful should be referred to a surgeon.

Counseling and prevention. Advise the parents and child to report any increase in discomfort and pain.

Follow-up. Assess at each well-child visit.

Consultations and referrals. Refer to a surgeon for spermatoceles that are painful.

Umbilical hernia

Treatments and medications. Defects greater than 1.5 cm should be referred to a surgeon for evaluation. Fascial defects of 0.5 to 1.5 cm in diameter are monitored during the first 4 years of life and usually heal spontaneously.

Counseling and prevention
- Reassure parents that surgical treatment is generally not required.
- Instruct the parents that the placement of coins or binders over the area does not accelerate healing.
- Instruct parents about the signs of an incarcerated or obstructed hernia, including tenderness or pain, redness that leads to intermittent or continuous crying, nausea, vomiting, abdominal distension, and lack of flatus and stool.
- Advise parents to report a change in mass size.

Follow-up. Assess at each well-child visit.

Consultations and referrals. Refer to a surgeon for signs and symptoms of strangulation or incarceration and fascial defects of 0.5 to 1.5 cm in diameter that do not heal within the first 4 years of life.

Infantile Colic

THERESA M. ELDRIDGE

Alert

Consult with or refer to a physician for the following:
- Projectile vomiting
- Signs and symptoms of dehydration
- Signs and symptoms of shock
- Bloody stools
- Signs and symptoms of congestive heart failure (e.g., diaphoresis, tachypnea, tachycardia, bradycardia or arrhythmia, cyanosis, pallor)
- Signs and symptoms of CNS involvement (e.g., meningitis, drug withdrawal, high-pitched cry, hyperirritability, lethargy, jitters).
- Signs of possible child abuse (e.g., unexplained bruising, failure to thrive, long bone fractures, retinal hemorrhages, evidence of increased intracranial pressure).

Etiology

Infantile colic is a poorly understood, benign, self-limited condition that is evident in persistent, unexplained crying and fussiness that lasts for longer than 3 hours a day and for more than 3 days a week. It is described as persistent crying beginning at 1 to 3 weeks of age and persisting until 3 to 6 months of age with either an abrupt or a gradual resolution. Keefe (1988, 1997) identified colic as a developmental sleep disorder characterized by recurrent episodes of fussiness, crying, and diminished soothability. These infants become overstimulated and lack the skills to self-soothe. The parent may not be able to appropriately respond to the infant's unclear cues, leading to a disruption in the parent-child relationship. Barr (1998) suggests that colic (excessive crying) is a normal behavioral process that reflects CNS development and is normal except that there is more of it. Others have indicated that infants with difficult temperaments or problems in the parental interaction may be the cause.

Infants who have recurrent episodes of excessive crying without an organic origin or cause have *idiopathic infant irritability.* As described previously, one possible cause is believed to be sleep-wake disturbances. Infants with sleep-wake disturbance exhibit the following characteristics:
- Inability to regulate their state (quiet sleep, active sleep, drowsy, quiet alert, active alert, crying)

- Becoming overtired and overstimulated easily
- Unable to self-soothe or reduce arousal level to calm self and go to sleep
- Increased night wakening
- Decreased total sleep (i.e., fewer, shorter naps), or increased sleep because of inability to deal with stimuli
- Decreased amount of quiet sleep
- Falling asleep only to awaken within 15 to 20 minutes
- Changing from sleep to awake without passing through all states
- Increased sensitivity to external stimuli

Some parents may also misinterpret the cues of their infant. They may not be able to recognize that their infant's cry is a way of communicating various needs, such as the child is hungry, wants to suck, or is tired. Whatever the cause, colic is a major parental concern.

Incidence

- Approximately 10% to 25% of healthy, full-term infants have colic.
- It occurs equally in breastfed and bottle-fed infants.
- It occurs equally in boys, girls, and all ethnic groups.
- It occurs equally in children of varying birth order (i.e., can occur in first, second, or third child).
- It has an onset between 1 to 3 weeks of age, with either abrupt or gradual resolution at 3 to 6 months of age.
- About 3% to 7% of infants have a cow's milk protein allergy. (Up to 50% of these are also allergic to soybean protein.)
- The prevalence of colic is twofold higher among infants of smoking mothers

Risk Factors

No predisposing risk factors are known.

Differential Diagnosis (Table 35-12)

Before arriving at an assessment of infantile colic or idiopathic infant irritability, the practitioner must rule out other possible organic causes. Following are some of the most serious concerns to be addressed. Other sections (Abdominal Pain, Vomiting, Diarrhea) provide more detailed information.

Infectious diseases. Infants who have an acute episode of inconsolable crying should be evaluated for a possible disease process such as acute otitis media, UTI, meningitis, or other infection (e.g., stomatitis).

Acute otitis media is usually associated with fever and clear or purulent nasal discharge. Physical examination shows inflamed upper respiratory tract and red tympanic membranes (see Ear Pain and Discharge in Chapter 34).

UTI is often missed, especially in the young infant. Infants who have inconsolable crying with or without fever may warrant a urinalysis and urine culture (see Painful Urination in Chapter 42).

Sepsis should be suspected when an infant has fever without an apparent cause. A septic work-up should be performed, including examination of blood, urine, and cerebrospinal fluid (see Fever in Chapter 43).

Meningitis in neonates occurs within the first week of life and is frequently associated with prematurity and premature or prolonged rupture of membranes. This early-onset meningeal infection is characterized by a rapidly progressing, severely ill-appearing infant who is hypotensive and may have signs of pneumonia (from group B streptococci). Late-onset meningitis

Table 35-12 Differential Diagnosis: Colic and Cow's Milk Allergy

CRITERIA	COLIC/INFANTILE IRRITABILITY	COW'S MILK ALLERGY
ICD-9 code	789.0	693.1
Subjective Data		
Onset/duration	Gradual or sudden at 1 to 3 weeks of age lasting 3 to 6 months	One day to 22 weeks; average age of onset, 1 week of age; however, onset can be at any age into adulthood
Gender	Equal in males and females	Higher incidence in boys in early infancy and then equal in later months
Fever	None	None
Vomiting	None	Found in one fourth to one half of all infants
Abdominal pain	History of drawing legs up, possible increased flatus, child acts as if in pain	Apparent abdominal cramps, abdominal distention
Diarrhea	None	Frequent, loose, often green with excess mucus, may have blood; steatorrhea often present
Constipation	Not related to colic but found in the normal distribution of infants	Constipation can be manifestation of allergy; may alternate with period of diarrhea
Intestinal bleeding	None	Gross bleeding may occur in first few weeks of life with blood streaks mixed in with stools
Irritability/decreased sleep	Cyclic, episodes of crying 3 or more hours per day; 3 or more days per week with higher intensity in afternoon and evening hours (diurnal); nonresponsive to comfort measures; sleep disturbance (see Box 35-2)	Increased irritability and decreased sleep, often also nonresponsive to comfort measures; irritability may occur 20 to 45 minutes after feeding or up to 2 hours after feeding; generally noncyclic but persistent
Proctalgia (painful defecation without constipation	None	May be found in infants with milk allergy
Feeding history	May be overfed with history of frequent feedings (every 2 hours) because of parents' inability to interpret child's cues; history of frequent formula changes or discontinuation of breast-feeding	Bottle-fed infants who also may be feeding frequently because of misread cues of irritability, but infant often acts hungry, takes formula and then cries with feeding; increased feedings usually increase the symptoms; breast-feeding infants who have allergy to milk in their mother's diet exhibit similar symptoms
Refusal of milk	None	Loss of appetite for cow's milk (may refuse feedings); often associated with decreased weight gain
Stomatitis	None	Report superficial ulcerations in oral mucosa; less often seen than with other allergies such as to tomatoes, nuts
Atopic dermatitis	None	Fifty percent or more of infants have lesions on forehead, cheeks, extensor surfaces of extremities, inguinal region, and buttocks, often without urticaria
Contact rash	None	May report blotchy erythema that is due to contact of milk on skin in infants, primarily around the mouth
Angioedema	None	May occur on skin, submucosa, subcutaneous upper respiratory tract and the gastrointestinal tract; may be seen with urticaria or alone; can cause respiratory distress or acute vomiting and abdominal pain
Rhinitis	None	Nasal stuffiness, sneezing, persistent watery or mucoid nasal discharge in 10% to 30% of allergic infants with onset in first few days or weeks after ingesting cow's milk formula
Chronic cough	None	Chronic cough associated with "noisy" breathing and gagging in approximately 20% of infants; may also have hypersecretion of mucus
Bronchitis/wheezing/recurrent pneumonia	None	History of recurrent bronchitis and wheezing beginning early in infancy; also history of recurrent pneumonia; pulmonary hemosiderosis occurs in 10% of cases
Serous otitis media	None	Serous otitis media often not discovered in young infants before superimposed secondary infection occurs and acute otitis media (AOM) develops; the relationship between recurrent AOM and otitis media with effusion still controversial to some practitioners
Anaphylaxis	None	Although rare, can occur within a few minutes after ingesting milk
Family history	No family history correlates	Usually a strong family history of allergies (often milk allergy) and asthma

Table 35-12 Differential Diagnosis: Colic and Cow's Milk Allergy—cont'd

CRITERIA	COLIC/INFANTILE IRRITABILITY	COW'S MILK ALLERGY
Objective Data *Physical examination*		
Temperature	Afebrile	Afebrile
Height/weight	Generally appropriate for age unless severe dysfunction of parent-child relationship or neglect/child abuse occurs	Poor growth frequent finding with infants, often below third percentile in height and weight
Other physical findings	Negative	Some infants may have the following on examination: Atopic dermatitis lesions, stomatitis, wheezing, urticaria, serous otitis media or acute otitis media, perioral contact dermatitis, rhinorrhea, hyperactive bowel sounds, hypertrophied tonsils with noisy upper airway congestion
Behavioral/ neurologic examination	Hypertonic, active infant; increased sensitivity to stimuli possible; marked response to Moro reflex, decreased self-soothing behaviors, decreased self-regulatory behaviors for state modulation (sleep, awake, and crying)	Normal
Observations	Parents may appear stressed, fatigued, resentful of infant; may exhibit disruption in parent-child interaction by a persistent lack of eye contact, physical touch, and decreased parent-infant attachment	Infant may initially appear healthy, but as symptoms increase child may become ill-looking; parents may also have similar feelings and behaviors as with an infant with colic, because of the infant's irritability
Laboratory data	None	Stool smear may be positive for occult blood and eosinophilia; blood may show positive eosinophilia; hypochromic microcytic anemia in infants with mild induced chronic pulmonary disease; thrombocytopenia can occur with severe allergy; skin prick test with cow's milk and hydrolysate formulas: Place a drop of formula on clear, nonscarred skin; prick with a pin; if positive (wheal greater than 3 mm at 15 minutes) to cow's milk and if skin prick negative to hydrolysate formula, it is unlikely infant will have allergic reaction to hydrolysate formula
X-ray	Negative	Some infants may have positive lung infiltrates with chronic pneumonia and pulmonary hemosiderosis (increased disposition of iron in the lungs)

is seen after the first week of life, with or without fever and with poor muscle tone, poor feeding, irritability, and lethargy.

Gastrointestinal tract disorders. Many infants were previously believed to have colic as a result of an immature GI system, constipation, abdominal distension resulting from gas, cow's milk allergy, lactose intolerance, or decreased gastric motility. Idiopathic infant irritability or infantile colic is not caused by any of these. However, an irritable infant should be evaluated to eliminate the serious GI tract problems listed below.

Intussusception is primarily seen in previously well infants of 2 to 4 months of age who have sudden onset of paroxysmal pain, often accompanied by vomiting. The infant rapidly becomes more ill and lethargic, and signs of shock may develop. Approximately 60% pass the diagnostic "currant jelly" stool. Examination reveals a tense abdomen with a sausage-shaped mass in the right upper quadrant and bloody mucus on rectal examination.

Meckel's diverticulum becomes evident with painless rectal bleeding, often without stool, in the child less than 2 years of age. Severe abdominal pain and vomiting may also occur.

GER onset is usually between 3 and 10 days of age with usually effortless regurgitation and vomiting in an otherwise healthy infant. Infants do not generally exhibit paroxysms of crying unless there is esophagitis or gastritis. These infants may

exhibit general irritability, often associated with feeding. Diagnosis of GER is made by history, negative findings on physical examination, and positive findings on upper GI tract radiography and esophageal pH probe. Apnea in young infants has been associated with GER, and infants may also be at risk for developing aspiration pneumonia.

GI tract upset can also be caused by gastroenteritis or cow's milk allergy. In breastfed babies a sensitivity to certain substances in the mother's diet (e.g., berries, tomatoes, onions, vegetables in the cabbage family, chocolate, spices, condiments, caffeine) can cause irritability, fussiness, and abdominal cramping.

Infants with colic or irritability often come to medical attention after a prolonged period of inconsolable, persistent crying. A thorough history and complete examination can often differentiate the infant with colic from the infant with abdominal distress that is attributable to other causes or a much more severe organic disease.

Trauma. Increased infant irritability can result from a foreign body (e.g., a hair in the eye), corneal abrasion, or hair tourniquet syndrome (human hair wrapped around a digit or penis, creating a tourniquet). The onset can be either sudden or gradual depending on the cause. Infants with these minor traumas (not associated with child abuse) or who may have

Box 35-2 Causes for Food Intolerance*

Enzyme deficiencies
  Lactose deficiency
  Sucrose deficiency
  Pancreatic (cystic fibrosis)
  Phenylketonuria
  Galactosemia
Pharmacologic reactions
  Chemicals in foods (e.g., caffeine)
  Tyramine (bananas, tomatoes, cheese)
  Tryptamine (plums, tomatoes)
  Alcohol
  Antibiotics
Additives and contaminants (e.g., food dyes, sulfites, nitrates and nitrites, monosodium glutamate)
Toxins, bacteria, and fungi
Psychologic causes (e.g., feeding aversion, eating disorders, child abuse)
Other disorders (e.g., collagen vascular disease, endocrine disorder)
Gastrointestinal diseases
  Hiatal hernia
  Peptic ulcer
  Gallbladder disease
  Neoplasm
  Intussusception
  Inflammatory bowel disease
  Pyloric stenosis
  Hirschsprung's disease
  Tracheal esophageal fistula
Cow's milk allergy

*This is not an all-inclusive list.

injuries such as testicular torsion or incarcerated hernia have a negative history of the recurrent, episodic bouts of fussiness and the behaviors that are usually associated with colic. Physical examination identifies the source of the trauma, and treatment or referral can be instituted.

Drug reactions. Infants may also have sudden irritability and fussiness after a reaction to the diphtheria, tetanus, and pertussis vaccine. There is often an associated fever and localized swelling and redness at the injection site. Infants who experience withdrawal from narcotics demonstrate irritability and crying. These infants often exhibit jitteriness and tremors, tachypnea, diarrhea, vomiting, a high-pitched cry, poor feeding, and fever. Symptoms may appear within the first 48 hours of life or as late as 4 to 6 weeks of age. History of maternal use of narcotics is significant in this instance (see Chapter 28).

Child abuse. A thorough history and physical examination should be performed on all infants to rule out the possibility of child abuse as the cause of irritability. Infants who have unexplained bruises and fractures and are not gaining weight or developing normally should be evaluated for nonaccidental trauma. A more detailed assessment is described in Physical Abuse and Neglect in Chapter 47. In addition, parents with a "colicky" infant often become exhausted from lack of sleep and feel powerless, resentful, and inadequate as parents. Escalation of these feelings may present a potential risk for child abuse, specifically for shaken baby syndrome.

Cardiovascular or hematologic disease. Infants who demonstrate extremely irritable behavior should be examined for possible cardiovascular disease, though it is rare (e.g., supraventricular tachycardia, congestive heart failure, anomalous left coronary artery originating from the pulmonary artery [ALCAPA]). Infants with sickle cell crisis may also have excessive crying and irritability as a result of vasoocclusive crisis. Any infant who has poor feeding, irritability, lethargy, pallor, cyanosis, diaphoresis, tachycardia, or signs of respiratory distress should be evaluated for possible cardiac disease. Infants with sickle cell disease or crisis usually exhibit anemia between 10 and 12 weeks of age with loss of splenic function between 4 months and 2 years of age with associated bacterial sepsis and meningitis (see Chapters 32 and 36).

Cow's milk allergy or intolerance. Cow's milk contains more than 25 protein components, which may cause specific antibody production in humans. Most allergic reactions to milk in children are attributable to whey and casein proteins. a-Lactalbumin, b-lactoglobulin, and serum albumin constitute the major whey proteins. When there is no immune mechanism involved, the adverse reaction is called "food intolerance." Food intolerances can also cause anaphylactic symptoms such as urticaria and wheezing. Immunoglobulin E (IgE)–mediated responses can include GI tract symptoms, hives, angioedema, rhinitis, asthma, and anaphylaxis.

It is difficult to determine whether infants are truly "allergic" or merely "intolerant" of cow's milk protein without extensive testing. Management is the same, regardless of the cause. It is important to consider other possible causes resembling food allergy (see Box 35-2).

Infants can become sensitized to milk protein in utero from the maternal diet and can have symptoms anytime after ingesting milk proteins. Infants who are breastfed may be sensitive to the maternal intake of milk proteins. The best method of determining milk allergy or intolerance is accomplished with a double-blind, placebo-controlled food challenge. All food challenges and skin tests should be performed in an environment that can provide emergency treatment for anaphylaxis. Other possible causes of vomiting and diarrhea are discussed in other chapters.

Management

Infantile colic or idiopathic infant irritability

Treatments and medications. Simethicone (Mylicon) and diphenhydramine hydrochloride (Benadryl) have been used by some health care practitioners but have not been found to be effective in alleviating symptoms and are based on the belief that colic is related to the GI tract and not a sleep disturbance. Herbal decoctions such as chamomile, licorice, fennel, balm mint, and peppermint have shown inconclusive effectiveness. The practitioner should collaborate with parents regarding their limited use. Antacids have occasionally been prescribed for infantile colic, but they are not effective, and chronic use of aluminum-containing antacids in infants has the potential risk for causing phosphate depletion and rickets.

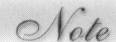

Note

Herbal decoctions or infusions (herbal "teas") can be dangerous. Some decoctions, such as Red Zinger and Mother's Milk tea, contain digitalis or theophylline derivatives, which can be harmful to infants. Also, there are no licensing or quality assurance requirements for herbs in some states. There are no established safe doses for infants.

Box 35-3 Behavior Management Program

Management of infant irritability (REST)

Regulation	Assist in regulating infant behaviors by learning their states and modulating them. Prevent overarousal and overstimulation
Entrainment	Infant behavior is synchronized with the environment. Light/dark, noise/quiet, and activity levels are all synchronized with the sleep/wake cycle of the infant.
Structure	Provide a predictable, structured pattern of events for the infant (e.g., established feedings, bathing, sleeping routines).
Touch	Chest-to-chest, skin-to-skin contact with a vertical, ventral positioning has been found to be useful for some infants in breaking the cycle of excessive crying. Slow up-and-down movements such as gentle bouncing and rocking (vestibular stimulation) have also been effective.

Interventions for parents (REST)

Reassurance	Parents need reassurance that their infant is not ill or in pain. They also need reassurance that this irrability is time-limited and that they are competent and capable parents.
Empathy	Provide empathy by listening and acknowledging the difficulty of having an irritable infant. Share experiences of others to help parents feel less isolated. Acknowledge their feelings about this infant.
Support	Provide support by helping parents get the support they need from family, friends, or other parents who have gone through this experience. Be available either by telephone or personal contact.
Time out	Support and encourage parents to take time for themselves. Assist parents in scheduling break times and time away from their infant. Encourage negotiation for babysitting time or relief time with family and friends.

Using this REST regimen has implications for the mother-child (parent-child) dyad as well. It is hoped that the outcomes will result in the following:

Reciprocity	Infant develops interactive capabilities, and the parent is able to appropriately read the infant's cues.
Engagement	Parent is able to interact appropriately with the infant and is able to read cues to know when the infant has had enough interaction or stimulation.
Synchrony	Parent and child are in synchrony with each other.
Turn-taking	Parents need to take turns with their infant and have appropriate interactions in response to each other's actions.

Counseling and prevention

- Educate parents about the cause of symptoms.
- Encourage the use of support groups for parents of infants with colic or idiopathic infant irritability.
- Counsel parents about their feelings of inadequacy, guilt, frustration, and stress.
- Reassure parents that colic will not harm the baby physically or psychologically, and that colic is self-limiting and will resolve.
- Encourage parents not to smoke.
- Provide parents with possible resources to help soothe infant:
  Pacifiers
  Hot water bottles (check temperature to avoid skin burns)
  Infant swings
  Tape recordings of heart sounds, womb sounds, white noise, or music
  Books and tapes on infant massage
  Car-ride simulators
  Rocking chairs
  Musical toys and lights for the nursery
- Counsel parents on using the behavior management program found in Box 35-3. This program was developed by Keefe (1988) and Keefe and Froese-Fretz (1991, 1997) as part of a funded research grant from the National Institutes of Health and the National Institute of Nursing.
- Remember that not all techniques work for all babies. Some infants become calm when being wrapped tightly in a blanket, whereas others react violently. Also, not all babies like lullabies; some parents report that rock-and-roll music works best for their infant. Specific suggestions for

Box 35-4 Infant Behavior Cues

Engagement

Quiets or becomes alert
Looks at parent's face
Turns eyes or head toward parent
Vocalizes (e.g., coos, babbles)
Smiles
Makes smooth body movements
Opens eyes wide
Brightens in the face

Disengagement

Turns head or eyes away
Cries or fusses
Arches back or shows increased agitation
Pulls away, squirms, or kicks
Frowns or compresses lips
Hiccoughs or spits up
Makes increased sucking noises
Makes hand-to-mouth movements
Turns red in the face or shows skin mottling
Falls asleep

identifying infant-behavior cues, calming strategies, and helping the irritable infant sleep are found in Boxes 35-4 to 35-6. Encourage parents to experiment until they find what works for their infant.

- Reassure parents that they cannot spoil their child by holding him or her and that letting their infant "cry it out" is not effective in managing the irritable infant.

Box 35-5 Infant Calming Techniques

Wait to see if the infant calms self before intervening. (Be sure the infant is unwrapped so hands and feet are available.)

Begin with one to three soothing actions at a time and repeat them over and over. Do each one for a minimum of 5 minutes. (Repetition is the key.)

Changing too frequently only increases stimulation instead of soothing.

Calming techniques include the following (do one at a time):

- Show the infant your face.
- Gently hold the baby's arms close to body.
- Hold the infant with firm pressure in a vertical position over the shoulder.
- Talk or sing to the infant in a soft voice.
- Turn on the water faucet and let the infant watch and listen.
- Play music (find the music your infant responds to).
- Turn on vacuum cleaner, fan, or other white noise (e.g., radio on but turned between stations).
- Decrease sensory stimuli: Close drapes, lower the lights, and go into quiet room.

- Wrap the infant snugly in blanket (or unwrap if this causes increased agitation).
- Repeatedly touch or stroke the same area of the body (e.g., back, head) rhythmically but firmly.
- Give the infant a pacifier, or assist the infant in finding hands or fingers to suck.
- Place the infant in a swing, take a car ride, or go for a walk in the stroller.
- Put the infant in the infant seat on top of the dryer while it is running (because the motion calms); be sure to stay with the infant to avoid falls.
- Walk up and down stairs.
- Rock in a rocking chair.

Develop a consistent routine for crying episodes and for nap times and bedtimes.

Never let an infant "cry it out"; the cyclic, intense crying only becomes worse.

Box 35-6 Establishing a Routine for Sleep in the Irritable Infant

Establish a bedtime routine that takes approximately 10 to 20 minutes (e.g., give the infant a warm bath, hold and rock the infant, sign a song). Then, place the infant in the crib when drowsy but awake. The infant should fall asleep in the crib, not parents' arms, so that the infant begins to learn self-regulating behaviors. Always use the same order and the same routine each time.

Once the child is in the crib, say goodnight and leave the room.

Control the environment (e.g., soft light left on, soft music in the background or total silence)

If the infant cries, allow the crying for 5 minutes, then return to the room and use one of the calming techniques suggested in Box 37-3 (or any other technique one wishes to use).

Use one calming technique for a minimum of 5 minutes. Then add a second technique for 5 to 10 minutes. Use up to three techniques as needed if the child does not calm down. One technique may be all that is needed if the child becomes quiet. After 10 to 15 minutes, place the child in the crib for 5 minutes.

Continue to repeat this cycle, never letting the child cry for more than 5 minutes before starting the soothing techniques (unless one can tell the infant is beginning to wind down with minimal fussing that may last 15 to 20 minutes before the infant finally goes to sleep.

Follow-up. Parents need frequent follow-up either by telephone or office visit. Instruct parents to return if signs or symptoms of illness develop and suggest they call the practitioner or child abuse prevention hotline if they feel out of control and about to abuse their infant.

Consultations and referrals

- Refer to a mental health professional any parents who are experiencing depression or family-relationship dysfunction and those at risk for child abuse.
- Refer the family to community resources for support and financial aid.

Cow's milk allergy

Treatments and medications

Dietary treatment

- Eliminate all dairy products from the diet.
- Use a suitable milk substitute
- Avoid other common allergens and cross-reacting foods.
- Remember that the formula of choice is casein hydrolysate, which is high in cost. Soybean formulas cost less, but approximately 10% to 50% of infants are also allergic to them. Breastfeeding mothers may need to eliminate dairy products from their diet.
- Introduce new foods one at a time at 1-week intervals when the infant is free of illness and allergic symptoms.
- Keep in mind that parents may try an oral milk challenge with supervision on their child when he or she is 1 year of age. If symptoms recur, eliminate dairy products from diet and rechallenge every 6 months. Most infants recover from milk allergy within 1 to 3 years. However, a small percentage of cases persist into adulthood.

Medications. Rhinitis can be treated with an oral antihistamine, but this is not recommended for infants under 6 months of age and should be used sparingly for children under 2 years of age (see Nasal Congestion and Obstruction in Chapter 41). For atopic dermatitis, see Rash in Chapter 37 and Allergies in Chapter 43. Pulmonary manifestations (e.g., bronchitis, pneumonia, wheezing) should be treated as indicated in Chapter 41 and the section on Asthma in Chapter 45. Disodium cromoglycate (cromolyn) taken orally has been shown to reduce intestinal symptoms.

Counseling and prevention

- Recommend that infants who have a family history of allergies be started on a milk substitute.
- Encourage and promote breastfeeding whenever possible.
- Mothers who are breastfeeding and have a family history of allergies may need to restrict or eliminate dairy products from their diet.
- Reassure parents that many children "outgrow" their allergy to cow's milk by 3 years of age.
- Educate parents about the causes of cow's milk allergy.
- Instruct parents about the dietary management of cow's milk allergy, common allergies, and cross-reacting foods.

- Teach parents to read product labels and avoid whey, casein, caseinate, sodium caseinate, lactalbumin, and soybean products (e.g., soybean oil, soybean lecithins, margarines).
- Encourage parents to keep a food diary, including the time, type of food, and reactions.
- Counsel parents to observe for signs and symptoms of stridor, wheezing, respiratory distress, and urticaria and to seek emergency medical assistance if they occur.
  Follow-up
- Call or schedule a return visit if the child becomes worse or has no improvement in 48 hours (which may indicate sensitivity to the milk substitute or other allergens).
- Call or schedule a return visit in 2 weeks for follow-up and weight check.
  Consultations and referrals. Refer to physician for the following:
- Infants with severe anaphylactic responses (e.g., stridor, pulmonary hemosiderosis, thrombocytopenia, severe enterocolitis)
- Indications of complications
- No response to treatment in 4 to 6 weeks

Mouth Sores

ELIZABETH F. GUNHUS

Alert

Consult with or refer to a physician for the following:
- Moderate to severe dehydration
- Hypersensitivity or reaction to a medication, especially with any "bull's eye" types of lesions that affect mucosal areas
- Suspected immune deficiencies
- Presence of chronic illnesses, including diabetes mellitus
- Malnutrition
- Mouth sores that remain unresponsive to treatment

Etiology

There is a multitude of causes that produce mouth sores and lesions of the oral mucosa. Viral, bacterial, or fungal pathogens produce oral lesions. Adverse drug reactions may precipitate the development of mouth sores. Smoking and the use of smokeless tobacco have also been identified as a cause of mouth sores and mucosal changes. Dental trauma and abscesses related to dental caries, overcrowding of teeth, or malocclusion are known to affect the entire mouth. There are some oral sores for which the cause remains unidentified.

Incidence

- Oral candidiasis is an infection that frequently occurs in early infancy.
- Seasonal peaks of streptococcal infections occur in late winter and early spring.
- Primary oral infection of herpes simplex most frequently occurs between 2 and 4 years of age.
- The peak incidence of herpangina occurs in summer and fall months in temperate climates.

Risk Factors

- Systemic disorders (e.g., immune deficiencies, diabetes)
- Starvation or malnutrition
- Aphthous ulcers (more common in individuals with IBD)
- Exposure to infectious contacts (e.g., day care, schools, family members)
- Poor oral hygiene practices
- Use of smokeless tobacco
- Recent course of medication, especially sulfonamides, penicillins, or phenytoin
- Dental trauma

Differential Diagnosis (Table 35-13)

Oral candidiasis is a fungal infection frequently affecting the mouth, tongue, and oral mucosa. Also referred to as *thrush,* the fungus *Candida albicans* is the cause of the infection. Oral candidiasis is frequent in newborns. It is also present with immune deficiencies, diabetes, and malnutrition. Administration of corticosteroid inhalers or systemic antibiotics may also lead to the overgrowth of *Candida* organisms. White plaques are noted on lips, tongue, and pharynx, often with a "milk-curd" appearance. The oral mucosa bleeds when plaques are removed.

Aphthous ulcers, or *canker sores,* are painful ulcerative lesions in the mouth. These ulcers are limited to the loose labial, buccal, and lingual oral mucosa. The cause of aphthous ulcers is unknown, but they may be induced by an autoimmune reaction. Nutritional deficiencies and IBD may precipitate lesions. The lesions initially appear as pinhead-sized vesicles on the oral mucosa. These further rupture into ulcers with a red base.

Herpetic gingivostomatitis is caused by an infection with herpes simplex virus, type 1. It is spread by direct contact with another infected individual. The primary oral infection most frequently occurs in early childhood. The incubation period is from 2 to 20 days. Latency occurs throughout the lifespan. Infants under 6 months of age appear to be protected from this infection by the presence of maternal antibodies. The vesicles are noted on the lips, buccal mucosa, anterior tongue, and palate, and these vesicles rupture into gray ulcers. Primary infections may also appear as an exudative pharyngitis after oral sexual contact.

Streptococcal gingivitis or *stomatitis* results from the growth of group A β-hemolytic *Streptococcus* organisms in the oral mucosa and pharynx. The illness becomes evident with a rapid onset of symptoms that include gingival erythema, inflammation of pharynx, and fever. This bacterial pathogen follows a seasonal pattern, with the greatest incidence of infection in late winter and early spring.

Varicella (chickenpox) is caused by the varicella-zoster virus. Varicella is known for a classic vesicular pruritic rash. Varicella lesions may appear on any of the body's mucosal surfaces, including the lips, buccal mucosa, and pharynx (see Varicella-Zoster Virus in Chapter 44).

Herpangina results from a enterovirus, primarily the coxsackieviruses. The greatest number of outbreaks occur during the summer and fall months. Transmission is usually through the oral-fecal route, but it may also result from direct contact with infected respiratory or ocular secretions. There is no prodrome, but there is a sudden onset of fever and oral lesions. The characteristic white ulcerations generally occur on the tonsillar pillars and posterior area of the pharynx.

Hand-foot-and-mouth disease is caused by coxsackievirus. Infections result in vesicular lesions in the mouth and oropharynx. Additional features include a characteristic exanthem affecting the palms and soles of the infected individual. Incubation period is from 5 to 7 days.

Acute necrotizing ulcerative gingivitis (*Vincent's stomatitis* or *trench mouth*) is a rare but serious infection that results in extensive involvement of the mouth, pharynx, and oral

Table 35-13 Differential Diagnosis: Mouth Sores

CRITERIA	VARICELLA	INFECTIOUS MONONUCLEOSIS	HAND-FOOT-MOUTH DISEASE	HERPANGINA	ORAL CANDIDIASIS
ICD-9 code	052.9	075.	074.3	074.0	112.0
Subjective Data					
Onset	Sudden	Gradual	Gradual	Sudden	Gradual
Duration	7 to 14 days	1 to 4 weeks	4 to 7 days	7 days	5 to 7 days
Fever	Yes	Yes	Yes	Yes	None
Oral symptoms	Pain	Dysphagia	Pain	Dysphagia, pharyngitis	White lesions, discomfort in mouth
Other signs/symptoms	Pruritic, nausea	Malaise	Pain at skin lesions, malaise	Anorexia, headache	Anorexia
Associated exanthem	Yes	Yes	Yes	No	Yes
Exposure	Infectious contact	Infectious contact	Infectious contact	Infectious contact	Maternal vaginal flora, contaminated nipples
Patient and family history	No varicella vaccine	Illness most common in teens and young adults	None	None	Incidence increased with immune deficiency, diabetes malnutrition
Objective Data					
Physical examination					
Vital signs	Fever	Fever	Fever	Fever	Stable
Lymphadenopathy	None	Cervical	None	Cervical	None
Mouth	Vesicles and ulcer on mucosal surfaces	Not affected	Vesicles and ulcer on palate	Vesicles and ulcers on palate	White plaques on lips, tongue, and pharynx; "milk-curd" appearance; mucosa bleeds with plaque removal
Ear, nose, throat	Rhinorrhea; pharyngitis	Exudative tonsillopharyngitis	None	Vesicles and ulcers on tonsillar pillars	White lesions on pharynx
Skin	Generalized vesicular lesions with red bases that rupture into ulcers and form crusts	Maculopapular rash with ampicillin therapy	Papules and vesicles on hands, palms, and soles; may affect anus	Not affected	Diaper area with bright red rash includes intertriginous areas and satellite lesions
Laboratory data	None	Epstein-Barr antibody test	None	None	Fungal culture when necessary for diagnosis

CRITERIA	APHTHOUS ULCERS	HERPETIC GINGIVOSTOMATITIS	STREPTOCOCCAL GINGIVITIS/STOMATITIS	ERYTHEMA MULTIFORME*	ACUTE NECROTIZING ULCERATIVE GINGIVITIS*	KAWASAKI'S DISEASE*
ICD-9 code	528.2	054.2	523.1/041.01	695.1	101.0	446.1
Subjective Data						
Onset	Sudden	Sudden	Sudden	Gradual	Gradual	Gradual
Duration	7 to 14 days	5 to 7 days	5 to 7 days	Prolonged	Prolonged	Prolonged
Fever	None	Yes	Yes	Yes	Yes	Yes; prolonged
Oral symptoms	Pain	Pain	Pain	Stomatitis	Severe pain; foul breath and taste; thick saliva, bleeding from lesions	Dysphagia; red lips and oral mucosa
Other signs/symptoms	None	Irritability	Throat pain, nausea/vomiting, headache	"Toxic" appearance, dehydration; myalgia	Malaise	Peripheral edema, conjunctivitis
Associated exanthem	No	No	Yes	Yes	No	Yes
Exposure	Unknown	Infectious contact	Infectious contact	May follow course of precipitating medication	May result from stress or local tissue trauma	None
Patient and family history	Increased incidence with ulcerative colitis	Infants under age 6 months protected by maternal antibodies	Poor dental hygiene may cause gingivitis	None	Poor oral hygiene practices; incidence increased with immune deficiencies	Most frequent under age 4 years
Objective Data *Physical examination*						
Vital signs	Subtle	Fever	Fever	Fever	Fever	Fever
Lymphadenopathy	None	Cervical and submental	Cervical	Generalized	Submaxillary nodes	Cervical nodes
Mouth	Pinhead-size vesicles on mucosa; rupture into ulcers with red base; membranous covering	Vesicles on lips, buccal mucosa, anterior tongue and palate; rupture into gray ulcers	Gingival tissue with erythema; inflammation of oral mucosa	Bullae on oral mucosa	Craterlike ulcers on gingiva with white pseudomembranous covering	Fissures lips with erythema; "strawberry tongue"
Ear, nose, throat	None	None	Inflammation of pharynx; white exudate on tonsils; petechiae on palate	Erosive bullous lesions on mucosal surfaces or eyes, nose and throat	Necrotic ulcers on pharynx	Infection of pharynx and conjunctiva
Skin	Not affected	Not affected	Sandpaper-like rash with desquamation of hands and feet	Papular to plaquelike lesions with "target" appearance of concentric rings of color	Not affected	Polymorphorous rash on trunk; periungual desquamation
Laboratory data	None	Viral culture when necessary for diagnosis	Oropharyngeal culture for group A *Streptococcus*	None	Microscopic examination of oral secretions for spirochete	None

Immediate referral to a physician.

mucosa. It most commonly occurs during the second and third decades of life, particularly in individuals with poor dental hygiene. The infection is caused by fusiform bacilli and spirochetal organisms. Microscopic examination of infected oral secretions reveals the pathogen.

Kawasaki's disease (which requires immediate referral to a physician) is an illness of idiopathic origin that results in childhood vasculitis of the small and medium-sized blood vessels. It is among the primary causes of acquired heart disease in children. Involvement of the lips, tongue, and oral pharynx is frequently associated with the presentation of the illness.

Erythema multiforme major, or *Stevens-Johnson syndrome* (which also requires immediate referral to a physician) is a serious illness, the presentation of which is frequently related to the recent use of medication. Sulfonamides, NSAIDs, penicillins, and anticonvulsants (phenytoin) have been shown to be precipitators of the illness. The classic presentation includes edema, erythema, and a burning sensation of the lips and buccal mucosa along with the characteristic cutaneous lesions involving two or more mucosal surfaces. Vesicular lesions and bullae in the mouth produce great pain. The extremities, trunk, neck, and scalp are frequently affected with macular lesions that progress into papules and then plaquelike figures with concentric rings of color resembling a target or bull's eye. Mucosal ulcerations may involve conjunctivae, nares, anorectal junction, vulva, and urethral meatus. The joints and kidneys and lungs may also be affected. Occasionally ocular involvement may lead to blindness.

Infectious mononucleosis is caused by the Epstein-Barr virus. Fever, malaise, and exudative pharyngitis are frequent presenting symptoms. The acute phase lasts 7 to 14 days. Group A *Streptococcus* organisms may occasionally cause a concurrent infection of the pharynx. Administration of ampicillin may potentially induce development of immunologically mediated rash. Hepatosplenomegaly is often present with the illness.

Management

Oral candidiasis

Treatments and medications

- Prescribe oral nystatin suspension (100,000 U/mL). The dosage for infants) 1 ml applied to each side of mouth and tongue four times daily. Older children may receive up to 4 ml to each side of the mouth four times daily. Continue medication for 2 or 3 days after all lesions resolve. Medication should be applied directly to the lesion when possible.
- Treat any concurrent diaper-area candidiasis.
- Treat any concurrent candidiasis of the maternal breast in a breastfeeding infant.

Counseling and prevention

- Counsel parents regarding appropriate sterilization of bottle nipples and pacifiers with boiling water. Any hard "teething" toys should also be cleaned.
- Educate parents that an infant's nipple or pacifier should not be "rinsed" in an adult's mouth. This could possibly inoculate the nipple with the *Candida* organism that is a part of the normal oral flora of any older person.
- Reinforce the importance of rinsing the mouth after the use of a corticosteroid inhaler.
- Educate families that oral candidiasis may occur after a course of antibiotics, which may alter the normal flora of the oral organisms and lead to an overgrowth of *Candida* organisms.

Follow-up. Instruct parents to call if there is no improvement in 72 hours or if symptoms worsen. Schedule a return visit in 2 weeks.

Consultations and referrals. Refer to a physician if the condition is not resolved after initial treatment; for a child with inadequate hydration status; or if compromised immune status is suspected.

Aphthous ulcers

Treatments and medications

- Recommend palliative treatment with 0.2% aqueous chlorhexidine gluconate mouthwash to maintain oral hygiene.
- Instruct the patient to use topical viscous lidocaine for pain relief, especially before eating.
- Remember that topical corticosteroid in mucosal adhering agent (0.1% triamcinolone in Orabase Baby [benzocaine]) may help reduce inflammation.
- Have the patient swish and swallow with a 1:1 mixture of diphenhydramine elixir (12.5 to 25 mg three or four times daily) and Maalox suspension.
- Rinse the mouth after eating to avoid development of secondary infections.

Counseling and prevention

- Advise the parents and child that sores may last as long as 14 days.
- Remember that ulcers may be precipitated by minor local trauma, stress, and anxiety.
- Instruct to the patient to follow a bland diet. Avoid spicy, salty, and citrus foods.

Follow-up. Instruct the parents to call if hydration status worsens.

Consultations and referrals. None are needed.

Herpetic gingivostomatitis

Treatments and medications

- Antipyretics for fever or pain (acetaminophen or ibuprofen)
- Adequate oral hydration, which may include apple juice, ice slurries, and Popsicles
- Bland diet
- Frequent rinsing of mouth to prevent secondary infections
- Intravenous fluids and the antiviral medication acyclovir for prolonged cases of illness with severe dehydration

Counseling and prevention

- Provide instructions on symptomatic treatment:
- Administer acetaminophen approximately 30 minutes before eating.
- Remember that the cold from ice slurries and Popsicles may help to numb affected areas.
- Instruct parents regarding the signs and symptoms of dehydration.
- Advise parents that the disease is self-limiting and resolves in 7 to 14 days with gradual crusting and then reepithelialization of lesions.
- Inform the family that reactivation of mouth sores may be induced by fever, local trauma, stress, or exposure to ultraviolet radiation. Prodrome of burning and tingling at affected site signals recurrences.
- Advise that thumbsucking or nail-biting with an active lesion on the lips or mouth could lead to infection of the paronychial region. Contact with lesions may also lead to autoinoculation of the eyes or genital areas, resulting in the spread of lesions.
- Counsel that transmission increases with open, draining lesions but may also occur with an asymptomatic carrier.

Follow-up. Instruct the parents to call in 24 to 48 hours to report progress and assess hydration status, and schedule a return visit in 1 week.

Consultations and referrals. Refer to a physician if hydration status is compromised or if illness is not resolved within 14 days.

Streptococcal gingivitis and stomatitis

Treatments and medications

- Penicillin V 250 mg by mouth twice daily for 10 days in children weighing 50 pounds or less, and 500 mg by mouth twice daily for 10 days in children or adolescents weighing more than 50 pounds
- Benzathine penicillin G intramuscular injection, 600,000 U in a single dose for children, and 1.2 million U in a single dose for those 12 years of age and older
- Erythromycin for individuals with penicillin allergies (erythromycin estolate, 20 to 40 mg/kg divided into two to four doses daily for 10 days)

Counseling and prevention

- Reinforce the importance of good oral hygiene practices, including brushing of teeth and timely dental treatment.
- Instruct on the need to maintain adequate fluid intake.
- Suggest that contaminated toothbrushes be replaced after the infection is resolved.
- Remember that the child should not attend school or group day care until 24 hours after antibiotic treatment has started or while the fever persists.
- Encourage frequent handwashing by the affected child.

Follow-up. Instruct the parents to call in 24 to 48 hours if there is no improvement, and schedule a return visit in 14 days.

Consultations and referrals. Refer to a physician if there are concerns regarding possible sequelae of acute rheumatic fever or glomerulonephritis.

Varicella. See Varicella-Zoster Virus in Chapter 44.

Treatments and medications

- Acetaminophen for fever
- Diphenhydramine 5 mg/kg orally divided every 6 hours for severe itching
- Topical preparations for relief of itching, including calamine lotion and oatmeal bath preparations
- Topical antibiotic ointment (e.g., bacitracin, Polysporin Ointment) as necessary for localized infections

Counseling and prevention

- Suggest frequent tepid baths for relief of itching.
- Suggest that Popsicles or ice slurries may help relieve local irritation of oral lesions.
- Keep in mind that the child should not return to school or group day care until all lesions are dry and crusted.

Follow-up. Instruct the parents to call in 48 hours if hydration status is compromised.

Consultations and referrals. Refer to a physician if immunodeficiency is present.

Herpangina

Treatments and medications. Administer antipyretics for fever and pain.

Counseling and prevention

- Advise parents that transmission is mainly by the fecal-oral route or by direct contact with infected respiratory or ocular secretions. Frequent handwashing and good personal hygiene diminish the risk of transmission.
- Educate on the signs and symptoms of dehydration and reinforce the importance of adequate fluid intake.
- Instruct the patient to follow a bland diet and avoid spicy, salty, or citrus foods.

Follow-up. Schedule a return visit if signs and symptoms of dehydration are present.

Consultations and referrals. Consult with a physician if severe pain is present. Refer to a physician if lesions are not resolved after 2 weeks.

Hand-foot-and-mouth disease

Treatments and medications. Administer antipyretics for fever or pain and ensure adequate fluid intake.

Counseling and prevention

- Advise that the duration is usually from 5 to 7 days.
- Educate parents that the disease is highly contagious and that it is spread through a fecal-oral route and also by respiratory secretions.
- Remember that the child should not attend school or group day care while febrile.
- Remind parents to maintain strict handwashing after diaper changes to prevent further transmission.
- Educate on the signs and symptoms of dehydration and reinforce the importance of adequate fluid intake.
- Advise the patient to follow a bland diet and avoid spicy, salty, or citrus foods until oral lesions are resolved.

Follow-up. Make telephone contact in 24 to 48 hours if there are concerns regarding hydration status.

Consultations and referrals. Refer to a physician if dehydration is evident.

Acute necrotizing ulcerative gingivitis (Vincent's stomatitis or trench mouth)

Treatments and medications

- 0.2% aqueous chlorhexidine gluconate mouthwash four times daily for empiric relief and to prevent secondary infections
- Maintenance of fluid intake for adequate hydration

Counseling and prevention. Instruct on improved oral hygiene to diminish the accumulation of food and bacteria in gingival crevices that causes gingivitis

Follow-up. Make a telephone call in 24 hours to assess hydration status and pain management.

Consultations and referrals. Refer to an oral surgeon for local curettage of affected gingival tissue, and consult with a physician for complaints of severe pain or if dehydration is present.

Kawasaki's disease

Treatments and medications. Administer antipyretics for fever and pain and ensure adequate fluid intake.

Counseling and prevention. Provide instructions regarding signs and symptoms of dehydration and need for sufficient fluid intake.

Follow-up. Schedule a return visit if signs or symptoms of dehydration develop or the child's condition worsens.

Consultations and referrals. Refer to a physician for management of disease.

Erythema multiforme (Stevens-Johnson syndrome). This requires immediate referral to a physician.

Treatments and medications

- Antipyretics for pain or fever (acetaminophen or ibuprofen)
- Maintenance of adequate fluid intake and close monitoring of hydration status
- Discontinuation of any medications that could contribute to the condition

Counseling and prevention

- Advise the patient and family that the condition may be exacerbated by several medications. Review all recent medications with a physician and discontinue use of all nonvital medications until advised by a physician.

- Educate parents regarding the signs and symptoms of dehydration and reinforce the importance of maintaining adequate fluid intake.

Follow-up. Schedule a return visit if the condition or hydration status worsens.

Consultations and referrals. Provide immediate referral to a physician for hospitalization. Also consult an ophthalmologist to assess for potential corneal involvement.

Infectious mononucleosis
Treatments and medications

- Antipyretics for fever or pain (acetaminophen or ibuprofen)
- Gargles and warm drinks for comfort of throat pain
- Penicillin if concurrent streptococcal infection of the pharynx is present (ampicillin may cause a rash)
- Limited physical activity

Counseling and prevention

- Educate on the signs and symptoms of dehydration and reinforce need for adequate fluid intake.
- Reinforce the need for adequate bed rest during the acute phase of the illness. Participation in physical activities should be allowed only as easily tolerated during the recovery phase.
- Advise avoidance of contact sports until illness and splenic involvement is resolved.
- Remember that tonsillar hypertrophy that impairs respiration requires hospitalization and steroid therapy.

Follow-up. Schedule a return visit if dehydration is present or there is no improvement of symptoms after 48 hours. Also schedule a return visit in 1 week.

Consultations and referrals. Refer to a physician if hepatomegaly or splenomegaly is present. Consult with a physician regarding signs or symptoms of dehydration.

Nausea and Vomiting

JANE A. FOX

Alert

Consult with or refer to a physician for the following:
- History of significant head trauma, with or without loss of consciousness.
- Signs of meningitis (e.g., bulging fontanel, listlessness, behavior change, nuchal rigidity)
- Suspicion of congenital obstruction or anomalies
- Absence of bowel sounds
- Suspicion of diabetic ketoacidosis, either new onset or in a child with insulin-dependent diabetes mellitus (as indicated by increased urination and thirst and ketonuria)
- Projectile vomiting
- Poison ingestion
- Onset of severe abdominal pain
- Signs of severe dehydration
- Jaundice
- Signs and symptoms of failure to thrive (FTT)
- Bloody or tarry stools
- Hematemesis
- Severe anorexia
- Persistent weight loss
- Vomitus with fecal odor or undigested food
- Chronic or persistent early morning vomiting, especially when associated with recurrent headaches

Etiology

Nausea is the unpleasant sensation that usually precedes vomiting. Irritation of nerve endings in the stomach or elsewhere in the body can produce the sensation of nausea. Messages are sent from these irritated nerves to the brain, which controls the vomiting reflex, and when the irritation becomes intense, vomiting occurs. Vomiting is the forceful ejection of gastric contents through the mouth. The vomiting center, located in the medulla, is influenced by irritation of the peritoneum or mesentery, obstruction of the intestine, action of toxins on the medulla, or primary CNS disorders.

The most common cause of vomiting in children is acute gastroenteritis. Other infections such as otitis media, UTI, and meningitis may also cause vomiting. Vomiting in infants is one of the most common complaints and can be associated with many disturbances. Often vomiting is the result of faulty feeding techniques, improper feeding preparations, or chalasia (relaxation of a body opening).

Vomiting may be caused by congenital anomalies, a foreign body, trauma, intoxication or drug overdose (e.g., on lead, salicylates), CNS lesions causing increased intracranial pressure, various endocrine and metabolic disorders, food poisoning, and pregnancy.

Incidence

- It is a common complaint.
- The incidence depends on origin or cause.
- Vomiting occurs in all age groups but is most common in infancy and childhood.
- GER is one of the most common GI problems in children and the most common reason for referral to pediatric gastroenterologists.
- Studies indicate that 25% to 80% of children with asthma have reflux. Reflux may be the underlying problem for a child with nighttime asthma symptoms, including cough.

Risk Factors

- Maternal polyhydramnios, which commonly occurs in children with congenital anomalies
- No stool within 48 hours after birth
- Family history of milk protein intolerance
- Poisoning
- Chemotherapy
- Recent surgery
- Medications (e.g., antibiotics, theophylline, digitalis)
- Pregnancy
- Drug overdose
- NSAID therapy

Differential Diagnosis (Table 35-14)

Vomiting is a symptom that can have many causes. It should be differentiated from regurgitation, which is the effortless, nonprojectile, nonforceful spitting up of small amounts of liquid or food after being fed. Vomiting can be a symptom of a life-threatening illness and must be evaluated carefully to determine the cause. It is important to observe the frequency, severity (forcefulness), and timing of the vomiting. Special attention should be given to the quantity and quality or appearance of the vomitus. The absence of bile in vomitus is suggestive of an obstruction proximal to the pylorus. Bile vomitus, which turns green when exposed to air, results from an obstruction below the second part of the duodenum. When vomitus has a fecal odor, it is suggestive of peritonitis or an obstruction of the

Table 35-14 Vomiting: Diagnostic Considerations

CONDITION	DIAGNOSTIC FINDINGS	EVALUATION	COMMENTS/MANAGEMENT
Infection/Inflammation			
Acute gastroenteritis	Acute onset with nausea, fever, diarrhea, and evidence of systemic illness	Fluid status, stool culture if needed	Nothing by mouth, if indicated; clear liquids, advance slowly
Posttussive/posterior nasal drip	Follows vigorous coughing; may be greatest at night when recumbent; associated cough, rhinorrhea	Chest x-ray study if needed	Therapeutic trial: Cough suppressant or decongestant
Otitis media	Fever, irritability, painful ear		Antibiotics; topical therapy for extreme pain
Esophagitis/gastritis	Variably "coffee ground," bloody; epigastric or substernal pain, discomfort; reflux	Endoscopy; upper GI series	Associated reflux, hiatal hernia; drugs; trial of antacids
Ulcer, peptic/duodenal*	Usually coffee ground; epigastric, abdominal pain; may be chronic or acute; possible anemia	Endoscopy; upper GI series	May be life threatening: Refer immediately
Hepatitis*	Associated liver tenderness; icterus	Liver function tests	Usually infectious; viral, Epstein-Barr virus
Peritonitis* Appendicitis* Cholecystitis*	Generalized or localized tenderness, guarding, rebound	White blood cell count, x-ray studies, urinalysis	Surgical exploration usually needed: Refer immediately
Pancreatitis*	Abdominal tenderness, pain, back pain	Amylase	GI rest, decompression; evaluate cause
Cystitis Pyelonephritis	Associated fever, dysuria, frequency, burning, variable costovertebral angle tenderness	Urinalysis, urine culture	Initiate antibiotics pending culture results
Meningitis* Central nervous system abscess* Subdural effusion/empyema*	Fever, systemic toxicity; changed mental status; local neurologic signs, variable signs of increased intracerebral pressure	Lumbar puncture; CT scan if needed	Antibiotics; neurosurgical consultation if indicated: Refer immediately
Congenital			
Pyloric stenosis*	Regurgitation progressing to projectile vomiting; palpable, olive-sized tumor in right upper quadrant; vigorous gastric peristalsis present; variable dehydration, poor weight gain	Upper GI series (delayed gastric emptying, narrow pyloric channel ["string sign"], ultrasound may substitute; electrolytes to assess hydration	Usually male 4 to 6 weeks of age; treat fluid deficits, then surgery (pyloromyotomy): Refer immediately
GI tract obstruction* Intestinal obstruction/stenosis/bands Imperforate anus Malrotation Meconium ileus/plug Volvulus, sigmoid/midgut Intussusception	Obstructive pattern beginning in newborn period: Greater than 20 ml in gastric aspirate; if proximal to ampulla of Vater: distention of epigastrium or left upper quadrant and gastric peristaltic wave; if distal to ampulla of Vater, vomitus contains bile, generalized distention	Abdominal x-ray study with contrast studies if needed; electrolytes to assess fluid status	Immediate decompression; correction of fluid deficits; surgical consultation: Refer immediately

Associated with cystic fibrosis

Life threatening

Life threatening |
Hydrocephalus*	Excessive growth of head circumference; irritability, lethargy, headache, bulging of fontanel	CT scan	May involve blockage of ventricular shunt; neurosurgical consultation; urgent care: Refer immediately
Trauma			
Concussion	Trauma; headache, minimally changed mental status; often projectile vomiting	Skull x-ray study, CT scan	Support; monitoring
Subdural hematoma*	Marked change in mental status, signs of increased intracranial pressure: headache, ataxia, sixth-nerve palsy, seizures; focal neurologic signs	CT scan	Immediate neurosurgical consultation; support: Intubate, hyperventilate, diuretics: Refer immediately

From Barkin, R.M. & Rosen, P. (1999). Emergency pediatrics: a guide to ambulatory care *(5th ed.). St Louis: Mosby.*
*Immediate referral to physician.
ABG, *Arterial blood gas;* CT, *computed tomography;* EDTA, *ethelenediamine tetraacetic acid.*

Continued

Table 35-14 Vomiting: Diagnostic Considerations—cont'd

CONDITION	DIAGNOSTIC FINDINGS	EVALUATION	COMMENTS/MANAGEMENT
Trauma—cont'd			
Foreign body*	History: May have dysphagia or total obstruction; may have respiratory distress	X-ray study; esophagoscopy	Refer to a physician if esophagus, attempt to remove by use of Foley catheter under fluoroscopy; if elsewhere, endoscopy or surgery, depending on foreign body
Intramural duodenal hematoma*	Following even minimal blunt trauma: nausea, bilious vomiting, pain, tenderness, ileus; may have abdominal mass	Upper GI series	May be delay in symptom presentation Refer immediately
Ruptured viscus*	Trauma followed by abdominal tenderness, rebound, guarding	Peritoneal lavage; x-ray study for free air	Immediate surgical intervention; fluids, antibiotics: Refer immediately
Subarachnoid hemorrhage*	Headache, stiff neck, progressive loss of consciousness; focal neurologic signs	CT scan; bloody spinal fluid	Neurosurgical consultation; supportive care: Refer immediately
Cerebral edema*	Signs of increased intracranial pressure: headache, ataxia, sixth-nerve palsy; altered mental status	CT scan	Diuretics, corticosteroids, hyperventilation, elevation: Refer immediately
Intoxication			
Alkali burns*	Associated mouth burns, difficulty swallowing	Endoscopy	Lye, bleaches most common; surgery consultation: Refer immediately
Salicylates*	Nausea, vomiting, tinnitus	Salicylate level	Stop medication; antacids, fluids: Refer immediately
Iron*	Hematemesis, shock, acidosis	Iron and ABG levels, complete blood cell count	Urgent treatment with deferoxamine: Refer immediately
Lead*	Usually chronic exposure; signs of increased intracranial pressure	Lead level	Dimercaprol, EDTA: Refer immediately
Digitalis*	Underlying heart disease; nausea, arrhythmias	Digitalis level; electrocardiogram	Stop digitalis; institute active treatment of dysrhythmia: Refer immediately
Vascular			
Migraine	Unilateral, throbbing headache, aura; family history		Consider therapeutic trial of ergotamine; analgesia, corticosteroids
Hypertensive encephalopathy*	Rapid increase in blood pressure; changed mental status; headache, nausea, anorexia	Evaluation of underlying disease	Rapid response when diastolic blood pressure brought below 100 mm Hg
Endocrine/Metabolic			
Acidosis*	Underlying cause; rapid, deep breathing	ABG levels	Correction: Refer immediately
Diabetic ketoacidosis*	Kussmaul breathing; history of diabetes; nausea, abdominal pain; ketones on breath	Electrolytes; ABG; glucose; ketone levels	Hydration, insulin, potassium: Refer immediately
Uremia*	Oliguria, often predisposing cause	Blood urea nitrogen, creatinine levels; tests for underlying conditions	Evaluate and treat underlying cause: Refer immediately
Inborn errors of metabolism Amino/organic acids*	Associated acute-onset vomiting and acidosis, progressive deterioration or poor growth and development	Urine and blood for amino and organic acids; electrolytes, ABG levels: Acidosis	Exacerbation precipitated by acute illness: Refer immediately
Fructose intolerance*	Associated with ingestion of sugar or fruits	Challenge test under controlled conditions	
Addison disease*	Dehydration, circulatory collapse; if chronic: weakness, fatigue, pallor, diarrhea, increased pigmentation	Low serum sodium and elevated potassium levels: blood and urine adrenocorticosteroids low	Adrenal genital syndrome in newborns: Refer immediately
Reye syndrome*	Associated liver failure, with marked change in mental status (often combative)	Liver function test results and ammonia level elevated	

Immediate referral to physician.
ABG, *Arterial blood gas;* CT, *computed tomography;* EDTA, *ethelenediamine tetraacetic acid.*

Table 35-14 Vomiting: Diagnostic Considerations—cont'd

CONDITION	DIAGNOSTIC FINDINGS	EVALUATION	COMMENTS/MANAGEMENT
Intrapsychic			
Attention getting	Inconsistent history; times usually related to getting attention	Psychiatric evaluation	Organic causes must be ruled out
Hysteria/ hyperventilation	Anxiety, nausea, and other psychosomatic symptoms; may hyperventilate	Psychiatric evaluation	Exclude organic causes
Neoplasm			
GI tract*	Related to location, type, and extent of neoplasm; insidious onset of symptoms	Specific for tissue considerations	Rare in children
Intracerebral*			Refer immediately
Miscellaneous			
Improper feeding techniques	Often regurgitation; bad nipple; improper position; usually occurs shortly after feeding; usually vomited material is undigested	Rarely need upper GI series to rule out abnormality	Implement support system; make sure child not overfed
Chalasia	May be small amounts; associated with feeding, usually within 30 to 45 minutes of feeding; child well, good growth	Upper GI series if needed	Trial of slow, careful, prone, upright feedings; child usually under 6 months of age; avoid overfeeding
Pregnancy	Increased intraabdominal pressure; usually first trimester		
Epilepsy	Aura or seizure may involve vomiting	Electroencephalogram	Refer to neurologist
Ascites*	Increased intraabdominal pressure	As related to cause; total serum protein, albumin levels	Refer to physician
Environmental			
Heat illness (hyperthermia)*	Abnormal mental status; variably febrile, leg cramps, dehydrated	Electrolyte levels	Fluids, cooling
Superior mesenteric artery syndrome	Compression of duodenum in child (adolescent female) leading to obstruction; usually recent marked weight loss	Upper GI tract series	Usually requires psychiatric therapy for underlying problems; support

*Immediate referral to physician.

lower bowel or colon. Bloody vomitus indicates that the blood has had little contact with gastric juices and bleeding is at or above the cardia or the stomach, whereas "coffee ground" vomitus indicates that blood has been altered by gastric juices, suggestive of slow bleeding from the esophagus, cardia, stomach, or duodenum.

When the patient's history is obtained, it should include any other associated symptoms such as fever, diarrhea, cough, coryza, abdominal pain, dysuria, polydipsia, jaundice, bloody stool, headache, alterations in mental status, constipation, and FTT. A family history of dietary intolerance and feeding techniques (i.e., amount of feeding, spitting up after feeding, frequency of burping) should be investigated. The history should be evaluated to determine precipitating factors such as trauma, recent illness, medications, and instability in the environment causing emotional disturbances.

Since vomiting can be caused by many factors, the physical examination must be complete and should include vital signs, assessment of hydration status, and evaluation of each organ system. Plot the child's height, weight, and head circumference on an appropriate growth curve to identify FTT or rapid increase in head growth. Assess mental status to determine focal neurologic signs, delayed neurologic development, possible seizure activity, hypotonia, retinal hemorrhages, irritability, lethargy, or ataxia. Document signs of infection, lymphade-

nopathy, or hepatosplenomegaly. The evaluation of vomiting is guided by the age of the child (Table 35-15). GER and gastroesophageal disease (GERD) are compared in Table 35-16.

Management
Acute gastroenteritis. See Diarrhea and Loose Stool.

Treatments and medications. Most causes of diarrhea and vomiting are self-limiting. Correct the existing dehydration and maintain fluid and electrolyte status. The infant is at risk for rapid dehydration. Treatment should include clear liquids for the first 24 hours. This may include Pedialyte or Ricelyte for infants and flat cola, ginger ale, or Gatorade at room temperature for older children.

After 24 hours, if the diarrhea has improved, an infant who takes only formula should receive half-strength formula (formula with twice as much water). An older child may be advanced to a diet that includes bananas, rice, applesauce, tea, and toast. If this diet is tolerated, the child may then return to a regular diet over the next 2 or 3 days. Children over 1 year of age should not be given cow's milk products (i.e., milk, cheese, ice cream, butter) for several days.

For antibiotic therapy, see Diarrhea and Loose Stool.
Counseling and prevention
- Explain the treatment plan to parents and assess their understanding of rehydration.

Table 35-15 Causes of Vomiting by Age

NEONATE (0-28 DAYS)	INFANT	CHILD (>2 YEARS)	ADOLESCENT
Gastrointestinal: Obstructive			
Intestinal atresia/stenosis	Incarcerated hernia	Foreign body	Foreign body
Malrotation of bowel	Foreign body	Duodenal hematoma	Malrotation of bowel
Volvulus	Malrotation/volvulus	Intussusception	
Meconium ileus/plug	Intussusception	Meckel diverticulum	
Hirschsprung's disease	Meckel diverticulum	Hirschsprung's disease	
Imperforate anus	Hirschsprung's disease	Incarcerated hernia	
Incarcerated hernia		Adhesions	
Pyloric stenosis			
Gastrointestinal: Infectious or Inflammatory			
Necrotizing enterocolitis	Gastroenteritis	Gastroenteritis	Gastroenteritis
Gastroesophageal reflux	Gastroesophageal reflux	Peptic ulcer disease	Peptic ulcer disease
	Peritonitis	Appendicitis	IBD
	Milk allergy	Pancreatitis	Appendicitis
		Paralytic ileus	Pancreatitis
		Peritonitis	Peritonitis
Neurologic			
Hydrocephalus	Hydrocephalus	Brain tumor	Brain tumor
Increased intracranial pressure	Brain tumor	Migraine	Increased intracranial pressure
Cerebral edema	Cerebral edema	Increased intracranial pressure	Motion sickness
Endocrine and Metabolic			
Inborn error of metabolism	Inborn error of metabolism	Diabetic ketoacidosis	Diabetic ketoacidosis
Adrenogenital syndrome	Adrenal failure	Adrenal insufficiency	Adrenal insufficiency
	Renal tubular acidosis		
Infection			
Sepsis	Sepsis	Sepsis	Sepsis
Meningitis	Meningitis	Meningitis	Meningitis
	Otitis media	Otitis media	Hepatitis
	UTI	UTI	UTI
	Pertussis	Foreign body	Foreign body
	Pneumonia	Pneumonia	
	Asthma		
Overdose			
	Lead	Lead	Digitalis
		Digitalis	Theophylline
		Theophylline	Salicylates
		Salicylates	
		Iron	
Other			
			Pregnancy
			Psychogenic
			Bulimia
			Anorexia

- Advise the avoidance of children with suspected gastroenteritis.
- Explain the importance of good handwashing after diaper changes or bathroom use to prevent spread.
- Instruct parents on the signs and symptoms of dehydration (e.g., dry mouth, no tears, decreased urination, weight loss, lethargy, irritability).

Follow-up. Provide telephone care for first 24 hours and schedule a return visit if the diarrhea increases in frequency and amount, does not improve after 24 hours of clear liquids or does not resolve entirely after 3 or 4 days, or if the stool contains blood.

Consultations and referrals. Refer to a physician for possible hospitalization if compliance of the family is questionable; excessive vomiting interferes with rehydration; there are signs and symptoms of moderate to severe dehydration; stool contains blood; or diarrhea persists after 3 or 4 days.

Overfeeding

Treatments and medications. Treatment is directed at educating the parents regarding the nutritional needs of the child.

Table 35-16 Comparison of Gastroesophageal Reflux and Gastroesophageal Disease

	GER	GERD
Age	Resolves by 12 to 18 months	Usually resolves by 2 years of age but may persist into childhood
Risk factors	Can occur in any newborn	Prematurity with respiratory complications; GI tract anatomic anomalies
Severity	Mild to moderate	Moderate to severe
Pathophysiology	Reflux only	Reflux with possible esophagitis or respiratory disorders
Laboratory evaluation	None	Possible pH probing or endoscopy
Treatment	Prone positioning	Prone positioning
		For older children, small, frequent, thickened feedings, dietary modifications, and weight reduction
		Possible referral for drug therapy
		Surgery if no improvement

Data from Bradley, R.B. (2001). Advance for Nurse Practitioners, 9*(8), 45.*

Counseling and prevention

- Educate parents in the basic foods and how to determine the amount necessary for appropriate growth. For the bottle-fed infant, instruct the parents that infants eat more than they require if they are fed whenever they cry. It is important to recognize the infant's needs for nonnutritive sucking and contact.
- Remember that some parents may be confused by "demand" feedings. It is more beneficial to adjust the feeding schedule to a reasonable amount of time between feedings.
- Advise that water may be used to supplement a feeding if the infant is thirsty; otherwise, it should be delayed until the next appropriate feeding time.
- Explain that if the infant is gaining weight appropriately, he or she is not underfed.

Follow-up. Schedule a return visit if the infant or child has any change in activity, becomes constipated, or has green stool or scant urine with a strong odor. An infant who is doing well should be seen in 1 week, and a recovering child should be seen in 2 weeks.

Consultations and referrals. If it is determined that vomiting is attributable to overfeeding, no referrals are necessary. If vomiting persists despite appropriate intervention and counseling, consult a physician.

Spitting up and regurgitation

Treatments and medications. Treatment is directed at giving parents support. Explain that this condition is normal for the first 6 months of life and sometimes continues until 1 year of life. Be sure that bottles have a proper nipple-hole size. Instruct parents to thicken feeds with rice cereal and to frequently burp the baby during feedings. Have the baby remain prone or with the head of bed elevated 30 degrees for approximately 30 minutes after feeds. Formula may be changed to either soybean, low-iron, or evaporated milk formula. However, changes are controversial and may lead to a misconception that the child has a sensitivity to a particular formula.

Counseling and prevention. Teach parents that regurgitation can be reduced by decreasing the amount of air swallowed during and after feedings. Suggest that they gently handle the infant after feedings and place infant on right side or abdomen immediately after eating. The baby's head should not be lower than the rest of the body while resting.

Table 35-17 Drugs (Prokinetic Agents) Used in the Treatment of Children with Gastroesophageal Reflux

DRUG	DOSAGE
Bethanechol chloride (Urecholine)	0.1 mg/kg per dose, orally, four times a day and given 15 to 30 minutes before a feeding or meal. *Use with caution if CNS disease, reactive airway disease, or cardiac disease is present.*
Metoclopramide (Reglan)	0.1 mg/kg per dose, orally, four times a day and given 15 to 30 minutes before a feeding or meal and at bedtime.
Cisapride* (Propulsid)	0.2 mg/kg per dose, orally, four times a day and given 15 minutes before a feeding or meal and at bedtime.

Drug of choice.

Follow-up. If regurgitation continues past 6 months of age, monitor monthly for weight gain.

Consultations and referrals. Refer to a physician any infant or child who is spitting up blood or not gaining weight, if the spitting up is projectile, if the child is over 12 months of age, or if coexistent esophagitis is suspected.

Gastroesophageal reflux

Treatments and medications

- Suggest small, frequent feedings to reduce gastric distension.
- Position the child on a 30-degree incline (with the head of the bed elevated) or prone throughout most of the day, especially after feedings. Consider thickening the infant's formula with cereal (1 tablespoon of dry rice cereal per oz of formula).
- In the child with severe GER, consider using medications to assist in the prevention of reflux (Table 35-17). Bethanechol (Urecholine) decreases vomiting by increasing esophageal sphincter pressure, and metoclopramide

(Reglan) increases gastric emptying. Cisapride (Propulsid) was recently approved in the United States for pediatric use and is prescribed over metoclopramide because it has fewer side effects.

Counseling and prevention

- Explain to parents that GER occurs in 1 of 500 live births and usually improves spontaneously by 6 to 9 months of age.
- Advise parents to give medications 30 minutes before meals. Explain the actions of any medications (e.g., bethanechol decreases vomiting by increasing esophageal sphincter pressure, metoclopramide and cisapride increase gastric emptying).

Follow-up. Schedule a monthly return visit to ensure that the child does not fall from the growth curve and to assess for esophagitis resulting from the recurrent reflux. Esophagitis should be suspected in any infant with reflux who exhibits irritability and abnormal posturing. Consider using antacids or cimetidine in these children.

Consultations and referrals. The children most at risk for complications are the neurologically impaired. Refer to a surgeon if severe reflux persists for more than 2 months after all medical therapy has been tried for possible surgical correction with a Nissen fundoplication. The medical therapy may be shortened and immediate referral to a surgeon given if recurrent aspiration or esophageal strictures form.

Esophagitis

Treatments and medications

- Institute a feeding regimen that includes frequent feedings of a bland diet, progressing to five meals a day with no bedtime meal.
- Avoid very hot foods, spices, alcohol, tobacco, caffeine-containing foods, coffee, and food high in residue.
- Avoid salicylates and anticholinergics. Food should be chewed well and slowly.
- Possibly elevate the head of the bed 15 to 20 cm.
- Advise the promotion of a relaxing atmosphere during mealtimes.
- Administer antacids (cimetidine or ranitidine), especially at bedtime, to reduce gastric secretions (Table 35-18).

Counseling and prevention. Advise parents of the dietary constraints. Parents should understand that the child should have five small meals to decrease the incidence of regurgitation and no meals at bedtime, which will decrease the risk of regurgitation while recumbent. The diet should contain bland food only. Avoid fried or spicy foods, alcohol, tobacco, coffee, and caffeine-containing foods.

Table 35-18 H₂-Receptor Blockers Used in Children and Adolescents with Esophagitis

DRUG	DOSAGE
Cimetidine (Tagamet)	5 to 10 mg/kg per dose, four times a day, with a maximum dose of 300 mg per dose, four times a day
Ranitidine (Zantac)	1 to 3 mg/kg per dose, two to three times a day, with a maximum dose of 150 mg per dose, two times a day

Follow-up. Initially schedule return visits every 2 weeks, increasing the intervals to assess for signs of strictures (e.g., dysphagia) and compliance with treatment.

Consultations and referrals. Refer to a physician for strictures. Surgery may be considered when conservative measures fail.

Perianal Itch and Pain

JANE A. FOX

Alert

Consult with or refer to a physician for the following:
- Foreign body (rectal or vaginal) that cannot be easily visualized and removed
- Signs and symptoms of suspected sexual abuse
- Sexually transmitted disease in young children
- Rectal thrombosis or rectal hemorrhage
- Hemorrhoidal strangulation
- Anal mass or neoplasm
- Rectal prolapse
- Intussusception

Etiology

Pruritus ani, an intense itching in the anal and perianal skin, is usually an acute symptom. Common clinical problems associated with perianal itch include skin disorders caused by allergies, contact dermatitis, eczema, anal fissures and fistulas, hemorrhoids, neoplasms, psoriasis, and seborrheic dermatitis. Infectious causes include pinworms and other worms, scabies, and pediculosis. Other causes include poor hygiene, chemical irritants (e.g., a bubble bath), alkalotic irritation from diarrhea, diabetes mellitus, chronic liver disease, trauma from scented toilet tissue, sexual abuse, and sexual intercourse or sexual contact with a person who has an anogenital infection.

Rectal pain can be a minor discomfort or an acute symptom. Common clinical problems associated with rectal pain include many of the causes associated with perianal itching. In addition, rectal pain can be caused by straining at defecation, an anal mass, a rectal prolapse, or an intussusception.

Incidence

- Pruritus ani is common in all ages.
- Pubic lice *(Phthirus pubis)* are most common in adolescents engaging in multiple sexual relationships, but they can occur in adults or in the eyelashes of infants and children who have been sexually abused.
- Pinworms *(Enterobius vermicularis)* produce a common parasitic infestation to which all ages are susceptible. The prevalence is higher in preschool and school-age children and adults in contact with infected children. Infestation rates are high in institutional and boarding school populations.
- Pubic lice and pinworms affect individuals of all socioeconomic classes.
- Hemorrhoids occur at all ages but are more common in adults.
- Anal fissure occurs at all ages but is more common in adults.
- Vaginal foreign body is common in prepubescent age groups.

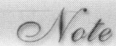

Risk Factors

- Poor hygiene
- Close contact with infected persons
- Constipation or hard stool
- Obesity
- Preexisting skin condition
- Pregnancy
- Neuromuscular disorders or immobility
- Sexual abuse and anal intercourse
- Trauma
- Communal living conditions or crowded households
- Warm climates

Differential Diagnosis (Table 35-19)

Pruritus ani may be caused by multiple dermatologic disorders such as anal fissures, parasitic or ectoparasitic infestations such as pinworms or pubic lice, poor hygiene, or trauma. The usual course is acute and resolves when the underlying cause is treated. Chronic pruritus ani is a symptom of a disease, not a diagnosis or disease in itself.

Pubic lice (crab lice) are a common cause of anorectal pruritus. *Phthirus pubis,* an ectoparasite, is completely dependent on the host's blood for survival. A mature adult often lays 3 to 6 eggs a day, which hatch into adulthood. Lice are found at the base of the hairs, and nits are present at the base of the hair shafts. Infestation is sometimes manifested as gray-blue purpuric lesions. In heavy infestations, excoriations and multiple bite and scratch marks are present in the pubic area, with gray-blue macules in the groin area adjacent to the infestations. Although lice are found in pubic hair, in young children they may attach to body hair and eyelashes. In this case always consider the possibility of sexual abuse (see also Lice in Chapter 37).

Pinworms are the most common cause of anorectal itching in children. Patients usually have nocturnal anal pruritus. Parents may report seeing worms in the stool. *Enterobius vermicularis,* a white, threadlike worm 1 cm in length, primarily inhabits the cecum and the adjacent bowel. The gravid female detaches from the cecal mucosa, migrates down the large bowel to the rectum, and passes out the anus onto the perianal skin, where eggs are laid. The eggs become infectious in about 2 to 4 hours. Humans become infected by ingesting embryonated eggs carried on the hands or inhaling eggs deposited in house dust, dirt, or room air. Autoinfection easily occurs by ingesting eggs picked up from the perianal skin through scratching or through insufficient hand washing after defecation. Reinfection by hand-to-mouth transmission is common.

Hemorrhoids, a varicosity that can be internal or external, are uncommon in children. External hemorrhoids, the more common of the two types, can be a cause of both anal pain and pruritus. They occur with chronic constipation or impaction and often become evident with bleeding and hemorrhoidal prolapse. Hemorrhoids are common during pregnancy.

Anal fissure is a common cause of painful defecation and the most common cause of rectal bleeding in infants. It frequently results from the passage of hard stool, and symptoms include pain, constipation, and bloody streaking in the stool.

Vaginal or anal foreign body is a common cause of anogenital discomfort or bleeding or vaginal discharge. Toilet tissue is a common foreign body in prepubescent girls. Often foreign bodies are placed in the vagina or rectum by normally inquisitive toddlers and children. A thorough history is important in ruling out child abuse when children have anogenital trauma.

Management

Pruritus ani

Treatments and medications

- Treat the predisposing factor (e.g., pediculosis [lice], parasites [pinworms], hemorrhoids, anal fissure) and remove, or refer for removal, any vaginal or anal foreign bodies.
- Advise the avoidance of tight-fitting clothing.
- Advise the wearing of cotton underpants.
- Advise the patient to cleanse the anal area with cotton moistened with water or plain unscented toilettes after each bowel movement.

Counseling and prevention

- Educate the parents and child on the cause of the symptom and treatment.
- Advise the parents and child that depending on the cause, the itching in the perianal skin usually resolves.
- Advise the parents and child that depending on the cause, the symptom may be persistent and recurrent, but comfort measures can be used.
- Instruct on comfort measures and control strategies, including:
  Avoid laxatives.
  Avoid topical agents.
  Practice good hygiene and good handwashing after toileting.
  Change the infant's diaper frequently and expose the inflamed anal area to room air.

Follow-up. Schedule a return visit if symptoms do not resolve with treatment plan.

Consultations and referrals. Refer to a physician if frequent rectal bleeding occurs; if symptoms persist or worsen; or if other causes are suspected (e.g., diabetes mellitus, liver disease, neoplasms).

Pubic lice

Treatments and medications. See Lice in Chapter 37. Treatments include:

- Pyrethrin (A-200 Pyrinate, Pyrinal, Pronto, RID) shampoo, gel, or liquid, all in combination with piperonyl butoxide. Apply to the hair for 10 minutes and then wash thoroughly. This may be repeated in 7 to 10 days. It is for topical use only, and avoid contact with the face or eyes.
- Gamma benzene hexachloride (Kwell, Lindane, Scabene) shampoo 1%. Leave on the hair 4 to 8 minutes before rinsing, and repeat in 7 days if lice or nits are still present. This is also available in lotion 1% or cream 1%. Apply to the skin, leave on 8 to 12 hours, and then wash off. (These have the highest potential neurotoxic effects.) Do not use for pregnant women, infants, or children under 10 years of age, and avoid contact with the face, urethral meatus, or mucous membranes.
- For eyelash infestation, careful manual removal of lice and nits or by application of petroleum ointment (Vaseline) three or four times a day for 8 to 10 days. Pediculicides should never be used to treat eyelash infestations.

Table 35-19 Differential Diagnosis: Perianal Itch or Pain (698.0)

CRITERIA	ANAL FISSURE	ANAL FOREIGN BODY	HEMORRHOIDS	VAGINAL FOREIGN BODY	PRURITUS ANI	PHTHIRUS PUBIS	PINWORMS
ICD-9 code	565.0	937.	455.6	939.2	698.0	132.2	127.4
Subjective Data							
Associated symptoms	Bloody, streaked stool; rectal pain; rectal bleeding; anal discomfort	Anal discomfort, anogenital bleeding	Rectal pruritus, constipation, straining with defecation, bowel incontinence, rectal bleeding, anal pain	Vaginal odor, vaginal bleeding, chronic vaginal discharge	Anal itching, rectal itching	Anogenital pruritus; multiple bite and scratch marks in the pubic area; "bugs" in pubic hair, around anus, axillae, abdomen, beard, eyebrows, or eyelashes	Perianal itching, perineal itching, nocturnal perianal pruritus, vulvovaginal itching, restlessness, sleeplessness Parents may report seeing tiny white worms crawling on the skin "within perianal region" Dysuria, vulvar itching
Objective Data *Physical examination*							
Inspection of anus, rectum, vagina	Tear in the anal mucosa; anal ulceration	Anorectal fissure, perianal chafing, perianal erythema, anal laceration	Dilated hemorrhoidal veins, dark anal protrusions, hemorrhoidal prolapse, hemorrhoidal thrombosis	Redness of vagina, foul-smelling discharge from vagina, bloody or nonbloody vaginal discharge, friability of vaginal wall	Anal erythema, anal fissures, candidiasis, excoriation, lichenification, tinea	Nits may be seen at the base of the hair shafts (see above); gray-blue macules may be seen in the groin area (purpuric lesions); ova may be seen as white ellipsoids attached to the hair shaft; bite marks on the abdomen, thighs, and genital area; excoriation from scratching; secondary infection in areas of excoriation; ova may be seen attached to the hair shafts on examination	Ova or creamy white, threadlike worms may be seen near the anal orifice; rectal excoriation; inflammation of the vulva; vaginal discharge; eczematous dermatitis of perianal and perineal areas; less commonly, a small white worm may be seen crawling on the skin in the perianal region on examination
Laboratory data	None	None	None	None	Stool for ova and parasites; skin scraping for yeast fungi	Lice or eggs (nits) may be observed on examination and confirmed by magnifying glass or microscope; Wood's lamp examination: Live nits, fluoresce white; empty nits, fluoresce gray	Diagnosis is made by microscopic identification of pinworm ova on transparent tape that has been pressed to the perianal skin. The tape should then be affixed, adhesive side down, to a microscope slide and sanned for the presence of eggs. (A drop of toluene placed between the tape and the slide can assist in making the preparation easier to read during examination under a low-power microscopic lens.)

Counseling and prevention

- Explain the cause of pubic lice infection to the parents and child.
- Reassure the parents and child that the infection is easily treated.
- Discuss the method of transmission from person to person.
- Support and comfort the child who has been sexually abused (see also Chapter 47).
- Teach the name, dose, frequency, administration, purpose, and side effects of medications.
- Explain the necessity to comply with treatment to prevent recurrence.
- Notify sexual contacts to seek treatment.
- Treat sexual contacts simultaneously.
- Advise to avoid close physical contact and sexual intercourse during infestation and treatment.
- Caution on not scratching.

Follow-up. Provide follow-up as needed for recurrence or secondary infection.

Consultations and referrals. Consult a physician for concomitant sexually transmitted disease; pregnant women; and infants and children when child abuse is suspected. Report to the appropriate authorities if sexual abuse is suspected.

Pinworms. See Parasitic Diseases in Chapter 44.

Treatments and medications. It is advisable to treat all members of the household simultaneously (except children under 2 years of age and pregnant women). Possible medications include:

- Pyrantel pamoate (Antiminth), 11 mg/kg (maximum of 1 g) orally as a single dose and repeated in 2 weeks. This is available in oral suspension form at 50 mg/ml. Shake well and give with milk, fruit juice, or food.
- Mebendazole (Vermox), 100 mg orally as a single dose (with the same dose for all body weights for all ages over 2 years) or 100 mg chewable tablet (which must be chewed thoroughly). Treatment is repeated in 2 weeks.
- Piperazine citrate (Vermizine), 65 mg/kg (maximum of 2.5 g/day) for 7 days, taken in the morning on an empty stomach. Treatment may be repeated in 2 weeks if necessary. This drug is contraindicated in cases of epilepsy.

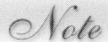

In children under 2 years of age, experience with pyrantel pamoate and mebendazole is limited; therefore the risks and benefits of this drug should be evaluated before administration. Consult a physician.

Counseling and prevention

- Explain the cause of pinworm infection to the parents and the child. Reassure the parents and child that the infection is common and that pinworm infestation is easily treated. Explain that the infection is not the result of an unclean home.
- Teach the name, dose frequency, administration, purpose, and side effects of medications.
- Explain that pinworm infection frequently recurs, particularly in large families.
- Stress personal hygiene to avoid autoinfection: frequent handwashing and handwashing after toileting and before eating.

- Advise parents that the child's fingernails should be trimmed and kept short and clean.
- Stress the need to avoid scratching the affected area. Recommend a daily bath or shower. Caution not to scratch the anus or put fingers near the mouth or nose.
- Instruct parents on how to collect a specimen: To collect the eggs, the adhesive side of transparent tape is pressed against the anus at bedtime or in the early morning. The specimen should be taken before the child gets out of bed, before washing, and before defecation.

Follow-up. Follow-up is not generally indicated. Schedule a return visit in 3 weeks if the patient is symptomatic or if symptoms recur.

Consultations and referrals. Consult a physician for pregnant women and children under 2 years of age.

Hemorrhoids

Treatments and medications. Sitz baths may help relieve discomfort. Cleanse the affected area with plain soap and water, and rinse thoroughly. Gently dry the affected area by patting or blotting with plain, soft toilet tissue or a soft cotton or terry cloth. For constipation, hard stool, or softening of stool, recommend oral docusate sodium (Colace), with a dosage based on age:

- *Less than 3 years of age*—10 to 40 mg/day divided into one to four doses
- *3 to 6 years of age*—20 to 60 mg/day divided into one to four doses
- *6 to 12 years of age*—40 to120 mg/day divided into one to four doses
- *Greater than 12 years of age*—50 to 240 mg every 24 hours divided into one to four doses

The liquid, but not syrup form, may be diluted in juice if the taste is unpleasant. Fiber supplements may also be recommended, and hydrocortisone ointment may be used. With this condition, taking a rectal temperature is contraindicated.

Counseling and prevention

- Teach dietary strategies to avoid constipation (see Constipation and Fecal Impaction) (e.g., high-fiber diet, increased fluids).
- Discuss the use of stool softeners.
- Recommend avoidance of prolonged sitting and straining during defecation.
- Encourage exercise.

Follow-up. Schedule follow-up care as needed.

Consultations and referrals. Refer to a physician for thrombosis, secondary infection, ulceration, or prolapsed rectum.

Anal fissure. See also Constipation and Fecal Impaction.

Treatments and medications. A sitz bath may offer temporary relief. Cleanse the affected area frequently with plain soap and water, and rinse thoroughly. Gently dry the affected area by patting or blotting with dry cotton; plain, soft toilet tissue; or a soft cotton or terry cloth. Expose the anal area to room air. Stool softeners (see Hemorrhoids) and fiber supplements may also be used. Taking a rectal temperature is contraindicated.

Counseling and prevention

- Teach dietary strategies to avoid constipation; increase fiber in the diet; and increase fluids.
- Discuss the use of stool softeners.
- Instruct to avoid straining during defecation.

Follow-up. Schedule follow-up as needed for well-child care.

Consultations and referrals. Refer to a physician if there is an increase in the size of the fissure; if severe pain exists, despite conservative measures; or if there are chronic fissures and skin tags.

Vaginal or anal foreign body

Treatments and medications. Treatment is determined by whether the foreign object can be visualized and whether the consistency of the object is sharp or solid. Irrigate the vagina with sterile water through a soft feeding tube to dislodge a visible foreign body. Observe passed stool and examine it for the presence of any noted foreign body.

Counseling and prevention. Stress the importance of not placing foreign objects or toilet tissue into the vagina or rectum.

Follow-up. Schedule follow-up care as needed, and for well-child care.

Consultations and referrals. Refer to physician for trauma to the hymenal membranes suggestive of the passage of a foreign object through the vaginal orifice; trauma, lacerations, or anal tears into the perineum suggestive of the passage of a foreign object into the rectum; or when anesthesia is required for comprehensive examination, instrumentation, and surgical removal of a foreign object and surgical repair of the perineum.

Stool Odor, Color, and Consistency Changes

JANE A. FOX

Alert

Consult with or refer to a physician for the following:
- Stool changes associated with weight loss
- Any newborn who does not pass meconium or plug within 48 hours of birth
- Abdominal pain with stool increased or decreased frequency, odor, or consistency changes
- Recurrent blood in stool
- Any signs of physical abuse
- Suspicion of intestinal obstruction

Etiology

The cause of changes in stool odor, color, and consistency can be divided into normal and abnormal variations. Normal variations take into account the age of the child, stage of growth and development, diet, medications, and stress or anxiety. Stool changes occur from birth until 2 years of age as a result of the maturation of the digestive system. Changes in stool patterns and consistency may be noted in adolescence as a result of dietary changes and rapid growth in the digestive system. Alteration in bowel function can have a multifactorial origin, including genetic, environmental, infectious, and immunologic causes.

Incidence

- The presentation of altered bowel habits may be transient, insidious, acute, or chronic.
- Incidence depends on the age, symptoms, and diagnosis.

Risk Factors

- Diet, including excessive intake (e.g., of fruit, juice), decreased intake (e.g., of fluids, fiber), and any changes
- Family history of altered bowel function or diseases
- Psychologic stressors
- Infections

- Drugs, especially antibiotics
- Cystic fibrosis
- Malabsorption syndrome
- IBD

Differential Diagnosis

Normal variations

Color and consistency. Normal variations of stool color and consistency depend on the age and diet of a child. What may be normal for one child may not be for another (this is especially true in early infancy). The history should include the child's normal stooling pattern, typical consistency, color, and odor (Table 35-20).

Frequency. In newborns, the number of daily stools varies with the number and type of feedings. More than 10 stools in any 24-hour period may be considered abnormal for some newborns but can be normal for others. In the first month of life the average frequency of stools becomes established. Breastfed infant tends to have more stools than formula-fed infants. A breastfed infant's stooling pattern may vary from one with every feeding to one every 3 days. The average can be one or two stools a day but can decrease to one every 2 or 3 days for some infants and can increase for others. Alterations in frequency of stooling in any child can be attributable to stress, diet, medications, or neurologic deficits.

Abnormal variations. Abnormal variations in stool may be caused by systemic disease, an inflammatory process in the bowel, or altered absorption. Differential diagnosis includes IBD, malabsorption syndrome, GI tract hemorrhage, infection, and constipation.

Table 35-21 describes abnormal variations in the stool and possible diagnoses. Box 35-7 lists various diagnoses according

Table 35-20 Normal Variations: Consistency and Color Changes by Age

AGE	DESCRIPTION OF STOOL
Newborn, days 1 to 4	Meconium: A thick, black-green, tarry, odorless stool; first stool should occur within 24 to 48 hours after birth
1 to 2 weeks	Transitional: Dark green, seedy, continues changing color towards yellow
2 weeks to 4 months	Dependent on the type of protein or formula ingested
	Breastfed: Light or bright yellow, loose, seedy to pasty
	Milk-based formula: Yellow to brown, becoming firm and formed
	Soy-based formula: Green, soft, distinctive odor
	Protein hydrolysate formula: Yellowish green, soft to loose with some mucus
4 to 6 months	Color and consistency influenced by the introduction of solid foods; presence of undigested foods may be seen in the stool
2 years and older	Changes evident as a result of the increasing variety of foods in the diet; in addition, food coloring found in gelatin, colored drinks, dark chocolate, beets, spinach, or blueberries may color the stool; the child begins to have some bodily control over defecation

Table 35-21 Abnormal Variations: Odor, Consistency, and Color Changes

ABNORMAL VARIATIONS	POSSIBLE INDICATION
Abnormal Odor	
Foul-smelling	Infection: Bacterial (*Salmonella, Shigella* species)
	Parasitic: *Giardia lamblia*
	Viral: Rotavirus
Yeast or acid smell	Carbohydrate malabsorption
Abnormal Consistency	
Watery, increased number	Diarrhea
Frothy, mucus	Cystic fibrosis
Hard, pellet-sized	Constipation
Mucus, oily, bulky	Malabsorption
Profuse, watery	Bacterial infection
Purulent	Colitis, IBD
Ribbonlike	Hirschsprung's disease
Steatorrhea	Liver disease, pancreatic insufficiency, Crohn's disease, cystic fibrosis, short-bowel disease, malabsorption syndromes, celiac disease
Water ring around stool	Malabsorption, lactose intolerance
Abnormal Color	
Blood in stool	See Tables 37-21 and Box 37-12 for possible diagnoses
Blood clots	Colitis, milk or soy allergy
Bloody diarrhea or rectal bleeding	Hemolytic-uremic syndrome (systemic disease); grossly bloody stools rare in viral enteritis but are common in bacterial enteritis; in newborns this also includes rotavirus
Blood streaking in formed stool (can occur intermittently)	Anal fissure (younger than 5 years of age)
Claylike or pale	Biliary atresia, bile acid insufficiency
"Currant jelly"	Intussusception
Green-black	Iron supplementation, blood or bismuth (Pepto-Bismol)
Hematochezia (passage of red blood through the rectum)	Colon or rectal bleeding; inflammatory bowel disease
Melena (dark, tarry stool)	Bleeding in the upper GI tract or small intestine; may indicate peptic ulcer or small-bowel disease
Occult blood	GI tract lesions; may cause anemia

Box 35-7 Differential Diagnosis: Gastrointestinal Tract Bleeding or Blood in Stool (578.9)

Newborn

Vitamin K deficiency
Anal fissure
Necrotizing enterocolitis
Milk allergy
Aspiration of maternal blood
Intestinal infection
Bacterial enteritis
Intussusception
Hemorrhagic disease of the newborn
Intestinal or liver trauma

Infant and Young Child

Intussusception
Anal fissure
Gastritis or peptic ulcer
Bacterial enteritis
Meckel's diverticulum
Intestinal polyps

Swallowed epistaxis
Esophagitis
Foreign body
Sexual abuse

Adolescent

Peptic ulcer
Intestinal polyps
Bacterial enteritis
Irritable bowel syndrome
Henoch-Schönlein disease or purpura
Hemolytic-uremic syndrome
IBD
Esophagitis
Sexual abuse
Mallory-Weiss syndrome
Anal fissure
Hemorrhoid

to age that must be considered when there is blood in the stool. The following conditions may cause a change in stool color, odor, and consistency.

Celiac disease is the inability of the small intestine to absorb gluten from wheat, oats, barley, or rye (Tables 35-22 and 35-23).

Constipation is a bowel dysfunction of infrequency, reduced water consistency, or difficulty in passing stool. Parents may consider the normal passage of stool in the infant or child as constipation because of observing changes of facial expression (like turning red), pulling up of the legs into the abdomen, or a change in frequency even though the stool is of a soft consistency (see Constipation and Fecal Impaction).

Diarrhea is a sudden increase in frequency of stools within a specific time or number of hours. The stool has a reduction in the regular consistency with an increase in water content (see Diarrhea and Loose Stool).

GI tract bleeding can occur in the upper GI tract, intestine, or rectum. Depending on the presentation, age of child, and disease, the signs and symptoms vary. For possible differential diagnoses, see Box 35-7.

Hirschsprung's disease is the congenital absence of the intramural ganglion cells, which results in functional obstruction of the colon. This disease should be suspected in any infant less than 1 month of age with failure to pass stool and who has progressive abdominal distension. This diagnosis should be considered in older children (1 to 6 months of age) with chronic constipation, abdominal distension, and FTT.

IBD occurs between 10 and 30 years of age. Ulcerative colitis and Crohn's disease (regional enteritis) are IBDs that cause abdominal pain and diarrhea. The cause of IBD is unknown, but it is considered an autoimmune disease involving the intestinal immune system (see Table 35-22 and Diarrhea and Loose Stool).

Intussusception is the telescoping of the intestines. The onset is usually at 3 to 18 months of age. It can occur in older children, with the underlying disease being intestinal polyp or Meckel's diverticulum. The presentation is intermittent, colicky abdominal pain lasting only 2 to 3 minutes at a time and stool containing blood and mucus, followed by vomiting and abdominal distension.

Irritable bowel syndrome usually occurs during adolescence and becomes evident with alternating diarrhea and constipation and abdominal pain. Stools may contain mucus, and pain

Table 35-22 Chronic Diarrhea

CRITERIA	IRRITABLE BOWEL	CROHN'S DISEASE	ULCERATIVE COLITIS
ICD-9 code	564.1	555.9	556.9
Age at onset	Adolescence; insidious	10 to 16 years; more common; insidious	Adolescence to 20 years; less common; insidious
Symptoms depend on location and bowel involvement	Alternating diarrhea with constipation, flatulence, and lower abdominal pain; in addition, functional dyspepsia, postprandial abdominal pain	Diarrhea, weight loss, abdominal pain, periumbilical cramping, anorexia, delayed sexual maturation, increased urgency to defecate, fever (50%), perianal disease (e.g., fistulas)	Early: Diarrhea, later with hematochezia; late: Systemic disease, growth delay, anorexia, GI distress, fever, abdominal tenderness, abdominal cramping, arthritis

Table 35-23 Malabsorption Syndromes

CRITERIA	COW'S MILK INTOLERANCE	GLUCOSE, GALACTOSE	DISACCHARIDE LACTOSE, SUCROSE	BILE ACID PANCREATIC INSUFFICIENCY	CELIAC DISEASE
ICD-9 code	271.3	271.3	271.8	577.8	579.0
Age at onset	3 to 6 months of age; acute or insidious	Congenital, rare, neonatal onset (acute) by day 4 of life	Congenital or secondary, any age	Depends on pancreatic function and deficiency	Usually before 2 years of age; can occur at 1 to 5 years of age
Symptoms	FTT, abdominal pain, vomiting, irritability, eczema, respiratory symptoms	Dehydration, vomiting, abdominal distention	Abdominal cramping, bloating and flatulence, malnutrition in infancy and dehydration	Abdominal distention, vomiting; in addition, cystic fibrosis present with FTT, meconium ileus, and pulmonary disease	Irritable, anorexia but occasionally an increase in appetite, abdominal distention and pain
Stool characteristics	Diarrhea, colitis or occult blood, possible allergy	Profuse, watery diarrhea; profuse, acid odor	Watery diarrhea with a ring around stool, acid odor, reducing substance positive	Infancy: Persistent diarrhea; older child: Bulky, foul smell, steatorrhea	Diarrhea (Acute or insidious, pale, loose, bulky)

is usually relieved with defecation (see Table 35-22 and Diarrhea and Loose Stool).

Malabsorption syndrome is the inability to absorb or digest nutrients, lipids, carbohydrates, or protein. There is no specific onset, and the syndrome depends on the type of malabsorption. The most common types are disaccharide deficiency and lactose intolerance (see Tables 35-22 and 35-23).

Meckel's diverticulum is bleeding that occurs when acid is secreted by ectopic gastric mucosa in the diverticulum, causing ulceration of the adjacent intestinal mucosa. It becomes evident suddenly before 2 years of age with painless rectal bleeding (with or without stool) and crampy abdominal pain.

Management

Normal variations

Treatment and medications. None are needed.

Counseling and prevention

- Review with parents the age-appropriate feeding of the infant or child.
- Educate on the normal bowel function of an infant, child, or adolescent, including stooling pattern and frequency.
- Evaluate diet and educate parents that certain foods affect bowel function and consistency. Stress the need to maintain regularity.

Follow-up. Schedule age-appropriate well-child care visits.

Consultations and referrals. Usually none is needed.

Gastrointestinal tract bleeding

Treatments and medications. Initially confirm occult blood in the stool and assess for possible blood loss or need for surgical intervention. If further investigation is required, consult with or refer to a physician. Treatment varies based on the diagnosis and severity (see Box 35-7). After diagnosis, consult a physician for ongoing therapy.

Counseling and prevention. Educate the parents and child on diagnosis and plan of treatment, including any medications and side effects.

Follow-up. Follow-up care is based on the diagnosis and treatment plan.

Consultations and referrals. Provide immediate referral to a physician or pediatric gastroenterologist for recurrent bleeding, abdominal pain, or suspicion of intestinal obstruction, or if surgical intervention is required. Any volume loss requires immediate investigation and direct hospital admission.

Inflammatory bowel disease. See Diarrhea in this chapter. Differentiation of Crohn's disease from ulcerative colitis may not be possible because of the area of colon involvement and inflammation (see Table 35-23).

Treatments and medications. Treatment is dependent on the exacerbation, remission, and severity of disease. Mild disease responds to medication, usually within 2 weeks. Moderate and severe disease with systemic involvement requires hospitalization and possible surgical intervention. Treatment includes:

- Bed rest
- Low-residue diet
- Correction of nutritional deficits
- A goal of controlling symptoms
- Medications (with physician consultation), including prednisone 1 to 2 mg/kg per day for 2 weeks, then tapered; sulfasalazine 50 to 75 mg/kg per day, introduced gradually and increased as tolerated until full dose is achieved. The maximum dosage is 3 to 4 g per day.

Counseling and prevention

- Remember that child and parent participation is required in management.

- Educate the parents and child that this is a lifelong disease having periods of exacerbation and remission.
- Help the parents and child learn what exacerbates illness and how to control stress.
- Educate on the use of medications and possible side effects.
- Provide nutritional counseling for optimal nutrition and to allow for catch-up growth.
- Offer counseling for psychologic adjustments to disease.
- Work toward the child's participation and willingness to become active in management.

Follow-up. Follow-up treatment depends on any exacerbation or remission. Schedule a return visit at least every 6 months.

Consultations and referrals. Refer to a physician or gastroenterologist for the initial diagnosis, evaluation, and treatment plan for recurrent bleeding, abdominal pain, or suspicion of intestinal obstruction. Any volume loss requires immediate investigation and direct hospital admission.

Irritable bowel syndrome. See also Diarrhea in this chapter.

Treatments and medications

- High-fiber, low-fat diet
- Psyllium preparations to add fiber
- Avoidance of carbonated drinks, chewing gum, artificial sweeteners with sorbitol, and legumes
- Medications (with physician consultation), including antispasmodics, anticholinergics, and simethicone

Counseling and prevention

- Advise the parents and child to anticipate stress and causes of exacerbation of symptoms.
- Instruct on stress reduction.
- Educate the parents and child that this is a lifelong disease having periods of exacerbation and remission.
- Instruct on the use of medications and possible side effects.
- Provide nutritional counseling for optimal nutrition and to allow for catch-up growth.
- Offer counseling for psychologic adjustments to disease.
- Work toward the child's participation and willingness to become active in management.

Follow-up. Follow-up treatment depends on exacerbation. Schedule a return visit at least every 6 months.

Consultations and referrals. Refer to a physician or gastroenterologist for the initial diagnosis, evaluation, and course of treatment (which initially may be for IBD). Provide immediate referral to a physician for recurrent bleeding, abdominal pain, or suspicion of intestinal obstruction.

Malabsorption syndrome

Treatments and medications

- A treatment plan individualized to the degree and type of malabsorption
- Performance of a challenge test by removal of the suspected deficiency from the diet and then reintroduction to see whether symptoms return
- A diet specific to the malabsorption identified (see Table 35-23)
- For an infant, a change of formula to an elemental formula (e.g., Alimentum, Nutramigen, Pregestimil)
- For a child or adolescent, avoidance of any food that exacerbates the symptoms
- Encouragement of parents or child to keep a food diary, including the introduction or elimination of milk, formula, protein, wheat, lactose, sucrose, or any food that correlates with the onset of symptoms

Counseling and prevention

- Provide nutritional and dietary counseling for the parents and child.

- Help parents and child understand the malabsorption or deficiency and what to expect if there is a primary or secondary intolerance.
- Instruct on the need to adhere to dietary restrictions.

Follow-up. Schedule a return visit after a challenge test and provide frequent follow-up as required for assessment of growth and nutritional status

Consultations and referrals. Refer to a physician or pediatric gastroenterologist for the following:

- Any alteration in growth
- Chronic diarrhea lasting more than 14 days
- Suspicion of cystic fibrosis

Resources

Websites

@Gastroenterology (atgastroenterology.com)

Gastrohep (www.gastrohep.com)

Healthlink USA Gastroenterology Links (healthlinkusa.com/gastroenterology.htm)

The Hernia Organization (www.hernia.org)

Johns Hopkins University (www.med.jhu.edu)

Keep Kids Healthy (www.keepkidshealthy.com or kidshealth.org)

Medscape Gastroenterology (gastroenterology.medscape.com)

National Library of Medicine (www.nlm.nih.gov/medlineplus/)

Pediatric Database (PEDBASE) (www.icondata.com/health/pedbase/files/hydrocel.htm)

University of Chicago Children's Hospital and Department of Pediatrics (www.ucch.org/sections/urology/inforesource/hernia-hydro.html)

Atlas containing multiple graphics of a variety of mouth and oral lesions (www.uiowa.edu/-oprm/AtlasMAC/)

Bibliography

American Academy of Pediatrics (2000). Group A streptococcal infections. In Pickering, L.K. (Ed.). *Red book 2000: Report of the Committee on Infectious Diseases* (25th ed.). Elk Grove Village, IL: American Academy of Pediatrics.

American Academy of Pediatrics (2000). *Helicobacter pylori* infections. In Pickering, L.K. (Ed.). *Red book 2000: Report of the Committee on Infectious Diseases* (25th ed.). Elk Grove Village, IL: American Academy of Pediatrics.

American Academy of Pediatrics (1994). Workgroup on cow's milk protein and diabetes mellitus: Infant feeding practices and their relationship to the etiology of diabetes mellitus. *Pediatrics 94,* 752-753.

Ashcraft, K.W. & Holder, T.M. (2000). *Pediatric surgery* (3rd ed.). Philadelphia: W.B. Saunders.

Balon, A.J. (1997). Management of infantile colic. *American Family Physician, 55,* 235-244.

Barr, R.G. (1998). Management of clinical problems and emotional care: Colic and crying syndromes in infants. *Pediatrics, 102,* 1282-1286.

Bergeson, P.S. (1993). Herbal teas for infant colic (letter). *Journal of Pediatrics, 123,* 670.

Berquist, W.E. (1998). New, improved *Helicobacter pylori* eradication therapy in children. *Journal of Pediatric Gastroenterology and Nutrition, 45*(4), 729-772.

Brazelton, T.B. (1969). *Infants and mothers.* New York: Dell.

Brazelton, T.B. (1962). Crying in infancy. *Pediatrics, 29,* 579-588.

Carey, W.B. (1984). Colic: Primary excessive crying as an infant and environment interaction. *Pediatric Clinics of North America, 31,* 993-1005.

Carey, W.B. (1972). Clinical application of infant temperament measurements. *Journal of Pediatrics, 81,* 823-828.

Cervisi, J., Chapman, M., Nicklos, B., et al. (1991). Office management of the infant with colic. *Journal of Pediatric Health Care, 5,* 184-190.

Cherry, J.D. (1998). Herpangina; pharyngitis (pharyngitis, tonsillitis, tonsillopharyngitis and nasopharyngitis). In Feigin, R.D. & Cherry, J.D. (Eds.). *Textbook of pediatric infectious diseases* (4th ed.). Philadelphia: W.B. Saunders.

Cox, J.A., & Ziegler, M.M. (1997). Lumps and bumps. In Schwartz, M.W., Curry, A.T., Sargent, J.A., Blum, N.J., & Fein, J.A. (Eds.). *Pediatric primary care: A problem oriented approach* (3rd ed.). St. Louis: Mosby.

Darmstadt, G.L. (2000). Vesiculobullous disorders: Disorders of the mucous membranes. In Behrman, R.E., Kliegman, R.M., & Jenson, H.B. (Eds.). *Nelson textbook of pediatrics* (16th ed.). Philadelphia: W.B. Saunders.

Dihigo, S.K. (1998). New strategies for the treatment of colic: Modifying the parent/infant interaction. *Journal of Pediatric Health Care, 12,* 256-262.

Doody, D.P. & Ryan, D.P. (1999). Genital pain. In Dershowitz, R.A. (Ed.). *Ambulatory pediatric care* (3rd ed.). Philadelphia: Lippincott-Raven.

Foglia, R.P. (1999). Groin hernia and hydroceles. In Dershowitz, R.A. *Ambulatory pediatric care* (3rd ed.). Philadelphia: Lippincott-Raven.

García, V.F. (2000). Umbilical and other abdominal wall hernias. In Ashcraft, K.W. & Holder, T.M. (2000). *Pediatric surgery* (3rd ed.). Philadelphia: W.B. Saunders

Garrison, M.M. & Christakis, D.A. (2000). Early childhood: Colic, child development, and poisoning prevention. *Pediatrics, 106,* 184-190.

Gill, F.T. (1998). Umbilical hernia, inguinal hernias and hydroceles in children: Diagnostic clues for optional patient management. *Journal of Pediatric Health Care, 12,* 231-235.

Goepp, J.G. (2000). Stomatitis. In Hoekelmann, R.A., Adam, H.A., Nelson, N.M., Weitzman, M.L., & Hoover Wilson, M. (Eds.). *Pediatric primary care* (4th ed.). St. Louis: Mosby.

Hill, D.J. & Hosking, C.S. (2000). Infantile colic and food hypersensitivity. *Journal of Pediatric Gastroenterology and Nutrition, 30,* S67-S76.

Hofman, A.D. & Greydanus, D.E. (1997). *Adolescent medicine* (3rd ed.). East Norwalk, CT: Appleton & Lange.

Irish, M.S., Pearl, R.H., Caty, M.G., & Glick, P.L. (1998). The approach to common abdominal diagnoses in infants and children. *Pediatric Clinics of North America, 45*(4), 729-772.

Keefe, M.R. (1988). Irritable infant syndrome: Theoretical perspectives and practice implications. *Advances in Nursing Science, 10,* 70-78.

Keefe, M.R. & Froese-Fretz, A. (1991). Living with an irritable infant: Maternal perspectives. *Maternal Child Nursing, 16,* 255-259.

Keefe, M.R., Froese-Fretz, A., & Kotzer, A.M. (1998). Newborn predictors of infant irritability. *Journal of Obstetric, Gynecologic, and Neonatal Nursing, 27,* 513-520.

Keefe, M.R., Froese-Fretz, A., & Kotzer, A.M. (1997). The REST regimen: An individualized nursing intervention for infant irritability. *Maternal Child Nursing, 22,* 16-20.

Keefe, M.R., Kotzer, A.M., Froese-Fretz, A., et al. (1996). A longitudinal comparison of irritable and nonirritable infants. *Nursing Research, 45,* 4-9.

Kohl, S. (1999). Postnatal herpes simplex virus. In McMillan, J., DeAngelis, C.D., Feigin, R.D., & Warshaw, J.B. (Eds.). *Oski's pediatric principles and practice* (3rd ed.). Philadelphia: Lippincott, Williams & Wilkins.

Long, S.S. (1999). Herpangina. In McMillan, J., DeAngelis, C.D., Feigin, R.D., & Warshaw, J.B. (Eds.). *Oski's pediatric principles and practice* (3rd ed.). Philadelphia: J.B. Lippincott; Williams & Wilkins.

Mahle, W.T. (1998). A dangerous case of colic: Anomalous left coronary artery presenting with paroxysms of irritability. *Pediatric Emergency Care, 14,* 24-27.

Muscari, M.E. & Milks, C.J. (1995). Assessing acute abdominal pain in adolescent females. *Pediatric Nursing, 21*(3), 215-220.

Noseworthy, J. (2000). Testicular torsion. In Ashcraft, K.W. & Holder, T.M. (Eds.). *Pediatric surgery* (3rd ed.). Philadelphia: W.B. Saunders.

Pietzak, M.M. & Thomas, D.W. (2000). Pancreatitis in childhood. *Pediatrics in Review, 21*(12), 406-412.

Plachter, N.B., Schulman, S.L., & Canning, D.A. (1999). Identification and management of urinary tract infections in the preschool child. *Journal of Pediatric Health Care, 13*(6), 268-272.

Pletcher, J.R. & Slap, G.B. (1998). Pelvic inflammatory disease. *Pediatrics in Review, 19,* 361-365.

Reijneveld, S.A., Brugman, E., & Hirasing, R.A. (2000). Infantile colic: Maternal smoking as potential risk factor. *Archives of Disease in Childhood, 83,* 302-303.

Steele, R.W. (1999). The epidemiology and clinical presentation of urinary tract infections in children two years of age through adolescence. *Pediatric Annals, 28*(10), 653-658.

Treem, W.R. (1994). Infant colic: A gastroenterologist's perspective. *Pediatric Clinics of North America, 41,* 1121-1138.

Weber, T.R. & Tracey, T. F. (2000). Groin hernias and hydroceles. In Ashcraft, K.W. & Holder, T.M. (Eds.). *Pediatric surgery* (3rd ed.). Philadelphia: W.B. Saunders.

Weizman, Z., Alkrinawa, S., Goldfarb, D., et al. (1993). Efficacy of herbal tea preparation in infantile colic. *Journal of Pediatrics, 122,* 650-652.

Wolke, D., Gray, P., & Meyer, R. (1994). Excessive infant crying: A controlled study of mothers helping mothers. *Pediatrics, 94,* 322-332.

World Health Organization (1993). *The management and prevention of diarrhea: Practical guidelines* (3rd ed.). Geneva: World Health Organization.

Chapter 36 *Hematologic System*

Anemia, p. 471
Jaundice in the Newborn, p. 480
Pallor, p. 483
Petechiae and Purpura, p. 486

Risk Factors*

- Two conditions put patients at risk for anemia:
  1. A decrease in the production of red blood cells (RBCs) from a deficiency of an essential nutrient (e.g., iron, vitamin B_{12}, or folic acid) or from a metabolic abnormality related to a structural problem in the bone marrow or an inherited defect in production
  2. The accelerated destruction or loss of RBCs, the condition being either acquired (e.g., acute or chronic blood loss) or inherited (e.g., sickle cell disease, thalassemia)
- A diet poor in iron sources (e.g., meat, iron-fortified cereals, formulas)
- Early or excessive use of cow's milk instead of iron-fortified formula or breast milk
- Prematurity or low birth weight (LBW)
- Low socioeconomic status
- Recent oxidant exposure
- Genetic history of thalassemia, sickle cell disease, or hemolytic disease
- Maternal-infant rhesus factor (Rh) incompatibility (e.g., mother Rh negative, infant Rh positive)
- Maternal-infant ABO blood type incompatibility (e.g., mother's blood type O, infant's blood type A or B)
- Exposure to viral infection or upper respiratory tract infection

Health Promotion

Promotion of Optimal Nutrition

- Promote breastfeeding (iron from human milk is more readily absorbed than iron in infant formulas) for the first 5 or 6 months of life or longer.
- For breastfed infants who need supplemental formula, recommend only iron-fortified formula.
- For breastfed infants who do not receive supplementary iron-rich foods (iron-fortified cereal by 6 months of life), recommend 1 mg/kg per day of iron drops.
- For breastfed infants who were preterm or had LBW, recommend 2 to 4 mg/kg per day of iron drops (maximum of 15 mg/day) starting at 1 month of age and continuing through the first birthday.
- For bottle-fed infants, use only iron-fortified formulas (12 mg of iron per liter) in the first year of life. Discourage cow's milk, goat's milk, and soybean milk. Constipation is not a documented side effect of iron-fortified formulas.
- Promote only iron-fortified cereals in the first 2 years of life.

- Recommend iron-fortified cereal among the first foods introduced, as early as 4 months of age if developmentally appropriate (i.e., no tongue-extrusion reflex). Two servings of iron-rich infant cereal per day meet an infant's iron requirement.
- By 6 months of age, encourage one feeding per day of foods rich in vitamin C (e.g., fruits, vegetables, juice) with the iron-rich food to improve absorption of iron.
- Suggest introducing plain, pureed meats after 6 months of age.
- Because of the risk of occult GI bleeding, avoid cow's milk until at least 12 months of life (cow's milk formula does not cause bleeding because of a modification of the protein in processing). After 12 months of age, promote whole milk up to 24 ounces per day. From 2 to 5 years of age, promote low-fat milk 24 ounces per day.
- Monitor all infants' nutritional status and hydration.

Routine Health Screening

- Childhood anemia screening recommendations from the Centers for Disease Control and Prevention (Box 36-1).
- Routine newborn screening for rare inborn errors of metabolism (e.g., glucose-6-phosphate dehydrogenase deficiency [G6PD], hypothyroidism, galactosemia, hemoglobinopathies like sickle cell disease and thalassemia). Newborn screening panel varies by state in the United States. Most states directly refer positive disease cases to regional pediatric treatment centers for follow-up study.
- Screening of all pregnant women for:
  Risk factors for infection (toxoplasmosis, rubella, cytomegalovirus [CMV], herpes simplex [TORCH]).
  Risk factors for hemoglobinopathies (e.g., lifetime history of anemia, persons of African, Mediterranean, Hispanic, or Asian descent).

Prevention of Rh Disease

- Check blood type and Rh factor in all mothers and newborns.
- Direct Coombs' test on all infants at risk for incompatibility.
- Administer human anti-D immunoglobulin (RhoGAM or Winrho) within 72 hours of abortion, amniocentesis, or delivery of Rh-positive infant. This is given in pregnancy to all Rh-negative, unsensitized women.
- Observe all newborns for icterus.

Subjective Data

- Demographics, including age, sex, race, and ethnic and geographic origins
- Reason for visit and description of problem, including parental concerns
- Onset of symptoms and surrounding circumstances
- Recent trauma (e.g., fractures, burns)

*Chapter overview written by Jacqueline G. Ioli.

Box 36-1 Childhood Anemia Screening

Screen using an in-office hemoglobin test or hematocrit. Alternatively, send a CBC count.

Infants and Preschoolers

Screen for risk factors of IDA between 9 to12 months of age, 6 months later, and annually from 2 to 5 years of age. Screen before 6 months of age if a child was preterm, had a LBW, or received low-iron formula over 2 months. Risk factors include:

- Low-income families, Women, Infants, and Children (WIC)-eligible children, and recently arrived refugee children
- Infants under 1 year of age on low-iron formulas for over 2 months or who have had cow's milk before 12 months of age
- Breastfed infants who do not consume a diet adequate in iron after 6 months of age (i.e., who receive insufficient iron from supplementary food)
- Toddlers who consume greater than 24 oz of cow's milk daily
- Children with special health care needs

If there are no high risk factors for IDA, screen at 9 to 12 months of age and 6 months later (at 15 to 18 months of age, when children are eating table food and off iron-fortified formula). Through a history at every visit, assess for dietary and other risk factors for anemia.

School-Age Children and Adolescent Males

Screen for history of IDA, low iron intake, and special health care needs.*

Adolescent Females

Screen for dietary risk factors for IDA (e.g., non–meat eaters, various fad diets, excessive milk intake, low vitamin C intake), heavy menses or other blood loss, history of IDA, and special health care needs.*

Screen every 5 to10 years if there are no risk factors. Screen yearly if there are risk factors.

Modified from Centers for Disease Control and Prevention. (1998). Morbidity and Mortality Weekly Report 47(RR-3), 1-36.
Children with special health care needs may have chronic illness, restricted diet, or blood loss, or may use of a medication that interferes with iron absorption.

- Recent infection, including human parvovirus B19–induced illness (also called *fifth disease*, or *erythema infectiosum*); Epstein-Barr virus (EBV); CMV; upper respiratory tract infection or other nonspecific viral infection; hepatitis A, B, or C virus; or human immunodeficiency virus (HIV)
- Associated signs and symptoms, including fatigue, inactivity, malaise, pain, irritability, changes in behavior or alertness, headache, dizziness, peripheral neuropathy (affecting legs more than arms), spastic weakness, ataxia, scleral jaundice, visual changes (diplopia, blurring, spots, cataracts), vertigo, tinnitus, chest pain, acute bleeding from urinary tract or lungs, epistaxis, bleeding of gums, hematuria, menstrual irregularities, occult bleeding (black, tarry stools; guaiac positive), gastrointestinal (GI) tract symptoms (e.g., indigestion, bloating, anorexia, vomiting, diarrhea), and endocrine symptoms (e.g., temperature intolerance, polyuria, polydipsia, polyphagia)
- Past health history, including hospitalizations; surgeries; chemotherapy or radiation therapy; chronic disease (inflammatory or malignant disease); transfusions; disease of the kidneys, liver, or thyroid; gallstones; or immunosuppression
- Immunization history
- Family health history, including any family history of genetic disorders, hemoglobinopathies, or anemia; death of any siblings; any family member's recent illness (e.g., jaundice, anemia, splenomegaly, or gallstones, especially before 30 years of age); and any history of gallbladder disease, enlarged spleen, bleeding, or platelet disorders
- Prenatal history, including maternal and paternal blood types and Rh status, delivery complications (e.g., uterine trauma, placental abruption, perinatal blood loss), maternal infections, previous pregnancies and outcomes, and maternal dietary habits, especially strict vegetarian (vegans) diet, macrobiotic diet, or maternal history of malabsorption
- Neonatal history, including prematurity, birth weight, Apgar scores, neonatal problems or congenital anomalies, perinatal infection, trauma or bruising, and neonatal jaundice
- Developmental history, including milestones and ages achieved and physical development
- Current medications, including prescription (e.g., oral contraceptives), nonprescription (e.g., vitamins or supplements or herbal remedies, antipyretics), and illicit drugs
- Allergies (e.g., to medications, foods, other substances)
- Social history, including economic factors
- Lead or chemical exposure
- Alcohol consumption
- Feeding history, including diet recall (24-hour recall or typical-day recall); identification of sources of iron, supplements, vitamins, and milk (e.g., breast, formula, powdered, cow, goat); availability of meat; and notation of any feeding difficulty or decreased appetite, anorexia, pica (including any nonfood substance such as dirt, clay, paper, paint chips, and ice), or food fads
- Elimination history, including pattern, color, and consistency

Objective Data

Physical Examination

A thorough physical examination is necessary for all infants and children with hematologic symptoms. It should include:

- *Measurements*—Vital signs, height and weight, rate of growth (with plotting on appropriate growth charts)
- *Skin*—Inspection for pallor, pinkness of nail beds, conjunctivae, mucous membranes, and lips, and checks for jaundice (also scleral icterus), petechiae, ecchymosis, rash, and ulcerations.
- *Head and neck*—Inspection of eyes for scleral icterus or hemorrhages; mucous membranes for signs of bleeding or petechiae; and hair texture and pattern for irregularities; palpation of lymph nodes and thyroid for any adenopathy
- *Heart*—Auscultation for tachycardia, arrhythmia, systolic murmur, or gallop, and notation of any increased pulsations, bruits, or cardiac enlargement
- *Chest*—Assessment of breast and axillary tissue for lymphadenopathy
- *Lungs*—Auscultation of breath sounds and notation of tachypnea, shortness of breath, chest pain, retractions, cough, or other signs of respiratory distress
- *Neurologic*—Observation of overall activity, level of consciousness, and mental status, with notation of any

hemiparesis or seizures; tests for vibration and proprioceptive sensation, and examination for meningeal signs and high-pitched cry
- *Musculoskeletal*—Observation of range of motion for weakness, stiffness, or painful or swollen joints, and inspection for bony deformities, triphalangeal thumbs, spoon nails, or edema of hands or feet

- *Abdomen*—Inspection, percussion, and palpation of abdomen for enlarged spleen and liver
- *Pelvic*—Rectal examination, with notation of the presence of occult blood in stools or urine, ulcerations, inflammation, or hemorrhoids; Tanner staging and pelvic examination (if appropriate)
- *Denver II test*

Table 36-1 Diagnostic Procedures and Laboratory Tests

TEST NAME	MEASURES	NORMAL
Hematocrit (Hct)	Volume of circulating RBCs	40%-65% @ 1-3 days of age 30%-40% @ 6 months to school age 40%-50% @ adolescence
Hemoglobin (Hgb) (g/dl)	Ability of RBCs to carry oxygen	14-22 @ 1-3 days of age 10-15 @ 6 months to school age 12-18 @ adolescence

Mean corpuscular volume (MCV) (μm^3)	Size of RBCs
	  Microcytic
	  Macrocytic
	  Normocytic
		110-128 @ birth
		71-85 @ 6 months
		75-90 @ 2-6 years
		78-95 @ 6 years
		80-100 @ adult
		Rule of thumb in children is 70 plus age in years

Mean corpuscular hemoglobin (MCH) (pg)	Amount of Hgb per RBC	27-32
Mean corpuscular hemoglobin concentration (MCHC) %	Portion of RBC occupied by hemoglobin	32%-36%
Reticulocyte count %	Function of bone marrow; percentage of immature RBCs	0.5%-2%
Smear (peripheral)	Automated or manual slide examination of cell shape, size, color, and the presence of aberrations: sickle cells, spherocytes, teardrop cells, schistocytes, target cells, shift cells, bite cells, elliptocytes	Red cell size should compare with lymphocyte shape, color Manual exam is performed by a hematologist
Quantitative hemoglobin (A, A_2, and F) electrophoresis (% of total hemoglobin)	Screen for hemoglobinopathies (sickle cell disease, Hgb C disease, thalassemia)	Over age 6 months: • Hgb A 95%-97% • Hgb A_2 2.0%-3.5% • Hgb F <2% • Hgb S >40% is evidence of disease • Typical in sickle trait is Hgb A = 62%, Hgb S = 38%
Serum ferritin assay Total iron-binding capacity (TIBC) ($\mu g/dl$)	Screen for iron deficiency	60-175 @ birth 100-400 in infant 250-400 to adult
Serum iron concentration ($\mu g/dl$)	Reflects intake in previous 24 hours	110-270 @ birth 30-70 @ 4-10 months 53-119 @ 3-10 years
Serum transferrin Serum ferritin concentration Serum ferritin determinates Iron saturation	Reflects iron stores	200-400 $\mu g/dl$ <10-12 $\mu g/L$ 20-120 $\mu g/dl$ >16%

Vitamin B_{12} and folate assays
  Serum vitamin B_{12}
  Serum folate
  Schilling test (vitamin B_{12} malabsorption)
	Screen for megoblastic, vitamin B_{12}/folate deficiency	
		130-785 pg/ml
		>2.8 ng/ml
		>8% excretion

Direct, and indirect Coombs' test	Screen for immune hemolysis	Negative
Bilirubin level	Screen for jaundice, byproduct of heme breakdown	See Jaundice later in this chapter

Other tests
  Bone marrow biopsy
  Fecal and urine tests for occult blood
	
	Screen for hypoplasia or infiltration
	Screen for GI or gastrourinary tract bleeding	

Serum lead levels*		<10 $\mu g/dl$ in child

*Treatment is recommended for levels greater than 20 $\mu g/dl$ (see Chapter 47).

Diagnostic Procedures and Laboratory Tests

The following laboratory results are essential for determining the type of anemia: *mean corpuscular volume* (MCV), *peripheral smear,* and *reticulocyte count*. Anemia is often classified according to the MCV (RBC size) as *normal, microcytic,* or *macrocytic*. Based on the results of these first three tests, narrow the diagnostic focus and follow with appropriate testing. A list of these tests is found in Table 36-1.

Anemia

JACQUELINE G. IOLI

Alert

Consult with or refer to a physician for acute anemia caused by erythroblastopenia (also called *aplastic crisis*) may occur when patient with sickle cell disease, thalassemia major, congenital hemolytic anemia, or other chronic hemolytic disease is exposed to human parvovirus B19 or other viral infection. Symptoms of aplastic crisis include weakness, pallor, and signs and symptoms of high cardiac output or failure.

The following acute complications of sickle cell disease also require immediate intervention:
- Bacterial sepsis or meningitis (particularly pneumococci)
- Splenic sequestration (sudden enlargement of spleen, spleen pooling of RBCs, acute anemia, hypovolemic shock)
- Aplastic crisis (pallor, lethargy, dyspnea)
- Vasoocclusive events:
  Acute chest syndrome (fever, pleuritic chest pain, pulmonary infiltrates, hypoxemia)
  Stroke
  Dactylitis (hand-and-foot syndrome often an initial symptom)
  Bone infarction (ischemic pain)

Etiology

Anemias can be categorized in two major ways: (1) decreased production or increased destruction of RBCs (i.e., hemolytic anemia), or (2) based on RBC size (i.e., microcytic, normocytic, macrocytic). In addition, each type of anemia can be acquired or inherited. Some anemias are pathologic; others represent an individual patient's normal baseline hemoglobin and RBC size. Anemia with concomitant alterations in platelet count or white blood cell (WBC) count (especially if neutropenia is present) is suggestive of possible aplastic anemia or malignancy and should be immediately referred to a pediatric hematologist-oncologist.

Incidence

Iron-deficiency anemia. The prevalence of iron deficiency and iron-deficiency anemia (IDA) in the United States (from the third National Health and Nutrition Examination Survey [1988-1994]) (Looker, et al. [1997]) is as follows:
- 1- to 2-year-old boys and girls:—iron deficiency at 9%, IDA at 3%
- 12- to 15-year-old girls—iron deficiency at 9%, IDA at 2%
- 16- to 19-year-old girls—iron deficiency at 11%, IDA at 3%
- 12- to 19-year-old boys—iron deficiency at less than 1%, IDA at less than 1%

IDA is uncommon in the neonatal period because fetal iron "endowment" lasts for the first 4 to 6 months of life in term infants of adequately nourished mothers. Thus preterm infants are at high risk.

Up to 30% of children in one public health service clinic had anemia, and about 25% had iron deficiency, as compared with a private practice where only 8% had anemia and 11% had iron deficiency. Inner-city infants fed iron-fortified formulas have a less than 1% incidence of iron deficiency, while inner-city infants fed low-iron formulas have a nearly 20% incidence of iron deficiency.

Megaloblastic anemias. Although specific incidence and prevalence data are not available for children, the National Health and Nutrition Exam Study noted that most Americans take in 200 to 300 μg/day of folate. The World Health Organization (WHO) (1987) recommends 200 μg/day.

Glucose-6-phosphate dehydrogenase deficiency. An estimated 400 million people worldwide are affected, making glucose-6-phosphate dehydrogenase (G6PD) deficiency the most common enzyme deficiency in the world. It is an X-linked genetic disorder (males are mostly affected). Because of the high prevalence of this disorder, homozygote females (i.e., the daughter of a male with the deficiency and a female with the trait) are not uncommon. The condition is most common in persons of African, Mediterranean (e.g., Italians, Greeks, Sephardic Jews [Jews of Spain and Portugal]), and Asian descent. The severity of the enzyme deficiency is highly variable and is worse among Mediterraneans and Asians as compared with persons of African descent. There is a geographic correlation between the worldwide distribution of G6PD and malaria, and having G6PD trait offers a mild protective effect against malaria in female carriers, though not in affected males.

β-Thalassemia major (Cooley's anemia). Common among children of Mediterranean descent, this also occurs in those of Asian descent. As with G6PD, there is a geographic correlation between worldwide distribution of the trait of β-thalassemia major and malaria. β-Thalassemia major usually becomes evident as hemolytic anemia within the first year of life and is often identified by the standard newborn screening for hemoglobinopathies that is now mandatory in most states in the United States.

Hereditary spherocytosis. The prevalence of hereditary spherocytosis (HS) is 1 in 200 among persons of northern European descent.

Inherited hemoglobin traits. The WHO estimates that 4.5% of the world population carries a hemoglobinopathy trait, and the global birthrate of affected infants is 2 in 1000, with almost three fourths of affected births occurring in Africa. Sickle trait does *not* cause anemia unless the child has a concomitant one or two α-globin gene deletion. Sickle trait is common in children of African, Mediterranean, and Hispanic descent, and 1 in 8 African Americans has sickle trait.

Hemoglobin E trait is the most common hemoglobinopathy worldwide. It is common in Asians, occurring in 34% of people in Cambodia, 375 people in Laos, 7235 people in Malaya, 14% to 42% of people in Thailand, and 25% of people in Vietnam. In California, the state newborn screening program finds that 1 in 12 of Southeast Asians and 1 in 4 Cambodian newborns has E trait.

Hemoglobin C trait is common in persons of western African ancestry but is also occasionally found in children of Hispanic descent. About 1 in 400 African Americans has hemoglobin C trait.

α-Thalassemia traits are common in persons of African, Mediterranean, and Asian descent. It is possible to have *both* an α- and a β-globin gene variant. The prevalence varies based on population and type of α-thalassemia trait; for example, for the one α-globin gene deletion, occurrence is 20% in Cambodia,

6% in south China, 10% in Cyprus, 7% in Greece, 20% in Laos, 34% in Sardinia, 8% to 10% in Thailand, and 30% in the African-American population; for the two α-globin gene deletion, occurrence is 8% in Cambodia, 5% in Hong Kong, 9% in southern China, 10% in Hmongs from Laos, 10% to 17% in Thailand, 8% in Vietnam, and 3% in the African-American population.

β-Thalassemia trait is common in persons of African, Mediterranean, and Asian descent. The prevalence varies based on population, for example, 2.5% in southern Italy but 12% to 13% in Sardinia, 8% in Greece, 0.001% in northern Europe but higher in Ireland and the Netherlands, 15% to 17% in Cyprus, 3% in Cambodia, 5% to 10% in Thailand, up to 10% in Iran, 8% in Pakistani Pathans, and 0.3% to 1% in the African-American population.

Risk Factors

- Diet poor in iron sources (e.g., meat, iron-fortified cereals, formulas)
- Early or excessive use of cows' milk instead of iron-fortified formula or breast milk
- Prematurity
- Heavy menses
- Anorexia, food fads, or overuse of goat's milk
- Family history of genetic hemoglobinopathies:
- Recent exposure to oxidant stress
- Elevated lead level (more than 10 μg/dl)

Differential Diagnosis (Table 36-2)

Iron-deficiency anemia. IDA, the most common anemia in children, is characterized as an acquired microcytic anemia of underproduction. Iron deficiency is primarily related to poor nutrition and is a preventable cause of irreversible brain injury, which affects intelligence quotient (IQ) and motor function. These deleterious effects are not completely reversible with iron therapy. Severe, chronic IDA is a subtle cause of neurocognitive dysfunction with behavior and learning problems that can persist up to 10 years after the anemia is corrected. IDA is the result of a series of intermediary steps. First, bone marrow iron stores are depleted. This can occur from poor maternal intake of iron or from prematurity as the infant passively receives most maternal stores during the last trimester of pregnancy. These stores are adequate for the first 4 to 6 months of life in term infants if maternal intake is adequate. As the iron stores become depleted, the RBC distribution width widens. If sufficient intake does not occur, a loss of transport iron, which manifests by a reduced serum iron level, occurs. Finally, iron-deficient erythropoiesis results in a low mean cell volume (MCV) and overt anemia. Poor dietary intake of iron and blood loss (e.g., from menorrhagia in adolescent females, GI losses caused by early excessive intake of cow's milk) are the most common etiologic agents; when chronic blood loss is part of the history, a bleeding history should also be obtained. Pica can result from iron deficiency; children who have pica are also at risk for lead toxicity (see Chapter 47). However, serum lead would have to be at near-seizure levels (i.e., over 100 μg/dL) to affect hematopoiesis. In addition, infection and chronic disease or inflammation must also be considered in the differential. If microcytosis persists despite iron sufficiency, inherited hemoglobin traits must be ruled out.

When IDA is suspected, either an in-office hemoglobin test *or* a complete blood cell (CBC) count should be obtained. If the patient is anemic for age and the history and physical examination are consistent with IDA, the patient should be treated with supplemental iron and scheduled for a return of-fice visit within a few days to a few weeks later depending on the family, examination, and degree of anemia. However, cardiovascular instability or hemoglobin less than 7 g should prompt consultation with a physician. If the anemia resolves with iron supplementation, the diagnosis is IDA. If the anemia does not resolve, one can perform more sophisticated testing, such as testing for total iron-binding capacity (TIBC), ferritin, and serum iron and performing hemoglobin electrophoresis to rule out inherited hemoglobin traits. The hemoglobin electrophoresis should be delayed until the patient is iron replete since hemoglobin A_2 production is decreased in iron-deficient hematopoiesis. If the electrophoresis is done when the patient is iron deficient, a diagnosis of β-thalassemia trait with its elevated hemoglobin A_2 could be missed. Serum ferritin is a reflection of body iron stores. The serum ferritin is an acute-phase reactant and thus can be falsely elevated in inflammatory states (e.g., infection, stress). Children may be iron deficient without being overtly anemic.

Vitamin B_{12} (cobalamin) and folate deficiency anemias. Commonly caused by nutritional deficiency or malabsorption, vitamin B_{12} (cobalamin) and folate deficiency anemias may occur with failure to thrive (FTT), various neurologic deficits, or general hematologic cytopenias. Although in adults these are acquired macrocytic anemias of underproduction, children may not become macrocytic. The most common cause of cobalamin deficiency in children is dietary deficiency in their mothers. Both vitamin B_{12} and folic acid are required for normal cell division. Consequently, a deficiency of either nutrient damages dividing cells. In the cells of the hematologic system, the manifestations of these deficiencies are large megaloblastic RBCs, an indication of ineffective hematopoiesis, and hypersegmented neutrophils. Both nutrients play critical but poorly understood roles in neural tube development in the fetus.

Vitamin B_{12} deficiency in particular adversely affects the nondividing cells of the neurologic system because of degeneration of myelin sheaths and disruption of the axons in the spinal cord, white matter of the brain, and peripheral nerves. Not surprisingly, vitamin B_{12} deficiency can be a cause of subtle neurocognitive dysfunction. In adults, suboptimal folate intake increases cancer risk. Further, elevated plasma homocysteine levels are found in folate deficiency, and this elevation is a known risk factor for atherosclerotic vascular disease in adults. Vitamin B_{12} (cobalamin) binds with intrinsic factors in the lower bowel, is metabolized in the mitochondria, and is required for the metabolism of methylmalonic acid (MMA). Vitamin B_{12} helps recycle folate in the homocysteine-to-methione reaction. Both RBC folate and serum folate levels are reduced by vitamin B_{12} deficiency. Correct diagnosis of either vitamin B_{12} deficiency or folate deficiency is critical because treating vitamin B_{12} deficiency with folate could cause improvement in the hematologic parameters with deterioration in the neurologic status as the neurologic damage from untreated vitamin B_{12} deficiency continues untreated.

Like many other nutritional deficiencies, the effects of folate or vitamin B_{12} deficiency are progressive. In its earliest phases, negative folate balance is characterized by normal RBC folate but decreased serum folate. As deficiency progresses, both serum and RBC folate levels are affected, and the condition progresses to folate-deficient hematopoiesis, progressively increasing RBC size, and hypersegmentation of neutrophils. Finally, clinical folate deficiency results with the classic picture of frank macrocytic anemia. However, macrocytosis (MCV

Table 36-2 Differential Diagnosis: Anemia in Primary Pediatric Care

CRITERIA	IRON-DEFICIENCY ANEMIA	VITAMIN B₁₂/FOLATE-DEFICIENCY ANEMIA	G6PD*	β-THALASSEMIA*/HEMOGLOBIN H DISEASE	MAJOR SICKLE CELL DISEASE*	HEREDITARY SPHEROCYTOSIS*	INHERITED HEMOGLOBIN TRAITS (E, C, β-THALASSEMIA)
ICD-9 code	280.9	266.2/281.2	282.2	282.4	282.60	282.0	
Subjective Data Age at onset	9-24 months; adolescence	9 months to 10 years (vitamin B₁₂); 4-7 months (folic acid)	Newborn period	0-12 months	8 months-5 years	Newborn, infancy	Newborn, adolescence
Dietary recall	Limited sources of meat; large amounts of cow's milk; lack of iron supplement; pica or anorexia may be present	Limited sources of vitamin B₁₂: Strict vegetarian or vegan diet; Infants of breastfeeding vegetarian mothers; infants refusing or delayed introduction of solid foods Folic acid: Excessive or exclusive use of goat's milk or powdered milk	Recent ingestion of fava beans or medication oxidant	Poor appetite	Anorexia	May exhibit poor feeding	Typical for age
Pain	Headache may be present	None	None	None	Severe pain crises: Muscular pain, arthalgia of long bones and joints, abdominal pain and rigidity; headache		None
Other symptoms	Active or occult blood loss from GI tract bleeding or menstrual bleeding	Diarrhea, anorexia, poor growth	Jaundice	Poor growth and development, jaundice, bony deformities, characteristic facies (prominent forehead and maxilla), lethargy	Growth retardation, shortness of breath, cough, faintness, or weakness; increased urine output	Jaundice	None
Exposure	Lead exposure	Vitamin B₁₂: Recurrent illness, intestinal disease or surgery may interfere with absorption Folic acid: Intestinal or liver disease; certain medications may interfere with folic acid absorption	Recent oxidant stress: Medications, fava beans, or recent infection	At risk for aplastic crisis with exposure to human parvovirus B19 or other viral infection (see Alert box)	See Alert box	See Alert box	None

*Refer to a physician.

Continued

Table 36-2 Differential Diagnosis: Anemia in Primary Pediatric Care—cont'd

CRITERIA	IRON-DEFICIENCY ANEMIA	VITAMIN B$_{12}$/FOLATE-DEFICIENCY ANEMIA	G6PD*	β-THALASSEMIA*/HEMOGLOBIN H DISEASE	MAJOR SICKLE CELL DISEASE	HEREDITARY SPHEROCYTOSIS*	INHERITED HEMOGLOBIN TRAITS (E, C, β-THALASSEMIA)
Subjective Data—cont'd							
Child/family history	Child history of chronic disease	Family history of pernicious anemia	Child history of neonatal hyperbilirubinemia	Family history α– or β-thalassemia Major or trait	Family history of sickle cell disease, sickle trait, or other unusual hemoglobin traits (C, E, β-thalassemia)	Family history of hemolytic disease in most cases; 20% to 25% of cases appear to be spontaneous; child history of neonatal jaundice	Family history of anemia (especially of unknown cause) or sickle cell disease or trait
Objective Data							
Physical examination							
Vital signs	May have tachycardia				Fever, tachycardia, tachypnea		Normal
Cardiac/hematologic	Pallor; systolic murmur may be heard; cardiac enlargement		Pallor, jaundice; cardiac compromise can occur in severe cases	Jaundice	Pallor, jaundice, cardiac dilation, edema, dactylitis, hematuria	Pallor, jaundice	Normal (murmur should not be attributed to inherited hemoglobin traits)
Growth and development	Reversible delay in development may occur	Growth and developmental delay; head circumference and weight below normal curve			Weight and height below curve		Normal
Neurologic	Irritability	Vitamin B$_{12}$: Many neurologic symptoms (decreased proprioception and vibration, hypotonia, hyperreflexia, choreoathetoid movements) Folic acid: Irritability may be noted		Decreased activity	Hemiplegia, seizures		Normal
Gastrointestinal/abdominal				Hepatosplenomegaly	Enlarged spleen	Enlarged spleen	Normal

Laboratory data						
MCV ↓ (<70 µg³); RDW ↑; anisocytosis and poikilocytes noted on smear; iron studies reveal low serum iron level and iron saturation (<16%); ↑ TIBC, ↓ ferritin saturation, ↑ FEP, ↑ TIBC; ↓ ferritin (<10 ng/ml), stools may be guaiac positive	MCV ↑ (>100 fl); reticulocyte count normal, serum vitamin B_{12} level below normal (normal, 140-700 pg/ml); Schilling test for absorption of vitamin B_{12} and serum folate shows low levels (normal, 7-32 ng/ml); hypersegmented neutrophils may be noted	MCV normal; serum iron level normal; Heinz bodies and "bite cells" noted; reduced G6PD in erythrocytes	Severe anemia (hemoglobin <5-6 g/dl); MCV ↓; reticulocyte count ↑, normal or ↑ iron studies, target cells noted on smear; hemoglobin electrophoresis confirms diagnosis: hemoglobin A decreased or absent, hemoglobin A_2 >3.5%, hemoglobin F may represent 90% of total hemoglobin	Severe anemia (hemoglobin 5-9 g/dl); MCV normal; reticulocytes ↑ (5%-15%); sickling and target cells noted on smear; Howell-Jolly bodies and nucleated red blood cells noted; hemoglobin electrophoresis is important in diagnosis: 75% to 100% hemoglobin S and elevated fetal hemoglobin	Anemia (hemoglobin 9-12 g/dl); MCV normal; reticulocytes ↑; spherocytes noted on smear; white blood cells, platelets normal; Coombs' test negative (positive Coombs' test indicates immune disease	MCV ↓ (<70) in α-, C, E, and β-thalassemia traits; MCV normal in sickle trait; hemoglobin may or may not be low (10-11 g) in C, E, and β-thalassemia traits; hemoglobin is normal in sickle trait. Typical hemoglobin electrophoresis: Sickle trait: A = 62%, S = 38% C trait: A = 50%, C = 50% E trait: A = 70%, E = 30% β-Thalassemia trait: A = 95%, A_2 = 5% α-Thalassemia trait: Normal; may have some hemoglobin F present

*Refer to a physician.
FEP, Free erythrocyte protoporphyrin; RDW, red cell distribution width.

above 92 fl) is rare in children with folate deficiency. In adults, folate deficiency can take 5 months to progress to this symptomatic stage. Likewise, vitamin B_{12} deficiency can progress through stages first beginning with low serum vitamin B_{12} and elevated serum MMA and homocysteine levels but no subclinical or clinical abnormalities. Subclinical abnormalities such as mild neurologic or hematologic changes occur next in addition to continued low B_{12} levels. Later, patients have mild to severe clinical symptoms with hematologic or neurologic abnormalities. Neurologic abnormalities may occur without anemia. Vitamin B_{12} deficiency can take up to 2 years to progress to a clinically evident state.

The most common cause of vitamin B_{12} and folate deficiencies in children is poor nutrition resulting from poor maternal nutrition or inadequate absorption in a breastfed infant. Diets low in folate and cobalamin may result in general malnutrition as would occur in extreme-poverty, vegetarian (even ovo-lacto), vegan, or macrobiotic diets. Malabsorption can also cause folate or vitamin B_{12} deficiency, as with surgical resection of the bowel, inflammatory disease, overgrowth of intestinal bacteria, infestation with fish tapeworm, Crohn's disease, recurrent illness, celiac disease, chronic infectious enteritis, or enteroenteric fistulas. Certain medications may interfere with folic acid absorption (e.g., anticonvulsants, methotrexate, trimethoprim-sulfamethoxazole, oral contraceptives).

However, rare inborn errors of vitamin B_{12} or folate transport or metabolism can occur. The most common of these errors is pernicious anemia caused by a lack of functional intrinsic factor as a result of chronic gastritis that secondarily causes poor absorption of vitamin B_{12}. It is important to avoid equating pernicious anemia with vitamin B_{12} deficiency. Most commonly, pernicious anemia is a disease of adults that develops slowly over a period of years either because of an autoimmune disorder that causes antibodies to the gastric parietal cells or because of excessive alcohol ingestion or cigarette smoking.

Cobalamin and folate levels should be measured (including both serum folate and RBC folate; serum levels represent the previous day's intake and may fluctuate) along with MMA and homocystine levels; elevation of these would reflect a lack of functional folate or cobalamin. Once treated, clinical improvement of neurologic symptoms may occur slowly over the next 6 months and may not return to the baseline value. Although children with vitamin B_{12} and folate deficiency do not commonly appear with macrocytosis, for children with elevated MCV (greater than 92 fl) the most common association is drug ingestion (e.g., anticonvulsants, zidovudine, immunosuppressives), congenital heart disease, Down syndrome, reticulocytosis, marrow failure, or myelodysplasia. Pernicious anemia is diagnosed with a Shilling test, also known as a cobalamin absorption test. This test should be ordered in conjunction with a hematologist and involves a radiolabeled dose of cyanocobalamin and a subsequent 24-hour urine collection.

Glucose-6-phosphate dehydrogenase deficiency. G6PD deficiency causes intermittent hemolytic anemia and could be characterized as both an inherited anemia and an acquired one. Most children with G6PD have normal lives and a normal-appearing CBC. Generally there is only a mild reduction in the RBC lifespan. G6PD is an enzyme responsible for protecting the RBC from oxidative stress. When sufficient G6PD is present, oxidative stress is balanced by the presence of the enzyme, and hemolysis is prevented. Without sufficient G6PD, mild to severe hemolysis occurs, 1 to 3 days after exposure to a trigger (e.g., fava [broad] beans, aspirin, sulfonamide drugs. People with G6PD are a heterogeneous group with varying amounts of G6PD present at any given time. The following oxidants may precipitate anemia: aspirin, acetaminophen, ascorbic acid, sulfonamide drugs, certain antibiotics (e.g., Macrodantin, Furadantin), naphthalene, thiazides, antimalarials, vitamin K, fava beans, recent infection. Differential diagnoses for G6PD includes IDA, history of neonatal hyperbilirubinemia, and immune anemia (positive Coombs' test).

Determining G6PD status is best done when a child is healthy because an elevated (over 5%) reticulocyte count in recovering from hemolytic anemia may yield false-negative results because reticulocytes and young RBCs are relatively high in G6PD. A quantitative G6PD analysis should be ordered. Avoid the qualitative analysis, which gives less information than the quantitative analysis; surprisingly, the qualitative analysis can also be more costly than the quantitative analysis. A CBC with reticulocyte count should also be performed. Cardiovascular instability or hemoglobin less than 7 g should be co-managed with a physician. It is not usual for the child to be the index case in the family.

Hereditary spherocytosis. Caused by a defect in the RBC membrane, HS is a common inherited hemolytic anemia. Instead of the normal, biconcave disk shape in the RBCs, the RBCs in HS are shaped like a sphere. These spherocytes have a less "stretchy" membrane as compared to that of normal RBCs. The RBC membrane in HS is like a plastic bag, easily deformed but not stretchy, making the cells subject to easy rupture (hemolysis). The organ where this increased destruction occurs is the spleen because the RBCs in HS survive well after splenectomy. Children with HS are a heterogeneous group; some require monthly blood transfusions, and others have rare to infrequent anemia symptoms. Differential diagnosis must include other causes of hemolysis, especially in the newborn period, and other RBC membrane defects or enzyme deficiencies (e.g., G6PD, pyruvate kinase). Children with HS can have manifestations similar to those of children with thalassemia major (anemia and splenomegaly) and thus should be evaluated in consultation with a physician.

Definitive diagnosis is made based on osmotic fragility testing (a laboratory evaluation usually not available outside the context of a hematologist, in which the response of a patient's RBCs are compared to a normal control's RBCs when exposed to increasing concentrations of water; RBCs in HS break sooner than the control), visual evaluation of the peripheral smear (spherocytes present) by a pediatric hematologist, and the CBC (MCHC is often elevated; the child may or may not have anemia). A family history is invaluable because HS is an autosomal dominant disorder; thus one parent has HS. It is not unusual for the child to be the index patient in the family.

Bone marrow failure. Bone marrow failure can be congenital or acquired. Neoplastic cells may replace bone marrow and inhibit erythrocyte production. Acute lymphoblastic leukemia is a common type of childhood leukemia that becomes evident as anemia with petechiae or purpura, lymphadenopathy, and splenomegaly. Bone marrow biopsy is important in differentiating anemia from malignancy. Bone marrow failure should be suspected when any two of the three cell lines (i.e., RBCs, WBCs, platelets) are affected on the CBC.

Inherited hemoglobin traits. Inherited β-hemoglobin traits (e.g., sickle trait, C trait, E trait, β-thalassemia trait, one or two α-globin gene deletions) are *not* disease states. However, these trait states may cause mild microcytic anemia (e.g., no lymphadenopathy, no splenomegaly, no exercise intolerance) with normal physical examination and normal serum iron studies (i.e., TIBC, ferritin).

Humans have two β-globin genes, one on each chromosome 11. β-Globin traits represent a compound heterozygote state with one "normal" gene for hemoglobin A and one unusual gene (C, E, and β-thalassemia traits are the most common). These states do have some mild medical and family planning considerations and are part of the differential diagnosis of IDA. Sickle trait is an inherited hemoglobin trait that does not cause anemia unless it is coinherited with an α-globin variant.

Inherited α-globin states occur because of alterations in any of the four α-globin genes; two are located on each chromosome 16 for a total of four α-globin genes. A one α-globin gene deletion is called α-*thalassemia silent carrier*. A two α-globin gene deletion is called α-*thalassemia trait*. The α-thalassemia traits do not cause symptoms but may cause a mild microcytic anemia.

For β-globin traits, the hemoglobin electrophoresis can clarify the diagnosis. *Sickle trait* is characterized by a hemoglobin electrophoresis with just over 60% A and just under 40% S; a form of sickle cell disease should be suspected if hemoglobin S is over 50%. Hemoglobin electrophoresis results vary with age. In the last trimester of pregnancy, the fetus begins to produce adult genetic complement of hemoglobin in very small amounts (usually less than 10%). Usually by 6 months of age, the full adult complement is produced. Avoid using a Sickledex or sickle prep as a test to determine sickle trait status. Some sickling disorders such as sickle cell $^{\beta+}$-thalassemia and sickle hemoglobin C disease are characterized by near-normal hemoglobin levels. Thus a sickle prep could yield a false-negative result leading to inappropriate management, particularly of fever and pain. In addition, the sickle prep should *not* be used in infants under 6 months of age whose fetal hemoglobin may still be somewhat elevated, and the hemoglobin S must be at least 20% to result in a positive sickle screen; again, a false-negative result could lead to inappropriate management. Because of cost considerations, many practitioners perform a sickle prep in at-risk populations (e.g., persons of African, Hispanic descent) about the time the screening CBC is done (9 to 12 months of age). If the sickle prep is positive, full hemoglobin electrophoresis should be performed.

Persons with hemoglobin E trait have a similar electrophoretic pattern to sickle trait (i.e., just over 60% A and just under 40% E); there may be slight microcytic anemia. Homozygous E comprises over 90% E and some hemoglobin F; these children have a baseline hemoglobin of about 10 g and are otherwise healthy. In hemoglobin C trait, hemoglobins A and C are each about 50%; again there may be slight microcytic anemia. β-Thalassemia trait (also called β-*thalassemia minor*) is characterized by the presence of elevated hemoglobin A_2 (over approximately 3.5%), such as A = 95%, A_2 = 5%. Persons with β-thalassemia trait have one normal gene and one "broken" gene and have only a mild microcytic anemia.

The α-thalassemia traits *cannot* be directly detected on the hemoglobin electrophoresis outside the newborn period with the presence of Bart's hemoglobin. However, one clue often is the persistence of hemoglobin F after 6 months of age. Definitive diagnosis of α-thalassemia traits must be made by globin gene analysis, which is often not readily available without the assistance of a reference laboratory. Since a one or two α-globin gene deletion does not cause disease, only a mild microcytic anemia in the face of normal iron studies and a near-normal electrophoresis, it may not be practical to send some children to a hematologist for definitive diagnosis. It is not unusual for the child to be the index case of the family. Particularly because of the difficulty in obtaining definitive testing, most adults are unaware of their α-hemoglobin trait status.

Thalassemias. β-Thalassemia major (Cooley's anemia) is characterized as an inherited microcytic anemia of underproduction. Genetically, β-thalassemia major is classified as homozygous recessive; thus there is a 25% chance with each pregnancy that two parents who are *both* affected with β-thalassemia trait will have a child with β-thalassemia major.

Children who have inherited two "broken" β-globin genes are unable to make adult hemoglobin and have β-thalassemia major. Children who inherit a β-thalassemia trait from one parent and another unusual β-globin hemoglobin trait (e.g., C, E) from the other have a form of β-thalassemia (hemoglobin C–β-thalassemia or hemoglobin E–β-thalassemia). These children may have a similar clinical course described as β-*thalassemia major* or a milder clinical course described as *thalassemia intermedia*. If a thalassemia trait is inherited with sickle trait, the resulting disorder is characterized as sickle-thalassemia, a subtype of sickle cell disease (see Chapter 45). Further, β-thalassemia traits are often described as *plus* or *zero* depending on whether the thalassemia gene makes a reduced amount of hemoglobin A or no hemoglobin A. Thus E β^+-thalassemia describes a thalassemia characterized by inheritance of one hemoglobin E gene and a thalassemia gene that makes some hemoglobin A. The presence of hemoglobin A has an ameliorating effect on the clinical picture; a child with E β^0-thalassemia can be expected to have a clinically more severe course possibly requiring chronic RBC transfusion. Thalassemia major is most frequently identified by state newborn screening programs because hemoglobin F only is found in a term newborn. In contrast, the most common finding would be FA.

Children with β-*thalassemia intermedia* are able to maintain their hemoglobin over 7 g/dl and may have any or all of the following symptoms: growth delay, delayed puberty, exercise intolerance, leg ulcers, inflammatory arthritis, iron overload (from enhanced oral absorption, hypersplenism and splenic pain, and bony deformities (maxillary hyperplasia, spinal cord compression) caused by extramedullary hematopoiesis.

Children who have untreated β-*thalassemia major* have ineffective erythropoiesis, fragile RBCs, and enhanced clearance of defective RBCs by the spleen. Their marrow is very active in trying to keep up with the demand for new RBCs, resulting in elevated platelet and WBC counts but a low reticulocyte count. Electrophoresis shows no hemoglobins A or A_2 and only hemoglobin F. The symptoms and signs of thalassemia intermedia occur in thalassemia major as well.

Hemoglobin H disease occurs when a child is missing three out of four α-globin genes. Although more rare than β-thalassemia major, hemoglobin H disease is a form of α-thalassemia that can have a similar clinical picture as β-thalassemia major or intermedia. In general, children with hemoglobin H disease have a stable anemia that may be worsened by hemolysis caused by viral infections and oxidant stress (similar to G6PD).

β-*Thalassemia major* occurs when all four α-globin genes are missing. The fetus cannot produce adequate fetal hemoglobin, and most often, early fetal death occurs or a severely hydropic and hypoxic fetus results. There is often maternal toxemia from postpartum hemorrhage. If these fetuses are identified early, they represent case reports of intrauterine transfusion resulting in the delivery of healthy but transfusion-dependent infants. Either β-thalassemia major or hemoglobin H disease should be suspected when a child under 12 months of age has anemia with splenomegaly and a hemoglobin electrophoresis without hemoglobin A present or with a very high amount of hemoglobin F for the age of the child. However, since children with anemia with splenomegaly could also be have hemolytic anemias or malignancies, they should be co-managed in consultation with a pediatric hematologist.

Management

Iron-deficiency anemia

Treatments and medications. The treatment is oral iron (i.e., iron sulfate, fumarate, gluconate). The usual dosage 4 to 6 mg/kg per day of elemental iron every 12 to 24 hours. The maximum dose 15 mg/day of elemental iron. Listed below are common forms of ferrous sulfate with the amount of elemental iron listed in parentheses:

- Drops (Fer-In-Sol)—75 mg/0.6 ml (15 mg/0.6 ml).
- Syrup (Fer-In-Sol)—90 mg/5 ml (30 mg/5 ml).
- Elixir (Feosol)—220 mg/5 ml (44 mg/5 ml); because of 5% alcohol content, this is not appropriate for children under 12 months of age.
- Tablets (generic)—324 mg/tablet (65 mg/tablet).

Be cautioned that multivitamin supplements are *not* a substitute for therapeutic doses of iron in severe iron deficiency.

To improve tolerance and compliance, change the preparation (from sulfate to gluconate) or change the dosing frequency or timing with meals (iron is absorbed best before meals but is tolerated best after meals). To enhance adherence, give a dose only once or twice per day.

The following substances inhibit iron absorption: tea, coffee, milk, vegetable fiber. Possible side effects include GI tract irritability, constipation, and diarrhea. Iron supplements must be kept out of reach of children because iron is a common cause of accidental poisoning. Parenteral iron or iron dextran is not usually indicated, and transfusion is reserved for cases of severe anemia (e.g., hemoglobin level less than 5 g/dl or cardiovascular instability).

Counseling and prevention

- Educate parents about dietary sources of iron, including iron-fortified baby cereal and breakfast cereal (in particular, cereals that are approved by the United States government's Women, Infants, and Children [WIC] program, information from which is posted in most United States grocery stores), meats and poultry, beans and dried peas, nutritional yeast, dried fruits, spinach, broccoli, greens, tomato juice, prune juice, watermelon, winter squash, enriched corn tortillas and taco shells, breakfast or snack type of bars, nuts (e.g., almonds, cashews), iron-fortified soybean beverages, infant-toddler and pediatric formulas, fortified tofu, seeds (e.g., pumpkin, sesame), and molasses.
- Encourage parents to include an iron-rich food at each meal with some form of vitamin C–rich food because vitamin C enhances absorption of iron; vitamin C–rich foods include asparagus, bell pepper, broccoli, cabbage, cantaloupe, cauliflower, citrus fruits, vitamin C–fortified apple juice, green chili sauce, salsa, potatoes, strawberries, spinach, tomatoes, and turnips.
- Provide examples of combination meals (with iron and vitamin C) (e.g., iron-fortified WIC cereal and orange or fortified apple juice, bean and beef taco [cooked in cast iron] with tomato and salsa, meat with vitamin C–rich fruit for dessert).
- Encourage parents to cook in cast iron cookware.
- Discuss the possible side effects of iron therapy (e.g., stomach upset, constipation or diarrhea, dark stools).

Follow-up

- Keep in mind that the reticulocyte count should increase rapidly (within 72 to 96 hours) after treatment begins.
- Repeat the hemoglobin check again in 1 week (in-office testing is adequate).
- Remember that hemoglobin levels should return to normal or near-normal within 1 month if the child receives the iron supplement. There are rare cases of malabsorption that can be ruled out by in-office challenge. The serum iron is measured, the iron preparation is administered under supervision, and the serum iron level is repeated 1 hour later. If the serum iron rises after iron therapy, poor adherence is an issue.
- To replenish iron stores, follow with an additional 1 to 2 months of iron replacement (not to exceed 6 months total) after laboratory results are within normal limits.
- Consider inherited hemoglobin traits if the patient is unresponsive to iron therapy in 1 month.

Consultations and referrals. Refer to a physician or hematologist if the patient is unresponsive to iron therapy, for cardiovascular instability, or if the clinical picture is complex. A dietitian can be consulted.

Vitamin B$_{12}$ (cobalamin) and folate deficiency anemias

Treatments and medications. Treat the underlying cause first; in particular, address any nutritional issues.

- Pernicious anemia—Cyanocobalamin (vitamin B$_{12}$) 30 to 50 μg/day intramuscular or subcutaneous for 2 or more weeks to a total dose of 1000 to 5000 μg and then 100 μg monthly as maintenance.
- Vitamin B$_{12}$ deficiency—Cyanocobalamin (vitamin B$_{12}$) 100 μg/day for 10 to 15 days (total dose of 1 to 1.5 mg) and then once or twice weekly for several months, tapered to 60 μg monthly. Monitor reticulocyte count, CBC count, and serum iron (iron deficiency may have been masked by the macrocytosis). Expect the MCV to decrease by 5 fl over the first 2 weeks of therapy. Expect elevated homocysteine or MMA levels to return to normal. In severe anemia, the child should be hospitalized for careful transfusions with potassium supplementation or diuretics as needed.
- Folic acid deficiency—Oral dose is 50 μg/day for infants and 1 mg/day for children and adults, 1 mg/day. Parenteral dose is the same as the oral dose, but avoid its use in premature infants because of alcohol content. High-dose folic acid therapy is contraindicated in cases of vitamin B$_{12}$ deficiency because it may mask neurologic manifestations of vitamin B$_{12}$ deficiency and thus delay diagnosis.

Counseling and prevention. Discuss with parents various dietary sources of vitamin B$_{12}$ (e.g., meat, eggs, dairy products, vitamin B$_{12}$–fortified soybean milk) and folate (e.g., green vegetables, lima beans, whole-grain cereals, liver, milk [preferably breast milk or pasteurized cow's milk, because heat-sterilized and evaporated milk are poor sources of folate]).

Follow-up. Should see some improvement of anemia and neurologic status should be seen within 1 week. Follow-up on weight gain, height, and development.

Consultations and referrals. Consult or refer to a dietitian. Consider neuropsychologic testing.

Glucose-6-phosphate dehydrogenase deficiency

Treatments and medications. Occasionally, transfusion is necessary.

Counseling and prevention

- Educate about drugs to be avoided, in particular sulfonamides (Bactrim, Septra), salicylates (aspirin, Pepto-Bismol), high-dose vitamin C (nutritional doses are safe), chloramphenicol, some antimalarials, some oral hypoglycemics, nitrofurantoin, phenacetin (Darvon), thiazide diuretics, phenothiazines, methylene blue, and dimercaprol (BAL).
- Stress the need to avoid broad (fava) beans; other beans may be eaten without problems. Language and translation may be an issue with some Mediterranean families. When in doubt, ask the family to bring in some of beans in question. Broad beans are dark brown in color and range in size from 0.5 cm to the more common 2.5-cm size.
- Stress the need to avoid accidental ingestion of benzene, naphthalene mothballs.
- Screen if there is a positive family history of G6PD, severe hemolytic anemia, or history of unexplained hyperbilirubinemia in neonatal period. Since Asians and Mediterraneans have the most severe reactions, consider screening these populations routinely. Since persons of African descent have less severe reactions, screening may be deferred unless indicated by a positive family history.

Follow-up. Follow-up as needed. Reinforce avoidance teaching at regular visits.

Consultations and referrals

- During hemolytic episodes, manage in consultation with a physician.
- Refer for genetic counseling if family desires.

β-thalassemia major and hemoglobin H disease

Treatments and medications. For thalassemia intermedia (i.e., non–transfusion dependent), transfusions may be needed only under conditions of stress. Avoid substances that cause oxidant stress (see G6PD). Suggest folic acid, 1 mg daily.

For thalassemia major (i.e., transfusion-dependent), there is a need for frequent transfusions (every 2 to 6 weeks). Iron overload occurs after about a year of monthly transfusions and requires chelation with deferoxamine. Splenectomy may be needed because of hypersplenism and increasing transfusion requirements (200 to 250 ml/kg per year). After splenectomy, children are at increased risk for infection from encapsulated organisms such as *Streptococcus pneumoniae* and *Haemophilus influenzae.* Many pediatric hematologists recommend antibiotic prophylaxis after splenectomy with penicillin VK, 125 mg twice a day (for those under 3 years of age) and 250 mg twice a day (for those over 3 years of age). In addition, standard dental prophylaxis (per the American Heart Association [AHA]) for subacute bacterial endocarditis prevention is often recommended.

Standard immunizations for age should be provided, including hepatitis A and B, pneumococcal, *H. fluenzae* type B (Hib), meningococcal, and yearly influenza vaccines.

Bone marrow transplantation is also a possible treatment option.

Counseling and prevention

- Teach patient and parents to monitor symptoms that indicate a need for transfusion (e.g., fatigue, night sweats) and signs and symptoms of severe anemia (e.g., fatigue, paleness, elevated heart rate, poor exercise tolerance).
- Counsel on long-term outcomes, the importance of chelation therapy, and avoidance of heart and liver damage from iron overload. Avoid iron supplementation, even in multiple vitamins.

Follow-up. Thalassemia major requires monthly follow-up evaluation with a pediatric hematologist, yearly hearing screens, endocrine evaluation (e.g., thyroid function and diabetes screen), and cardiac screen (often with echocardiogram and electrocardiogram [ECG]).

Consultations and referrals

- Consult with physician or hematologist for diagnosis, treatment, and follow-up care.
- Refer for genetic counseling and prenatal testing (e.g., chorionic villi sampling, amniocentesis) all women with thalassemia trait or disease.

Hereditary spherocytosis

Treatment and medications. Wide clinical heterogeneity is associated with hereditary spherocytosis (HS). Baseline hemoglobin value should be assessed every 1 to 2 years. Folic acid, 1 mg daily, though it should theoretically improve RBC production, can be prescribed to a family who wishes to give it. Because there is no evidence to support improved outcome in HS, folate supplementation should *not* be considered mandatory. Occasionally, RBC transfusions may be necessary on an as-needed basis for a child who has an acute virus-associated hemolytic crisis. Children with chronic hemolytic anemias may experience aplastic crisis during infection with parvovirus B19 (erythema infectiosum, or fifth disease). In addition, there are young children with HS with a high degree of hypersplenism who may require monthly transfusion therapy. Splenectomy would eliminate the need for frequent transfusions, because the spleen destroys the fragile RBCs. However, many hematologists and parents prefer to defer splenectomy to as close to the fifth birthday as possible to allow the spleen to assist in antibody formation. Because of the possibility of splenectomy, children with HS should have all standard immunizations including Hib, pneumococcal, and meningococcal vaccines. Should iron overload develop, deferoxamine should be used. Another complication of HS and all chronic hemolytic anemias is cholelithiasis. About one third of children with chronic hemolytic anemias require cholecystectomy before 21 years of age.

Counseling and prevention. Discuss with parents the importance of medical follow-up observation for unusual paleness (possible acute anemia) and epigastric pain (possible cholelithiasis) and the avoidance of therapeutic doses of iron. Children with HS who have mild anemia will not improve with therapeutic doses of iron.

Follow-up. Perform a yearly CBC count with differential and reticulocyte count to establish a baseline hemoglobin value, as well as ultrasonography of the gallbladder for suspected cholelithiasis.

Consultations and referrals

- Hematology for management of acute anemia
- Surgery for cholelithiasis
- Genetics for family planning counseling.

Inherited hemoglobin traits

Treatments and medications. None are needed because these are not disease states. Avoid iron overload, though nutritional doses of iron are appropriate if clinically indicated.

Counseling and prevention. Discuss with parents the importance of avoiding iron overload. Explain that these traits were inherited by the child from a parent; thus both the child and parents are at risk for having children with disease states (e.g., sickle cell disease, thalassemia major).

Follow-up. Reinforce avoidance teaching at family planning visits.

Consultation and referrals. Refer for genetic counseling.

Jaundice in the Newborn

JACQUELINE G. IOLI

Alert

Consult with or refer to a physician for the following:
- Jaundice (bilirubin level greater than 5 mg/dl) in the first 24 hours of life
- Jaundice persisting for more than a week
- Jaundice appearing after the first week of life
- Hyperbilirubinemia (bilirubin level greater than 20 to 24 mg/dl)
- Signs and symptoms of bilirubin encephalopathy or kernicterus (e.g., lethargy, poor feeding, temperature instability, hypotonia, seizure activity, high-pitched cry)
- Jaundice associated with signs or symptoms of sepsis
- Erythroblastosis fetalis (a rare consequence of Rh disease), with hydrops and severe anemia (hematocrit of 15% to 20%)
- Direct, conjugated bilirubin levels greater than 2 mg or 15% of total bilirubin
- Dark urine, clay-colored stools
- Hepatomegaly

Etiology

Because healthy term infants are now routinely discharged from the hospital within 48 hours of birth, management of jaundice in the newborn period is increasingly the responsibility of primary care providers (PCPs) who must provide early recognition and treatment. Further, jaundice is the most common cause of infant readmission to the hospital in the first week of life.

Incidence

- Over 50% of all newborns may have some degree of icterus (up to 80% of preterm).
- Only 3% of full-term infants have severe jaundice (i.e., bilirubin level of 15 mg/dL).
- Peak prevalence is between 2 and 5 days of life.
- It is more common in infants of Asian or Mediterranean descent.
- Breast milk jaundice has a later onset (days 4 to 7) and occurs in 10% to 30% of breastfed infants in the first 2 to 6 weeks of life.

Risk Factors

- Rh incompatibility (e.g., mother Rh negative, infant is Rh positive)
- ABO incompatibility (e.g., mother blood type O, infant blood type A or B)
- Positive Coombs' test result
- Breastfeeding
- Males of Asian, African, or Mediterranean descent (who have increased risk of G6PD)
- Polycythemia
- Bruising, hematomas, hemorrhages, or birth trauma
- Infant of diabetic mother
- Delayed meconium stooling
- Dehydration
- Maternal infection
- Perinatal asphyxia
- Prematurity
- Cystic fibrosis
- Family history of jaundice, anemia, or cholelithiases before 30 years of age (ABC enzyme deficits)

Differential Diagnosis (Table 36-3)

Bilirubin is a natural product of hemoglobin degradation and accumulates in the neonate because of enhanced production, delayed clearance, or a combination of both. Normal RBC destruction accounts for over three fourths of daily bilirubin production in healthy neonates. In addition, bilirubin is reabsorbed from the intestines before excretion in the bowel. Production of bilirubin is affected by stress states, fever, bacterial toxins, and starvation. Overproduction of bilirubin occurs during hemolysis of RBC in isoimmune Rh/ABO disease by maternal antibodies. Because of ongoing destruction, the neonate's metabolism may not be able to keep up with the degree of production. Polycythemic infants (hematocrit over 65%) also produce large amounts of bilirubin.

Bilirubin is divided into two types: conjugated, water-soluble bilirubin (direct bilirubin) and unconjugated, fat-soluble bilirubin (indirect bilirubin). The indirect, or unconjugated, bilirubin can be further categorized based on whether it is bound to albumin. It is this unconjugated, fat-soluble (measured by the indirect bilirubin) bilirubin that is potentially toxic. In particular, unconjugated bilirubin may be bound to albumin or unbound. Unconjugated, unbound bilirubin can cross the blood-brain barrier to cause transient or permanent neurologic damage. In addition, some newborns have disrupted blood-brain barriers and are more susceptible to this sort of injury (e.g., hypoxia, hypercapnia, hyperosmolarity, hyperthermia, septicemia). Unbound bilirubin is technically difficult to measure; thus it must be indirectly assessed by the serum levels of both indirect bilirubin and albumin. In contrast, conjugated bilirubin is stable and water soluble and is the form that is secreted in urine and stool.

Physiologic jaundice. The most common type of hyperbilirubinemia is physiologic jaundice, defined as a bilirubin level of 1 to 3 mg/dl at birth with a rise of less than 5 mg/day, peaking on day 3 of life in term infants and days 5 and 6 in preterm infants with a maximum level less than 13 mg/dl. Babies with physiologic jaundice are asymptomatic, other than having icteric coloring. Physiologic jaundice is a normal finding in otherwise healthy newborns. In the absence of ABO/Rh incompatibility, with negative Coombs' test results, and when there is no evidence of hemolysis or sepsis, jaundice in the newborn is likely benign. It occurs naturally in part because of the breakdown of excess fetal hemoglobin and the immaturity of the newborn's liver.

Jaundice associated with breastfeeding. Jaundice is more common in breastfeeding infants; their bilirubin levels may rise slightly higher and resolve somewhat more slowly than bottle-fed infants with physiologic jaundice. Jaundice associated with breastfeeding that becomes evident without hemolysis or incompatibility is usually a benign condition associated with poor intake or dehydration and delayed stooling. In some cases it may be attributed to enhanced intestinal absorption of unconjugated bilirubin (enterohepatic shunting) during the digestion of breast milk. There are several hypotheses regarding the cause of breast milk jaundice and the slightly increased incidence of jaundice with breastfeeding. However, kernicterus has not been reported in association with simple jaundice in breastfeeding infants.

Table 36-3 Differential Diagnosis: Jaundice in the Newborn

CRITERIA	PHYSIOLOGIC JAUNDICE	ABO/RH INCOMPATIBILITY	SEPSIS/ INFECTION*	GENETIC DISORDER†	OBSTRUCTION OF GI BILIARY TRACT*
ICD-9 code	774.6	773.0	771.8	277.4	576.2
Subjective Data					
Family history	May have history of previous children with physiologic jaundice	Jaundice or hemolytic disease in other children	Perinatal infections	Males of African, Asian, and Mediterranean descent Family history of anemia, jaundice, and cholelithiasis before age 30	May have family history of obstruction
Objective Data					
Physical examination					
Vital signs	Stable		Fever/temperature instability, tachypnea, apnea		May have nonspecific signs and symptoms of sepsis
Skin	Mild to moderate icterus	Icterus spreading to lower extremities	Icterus, petechiae, pallor, pustules, mottling	Icterus spreading to lower extremities	Icterus
Associated findings	May be slightly lethargic	Enlarged spleen		Enlarged liver, spleen	Abdominal distention, pain
Laboratory data					
Bilirubin levels, onset and duration	Day of life 2 to 3: <0-13 mg/dl; resolves spontaneously within a week	>5 mg/dl at birth or within first 24 hours; rate of rise >5 mg/dl per day	>5 mg/dl at birth or within first 24 hours; rate of rise >5 mg/dl/day; or onset after day 3 of life	Onset after 1 week of age	Onset after 1 week of age; prolonged jaundice >2 to 3 weeks; direct, conjugated bilirubin levels >2 mg/dl or 15% of total bilirubin
Other laboratory data	Hematocrit stable	Hematocrit dropping; mother's blood type O and/or Rh negative and baby's blood type incompatible; Coombs' test positive; reticulocytosis	Elevated white blood cell count; cultures positive	Severe hemolysis; smear may indicate spherocytes (hereditary spherocytosis, thalassemia); urine/blood screening positive for hemoglobinopathies; Coombs' test negative	Results of liver function tests may be elevated

*Immediate referral to a physician.
†Refer to a physician.

Pathologic jaundice. In general, bilirubin levels associated with pathologic jaundice rise quickly, are persistent, and are associated with other symptoms. Characteristics of pathologic jaundice include jaundice in the first 24 hours of life, total serum bilirubin increases of over 5 mg/dl per day, total serum bilirubin over 13 mg/dl in a term infant but 15 mg/dl in a preterm infant, direct serum bilirubin over 1 to 2 mg/dl, and jaundice lasting over 1 week in a term infant but 2 weeks in a preterm infant. Bilirubin encephalopathy and kernicterus describe the neurologic damage that can occur with hyperbilirubinemia. Classically, kernicterus is a syndrome of irreversible injury characterized by brain damage caused by excessive bilirubin accumulation. Neonates may have seizures, opisthotonos, hypertonia or hypotonia, high-pitched cry, and fever. Long-term infants affected with kernicterus may have spasticity, paresis of upward gaze, hearing loss, and cerebral palsy. Kernicterus is most common in preterm infants, especially those of less than 32 weeks gestation, and occurs in only 2% of healthy term infants. Pathologic jaundice should be referred to a physician (see Alert box). The most common cause of pathologic jaundice is hemolytic disease of the newborn, often a result of Rh incompatibility. Jaundice associated with ABO incompatibility is usually mild and requires minimal treatment. Coombs' test is essential in detecting the presence of antibodies that are bound to the infant's RBCs in the case of blood group incompatibility. Jaundice can also be a symptom of underlying disease such as sepsis or congenital infection (e.g., toxoplasmosis, CMV). Infection, asphyxia, and prematurity all increase the permeability of the blood-brain barrier, resulting in greater risk of bilirubin encephalopathy. Although rare, genetic hemolytic disease increases the bilirubin load as a result of the premature destruction of RBCs. Genetic disorders (e.g., G6PD, hypothyroidism, galactosemia, hereditary spherocytosis, other RBC enzyme defects) often become evident as hyperbilirubinemia in newborns. Obstructions of the GI or biliary tract inhibit excretion of bilirubin. Jaundice may be a symptom of underlying biliary atresia, Hirschsprung's disease, ileus, or cholestasis. Jaundice may also indicate neonatal hepatitis. Other possible causes include rare genetic syndromes and EBV.

Assessment of jaundice. Assess for jaundice by applying brief, gentle finger pressure to the skin of the neonate on the forehead or nose, chest, and leg. Jaundice progresses in a cephalocaudal manner as bilirubin levels rise. Thus a very rough estimate of serum bilirubin can be made by the following: jaundice of the head and neck is associated with an indirect bilirubin of 8 mg/dl, jaundice of the umbilicus with levels from 5 to 12 mg/dl, that above the knees with bilirubin from 8 to 16 mg/dl, that in the knees to ankles with levels 11 to 18 mg/dl, and that of the feet with levels of 35 mg/dl. The visual assessment should occur in a room with good lighting, and the entire body surface should be inspected. Cephalohematoma, or bruising, predisposes to hyperbilirubinemia. Stooling patterns should be assessed carefully because most bilirubin is excreted in the stool, and delays in stooling are associated with ever-increasing bilirubin levels. Hepatosplenomegaly is an unexpected finding and may occur in infection states or hemolytic anemias. General neurologic status, feeding ability, and temperature should be assessed. Hydration status should be assessed by the number of wet diapers per day (six to eight is normal) and whether the mucus membranes are moist, because dehydration is associated with hyperbilirubinemia.

Laboratory analysis. Conjugated serum bilirubin (indirect bilirubin) values above a range of 10% to 20% of the total serum bilirubin levels are suggestive of liver disease. Interestingly, bilirubin is a potent antioxidant and may protect from injury from oxidant stress as could occur in ischemia and retinopathy of prematurity. There is not sufficient current data to establish a maximum safe serum bilirubin level. At this time, only low levels of bilirubin are considered safe. Direct Coombs' testing should be performed to rule out an immune-mediated anemia. Direct bilirubin should be measured to rule out liver disease.

Management

The treatment of jaundice should be individualized. Decisions are based on thorough assessment of the infant, including gestational age, severity of laboratory findings, infant's age at onset, rate of rise of bilirubin, and possible causes. Any cases of suspected pathologic jaundice should be referred to a physician.

Physiologic hyperbilirubinemia

Treatments and medications. Most cases of physiologic jaundice require no treatment other than monitoring.

Phototherapy (Table 36-4). Place the infant approximately 16 to 18 inches from fluorescent blue-spectrum lights in tube or bulb form. A fiberoptic blanket (Wallaby system) may also be used. One or more lights may be used in combination as "double phototherapy" for maximum skin exposure. (Phototherapy light converts bilirubin in the skin to a form that can be excreted in stool and urine.) The infant's eyes must be shielded and the temperature monitored to reduce the risks of corneal damage and hyperthermia. Good home phototherapy candidates are term infants over 48 hours old with a serum bilirubin level over 14 mg/dl but less than 18 mg/dl with normal physical examination and normal CBC counts. The family must be agreeable to home therapy, and a reliable home care company must be in place to train the parents in use of the phototherapy unit and provide nursing support and assessment. Related measures include:

- Increase fluid intake by 10% to 25% to compensate for insensible water loss. At home, infants can have these

Table 36-4 Managing Hyperbilirubinemia in the Term (>2500 g) Infant

AGE (HOURS)	UPPER LEVEL BILIRUBIN (MG/DL)	TREATMENT	
		NO HEMOLYSIS	HEMOLYSIS LIKELY
<24	5	Investigate	Phototherapy
24-48	13	Monitor	Phototherapy
48-72	17	Phototherapy	Exchange transfusion
72+	22	Phototherapy/exchange transfusion	Exchange transfusion

fluid needs met with breast milk or infant formula. Loose stools, skin changes (e.g., rash, tan), and sensory deprivation may be temporary side effects.

- Promote parent-infant interaction by allowing short periods out from phototherapy with the eye shields removed. Encourage parents to participate in care and feedings. Home phototherapy allows more parent interaction.
- Monitor bilirubin levels for results within 12 to 24 hours after treatment has begun (phototherapy alone may reduce bilirubin by 3 to 6 mg/dl). Check bilirubin levels every 8 to 24 hours and at least once every 24 hours after phototherapy has ended. Hospital discharge need not be delayed because rebound is seldom more than 1 mg/dl. Phototherapy may be discontinued when serum bilirubin levels are 14 to 15 mg/dl.
- Keep in mind that exchange transfusion is rarely needed except for severe cases (such as healthy infants over 2500 g with bilirubin over 25 mg/dl or high-risk infants over 2500 g with bilirubin over 18 mg/dl). High-risk infants are those with Apgar scores under 7, hypoxia, acidosis, hypothermia, hypoglycemia, sepsis, hypoalbuminemia, or clinical deterioration for any reason.
- Note that interruption of breastfeeding is not necessary in healthy term infants. Acceptable treatment may include observation, phototherapy, supplemental formula feeding, or a combination of these. If breastfeeding is interrupted for 72 hours and bilirubin does not decrease, the infant does *not* have breast milk jaundice. The risk for interrupting breastfeeding is that the interruption can become permanent and the benefits are negligible.
- Remember that investigational drug therapy may include phenobarbital, albumin, and metalloprotoporphyrins.

Counseling and prevention

- Teach the parents about jaundice, including the cause and treatments, the fact that it is self-limiting, and that it is common in the newborn period.
- Instruct all parents to recognize jaundice (see the Note box following this section).
- Instruct parents to monitor a new infant for changes in activity (e.g., lethargy), poor feeding, or any other signs of sepsis (e.g., fever or hypothermia, respiratory difficulty, diarrhea, vomiting).
- Encourage parents to feed the infant frequently with breast milk or formula only (avoiding supplemental plain water) to maintain good hydration. Early feedings or non-nutritive sucking or feeding encourages gastrocolonic reflex. These are the most important interventions in decreasing bilirubin.
- Avoid cessation of breastfeeding (and encourage pumping if necessary).
- Encourage natural ultraviolet (UV) radiation exposure for newborns at risk (e.g., place the infant near a sunny window). This method is based on early observations of improvement in jaundice by British nurses. However, it is not a substitute for phototherapy and may expose infants to unwanted UV radiation from the sun, with risks to the skin and eyes. The infant needs a large portion of skin exposed, and this would not be appropriate for infants with temperature instability.
- Keep in mind that early phototherapy is often useful in preventing the need for exchange transfusion.

Follow-up

- Follow-up with a visit to all newborns discharged from the hospital in less than 48 hours for hyperbilirubinemia within 2 or 3 days.
- Recheck bilirubin levels even after phototherapy is discontinued for rebound hyperbilirubinemia.

Consultations and referrals. Jaundice should be evaluated in consultation with a physician.

Note

- Icterus spreads from head to toe and centrally to peripherally.
- Icteral color extending to the toes indicates a high bilirubin level.
- Icterus is easily seen to the naked eye when bilirubin level is 5 to 8 mg/dL.
- Blanching bony prominences highlight yellow coloring of the skin.
- In infants with dark skin, icterus is best seen in the mucosal membranes and sclerae.

Pallor

JENNIFER PIERSMA D'AURIA

Alert

Consult with or refer to a physician for the following:
- Newborn with pallor
- Altered level of consciousness
- Signs and symptoms of shock, respiratory illness, blood loss or purpura with pallor
- History of hemoglobinopathy or deficiency of RBC enzymes

Etiology

Pallor is a common symptom during childhood. It is most commonly caused by constitutional factors, including hereditary or familial trait, limited exposure to sunlight, allergies or atopy, and normal fatigue. Acute pallor frequently accompanies minor childhood illnesses, especially respiratory and GI tract infections. Acute pallor may also be associated with fear of health-related procedures in children and adolescents. Less common causes of acute pallor include closed head trauma, serious infectious processes (e.g., bacteremia, pyelonephritis), shock, and paroxysmal disorders (e.g., seizures, migraines). Pallor may also be associated with a variety of pathologic processes that cause low hemoglobin concentration, vasoconstriction of subcutaneous blood vessels, and edema formation. Chronic diseases such as inflammatory diseases (e.g., rheumatoid arthritis, inflammatory bowel disease [IBD]), disorders associated with edema (e.g., nephrosis, hypothyroidism), cystic fibrosis, and juvenile diabetes mellitus may be associated with pallor. Temper tantrums and breath-holding spells may be accompanied by either pallid (acyanotic) or cyanotic spells.

Incidence

- Heredity is regarded as the most common cause of pallor.
- Pallor is more common in children who live in northern climates during the winter months.

- Pallor is commonly found in children with allergies or atopic dermatitis.

Risk Factors

- Age and gender (e.g., children under 3 years of age and adolescent girls at increased risk for IDA)
- Incompatibility between fetal and maternal Rh, ABO, or other blood-group antigens
- Ethnic background (e.g., sickle cell anemia occurs most commonly in African Americans, thalassemia occurs most frequently in African Americans and children of Mediterranean and Southeast Asian descent)
- Family history of pallor as a hereditary or familial trait, allergies (atopy), high incidence of cancer, inherited hematologic disorder (may have history of jaundice, anemia, splenectomy or cholecystectomy, sickle cell anemia, thalassemia, G6PD), paroxysmal disorders (e.g., migraine, seizures), cystic fibrosis, diabetes mellitus, hypothyroidism, or rheumatoid arthritis
- Children who live in northern climates during winter months
- Children who spend time indoors reading books, watching television, or playing video or computer games
- Children who play indoor as opposed to outdoor sports
- State of physical or mental overwork
- Children with a history of chronic illnesses (e.g., allergy [atopy], juvenile rheumatoid arthritis, IBD, cancer, cardiorespiratory disorders, systemic lupus erythematosus, cystic fibrosis, juvenile diabetes mellitus, hypothyroidism, chronic pyelonephritis, hemolytic disease)
- Environmental history of pica or exposure to lead
- Poor dietary intake of iron, or folate or vitamin B_{12} deficiency

Differential Diagnosis

The practitioner must keep in mind that pallor is generally not the chief complaint. If there is disease present, other signs and symptoms will be present. During the history it is important to ask the parent or child what he or she thinks is the cause of pallor. Frequently parents and older children may have underlying concerns about pallor because they associate it with anemia or leukemia. Several factors may complicate the assessment of pallor during physical examination. They include fluorescent lighting, dark skin tones, and concurrent disorders (e.g., cyanosis, jaundice), which may mask pallor. Table 36-5 outlines diagnostic criteria for developing a differential diagnosis of pallor.

Constitutional factors. Constitutional factors account for the majority of cases of acute pallor that are encountered in primary care pediatrics. They include hereditary or familial traits, limited exposure to the sun, allergy (atopy), normal fatigue, and fear related to health-care procedures.

Minor childhood infection. Minor episodes of respiratory and GI tract illness in children may be associated with acute pallor, fatigue, and listlessness. Generally symptoms other than mild pallor precipitate the office or clinic visit. Pallor is generally limited to the acute stage of the infectious process (refer to Chapters 35 and 41).

Anemia. Parents and children may commonly associate pallor with anemia. Although IDA is a significant cause of pallor in children under 3 years of age and adolescent girls, anemia in general is not the most common cause of pallor in pediatric primary care (see the section on Anemia earlier in this chapter).

Management

Familial trait
Treatments and medications. None are indicated.
Counseling and prevention

- Reassure the child and parents that this condition is within the range of normal.
- Explain the role of melanin in producing differences in skin tones.
- Discuss pallor in relation to body image.
- Increase time outdoors (if desired) and stress the need to use a sun-blocking lotion.
Follow-up. None are indicated.
Consultations and referrals. None are indicated.

Limited exposure to the sun
Treatments and medications. If there are no medical contraindications, increase time outdoors (if desired).
Counseling and prevention

- Reassure the child and parents that this condition is within the range of normal.
- Discuss the importance of fresh air and exercise for physical and emotional health.
- Warn about UV radiation exposure and stress the need to use sunscreen with a minimum sun-protective factor (SPF) of 15.
- Educate the child and parents that indoor exercise and outdoor sports are equally beneficial.
- Caution about the overuse of sedentary activities (e.g., video and computer games).
Follow-up. None are indicated.
Consultations and referrals. None are indicated.

Allergy or atopy
Treatments and medications. If there are no contraindications, increase time outdoors (if desired).
Counseling and prevention

- Reassure the child and parents that this condition is within the range of normal.
- Discuss the predisposition of children with allergies or atopic dermatitis to have pallor and allergic facies.
- Discuss pallor in relation to body image.
Follow-up. Follow-up as indicated for the underlying disorder.
Consultations and referrals. Provide as indicated for the underlying disorder.

Normal fatigue
Treatments and medications. None are needed.
Counseling and prevention

- Reassure the child and parents that fatigue is not pathologic.
- Discuss sleep, rest, and nutrition principles.
- Discuss measures to promote relaxation and reduce anxiety or stress.
Follow-up. Schedule a return visit if fatigue becomes a chronic problem or other signs and symptoms occur.
Consultations and referrals. Refer to a physician if pallor becomes a chronic problem as a result of psychosocial stressors or physiologic disorder.

Fear of health-related procedures
Treatments and medications

- Establish a trusting relationship with the child.
- Do not ridicule the child.
- Do not reinforce the fear.
- Perform only necessary treatments and procedures.
- Prepare the child for what is happening in advance as well as throughout the procedure.

Table 36-5 Differential Diagnosis: Pallor (782.61)

CRITERIA	FAMILIAL TRAIT	LIMITED EXPOSURE TO SUN	ALLERGY/ATOPY	NORMAL FATIGUE	FEAR OF HEALTH-RELATED PROCEDURES
ICD-9 code		368.13	995.3	780.79	300.29
Subjective Data					
Onset/duration	Long-standing	May be seasonal, especially during winter months in northern climates	Long-standing	Acute, may be prolonged	Acute or may have a history of specific fears related to health-related procedures
Child medical history		Frequently spends time indoors due to a chronic illness, hospitalization	Allergic or atopic disease, allergic facies		May have history of frequent, minor, acute illness, chronic illnesses associated with procedures or treatments (e.g., needles, breathing treatments)
Family history	Family members described as pale		Allergic or atopic disease	May have current family stress (e.g., divorce, move)	Other family members may also have associated fears that are conveyed to the child
Child's review of systems	No fever, weight loss, cough, rash, change in activity, bruising, jaundice, allergy/atopy	If chronic illness, signs and symptoms may be disease related	Symptoms consistent with allergy or atopy	May report stress-related symptoms	May report stress-related symptoms
Diet history		No risk of iron deficiency, especially if <3 years of age or adolescent girl			
Child's daily habits and activities		May spend time indoors, reading books, watching television, or playing video-computer games; may prefer indoor versus outdoor sports		State physical or mental overwork such as competitive sports, cramming for tests, poor eating habits, late-night hours; problems with school, peers, drugs, home	
General appearance	Active and alert; appears pale	Active and alert; appears pale	Appears pale, may have allergic facies	Appears pale; may appear tired or fatigued	Pallor appears suddenly; fearful or anxious facial expression
Growth parameters	Growth rate maintained	Growth rate maintained	Growth rate maintained (may depend on severity)	Growth rate maintained	
Other findings	Within normal limits	Within normal limits; if chronic illness, findings not related to anemia of a chronic disorder	May be consistent with allergy or atopy	Within normal limits	May have increased heart rate, respiratory rate, blood pressure, rest of physical examination normal
Objective Data *Laboratory data*	Hematocrit and hemoglobin tests may be necessary; if done, results will be within normal limits for age				None

- Encourage parents to be present during the procedure (if they desire to be and the child wants them there).
- Reinforce parental attempts to comfort the child.
- Provide distraction (e.g., toys, songs, counting) throughout the procedure.
- Teach and support the use of cognitive strategies (e.g., relaxation, imagery, self-talk).
- Debrief the child after the procedure.
  Counseling and prevention
- Involve the parents and child in discussion about the fear. Give detailed explanations to older children.
- Reassure the child and parents that fear may be very real but that efforts will be taken to protect the child or minimize intrusive procedures.
- Discuss and reinforce strategies to reduce anxiety or stress associated with the health care procedure (e.g., distraction, relaxation, imagery).
- Involve the child and parents in an evaluation of coping strategies and modifications of plan.

Follow-up. Record the child's fears and any effective coping strategies for future health care encounters.

Consultations and referrals. Refer to a mental health professional if persistent fears become exaggerated or disruptive and cannot be managed by the child or parents.

Petechiae and Purpura

JACQUELINE G. IOLI

Alert

Consult with or refer to a physician for the following:
- Petechiae with fever
- Petechiae without fever but with an unexplained origin or cause
- Progressive purpura without fever
- Bleeding or possibility of disseminated intravascular coagulation
- Suspected child abuse

Etiology

The presence of petechiae often indicates a platelet disorder because large ecchymoses, especially those with hard centers, are highly suspicious for a coagulation disorder. The most common cause of petechiae in children is idiopathic (or immune) thrombocytopenic purpura (ITP). A less common cause of petechiae in childhood is Henoch-Schönlein purpura (HSP). Whenever petechiae are seen, infectious thrombocytopenia must also be considered as a cause. Trauma and nonspecific vasculitis should be considered in some cases. Any case of petechiae in childhood may also be a symptom of leukemia.

Incidence

- Idiopathic thrombocytopenic purpura is most common between 2 and 5 years of age; usually follows viral infection (rubella, varicella, EBV). An estimated 100,000 people in the United States have ITP, with 20,000 new cases per year.
- HSP occurs more frequently in boys 2 to 7 years of age.
- HSP occurs more frequently in the spring and fall with a history of upper respiratory tract infection in the previous 1 to 3 weeks.

Risk Factors

- Viral infection
- Upper respiratory tract infection

Differential Diagnosis (Table 35-6)

Idiopathic thrombocytopenic purpura. ITP is a benign, self-limited disorder of previously healthy children. It is characterized by production of antiplatelet antibodies that cause thrombocytopenia by binding to platelets. These antibody-platelet complexes are destroyed in the spleen, causing thrombocytopenia. ITP may be seen after a recent viral illness such as rubella, varicella, measles, or EBV. Despite thrombocytopenia, the surviving platelets in the circulation are young and relatively "sticky"; thus there is less bleeding than would be expected for the degree of thrombocytopenia, and severe bleeding is quite rare (e.g., intracranial, GI). Sudden onset of petechiae with mucocutaneous bleeding is the hallmark sign of ITP. Complications from ITP (e.g., serious bleeding) are rare. ITP is a diagnosis of exclusion. The CBC count should reflect isolated thrombocytopenia without anemia or neutropenia, and the physical examination should be normal, without hepatosplenomegaly or lymphadenopathy. Many practitioners obtain a prothrombin time/partial thromboplastin time (PT/PTT), but these are expected to be normal. Checking the bleeding time is unnecessary and will most likely be prolonged in any child with a platelet count under 50,000. Antiplatelet antibody testing is not clinically useful in acute ITP but may be of some academic interest. Since ITP can be secondary to HIV infection, HIV testing should be considered if appropriate risk factors are present. Some controversy exists in the pediatric hematology community about how aggressively ITP should be treated or even if it should be treated at all. ITP is characterized by spontaneous remissions without treatment.

Vascular nonthrombocytopenic purpura, or Henoch-Schönlein purpura. HSP is a nonthrombocytopenic purpura and is a common form of vasculitis in childhood. Antigen-antibody complexes occur throughout the body, with an unknown cause or mediated by toxins from virus or by drugs. In 50% of cases, HSP follows an upper respiratory tract infection. The hallmarks of the physical examination are palpable purpura (especially of the buttocks and lower extremities) and polyarthritis. In addition, the neurologic system can be affected (e.g., headache, changes in mental status or irritability, seizures), as can the GI system can in two thirds of cases (e.g., heme-positive stools, abdominal pain); about 40% of children have renal involvement (e.g., nephrotic syndrome, renal failure in only 5%). Remission usually occurs within a month without intervention. Helpful laboratory studies in the making of the diagnosis include CBC count, electrolytes, blood urea nitrogen (BUN) and creatinine, liver function, erythrocyte sedimentation rate (ESR), antinuclear antibody (ANA), rheumatoid factor, complement C3 and C4, PT/PTT, blood cultures, immunoglobulin A (IgA), and urinalysis.

Infectious thrombocytopenia. Purpura and petechiae associated with fever are classic signs of meningitis and other serious viral or bacterial illness. Infectious thrombocytopenia can occur with many bacterial or viral illnesses, including septicemia, bacteremia, HIV infection, rubella infections, echovirus 9, meningococcemia, and rickettsial infections. In these cases, petechiae are a sign of more serious illness that must be managed in a hospital setting. As a general rule, more severe, widespread petechiae indicate more serious illness.

Trauma. Trauma can produce petechiae. This can be self-induced, but the possibility of nonaccidental trauma must also

Table 36-6 Differential Diagnosis: Petechiae/Purpura in Primary Pediatric Care

CRITERIA	IDIOPATHIC THROMBOCYTOPENIC PURPURA	HENOCH-SCHÖNLEIN*	INFECTIOUS THROMBOCYTOPENIA†	TRAUMA-INDUCED PETECHIAE*
ICD-9 code	287.3	287.0	287.5	772.6
Subjective Data				
Onset or distribution	Acute onset; lasts a few months	Irregular purpuric lesions on lower extremities, buttocks; 2 weeks to 1 month	Severe rash spreading throughout body	Fade within a few days, no new lesions
Pain	None	Arthritic pain of joints, colicky abdominal pain	Neck pain, myalgia, arthralgia	
Other symptoms	Mucocutaneous bleeding; epistaxis, otherwise healthy	Gastrointestinal tract symptoms, arthralgia, hematuria	Other signs of illness are usually present (e.g., vomiting, anorexia)	No other signs of bleeding
Exposure	Recent viral illness (rubella, varicella, measles, Epstein-Barr virus); may be drug-induced immune reaction	Often follows an upper respiratory tract infection		No symptoms of underlying disease; may be associated with violent coughing
Objective Data **Physical examination**				
Petechiae/rash	Petechiae and ecchymosis, especially on lips and buccal mucosa	Raised rash, usually confined to lower extremities and buttocks	Severe rash with general distribution	Confined to local areas
Vital signs	Afebrile	May be normal	Fever, tachycardia, hypotension	Afebrile
Neurologic signs	None	Rare	Changes in mental status; meningococcemia signs: Stiff neck, positive Brudzinski and Kernig signs, irritability, lethargy	None
Associated findings		Nephritis, hematuria, edema		None
Laboratory data	Platelet count low (<50,000 cells/mm³) all other laboratory results essentially normal	Platelet count normal; bleeding time normal; WBC count normal; urine and stool may be positive for occult blood; laboratory findings may reveal renal insufficiency	Elevated WBC count, cultures of body fluids positive	Not usually needed

*Immediate referral to a physician.
†Refer to a physician.

be considered. Violent coughing, crying, cupping, coining, or any kind of mechanical pressure can produce petechiae. This type of petechiae usually fades within a few days, no new lesions occur, no other signs of bleeding are evident, the family history is negative for bleeding, bruisability, or menorrhagia, and there are no signs or symptoms of underlying disease. Petechiae resulting from excessive crying, coughing, or distress are usually limited to the area above the nipple line (i.e., upper chest, neck, face). These cases require only continuous reassessment and observation as long as the platelet count is within normal limits.

Other diseases. Other differential diagnoses may include acute lymphoblastic leukemia, systemic lupus erythematosus, von Willebrand disease or platelet function defect, hemolytic-uremic syndrome (usually following gastroenteritis), and Rocky Mountain spotted fever.

Management

Idiopathic thrombocytopenic purpura
Treatments and medications

- Keep in mind that over 90% of patients have spontaneous remission within 9 to 12 months.
- Remember that children over 10 years of age, especially females, have a higher risk of chronic ITP than younger children and males in general.
- Provide comfort and palliative care; acetaminophen as needed.
- Observe for risk of hemorrhage.

For a platelet count less than 20,000 cells/mm³ or symptomatic thrombocytopenia consider:

- Prednisone 2 mg/kg per day administered orally for 10 days, then tapered over 10 days to decrease bleeding tendency
- Possible bone marrow aspiration before corticosteroid therapy is started to rule out malignancy
- Intravenous γ-globulin therapy 1g/kg per day for 1 to 3 days
- Splenectomy in severe or chronic cases (symptoms lasting 6 months to 1 year without remission)

Counseling and prevention

- Explain to the parents and child the normal course of the disease.
- Instruct parents to call if there are any bleeding episodes, especially epistaxis, and *any* trauma to the head, neck, chest, back, or abdomen.
- Counsel about prevention of further bleeding or trauma (e.g., gentle handling; avoidance of sports, aspirin or other salicylate products [bismuth salicylate or Pepto-Bismol], nonsteroidal antiinflammatory drugs [NSAIDS]).

Follow-up. Instruct the parents to call or schedule a return visit immediately if there are signs of bleeding. Have the patient return for a platelet count check weekly until stable, then monthly until stable, and then after the first viral illness. Determine the frequency of assessments with the hematologist.

Consultations and referrals

- Notify the school nurse of the ITP.
- Refer all cases to a hematologist.
- Immediately refer to physician for the following findings: purpura with fever, systemic or prolonged thrombocytopenia, neutropenia, any abnormal WBCs (lymphoblasts or myeloblasts on smear), anemia, bone pain, congenital anomalies.

Vascular, nonthrombocytopenic purpura, or HSP
Treatments and medications

- Referral to a physician for supportive care and guidance in co-management
- Spontaneous resolution usually in 1 to 3 months
- Prednisone (also see Treatments and Medications for ITP)

Counseling and prevention. Explain the usual course of the disease to the child and parents and educate about possible complications.

Follow-up. Observe closely for complications, including renal failure, hemorrhage, central nervous system (CNS) manifestations, or intestinal obstruction or perforation.

Consultations and referrals. All suspected cases of HSP should be referred to or co-managed with a physician.

Infectious thrombocytopenia
Treatments and medications. Cultures of cerebrospinal fluid, blood, urine, skin lesions may be performed

Counseling and prevention. None is indicated.

Follow-up. None is indicated.

Consultations and referrals. Refer to a physician. Provide immediate hospitalization for antibiotic therapy and intensive supportive care.

Resources

Australian Iron Status Advisory Panel (www.ironpanel.org.au/AIS/AISdocs/index.html)
Cooley's Anemia Foundation (www.thalassemia.org)
Dietician.com (www.dietician.com)
An Introduction to G6PD Deficiency (rialto.com/g6pd/)
ITP People Place (www.ITPpeople.com)
Joint Center for Sickle Cell and Thalassemic Disorders at Harvard University and Massachusetts General Hospital (cancer.mgh.harvard.edu/medOnc/sickle.htm)
KidsGrowth.com (www.kidsgrowthmarketplace.com)
Nutrition Education for New Americans Project (monarch.gsu.edu/nutrition/)
Recommendations to Prevent and Control Iron Deficiency in the United States (wonder.cdc.gov/wonder/prevgid/m0051880/m0051880.htm)
Thalassemia.com (Children's Hospital Oakland) (www.thalassemia.com)

Bibliography

Augustine, M.C. (1999). Hyperbilirubinemia in the healthy term newborn. *The Nurse Practitioner, 23*(4), 24-43.
Buchannan, G.R. (1999). The tragedy of iron deficiency during infancy and early childhood. *Journal of Pediatrics, 135*(4), 413-415.
Centers for Disease Control and Prevention. (1998). Recommendations to prevent and control iron deficiency in the United States. *Morbidity and Mortality Weekly Report 47*(RR-3), 1-36.
Deacon, J. & O'Neill, P. (1999). Core curriculum for neonatal intensive care nursing (2nd ed.). Philadelphia: W.B. Saunders.
Dixon, L. R. (1997). The complete blood count: Physiologic basis and clinical usage. *Journal of Perinatal and Neonatal Nursing, 11*(3), 1-18.
Friedman, D.L. (2000). Pallor. In Schwartz, M.W. (Ed.). *The 5 minute pediatric consult*. Philadelphia: Lippincott, Williams & Wilkins.
Harley, J.R. (1997). Disorders of coagulation misdiagnosed as nonaccidental bruising. *Pediatric Emergency Care, 13*(5), 347-349.

Korones, D.N. & Cohen, H.J. (1997). Anemia and pallor. In Hoekelman, R.A., Friedman, S.B., Seidel, H.M., & Weitzman, M.L. (Eds.). *Pediatric primary care*. St. Louis: Mosby.

Kwiatkowski, J.L., West, T.B., Heidary, N., Smith-Whitley, K., & Cohen, A.R. (1999). Severe iron deficiency anemia in young children. *Journal of Pediatrics, 135*(4), 514-516.

Looker, A.C., et al. (1997). Prevalence of iron deficiency in the U.S. *Journal of the American Medical Association, 277* (12), 973-976.

Lozoff, B., Jimeniz, E., Hagen, J., Mollen, E., & Wolf, A.W. (2000). Poorer behavioral and developmental outcome more than 10 years after treatment for iron deficiency in infancy (electronic article). *Pediatrics, 105*(4), e51.

Oski, F.A. (1993). Iron deficiency in infancy and childhood. *The New England Journal of Medicine, 293*(3), 190-193.

Rosenblatt, D.S. & Whitehead, V.M. (1999). Cobalamin and folate deficiency: Acquired and hereditary disorders in children. *Seminars in Hematology, 36*(1), 19-34.

Schwoebel, A. & Sakraida, S. (1997). Hyperbilirubinemia: New approaches to an old problem. *The Journal of Perinatal and Neonatal Nursing, 11*(3), 78-97.

Swain, R.A. & St. Clair, L. (1997). The role of folic acid in deficiency states and prevention of disease. *The Journal of Family Practice, 44*(2), 138-144.

Taketomo, C.K., Hodding, J.H., & Draus, D.M. (1998). *Pediatric dosage handbook* (5th ed.). Cleveland, OH: Lexi-Comp.

Tunnessen, W.W. (Ed.). (1999). *Signs and symptoms in pediatrics* (3rd ed.). Philadelphia: J.B. Lippincott.

Walters, M.C. & Abelson, H.T. (1996). Pediatric hematology: Interpretation of the complete blood count. *Pediatric Clinics of North America, 43*(3), 600-620.

Wickramasinghe, S.N. (1999). The wide spectrum and unresolved issues of megaloblastic anemia. *Seminars in Hematology, 36*(1), 3-18.

World Health Organization. (1987). *Requirements of vitamin A, folate, and vitamin B_{12}*. Geneva, Switzerland: World Health Organization.

Chapter 37 *Integumentary System*

Abscesses (Boils), p. 496
Acne, p. 499
Birthmarks, p. 504
Bites: Insect, Animal, and Human, p. 508
Corns and Calluses, p. 513
Diaper Rash, p. 514
Hair Loss, p. 518
Heat Rash, p. 520
Hives (Urticaria), p. 521
Lice (Pediculosis), p. 522
Minor Trauma: Abrasions, Lacerations, Bruises, and
    Puncture Wounds, p. 525
Nail Injury and Infection, p. 526
Rash, p. 528
Scaly Scalp, p. 533
Sunburn, p. 535
Warts (Verrucae), p. 537
Weeping Lesions (Impetigo), p. 540

Risk Factors*

- Infancy and adolescence
- Low birth weight (LBW), including prematurity
- Immunization status incomplete
- Decreased mobility
- Emotional and physical stress
- Obesity
- Medication use (e.g., of photosensitizing drugs, corticosteroids)
- History of recurrent skin infections
- Recent streptococcal infection
- Sustained hypoxia (evidenced by nail clubbing), which may indicate cardiac dysfunction, cardiac malformations, bronchopulmonary dysplasia, or severe anemia
- Family or child history of allergies, atopic dermatitis (eczema), psoriasis, or melanoma
- Systemic disorders (e.g., immunosuppression, diabetes)
- Anemia
- Poor hygiene
- Crowded living conditions
- Trauma
- Poor nutrition
- Blistering, repeated burns and exposure, or fair eye and skin color (which lead to increased risk of sunburn)
- Drug abuse, especially of intravenous drugs
- Environmental exposure
- Insect bites

*Chapter overview written by Jane A. Fox and Loren O'Connor Dempsey.

Health Promotion

Prevention of Infections and Promotion of Skin Integrity

- Teach parents the importance of immunization status, nutrition, hygiene, sleep requirements, and exercise as they relate to health promotion.
- Teach the proper handwashing technique, including the washing of hands before eating and after toileting.
- Teach the washing of the face and body with a washcloth to dislodge oil and dirt.
- Advise the use of moisturizing soap and water for routine bathing and handwashing.
- Teach parents the role of antibacterial products and advise limited use of antimicrobial soaps to avoid overly dry skin, except during periods of infectivity with known or suspected pathogens.
- To prevent dry skin, instruct parents on washing the child with tepid, not hot, water, to preserve body oils. Pat dry and avoid rubbing. Use mild soaps such as Dove (unscented), Aveeno, or Basis. Use a liberal application of moisturizers; unscented products are best (e.g., Aveeno, Eucerin, Vaseline Intensive Care, Nutraderm 30, Lubriderm, Alpha-Keri, Cetaphil), keeping in mind that generic moisturizers are less expensive. Apply while skin is damp from the bath.
- Discuss the risks and infection control measures if the patient is considering body piercing, tattooing, or branding.

For infants

- Encourage parents to have infants immunized.
- Suggest careful cleansing when changing a diaper to prevent diaper rash. Advise parents to allow air-drying of the diaper area when possible, and to change the diaper as soon as possible if soiled with stool.
- Teach about proper diaper disposal and careful handwashing.
- Avoid heavily perfumed soaps, moisturizers, and shampoos.
- Launder baby items with gentle detergents (e.g., Dreft, Ivory Snow). Keep in mind that generic store brands are less expensive.
- Double-rinse laundry in the washer if the infant is sensitive to soaps.
- Wash the infant's face (and neck) with plain water after spit-ups to avoid skin irritation.
- Avoid the use of talcum-powder products. Talcum is composed of large particles that, when inhaled, stick in the pulmonary tree and create a potential risk for respiratory distress or infection.
- Dress the infant in cotton clothing whenever possible.
- Avoid sun exposure for an infant (see Sunburn Prevention). An infant should wear a hat and sunglasses if exposed to the sun.

For toddlers and school-age children
- Keep immunizations current.
- Help the child develop good hygiene habits, including washing hands before eating and after toileting.
- Teach the child to wash the face with an appropriate soap and washcloth to dislodge oil and dirt.
- Have the child avoid play in open sandboxes that may be a reservoir for animal feces and urine.
- Teach the parents and older child to apply sunscreens liberally over sun-exposed skin surfaces before engaging in outdoor play. Limit sun exposure during peak hours (10 AM to 2 PM). Advise the use of wide-brimmed hats, protective clothing, and sunglasses.
- Teach parents the limited role of tents, tree canopies, and so on in limiting ultraviolet (UV) radiation exposure.
- Teach tick- and insect-bite prevention and the use of insect repellents.

For adolescents
- Keep immunizations current.
- Help develop good hygiene habits, including washing hands before eating and after toileting; showering daily, especially after exercise, with tepid (not hot) water to preserve body oils; patting dry to avoid rubbing; and applying moisturizers while skin is moist to improve absorption.
- Teach the teenager to wash the face with an appropriate soap and washcloth to dislodge oil and dirt. Over-the-counter (OTC) acne products may be used as a first-line defense against acne. Advise the teenager and parents to schedule an office visit if acne develops to ensure early intervention. OTC products are not as effective as prescribed treatments. (See Acne later in this section.)
- Instruct on the importance and proper use of sunscreens (see Sunburn in this chapter).
- Instruct the patient to avoid UV radiation exposure if using the following: cosmetic preparations containing furocoumarin; systemic antibiotics, especially doxycycline, tetracycline, sulfonamide, and nalidixic acid; antifungal preparations, especially griseofulvin.
- Discuss with parents and adolescents the need to read information given with OTC medications to decrease risk of sun-sensitive reactions. Advise the parents and adolescent to develop a habit of discussing side effects of prescription and OTC drugs with their pharmacist and health care practitioner.
- Teach tick- and insect-bite prevention.
- Advise wearing shoes outdoors.
- Teach the teenager about sexually transmitted diseases (STDs) or infestations spread through skin-to-skin contact (e.g., herpes, genital warts, scabies, crabs). Barrier contraception (e.g., male and female condom, dental dam) do not ensure avoidance because these infections commonly occur at sites not protected by the barrier.
- Discuss the risks of body tattooing, body piercing, and branding.

Prevention of Atopic Dermatitis
- Change diaper when wet or soiled with stool to avoid irritation in the diaper area. Wipe the area with plain water for any urine (because it is sterile) and with a mild soap after a bowel movement. Mineral oil may be used in place of water as a cleanser for short periods of time if infant's skin is inflamed and breakdown is eminent. Use of this moisturizing product may prevent diaper dermatitis.
- Avoid the use of soap on the baby's face. No treatment is necessary for neonatal acne. If there is a strong history of allergies within the family, suggest the use of unscented soaps (e.g., Basis, Aveeno, Dove).
- Identify and avoid triggering substances.
- Suggest the use of mild moisturizers (e.g., Eucerin, Aveeno, Nutraderm) or other unscented body lotions if the patient is prone to dry skin.
- Keep in mind that hydration is the optimal therapy. Soak the skin in water and then immediately seal in the moisture with an occlusive substance. Use tepid, not hot, water; pat dry with a towel; and immediately apply emollient. Emollients with a water-in-oil or fatty hydrophobic base are the best choices. Moisturizing ointments or creams should be applied three or four times a day or whenever the skin feels dry. Lotions are the least helpful of the moisturizers. An emollient should be applied after handwashing. Topical steroids are the mainstay of treatment.

Prevention of Sunburn
- Warn the parents and teenager that UV radiation exposure, especially exposure that results in burns, has been linked to skin cancer in adulthood. Inform parents and teens that protection from UV radiation is the primary goal in sunburn protection. Daily use of sunscreens and eye protection is the best protection against UV radiation skin and eye damage.
- Inform the parents and teenager about the risks of sun beds and sunlamps (including the risk of retinal damage).
- Inform the parents and teenager that open spaces such as snow, water, and sand-covered areas reflect and intensify UV radiation.
- Ask the teenager about the desire for sun tanning and provide pointed preventive education to reduce the risks of UV radiation skin and eye damage.
- Teach the parents and teenager how to apply sunscreen properly. The product must be applied thickly and evenly to all sun-exposed skin surfaces. Apply before the child is dressed at home, at least 30 minutes before exposure.
- Use a para-aminobenzoic acid (PABA)–free sunscreen with a skin protection factor (SPF) of at least 15, protecting against UV A and B rays, at all times. Inexpensive products are as effective as costly ones, provided that they meet the basic protective criteria. There are two different types of sunscreens. Physical sunscreens have an active agent of zinc or titanium dioxide and physically block the damaging rays of the sun. They may be preferred to chemical products, especially in young children, because they are less irritating and less all allergenic. Chemical sunscreens contain compounds that absorb some of the damaging rays of the sun. These products may contain PABA, which absorbs UV B rays, or benzophenones, which provide complete UV B protection and partial UV A protection. The dibenzoylmethanes are the most effective UV A screens currently available in the United States (e.g., UVA Shade Guard).
- Pay special attention to nose, face, eyes, and lips. Choose a product that is waterproof, and follow the product guidelines for reapplication. Reapply sunscreen at least every 4 hours and after prolonged swimming, 30 minutes of perspiring, or rubbing with a towel.

- Recommend avoiding exposure by the use of sunglasses with lenses that absorb 99% to 100% of UV radiation and use of a baseball cap or another hat with a brim. Avoid the sun between 10:00 AM and 4:00 PM whenever possible.
- Dress children in lightweight tightly woven long sleeves and long pants when possible. Cotton clothing fitting these criteria is readily accessible, and UV radiation–protective clothing or sunsuits can be found in specialty stores. Parents should be advised to carefully investigate specialty clothing to ensure their child's safety. Sunscreens should always be used with protective clothing.
- In infants less than 6 months of age, remember that UV radiation avoidance and clothing must be used as first-line sun protection, and infants in this age group should be kept out of the sun at all times. Parents should be advised that application of sunscreen to small areas of the body (e.g., hands, face, neck) is reasonable as an adjunct to the other measures.
- Inform parents that reflective canopies such as umbrellas and trees may aid in sun avoidance but provide limited reduction in actual UV radiation exposure (estimated at 50%).

Prevention and Early Identification of Melanomas

Melanoma is increasing in adolescents and adults at a higher rate than any other cancer. Identify those at risk for developing melanoma and offer appropriate education. Those with red hair and freckles who do not use adequate sun protection have the greatest risk. Blistering sunburns and intermittent intense sun exposure during childhood are major risk factors. Another risk factor is an increased number of pigmented nevi, which usually result from increased sun exposure. A family history of melanoma and those children with two or more family members who have had primary malignant melanomas are particularly at risk. Melanomas may develop in childhood in those individuals with one of the rare genetic or premature aging syndromes.

Early identification of melanomas is critical. To assess for and help prevent melanomas:

- Do routine mole checks yearly or more frequently depending on the number of risk factors in any child with risk factors and for all patients once puberty begins.
- Teach parents and the adolescent to distinguish between melanoma and benign nevi.
- Teach the ABCDs of melanoma detection (Box 37-1), which are important but have limitations when applied to children.
- Refer patients with suspicious moles to a dermatologist.
- Educate parents, children and adolescents on prevention. See Prevention of Sunburn.

General Guidelines for Topical Skin Preparations

Topical medications and moisturizers are often prescribed. Practitioners need to be aware of the differences between products to ensure appropriate selection. The effective absorption of a product is affected by age, location of injury or infection, condition of skin (intact or broken down), natural occlusion of site (e.g., axilla, inguinal areas), allergies, other medications, and application method.

Important reminders include:

- Initiate therapy with the lowest concentration available.
- Remember that generic products are generally as effective and less expensive.
- In hot weather, choose the least occlusive product available (e.g., cream or lotion versus ointment). Table 37-1

Box 37-1 The ABCDs of Melanoma Detection

A = Asymmetry—The pigmented lesion has an irregular shape.

B = Border and bleeding—The border is not sharp but notched and uneven. Any pigmented nevus that bleeds may be suggestive of melanoma and needs to be removed.

C = Color—A pigmented lesion that goes from light brown to dark brown is not cause for concern. However, if areas of red, white, or blue appear in a pigmented lesion, the patient should be referred to a dermatologist.

D = Diameter—Pigmented lesions larger than 10 mm are significant because they are more likely to be melanoma. Most benign pigmented nevi in prepubertal children are only 2 to 6 mm.

Data from Morelli, J.G. & Weston, W.L. (1999). Contemporary Pediatrics, 16(6), 65.

---

lists topical corticosteroids that the practitioner may commonly use. Clinicians are advised to consult current drug indices before prescribing.

Topical corticosteroids. Topical corticosteroids are classified according to potency (see Table 37-1). Potency is determined by activity in a vasoconstrictor assay. The most effective is the one that eradicates symptoms with minimal side effects. Most childhood skin eruptions require the use of corticosteroids. Generally a low-medium potency preparation is adequate. Factors to consider when one is selecting an appropriate topical corticosteroid are:

- *Age*—For children with mild to moderate disease, hydrocortisone 1% to 2.5% is usually effective. High-potency topical corticosteroids should be used with caution in children because of possible adverse side effects. Although rare, prolonged use has been associated with stunted growth. The most common adverse effect is thinning of the skin. Those receiving chronic therapy should take frequent breaks from their topical therapy (e.g., no topical corticosteroids for 1 week each month).
- *Site*—Higher potency preparations may be required for areas of thicker skin such as the palms of the hands or soles of the feet. Lower potency preparations should be used in thin skin areas such as the face and skin folds. Even the least potent topical corticosteroid should be used with extreme caution around the eyes.
- *Preparation type*—Ointments have a greater occlusive effect, resulting in better penetration and greater potency. Creams, lotions, and gels are easier to apply. Topical steroids should not be used as a preventive measure. New corticosteroids such as fluticasone have a design to maximize penetration and the antiinflammatory benefits while minimizing adverse side effects.
- *Extent of the dermatitis*—High-potency corticosteroids should not be used when inflammation is widespread to avoid risk of systemic side effects.
- *Application method*—Application should be made one or two times daily (with recent studies having indicated no significant difference in efficacy in an application between one and two times a day) in the direction of hair growth to cover the area affected. Bathe or shower before application to improve penetration.

Table 37-1 Topical Corticosteroids

GROUP	GENERIC NAME	TRADE NAME	
1	Betamethasone dipropionate, augmented 0.05%	Diprolene 0.05%	High potency
		Diproline AF 0.05%	
	Clobetasol propionate 0.05%	Temovate 0.05%	
		Dermovate 0.05%	
2	Diflorasone diacetate 0.05%	Psorcon 0.05%	
	Halobetasol propriate	Ultravate 0.05%	
	Amcinonide	Cyclocort ointment 0.1%	
	Betamethasone dipropionate	Diporone ointment 0.05%	
	Diflorasone diacetate	Florone ointment 0.05%	
		Maxiflor ointment 0.05%	
	Halcinonide	Halog cream 0.1%	
		Halciderm 0.1%	
	Fluocinonide	Lidex cream 0.05%	
		Metosyn 0.05%	
		Lidex ointment 0.05%	
3	Desoximetasone	Topicort cream 0.25%	
	Mometasone furoate	Elocon ointment 0.1%	
	Betametasone dipropionate	Diprosone cream 0.05%	
	Betametasone benzoate	Benisone gel 0.025%	
	Betametasone valerate	Valisone ointment 0.1%	
		Betacap 0.1%	
4	Fluticosone propionate	Cutivate ointment 0.05%	
	Triamcinolone acetonide	Aristocort ointment 0.1%	
	Fluradrenolide	Cordran ointment 0.05%	
	Triamcinolone acetonide	Kenalog ointment 0.1%	
		Adocortyl 0.1%	
5	Fluocinolone acetonide	Synalar cream 0.025%	
	Desonide	Tridesilon ointment 0.05%	
	Triamcinolone acetonide	Aristocort cream 0.1%	
	Fluradrenolide	Cordran SP cream 0.05%	
	Fluocinolone acetonide	Fluonid cream 0.01%	
		Synalar 0.025%	
		Synalar cream 0.01%	
6	Triamcinolone acetonide	Kenalog cream 0.1%	
	Betamethasone valerate	Valisone cream 0.1%	
	Hydrocortisone valerate	Westcort cream 0.2%	
	Hydrocortisone butyrate	Locoid cream 0.1%	
	Hydrocortisone 1%, urea 10%	Alphaderm cream 1%	
	Flumetasone pivalate	Locorten cream 0.03%	
	Desonide	Tridesilon cream 0.05%	
	Alclometasone dipropionate	Aclorate cream 0.05%	
		Modrasone 0.05%	
7	Hydrocortisone 1%	Hytone cream 1%	
		Cobadex 1%	
		Dioderm 1%	
		Mildison 1%	
		Hydrocortisyl 1%	
		Hytone ointment 1%	
	Dexamethasone	Hexadrol cream 0.04%	
	Methylprednisolone acetate	Medrol ointment 0.25%	
	Prednisolone	Meti-derm cream 0.5%	
8	Hydrocortisone 0.5%	Cortaid cream	Low potency

From Cohen, B.A. (1999). Pediatric dermatology (2nd ed.). London: Mosby International.

- *Adverse effects*—The most common adverse effects from the use of topical corticosteroids are thinning of the skin and hypopigmentation.

Emollients. Emollients (lubricants) are any product that reduces friction and leaves a smooth occlusive film that prevents drying. Ointments provide the best lubrication for those with chronic dermatitis especially during the winter months (Box 37-2).

Lotions. Lotions are suspensions of water and medicated powder. Water evaporates, cooling and soothing the skin and leaving medicated powder behind to protect the skin. Lotions

Box 37-2 Lubricants

Petrolatum   Ointment/oily
Aquaphor ointment base
Mineral oil
Eucerin cream
Acid mantle cream
Sheperd's skin cream
Keri lotion
Lubridem lotion
Carmol 10% lotion
Lacticare lotion
Moisturel skin lubricant-moisturizer
Neutroderm lotion
Complex 15 phospholipid moisturizing
   cream and lotion
Cetaphil lotion
Purpose lotion
Oil of Olay (oil free)
Neutrogena moisture   Oil free

From Cohen, B.A. (1999). Pediatric dermatology (2nd ed.). London: Mosby International, Ltd.

may also act as a vehicle for other agents. They are used commonly for acute dermatitis and are excellent for infants. Some lotions (e.g., calamine) must be shaken before use to distribute the medicated powder. Emulsion lotions contain oil, and they enhance drying and are less occlusive than ointments or creams; these lotions include Cetaphil, Keri, Nutraderm 30, Lubriderm, and Alpha-Keri. Antifungal agents and corticosteroids are available in this form.

Ointments. Ointments are a combination of water and oil or pure oil (petrolatum) that hold material on the skin for a prolonged time. The water evaporates, leaving an occlusive film. Products include Aquaphor, Eucerin, Desitin, A&D ointment, and Balmex. Ointments are ideal for barriers, prophylaxis, and dry skin areas. Medication is absorbed by the skin more slowly with ointments. They are least likely to cause allergic reactions or irritation to the skin. They should not be used in intertriginous areas (e.g., axilla, between toes) because such use may increase maceration.

Creams. Creams are a combination of oil (e.g., lanolin, petrolatum) droplets in water. The water evaporates, leaving a film on the skin. As the proportion of oil increases, the preparation becomes more of an ointment. Creams carry medication into the skin and are preferable for intertriginous areas. They may be drying and are sometimes sensitizing. Examples include Lubriderm, Nivea, Keri cream, Eucerin, and Aquaphor cream. Antifungal agents and hydrocortisone are available in this form.

Gels. Gels are composed of water and precipitated colloids. Gels are best for hairy areas including the scalp. Examples include benzoyl peroxide, corticosteroids, tars, and keratolytics.

Oils. Oils are fluid fats. They hold medications to the skin for a long period. Oils are ideal for barriers but are generally not recommended because they are occlusive. Examples include mineral oil, baby oil, and cooking oils.

Aerosols. Aerosols and sprays act in a similar manner to lotions and gels. The active ingredients are incorporated into an aqueous solution allowing for easy dispersion over the skin surface. They are particularly useful on the scalp.

Powders. Powders are an aggregation of fine particles. They enhance evaporation and reduce friction, and they are soothing, absorb fluids, and reduce surface moisture. Powders should be avoided in infants because of the risk of inhalation. They also may cake in skin creases, causing excoriation. Talcum does not absorb water and is the most lubricating. Cornstarch absorbs water but is less lubricating and tends to cake and irritate the skin, creating an excellent medium for bacteria and fungi growth (avoid in the diaper area). Medicated powders such as Caldesene are water absorbent and have antibacterial and antifungal features.

Pastes. Pastes are a combination of oil and powder. They are useful in diaper dermatitis.

Shampoos. Shampoos are liquid soaps or detergents that are used for cleansing the hair. They must be well rinsed from the hair, and the eyes of children should be well protected. Mild shampoos with no added perfumes are useful for those with atopic dermatitis or dry scalp; these products include Neutrogena, Castille soap, and children's shampoos. Tar shampoos may be indicated for treatment of psoriasis and seborrhea.

Wet dressings. The goal in therapy is to allow for evaporation of fluid from the skin surface with resulting débridement of crusts and decreased pruritus. Wet dressings can be made with tap water, saline solution (1 teaspoon of table salt to 1 pint of warm water), or Burrow's solution (1 Domeboro tablet to a pint of warm water). Solution should be applied with soft, clean linens such as a handkerchief or old, clean sheets. The dressing should remain moist for the duration of compression (20 minutes for up to four times daily). This is effectively done with frequent changing and rewetting of cloths. Medications should be applied after compression because they are best absorbed by the skin at that time.

Baths. Oatmeal and baking soda baths are recommended for extensive viral or allergic skin eruptions.

Subjective Data

A complete history of the problem with expanded emphasis on past history for new patients should be obtained. It should include:

- Demographics, including age, sex, and race
- Reason for visit, description of problem, and child and parental concerns
- Onset of symptoms and associated circumstances, with description of rash by parents and child
- Course of illness (e.g., acute, recurrent, chronic)
- Recent trips (e.g., camping) or exposure to others with an infectious disease or rash, including household contacts with a similar rash
- Use of soaps, cleaning products, lotions, shampoos, and hairstyling products.
- Recent change in environment (e.g., use of lawn chemicals, crafts, outdoor activities)
- Associated symptoms (e.g., fever, pain, tenderness, erythema, weeping lesions, odor, pruritus, swollen glands, eye pain, rash, flaking skin, loss of hair, changes in appearance)
- Past medical history, including any atopic dermatitis (eczema), allergic rhinitis, severe burns, photosensitivity reactions, drug reactions, exposure to viral hepatitis, allergies to foods or environmental agents, trauma, fungal or bacterial infections, or excessive sweating
- Medications, both prescribed and over the counter (OTC)
- Allergies, including descriptions of reactions and known allergies

Table 37-2 Terminology of Skin Lesions

LESION	DESCRIPTION
Macule	Small (less than 1 cm [0.4 inch], flat mass; differs from surrounding skin (e.g., freckle)
Papule	Small (less than 1 cm [0.4 inch], raised solid mass (e.g., small nevus)
Nodule	Solid, raised mass; slightly larger (1 to 2 cm [0.4 to 0.8 inch]) and deeper than a papule
Tumor	Solid, raised mass; larger than a nodule; may be hard or soft
Wheal	Irregularly shaped, transient area of skin edema (e.g., hive, insect bite, allergic reaction)
Vesicle	Small (less than 1 cm [0.4 inch], raised, fluid-filled mass (e.g., herpes simplex, varicella)
Bulla	Raised, fluid-filled mass; larger than a vesicle (e.g., second-degree burn)
Pustule	Vesicle containing purulent exudate (e.g., acne, impetigo, staphylococcal infections)
Scale	Thin flake of exfoliated epidermis (e.g., psoriasis, dandruff)
Crust	Dried residue of serum, blood, or purulent exudate (e.g., eczema)
Erosion	Moist lesion resulting from loss of superficial epidermis (e.g., rupture of lesion in varicella)
Ulcer	Deep loss of skin surface; may extend to dermis and subcutaneous tissue (e.g., syphilitic chancre, decubitus ulcer)
Fissure	Deep, linear crack in skin (e.g., athlete's foot)
Lichenification	Thickened skin with accentuated skin furrows (e.g., sequela of eczema)
Striae	Thin white or purple stripes, commonly found on abdomen; may result from pregnancy or weight gain
Petechia	Flat, round, deep-red or purplish mass (less than 3 mm or [0.1 inch]); purpuric lesion
Ecchymosis	Mass of variable size and shape; initially purplish, fading to green, yellow, then brown; purpuric lesion

Modified from Engel, J. (1993). Pocket guide to pediatric assessment (2nd ed.). St Louis: Mosby.

- Sexual history (which should be taken at each visit with an adolescent), with sensitivity to adolescent concerns about privacy (e.g., ask teenager for sexual history while parent is out of the room; know and advise teenager of confidentially law in state of practice). Include complete sexual history, including age of first sexual experience, last sex, description of sex (e.g., oral, anal, vaginal, heterosexual, bisexual, lesbian, gay), any safe sex practices, number of lifetime partners, history of routine preventive care (e.g., Papanicolaou [Pap] tests, STD or human immunodeficiency virus [HIV] screening) and name and phone number of specialty provider, history of STD infection and treatment, involvement of parents or other adults in support of reproductive health care needs, and evaluation of the teenager for ability to cope with stresses associated with sexual relationships (refer for mental health counseling as appropriate) For new patients, include the following:
- Prenatal history
- Neonatal history, including birth weight, gestational age, and neonatal complications
- Hospitalizations, including where, when, reasons, treatments, and resolution of problems
- Chronic conditions
- Immunization history, including doses received and reactions
- Family history, including genetic disorders, chronic disease, allergies, and hair loss
- Social history, including family composition, living conditions, economic status, pets, peer relations, emotional or behavioral problems, attendance in school or day care, and cultural practices

Objective Data

Physical Examination

- Perform a complete physical examination in infants and young children. In older children adapt the physical examination according to symptoms.
- Take temperature.

- Examine the skin in natural light. Notice temperature, moisture, color, turgor, and texture.
- Inspect all skin surfaces, including the scalp, hair, nails, face, oral mucosa, neck folds in infants, and anogenital region.
- Inspect terminal hair (on scalp, eyebrows, axillae, pubic areas) and vellus hair (fine body hair).
- Identify patches of hair loss, and inspect for differences from similar hair in the same region. Observe for erythema, edema, exudate, and trauma to skin surfaces from pruritus.
- Palpate lymph nodes if enlarged. Notice location and size.
- Examine lesions (with a magnifying glass if it is helpful). Notice type, location, color, distribution, pattern. Measure size and describe the lesions. (Table 37-2 presents the terminology of skin lesions.)

Diagnostic Procedures and Laboratory Tests

Diagnostic testing is dictated by history, physical examination, and age of the patient.

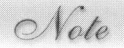

Note

Objective examination is a must in the majority of acute skin conditions. Systemic manifestations of rash may require rapid laboratory evaluation in a hospital setting (as with meningitis). Skin rashes that may be precursors to chronic conditions (e.g., butterfly rash on the face in cases of systemic lupus erythematosus) may require consultation with specialty providers. Seek consultation as appropriate.

A complete blood cell (CBC) count should be obtained on children whose rashes reflect systemic involvement, to rule out bacterial and viral infections. A key marker in parasitic and allergic conditions is an increase in the total number of eosinophils. Elevated total white blood cell count with neutrophilia may ensue after bacterial invasion and tissue damage. The increased production of mature and immature neutrophils that occurs with pronounced bacterial infections is termed a "shift to the left" in the differential. Practitioners are guided in therapeutic modalities by this response.

Erythrocyte sedimentation rate (ESR) is a marker for inflammatory processes occurring within the body. Although nonspecific, an elevated "sed rate" confirms the suspicion that the body has become stressed in some fashion.

Serum Venereal Disease Research Laboratory (VDRL) test or rapid plasmin reagin test is indicated to evaluate for syphilis. Rashes such as those found in pityriasis rosea, tinea, and syphilis become evident in similar fashion with a scaly herald patch (erythematous) with variable pruritus. Testing is also recommended for patients who have genital warts. This test requires a venous sample of blood taken with care to avoid hemolysis. Preparation includes avoidance of alcohol for 24 hours before collection. Test results are recorded as reactive or nonreactive. A positive test result requires prompt care. False-positive results have been reported with mononucleosis, hepatitis, systemic lupus erythematosus, rheumatoid arthritis, and other conditions. Careful history and physical examination are essential.

Fungal examinations and cultures are used to determine if fungus has invaded the skin, scalp, or nail. Specimen collection requires careful inspection of the affected surface for inoculation. Gentle scrapings with a No. 15 scalpel blade or individual hairs broken off at the follicular base are incubated. Collection and processing of fungal cultures varies by laboratory. Consult reference laboratory guidelines before collection of specimens. One of the most helpful diagnostic procedures is the potassium hydroxide preparation. This involves a wet mount of skin scrapings for microscopic examination. 20% potassium hydroxide (KOH) is used to change the visual properties of skin samples to make the scales more transparent.

Dermatophyte test medium (DTM) contains phenol red, an indicator that changes from yellow to red over the course of several days, allowing quick diagnosis. However, DTM has a high rate of false-positive results.

A visual Wood's lamp examination, once believed to be the standard for diagnosis of tinea, provides the examiner with a source of black light (UV radiation). This light source improves visualization of surface alterations (spots and color) in fair-skinned individuals. It is no longer the method of choice for diagnosis of skin dermatosis. It had been useful in the diagnosis of tinea capitis but now the most common fungus associated with tinea capitis is *Trichophyton tonsurans,* which does not fluoresce. Wood's light is valuable in diagnosing tinea versicolor, which fluoresces a green-yellow color.

Wound culture, or pus culture, is used to determine the presence of infection (not the cause) and to identify predominant organisms. Purulent material is aspirated with a syringe and needle from the wound, or sterile swabs are used to absorb purulent material from a draining wound. Swabs are then placed in a culture tube and refrigerated until transport to the laboratory. Culture should be done, if possible, before antibiotic therapy. Care must be taken to avoid contamination of the specimen. A normal culture shows no growth.

Note

Encapsulated pockets of pus, when cultured, may be sterile (no growth of known organisms). Encapsulated pus pockets that do not respond to incision and drainage may need surgical removal.

Skin biopsy and shave or punch biopsy are used to investigate skin lesions of unknown origin. Each requires consultation with a dermatologist. Shaving is used to examine superficial lesions such as rashes and scales. It usually provides a nonspecific diagnosis. Punch and biopsy are tests that are used to evaluate deep lesions and nodules, and a diagnostic report is usually generated directing treatment options.

Serologic testing for Lyme disease (erythema migrans not visualized) requires a venous sample of blood for enzyme-linked immunosorbent assay (ELISA) studies for both immunoglobulin G (IgG) and immunoglobulin M (IgM) antibodies at least 3 weeks after tick bite and before antibiotic therapy is started. Both tests must be interpreted with special attention to the clinical stage of the disease suspected. False-positive and false-negative results are common. Healthy asymptomatic individuals have also been noted to seroconvert. The immunoblot technique (Western blot) has been used for those with borderline ELISA serologic features and whose clinical presentation is inconclusive. (See Lyme Disease in Chapter 44.)

Individuals can be assessed for the risk of developing rubella, commonly referred to as *German measles,* through a simple blood test, or rubella titer. Practitioners must pay close attention to the immunization record of their parents to ensure promotion of health standards. Collection of a rubella titer assists the practitioner in the decision to immunize a child whose records have been lost and in whom immunization is uncertain. Standard prenatal care for adolescents must include a titer for this virus to provide the mother appropriate guidance. German measles is known to cause serious birth defects in unborn children.

The Tzanck smear is an important diagnostic tool in the evaluation of blistering skin disorders. It is most commonly used to differentiate viral diseases (e.g., herpes simplex virus [HSV]) from nonviral diseases. The roof of a blister is removed, and the moist cloudy debris is obtained by scraping of the base. The debris is spread on a glass slide, air-dried, and stained with a Giemsa or Wright stain. Viral blisters appear as a multinucleated giant cell under the microscope.

Food hypersensitivity may be identified by use of skin tests and specific immunoglobulin (IgE) antibodies. A negative skin prick test eliminates immediate food hypersensitivity. The skin prick test is a good preliminary test to exclude food antigens. (See also Allergies in Chapter 43.)

Abscesses (Boils)

LOREN O'CONNOR DEMPSEY

Alert

Consult with or refer to a physician for the following:
- Patient's age less than 1 year
- History of immunosuppression
- Known diabetes
- Signs and symptoms of cellulitis
- Lesions of the face, scalp, or neck (which may require aggressive therapy)
- Lesions that are confluent (which may require aggressive therapy)
- Lesions that are unresponsive to treatment
- Malnutrition

Etiology

Abscesses are the result of bacterial invasion of the skin and surrounding hair follicles. Staphylococci and streptococci organisms, the most prominent cause, enter the body at the site of damaged skin, hair follicles, or sebaceous glands. There is a direct correlation between lesion size, bacteria multiplication, and immune response. Red, painful lesions are formed when polymorphonuclear leukocytes and bacteria are trapped under the skin. Lesions may be as large as 5 cm in diameter. The healing process ensues after rupture or reabsorption of the lesion. Incision and drainage may be necessary to facilitate this process.

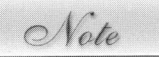

Abscesses contain highly communicable contents. Contact precautions must be maintained.

Incidence

- These occur most commonly in older children.
- Areas of the body at increased risk include hairy body surfaces; extremities prone to trauma, friction, or chemical irritation; and the head, neck, axillae, groin, buttocks, face, and scalp.

Risk Factors

- Impaired skin integrity
- Prior abscesses
- Exposure to an individual with a draining lesion
- Immunosuppression, corticosteroid therapy, leukopenia, or hypogammaglobulinemia
- Diabetes, which increases the potential for prolonged healing

Differential Diagnosis (Table 37-3)

Superficial folliculitis is an inflammation of a hair follicle resulting in a pustule. It is most commonly caused by *Staphylococcus aureus.* Injury, chemical irritation, poor hygiene, and occlusion of the skin may predispose individuals to outbreaks.

Furuncles, also known as *abscesses* or *boils,* are deeprooted, inflamed nodules under the skin. The condition begins with invasion of a hair follicle or sebaceous gland and leads to subcutaneous accumulation of pus and necrotic tissue. Healing occurs after natural absorption or rupture. The most common cause is *S. aureus.*

Carbuncle is the term used to describe two or more furuncles that are interconnected (confluent). Distinguishing factors include multiple drainage sites, location deep in the dermis, slow onset, and mobility of infectious material within the lesions.

Management

Superficial folliculitis

Treatments and medications

- Prescribe systemic medications if needed. The drug of choice is dicloxacillin (see Furuncles and Carbuncles for dosages). Medication is not needed unless the patient is immunocompromised, diabetic, or has a particularly severe case.
- For local care, clean the affected skin with an antibacterial soap (e.g., Dial) and water before topical application of medications. Use a topical ointment or solution such as mupirocin (Bactroban) 2% ointment applied three times a day for 10 days (the drug of choice), or erythromycin solution 2% applied twice daily for 10 days. Cover the site with a loose cotton dressing and change as necessary.

Counseling and prevention

- Instruct parents about proper cleansing techniques and application of topical medications and dressings.
- Instruct the parents and child on prevention of spread to others (e.g., meticulous handwashing, proper disposal of dressings).
- Discuss proper handling of drainage and linens. Wash hands before and after handling drainage and linens. Children must not share a bed or towel until lesions have cleared. Clothing, towels, washcloths, and bedding should be washed daily, and all washable items should be cleansed in hot water with chlorinated bleach.
- Instruct parents not to squeeze or lance lesions; this promotes entry of bacteria into the surrounding tissues and bloodstream and exposes others to pus. Drainage is highly contagious.
- Inform parents that lesions will either come to a head and express contents (pus) or be reabsorbed by the body. Lesions that drain must be covered.
- Explore the child's participation in contact sports. Advise parents to contact the school to determine whether shared equipment has been properly cleaned. Possible carrier sites include weight-lifting apparatus, wrestling mats, and football equipment.
- Inform parents that recurrence, despite appropriate treatment, is possible.
- Discuss with the parents and child the importance of daily showering and shampooing to decrease the staphylococci count on the skin surface.
- Discuss with the parents and child the importance of good nutrition.
- Inform parents that within 2 or 3 days lesions should improve significantly, healing in a week to 10 days.
- Teach parents the signs and symptoms of systemic involvement or worsening infection (e.g., fever greater than 100.5° F, red streaking from lesion, symptoms of cellulitis).
- Instruct parents that children with lesions that are weeping or cannot be covered should be kept out of day care, school, and other social situations in which contact with others cannot be avoided.

Follow-up. Have parents call in 1 week, and schedule a return visit if:

- Lesions do not improve or come to a head within 7 days
- Systemic symptoms develop (e.g., fever greater than 100.5° F)
- Lesions develop on the face
- Red streaking is noted on skin near the lesion

Consultations and referrals. Usually none are needed. Refer to a physician for the following:

- Patient under 1 year of age
- Symptoms of systemic infection, immunosuppression, diabetes or other medical condition that may require aggressive therapy
- Recurrent abscesses despite appropriate therapy

Refer to community supports or social services if family resources for housing or nutritional support are inadequate, and notify the school nurse if appropriate.

Table 37-3 Differential Diagnosis: Abscesses (Boils)

CRITERIA	SUPERFICIAL FOLLICULITIS	FURUNCLES	CARBUNCLES
ICD-9 code	704.8	680.9	680.9
Subjective Data			
Description of problem	Child or parent may report small, raised areas around hair shaft	Child or parent reports one tender to painful red lump under the skin	Child or parent reports deep, painful lumps (two or more) under the skin in the same area
Predisposure for lesions	May report exposure to substances that occlude the skin surface: tar compounds, oils, occlusive dressings; participation in contact sports; exposure to a person with a draining lesion	May report exposure to substances that occlude the skin surface: tar compounds, oils occlusive dressings; participation in contact sports; exposure to a person with a draining lesion. Carriage of *Staphylococcus* in the nares.	May report exposure to substances that occlude the skin surface: tar compounds, oils, occlusive dressings; participation in contact sports; exposure to a person with a draining lesion
Fever	Usually none	Possible	Yes
Onset	Rapid	Varies	Slow to develop
Patient or family history	May report history of recurrent dermatoses; poor diet, homelessness, inadequate access to or use of hygienic utilities (shower, bath)	May report history of recurrent dermatoses; poor diet, homelessness, inadequate access to or use of hygienic utilities (shower, bath)	May report history of recurrent dermatoses; poor diet, homelessness, inadequate access to or use of hygienic utilities (e.g., shower, bath)
Objective Data			
Physical examination			
Vital signs	Normal	Usually normal; fever may be present	Fever typical
Typical location	Scalp, arms, legs, back, neck, face, buttocks	Groin, waistline, axillae, thighs, perineum, buttocks	Neck, shoulders, outer thigh, hips
Description			
Size	1 to 4 mm in diameter	Up to 5 cm in diameter	Up to 5 cm in diameter
Appearance	Yellow pustule(s) at follicular base	Subcutaneous nodule; skin covering is moderately to severely erythemic; firm texture	Deep-rooted nodules with multiple drainage sites; lesions are generally indurated with mild erythema; pus will move from one lesion to another with palpation (confluent)
Number of lesions	Singular to small groups	Usually singular	Two or more that are confluent
Depth of lesions	Superficial	Varies	Usually involves deep tissues
Lymph nodes	Normal	May have lymphadenopathy in nodes near lesions	May have lymphadenopathy in nodes near lesions
Laboratory data	Usually not necessary; Gram stain and culture with antibiotic sensitivity testing in cases of severe resistance; staphylococcal organisms generally isolated; gram-negative organisms *(Klebsiella, Proteus)* have been linked to patients on long-term antibiotic therapy (acne therapy)	Gram stain and culture with antibiotic sensitivity testing in cases of severe resistance; staphylococcal organisms generally isolated	Gram stain and culture with antibiotic sensitivity testing in cases of severe resistance; staphylococcal organisms generally isolated

Furuncles and carbuncles

Treatments and medications. For local care, apply warm compresses for 10 to 20 minutes three or four times a day. Cleanse the affected skin surface with an antibacterial soap (e.g., Dial) before topical application of medications. Use mupirocin 2% ointment applied three times a day for 10 days (the drug of choice), or erythromycin solution 2% applied twice daily. Cover the site with a loose cotton dressing and change as necessary. If the patient is seen in the early stage (i.e., is nondraining), begin therapy with penicillinase-resistant penicillin for minimum of 10 days.

Medications of choice include the following:
- Dicloxacillin 12 to 25 mg/kg divided four times a day, or 250 mg four times a day (for middle and late teenagers)
- Cefadroxil (Duricef) 30 mg/kg per day in two divided doses (serum half-life prolonged in those under 1 year of age), or 1 g orally or 500 mg twice daily (for middle and late teenagers)

- Cephalexin (Keflex) 25 to 50 mg/kg divided four times a day (maximum dose of 100 mg/kg per day), or 500 mg orally two times a day (for middle and late teenagers)
- Erythromycin (as a base) 30 to 50 mg/kg per day divided three or four times a day (maximum dose of 100 mg/kg per day), or 500 mg orally two times a day (for middle and late teenagers; 1 g/day maximum when dosing two times a day)

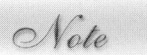

Cases in which lesions are already draining and healing appears to have begun can be treated locally.

Systemic antibiotics must be used if lesions are confluent. Incision and drainage is commonly required for cases unresponsive to antibiotics but is not used in the early phase of lesion development, when systemic antibiotic therapy is the standard of treatment. When a lesion comes to a head, it may be excised with a scalpel blade to speed healing and obtain a wound culture (consult with a physician). Surgical excision may be necessary in severe, recurrent cases.

Counseling and prevention
- See Superficial Folliculitis.
- Inform parents that the entire course of oral antibiotic therapy must be completed.
- Counsel about possible side effects of medications.
- Inform parents that healing of the lesion (crusting) is expected 2 or 3 days after rupture or reabsorption. The site may not heal completely for 2 to 3 weeks.
- Inform parents that surrounding skin may take a few months to return to normal color and texture.

Follow-up. Schedule a return visit in 1 week for severe cases or confluent lesions. Make a telephone call in 1 week in cases for which topical therapy alone is indicated. Schedule a return visit if:
- Lesions do not improve or come to a head within 7 days
- Systemic symptoms develop (e.g., fever greater than 100.5° F)
- Lesions develop on the face
- Red streaking is observed on skin near lesion
- Side effects of antibiotic therapy occur, or treatment is not tolerated
- Condition worsens despite treatment

Consultations and referrals. Refer to a physician for the following:
- Patients less than 1 year of age
- Need for incision and drainage are needed
- Immunosuppression, diabetes, or other medical conditions necessitating aggressive treatment
- Recurrent abscesses, despite appropriate therapy
- Cellulitis.

Remember that severe cases with systemic lymphadenitis, fever, and malaise may require intravenous antibiotics therapy. Notify the school nurse, if appropriate, and refer to community support or social services if family resources for housing or nutritional support are inadequate.

Acne

JANE A. FOX

Alert

Consult with or refer to a dermatologist if severe nodulocystic acne is present or the patient is unresponsive to therapy within 3 months

Etiology

Acne is a disorder of the sebaceous follicles. It is caused by many factors. Androgens in puberty stimulate the sebaceous glands and because of their effect on the pilosebaceous unit (hair and sebaceous glands) play an important role in the pathogenesis of acne. Lesions are caused by obstruction of the pilosebaceous units, which are found in large numbers on the face, upper chest, and back and are rich in sebum. Sebum is an oily substance produced by the sebaceous glands in increased amounts because of elevated levels of androgens. Sebum is also produced in high amounts after birth because of circulating maternal hormones. These hormones are cleared by 6 to 12 months of age but increase again by 6 to 8 years of age, peaking during adolescence. The plugging of the pilosebaceous follicles is another cause of acne vulgaris. Abnormally adherent keratinocytes cause plugging of the follicular duct followed by accumulation of sebum and keratinous debris resulting in the formation of the primary lesion of acne, the comedo. Inflammation of comedones produces papules, pustules, and nodules. *Propionibacterium acnes* is part of the normal skin flora and proliferates in the mixture of sebum and keratinized cells in the pilosebaceous follicles. *P. acnes* metabolizes the triglycerides in sebum to free fatty acids that are extremely irritating to the skin. *P. acnes* also secretes chemotactic factors that attract polymorphonuclear cells to the area and may contribute to damage and rupture of the follicular wall.

Precipitating factors for acne may include familial predisposition; stress; lack of sleep; menses; hot, humid weather; occlusive cosmetics and creams; or an occupation that includes working with frying oils or grease. An excessive production and accumulation of sebum appears directly related to androgenic hormones and the pathogenesis of acne. Testosterone is converted to dihydrotestosterone in the skin, which increases the size and productivity of the sebaceous glands.

Incidence

- Acne affects 30% to 90% of adolescents.
- By their mid-teens, 40% of adolescents will require acne treatment.
- Acne generally disappears by the early twenties in men, later in women.
- Severe disease affects males 10 times more frequently than females.
- Acne commonly occurs on the face, back, and chest.
- Comedonal acne occurs in up to 20% of newborns.

Risk Factors

- History of using oil-based cosmetics, foundation, and moisturizers
- Environmental irritants (e.g., hot, humid conditions)
- Mechanical trauma (e.g., picking, squeezing)
- Menstrual cycle (progesterone dominant)

- Stress
- Hereditary factors
- History of prolonged use of broad-spectrum antibiotics
- Corticosteroid therapy

Differential Diagnosis (Table 37-4)

Acne neonatorum becomes evident as tiny yellow papules on the forehead, cheeks, and nose of infants during the first months of life as a result of sebaceous gland hyperactivity under the influence of maternal hormones.

Prepubescent acne becomes evident as comedones and erythematous papules on the face in the prepubescent period.

Acne vulgaris, the most common type of acne, involves several types of lesions, any of which may predominate. These include open and closed comedones, inflammatory papules and pustules, and nodulocystic lesions. Acne vulgaris may be categorized as mild to moderate to severe. Mild acne is characterized as closed comedones (whiteheads), open comedones (blackheads), and occasional pustules. Moderate acne is characterized as comedones (open and closed), papules, and pustules. Severe acne includes comedones (open and closed), erythematous papules, pustules, and cysts.

Management

General measures. Therapy should be based on type, severity, and location of lesions. It is important to adequately treat acne, even mild cases, because the potential negative psychologic consequences may be much greater than its cosmetic consequences.

Topical agents are effective for mild and moderate acne vulgaris, especially when the condition is limited to the face. They are useful as an adjunct for patients requiring systemic therapy. Their main advantage is avoiding possible side effects associated with systemic therapy. Various prescription and OTC products are available.

Benzoyl peroxide (BPO) (Table 37-5) is the most frequent topical preparation used for the treatment of acne. It is effective against inflammatory and noninflammatory lesions and may be useful as monotherapy for mild acne. It has antimicrobial effects to reduce the colonization of *P. acnes* on the skin surface; decreases surface free-fatty-acid concentrations, which may result in the decrease of retention hyperkeratosis and microcomedones; and also has an antiinflammatory effect by reducing the number of oxygen free radicals. It is available in concentrations of 2.5% to 10% and comes in a variety of formulations (e.g., gels, lotions, washes, creams). BPO may be applied once or twice a day, with skin irritation being one possible side effect. BPO preparations can bleach clothing.

Topical retinoids (see Table 37-5) are an extremely effective class of medication for the treatment of acne vulgaris. They have strong comedolytic and anticomedogenic activity and indirect antibacterial effects. They unblock pores and reduce skin bacteria. Tretinoin is the prototype drug in this class, and it comes in cream, liquid, and gel formulations. Topical retinoids are usually applied daily, generally at night to limit the risk of phototoxicity (a rare side effect). The most common side effects are erythema, dryness, and burning. To minimize side effects, instruct the patient to apply the medication only to thoroughly dried skin. Suggest washing and then allowing 30 to 45 minutes of air-drying. Advise the patient to apply only the minimum amount necessary (a pea-sized amount for entire face is generally adequate). Liquid and gel forms of tretinoin are more drying than the cream. Begin the lower strength cream and gradually increase the concentration of the product as the patient tolerates it. Patients receiving topical retinal therapy must always apply a sunscreen with SPF of 15 to 30 to avoid phototoxicity. Tretinoin is also a pregnancy category C drug, so women of childbearing age must be counseled on the reported risks.

Topical antibiotics reduce *P. acnes* on the skin surface and within the hair follicles. The most commonly prescribed in acne therapy are clindamycin, erythromycin, and sulfonamides. They do not have comedolytic effects and are best used in combination regimen. They are usually applied to affected areas once or twice a day.

Acne neonatorum

Treatments and medications. The disease is usually mild and of short duration. It is a common, benign condition and should resolve spontaneously in 1 to 3 months.

Counseling and prevention

- Describe condition and progression of symptoms.
- Reassure about parenting capability.
- Advise against use of oil-based lotions and creams on face or hair.

Follow-up

- Have parents call in 72 hours to report condition, and again in 10 days.
- Schedule a return visit if condition worsens or as needed for parental reassurance and well-child care.

Consultations and referrals

- Refer to a dermatologist all severe cases and those of long duration.
- Refer to an endocrinologist if an underlying endocrine abnormality is suspected.

Prepubescent acne

Treatments and medications

- See the strategies for Acne Vulgaris (Mild, Moderate, and Severe).
- Wash face twice daily.

Counseling and prevention

- Instruct on the treatment regimen.
- Instruct parents to observe when the face gets greasier; facial washings should be done at this time.
- Assist parents in identifying or predicting stressful situations for the child so that they may be avoided or the stress lessened when possible.

Follow-up

- Have parents call to report progress every 2 weeks.
- Schedule return visits as needed for reassurance, health teaching, and well-child care.

Consultations and referrals. Refer to a dermatologist any severe cases and any cases unresponsive to the prescribed therapy.

Acne vulgaris: mild

Treatments and medications

- Wash the face gently no more than two times daily with a mild soap such as Dove, Aveeno, or Basis.
- Apply a topical agent such as 2.5% benzoyl peroxide gel keratolytic daily or 5% every other day. If no sensitivity is noted within 2 weeks, application may be increased to twice a day. If no response is noted within 1 month, increase the benzoyl peroxide preparation to 10% and apply daily. Gradually increase application to twice a day if no sensitivity occurs. For best results in preventing acne, topical agents should be applied as a thin layer over the entire affected area, not as "spot therapy" for individual lesions.

Table 37-4 Differential Diagnosis: Acne

CRITERIA	ACNE NEONATORUM	PREPUBESCENT ACNE	ACNE VULGARIS
ICD-9 code	706.1	706.1	706.1
Subjective Data			
Age of onset	Usually occurs in infant less than 3 months of age but may occur in child up to 2 years of age	Usually appears between 6 and 8 years of age	Usual onset between 9 and 20 years of age; most severe in girls 14 to 17 years and boys 16 to 19 years
Description of problem	Parents may report "pimples" on face of infant or child	Parents state that child has "pimples, black-heads, or whiteheads"	Chief complaint usually pimples, blackheads, whiteheads, bumps, or "zits"
Aggravating factors	History of parents using baby oil products such as lotions and creams on infant's face, head; sweat	History of child using oil-based facial lotions, soap; hot, humid weather; poor hygiene; mechanical trauma	Same as prepubescent acne; also history of stress, menstrual cycle, use of cosmetics, foundation; occupation associated with frying oils and grease
Past medical history	If numerous pustules are present, there may be underlying endocrinologic abnormality	History of prolong use of broad-spectrum antibiotics	History of prepubescent acne; history of overextended use of broad-spectrum antibiotics; history of using birth control pills; poor sleeping habits
Past family history	Family history may reveal one or both parents having severe acne	Family history of acne in one or both parents or siblings	Family history of acne
Objective Data ***Physical examination*** Skin examination			
Description of lesions	Most common lesions appear as tiny yellow papules; lesions may appear as erythematous papules, papulopustules, and comedones	Comedones, erythematous papules, papulopustules, even nodulocystic lesions noted	Comedones (whiteheads and blackheads), inflammatory papules, pustules, nodules, cysts, scars may be noted
Location of lesions	Cheeks are the most common site, but forehead and chin may be involved	Forehead and chin, but may appear anywhere on the face	Face, back, shoulders, upper chest, neck

Table 37-5 Treatment Options for Acne

PRODUCT	INDICATION	DOSE	SIDE EFFECTS	COMMENTS
Topical Therapies				
Benzoyl peroxide	Noninflammatory and inflammatory lesions	One or two times/day. Decrease frequency if irritation develops. Alternate AM-PM, use if used with another topical agent	May cause skin irritation. May increase sensitivity to sun	Most frequently used topical. It is a peeling agent that dries the skin and helps stop the growth of bacteria.
Antibiotics: tetracycline, erythromycin, clindamycin	Inflammatory acne; clindamycin and erythromycin are the most effective	Two times/day. If irritation develops, drop to once a day or alternate days.	May cause skin irritation. May increase sensitivity to sun. Tetracyclines may cause yellow staining of clothing and skin	
Retinoids: tretinoin (Retin-A, Avita)	Most effective topical agent available	Start with lowest strength (0.025% cream, 0.01% gel, 0.05% solution to minimize irritation). Progress as tolerated	Skin irritation, drying, itching. Increased sensitivity to sun; sunscreen with SPF 15 or greater recommended	A peeling agent that loosens skin plugs. Most effective for blackheads and whiteheads.
Adapalene (Differin)	Acne vulgaris	0.1% gel	Skin irritation, drying, itching	
Systemic Treatments				
Antibiotics				
Tetracycline	Inflammatory acne and cases resistant to topicals	250-500 mg two times/day	GI upset, vaginal candidiasis	Use only in patients over 8 years of age. Antacids, dairy produts and food may decrease absorption. Potential drug interaction with penicillin, anticoagulants, oral contraceptives.
Doxycycline	Same as above	100 mg two times/day	GI upset, photosensitivity; may be taken with food	Use only in patients over 8 years of age. Antacids and dairy products may decrease absorption. See tetracycline.
Minocycline	Same as above	50-100 mg two times/day	Vestibular disturbances, blue-gray pigmentation in areas of cutaneous inflammation	Has been associated with severe but rare side effects. See tetracycline and doxycycline.
Erythromycin	Same as above	500 mg two times/day	GI upset; emergence of resistant *Propionibacterium acnes* strains common	Potential drug interaction with theophylline, digoxin, anticoagulants, terfenadine, astemazole.
Co-trimoxazole (trimethoprim-sulfamethoxizole)	Same as above	160-800 mg two times/day	Rash, hypersensitivity reactions, bone-marrow suppression	
Retinoids				
Isotretinoin (Accutane)	Resistant or cystic acne	Refer to dermatologist	Severe birth defects, elevated lipids, muscle aches, joint pain, photosensitivity	Refer to dermatologist.
Oral contraceptives	Androgen-induced acne	Daily	Avoid contraceptives with lorgestrel or levonorgestrel; they may increase acne	Do not prescribe OCPs with lorgestrel or levonorgestrel because they may increase acne. Refer to gynecologic practitioner.

Data from Pogue, S.J. (1999). Advance for Nurse Practitioners, 7(4), 55.

- For more persistent cases, a comedolytic agent may be added (e.g., topical retinoic acid cream [Retin-A] 0.025% to 0.05% daily). If no sensitivity is noted within 2 weeks, application may be increased to twice a day. If no response is noted within 1 month, increase the retinoic acid preparation to 0.1% cream or 0.025% gel daily. Gradually increase application to twice a day if no sensitivity occurs.

Counseling and prevention

- Carefully explain the cause and prolonged course of the disease and that it is not curable but is controllable.
- Explain the treatment regimen and the importance of the patient's active and willing participation. Include a written, detailed description of the home treatment schedule (e.g., names of the topical agents to be applied, frequency, dosages, amount, time). Instruct to apply medication lightly to the affected area and not rub in vigorously. Apply as a thin layer to the affected area, rather than using "spot therapy."
- Instruct on proper skin cleansing. Wash face or other affected areas with warm, soapy water no more than three times daily for 1 minute. Rinse well with warm water. Use a clean washcloth with each washing. Avoid abrasive agents.
- Inform of any possible side effects of the prescribed treatment. If noticeable erythema and pruritus develop in response to topical medication, discontinue use temporarily for 1 week and then resume with less frequent application. A feeling of warmth and slight stinging with application should be expected.
- Inform the patient that after local treatment is instituted, acne may appear worse before it improves.
- Advise there will be a delay in noticeable improvement for 4 to 8 weeks.
- Stress the need to eat a normal, well-balanced diet. Address misconceptions about diet control.
- Instruct that overexposure to sunlight can have adverse effects, alone or in combination with retinoic acid. It may be necessary to discontinue these medications in the summer. A sunscreen must be used.
- Instruct not to pick or squeeze lesions; this habit retards healing and causes scarring.
- Advise to shampoo frequently and to change pillowcase daily.
- Instruct that "facials" may exacerbate acne.
- Stress the importance of using water-based cosmetics, and explain that acne medication can be applied under cosmetics and sunscreens. Oil-based cosmetics, face creams, and hairstyling mousse should be avoided.

Follow-up

- Remember that return visits must be individualized according to severity of the acne and the emotional needs of the patient.
- Remember that return visits are necessary before application times and strengths of topical antimicrobial and comedolytic agents are increased.
- On average, schedule return visits every 2 to 4 weeks.
- Schedule a return visit if noticeable erythema or pruritus develops in response to topical medication.

    Consultations and referrals. Usually none are needed.

Acne vulgaris: moderate

Treatments and medications

- See the strategies for Acne Vulgaris: Mild.

- Perform a complete comedone extraction. The face should be thoroughly washed with warm, soapy water before and after removal of comedones.
- Apply hot soaks to pustules five or six times a day.
- For systemic therapy, prescribe tetracycline (the drug of choice) 250 mg orally four times a day, or 500 mg orally twice a day for 1 month. If no improvement is noted, increase tetracycline to 1.5 g/day for 2 weeks, and then to 2 g/day for 2 weeks. With considerable improvement, decrease tetracycline to 250 mg twice a day. Do not use in children 8 years of age and younger because tetracycline-class antibiotics may cause permanent yellow-gray-brown staining of the teeth. Photosensitivity is also a concern. Dairy products and antacids may inhibit absorption. Tetracycline should be taken 1 hour before or 2 hours after meals. Systemic therapy may be combined with topical therapy. If a significant inflammatory process is evident, topical antibiotics or a combination of erythromycin and benzoyl peroxide (Benzamycin) may be effective.
- One treatment option for females with mild to moderate acne is estrogen therapy through the use of birth control pills. One birth control pill approved by the Food and Drug Administration (FDA) for treating acne is norgestimate—ethinyl estradiol (Ortho Tri-Cyclen).

Counseling and prevention

- See the strategies for Acne Vulgaris: Mild.
- Inform about the side effects of tetracycline. The patient must restrict exposure to sunlight and take medication on an empty stomach 1 hour before or 2 hours after meals. Dairy products interfere with absorption. The patient should not take medication if there is any question of pregnancy. Candidiasis may occur in girls.
- If the patient is taking birth control pills, she may need to change to one that does not contain norgestrel, norethindrone, or norethindrone acetate.
- Instruct on the extraction of comedones. Purchase a comedo extractor at a local pharmacy. Place the hole at the end of the extractor over comedo and gently press against the skin with a mild sliding motion. The face should be thoroughly washed with warm, soapy water before and after removal. Hot towels may be placed on skin before extraction. The extractor should be carefully washed with soap and water before and after use and kept in alcohol between uses.
- Advise that the condition usually worsens before it improves, because the comedones come to the surface.

Follow-up

- Make a telephone call in 72 hours to determine the effectiveness of and compliance with treatment.
- Schedule a return visit in 2 weeks to assess effectiveness of tetracycline therapy.
- Schedule return visits approximately every 2 weeks according to individual needs (e.g., if tetracycline dose must be gradually increased). Visits may be decreased to once a month if improvement is noted.

Consultations and referrals

- Refer to a dermatologist if acne remains unresponsive to therapy or condition worsens; for those patients with nodulocystic lesions, draining cysts and sinuses, scars, diabetes, or secondary bacterial infections; and for those patients who are pregnant.
- Refer to a mental health professional if counseling is needed for problems in body image or low self-esteem.

Acne vulgaris: severe

Treatments and medications

- See the strategies for Acne Vulgaris: Mild and Acne Vulgaris: Moderate.
- Limit refills on tetracycline to ensure follow-up visits.
- In severe cases of acne where other treatments have failed, consider isotretinoin (Accutane). This should be prescribed by a dermatologist. There has been much controversy on the use of this medication because of its possible link to depression and suicide in adolescents.

Counseling and prevention. See the strategies for Acne Vulgaris: Mild and Acne Vulgaris: Moderate.

Follow-up. See the strategies for Acne Vulgaris: Mild and Acne Vulgaris: Moderate.

Consultations and referrals. Refer to a dermatologist.

Birthmarks

JANE A. FOX

Alert

Consult with or refer to a dermatologist for the following:
- Port-wine stains in the trigeminal distribution
- Hemangiomas that compromise vital structures (e.g., eyes, ear canals, airways)
- Periorbital hemangiomas or infection
- Lesions that are subject to repeated trauma, causing ulceration
- Atypical lesion, or one with recent change in color border, diameter (greater than 0.6 cm), or asymmetry
- More than five café-au-lait spots
- Lesion greater than 20 cm in diameter and located on the buttocks, scalp, or paravertebral area in the distribution of a garment

Etiology

Hemagiomas are a benign growth of epithelial cells that usually arises in the neonatal period a few weeks after birth. Vascular nevi are ectatic blood vessels. The lesions are usually confined to the skin but are occasionally associated with systemic conditions. Examples are salmon patches, port-wine stains, and hemangiomas. Melanocytic lesions have an increased number of melanocytes. Examples include freckles, café-au-lait spots, mongolian spots, junctional nevus, compound nevus, intradermal nevus, spindle cell nevus, giant congenital nevus, dysplastic nevus, and malignant melanoma.

Incidence

- Hemangiomas are the most common type of soft-tissue growth in infancy
- Vascular nevi occur in 20% to 40% of newborns.
- Melanocytic lesions (e.g., café-au-lait spots) occur in 10% to 19% of the population.
- Mongolian spots occur in 90% of Native American, African-American, and Asian infants.

Risk Factors

- Family history of café-au-lait spots
- Family history of freckles
- Family history of hemangiomas
- Prematurity
- Female gender
- Mother who underwent chronic villus sampling

Differential Diagnosis (Tables 37-6 and 37-7)

Salmon patches are irregularly shaped pink, salmon, or light red macules, usually located on the neck, glabella, or upper eyelids.

Port-wine stains are irregularly shaped red to purple macules. The lesions are usually confined to the skin but may be associated with systemic disorders.

Hemangiomas are vascular nodules to plaques that are strawberry red to deep purple. They are usually located on but not limited to the head and shoulders.

Freckles are round macules that are tan to dark brown. They are usually less than 0.05 cm in diameter and are located on but not limited to sun-exposed areas.

Café-au-lait spots are oval or irregularly shaped macules that are light to dark brown and are located on any part of the body.

Mongolian spots are poorly circumscribed, large, blue-black macules that are located on the buttocks and lumbosacral area.

Junctional nevi are dark brown to black macules that are located on any part of the body.

Compound nevi are slightly raised papules with warty or smooth surfaces that are located on any part of the body. They can be pale to dark brown or red.

Intradermal nevi are dome-shaped papules with smooth, uniform surfaces and are located on any part of the body.

Spindle cell nevi are dome-shaped papules with smooth, firm surfaces and are located on but not limited to the face and legs. They can be pink, red, or brown to dark brown.

Giant congenital nevi are dark brown to black pigmented lesions greater than 20 cm in diameter that are usually located on the buttocks, scalp, or paravertebral area in the distribution of a garment.

Dysplastic nevi are raised papules with atypical features and are located on the trunk, feet, scalp, or buttocks. They are pink, tan, or brown.

Table 37-8 describes several diagnoses that require a medical referral or consultation.

Management

Salmon patches

Treatments and medications. None are indicated.

Counseling and prevention

- Advise parents that the lesion is benign.
- Inform parents that eye and face lesions completely fade between 3 and 6 months of age and that lesions at the nape of the neck does fade but may persist into adulthood.

Follow-up. None is indicated.

Consultations and referrals. None are indicated.

Port-wine stains

Treatments and medications. None are required. Pulsed-dye laser surgery may be done (and several treatments may be necessary) as elective surgery for facial disfigurement; this is usually performed by 5 years of age.

Counseling and prevention

- Inform parents that a port-wine stain does not improve.
- Instruct on ways to cover the stain for cosmetic purposes.

Follow-up

- Provide follow-up care as needed.
- If lesion is in the distribution of the trigeminal nerve, observe for signs or symptoms of Sturge-Weber syndrome (e.g., seizures, mental retardation, glaucoma, hemiplegia). If the lesion is over an extremity, observe for hypertrophy.

Consultations and referrals

- Refer to a physician if Sturge-Weber or Klippel-Trénaunay syndrome is suspected.

Table 37-6 Differential Diagnosis: Vascular Birthmarks

		VASCULAR MALFORMATIONS	
CRITERIA	HEMANGIOMA	SALMON PATCH	PORT-WINE STAIN
ICD-9 code	228.0		757.32
Subjective Data			
Age of onset	Soon after birth	Birth	Birth
Sex/race	Any	Any	Any
Description of problem	Parents may report "birthmark" that first appeared as a blanched area	Parents may report that "birthmark" fades with age but reappears during crying episodes; that "birthmark" blanches with pressure	Parents may report that "birthmark" grows in proportion to growth of child; that "birthmark" darkens and thickens with age
Associated symptoms	Usually none	None	None
Family history	None	None	None
Objective Data			
Physical examination			
Skin examination			
Inspection	Vascular nodule	Flat macule	Flat vascular macule
Location	Located on but not limited to head and shoulders	Neck, glabella, or upper eyelids	Located on but not limited to face and neck
Size/shape	Variable size	Variable size; blotchy, irregular shape; may be transient	Usually unilateral
Description	Strawberry red; may enlarge rapidly during the first 8 months then change to blue-red in color	Pink, salmon, or light red; macule located on the neck is sometimes referred to as a "stork bite" and on the upper eyelids as "angel kisses"	Sharply demarcated; pale pink, to deep red or purple
Palpation	Rubbery, smooth surface; may be slightly raised	Flat	Flat

- Refer to a dermatologist for possible removal of any facial disfigurement or at parents' or child's request.

Hemangiomas

Treatments and medications. None are indicated unless there is compromise of a vital function (e.g., sight, respiration, nutrition), cardiac decompensation, thrombocytopenia, or significant ulceration or deformity (in which case, refer to a physician). Treatment might include prednisone 2 to 4 mg/kg per day tapered over 2 to 4 months; interferon alfa-2a; and laser surgery for any deformity.

Counseling and prevention

- Inform parents that lesions may grow rapidly before spontaneous resolution.
- Inform parents that 50% of lesions resolve spontaneously by 5 years of age and 70% by 7 years of age.
- Advise parents that observation is the best treatment unless the lesion compromises a vital function.
- Instruct parents to observe for changes and call if any are noted.

Follow-up

- Provide observation at well-child visits to monitor growth or resolution.
- Schedule a return visit if enlargement is noted by parents.

Consultations and referrals. Provide immediate referral to a physician if the lesion compromises a vital function (see Table 37-7). Also refer to a physician if the lesion is growing or if the child has symptoms of Kasabach-Merritt syndrome (see Table 37-8).

Freckles

Treatments and medications. None are indicated.

Counseling and prevention

- Inform parents that the lesion or lesions are benign.

- Discourage sun exposure.
- Encourage the parents and child to use sunblocking lotion with an SPF of 15 and UV A and B protection when sun exposure is anticipated..
- Recommend that the child wear a hat, sunglasses, and a shirt while exposed to the sun.

Follow-up. None is indicated.

Consultations and referrals. None are indicated.

Café-au-lait macules

Treatments and medications. None are indicated.

Counseling and prevention. Inform parents that if less than five lesions are present, the condition is benign.

Follow-up. Provide periodic observation at well-child visits for tumors of the skin or neurologic involvement.

Consultations and referrals. Refer to a physician if the child has more than five lesions or for the presence of cutaneous tumors or neurologic involvement.

Mongolian spots

Treatments and medications. None are indicated.

Counseling and prevention

- Inform parents that the lesion is benign.
- Counsel parents that the lesion fades with time and usually disappears by 5 years of age, but also that it may persist in adulthood.
- Advise parents that lesions are not bruises. Mongolian spots are almost always present in infants of Asian, Native American, and African-American heritage.

Follow-up. None is indicated.

Consultations and referrals. None are indicated.

Junctional and compound nevi

Treatments and medications. Usually none are needed. Total excision is required if lesions change in size or color.

Table 37-7 Differential Diagnosis: Birthmarks (Melanocytic Lesions)

CRITERIA	FRECKLES (EPHELIDES)	CAFÉ-AU-LAIT SPOT	MONGOLIAN SPOTS	JUNCTIONAL NEVI	COMPOUND NEVI	INTRADERMAL NEVI	SPINDLE CELL NEVI	DYSPLASTIC NEVI
ICD-9 code	709.09	709.09	757.33	←——— Code neoplasm, skin, benign by site ———→				
Subjective Data								
Age of onset	Early childhood	Birth or early infancy	Birth	Birth	Childhood or adolescence	Adulthood but may develop during childhood	Childhood	At puberty, but may appear as early as 5 to 8 years of age
Sex/race	Highly prevalent in children with blue eyes, red or blond hair	Any	Highly prevalent in Native American, African-American, and Asian infants	Any	Any	Any	Any	Any
Description of problem	Parents report freckle is accentuated by sun exposure and lighter in absence of sun exposure	Parents report that "birthmarks" increase in number with age	Parents report that "birthmark" looks like a bruise	Parents report changes in size and appearance of "birthmark" as the infant ages	Parents report that "birthmarks" increase in number with age	Parents report that number, size, and appearance increase with age	Parents report that size and appearance change with age	
Associated symptoms	None	None	None	None	None	None	None	Child may be predisposed to melanoma
Family history	Yes	May have familial history of neurofibromatosis	Yes	No	No	No	No	No
Objective Data **Physical examination** Skin								
Inspection	Flat macule	Flat macule	Flat macule	*(Could progress to compound)* Flat macule	*(Could progress to intradermal)* Slightly raised papule	Raised papule	Raised papule	Raised papule
Location	Located on but not limited to sun-exposed areas	Located on any part of the body	Located on the buttocks, lumbo-sacral area, and sometimes the shoulders	Located on any part of the body including genitalia and mucous membranes	Located on any part of the body	Located on any part of the body	Commonly located on but not limited to the face, legs	Commonly located on trunk, feet, scalp, buttocks
Size/shape	Variable size, usually less than 0.05 cm	Variable size and number; irregular or oval shape	Often very large; single or multiple lesions	Variable		Dome-shaped	Dome-shaped	
Description	Usually rounded but may have an irregular shape; tan to dark brown	Well circumscribed; light brown on light skin, dark brown on dark skin	Poorly circumscribed; blue-black	Borders are distinct; usually hairless; dark brown to black	May be hair bearing (dark, coarse hairs); pale brown to dark brown to reddish brown	Hair bearing; coarse central hairs	Hairless; borders may be irregular or sharply demarcated; pink, red, brown, or dark brown	Irregular borders; atypical features; indistinct margins 6 to 15 mm in size; pink, tan, or brown
Palpation	Flat	Flat	Flat	Flat or slightly elevated	May be raised; warty or smooth surface	Smooth, uniform surface	Smooth, firm surface	Rough surface

Table 37-8 Assessment and Management of Diagnoses Requiring Medical Referral or Consultation

DIAGNOSIS	CLINICAL MANIFESTATIONS	MANAGEMENT
Sturge-Weber syndrome	Port-wine stain in the distribution of the trigeminal nerve or covering the entire half of the face	Refer to physician
		Emotional support
	Highest association with Sturge-Weber is port-wine stain involving bilateral eyelids	Medications as needed for management of seizures and glaucoma
	Clinical symptoms include seizures (beginning as focal motor and then generalized), mental retardation, hemiparesis or hemiplegia contralateral to the lesion, glaucoma	Physical therapy for hemiparesis
		Follow-up by practioner in consultation with physician
Klippel-Trénaunay-Weber syndrome	Congenital vascular malformation associated with localized overgrowth of bone and soft tissue (may include port-wine stain or hemangioma)	Refer to physician
		Emotional support
		Treatment is usually unsuccessful
	Generally involves a lower extremity	Compressive bandages
	Hypertrophy of extremity	Surgery to prevent limb hypertrophy
	Superficial venous varicosities may occur	Radiation therapy is rarely used
	Angiomas of gastrointestinal tract and bladder	
Kasabach-Merritt syndrome	Large hemangioma	Refer to physician
	Rapidly enlarging hemangioma	Emotional support
	Pallor	Prednisone 2 to 4 mg/kg/day orally with frequent evaluations
	Ecchymoses	
	Petechiae	Interferon alfa-2a (may be used in combination with prednisone)
	Bleeding lesion	
	Thrombocytopenia	Compressive bandages
	Anemia	Surgical debulking of lesion
	Disseminated intravascular coagulopathy	Embolization
	Amblyopia or visual obstruction	Irradiation
	Cardiac decompensation (high cardiac output failure)	Platelet transfusion
	Difficulty with urination or defecation	Fresh frozen plasma
		Cryoprecipitates
		Digitalis, diuretics
		Follow-up by physician as needed
Neurofibromatosis (NF)	Family history of NF (only 50% of cases)	Refer to physician
	Presence of five or more café-au-lait macules greater than 0.5 cm after puberty	Emotional support
		Genetic counseling
	May have tumors arising on skin	Pain management
	Skeletal deformities (bowing of shins, may be missing the sphenoid bone)	Observation for NF sarcomas
		Follow-up by physician as needed
	May have seizures, pheochromocytoma, precocious puberty, kyphoscoliosis, bone cysts, pathologic fractures, bone hypertrophy, ependymomas of spinal cord, or malignant astrocytomas	
Giant pigmented nevi	Congenital pigmented lesion greater than 20 cm located on buttocks, scalp, and paravertebral area in the distribution of a garment	Consult with physician
		Refer to dermatologist
		Emotional support
	Dark brown to black	Total excision
	Irregular borders	Follow-up by dermatologist as needed
	Varied color and thickness	
	May be hair bearing after a few years of life	
	May show malignant change in color, borders, size, thickness, bleeding, and ulceration	
Malignant melanoma	Highly prevalent in adults	Immediate referral to dermatologist
	New lesion or recent change in existing pigmented lesion	Total excision
	Recent changes: Color, border, size, thickness	Emotional support
	Variegated colors (red, white, blue)	Careful observation of remaining nevi by parent or child
	Irregular or smooth surface	
	Usually hairless	Follow-up by dermatologist
	Bleeding, crusting, ulceration, and pain are signs of advanced disease	

Counseling and prevention
- Inform parents that the number of lesions may increase with the age of the child.
- Suggest that the child avoid exposure to sunlight and irritation.
- Instruct parents that removal may be indicated if there is a change in size or color or if lesion is repeatedly irritated (in which case total excision is required).
  Follow-up. Provide periodic observation at well-child visits for changes in the lesion.
  Consultations and referrals. Refer to a dermatologist if the lesion changes in size or color. The parents or child may request elective removal for cosmetic purposes.

Intradermal nevi
Treatments and medications. None are indicated.
Counseling and prevention
- Inform parents that the lesion is benign.
- Counsel parents that lesions will involute and may be replaced by fibrous or fatty tissue.
  Follow-up. None is indicated.
  Consultations and referrals. None are indicated.

Spindle cell nevi
Treatments and medications. None are indicated.
Counseling and prevention
- Inform parents that the lesion is benign.
- Advise parents that the lesion may persist into adulthood.
- Instruct parents to observe for any changes and call if any are noted.
  Follow-up. None is indicated.
  Consultations and referrals. Refer to a dermatologist if the lesion is dark brown to confirm diagnosis.

Dysplastic nevi syndrome
Treatments and medications
- Remember that patients with multiple nevi should have biopsy of several of the most atypical-appearing lesions to confirm the diagnosis.
- Remember that total excision of any lesion suspected of being a melanoma is necessary.
  Counseling and prevention
- Instruct parents that lesions are benign. However, the child may be predisposed to malignant melanoma.
- See Prevention of Sunburn.
  Follow-up. Follow-up every 6 months, or earlier if lesions change.
  Consultations and referrals. Refer to a dermatologist to determine whether biopsy is necessary to confirm diagnosis or if melanoma is suspected.

Bites: Insect, Animal, and Human

JANE A. FOX

Alert

Consult with or refer to a physician for the following:
- Systemic reaction
- Venomous snake bite
- Any bite or laceration requiring stitches
- A bite from an animal or insect that is potentially poisonous
- Past history of an allergic reaction to insect bites
- Human bite from a person who has HIV
- Wounds in patients with peripheral vascular insufficiency
- Patients who are asplenic or immunocompromised
- Unknown or inadequate immunization status
- Human or animal bite involving the face
- A bite that penetrates a joint or the periosteum
- Signs and symptoms of cellulitis with gray malodorous discharge

Etiology

A bite can be inflicted by an insect, animal, or human. Infection of the surrounding soft tissue is the most common complication of these bites. Some bites cause local inflammation or systemic symptoms or may transmit serious systemic disease.

Incidence

- Mosquito bites are the most common type of insect bites in children.
- There is a higher incidence of insect, especially tick, bites on children during warm weather. Less clothing is worn in warmer climates; thus more areas of the skin are exposed.
- There is a higher incidence of flea bites of children who live with cats and dogs.
- Fire ant bites affect more children in the southeastern United States than elsewhere.
- Spider bites affect more children living in rural areas.
- Animal bites occur commonly, with children being the victims approximately 75% of the time.
- Over 1 million dog bites occur each year.
- The ratio of dog to cat bites is 10:1.
- Approximately 10 children per year are killed by dog attacks, usually by family or neighborhood dogs.
- Boys are twice as likely to be bitten by dogs as girls, whereas girls are twice as likely to be bitten by cats. Peak age is 5 to 14 years and usually occurs in the spring and summer.
- Human bites are not so common as other bites but are potentially more serious.
- Cat bites become infected more frequently than dog bites (20% to 50% and 5% to 10%, respectively) because they usually produce punctures that inoculate bacteria deep into the wound, close quickly, and are difficult to clean and débride.
- The rate of infection is highest for bites to the hand and lowest for bites to the face.
- The longer the delay in seeking medical attention for a bite, the higher is the incidence of infection.
- Snake bites are more common in boys and usually occur as a result of handling or trying to catch a snake.
- Most snake bites occur in the southern United States.
- About 5% to 10% of snakes that are most commonly encountered include pit vipers, water moccasins, copperheads, and coral snakes.

Risk Factors

- Warm climates and the seasons of spring and summer
- History of owning a dog or cat
- Exposed skin
- Living or visiting in a rural area
- Wearing brightly colored clothes
- History of aggravating a dog or cat (e.g., pulling the tail)
- Wearing scented cosmetics or perfumes
- Not wearing adequate foot protection

Differential Diagnosis (Table 37-9)

Insect bites may be caused by a variety of insects including ticks, spiders, mosquitoes, fleas, fire ants, wasps, and bees. Each bite may produce a variety of systemic effects, reflecting

Table 37-9 Differential Diagnosis: Bites (Insect, Animal, Human, Snake)

CRITERIA	INSECT BITE	ANIMAL BITE	HUMAN BITE	SNAKE BITE
ICD-9 code	Injury by site	Wound by site	Wound by site	989.5
Subjective Data				
Age/sex	Any age or sex	Any age; peak age is 5 to 14 years with the highest incidence among boys	Any age or sex	Any age or sex; most common in boys over 15 years of age
Description of problem	Report bite marks from tick, spider, mosquito, flea, fire ant, wasp, or bee	Report bite from dog or cat	Report human bite mark	Report a snake bite
Location of bite	Anywhere on exposed skin	Located anywhere on body	Located anywhere on body	Located anywhere on body, but most common on feet, legs, arms, fingers
Associated symptoms:				
Pain	Pain depends on type of bite	Painful	Painful	Painful
Fever	Febrile if infection is present; depends on the insect's systemic sequelae	Febrile if infection is present	Febrile if infection is present	Febrile if infection is present
Predisposing factors	Wearing brightly colored clothes, scented perfumes, or cosmetics; warm climates; spring and summer seasons; exposed skin; not wearing adequate foot protection	Aggravating a dog or cat (e.g., pulling the tail)	Fist-fighting	Area where snakes are present (e.g., Southern states)
Past medical history	History of allergies to insect bites, especially wasps and bees			
Immunization history (especially, tetanus)		May be incomplete; no booster in 5 years		
Social or family history	Family history of allergies to bees, wasps, insect bites; living in or visiting rural areas	Family or neighbor ownership of dog or cat		
Review of systems indicating systemic complication	Tick: Paralysis, relapsing fever Spider: Headache, fever, nausea, vomiting, joint pain, cyanosis, seizures Mosquito: Fever, adenopathy Flea: No complications Fire ant: Urticarial reaction Wasp/bee: Vomiting, diarrhea, dizziness, muscle spasms, convulsions, wheezing, fever	Dog: Erythema, swelling, tenderness, fever, rabies, arthritis Cat: Same as dog bite	Human bite: Fever, erythema, swelling, tenderness, human immunodeficiency virus (HIV)	Venomous snake: Edema of the arm or leg, ecchymoses, lymphadenopathy, nausea, vomiting, sweating, chills, numbness
Objective Data *Physical examination*				
Temperature	Tick: Usually afebrile, unless systemic infection present (see below) Spider: Usually afebrile, unless systemic infection is present (see below) Mosquito: Afebrile Flea: Afebrile Fire ant: Afebrile Wasp/bee: Usually afebrile unless a delayed serum-sickness reaction occurs (see below).	Dog: Usually afebrile, unless infection is present (see below) Cat: Usually afebrile unless infection is present	Afebrile unless infection is present	Afebrile unless infection is present
Inspection of skin/location of bite	Tick: Located on body where skin is exposed, usually on extremities Spider: Located on body where skin is exposed, usually on extremities Mosquito: Located on body where skin is exposed Flea: Located on body where skin is exposed or body sites where clothing is snug Fire ants: Located on body where skin is exposed, especially the feet Wasp/bee: Located on body where skin is exposed	Dog: Located anywhere on body, especially on hands or arms; in infants, usually the scalp Cat: Located anywhere on body, especially on hands or arms	Located anywhere on body, especially on the hand and fist	Peripheral injuries account for over 90% of bites

Continued

Table 37-9 Differential Diagnosis: Bites (Insect, Animal, Human, Snake)—cont'd

CRITERIA	INSECT BITE	ANIMAL BITE	HUMAN BITE	SNAKE BITE
Physical examination—cont'd				
Pain on palpation	Tick: Usually painless Spider: Painful Mosquito: Pruritic, not painful Flea: Pruritic, not painful Fire ant: Painful Wasp/bee: Painful	Dog: Usually painful Cat: Usually painful	Usually painful	Painful
Description of bite site	Tick: Visible in the skin; patchy hair loss in the area of the bite may occur Spider (brown recluse spider): erythema develops at the bite site 2 to 8 hours after the bite, followed by bleb or blister formation, with a surrounding area of pallor; over 48 to 72 hours central induration occurs, and a dark violet color develops; the area then ulcerates and a black eschar forms within a week; it heals over 6 to 8 weeks Mosquito: Presence of erythematous papules; urticaria results Flea: Irregularly grouped urticarial papules with a central hemorrhagic punctum; the lesions may occasionally be vesicular, pustular, or bullous; may resemble chickenpox Fire ant: Wheals develop on exposed areas, followed by vesicles and pustules with a central punctum; scarring usually occurs Wasp/bee: Edema noted at the site with the stinger usually visible at the central point	Dog: Open wound with possible bleeding; soft-tissue damage and swelling present; puncture marks by the dog's teeth Cat: Deep puncture wound with possible bleeding, soft tissue damage, and swelling	Open wound with possible bleeding; soft-tissue damage and teeth marks present	Fang marks are displayed with subsequent burning, swelling, and erythema; this may progress rapidly to hemorrhage and necrosis
Examination for possible systemic complications	Tick: Rocky Mountain spotted fever, Lyme disease, tick bite, paralysis, and relapsing fever Spider: Venom from the brown recluse spider may cause headache, fever, nausea, vomiting, joint pain, cyanosis, hypotension, and seizures; complications result in renal failure, disseminated intravascular coagulation, and (rarely) death Mosquito: Regional adenopathy and fever may be associated systemic complications if secondary infection occurs Flea: None Fire ant: Systemic urticarial reactions may occur Wasp/bee: Toxic reactions may occur with multiple stings (10 or more); symptoms include vomiting, diarrhea, dizziness, muscle spasms and rarely convulsions; anaphylactic reactions such as wheezing and urticaria occur in sensitive individuals; delayed serum-sickness reaction occurs 10 to 14 days after the sting with morbilliform rash, urticaria, myalgia, arthralgia, and fever	Dog: Cellulitis may develop with the onset of erythema, swelling, and tenderness; lymphadenitis may also develop; other complications include rabies, crush injuries, osteomyelitis, septic arthritis, and tenosynovitis Cat: Same as dog bite; cat-scratch disease may produce regional lymphadenitis of an extremity 14 days after the scratch	Systemic infection includes cellulitis with potential closed space infections and abscess formation, as well as osteomyelitis and septic arthritis; the HIV virus may also be transmitted	Vomiting, sweating, chills, numbness, paresthesias of the tongue and perioral region, dysphagia, bleeding, and hypotension; complications: Disseminated intravascular coagulation and hemolysis, respiratory failure, renal failure, seizures, shock, and possible death

individual sensitivity and the number of bites inflicted by the offending insect. The most critical diagnostic clues are systemic and dermatologic characteristics.

Animal bites are commonly caused by dogs and cats. There are, however, other animal bites that are a danger to children, including raccoon, rat, and snake bites. The most critical diagnostic clues include systemic and dermatologic characteristics. Cellulitis and abscesses are the two most common infections. Rabies, though rare, is the ever-present, dreaded outcome of an animal bite. Infection of tendons, periosteum, and joint spaces is also a serious potential complication. *Pasteurella multocida* is present as a normal mouth flora in 10% to 60% of dogs and 50% to 70% of cats and is the causative agent in 20% to 50% of infections from dog bites and 80% from cats. It is a virulent pathogen, usually producing clinical signs of infection within 24 hours after the bite. Dog bites may also become infected with *S. aureus*.

Human bites are most often associated with a clenched fist striking an opponent's mouth. The most critical diagnostic clue includes its systemic and dermatologic characteristics. Over 40 organisms have been identified in mouth flora that are potential pathogens causing infection, the most common being *S. aureus* and (the most feared) HIV.

Snake bites can be inflicted by venomous and nonvenomous snakes. It is often difficult to distinguish between them. A venomous snake bite is a medical emergency and requires immediate transport to the nearest emergency facility. Venomous snakes, the most common being pit vipers, usually have long, hollow fangs, vertically elliptic pupils, a rattle, and a very short maxilla hinged to the prefrontal bone. Nonvenomous snakes have round pupils and no pit, rattle, or fangs. Most snake bites are peripheral (e.g., those on legs, feet, hands, or fingers).

Management

Tick bites. See also Lyme Disease in Chapter 44.
Treatments and medications
- Remove the tick. Do not squeeze, squash, or puncture the body of the tick, since the fluids may contain infective agents.
- Remember that embedded ticks usually can be withdrawn by covering the tick with alcohol, mineral oil, or ointment.
- Use a blunt, curved forceps or tweezers. Grasp the tick close to the surface and pull upward in a steady motion.
- Do not handle the tick with bare hands.

Counseling and prevention
- Explain to parents what ticks are, their appearance, and the need to complete a careful, daily inspection for ticks at bath time.
- Inform parents that tangled woods and high grass are most hospitable to ticks and should be avoided.
- Suggest wearing protective light-colored clothing to reduce potential exposure to ticks. Tuck pant legs into socks and tuck long-sleeve shirts into pants.
- Inform parents that the peak season of tick activity is late spring and early summer.
- Instruct parents how to remove ticks. Wash the skin with soap and water, then use a tweezer to pull the tick back with a slow steady force. Once the tick is removed, again wash the skin with soap and water.
- Advise parents to save the tick once it is removed. Fix the tick to adhesive tape and place in sealed jar.
- Instruct the parents and child on the signs and symptoms of Lyme disease (if bitten by a deer tick) and the signs and symptoms of Rocky Mountain spotted fever if indicated.

Follow-up. Follow-up care is usually not necessary if the tick is removed and no complications are noted.
Consultations and referrals. Refer immediately to a physician if Rocky Mountain spotted fever is suspected or systemic complications are noted.

Spider bites
Treatments and medications
- For local wound care at the site of the bite, apply ice and then cool, wet compresses.
- Prescribe acetaminophen 10 mg/kg orally every 4 hours for pain control.
- If systemic signs develop, provide hydrocortisone 5 mg/kg intravenously every 6 hours. Consult a physician because hospitalization may be required.

Counseling and prevention
- Inform parents that tangled woods and high grass are hospitable to spiders.
- Inform parents that protective clothing such as pants, long-sleeve shirts, and shoes reduce potential exposure to spiders.

Follow-up
- Have the patient return in 2 to 4 days for local wound care and reevaluation.
- Have the patient go to nearest emergency room if systemic reactions occur (usually within 24 hours).

Consultations and referrals. Refer immediately to a physician if anaphylaxis or systemic reactions occur.

Mosquito bites
Treatments and medications
- Apply calamine lotion to bites.
- Prescribe diphenhydramine 5 mg/kg per day orally every 6 hours if needed for itching.
- Use a topical corticosteroid such as hydrocortisone 1% on the affected area or areas twice a day.

Counseling and prevention
- Instruct parents that mosquito bites can be prevented. Suggest applying Avon's Skin So Soft or citronella lotion when going outside.
- Inform parents that protective clothing should reduce exposure to mosquitoes.

Follow-up. Usually no follow-up is necessary unless there is secondary infection.
Consultations and referrals. Usually none are needed. Refer to a physician if systemic complications are observed (e.g., regional adenopathy and fever).

Flea bites
Treatments and medications. See Mosquito Bites.
Counseling and prevention. Inform parents that fleas may live as long as 2 years and survive for months without blood. Fleas live in upholstery, carpeting, and debris in corners and floor cracks. Instruct parents that therapy includes elimination of the fleas by treating animals and by spraying carpets, upholstery, floors, and corners with gamma benzene hexachloride. Recommend that they change or empty vacuum cleaner bags outdoors.
Follow-up. Have the parents call if the condition worsens.
Consultations and referrals. None are indicated.

Fire ant bites
Treatments and medications
- Prescribe acetaminophen 10 mg/kg per dose orally every 4 hours for pain.
- Remember that lesions are self-limited but often leave scarring.
- Remember that systemic urticarial reactions may require systemic antihistamines and epinephrine.

Counseling and prevention. Inform parents that protective clothing, especially shoes, should reduce potential exposure to fire ants.

Follow-up. Have the parents call immediately if systemic complications occur.

Consultations and referrals. Refer immediately to a physician if a systemic reaction occurs.

Wasp and bee stings
Treatments and medications

- Cleanse and remove the stinger with a scraping motion.
- Apply cold compress. This may provide symptomatic relief.
- Prescribe diphenhydramine 5 mg/kg per day orally divided every 6 hours to reduce local and systemic signs and symptoms.
- For systemic signs of anaphylaxis, treat with epinephrine, nebulized beta-agonist agents, and corticosteroids (and refer to a physician).

Counseling and prevention

- Inform parents that children should avoid clothing with bright colors and flowery patterns, as well as perfumes, hair spray, and colognes that attract insects.
- If a parent has a child who has had a severe reaction to bee stings, instruct on the use of a bee sting kit that contains epinephrine and syringes. This kit should be carried by those who have had severe local or systemic reactions.

Follow-up. Have the patient and parents make a telephone call immediately and go to nearest emergency room if systemic reaction occurs.

Consultations and referrals

- Refer to a physician immediately if a severe reaction occurs. The patient may need to be hospitalized for continued emergent care.
- Refer to a physician if delayed serum sickness is noted 10 to 14 days after the sting.

Dog bites
Treatments and medications

- Copiously irrigate the wound with 150 to 1000 ml of normal saline. This reduces the total bacterial load of the wound. Add 1% povidone-iodine (Betadine) to the normal saline.
- Débride the wound to further reduce the risk of infection. Foreign bodies must be meticulously removed, and jagged edges must be trimmed for a better cosmetic result.
- Irrigate the wound again with normal saline after débridement.
- Suture the wound if needed for cosmetic and functional reasons. Hand injuries, wounds involving extensive soft-tissue injury or damage to deep tissues, puncture wounds, and wounds older than 24 hours should not be sutured.
- Begin prophylactic antibodies for hand bites, deep facial bites, or other bites likely to become infected. Penicillin 15 to 56 mg/kg per day orally divided four times a day for 5 days or, if there is an allergy to penicillin, erythromycin 30 to 50 mg/kg per day orally every 6 hours for 5 days. Rabies prophylaxis must be administered if the animal is proved to have rabies or is suspected of having rabies.
- Administer tetanus toxoid if the child is not completely immunized or has not had a booster dose within 5 years for a contaminated wound or 10 years for superficial bite, or if immunization status is unknown.

Counseling and prevention

- Instruct the parents and child about the hazards of playing with unfamiliar animals. Do not allow a child to place the face near a dog. Do not leave a child unattended with dogs. Obey leash laws, and be particularly careful with large dogs.
- Teach parents responsible pet ownership and care.
- Instruct parents on the signs and symptoms of infection.

Follow-up

- If a bite is sutured, schedule a return visit within 24 hours.
- Have parents call immediately if the wound becomes red, tender, or swollen, or develops a discharge.
- If the child is placed on antibiotic therapy, schedule a return visit after 5 days for reevaluation.

Consultations and referrals

- Refer to a physician if suturing is required; prophylactic rabies treatment is needed; the bite is on the scalp, face, hand, or joint area; or the child has peripheral vascular insufficiency or is asplenic or immunocompromised.
- Report to an appropriate agency, if abuse is indicated.

Cat bites. See Dog Bites.

Human bites
Treatments and medications

- Provide irrigation and débridement (see also Animal Bites).
- Never suture a human bite because of the high risk of infection.
- Remember that antibiotics should be administered as noted for animal bites (see Dog Bites).

Counseling and prevention. Instruct the parents and child on the signs and symptoms of infection.

Follow-up

- Have parents call immediately if the wound becomes red, tender, swollen, or develops a discharge.
- Schedule a return visit after 5 days of antibiotics.

Consultations and referrals. Refer to a physician if infection is present (hospitalization may be required); if there is a bite on the scalp, face, hand, or joint area; if the patient has peripheral vascular insufficiency or is asplenic or immunocompromised; or if the bite is from an HIV-positive person.

Snake bites (venomous)
Treatments and medications

- Remember that, if possible, the snake should be killed and identified, with careful handling of the head because it can still deliver venom for up to 1 hour after death.
- Initially apply a broad, firm constructive bandage proximally to the bitten area and around the limb.
- Splint the extremity to reduce motion.
- Immediately transfer to a hospital or emergency facility for administration of antivenin. Antivenin should be administered intravenously. A patient with serious bites must be given antivenin, regardless of any sensitivity to horse serum. Reactions to the antivenin can be managed by slowing down or temporarily stopping infusions and pretreatment with diphenhydramine and histamine blockers. The amount of antivenin administered relates to the category of the patient as determined by symptoms.
- Remember that no therapy is required if there are no findings beyond fang marks.
- Complete CBC and platelet counts; coagulation fibrinogen and fibrin split products studies; urinalysis; and blood urea nitrogen, serial electrolyte, and creatinine level tests.

Counseling and prevention

- Explain to the parents and children the distinguishing features of venomous and nonvenomous snakes.
- Provide emergent treatment is essential after a snake bite.
- Instruct on environmental awareness. The most commonly encountered venomous snakes are pit vipers, water moccasins, copperheads, and coral snakes. The larger the snake, the more venom it produces.
- Advise parents to use extreme caution if snakes (especially venomous snakes) are kept in the home as pets.

Follow-up. Follow-up care depends on the systemic complications of the snake bite.

Consultations and referrals. Refer immediately to a physician all patients with venomous snake bites. Admit them to the hospital for supportive care.

Corns and Calluses

JANE A. FOX

Alert

Consult or refer to a physician for the following:
- Corns or calluses resistant to conventional therapy
- Diabetic patients

Etiology

The most common causes of corns and calluses are mechanical in origin. A corn is the painful thickening of the skin that develops over a bony prominence. Corns usually occur on the foot, where there is recurrent pressure and chronic friction. This pressure can be caused by ill-fitting footwear, unequal weight distribution, excessive body weight, or abnormalities in the bone structure of the feet. A callus is a painless thickening of the epidermis that can occur anywhere on the body where there is external pressure or friction. Calluses are most commonly found on the feet and hands.

Incidence

- This condition affects 10% of school-age children.
- Peak incidence is during adolescence.
- It has a worldwide occurrence and a high incidence of recurrence.

Risk Factors

- Tight or poorly fitting shoes
- History of wearing high-heeled and pointy-toed shoes for long periods
- Weight-bearing on feet for long periods
- Jogging

Differential Diagnosis (Table 37-10)

Corns are a painful conical thickening of skin that results from recurrent pressure on normally thin skin. The apex of the cone points inward and causes pain. Characteristically corns occur over bony prominences. When they occur in moist areas, they are called "soft corns."

Calluses are areas of greatly thickened skin that develop in a region of recurrent pressure. Calluses involve skin that is normally thick, such as the sole of the foot or the palms of the hand, and are usually painless.

Management

Corns

Treatments and medications
- Soak the affected foot in warm water to soften the skin. Pare the corn with a surgical blade to remove it.
- Apply a thin, soft, felt pad with a hole at the site of the corn.
- Correct the mechanical abnormalities of the shoe with a shoe insert.
- Relieve the friction point in footwear.

Counseling and prevention
- Discuss the importance of wearing correctly fitting footwear.
- Instruct on home care of the corn, including the use of a pumice stone for paring.

Table 37-10 Differential Diagnosis: Corns and Calluses

CRITERIA	CORNS	CALLUSES
ICD-9 code	700.0	700.0
Subjective Data		
Pain	Pain on weight-bearing	Burning sensation
Location of pain	Pain located over bony prominences	Burning sensation located at callus site
Social or family history	History of buying new shoes; wearing high-heeled or pointy-toed shoes	History of repeated friction on hands, fingers, or of long hours standing at work or jogging for long periods of time; history of diabetes
Objective Data		
Physical examination		
Pain	Pain and point tenderness noted on palpation	Painless to pressure
Location of pain	Pain located over bony prominences	
Skin examination	Hard, dry skin in small areas over bony prominences; hard skin has a small diameter and is translucent	Dry skin with general thickening of skin over a large area, especially the soles of the feet
Laboratory data	None	None

Follow-up. Schedule a return visit in 4 to 6 weeks for reevaluation.

Consultations and referrals. Refer to a podiatrist for evaluation and possible fitting of shoe inserts for correction of abnormalities.

Calluses

Treatments and medications

- Soak the affected area in warm water to soften the skin. Pare the callus with a surgical blade to remove it.
- Apply a keratolytic agent, such as a compound of salicylic acid, acetone, and collodion, to the callused skin. Every night cover the paste with a piece of adhesive and then remove in the morning. Continue this until the hard callus is resolved.

Counseling and prevention

- Discuss the importance of properly fitting footwear.
- Instruct on the use of a pumice stone on the callus.
- Discuss the use of liberal amounts of skin cream to keep skin soft.

Follow-up. Schedule a return visit in 4 to 6 weeks for reevaluation.

Consultations and referrals. None are indicated.

Diaper Rash

JANE A. FOX

Alert

Consult with or refer to a physician for the following:
- Diaper rash that is unresponsive to all treatment options
- Systemic symptoms (e.g., fever or malaise without identified source)
- Severe rash in an infant less than 2 months of age
- Sudden onset of rash that is rapidly spreading
- Rash that is painful to the touch or painful with voiding or stooling (possibly a result of staphylococcal scalded skin syndrome)
- Blistering and deep ulcerations (as seen with HSV)
- Bleeding from a preexisting hemangioma
- Unclear diagnosis of a persistent or unusual diaper rash

Etiology

Diaper dermatitis is not a specific disease but rather a variety of inflammatory disorders affecting the lower aspect of the abdomen, genitalia, buttocks, and upper portion of the thigh. Diaper dermatitis represents a primary reaction to irritation by urine, feces, moisture, or friction. The diaper area is occluded by mechanical means such as plastic or rubber pants or diapers. Moisture becomes trapped, resulting in alteration of the stratum corneum layer, maceration, and cutaneous erosion. Contact irritation is produced by friction and wetness in the inguinal area. In addition to irritation and moisture, poor hygiene may enhance the growth of bacteria or fungi. Allergies to plastic diapers, laundry detergent, or topical ointments, diarrhea, recent oral antibiotics may also exacerbate diaper dermatitis in infants. Once established, the irritated area can become colonized by bacteria or fungi that cause secondary changes.

Incidence

- This is most common before 2 years of age.
- The peak age is between 9 and 12 months of age.

- Irritant contact dermatitis is the most common type of diaper dermatitis.

Risk Factors

- Prolonged contact with urine and feces
- Poor hygiene
- Friction caused by diapers or plastic pants
- Synthetic components of paper diapers, rubber or plastic pants, diaper wipes, or laundry products
- Caregiver neglect
- Maternal candidiasis
- Family history of allergies
- History of antibiotic use
- Bottle feeding (breastfed infants may have less severe diaper dermatitis)

Differential Diagnosis (Table 37-11)

Primary irritant dermatitis, or *contact dermatitis,* is usually not seen until after 3 months of age. It is caused by trapped moisture and friction at the site of contact with the diaper. Ammonia and its irritant products from bacterial enzyme catabolism may contribute to the irritation. Tightly applied diapers, especially with occlusive edges, and rubber or plastic pants that overlie diapers increase the risk of irritant contact dermatitis. The eruptions usually occur where the skin is in greatest contact with the diaper: the convex areas of the buttocks, lower abdomen, medial area of the thighs, mons pubis, labia majora, and the scrotum. The skin folds are usually spared unless oils or lotions are the offending agents. Lesions are red with edema, and papules are commonly noted. Scaling may be present.

Allergic contact dermatitis is unusual in infants but has been reported after the use of contact sensitizers such as neomycin and preservatives in cream. The diaper rash from a topical medication often becomes evident as an exacerbation of the rash previously treated. Itchy, papular, vesicobullous, or weeping eruption that is confined to areas that have been in contact with an irritant or allergen is noted.

Candida (Monilia) albicans is the most characteristic of the diaper rashes. The infant may have concomitant oral thrush or *Candida* organisms in the gastrointestinal (GI) tract or may have been exposed to maternal vaginal candidiasis. Many infants with candidal infections have a recent history of antibiotic use. Lesions are fiery-red patches with fine peripheral scales and satellite papules. Involved area may look like skin has peeled, but the rash is usually not painful. The inguinal folds and genitalia are usually involved with satellite oval lesions also on thighs and trunk.

Seborrheic diaper dermatitis commonly occurs in the diaper area of infants beginning at 3 or 4 weeks of age and resolves by 3 to 4 months of age. The rash is characterized by a well-circumscribed, erythematous rash with satellite lesions and yellowish oily scales. The skin folds are involved. Other sites such as the scalp (cradle cap), face, retroauricular areas, axillae, neck folds, and umbilicus may be affected.

Bullous impetigo diaper rash is a bacterial infection caused by *S. aureus* and group A β-hemolytic streptococci (GABHS). The vesicles and bullae in the diaper area tend to be flaccid and rupture easily, leaving a denuded red base.

Management

Primary irritant contact dermatitis

Treatments and medications.

- Remember that the treatment of diaper dermatitis is most successful if the cause of the rash is determined. Since

Table 37-11 Differential Diagnosis: Diaper Dermatitis

CRITERIA	PRIMARY IRRITANT DERMATITIS	ALLERGIC CONTACT DERMATITIS	CANDIDA (MONILIA) ALBICANS	SEBORRHEIC DIAPER DERMATITIS	BULLOUS IMPETIGO DIAPER RASH
ICD-9 code	692.9	692.9	112.9	690.12	684.
Subjective Data					
Age of onset	After 3 months of age	Unusual in infants	All ages	Infants beginning at 3 or 4 weeks of age	Unspecified age
Description of problem	Parents report "shiny redness and sores on buttocks with a strong ammonia odor"	Parents report "previous rash has returned with tiny sores and redness"	Parents report "patches of very red rashes" involving the inguinal folds	Parents report "yellow, greasy rash starting in inguinal folds; scaly"; may state that rash is also on other parts of body, such as head, face axillae, neck folds, and umbilicus	Parents report "red buttocks with yellow, crusting sores"
Fever	None	None	None	None	May be present because of possible systemic infection
Mouth sores	None	None	White plaques (thrush) may be present	None	None
Past medical history	May have had history of gastrointestinal virus that caused large episodes of diarrhea	History of allergies	History of Candida organisms in the gastrointestinal tract, or infant exposed to maternal vaginal candidiasis		History of bacterial infection (caused by S. aureus)
Medication history		May report recent use of contact sensitizers such as preservatives in cream (topical medications)	Possible recent history of antibiotic use	None	None
Elimination history	History of frequent diarrheal stool		May have frequent diarrheal stool from antibiotic use		
Diaper use	History of tightly applied diapers, especially with occlusive edges and use of rubber or plastic pants that overlie diapers; infrequent changes of diapers	May report use of paper diapers or rubber or plastic pants, OTC diaper wipes, harsh laundry products, perfumed soaps, creams, and powders	Report of long naps and sleeping through the night without changing moist diaper		
Associated symptoms	Painful to infant if contaminated with urine or feces	Mild irritability	Mild irritability	Nonpruritic	Characterized by noticeable pruritus
Family history	Possible caregiver neglect; history of change in family situation; other children with rashes or poor hygiene	Child or family history of allergies; history of food allergies	History of maternal vaginal candidiasis		Possible family member or caregiver history of bullous impetigo; bullous impetigo is very contagious by skin-to-skin contact

Continued

Table 37-11 Differential Diagnosis: Diaper Dermatitis—cont'd

CRITERIA	PRIMARY IRRITANT DERMATITIS	ALLERGIC CONTACT DERMATITIS	CANDIDA (MONILIA) ALBICANS	SEBORRHEIC DIAPER DERMATITIS	BULLOUS IMPETIGO DIAPER RASH
Objective Data					
Physical examination					
Temperature	Afebrile	Afebrile	Afebrile	Afebrile	Febrile: may be caused by associated systemic infection
Skin examination					
Location of lesions	Buttocks, appears on convex surfaces with sparing of the inguinal folds	Buttocks	Buttocks, inguinal folds	Starts in the folds and extends to the convex surfaces of the buttocks; skinfolds involved	Buttocks area: exfoliation typically begins around orifices, including the perineal areas
Description of lesions	Diffuse redness under diaper area; shiny, erythematous appearance; pustules, nodules, and erosions are frequently found; erythematous papules may be present, especially at the periphery of the rash	Sharply demarcated areas that were exposed to the sensitizing agent; begins as tiny superficial vesicles that rupture and appear eczematous within 2 days after onset of eruption	Beefy, red rash with sharp borders and satellite pustules and papules beyond the borders; possible perianal erythema with papules and pustules (suggestive of candidal infection with seeding from the GI tract)	Sharply demarcated rash with satellite lesions and yellowish, oily scales	The rash begins as tender patches of erythema. Superficial vesicles and pustules develop and rapidly rupture to form yellow crusts overlying the erythema
Oral examination	Normal	Normal	Thrush present in infant's mouth	Normal	Normal
Laboratory data	None	None	None	None	None

friction and occlusion are detrimental in all forms of dermatitis, the diaper area should be kept dry and occlusive pants eliminated. The diaper area should be dried gently and exposed to air to dry completely after urination, but washing of the diaper area after each urination is excessive and may be irritating. Cleansing after bowel movements is necessary, but only mild soaps such as Dove, Cetaphil, Ivory Moisture Care, or Basis should be used. Commercial wipes should not be used if they prove irritating especially if diaper dermatitis is erosive.

- Use ointments such as zinc oxide (Desitin), Balmex, Johnson & Johnson diaper ointment, Triple Paste, or A&D ointment to reduce friction and protect the skin from irritants.
- Give the infant 2 to 3 oz of cranberry juice a day, which may help to lower the pH of the urine, thereby decreasing the enzyme action that produces irritation.
- For moderate to severe irritant diaper dermatitis and when protective agents are unsuccessful, topical low-potency corticosteroids may be prescribed. Use only nonhalogenated corticosteroids (e.g., hydrocortisone) in the diaper area, applying two times a day for no longer than 2 weeks at a time. Antiinflammatory medication must be applied first before any protective paste or ointment.
- Do not prescribe products that combine antiyeast and fluorinated corticosteroids (e.g., triamcinolone with nystatin).

Counseling and prevention

- Instruct parents on prevention of diaper rash.
- Discuss with parents that frequent diaper changes are important to reduce the irritable effects of prolonged contact of urine and feces on the buttocks. If infant has diaper dermatitis, recommend changing the diaper at least every 2 hours during the day and once at night.
- Discuss possible benefits of using superabsorbent diapers.
- Suggest whenever practical to leave the infant without a diaper. Instruct parents to omit use of diapers as often as possible.
- Explain the causes of diaper dermatitis to parents.
- Advise elimination of rubber pants and tight-fitting diapers.

Follow-up. Make a telephone call or schedule a return visit if there is no improvement in 2 days, or immediately if rash worsens.

Consultations and referrals. Usually none are indicated.

Allergic contact dermatitis

Treatments and medications

- See strategies for Primary Irritant Contact Dermatitis.
- Remember that this condition is best treated with avoidance of the offending agent, type of diaper, laundry detergent, diaper wipes, or plastic or rubber pants.
- Apply 1% hydrocortisone cream to affected area twice a day. Use with caution in diaper areas because it causes striation of skin.

Counseling and prevention

- See the strategies for Primary Irritant Contact Dermatitis.
- Instruct parents on home laundering of diapers. Wash diapers with a mild soap such as Ivory. Do not use bleach, fabric softeners in wash, or softener sheets in dryer. Put diapers through the rinse cycle twice.
- Instruct parents to eliminate plastic or rubber pants. If they must use them, suggest folding the plastic away from the body.

Follow-up. Have the parents call or schedule a return visit if no improvement in 2 days, or immediately if rash worsens.

Consultations and referrals. Refer to a dermatologist if the patient is unresponsive to treatment.

Candida (Monilia) albicans

Treatments and medications

- Keep the affected area dry.
- Apply to the affected area a topical antifungal preparation such as:
  Clotrimazole (Lotrimin) cream twice a day
  Miconazole (Monistat-Derm) twice a day
  Nystatin (Mycostatin) cream liberally twice a day
- Continue the topical agent for at least 1 week after rash has cleared.
- If thrush is present or the GI tract is suspected of being the source of candidal organisms, administer nystatin oral solution, 200,000 U, four times a day for 7 days.

Counseling and prevention

- Instruct parents to keep the area dry.
- See the strategies for Primary Irritant Contact Dermatitis.
- Instruct parents to continue the topical medication for at least 2 full days after the disappearance of the rash.
- Instruct parents on prevention of diaper rash.

Follow-up. Have the parents call or schedule a return visit if rash worsens or if there is no improvement in 3 to 5 days.

Consultations and referrals. Refer to a dermatologist if *C. albicans* is not responsive to antifungal therapy.

Seborrheic diaper dermatitis

Treatments and medications

- See the strategies for Primary Irritant Contact Dermatitis and Allergic Contact Dermatitis.
- Remember that ketoconazole cream is the initial treatment of choice, but 1% hydrocortisone cream applied twice a day to the affected area may be helpful. Use hydrocortisone cream with caution in diaper areas because it will cause striation of skin.

Counseling and prevention

- See the strategies for Primary Irritant Contact Dermatitis and Allergic Contact Dermatitis.
- Instruct parents not to use a fluorinated corticosteroid preparation in groin area because of the high risk of local side effects, especially skin atrophy.

Follow-up. Have the parents call or schedule a return visit if no improvement is noted in 2 days or if rash worsens.

Consultations and referrals. Refer to a dermatologist if rash is unresponsive to antiinflammatory therapy.

Bullous impetigo diaper rash. See also Weeping Lesions later in this chapter.

Treatments and medications

- Remove crusts by gently washing with warm water and an antiseptic soap or cleanser such as povidone-iodine, chlorhexidine gluconate (Hibiclens), or hexachlorophene (pHisoHex). Rinse well.
- Remember that topical or systemic treatment usually depends on the age of the child.
- Apply one of the following antibiotic ointments to the affected area:
  Neosporin for crusted lesions four times a day
  Mupirocin (Bactroban) for bullous lesions three times a day
- If clearing has not begun after 2 days and other lesions have appeared, begin systemic treatment with dicloxacillin 25 mg/kg per day divided four times a day, or erythromycin 30 to 50 mg/kg per day divided four times a day for 7 to 10 days.

Counseling and prevention
- Explain to parents that bullous impetigo diaper rash is caused by bacteria (*S. aureus* or *Streptococcus* organisms).
- Emphasize that this infection is contagious by skin-to-skin contact. The parents and caregivers must adhere to strict handwashing.
- Explain to parents that topical medication might not cure the rash, and that systemic antibiotic therapy may be necessary.

Follow-up
- Make a telephone call or schedule a return visit if improvement to initial topical antibiotic treatment is not apparent in 3 to 5 days or if more lesions have appeared. Systemic treatment is then needed.
- Schedule a return visit after antibiotics are completed to assess rash. Have the parents call if the infant becomes febrile.

Consultations and referrals. Refer to a dermatologist if the rash worsens while on systemic antibiotic therapy.

Hair Loss

VICTORIA VECCHIARIELLO

Alert

Consult with or refer to a physician for the following:
- Patches of hair loss accompanied by a history that may indicate child abuse
- Psychologic problems related to hair loss, particularly in adolescents
- Hair loss accompanied by structural or systemic abnormalities

Etiology

Alopecia, or hair loss, is a common dermatologic disorder. Causes may include trauma, environmental factors, fungal infections, familial predisposition, autoimmune diseases, medications, and psychosomatic factors.

Incidence

- Hair loss is a common finding during the first year of life when an infant is placed in the same position on a continuous basis.
- During the first year of life, hair is usually replaced by thicker and darker hairs.
- Vellus hairs are replaced with terminal hairs at puberty as a result of increased androgen levels.
- Tinea capitis is the most common dermatophyte infection in childhood.
- Tinea capitis occurs most commonly in the 4- to 7-year-old age group.

Risk Factors

- History of trauma
- Prior fungal infections
- History of allergies and contact dermatitis
- Poor nutrition
- Stress
- Familial predisposition
- Chemotherapeutic agents

Differential Diagnosis (Table 37-12)

Alopecia areata is the abnormal cessation of the hair growth cycle resulting in sudden hair loss. Although the cause is still unknown, this process is believed to be of immunologic origin. Nail abnormality may accompany this disorder.

Tinea capitis is a fungal infection of the hair and scalp. Also known as *ringworm*, *Trichophyton tonsurans* is the responsible organism for 95% of tinea capitis in North America. It weakens the hair shaft, causing breakage and hair loss. Other signs may include scaling and possible enlarged postauricular lymph nodes. *Microsporum canis,* which is usually transmitted by a pet cat, causes a very small percentage of cases.

Traction alopecia is hair loss resulting from traction or trauma to the hair shaft. This may cause shaft fractures as well as follicular damage. The most common causes are repetitive hairstyling or product use.

Trichotillomania is hair loss usually caused by repetitive pulling or twisting of the hair. This habitual action causes fractures to the longer hair shafts.

Management

Alopecia

Treatments and medications. None are indicated. Hair regrows spontaneously.

Counseling and prevention
- Inform the parents and child that new patches of hair loss may occur before regrowth occurs.
- Reassure the parents and child that spontaneous regrowth of hair occurs in 95% of cases within 1 year.
- Inform the parents and child that no interruption of school or activities is necessary.
- Address psychologic effect of hair loss, particularly with adolescents.

Follow-up. Schedule a return visit in 2 to 3 months to monitor hair growth and provide reassurance to the child and family.

Consultations and referrals
- Consult with a dermatologist if hair loss persists longer than 6 months or worsens at any time.
- Refer to a dermatologist for management of treatment with corticosteroids.

Tinea capitis. Also see Fungal Infections (Superficial) in Chapter 44.

Treatments and medications. Despite growing resistance, the first line of treatment remains griseofulvin. Griseofulvin taken orally is available in liquid and capsule forms, usually given 2 weeks beyond clinical resolution. Griseofulvin is best absorbed if taken with fatty foods (e.g., whole milk, ice cream). It is necessary to monitor liver function during therapy. When griseofulvin is not effective or the patient is unable to tolerate therapy, use ketoconazole for patients 2 years of age and older. Keep in mind that ketoconazole is available in tablet form only.

A topical antifungal agent (e.g., clotrimazole cream 1%) applied to affected site two times a day for 1 week may decrease the risk of cross-contamination to self and others. This medication is not effective against the fungus that causes ringworm of the scalp because it is unable to penetrate deep into the hair shaft. New antifungals, to used for 2 to 4 weeks with the dosage adjusted according to the age and weight of the child, include terbinafine (Lamisil, Novartis), itraconazole (Sporanox), and fluconazole (Diflucan). These show promise but are not currently indicated for use in children to treat tinea capitis. Fluconazole is FDA approved for use in children but not for tinea capitis.

Ketoconazole shampoo (Nizoral) used daily may shorten the course or improve response to oral agents. Selenium sulfide 2.5% (Selsun) shampoo used twice weekly may be helpful in decreasing spore shedding and spreading to other areas or contacts. Family members should also use the shampoo. A

Table 37-12 Differential Diagnosis: Hair Loss (704.0)

CRITERIA	ALOPECIA AREATA	TINEA CAPITIS	TRACTION ALOPECIA	TRICHOTILLOMANIA
ICD-9 code	704.01	110.0	704.09	312.39
Subjective Data				
Age/sex	None specific	Most frequent in school-age children	More common in young girls and infants; particularly those of African-American descent	Usually seen in school-aged children or adolescents
Onset or duration of hair loss	Abrupt loss of hair	Transient hair loss	Transient hair loss	Usually abrupt
Persistent history of associated symptoms	History of poor nutrition	Report broken hairs, partial hair loss, scaly scalp	Report of immobility, rubbing; frequent use of hair care products or hairstyling techniques	History of trauma or self-inflicted hair pulling; psychiatric problems
Allergy history	Possible	No	No	No
Objective Data *Physical examination*				
Inspection of hair	Defined oval or round patches of hair loss	Broken hairs at affected areas	Broken hairs of different lengths; area of hair loss usually oval or linear	Broken hairs of different lengths; irregular patches of hair loss
Condition of scalp	Smooth scalp with no inflammation	"Black dots" may be noted at affected site; in the latter phase scalp may have golden crust, inflammation, or scaling	Inflamed, follicular papules may be observed	Petechiae may be present or folliculitis
Other signs	May have hair loss on other body sites; nail pitting may accompany this disorder	Dull hair may be observed	Folliculitis	Eyebrows and lashes may be involved
Laboratory data	None	Fungal cultures show *Trichophyton tonsurans*	None	None

1% oil of eucalyptus ointment applied to affected areas may provide relief.

Counseling and prevention
- Instruct that griseofulvin must be taken orally with fatty foods to aid absorption.
- Advise that household members and contacts should be examined closely to determine whether treatment is warranted. Suggest family members use prescribed shampoo.
- Instruct the parents and child on prevention of spreading of fungus, including not sharing hair products (e.g., combs, brushes, hats), clothing, or bedding.
- Instruct the child to shower daily.
- Launder clothing and linen in hot water.
- Remember that the child may return to school 48 hours after griseofulvin therapy has been started.
- Instruct parents to check pets; if skin rash or sores are seen, the animal should be examined by a veterinarian.
- Instruct parents to call if there are signs of secondary infection (e.g., pus or yellow crusting in the affected area); if scalp becomes swollen, boggy, or tender; or if there is no improvement after 2 weeks of treatment.
- Reassure parents that removal of hair (shaving) is unnecessary.

Follow-up
- Schedule a return visit in 4 weeks for a repeat fungal culture and evaluation of therapy.
- Remember that a follow-up visit every 4 weeks is necessary until hair growth begins.

- Remember that liver enzymes must be evaluated every 4 to 6 weeks during griseofulvin therapy.

Consultations and referrals. Consult with a dermatologist if therapy is not effective or frequent hair loss persists. Notify the school nurse.

Traction alopecia
Treatments and medications. Advise avoidance of tight hairstyles (e.g., corn rows, ponytails, braiding). Discontinue use of rollers and hot combs.

Counseling and prevention
- Instruct parents to avoid keeping the infant in one position and suggest the need to provide the infant with stimulation.
- Instruct the parents and child to avoid tight hairstyles and products.
- Keep in mind that no interruption of school or activities is necessary.
- Reassure the parents and child that spontaneous regrowth of hair usually occurs if compliant with the treatment regimen.

Follow-up. Schedule a return visit in 2 to 3 months to monitor hair growth and provide reassurance to the child and family.

Consultations and referrals. Consult with a dermatologist if hair loss persists.

Trichotillomania
Treatments and medications. Apply petrolatum to the hair to decrease pulling and twirling of the hair while the child is at home so that child will not suffer from social isolation.

Counseling and prevention
- Advise parents that child is not doing this on purpose.
- Encourage the child to seek diversional activities (e.g., arts and crafts, sports) to keep the hands busy.
- Keep in mind that the child may seek professional counseling to break habit of hair pulling or discover a reason for it.
- Attempt to decrease stress in the child's life by exploring any stressful situation and attempting to help the child cope with it.

Follow-up. Schedule a return visit in 1 month to evaluate the situation and any hair growth or loss.

Consultations and referrals. Refer to a mental health professional as necessary.

Heat Rash

VICTORIA VECCHIARIELLO

Alert

Consult with or refer to a physician for signs and symptoms of heat stroke, including hot flushed skin, fainting, delirium, unconsciousness, and temperature greater than 105° F. This is a medical emergency.

Etiology

Heat rash is caused by the temporary occlusion of sweat ducts, resulting in their rupture. Excess sweat, heat, and occlusion are essential to the formation of this rash. The areas most frequently affected include most flexoral surfaces; the neck, face, axillae, groin; and the chest in newborns. Skin closely covered with clothing is at increased risk as well.

Incidence

- Most children have episodes of heat rash when certain conditions are present, such as excessive clothing or obesity.
- High heat and humidity during the summer months increase the risk.

Risk Factors

- Infancy
- Tight or excessive clothing in warmer weather
- Damp clothing over flexoral surfaces
- Obesity

Differential Diagnosis (Table 37-13)

Contact dermatitis is an eczematous inflammatory reaction of the skin caused by direct contact or repeated exposure with environmental agents.

Miliaria rubra, or *heat rash,* is identified as minute papules and papulovesicles surrounded by erythema, which are usually pruritic. The most prominent source of infection is identified as *S. aureus.*

Viral exanthem is a common, acute illness of childhood. A variety of symptoms such as fever, sore throat, or arthralgia may precede this multiform rash.

Table 37-13 Differential Diagnosis: Heat Rash (Miliaria Rubra)

CRITERIA	CONTACT DERMATITIS	MILIARIA RUBRA	VIRAL EXANTHEM
ICD-9 code	692.9	705.1	057.9
Subjective Data			
Age	None specific	Most common in newborns but occurs in infants and children	Most common in school-age children
Onset or duration	Sudden onset of rash; persists with prolonged contact of agent	Sudden onset of rash; most usual in hot, humid weather	Rash may be preceded by fever, lethargy, and decrease in appetite; usually sudden onset
Pruritus	Present	Present	Possible
Contact or exposure	May report contact with environmental agent	Parents may report use of excessive heat in the winter	May report contact with others who have similar rash
Allergy history	Present	None	None
Associated symptoms	Edema, erythema	Usually none	Lethargy, recent fever, diarrhea, nausea and vomiting, decrease in appetite
Objective Data			
Physical examination			
Temperature	Normal	Normal	Normal but may have fever
Examination of skin			
Location of lesions	None specific	Areas where sweat glands are concentrated, usually the chest, flexural surfaces, axillae, groin, and neck	Generalized
Distribution	Usually localized to area of contact with offending agent	May be isolated or found in patches	Can be generalized or localized eruptions
Description	Erythematous papules, oozing, scaling, and crusting of lesions	Erythematous pinpoint papules or vesicles on an erythematous base	Multiform rash; macules, papules, vesicles, pustules, petechiae, erythema, and purpura may be seen
Laboratory data	Usually none	None	None

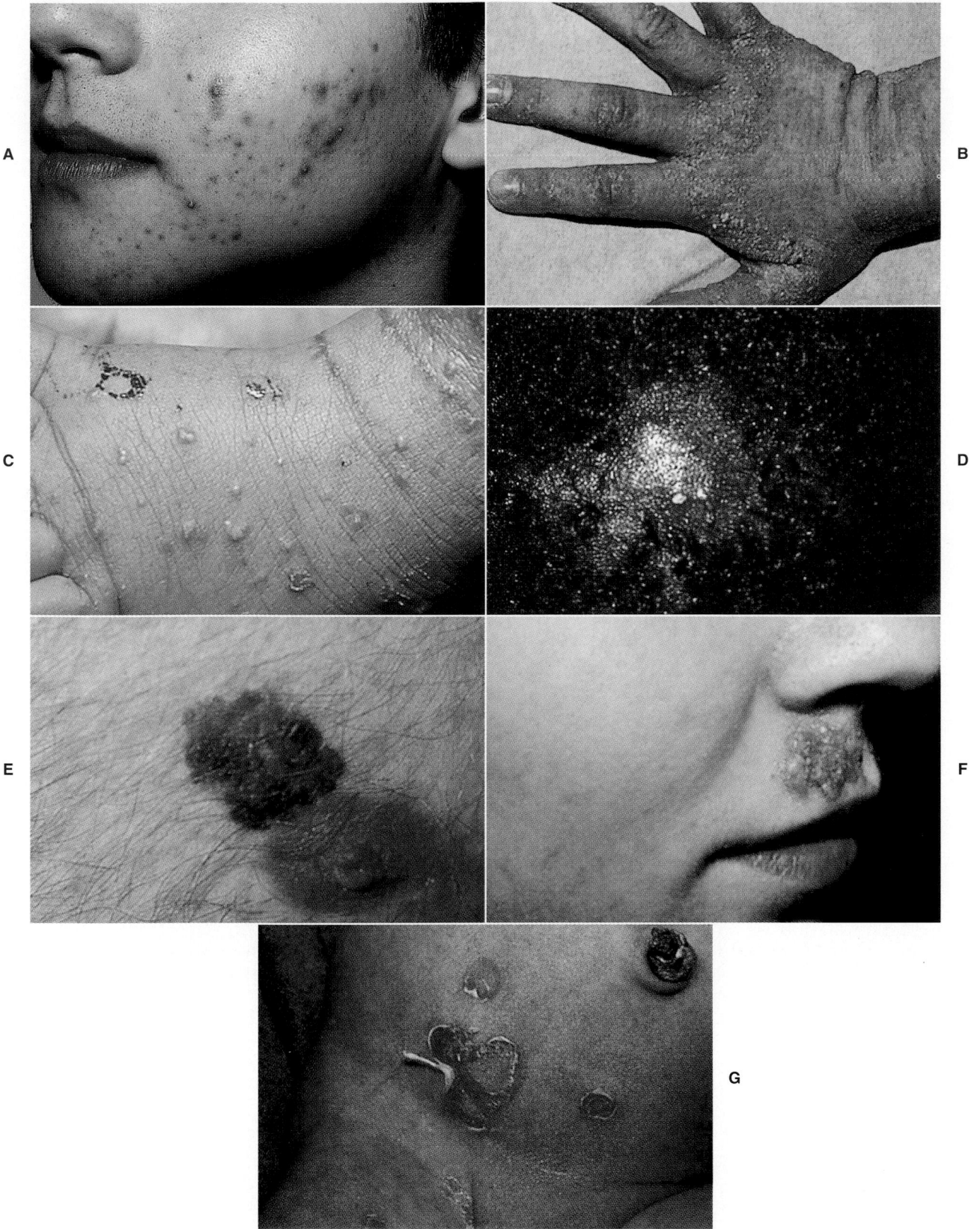

A, Acne. B, Scabies. Involvement of the dorsa of the hand and interdigital webs. C, Scabies. D, Boggy, red scalp nodule with superficial pustules in kerion. E, Malignant melanoma. F, Impetigo. Honey-colored moist crust just above the upper lip. G, Bullous impetigo. (A, From Callen, J.P., et al. [2000]. *Color atlas of dermatology* [2nd ed.] Philadelphia: W.B. Saunders. B, D, E, F, and G, From Weston, W.L. & Lane, A.T. [1996]. *Color textbook of pediatric dermatology* [2nd ed.]. St. Louis: Mosby. C, From Cohen, B.A. [1999]. *Pediatric dermatology* [2nd ed.]. St. Louis: Mosby.)

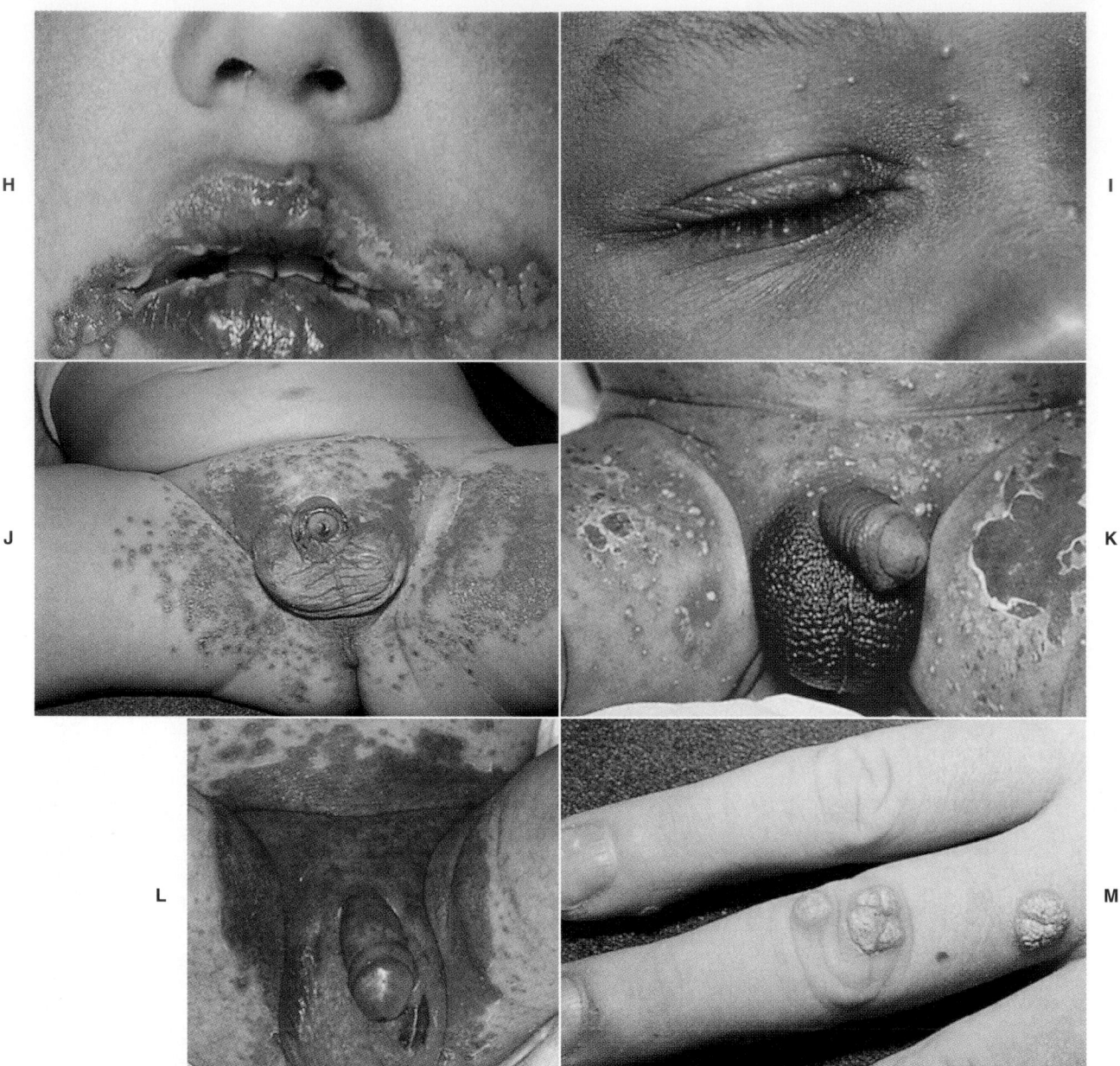

H, Primary HSV-1 gingivostomatitis in an infant. **I,** Mollolscum contagiosum. **J,** Diaper candidiasis. **K,** Staphylococcal diaper dermatitis. **L,** Seborrheic diaper dermatitis. **M,** Warts. (**H, I,** and **M,** From Weston, W.L. & Lane, A.T. [1996]. *Color textbook of pediatric dermatology* [2nd ed.]. St. Louis: Mosby. **J, K,** and **L,** From Cohen, B.A. [1999]. *Pediatric dermatology* [2nd ed.]. St. Louis: Mosby.)

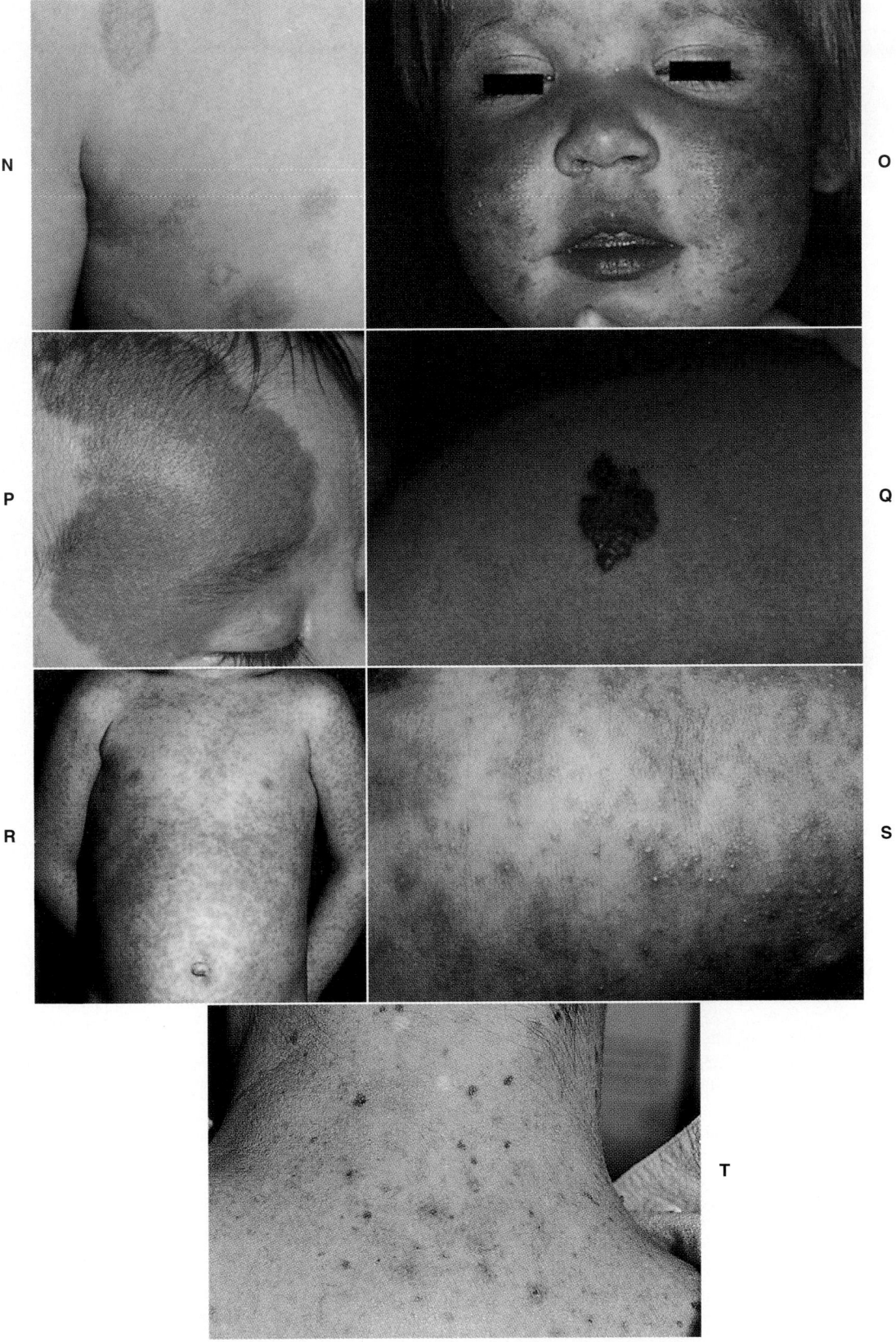

N, Pityriasis rosea. **O,** Sunburn. **P,** Port-wine stain. **Q,** Hemangioma. **R,** Drug eruption. **S,** Erythema toxicum neonatorum. **T,** Pediculosis capitis. (**N, O, Q,** and **R,** From Weston, W.L. & Lane, A.T. [1996]. *Color textbook of pediatric dermatology* [2nd ed.]. St. Louis: Mosby. **P** and **S,** From Cohen, B.A. [1999]. *Pediatric dermatology* [2nd ed.]. St. Louis: Mosby. **T,** From Callen, J.P., et al. [2000]. *Color atlas of dermatology* [2nd ed.] Philadelphia: W.B. Saunders.)

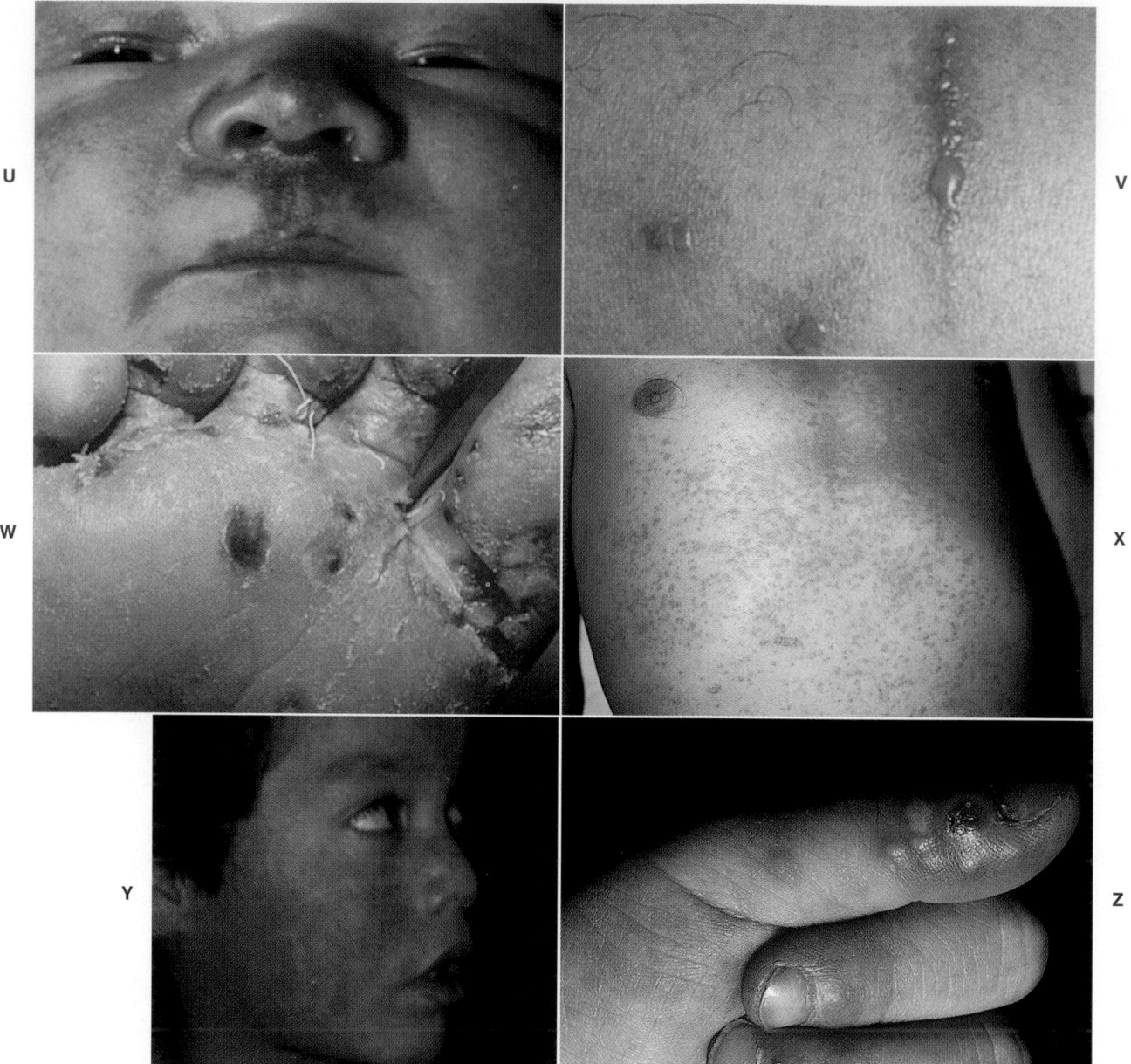

U, Salmon patches. **V,** Poison ivy. **W,** Tinea pedis. **X,** Viral exanthem. **Y,** Erythema infectiosum (parvovirus B19). **Z,** Herpetic whitlow. (**U, V,** and **W,** From Cohen, B.A. [1999]. *Pediatric dermatology* [2nd ed.]. St. Louis: Mosby. **X** and **Z,** From Callen, J.P., et al. [2000]. *Color atlas of dermatology* [2nd ed.] Philadelphia: W.B. Saunders. **Y,** From Weston, W.L. & Lane, A.T. [1996]. *Color textbook of pediatric dermatology* [2nd ed.]. St. Louis: Mosby.)

Management

Contact dermatitis

Treatments and medications

- If possible, remove the offending agent (e.g., soap, clothing, plants).
- For mild cases, recommend calamine lotion be applied to the affected area or areas.
- For severe cases, prescribe topical corticosteroid preparations to be applied to the affected area or areas until rash resolves.
- Possibly give oral antihistamines to alleviate pruritus.

Counseling and prevention

- Teach parents that application of medication to the site after the rash clears disrupts the skin's normal flora.
- Instruct parents to clean the area between each application of corticosteroids.
- Instruct parents to use mild soaps and fragrance-free detergents (e.g., Dove, Tide, Ivory Snow).
- Discontinue the use of fabric softener.
- Recommend the parents bathe the child every other day.
- Advise parents to avoid wool clothing and other possible irritants for the patient.
- Teach parents the signs and symptoms of superinfection (e.g., weeping lesions, fever, edema, intense erythema, pain).

Follow-up

- Make telephone contact in 4 to 6 days.
- Schedule a return visit if rash worsens or if there is no improvement despite therapy.

Consultations and referrals. Refer to a physician any infant less than 2 months old with a superinfection or any patient if the condition does not improve despite follow-up treatment.

Miliaria rubra

Treatments and medications

- Tepid baths for infants and cool compresses for older children
- Maintenance of a cool, dry environment
- Dressing of children in lightweight cotton clothing
- Avoidance of overdressing and tight clothing
- For severe heat rash, application of topical corticosteroids to affected area or areas

Counseling and prevention

- Instruct parents to avoid plastic undergarments and covers.
- Advise parents to avoid the use of ointments that contain petrolatum jelly; these products occlude the skin and promote heat rash.
- Instruct parents to clean the area or areas between each application of hydrocortisone.
- Instruct parents to pat powder on a hand first and then on the area to avoid inhalation.

Follow-up

- Make telephone contact in 4 to 6 days.
- Schedule a return visit if the rash worsens or there are changes despite therapy.

Consultations and referrals. Refer to a physician if condition does not improve despite treatment.

Viral exanthem

Treatments and medications. Treatment is symptomatic. Encourage fluids, rest, and acetaminophen 10 to 15 mg/kg per dose every 4 to 6 hours as needed for fever.

Counseling and prevention. Reassure parents that the rash generally resolves after 2 to 3 days.

Follow-up

- Make telephone contact in 4 to 6 days.
- Schedule a return visit if the rash worsens or there are changes despite therapy.
- Schedule a return visit for increased or persistent fever.

Consultations and referrals. Refer to a physician if the condition does not improve despite treatment.

Hives (Urticaria)

VICTORIA VECCHIARIELLO

> **Alert**
>
> Consult with or refer to a physician for the following:
> - Child who does not respond to treatment within 24 hours or whose condition worsens.
> - Signs of an anaphylactic reaction (e.g., flushing, generalized pruritus, increased warmth) followed by urticaria, respiratory distress, abdominal pain, angioedema, dysphagia, vomiting, lightheadedness, or alteration or loss of consciousness

Etiology

Urticaria (hives) is most commonly caused by a hypersensitivity reaction to an offending agent. Other factors include IgE antibody response and complement activation. The response of the immunologic system causes the release of histamine and leukotrienes, resulting in urticaria. Offending agents that cause urticaria include:

- *Drugs*—Especially penicillins, sulfonamides, nonsteroidal antiinflammatory drugs (NSAIDs)
- *Foods*—Including nuts, seafood, strawberries, eggs, milk products
- *Inhalants*–Pollens, molds, plants, animal dander
- *Bites and stings*—From bees, wasps, mosquitoes, cockroaches, spiders, jellyfish, mites, fleas, rats, domestic animals
- *Infections*—Streptococcal and other bacterial infections that are chronic (e.g., sinus or dental infections, viral hepatitis, infectious mononucleosis, coxsackievirus)
- *Parasites*—Trichinosis, giardiasis, roundworms
- *Genetic*—Familial cold-heat urticaria
- *Environmental*—Solar induced, presence of stress (primarily in adolescents)

Incidence

- Hives are common in the pediatric population.
- Approximately 20% of children have hives at some point in their lives.
- Chronic eruption is more common in adults than children, as well as in those with an allergy history.

Risk Factors

- History of allergies, asthma, or atopic diseases
- History of exposure to viral hepatitis

Differential Diagnosis (Table 37-14)

Urticaria, or *hives,* is a spontaneous eruption of maculopapular lesions consisting of localized edema (wheal) with erythema, accompanied by pruritus. Most cases of urticaria are diagnosed by a positive history. The most common causes of urticaria are food or drug allergy, insect bites, poison ivy, and poison oak.

Table 37-14 Differential Diagnosis: Hives (Urticaria)

CRITERIA	URTICARIA	SYSTEMIC JUVENILE RHEUMATOID ARTHRITIS*
ICD-9 code	708.9	714.30
Subjective Data		
Onset or duration	Usually sudden after contact with offending agent; most often lasts less than 24 hours	Usually occurs during febrile episodes; may be sudden
Age and sex	Not specific; most children have at least one episode in their lives	Childhood; females more prone than males
Pruritus	Yes; may be intense	Not likely
Patient or family history	History reveals exposure to new agents: soaps, cosmetics, foods, medicines, or animals	May report superficial mild trauma
Associated symptoms	None specific	Fever irritability, arthralgia
Objective Data		
Physical examination		
Skin examination		
Location of lesions	None specific	Usually on trunk and proximal extremities; palms and soles may also be affected
Distribution of lesions	Can be generalized or localized eruptions; usually generalized with insect reactions; localized with plant contact	Generalized
Description of eruption	Various sizes; may be small or large erythematous wheals	Macular or papular with an area of central clearing usually salmon-colored or red; has irregular margins

*Refer to a physician.

Systemic juvenile rheumatoid arthritis is the most common collagen vascular disease in childhood. Along with fever, irritability, and arthritis, a red macular rash with irregular borders accompanies this disease.

Management

Urticaria

Treatments and medications

- Removal of offending agent if identified
- For relief of pruritus, ice application, cool compresses, calamine lotion, or topical corticosteroid preparations
- Oral antihistamines, with cetirizine (Zyrtec) preferred over hydroxyzine (Atarax) or diphenhydramine (Benadryl) for patients older than 2 years of age because of the nonsedating component and longer half-life
- If a severe reaction has occurred, consult a physician, who may consider a preventive prescription for self-administered epinephrine.

Counseling and prevention

- Explain to the parents and child any identified causes (if known) and the need for avoidance of them.
- Reassure the parents and child that condition is usually self-limited, with spontaneous resolution within 48 hours.
- If food allergy is identified, counsel the parents and child regarding food groups and need for careful inspection of menu choices.
- Advise parents to notify all caregivers and the child's school of known food allergies.
- If an insect bite is identified as the cause, encourage the use of insect repellent and screens for windows and doors. Recommend avoidance of bright-colored or flower-patterned clothing, scented hair spray, perfumes, and scented body lotions while outdoors.

Follow-up. Perform an immediate recheck if symptoms persist or worsen, despite treatment, after 24 hours.

Consultations and referrals

- Refer to the emergency room any child with a severe reaction who does not respond.
- within 24 hours to treatment or whose condition worsens.
- Refer a child with recurrent episodes to a pediatric allergist.

Systemic juvenile rheumatoid arthritis

Treatments and medications. The goal of treatment is to relieve symptoms. NSAIDs are preferred, and physical therapy is needed to maintain joint function.

Counseling and prevention

- Counsel the parents and child that this is a chronic disease with exacerbations.
- Teach the parents and child the importance of exercise and heat application.

Follow-up. Make telephone contact to maintain a relationship with the child and family.

Consultations and referrals

- Refer to a pediatric rheumatologist.
- Refer to local support groups.
- Refer to a mental health professional as needed.
- Refer for physical therapy.
- Notify the school nurse and gym teacher of possible activity limitations.

Lice (Pediculosis)

JANE A. FOX

Alert

Consult with or refer to a physician for the following:
- Infant with lice
- Pregnant or nursing woman
- Child with pubic lice

Etiology

Lice are small, wingless insects that depend on the blood of their host for survival. Lice are highly contagious and are transmitted by direct contact with infected individuals or through infested brushes, combs, hats, bedding, and clothing. Human lice are not transmitted by animals. The ova or eggs ("nits") hatch in 4 to 14 days. Head lice can survive only 1 or 2 days away from the blood supply through the scalp. However, body lice survive away from a blood supply for more than 10 days. Different types of lice include *Pediculus humanus capitis* (head louse), *Pediculus humanus corporis* (body louse), and *Phthirus pubis* (pubic or crab louse).

Incidence

Pediculosis capitis

- This is prevalent in school-age children and young children who attend day care, but it can occur at any age.
- It is more common in girls than in boys.
- Conservative estimates of head lice are over 6 million American cases a year.
- African Americans have a lower incidence of infestation than other races.
- Crowded conditions and poor hygiene are associated factors.
- Transmission occurs by direct contact through infected persons, or contact through combs, brushes, hats, and bedding.
- It affects all socioeconomic groups.

Pediculosis corporis

- It is greatly influenced by personal hygiene.
- It is rare in children and affluent populations.

Pediculosis pubis

- This is prevalent in adolescents and young adults.
- African Americans and Caucasians have equal incidence rates.
- It is transmitted through sexual contact and (sometimes) contaminated items, including towels.
- It may infest eyelashes (this is seen almost exclusively in children); eyebrows; and body, facial, and axillary hair, but pubic hair is the most common site of infestation.

Risk Factors

- Recent contact with an infested person
- Children who attend day care or nursery school
- Sexually active adolescents with multiple partners
  Factors that contribute to resistant pediculosis include:
- Inappropriate use of pediculicides in nonlice cases (e.g., for dandruff)
- Overuse of OTC treatments for nonviable nits or dead lice
- Misuse of pediculicides (e.g., not following instructions for use) or use of pediculicides as prophylaxis

Differential Diagnosis

When diagnosing pediculosis capitis (Table 37-15), consider dandruff, hair casts, hair spray, and dirt. With pediculosis corporis and pubis, rule out scabies, eczema, and insect bites. Pediculosis pubis in a child should alert the practitioner to possible sexual abuse. Infestation of eyelashes in a young child should always be diagnosed as sexual abuse. (Pediculosis capitis never involves eyelashes.)

Management

Pediculosis capitis

Treatments and medications. Permethrin 1% (Nix) cream rinse is applied to shampooed, rinsed, and towel-dried hair. Leave on for 10 minutes and then rinse thoroughly. It is available OTC. This treatment has a high cure rate because of high ovicidal activity, and it has a low potential for toxicity. A single treatment is usually adequate, but treatment may be repeated in 7 to 10 days. Do not prescribe for pregnant women or infants under 2 months of age.

Natural pyrethrin-based products (e.g., Rid) include a 10-minute shampoo applied to thoroughly wet hair. Massage in, leave in for 10 minutes, and rinse thoroughly. It is available OTC. This treatment has low ovicidal activity, and treatment should be repeated in 7 to 10 days. Do not prescribe for pregnant women.

Lindane 1% (e.g., gamma benzene hexachloride, Kwell) is a 4-minute shampoo applied to dry hair until it becomes wet. Leave on for 4 minutes, add water, lather, and rinse thoroughly. This is available only by prescription. This treatment has low ovicidal activity, and treatment should be repeated in 7 to 10 days, if needed. This treatment has the highest potential for neurotoxicity: Do not prescribe for pregnant women, infants, or young children. The Centers for Disease Control and Prevention (CDC) recommends the use of other scabicides for children under 10 years of age.

Treat secondary infections topically with mupirocin. Systemic antibiotics effective against staphylococci and streptococci may be needed in some cases. Nits can be removed, if desired, with an application of mineral oil, 1:1 mixture of white vinegar and water (applied to the hair for 20 minutes), or 8% formic acid. Hair is then combed with a fine-toothed comb. A metal lice comb can be effective in removing nits and dead lice. If the infestation is heavy, a haircut may be better than tedious removal of nits.

Soak all combs and brushes in hot water with pediculicide shampoo for 15 minutes. Infested clothes, hats, coats, and bed linens should be dry cleaned or washed and dried in a hot cycle of the washing machine and dryer and ironed with a hot iron. Sealing infested items in plastic bags for 10 to 14 days is also effective. Avoid pediculicidal sprays.

A child may return to school or a day care center the day after treatment. About 8 to 10 days after initial treatment a second treatment using the same OTC medication is recommended to ensure that nits are killed after hatching. On recheck in 8 to 10 days after two OTC treatments, if live lice are noted, second-line therapy with a prescription pediculicide should be initiated. Malathion lotion 0.5% in combination with nit combing is recommended. A second treatment with malathion can be applied 7 to 10 days after initial treatment, if needed.

Counseling and prevention

- Educate on the prevention of lice transmission.
- Encourage contacts and housemates to be examined and treated if infested.
- Educate on the use of pediculicidal agents. Apply agents only as prescribed and avoid contact with eyes. Evaluate in 7 days and re-treat if lice or nits are present.
- Avoid pediculicidal sprays.
- If second-line therapy is needed, carefully review the package instructions with parents or caregivers. Be sure they understand. Remind them that malathion is flammable, so the child should not be exposed to electric heat sources or an open flame (including cigarettes). Avoid any contact with the eyes and mouth.

Table 37-15 Differential Diagnosis: Lice

CRITERIA	PEDICULOSIS CAPITIS (HEAD LICE)	PEDICULOSIS CORPORIS (BODY LICE)	PEDICULOSIS PUBIS (PUBIC LICE)
ICD-9 code	132.0	132.1	132.2
Subjective Data			
Presenting symptoms	Itching of scalp; "bugs" on head; dandruff that does not fall off	Itching of body (worse at night)	Itching of anorectal area (worse at night); "walking dandruff"; "bugs" in pubic hair, eyebrows, eyelashes, axillae, or facial hair
Age	Most common in school-age children	Rare in children	Adolescent who is sexually active; rare in prepubescent child
Exposure history	Recent contact with infected individual at home or school	Yes	Yes; may also have recent exposure to or history of other STDs
Objective Data			
Physical examination			
Visualization of nits or lice (use magnifying glass)	Glistening, tiny gray-white nits are visualized attached to hair shaft; very difficult to remove; head lice (2 to 3 mm long) found at base of hair or at nape of neck and behind the ears	Small, red papules, in early cases; lice and nits visualized in seams of clothing	Presence of lice or nits on pubic hair shaft, axillary hair, eyebrows, eyelashes, or facial hair; white nits attached to hair shaft, difficult to remove
Inspection of surrounding area	Bite and scratch marks on scalp; excoriation of skin from scratching	Excoriation with bloody crusts along scratch lines (especially upper back, axillae, waist); secondary bacterial infection common; if prolonged infestation, lichenization of skin	Multiple bite and scratch marks on abdomen, thighs, or anorectal area; maculae caeruleae: Sign of heavy lice infestation is the presence of bluish or slate-colored macules on the chest, abdomen, or thighs; excoriation of skin caused by scratching; secondary infection possible at excoriated sites
Lymphadenopathy	Occipital and cervical in severe cases as result of secondary infection	Axillary and inguinal in severe cases	Inguinal
Other	A generalized macular-papular eruption has been reported to be associated with infestation of head lice		
Laboratory data	Usually none; Wood's lamp, nits fluoresce	Usually none; Wood's lamp, nits fluoresce	Test for other STDs, especially gonorrhea and syphilis

- Vacuum carpets, car seats, furniture, and play areas.
- Advise washing recently used clothes, towels, and bedding at 130° F or drying on high heat. If the child sleeps with a stuffed animal or blanket, wash it in hot water (130° F) or dry on high heat.
- Clean the child's brushes, combs, and hair accessories (e.g., clips, barrettes) in hot water.
- Discourage the child from borrowing hats, brushes or combs, hair accessories, headphones, towels, pillows, or helmets from others.

Follow-up
- Recheck in 3 to 5 days if child has a secondary infection; otherwise, recheck in 7 days and retreat if lice or nits are present. Recheck 8 to 10 days after the second OTC treatment.
- Schedule a return visit if symptoms worsen.

Consultations and referrals
- Consult with a physician if infant or pregnant (or nursing) woman has lice.
- Send a note to the school or day care nurse.

Pediculosis corporis

Treatments and medications
- Improve hygiene.
- Wash clothes and bed linens in hot water with detergent; use hot dryer and hot iron or dry clean.
- Remember that ectoparasiticidal agents are generally not needed, but for severe cases the agents used to treat pediculosis capitis are effective.
- Treat secondary infections as indicated.
- Vacuum carpets, car seats, furniture, and play areas.
- Avoid pediculicidal sprays.

Counseling and prevention
- Explain that body lice are transmitted by direct contact with infested clothing and bedding (they line the seams of clothing or bedding).
- Encourage housemates and contacts to be examined and treated if infested.

Follow-up. See the strategies for Pediculosis Capitis.

Consultations and referrals
- Consult with a physician if an infant or pregnant (or nursing) woman has lice.
- Send a note to the school or day care nurse.

Pediculosis pubis

Treatments and medications
- Remember that ectoparasiticidal agents that are used to treat pediculosis capitis are effective. Re-treat in 7 to 10 days after the initial treatment.
- For eyelash infestation, apply petroleum ointment three or four times a day for 8 to 10 days; manual removal of nits is required in accordance with the American Academy of Pediatrics (AAP).
- Encourage treatment of all sexual contacts.
- Treat any secondary infections.
- Avoid pediculicidal sprays.
- Vacuum carpets, car seats, furniture, and play areas.

Counseling and prevention. Inform that transmittal is through sexual contact in adolescents. For young children, transmittal is by close contact with an infested adult.

Follow-up. See the strategies for Pediculosis Capitis.

Consultations and referrals. Report to the appropriate agency for any infested young child, because sexual abuse must be suspected.

Minor Trauma: Abrasions, Lacerations, Bruises, and Puncture Wounds

JANE A. FOX

Alert

Consult with or refer to a physician for the following:
- Deep or contaminated lacerations
- Lacerations involving damage to bones, tendons, or motor and sensory nerves
- Lacerations involving major vessels
- Child with a wound requiring sutures
- Large puncture wounds
- Signs and symptoms of wound infection
- Inadequate immunization history, including tetanus
- Lacerations involving the face
- Severe bruising involving the eyes
- Accidental needle punctures from a person who is positive for HIV or with an unknown HIV or hepatitis status
- Suspected child abuse
- Suspected bleeding disorder

Etiology

Abrasions are an injury in which the outer skin layer is scraped off. There is little or no bleeding, and healing is quick. With a deep abrasion there is loss of the epidermis exposing the underlying tissue to infection and desiccation. Lacerations are incised wounds that are caused by sharp instruments such as a knife, razor, or glass. Tear wounds are produced by blunt trauma, especially by a blunt instrument under force or a child falling against a blunt object. Puncture wounds are caused by a sharp instrument such as a needle, knife, or nail. Bruises (contusions) are damaged vessels within the tissue causing interstitial hemorrhage. Bruises are caused by blunt trauma to the body without a break in the skin.

Incidence

- Puncture wounds most frequently occur to a child's feet.
- A higher percentage of bruising and lacerations is noted in boys than in girls.

Risk Factors

- Involvement in sporting activities, especially very physical sports (such as football, hockey)
- Risk-taking
- Being a gang member
- Family history of child abuse
- History of coagulation factor VIII deficiency, hemophilia, or coagulation disorders
- History of walking barefoot

Differential Diagnosis

Abrasions occur when the outer skin layer is scraped away.

Lacerations are a break in dermal and epidermal integrity most often caused by penetrating injuries. Symptoms vary and depend on cause, elapsed time, pain, loss of movement of injured part, sensory loss contamination, depth of injury, and tetanus prophylaxis.

Contusions (bruises) are compressive injuries from a blunt object. Interstitial hemorrhage, which is attributable to damaged tissue vessels, causes the bruising and local tissue ischemia. Symptoms vary and depend on the cause, elapsed time, pain, loss of movement in the injured part, or sensory loss.

Puncture wounds are usually deep, with a small entry point. Symptoms vary and depend on the cause, elapsed time, pain, sensory loss, loss of movement in the injured part, contamination, tetanus prophylaxis, or depth of injury.

Management

Abrasions

Treatments and medications. Carefully cleanse the wound. If foreign material remains, abrade the area with a sterile surgical brush or a gauze sponge soaked in saline. Do not use detergent-containing solutions. Cover with an antibiotic ointment (e.g., Bacitracin) or with a nonadherent dressing.

Counseling and prevention
- Discuss the treatment plan.
- Review injury prevention if appropriate.
- Review the signs and symptoms of infection.

Follow-up. Usually none is indicated. If deep abrasions, schedule a return visit in 2 days to check wound and then every 3 or 4 days to monitor healing.

Consultations and referrals. None are indicated.

Lacerations

Treatments and medications
- Stop the bleeding by applying direct pressure to the laceration with sterile gauze. Elevate the extremity for a brief period.
- Determine whether any neurovascular compromise distal to the injury site is present.
- Palpate the underlying bone at the site of the injury to identify an open fracture that requires urgent surgical evaluation for débridement and closure.
- Irrigate the wound with saline solution.
- Clean the wound with an antibacterial agent such as povidone-iodine solution.
- Inspect the wound for any foreign body.
- If the wound is clean and superficial and there is no tension on the skin, close the wound with Steri-Strip tape or a butterfly bandage painted with providone-iodine and cover with a dry, sterile bandage for 72 hours. There is no need for a prophylactic antibiotic.
- If the wound is deep, it should be sutured with nylon, a monofilament suture material. Sutures should remain intact for 1 week.
- If the wound is considered "dirty," start prophylactic antibiotics (e.g., penicillin 15 to 56 mg/kg per day in four divided doses for 5 days, or amoxicillin-clavulanate [Augmentin] 20 to 40 mg/kg per day in three divided doses for 5 days).
- Administer tetanus toxoid booster if immunization status is unknown or incomplete or date of the last tetanus vaccination is more than 5 years from the present.

Counseling and prevention
- Instruct the child and parents to keep the bandage dry and clean.
- Inform the child and parents that Steri-Strip tape should be kept in place for 5 to 7 days and sutures for 7 days.
- Instruct the child and parents regarding tetanus immunization and document accordingly.

- Identify to parents the signs and symptoms of infection.
- Advise on appropriate safety precautions.

Follow-up
- Schedule a return visit in 24 to 48 hours for dressing change and reevaluation.
- Schedule a return visit or have the parents telephone immediately if there is a malodorous dressing, increased pain, discharge from the wound, fever, or erythema.
- Depending on suture placement, follow-up accordingly for suture removal.

Consultations and referrals. Refer to a physician for lacerations with concomitant neurovascular or musculoskeletal injuries (which may be a surgical emergency). If the wound is grossly contaminated or deep, a physician should be consulted regarding surgical débridement or suture closure.

Puncture wounds. See Lacerations. Also, refer to a physician for deep or grossly contaminated open puncture wounds for possible sutures or débridement.

Contusions

Treatments and medications
- Apply ice immediately or within the first 6 hours and continue intermittent ice pack
- applications for the following 24 to 48 hours. Ice decreases pain by reducing nerve impulses, limits hemorrhage by vasoconstriction, and prevents further tissue damage by decreasing catabolism.
- Rest the injured area for the first 24 to 72 hours to minimize further bleeding into the injured tissue.
- Apply a compression dressing, if needed, to decrease swelling.

Counseling and prevention
- Instruct on appropriate safety precautions.
- Instruct on the treatment plan.

Follow-up. Unless there are specific indications such as an expanding hemorrhage or infection, no follow-up care is indicated.

Consultations and referrals. Provide immediate referral to a surgeon if fracture of bones is suspected or there is neuromuscular or neurovascular compromise.

Nail Injury and Infection

LOREN O'CONNOR DEMPSEY

Alert

Consult with or refer to a physician for the following:
- Infections unresponsive to treatment
- Nonsuperficial injuries or infections with possible bone or soft-tissue involvement
- Immunosuppressed children
- Diabetic children
- Signs and symptoms of medication toxicity
- Red streaking
- Child abuse

Etiology

Inflammation of the skin surrounding the nail is termed *paronychia,* or *periungual abscess.* Trauma to the cuticle bed alters the normal skin barrier, allowing for microbial invasion. Paronychia may be acute or chronic. Causative organisms most commonly identified are *S. aureus* (acute) and *C. albicans* (chronic).

Incidence

- Infants are prone to candidal paronychia because of frequent finger-sucking.
- Bacterial nail infections are rare in young children and usually occur in the late school-age population.
- Adolescent girls are at increased risk if nail care equipment is not clean.

Risk Factors

- Nail-biting or picking at cuticles
- Finger-sucking
- Dry cuticles or hangnails
- Splinters or other trauma affecting the edges of the nail
- Trauma to fingers (near the nail), resulting in hematoma

- Manicures involving cutting of the cuticle with infected equipment

Differential Diagnosis (Table 37-16)

Paronychia describes the infectious invasion of the nail margins that causes redness, swelling, and suppuration. Paronychia can be acute (bacterial) or chronic (fungal). Several systemic diseases in children are associated with paronychia. The diseases include mucocutaneous candidiasis, acrodermatitis enteropathica, histiocytosis X, and Reiter syndrome.

Herpetic whitlow describes a localized HSV infection involving the fingertip near but not localized to the nail. About 10% of cases involve children who suck on their fingers, which become infected with herpes HSV type 1. About

Table 37-16 Differential Diagnosis: Nail Injury or Infection

CRITERIA	BACTERIAL PARONYCHIA	FUNGAL PARONYCHIA	HERPETIC WHITLOW
ICD-9 code	681.9	681.9	054.6
Subjective Data			
Age	Any age	Any age	Any age
Onset	Over a few days	Over a few days	Over several days
Fever	None reported	None reported	May be reported
Associated symptoms	May report swelling and redness around nail; pus under skin	May report swelling and redness around nails; pus under skin	May report swelling, blisters, redness on fingertip, which may include the skin around the nail, malaise
Pain	May report mild to moderate discomfort	May report minimal to mild discomfort	Report moderate to severe pain
Exposure	May report exposure to a draining lesion (schoolmate, teammate, etc.)	May report white oral patches or bright red diaper rash	May report sexual contact with a person known to have herpes simplex virus type 1 or 2: *Be alert for child abuse*
Client or family history	History of immunosuppression possible	History of immunosuppression possible	May report frequent cold sores (herpes simplex virus type 1), genital lesions (herpes simplex virus type 2); history of herpetic carrier state possible
Objective Data ***Physical examination***			
Vital signs	Normal	Normal	Fever may occur
Skin/nail examination	Intense erythema and edema at paronychial folds; pus, fissures and maceration possible; pain noted on palpation	Moderate erythema and edema at paronychial folds; clear fluid; may become turbid; rarely purulent; chronic condition results in thickened, discolored paronychial folds; discomfort may occur with palpation	Moderate to severe edema of affected area; singular or grouped vesicles on an erythematous base; deep tissue involved: lesions may be seen in various states of eruption (vesicular, ulcerative, crusting); intense pain and guarding with palpation
Location	Usually involves lateral and posterior aspects of nail bed uniformly	Usually involves lateral and posterior aspects of nail bed uniformly	Not uniform in appearance; usually involves fingertip and part of the nail bed
Laboratory data	None usually; Gram stain and culture with antibiotic sensitivity testing if severe involvement occurs or in cases resistant to topical therapy; culture should always be obtained if oral antibiotic therapy is to be started; staphylococci most commonly isolated	None usually; Gram stain and culture with antibiotic sensitivity testing if severe involvement occurs or in cases resistant to topical therapy; culture should always be obtained if oral antibiotic therapy is to be initiated; *Candida albicans* most commonly isolated	Diagnosis generally made on clinical presentation; culture and Tzanck smear obtained for confirmation; serologic tests of herpes virus may be done to determine appropriate treatment of recurrent episodes; herpes simplex virus type 1 or 2 most commonly isolated

90% of cases involve HSV type 2 and are the result of sexual transmission.

Management

Bacterial and fungal paronychia. The goal in the treatment of paronychia is to dry out the affected areas and kill the bacteria or fungus causing the infection.

Treatments and medications

- Advise wet soaks made with Burrow's solution or saline to be applied four times a day.
- Between soaks, keep the lesion covered with a loose, dry bandage to prevent spread of infectious material.
- Remember that bacterial paronychia may be treated with clindamycin (Cleocin T) solution applied to affected areas twice daily. Cleocin T solution has an alcohol base, which aids in nail-base drying, as well as an unpleasant taste. Consider alternative treatment with systemic antibiotics if the infection is severe or the affected area is grossly macerated. Drainage should be cultured to determine antibiotic sensitivity if systemic antibiotic therapy is warranted, and medications must be reevaluated once sensitivity is determined by culture.
- For children (40 kg and less), consider prescribing:
  Erythromycin base 30 to 50mg/kg per day, divided into two to four doses a day and with a maximum dose of 100 mg/kg per day
  Dicloxacillin 12.5 mg/kg daily given in divided doses every 6 hours
- For adolescents (and children over 40 kg), consider prescribing:
  Erythromycin base 500 mg twice a day
  Dicloxacillin 125 mg every 6 hours
- Remember that chronic paronychia may be treated with the application of an antifungal agent.
- For children and adolescents, consider prescribing:
  Clotrimazole 1% solution to be applied twice daily
  Nightly application of nystatin cream or ointment 100,000 U/g (covered with an adhesive bandage to promote absorption)
- Consider acetaminophen 10 to 15 mg/kg per dose every 4 to 6 hours for pain.

Counseling and prevention

- Instruct the parents about the signs and symptoms of worsening infection.
- Teach the parents and child to apply wet soaks with clean gauze or cotton washcloths.
- Discuss with the parents and child the aggravating cause or causes of this condition, that being nail-biting or sucking of fingers.
- To decrease unintended trauma to fingers, cover the child's hands with clean cotton socks or gloves at bedtime and provide the child with activities that keep the hands busy.
- Give an infant or toddler a pacifier.

Follow-up

- Schedule a return visit necessary if fever develops, red streaking occurs, or the condition worsens despite treatment.
- Schedule a return visit in 2 weeks for an uncomplicated case.

Consultations and referrals. Refer or consult with a physician if incision and drainage are necessary, if red streaking is noted from the nail bed, or if condition worsens despite treatment. Widespread infections involving the hands and feet warrant evaluation for systemic disease.

Herpetic whitlow

Treatments and medications

- Advise wet soaks made with Burrow's solution five or six times daily to promote healing and relieve pain.
- Apply topical acyclovir (Zovirax 5%) cream after soaks six times a day.
- Cover the site with an occlusive dressing such as Tegaderm or plastic wrap to promote medication absorption if possible.
- Remember that severe initial outbreaks may be treated orally with acyclovir. For children (over 2 years of age), prescribe 20 mg/kg per dose orally four times a day for 5 days (maximum dosage of 800 mg/dose). For adolescents (over 40 kg), prescribe 400 mg orally three times a day for 7 to 10 days. Acetaminophen 10 to 15 mg/kg every 4 to 6 hours for pain may also be given.

Counseling and prevention

- Teach the parents and child how to make and apply compresses.
- Inform the parents and child that pain from lesions usually subsides after approximately 1 week. Resolution may take up to 3 weeks.
- Inform the parents and child of the following:
  Drainage from the lesions should be handled with gloves to prevent transference of infectious material.
  Draining lesions must be covered with a loose gauze dressing.
  Ointments should be applied with a finger cot or glove, never directly with a finger.
  Acyclovir may produce side effects such as nausea, headache, lethargy, and vomiting.

Follow-up

- Schedule a return visit in 1 week.
- Inform the parents and child to call if red streaking is noted around lesion or lesions or if condition worsens despite treatment.

Consultations and referrals. Refer to a physician for the following:

- Severe cases in which intravenous antiviral medications may be warranted
- Child with a history of immunosuppression or diabetes

Rash

JANE A. FOX

Alert

Consult with or refer to a physician for the following:
- Signs and symptoms of anaphylactic shock (which is a medical emergency)
- Petechiae (that do not blanch), purpura, or febrile-related convulsions
- Severe dehydration
- Extensive rash and pruritus that are unresponsive to appropriate treatment
- Significant lesions involving the eyes and genitalia
- Pregnancy
- Red or cola-colored urine
- Child who is immunocompromised or on immunosuppressive therapy
- Lesions that appear burnlike (e.g., scaled skin)
- Lesions that are red or blue or tender to the touch
- Lesions that have red streaking
- Rashes with accompanying fever, conjunctival erythema, and cervical adenopathy (Kawasaki's disease)

Etiology

Skin eruptions occur frequently in children and are of great concern to parents. With experience and guidance by the practitioner, parents can learn to differentiate between rashes (exanthems) that require an office visit and common, self-resolving lesions.

Rashes are caused by a wide variety of stimulants. Exposure to bacteria, fungi, parasites, and viral infections is often the cause, along with stress, allergies, trauma, and insect bites.

Incidence

- Rashes are a frequent occurrence in all age groups.
- Exposure to poison ivy, poison oak, or poison sumac is the most common cause of contact dermatitis in children in the United States.

Risk Factors

- Known exposure
- History of similar symptoms, skin condition (e.g., atopic dermatitis), environmental exposure, allergies, or asthma
- Family history of allergies
- Inadequate or incomplete immunizations
- Viral or bacterial infections
- Outdoor play in wooded areas
- Day care environment
- Immunosuppressive therapy

Differential Diagnosis

A practitioner should approach the diagnosis of rash with care (Table 37-17). The term "rash" is used to describe a skin eruption and is not descriptive of any specific lesion. Life-threatening diseases (e.g., lesions that are purple or look like blood and do not blanch, such as those caused by meningococcemia, toxic shock syndrome, sepsis with thrombocytopenia, or disseminated intravascular coagulation [DIC]), diseases that include signs and symptoms of cellulitis, and diseases that are highly contagious (e.g., measles, varicella) must be quickly identified. In addition, it is necessary to differentiate between a manifestation of a systemic disease and localized integumentary disease. Elicit a careful history (see Subjective Data in this chapter), including information on the rash such as onset, progression, distribution, associated symptoms (e.g., fever, pruritus), exposure, and allergies. Perform a careful examination. Rashes can be classified based on their structure into three groups to help with the diagnosis.

Papulosquamous rashes have raised, scaly lesions. They are usually localized, often highly pruritic, and are not associated with fever unless a secondary infection is present as a result of scratching. The site of the eruption often varies according to the age of the child. Other family members may have similar symptoms. A history of allergies in the child or family is often present. The most common causes of papulosquamous rashes in children are atopic dermatitis and scabies.

Maculopapular rashes are usually erythematous with flat or slightly raised lesions. They may involve the face, trunk, and extremities, and occasionally lesions are found in the mouth (enanthems). These rashes are usually associated with fever and often lymphadenopathy, rhinorrhea, and conjunctivitis. Immunization status may be incomplete or inadequate. These rashes can be caused by numerous viruses, bacteria, and rickettsias, and they are associated with many diseases, including measles (rubeola), rubella, roseola, erythema infectiosum, Kawasaki's disease, scarlet fever, and pityriasis rosea, as well as diseases caused by enteroviruses. Maculopapular eruptions are also associated with allergic reactions to medications, especially antibiotics. Antibiotic reactions are usually not accompanied by fever.

Vesicular rashes have distinctive lesions that are raised and fluid filled. The differential diagnosis is usually based on location (which can be anywhere on the body), distribution of the lesions, and the presence of fever. The lesions, depending on origin, may be pruritic. Other associated symptoms may include upper respiratory tract symptoms and a decreased appetite, especially if lesions are in the mouth on the mucous membranes. The history may be suggestive of exposure with affected contacts, outdoor activities, and a specific prodrome. Several conditions cause vesicular lesions (e.g., varicella, coxsackievirus, herpes simplex–herpes zoster, scabies, poison ivy, poison oak, poison sumac, tinea, dyshidrotic eczema, staphylococcal scalded skin syndrome, herpetic whitlow).

Disease-specific differential diagnoses

Coxsackievirus (hand-foot-and-mouth disease). This condition becomes evident with a brief history of malaise, low-grade fever, sore mouth, and anorexia. About 1 to 2 days after this prodromal phase, oral lesions appear, followed by erythematous macules on the hands, fingers, feet, toes, and interdigital surfaces. Approximately 90% of patients with coxsackievirus have oral lesions, and two thirds of patients have the classic exanthem. This condition is highly contagious, with an incubation phase of 2 to 6 days. Peak incidence is late summer and early fall (see also Mouth Sores in Chapter 35).

Erythema infectiosum (fifth disease). This condition is commonly referred to as "slapped cheek disease." Human parvovirus B19 is the cause of this condition, which peaks in late winter and early spring and is spread via respiratory droplets. Prodrome may include headache, nausea, and body ache. The rash first appears over both cheeks as erythematous, warm, nontender patches that have characteristic circumscribed borders and a macular or maculopapular appearance. Over 3 to 7 days the cheek rash fades and a lacelike, pale pink rash appears on the extensor surfaces of the arms and legs, gradually spreading to the trunk and buttocks.

Kawasaki's disease. Kawasaki's disease is characterized by abrupt fever lasting 5 or more days. Bilateral conjunctivitis, inflammation of the oral and pharyngeal mucous membranes, development of a "strawberry tongue," and cervical lymphadenopathy are manifestations of this syndrome. The rash may become evident as multiform. Referral to a physician is indicated, and hospitalization is required. Potential sequelae include cardiac involvement.

Roseola infantum. See Roseola in Chapter 44.

Measles (rubeola). See Rubeola in Chapter 44.

Varicella. See Varicella-Zoster Virus in Chapter 44.

Periorbital buccal cellulitis. This condition is most commonly caused by *Haemophilus influenzae* type B organism. Fever, lethargy, and bacteremia precede this noncircumscribed cellulitic rash in the periorbital region. Associated symptoms may include edematous cheeks with reddish purple discoloration. Consult with a physician.

Pityriasis rosea. This condition is caused by a virus that is usually seen in adolescence. Initially a herald patch (a round, scaly patch of skin on the trunk) appears, followed soon after by small, round papules with a scaly surface in a Christmas-tree configuration. Prodromal symptoms include lethargy and headache. This exanthem resolves over an extended period of time in its initial presentation.

Scarlet fever. Scarlet fever is caused by GABHS. The usual course is abrupt onset of fever, chills, headache, sore throat,

Table 37-17 Differential Diagnosis: Pediatric Infections with Dermatologic Manifestations

CLINICAL ENTITY	CAUSATIVE AGENT	AGE	CLINICAL SYNDROME	TYPE OF RASH	DISTRIBUTION	SIMILAR ENTITIES	TREATMENT
Roseola infantum (exanthema subitum) (MP)	Human herpesvirus, 6 or 7	6 months to 4 years	Fever, irritability, rapid lysis of fever with appearance of rash	Discrete macular or papular rash	Trunk with extension to neck, extremities, face	Enteroviral infection; *Mycoplasma*; drug eruption	Symptomatic: Acetaminophen, tepid baths, encourage fluids
Erythema infectiosum (fifth disease) (MP)	Parvovirus B19	School-age children; infants, adults less common	Flulike illness	Bilateral erythema of cheeks; "slapped cheeks"; lacyreticular exanthem	Face, trunk, extremities; palms, soles spared	Scarlet fever; rubella	Symptomatic: Acetaminophen
Measles (MP)	Measles virus	All ages	Fever, cough, coryza, conjunctivitis	Koplik spots, maculopapular eruption of upper trunk, face spreads to lower trunk, extremities; becomes confluent	Starts on face, moves downward	Enteroviral infection; *Mycoplasma*; drug eruption	Symptomatic: Vitamin A administration to those deficient
Pityriasis rosea (MP)	Unknown	Rare in infants; most common in adolescents, young adults	Headache, malaise, sore throat	Initially a "herald patch"; lesions are oval, salmon-colored with an erythematous border	Spreads peripherally, "Christmas tree" configuration	Tinea corporis; seborrheic dermatitis; secondary syphilis	Symptomatic: cool compress, diphenhydramine
Scarlet fever (MP)	Group A β-hemolytic streptococci (GABHS)	Toddlers >3 years of age, school-age children	Fever, sore throat, vomiting, abdominal pain; child may appear toxic	"Strawberry tongue" (bright red with sandpaper texture) that blanches with pressure, Pastia's lines	Begins in skin crease, spreads rapidly to trunk, extremities; face	Rubeola; rubella; roseola; fifth disease; Kawasaki's disease	Penicillin G; acetaminophen; warm saline gargles
Kawasaki's disease* (MP)	Unknown	Peak 6 months to 2 years	Fever, bilateral conjunctival infection, mucous membrane changes, peripheral extremity changes, cervical lymphadenopathy	Nonvesicular, polymorphic, "strawberry tongue"	Primarily truncal	Scarlet fever; staphylococcal scalded skin syndrome; rubeola; juvenile rheumatoid arthritis	Supportive care; antiinflammatory; immunoglobulin therapy
Hand-foot-mouth disease (V)	Primary: Coxsackievirus A; secondary: Coxsackievirus B, enterovirus	<10 years	Fever, anorexia, oral pain	Oral: Discrete, ulcerative; skin: Maculopapular, vesicular	Anterior mouth, hand, feet; occasionally neck, face	Aphthous stomatitis; varicella; herpes simplex	Symptomatic: Acetaminophen, warm saline rinses, tepid baths, encourage fluids

Condition	Cause	Age	Systemic Symptoms	Lesion Description	Distribution	Differential Diagnosis	Treatment
Varicella (V)	Varicella–zoster virus	90% of cases, <15 years	Fever, pruritus, malaise	Maculopapular, then vesicles on erythematous base, which rupture; crusting	Diffuse, includes scalp, oral mucosa	Insect bites; Herpes simplex	Symptomatic: Aveeno oatmeal baths, diphenhydramine, acetaminophen, warm saline rinses
Staphylococcal scalded-skin syndrome (V)	Staphylococcus aureus	Infants	Fever, irritability, septicemia (rare), eye and nasal discharge	Tender, diffuse; erythematous rash progressing to bullae; positive Nikolsky sign, exfoliation	Diffuse	Bullous impetigo; erythema multiforme; toxic epidermal necrolysis; pemphigus; epidermolysis bullosa; Kawasaki's disease	Intravenous therapy with a penicillinase-resistant penicillin
Poison ivy/ poison oak/ poison sumac (V)	Exposure to genus Toxicodendron (formerly Rhus)	Childhood, adolescence	None	Highly pruritic, vesicular, red eruption	Often linear; legs most common but anywhere on body	Atopic dermatitis; medication reaction; varicella; impetigo; herpes zoster	Symptomatic: Relief of pruritus hydroxine or diphenhydramine; cool compresses to lesions; severe cases: Systemic corticosteroids 1–2 mg/kg per day of prednisone
Impetigo (V)	GABHS, S. aureus	Any age	None	Lesions usually start in traumatized area as erythematous papule and then groups of vesicles, pustules that rupture to cause honey-colored crusts	Anywhere on body, most common on exposed areas, full extremities	Herpes simplex; folliculitis	For only a few lesions, topical antibiotic ointment; mupirocin; possible systemic treatment: Dicloxacillin
Periorbital buccal cellulitis*	Primary: Haemophilus influenzae type B; secondary: S. pneumoniae; S. aureus; β-hemolytic streptococci	3 to 36 months	Fever, bacteremia	Unilateral, indurated cellulitis; indistinct borders, violaceous hue	Periorbital, cheek	Orbital cellulitis; parotitis	High-dose antimicrobial therapy
Fungal infections Infestations							See Fungal Infections (Superficial) in Chapter 44 See Scabies in Chapter 44; see Lice in this chapter

*Refer to a physician.
MP, Maculopapular; V, vesicular.

lethargy, nausea, and vomiting. The rash (small, papular red lesions with a sandpaper-like texture) appears 12 to 48 hours after the initial symptoms. The skin appears sunburned and blanches with pressure. A "strawberry tongue" may accompany this syndrome (see also Sore Throat in Chapter 41).

Staphylococcal scalded-skin syndrome. This syndrome is caused by phase II coagulase-positive staphylococci. Primary infections are mild impetigo and conjunctivitis. Fever, irritability, and vomiting follow this tender rash, which rapidly spreads from head to toe.

Contact dermatitis. Also see Allergies in Chapter 43. The most common cause of contact dermatitis is exposure to poison ivy, poison oak, or poison sumac (members of the genus *Toxicodendron,* formerly *Rhus*). The patient usually has intensely pruritic, linear streaks of erythema and vesicles. The legs are most commonly involved, but the rash may occur on any part of the body. There may be a history of exposure. Autoinoculation occurs as the resin from the plant is carried to other body parts (e.g., face, neck, genitalia).

Fungal infections. See Fungal Infections (Superficial) in Chapter 44.

Management

Treatments and medications

Weeping rash. The strategy for care is aimed at drying these highly pruritic lesions. Have the patient take cool baths or apply wet compresses (soaks) up to four times daily. Soaks can be made from colloidal oatmeal, Aveeno, or Domeboro powder or tablets. Add one packet or one tablet to 1 pint of lukewarm water (1:40 Burrow's solution).

To prepare wet soaks:

- Tear clean cotton bedding, a thin towel, or a cotton T-shirt into long strips.
- Soak the strips in the chosen solution (e.g., oatmeal, Aveeno, Domeboro).
- Apply four to six layers to the affected skin surface and leave in place for 20 minutes.
- Apply drying lotion (e.g., calamine) after each soak.

After weeping or blistering has ceased, medicate with topical corticosteroid ointments in a thin layer. Use hydrocortisone ointment 1% two times a day on the face and intertriginous areas, and hydrocortisone ointment 2.5% four times a day on the body.

Dry rash. Strategies for care are aimed at decreasing pruritus and hydrating the skin surface.

- Decrease the frequency of bathing to three times a week.
- Wash the child with tepid bath water, then pat dry (do not rub).
- Advise the use of high-fat soaps (e.g., Dove, Basis, soap substitutes such as Cetaphil).
- Advise frequent lubrication of skin surface (three or four times a day) in winter months. The patient may use Eucerin cream, Moisturel cream, Aquaphor ointment, Keri creme, or Aveeno cream. Instruct the patient to apply lubricant after bathing; this results in increased penetration.
- Medicate affected skin surfaces with topical corticosteroid in a thin layer. Use hydrocortisone ointment 1% two times a day on the face and intertriginous areas, and hydrocortisone ointment 2.5% three times a day on the body.
- To relieve pruritus, prescribe diphenhydramine, 5 mg/kg in 24 hours and divided into doses every 6 to 8 hours, or

hydroxyzine 2 mg/kg in 24 hours, divided into doses every 6 to 8 hours

- For pain relief, prescribe acetaminophen, 10 to 15 mg/kg per dose every 4 to 6 hours, or ibuprofen 5 mg/kg per dose every 6 to 8 hours. Provide warm saline rinses for painful oral lesions. Provide cold, bland liquids (e.g., Jell-O, ice pops, Italian ice), and apply cool compresses to affected skin.
- Teach avoidance of exposure to UV rays.
- Dress the child in loose-fitting cotton clothing and use cotton sheets and bedding.
- Keep the child in a cool environment.
- Keep the child's nails trimmed short.
- Place cotton socks or gloves over the child's hands during sleep if the rash is pruritic.
- Advise frequent handwashing.

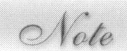

Aspirin is not an appropriate therapy for children with viral exanthems because of the risk of Reye syndrome.

Counseling and prevention

- Teach parents about any medications, including name, dose, schedule, and side effects.
- Encourage appropriate and timely vaccinations.
- Teach the parents and child to recognize and avoid certain plants if allergic to poison ivy, poison oak, or poison sumac. Teach the saying, "Leaves of three, let them be."
- If there is a known exposure, wash the exposed skin areas with soap and water. Dry with paper towels and discard.
- Avoid exposure to persons with exanthems.
- Instruct parents on the communicability of an exanthem.
- Advise parents to isolate children with exanthems from pregnant women, immunocompromised persons, and other children.
- Teach parents the appropriate application of cool compresses and use of saline rinses.
- Teach parents the signs and symptoms of dehydration and superinfection.
- Suggest precautions to prevent or limit spread to others, including frequent handwashing, individual towels and washcloths, covering the couch with a clean cotton sheet, and applying medication with gauze, tissue, or glove-covered hands.
- If the cause poison ivy, poison oak, or poison sumac, inform the parents and child that vesicle fluid does not contain the antigen and is not contagious. Instruct the parents never to burn poison ivy vines.

Follow-up

- Make a telephone call in 48 hours to monitor progress.
- Schedule an immediate return visit if the child's symptoms change or worsen.
- Schedule a return visit in 1 week to monitor progress.

Consultations and referrals. Provide immediate referral to a physician for children with seizure or febrile-related convulsions. Also, refer to or consult with a physician for the following:

Patient less than 2 months of age or less than 1 year with severe rash

Immunosuppressed patient or a patient receiving immunosuppressive therapy

Petechiae or purpura
Concurrent burns or uncontrolled eczema
Severe dehydration
Red or cola-colored urine

Scaly Scalp

VICTORIA VECCHIARIELLO

Alert

Consult with or refer to a physician for the following:
• Child who is unresponsive to appropriate treatment or after treatment options fail
• Immunocompromised child
• Systemic involvement

Etiology

Scaling of the scalp is a chronic inflammatory disease, the cause of which is unknown. This disorder is most common in the pediatric age group. It may be exacerbated by stress, excessive perspiration, or poor hygiene.

Incidence

• This is prominent in newborns and adolescents.
• Histiocytosis X is usually diagnosed at a very young age.

Risk Factors

• Excessive perspiration
• Eczema
• Allergies
• Immunosuppression
• Neonatal and adolescent period

Differential Diagnosis (Table 37-18)

Seborrheic dermatitis is an inflammatory, eczematous dermatitis sometimes confused with atopic dermatitis. Areas prone to involvement are hair-bearing and intertriginous areas of the body. The usual location is the scalp, where the condition is commonly referred to as *cradle cap*. This condition occurs primarily in newborns and at puberty. HIV must be considered in adolescents with this condition.

Folliculitis is an inflammation of a hair follicle, most commonly caused by *S. aureus* and resulting in a pustule. It is particularly problematic in the scalp, where follicles have been occluded by hair grease. Tight braiding of hair increases the risk for this condition. On inspection of the scalp, superficial pustules with surrounding erythema are visualized (see Abscesses [Boils] in this chapter).

Dandruff is the normal process of skin rejuvenation and may be observed as small white flakes or greasy scalp scales.

Tinea capitis is a fungal infection of the scalp. The distinguishing features are thickened, broken-off hairs, erythema, and scaling of the scalp (see Fungal Infections [Superficial] in Chapter 44).

Pediculosis capitis (infestation with head lice) is most commonly seen on hair at the nape of the neck. "Nits" (ova) may be visualized on the hair shaft. The child usually has severe itching of the scalp, excoriation from scratching, and secondary bacterial infections. Occipital and cervical adenopathy is common (see Lice in this chapter).

Langerhans' cell histiocytosis (which requires immediate referral to a physician), also known as *Letterer-Siwe disease*, constitutes a class I histiocytosis. This type of disorder is usually rare. A proliferation of Langerhans' cells is noted in combination with other cells in various proportions. Through the course of the disease, the lesions become fibrotic and necrotic. The disorder becomes evident in infancy, mimicking seborrheic dermatitis with scaly, erythematous patches on the scalp and in skin folds. It often mimics diaper rash, but the presence of petechiae is a warning sign. Major differences include depth of ulcerations and formation of vesicles with associated gingival and visceral alterations. Multisystem involvement may include lung infection, hepatosplenomegaly, bone marrow alterations, pancytopenia, and osteolytic bone disease. Fever from secondary bacterial infection may also occur.

Management

Seborrheic dermatitis

Treatments and medications. Daily care during acute episode includes application of a small amount of mineral oil to the scalp for 1 hour and then combing the hair gently with a soft brush. Wash hair with an antidandruff shampoo. (Products that contain selenium sulfide, tar, or salicylic acid are best.) If lesions are inflamed, topical corticosteroids promote comfort and healing.

Counseling and prevention
• Instruct the parents and child how to care for an acute episode. Continue daily care for at least 2 days after lesions clear and then twice weekly.
• Reassure the parents and child that condition will resolve.
• Advise the parents and child to avoid hair products that are oily or contain alcohol, which may dry the scalp.
• Teach the parents and child the symptoms of secondary bacterial infections, including swelling, redness, and drainage from ulceration.

Follow-up
• Advise parents to call if there are symptoms of secondary bacterial infection.
• Make telephone contact in 1 week to monitor progress.
• Schedule a return visit in 2 weeks to ensure resolution.
• Schedule a return visit if secondary infection occurs or condition worsens despite appropriate therapy.

Consultations and referrals. Refer to a pediatric dermatologist if treatment options fail.

Dandruff

Treatments and medications. Advise daily use of an antidandruff shampoo such as Selsun Blue, Sebulex, or Head & Shoulders.

Counseling and prevention
• Reassure the parents and child that dandruff is a normal skin process that can be well controlled with daily care.
• Instruct the parents and child to brush the child's hair well before shampooing.
• Advise the parents and child that antidandruff shampoo should be continued on a daily basis to prevent acute episodes of dandruff.
• Advise the parents and child to clean any hairbrush weekly.

Follow-up. Provide follow-up care as necessary.

Consultations and referrals. Refer to a pediatric dermatologist if treatment fails.

Langerhans' cell histiocytosis. This requires immediate referral to a physician.

Table 37-18 Differential Diagnosis: Scaly Scalp

CRITERIA	SEBORRHEIC DERMATITIS	SUPERFICIAL FOLLICULITIS	DANDRUFF	TINEA CAPITIS	LANGERHANS' CELL HISTIOCYTOSIS FORM OF HISTIOCYTOSIS X*
ICD-9 code	690.10	704.8	690.18	110.0	277.8
Subjective Data					
Age	Birth to 3 months and puberty	Any age	Any age	Most frequent in school-age children	Any age (most common under 2 years of age)
Presenting complaint(s)	Child or parent may report patch(es) of dry or ulcerated skin usually on scalp or in skin folds	May report small raised areas on scalp around hair shaft	Child or parent reports white flaking from scalp	Broken hairs, scaly scalp, fungal infection	Child or parent reports patches of dry or ulcerated skin; usual location: scalp, diaper area, palms, soles
Pruritus	Not likely	May report itching	Child or parent reports mild to none at all	None	Usually none reported
Patient and family history	History of allergies, food intolerances, allergic dermatitis; history of immunosuppressive condition such as cancer, HIV	History may reveal recurrent dermatoses; poor diet; homelessness or inadequate access or use of hygienic utilities (e.g., shower, bath); exposure to substances that occlude the skin surface (e.g., tar compounds, oils, occlusive dressing); hair braiding; exposure to a person with a draining lesion		May report that other family members have similar problem	Skin eruption is a common presentation of histiocytosis X; may report multisystem symptoms
Objective Data					
Physical examination					
Presenting location	Scalp, face, skin folds, behind ears; any skin surface with sebaceous glands	Scalp, arms, legs, buttocks	Usually seen on scalp; white flakes on clothing	Scalp	Scalp, behind ears; axillary, perianal and diaper areas; palms and soles may be affected, which assists in differentiation from seborrheic dermatitis; concomitant lesions in gingival and visceral skin surfaces
Inspection of skin/description of lesion	Erythematous scaly, crusty patches of skin; yellow and oily secretions; may note excoriation from scratching; crusting, waxlike buildup on affected skin surfaces	Small, dome-shaped pustule(s) at follicular base 1 to 4 mm in size, singular or in small groups on an erythematous base	Small, white flakes; greasy, scalp scales	"Black dots" may be noted at affected site; in the later phase, scalp may have golden crust; inflammation, scaling, dull hair may be noted; broken hairs at affected areas	Erythematous scaly patches of skin with associated petechiae, pustules, ulcerations, and hemorrhagic papules
Lymphadenopathy	Adolescents may report "flaking"	None	None	None	May be generalized or in areas with acute lesions
Associated signs	None None	None	None	None	May note hepatosplenomegaly, jaundice, exophthalmos, pulmonary alterations, bone lesions, growth retardation
Laboratory data	None	Usually not necessary; Gram stain and culture with antibiotic sensitivity testing in cases of severe resistance (see Management in text); staphylococcal organisms generally isolated	None	Fungal cultures positive for *Trichophyton tonsurans*	Diagnosis requires complete blood cell count with differential to evaluate for anemia and thrombocytopenia; refer patient for biopsy of abnormal bone, skin, bone marrow, lymph nodes, and liver

*Immediate referral to a physician.

Sunburn

LOREN O'CONNOR DEMPSEY

Alert

Consult with or refer to a physician for the following:

- Signs and symptoms of sunstroke (a medical emergency):
  Temperature greater than 105° F (40° C)
  Syncope, fainting, and poor perfusion
  Central nervous system (CNS) dysfunction with possible
     seizures, combative state, disorientation, weakness, nausea
     and vomiting, headache, thirst, or muscle cramping
  Sweating in the presence of elevated temperature
- Infant with severe sunburn
- Extensive burns, which may require corticosteroid therapy
- Children with signs of actinic keratitis after UV radiation
  exposure, or with eye pain or photophobia.

Etiology

UV radiation produced by the sun causes permanent dermatologic changes. UV radiation B (less than 0.5% of UV radiation reaching earth) is responsible for most acute and chronic skin damage and is most intense in the summer, at midday, at high altitudes, and along the equator. Sunlight is reflected (up to 85%) by sand, concrete, snow, and water, and such reflection intensifies exposure. Six sun-reactive skin types (Table 37-19) and a UV radiation predictive exposure index have been developed (Table 37-20) to educate and inform the public about sunburn. The index is reported daily on both radio and television by weather forecasters during the summer months.

Erythema and pain associated with sunburn (first-degree burns) are caused by vasodilatation of blood vessels in the dermis. A change in the permeability of the dermis results in edema. Sunburn is directly correlated to skin type, amount of exposure, ability to produce melanin before and after sun exposure, and protective devices that are used. Melanin is the body's protective response to sun exposure and is produced in limited quantities, which varies by skin type. Tanning begins during sun exposure and continues for 7 to 10 days as the body produces new melanin. Tanning beds induce melanin production (tanning) by exposing the skin to primarily UV radiation A and have been linked with an increased risk of melanoma in some studies. The risk of retinal damage has also been identified.

Skin cancers have been linked to cumulative UV radiation exposure, with the highest risks associated with lengthy exposures that are episodic in nature. Childhood burns increase the risk of skin cancer in adulthood.

Additional risks of UV radiation exposure include: (1) skin aging, (2) damage to the eyes, including retinal injury (infants and children under 10 years of age are at greatest risk) and macular degeneration, and (3) immune system suppression, believed to play a role in skin cancer development and vaccine response. Further research may link UV radiation to allergies, asthma, and autoimmune disease.

Incidence

- Approximately 80% of lifetime UV radiation exposure is estimated to occur before 18 years of age.
- Sunburn can occur in any child, regardless of skin type, after exposure to UV radiation.
- Sunburn occurs more quickly and more severely in fair-skinned children whose bodies do not produce large quantities of melanin.

Table 37-19 Classification of Sun-Reactive Skin Types*

SKIN TYPE	HISTORY OF SUNBURNING OR TANNING
I	Always burns easily; never tans
II	Always burns easily; tans minimally
III	Burns moderately; tans gradually and uniformly (light brown)
IV	Burns minimally; always tans well (moderate brown)
V	Rarely burns; tans profusely (dark brown)
VI	Never burns; deeply pigmented (black)

Data from the American Medical Association Council on Scientific Affairs (1989). JAMA, 262, 380-384.
Based on 45 to 60 minutes of sun exposure after winter or no sun exposure

Table 37-20 Exposure Levels Predicted by the Ultraviolet Index*

INDEX VALUE	EXPOSURE LEVEL	TIME IN SUN NEEDED FOR BURN
0 to 2	Minimal	1 hour
3 to 4	Low	30-60 minutes
5 to 6	Moderate	20-30 minutes
7 to 9	High	minutes
10 to 15	Very high	Less than 13 minutes

Data from National Association of Physicians for the Environment (1994, June). UV index fact sheet. Bethesda, MD: National Association of Physicians for the Environment.
These UV effects are on unprotected skin type II, which usually burns easily and tans minimally.

- One in five Americans will suffer from some form of skin cancer in his or her lifetime.
- Each blistering sunburn doubles the risk of developing malignant melanoma.
- About 8% of all cases of skin cancer surround the eyes and eyelids, and one third occur on the nose.

Risk Factors

- Age less than 6 months
- Light-colored skin, hair, or eyes; freckles; vitiligo; or an excessive number of nevi
- UV exposure without protection
- Exposure to UV radiation during peak sun hours (10:00 AM to 2:00 PM)
- Acne treatment
- Children undergoing chemotherapy or radiation treatment
- Systemic medication therapy
- Xeroderma pigmentosum (XP) syndrome
- Systemic lupus erythematosus
- Familial dysplastic nevus syndrome
- Children with two or more family members with melanoma

Differential Diagnosis (Table 37-21)

Sunburn is a common reaction to exposure to the UV rays of the sun that results in varied degrees of erythema, edema, and potential blistering.

Table 37-21 Sunburn

CRITERIA	SUNBURN	PHOTOSENSITIVE SKIN REACTIONS	VIRAL EXANTHEMS
ICD-9 code	692.71	692.82	057.9
Subjective Data			
Reported duration of ultraviolet (UV) radiation exposure	30 minutes to 4 hours	15 minutes to 1 hour	Varies
Associated history	Child or parent reports UV exposure with either inadequate or lack of sunscreen protection; child or parent may report hobbies or leisure activities associated with open spaces such as the beach, snow, or water-covered environments; outdoor activities between the hours of 10:00 AM and 2:00 PM	Child or parent may report use of one or more of the following medications: Sulfonamides Tretinoin Tetracyclines Thiazides	Child or parent may report symptoms of a viral infection such as malaise; child or parent may report rash that had cleared and has now resurfaced after the affected skin surface was exposed to UV; rash generally appears 24 to 48 hours after sun exposure
Objective Data *Physical examination*			
Vital signs	Normal; children with sunstroke may have temperature elevations up to 105° F (this is a medical emergency)	Normal	Normal; mild temperature elevation may be seen with concurrent systemic viral symptoms
Skin examination	Erythema, edema, and blistering on exposed skin surfaces; Skin damage depends on duration and type of UV exposure	Erythema and tenderness; blistering may occur if UV exposure is prolonged	Erythema and tenderness noted in skin surfaces exposed to UV; previously cleared rash may return; macules and papules may be seen
Laboratory data	None	None	None

Photosensitive skin reactions are a result of the body's reaction to UV radiation in the presence of particular drugs, lotions, or perfumes.

Viral exanthems are skin eruptions that reappear in the presence of UV radiation, producing a superficial exanthem. This eruption is generally confined to the area of skin exposed to UV radiation and assumes an appearance similar to the once-cleared rash. Patients generally report a recent past history of malaise (viral in origin) that may have initially become evident with a rash.

Management

Sunburn

Treatments and medications

- Rehydrate the child with plenty of free fluid (e.g., water, juice).
- Advise the use of NSAIDs to relieve discomfort. Prescribe ibuprofen 5 to 10 mg/kg every 6 to 8 hours with a maximum of 40 mg/kg per day (not recommended in children under 6 months of age).
- For painful burns, apply cool-water compresses to affected areas.
- Advise the use of Burrow's solution compresses for 20 minutes four to six times a day.
- Remember that use of aloe gels may provide short-term relief.
- Keep the child in a cool environment. Use of cotton sheets and loose-fitting cotton clothing may increase comfort.
- Avoid additional exposure to UV radiation. Keep out of sun.

- Avoid use of all soap and perfume products or first-aid creams that contain benzocaine (which may cause an allergic rash).
- Apply perfume-free lotions (e.g., Aveeno, Eucerin, Vaseline Intensive Care) to ease dryness and decrease itching.

Counseling and prevention

- Explain the treatment plan to the parents and child, including medication dosing and possible side effects, application of wet soaks, and the need to increase fluid intake.
- See Prevention of Sunburn earlier in this chapter.

Follow-up. Follow-up is usually not necessary. Schedule a return visit or make a telephone call if blisters from sunburn become infected.

Consultations and referrals

- Provide immediate physician referral for children with third-degree burns or burns covering a large part of the body, or signs of actinic keratitis.
- Keep in mind that physician consultation may be necessary if blisters become infected.
- If burns are a result of neglect or abuse is suspected, report to the authorities (this is mandatory).

Photosensitive skin reactions

Treatments and medications

- Keep the child out of the sun.
- Use cool compresses to relieve discomfort as necessary.
- See Sunburn in this chapter.

Counseling and prevention

- Instruct the parents (when prescribing medications) if the child must avoid the sun.
- Teach parents signs and symptoms of superinfection.

Follow-up. Follow-up is usually not necessary. Schedule a return visit if blisters become infected or the condition worsens.

Consultations and referrals

- Provide immediate physician referral for children with third-degree burns or burns covering a large part of the body.
- Keep in mind that physician consultation may be necessary if blisters become infected.
- If burns are a result of neglect or abuse is suspected, report to the authorities (this is mandatory).

  Viral exanthems. See Rash in this chapter.

Warts (Verrucae)

LOREN O'CONNOR DEMPSEY

Alert

Consult with or refer to a physician for:

- Diabetes mellitus
- Unusual warts with hair growth, unusual pigmentation, induration (except molluscum contagiosum), fixed location, or ulceration
- Patients with impaired circulation
- History of immunosuppression
- Anogenital warts in young children
- Warts that are unresponsive to treatment
- Confluent plantar warts

Etiology

Warts are common, benign skin tumors that are caused by over 60 different types of human papillomavirus (HPV). Once inoculated onto the skin surface through direct contact, this deoxyribonucleic acid (DNA) virus causes abnormal epidermal growth, forming a warty mass on the skin surface. The incubation period is 1 to 6 months, with spontaneous resolution of the virus in 25% of cases in 3 to 6 months and 65% of cases in 2 years. Warts are superficial lesions without roots, remain isolated to the skin, and are most commonly seen on the hands, fingers, and feet. Growths may be sharply circumscribed, raised groups of papillomas, or singular and flat. Color varies; lesions may be pink, yellow, brown, or gray. They may be crusty with irregular, rough surfaces or smooth. Periungual, subungual, and mucous membrane growths are more common in persons who bite their nails.

Incidence

- Warts are common in children and young adults.
- Warts affect about 10% of school-age children.
- Molluscum contagiosum is common in infants, preschoolers, and sexually active adolescents.
- There is a higher incidence of warts in those who are immunocompromised.
- Peak incidence for condylomata acuminata (genital warts) is 18 to 24 years of age.
- There is a 60% transmission rate for venereal or genital warts.

Risk Factors

- Finger-sucking, nail or hangnail biting, and trauma
- Frequent exposure to locker room or gym floors, going barefoot, or being around a swimming pool
- History of immunosuppression, immunosuppressive therapy, acquired immune deficiency syndrome (AIDS), or lymphoma
- Unprotected sex or direct contact with an infected individual
- Multiple sex partners
- History of atopic eczema (this factor is challenged in current research)

Differential Diagnosis (Table 37-22)

Common warts (verrucae vulgaris) may resemble molluscum contagiosum, seborrheic keratosis (horny growths), nevus, clavus, acrochordon, and squamous cell cancer. Accurate lesion diagnosis is essential in the treatment of warts. When in doubt, clinicians should seek specialty evaluation. Common warts begin as small, smooth papules that grow over a period of several weeks into dome-shaped, hyperpigmented growths. Black dots, easily exposed by paring of the top of the wart, are the result of thrombosed capillaries. These warts are often found around (periungual) and under the nail (subungual).

Plantar warts are caused by HPV type 1 and are commonly found on the heel or ball of the foot. These warts cause significant pain and grow much larger than they appear. Weight-bearing skin surfaces are at increased risk for this type of wart. Look for disruption in the normal skin pattern (lines) and thrombosed capillaries (black dots that can be revealed with gentle shaving of the outermost horny layer of the lesion). Corns and calluses do not have these distinguishing features. Plantar warts are transmitted through direct contact with any surface exposed to the virus (e.g., floors, benches, exercise mats). Plantar warts that appear in clusters around a larger wart are termed "mosaic warts" and are difficult to treat (refer to a dermatologist). Differential diagnosis of plantar warts includes corns, callus, and palmar or plantar keratoses (horny growths).

Molluscum contagiosum begins as small papules 3 to 12 weeks after exposure and grows to up to 5 mm in size. As the wart matures, a sharply circumscribed, waxy papule develops. The center of this lesion becomes umbilicated with a soft, white center. Papules may appear in a linear pattern, since the virus is spread through scratching. Crops of molluscum are not uncommon. This lesion, caused by the poxvirus, is contagious and may be found anywhere on the body except the palms of the hands and soles of the feet. Frequently affected are the axillae, trunk, face, and genitals.

Verrucae planae (singular is *verruca plana*) are small, subtle, flat warts caused by HPV types 3, 10, and 28. These warts are commonly seen on the face, arms, and legs. Flat warts may be pink, light brown, or light yellow. They generally occur in clusters, are spread by scratching, and are often resistant to treatment. Verrucae planae may resemble epidermal nevi, lichen nitidus, and lichen planus.

Verrucae filiformes (singular is *verruca filiformis*) are small, fingerlike, flesh-colored warts that are commonly found on the face, neck, eyelid, and nasolabial region. Easily spread, this growth is difficult to treat. Referral for removal by excision is warranted.

Condylomata acuminata (singular is *condyloma acuminatum*) are soft, fleshy-colored genital warts with a cauliflower-like appearance. These lesions are often found in the anogenital region and mucous membranes. Acetic acid 3% to 5% (white vinegar is 5% acetic acid) applied directly to the growth will

Table 37-22 Differential Diagnosis: Warts

CRITERIA	VERRUCAE VULGARES (COMMON WARTS)	PLANTAR WARTS	MOLLUSCUM CONTAGIOSUM	VERRUCAE PLANA (FLAT WARTS)	VERRUCAE FILIFORM (FILIFORM WARTS)	CONDYLOMATA ACUMINATUM (GENITAL WARTS)
ICD-9 code	078.10	078.19	078.0	078.10	078.10	078.11
Subjective Data						
Age	Any age; common at 12 to 16 years of age	Any age; common at 12 to 16 years of age	Any age; common at 12 to 16 years of age	Any age	Any age	Any sexually active person
Gender preference	Female > male	Female > male	None	None	None	None
Description of problem	May report pain with pressure (e.g., holding pencil)	May report pain with walking	Most patients are asymptomatic; many report bumps on the skin	May report flat lesions on face	May report finger-like growth on face or neck	May report uncomfortable growth in vaginal region, on penis, or in rectum
Past health history	Possible history of immunosuppression, widespread atopic dermatitis, acquired immunodeficiency syndrome, lymphoma, diabetes, neonatal exposure at delivery					
Social habit history	May report nail biting, finger sucking	May report frequent exposure to locker or gym room floors				May report multiple sex partners, unprotected sex, child or sexual abuse
Objective Data *Physical examination* Skin examination						
Common location	Hand or fingers most common; any skin exposed to trauma	Plantar surface of feet and hands	Face, trunk, axillae, genitals, inner thigh, abdomen	Face and neck most common; extensor aspect of forearm, hands	Face, neck	Warm, moist intertriginous areas of the body and genital region; foreskin, penis; vagina and labial mucosae
Number of lesions	Singular or in crops	Singular or grouped to form mosaic pattern	Alone or in clusters	Singular or grouped	Alone or in clusters	Grouped
Lesion size	Varies	Varies	1 to 5 mm	1 to 5 mm	Up to 1 cm in length	Varies
Appearance	Growth begins as a smooth translucent papule; sharply circumscribed, dome-shaped, hyperpigmented growth emerges over several weeks	Immature lesion is flat or slightly elevated; the majority of this wart grows beneath the skin surface; interrupts skin line; thrombosed capillaries	Discrete, pearly white or skin-toned papules that evolve into umbilicated, waxy papules with white core, sharply circumscribed	Discrete, flesh-colored or tan papules	Soft, flesh-colored, fingerlike growths	Soft, skin-toned vegetative growth; small warts may be hyperpigmented; cauliflower-like appearance
Laboratory data	None	None	Molluscum contagiosum bodies expressed from the umbilicated core can be seen microscopically; not necessary for diagnosis	None	None	Pap smear to rule out cervical warts; offer work-up for sexually transmitted disease, including testing for human immunodeficiency virus infection, chlamydiosis, gonorrhea, herpes, and syphilis
Causative organism	HPV types 1, 2, 4	HPV type 1	Poxvirus	HPV types 3, 10, 28	HPV type 2	HPV types 6, 11

cause the surface to turn white, aiding the clinician in diagnosis. Condyloma acuminatum may look like condyloma latum, a sign of secondary syphilis. Condyloma latum differs from condyloma acuminatum in that latum appears as a flat mucus patch with distinct borders covered with gray exudate. Consider sexual abuse in all children having either of these lesions.

Management

General measures. Warts are a benign skin condition. Therefore therapy should not be harmful to the patient, scarring is unnecessary, and side effects should be minimal. Consider observation alone in children under 2 years of age.

Common warts (verrucae vulgares) and plantar warts

Treatments and medications. Treatment of plantar warts is indicated only if the patient is symptomatic. Salicylic acid is contraindicated in known diabetics; cases of unusual warts with hair growth, birthmarks, or moles; and patients with impaired circulation. Keratolytic therapy is the treatment of choice. This includes topical application of salicylic acid (OTC forms are Duofilm and Occlusal-HP). Duofilm and Occlusal-HP contain 17% salicylic acid in a solution. Abrade the surface of the wart with a pumice stone, emery board, or sandpaper. Soak the affected site with very warm water for 10 minutes to facilitate penetration of medicine by softening the keratin surface. Apply 1 drop of salicylic acid solution and allow to dry. Repeat until the wart is completely covered. Occlude the site with adhesive tape to increase absorption of medication and leave the tape in place for 24 hours. Nightly application for several weeks (up to 12) is necessary. If the patient develops soreness, advise a break from therapy.

A salicylic acid patch (Trans-Ver-Sal; 15% salicylic acid) is available in 6-mm and 12-mm pads. Clean the site; abrade with emery board, sandpaper, or pumice stone; moisten the site with water; and apply a patch that is trimmed to the wart's size. Avoid contact with normal skin. Secure with adhesive tape. Apply nightly and remove in the morning.

For large plantar warts, use salicylic acid plasters. Mediplast (40% salicylic acid) is available in 4 × 3 inch sheets. Cut the plaster to the wart's size and apply to the site, securing with adhesive tape. Remove 24 to 48 hours later, clean the area, and abrade the wart with an emery board, pumice stone, or sandpaper to remove the soft, white center (keratin). Removal of this central aspect of the lesion leads to rapid pain reduction in the first few days of treatment. Daily or every-other-day application of this plaster for several weeks is necessary for successful treatment. Although plasters work more slowly than salicylic acid solutions, this treatment is often preferred because it is less irritating than liquid or gel solutions.

Counseling and prevention

- Teach the parents and child that warts are caused by a virus, often after trauma.
- Teach parents that virus can be spread to others through direct contact and that care should be taken to keep affected areas covered.
- Teach the parents and child to cover the child's feet in public places (e.g., pools, locker rooms, exercise mats) to prevent new infection and reduce transmission of the existing virus.
- Advise that the virus generally resolves within 2 years (65% of cases) if left untreated, but recurrence is common in 20% to 30% of all cases.
- Avoid pressure and trauma to the feet through properly fitting shoes.

- Advise the parents and child that treatment, though relatively effective, may not completely resolve all warts. Nightly application for up to 12 weeks may be necessary. Clinical improvement is expected in 2 to 4 weeks. The treatment is nonscarring and safe when used as directed.
- Teach the parents and child proper application of medication, with precautions being taken to avoid contact with the eyes or mucous membranes. Discontinue treatment if excessive irritation develops. Teach the parents and child the symptoms of secondary bacterial infections, including swelling, redness, drainage, and fever of more than 100.5° F.

Follow-up. Usually none is indicated. Advise the parents to call if there are symptoms of secondary bacterial infection.

Consultations and referrals. Refer to a pediatric dermatologist if treatment options fail, if warts are widespread and curettage is necessary, if the parents and child are not satisfied with topical treatment, or for mosaic plantar warts.

Molluscum contagiosum

Treatments and medications. Treatment of the individual lesion helps prevent autoinoculation and person-to-person transfer of the virus. Topical therapy with a blistering agent (e.g., Occlusal-HP, Duofilm) is the treatment of choice for mild cases of this warty virus. Patients who have widespread lesions, are immunocompromised, or have extensive atopic dermatitis should be referred for removal by curettage or cryotherapy with liquid nitrogen or dry ice.

Topical application of salicylic acid (OTC forms are Duofilm and Occlusal-HP) can be done. Duofilm and Occlusal-HP contain 17% salicylic acid in a solution. Soak the affected site in very warm water for 10 minutes to facilitate penetration of medicine by softening the keratin surface. Apply 1 drop of salicylic acid solution and allow to dry. Repeat this procedure until the wart is completely covered. Occlude the site with adhesive tape to increase absorption of medication. Remove after 12 hours and replace until core is expelled. The curdlike core should be expressed in 3 to 5 days, after which treatment can cease.

Counseling and prevention

- Advise the parents and child that the natural course of this virus is spontaneous resolution, which varies widely from 2 weeks to 1½ years.
- Advise the parents and child that molluscum contagiosum is easily spread from person to person by direct or indirect contact. Avoid direct contact with the skin surface until the core is expressed.
- Suggest that good handwashing is essential to prevent spread and secondary bacterial infection.
- Suggest that clean, white cotton socks worn over the hands at night may prevent the child from picking at lesions.
- Teach parents that a scaly red ring of dry skin may occur around lesions as the virus resolves.
- Teach the parents and child the symptoms of secondary bacterial infection, including swelling, redness, drainage, and fever (100.5° F or greater).
- Advise parents to call if symptoms of secondary bacterial infection develop or if extensive irritation occurs from topical therapy.

Follow-up. Schedule a return visit in 1 week.

Consultations and referrals. Refer to a pediatric dermatologist if there are widespread lesions, the patient is immunocompromised, or the lesions are unresponsive to treatment.

Flat warts (verrucae planae)

Treatments and medications. Refer to a dermatologist for treatment of the lesions.

Counseling and prevention

- Inform the parents and child that virus is spread through direct contact. The child should avoid picking and scratching warts.
- Advise frequent handwashing.
- Suggest that cotton socks may be worn over the hands at night to decrease scratching.

Follow-up. Follow-up is determined by a dermatologist.

Consultations and referrals. Refer to a dermatologist for treatment.

Filiform warts (verrucae filiformes)

Treatments and medications. Refer to a dermatologist for treatment by electrosurgery or cryosurgery.

Counseling and prevention

- Advise the parents and child that warts are easily removed but have a high rate of recurrence, lasting years.
- Encourage reduced spread of the virus by avoidance of shaving the affected site (e.g., face, leg).

Follow-up. Monitor for recurrence with routine checkup.

Consultations and referrals. Refer to a dermatologist for treatment.

Condylomata acuminata

Treatments and medications. Refer to an adolescent medicine specialist, dermatologist, or gynecologist-midwife for evaluation and management. The goal of treatment is to remove visible genital warts and those that are symptomatic because there is no evidence indicating that available therapies affect the natural history of HPV. HPV can survive in the basal layer of the skin, acting as a viral reservoir; therefore absence of visible lesions may not decrease infectivity. Clinicians should seek evaluation by an experienced health care provider to ensure comprehensive screening for all STDs, especially cervical dysplasia and syphilis. Currently, available treatments include those that are patient applied (e.g., podofilox, imiquimod) and provider administered (e.g., cryotherapy podophyllin resin, trichloroacetic acid, interferon, laser surgery).

Counseling and prevention

- Inform the parents and child that the lesions are spread through direct contact with an infected person (60% transmission rate).
- Teach adolescents about the maturation of the cervix, specifically the presence of a wide transformation zone, which, until involuted, places the teenager at a higher risk for acquiring STDs.
- Inform adolescents that some strains of HPV have been directly linked to cervical cancer.
- Instruct that barrier protection (condoms) must be used during sexual intercourse to reduce transmission of the virus; however, barrier protection may not be enough because lesions typically occur at sites not protected by condoms and can survive in skin layers once infected by an HPV lesion.
- Advise that growth of existing lesions may be stimulated by trauma, pregnancy, tobacco use, current infection, oral contraceptive use, and immunosuppression.
- Inform the patient that 25% of genital warts recur in 3 months.
- Advise that girls and women with genital warts require a Pap smear to rule out cervical warts.
- Offer a rapid plasmin reagin test and screening for all STDs, including HIV.

Follow-up. Provide follow-up as directed by the consulting provider.

Consultations and referrals. Refer to an adolescent medicine specialist, dermatologist, or gynecologist-midwife for treatment. Report to the appropriate authorities if sexual abuse is suspected.

Weeping Lesions (Impetigo)

VICTORIA VECCHIARIELLO

Alert

Consult with or refer to a physician for the following:
- Signs and symptoms of acute glomerulonephritis resulting from nephrogenic strains of streptococci
- Ecthyma, a streptococcal infection with extension through the epidermis resulting in a firm, dry crust with surrounding erythema and elevated margins.

Etiology

Most cases of nonbullous impetigo and all cases of bullous impetigo are caused by *S. aureus*. The remainder of cases of nonbullous impetigo are attributable to GABHS or a combination of these organisms. GABHS colonize the skin directly by binding to sites on fibronectin that are exposed to trauma. In contrast, *S. aureus* first colonizes the nasal epithelium, and then from this reservoir, colonization of the skin occurs.

Incidence

- It is seen in children of all age groups and accounts for 10% of all skin problems seen in pediatrics.
- It is found most commonly on face, the nares, and the extremities.

Risk Factors

- Poor hygiene
- Antecedent lesions such as chickenpox, scabies, insect bites, trauma (skin bruising), or burns
- Humidity and warm temperature
- Communicable up to 48 hours after antibiotic therapy is initiated
- Living in areas of high insect infestation
- Age
- Preexisting skin condition (e.g., atopic dermatitis)
- Crowding or poor living conditions

Differential Diagnosis (Table 37-23)

Impetigo is a superficial, contagious skin infection. It is one of the most common skin infections in children. It usually begins with a superficial vesicular or pustular lesion and develops through exudative and crusted stages. The incubation period is 2 to 10 days (usually 1 to 3 days). It is transmitted by direct and sometimes indirect contact. Impetigo has two forms, nonbullous and bullous.

Nonbullous impetigo, or *classic impetigo,* is characterized by honey-colored, crusted lesions. The lesion usually begins in a traumatized area (such as a scratch, insect bite) as a small vesicle. This vesicle quickly develops into a pustule and ruptures, forming honey-colored crusts and scabs. There is usually pruritus. The lesions may appear anywhere on the body but are

Table 37-23　Differential Diagnosis: Impetigo

CRITERIA	NONBULLOUS IMPETIGO	BULLOUS IMPETIGO
ICD-9 code	684.	684.
Subjective Data		
Age	Any age	Any age
Description of problem	Reports clear sores on red, irritated skin; once vesicle enlarges and ruptures, a honey-colored crust is formed; this is spread quickly	Reports rapidly formed sores that are filled with clear to cloudy fluid; once vesicle ruptures, it leaves a shiny red base
Location of sores	May occur anywhere on body	May occur anywhere on body
Aggravating factors	Pruritus	Prutitus
Predisposing factors	History of minor trauma: Insect bites, scabies, scratches, chickenpox; history of exposure to impetigo; poor hygiene; preexisting skin condition	History of minor trauma: Insect bites, scabies, scratches, chickenpox; history of exposure to impetigo; poor hygiene; preexisting skin condition
Family history	Family member has impetigo	Family member has impetigo
Objective Data		
Physical examination		
Skin examination		
Description of lesions	Lesion appears as clear vesicle on erythematous base and rapidly becomes pustular; pustule ruptures, enlarges, and spreads; characteristic honey-colored adherent crust is formed; satellite lesions are common	Lesions are rapidly formed: Fragile bullae filled with clear fluid, which progresses to cloudy fluid before rupture; these bullae heal centrally, leaving a crusted annular formation; recently ruptured bullae have an erythematous shiny base; older lesions are dry and nonerythematous
Location of lesions	May occur anywhere on body; face, hands, perineum most likely	May occur anywhere on body; skin folds most common
Lymph nodes	Regional lymphadenopathy common	Regional lymphadenopathy usually absent
Laboratory data	Usually none but may obtain culture and Gram stain beneath crusts; if recurrent infection, nasal swab to determine staphylococcal carrier status	Obtain swab from bullous fluid for Gram stain and culture

most common on exposed areas (e.g., face, extremities). From the initial area of infection, there may be spread to other parts of the body.

Bullous impetigo, the least common form of impetigo, often begins in the skin folds of the neck or groin. It is characterized by the presence of bullae (less than 3 cm in diameter) on intact skin. Vesicles enlarge into flaccid, transparent bullae containing straw-colored or cloudy, yellow fluid. These bullae rapidly rupture and become erosions and crusts. There is no surrounding erythema. Infants and young children are most commonly affected. Ecthyma may occur simultaneously with impetigo. It is characterized by a firm, dry, dark crust surrounded by erythema and induration. If direct pressure is applied to the crust, purulent material from beneath the crust is expelled. The skin of the legs is most commonly affected.

Nummular dermatitis has dozens of lesions symmetrically distributed, whereas impetigo has only a few nonsymmetric lesions.

Herpes simplex usually has a group of distinct lesions that even when crusted show a group of individual papules and vesicles beneath. It can mimic impetigo on the cheek and forehead. A Tzanck smear, HSV antibody test, or bacterial and viral culture will differentiate the two.

Kerion, an erythematous boggy nodule with superficial pustules, results from a dermatophyte infection and may have moist crusts and appear like impetigo. It is usually hairless and will lead to permanent hair loss if untreated. A kerion may appear 2 to 8 weeks after an infection begins and is an exaggerated host response to the invading fungus.

Management
Nonbullous and bullous impetigo
Treatments and medications
- Keep in mind that removal of crusts by a gentle soaking with warm water compresses or antiseptic soap or cleanser has not been shown to be effective.
- If only a few lesions are present, apply mupirocin ointment to affected lesions three times a day for 7 to 10 days or until all lesions have cleared. Mupirocin is highly effective against gram-positive pathogens, especially *S. aureus* and group A streptococci. Reevaluate in 3 to 5 days if there is no response.
- If there is widespread, deep involvement or failure with topical preparations, initiate systemic treatment. A β-lactamase–resistant drug such as dicloxacillin (the drug of choice) or erythromycin should be chosen. Avoid erythromycin if there is widespread erythromycin resistance in the community. A first- or second-generation cephalosporin is also effective.
- If response to systemic treatment is inadequate, culture a lesion and alter treatment according to the culture results.

Counseling and prevention
- Instruct the parents and child to continue medication for 10 full days; do not stop because lesions have cleared.
- Explain to the parents and child that the incubation period is usually 1 to 3 days and that impetigo spreads cutaneously as well as systemically.
- Advise the parents and child on the importance of good handwashing and on using separate towels and washcloths

to prevent spread. Wash linens and clothing in hot water. Assess sleeping arrangements and make appropriate changes during the communicable stage.

- Keep fingernails short to minimize the spread caused by scratching.
- Instruct parents to check other friends or family members for impetigo.
- Explain to parents that the child should not return to school until 24 hours after treatment has started.
- Explain to parents that the transmission of impetigo is by direct and sometimes indirect contact.
- Advise that treatment with antibiotic therapy should begin before the child returns to school or a day-care center.
  Follow-up
- Schedule a return visit if the condition worsens or if there is no response to treatment in 5 to 7 days. Obtain culture and sensitivity and treat accordingly.
- Keep in mind that a return visit in 10 days may be useful to evaluate the response to treatment and determine any spread to contacts.
- Have parents call immediately if dark-colored urine, decreased urinary output, or edema is noted.
  Consultations and referrals
- Refer to a nephrologist if there are signs or symptoms of acute glomerulonephritis.
- Refer to a dermatologist if after culture, sensitivity testing, and appropriate treatment, the response is less than expected.

Resources

Websites
All about Allergies (www.allergies.about.com)
American Academy of Dermatology (AAD) (www.aad.com)
The American Society of Dermatology (ASD) (www.asd.org)
Dermatology Online Journal (dermatology.cdlib.org)
Health Information Service of the National Library of Medicine and National Institutes of Health (www.medlineplus.com)
MDAdvice.com (www.mdadvice.com)
Medscape Dermatology (dermatology.medscape.com/Home/Topics/Dermatology/Dermatology.html)
Medscape Primary Care Dermatology Atlas (ID.medscape.com/LII/DermAtlas/index.cfm)
Morbidity and Mortality Weekly Report (www.cdc.gov/mmwr/mmwr.html)
National Alopecia Areata Foundation (www.alopeciaareata.com)
Physicians for the Environment (www.napenet.org/index.html)
SupportPath.com (www.supportpath.com)
United States Environmental Protection Agency (www.epa.gov/ozone/uvindex/uvover.html)

Bibliography

Achauer, B.M. & VanderKam, V.M. (2000). Treating vascular birthmarks with laser surgery. *Contemporary Pediatrics, 17*(3), 91-109.

American Academy of Pediatrics (2000). *2000 Red book: Report of the Committee of Infectious Diseases* (25th ed.). Elk Grove Village, IL: American Academy of Pediatrics.

American Academy of Pediatrics (1999, August). Policy statement: Ultraviolet light: A hazard to children (RE9913). *Pediatrics, 104*(2), 328-333.

American Medical Association Council on Scientific Affairs (1989). Harmful effects of ultraviolet radiation. *Journal of the American Medical Association, 262,* 380-384.

Amsleier, S.L. & Paller, A.S. (1997). Getting to the bottom of diaper dermatitis. *Contemporary Pediatrics, 14*(11), 115-129.

Arndt, K.A., et al. (1997). *Primary care dermatology.* Philadelphia: W.B. Saunders.

Behrman, R., Kliegman, R., & Jenson, H. (2000). *Nelson textbook of pediatrics* (16th ed.). Philadelphia: W.B. Saunders.

Boiko, S. (2000). Making rash decisions in the diaper area. *Pediatric Annals, 29*(1), 50-56.

Bower, M.G. (2001). Managing dog, cat, and human bite wounds. *The Nurse Practitioner, 26*(4), 36-45.

Braverman, I. (1998). *Skin signs of systemic disease* (3rd ed.). Philadelphia: W. B. Saunders.

Bruckner, A.L. & Weston, W. L. (2001). Beyond poison ivy: Understanding allergic contact dermatitis in children. *Pediatric Annals, 30*(4), 203-206.

Burke, C.C. (2000). Sins of the sun. *Advance for Nurse Practitioners, 8*(5), 33-47.

Centers for Disease Control and Prevention (1998, January 23). Guidelines for treatment of sexually transmitted diseases. *Morbidity and Mortality Weekly Report, 47*(RR-1), 1-118.

Champion, R., et al. (1998). *Textbook of dermatology* (6th ed.). Oxford, England: Blackwell Science.

Cohen, B.A. (2000). *Pediatric dermatology* (2nd ed.). Philadelphia: W.B. Saunders.

Darmstadt, G.L. (1999). A guide to abscesses in the skin. *Contemporary Pediatrics, 16*(4), 135-145.

Dershewitz, R. (1999). *Ambulatory pediatric care* (3rd ed.). Philadelphia: Lippincott-Raven.

Freedberg, I., et al. (1999). *Fitzpatrick's dermatology in general medicine* (5th ed.). New York: McGraw-Hill.

Garzon, M.C. & Frieden, I.J. (2000). Hemangiomas: When to worry. *Pediatric Annals, 29*(1), 58-67.

Gern, J. & Busse, W. (1999). *Contemporary diagnosis and management of allergic diseases and asthma* (3rd ed.). Newton, PA: Handbooks in Healthcare.

Gilbert, D.N., et al. (2000). *The Sanford guide to antimicrobial therapy* (13th ed.). Hyde Park, VT: Jeb. C. Sanford.

Hay, W., et al. (1999). *Current pediatric diagnosis and treatment* (14th ed.). Stamford, CT: Appleton & Lange.

Hansen, R.C. (2000). Guidelines for the treatment of resistant pediculosis. *Contemporary Pediatrics* (supplement), 4-10.

Herman, B.E. & Skokan, E.G. (1999). Bites that poison: A tale of spiders, snakes, and scorpions. *Contemporary Pediatrics, 16*(8), 41-65.

Krowchuk, D.P. & Lucky, A.W. (2001). Managing adolescent acne. *Adolescent Medicine, 12*(2), 355-374.

Lehman, H., Andrews, J., Robinson, K., et al. (2001). *Management of acne: summary, evidence report/technology assessment* (AHRQ, 17 Publication No. 01-E018.) Rockville, MD: Agency for Health Care Research and Quality. Available online at www.ahrq.gov/clinic/acnesum.htm or www.ahrq.gov/clinic/epcix.htm (full report)

Mancini, A.J. (2000). Acne vulgaris: A treatment update. *Contemporary Pediatrics, 17*(12), 122-133.

Mendenhall, A.K. & Eichenfield, L.F. (2000). Back to basics: Caring for the newborn's skin. *Contemporary Pediatrics, 17*(8), 98-114.

Morelli, J.G. & Weston, W.L. (1999). Sun, kids, moles, and melanoma. *Contemporary Pediatrics, 16*(6), 61-76.

National Association of Physicians for the Environment (1994, June). *UV index fact sheet.* Bethesda, MD: National Association of Physicians for the Environment.

Nicol, N.H. (2000). Managing atopic dermatitis in children and adults. *The Nurse Practitioner, 25*(4), 58-79.

Orchard, D. & Weston, W.L. (2001). The importance of vehicle in pediatric topical therapy. *Pediatric Annals, 30*(4), 208-210.

Pogue, S.J. (1999). Acne in adolescents. *Advance for Nurse Practitioners, 7,* 53-56.

Raimer, S.S. (2001). The safe use of topical corticosteroids in children. *Pediatric Annals, 30*(4), 225-229.

Scher, R.K. & Daniel, C.R. (1997). *Nails: Therapy, diagnosis, surgery* (2nd ed.). Philadelphia: W.B. Saunders.

Scheman, A. & Severson, D. (1999). *Pocket guide to medications used in dermatology* (6th ed.). Philadelphia: Lippincott, Williams & Wilkins.

Sidbury, R. & Paller, A.S. (2000). The diagnosis and management of acne. *Pediatric Annals 29*(1), 17-24.

Chapter 38 *Musculoskeletal System*

Amy Verst

Athletic Injuries, p. 556
Back Pain, p. 559
Disturbance in Gait: Limp, p. 561
Disturbance in Gait: Toeing-In, p. 566
Foot Deformity and Pain, p. 568
Growing Pains, p. 569
Hip Pain and Click, p. 569
Joint Pain and Swelling, p. 570
Leg Deformity, p. 572
Spine Deformity, p. 574

Risk Factors

- Family history of musculoskeletal disorders
- Genetic disorders
- Participation in recreational or organized athletic activity
- Ill-fitting equipment (e.g., wrong-sized helmet or shoulder pads)
- Coaches not certified in first aid and cardiopulmonary resuscitation (CPR)
- Unsafe playing fields (e.g., concrete parking lots, unclean fields, uneven fields, wet gymnasium floors)
- Not wearing safety equipment (e.g., mouth guard, shin guards, helmet)
- Improper footwear (e.g., running shoes for basketball, metal [not plastic] cleats, shoes too small or big, soles worn down)
- Improper training techniques (e.g., beginning season with intense training, running high mileage, encouraging extensive weight loss, practice that lasts over 2 hours a day, pitching over 6 innings a week)
- Lack of flexibility, especially in hamstring muscles
- Excessive dieting, including eating disorders
- Reckless athlete
- Highly motivated athlete
- Nonmotivated athlete
- Obesity
- Use of steroid preparations for weight gain
- Past history of injury (usually not properly rehabilitated)
- Unsupervised play time and area
- Children with any one of the following:
  Low birth weight (LBW)
  Congenital musculoskeletal defect
  Constitutional delay of growth
  Retarded bone growth
  Antecedent history of transient synovitis
  Delayed puberty
  Valgum or varum of the knee or elbow
  Hyperextended joints

Health Promotion

General Measures

- Educate parents and children about a healthy diet and the prevention of obesity. Proper nutrition is essential for normal growth and development of bones and muscles.
- Stress the importance of daily exercise (discussed later in this section). Encourage less television viewing and computer games and more outside activities.
- Discuss developmentally appropriate activities.
- Teach parents that safe play areas, inside and outside, must be provided for all children (see Chapter 14).
- Remember that early identification and treatment of skeletal abnormalities may prevent future problems.
- Advise parents that they should not pull, jerk, or swing infants by their arms because doing so can cause dislocation of the radial head.
- Encourage parents to help their child maintain good posture. Discuss why good posture is important (i.e., when the body is properly aligned, it allows the musculoskeletal system to function with efficiency and minimal effort). Stress the benefits of good posture (e.g., nonfatigue decreases possibility of strain to joints and ligaments, results in a better appearance, provides for proper functioning of the weight-bearing joints, can be maintained for long periods of time).
- Instruct parents in the selection of footwear. Shoes are needed when the infant first begins to walk. High-top or other expensive shoes are not needed unless a foot problem exists. Sneakers or moccasins are good choices. The shoes should be inexpensive because they need to be replaced frequently. Proper fit is very important. The shoes should permit full motion of the foot, and the soles should not be slippery.
- Review proper footwear periodically at well-child visits.

Promotion of Athletic Activity

Encourage all children to exercise. Discuss the benefits of exercise at well-child visits. Assess current activity level. Encourage age-appropriate activities (e.g., biking, hiking, swimming, team sports). Most athletic injuries can be prevented with proper conditioning techniques. Full painless range of motion (ROM) is imperative for all athletes, and the development of strength through all planes of motion is one of the goals of preactivity conditioning. Once injured, athletes need to be rehabilitated to the level of strength attained before the injury.

Encountering an athlete who is injured can be very difficult. Most athletic participants are involved in activity because they love it. Injuries prevent athletes from doing something that is very important to them. Adolescent athletes may feel athletic performance defines their personality. Many participants release stress through athletic activity. When they are injured, the stress-coping mechanism that had worked so well for them is gone.

Rehabilitation of an athlete can be very rewarding. The time spent with the athlete allows for a discussion of many health-promotion topics. The opportunity to develop a relationship with a health professional is one that many adolescents need but never have the chance to do. Rehabilitation involves the injured area but includes the total body. For many athletes, rehabilitation helps them achieve a higher level of aerobic conditioning and total body strength.

Prevention of Athletic Injuries

Instruct the child, parent, or coach to follow these guidelines for athletic activity (and see also Chapter 14):

- Athletes should always warm up and cool down; each of these periods should involve a routine of stretching the entire body in head-to-toe sequence and also concentrate on the joints and muscles required for the athletic activity.
- Athletic conditioning should be gradual. Athletes should train using the 10% principle (i.e., no more than a 10% increase in the quantity of training should occur from 1 week to another).
- The timing of athletic conditioning is important. Conditioning should start before practices and games begin.
- Practice should focus on quality and not quantity, with no more than 2 hours of practice a day, including weight-room work and field work.
- Establishing a routine of activity is important, as is not playing or practicing when extremely tired.
- Athletes should work at their individual capacity level. Perceived exertion is a good measure of the intensity of the workout.
- All equipment should fit the athlete. This includes shoes, helmets, and shoulder pads.
- Athletes who are highly motivated should be observed for overuse training patterns. Athletes who are not motivated should be observed for lack of conditioning. Athletic conditioning should include specialization to the activity (e.g., volleyball conditioning should include shoulder strengthening).
- All safety equipment is mandatory for participation—mouth guards, helmets, shin guards, gloves, shoulder pads.
- Weight loss should not exceed 2 pounds a week.
- Reckless play (e.g., spearing, slide tackling from behind, foul play) should be discouraged.
- The team or organization should be encouraged to have qualified health care personnel at practice and games.
- One should never begin an activity until an injury is fully rehabilitated.
- Protective braces have been shown to reduce the severity of athletic injuries.
- Weight categories for athletic activities, not categories based on age, are recommended.
- Weight training should focus on conditioning, not strength or power; (i.e., the repetitions should be high with low weight).
- All athletes must have a preparticipation physical examination within 6 months of the activity.
- Fluid breaks should be mandatory every 45 minutes (more often in warm weather or with young children).

Guidelines for Safe Stretching and Strengthening of Muscles

Stretching and strengthening are keys to total body fitness and the prevention of activity-related injuries. Stretching basics include the following:

- Warm up with a light jog.
- Hold each stretch for 20 to 30 seconds, and do not bounce.
- Hold stretches at the point of pull, not pain.
- Stretch all muscle groups from head to toe and then specialize to the given activity.
- Remember that stretching should last 10 to 15 minutes before the activity and 5 minutes at the conclusion of the activity.
- Do not compare one person's ability to stretch with another's.

Strengthening is not the same as weight training. Athletes can develop strength in the muscle groups without having access to weight machines. Isokinetic and isometric exercises are the basis of strength training. Accommodating resistance exercise uses total involvement of the muscle fibers through ROM. Exercises such as leg lifts, calf raises, push-ups, and sit-ups strengthen the body and can be performed every day. Many adolescents and preadolescents prefer to use weight machines or free weights. If so, the weight room must be supervised, and the concentration should be on conditioning, not power. It should be enforced that weights are not toys, and devastating accidents can occur. Weight lifting should be done on an every-other-day schedule.

Athletes must be advised to develop both upper and lower body strength. Most girls have weak upper body muscle, and most boys desire the esthetics of a strong upper body. Both groups generally ignore lower body exercises and concentrate on upper body activities.

Prevention of Infection and Promotion of Healing

- Instruct the child to complete all antibiotic therapy as prescribed.
- Evaluate all braces for proper fit and for areas of skin breakdown.
- Teach proper cast care:
  Keep the cast dry.
  Do not bang or hit the cast.
  Do not put anything down inside the cast (e.g., pencils, coat hangers).
  Do not continue athletic activities when wearing a cast (unless it is cleared with the physician).
  Report any foul smell from the cast or any change in sensation, color, or temperature of the extremity in the cast.

Subjective Data

The history should be appropriately adapted by the practitioner according to the presenting problem but should possibly include:

- Demographics, including age, sex, race, and socioeconomic status
- Reason for the visit and description of the problem
- Onset and surrounding circumstances
- Recent trauma or infection
- Parental and child concerns about mobility, gait, gross and fine motor development
- Associated signs and symptoms (describing each), including pain, rash, fever, irritability, tenderness, swelling, color changes, bruising, erythema, posturing of joint, position of comfort, loss of ROM, and swollen glands (popliteal, epitrochlear, inguinal, and axillary)
- Past health history, including hospitalizations and surgeries
- Any joint and bone infection, trauma, or disease (including any treatment)
- Chronic or infectious diseases

- Prenatal history, including multiple births and oligohydramnios
- Neonatal history, including prematurity or LBW, hospitalization (and how long), delivery position (e.g., breech), and in utero positioning
- Developmental history, including milestones (especially gross and fine motor) and the ages at which they were achieved
- Medications (prescription or nonprescription), including steroids
- Allergies
- Immunization data
- Family history, including torsional deformities, genu varum or valgus, foot deformities, genetic disorders, chronic diseases, joint and bone problems, gait problems, and allergies
- Social history, including family composition, interpersonal relationships, living conditions (e.g., stairs, throw rugs, narrow halls), economic status, pets, peer relationships, emotional and behavioral problems, attendance in day care or school (with grades, if applicable), and participation in sports (recreational or scholastic, and which specific sports)
- Past results of goniometer testing (a measurement of ROM of joints)
- Past laboratory and radiographic examination data
- Activity level and preferred sleeping position

Objective Data

Physical Examination

The physical examination should be appropriately adapted by the practitioner according to the presenting problem. Perform a systematic evaluation, including inspection, palpation, ROM, resistive strength, sensation, deep tendon reflexes, and special tests, of the musculoskeletal system by assessing the patient in a head-to-toe manner. Remember to compare the affected joint to the unaffected joint (when applicable) when inspecting the cervical spine; shoulder complexes; elbows; wrists, hands, and fingers; lumbar spine; hips; knees; and ankles, feet, and toes.

Inspection. The child should wear minimal clothing (e.g., shorts and a tank top with shoes off).
- *General*—When developmentally appropriate, assess gross motor function. Does the infant or child walk and run with a balanced, even gait? Can he or she climb on and off the examination table?
- *Skin*—Inspect for rashes, bruising, abrasions, puncture sites, edema, and erythema.
- *Spine*—While the child is standing, observe for curvature and level of shoulders, scapula, and hips (i.e., a scoliosis examination).
- *All other joints*—Observe for gross deformity (with comparison to the opposite limb), edema, atrophy, asymmetry, angular deformity, and color changes. Include a skin assessment.

Palpation. The practitioner can palpate each joint and limb for areas of tenderness, changes in temperature, or defects in soft tissue or bone. Begin with the bony prominences and then the soft-tissue landmarks.

Range of motion
- *Active*—The practitioner should have the patient perform active ROM of each joint to the fullest extent and record each measurement with a goniometer (for greatest accuracy).

- *Passive*—If a deficits exist, the practitioner should attempt gentle passive ROM and record each measurement with a goniometer.

Muscle strength. The examiner can test resistive strength of each movement by applying counterpressure with a hand and comparing to the other side. Grade 5 is full strength and normal, 3 is full ROM with gravity (muscle strength is fair), and 0 is no voluntary movement.

Sensation. Evaluate sensation of the upper and lower extremities with soft touch.

Deep tendon reflexes. Evaluate all deep tendon reflexes.

Special tests. Perform symptom-specific tests as indicated.
- *Infant hip examination*—This should be done at birth, 2 to 3 weeks of age, and 4 to 6 weeks of age to rule out developmental dysplasia of the hip (DDH).
- *Complete ROM of the hip*—With DDH, the infant has limited abduction caused by shortened and contracted hip adductor muscles.
- *Ortolani maneuver (reduction test)*—The infant should be relaxed and lying supine. The hips and knees should be flexed to 90 degrees. Each hip should be examined separately. The thigh is grasped with the middle finger over the greater trochanter and simultaneously lifted and abducted. A positive result is reduction of the femoral head into the acetabulum causing a palpable "clunk" (Fig. 38-1).
- *Barlow test (dislocation test)*—This is the reverse of the Ortolani maneuver. As the practitioner attempts to dislocate the femoral head, hands are placed the same as described previously and the thighs are adducted with gentle downward pressure. A positive result is the palpable dislocation of the femoral head (Fig. 38-2).
- *Skinfolds test*—The skinfolds should be evaluated for symmetry with the infant prone. A positive result is unequal skinfolds (more on the affected side) (Fig. 38-3).

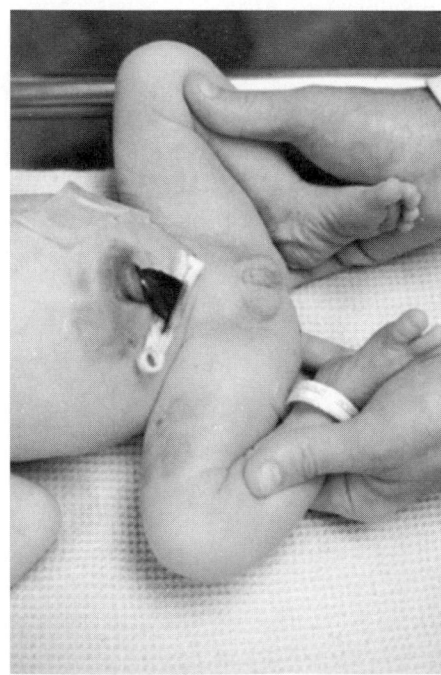

Fig. 38-1 Ortolani maneuver. (From Seidel, H. [1999]. *Mosby's guide to physical examination* [4th ed.]. St. Louis: Mosby.)

After 2 months of age, the Ortolani and Barlow tests are not accurate measurements. The following tests should be performed:

- *Complete ROM test*—This test should be performed at each visit for the first year of life and if a child has a limp or hip pain.
- *Skinfolds test*—This test may be performed at any age.
- *Leg length test*—A paper tape measure is used to evaluate leg length. Measure from the iliac crest to the medial malleolus. Compare measurements between extremities. Evaluate the level of the iliac crests posteriorly while the child is standing and sitting.
- *Allis sign*—With the child supine and the knees bent, the knee of the affected side is lower because the femoral head is posterior to the acetabulum (Fig. 38-4).

- *Trendelenburg test*—With the child standing and the practitioner inspecting the level of the iliac crests posteriorly, the weight is transferred to one leg (i.e., child stands on one leg). A positive result is when the child is standing on affected leg only, the normal side (iliac crest) droops down because the affected side hip adductors are weak and cannot hold the pelvis level (Fig. 38-5).

Evaluation for torsional deformity of an infant or child

Hip rotation. With the infant or child prone and the knee flexed, the thigh or leg falls laterally from the vertical position as far as it will go (internal rotation), and the angle is measured and recorded (Fig. 38-6, *A*). For external rotation the thigh or leg is folded inward and across the midline, and the angle is recorded (Fig. 38-6, *B*); normally the two measurements equal 100 degrees.

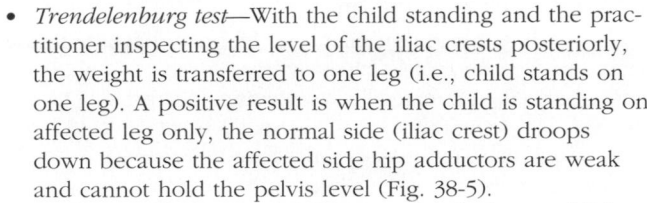

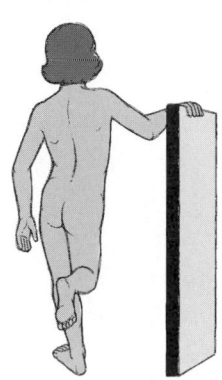

Fig. 38-5 Positive Trendelenburg sign or gait (if child is weight-bearing). (From Wong, D. [1999]. *Nursing care of infants and children* [6th ed.]. St. Louis: Mosby.)

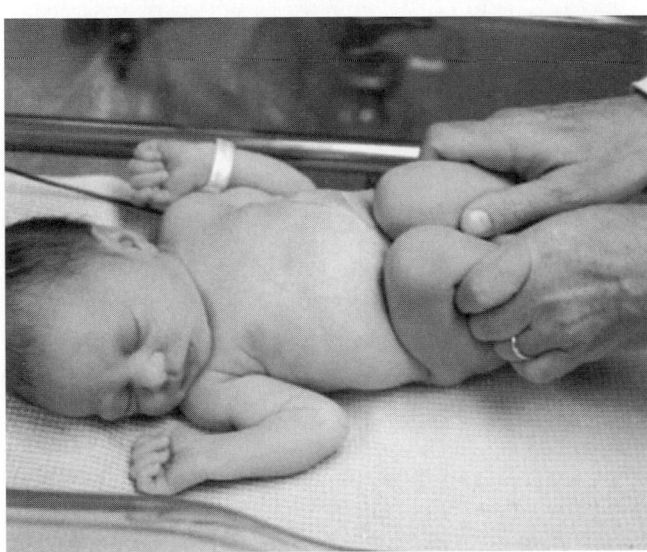

Fig. 38-2 Barlow test. (From Seidel, H. [1999]. *Mosby's guide to physical examination* [4th ed.]. St. Louis: Mosby.)

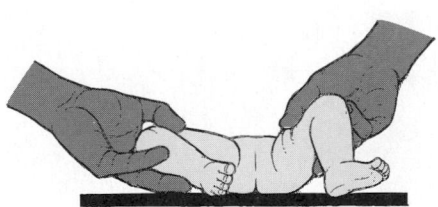

Fig. 38-3 Signs of hip dislocation: limitation of abduction and asymmetric skinfolds. (From Wong, D. [1999]. *Nursing care of infants and children* [6th ed.]. St. Louis: Mosby.)

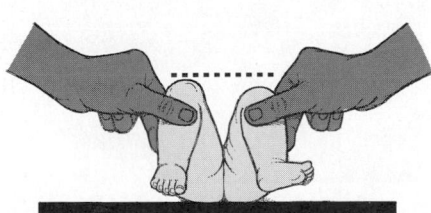

Fig. 38-4 Allis sign. (From Wong, D. [1999]. *Nursing care of infants and children* [6th ed.]. St. Louis: Mosby.)

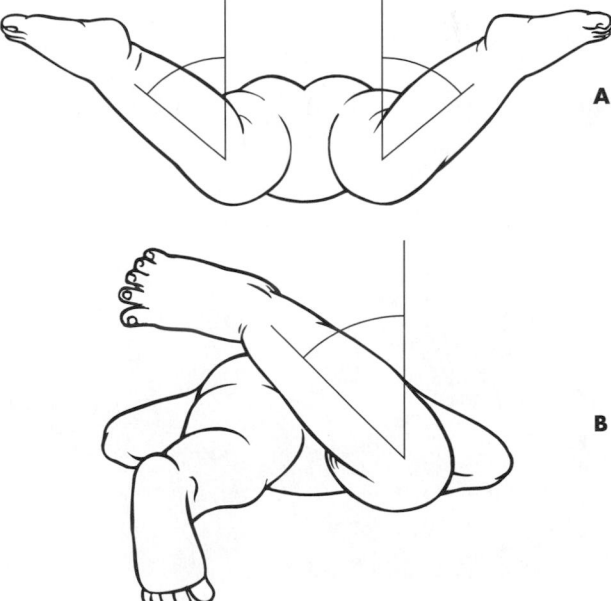

Fig. 38-6 Hip rotation. A, Internal. B, External.

Thigh-foot angle (axis). The thigh-foot angle (axis) defines the degree of tibial torsion an infant or child may have. With the patient prone, the foot is passively dorsiflexed to 90 degrees. Inspect the angle created by comparing the forefoot to the hindfoot. A toeing-out foot is expressed in positive (+) degrees; toeing-in is expressed in negative (−) degrees.

Foot axis or shape. Examination of the foot is made by comparing the axis of the hindfoot to the axis of the forefoot. Normally the two should make a straight line. An obtuse angle is made in metatarsus adductus (Fig. 38-7).

Angle of gait. The examiner should estimate the average angle of each step made while watching the child walk.

Intercondylar distance. The distance between the medial femoral condyles is measured while the child is standing with the feet together. This measurement is used to evaluate genu varum, or bowlegs.

Intermalleolar distance. The distance between the medial malleoli of the ankles is measured while the child is standing and the knees are together. This measurement is used to evaluate genu valgum, or knock-knees.

Scoliosis evaluation. See Preparticipation Physical Examination. All children being evaluated should be barefoot and

unclothed from the waist up. The bony landmarks and skinfolds of the back must be fully visualized.

Inspection. The child should stand with his or her back to the examiner. The child's feet should be together with the arms hanging freely at the sides. The examiner assesses shoulder and hip heights for symmetry. The back should have symmetric rib humps and skin creases. Next ask the child to bend forward with the arms together as if diving into a pool. The practitioner should examine the child's back from the posterior and lateral views for symmetric rib humps. Posturally, the child can have uneven shoulder and hip heights without any lateral curvature of the spine.

Athletic injury evaluation. See also Chapter 14.
Shoulder evaluation
- *Drop arm test*—With the thumbs pointing down, the child abducts the arm as far as possible and then lowers it to 90 degrees. A light tap is given on the wrist, causing the affected arm to fall. A torn rotator cuff may be indicated.
- *Apprehension test*—The child's affected arm is abducted to 90 degrees. With the examiner's hand on the humeral head and the other at the wrist, the shoulder is slowly and gently externally rotated as far as the child allows. A palpable subluxation or facial grimace is positive for recurrent shoulder dislocation.

Elbow and wrist or hand evaluation
- *Lateral stress test*—The arm or wrist is held in passive extension with one hand on the joint line medially and the other at the wrist. A medial stress is applied with the hand on the joint line. A positive result is laxity laterally, indicating a sprain.
- *Medial stress test*—The arm or wrist is held in passive extension with one hand on the joint line laterally and the other at the wrist while a lateral stress is applied. A positive result is laxity medially, indicating a sprain.

Knee evaluation
- *Lateral and medial stress tests*—The test is performed as in the elbow, wrist, and hand evaluation, but with the knee (Fig. 38-8).

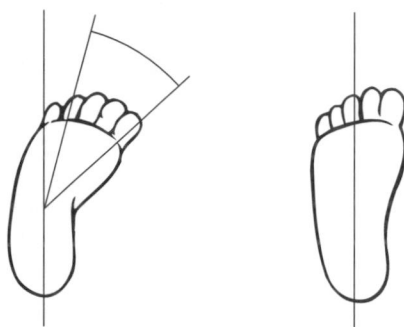

Fig. 38-7 Examination of foot axis.

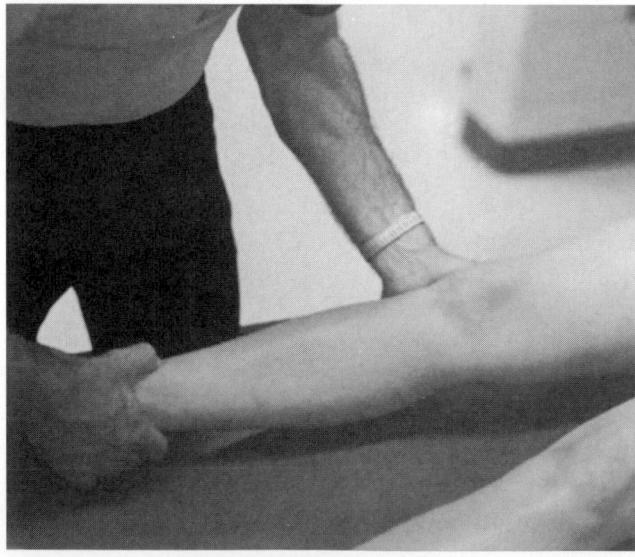
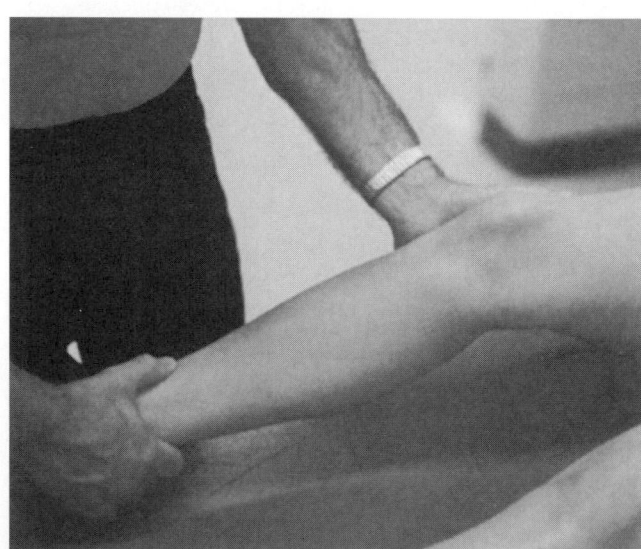

Fig. 38-8 A and **B,** Medial stress test. (From Booher, J.M. & Thibodeau, G.A. [1994]. *Athletic injury assessment* [3rd ed.]. St. Louis: Mosby.)

- *Anterior drawer test*—With the child supine on the examination table, the affected knee is bent at 90 degrees with the foot straight. The practitioner stabilizes the foot by partially sitting on it and places their hands around the upper portion of the tibia. An anterior force (pulling the tibia toward you) is applied to stress the anterior cruciate ligament. A positive result is the sliding forward of the tibia, indicating a torn anterior cruciate ligament (ACL).
- *Lachman test*—With the child supine on the examination table, the affected knee is at 15 degrees of flexion with the leg externally rotated. The practitioner stabilizes the leg by grasping the distal end of the thigh with the other hand grasping the proximal aspect of the tibia, attempting to move it anteriorly. A positive result with movement of the tibia indicates a torn ACL.
- *Patellar apprehension test*—The child is supine with a rolled towel under the affected knee. The patella is pressed downward into the femoral groove. It is then moved forward and backward. A positive result is pain or a grinding sound.

Ankle evaluation

- *Lateral and medial stress test*—The test is performed as in the elbow, wrist, and hand evaluation but with the ankle complex (Fig. 38-9).
- *Anterior drawer test*—The test is performed as in the knee evaluation but with the ankle complex (Fig. 38-10).

Preparticipation physical examination. This examination should include the following:

- Detailed health history, especially related to cardiovascular disease, congenital defects, musculoskeletal injuries, and drug use (e.g., growth hormone, anabolic steroids)
- Height and weight
- Eye examination, including acuity, PERRLA (pupils equal, round, and reactive to light and accommodation), and the presence of glasses or contact lenses
- Cardiovascular examination, keeping in mind that cardiovascular conditions limit athletic participation more often than any other condition and hypertrophic cardiomyopathy causes the most nontraumatic deaths among athletes. Evaluate blood pressure (BP), pulses (e.g., brachial, femoral), and heart sounds with the athlete standing and supine, and while the patient is performing a Valsalva maneuver

- Pulmonary examination, including chest shape and lung sounds
- Abdominal examination, including masses, organomegaly, and kidney function (noting the presence of both kidneys)
- Skin, including rashes, lesions, acne, scabies, lice, and athlete's foot
- Genitalia, including hernia, Tanner staging, and the presence of both testicles (in males)
- Musculoskeletal examination (Figs. 38-11 to 38-23)

Text continued on p. 555

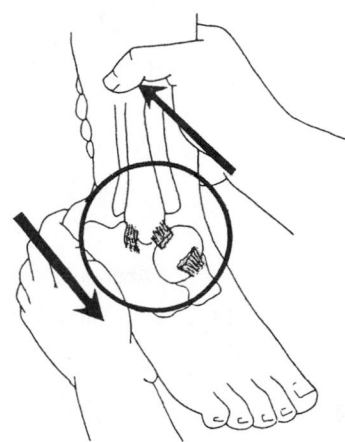

Fig. 38-10 Anterior drawer test. (From Arnheim, D.D. & Prentice, W.E. [2000]. *Principles of athletic training* [10th ed.]. Boston: McGraw-Hill.)

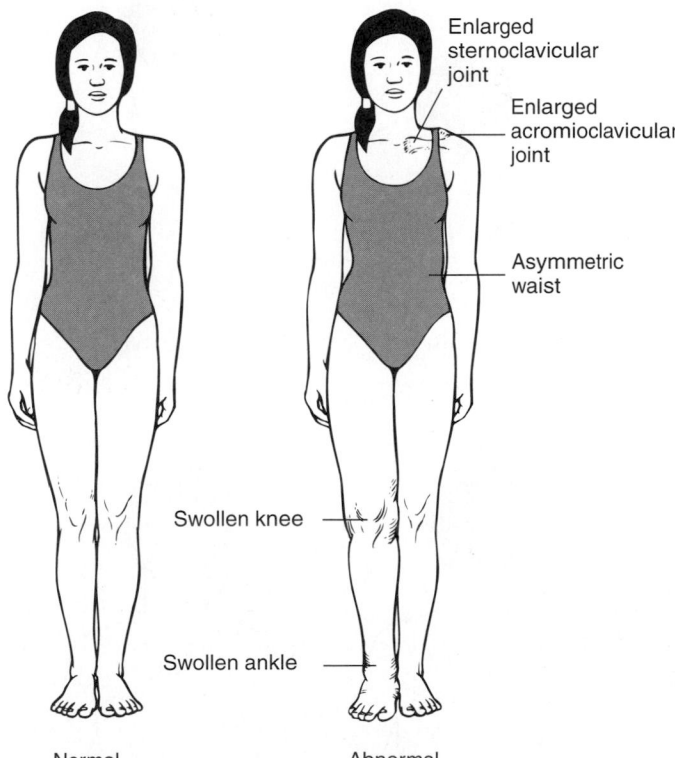

Fig. 38-11 Symmetry of upper and lower extremities and trunk (patient facing examiner).

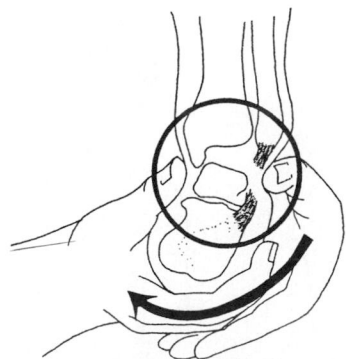

Fig. 38-9 Lateral stress test. (From Arnheim, D.D. & Prentice, W.E. [2000]. *Principles of athletic training* [10th ed.]. Boston: McGraw-Hill.)

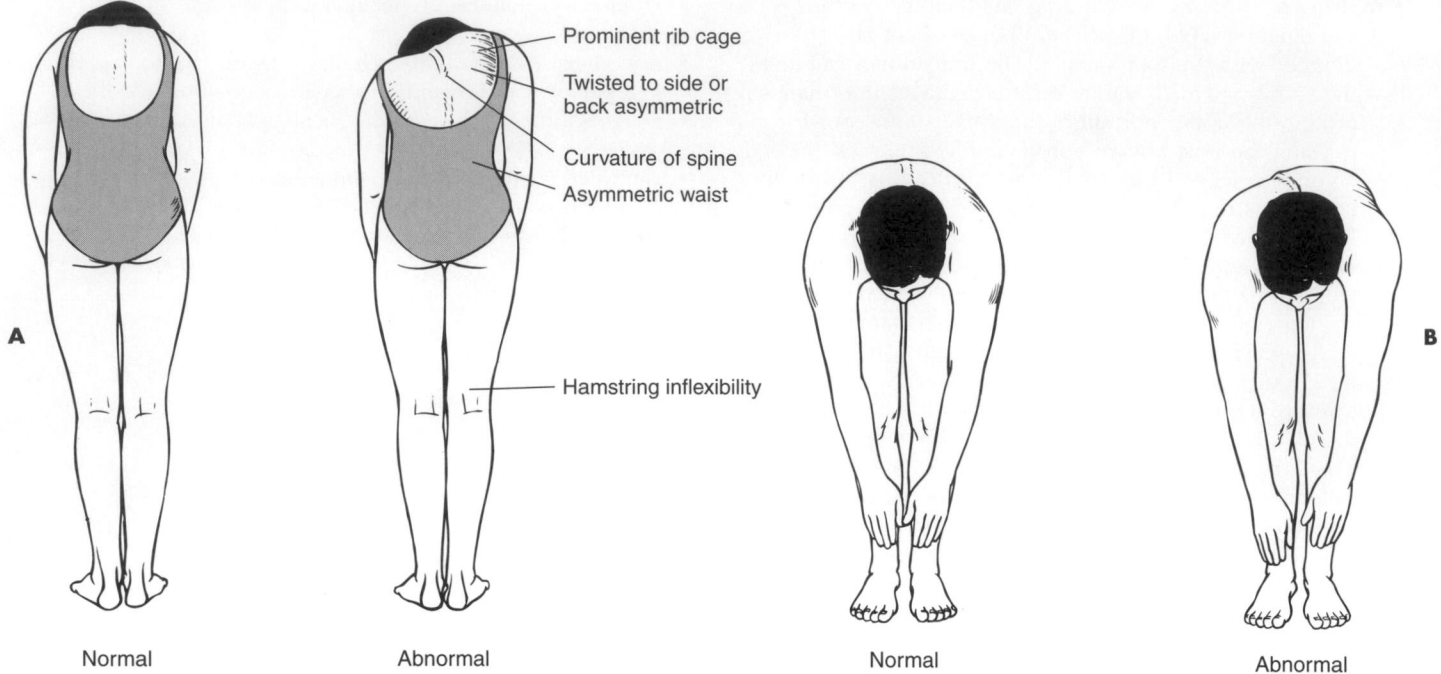

Fig. 38-12 Back flexion. **A,** Patient facing away from examiner. **B,** Patient touching toes, facing examiner.

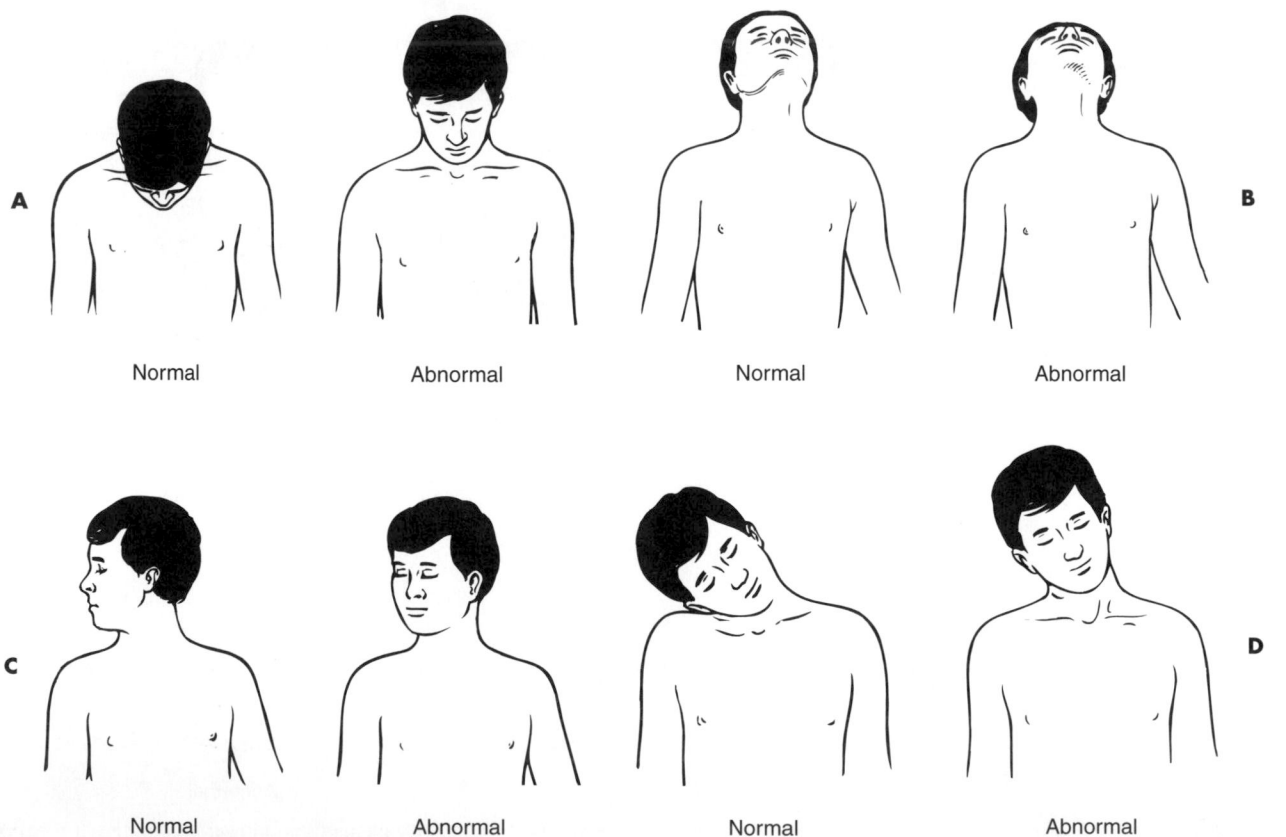

Fig. 38-13 Neck ROM. **A,** Flexion. **B,** Extension. **C,** Left and right lateral rotation. **D,** Left and right lateral flexion.

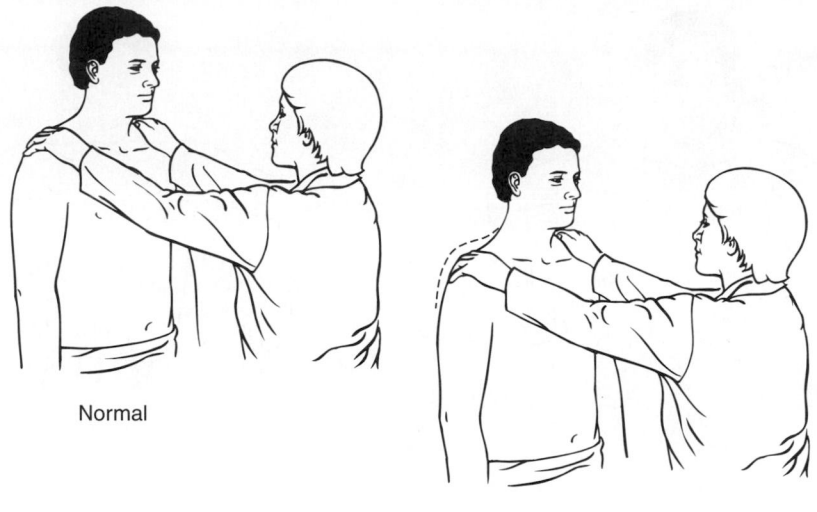

Normal

Abnormal

Fig. 38-14 Resisted shoulder shrug—trapezius strength.

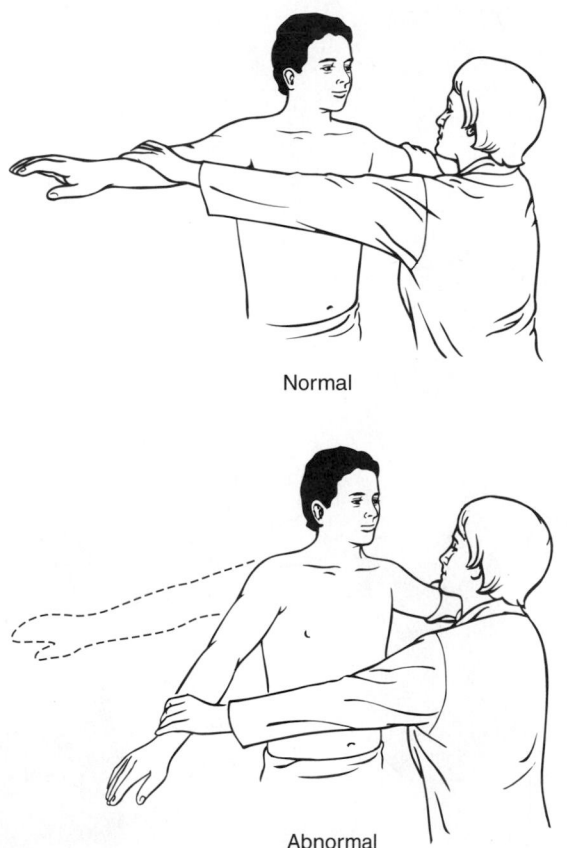

Normal

Abnormal

Fig. 38-15 Resisted shoulder abduction—deltoid strength.

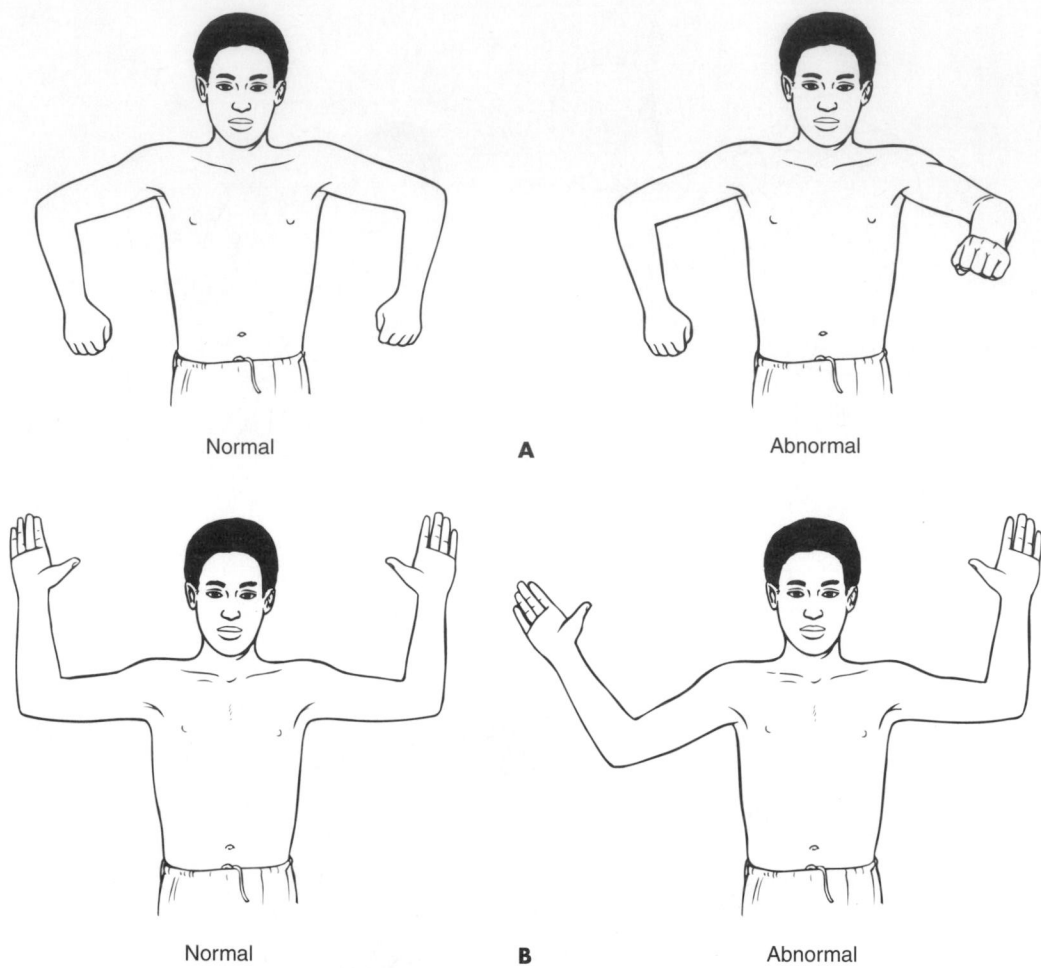

Fig. 38-16 Shoulder ROM. A, Internal rotation. B, External rotation.

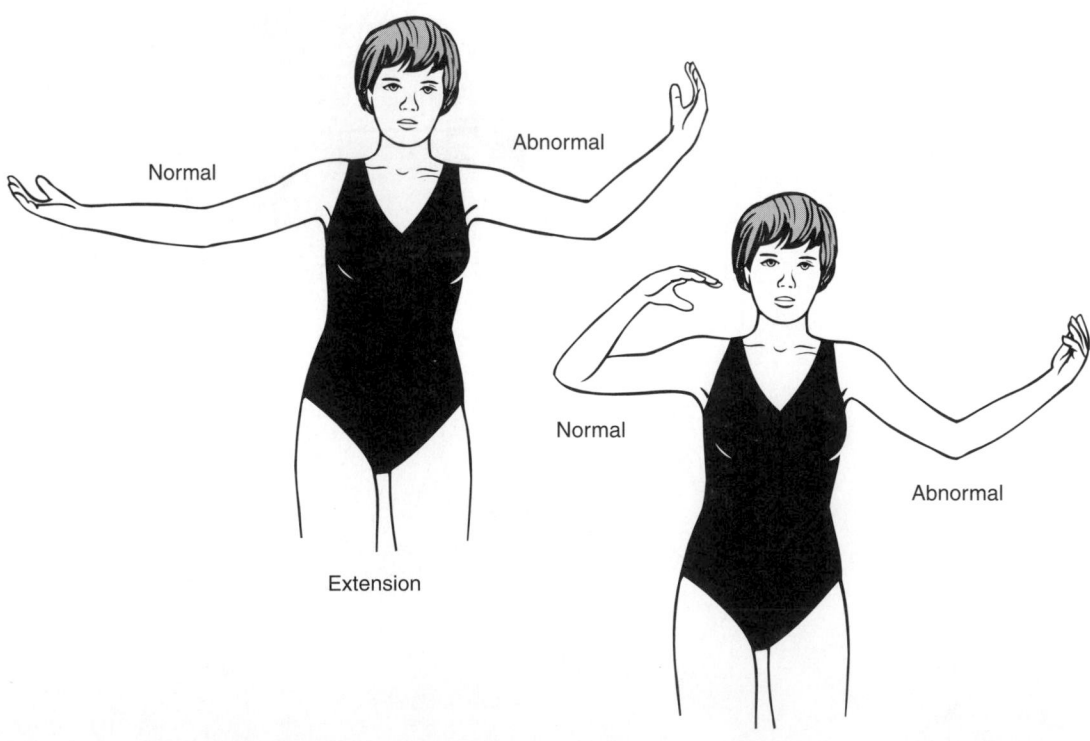

Fig. 38-17 Elbow ROM—extension and flexion.

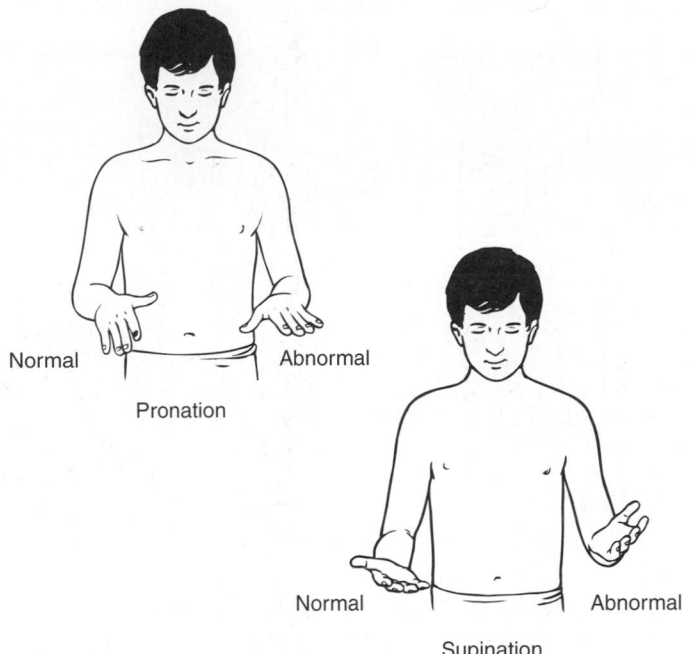

Normal   Abnormal

Pronation

Normal   Abnormal

Supination

Fig. 38-18 Elbow ROM—pronation and supination.

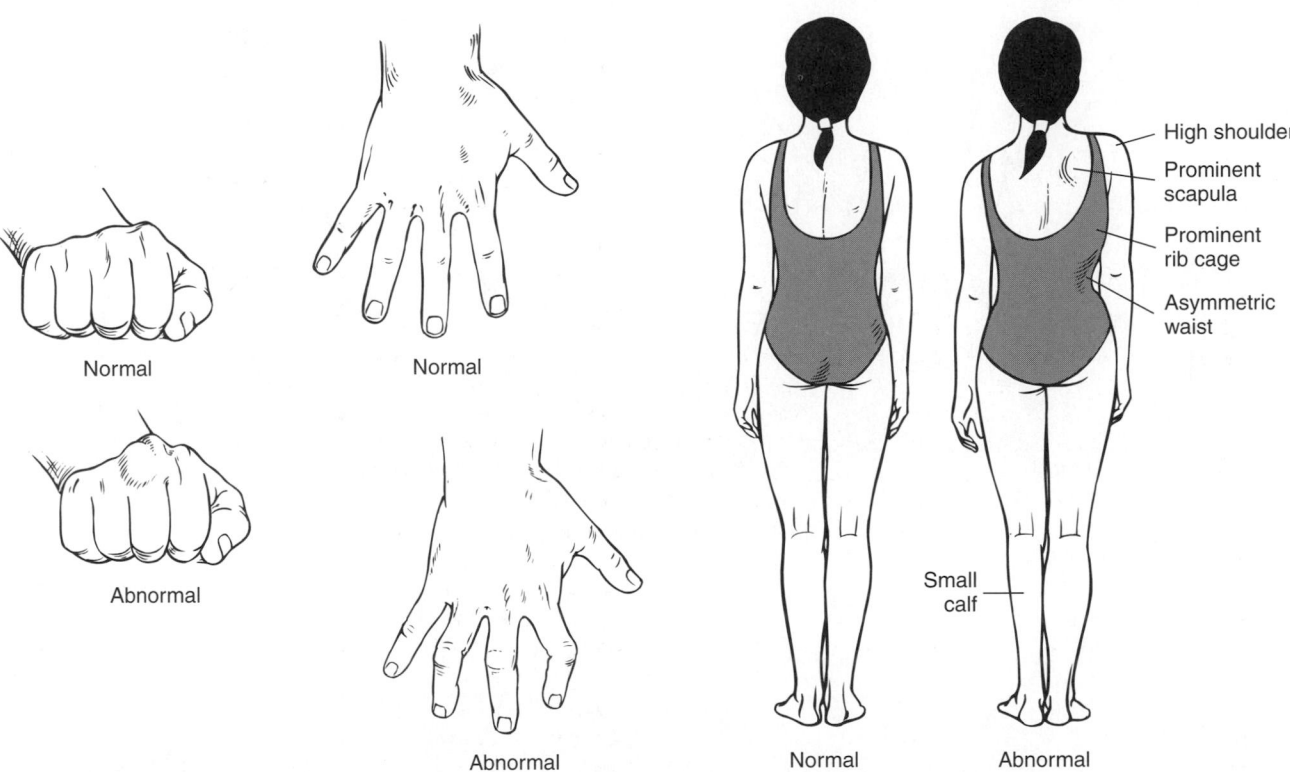

Fig. 38-19 Hand and finger ROM (patient making a fist and spreading fingers).

Fig. 38-20 Symmetry of upper and lower extremities and trunk (patient facing away from examiner).

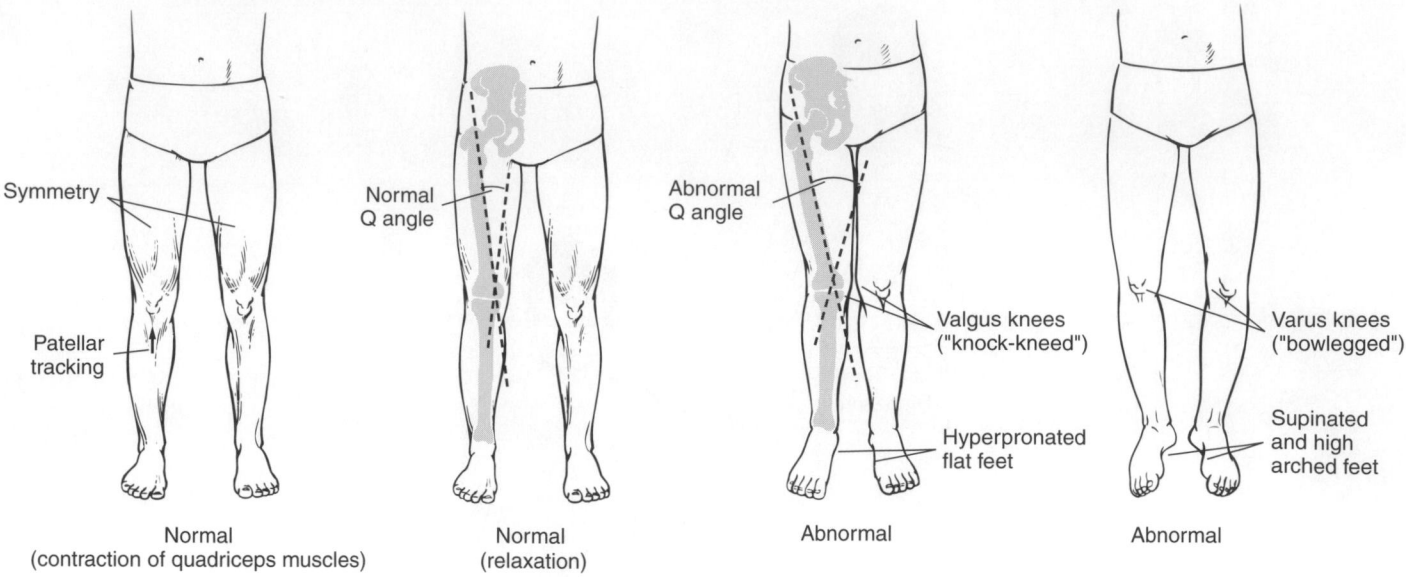

Fig. 38-21 Examination of lower extremities.

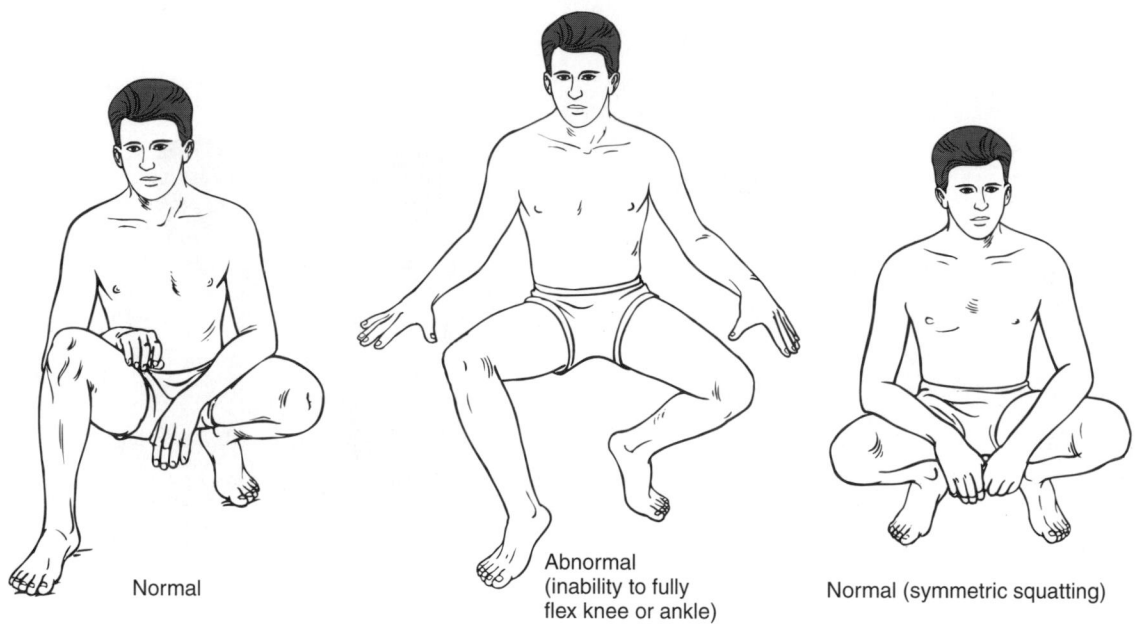

Fig. 38-22 Squat and "duck walk."

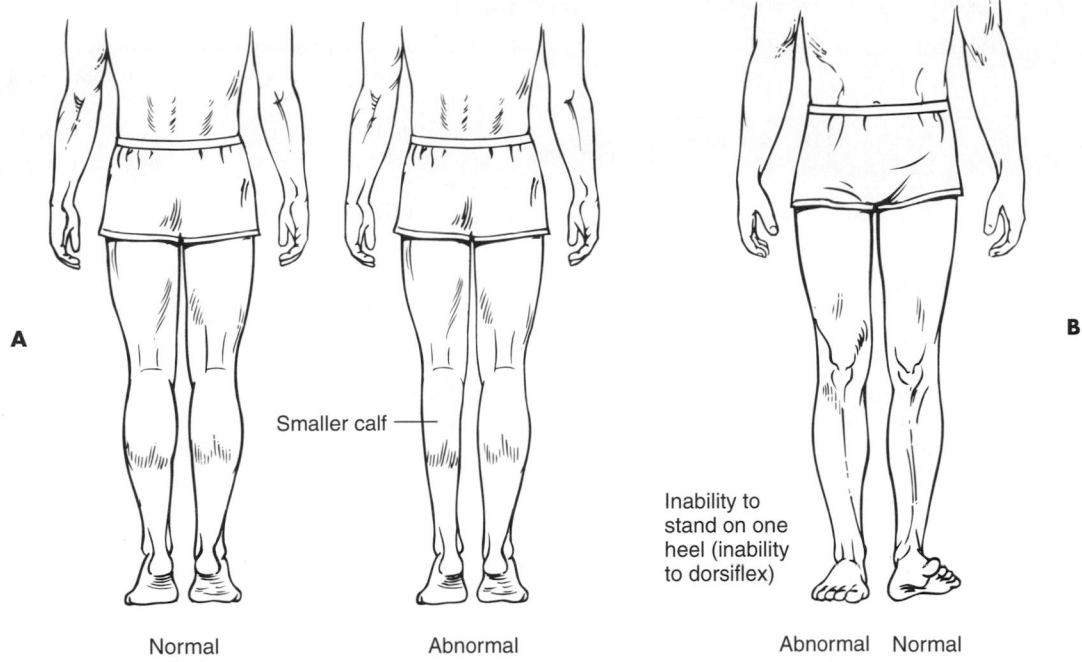

Fig. 38-23 Examination of lower extremities. **A,** Patient standing on toes, facing away from examiner. **B,** Patient standing on heel, facing examiner.

Diagnostic Procedures and Laboratory Tests

Diagnostic tests are dictated by the age of the child and the history and physical examination findings. They include:

- *Radiologic examination of the injured area and contralateral area*—Almost all musculoskeletal complaints should have a radiographic evaluation to view the open growth plate, rule out a fracture or tumor, and compare the affected area to the nonaffected area for comparison of landmarks.
- *Complete blood cell (CBC) count with differential blood count*—In respect to the musculoskeletal system, a CBC count is performed to rule out an infectious cause. The differential count of the white blood cell (WBC) count is evaluated for "shifts" indicating bacterial or viral causes.
- *Complete blood cell (CBC) count with differential blood count*—In respect to the musculoskeletal system, a CBC count is performed to rule out an infectious cause. The differential count of the white blood cell (WBC) count is evaluated for "shifts" indicating bacterial or viral causes.
- *Erythrocyte sedimentation rate (ESR, or sed rate)*—This blood test evaluates the presence of inflammation. It is indicated to rule out arthritis or another chronic inflammatory process.
- *Antinuclear antibody (ANA) test*—This blood test is used to screen for autoimmune disease or system lupus erythematosus, or both. Certain medications (including penicillin, procainamide, and hydralazine) can cause false-positive results.
- *Human leukocyte antigen B27 (HLA-B27 test)*—This blood test identifies the presence of the antigen HLA-B27. It is believed that this antigen is a marker of disease susceptibility. HLA-B27 has a high correlation with ankylosing spondylosis and Reiter syndrome.

- *Aspiration of fluid from a joint*—Joint aspirate may be serous, serosanguinous, or purulent. Hemarthrosis (bleeding into the joint) often indicates a more serious injury, whereas purulent drainage indicates infection and must be cultured.
- *Magnetic resonance imaging (MRI)*—An MRI is used to evaluate torn ligaments or damage to cartilage.
- *Laparoscopy*—A laparoscopic examination may be performed at any joint to evaluate the extent of torn ligaments or cartilage. It is also used to remove torn cartilage and repair partially torn ligaments.
- *Ultrasonography*—This procedure evaluates structures within a joint. It is useful in locating loose bodies within a joint space.
- *Range-of-motion testing with a goniometer*—A goniometer is a simple instrument that measures the ROM of a joint. The goniometer is placed in alignment with the axis of rotation of the joint and moved as the joint moves. The measurements allow evaluation of ROM.
- *Myelography (myelogram)*—This is a radiographic study usually done with contrast medium to evaluate spinal disorders (e.g., identify an obstruction or abnormality that may impinge on the spinal cord or nerve roots). This test is frequently combined with computed tomography (CT) scan.
- *Electromyography (EMG)*—Recording the electric potential of various muscles in both a resting state and during voluntary contraction is a test that is helpful in differentiating nerve involvement from a muscle disorder when there is weakness or paralysis.
- *Computed tomography scan*
- *Arthrogram*

Athletic Injuries

Alert

Consult with or refer to a physician for the following:
- Obvious deformity after traumatic event
- Injury that results in loss of consciousness, transient paralysis, or paresthesia
- Athlete suspected of an eating disorder or with excessive weight loss
- Use of anabolic steroids

Etiology

Accidental insults are the cause of most athletic injuries. Improper training is the second leading cause of athletic injuries. Fatigue and improper nutrition also contribute to many athletic injuries. (For more information on athletic injuries, see also Chapter 14.)

Incidence

- Over 20 million children participate in organized athletics.
- As many as 1 in 14 adolescents are treated for an athletic injury.
- Sex-related injury patterns are sports-related (e.g., girls' softball and soccer have more injuries than boys' baseball and soccer).
- Football causes the most athletic injuries, whereas baseball causes the least.
- The lower extremities are injured more often than the upper extremities in most sports.

Risk Factors

- Improper training
- Being underweight or overweight
- Heavier body type (more prone to injuries)
- Poor flexibility (tight muscles cause sprains and strains)
- Poor muscle strength (causing instability of a joint)
- Use of anabolic steroids

Table 38-1 Differential Diagnosis: Common Shoulder Injuries

CRITERIA	ROTATOR CUFF TEAR*	SEPARATED SHOULDER*	SHOULDER DISLOCATION*	BRACHIAL PLEXUS STRETCH
Defining characteristics	Strain of one or more of the rotator cuff tendons	Sprain of one or more of the ligaments of the acromioclavicular joint or the sternoclavicular joint	Dislocation of the humeral head posterior or anterior	Stretch of the brachial plexus that results in burning and transient loss of function (15 sec to 2 min)
ICD-9 code	840.4	831.00	831.00	953.4
Subjective Data				
Age/onset	Any age/acute or gradual	Any age/acute	Any age/acute	Any age/acute
Mechanism of injury	Violent pull to the arm, abnormal rotation, fall on outstretched arm	Direct blow to tip of shoulder	Direct blow to posterolateral aspect of the shoulder, arm tackle, violent pull	Depression of the shoulder with the head and neck forced to the contralateral side
At risk	Throwing activities, freestyle and butterfly swimmers, wrestlers, wheelchair athletes	Collision sports, players with poor-fitting shoulder pads	Collision sports, wrestling, wheelchair sports	Collision sports, athlete with previous brachial plexus stretch (burner)
Objective Data				
Musculoskeletal examination				
Inspection	Swelling, bruising	Swelling, bruising, may have obvious deformity	Flattened deltoid contour, arm carried in slight abduction and external rotation	Affected arm hanging at the side (immediately after injury); no obvious deformity
Palpation	May feel defect in tendon	Prominence of clavicular head, defect felt in ligaments	Humeral head out of socket	No obvious deformity
Range of motion	Limited, depending on tendon affected	Limited, related to pain	Limited	Full ROM
Special tests	Drop arm test	None	Apprehension test	Sensation testing, deep tendon reflexes
Laboratory data	Radiographs: Should have normal findings	Radiographs: Should have widening of joint space	Radiographs: May have normal findings or show dislocated humeral head	None

*Refer the child to an orthopedist.

- Inadequate rehabilitation (e.g., returning to play too early)

Differential Diagnosis (Tables 38-1 to 38-5)

For *fractures*, see Joint Pain and Swelling later in this chapter and Orthopedic Fractures in Chapter 48. For *sprains* and *strains*, see Joint Pain and Swelling.

Overuse injuries are the result of improper training techniques or the repetitive activities of athletics (e.g., running, throwing, jumping). The repetitive stress on the bones and soft tissues causes microtrauma. Stress fractures, Little League elbow, tendinitis, and osteochondritis dissecans are the most common overuse injuries.

Table 38-2 Differential Diagnosis: Common Elbow Injuries

CRITERIA	LITTLE LEAGUE ELBOW	PANNER DISEASE*	OSTEOCHONDRITIS DISSECANS OF THE ELBOW*
Defining characteristics	Inflammation, fragmentation and avulsion of the apophysis, loose bodies, osteochondritis dissecans	Lesion of the capitellum that begins with degeneration and regeneration	Lesion of the capitellum that causes the subchondral bone to flake and form loose bodies
ICD-9 code	718.82	732.3	732.78
Subjective Data			
Age/onset	8-16 years of age/gradual	7-12 years of age/gradual	13-16 years of age/gradual
Mechanism of injury	Repetitive valgus stress	Excessive force when throwing	Repetitive throwing
At risk	Throwing activities	Throwing activities	Throwing activities
Objective Data			
Musculoskeletal examination			
Inspection	No obvious deformity	Swelling of area	Flexion contracture
Palpation	Point tenderness at the medial epicondyle	No obvious findings	No obvious findings
Range of motion	Full ROM, painful, resists flexion or pronation	Extension may be limited	Elbow may lock/catch with ROM
Special tests	Lateral and medial stress tests	Lateral and medial stress tests	Lateral and medial stress tests
Laboratory data	Radiographs: Show loose bodies and fragmentation	Radiographs: Show a lesion of the capitellum	Radiographs: Show loose bodies and flaking of the bone

*Refer the child to an orthopedist.

Table 38-3 Differential Diagnosis: Common Wrist and Hand Injuries

CRITERIA	WRIST SPRAIN	WRIST FRACTURE*	JAMMED FINGER
Defining characteristics	Ligamentous injury to the wrist	Break in a bone of the wrist and hand	Ligamentous injury with or without dislocation
ICD-9 code	842.00	814.00	959.5
Subjective Data			
Age/onset	Any age, rare in skeletally immature/acute onset	Any age, radial and ulnar fracture in young child, scaphoid fracture in adolescence/acute onset	Any age/acute onset
Mechanism of injury	Fall on outstretched hand	Fall on outstretched hand	Axial load to tip of finger
At risk	All athletic activities	All athletic activities	All athletic activities
Objective Data			
Musculoskeletal examination			
Inspection	Swelling, bruising	Swelling, bruising, may have obvious deformity	Swelling, bruising, may have obvious deformity
Palpation	May feel defect in ligaments	May feel crepitus, obvious deformity	May feel crepitus, defect in ligaments
Range of motion	Limited by pain	Limited by deformity	Limited by pain
Special tests	Lateral and medial stress tests	None	Lateral and medial stress tests
Laboratory data	Radiographs: Used to rule out fracture	Radiographs: Shows type of fracture	Radiographs: Used to rule out fracture

*Refer the child to an orthopedist.

Table 38-4 Differential Diagnosis: Common Hip Injuries

CRITERIA	HIP POINTER	GROIN PULL
Defining characteristics	Contusion to the iliac crest	Strain of the adductor muscle group
ICD-9 code	922.2	848.8
Subjective Data		
Age/onset	Any age/acute	Any age/acute
Mechanism of injury	Direct blow to unpadded iliac crest	External rotation of abducted leg, quick change of movement
At risk	Contact and collision sports	Sports requiring quick directional changes
Objective Data		
Musculoskeletal examination		
Inspection	Swelling, bruising	None
Palpation	No obvious deformity	Localized tenderness, may feel defect in muscle
Range of motion	Trunk rotation and flexion of the hip painful	Passive abduction painful
Special tests	None	None
Laboratory data	Radiographs: Used to rule out fracture	None

Table 38-5 Differential Diagnosis: Common Knee Injuries

CRITERIA	SPRAINS*	OSGOOD-SCHLATTER DISEASE	CHONDROMALACIA PATELLAE*	OSTEOCHONDRITIS DISSECANS OF THE KNEE*	PATELLOFEMORAL SYNDROME
Defining characteristics	Stretch injury to a ligament of the knee	Overgrowth of the tibial tubercle at the insertion of the patellar tendon with partial avulsion of the tibial tubercle	Degenerative softening of the cartilage that results in fragmentation	Vascular necrosis of subchondral bone that results in loose bodies	Collection of symptoms relating to patellofemoral pain
ICD-9 code	844.9	732.4	717.7	732.78	719.46
Subjective Data					
Age/onset	Any age/acute	Prepubescence/gradual onset	Adolescence/gradual onset	Adolescence/gradual onset	Adolescence/gradual onset
Mechanism of injury	Forced valgus or varus stress, rotation injury	Overuse	Overuse	Overuse	Overuse
At risk	Contact, collision sports	Repetitive knee extension and flexion	Athlete with abnormal patellar tracking, abnormal Q angle	Male athletes	Female athletes with wide Q angle
Objective Data					
Musculoskeletal examination					
Inspection	Swelling, bruising	Large tibial tuberosity	No obvious deformity	No obvious deformity	Prepatellar swelling, subtle atrophy
Palpation	May feel defect in ligament	Tenderness at tibial tuberosity	Crepitus	None	Inhibition or crepitus
Range of motion	Limited by pain	Full ROM	Full ROM with grating sensation	Full ROM with locking or catching	Full ROM
Special tests	Lateral and medial stress tests, anterior drawer test, Lachman test	None	Patellar apprehension	Patellar apprehension	Patellar apprehension
Laboratory data	MRI: Shows torn ligaments	Radiographs: May show radio dense fragments separated from tibial tuberosity	None	Radiographs: Show loose bodies, flaking of bone	None

*Refer the child to an orthopedist.

Management

Treatments and medications. Overuse injuries usually respond to conservative treatment. Rest, ice, and a gradual return to athletic activities are the components of a successful treatment plan. Nonsteroidal antiinflammatory drugs (NSAIDs) may be prescribed to reduce inflammation and pain. (See also the discussion of trauma in Disturbance in Gait: Limp.)

Counseling and prevention. See Promotion of Athletic Activities.

Follow-up. Follow-up is dependent on the area affected and the physician's protocol.

Consultations and referrals. Refer to an orthopedist any children who do not respond to conservative treatment and those with severe symptoms.

Back Pain

Alert
Consult with or refer to a physician for the following:
• Any child with a structural lateral curvature of the spine or kyphosis
• Paresthesias or paralysis
• Excruciating flank pain radiating to the genitalia or down the leg
• Inability to perform a straight leg lift

Etiology

Back pain can be produced by stretching or incomplete tearing (see the discussion of sprains and strains in Disturbance in Gait: Limp) of the muscles, tendons, or ligaments of the back. Gross structural change is not evident. Common causes of back sprains and strains include improper body mechanics when one is lifting heavy objects, strenuous participation in athletic activities, and abnormal posture.

A traumatic incident such as a fall or blow to the back may also cause pain. This is a common occurrence in contact sports, especially football and wrestling. Limited contact and no-contact sports may also cause a back injury. Gymnastics and diving produce heavy loads on the immature spine of a child.

Back pain may signal an infectious process (e.g., diskitis). Referred pain to the back is common and may be the result of a urinary tract infection (UTI), menstrual cramps, or appendicitis. Children with back pain need to have a thorough examination. Unlike adults, the cause for back pain in children is usually organic. In children who have had back pain for at least 2 months, over 80% have a specific lesion.

Incidence

- Back pain in children is rare, but the cause is usually organic.
- Osteoid osteoma is the third most common benign bone tumor, but it is uncommon in young children.
- Spondylolysis and spondylolisthesis is more common among gymnasts and football linemen.

Risk Factors

- Athletic activities that result in an axial load, with or without extension and torsion
- Poor posture
- Children with improper back mechanics
- Obesity
- Adolescents who work out with free weights (unsupervised)
- Athletes who do not properly warm up and stretch out

Differential Diagnosis (Table 38-6)

Ligamentous strain of the lower back occurs most often as the result of improper back mechanics. It is also common in athletes who do not warm up and stretch out before a practice or game. A strain causes an area of the musculature to be stretched forcefully, partially tearing it. Radiologic examination is normal.

Spondylolysis is defined as a defect in the pars interarticularis and usually occurs with spondylolisthesis. *Spondylolisthesis* is the forward slippage or displacement of one vertebra onto another. It occurs most often at the level of L5-S1. Spondylolisthesis may be graded from 1 (less than 25% displacement) to 5 (complete displacement). The diagnosis for either deformity is confirmed by radiologic examination.

Diskitis is inflammation of an intervertebral disk. The inflammation causes a bulging annulus, not a herniated nucleus. The condition may be infectious or not. *Staphylococcus* is the most common causative agent if the child exhibits a systemic process. Diskitis is benign and self-limiting.

A *herniated disk* causes inflammation and compression on the nerve root at the level affected. The nucleus of the disk herniates related to heavy loading forces or chronic disease. Disk disease is uncommon in the pediatric age group. Adolescents have disk disease most often, though rarely. Diagnosis is confirmed by myelogram.

Osteoid osteoma is most often found in people 20 to 30 years of age. It is uncommon in young children. If it does occur, it affects the long bones and spine most often.

Referred pain to the back occurs frequently. Causative agents may include pelvic inflammatory disease, pneumonia, osteomyelitis, appendicitis, UTI, or gastrointestinal (GI) disease. The practitioner must pay close attention to the history and physical examination data to arrive at a diagnosis.

Management

Lower back strain

Treatments and medications. For an acute strain, follow the treatment plan for trauma in Disturbance in Gait: Limp.

Counseling and prevention

- Instruct that proper warm-up and cool-down exercises reduce the number of strains sustained by athletes.
- Explain that athletes who work with weights should be properly supervised and taught proper lifting mechanics to prevent injury.
- Teach regarding medications (e.g., the importance of taking analgesics before pain is severe, the importance of taking prescribed medications correctly). Instruct in the name of the medication and its dosage, frequency, and side effects.
- Instruct in body positions (e.g., sit straight in a chair, maintain good posture).
- Instruct on the importance of weight reduction, if indicated. Discuss the relation between increased weight and back strain or injury.
- Demonstrate correct body alignment for lifting.
- Demonstrate exercises to strengthen back and abdominal muscles after acute pain subsides.

Table 38-6 Differential Diagnosis: Back Pain

CRITERIA	STRAIN	SPONDYLOLYSIS/ SPONDYLOLISTHESIS*	DISKITIS	HERNIATED DISK*	OSTEOID OSTEOMA*	REFERRED PAIN
ICD-9 code	847.9	756.11/756.12	722.90	722.2	213.9	
Subjective Data						
Age	Any age	Rare before 10 years of age	Any age	Any age; rare in children and adolescents	Rare in childhood; 20-30 years of age	Any age
Onset	Acute	May have congenital deformity that is injured acutely	Sudden	Variable	Gradual	Sudden
Description of problem	States lower back pain	States lower back pain	States back pain	States back pain with radiation to legs	States back pain	States back pain with other symptoms
Associated symptoms	Afebrile, acute pain	Afebrile, low back pain	Fever, diffuse nonradiating pain	Afebrile, sciatica pain, incontinence	Afebrile, nonradicular pain at night, incontinence	Often febrile, diffuse pain, radiation of pain dependent on cause
History of trauma	Yes	Possible	Possible	Possible	No	Possible
Athletic activity	Yes	Yes	No	Possible	No	Possible
Family history	No	Yes	No	No	No	No
Objective Data						
Musculoskeletal examination						
Inspection	No obvious deformity	Lumbar lordosis posture	No obvious deformity	No obvious deformity	No obvious deformity	No obvious deformity
Palpation	No point tenderness but certain area is tender	Usually have point tenderness at L5-S1	Usually have point tenderness at affected disk space	Usually have point tenderness at affected disk space	No palpable deformity	No point tenderness
Range of motion	Limited by pain	Tight hamstring muscles	Will not flex the spine	Limited by pain	Full ROM	Full ROM
Special tests	Straight leg lift	Straight leg lift	None	Straight leg lift	None	None
Laboratory data	AP lateral and oblique radiographs: No abnormal findings	AP lateral and oblique radiographs, bone scan if radiographs normal: Reveals forward slip with or without fracture	CBC with differential: Elevated WBC; ESR: Elevated; AP lateral radiographs: Reveals narrowed disk spaces	AP lateral radiographs: No abnormal findings; MRI: Shows herniated disk	AP lateral radiographs, bone scan, CT: Reveal bone tumor	CBC with differential: May be elevated; urine culture and sensitivity: May be positive with UTI; chest radiograph: May show pneumonia

*Refer the child to a physician.
AP, Anteroposterior.

Follow-up

- Schedule a return visit in 1 week after injury for rehabilitation exercises. Approximately 4 weeks after the injury, schedule a return visit to evaluate proper rehabilitation.
- Advise parents to telephone immediately if symptoms worsen.

Consultations and referrals

- Refer the child to a physician if the pain persists 1 week or if there is severe pain.
- Inform the school nurse or employer of limitations.

Spondylolysis and spondylolisthesis

Treatments and medications. The child is placed in a brace and taught antilordotic exercises. Many athletes can play in a brace if pain free. An NSAID may also be prescribed.

Counseling and prevention

- Advise that athletes who perform repetitive flexion and hyperflexion are at the highest risk.
- Encourage compliance with bracing and exercises.
- Teach the need for frequent assessment for skin breakdown.

Follow-up. Follow-up per physician's protocol.

Consultations and referrals. Refer the child to an orthopedist if the diagnosis is suspected.

Diskitis

Treatments and medications

- If there are systemic symptoms, treat with an antibiotic sensitive to *Staphylococcus* organisms.
- If there are no other symptoms, treat for pain with an age-appropriate dose of acetaminophen or ibuprofen.

Counseling and prevention. Teach the parents and child that diskitis is self-limiting and benign. It does not cause meningitis.

Follow-up. Schedule a return visit at the conclusion of antibiotic treatment. If the pain persists or is severe or if the fever is high, schedule an immediate visit.

Consultations and referrals. Refer the child to a physician if the pain is severe or systemic symptoms occur.

Herniated disk

Treatments and medications. Usually treatment is conservative with traction, steroids, and physical therapy. Surgical intervention may be needed to correct the herniated disk if conservative treatment fails.

Counseling and prevention. Athletes who receive an axial load while extending or rotating are at the highest risk for a herniated disk. This group includes football linemen, wrestlers, divers, and gymnasts. Inform coaches and parents of this risk.

Follow-up. Follow-up per physician's protocol.

Consultations and referrals. Refer the child to a neurosurgeon if the diagnosis is suspected.

Osteoid osteoma

Treatments and medications. Salicylates are the medication of choice to treat the pain associated with osteoid osteoma. Surgical intervention is done to resect the osteoma.

Counseling and prevention

- Explain the cause, treatment, and recovery to the parents and child.
- Explain that athletic activity may be limited to noncontact sports after resection.

Follow-up. Follow-up per physician's protocol.

Consultations and referrals. Immediately refer the child to a physician or orthopedist if the diagnosis is suspected.

Referred pain

Treatments and medications. Treatment and medications are dependent on the cause of the pain.

Counseling and prevention. Counseling and prevention is dependent on the cause of the pain.

Follow-up. Follow-up is dependent on the cause of the pain.

Consultations and referrals. Refer to a physician any child with severe pain that is not relieved with acetaminophen or ibuprofen or systemic symptoms with no identified causative agent, or any child in which the cause of pain cannot be determined.

Disturbance in Gait: Limp

Alert

Consult with or refer to a physician for the following:

- High fever with painful limp
- Functional derangement, limp, and pain
- Suspected slipped capital femoral epiphysis (SCFE) (which requires immediate hospitalization to prevent further slip)
- Recent onset of limp with joint findings (suspect septic arthritis and attempt to promptly differentiate diagnosis to reduce morbidity of the femoral head and neck)
- History significant for nonintentional injury (suspect physical abuse)

Etiology

A limp represents a disturbance of gait. It is never a normal symptom and should not be considered unimportant or accepted without a thorough investigation to determine its cause. A limp is a common reason for visiting a health professional. Parents often become concerned about a limp if it occurs for more than a short period of time and will seek health care.

Many illnesses and injuries may cause a child to limp. The entire lower extremity and lower abdomen must be examined to rule out systemic disease or acute injury. The practitioner must differentiate between a limp that is painful and a limp that is not. Most painful limps are associated with an acute onset and are usually the result of trauma, infection, or inflammatory disease. Limping that is painless is usually accompanied by weakness of the muscles supporting the hip. The weakness can be related to past trauma or a neuromuscular disease. Box 38-1 lists causes of both painful and painless limp.

Incidence

- A child may develop a limp at any age.
- Transient (toxic) synovitis is most common in girls 2 to 12 years of age and boys 5 to 10 years of age.
- Legg-Calvé-Perthes (LCP) disease is most common in Caucasian boys 4 to 9 years of age.
- SCFE is more common in African-American boys before epiphyseal plate fusion (10 to 17 years of age).
- Developmental dysplasia of the hip (DDH) is most common in first-born, breech-position, female infants.

Risk Factors

- Participation in contact sports
- LBW
- Child with constitutional delay of growth
- Child with retarded bone age
- Child with antecedent history of transient synovitis
- Positive family history of LCP disease

Box 38-1 Causes of a Limp

Painless Limp

Neurologic conditions—Flaccid paralysis, spasticity, ataxia, spinal diseases

Muscle disease—Muscular dystrophy, arthrogryposis

Joint disorders—Contractures, congenital hip dysplasia, hyperextensible joints

Bone disorders—Knock-knees, leg discrepancy, Blount disease, tibial torsion, SCFE, coxa vara, epiphyseal dysplasias, spondylolisthesis

Hysteria or mimicry

Painful Limp

Trauma—Intentional or nonintentional injuries that may result in sprains, strains, tendinitis, fractures, bruises, injections

Infections—Septic joint, osteomyelitis, pyomyositis, epidural abscess

Intraabdominal processes—Appendicitis, retroperitoneal masses, iliac adenitis

Inflammatory disorders—Toxic synovitis, inflammatory bowel disease, rheumatic fever, juvenile arthritis, systemic lupus erythematosus

Aseptic necrosis and osteochondritis—Legg-Calvé-Perthes disease, Osgood-Schlatter disease, chondromalacia patellae, osteochondritis dissecans

Neoplasms—Leukemia, malignant and benign bone tumors

Hematologic disorders—Hemophilia, sickle cell disease, phlebitis, scurvy

Dermatologic disorders—Ingrown toenail, callus, plantar wart, puncture on sole, blisters

Other disorders—Henoch-Schönlein purpura, serum sickness

Differential Diagnosis

Painful limp (Table 38-7)

Trauma can occur at any age and is the leading diagnosis for painful limp. Physically induced (traumatic) injuries include sprains, strains, and fractures. All musculoskeletal complaints should be evaluated for trauma as the causative agent. Children involved in athletic activities frequently come to the office with an traumatic injury. However, all children are very active and may become injured. (For more information on fractures, sprain, and strain, see Joint Pain and Swelling.)

Septic arthritis is a bacterial infection of the joint space caused most often by *Haemophilus influenzae*. Pneumococci, streptococci, gonococci, and salmonellae are also common causative agents. Infants or children show symptoms of a sudden onset of fever, joint pain (affected joint only), and painful limp. The child should be immediately referred to a physician.

The most common cause of nontraumatic limp in childhood, *transient (toxic) synovitis* is a relatively benign and self-limiting disorder. It frequently follows an upper respiratory tract infection and is the most common cause of hip pain in childhood. Transient synovitis is a diagnosis of exclusion. The infant or child has a gradual onset of symptoms that include flexion of the affected joint, unilateral limp, and slightly raised temperature. The child should be immediately referred to a physician to rule out septic arthritis.

Juvenile arthritis (JA) is an inflammatory disorder with no known causative agent. It is a persistent noninfectious arthritis that lasts more than 6 weeks. JA begins with insidious inflammation of affected joints and leads to joint effusion and destruction. Systemic JA (Still's disease) is characterized by a high fever, rash, lymphadenopathy, and polyarthritis. Complications such as serositis of the pleura, pericardium, and peritoneum may occur. JA is a chronic health condition.

Legg-Calvé-Perthes disease is aseptic or avascular necrosis of the femoral head. It is potentially serious if not recognized early because the femoral head may die from lack of blood flow. The child shows an insidious onset of limp with knee pain. Pain may also be felt in the groin or lateral area of the hip. The disease lasts 1 to 3 years in most children. If the child is in the chronic stage of the disease, the limp is no longer painful.

Slipped capital femoral epiphysis is a disruption in the anatomic relationship of the femoral head and femoral neck. The femoral head may slip off the femoral neck, disrupting the blood supply and causing death of the femoral head. SCFE is a serious condition of obese preadolescents. A painful limp is noted with pain in the knee, groin, buttock, or lateral area of the hip. A chronic low-grade slip may not cause a painful limp.

Painless limp (Table 38-8)

Developmental dysplasia of the hip involves abnormal development or dislocation of the hip. It is a congenital condition but may not be recognized until ambulation occurs. The child then shows a painless limp related to a dislocated hip. The chronically dislocated femoral head causes the acetabulum to be flat rather than round. It is important to diagnose this disorder early to allow the acetabulum and femoral head to become remodeled.

Leg-length discrepancy, the shortening of a lower extremity, can occur at the level of the femur, tibia, or both. Many conditions may cause a leg-length discrepancy, including DDH, LCP, osteomyelitis, epiphyseal plate injury, or a tumor.

Duchenne muscular dystrophy is a sex-linked recessive disorder that results in progressive weakness and atrophy of specific muscle groups. Children with this disease rarely survive past the third decade. One of the first symptoms is difficulty rising from the floor. The Gower maneuver is observed when the children put their hands on their knees and literally walk their hands up their legs until standing erect. (See Duchenne Muscular Dystrophy in Chapter 46.)

Cerebral palsy is a nonspecific term applied to disorders characterized by impaired movement and posture and early onset. It is nonprogressive and may be accompanied by other deficits. (See Cerebral Palsy in Chapter 46.)

Management

Painful limp

Trauma. For fracture, sprain, or strain, see Joint Pain Swelling.

Table 38-7 Differential Diagnosis: Painful Limp

CRITERIA	TRAUMA	SEPTIC ARTHRITIS*	TRANSIENT SYNOVITIS*	JUVENILE ARTHRITIS	LCP DISEASE ACUTE*	SCFE ACUTE*
ICD-9 code		711.00	727.00	714.30	732.1	732.2
Subjective Data						
Age	Any age	Any age	5-10 years	2-16 years	4-9 years	10-17 years
Onset	Abrupt	Sudden	Gradual	May be insidious or sudden	Insidious	Insidious unless associated with trauma
Description of problem	States pain after traumatic incident	States painful, red, swollen joint with fever	States painful joint	States pain in one or more joints, afternoon fevers	States pain in hip, may refuse to walk	States hip pain
Associated symptoms: pain/fever	Afebrile, painful affected area	Fever, pain in affected joint	Afebrile or low-grade fever, pain with movement of the affected joint	Intermittent high fever, pain of affected joints	Afebrile, knee, groin, or lateral hip pain	Afebrile, knee, groin, buttock, or lateral hip pain
History of trauma	Yes, and trauma may be acute or chronic with repetitive stress	None	None	None but traumatic event may precipitate symptoms	None, but traumatic event may exacerbate symptoms	None, but traumatic event may exacerbate symptoms
Family history	None	None	None	Genetic factors such as human leukocyte antigen (HLA) type may play a role	Yes	Genetic factors may play a role
Athletic activity	Yes, contact and limited contact sports implicated most often	None	None	None, unless as traumatic event	None, unless as traumatic event	None, unless as traumatic event
Objective Data						
Temperature	Afebrile	Elevated	Afebrile or low-grade fever	Elevated	Afebrile	Afebrile
Musculoskeletal examination						
Inspection	Affected area may have swelling, bruising, deformity, abrasions	Child appears seriously ill, redness and swelling of affected area noted	No obvious signs	Nonpuritic, pale red, macular rash noted on the trunk and extremities; affected joints swollen	No obvious signs	No obvious signs
Palpation	May be able to palpate defect in bone or soft tissue	Affected area warm	No obvious signs	Affected joints warm	No obvious signs	No obvious signs

*Immediate referral to a physician.

Continued

Table 38-7 Differential Diagnosis: Painful Limp—cont'd

CRITERIA	TRAUMA	SEPTIC ARTHRITIS*	TRANSIENT SYNOVITIS*	JUVENILE ARTHRITIS	LCP DISEASE ACUTE*	SCFE ACUTE*
Musculoskeletal examination—cont'd						
Range of motion	ROM of affected area may be slightly or severely limited by pain, swelling, or deformity	Full ROM possible but painful	Full ROM possible but painful	ROM may be limited by flexion contractures	Limited passive internal rotation and abduction of the hip joint; hip flexion contracture and atrophy of leg muscles in long-standing cases	Unable to properly flex the hip because the femur will abduct and rotate externally
Special tests	Dependent on area affected and injury suspected	None	None	None	None	None
Laboratory data						
Radiograph	May have fracture of growth plate or avulsion fracture	No abnormalities	No abnormalities	May have arthritic changes of the joint	Shows disease progression and sphericity of the femoral head	Shows the degree of slippage between the femoral head and neck
CBC with differential	Not indicated	Elevated	Normal or slightly elevated	Usually elevated with left shift	Not indicated	Not indicated
ESR	Not indicated	Elevated	Normal or slightly elevated	Highly elevated	Not indicated	Not indicated
Joint aspiration	Not indicated	Pyogenic infection with positive joint or blood culture	Normal fluid	Not indicated	Not indicated	Not indicated
Other	None	None	None	Rheumatoid factor, HLA-B27 antigen, ANA	None	None

*Immediate referral to a physician.

Table 38-8 Differential Diagnosis: Painless Limp

CRITERIA	DEVELOPMENTAL DYSPLASIA OF THE HIP*	LEG-LENGTH DISCREPANCY	DUCHENNE MUSCULAR DYSTROPHY*	CEREBRAL PALSY*
ICD-9 code	755.63	755.30	359.1	343.9
Subjective Data				
Age	Most have as newborns but may have at any age	Any age	3-7 years	Any age
Onset	Gradual or present at birth	Gradual	Gradual	May be sudden or insidious
Description of problem	No mobility problem noticed in infancy, limp in child may be described when begins walking	States limp; shoe soles may be worn unequally	States weak muscles	States tight muscles, may describe seizure activity
Associated symptoms	Afebrile, painless, may have ligamentous laxity	Afebrile, painless	Afebrile, painless, progressive muscle weakness of pelvis and shoulder girdle	Afebrile, painless, hypertonic muscle contractions
History of trauma	None	None	None	None
Family history	None	None	Sex-linked recessive; all male offspring affected	None
Athletic activity	None	None	None	None
Objective Data				
Musculoskeletal examination				
Inspection	Asymmetric thigh folds, level of the pelvis unequal, depends on age	Level of the pelvis unequal	Distorted posture with protuberant abdomen, exaggerated lumbar lordosis	Flexion contractures, spastic movements are common
Palpation	May be able to palpate femoral head out of acetabulum	No obvious deformity	No obvious deformity	Flexion contractures
Range of motion	Limited abduction of the affected hip	Full ROM	Full ROM but resistive strength decreased	ROM limited by flexion contractures
Special tests	Ortolani, Barlow, ROM, Trendelenburg tests (see Objective Data, earlier in chapter)	Trendelenburg test, measurement of extremities (see Objective Data, earlier in chapter)	Assess for Gower maneuver	None; somewhat a diagnosis of exclusion
Laboratory data				
Radiography	Used to assess relationship of the femoral head to the acetabulum	Plain radiograph not indicated	Not indicated	Not indicated
Ultrasonography	Assess hip stability and acetabular development	Not indicated	Not indicated	Not indicated
Other	None	Teleroentgenogram (< 5 years), orthoroentgenogram, or scanogram reveal discrepancies in bone length	Serum muscle enzymes (creatine kinase [CK]), muscle biopsy, and electromyogram	None

*Refer the child to a physician.

Septic arthritis

Treatments and medications. Hospitalize the child for intravenous administration of antibiotics. The length of stay is dependent on the response to antibiotic therapy.

Counseling and prevention. Prepare the parents and child for the hospitalization, procedures, and course of treatment.

Follow-up. Follow-up as per the physician's protocol.

Consultations and referrals. Refer the child immediately to a physician.

Transient synovitis

Treatments and medications. If there is high fever or severe symptoms, hospitalize the child to differentiate between transient synovitis and septic arthritis. Analgesics and rest are the main treatment therapies. Administer ibuprofen every 4 to 6 hours around the clock during the course of the illness with activity as tolerated.

Counseling and prevention. Teach the parents that the illness lasts from 3 to 5 days and is benign and self-limiting.

Follow-up. Follow-up per the physician's protocol. Usually the child is seen every other day while symptoms persist to evaluate resolution or progression.

Consultations and referrals. Refer the child to a physician to rule out septic arthritis.

Juvenile arthritis

Treatments and medications. Aspirin is the drug of choice for JA. Administer 60 to 100 mg/kg per day divided into four daily doses. Other NSAIDs may be used because of fewer GI side effects and less frequent administration. Physical therapy helps increase or maintain strength and ROM and prevent contractures.

Counseling and prevention

- Inform the parents and child that JA is a chronic disease that has exacerbations and remissions. The child should be encouraged to attain the highest level of independence that can be managed.
- Keep in mind that a home routine that balances time for rest, therapies, school, adequate nutrition, and normal family activities is best.
- Remember that pain control can be achieved with ibuprofen in the beginning stages of the disease.

Follow-up. Follow-up per the physician's protocol.

Consultations and referrals. Refer the child to a physician for diagnosis and initial treatment.

Legg-Calvé-Perthes disease

Treatments and medications. The goal of treatment is to restore ROM while maintaining the femoral head within the acetabulum. Buck's traction, an orthotic appliance, or surgery may be necessary.

Counseling and prevention

- Explain to the parents and child that the treatment regimen is dependent on the extent of the disease process.
- Inform the parents and child that LCP disease lasts 1 to 3 years and is potentially serious if not treated properly.
- Encourage compliance with appointments and treatments for the best outcome.

Follow-up. Follow-up per the physician's protocol.

Consultations and referrals. Refer the child immediately to an orthopedic physician to preserve the femoral head.

Slipped capital femoral epiphysis

Treatments and medications. The treatment goal is to prevent further slippage. No ambulation is allowed. The slip may be treated with traction, a screw insertion, or an open bone graft.

Counseling and prevention

- Inform the parents and child that SCFE is a potentially serious condition.
- Encourage compliance with appointments and treatments for the best outcome.
- Stress that ambulation with crutches is necessary to prevent further slip.

Follow-up. Follow-up per the physician's protocol.

Consultations and referrals. Refer the child immediately to an orthopedic physician to prevent further slippage.

Painless limp

Developmental dysplasia of the hip

Treatments and medications. A Pavlik harness is used to maintain a position of flexion and abduction in infants 1 to 6 months of age. Casting, surgical reduction, or traction may be indicated if the harness does not help.

Counseling and prevention

- Stress that DDH must be addressed early in infancy for the best outcome. Encourage the parents to be compliant with the harness or traction devices. Once the deformity is corrected, no further bracing is required.
- Instruct the parents that the infant should be allowed to sleep supine or side-lying, not prone.

Follow-up. Follow-up as per the physician's protocol.

Consultations and referrals. If the diagnosis is suspected, referral to a physician is necessary.

Leg-length discrepancy

Treatments and medications. Discrepancies greater than 2 cm at maturity require treatment. Conservative treatment involves a lift for the affected shoe. Surgical intervention may be required if the defect is large.

Counseling and prevention

- Encourage compliance with therapies and shoe lifts.
- Advise that activity should not be limited if pain free.

Follow-up. Follow-up per the physician's protocol.

Consultations and referrals. Refer to a physician for large discrepancies or those children with severe symptoms.

Duchenne muscular dystrophy. See Duchenne Muscular Dystrophy in Chapter 46.

Cerebral palsy. See Cerebral Palsy in Chapter 46.

Disturbance in Gait: Toeing-In

Alert

Consult with or refer to a physician for the following:
- Child who walks toeing-in and walks on the toes
- Heel cord tightening or shortening
- Rigid forefoot or clubfoot
- Neurologic deficit
- Unilateral or asymmetric involvement

Etiology

Toeing-in is a common gait disturbance described by parents. Internal (medial) tibial torsion is the most common cause of toeing-in in children less than 2 years of age. It is secondary to fetal position in utero. For children older than 2 years of age, internal femoral torsion (anteversion) is the most common cause of toeing-in. The child with femoral torsion often has generalized ligamentous laxity and may have acquired femoral torsion with abnormal sitting habits. Neural tube defects and spinal curvatures or other neurologic disease are rare causes.

Incidence

- About 1% of children with internal femoral torsion have a severe deformity.
- True tibial torsion persisting after 6 years of age is rare.
- Metatarsus adductus is the most common congenital foot deformity.
- About 10% of the children with metatarsus adductus also have DDH.
- Equinovarus is two times more common in boys and is associated with neuromuscular abnormalities (e.g., spina bifida).

Risk Factors

- Neuromuscular disorder
- Family history
- Sleeping in prone position
- Intrauterine position or compression
- Sitting in "tailor position" or "TV squat" (sitting on haunches with legs tucked under and feet turned in or out)

Differential Diagnosis (Table 38-9)

Internal femoral torsion, or *femoral anteversion,* is a torsional deformity that occurs at the level of the hip. It represents a failure of progression and persistence into childhood and adult life of the normally anteverted position of the femur. The cause

Table 38-9 Differential Diagnosis: Toeing-In

CRITERIA	INTERNAL FEMORAL TORSION	INTERNAL TIBIAL TORSION	METATARSUS ADDUCTUS*	EQUINOVARUS*
ICD-9 code	736.89	736.89	754.79	754.51
Subjective Data				
Age	Less than 8 years	Less than 6 years	Infancy	Infancy
Onset	Insidious	Insidious	Congenital	Congenital
Description of problem	States toeing-in	States toeing-in	States toeing-in	States toeing-in
Associated symptoms	None	None	DDH, internal tibial torsion	Neuromuscular disorder
Family history	None	Yes	Yes	None
Objective Data				
Musculoskeletal examination				
Inspection	Internal rotation of affected leg, flat feet, increased lumbar lordosis	Lateral malleolus at same level as or anterior to medial malleolus when the leg is straight with the patella facing forward	Sole of the affected foot medially concave and laterally convex; forefoot medially deviated and adducted and supinated	Adduction of the affected forefoot with plantar flexion and inversion of the heel; the calf muscles thin and atrophic
Palpation	No obvious deformity	No obvious deformity	May be rigid or supple	May be rigid
Range of motion	Internal rotation greatly exceeds external rotation	Full ROM of hip, knee, ankle	May have full ROM or limited or absent ROM	Limited dorsiflexion related to Achilles tendon contracture
Special tests	None	Thigh-foot Axis	Ruler placed along the lateral border of the foot does not touch the forefoot	None
Laboratory data	None	None	Serial radiographs to evaluate the progression of manipulation of rigid forefoot	Serial radiographs to evaluate the progression of manipulation with serial casting

*Refer the child to an orthopedist.

is unknown, but some believe it is related to sitting position (tailor position). In the prone position the child has greater external rotation of the thigh.

Internal tibial torsion is often present with toeing-in gait. It is caused by many factors, including heredity, intrauterine position, and sleeping position. It rarely persists past 6 years of age. In this condition the tibial tubercle is rotated medially. The thigh-foot angle is recorded in degrees, with positive degrees indicating toeing-out and negative degrees indicating toeing-in.

Metatarsus adductus, a congenital anomaly of the forefoot that causes the metatarsals to point medially, may be rigid or supple. If the foot is rigid, it cannot be passively corrected to the midline or neutral position. If the foot is supple, it can be passively corrected to at least the midline or neutral position.

Equinovarus, or *clubfoot,* is a congenital anomaly of the foot that causes adduction of the forefoot, equinus positioning of the foot, and inversion of the heel. In equinovarus the distal end of the tibia has growth arrest related to intrauterine compression. The fibula continues to grow and pushes the foot over while the Achilles tendon is shortened by lack of dorsiflexion of the foot. Serial casting with manipulation begins at birth. Corrective surgery may also be indicated.

Management

Internal femoral torsion

Treatments and medications. Surgical management is indicated for 1% of children. Braces and cables have no effect on femoral anteversion.

Counseling and prevention
- Reassure the parents and child that 99% have spontaneous resolution by 8 years of age.
- Counsel the child to sit with ankles crossed or in yoga position.

Follow-up. Evaluate at all well-child visits.

Consultations and referrals. Refer to a physician if the child is older than 8 years of age or if the child's condition worsens.

Internal tibial torsion

Treatments and medications. Correction is accelerated when night splints that keep the foot in a neutral position are worn. However, most children have spontaneous correction with growth and need no treatment.

Counseling and prevention
- Reassure the parents and child that resolution of symptoms occurs by 6 years of age.
- Instruct the parents to allow the infant or child to sleep supine, not prone.
- Recommend that the child not sit on his or her feet.
- Encourage compliance with all appointments for close follow-up evaluation.

Follow-up. Evaluate at all well-child visits.

Consultations and referrals. Refer the child to an orthopedist if the deformity is excessive, the condition worsens, or the deformity persists past 6 years of age.

Metatarsus adductus

Treatments and medications
- For supple metatarsus adductus, teach parents to stretch the forefoot in all planes of motion with each diaper change.

- For rigid metatarsus adductus, explain that serial casting or bracing is done until 2 years of age. The child is then placed in straight-laced and outflare shoes until there is no chance of recurrence. If the child is older than 2 years of age at diagnosis, surgical intervention is required.
Counseling and prevention
- Explain to the parents that the earlier the treatment is, the better the results are. Treatment is very important. If the condition is left untreated, it may persist for life and become a disabling condition.
- Teach the parents cast or brace care. The cast or brace is worn until the deformity is corrected, but no further bracing is needed after correction.
- Demonstrate stretching exercises to the parents and have them perform a return demonstration (for supple metatarsus adductus).
Follow-up. Follow-up per the physician's protocol
Consultations and referrals. Refer cases of rigid metatarsus adductus to an orthopedist.

Equinovarus
Treatments and medications. Serial casting with manipulation begins at birth and lasts until 3 to 6 months of age. If further correction is required, surgery is indicated.
Counseling and prevention
- Encourage the parents to keep all physician appointments. It is very important to have casts changed regularly because the infant is growing rapidly. Treatment should be maintained until the best result is achieved to prevent lifetime deformity. The child is then placed in straight-laced and outflare shoes until 2 years of age.
- Teach the parents cast care. Casts must be worn until the deformity is corrected, and then no further casting is required.
Follow-up. Follow-up per the physician's protocol.
Consultations and referrals. Immediately refer the child to an orthopedist.

Foot Deformity and Pain

Alert

Consult with or refer to an orthopedist for cases of rigid deformity or conditions that do not improve with conservative treatment

Etiology

During the evaluation of a foot deformity of an infant, the practitioner must make the distinction between posturing of the foot and actual foot deformity. The habitual position in which the infant holds the foot is called *posturing*. Upon manipulation by the examiner, the foot can be palpated through normal ROM and positioned in a normal shape. With a true foot deformity, the foot cannot be manipulated into a normal shape. The foot is found to be rigid when palpated. Most foot deformities are congenital. Other causes of foot deformity include infections, tumors, and a misaligned healed fracture.

Incidence

- See Disturbance in Gait: Toeing-In.
- Flexible flatfoot is common in infants and toddlers.

Risk Factors

- Neuromuscular condition
- Intrauterine positioning
- Breech birth
- Family history

Differential Diagnosis (Table 38-10)

Pes planus, or *flatfoot,* is observed in the pronated foot. A loss of the medial longitudinal arch is seen with weight bearing. The foot may be flexible or rigid. In flexible flatfoot the arch disappears when bearing weight but reappears when the child is standing on

Table 38-10 Differential Diagnosis: Foot Deformity or Pain

CRITERIA	PES PLANUS	PES CAVUS*
ICD-9 code	734.	754.71
Subjective Data		
Age	Flexible flatfoot common in infants and toddlers, can present at any age	Most appear in middle childhood
Onset	Gradual	Gradual
Description of problem	States flatfeet	States high arches
Associated symptoms	Pronated foot, may complain of foot pain, back pain	Inverted cant of heel with or without Achilles tendon shortening
Family history	Familial pattern of rigid flatfoot	None
Objective Data		
Musculoskeletal examination		
Inspection	Pronated foot with loss of medial longitudinal arch with weight bearing	Exaggerated medial longitudinal arch with an inward cant of the heel
Palpation	May be flexible or rigid	Foot is taut
Range of motion	Full ROM with flexible; limited ROM with rigid	Limited ROM
Special tests	None	None
Laboratory data	None	None

*Refer the child to an orthopedist.

his or her toes. A diagnosis of flatfoot is not made until after 6 years of age. Pes planus is caused by ligamentous laxity and fat development in the area of the medial longitudinal arch.

Pes cavus, or *high arches,* occurs with an exaggerated medial longitudinal arch that is associated with an inward cant of the heel. This position may shorten the Achilles tendon and put the child at risk of an inversion ankle sprain. It may be a progressive deformity that leads to compromise of foot function. High arches are commonly noted in middle childhood.

For *metatarsus adductus* and *equinovarus,* see Disturbance in Gait: Toeing-In, as well as Table 38-9.

Equinovarus. See Disturbance in Gait: Toeing-In, as well as Table 38-9.

Management

Pes planus

Treatments and medications. Treat conservatively with a commercially available medial longitudinal arch support. Further treatment is warranted for cosmetic purposes if desired by the parents or child.

Counseling and prevention

- Reassure parents that all infant's feet normally appear flat. It is difficult to make a definite diagnosis until the child is approximately 6 years of age.
- Suggest that some pain may be relieved by the use of orthotics, or "cookies," in the shoes. Remember that orthotics do not correct pes planus, and ongoing use is required.
- Instruct the parents that the best treatment is exercise to strengthen the foot-supporting muscles (e.g., with calf raises, toe flexing and extending).
- Reassure the parents and the child that flatfeet should not prevent participation in activity.

Follow-up. Follow-up is not indicated unless the child is having severe pain. Assess at well-child visits.

Consultations and referrals. Referral is not indicated unless the child is having severe pain.

Pes cavus

Treatments and medications. Treatment is aggressive to prevent further deformity. Surgical intervention is usually indicated.

Counseling and prevention. Prompt referral is necessary to prevent further deformity.

Follow-up. Follow-up per the physician's protocol.

Consultations and referrals. Refer the child to an orthopedist for evaluation.

Metatarsus adductus. See Disturbance in Gait: Toeing-In.

Equinovarus. See Disturbance in Gait: Toeing-In.

Growing Pains

Alert

Consult with or refer to a physician in the following situations:
- Severe systemic symptoms
- Hemarthrosis
- Suspected SCFE
- Obvious deformity

Etiology

Growing pains may be difficult to diagnose and is a diagnosis of exclusion. The child has no history of traumatic insult, no loss of ambulation or mobility, no systemic disease, and no edema or erythema. All laboratory studies are normal. Related factors include rapid growth, puberty, fibrositis, weather, and psychologic factors.

Incidence

- The prevalence increases after 5 years of age.

Risk Factors

- Rapid growth

Differential Diagnosis (Table 38-11)

Growing pains is a term used to describe pain experienced in the lower limbs. The pain is noted to be bilateral, intermittent, and localized to the muscles of the legs and thighs. It occurs late in the day, in the evening, or at night, and is a diagnosis of exclusion

For *trauma, infection,* and *slipped capital femoral epiphysis,* see Table 38-7.

In regard to hematologic causes, *hemophilia* and *sickle cell anemia* are considered in the differential diagnosis (see Table 38-11). See Hemophilia in Chapter 45 and Anemia in Chapter 36.

For *Osgood-Schlatter disease,* see Table 38-5.

For *osteochondritis dissecans,* see Tables 38-2 and 38-5.

Management

Growing pains

Treatments and medications. The practitioner may prescribe an antiinflammatory medication. Age-appropriate doses of ibuprofen taken regularly help with the pain. Massage to the area and a heating pad applied to the area are also helpful.

Counseling and prevention

- Teach the parents and child how to use a heating pad. Do not apply directly to the skin; do not take the heating pad to bed; and do not use the highest setting for long periods of time.
- Teach the child and parents how to massage the area.
- Allow rest with painful episodes. Encourage activity as tolerated when pain free.

Follow-up. Follow-up as needed for well-child care or if the pain becomes severe or the child develops systemic symptoms.

Consultations and referrals. Consult a physician if the pain does not improve over several weeks or if the pain is severe.

Hip Pain and Click

Alert

Consult with or refer to a physician for the following:
- Toddler who begins ambulation with a limp
- Signs of infection in the hip (e.g., swelling, redness, warmth, pain, fever)
- Traumatic injury

Etiology

The hip is a ball (femoral head) and socket (acetabulum) joint that involves an interdependent relationship of the two for normal development. Any cause of disruption in the relationship between the femoral head and acetabulum results in abnormal hip development. The hip is vulnerable to injury by disruption of the blood supply to the femoral head. The normal blood supply to the femoral head lies on the surface of the femoral neck and enters the epiphysis peripherally. Damage to this blood supply is common in septic arthritis, trauma, and other vascular insults. The causes of hip pain may include trauma, infection, or congenital deformity.

Table 38-11 Differential Diagnosis: Growing Pains

CRITERIA	GROWING PAINS	SICKLE CELL ANEMIA*	HEMOPHILIA*
ICD-9 code	781.99	282.60	286.0
Subjective Data			
Age	5 years, most common 11-13 years of age	Congenital, onset of symptoms unusual <3-4 months of age	Congenital
Onset	Gradual	Congenital	Congenital
Associated symptoms: pain/fever	Pain or ache localized to the lower extremities; afebrile	Pale, fatigue, severe pain in joints with crisis, small stature	Pain in joints related to hemarthrosis
History of trauma	No	No	Possible
Family history	No	Yes, recessive transmission	Yes, X-linked recessive transmission
Athletic activity	No	No	Possible
Objective Data			
Musculoskeletal examination			
Inspection	No obvious deformity or erythema	No obvious deformity of joints, may have respiratory distress	Affected joint severely swollen
Palpation	No obvious findings	No obvious findings	Tense skin over joint related to hemarthrosis
Range of motion	Full ROM	Full ROM, may be painful	Limited by swelling
Special tests	None	None	None
Laboratory data	Radiograph of affected area, CBC with differential, ESR: All results normal	Sickle cell screen: Abnormal	Hemophilia screen: Abnormal

*Refer the child to a physician.

Incidence

See Disturbance in Gait: Limp, earlier in this chapter.

Risk Factors

See Disturbance in Gait: Limp, earlier in this chapter.

Differential Diagnosis

For *trauma, Legg-Calvé Perthes disease, slipped capital femoral epiphysis, septic arthritis of the hip,* and *toxic synovitis of the hip,* see Table 38-7. For *developmental dysplasia of the hip* and *leg-length discrepancy,* see Table 38-8.

Management

Trauma. See Painful Limp.
Developmental dysplasia of the hip. See Painless Limp.
Leg-length discrepancy. See Painless Limp.
Legg-Calvé-Perthes disease. See Painful Limp.
Slipped capital femoral epiphysis. See Painful Limp.
Septic arthritis of the hip. See Painful Limp.
Toxic synovitis of the hip. See Painful Limp.

Joint Pain and Swelling

Alert

Consult with or refer to a physician for the following:
- Acute pain or symptoms of a systemic infection
- Polyarthritis, with or without a new onset murmur
- Open and draining wounds
- Joint that is no longer mobile
- Recent history of streptococcal infection
- History of Lyme disease, tick bite, or rash
- Chronic illness (e.g., hemophilia, sickle cell anemia, JA)
- Suspected physical abuse

Etiology

Joint pain or swelling is caused by many agents. Accidental injuries to the joints are common in children. A fall or twist of an immature joint commonly causes a fracture because the epiphyseal plate is weaker than the ligaments in a child. Joint pain or swelling may be associated with JA, sickle cell crisis, or hemophilia.

Incidence

- The clavicle is the most frequently fractured bone in children under 10 years of age.
- Fractures of the upper extremities are seven times more common than those of the lower extremities.
- Sprains are the most common sports-related injury.
- The knee is the most frequently injured joint in football.

Risk Factors

- Family history of JA
- Athletic participation, especially if there are no warm-up or cool-down periods
- Fatigued athlete
- Skeletally immature athlete
- Ligamentous laxity
- Chronic illness

Differential Diagnosis (Table 38-12)

A *fracture* is a break in the continuity of a bone. Although the bones of a child are more porous and can accept more force than an adult's bones, fractures are common in children. The epiphyseal plate (growth plate) is injured often because it is the weakest part of the bone. The epiphyseal plate will fail before the ligaments or tendons in a skeletally immature child; this is known as a *Salter-Harris fracture.* Stress fractures and avulsion fractures are also common.

Table 38-12 Differential Diagnosis: Joint Pain or Swelling

CRITERIA	FRACTURE*	SPRAIN OR STRAIN	MENISCAL INJURY*	CONTUSION
ICD-9 code	829.0	848.9	959.7	
Subjective Data				
Age	Any age	Any age	More common in adolescents	Any age
Onset	Acute	Acute	Sudden	Acute
Description of problem	States pain or swelling after traumatic incident	States pain or swelling after traumatic incident	States pain or swelling of joint after traumatic incident	Bruising of area after traumatic incident
Associated symptoms	Localized pain, swelling	Diffuse pain, swelling, bruising of area	Diffuse pain of the knee, limited swelling	Diffuse pain, swelling, bruising
History of trauma	Yes	Yes	Yes	Yes
Athletic activity	Yes	Yes	Yes	Yes
Objective Data				
Musculoskeletal examination				
Inspection	May have obvious deformitiy, severe swelling	Moderate-severe swelling, bruising	Limited swelling	Swelling, bruising
Palpation	May feel crepitation as palpate area	May feel interruption of ligament or tendon	May feel large discoid meniscus	May feel a hematoma or calcification (chronic)
Range of motion	Limited by pain or deformity	Limited by pain or deformity	Limited if meniscus torn and trapped	Full ROM or limited by swelling or calcification
Special tests	Tests for stability	Lateral and medial stress tests, anterior drawer test	Lateral and medial stress tests, anterior drawer test, Lachman test	None
Laboratory data	Radiograph of area and contralateral joint: Reveals type and extent of fracture	Radiograph of area and contralateral joint: Should have normal findings; may observe separation of tibia and fibula with syndesmotic ankle sprain	Radiograph of bilateral knees: Evaluate structural abnormalities	Radiograph: Suspicion of calcification

*Refer the child to an orthopedist.

A *sprain* is a stretch or tear injury involving a ligament. Ligaments attach bone to bone and are frequently injured in skeletally mature athletes. Ankle sprains are the most common injury. Sprains are graded on a scale from I to III depending on the severity:

- *Grade I*—Mild stretching of the ligament, tendon, or muscle; stable joint; full ROM; minimal pain and swelling; normal weight-bearing
- *Grade II*—Partial tear of the ligament, tendon, or muscle; stable joint; decreased active ROM; moderate swelling or pain; weight-bearing difficult
- *Grade III*—Complete tear of the ligament, tendon, or muscle; unstable joint; unable to perform active ROM; severe pain and swelling; no weight-bearing

A *strain* is a stretch or tear injury involving a muscle or its tendon. Tendons attach muscle to bone and are frequently injured with overuse. Strains are graded on a scale from I to III depending on the severity. (See the preceding scale for sprains.)

Meniscal injuries can occur at any joint but are most common in the knee. The meniscus is a crescent-shaped disk of fibrocartilage attached to an articular surface. It can be torn with a traumatic insult. These injuries are rare before 12 years of age. There is usually a recent history of a knee injury with resulting locking of the knee.

A *contusion* is an injury that does not break the skin. It is also known as a bruise. Contusions can occur at any joint or to any muscle body. A deep muscle bruise can be painful enough to limit a child's athletic performance.

For *juvenile arthritis*, see Disturbance in Gait: Limp.

Management

Fractures

Treatments and medications. Most fractures are treated with cast immobilization. Pain control is achieved with acetaminophen or ibuprofen. Ice should be applied to a new fracture for the first 48 hours. This can be done with a cast in place.

Counseling and prevention

- Teach the parents and child cast care.
- Advise that fractures are reduced in athletes who wear commercial ankle braces.
- Instruct that athletes should not return to competition until fully rehabilitated.

Follow-up. Follow-up per the physician's protocol.

Consultations and referrals. Refer any child with a fracture to an orthopedist. For prepubescent patients, implement the Ottawa Ankle Rules (OAR). An ankle radiographic series is necessary only if a patient has pain near the malleoli and: (1) cannot walk four steps immediately after injury, or (2) has bone tenderness at the posterior edge or tip of either malleolus. A foot radiographic series is necessary only if a patient has midfoot pain and: (1) cannot walk four steps immediately after injury and on examination, or (2) has bone tenderness at the navicular or the base of the fifth metatarsal. Children with persistent pain and swelling of a joint or prepubescent athletes should have a repeat radiographic evaluation to rule out a stress fracture.

Sprain and strain

Treatments and medications. For immediate treatment (first 24 to 48 hours): follow the PRICE protocol:

- *Protection*—Make sure the area is fully protected from further injury. This may involve a splint, elastic wrap, or brace.
- *Rest*—Allow the injured area to rest. Use crutches or a splint if necessary and do no or limited activity.
- *Ice*—Apply ice to the area immediately after the injury. Continue to use ice applications for the first 24 to 48 hours. Place the ice on the injured area for 15 minutes and then remove. Do this at least three times a day. Always apply ice after activity.
- *Compression*—Apply an elastic bandage or wrap to decrease the swelling. Do not allow the patient to sleep with the bandage on.
- *Elevation*—Elevate the area to decrease the swelling.

About 48 hours after the injury, ibuprofen can be given every 4 to 6 hours for pain and inflammation reduction. Use of a brace versus a cast is dependent on the injury and activity level of the athlete. Rehabilitation can begin after 48 hours if no fracture is present. The goal is to achieve pain-free active ROM and weight-bearing activity by the following measures:

- Treatment modalities as indicated (e.g., ice, ultrasonography)
- ROM and general stretching exercises
- Strengthening exercises (e.g., general body exercises, resistive strengthening of injured area)
- Proprioceptive training
- Activity-specific training
- Protective taping or bracing for return to activity

Counseling and prevention

- See Prevention of Athletic Injuries, earlier in this chapter.
- Instruct the parents and child that a compression wrap should not be worn when sleeping.
- Caution the parents and child against the use of ibuprofen if the child has aspirin sensitivity and in the first 48 hours after injury.
- Advise the parents and child that if pain and swelling continue to worsen or if the child is unable to perform the beginning phases of rehabilitation exercises, a return visit is required.
- Instruct the parents and child on return-to-play criteria if injured during a game or practice or after rehabilitation. The child must show or have the following: full ROM, minimal to no swelling, no bony crepitus on palpation, no limp or altered gait, the ability to run or sprint straight ahead and perform cuts, the ability to perform sport-specific drills (e.g., running backward, crossover), the ability to perform the one-hop test (hop up and down on the affected extremity), the ability to defend and protect self from further injury.

Follow-up

- Instruct the parents to call or make a return visit immediately if there is a change in sensation of the affected extremity.
- Schedule a return visit in 1 week for evaluation and assessment of progress.
- Schedule a return visit approximately 6 weeks after the injury to assess full rehabilitation. (The visit may be earlier if the injury was mild or the child is highly motivated to return to activity.)

Consultations and referrals. Consult an orthopedist if a more serious injury is suspected.

Meniscal injury

Treatments and medications. Surgical intervention is indicated if the joint is locking or very painful.

Counseling and prevention. Advise that the severity of knee injuries is reduced when prophylactic knee braces are worn.

Follow-up. Follow-up per the physician's protocol.

Consultations and referrals. Most knee injuries should be referred to an orthopedist because of the complexity of the knee joint.

Contusion

Treatments and medications. Follow PRICE protocol outlined earlier in this chapter. Teach the child or adolescent how to perform ice massage to the affected area.

Counseling and prevention

- Advise the parents and child that proper use of pads can reduce the severity of contusions.
- Instruct the parents and child to report hardening of the bruised area immediately.

Follow-up. Schedule a return visit in 1 week after injury to assess healing of the contusion.

Consultations and referrals. Referrals are rarely indicated; if the child develops a hardening of the area, indicating calcification, refer to a physician for evaluation.

Leg Deformity

Alert

Consult with or refer to a physician for the following:
- Obvious deformity where correct alignment cannot be achieved passively
- Unilateral or asymmetric involvement
- Neurologic dysfunction
- Muscle atrophy
- Intermalleolar distance greater than 2 inches or intercondylar distance increasing by more than $1/2$ inch in 6 months

Etiology

Children are often brought to the practitioner for the evaluation of a leg deformity. Many conditions cause leg deformities. Congenital abnormalities related to intrauterine position or compression are common. Most congenital conditions have a component that involves heredity. Other conditions may also contribute to the deformity (e.g., joint laxity). Tumors, infection, neuromuscular diseases, and malaligned healed fractures are rare causes of leg deformity.

Incidence

- Genu valgum is very rare.
- Genu varum is often difficult to distinguish from Blount disease.
- Blount disease is most common in obese, African-American, female infants and obese, tall, African-American male adolescents.
- A practitioner should consider rickets in a malnourished child or a child in renal failure

Risk Factors

- Athletes with genu varum or valgum (at risk for ligamentous injury of the knee)
- Children with malnutrition (vitamin D deficiency) (at risk for rickets)
- Family history of genu valgum or genu varum

Differential Diagnosis (Table 38-13)

Commonly known as *knock-knees, genu valgum* occurs when the legs distal to the knee are tilted toward the midline of the body. It is considered normal until 7 years of age unless the intermalleolar distance is more than 2 inches or changing at a rate of ½ inch over 6 months or is unilateral. Genu valgum may be related to intrauterine position. The development of genu valgum may be related to the body's overcorrection of bowlegs seen in infancy.

Commonly known as *bowlegs, genu varum* occurs when the extremity distal to the knee is tilted away from the midline. It is considered normal until 2 years of age unless the intercondylar distance is greater than 2 inches or changing at rate of ½ inch over 6 months.

Blount disease (tibia vara) is the most common pathologic disorder producing a progressive genu varum deformity. It is characterized by abnormal growth of the medial aspect of the proximal tibial epiphysis and results in varus angulation beneath the knee. Blount disease is associated with internal tibial torsion.

A condition caused by a deficiency of vitamin D, *rickets* is characterized by short stature and bending and distortion of the bones under muscular action. Fontanel closure is also delayed in infants with rickets.

For *leg-length discrepancy,* see Table 38-8

Management

Genu valgum

Treatments and medications. Genu valgum may need surgical intervention to correct the deformity.

Counseling and prevention. Reassure the parents and child that a knock-kneed appearance is normal until 7 years of age.

Follow-up. Follow-up per the physician's protocol. The practitioner should reevaluate at each well-child visit.

Consultations and referrals. Refer to an orthopedist any child with a unilateral deformity, those over 7 years of age, and those with an intermalleolar distance greater than 2 inches.

Genu varum

Treatments and medications. Genu varum is commonly treated with a long leg brace with a lateral pull strap, a frame brace, or a Blount brace. If it is severe or unilateral, genu varum may require surgical intervention

Counseling and prevention. Reassure the parents that a bowlegged appearance is normal until 2 years of age. Blount disease should be considered if severe deformity persists past 2 years of age.

Table 38-13 Differential Diagnosis: Leg Deformity

CRITERIA	GENU VALGUM	GENU VARUM	BLOUNT DISEASE*	RICKETS*
ICD-9 code	736.41	736.42	732.4	268.0
Subjective Data				
Age	Normal until 7 years of age, presents at any age	Normal until 2 years of age, may present at any age	Presents at any age, most common in infancy or adolescence	Presents at any age, most common in infancy and childhood
Onset	Gradual	Gradual	Gradual	Gradual
Description of problem	States walks with knock-knees	States walks with bowed legs	States walks with bowlegs	States walks with bowed legs
Associated symptoms	None	None	Obesity	Vitamin D deficiency, malnutrition, muscle pain, sweating of the head
Family history	None	None	None	None
Objective Data				
Musculoskeletal examination				
Inspection	Legs distal to the knees tilted toward the midline of the body	Legs distal to the knees tilted away from the midline of the body	Legs distal to the knees tilted toward the midline of the body	Legs distal to the knees tilted away from the midline of the body
Palpation	No obvious deformity	No obvious deformity	Overgrowth of the medial aspect of the proximal tibial epiphysis	Nodular enlargements on the ends and sides of the bones
Range of motion	Full ROM	Full ROM	Full ROM	Full ROM, may be limited by abnormal shape of bones
Special tests	Intermalleolar distance	Intercondylar distance	None	None
Laboratory data	Standing AP and lateral radiographs, measure tibiofemoral angle (>15 degrees of valgus)	Standing AP and lateral radiographs, measure tibiofemoral angle (>25 degrees of varus)	Standing AP and lateral radiographs, measure tibiofemoral angle (>15 degrees of varus)	Standing AP and lateral radiographs, measure tibiofemoral angle (>15 degrees of varus)

Refer the child to a physician.

Follow-up. Follow-up per the physician's protocol. Practitioners should reevaluate the intercondylar distance at each well-child visit.

Consultations and referrals. Refer to an orthopedist any child over 2 years of age, those with an intercondylar distance of greater than 2 inches, and those with unilateral involvement.

Blount disease

Treatments and medications. Orthotics and braces are used to treat an infant or young child; surgical intervention is often required for an adolescent.

Counseling and prevention. Teach the parents cast- or brace-care techniques. Compliance to treatment is important for maximum remodeling of the bone.

Follow-up. Follow-up per the physician's protocol. Practitioners should reevaluate the intercondylar distance at each well-child visit.

Consultations and referrals. Refer to an orthopedist any child over 2 years of age, those with severe or unilateral genu varum, and those with an intercondylar distance of greater than 2 inches.

Rickets

Treatments and medications. Vitamin D and sunlight combined with an adequate diet are curative unless the parathyroid glands are not functional or the child has hypophosphatemic vitamin D–resistant rickets.

Counseling and prevention. Instruct the parents on the need to provide a balanced diet and vitamin supplements as needed.

Follow-up. Follow-up per the physician's protocol.

Consultations and referrals. Refer to a physician any child with suspected rickets.

Leg-length discrepancy. See Painless Limp, earlier in this chapter.

Spine Deformity

Alert

Consult with or refer to a physician for the following:
- Paresthesia or paralysis
- Weakness upon standing
- Structural curve observed before puberty
- Respiratory symptoms related to structural curve
- Lateral curvature of the spine

Etiology

A deformity of the back may be caused by several factors. Congenital conditions such as Down syndrome or muscular dystrophy may be associated with deformities of the back. Scoliosis has a familial trait. Traumatic insults rarely cause a back deformity.

Incidence

- Of the first-degree female relatives of affected girls with scoliosis, 7% to 12% develop a curve.
- About 15% of children with Down syndrome have atlantoaxial instability.

Risk Factors

- Down syndrome (at risk for atlantoaxial instability)
- Family history of scoliosis
- Females at risk for a more severe scoliotic curve than males
- Congenital defect (e.g., cervical stenosis)

Differential Diagnosis (Table 38-14)

Idiopathic scoliosis is the most common form of scoliosis and is more prevalent in females. A 10-degree lateral and rotational curvature of the spine is considered the threshold for scoliosis. Larger curves progress to a greater degree than smaller curves. Most patients are unaware of the curvature even when the curve is extensive.

Scheuermann kyphosis, or *Scheuermann disease,* is an abnormal increase in the posterior convexity of the thoracic spine. It is the most common cause of structural kyphosis of the thoracic and thoracolumbar spine. The cause is unknown but involves a change in the matrix of the vertebral plate, leading to alterations in the ossification process. There is a strong hereditary tendency. In Scheuermann kyphosis the deformity persists with the child in a prone position. A child with Scheuermann kyphosis may also have tight hamstrings, poor posture, and back pain located over the apex of the kyphosis.

Atlantoaxial instability is a widening of the space between the atlas and the axis. It can be demonstrated radiographically in 15% of children with Down syndrome and can cause devastating injury if not treated properly.

Spondylolysis and spondylolisthesis. See Back Pain, earlier in this chapter.

Management

Idiopathic scoliosis

Treatments and medications. The treatment is dependent on the severity of the curve and the child's age. Exercises, electrical stimulation, bracing, or surgery may be indicated.

Counseling and prevention

- Remember that the only prevention of severe deformity is by early recognition and treatment. Close follow-up and aggressive treatment are important in remodeling of the bones. Screening before 10 years of age should include both boys and girls. (See Objective Data, earlier in this chapter.)
- Encourage compliance with bracing and exercises. Bracing slows or arrests the deformity but does not completely correct it. Once the child has reached bone maturity, further bracing is not required.
- Encourage frequent assessment of skin integrity if the child is wearing a brace.
- Recommend that activity not be limited if pain-free in the brace.

Follow-up. Follow-up per the physician's protocol.

Consultations and referrals. Refer to an orthopedist or physician any child with a lateral curvature of the spine.

Scheuermann kyphosis

Treatments and medications. Surgical intervention is rarely indicated. Electrical stimulation, bracing, and pain control are the common treatments.

Counseling and prevention

- Instruct on pain-control measures, administration of ibuprofen every 4 to 6 hours around the clock or as needed, and rest.
- Discourage activities that require standing for long periods of time because of the pain associated with standing.
- Encourage the maintenance of normal posture.

Table 38-14 Differential Diagnosis: Spine Deformity

CRITERIA	IDIOPATHIC SCOLIOSIS*	SCHEUERMANN KYPHOSIS*	ANTLANTOAXIAL INSTABILITY*
ICD-9 code	737.30	737.1	723.9
Subjective Data			
Age	Can occur at any age, most commonly seen in preadolescence and adolescence	10-12 years of age	Congenital
Onset	Gradual	Gradual	Congenital
Description of problem	Usually unnoticed by child or parent	States "hump on back"	Usually unnoticed by child or parent
Associated symptoms	May have back pain (rare)	Localized back pain, protuberant abdomen	Down syndrome
Family history	Yes, possible	None	None
Objective Data			
Musculoskeletal examination			
Inspection	See Objective Data, earlier in this chapter.	Examiner posterior with child upright with feet together and arms at sides: Thoracic kyphosis, scapular winging noted; with child prone: persistence of thoracic kyphosis	No obvious deformity
Palpation	No additional findings	No additional findings	No obvious deformity
Range of motion	May be limited dependent on severity of curve	May be limited dependent on severity of curve	Full ROM
Special tests	Measure with scoliometer	None	None
Laboratory data	AP erect radiograph of the spine from occiput to sacrum: Evaluates the degree of deformity	AP and lateral radiographs: Evaluate the degree of deformity	Radiographs of cervical spine in neutral, flexion, and extension positions: Evaluate the degree of deformity

*Refer the child to a physician.

- Encourage brace use. Bracing can correct the deformity. Continued bracing is not required after the deformity is resolved. If brace use is limited, spinal fusion may be necessary.
  Follow-up. Follow-up per the physician's protocol.
  Consultations and referrals. Refer to a physician if the diagnosis is suspected.

Atlantoaxial instability

Treatments and medications. Surgical intervention to stabilize the vertebrae may be indicated.

Counseling and prevention. All children with Down syndrome who compete in high-risk sports such as gymnastics, diving, butterfly stroke, and swimming events that have a diving start must have lateral view radiographs of the neck in flexion, extension, and neutral positions.

Follow-up. Children with radiographic evidence of atlantoaxial instability should have a yearly neurologic examination.

Consultations and referrals. Children with Down syndrome who compete in athletics should be referred for radiographic evaluation of atlantoaxial instability.

Spondylolysis and spondylolisthesis. See Back Pain, earlier in this chapter.

Resources

Websites
Family Practice Notebook (www.fpnotebook.com)
Orthoseek (www.orthoseek.com)
Wheeless's Textbook of Orthopaedics (www.medmedia.com)

Bibliography

American Academy of Family Physicians, American Academy of Pediatrics, American Medical Society for Sports Medicine, American Orthopaedic Society for Sports Medicine, American Osteopathic Academy of Sports Medicine. (1997). *Preparticipation physical evaluation* (2nd ed.). Minneapolis: McGraw-Hill Healthcare.

Arnheim, D.D. & Prentice, W. (2001). *Principles of athletic training* (10th ed.). Boston: McGraw-Hill.

Maron, B.J., Thompson, P.D., Puffer, J.C., et al. (1996). Cardiovascular preparticipation screening of competitive athletes: A statement for health professionals from the Sudden Death Committee (clinical cardiology) and Congenital Cardiac Defects Committee (cardiovascular disease in the young, American Heart Association). *Circulation, 94*(4), 850-856.

Patel, D.R., Greydanus, D.E., & Pratt, H.D. (2001). Youth sports: More than sprains and strains. *Contemporary Pediatrics, 18*(3): 45-74.

Powell, J.W. & Barber-Foss, K.D. (1999). Injury patterns in selected high school sports: A review of the the 1995-1997 seasons. *Journal of Athletic Training, 34*(3), 277-284.

Staheli, L. (1998). *Fundamentals of pediatric orthopedics* (2nd ed.). Philadelphia: Lippincott-Raven.

Verst, A.L. (2001). Get in the game: Principles of the preparticipation physical. *Advance for Nurse Practitioners, 8*(8), 66-71.

Chapter 39 *Neuropsychiatric System*

Depression, p. 584
Headaches, p. 587
Large Head and Small Head, p. 590
Seizures, Breath-Holding Spells, and Syncope, p. 595
Suicide Attempts and Suicide, p. 605
Tics, p. 607

Risk Factors*

- Maternal drug use (e.g., of illicit drugs, alcohol)
- Maternal malnutrition
- Maternal illness during pregnancy, including measles, chickenpox, human immunodeficiency virus (HIV) infection, TORCH (toxoplasmosis, other agents, rubella, cytomegalovirus, herpes simplex) infection, syphilis, toxemia, viral infection, and diabetes mellitus.
- Maternal prescription drug use during pregnancy (e.g., of anticonvulsants)
- Premature birth
- Family history of chromosomal abnormalities, mental illness, neurologic disease, neurocutaneous disease, epilepsy, migraine headaches, cancer, neuromuscular disease, mental retardation, or neural tube defects
- Birth trauma
- Accidental injury (e.g., head trauma, near-drowning)
- Ingestion of lead or other toxic substances
- History of meningitis
- Chronic illness (e.g., diabetes, HIV, asthma)
- Incomplete or lack of immunizations
- Mental retardation
- Child abuse
- Chromosomal abnormalities (e.g., Down syndrome)
- Drug abuse

Health Promotion

Prenatal

Preventive
- Early prenatal care
- Prenatal vitamins (folic acid in particular), which are crucial in the first trimester of pregnancy
- Early access to prenatal care and inclusion in school health curriculum
- Avoidance of medication unless it is prescribed and supervised by a health professional

Early diagnosis
- See Chapter 5
- Amniocentesis
- Chorionic villus sampling

Infancy, Childhood, and Adolescence

Immunizations
- Immunize per the schedule recommended by the American Academy of Pediatrics (AAP) (see Chapter 13)

- Educate families regarding potential immunization side effects and the administration of acellular pertussis

Parenting preparation
- Family planning (see Chapters 3 and 11)
- Identification of normal and abnormal behavior, including age-appropriate developmental milestones and discipline (see Discipline in Chapter 19)
- Fostering a positive self-esteem, including provision of a nurturing environment free of violence, encouragement of strengths, working with weaknesses, and development of positive coping mechanisms

Safety promotion and prevention of injury
- See Chapter 14
- Household, bicycle, car, and pool safety
- Sports safety, including proper equipment and instruction (see also Chapter 38)

Screening
- Early identification and intervention
- Lead levels (see Lead Poisoning in Chapter 47)
- Potential for child abuse (see Physical Abuse and Neglect in Chapter 47)
- Mental illness, including depression and potential suicide (see Suicide and Depression, later in this chapter)

Other areas of anticipatory guidance
- Avoidance of adolescent pregnancy and use of safe sex practices
- Encouragement of regular physical exercise
- Stress reduction
- Abstinence from tobacco, drugs, and alcohol
- Avoidance of illegal substances (e.g., illicit drugs)
- Inclusion of the preceding topics in school curriculum
- Stress management, including exercise and after-school programs
- Available family support groups dealing with specific disabilities and disorders as well as health promotion (see Resources at the end of this section)

Subjective Data

Diagnosing neuropsychiatric problems begins with a systematic, directed history. Critical to taking a detailed history is the reliability of the historian. The primary problem is usually embodied in the chief complaint. In addition to the parents, every effort should be made to interview the child (as appropriate, considering the child's age and cognitive development).

The history should include information on demographics, including age, sex, and race. It should also thoroughly describe the chief complaint, including:
- Description of problem
- Date of onset, and whether it was acute or insidious
- Characteristics, including quality, location, intensity, frequency and temporal quality (e.g., continuous, intermittent, rhythmic), duration, and relationship to other events

*Chapter overview written by Nancy E. Alfieri.

- Precipitating or alleviating factors (e.g., sleep, exercise, darkness)
- Associated symptoms, including bed-wetting (a sign of nighttime seizures); loss of consciousness; aura; anxiety or nervousness; headache; changes in sleep, appetite, or general behavior; deterioration in school performance; mood swings; speech changes; ataxia, clumsiness; tremors, weakness, or tics; hallucinations; memory changes; and depression
- Previous diagnostic procedures and results
- Previous treatments and home remedies, and their effectiveness
  The past medical history should include information on:
- Previous illnesses, including meningitis, chronic illness (diabetes mellitus, mental retardation, cerebral palsy, sickle cell anemia, cancer, epilepsy), and psychiatric disorder

- Previous injuries, including head injury (with date of injury, description of any accident including loss of consciousness, associated symptoms, treatment, and sequelae)
- Hospitalizations
- Medications
- Growth parameters, including previous measurements
- Most recent hearing and vision examination dates and results
- Risk factors (see the previous section on Risk Factors)
- Prenatal and birth history
- Neonatal history, with specific attention intraventricular hemorrhage (IVH), intracranial infection, syphilis, hydrocephalus, cyanosis, anemia, seizures, and feeding history
- Behavior, including a general disposition, personality changes and activity level, as well as a parent/caregiver questionnaire, the Child Symptom Inventory (Fig. 39-1)

CHILD SYMPTOM INVENTORY - 4: TEACHER CHECKLIST

CHILD'S NAME	AGE	GENDER
SCHOOL	GRADE	DATE

NAME OF PERSON COMPLETING THIS FORM:_____ POSITION:_____

LENGTH OF TIME YOU HAVE KNOWN STUDENT:_____ LENGTH OF TIME EACH DAY WITH STUDENT:_____

TYPE OF CLASS (E.G., REGULAR 2ND GRADE, RESOURCE ROOM, 6TH GRADE ENGLISH):_____

CURRENT SPECIAL EDUCATION SERVICES (E.G., RESOURCE ROOM, SPEECH THERAPY):_____

CURRENT SPECIAL EDUCATION LABEL (E.G., LEARNING DISABILITY):_____

CURRENT ACADEMIC PERFORMANCE: CHECK APPROPRIATE GRADE LEVEL (G.L.)

SUBJECT	2 OR MORE YRS. BELOW G.L.	1 TO 2 YEARS BELOW G.L.	AT OR ABOUT G.L.	1 TO 2 YEARS ABOVE G.L.	2 OR MORE YEARS ABOVE G.L.
READING					
WRITING					
SPELLING					
ARITHMETIC					

DIRECTIONS: CHECK WHICH RATING BEST DESCRIBES THIS CHILD'S OVERALL BEHAVIOR IN OR AROUND SCHOOL. ANSWER EACH QUESTION TO THE BEST OF YOUR ABILITY.

CATEGORY A		NEVER	SOME-TIMES	OFTEN	VERY OFTEN
1.	FAILS TO GIVE CLOSE ATTENTION TO DETAILS OR MAKES CARELESS MISTAKES				
2.	HAS DIFFICULTY PAYING ATTENTION TO TASKS OR PLAY ACTIVITIES				
3.	DOES NOT SEEM TO LISTEN WHEN SPOKEN TO DIRECTLY				
4.	HAS DIFFICULTY FOLLOWING THROUGH ON INSTRUCTIONS AND FAILS TO FINISH THINGS				
5.	HAS DIFFICULTY ORGANIZING TASKS AND ACTIVITIES				
6.	AVOIDS DOING TASKS THAT REQUIRE A LOT OF MENTAL EFFORT (SCHOOLWORK, HOMEWORK, ETC.)				
7.	LOSES THINGS NECESSARY FOR ACTIVITIES				
8.	IS EASILY DISTRACTED BY OTHER THINGS GOING ON				
9.	IS FORGETFUL IN DAILY ACTIVITIES				

Fig. 39-1 Child Symptom Inventory. (From Gadow, K.D. & Sprafkin, J. [1994]. Stony Brook, N. Y.: Checkmate Plus; www.checkmateplus.com.)

Continued

CATEGORY A		NEVER	SOME-TIMES	OFTEN	VERY OFTEN
10.	FIDGETS WITH HANDS OR FEET OR SQUIRMS IN SEAT				
11.	HAS DIFFICULTY REMAINING SEATED WHEN ASKED TO DO SO				
12.	RUNS ABOUT OR CLIMBS ON THINGS WHEN ASKED NOT TO DO SO				
13.	HAS DIFFICULTY PLAYING QUIETLY				
14.	IS "ON THE GO" OR ACTS AS IF "DRIVEN BY A MOTOR"				
15.	TALKS EXCESSIVELY				
16.	BLURTS OUT ANSWERS TO QUESTIONS BEFORE THEY HAVE BEEN COMPLETED				
17.	HAS DIFFICULTY AWAITING TURN IN GROUP ACTIVITIES				
18.	INTERRUPTS PEOPLE OR BUTTS INTO OTHER CHILDREN'S ACTIVITIES				
CATEGORY B					
19.	LOSES TEMPER				
20.	ARGUES WITH ADULTS				
21.	DEFIES OR REFUSES WHAT YOU TELL HIM/HER TO DO				
22.	DOES THINGS TO DELIBERATELY ANNOY OTHERS				
23.	BLAMES OTHERS FOR OWN MISBEHAVIOR OR MISTAKES				
24.	IS TOUCHY OR EASILY ANNOYED BY OTHERS				
25.	IS ANGRY AND RESENTFUL				
26.	TAKES ANGER OUT ON OTHERS OR TRIES TO GET EVEN				
CATEGORY C					
27.	PLAYS HOOKEY FROM SCHOOL				
29.	LIES TO GET THINGS OR TO AVOID RESPONSIBILITY ("CONS" OTHERS)				
30.	BULLIES, THREATENS, OR INTIMIDATES OTHERS				
31.	STARTS PHYSICAL FIGHTS				
33.	HAS STOLEN THINGS WHEN OTHERS WERE NOT LOOKING				
34.	HAS DELIBERATELY DESTROYED OTHERS' PROPERTY				
36.	HAS STOLEN THINGS FROM OTHERS USING PHYSICAL FORCE				
38.	HAS USED A WEAPON WHEN FIGHTING (BAT, BRICK, BOTTLE, ETC.)				
40.	HAS BEEN PHYSICALLY CRUEL TO PEOPLE				
CATEGORY D					
42.	IS OVERCONCERNED ABOUT ABILITIES IN ACADEMIC, ATHLETIC, OR SOCIAL ACTIVITIES				
43.	HAS DIFFICULTY CONTROLLING WORRIES				
44.	ACTS RESTLESS OR EDGY				
45.	IS IRRITABLE FOR MOST OF THE DAY				
46.	IS EXTREMELY TENSE OR UNABLE TO RELAX				

Fig. 39-1, cont'd For legend, see p. 577.

- Developmental milestones, including age and order of achievement
- Speech
- School performance, including attendance, grade level, academic grades, behavior, and a teacher questionnaire, the Child Symptom Inventory (see Fig. 39-1)
- Immunization history
- Diet history, including intake (for 24 hours and 1 week), appetite, variety, coordination, and drooling
- Social history, including living conditions, economic status, hobbies, habits (e.g., tobacco, alcohol, drugs), major changes in primary caregiver, major losses, and employment (e.g., of parents, adolescent)
- Family history of medical and psychiatric illnesses

Finally, the review of systems should include careful attention to the following areas:
- *Cerebral function*—Memory changes, behavioral changes, speech changes
- *Cranial nerves*—Loss of smell, abnormal eye movements, visual changes, headache, facial drooping, facial weakness, absence of blinking, drooling, hearing loss, vertigo, tinnitus, hoarseness, difficulty swallowing, frequent choking, abnormal tongue movements
- *Motor*—Abnormal movements, muscle weakness, change in gait (e.g., clumsiness, dragging of a leg or foot), coordination and balance difficulties, decrease in range of motion (ROM)
- *Sensory*—Numbness, tingling, pins and needles, loss of position sense
- *Reflexes*—Deep tendon, foot drop, upturning great toe

CATEGORY E		NEVER	SOME-TIMES	OFTEN	VERY OFTEN
49.	SHOWS EXCESSIVE FEAR TO SPECIFIC OBJECTS OR SITUATIONS (ANIMALS, HEIGHTS, STORMS, INSECTS, ETC.)				
50.	CANNOT GET DISTRESSING THOUGHTS OUT OF HIS/HER MIND (WORRIES ABOUT GERMS OR DOING THINGS PERFECTLY, ETC.)				
51.	FEELS COMPELLED TO PERFORM UNUSUAL HABITS (HAND WASHING, CHECKING LOCKS, REPEATING THINGS A SET NUMBER OF TIMES)				
52.	HAS EXPERIENCED AN EXTREMELY UPSETTING EVENT AND CONTINUES TO BE BOTHERED BY IT				
53.	DOES UNUSUAL MOVEMENTS FOR NO APPARENT REASON (EYE BLINKING, TWITCHING, LIP LICKING, HEAD JERKING, ETC.)				
54.	MAKES VOCAL SOUNDS FOR NO APPARENT REASON (COUGHING, THROAT CLEARING, SNIFFLING, GRUNTING, ETC.)				

CATEGORY F					
55.	HAS STRANGE IDEAS OR BELIEFS THAT ARE NOT REAL (CHILD'S FOOD IS POISONED, PEOPLE ARE TRYING TO GET HIM/HER, ETC.)				
56.	HAS AUDITORY HALLUCINATIONS--HEARS VOICES TALKING TO OR TELLING HIM/HER TO DO THINGS				
57.	HAS EXTREMELY STRANGE AND ILLOGICAL THOUGHTS OR IDEAS				
58.	LAUGHS OR CRIES AT INAPPROPRIATE TIMES OR SHOWS NO EMOTION IN SITUATIONS WHERE MOST OTHERS OF SAME AGE WOULD REACT				
59.	DOES EXTREMELY ODD THINGS (EXCESSIVE PREOCCUPATION WITH FANTASY FRIENDS, TALKS TO SELF IN A STRANGE WAY, ETC.)				

CATEGORY G					
60.	IS DEPRESSED FOR MOST OF THE DAY				
61.	SHOWS LITTLE INTEREST IN (OR ENJOYMENT OF) PLEASURABLE ACTIVITIES				
62.	HAS RECURRENT THOUGHTS OF DEATH OR SUICIDE				
63.	FEELS WORTHLESS OR GUILTY				
64.	HAS LOW ENERGY LEVEL OR IS TIRED FOR NO APPARENT REASON				
65.	HAS LITTLE CONFIDENCE OR IS VERY SELF CONSCIOUS				
66.	FEELS THAT THINGS NEVER WORK OUT RIGHT				

69.	HAS EXPERIENCED A BIG CHANGE IN HIS/HER NORMAL ACTIVITY LEVEL (CIRCLE YES OR NO)	NO		YES	
70.	HAS EXPERIENCED A BIG CHANGE IN HIS/HER ABILITY TO CONCENTRATE (CIRCLE YES OR NO)	NO		YES	
71.	HAS EXPERIENCED A BIG DROP IN SCHOOL GRADES OR SCHOOLWORK (CIRCLE YES OR NO)	NO		YES	

3

Fig. 39-1, cont'd For legend, see p. 577.   *Continued*

Objective Data

The majority of objective data is collected by close observation, whereas the subjective data are simultaneously collected. The practitioner should create a natural environment for the child to behave in and perform the least upsetting tasks first. The practitioner should also be sensitive to the child's personality and mood. The neurologic examination described in this chapter is presented in a systemic manner; however, it is not performed in this manner until the child is at least of school age. By initially practicing the examination in the order presented, the practitioner can later adapt the examination to the child's age and behavior without omitting parts.

Physical Examination

• *General appearance and behavior*

• *Height, weight, and head circumference*—These should be plotted on an appropriate graph (see Appendix A). For head circumference, measure head circumference every month for the first year of life, every 3 months during the second year, twice a year from 3 to 5 years of age, and then annually. The average head circumference at birth is 35 cm. At 1 month of age, head circumference should increase by 2 cm; by 4 months, 6 cm; by 6 months, 7 cm; and by 12 months, 12 cm. Also note the shape of the head.

• *Fontanels*—Anterior fontanel average diameter is 2.5 cm but can be up to 4.5 cm. About 90% of them are closed by 19 months of age. The posterior fontanel average diameter is 0.5 cm but can be up to 1 cm. It is not palpable after 4 to 8 weeks of age.

CATEGORY H		NEVER	SOME-TIMES	OFTEN	VERY OFTEN
72.	HAS A PECULIAR WAY OF RELATING TO OTHERS (AVOIDS EYE CONTACT, ODD FACIAL EXPRESSIONS OR GESTURES, ETC.)				
73.	DOES NOT PLAY OR RELATE WELL WITH OTHER CHILDREN				
74.	NOT INTERESTED IN MAKING FRIENDS				
75.	IS UNAWARE OR TAKES NO INTEREST IN OTHER PEOPLE'S FEELINGS				
76.	HAS A SIGNIFICANT PROBLEM WITH LANGUAGE DEVELOPMENT				
77.	HAS DIFFICULTY MAKING SOCIALLY APPROPRIATE CONVERSATION				
78.	TALKS IN A STRANGE WAY (REPEATS WHAT OTHERS SAY; CONFUSES WORDS LIKE "YOU" AND "I"; USES ODD WORDS OR PHRASES, ETC.)				
79.	IS UNABLE TO "PRETEND" OR "MAKE BELIEVE" WHEN PLAYING				
80.	SHOWS EXCESSIVE PREOCCUPATION WITH ONE TOPIC				
81.	GETS VERY UPSET OVER SMALL CHANGES IN ROUTINE OR SURROUNDINGS (CLASS SCHEDULE, ETC.)				
82.	MAKES STRANGE REPETITIVE MOVEMENTS (FLAPPING ARMS, ETC.)				
83.	HAS STRANGE FASCINATION FOR PARTS OF OBJECTS				

CATEGORY I					
84.	TRIES TO AVOID CONTACT WITH STRANGERS; ABNORMALLY SHY				
85.	IS EXCESSIVELY SHY WITH PEERS				
86.	IS GENERALLY WARM AND OUTGOING WITH FAMILIAR ADULTS				
87.	WHEN PUT IN AN UNCOMFORTABLE SOCIAL SITUATION, CHILD CRIES, FREEZES, OR WITHDRAWS FROM INTERACTING				

OTHER PROBLEMS OR COMMENTS (ATTACH ADDITIONAL PAGE IF NEEDED):_____

_____

_____

_____

_____

_____

_____

_____

_____

_____

_____

_____

_____

THANK YOU!

☑ **CHECKMATE PLUS, LTD.**
P.O. BOX 696, STONY BROOK, NY 11790-0696

Fig. 39-1, cont'd For legend, see p. 577.

- *Cranial sutures*
- *Eyes*—Shape, position, PERRLA (pupils equal, round, reactive to light and accommodation), extraocular movement (EOM), red reflex, and visual acuity should be noted.
- *Ears*—Shape, position, tympanic membranes, mobility, and hearing acuity should be noted.
- *Skin*—Hypopigmented or hyperpigmented spots, nevus, hemangioma, and signs of physical abuse should be noted.
- *Heart*—Heart sounds should be auscultated.
- *Lungs*—Breath sounds should be auscultated.
- *Abdomen*—Liver and spleen should be palpated (for organ enlargement, seen in storage diseases of the brain).
- *Spine*—Curvature, bend test, dimples, hair tufts, tenderness, and ROM should be noted.

Neurologic examination
- *Cerebral function*—The Denver II should be administered to all children 6 years of age and younger. Assess the child's general behavior, level of consciousness, orientation, and intellectual performance, including knowledge, judgment, calculation, memory (immediate, recent, and remote), thought content, mood, and behavior.
- *Cranial nerves*—The cranial nerves (CNs) are examined primarily by observation. Use bright objects to capture the interest of the child. Always evaluate red retinal reflex in infants. Observe facial movements during the examination and make faces and laugh to evaluate symmetry. Observe the infant sucking and the child drinking from a cup. Evaluate the olfactory, optic, oculomotor, trochlear, abducens, trigeminal, facial, auditory, glos-

sopharyngeal, vagus, spinal accessory, and hypoglossal nerves.

- *Motor function*—Muscle tone and bulk (active and passive, ROM, and muscle size and shape), muscle strength (symmetry), and abnormal muscle movements should be assessed. A general screen of the motor system may be performed by having the child do age-appropriate tasks (Boxes 39-1 and 39-2). If abnormalities are not identified, the motor system can be considered intact. However, if abnormalities are detected, assess the following areas:

  Sit, stand, hop, and arise from a chair or the floor

  Romberg sign (ask child to stand with feet close together, arms and hands outstretched, and eyes closed. Observe for swaying, drifting of the arms, and adventitious movements, particularly of face, arms, and hands)

  Finger to finger to nose

  Heel-knee test

  Gait, including forward, backward, up and down stairs, toe walk, heel walk, and tandem walk (for children 5 years of age or older)

  Run (which exaggerates neurologic impairments)

  Rise from the floor from supine position (look for muscle use of neck, trunk, arms, and legs, and Gower's sign; if Gower's sign is present, the child will arise by climbing up legs or pushing off to stand)

  For motor evaluation in infants:

    Traction maneuver—Infant is lying supine. Practitioner grasps each hand and gently pulls the infant slowly to a sitting position. Observe for head and trunk tone.

    Vertical suspension—A hypotonic infant slips through the practitioner's hands, while a hypertonic infant clenches fists, extends legs, crosses legs, or scissors legs.

    Horizontal suspension—A hypotonic infant droops over the practitioner's hand, while a hypertonic infant extends the head, neck, and back.

- *Cerebellar function*—Balance and coordination are tested during the motor function examination. Additional methods of testing cerebellar function include the following:

  Hand-patting (alternating pronation and supination of one hand while the other remains stationary)

  Repetitive finger-tapping (thumb to forefinger)

  Foot-tapping

- *Sensory function*—Sensory examination is of little value in a child younger than 5 years of age. However, a basic screening test can be performed on all children. The examination is divided into two parts: assessments concerned with primary sensation and those concerned with cortical and discriminatory forms of sensation. Lesions in the sensory pathway produce various sensory loss. Knowledge of the dermatomes aids in identifying the location of neurologic lesions (Fig. 39-2).

- *Reflexes*—Reflex examination should be performed systematically, assessing for symmetry and strength (Box 39-3). Also include the mass and cross-adductor reflexes in infants.

- *Neurologic soft signs*—The significance of variations from the norm has yet to be proved. Examples include, but are not limited to, clumsiness, language disturbances, mirroring movements (also known as "motor overflow"), and short attention span. These signs usually appear in preschool children of varying cognitive levels. Neurologists

disagree on their significance. Some believe that they are predictors of future school problems.

A screening neurologic examination is outlined in Box 39-4.

Diagnostic Procedures and Laboratory Tests

Many diagnostic procedures and laboratory tests are performed when one is diagnosing neuropsychiatric problems (Table 39-1). The results of these examinations are supplemental. They must be put into context with the individual's clinical presentation.

- *Anticonvulsant serum levels*—Use of a serum levels can measure the amount of anticonvulsant medication in the blood. It is important to document the time of blood drawing and the time medication was last taken. This level is routinely measured every 4 to 6 months.

- *Imaging*—Different types of imaging include magnetic resonance imaging (MRI), magnetic resonance spectroscopy (MRS). and magnetic resonance angiography (MRA). MRS and MRA yield very specific, detailed information, but are almost exclusively available only in tertiary care centers.

Box 39-1 Age-Appropriate Gross Motor Development

AGE	SKILL
3 months	Holds head and chest up when prone
	Has little or no head lag when pulled to sit
4 months	Sits with support
	Good head control
8 months	Sits without support and maintains balance
10 months	Pulls to stand
12 months	Walks with support
15 months	Walks without support
30 months	Jumps
36 months	Stands on one foot momentarily
48 months	Hops on one foot
	Throws ball overhead
60 months	Skips

Box 39-2 Age-Appropriate Fine Motor Development

AGE	SKILL
4 months	Reaches for objects with whole hand
6 months	Transfers object from hand to hand
10 months	Drinks from a cup with assistance
11 months	Has a pincer grasp
14 months	Scribbles with a crayon
18 months	Feeds self
	Takes off clothes
24 months	Turns single pages of a book
30 months	Imitates circular strokes
48 months	Uses scissors to cut out paper
60 months	Dresses and undresses

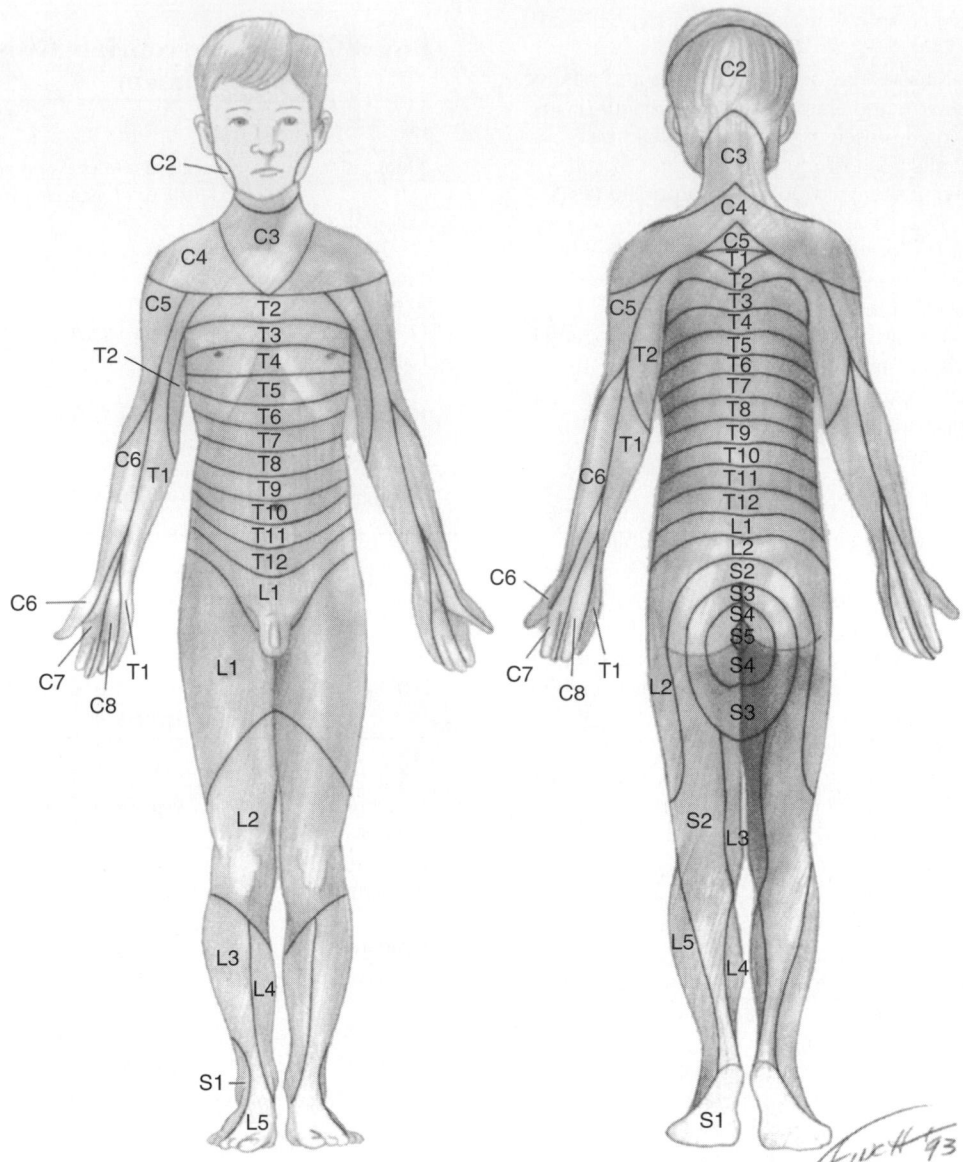

Fig. 39-2 Radicular cutaneous fields. (From Swaiman, K. [1999]. *Pediatric neurology: Principles and practice* [3rd ed.]. St. Louis: Mosby.)

Box 39-3 Reflexes

DEEP TENDON REFLEXES	SPINE LOCATION
Biceps	C5, C6
Brachioradialis	C5, C6
Triceps	C6-C8
Patellar	L2-L4
Achilles tendon	L5-S2

SUPERFICIAL REFLEXES	SPINE LOCATION
Abdominal upper	T8-T10
Abdominal lower	T10-T12
Plantar	L4-S2
Cremasteric	L1, L2

- *Electroencephalogram*—Electroencephalography (EEG) measures electrical activity in the brain and is ordered when seizures are suspected. It is noninvasive, requires 1 to 1.5 hours, and necessitates sedation (drug of choice: chloral hydrate, 50 to 75 mg/kg; pharmacologic sedation is not recommended for infants less than 3 months of age; procedure should be scheduled around child's sleep times). A seizure may not be seen on EEG.
- *Electromyography*—Electromyography (EMG) is used in diagnosing neuromuscular disease. One performs it by inserting needle electrodes into the muscle and recording the potentials on a cathode-ray oscillograph during relaxation, slight contraction, and intense contraction. The procedure is painful and rarely performed successfully in children less than 7 years of age.

Box 39-4 Screening Neurologic Examination

Requirements—General examination provides no specific evidence of a disorder that may involve the brain, and there are no neurologic symptoms.

Mental status—This includes state of consciousness (e.g., alert, lethargic), affect (e.g., cheerful, shy, angry), speech, and intelligence (as assessed by the content of a social conversation)

Cranial nerves
- II: Visual acuity is noted (Snellen Chart).
- VII: Symmetry of the face during speaking and while smiling or laughing is observed.
- VIII: Child should respond promptly to conversational cues and should hear fingers rubbed beside one and then both ears.
- IX, X: Palatal elevation should be symmetric.
- XII: Unilateral tongue atrophy or fasciculations should not be present.

Motor
- Gross motor skills and balance are observed as the child walks into and around the examining room and gets onto and off the examining table.
- Fine motor coordination is required for facile buttoning, pulling up socks, and tying shoes.
- Asymmetries of outstretched arms are observed.
- Finger-nose-finger test is performed.
- Limping, asymmetric gait, asymmetries of arm swing when walking, and asymmetric hand usage are noted.
- Tremors, tics, myoclonic jerks, excessively slow movements (bradykinesia), apparently stiff movements, and fixed postures are all abnormal.

Tendon reflexes and plantar responses—Symmetry should be noted.

Sensation—In the absence of symptoms, sensory testing is not helpful for the child with a learning disorder.

From Kandt, R. (1984). Neurological examination of children with learning disorders. Pediatric Clinics of North America, 31(2), 297-314.

- *Lumbar puncture*—Perform a lumbar puncture if any suspicion of meningitis exists. The results are indicated in Appendix D.

Resources

Organizations
The Family Village, Waisman Center, University of Wisconsin-Madison, 1500 Highland Avenue, Madison, WI 53705-2280; e-mail at familyvillage@waisman.wisc.edu; www.familyvillage.wisc.edu

National Information Center for Children and Youth with Disabilities (NICHCY), PO Box 1492, Washington, DC 20013-1492; (800) 695-0285 or (202) 884-8200; e-mail at nichey@aed.org; www.nichcy.org

Websites
Bright Futures (www.brightfutures.org)

Table 39-1 Ordering Diagnostic Procedures and Laboratory Tests

DEVELOPMENTAL ASSESSMENT TOOLS AND LABORATORY TESTS	DISORDER SUSPECTED
Developmental Assessment Tools	
Denver II	Developmental age and chronologic age incongruency
Bayley Scale of Infant Development	
Stanford-Binet test	
Weschler Intelligence Scale for Children (WISC-R)	
Early Language Milestone Scale	Language disturbances
Vineland Early Childhood Inventory	Parental rating scales identifying behavioral concerns
Laboratory Tests	
CBC count, differential, and platelets	Infection, anemia, thrombocytopenia
Serum chemistry	Electrolyte imbalance and liver function
Urinalysis	Infection
Urine amino acids	Metabolic disease
Urine organic acids	
TORCH titers	Infection
Blood cultures	
Toxicology screen	Illicit drug use
Anticonvulsant serum levels	Medication metabolism, compliance
Lead level	Lead intoxication
Chromosomes	Genetic Abnormalities— Fragile X syndrome, mental retardation, Lyme disease
DNA for fragile X	
Lyme titers	
Thyroid screen	Hypothyroidism, hyperthyroidism
Any other test indicated by history and physical examination	
Radiologic Tests	
Skull radiography	Skull fracture, craniosynostosis, craniopharyngioma
Ultrasonography (e.g., of infants, head)	Hydrocephalus, intraventricular hemorrhage, fetal abnormalities
CT scan	Brain tumors, brain atrophy, subdural hematoma, hydrocephalus, subependymal bleed, intracranial calcification
MRI	
MRS	Metabolic disorders
MRA	AV aneurysm, malformation
Amniocentesis	Genetic abnormalities
Chorionic villus sampling	
EEG	Seizures
EMG	Neuromuscular diesase
Lumbar puncture	Meningitis
Vision testing	Visual disturbances
Audiometric studies	Hearing loss
Psychologic testing	Mental illness

Depression

SUSAN M. WATSON

Alert

Consult with or refer to a physician or mental health professional for the following:

- Depressed mood, including feeling sad, bored, angry, irritable, worthless, or inappropriately guilty each day for a period of at least 2 weeks
- Loss of interest or pleasure in previously enjoyed activities, apathy, or inability to concentrate
- Social withdrawal, isolation, and loss of friends
- Decline in academic performance or truancy
- Unexplained, frequent somatic complaints (e.g., abdominal pain, headaches)
- Psychomotor agitation or retardation
- Suicide thoughts or attempts, or recurrent thoughts about death
- Sudden interest in weapons and firearms
- Weight change without intent (gain or loss)
- Changes in sleep patterns (insomnia or excess sleep)
- Fatigue and loss of energy
- Alcohol or substance abuse
- Evidence of self-mutilation or injury

Etiology

The exact cause of depression in childhood and adolescence is unknown. It is probable that several interrelated factors are responsible. Depressed children and adolescents are more likely to have one or more parents who are depressed, and they are more likely to be exposed to family discord. Depressed children and adolescents often have experienced stressors such as significant loss, abuse, or trauma. Examples of loss include death, separation, rejection, or disappointment in not succeeding in a social or academic task.

A positive self-esteem is correlated to being able to cope with the normal losses and disappointments that occur. With a low self-esteem there is greater potential for depression. The adolescent's self-esteem is generated from a sense of achievement in relation to aspirations and the effect of responses from the significant people in their lives. The normal developmental tasks of adolescence are difficult. It is when the adolescent feels overwhelmed and is unable to cope with these demands that depression may occur.

Depression in children may also occur as a result of chronic illness or disability, as a side effect of medications or recreational drugs, and from accidental ingestion of toxic substances (e.g., lead).

In some cases a biochemical imbalance also has been demonstrated. Researchers have identified low functional levels of norepinephrine and serotonin in depressed individuals and believe that they are important genetic markers.

Incidence

- The prevalence of major depression in childhood ranges from 1.8% to 2.5%. The prevalence of major depression in adolescence ranges from 4.7% to 8.3%.
- The prevalence of dysthymia in adolescence is 3.3%.

- The prevalence of any depression is greater than 6% in children 9 to 17 years of age.
- Children are three times more likely to develop depression with a parental history of depression.
- The mean age for the first onset of major depression is 14 years.
- Before puberty, depression occurs equally in boys and girls.
- Adolescent females are two to four times more likely to be diagnosed with depression than males.
- Adolescent depression tends to recur and persist into adulthood in 60% to 70% of cases.
- About 40% to 70% of adolescents with major depression have one or more comorbid disorders.
- Approximately 20% to 40% of depressed adolescents exhibiting psychotic features are at an increased risk of developing a bipolar disorder within 5 years.
- Bipolar disorders are equally common in boys and girls regardless of age.

Risk Factors

- History of a parent or parents with depressive illness
- History of physical or sexual abuse
- History of significant loss or change of lifestyle, including the death of parent, sibling, friend, or close relative; divorce; abandonment; and rejection (e.g., romantic breakups)
- Presence of a chronic illness (such as sickle cell anemia, diabetes mellitus, cystic fibrosis)
- Presence of chronic condition or disability (such as attention deficit–hyperactivity disorder [ADHD] or learning disability)
- Significant family dysfunction, including domestic violence, economic stressors, substance abuse (e.g., drugs, alcohol, smoking), physical or sexual abuse or neglect, and trauma related to natural disasters or school violence

Differential Diagnosis

Clinical symptoms of major depression may be insidious in onset. Depressed children and adolescents feel sad. This sadness can be obvious, such as a general unhappiness or tearfulness, or it can be masked by anger. Depressed children frequently have somatic complaints. Comorbid anxiety is common among prepubertal children.

Adolescents feel things intensively, and their feelings are often felt by those around them. It is sometimes difficult to distinguish depression from adolescent mood swings and symptoms caused by an illness. Depressed adolescents feel they have nothing to look forward to or that they will never reach their goals. They consider themselves unsuccessful and unattractive and therefore not worthy of acceptance. They, like their younger counterparts, withdraw from social and academic activities.

Their loss of energy can be profound. Just getting out of bed may be too much. The fatigue may interfere with schoolwork, sports, or afterschool activities. There is a tendency to seek sleep as an escape, but often the sleep is interrupted, and the fatigue is made worse. However, the depressed child may also prove to be more restless and even disruptive. For some adolescents there is a surge of energy. To avoid dealing with their depression, these adolescents occupy every hour of the day with activity. Some depressed adolescents turn to risk-taking behaviors to cope with the discomforts of depression. Reckless driving, stealing, truancy, and promiscuity are just a few examples of ways such adolescents attempt to deal with their pain. Others self-medicate with abusive substances such as cigarettes, recreational drugs, and alcohol. Self-injurious behavior such as cutting or burning of the skin is also observed but is less common.

Depression is classified by the American Psychiatric Association (1994) as major depressive episode, dysthymic disorder, or adjustment with depressed mood.

A *major depressive episode* is defined as a depressed or irritable mood (e.g., sad, blue, bored, angry) with greatly decreased interest or pleasure in almost all the usual activities, most of the day, nearly every day, lasting for 2 weeks (by self-report or observation) and representing a change from previous functioning. At least four of the following seven symptoms (three for children under 6 years of age) must also be present:

1. Significant weight loss or gain (more than 5% of body weight in a month) or failure to make expected weight gain
2. Insomnia or hypersomnia
3. Psychomotor agitation or retardation, observable nearly every day
4. Fatigue or loss of energy nearly every day
5. Feelings of worthlessness or excessive guilt nearly every day
6. Diminished capacity to think or concentrate or indecisiveness nearly every day
7. Recurrent thoughts of death, recurrent suicidal ideation or behavior

In *dysthymic disorder,* the symptoms are less severe but more persistent than those of major depression. It involves a depressed or irritable mood for most the day, on most days, for at least a year. It also includes the presence of two or more of the following: poor appetite or overeating, insomnia or hypersomnia, low energy or fatigue, poor concentration, and hopelessness.

An *adjustment disorder* is characterized by less severe mood disturbances than a dysthymic disorder. It is generally a mild, self-limiting disturbance that occurs within 3 months of the onset of a life stressor (e.g., death, divorce). The distress significantly impairs social or academic functioning. Once the stressor (or its consequences) has terminated, the symptoms do not persist for more than 6 months.

Mania and depression are demonstrated in a mixed state with *bipolar disorder.* At times the child or adolescent displays mania, including euphoria and grandiosity, and at other times depression or hypomania. Mania may also be expressed by anger and irritability. There may be a decreased need for sleep, pressured speech, and poor judgment.

The symptoms of depression are often difficult to distinguish from and may be related to various medical conditions. The symptoms of depression and certain medical conditions often overlap. Thus a medical cause for the depression needs to be ruled out. For example, the adolescent who is hypothyroid complains of appetite changes, fatigue, and weight gain. Severely anemic patients often lack energy and have poor concentration abilities. Patients with chronic fatigue syndrome are usually tired and may withdraw from activities and seek sleep frequently.

Box 39-5 Evaluation of Adolescent Depression: Comprehensive History

Description of Present Complaint

What is the reason for the visit? (Interview patient and parents separately)

What is the concern?

When was the onset?

How frequently does it occur?

Are there any disruptions in normal functioning?

Has this ever happened before?

Is there a past history of feeling depressed? Has there been previous contact with a mental health professional? What was the treatment?

Are there any other symptoms associated with depression?

Are you (the child or teenager) anxious, preoccupied, worried, sad, irritable?

Family History

Is there any history of mental illness, depression, or anxiety?

Is there any history of substance abuse?

Is there a history of violence in the home?

Have you (the child or teenager) been exposed to violence in your environment?

School History and Social History

Is there any change in school performance or attendance?

Are there any complaints from teachers?

Is there less interest in or less contact with friends, sports, or activities?

Is there any refusal to see friends or participate in their activities?

Has there been any contact with law-enforcement agencies?

Is there any use of alcohol, drugs, or cigarettes?

Are you (the teenager) sexually active? Any recent romantic breakups?

Review of Symptoms

Has there been any suicide ideation or attempt?

What is the past medical history?

Is there any history of physical or sexual abuse?

Some children develop depression secondary to the effects of chronic medical conditions such as neoplasms, infection, or metabolic, nutritional, endocrine, immunologic, or CNS disorders. Certain substances can also produce secondary depression; these include medications such as oral contraceptives, methylphenidate, clonidine, phenobarbital, and steroids; environmental toxins including lead; and alcohol and recreational drugs.

A complete history (Box 39-5) and physical examination, including laboratory tests (complete blood cell [CBC] count, urinalysis, blood chemistry determination, thyroid profile, any other tests pertinent to the history and physical examination) should be performed on any child or adolescent with symptoms of depression.

A variety of depression scales and questionnaire tools are available for use with children suspected of having depression, among them the Child Behavior Checklist (CBCL, recommended for those 4 to 18 years of age) and the Children's Depression Inventory (CDI, for those 7 to 17 years of age).

Management

Once a medical cause is excluded and a depressive disorder is the primary diagnosis, a mental health professional should evaluate the patient.

Treatments and medications. Examples of mental health interventions may include psychoeducation, psychotherapy, or pharmacotherapy.

- Individual psychotherapy should be considered for all patients with moderate to severe depression. Therapists who work with young children or those unable to verbalize their feelings use play-therapy techniques. Cognitive-behavioral therapy has been shown to relieve depression in children and adolescents. In cognitive therapy, the goals are to improve the adolescent's interpersonal skills and alter negative self-perceptions. Group therapy and family therapy can also be helpful. Parents should be assisted in identifying how they can help their child overcome feelings of low self-esteem and helplessness.
- Selective serotonin reuptake inhibitors (SSRIs) are considered first-line drug treatment for child and adolescent depression because of their efficacy and safety. Commonly used SSRIs include fluoxetine (Prozac), sertraline (Zoloft), and paroxetine Hcl (Paxil). Serotonin norepinephrine reuptake inhibitors (SNRIs) such as venlafaxine (Effexor) are also used. Second-line medications include bupropion (Wellbutrin) (a dopamine and norepinephrine inhibitor) and mirtazapine (Remeron) (a tetracyclic).
- Tricyclic antidepressants (TCAs) such as imipramine (Tofranil), desipramine (Norpramin), and nortriptyline (Pamelor) are used infrequently because of significant side effects and the need for frequent blood level monitoring.
- Even less commonly used are monoamine oxidase inhibitors (MAOs), which generally have a serious side-effect profile and interact with many other medications and foods.
- Mood stabilizers (e.g., lithium compounds) are frequently used to treat mania in bipolar children and adolescents. Lithium can also be used in combination with antidepressants. Most of these medications are not approved for use in children and are most often prescribed and monitored by a skilled child psychiatrist. Psychiatric medications in general should always be slowly tapered off before discontinuance.
- Psychotherapy is usually started after the child or adolescent begins to respond to drug therapy. After remission of symptoms, continuation of treatment with medication and psychotherapy for at least several months is usually recommended, given the high risk of relapse and recurrence of depression.
- In general, most depressed children or adolescents can be managed as outpatients by the mental health professional in collaboration with the primary care practitioner (PCP).
- Inpatient management may be indicated for those displaying any signs of psychotic or manic behaviors. Hospitalization may be necessary with suicidal patients or those involved with alcohol and drugs, which may interfere with outpatient care.

Counseling and prevention

- Stress the importance of therapy for the patient and family.
- Educate the patient and family about the purpose of any medications prescribed by the mental health professional. The patient needs to be comfortable with the dosage and administration and be aware of any potential side effects.
- Educate the family about the symptoms of depression and the importance of adherence to and involvement in therapy. The family needs to contact the PCP or therapist with any new symptoms or recurrence of any previous symptoms.
- Discuss the warning signs of suicide and the association of suicide and depression with the family. The family should be alert to any persistent talk of death, hopelessness, persistent sadness, poor self-esteem, or lack of interest in friends or previously enjoyed activities. Advise the parents to call with any concerns.
- Suggest that the family notify the school nurse.
- Educate school personnel regarding warning signs of depression (e.g., change in school performance, isolation from activities and friends, sadness, boredom, anger). The practitioner needs to be available to the school staff to answer any of their concerns or questions.
- Advise school officials to notify the parents of any signs of new problems (e.g., missed classes).
- Instruct the parents that all use and availability of drugs and alcohol in the family needs to be discontinued. All weapons must be removed from the home.

Follow-up

- Maintain close contact with the child or adolescent, the family, and the mental health professional. Call the patient and the mental health professional and check on the status of the treatment and symptoms weekly.
- Have the parents or patient call immediately if the patient is experiencing any side effects from treatment.
- Monitor the child or adolescent for any warning signs of relapse (see the Alert box).

Consultations and referrals

- Remember that the provision of care for a diagnosis of major depression is beyond the scope of practice for most PCPs.
- Refer the child or adolescent and the family to a mental health professional for a more detailed and expert evaluation and treatment plan, with immediate referral to a hospital if the child is deemed at risk for suicide.
- Refer the child and family to available support groups in local hospitals or community centers.
- Make local hotline numbers and Internet resources available to the patient and family.
- Notify the school nurse, if appropriate.

Resources

Websites

American Academy of Child and Adolescent Psychiatry (www.aacap.org)
American Psychiatric Association (www.psych.org)
American Psychological Association (www.apa.org)
Child and Adolescent Bipolar Foundation (www.bpkids.org)
National Depressive and Manic-Depressive Association (www.ndmda.org)
National Institute of Mental Health (www.nimh.nih.gov)
National Mental Health Association (www.nmha.org)

Headaches

BARBARA GOLDEN

Alert

Consult with or refer to a physician for the following:
- Signs or symptoms of increased intracranial pressure (ICP)
- History of headache after changes in position of the head, especially when the child arises from sleep
- Headache associated with seizures, ataxia, lethargy, weakness, and nuchal rigidity
- Pain precipitated by strain, cough, or sneeze
- Pain relieved when the child lies down
- Headache associated with vomiting but without nausea
- History of localized morning headache
- Concurrent history of blurred vision
- Photophobia
- Meningeal signs
- Impaired level of consciousness
- Papilledema
- Diplopia
- Child younger than 5 years of age (for which an organic cause is likely)

Etiology

Most headaches in children are the result of vessel dilatation or migraine. However, headaches secondary to changes in ICP can be a result of brain tumors, hematomas, abscesses, central nervous system (CNS) leukemia, or arteriovenous (AV) malformations. Headaches also can be caused by ocular problems, sinusitis, hypertension, trauma, alcohol ingestion, allergic reactions, or psychologic factors (e.g., depression).

Incidence

- Headaches are a common, frequently benign, symptom in late childhood or early adolescence.
- Headaches are unusual and more indicative of serious underlying disease in pre–school-age children.
- Headache prevalence is 37% to 51% by 7 years of age and 51% to 82% from 7 to 15 years
- Migraine is a familial disorder, and there is a positive family history in over 70% of migraine patients. Tension-type headaches are frequently seen in dysfunctional families or those with psychosomatic disorders.

Risk Factors

- Family history of headaches
- Infection (e.g., sinusitis)
- Emotional or physical stress, missed meals, sleep deprivation
- Stress associated with school performance (profile of "high achiever"), peer pressure
- Suppressed feelings of anger, aggression, resentment, guilt
- Psychogenic depression
- Foods and substances such as cheese, chocolate, and caffeine
- Alcohol
- Allergies
- Menstruation
- Birth control pills
- Refractive errors
- Hypoglycemia

Differential Diagnosis

The practitioner should rule out CNS disorders (e.g., meningitis, tumor) and systemic disease with a careful history, and perform physical and neurologic examination before diagnosing and managing headaches (Table 39-2). It is helpful to classify headaches. Five patterns can be identified: acute, acute recurrent, chronic progressive, chronic nonprogressive, and mixed (Table 39-3).

An *acute headache* is a single event with no history of previous similar events. The differential diagnosis for acute generalized headache involves a variety of disorders including CNS infections, subarachnoid hemorrhage, trauma, systemic illness, and hypertension. Diagnosis should be made quickly, especially if the patient is clinically ill. Sinusitis, otitis, ocular and dental problems, and head trauma may cause acute localized headache.

Acute recurrent headaches are periodic events separated by pain-free intervals. When associated with symptoms such as nausea, vomiting, phonophobia, photophobia, and when relieved by sleep, these headaches are usually migrainous. Some migraines are precipitated by particular triggers, including anxiety, fatigue, stress, exercise, and diet. Foods frequently associated with migraine are chocolate, preserved meats with nitrites, and those foods and drinks containing caffeine. Subclassifications of migraine include ophthalmoplegic migraines and others that disturb brainstem function. Symptoms may include vertigo, vomiting, anorexia, behavioral changes, and ataxia (Box 39-6).

Table 39-2 Differential Diagnosis: Headache (784.0)

TYPE OF HEADACHE	LOCATION OF PAIN	QUALITY OF PAIN	ASSOCIATED SIGNS AND SYMPTOMS	SIGNIFICANT HISTORY
Acute	About the head, neck, and face	Severe, intermittent, debilitating	May be clinically ill (with fever, pain, swelling, ataxia, convulsions, or hypertension)	Infection, change in mental status, or head trauma
Acute recurrent (migraine)	Unilateral, frontal, temporal, and retroorbital	Throbbing, pulsating	Nausea, vomiting and scotomas (e.g., visual disturbances, field cuts, abdominal pain)	Family history; precipitated by triggers (e.g., diet, sleep deprivation, stress, exercise)
Chronic progressive	About the head	Dull, aching	Symptoms of ICP, vertigo, ataxia, and behavioral changes	Headaches worsen in frequency and severity
Chronic nonprogressive (tension-type)	Bilateral, neck, and occipital	Dull, mild to moderate	Fatigue and nausea	Normal neurologic examination; common in adolescent females; related to stress

Table 39-3 Examples of Syndromes that Cause Headaches

ACUTE GENERALIZED	ACUTE LOCALIZED	ACUTE RECCURENT	CHRONIC PROGRESSIVE	CHRONIC NONPROGRESSIVE
Fever	Sinusitis	Migraine	Tumor	Muscle contraction
Systemic infection	Otitis	Complex migraine	Pseudotumor	Conversion
CNS infection	Ocular abnormality	Migraine variants	Brain abscess	Malingering
Toxins (e.g., lead,	Dental disease	Cluster	Subdural hematoma	After concussion
carbon dioxide)	Trauma	Paroxysmal hemicrania	Hydrocephalus	Depression
After seizure	Occipital neuralgia	After seizure	Hemorrhage	Anxiety
Electrolyte imbalance	Temporomandibular	Tic doloreux	Hypertension	Adjustment reactions
Hypertension	joint dysfunction	Exertional	Vasculitis	Hemicrania continua
Hypoglycemia				
After lumbar puncture				
Trauma				
Embolic				
Vascular thrombosis				
Hemorrhage				
Collagen disease				
Exertional				

From Swaiman, K. (1999). Pediatric neurology: Principles and practice (3rd ed.). St. Louis: Mosby.

Box 39-6 Migraine Patterns and Migraine Equivalents

Benign Paroxysmal Torticollis

Onset during infancy, with or without pallor, vomiting, and behavioral changes
Lasts hours to days
Frequency and duration decline with age
Resolves by 2 to 5 years of age

Benign Paroxysmal Vertigo

Onset at 1 to 3 years of age, with vertigo, unsteadiness, pallor, and fear
Typically lasts 1 to 5 minutes
Resolves 1 to 2 years after onset

Cyclic Vomiting and Abdominal Migraine

Onset is at 4 to 10 years of age
Episodic nausea, vomiting, abdominal pain, and pallor
Typically lasts 30 to 60 minutes
Resolves 1 to 2 years after onset

Acute Confusional Migraine

Onset at 5 to 15 years of age, often preceded by minor head trauma
Causes confusion, agitation, memory disturbances, and mild headache
Lasts 6 to 8 hours

Migraine without Aura

Headaches that last 4 to 72 hours
Has two of the following qualities: unilateral location, pulsating quality, moderate to severe intensity, and aggravation by physical activity
Causes nausea, vomiting, and phonophobia and/or photophobia
Causes a desire to sleep, with relief upon waking

Migraine with Aura

Has one or more reversible symptoms (e.g., visual disturbances, weakness, sensory abnormalities lasting 4 to 60 minutes)
Headache follows the aura
Similar to migraine without aura

Ophthalmoplegic Migraine

Causes eye pain, some form of CN III palsy, ptosis, and unilateral pupillary dilatation

Basilar Migraine

Causes paroxysmal acute ataxia, alternating weakness, vertigo, or loss of consciousness
More common in girls than boys

Chronic progressive headaches are those that worsen in frequency and severity over time. They may be accompanied by symptoms of ICP such as vomiting, lethargy, change in mental status, ataxia, weakness, or visual disturbances. Such headaches may be attributable to an organic process such as hydrocephalus or brain tumor.

Chronic nonprogressive headaches, also known as *tension-type headaches,* occur more frequently than migraines, may be chronic or episodic, and are mild to moderate in severity. Patients usually have a normal neurologic examination. Headache is frequently related to stress or emotional problems and is more frequent in adolescent females.

A *mixed-headache syndrome* is a combination of acute recurrent headache and chronic nonprogressive headaches, usually occurring in adolescents. Known triggers include stress, sleep deprivation, missed meals, and anxiety.

Specific questions may provide valuable information on which to base a diagnosis. The practitioner should be alert for sings of increased ICP, chronic medical conditions, and school absences (Box 39-7).

Box 39-7   Headache History Data

How many different kind of headaches do you have?
How often do headaches occur?
Can you describe an episode?
How long does a headache last?
Where does it hurt?
What time of day do headaches occur?
Are there any unusual occurrences before a headache?
What makes the headache better or worse?
Can you think of anything that causes the headaches?
Does anyone else in the family have headaches?

Laboratory tests should be ordered based on the history and the physical and neurologic examination. Routine blood work (i.e., CBC count, erythrocyte sedimentation rate [ESR], general blood chemistry, antinuclear antibody [ANA] profile, urinalysis) and neuroimaging studies are not usually helpful in diagnosing patients with migraine or tension-type headaches. If there is a nonemergent situation where neuroimaging is warranted (e.g., sinusitis), MRI is more valuable than CT.

Once the diagnosis is confirmed, treatment can be started. Keeping a headache calendar for 4 to 8 weeks is helpful in identifying effective treatments and headache triggers.

Management

Management of headaches varies with and is dependent on the cause.

Tension-type headaches

Treatments and medications. Medications include:

- Acetaminophen 10 to15 mg/kg per dose every 4 to 6 hours, with a maximum of five doses per 24 hours.
- Ibuprofen 5 to 10 mg/kg per dose every 6 to 8 hours.
- Naproxen sodium 5 to 10 mg/kg per dose every 8 to 12 hours.
- Amitriptyline 25 to 50 mg every hour of sleep.

Behavior modification therapy may also be used. Biofeedback has been effective in reducing the incidence and severity of acute recurrent and tension-type headaches by helping patients gain a sense of control. Relaxation, breath control, and visual imagery are among techniques easily taught to children. Electromyographic and thermal biofeedback training encourages children to assume self-responsibility and control of the headaches. Successful biofeedback therapy can supplant, reduce, or eliminate the use of daily medication.

Counseling and prevention

- Reassure the parents and child that the pain is not caused by a brain tumor or structural abnormality.
- Educate regarding tension-type headaches and their favorable prognosis
- Discuss the need for good general health habits, as well as regular eating and sleeping.
- Assess stress levels at home and school and suggest ways to reduce stress.
- Advise the parents and child to keep a headache diary, documenting the date and time of headache, associated symptoms, any known triggers, and relief measures.
- Encourage positive psychosocial relationships with peers, teachers, and family members.
- Educate regarding medications.

Follow-up

- Call in 2 weeks to monitor progress.

- Schedule a return visit in 4 weeks if medication was prescribed. Go over the patient's headache diary.

Consultations and referrals

- Consult a physician if the pain worsens or does not improve with appropriate treatment
- Consult a neurologist if headaches are nocturnal or painful with coughing, or if the patient exhibits ataxia, CN involvement, or signs of increased ICP.

Acute recurrent headaches (migraines)

Treatments and medications. Abortive preparations include (Table 39-4):

- Ibuprofen 5 to 10 mg/kg per dose every 4 to 6 hours. Ibuprofen is twice as likely to abort the headache if it is given at the onset of the headache.
- Acetaminophen 10 to 15 mg/kg per dose every 4 to 6 hours. Suppositories may be given if patient is vomiting.
- Naproxen sodium 5 to 10 mg/kg per dose every 12 hours.
- Fiorinal 1 or 2 capsules every 4 hours. Total daily dose should not exceed 6 capsules.
- Sumatriptan: by mouth, 50 mg to children 6 to 12 years of age, 100 mg for those over 12 years of age; intranasally: 20 mg per dose in children 16 years of age and older; subcutaneously: 0.06 mg/kg per dose in children 16 years of age and older.

Prophylactic preparations include (see Table 39-4):

- Amitriptyline. For adolescents, give 25 to 50 mg every hour of sleep.
- Valproic acid 20 to 40 mg/kg per day. This is available in tablets, sprinkles, syrup, and extended-release forms.
- Cyproheptadine 0.25 to 0.4 mg/kg per day. The dose may be divided twice a day, and the medication is available in tablet and syrup forms.
- Propranolol 10 to 40 mg two or three times a day. A long-acting preparation is available.
- Naproxen sodium 5 to 10 mg/kg two times a day.

Behavior modification as described for Tension-Type Headaches may also be used, and during a headache, the child should be allowed to sleep in a quiet darkened room.

Counseling and prevention

- Reassure the parents and child that the pain is not caused by a brain tumor or structural abnormality.
- Suggest the avoidance of fatigue or excitement. Suggest a regular schedule of eating, sleeping, and school activities.
- Educate the child to recognize precipitating factors (triggers) and to understand the importance of abortive therapies at headache onset.
- Encourage the use of a headache calendar.

Follow-up

- Follow up by telephone in 2 to 4 weeks to monitor improvement.
- Schedule a return visit immediately if the child's condition worsens.

Consultations and referrals

- Refer the child to a neurologist if the condition worsens or there is no improvement with appropriate treatment.
- Refer the child for behavior modification therapy if indicated, and to available support groups.

Chronic progressive headaches. Headaches associated with vomiting, focal weakness, ataxia, change in mental status, lethargy, visual disturbances, or seizure may indicate increased ICP. These symptoms may indicate hydrocephalus, pseudotumor cerebri, brain tumor, abscess, or chronic subdural hematoma. Refer immediately to the emergency department.

Table 39-4 Medication Management for Acute Recurrent Headache Relief

MEDICATION	DOSE	COMMENTS
Abortive		
Acetaminophen	10-15 mg/kg per dose every 4-6 hours	Available in chewable tablets, liquid, drops, tabs, caplets, and suppositories
Ibuprofen	5-10 mg/kg per dose every 6-8 hours	Available in chewable tablets, liquid, drops, tabs, and caplets May cause GI upset, so give with food
Naproxen sodium	5-10 mg/kg per dose every 12 hours	Available in tablets and liquid May cause GI upset, so give with food
Butalbital (with acetaminophen or aspirin)	1-2 capsules every 4 hours, not to exceed 6 in 24 hours	Contains caffeine
Sumatriptan	25 to 100 mg orally 20 mg intranasally 6 mg subcutaneously	Age 16 years and older Nose and throat irritation Increased blood pressure, heaviness in chest. Do not use with MAO inhibitors
Prophylactic		
amitriptyline	25-50 mg every hour of sleep	Age 12 years and older May cause arrhythmia
Valproic acid	20-40 mg/kg per day	Available in tablets, sprinkles, liquid, and extended-release form May increase appetite, cause GI upset, increase appetite, elevate liver functions, and decrease platelets
Cyproheptadine	0.25-0.4 mg/kg per day or twice a day	Available in tablets or liquid May cause drowsiness and increased appetite
Propanol	2-4 mg/kg per day	Available in long-acting form Not for use in asthmatics May cause hypotension
Naproxen sodium	5-10 mg/kg per dose every 12 hours	Same as naproxen sodium (above)

Resources

Organizations

The American Council for Headache Education, 19 Mantua Road, Mt. Royal, NJ 08061; (800) 255-ACHE; www.achenet.org

The National Headache Foundation, 428 W. St. James Place, 2nd Floor, Chicago, IL 60614-2750; (888) NHF5552; www.head-aches.org

Large Head and Small Head

CATHERINE ASCHER

Alert

Consult with or refer to a physician for the following:
- Signs or symptoms of increased ICP (Box 39-8)
- Successively plotted head circumference measurements that cross two graph lines up or down
- Successively plotted head-circumference measurements that are greater than 2 standard deviations above or below the mean on a standardized growth chart
- Head circumference that is not growing faster than height and weight
- Head circumference that is growing more than 1 cm per week
- Head circumference that levels off at 5 or 6 months of age

Etiology

Head circumference, also called *occipitofrontal circumference* (OFC), is the measurement of the head above the eyebrows and above the ears over the most prominent portion of the occiput. A paper or metal tape should be used (a cloth tape could stretch). Several measurements should be done to ensure accuracy. Measurements should be plotted on a standardized curve. Standardized head circumference charts are available based on age and gender. Special charts are available for premature babies (see Appendix A.)

The average head circumference at birth is 35 cm, or 2 cm greater than the chest circumference. Male head circumferences are generally 1 to 2 cm greater than those of females. Head circumference increases linearly with height as the child grows. Head growth is faster in preterm infants than in full-term infants. Preterm head growth, dependent on mechanical ventilation and caloric deprivation, is divided into three phases: (1) initial period of growth arrest, or suboptimal head growth, (2) catch-up, and (3) growth along the standardized curves. It is imperative to use a standard plotting curve designed specifically for preterm infants.

Microcephaly denotes a small head size, as in 2 standard deviations below the mean (or the 2nd percentile) for age and gender. *Megalocephaly* (also known as *macrocephaly*) denotes a large head size, as in 2 standard deviations above the mean for age and gender. Microencephaly refers to a small brain size, and megalencephaly refers to a large brain size. A microcephalic child must be microencephalic by definition, but a macrocephalic child may have a normal brain, a microencephalic or megaloencephalic brain depending on the cause of the macrocephaly. The brain grows most rapidly in the first 6 months of life, with almost all growth completed by 2 years of age. The growth of the skull is caused largely by the growth of the brain. Boxes 39-9 and 39-10 list common causes for microcephaly and macrocephaly.

Three major components influence head circumference: (1) intracranial volume (brain, cerebrospinal fluid [CSF], blood volume,

Box 39-8 Increased Intracranial Pressure in Infants

Early Versus Late Signs

Early

Restlessness
Disorientation
Lethargy
Irritability
Sluggish pupillary reaction
Blurred vision
Headache

Late

Irregular respirations
Increased blood pressure
Decreased pulse
Increased temperature
Dilated, fixed pupils
Papilledema
Projectile vomiting

Acute Versus Chronic Signs

Acute

Irritability
Sleeplessness
Poor feeding or poor suck
Full, tense anterior fontanel
Increased head circumference
Splitting of cranial sutures
Hypertonia
Hypotonia

Chronic

Prominent forehead and scalp veins
Shiny skin on head or scalp
Nystagmus
Seizures
Large, open posterior fontanel

Box 39-9 Common Causes for Microcephaly and Microencephaly

1. Infections
   Cytomegalovirus
   Herpes simplex
   Rubella
   Varicella
   Coxsackie virus B
   Acquired immunodeficiency syndrome
   Toxoplasmosis
   Syphilis
   Postmeningitis
2. Drugs
   Alcohol
   Tobacco
   Marijuana
   Cocaine
   Heroin
   Anticancer
   Antiepileptic
   Prescription
3. Anoxia
   Generalized cerebral anoxia
   Post–status epilepticus
   Porencephaly or hydraencephaly
   Carbon monoxide poisoning
   Placental insufficiency
4. Heredity
   Normal, variation in occipitofrontal circumference (OFC), asymptomatic
   Mendelian pattern, symptomatic: autosomal dominant, autosomal recessive, or X-linked
   Craniosynostosis
   Heredofamilial degenerative diseases
      Pelizaeus-Merzbacher disease
      Neuronal ceroid-lipofuscinosis (Batten's disease)
   Aminoacidurias, organic acidurias

Miscellaneous syndromes, frequently with dwarfism (achondroplastic type excluded):
   Smith-Lemli-Opitz syndrome
   de Lange syndrome
   Rubenstein-Taybi syndrome
   Dubowitz syndrome
   Proportionate short stature syndromes
5. Chromosomal
   Down syndrome and other trisomies
   Ring chromosomes
   Deletions
   Sex chromosome aneuploidy
6. Malformations
   Microcephaly vera
   Atelencephaly
   Holoprosencephaly
   Lissencephaly
   Encephalocele
7. Trauma
   Birth trauma
   Child abuse
8. Perinatal metabolic and endocrine imbalances
   Hypoglycemia
   Hypothyroidism
   Hypopituitarism
   Hypoadrenocorticism
9. Malnutrition
10. Prenatal maternal
    Illness
    Systemic illness
    Anemia
    Malnutrition
    Toxic exposures

From Swaiman, K. (1999). Pediatric neurology: Principles and practice (3rd ed.). St. Louis: Mosby.

Box 39-10 Most Common Causes for Megalocephaly

1. Hydrocephalus
   Noncommunicating
      Chiari malformations
      Aqueductal stenosis
      Dandy-Walker malformation
      Walker-Walker syndrome (lissencephaly and Dandy-Walker)
   Neoplasms, supratentorial and infratentorial
   Arachnoid cyst, infratentorial
   Holoprosencephaly with dorsal interhemispheric sac
   [DeMyer, 1987]
   Communicating
      External or extraventricular obstructive hydrocephalus
         (dilated subarachnoid space)
      Arachnoid cyst, supratentorial
      Meningeal fibrosis or obstruction
         Postinflammatory
         Posthemorrhagic
         Neoplastic infiltration
      Vascular
         Arteriovenous malformation
         Intracranial hemorrhage
         Dural sinus thrombosis
         Galenic vein aneurysm
      Choroid plexus papilloma
      Neurocutaneous syndrome
         Incontinentia pigmenti
   Destructive lesions
      Hydranencephaly
      Porencephaly
   Familial, autosomal-dominant, autosomal-recessive, or
   X-linked
2. Megalencephaly
   Anatomic
   Metabolic
   Hydrodynamic

   Megalencephaly with hydrocephalic complication: achondroplasia and mucopolysaccharidoses
3. Subdural fluid
   Hematoma
   Hygroma
   Empyema
4. Brain edema (toxic-metabolic)
   Intoxication
      Lead
      Vitamin A
      Tetracycline
   Endocrine
      Hypoparathyroidism
      Hypoadrenocorticism
   Galactosemia
   Spongy degeneration of the brain
   Idiopathic (pseudotumor cerebri)
5. Thick skull
   Familial variation
   Anemia
   Myotonia dystrophica
   Cranioskeletal dysplasia:
      Rickets
      Osteopetrosis
      Osteogenesis imperfecta
      Orodigitofacial dysostosis
      Craniometaphyseal dysplasia of Pyle
      Cleidocranial dysostosis
      Hyperphosphatasemia
      Epiphyseal dysplasia
      Russell dwarf
      Pycnodysostosis
      Leontiasis ossea
      Progressive diaphyseal dysplasia
      Proteus (elephant man) syndrome

From Swaiman, K. (1999). Pediatric neurology: Principles and practice (3rd ed.). St. Louis: Mosby.

and space-occupying lesions), (2) the ability of the cranial sutures to expand, and (3) the thickness of the skull bones and scalp. Gender, age, and disease states influence these components.

Incidence

- *Microcephaly*—About 2.5% of the population are affected.
- *Megalocephaly*—About 2.5% of the population are affected.
- *Hydrocephalus*—Approximately 4000 infants are born with this every year, and another 6000 infants and children develop hydrocephalus before 2 years of age.
- *Caput succedaneum*—This is very common with vaginal deliveries.
- *Cephalohematoma*—Occurring in 0.4% to 2.5% of live births, this condition is nearly two times more common in males than in females. It is more frequent in primiparas. The incidence is increased with the use of forceps during delivery.
- *Subcutaneous scalp hematomas and subgaleal hematomas*—This is uncommon.
- *Craniosynostosis*—This condition occurs in approximately 1 in 2500 live births.
- *Plagiocephaly*—In 1992, the AAP issued a statement advising parents to position a sleeping infant supine to decrease the risk of sudden infant death syndrome (SIDS). Since that time, there has been a dramatic increase in plagiocephaly.

Risk Factors

- Prenatal maternal history of diabetes, viral illness, ionizing radiation, uremia, phenylketonuria (PKU), malnutrition, carbon monoxide, prescription drugs, illicit drug use, or smoking
- Premature infants (related to intraventricular hemorrhage, anoxia, infections, and metabolic diseases)
- Family history of microcephaly, megalocephaly, neurocutaneous disease, or chromosomal abnormalities (e.g., Down syndrome)
- AV malformation
- Malnutrition
- Trauma
- Tumor
- Child abuse
- Mental retardation

Differential Diagnosis (Table 39-5)

A useful approach to *microcephaly* is to categorize it into asymptomatic and symptomatic. *Asymptomatic benign microcephaly* is defined as a head circumference that falls 2 standard deviations below the mean (in accordance with a standardized chart) in an otherwise normal child. No other abnormalities may be present. Subsequent neurologic examinations and de-

ICD-9 code   767.1   761.1   756.0

Table 39-5 Differential Diagnosis: Large Head and Small Head

CRITERIA	CAPUT SUCCEDANEUM	CEPHALHEMATOMA	CRANIOSYNOSTOSIS*
ICD-9 code	767.1	761.1	756.0
Subjective Data			
Age	First day of life	Several days to 1 week old	Less than 6 months old
Birth history	Vaginal delivery ± prolonged difficult labor	Vaginal delivery Prolonged, difficult labor ± forceps delivery	Cesarean section or vaginal delivery
Onset			
Manner of onset	Birth	Acute	Subacute-chronic
Course since onset	Improving	Worse	Worse
Objective Data			
Physical examination			
Head and scalp	Discoloration, ecchymosis ± petechial hemorrhages	No discoloration	No discoloration
Skull	Diffuse edema that is soft, boggy ± pitting May cross cranial suture lines Most common location: vertex	Firm, tense, well-demarcated edema with ridged margins, recessed center Does not cross suture lines Limited to bone's edge Most common location is over parietal bone	No edema
Cranial sutures	± Overriding No ridging	Usually no overriding No ridging	No overriding Ridging
Cranial fontanel	Open and flat	Open, flat	Early closure
Other findings	None	None	Rare: asymmetrical craniofacial appearances; ± head tilt; proptosis; strabismus; papilledema or optic atrophy; syndactylism
Laboratory data	None	None	Skull radiographs

Refer to a pediatric neurologist.
± indicates symptom or sign may or may not be present.

velopment must be normal. There may be a family history of microcephaly with small stature and normal functioning. The practitioner should consult with a physician regarding these children. A child with a head circumference less than 2 standard deviations from the mean and abnormal neurologic findings is considered symptomatic, necessitating a search for the etiologiç agent. Specific abnormal neurologic findings include early cranial suture closure without palpable ridging, abnormal facial features, and delayed visual fixation, head control, eye-hand use, and vocalization.

In *megalocephaly,* or *macrocephaly,* it is necessary to determine whether the head-circumference measurements parallel the normal curve or are accelerating. Developmentally it must be determined whether the child is regressing or appropriately progressing. It is also important to inquire about other family members having a large head and their somatotype. Regression is indicative of an ongoing pathologic process. If the megalocephaly has been acquired since birth or the last visit, assess the child for signs and symptoms of increased ICP. The most common causes of megalocephaly are hydrocephalus, megalencephaly, subdural collection of fluid, edema of the brain, and skull dysplasia.

Hydrocephalus is an imbalance in the production and or absorption of cerebrospinal fluid within the ventricular system. Excess fluid can cause an enlargement of the ventricles and signs and symptoms of increased ICP. The cause may be unknown. Known causes include infection (prenatal or postnatal), congenital structural malformations, vascular abnormaities, mass lesions, and bleeding. Hydrocephalus is often associated with myelomeningocele in infants. Symptoms on examination may include frontal bossing, sunsetting eyes (downward position of the eyes), and a full or bulging fontanel.

Caput succedaneum is scalp edema resulting from compression by the birth canal. *Chignon* is edema caused specifically by vacuum extraction.

A *cephalhematoma* is caused by a subperiosteal collection of blood over one or more flat bones of the skull, secondary to the separation of the periosteum from the underlying bone. It does not cross the suture line because it is contained by the periosteum.

Subcutaneous scalp hematomas and *subgaleal hematomas* may cross the sutures and are not confined by the periosteum. They may be life threatening because of the increased vasculature of the head relative to total blood volume. They generally appear in the first day of life with decreased red blood cells on a CBC count, lethargy, and hypotonia.

Craniosynostosis is the premature fusion of the cranial sutures, usually beginning in utero. It most commonly involves one suture. The four primary sutures affected are metopic, coronal, sagittal, and lambdoidal. Sagittal synostosis is the most commonly affected suture occurring in approximately 50% of cases and is more common in boys. The child has an elongated head with frontal bossing (and possibly occipital bossing). A premature child may have a similarly shaped head, but it resolves spontaneously over the first 3 months of life. Restricting growth at one or more sutures may result in skull deformity, craniofacial abnormalities, and increased intracranial pressure. The causes of craniosynostosis ranges from unknown to chromosomal abnormalities (e.g., Crouzon and Apert syndromes) or metabolic disturbances.

Plagiocephaly is positional molding of the skull. It must be differentiated from craniosynostosis.

Management

Microcephaly

Treatments and medications. No treatments or medications are indicated.

Counseling and prevention

- Inform the parents that the condition might affect the child's development.
- Remember that identifying the etiologic agent may assist in preventing microcephaly in subsequent children.
- If a genetics evaluation is considered, support the family through the experience.

Follow-up

- Provide follow-up care on a well-child schedule.
- Monitor head circumference and plot on an appropriate chart.
- Measure and chart the head circumference of both parents.

Consultations and referrals. Refer all children with microcephaly to a neurologist initially for evaluation, and refer back immediately for any sign of developmental delay or any abnormality in the neurologic examination (Box 39-11).

Megalocephaly

Treatments and medications. Treatment is dependent on the cause. The child should be carefully examined. The fontanels should be carefully evaluated for size, contour, and tension; sutures should be palpated; fundi should be visualized to rule out papilledema; and the skin should be examined for neurocutaneous stigmas. A MRI should be ordered in nonemergent situations. If the reason for the megalocephaly is unclear, the child should be screened for inborn errors of metabolism. If some cases, vitamin A levels and lead levels may be useful. Chromosome analysis and fragile-X deoxyribonucleic acid (DNA) examination should be considered.

Counseling and prevention

- Teach parents the signs of increased ICP.
- Advise parents to report these signs immediately.

Follow-up

- Provide follow-up care on a well-child schedule.
- Monitor head circumference and plot on an appropriate chart.
- Chart the head circumference of both parents.

Box 39-11 Information to Include in a Referral

Reason for referral

Clinical manifestations

Successive head circumference measurements plotted on a standardized graph

Successive height and weight measurements plotted on a standardized graph

Past medical history, including birth history, perinatal infections, illnesses, and head trauma

Head circumference of parents and siblings (if available)

Developmental assessment

Any previous diagnostic procedures (e.g., MRI, computed tomography [CT] scan)

Consultations and referrals

- Refer all children with megalocephaly initially to a neurologist for evaluation, and refer back immediately for any sign of developmental delay or any abnormality in the neurologic examination.
- Refer for genetic counseling as indicated.

Hydrocephalus

Treatments and medications. Treatment is to relieve any obstructions that may be present (e.g., in aqueductal stenosis), and often a shunt is necessary to bypass the excess fluid to a cavity (e.g., the peritoneum) that can accommodate it. A child with a shunt requires close supervision. Shunts may require revisions as the child grows. Shunts can become obstructed, possibly causing signs of increased ICP. Shunt infections are also possible.

Counseling and prevention

- Remember that prevention depends on the cause.
- Educate parents on the signs and symptoms of increased ICP and on reporting them immediately.
- If child is shunted, advise parents to immediately report fever.

Follow-up

- Provide follow-up care on a well-child schedule.
- Monitor head circumference and plot on an appropriate chart.
- Collaborate closely with a pediatric neurology-neurosurgery team.

Consultations and referrals

- Refer all cases of suspected hydrocephalus immediately to a pediatric neurologist.
- If there are any signs of increased ICP, refer to the emergency room.
- Refer for genetic counseling as needed.

Caput succedaneum

Treatments and medications. Caput succedaneum resolves on its own within the first day to week of life. It is not associated with any complications and requires no intervention.

Counseling and prevention

- Reassure parents that swelling will resolve on its own in a day to a week.
- Advise parents there are no expected complications.

Follow-up. Provide follow-up care on a well-child schedule

Consultations and referrals. Generally none are needed.

Cephalhematoma

Treatments and medications. Evacuation of the lesion is contraindicated and requires no intervention. Resolution (absorption of the blood) takes several weeks to months, and it may calcify.

Counseling and prevention. Reassure parents that the hematoma will reabsorb in a few weeks to months

Follow-up

- Schedule a return visit monthly to monitor resolution.
- Assess for rare complications such as jaundice, anemia, and osteomyelitis.

Consultations and referrals. Refer immediately to a physician if there are any complications.

Subcutaneous scalp hematomas and subgaleal hematomas

Treatments and medications. Surgery may be necessary.

Counseling and prevention

- Remember that prevention depends on the cause.
- Support the parents through the treatment experience.
- Explain the condition.

Follow-up. Once the condition has resolved, provide follow-up care on a well-child schedule.

Consultations and referrals. Collaborate closely with a pediatric neurology-neurosurgical team.

Craniosynostosis

Treatments and medications

- Anteroposterior and lateral radiographs of the skull or a CT of the head with three-dimensional reconstruction should be obtained if necessary.
- Surgery is usually the treatment of choice.
- Goals of treatment are to ensure normal brain growth, to prevent increased ICP, to prevent compromise of visual and auditory function, and to provide cosmetic improvement.

Counseling and prevention

- Remember that prevention depends on the cause.
- If genetic evaluation is indicated, support the parents through the experience.
- Educate parents to signs and symptoms of increased ICP and to report them immediately.

Follow-up. Provide follow-up care on a well-child schedule. Monitor head circumference and plot on a curve.

Consultations and referrals

- Refer to a pediatric neurologist for initial evaluation.
- Refer to the emergency room for any signs of increased ICP.
- Collaborate closely with a pediatric neurology-neurosurgery team.

Plagiocephaly

Treatments and medications. Helmet therapy may be needed in severe cases. A special soft helmet is worn 23 hours a day for several months. This is most effective before 9 months of age.

Counseling and prevention

- Reassure parents that the condition is not harmful.
- Educate parents to change their child's position regularly.
- If a helmet is used, advise the parents or caregiver to monitor skin for signs of irritation or breakdown.

Follow-up. Provide follow-up care on a well-child schedule

Consultations and referrals. Refer to a pediatric neurologist for initial evaluation.

Resources

Organizations

Hydrocephalus Association, 870 Market Street, Suite 705, San Francisco, CA 94102; (888) 598-3789; www.hydroassoc.org

Microcephaly Network, 362 Jean Talon, St. Vanier, ON Canada K1L6T9; (613) 742-5936

National Hydrocephalus Foundation, 12413 Centralia Road, Lakewood, CA 90715; (888) 260-1789; www.nhfonline.org/

Websites

HYCEPH-L (e-mail group) (to subscribe, send a message to listserv@listserv.utoronto.ca. In the body of the message type: Subscribe HYCEPH-L Yourfirstname Yourlastname)

MICROCEPHALY (e-mail group) (to subscribe, send a message to marce@infospinner.com and request to be added to the list.

Seizures, Breath-Holding Spells, and Syncope

CATHERINE ASCHER

Alert

Consult with or refer to a physician for the following:
- Status epilepticus
- Infantile spasms

- Signs and symptoms of meningitis (e.g., fever, full bulging fontanel, high-pitched cry, stiff neck, headache, petechial rash, irritability, lethargy)
- First-time seizure, with or without fever
- Papilledema
- Dilated or fixed pupils
- Abnormal neurologic examination
- Pertussis vaccine in the previous 24 hours
- History of significant head trauma
- Raccoon eyes
- CSF draining from the ears or nose
- Chronic illness (e.g., diabetes mellitus, sickle cell disease, mental retardation, HIV infection, asthma)
- Hematocrit level below normal
- Ingestion of toxic substance
- Allergy to aspirin
- Neurocutaneous disease (e.g., neurofibromatosis, tuberous sclerosis, Sturge-Weber syndrome)
- Premature birth
- Lead intoxication

Etiology

A seizure is an electrical disturbance in the brain that manifests as changes in motor, sensory, or cognitive function. Signs and symptoms may include stiffening (tonic), shaking (clonic), staring, changes in behavior, confusion, and loss of consciousness. A seizure may be idiopathic or a result of pathologic processes such as infections, trauma, metabolic disease, endocrinologic dysfunction, congenital structural abnormalities, vascular abnormalities, neoplastic processes, and degenerative disorders. Box 39-12 identifies possible etiologic agents by the age of seizure onset. The underlying cause for the seizure will direct treatment. If the seizure is a result of acute infection such as meningitis or low blood glucose (hypoglycemia), the seizure is categorized as provoked.

Box 39-13 lists some common drugs that can provoke a seizure. If the underlying cause is treated, the seizures should not reoccur. If the seizures are idiopathic (have no identifiable cause), as occurs in 60% of all seizures in children, there is a 50% chance of having another seizure. If two or more unprovoked seizures occur, this is defined as epilepsy. A child with epilepsy must, by definition, have seizures, but not every child with a seizure has epilepsy.

Incidence

- About 50% of all seizures occur in children under 10 years of age.
- The prevalence worldwide is 5%.
- By 14 years of age, 1% of children experience a febrile seizure.
- At some point in life, up to 1 in 20 of the population will have at least one seizure.
- Seizures are slightly more common in males than females.
- Seizures are slightly more common in lower socioeconomic groups.
- The incidence of seizures is greater in African Americans than in Caucasians.
- Febrile seizures occur in up to 5% of young children. The onset is most common between 3 months and 5 years of age, with the peak incidence between 10 and 20 months. They are most common in boys and have a slightly higher incidence in Caucasians than in African Americans and those with a family history of febrile seizures.

Box 39-12 Etiology of Seizures by Age Group

Neonate

Intracranial hemorrhage
Meningitis
Other intracranial infections
Hypoxia
Electrolyte imbalance
Structural abnormality
Metabolic disorders
Epileptic disorders:
    Benign neonatal convulsions
    Early myoclonic encephalopathy

Infancy

Febrile seizures
Meningitis
Child abuse
Trauma
Electrolyte imbalance
Cerebral palsy
Epileptic disorders:
    Infantile spasms (West syndrome)
    Benign myoclonic epilepsy in infancy
    Severe myoclonic epilepsy in infancy

Childhood

Meningitis
Ingestion, poisoning
Child abuse

Drowning
Mental retardation
Diabetes mellitus
Sickle cell disease
Neurocutaneous disease
Intracranial infection, HIV infection, herpes simplex virus (HSV) infection
Brain tumor or neoplasm
Epileptic disorders:
    Myoclonic astatic epilepsy
    Lennox-Gastaut syndrome
    Childhood absence epilepsy
    Epilepsy with myoclonic absences
    Benign rolandic epilepsy
    Landau-Kleffner syndrome

Adolescence

Meningitis
Drug abuse
Head trauma
Chemical inhalation
Brain tumor or neoplasm
Epileptic disorders:
    Juvenile absence epilepsy
    Juvenile myoclonic epilepsy of Janz
    Tonic-clonic seizures on awakening
    Benign partial seizures of adolescence

Box 39-13   Possible Seizure-Inducing Drugs

Antihistamines
Asthma medications (e.g., theophylline)
Stimulants used in the treatment of hyperactivity (e.g., methylphenidate [Ritalin], Adderall , dextroamphetamine [Dexedrine])
Chemotherapeutic agents (e.g., methotrexate, chlorambucil, and L-asparaginase)
Immunosuppressives (e.g., cyclosporine, methylprednisolone [Solu-Medrol])
Antiinfective drugs (e.g., imipenem, penicillin [in high doses], metronidazole, lindane)
Psychiatric medications (e.g., phenothiazides, clozapine, tricyclic antidepressants)
Benzodiazepines and anticonvulsant medications (during withdrawal of medications)
Intravenous contrast
Topical anesthetics (e.g., lidocaine [in high doses])
Alcohol (when withdrawn)
Illegal drugs:
Cocaine or crack
Marijuana
LSD
Psychedelics
Opiates
Ectasy (MDMA)
Flunitrazepam (Rohypnol) (a "date rape drug")
Gamma hydroxy butyrate (GHB) (the newest "date rape drug")

- For information on breath-holding spells, see Chapter 19.
- About 20% of the population experience fainting once in their lives.
- Status epilepticus affects as many as 60,000 people yearly. It is most common in children under 3 years of age.
- Infantile spasms usually occur within the first year of life, with the peak incidence between 4 and 6 months of life. The annual incidence is less than 0.45 per 1000 live births.

Risk Factors

- Family history of epilepsy, neurocutaneous disease, sickle cell disease, febrile convulsions, breath-holding spells, or fainting
- Premature birth
- Birth trauma
- Perinatal intracranial infection
- Lack of immunization
- Delay in achievement of developmental milestones
- Previous abnormal neurologic examination
- Chromosomal disorders
- Illicit drug use
- Chronic illness (e.g., asthma, diabetes, HIV infection)
- Meningitis and encephalitis

Differential Diagnosis

The practitioner must keep in mind that a seizure may be a symptom of an underlying disorder (Tables 39-6 and 39-7). In addition, children may exhibit movements that mimic seizures such as tremors (which stop when the extremity is held), tics (involuntary movements such as eye blinking or sniffing), and pseudoseizures (which are psychogenic).

Table 39-6 Differential Diagnosis: Meningitis and Febrile Seizures

CRITERIA	MENINGITIS*	FEBRILE SEIZURES
ICD-9 code	322.9	780.31
Subjective Data		
Age	Any age, peak incidence 6-12 months	3 months to 5 years
State of consciousness	Depressed or irritated	Alert, active
Onset	Usually abrupt but may be gradual	Acute
Associated symptoms		
Headache	±; rare in children <3 years of age	±
Photophobia	±	−
Vomiting	±†	±†
Diarrhea	±†	±†
Cough	±†	±†
Rhinitis	±†	±†
Fever	±; infants may not exhibit fever	+ > 39.0° C (102.2° F)
Chills	±	±
Rash	± purpuric rash within the first several days of illness	± Macular papular rash related to associated illness
Anorexia	±	−
Arthritis	±	−
Description of event	Generalized or focal seizure 2 or 3 days into illness	Generalized tonic clonic seizure lasting <10 minutes
Behavior after event	Variable, ranging from lethargy to irritability	Normal
Course since onset	Unchanged or worse	Unchanged or improved
Immunization history	*Haemophilus influenzae* type b conjugate vaccine often not received	Complete for age
Recent illness	Upper respiratory or GI illness, otitis media, viral illness	Upper respiratory or viral illness, otitis media
Family history	None	±Family history of febrile seizures
Objective Data		
Physical examination		
General appearance	Appears ill	Appears well
Resting position	Fetal position, tripod position, opisthotonos	Sitting, lying, or standing comfortably
Fontanel	Full, bulging	Flat
Neck	Stiffness, decreased range of motion, ±Kernig sign, ±Brudzinski sign	Full range of motion, −Kernig sign, −Brudzinski sign
Skin	Petechiae, purpura	Maculopapular
Eyes, ears, nose, throat	±Orbital cellulitis; ±conjunctivitis; ±otitis media; ±pharyngitis	−Cellulitis; ±conjunctivitis; ±otitis media; ±pharyngitis
Neurologic examination		
Level of consciousness	Depressed, irritated	Within normal limits (WNL)
Cranial nerves	Papilledema (unusual before 15 months); orbital palsies; hearing deficit	WNL
Motor	±Ataxia	Normal gait
Sensory	Normal	Normal
Deep tendon reflexes (DTRs)	Hyperactive or hypoactive reflexes; ±Babinski reflex	Normal
Laboratory data		
EEG	± Slowing	Normal
Lumbar puncture	±; initially may be WNL (first couple hours)	
Color of CSF	Cloudy	Normal
Cell count	Increased 300-10,000	Normal
Protein	Increased	Normal
Glucose	May be decreased	Normal
Gram stain	±	−
Culture	Common organisms include *Haemophilus influenzae* type b, *Neisseria meningitidis*, group B streptococci, and *Streptococcus pneumoniae*	
CSF pressure	May be increased	Normal
CBC count		
Red blood cell	Normal	Normal
White blood cell	May be increased	May be increased
Platelets	Normal	Normal
Blood culture	±	±

Immediate referral to a physician.
†*Related to associated, concurrent illness.*
+ indicates symptom or sign is present; − indicates symptom or sign is not present; ± indicates symptom or sign may or may not be present.

Table 39-7 Differential Diagnosis: Seizures, Breath-Holding Spells, and Syncope

CRITERIA	BREATH-HOLDING	SYNCOPE	SEIZURES*
ICD-9 code	312.81	780.2	780.39
Subjective Data			
Age	First episode usally before 2 years of age	Usually in school-aged child or adolescent	Any age
Onset			
Manner of onset	Sudden, always initiated by crying	Sudden, patient always sitting or standing at onset	Abrupt
Previous episodes	±	±	±
Precipitating events			
Fever	−	−	±
Acute illness	−	−	±
Trauma	±	−	±
Pain	±	−	−
Aura	−	Nausea, visual changes	±Nausea, visual changes, headache, photophobia, numbness, tingling
Emotional stress	±Temper tantrum	Fright, overheating	±
Fatigue	−	±	±
Video games	−	−	−
Exercise	−	±	−
Description of event			
Responsiveness	±Loss of consciousness	Loss of consciousness	±Loss of consciousness
Memory of event	Unable to assess because of child's age	None	±
Length of attack	5-10 seconds, up to 1 minute	< 10 seconds	Usually <10 minutes; if longer, considered a medical emergency
Movements	±Twitching	±Tonic-clonic	Variable: Twitching, tonic, clonic, tonic-clonic, eye fluttering, eye deviations, lip smacking, dropping attacks
Cyanosis	±	−	±
Excessive salivation	−	−	±
Associated events			
Loss of bowel control	−	−	±
Loss of bladder control	−	−	±
Vomiting	−	−	±
Bed-wetting	−	−	±Caused by noctural seizures
Course since onset			
Recovery time	Usually within 2-3 minutes	Less than 30 seconds	Variable, several seconds to several hours
Recurrent attacks	Common	Common	50% after first attack; 75% chance after second episode
Medications	None	None	(see Box 39-11)
Past medical history			
Perinatal history	No significance	No significance	Premature birth, maternal illness during pregnancy, neonatal complications (e.g., intracranial hemorrhages, hyperbilirubinemia)
Stillbirths	No significance	No significance	±
Immunizations	No significance	No significance	Pertussis within the previous 72 hours
Head trauma	No significance	No significance	±
Family history			
Epilepsy	−	−	±
Febrile seizures	−	−	±

Refer to a physician or neurologist.
+indicates symptom or sign is present; −indicates symptom or sign is not present; ±indicates symptom or sign may or may not be present.
N/A, Not applicable; WNL, within normal limits.

The practitioner should be alert to signs, symptoms, and conditions necessitating consultation or referral to a physician (see the Alert box). In particular, the practitioner must be alert to two medical emergencies: status epilepticus and infantile spasms.

Status epilepticus is defined as either a prolonged seizure, lasting greater than 30 minutes, or a cluster of seizures where the child does not recover consciousness in between. It is a medical emergency, so obtain emergency care by dialing 911 or the local emergency number.

Table 39-7 Differential Diagnosis: Seizures, Breath-Holding Spells, and Syncope—cont'd

CRITERIA	BREATH-HOLDING	SYNCOPE	SEIZURES*
Subjective Data—cont'd			
Family history—cont'd			
Neurocutaneous disorders	−	−	±
Sickle cell	−	−	±
Diabetes mellitus	−	−	±
Chromosomal abnormalities	−	−	±
Breath-holding	±	−	−
Developmental history			
Achievement of milestones			
Age-appropriate	±	+	±
Appropriate order	±	+	±
Objective Data			
Physical examination			
Vital signs	WNL	±Orthostatic hypotension; ±thready pulse	WNL
General appearance	Alert, awake, active	Awake, alert	Dysmorphic features suggestive of chromosomal abnormalities
Skin			
Café-au-lait spots	−	−	±
Hypopigmented lesions	−	−	−
Pallor	−	−	−
Head			
Head circumference	WNL	WNL	Increased, decreased, or WNL
Fontanel	Flat	Closed	Bulging seen with increased ICP
Cranial structures	No splitting or ridging	Closed	Splitting may be seen with increased ICP
Neck			
Range of motion	Full	Full	Full, stiffness with meningitis
Chest			
Adventitious breath sounds	−	−	±
Cardiovascular	WNL	WNL	WNL
Neurologic examination			
Level of consciousness	Awake, alert, and oriented to person, place, and time	Awake, alert, and oriented to person, place, and time	Variable, lethargy, irritability, awake, and alert
Cranial nerves	WNL	WNL	WNL
Motor	WNL	WNL	WNL
Sensory	WNL	WNL	±Hyperactive reflexes
Deep tendon reflexes	WNL	WNL	±Hypoactive reflexes; ±Babinski reflex
Laboratory data			
CBC count	WNL	WNL	±Decreased hematocrit
Electrolytes	WNL	WNL	±Na, <135 mEq/L ±Ca <8.5 mg/dl ±Glucose <60 mg/dl
Anticonvulsant levels (serum)	N/A	N/A	Subtherapeutic (see Table 39-8)
EEG	WNL	WNL	Range from normal to abnormal
Imaging	Not usually ordered	Not usually ordered	±Abnormal findings

Infantile spasms (known as *West syndrome* if accompanied by mental retardation and hypsarrhythmia on EEG) are seizures clinically characterized as a brief head nodding associated with extension or flexion of the trunk and extremities. The rapidity of the movements is suggestive of a startle reaction. They are also referred to as "*salaam* convulsions." They occur in clusters, as many as a hundred a day. Infantile spasms is a medical emergency, so refer immediately to a pediatric neurologist. *Infantile spasms* may be associated with a syndrome such as tuberous sclerosis, or they may be

Box 39-14 International Classification of Seizure Type

Partial Seizures

Simple partial seizures
- With motor signs
- With somatosensory or special sensory hallucinations
- With autonomic symptoms
- With psychic symptoms
  Complex partial seizures
- Simple partial seizure followed by impairment of consciousness
- With impaired consciousness at onset
  Partial seizures evolving to secondary generalized seizures
- Simple partial seizures evolving to generalized seizures
- Complex partial seizures evolving to generalized seizures
- Simple partial seizures evolving to complex partial seizures

Generalized Seizures

Absence seizures
- Atypical absence seizures
  Myoclonic seizures
  Clonic seizures
  Tonic seizures
  Tonic-clonic seizures
  Atonic seizures

Unclassifiable Epileptic Seizures

From Swaiman, K. (1999). Pediatric neurology: Principles and practice (3rd ed.). St. Louis: Mosby.

Box 39-15 Differentiating between Jitteriness and Seizures in the Neonate Experiencing Drug Withdrawal

JITTERINESS	SEIZURES
No abnormal ocular movements	Often with subtle abnormal ocular movements
No autonomic effects	Autonomic changes (e.g., drooling, tachycardia, pupillary changes)
Sensitive to stimuli	Not affected by stimuli
Tremulous, rhythmic movements	Jerky movements
Movements stopped upon touch	Movements cannot be stopped
Occur at no specific times	Usually occur within 3 days of birth

idiopathic. Prognostically it is important to notice if any developmental delays occurred before the onset of seizures. Up to 80% of children with infantile spasms may develop some degree of mental retardation. All patients with infantile spasms, which are symptoms of an underlying condition, are associated with developmental delay, but up to half of those that are cryptogenic in origin may have normal development.

Seizures are classified as either *partial* (arising in one hemisphere) or *generalized* (arising in both sides simultaneously) (Box 39-14). Partial seizures occur in a localized area of the brain. They are characterized by asymmetric abnormal movements such as shaking one arm or brief changes in behavior. An aura, or peculiar sensation, may be experienced just before a seizure. Partial seizures may spread and take on characteristics of a generalized seizure. Staring episodes can either be manifestations of partial seizures or may be generalized as in absence seizures.

Generalized tonic-clonic seizures usually begin with the eyes rolling upward followed by loss of consciousness, falling to the ground, and stiffening of the body in a symmetric manner. Rhythmic shaking movements then ensue. At this time the child may lose control of his or her secretions and bowel and bladder function. The jerking movements usually wax and wane until the seizure ends with a few seconds or a few minutes. After the seizure (postictally) the child may be drowsy and may sleep for as long as several hours.

Absence seizures are characterized by an abrupt loss of consciousness with or without eye fluttering. The child ceases activity without a change in postural tone. It lasts 5 to 10 seconds. Activity is resumed without drowsiness or confusion. The frequency of attacks may range from 20 to several hundred daily. Teachers often bring attention to the seizures by reporting that the child is dazed, not paying attention, or staring off into space. These seizures are generalized, and the EEG generally demonstrates 3 Hz spike and wave discharges.

Myoclonus is a sudden, brief involuntary contraction of inhibition of a single muscle or muscle group. Myoclonic seizures are characterized by synchronous jerks of the body or segment of the body.

Atonic seizures, or *drop attacks,* are sudden, momentary loss of muscle tone and postural control. They are characterized by sudden falls to the floor if the child is standing or head drops if the child is sitting.

Febrile seizures are brief generalized seizures occurring in association with an elevated temperature. Considering fever to be the most common cause of seizure in children, it is imperative to differentiate a benign seizure from meningitis (see Table 39-6). Nonepileptic paroxysmal phenomenon (see Table 39-7) may mimic seizures.

Jitteriness, a condition seen most commonly in drug withdrawal, is a shaking movement of the extremities that can be stopped with touch (Box 39-15).

A *breath-holding spell* is a paroxysmal event in which children hold their breath, generally after prolonged crying or after being startled or frightened. The child becomes apneic, loses muscle tone, and eventually loses consciousness. After they lose consciousness, breathing resumes. If the event is prolonged and hypoxia occurs, a brief convulsion could occur. (See also Breath-Holding in Chapter 19.)

Syncope, or *fainting,* is defined as a transient loss of consciousness resulting from inadequate cerebral perfusion.

Collecting a history by asking skillful, directed, age-appropriate questions and looking for clues is essential in making a diagnosis. The age of the child, the events preceding the episode, the child's memory of the episode, and the state of consciousness after the episode are all important clues. The diagnosis will heavily rely on the subjective data collected.

Box 39-16 Seizure First Aid (What to Do during a Seizure)

Stay calm.

Turn the child on his or her side.

Loosen any tight clothing on the child.

Do not put anything in the child's mouth.

Move hard objects away so the child does not get hurt.

Stay with the child until the seizure stops.

Note the time the seizure begins and ends.

Call 911 if the seizure does not stop within 10 minutes or the child stops breathing.

Management

Status epilepticus

Treatments and medications

- Remember the ABCs; manage the child's airway, breathing, and circulation. This is a medical emergency.
- Carry out seizure first aid (Box 39-16).
- Obtain intravenous access. In extreme situations, an intraosseous route may be used. Administer diazepam 0.2 to 0.5 mg/kg over 2 to 3 minutes, intravenously or rectally. This may be repeated every 5 to 10 minutes if the seizure continues. The maximum dose for a child is 5 mg. Possibly administer longer-acting anticonvulsant medication (Table 39-8). Determine anticonvulsant serum levels (as appropriate).

Counseling and prevention

- Advise parents that prolonged seizures, such as those with status epilepticus, can cause residual effects.
- If the patient is epileptic, review the administration of antiepileptic medication and reinforce the danger of abruptly discontinuing the medication.
- Discuss how to monitor for drug side effects and reinforce medication teaching.

Follow-up. Provide follow-up for well-child care as determined by a neurologist.

Consultations and referrals

- Establish contact with the child and family during hospitalization to maintain continuity of care.
- Refer the child to a neurologist for management of the disease.
- Refer the child to a visiting nurse service to assess compliance with the treatment plan.
- Refer the parents to support groups.

Infantile spasms

Treatments and medications. Infant spasms are a medical emergency. The standard in treating infantile spasms is intramuscular adrenocorticotropic hormone (ACTH). The medication is in short supply and is available only by compassionate use through the National Organization of Rare Diseases (NORD). Hospitalization is necessary to start treatment, which is then done by the parents or caregivers.

Other medications used include clonazepam, valproate, topiramate, zonisamide, and vigabatrin (Sabril, which is not approved by the Food and Drug Administration [FDA] but is available through Canada and Europe). Carefully monitor the child's development and response to treatment.

Counseling and prevention

- Advise parents that the morbidity is very high. Prognosis is dependent on the cause (idiopathic infantile spasms seem to have the best outcome), preexisting neurologic condition (none is most favorable), and the time between the onset of seizures and treatment (treatment initiated within 1 month of onset may have more favorable outcome).
- Teach the parents intramuscular injection techniques and the side effects of the medications because the child will most likely be sent home on a regimen of intramuscular ACTH. Side effects of ACTH may include hypertension, hyperglycemia, irritability, and gastrointestinal (GI) bleeding.

Follow-up. See the patient for well-child care. Follow-up evaluation is determined by the neurologist.

Consultations and referrals

- Refer the child to a neurologist for management.
- Refer the child to a visiting nurse service to assess compliance with the treatment plan.
- Refer the parents to support groups.
- Collaborate with the neurologist in implementing the treatment plan, monitoring the side effects of medication, determining the response to treatment, and evaluating the need for rehabilitation services.

Reactive or provoked seizures

Treatments and medications. Treat the underlying cause.

Counseling and prevention. Counsel the family as appropriate about the underlying cause.

Follow-up. Follow-up as indicated by the cause and for well-child care.

Consultations and referrals. If treatment of the underlying cause fails to control the seizure, refer the child to a pediatric neurologist.

Nonreactive or unprovoked seizures

Treatments and medications. For a single unprovoked seizure, if the neurologic examination and EEG are normal and there are no risk factors for epilepsy, no treatment may be necessary. If the neurologic examination or EEG is abnormal or there are risk factors, anticonvulsant drug therapy should be considered.

For a second unprovoked seizure (epilepsy), consider anticonvulsant drug therapy. Monotherapy (single drug) is the goal. If monotherapy fails, two concurrent antiepileptic drugs may be prescribed by the neurologist. The duration of therapy is dependent on the neurologic findings, cause, and EEG findings. If the child is seizure free for 1 to 2 years of age, the neurologist may reevaluate the treatment plan and consider discontinuation of drug therapy. Less common treatments, reserved for intractable seizures, include a ketogenic diet, the vagal nerve stimulator, and epilepsy surgery.

Counseling and prevention

For a single unprovoked seizure:

- Inform the parents that the risk of recurrence is approximately 50%, usually within 3 months of the initial seizure.
- Advise that anticonvulsant therapy has potential side effects; therefore the benefit of therapy does not outweigh the risk and is not recommended unless there are risk factors or an abnormal EEG or neurologic examination.
- Instruct the parents or caregiver in seizure first aid (see Box 39-16).
- Teach the parents and child how to access medical care. For a second unprovoked seizure (epilepsy):
- Inform the parents that the likelihood of recurrence is 75% without treatment.
- Advise the parents and child that monotherapy is effective in up to 80% of all epilepsy cases.

Table 39-8 Anticonvulsant Medications

TRADE (GENERIC)	INDICATIONS*	AVAILABLE FORMS	DOSING
Carbatrol (extended-release carbamazepine)	Seizures in children and adults	200-mg and 300-mg capsules	5-10 mg/kg per day to start divided tid Maximum of 35 mg/kg per day
Cerebyx (fosphenytoin)	Status epilepticus; seizures	2-ml and 10-ml vials of 50 mg phenytoin equivalent (PE)/ml IM/IV	Loading dose of 10-20 PE/kg/IV Maintenance 4-6 PE/kg per day
Depakene/Depakote (valproic acid/divalproex sodium)	Seizures in children 10 years and older and adults	250-mg/5-ml syrup; 125-mg sprinkles; 250-mg and 500-mg tablets	0.1 mg-0.2 mg/kg bid/tid 10-15 mg/kg per day qd/tid Maximum 60 mg/kg per day
Diastat (diazepam rectal gel)	Cluster seizures and status epilepticus	2.5-mg, 5-mg, and 10-mg rectal gel	0.2 mg-0.5 mg/kg by age
Dilantin (phenytoin)	Seizures in children and adults	30-mg and 100-mg capsules; 50-mg chewable; 125-mg/5-ml suspension	5-10 mg/kg per day bid
Gabatril (tiagabine)	Partial seizures in children 12 years and older and adults	4-mg, 12-mg, and 16-mg tablets	4-32 mg/day bid/qid
Keppra (levetiracetam)	Add on for partial seizures in adults	250-mg and 500-mg tab	500-3000 mg/day bid
Klonopin (clonazepam)	Seizures in children and adults	0.5-mg, 1-mg and 2-mg tablets	0.01-0.03 mg/kg per day bid/tid to start
Lamictal (lamotrigine)	Add on for partial seizures in children 16 years and older and adults	5-mg and 25-mg chewable tablets; 25-mg, 50-mg, 100-mg, 150-mg, and 200-mg tablets	0.15-0.6 mg/kg per day qd to start Maintenance of 1-15 mg/kg per day bid
Mysoline (primidone)	Seizures in children 8 years and older and adults	50-mg and 250-mg tablets; 125-mg chewable; 250-mg/5-cc suspension	10-25 mg/kg per day tid/qid Maximum of 1500 mg/day
Neurontin (gabapentin)	Add on partial seizures in children 12 years and older and adults	100-mg, 300-mg, and 400-mg tablets	300-mg po qd to start Maximum of 3600 mg/day tid
Phenobarbital (phenobarbital)	Seizures in children and adults	15-mg, 30-mg, 60-mg, and 100-mg tablets; 20-mg/5-ml elixir	3-5 mg/kg per day bid
Sabril (vigabatrin)	Infantile spasms (not FDA-approved in the United States)	500-mg tablets and 500-mg sachets	500-mg per day to start Maximum of 1-2 gm/day bid
Tegretol (carbamazepine)	Seizures in children and adults	100-mg chewable tablets; 200-mg tablets; 100-mg/5-ml suspension	5-10 mg/kg per day bid/qid Maximum of 20 mg/kg per day
Tegretol XR (extended-release carbamazepine)	Seizures in children and adults	100-mg, 200-mg, and 400-mg capsules	5-10 mg/kg per day bid/qid Maximum of 20 mg/kg per day
Topamax (topiramate)	Add on partial seizures children 2 years of age and older and adults	25-mg, 100-mg, 200-mg tablets; 15-mg and 25-mg sprinkle caps	1-3 mg/kg/qd to start Maintenance of 5-9 mg/kg per day bid
Trileptal (oxcarbazepine)	Add on partial seizures children 4 years of age and older and adults	150-mg, 300-mg, and 600-mg tablets	8-10 mg/kg per day to start Maximum of 900-1800 mg per day
Zarontin (ethosuximide)	Absence seizures in children and adults	250-mg tablets; 250-mg/5-ml syrup	3-8 mg/kg per day by age
Zonegran (zonisamide)	Partial seizures in adults	100-mg capsules	100-mg po qd to start Maximum of 600 mg/day

*Check a drug reference for pregnancy category and counsel females of child-bearing age of potential teratogenic effects.
**Consult a drug reference book for a complete list of interactions.

- Instruct the parents or caregiver in seizure first aid (see Box 39-16).
- Advise the parents and child about seizure management (Box 39-17).
- Teach the parents and child about medication administration, the need for trade name products, their side effects, and how to monitor the side effects.
- Discuss the effects of epilepsy on daily living and maturational issues (e.g., pregnancy, driving, career choices).

Follow-up
- Provide follow-up for well-child care. The practitioner should evaluate, at the time of the routine checkup, the patient's compliance with and implementation of the treatment plan prescribed by the neurologist, the patient's acceptance of the diagnosis, and the integration of the condition into daily living.
- If anticonvulsant therapy is prescribed, follow-up care should be done in consultation with the neurologist.

LEVELS	SIDE EFFECTS	INTERACTIONS**
4-12 μg/ml	Drowsiness, dizziness, ataxia, blurred vision, nausea, CBC changes, rash	Biaxin/erythromycin increases levels and may decrease birth control effect
10-20 μg/ml of phenytoin	Nystagmus, dizziness, somnolence, hypotension	Read vial carefully because dose is in phenytoin equivalents (should be diluted)
50-120 mg/dl	Drowsiness, nausea, CBC changes, liver damage, increased appetite	Avoid CNS depressants Avoid antacids within 2 hours of dose
N/A	Sedation, hypotension, bradycardia respiratory depression	Avoid CNS depressants Avoid antacids within 2 hours of dose
10-20 mcg/ml	Dizziness, drowsiness, nystagmus, ataxia, gingival hyperplasia	Avoid grapefruit juice
Not clinically useful	Dizziness, drowsiness, nystagmus, ataxia, fatigue	Avoid CNS depressants Avoid antacids within 2 hours of dose
N/A	Dizziness, drowsiness, asthenia, infection	Avoid CNS depressants Avoid antacids within 2 hours of dose
10 ng/ml and 80 ng/ml Not clinically useful Not clinically useful	Drowsiness, dizziness, ataxia, blurred vision, constipation, drooling, urinary retention Rash, Steven's Johnson syndrome, nausea, dizziness, blurred vision	Avoid CNS depressants Avoid antacids within 2 hours of dose Avoid CNS depressants Avoid antacids within 2 hours of dose
4-8 mg/dl primidone 15-40 mg/dl phenobarbital	Drowsiness, dizziness, hyperactivity, rash	Avoid CNS depressants Avoid antacids within 2 hours of dose
N/A	Dizziness, drowsiness, fatigue, nystagmus, ataxia	Avoid CNS depressants Avoid antacids within 2 hours of dose
15-40 mg/dl	Dizziness, drowsiness, rash, hyperactivity, fever	Avoid CNS depressants Avoid antacids within 2 hours of dose
N/A	Visual field cuts, dizziness, drowsiness, behavior changes	Avoid CNS depressants Avoid antacids within 2 hours of dose
4-12 μg/ml	Dizziness, drowsiness, CBC changes, nausea, ataxia, mood changes	Biaxin/erythromycin increases levels and may decrease birth control effect
4-12 μg/ml	Dizziness, drowsiness, CBC changes, nausea, ataxia, mood changes	Biaxin/erythromycin increases levels and may decrease birth control effect
N/A	Cognitive dysfunction, kidney stones, weight loss, dizziness, diarrhea	Avoid CNS depressants Avoid antacids within 2 hours of dose
N/A	Dizziness, drowsiness, hyponatremia, headache, rash	Avoid CNS depressants Avoid antacids within 2 hours of dose
50-100 μg/ml	Nausea, vomiting, CBC changes, headache, drowsiness, dizziness	Avoid CNS depressants Avoid antacids within 2 hours of dose
N/A	Somnolence, headache, anorexia, dizziness, headache, mental slowing	Avoid CNS depressants Avoid antacids within 2 hours of dose

Consultations and referrals
- Consult with a physician for any first-time seizure.
- Refer the patient to a neurologist if seizures recur. If anticonvulsant therapy is prescribed, follow up with the neurologist. The practitioner should evaluate, at the time of the routine checkup, the patient's compliance with and implementation of the treatment plan prescribed by the neurologist, the patient's acceptance of the diagnosis, and the integration of the condition into daily living. Consult with a neurologist regarding the treatment plan

Febrile seizures
Treatment and medications
- Manage seizures as discussed in Box 39-17.
- Consider giving a prescription for Diastat (diazepam for rectal use) in consultation with a pediatric neurologist if the seizures are very frequent. Instructions for use vary from administration at the onset of fever to administration at the first sign of seizure.
- Implement fever control (see Fever in Chapter 43).

Box 39-17 Seizure Prevention and Teaching

Precautions for the Child and Parents

Always wear medical identification.

Never swim alone.

Supervise small children in the bathtub.

Let someone know when showering.

Wear protective headgear as needed.

Notify school personnel of the condition.

Do not drive a car or operate machinery if actively having seizures.

Never drink alcoholic beverages.

Take oral contraceptives under a neurologist's supervision.

Because of the teratogenic effects of anticonvulsants, seek a neurologist's guidance when planning pregnancy.

Remember that bicycling and horseback riding should be supervised.

Remember that the individual, family members, school personnel, and outside caregivers (e.g., babysitter, nurse) should know seizure first aid.

Avoid activities involving heights (e.g., rope climbing, rock climbing).

Precautions for the Practitioner

Always prescribe trade-name anticonvulsants.

Instruct the child and parents to bring medications to all health-care visits.

Teach the child and parents the signs and symptoms of toxicity and the common side effects of medications.

Advise the child and parents to never stop medication without the supervision of a neurologist.

Counseling and prevention

- Inform the parents that the overall risk of recurrence is 50%, of which 90% of seizures recur within 2 years of the initial episode.
- Keep in mind that recurrence is most common in children with a first episode during the first year of life.
- Remember that the risk of epilepsy is slightly greater for these patients than for the general population but remains low (approximately 3% to 5%).
- Instruct the parents on the treatment plan for fever.
- Advise the parents to call if seizure recurs.
- Offer reassurance and support.

Follow-up. Make a telephone call within 24 hours to offer support.

Consultations and referrals

- Refer the child to a physician if the sequence of events is atypical.
- Consult with a physician if it is the first episode.
- Refer the child to a physician if the neurologic examination is abnormal, the child has any risk factors for epilepsy, or the seizure is atypical. An atypical febrile seizure is characterized as lasting longer than 10 minutes, exhibiting movements indicative of a partial seizure, having a prolonged recovery period greater than 2 hours, or occurring in a child who appears very ill or has a severe developmental delay or abnormal neurologic examination.

Breath-holding spells. See also Breath-Holding in Chapter 19.

Treatments and medications. None are indicated. Screen for iron-deficiency anemia, which may be associated with breath-holding spells.

Counseling and prevention

- Instruct the parents that the attack is harmless and always stops by itself.
- Suggest to the parents that they apply a cold cloth to the child's forehead until breathing starts again. Do not use smelling salts.
- Have the parents time the length of the attack with the second hand of a watch.
- Tell parents not to try to resuscitate. It may be harmful, and it is unnecessary.
- After the attack, advise the parents to give the child brief support with a hug.
- Assist the parents in identifying precipitating factors and using avoidance or distraction.
- Advise that attacks are more frequent when parents respond by running and picking up the child every time crying starts or when parents give in to their child immediately after the attack. Encourage parents to avoid this reinforcing behavior.

Follow-up. Schedule a return visit immediately if attacks occur four or more times a week, last longer than 60 seconds, or undergo a change in the sequence of events.

Consultations and referrals. Refer the child to a physician if there is any suspicion of a seizure (i.e., the patient is younger than 3 months of age, experiences clonic jerks more than three times per week, or holds breath longer than 60 seconds) or if the sequence of events is not classic.

Syncope

Treatments and medications. Use ammonia or smelling salts.

Counseling and prevention

- Advise the parents that immediately after the episode the child should lie down for 10 minutes. Assist the parents and child in identifying precipitating factors.
- Encourage a balanced diet, including the need for proper hydration.
- Discuss present coping mechanisms and their effectiveness.
- Assist the child and parents in exploring other coping mechanisms.

Follow-up. Schedule a return visit if the episode occurs again.

Consultations and referrals

- Refer the child to a physician if there is any suspicion of a cardiac problem or a family history of sudden death or the condition is repetitive.
- Remember that therapy and prognosis greatly vary among these conditions. Collecting a history by asking skillful, directed, age-appropriate questions and looking for clues is essential in making a diagnosis. The age of the child, the events preceding the episode, the child's memory of the episode, and the state of consciousness after the episode are all important clues. The diagnosis will heavily rely on the subjective data collected.

Resources

Epilepsy Foundation of America, 4351 Garden City Drive, Landover, MD 20785; (301) 459-3700; www.efa.org

Suicide Attempts and Suicide

SUSAN M. WATSON

Alert

Consult with or refer to a physician or mental health professional for the following:

- Previous suicide attempt or any suicide ideation or thoughts of death
- Any suicide plan or availability of a weapon
- Giving away of possessions or writing notes about death
- Symptoms of depression or other psychiatric disorders
- Feelings of low self-esteem
- Antisocial behaviors (e.g., poor impulse control, truancy, delinquency, isolation, self-injurious behavior)
- Substance abuse
- Family dysfunction or poor family interactions
- Feelings and statements reflecting hopelessness (e.g., "My family is better off without me.")

Etiology

There is no one comprehensive theory to explain the cause of childhood or adolescent suicide. The cause appears to involve a combination of genetic, developmental, social, psychologic, and environmental factors. For example, most victims of suicide have been shown to have had a psychiatric illness. The most common mental illnesses associated with suicide are depression and bipolar illness. Those without a psychiatric diagnosis frequently have experienced severe anxiety, exhibited violent, impulsive behaviors, displayed deficient social skills, related poorly to family and friends, and have had few or no plans for the future. Completed suicides and suicide attempts are most often preceded by a "precipitant." Examples of some common precipitants include a recent or long-existing loss, family dysfunction, family or school violence, rejection, pregnancy, a sexually transmitted disease (STD), or physical or sexual abuse. Significant alcohol or drug use may be another contributing factor.

Environmental factors associated with suicide attempts, successes, or gestures include exposure to suicide in family and friends and the availability of weapons or drugs. The child or adolescent can be exposed to suicide by a classmate, a relative, or the media. Suicide imitators, or "copycat suicides," are common among adolescents, especially if they are already vulnerable. In recent years guns, knives, and a variety of drugs are readily available to children and adolescents. The availability of such destructive instruments has been associated with the increase in more violent suicidal actions.

Family history also plays a major role in the cause of suicide. Among child and adolescent suicide attempters and victims, there is a strong family history of mental illness, substance abuse, and suicidal actions and attempts. There seems to be more family conflict, ineffective communication skills, poor coping skills, and little support in families of suicide attempters and completers.

Incidence

- Suicide is the third most common cause of death in 15- to 19-year-olds in the United States, accounting for 13% of the total mortality in this age group.
- Over the past 30 years the suicide rate among adolescents has more than tripled.
- According to a survey in 1998 for students in grades 9 to 12, 24% have considered suicide, 17.7% have a specific plan, and 8.7% have attempted suicide
- Among suicidal attempters there is a strong history of alcohol and drug use.
- The suicide rate (successful) is six times higher in 15- to 19-year-old males than females; males tend to choose more lethal methods.
- The rate for suicide attempts (unsuccessful) is twice as great in females 15 to 19 years of age as in males; females tend to choose less lethal methods
- Suicide behaviors occur in all races and socioeconomic groups, but rates are highest in Native American adolescent males and lowest in African-American adolescent females.
- In grades 7 to 12, 20% to 28% of bisexual and homosexual youth attempt suicide.
- The most common method (more than 67% of cases) used in completed suicides is firearms (handguns), of which 90% are fatal, followed by hanging, jumping, carbon monoxide poisoning, explosives, and poisoning.
- Males tend to choose the more lethal and more violent forms, including firearms, hanging, and explosives; females more frequently choose poisonings.
- Common poisoning agents used include aspirin, hypnotics, sedatives, and painkillers.
- The most common methods used in suicide gestures are poisoning and wrist-cutting.
- Suicide is probably underreported because of the confusing nature of single-driver, single-car lethal accidents.

Risk Factors

- Previous suicide attempts (risk for reattempt is greatest in the first 3 months after the attempt)
- Psychiatric illness (e.g., major depressive or conduct disorder)
- Suicidal ideation, with or without a plan
- Relative or relatives with an affective disorder or a suicide success or attempt
- Patient or family substance and alcohol abuse
- Family discord (e.g., divorce, violence, abuse, conflict, no support, poor communication)
- Psychosocial traits (e.g., impulsiveness, truancy, hostility, hopelessness, poor social skills, isolation)
- Availability of weapons or drugs or medications
- Exposure to a suicide by family member or friend, or in community (e.g., school shooting, by the media)
- Chronic pain or debilitating illness and disability
- Academic failure
- Break-up of adolescent romantic relationship
- Living out of the home (e.g., at a correctional facility, group home)
- Legal difficulties
- Gay or bisexual preference

Differential Diagnosis

A suicide or suicide attempt is a true crisis. The completed suicide, a suicide gesture, or suicidal ideation are all interrelated. They differ only in the degree of severity: death or near-death. A completed suicide is a tragic ending resulting in death. A suicide attempt is an intentional, self-harming act that does not result in death. It may represent the ultimate attempt to communicate. Suicidal gestures are believed to reflect ambivalence. There seems to be a desire to die, yet there is a call for help. Suicidal ideations are thoughts or wishes about self-harm or ending one's life. These thoughts may or may not involve a suicide plan, including the method. The thoughts may be vague or well thought out. Suicidal thoughts are often associated with a preoccupation of death. All threats, attempts, and gestures are desperate acts that require serious attention.

Although a suicide usually cannot be predicted, the practitioner should be aware of risk factors (see previous section) associated with suicide attempts and thoughts. The practitioner is in an excellent position to detect self-destructive behaviors and thoughts. In a primary care setting the practitioner is often the child's or adolescent's first contact and therefore needs to be alert to the warning signs and be able to identify who is at risk (see Alert box and Risk Factors). Fortunately, in most cases involving suicide the practitioner is faced with attempts and thoughts rather than the final act.

Anyone determined to be "at risk" for suicide requires a comprehensive evaluation with questions aimed at identifying any signs of ideation. The practitioner should not hesitate to ask direct questions regarding suicide (Box 39-18). Questions about suicide will not initiate thoughts or actions. It has been shown such questions may give the vulnerable child or adolescent the opportunity to talk about a very frightening issue.

A comprehensive history and physical examination are necessary. Assess suicidal risk with questions regarding changes in appetite or sleep, social isolation, violent or rebellious behavior, running away, neglect in appearance, giving away possessions, or thoughts of death (see Box 39-18). The degree of parental involvement with the child or adolescent needs to be assessed. Whenever suicidal risk is determined, parents must be informed despite any issues of confidentiality previously established with the adolescent. The family history should be assessed regarding the presence of any risk factors or any potential precipitating factors, including family discord, family violence, family substance abuse, divorce, death, or history of mental illness. The past medical and psychiatric history, including depression, must be explored. Any behavioral or interpersonal concerns like police arrests, school problems, substance abuse, poor self-esteem, and personal or romantic loss need to be identified. The physical examination is normal except there may be a change or decline in personal appearance or hygiene. Laboratory work-up is generally not necessary.

Management

All suicide gestures must be referred to a mental health professional for a more detailed evaluation and treatment. Prompt mental health intervention should be pursued in any child or adolescent determined to be at risk for suicide. Any child or adolescent who has persistent suicidal ideations or has a history of a previous attempt should also be referred to a mental health professional.

Treatments and medications. The suicidal patient is managed by a mental health professional. A child or adolescent making suicidal gestures or having suicidal thoughts may require hospitalization (Box 39-19). The length of the admission depends on the result of the evaluation and on the family dynamics. Treatment generally focuses on providing a safe environment, identification and treatment of any mental illness, and the identification and resolution of personal and family conflict.

Counseling and prevention

- Listen to the patient and never dismiss his or her problems as trivial.
- Look for nonverbal clues (e.g., poor eye contact).
- Reassure the child or adolescent that he or she is not alone.
- Be direct and honest with the patient and family. Let them know that you are concerned and why.

Box 39-18 Suicide Risk Evaluation

1. Has a member of the patient's family ever attempted suicide?
2. Has the patient been treated for a mental illness?
3. Does the patient have a chronic, debilitating medical illness?
4. Does the patient have a history of self-destructive behavior (e.g., recklessness, propensity for accidents, alcohol abuse, drug abuse, self-abuse)?
5. Has the patient ever attempted suicide?
6. Has the patient experienced a loss (e.g., of a friend, loved one, pet) within the previous 3 months?
7. Is the patient socially isolated, without friends or support?
8. Is the patient exhibiting signs of psychosis now?
9. Is the patient clinically depressed?
10. Does the patient say he or she wishes to die?
11. Has the patient experienced a recent elevation in mood?
12. Does the patient regret that his or her suicide attempt failed?
13. Does the patient plan to try suicide again?
14. Does the patient hear voices telling him or her to kill self?
15. Has the patient decided to kill self?
16. Does the patient have a plan of action for suicide?

Interpreting the Results

High risk—"Yes" to any question numbered 12-16
Moderate risk—"Yes" to any four questions numbered 3-11, provided that all answers to questions 12-16 are "No"
Low risk—"Yes" to less than four questions numbered 3-11, provided that all answers to questions 12-16 are "No"
No risk—"No" to all questions numbered 3-16

Box 39-19 Indications for Hospitalization

Acute risk
- Medical complications associated with the attempt
- High intent and lethal method
- No compliance with therapy after previous attempt

Psychiatric illness
- Depression
- Psychosis

Suicidal thoughts, with a well-thought-out plan and ambivalence regarding wanting to live

Dysfunctional and nonsupportive family
- Parental psychiatric illness
- Environment unsafe for the patient because of abuse or parental alcohol or drug use

Substance-abusing patient

- Assure the patient and family that thinking about suicide does not mean that a person is "crazy," but it does mean intervention is needed.
- Instruct the family and patient on the need to eliminate all weapons and drugs from the home. No driving should be allowed for 24 hours.
- Educate the family and school on the warning signs and the fact that suicide can be prevented.
- Remember that the school and family need to be alert to changes in behavior. Involvement in risky behaviors (e.g., sexual activity, substance use, daredevil tricks), giving away of possessions, unusual purchases (e.g., ropes, hoses, razors, weapons), sudden happiness after prolonged depression, verbal threats (e.g., "Things will be better without me"), and depressive symptoms (e.g., sleep and appetite changes, somatic complaints, school and social changes) need attention.
- Support and encourage compliance with the mental health intervention for both the patient and family.
- Stress the importance of family communication.
- Stress the importance of individual and or family therapy.
- Give the patient and family suicide hotline numbers in their community.

Follow-up
- Maintain close contact with the patient, family, and mental health professional.
- Make a telephone call to maintain close contact, show an active interest in the patient, and promote compliance with treatment. The practitioner is the primary provider and most familiar with the patient and family, therefore being in the best position to promote compliance with the mental health intervention.
- Remember that any sign of a recurring problem requires immediate intervention (see Alert box).

Consultations and referrals
- Keep in mind that referral to a mental health professional is necessary for anyone who expresses suicidal ideation or has attempted suicide. Never take any chances. It may be possible that someone who exhibits suicidal behavior may have no intention of ending his or her life. But never wait to find out. If the patient is at risk, a referral is warranted.
- Refer the patient and family to local support groups.
- Provide the patient and family the numbers for local mental health hotlines (e.g., suicide hotlines). Provide internet resource information sites.

Resources

Hotlines
Suicide Prevention Hotline: (800) 827-7571
National Youth Crisis Hotline: (800) 422-HOPE
Websites
Association of Suicidology (www.suicidology.org)
Kids in Trouble (www.geocities.com/EnchantedForest/2910)
National Directory of Support Groups for Survivors of Suicide (www.suicidology.org/survivorssupport.htm)
Road2Healing (e-mail group) (www.yahoogroups.com) (list messages go to road2healing@yahoogroups.com
SCABS: Second Chance At Beating Suicide (e-mail group) (www.yahoogroups.com) (list messages go to 2ndchance@yahoogroups.com)
Survivor Teens of Loved One's Suicide (STOLOS) (e-mail group) (www.yahoogroups.com) (list messages go to STOLOS@yahoogroups.com)

Tics

BARBARA GOLDEN

Alert

Refer to a physician when other movements are present besides tics:
- Myoclonus (sudden, shocklike contractions of a muscle or muscle group)
- Tremor (regular, rhythmic, involuntary muscle movement)
- Chorea (brief burst of rapid, jerky movements, unpredictable, and rarely repetitive)
- Dystonia (involuntary slow twisting movements of large muscle groups of the trunk, neck, and limbs)
- Hemiparesis

Etiology

The most common cause of tic disorders is heredity. Hereditary tics are most often seen in male children. Often a careful history and discussion with the parents about family members reveals a dominant inheritance. Tics may also occur sporadically, when no other family members are affected.

Secondary causes of tic disorders are uncommon. They include birth injuries of various types, head trauma, encephalitis, and metabolic disorders.

Incidence

- Tic disorders affect between 1 and 10 per 10,000 persons
- Transient tic disorder (duration of less than 1 year) occurs in approximately 5% to 24% of schoolchildren.
- Tic disorders are more common in males than in females (3:1).
- An estimated one third of cases resolve by late adolescence.
- Tic disorders are more common in mentally retarded children.

Risk Factors

- Positive family history of tics
- School age
- Male gender
- Emotional stressors (e.g., death, divorce, illness)
- Mental retardation
- Psychostimulant treatment for ADHD

Differential Diagnosis

Tics are involuntary, sudden, rapid, repetitive, nonrhythmic stereotyped movements or vocalizations. They vary in duration and degree of complexity. Common characteristics of tics include brief voluntary suppression; exacerbation by anxiety, excitement, anger, or fatigue; reduction during absorbing activities or sleep; and fluctuation over time. There are three categories of tics: *motor, vocal* (each subdivided into simple and complex), and *sensory* (Box 39-20).

Simple motor tics are brief rapid movements that involve one muscle group (such as eye blink, head jerk, shoulder shrug). *Complex motor tics* are abrupt movements that involve either a cluster of simple tics or a more coordinated sequence of movements that serve no purpose (e.g., touch, clap, jump, smell). These should not be confused with compulsions, which are usually preceded by a conscious need to perform the action.

Box 39-20 Examples of Tic Behaviors per Classification

Simple motor tics—Eye blinking, eyebrow raising, facial grimace, head turning, nose wrinkling
Complex motor tics—Smelling objects, jumping, tapping, clapping hands
Simple vocal tics—Sniffing, grunting, throat clearing, coughing, humming
Complex vocal tics—Stuttering, repeating phrases of syllables, echolalia, palilalia, coprolalia
Sensory tics—Feeling cold, warm, pressure, tickling

Box 39-22 Diagnostic Criteria for Chronic Motor or Vocal Tic Disorder

Single or multiple motor or vocal tics, but not both, present at some time during the illness.
Tics occur many times a day nearly every day or intermittently throughout a period of more than 3 consecutive months.
Onset before 18 years of age
Disturbance not attributable to the direct physiologic effects of a substance or a general medical condition
Criteria not met for Tourette syndrome

Modified from the American Psychiatric Association (2000). The diagnostic and statistical manual of mental disorders (DSM -IV-TR) (4th ed.). Washington, DC: American Psychiatric Association.

Box 39-21 Diagnostic Criteria for Transient Tic Disorders

Presence of single or multiple motor or vocal tics
Tics occur many times a day, nearly every day for at least 4 weeks, but for no longer than 12 consecutive months
Onset before 18 years of age
Distribution not attributable to the direct physiologic effects of a substance or general medical condition
Criteria never met for Tourette syndrome or chronic motor or vocal tic disorder

Modified from the American Psychiatric Association (2000). The diagnostic and statistical manual of mental disorders (DSM -IV-TR) (4th ed.). Washington, DC: American Psychiatric Association.

Box 39-23 Diagnostic Criteria for Tourette Syndrome

Both multiple motor and one or more vocal tics present at some time during the illness, though not necessarily concurrently
Tics occur many times a day nearly every day or intermittently throughout a period of more than 1 year; during this period, never a tic-free period of more than 3 consecutive months
Onset before 18 years of age
Disturbance not attributable to the direct physiologic effects of a substance or a general medical condition

Modified from the American Psychiatric Association (2000). The diagnostic and statistical manual of mental disorders (DSM -IV-TR) (4th ed.). Washington, DC: American Psychiatric Association.

Simple vocal tics represent singular sounds such as sniffing, yelping, or throat clearing. Vocal tics are often discovered by careful history taking and may have been previously diagnosed as allergy symptoms. *Complex vocal tics* may be a string of words, syllables, phrases, echolalia (repeating other people's words), palilalia (repeating one's own words), or coprolalia (saying obscene words).

Sensory tics are described as an uncomfortable or abnormal sensation (e.g., warmth, cold, tickle), often localized to a specific body area.

Tics are further classified on the basis of age of onset, duration, and chronicity. The *Diagnostic and Statistical Manual of Mental Disorders* (DSM-IV) lists criteria for four categories of tic disorders: transient tic disorder (Box 39-21), chronic motor or vocal tic disorder (Box 39-22), Gilles de la Tourette syndrome (Box 39-23), and tic disorder not otherwise specified.

Gilles de la Tourette syndrome, or *Tourette syndrome* (TS), also must be considered when one is evaluating a patient with tics. TS is a chronic disorder characterized by involuntary motor and vocal tics that wax and wane for a period greater than 1 year. Symptoms begin before 18 years of age. In addition to tics, children with TS often have other psychopathologic conditions such as ADHD, obsessive-compulsive disorder (OCD), learning disabilities, and behavior problems. Half of children with tics have an attention deficit disorder, and a third have an OCD.

Attention deficit–hyperactivity disorder is characterized by hyperactivity, shortened attention span, restlessness, difficulty focusing, and impaired impulse control. ADHD is often treated with classroom accommodations, behavior modifications, and stimulant medications. Stimulants should be used with caution because they have the potential to accentuate tics.

Obsessive-compulsive disorder is characterized by ritualistic thoughts and actions. These may include handwashing, touching things, counting objects, and obsessive thoughts stemming from various fears such as violence or disease. OCD is most often treated with cognitive behavioral therapy or selective serotonin reuptake inhibitors (SSRIs).

The nurse practitioner (NP) must be certain not to confuse tics with other movementdisorders. The hallmark feature of tics is that they can be voluntarily suppressed, if only briefly. Essential myoclonus, which often affects the shoulders, cannot be suppressed. Dystonic disorders are typically characterized by sometimes painful, uncontrolled twisting or severe muscle tension.

An abrupt onset or repeated rapid worsening of tics and obsessive-compulsive features has been found to be associated with evidence of group A β-hemolytic streptococcal (GABHS) infections. This is known as PANDAS (pediatric autoimmune neuropsychiatric disorder associated with streptococcal infection). Prompt referral for treatment is imperative.

No diagnostic tests confirm the presence of tics or TS, nor is any of the treatment curative.

Management

Treatments and medications

- Most tic disorders are so mild that they do not require treatment.
- An older child may be instructed to inhibit tics during times when it would be socially inappropriate and then release them when alone.

Table 39-9 Medications Used to Treat Tic Disorders

MEDICATION	DOSE	ADMININSTRATION	COMMON ADVERSE REACTIONS	PRECAUTIONS	CONTRAINDICATIONS
Clonidine (antihypertensive)	0.1-0.3 mg/day 0.025 mg to start	Oral tablet— divided bid or tid Transdermal patch, changed weekly	Drowsiness, dry mouth, constipation, orthostatic hypotension	Begin slowly and taper slowly; monitor blood pressure	Hypersensitivity to medication
Guanfacine (antihypertensive)	Not FDA-approved for use in children 0.5-3 mg/day 0.5 to start	Oral tablet qd or bid	As above	As above	As above
Pimozide (neuroleptic)	0.05-0.2 mg/kg/day in children 12 years and older	Oral tablet bid or tid	Parkinsonian-like symptoms, sedation, tardive dyskinesia, prolonged QT interval, dry mouth, constipation, neuroleptic malignant syndrome*	Avoid alcohol and other CNS depressants; order baseline ECG; taper slowly; tardive dyskinesia may be a lifelong condition	Hepatic or renal dysfunction, congenital long QT interval, cardiac arrhythmias
Haloperidol (neuroleptic)	Initially 0.5 mg/day, not to exceed 3 mg/day	Oral tablets every 12 hours	Tardive dyskinesias, blurred vision, dry mouth, drowsiness, dizziness, neuroleptic malignant syndrome*	Avoid alcohol and other CNS depressants; tardive dyskinesia may be a lifelong condition; taper slowly	CNS depression, glaucoma
Risperidone (neuroleptic)	Not FDA-approved for use in children 0.25-3 mg/day bid, not to exceed 3 mg/day	Oral tablets or liquid bid or tid	As above Weight gain, sedation	As above	Hyperprolactinemia

*Symptoms include fever, tachycardia, tachypnea, diaphoresis, and muscle tightness. Syndrome may be fatal if not recognized early and treated.

- Cognitive-behavioral therapy has been shown to be an effective treatment for OCD, usually in children 7 years of age and older. This entails confronting fears through gradual exposure with the help of a specially trained therapist.
- Pharmacologic therapy is an option (Tables 39-9 and 39-10). Medication is reserved for those with psychosocially or functionally disabling symptoms, only after psychiatric or neurologic consultation.
- If the child is receiving stimulant medications, it is best to reduce the dose or discontinue the drug.
- Alpha-agonists (e.g., clonidine, guanfacine are the initial drugs of choice because side effects are limited to sedation.
- Neuroleptic medications (e.g., haloperidol [Haldol], pimozide, risperidone) may cause sedation as well (less so with risperidone). They can also induce other movement disorders such as acute dystonic reaction, which is bizarre muscle spasms of the head, neck, and tongue. This can be reversed with an antihistamine (diphenhydramine). Tardive dyskinesias may be induced as well. These are abnormal, involuntary movements of the tongue and face, are not easily treated, and may be permanent and disabling.
- Benefits of neuroleptics and alpha-adrenergic receptor agonists, which are started with very low doses, may not be seen for weeks after therapy is started.

Counseling and prevention

- Counsel the parents to pay as little attention as possible to tics so as not to increase tension or create the opportunity for secondary gains.
- Stress to the child and family that tics rarely cause significant discomfort or damage.

- Reassure parents that if the history and physical examination are otherwise normal, it is highly unlikely, based on the nature of tic disorders, that an underlying brain tumor or other serious medical problem could be the cause.
- Instruct the parents and child about the normal waxing and waning course of tics; they may disappear for months only to reappear. Most tics do not persist into adulthood.
- Present teachers and fellow students with educational materials regarding tic disorders.
- Educate parents about the side effects of prescribed medications, especially tardive dyskinesia and dystonic reaction. Instruct parents on the need to safely store medications.
- Alert parents about various comorbid conditions such as ADHD, learning disorders, and OCD.
- Diagnose and treat suspected strep infections without delay.

Follow-up. Frequency of follow-up visits is based on the severity of the tic disorder, trials of new medications, and the level of parent anxiety. After neurologic or psychiatric consultation, a visit is recommended to discuss diagnosis and treatment. Children receiving neuroleptic drugs require regular scheduled visits and telephone consultation to assess for side effects.

Consultations and referrals

- Refer the child to a pediatric psychiatrist or psychologist to help identify and treat stressors in the child's life and to help modify the child's behavior if comorbid problems are present. This should be done before medication therapy.
- Refer the child to a pediatric neurologist if any other movements are present.

Table 39-10 Medications Used to Treat Comorbid Features of Tic Disorders

DISORDER/DRUG	DOSE	ADMINISTRATION	COMMON ADVERSE REACTIONS	PRECAUTIONS	CONTRAINDICATIONS
OCD/SSRIs:					
Fluvoxamine	Ages 8-17 years, 25 mg every hour of sleep to start	Oral: tablets Increase by 25 mg every 4-7 days Doses over 50 mg are divided bid Maximum is 200 mg daily	Somnolence, headache, nausea and vomiting, agitation, insomnia	History of seizures Hepatic disease	Avoid benzodi-azepines
Sertraline	Ages 6-12 years, 25 mg/day Ages 13-17 years, 50 mg/day	Oral: liquid, tablets Increase by 25 mg every 4-7 days Maximum is 200 mg daily	Palpitations As above	History of seizures	MAO inhibitors
ADHD/Stimulants					
Methylphenidate	Begin at 5 mg, increasing by 5 mg as needed, every 4 hours for school-aged children	Oral: tablets, short- and long-acting (4-12 hours)	Headache, abdominal pain, tachycardia, loss of appetite, insomnia, tics	Not to be taken with fruit juice or chewed	Tic disorders, anxiety, agitation
Dexedrine	Begin at 2.5 mg (ages 3-5 years) As above for school-aged children	Oral: tablets, span-sules Short- and long-acting (4-6 hours)	As above	As above	As above
Adderall	As above	Oral: tablets (scored) (6 hours)	As above	As above	As above

Resources

Tourette Society Association (TSA), 42-20 Bell Boulevard, Bayside, NY 11361-9596; (718) 224-2999; www.tourettehelp.com

Bibliography

American Academy of Pediatrics, Committee on Adolescence (2000). Suicide and suicide attempts in adolescents, *Pediatrics, 105*(4), 871-874.

American Psychiatric Association (2000). *The diagnostic and statistical manual of mental disorders (DSM -IV-TR)* (4th ed.). Washington, DC: American Psychiatric Association.

American Psychiatric Association (1994). *Diagnostic and statistical manual of mental disorders*, (4th ed.). Washington, DC: American Psychiatric Association.

Annequin, D., Tournaire, B., & Massiou, H. (2000, June). Migraine and headache in childhood and adolescence. *Pediatric Clinics of North America, 47*, 617-631.

Castiglia, P. (2000). Depression in adolescents. *Journal of Pediatric Health Care, 14*(4), 180-182.

Castiglia, P. (1997). Tourette syndrome. *Journal of Pediatric Health Care, 11*(4), 189-191.

Clarksean, L. (1998, August). Tic disorders in children. *Advance for Nurse Practitioners*, 69-71.

Devinsky, O. (1999). *A guide to understanding and living with epilepsy* (2nd ed.). Philadelphia: F.A. Davis.

Divertie, V. (1996, September-October). Recurrent headaches in children. *American Journal of Maternal Child Nursing, 21*, 235-240.

Forsyth, R. & Farrell, K. (1999). Headaches in childhood. *Pediatrics in Review, 20*, 39-45.

Freeman, J.M., Vining, E.P.G., & Pillas, D.J. (1997). *Seizures and epilepsy in childhood: a guide for parents.* Baltimore: Johns Hopkins University Press.

King, R., Leonard, H., & March, J. (1998). Summary of the practice parameters for the assessment and treatment of children and adolescents with OCD. *Journal of the American Academy of Child and Adolescent Psychiatry, 37*, 1110-1116.

Lynch, J. (1998). Prescribing medications for mood disorders. *Advance for Nurse Practitioners, 6*(3), 22-26.

McGee, S. & Burkett, K.W. (2000). Identifying common pediatric neurosurgical conditions in the primary care setting. *Nursing Clinics of North America, 35*(1).61-85.

Melnyk, B. & Moldenhauer, Z. (1999). Current approaches to depression in children and adolescents. *Advance for Nurse Practitioners, 7*(2), 24-29, 97.

Murphy, S. (2000). Deaths: Final data for 1998 (DHHS Pub. No. [PHS] 2000-1120). *National Vital Statistics Report, 48*(11).

National Institute of Mental Health (2000, revised). *Depression in children and adolescents: A fact sheet for physicians* (NIH Pub. No. 00-4744). Bethesda, MD: National Institute of Mental Health.

Rivera, R.F. & Laureta, E. (1999). Emergency management of seizures: What fits for fits. *Contemporary Pediatrics, 16* (7), 49-63.

Rosenblum, R.K. & Fisher, P. (2001). A guide to children with acute and chronic headaches. *Journal of Pediatric Health Care, 15*(5), 229-235.

Sherry, S. & Jellinik, M. (1996). The many guises of depression. *Contemporary Pediatrics, 13*(5), 64-86.

Swaiman, K. (1999). *Pediatric neurology: Principles and practice* (3rd ed.). St. Louis: Mosby.

Chapter 40 *Reproductive System*

Ambiguous Genitalia, p. 616
Breast Masses and Changes, p. 616
Genital Lesions, p. 618
Menstrual Irregularities, p. 621
Penile Discharge, p. 625
Penile Irritation, p. 627
Pregnancy, p. 628
Undescended Testes (Cryptorchidism), p. 632
Vulvovaginal Symptoms, p. 634

Risk Factors*

- Male premature birth (risk for undescended testicles)
- Positive family history of menstrual irregularities
- Sexually active adolescents
- Unprotected sexual activity
- Multiple sexual partners
- Positive history of sexually transmitted disease (STD)
- Family or child with history of sexual abuse
- Substance abuse

Health Promotion

It is vital for parents and children to feel comfortable providing accurate information related to sexuality and sexual development to the practitioner. It is helpful to encourage parents to communicate openly with their children and answer children's questions about the reproductive system and its function with simple facts using correct terminology. Because parents' comfort with discussion of issues related to sexuality and sexual development varies, it is helpful to routinely discuss these issues during anticipatory guidance. It is best for the practitioner to be honest and straightforward in manner when discussing issues of sexuality and sexual development with patients and parents.

Confidentiality and trust are key components in eliciting accurate information from adolescents. It is vital to their well-being for the practitioner to be aware of the adolescent's circumstances related to reproductive health.

For more information, see also Chapter 17.

Encouragement of Healthy Habits

- Promote open and factual discussion between parents and children about issues of the reproductive system. Encourage parents to use anatomic terms and correct language.
- Teach parents and children to maintain good hygiene (e.g., routine bathing, clean clothing daily, washing hands after toileting, cleansing after toilet use).
- Educate parents and children about the signs of sexual abuse.
- Educate parents and children about safe sex and prevention of STDs. Discuss options, including condom use and abstinence.
- Educate adolescents who are sexually active to recognize the signs and symptoms of STDs.
- Educate girls at the onset of breast development to complete breast self-examination on a monthly basis (Fig. 40-1).
- Educate parents and adolescents that girls should begin having Papanicolaou (Pap) smears at the onset of sexual activity or at 18 years of age.
- Educate adolescent males to conduct a self-testicular examination on a monthly basis.

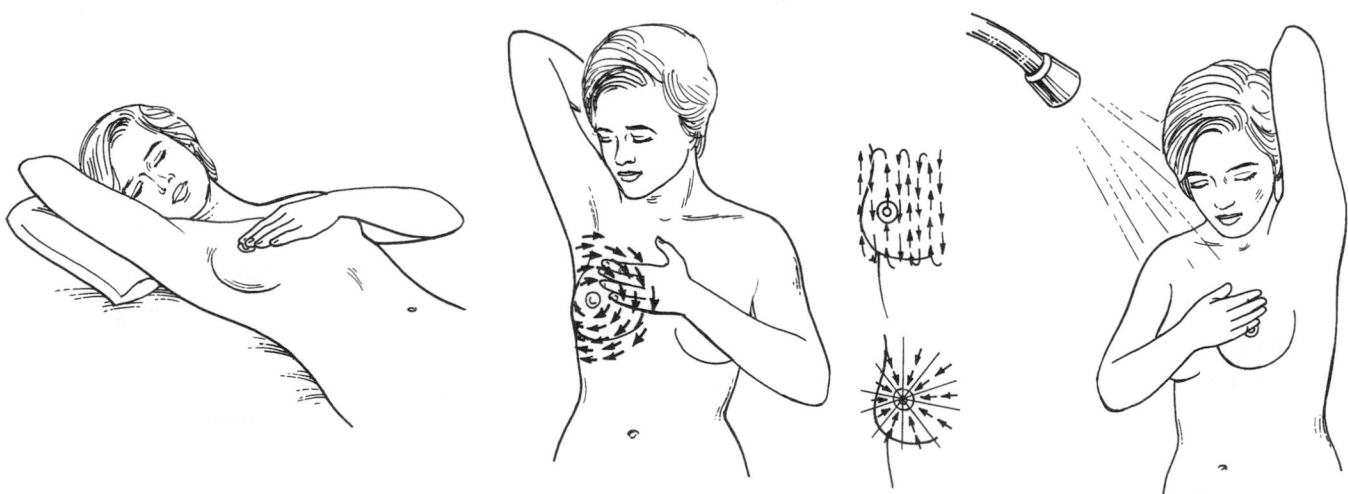

Fig. 40-1 Breast self-examination instructions. (From Lowdermilk, D.L. [2000]. *Maternity and women's health care* [7th ed.]. St. Louis: Mosby.)

*Chapter overview written by Margaret A. McCabe.

Issues of Teenage Pregnancy

- Educate teenagers about pregnancy and the risks associated with unprotected sexual activity (i.e., STDs, pregnancy).
- Inform teenagers of the risk behaviors associated with STDs and pregnancy, including substance use, a tendency to think in the present, and peer pressure.
- Offer teenagers birth control options if they are sexually active or are thinking about becoming sexually active.
- Educate teenagers regarding the risks of multiple sexual partners.
- Identify pregnant teenagers early, with immediate referral for obstetric care.
- Present options to pregnant teenagers, including continuing the pregnancy and becoming a parent, terminating the pregnancy, and continuing the pregnancy followed by adoption.

Subjective Data

Well-child care at all ages should include a history and examination of the external genitalia. Depending on the child's age, the subjective data may be given by the parents, the child, or both parents and child. The history related to a specific concern or symptom should include the location, chronology, severity or amount, aggravating and alleviating factors, associated symptoms (including behavior changes), and the patient's or family's perception of the problem. Elicit a complete history with careful attention to the following:

- Age
- Onset and duration of problem
- Description of the problem, including a review of signs and symptoms (including presence of vaginal or penile discharge, itching, or redness); presence of lesions; burning on urination; and abdominal discomfort
- Indicators of sexual development (may be behavioral or physical; the purpose is to gather information according to the patient's or parents' perspective)
- Past medical history, both general and related to the reproductive system (e.g., parity, menarche, last menses, menstrual cycle pattern, associated discomfort, STDs, pregnancies [number and outcome])
- History of urinary tract infections (UTIs) or cystitis
- Family history related to the reproductive system, including infertility, sexual abuse, anorchia, genetic anomalies, mother's menarche, breast changes, cancers of breast, ovaries, uterus, cervix, and testes
- History of sexual activity, including opposite-sex or same-sex partner, age of sexual debut, number of partners, past history of STDs, and other risk factors
- Birth control, including pattern of current use, method, satisfaction or dissatisfaction, use of barrier methods with nonbarrier methods, and perception of safe sex practices

Objective Data

Physical Examination

The age of the child affects the practitioner's approach to the examination of the reproductive system. For all age groups the procedure should be explained thoroughly with the opportunity for questions and exploration of the equipment that will be used (e.g., light, specula, cotton swabs). Infants and children require the support of a parent during the examina-

tion. The amount of parental involvement depends on the child and the parent and may range from verbal assistance to the mother actually positioning herself on the examination table with the child on top of her to assist the child through the examination. The examination of a female includes inspection and palpation of the breasts and inspection of the external genitalia; it may also include visualization of the vagina and cervix and rectoabdominal palpation. The examination of a male includes inspection and palpation of the breasts, inspection of the external genitalia (including retracting the foreskin if necessary), and palpation of the testes. The Tanner stages should be used to characterize maturation of external genitalia (Box 40-1). Adolescents may prefer to be examined in private, with the information related to the examination being kept confidential. This preference needs to be honored by the practitioner.

Examination of the male genitalia

- *Penis*—Examine the skin for lesions, the foreskin for hygiene and retractability, and the glans for the location of the urinary meatus.
- *Scrotum*—Inspect the skin and scrotal contours. Palpate the testes by blocking the inguinal canal and palpating between the thumb and first two fingers. Palpate the spermatic cord by blocking the inguinal canal and palpating between the thumb and first two fingers from the epididymis to the superficial inguinal ring. Observe for testicular descent, testicular size and shape, scrotal nodules or masses, and swelling. Elicit the cremasteric reflex (movement of testes when skin on front inner thigh is stroked).
- *Hernias*—Inspect inguinal and femoral areas for bulges, and palpate the inguinal canal.

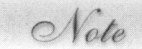

Note

The child may be standing, squatting, or seated cross-legged to enhance the practitioner's ability to palpate the testicles.

Examination of the female genitalia

- *Hernias*—Inspect and palpate for hernias.
- *External examination*—External examination includes the labia, clitoris, urethral orifice, and vaginal opening (Fig. 40-2). Inspect any inflammation, ulceration, discharge, swelling, nodules, or lesions. Palpate the following:
  Bartholin glands: Insert the index finger in vagina and palpate posterior sides between thumb (outside) and index finger (inside).
  Urethra: Insert the index finger in superior portion of the vagina and gently milk urethra.
- *Internal examination (speculum examination)*—See Fig. 40-3. Inspect the cervix for color, position, surface, ulcerations, nodules, masses, bleeding, and discharge. Obtain specimens, including an endocervical brush at the cervical os, a scraping of the cervical surface, and cervical cultures for *Neisseria gonorrhoeae* and *Chlamydia trachomatis*. While removing the speculum, inspect the vaginal mucosa for color, inflammation, discharge, ulcers, and masses.

  For bimanual palpation, insert a lubricated index and middle finger of one hand into the vagina while using the

Box 40-1 Secondary Sex Characteristics (Tanner Stages)

Breast Development

Stage I   Preadolescent; elevation of papilla only
Stage II   Breast and papilla elevated as small mound; areolar diameter increased
Stage III Breast and areola enlarged; no contour separation
Stage IV   Areola and papilla form secondary mound
Stage V   Mature; nipple projects areolar part of general breast contour
Note: Stages IV and V may not be distinct in some patients.

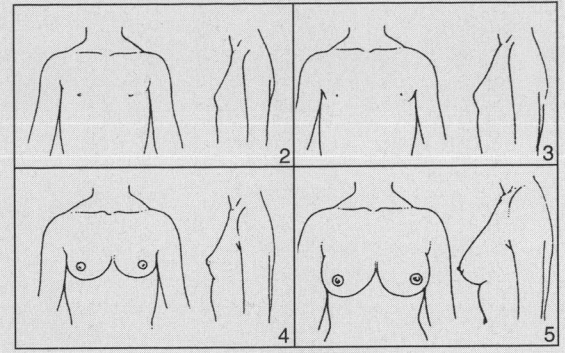

Genital Development (Male)

Stage I   Penis, testes, and scrotum preadolescent
Stage II   Enlargement of scrotum and testes, texture alteration; scrotal sac reddens; penis usually does not enlarge
Stage III Further growth of testes and scrotum; penis enlarges and becomes longer
Stage IV   Continued growth of testes and scrotum; scrotum becomes darker; penis becomes longer; glans and breadth increase in size
Stage V   Genitalia adult in size and shape

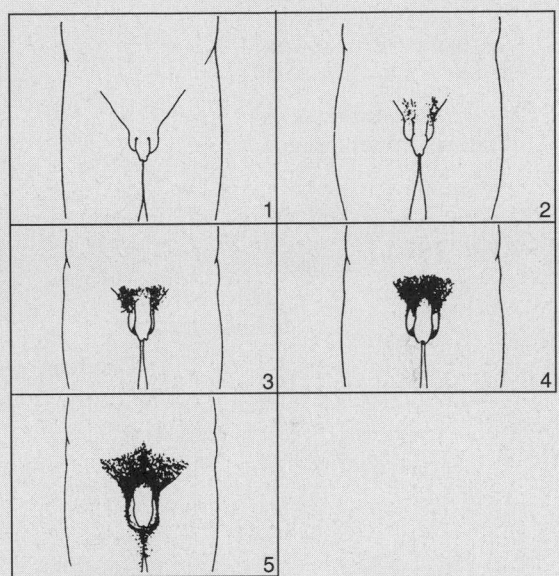

Pubic Hair (Male and Female)

Stage I   None; preadolescent
Stage II   Sparse growth of long, slightly pigmented downy hair, straight or only slightly curled, chiefly at base of penis or along labia
Stage III Considerably darker, coarser and more curled; hair spreads sparsely over junction of pubes
Stage IV   Hair resembles adult in type; distribution still considerably smaller than in adult. No spread to medial surface of thighs.
Stage V   Adult in quantity and type with distribution of the horizontal pattern
Stage VI   Spread up linea alba: "male escutcheon"

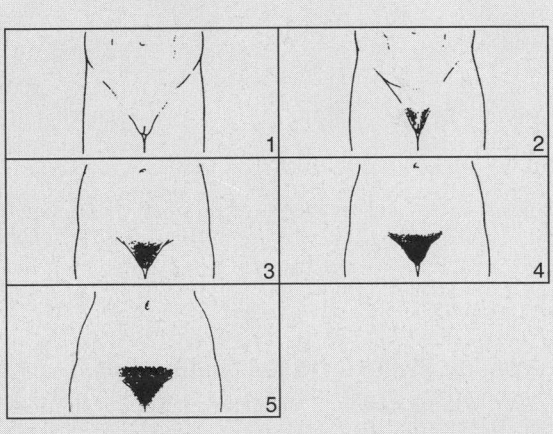

Data adapted from Tanner, J.M. (1962). Growth at adolescence (2nd ed.). Oxford, England: Blackwell Scientific.
Figures from Neinstein, L.S. (1991). Adolescent health care: A practical guide (2nd ed.). Baltimore: Urban & Schwarzenberg.

other hand for abdominal palpation of the uterus and ovaries. Check for the following:
Cervix: Position, shape, consistency, mobility, tenderness
Uterus: Size, shape, consistency, mobility, tenderness, masses
Adnexa: Size, shape, consistency, tenderness

For rectovaginal palpation (Fig. 40-4), insert a lubricated index finger into the vagina and a middle finger into the rectum.
Breasts—Inspect for surface skin changes, dimpling, and discharge from nipples. Palpate using concentric circles or a grid (see Fig. 40-1)

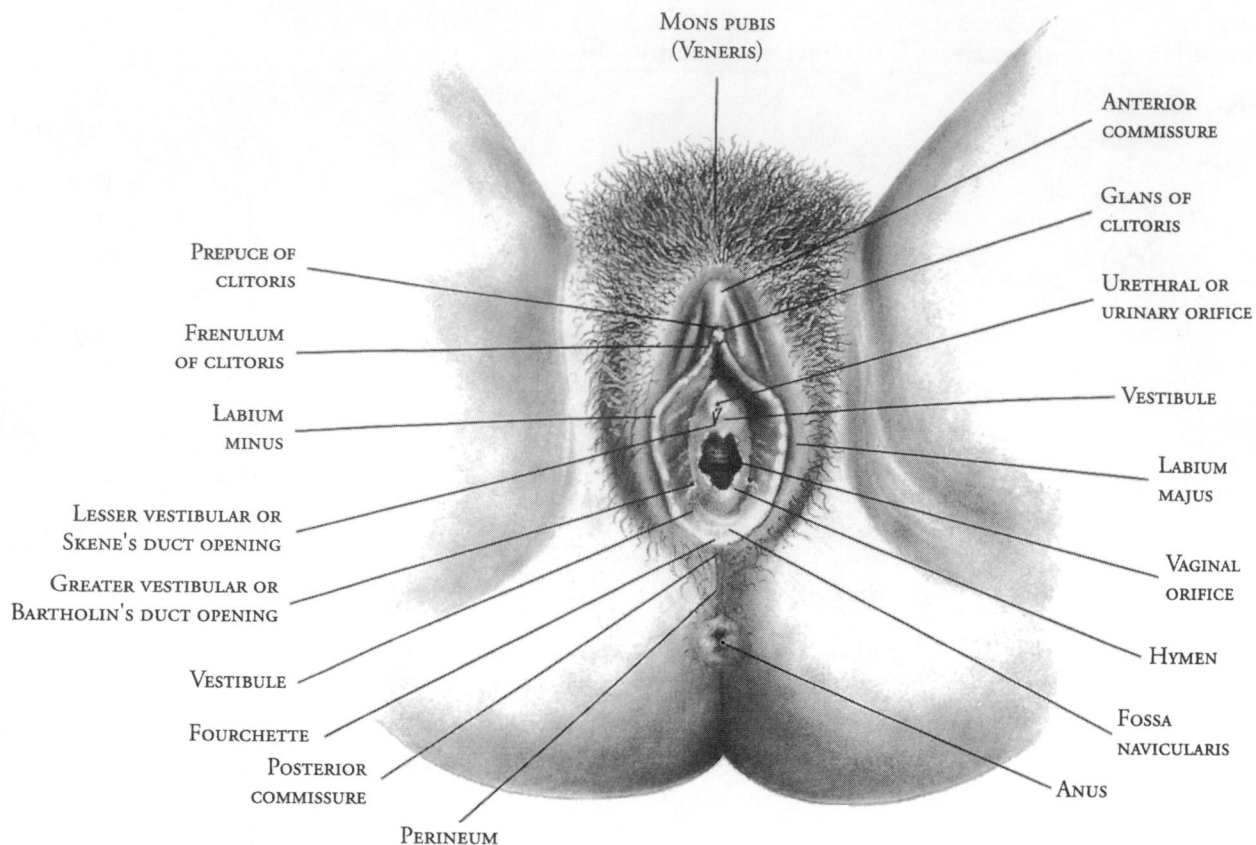

MONS PUBIS
(VENERIS)

PREPUCE OF
CLITORIS

FRENULUM
OF CLITORIS

LABIUM
MINUS

LESSER VESTIBULAR OR
SKENE'S DUCT OPENING

GREATER VESTIBULAR OR
BARTHOLIN'S DUCT OPENING

VESTIBULE

FOURCHETTE

POSTERIOR
COMMISSURE

PERINEUM

ANTERIOR
COMMISSURE

GLANS OF
CLITORIS

URETHRAL OR
URINARY ORIFICE

VESTIBULE

LABIUM
MAJUS

VAGINAL
ORIFICE

HYMEN

FOSSA
NAVICULARIS

ANUS

Fig. 40-2 External female genitalia. (From Lowdermilk, D.L. [2000]. *Maternity and women's health care* [7th ed.]. St. Louis: Mosby.)

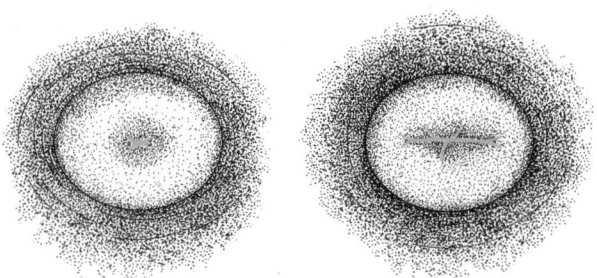

Fig. 40-3 External cervical os as seen through speculum. **A,** Non-parous cervix. **B,** Parous cervix. (From Lowdermilk, D.L. [2000]. *Maternity and women's health care* [7th ed.]. St. Louis: Mosby.)

Diagnostic Procedures and Laboratory Tests

• *Papanicolaou smear*—A Pap smear should be done annually during the speculum examination of a girl who is sexually active or a woman who is 18 years of age or older. High-risk individuals, including teenagers with multiple partners or a history of STDs, should be screened more frequently. This cytologic screening can identify abnormal cell growth on the cervix. The procedure for collection of cells is as follows. During the speculum examination, a spatula is used to scrape the cervix in a circular motion, and the material from both sides of the spatula is blotted on a glass slide. Next, an endocervical specimen is collected with a cytobrush or saline-moistened cotton-tipped applicator that is inserted into the os and rotated. This

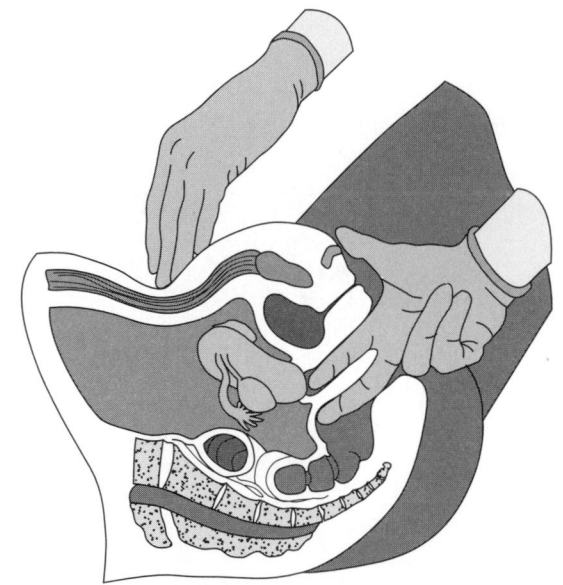

Fig. 40-4 Rectovaginal palpation. (From Seidel, H. [1999]. *Mosby's guide to physical examination* [4th ed.]. St. Louis: Mosby.)

sample is rolled onto another part of the glass slide. The slides should be fixed immediately. The results of the Pap smear are classified as indicated in Table 40-1.

• *Cervical mucus examination*—Examination of cervical mucus is used to evaluate estrogen status. The procedure for

Table 40-1 Comparison of the Bethesda Classification, CIN Classification, and Papanicolaou Reporting*

BETHESDA SYSTEM	CIN CLASSIFICATION	PAPANICOLAOU
Low-grade SIL	HPV change	Atypia: koilocytotic, warty, condylomatous
	CIN I	Mild dysplasia
High-grade SIL	CIN II—moderate dysplasia	CIN III—severe dysplasia, carcinoma in situ
	CIN III	

*From Hatcher, R. et al. (1994). Contraceptive technology (16th ed.). New York: Irvington Publishers.
CIN, *Cervical intraepithelial neoplasia;* SIL, *squamous intraepithelial lesions.*

collection is to swab the cervix with a large cotton-tipped applicator, which is discarded. Then a saline-moistened applicator is used to collect a sample of cervical mucus. The mucus is spread on a glass slide and allowed to air dry for about 5 minutes. Under the microscope a ferning pattern occurs during the late proliferative phase of the menstrual cycle. Ferning does not occur in the presence of progesterone. Cervical mucus is profuse, clear, and elastic during preovulation and ovulation. Immediately after ovulation the character changes to thick and sticky.

- *Wet preparations*—The wet preparation method is used to identify the cause of vaginal discharge. The procedure for collection of vaginal discharge for the prepubertal child is to use a saline-moistened Calgiswab (calcium alginate swab) or eyedropper to collect secretions from the vagina. In the adolescent a cotton-tipped applicator is inserted into the vagina to collect secretions. The applicator is rolled first in 1 drop of saline on a glass slide and then in 1 drop of 10% potassium hydroxide (KOH) on a glass slide; both specimens are then covered with a cover slip. The slides are examined under the microscope with low and then high power being used (Table 40-2). A swab with discharge containing leukocytes mixed with KOH smells "fishy," yielding a positive "whiff test."
- *pH*—Possible pH levels include:
  Prepubertal vagina: 7 (neutral)
  Pubertal adolescent: 4.5 (acid)
  Bacterial vaginosis or trichomoniasis: 4.5
- *Cultures*—For *Neisseria gonorrhoeae,* a cotton-tipped applicator is inserted into the cervical os and rotated (for a female) or a Calgiswab is inserted about ½ inch into the urethral opening and rotated (for a male) and then streaked on culture media. For *C. trachomatis,* a polyester fiber (Dacron)-tipped applicator is inserted into the cervical os and rotated (for female) or a Calgiswab is inserted about ½ inch into the urethral opening and rotated (for a male) and then inserted into a culture medium. Other screening methods such as enzyme immunoassays (EIA), direct immunofluorescent smears (DFS), or deoxyribonucleic acid (DNA) probes (which are primarily for adult women) may be used following basically the same procedure for specimen collection. *Aerobic cultures* of the vagina may be useful in the diagnosis and treatment of vaginitis in prepubertal girls because respiratory pathogens are a common cause of vaginitis in this age group. *Viral cultures* may also be collected from open lesions using a cotton-tipped applicator and an appropriate collection medium.

Table 40-2 Examination of Slides

SLIDE TYPE	FINDING	INDICATION
Saline	Trichomonads	*Trichomoniasis*
	Leukocytes	Bacterial vaginosis
	Clue cells	Bacterial vaginosis
KOH	Yeast and pseudohyphae	*Candida* vaginitis

- *Pregnancy test*—A variety of reliable over-the-counter (OTC) rapid urine pregnancy tests are available. Urine pregnancy screens are frequently used in clinical settings. It is important to know the sensitivity of the test used in the clinical site. Serum is used for qualitative and quantitative measurement of human chorionic gonadotropin (HCG). Quantitative HCG levels are important in cases of ectopic pregnancy, spontaneous abortions, molar pregnancies, and choriocarcinomas. Serum is preferred for serial measurements of HCG. HCG levels increase rapidly during the first trimester of pregnancy and peak at 10 to 14 weeks of pregnancy.
- *Buccal smear*—A buccal smear is a cytology screen used to quickly identify possible karyotype. One can obtain a specimen by scraping the buccal mucosa with a tongue depressor. The material is streaked onto a glass slide and fixed. The specimen is examined for Barr bodies; a normal range of Barr bodies indicates a normal female karyotype, 46,XX. Absent Barr bodies indicates 46,XY or 45,X karyotype.
- *Bone age*—One can determine a bone age by comparing wrist and hand radiographs to existing standards. The result is then compared to the patient's chronologic age.
- *Ultrasonography*—Pelvic ultrasound examination is useful in identifying anatomic structures of the pelvis. Transvaginal ultrasonography may be used to identify early pregnancy, ectopic pregnancy, spontaneous abortion, pelvic masses, pelvic inflammatory disease (PID), and uterine abnormalities.
- *Urinalysis*—A first-catch specimen should be collected from males. This specimen includes urine from the onset of the urine stream and may be used for a routine urinalysis; presence of white blood cell enzyme may be an indicator of the presence of an STD. A clean-catch specimen from a female may provide useful information, such as the presence of red blood cells, white blood cells, bacteria, and white blood cell enzyme.

Ambiguous Genitalia

MARGARET A. McCABE

Alert

Refer to a physician any neonate with apparently questionable genitalia.

Etiology

The underdevelopment of male genitalia or overdevelopment of female genitalia is related to hormonal influences in utero. It may be a maternal or fetal influence.

Incidence

- The incidence is about 1 in 2000 newborns
- Approximately 100 to 200 newborns are treated each year in the United States

Risk Factors

- Maternal history of congenital adrenal cortical hyperplasia; virilizing tumor; androgen, danazol, or synthetic prostaglandin use during pregnancy
- Positive family history of congenital adrenal cortical hyperplasia or aunts with amenorrhea and infertility.

Differential Diagnosis

In *congenital adrenal cortical hyperplasia,* inadequate cortisol synthesis leads to increases in adrenocorticotropic hormone (ACTH), resulting in increased adrenal androgen production, which produces the effect of ambiguous genitalia in female neonates.

Female pseudohermaphroditism may be caused by maternal drug use, maternal congenital adrenal hyperplasia (CAH), or virilizing tumor, resulting in ambiguous genitalia.

Male pseudohermaphroditism may be caused by defects of testicular differentiation, deficit in placental luteinizing hormone (LH), Leydig cell agenesis, or receptor deficits.

True hermaphroditism is evident when an infant possesses both ovaries and testes. This is rare. External genitalia may appear fully masculine to almost completely feminine.

Chromosomal abnormalities that may cause ambiguous genitalia include Klinefelter syndrome (XXY) and Turner syndrome (XXX).

Management

Treatments and medications. Treatment varies by cause and is managed by a physician.

Counseling and prevention
- Reassure the parents that there is an explanation for this occurrence and that their child has a genetically identifiable sex.
- Explain the testing procedures, the type of information they yield, and the length of time they take to complete.
- Provide a supportive environment to openly discuss how the parents can explain this issue to other family members and friends.

Follow-up. Provide follow-up care as determined by the physician and at well-child visits.

Consultations and referrals. Refer the child to an endocrinologist and a geneticist for evaluation.

Breast Masses and Changes

MARGARET A. McCABE

Alert

Consult with or refer the child to a physician for any mass that is persistent, discrete, nonmobile, hard, enlarging, tender, or associated with a retracted nipple.

Etiology

The age at which most girls begin breast development is 9 to 13 years. Breast development may occur in males, usually between 13 and 14 years of age.

Incidence

- Accessory nipples are found in 1% to 2% of healthy patients.
- It is estimated that fibrocystic changes occur in 50% of women clinically and 90% histologically.
- Malignant breast tumors are very rare in children.
- Fibroadenomas account for 94% of breast tumors in adolescents from 12 to 21 years of age.
- Gynecomastia (breast development in males) affects about 50% of 13- to 14-year-old males.

Risk Factors

- Past history of benign breast mass
- Positive family history of breast disease, including cancer
- Menarche younger than 12 years of age

Differential Diagnosis (Table 40-3)

Asymmetry of breast tissue occurs when one breast is larger than the other. *Hypertrophy* of breast tissue occurs when there is a large volume of breast tissue.

Accessory nipples of the breast are a benign congenital anomaly that occurs along the nipple line.

Nipple discharge may indicate infection or tumor and may be caused by certain pharmacologic agents, or it may be caused by chest wall trauma, pregnancy, exercise, or stress.

Fibrocystic mass (benign) occurs with diffuse changes that include thickenings and lumps in the breast, which may become tender and enlarged before menses each month.

Fibroadenoma (benign mass) is a firm, rubbery, mobile, discrete mass.

Infection occurs in breast tissue as a result of trauma, a localized bacterial infection, or during lactation.

Tenderness can occur as a normal part of the menstrual cycle.

Gynecomastia is the benign proliferation of breast tissue in males.

Management

Asymmetry

Treatments and medications. Serial measurement of areola, glandular breast tissue, and overall breast size is recommended.

Counseling and prevention
- Remember that breast development usually stops between 15 and 18 years of age.
- Remember that asymmetry decreases with age; it does not become more noticeable with age.
- Instruct on routine self-breast examination (see Fig. 40-1). Observe a return demonstration.

Follow-up. Provide follow-up care at yearly intervals and for well-child care, sooner if the patient or parents are concerned.

Consultations and referrals. None are necessary.

Hypertrophy

Treatments and medications. The patient may consider breast reduction at the completion of breast growth (15 to 18 years of age).

Counseling and prevention. Instruct about routine breast self-examinations.

Follow-up. Follow-up with routine care and well-child visits as appropriate for the age of the patient.

Consultations and referrals. Generally none are necessary. If the patient does consider breast reduction, referral to a plastic surgeon is necessary.

Accessory nipples or breasts

Treatments and medications. No treatment is necessary except for cosmetic reasons.

Counseling and prevention

- Inform the patient and parents that this is a variation, not a problem, and there is no medical indication for intervention.
- Instruct the patient to assess at routine intervals and report changes as with other mammary tissue.
- During lactation, breast tissue may enlarge and the nipples may leak milk, especially under slight expression.

Follow-up. Assess at routine well-child visits.

Consultations and referrals. None are needed, except if the patient and family consider cosmetic surgery. At this point the patient should be referred to a plastic surgeon.

Nipple discharge

Treatments and medications. The patient may need to be treated with an antibiotic if the cultured discharge indicates bacterial infection. The choice of antibiotic depends on the culture result.

Counseling and prevention

- Discuss the cause of the discharge and reassure the patient that discharge related to infection can be easily treated.
- Remember that patients with dark or blood-tinged discharge should be counseled to keep referral appointments with a gynecologist.
- Instruct about medications, if prescribed.

Follow-up

- If the discharge is related to infection, schedule a return visit in 1 to 2 weeks after treatment.
- Follow-up laboratory results if necessary.
- Follow-up specialty referral if necessary.

Consultations and referrals. Refer the patient to a gynecologist if there is blood-tinged discharge.

Fibrocystic mass (benign)

Treatments and medications

- Recommend a trial elimination of caffeine, the patient may expect improvement in 2 to 3 months.
- Reevaluate the lesion after the next menses. If it has decreased or is gone, it is probably a cystic change. If the lesion is still present, a needle aspiration may be done. Cysts yield fluid, while fibroadenomas yield a gritty substance. Send the cells for cytology.
- Refer the patient for excisional biopsy when the mass is persistent, discrete, nonmobile, hard, enlarging, or tender.

Counseling and prevention

- Instruct that fibrocystic masses may recur or a new one may form.
- Educate the patient about the importance of routine breast self-examinations and yearly gynecologic examinations.

Follow-up

- Schedule a return visit 1 week after the next menses for reevaluation.
- Schedule a return visit 3 months after an aspiration or biopsy.

Consultations and referrals. Refer to a gynecologist any patient with a persistent cystic mass for possible aspiration, as well as any patient with a breast mass associated with nipple retraction.

Fibroadenoma (benign mass)

Treatments and medications. The patient may need to be referred to a gynecologist for aspiration or excisional biopsy.

Counseling and prevention

- Advise that these masses tend to recur.
- Instruct about the importance of routine breast self-examinations and yearly gynecologic examinations.

Follow-up

- Schedule return visits at monthly intervals to assess mass size.
- Reevaluate the mass 3 months after aspiration or biopsy.
- Perform yearly gynecologic examinations.

Consultations and referrals. Refer to a gynecologist any patient with a mass with an undetermined cause, a mass that increases in size, or a breast mass associated with nipple retraction.

Infection

Treatments and medications

- Treat with a cephalosporin, such as cefadroxil 30 mg/kg per day in two divided doses for 10 to 14 days.
- Apply warm compresses to the area as needed for comfort.

Counseling and prevention

- Instruct the patient to clean the area with soap and water daily.
- Advise the patient to change her bra frequently.
- If the area is draining and a dressing is being used, instruct the patient in how to clean the area, change the dressing, and maintain clean technique.
- Instruct the patient in routine breast self-examinations.

Follow-up. Schedule a return visit 1 to 2 weeks after treatment. The patient should seek a follow-up visit if symptoms recur.

Consultations and referrals. Refer to or consult with a physician if the infection is moderate to severe or if the infection is not responsive to antibiotic therapy.

Tenderness

Treatments and medications

- Advise the patient to wear a comfortably fitting support bra.
- Recommend a trial elimination of caffeine, after which the patient may expect possible improvement in 2 to 3 months.
- Administer low-dose ibuprofen, 200 to 400 mg every 6 hours as needed.

Counseling and prevention

- Reassure the patient and parents (if appropriate) that this is a benign condition.
- Instruct the patient in routine breast self-examinations.

Follow-up. See the patient at routine well-child intervals.

Consultations and referrals. None are necessary.

Gynecomastia

Treatments and medications. If the condition is drug induced, discontinue drug use if possible. Indications for surgical treatment include pain, tenderness, and severe embarrassment.

Counseling and prevention

- Reassure the patient and parents that this is a benign condition.
- Advise that obesity may contribute to the size of the breasts.
- Discuss surgical options with the patient and parents.

Table 40-3 Differential Diagnosis: Breast Changes

CRITERIA	ASYMMETRY	HYPERTROPHY	ACCESSORY NIPPLES OR BREASTS	NIPPLE DISCHARGE
ICD-9 code	757.6	611.1	757.6	611.79
Subjective Data				
Age	Early in breast development	Puberty	Congenital occurrence may be identified at any age	Adolescent
History: past and present	None	None; breast discomfort; back pain	None; discharge during lactation	May have thyroid, pituitary or hypothalamic disease; vigorous exercise
Description of problem	Asymmetrical breast development	Large breasts with associated breast discomfort	May appear as dark spot on skin in nipple line	Discharge from one or both nipples
Associated symptoms	No discomfort	Back pain	Area may respond to hormonal changes during puberty and pregnancy causing tissue enlargement or lactation	May flow spontaneously or need to be expressed
Objective Data **Physical examination**				
General		Postural kyphosis		Assess thyroid
Breasts	Breast development appears unequal on visual inspection	Large amount of breast tissue	May include glandular tissue, areola, and nipple but commonly only small areola and nipple; located along embryologic milk line from axilla to groin	Small amount yellow or clear serous material normal; dark or blood-tinged discharge abnormal; green discharge abnormal
Internal genitalia	Normal	Normal	Normal	Irregular or cystic ovaries; enlarged uterus abnormal
Laboratory data	None	None	None	Pap smear; serology, thyroid function screen, prolactin level

Follow-up
- Provide follow-up care if further testing is needed or to evaluate the effects of changes in drug use.
- See the patient for routine well-child visits.
  Consultations and referrals
- Refer to a physician any patient with asymmetric breast development.
- Schedule a surgical consultation for patients and parents considering surgical intervention.

Genital Lesions

MARGARET A. McCABE

Alert

Consult with or refer to a physician for the following:
- Severe lesions
- Systemic involvement
- Late (tertiary) syphilis
- Prepubescent child

Etiology

In the United States the primary causes of genital ulcers are herpes simplex (herpes simplex virus type 2 [HSV-2]), syphilis *(Treponema pallidum),* and chancroid *(Haemophilus ducreyi).*

Incidence

- The incidence of syphilis is 20 to 30 per 100,000.
- Lesions have more than one cause in 3% to 10% of patients.
- Genital herpes is the most common cause of genital lesions in the United States, with at least 45 million cases of HSV-2 having been diagnosed in the United States.

Risk Factors

- Unprotected sex
- Multiple sex partners
- Substance abuse
- Previous history of genital lesions

Differential Diagnosis (Table 40-4)

Genital herpes simplex is characterized by ulcerative lesions on the genital area. It is a viral disease that is recurrent and incurable. Two serotypes have been identified, HSV-1 and

FIBROCYSTIC MASS (BENIGN)	FIBROADENOMA (BENIGN MASS)	INFECTION	TENDERNESS	GYNECOMASTIA (BENIGN)
610.1	611.72	611.0	611.71	611.1
Adolescent	Adolescent	Newborn period; adolescent	Early in breast development; early pregnancy	Newborn period; early adolescence; male
Previous history	Previous history	History of trauma; recent history of breast-feeding; history of shaved or plucked breast hair	Exercise history—trauma; premenstrual syndrome; history of fibrocystic disease	May report drug use: hormones, steroids, certain antibiotics; chemotherapeutics, cardiovascular drugs, psychoactive agents, recreational substances
Tenderness or cyclic tenderness	Firm, rubbery mass detected by patient on self-examination Fever; erythema	Localized tenderness	Localized or diffuse breast tenderness	Breast tissue enlargement
Appears normal Normally dense breast tissue	Appears normal Firm, rubbery, mobile, clearly defined edge; occurs more frequently in lateral breast quadrants	Appears normal Tender; erythema, warm to touch; yellow to green discharge from nipples	Appears normal Normal except tender on palpation	Appears normal Often unilateral, glandular tissue (firm, rubbery) palpable symmetrically under nipple and areola
Normal	Normal	Normal	Normal	Not applicable
Culture of aspirate, ultrasonography; biopsy	Culture of aspirate; ultrasonography; biopsy	Culture of discharge	None	Possible endocrine studies

HSV-2. About 5% to 30% of initial episodes are caused by HSV-1, which has a recurrence much less frequent than that of HSV-2. The primary infection is usually more symptomatic than recurrent infections. Systemic symptoms are common and include fever, headache, malaise, and myalgia. HSV-2 is characterized by clusters of papules, vesicles, pustules, or ulcers in the genital area. The lesions usually last 5 to 7 days.

Syphilis is a systemic illness. The primary stage, within the first year of infection, is characterized by a chancre; the secondary stage is characterized by cutaneous lesions; the tertiary stage is characterized by cardiac, neurologic, ophthalmic, auditory, or gummatous lesions.

Chancroid is characterized by one or more painful lesions on the genital area. High rates of human immunodeficiency virus (HIV) infection have been reported among patients with chancroid.

Condylomata acuminata, or *genital warts,* is an STD caused by the human papillomavirus (HPV). There are more than 20 types of warts that can infect the genital tract. Frequently infections are asymptomatic, subclinical, or unrecognized.

Management

Genital herpes simplex

Treatments and medications

- Suggest sitz baths for comfort and hygiene.
- Apply a topical anesthetic gel (e.g., lidocaine 2%) for comfort.
- For the initial infection, prescribe acyclovir 200 mg orally five times a day for 7 to 10 days, or acyclovir 400 mg orally three times a day for 7 to 10 days.
- For an episodic recurrent infection, prescribe acyclovir 400 mg orally three times a day for 5 days, or acyclovir 200 mg orally five times a day for 5 days, or acyclovir 800 mg orally two times a day for 5 days.
- For daily suppressive therapy in severe recurrent cases, prescribe acyclovir 400 mg two times a day for 1 year and then discontinue to evaluate the recurrence pattern.
- Remember that HIV-infected patients may require increased doses of medication.
- Apply a cool compress to the affected area as needed for relief of discomfort.
- Advise the patient to avoid tight, restrictive clothing.

Counseling and prevention. See Sexual Abuse in Chapter 47.

Table 40-4 Differential Diagnosis: Genital Lesions

CRITERIA	GENITAL HERPES SIMPLEX	SYPHILIS	CHANCROID	CONDYLOMATA ACUMINATA
ICD-9 code	054.10	091.0	099.0	078.11
Subjective Data				
Age	Any	Any	Any	Any
History: past and present	Sexual contact; history of exposure	Sexual contact; history of exposure	Sexual contact; history of exposure	Positive maternal history in child 1-20 months of age; sexual contact, possibly unknown
Description of problem	Pain, pruritus, dysuria	May be symptom free	Lesion on genital area	Itching; painful urination
Associated symptoms	Systemic symptoms, headache, fever, myalgia, malaise Vulvar or vaginal pruritus, pain; dysuria; urethral or vaginal discharge; painful, pruritic vesicles that rupture in 1-3 days	Lesion on genital area	Discomfort related to ulcers	
Objective Data				
Physical examination (general)	Appears normal; Lymphadenopathy; extragenital vesicles on buttocks, groin, thighs, pharynx, fingers, and conjunctivae, may have progressed to ulcerative lesions	Rash, mucocutaneous lesions, and adenopathy (secondary infection); cardiac, neurologic, ophthalmic, auditory, or gummatous lesions (tertiary infection)	Tender inguinal adenopathy	Rarely in mouth, urethral meatus, and conjunctivae
Temperature	Normal to elevated	Normal	Normal	Normal
External genitalia	Urethral or vaginal discharge; vesicles, perianal area, extragenital sites on buttocks, groin, thighs; vesicles rupture in 1-3 days	Genital lesions—penis, labia, vulva (primary infection)	One or more painful genital ulcers	Moist, cauliflower-like warts on mucous membranes and mucocutaneous junctions of the anogenital and inguinal areas; may appear white and macerated
Internal genitalia	Appears normal	Appears normal	Appears normal	Appears normal
Laboratory data	Serologic testing, RPR negative; viral culture (HSV)	Positive serologic testing, RPR positive or VDRL (serial) HIV screen	Serologic testing, RPR negative; culture positive for *H. Ducreyi* HIV screen	Biopsy of lesion; positive HPV

RPR, *Rapid plasma reagin.*

For young children

- Ensure that the parents understand the treatment regimen and medication schedule.
- Educate the parents to aid in understanding that the transmission of HSV-2 is by sexual contact.
- Inform the parents about the process of reporting sexual abuse in their state of residence.
- Reassure the parents that the intent is to protect the child and help the perpetrator to modify or stop his or her actions.
- Encourage the parents to answer children's questions related to the illness factually and honestly.
- Discuss the implications of HIV screening.
- Discuss the benefits of human services, social work, and psychology referral.

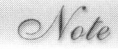
Note

Adolescents have the right to confidentiality in health-care issues related to sexuality. Parents may be informed of treatment and included in counseling if desired by the adolescent.

For adolescents

- Be sure that the patient understands the treatment regimen.
- Educate the patient to aid them in understanding that the transmission of herpes is by sexual contact.
- Discuss the importance of evaluation and treatment for contacts.
- Encourage open, honest communication with contacts.

- Teach the patient to use condoms to prevent exposure to infection.
- Instruct the adolescent on the need to abstain from sexual activity or use condoms until a cure is achieved.
- Discuss high-risk behaviors and their implications for health.
- Discuss the importance of referral for HIV assessment.
- If sexual abuse is suspected, inform the adolescent and parents about the process of reporting sexual abuse in their state of residence.
- Reassure the adolescent and parents that the intent is to protect the adolescent and help the perpetrator.
- Encourage the adolescent and parents to have open communication related to the illness.
- Discuss the implications of HIV screening.
- Discuss the benefits of human services, social work, and psychology referral.

Follow-up. A return visit is not required if the medication is used properly and the symptoms subside. If the patient is at risk for noncompliance, a return visit is recommended in 1 to 2 weeks. The patient should seek follow-up if symptoms recur. Annual gynecologic examinations with Pap smears are recommended for adolescent girls.

Consultations and referrals
- Possibly refer severe cases to a physician for management.
- Report suspected child abuse to the appropriate agency.
- Remember that cases that involve suspected child abuse should be followed closely by medical and social services professionals.
- Refer the adolescent for HIV assessment.
- Refer all sexual contacts for evaluation and counseling, even if asymptomatic.

Syphilis

Treatments and medications
- For primary, secondary, and early latent syphilis, administer penicillin G benzathine 2.4 million U intramuscularly in one dose for an adult or 50,000 U/kg up to the adult dose intramuscularly in one dose for a child. For nonpregnant, penicillin-allergic patients, prescribe doxycycline 100 mg orally two times a day for 14 days for adults.
- For late latent or latent syphilis, administer penicillin G benzathine 2.4 million U intramuscularly at 1-week intervals three times for adults or 50,000 U/kg up to the adult dose intramuscularly at 1-week intervals three times for children. For nonpregnant, penicillin-allergic adults, prescribe doxycycline 100 mg orally two times a day for 2 weeks if the infection is known to be less than 1 year; otherwise treat for 4 weeks.

Counseling and prevention. For young children and adolescents, see the discussion of Genital Herpes Simplex earlier in this section.

Follow-up. For primary and secondary syphilis, clinical and serologic follow-up evaluation are needed at 6 months and 12 months after treatment. Treatment failure occurs if signs and symptoms persist or recur after treatment or if titers fail to decrease fourfold from the baseline value within 6 months after treatment. These patients should be retreated according to the guidelines for latent syphilis.

For latent syphilis, clinical and serologic follow-up evaluation are needed at 6 months and 12 months after treatment. If the titer fails to decrease fourfold within 12 to 24 months or if the patient develops symptoms, referral for neurologic evaluation and retreatment is appropriate.

Consultations and referrals
- Refer patients with signs and symptoms of neurologic or ophthalmic disease for further work-up study.
- Refer late syphilis cases to a physician.
- Refer contacts for evaluation and treatment.
- Possibly refer severe cases to a physician for management.
- Report suspected child abuse to the appropriate agency.
- Remember that cases that involve suspected child abuse should be followed closely by medical and social services professionals.
- Refer the patient for HIV assessment.

Chancroid

Treatments and medications. Prescribe azithromycin 1 g orally in one dose, or ceftriaxone 250 mg intramuscularly in one dose, or erythromycin 500 mg orally four times a day for 7 days. HIV-infected patients may require longer courses of therapy.

Counseling and prevention. For young children and adolescents, see the discussion of Genital Herpes Simplex earlier in this chapter.

Follow-up. Schedule a return visit 3 to 7 days after initiation of therapy for evaluation of the lesion, at which time improvement should be evident. If there is no improvement, consider the possibility of coinfection with HIV or another STD or treatment noncompliance.

Consultations and referrals
- Refer contacts for evaluation and treatment.
- Possibly refer severe cases to a physician for management.
- Report suspected child abuse to the appropriate agency.
- Remember that cases that involve suspected child abuse should be followed closely by medical and social services professionals.
- Refer the patient for HIV assessment.

Condylomata acuminata. See Warts in Chapter 37.

Treatments and medications
- Treat any coexisting vaginitis.
- Use cryotherapy with liquid nitrogen (possibly with repeated application in 1 to 2 weeks), or use TCA 80% to 90% applied directly (repeated weekly as needed), or prescribe podofilox 0.5% solution or gel applied to the affected area two times a day for 3 days, followed by 4 days of no treatment (repeated as needed for a total of four cycles).

Counseling and prevention. See the earlier discussion of Gonorrhea.

Follow-up
- Schedule a return visit in 1 week for a repeat application until the lesion is gone, up to three times.
- Have the patient should seek follow-up evaluation if symptoms recur.
- Recommend annual gynecologic examinations with Pap smears.

Consultations and referrals. See the earlier discussion of Gonorrhea.

Menstrual Irregularities

LINDA C. ANDRIST

Alert

Consult with or refer to a physician for the following:
- Bleeding associated with systemic illness such as coagulation disorders
- Suspected ectopic pregnancy

- Any evidence of vaginal bleeding in a child under 9 years of age (rule out possible sexual abuse and foreign body)
- Primary amenorrhea (absence of menses by 16 years of age regardless of presence of normal growth and development of secondary sex characteristics)
- Amenorrhea associated with an eating disorder
- Any excessive bleeding or hemorrhage

Etiology

For most females between 12 and 50 years of age, menstruation is a normally occurring cyclic event. The menstrual cycle is repeated 300 to 400 times in the life of a female. The frequency of cycles vary from 21 to 40 days, with bleeding lasting between 3 and 8 days. Blood loss during one menstrual cycle averages 30 to 80 ml. Menstruation usually occurs without major difficulties.

Complicated neuroendocrine changes occur each month to ensure the regularity of the menstrual cycle. The interaction between the hypothalamus gland (producing gonadotropin-releasing hormone [GnRH]), pituitary gland (producing follicle-stimulating hormone [FSH] and luteinizing hormone [LH]), ovaries, and endometrium is complex. If their interactions do not take place in a sequential fashion, menstrual irregularities can occur.

Menstrual irregularities in the adolescent can result from: (1) pregnancy-related conditions, (2) anovulation, (3) coagulation disorders, (4) systemic disorders, (5) trauma, (6) lower reproductive tract infections, and (7) exogenous hormonal usage. Rarely, menstrual irregularities in an adolescent are the result of neoplasms such as endometrial hyperplasia, hormonally active ovarian tumors, leiomyoma, and vaginal tumors. The amount of bleeding from menstrual irregularities can vary from amenorrhea to menometrorrhagia (Table 40-5).

Incidence

- Within the first year of menarche, 55% of menses are anovulatory.
- Of the adolescent female population, 8.5% may have amenorrhea (excluding pregnancy).
- Amenorrhea or oligomenorrhea may occur in 10% to 20% of vigorously exercising women and up to 66% of female athletes.
- Of adolescents with menorrhagia, 20% may have a coagulation disorder.
- Most females with eating disorders (e.g., anorexia nervosa, bulimia) experience endocrine disturbances leading to menstrual irregularities or amenorrhea.
- Primary dysmenorrhea is present in 50% to 75% of women of reproductive age.

Risk Factors

- Coagulation disorders
- Excessive exercise
- Eating disorders
- Pregnancy
- Ectopic pregnancy
- STDs
- Use of hormonal preparations
- Sexual abuse
- Trauma of the genitalia
- Hormonal imbalances

Differential Diagnosis (Table 40-6)

Pregnancy should be considered in any female who has *amenorrhea,* even if the adolescent states that she is not sexually active. In addition, if the adolescent has previously delivered and is currently breastfeeding the infant, amenorrhea may be the manifesting symptom during lactation.

Eating disorders such as anorexia nervosa and bulimia nervosa may result in amenorrhea. Amenorrhea associated with eating disorders is the consequence of low estrogen levels re-

Table 40-5 Descriptive Terms of Menstrual Irregularities

TERM	DEFINITION
Amenorrhea	Absence of menses
Primary	Lack of secondary sexual characteristics and no menses by 14 years of age or no menses before 16 years regardless of development of secondary sexual characteristics
Secondary	Absences of menses for three to six cycles in a female who has had previous menstruation
Oligomenorrhea	Menses at intervals > 35 days
Polymenorrhea	Menses at intervals ≤ 21 days
Intermenstrual bleeding	Bleeding between normal menses
Menorrhagia	Bleeding rarely, yet excessive in duration or flow
Metrorrhagia	Irregularly bleeding
Menometrorrhagia	Frequent, irregular, excessive bleeding
Dysmenorrhea	Painful menses

Table 40-6 Differential Diagnosis of Menstrual Irregularities

DIAGNOSIS	AMENORRHEA/ OLIGOMENORRHEA	ABNORMAL BLEEDING
Pregnancy	X	X
Eating disorders	X	
Excessive exercise	X	
Endocrine imbalances	X	
Hormonal preparations	X	X
Polycystic ovarian syndrome (PCOS)	X	
Anovulatory uterine bleeding		X
Coagulation disorders		X
Reproductive tract infections		X
Systemic diseases		X
Trauma		X

X indicates that characteristic is present.

sulting from the decreased pituitary secretion of FSH and LH. In most females, weight loss precedes the symptom of amenorrhea. If the female already has an eating disorder, menarche may be delayed. (See Anorexia and Bulimia in Chapter 45.)

Excessive exercise may result in amenorrhea or *oligomenorrhea* that arises from the same hypoestrogenic state as in eating disorders. Female athletes also may have an associated eating disorder that includes restrictions of calories and over-exercising to burn calories. The "female athlete triad" is used to describe the interrelatedness of disordered eating, amenorrhea, and premature osteoporosis often associated with female athletes. Estrogen levels in these athletes can decrease to post-menopausal levels with irreversible bone loss. Amenorrheic athletes are at increased risk for stress fractures and other musculoskeletal injuries.

Endocrine imbalances have been associated with amenorrhea or oligomenorrhea. Hypothyroidism and the elevation of thyrotropin-releasing hormone (TRH) stimulates an increase in the release of prolactin (PRL) from the pituitary. The increase in PRL can result in amenorrhea. If the PRL level does not return to normal after treatment of hypothyroidism, pituitary microadenoma should be investigated.

Hormonal preparations, especially progesterone injections used for birth control, may result in amenorrhea. Amenorrhea is a common side effect with Depo-Provera (depot medroxyprogesterone acetate [DMPA]) injections and is not a cause for concern as long as the adolescent has taken the injections every 12 weeks.

Polycystic ovary syndrome (PCOS) is a condition in which there is noncyclic gonadotropin and androgen production with chronic anovulation. PCOS has been associated with Stein-Leventhal syndrome, with the clinical picture of obesity, hirsutism, oligomenorrhea, and enlarged ovaries with multiple small cysts. Any female appearing with chronic anovulation and hyperandrogenism satisfies the criteria for PCOS.

Anovulatory uterine bleeding, or *bleeding secondary to anovulation*, is one of the most common causes of abnormal bleeding in the adolescent and is a common cause of abnormal bleeding just after menarche. Anovulatory uterine bleeding is usually the result of a hormonal disturbance based on the failure of ovarian follicular maturation with resulting lack of progesterone production, limitation of endometrial growth, and synchronous shedding. The result of this hormonal disturbance is irregular spotting and episodes of profuse bleeding. Also called *dysfunctional uterine bleeding* (DUB), this is a diagnosis of exclusion and should be used only after other causes of abnormal bleeding have been ruled out.

Pregnancy should be investigated in any female who has abnormal bleeding. Bleeding during pregnancy may indicate ectopic pregnancy or spontaneous abortion. In addition, the adolescent should be questioned about whether she has recently undergone a voluntary abortion. Hemorrhage, shock, and loss of the pregnancy are the most common complications of bleeding during early pregnancy.

Coagulation disorders (von Willebrand disease) may be an underlying cause of increased bleeding in the adolescent. If the female has severe menorrhagia during the first menses, a coagulation disorder should be considered.

Reproductive tract infections are a common cause of abnormal bleeding. Reproductive tract infections are asymptomatic in many females, but some may experience abnormal vaginal bleeding, especially after intercourse. Although it is difficult to isolate a specific organism, *C. trachomatis* or *N. gonorrhoeae* may be the causative agent.

Systemic diseases such as diabetes mellitus, hepatic dysfunction, renal dysfunction, and thyroid dysfunction may be associated with abnormal bleeding. Appropriate laboratory testing should be conducted to rule out such disorders.

Trauma in the form of an accidental injury, coital trauma, or sexual abuse could be the cause of abnormal bleeding in children and adolescents. Younger children may have accidental injury resulting in vaginal bleeding because of a fall (bicycle accident) or from placing a foreign object in the vagina. Sexual abuse should be ruled out in all children with vaginal bleeding.

Exogenous hormone use may result in abnormal bleeding in the adolescent. Incorrect use of birth control pills or missing pills may result in breakthrough bleeding or irregular bleeding. Progesterone implants as a means of birth control frequently will result in irregular menses and spotting.

Dysmenorrhea is pain before or during menstruation. Dysmenorrhea is most commonly described as painful cramping in the lower abdomen or pelvis. The pain may be severe and may radiate to the back or down the medial area of the thighs. Primary dysmenorrhea may occur once ovulatory cycles are established and is caused by excessive prostaglandin release. Symptoms related to prostaglandin excess are diaphoresis, tachycardia, headache, nausea, vomiting, and diarrhea. Secondary dysmenorrhea is caused by pelvic pathologic conditions such as endometriosis and generally manifests later in a woman's life.

Management

Amenorrhea and oligomenorrhea
Treatments and medications

- Always rule out pregnancy before initiation of any treatment plan or medications.
- If laboratory tests indicate an underlying condition such as hypothyroidism, pituitary microadenoma, pregnancy, or premature ovarian failure, either refer or initiate appropriate treatment if within the scope of practice.
- If laboratory results are normal, administer a progestin challenge test. Give medroxyprogesterone acetate (MPA) 10 mg for 5 to 10 days. Withdrawal bleeding should occur within 2 to 7 days of completion of MPA, indicating that amenorrhea is most likely the result of anovulation. If withdrawal bleeding does not occur, administer a trial dose of estrogen followed by progestin (conjugated estrogens 1.25 mg orally for 21 days, and add MPA 10 mg orally the last 5 days of estrogen). If withdrawal bleeding occurs after this regimen, defects of the outflow track are eliminated. A serum FSH and LH will help diagnose ovarian failure, pituitary disease, and PCOS; however these conditions are rare in adolescents. The cause of amenorrhea in adolescents is probably related to low endogenous estrogen levels associated with hypothalamic-pituitary dysfunction.

  If withdrawal bleeding fails to occur after estrogen and progestin challenge, there may be an organ problem with the uterus such as Asherman syndrome. In the case of no withdrawal bleeding, the patient should be referred to a reproductive endocrinologist.

  After initiation of withdrawal bleeding, the drug of choice is a low-dose combination oral contraceptive or

Lunelle (a combined hormonal monthly injection) to prevent endometrial hyperplasia and to provide contraception, if appropriate. (See Birth Control in Chapter 17.)

- Keep in mind that the commonly accepted practice of performing a clinical breast and pelvic examination with a Pap smear is currently being questioned. The consensus of major organizations involved in the field of birth control supports the provision of hormonal contraceptives after a thorough medical history and blood pressure evaluation.

Counseling and prevention. If the patient is pregnant, counseling may be indicated regarding options (i.e., continue with pregnancy, abortion, adoption).

- Counsel the adolescent and parents about why the patient is taking oral contraceptives or Lunelle, especially if the adolescent is not sexually active.
- Teach the proper use of oral contraceptives. Counsel the adolescent and parents about why the patient is taking oral contraceptives or Lunelle, especially if the adolescent is not sexually active. The adolescent should take one pill per day at the same time of day. If one pill is missed, the patient should take it as soon as she notices it has been missed. If not noticed until the next day, she may take both pills at the same time. If she misses two pills, take two pills one day and two pills the next day. A backup method of birth control (e.g., condoms) is strongly advised in this situation. If more than two pills are missed, she should contact the practitioner, at which time emergency contraception can be discussed. She should have menses on the week of inactive pills (green pills). Any bleeding is considered a period, even if it seems like spotting to the patient. If the patient is on Lunelle, her regular withdrawal bleed may occur 2 weeks after her injection. If there is no menses, she should call the practitioner.
- Advise that side effects of combined hormonal methods include minor symptoms such as nausea, breast tenderness, bloating, weight gain, headaches, breakthrough bleeding, and acne, as well as major (but rare) symptoms such as heart attack, stroke, and blood clots. The patient should telephone the practitioner if she experiences blurred vision, chest pain, abdominal pain, or leg pain.
- If the patient is using Lunelle, give her a calendar to remind her when to come back for her monthly injection. Lunelle must be given every 28 to 30 days and no later than 33 days since the previous injection.
- If amenorrhea is found to be secondary to exercise, counsel the adolescent about decreasing exercise intensity or quantity and encourage weight gain. If amenorrhea is suspected to be caused by anorexia nervosa, the patient should be referred for counseling.

Follow-up

- If the adolescent was started on hormonal therapy, schedule a return visit in 3 months to determine the effectiveness of the medication.
- Recheck if withdrawal bleeding does occur after progestin challenge or challenge with estrogen and progestin.
- Schedule a return visit if questions or additional problems develop.
- Schedule a return visit for an annual examination in 1 year.

Consultations and referrals

- Consult a physician if there is pregnancy, a severe eating disorder, or a systemic disorder.
- Refer to a physician any adolescent with primary amenorrhea or secondary amenorrhea caused by complex endocrine or metabolic diseases or a coagulation disorder.

Referrals should be to a pediatric endocrinologist or to a gynecologist with a special interest in treating children and adolescents with menstrual irregularities.

Abnormal bleeding

Treatments and medications. No treatment is indicated in an adolescent with mildly abnormal bleeding and adequate hemoglobin levels. Manage with reassurance, supplemental iron, and frequent follow-up care.

In regard to medications, combined hormonal methods (e.g., oral contraceptives, Lunelle) promote atrophy of the endometrial lining, thus decreasing menorrhagia, and provide the progestin lacking when anovulation is the cause of the metrorrhagia.

An alternative drug regimen may include:

- Cyclic progestin: Administer MPA 10 mg/day for 10 to 14 days every 1 to 2 months to prevent endometrial hyperplasia and irregular bleeding caused by unopposed estrogen stimulation Administer DMPA 150 mg intramuscularly every 3 months. Patients taking DMPA may continue with abnormal bleeding, yet a majority achieve amenorrhea within 1 year of use.
- Nonsteroidal antiinflammatory drugs (NSAIDs): Administer mefenamic acid (Ponstel) 500 mg orally three times a day or naproxen (Naprosyn) 500 mg orally immediately and then 250 mg orally three times a day, beginning the first day of menses. Take with food. These are indicated because the antiprostaglandin effect may decrease the endometrial blood flow.
- Iron therapy: Initiate iron therapy if iron-deficiency anemia exists. Prescribe ferrous sulfate 300 mg orally with orange juice 30 minutes after meals.
- Keep in mind that higher-dose hormonal therapy is indicated for females bleeding acutely but not requiring hospitalization. Adolescents needing higher-dose hormonal therapy should be referred to a gynecologist.
- Remember that antibiotics are indicated if bleeding is secondary to reproductive tract infections.

Ultrasound evaluation should be considered if leiomyoma is suspected as the cause for abnormal bleeding, while the rate of current bleeding and the severity of existing anemia determine hospitalization.

Counseling and prevention

- Counsel the adolescent and parents about why she is taking hormones.
- Teach the proper use of hormonal contraceptives or MPA and when to return for hormonal injections.
- Instruct the adolescent in keeping a "bleeding calendar," which assists the practitioner in determining exactly when bleeding is occurring in respect to the menstrual cycle. This is especially important if the patient is already taking hormonal preparations.
- Teach the importance of a "pad count," which helps the practitioner assess the amount of bleeding.

Follow-up

- If no treatment was initiated, provide follow-up care every 1 to 2 months by telephone or return visit to evaluate if there has been any increase in bleeding, as an indication to monitor bleeding, and to provide support and reassurance.
- If hormonal therapy was started, have the patient schedule a return visit in 3 months to determine the effectiveness of the medication.
- Instruct the adolescent to telephone or schedule a return visit if abnormal bleeding increases in intensity, amount, or passage of large clots, or if there is no withdrawal bleeding during the inactive week of oral contraceptives.

- Schedule a return visit for an annual examination in 1 year.
Consultations and referrals
Consult a physician in the following situations:
- Severe abnormal bleeding
- Suspected sexual abuse
- Hospitalization being considered
Refer the patient to a physician in the following situations:
- Need for higher-dose hormonal therapy
- Severe abnormal bleeding associated with a coagulation disorder
- Suspected leiomyoma or pelvic disorder
- Pregnancy, especially if ectopic pregnancy is suspected
- Treatment has not been successful
Referrals should be to a pediatric endocrinologist or to a gynecologist with a special interest in treating children and adolescents with menstrual irregularities.

Primary dysmenorrhea

Treatments and medications. Treatment for dysmenorrhea is related to decreasing prostaglandin production and release in the endometrium. If the patient agrees, she may be treated with a trial of NSAIDs or combined hormonal contraceptives. NSAIDs are the first-line drugs of choice in adolescents not requiring contraception. This class of drugs relieves the pain by preventing the synthesis of prostaglandin, therefore stopping uterine hypercontractility and ischemia and restoring normal function. Although most NSAIDs will be effective for dysmenorrhea, the NSAIDs most commonly prescribed are outlined in Table 40-7.

Start NSAIDs 5 to 7 days before the expected menses and continue for the first 2 to 3 days of the flow. Take NSAIDs with food. Use one drug for a minimum of two to four cycles before evaluating effectiveness. The anticipated outcome is pain relief. If pain is not relieved, another NSAID may be initiated.

If no relief is obtained after using another drug for 2 to 4 months, initiate combined hormonal contraceptives. Low-dose combination oral contraceptives or the combination hormonal injection (Lunelle) reduces the pain of dysmenorrhea by suppression of ovulation and endometrial proliferation.

Counseling and prevention
- Counsel the patient on lifestyle factors that can facilitate a sense of control and alleviate a sense of frustration:
Exercise to increase endorphins, decrease prostaglandin, and increase the estrone-estradiol ratio, which decreases endometrial proliferation and shunts blood away from the uterus, thus decreasing pelvic pain and congestion
Nutrition (e.g., limited salty foods, increased fiber, increased water as a natural diuretic)
Heat therapy (e.g., warm bath or heating pads to decrease muscle spasms and provide comfort)
Relaxation techniques to supplement medications and enhance the patient's ability to deal with the pain
- Counsel the adolescent and parents about why the patient is taking combined hormonal therapies.
- Teach the proper use of oral contraceptives and advise the patient on when to return for her next combined hormonal injection.

Follow-up. If there is no pain relief after 2 to 4 months, call to discuss initiation of a new NSAID. If there is no relief with the second drug, a return visit is indicated.
Consultations and referrals
- Consult with a physician if the treatment regimen does not alleviate the pain.
- Refer the patient to a physician if symptoms are too severe to allow for a trial of medications.

Penile Discharge

MARGARET A. McCABE

Alert

Consult with or refer to a physician for the following:
- Unclear diagnosis
- Symptoms that are resistant to appropriate therapy
- Suspicion of child abuse

Etiology

Urethritis is an inflammation of the urethra accompanied by discharge of mucoid or purulent substance. The two most common bacterial agents that cause urethritis among men are *N. gonorrhoeae* and *Chlamydia trachomatis*.

Incidence

C. trachomatis causes 23% to 55% of cases of nongonococcal urethritis (NGU).

Risk Factors

- Positive past history of STD
- Family or individual history of sexual abuse
- Sexual activity (increased risk when sex is unprotected or with multiple partners)
- Delay in seeking health care
- Recent behavioral changes in patient

Differential Diagnosis (Table 40-8)

Nongonococcal urethritis is caused by organisms other than *N. gonorrhoeae*. These organisms are sexually transmitted, infecting the urethra and causing penile discharge. *N. gonorrhoeae* is sexually transmitted and infects the urethra causing penile discharge. *Trauma* to the urethra can irritate or break the surrounding epithelium and cause penile discharge, which is often bloody. The cause of such trauma can vary; therefore a thorough history is necessary.

Management

Nongonococcal urethritis

Treatments and medications. For children under 45 kg prescribe erythromycin 50 mg/kg per day orally divided into four doses daily for 10 to 14 days. For patients over 45 kg and

Table 40-7 Common NSAIDs Used for Dysmenorrhea (Oral Route of Administration)

DRUG	DOSE	FREQUENCY	MAXIMUM DAILY DOSE
Ibuprofen	200-400 mg	Every 6-8 hours	1200 mg
Naproxen sodium	500 mg then 275 mg	Once (stat.) every 6-12 hours	1375 mg
Ketoprofen	25-50 mg	Every 6-8 hours	300 mg

Table 40-8 Differential Diagnosis: Penile Discharge

CRITERIA	NONGONOCOCCAL URETHRITIS	*NEISSERIA GONORRHOEAE*	TRAUMA
ICD-9 code	099.40	098.19	607.9
Subjective Data			
Age	Any	Any	Any
History: past and present	Sexual contact	Sexual contact	Vigorous exercise; known traumatic event
Description of problem	Dysuria	Dysuria	Dysuria
Associated symptoms	Urethral discharge	Urethral discharge	Tenderness
Objective Data			
Physical examination			
Temperature	Normal	Normal	Normal
General appearance	Appears normal	Appears normal	Appears normal
External genitalia	Possible red, irritated urinary meatus	Red, irritated urinary meatus	Erythema, bruising; possible abrasion
Penile discharge	Mucopurulent or purulent	Mucoid	Bloody
Laboratory data	Urinalysis positive for leukocytes; Gram stain to determine causative organism	Culture positive for *N. gonorrhoeae*	None

8 years of age or older prescribe azithromycin 1 g orally in a single dose or doxycycline 100 mg orally two times a day for 7 days or erythromycin 500 mg orally four times a day for 7 days.

Counseling and prevention

For young children

- Ensure that parents understand the treatment regimen and medication schedule.
- Educate the parents to aid them in understanding that the transmission of NGU is by sexual contact. (See Sexual Abuse in Chapter 47.)
- Inform the parents about the process of reporting sexual abuse in their state of residence.
- Reassure the parents that the intent is to protect the child and help the perpetrator to modify or stop his or her actions.
- Encourage the parents to answer children's questions related to the illness factually and honestly.
- Discuss the benefits of human services, social work, and psychology referral.

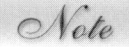

Adolescents have the right to confidentiality in health-care issues related to sexuality. Parents may be informed of treatment and included in counseling if desired by the adolescent.

For adolescents

- Stress the need to refer contacts for evaluation and treatment.
- Encourage open, honest communication with contacts.
- Teach patients to use condoms to prevent exposure to infection.
- Instruct patients on the need to abstain from sexual activity or use a condom until cure is achieved.

- Discuss high-risk behaviors and their implications for health.

Follow-up. Children and adolescents who have been treated for an STD need a follow-up culture 2 to 3 weeks after treatment. They also need to schedule an appointment if symptoms do not subside after treatment or if symptoms recur. Children whose case involves suspected child abuse should be followed closely by medical and social services professionals.

Consultations and referrals

- Report suspected child abuse to the appropriate agency.
- Refer the parents and child to community support groups.
- Refer the child for HIV assessment.
- Refer the patient to a mental health professional if there are high-risk behaviors.

Neisseria gonorrhoeae

Treatments and medications. For children under 45 kg administer ceftriaxone 125 mg intramuscularly in one dose. For adolescents administer ceftriaxone 125 mg intramuscularly in one dose, or cefixime 400 mg orally in one dose, or ciprofloxacin 500 mg orally in one dose, or ofloxacin 400 mg orally in one dose. For all of these, add azithromycin 1 g orally in a single dose.

Counseling and prevention. For young children and adolescents, see the discussion of Nongonococcal Urethritis earlier in this chapter.

Follow-up. Patients who have symptoms that persist after treatment should have a repeat culture. Children whose case involves suspected child abuse should be followed closely by medical and social services professionals.

Consultations and referrals. See the discussion of Nongonococcal Urethritis earlier in this chapter.

Trauma

Treatments and medications

- Discern the source of the trauma.
- Apply mupirocin ointment three times a day on the affected area.

Table 40-9 Differential Diagnosis: Penile Irritation

CRITERIA	PHIMOSIS	ADHESIONS OF THE FORESKIN	BALANOPOSTHITIS
ICD-9 code	605.	752.69	607.1
Subjective Data			
Age	Any	Any, usually resolves by 3 years of age	Any
History: past and present	May have past history of same problem	May have past history of same problem	May have past history of same problem
Description of problem	Unable to retract foreskin; foreskin is scarred	Unable to retract foreskin; foreskin remains supple	Tender foreskin and glans
Associated symptoms	Painful urination; poor urinary stream; tender foreskin; hematuria		Painful urination; frequent urination; penile discharge
Objective Data			
Physical examination			
Temperature	Normal	Normal	May be elevated
General appearance	Normal	Normal	Normal
External genitalia	Scarred foreskin; tip of foreskin whitish; small opening in foreskin; unable to retract foreskin over glans	Tip of foreskin may have small opening; unable to retract over glans; no scarring of foreskin	Foreskin and glans appear tender, warm, erythematous, edematous
Other findings	Negative	Negative	Negative
Laboratory data	Urinalysis positive for blood	Urinalysis normal	KOH may be positive; hyphae; wet prep may be positive: trichomonads

Counseling and prevention
- Teach good hygiene practices (e.g., wash the area with soap and water each day, retracting the foreskin if necessary).
- Teach the patient and parents to observe for symptoms of localized infection (e.g., erythema, warmth, purulent discharge).
- If child abuse is suspected, inform the parents about the process of reporting sexual abuse in the state of residence.
- Reassure the parents that the intent is to protect the child and help the perpetrator to modify or stop his or her actions.

Follow-up. The schedule for follow-up depends on the severity of trauma. For mild to moderate trauma, schedule a return visit in approximately 5 to 7 days. Severe trauma may require further follow-up. If the patient was referred for suspected abuse, close observation of the family is necessary by medical providers and social service workers.

Consultations and referrals
- Consult with or refer to a physician if trauma is severe or if the patient has symptoms of progressing infection.
- Report suspected child abuse to the appropriate agency.

Penile Irritation

MARGARET A. McCABE

Alert

Consult with or refer to a physician for the following:
- Unclear diagnosis
- Symptoms that are resistant to appropriate therapy
- Problems with urinary stream
- Suspicion of child abuse

Etiology

Tight or unretractable foreskin is a normal variation until 6 years of age. Penile irritation can be caused by poor hygiene or infection from bacteria or fungi.

Incidence

- Phimosis occurs in 2% to 10% of uncircumcised males.
- By 3 years of age, 90% of foreskin adhesions resolve.
- Children with balanoposthitis can have secondary infection caused by groups A and D streptococci, *Pseudomonas aeruginosa, Candida albicans,* and *Trichomonas vaginalis.*

Risk Factors

- Past history of phimosis
- Poor hygiene
- Uncircumcised male

Differential Diagnosis (Table 40-9)

Hypospadias is a common congenital defect in which the urinary meatus is on the underside of the penis. There is no urinary incontinence. Chordee (or gryposis penis), a vertical bend in the penis, is also frequently present.

Epispadias is a less common congenital defect causing the urethra to open on the dorsum of the penis. This is considered to be a variant of entrophy of the bladder.

Phimosis is the scarred unretractable foreskin in an uncircumcised male.

Adhesions of the foreskin are tissue growths between the foreskin and glans that make it difficult to retract the foreskin. The foreskin remains supple. It usually resolves by 6 years of age.

Balanoposthitis is inflammation of the glans and foreskin, usually as a result of poor hygiene, which may be a source of secondary infection from bacterial or fungal growth. The patient usually has soreness, irritation, and penile discharge. A smear of the discharge and culture can identify the causative organism.

Management

Hypospadias and epispadias. See Bladder and Urethral Anomalies in Chapter 42.

Phimosis

Treatments and medications. Phimosis may require circumcision.

Counseling and prevention. Inform the parents that many boys do not have a retractable foreskin but that true phimosis may need surgical correction or circumcision.

Follow-up. Observe the child at well-child visits. Inform the parents to call the office if the child has difficulty with urination or infection.

Consultations and referrals. Refer the patient to a surgeon if he has difficulty with urination, repeated infection, or bulging of the foreskin with urination, or if the patient or parents desire referral.

Adhesions of the foreskin

Treatments and medications. Retract the foreskin, clean the area, and return the foreskin to appropriate position daily.

Counseling and prevention

- Inform the parents that the problem often resolves as early as 3 years of age and normally resolves by 6 years of age.
- Advise the parents to call if the child experiences pain or discomfort from the condition.

Follow-up. Observe at well-child visits.

Consultations and referrals. Refer to a surgeon any children older than 3 years of age with severe adhesions or those who experience pain or discomfort as a result of the adhesions.

Balanoposthitis

Treatments and medications

- Elevate the penis to decrease edema.
- Use warm soaks for the penis.
- Administer broad-spectrum systemic antibiotics if the infection is severe. For *C. albicans,* apply topical nystatin cream two times each day until resolved. For *T. vaginalis,* treat with metronidazole (Flagyl) (adult dose, 500 mg orally two times a day for 7 days or 2 g orally in one dose; pediatric dose, 125 mg [15 mg/kg per day] three times a day for 7 days).

Counseling and prevention

- Instruct the patient about the medications and treatment plan.
- Stress the importance of good hygiene, washing daily, and wearing clean clothes daily.

Follow-up. Provide follow-up care by telephone or an office visit after the course of antibiotics and then at routine well-child visits.

Consultations and referrals. A chronic problem may require surgical referral for circumcision.

Pregnancy

KATHERINE SIMMONDS

Alert

Consult with or refer to a physician immediately for the following:
- Vaginal bleeding

- Lower abdominal pain or cramping
- Abnormal vaginal discharge
- Persistent, severe nausea or vomiting
- Severe headache
- Edema of hands and face
- Visual disturbances
- Dysuria, flank pain, chills, or fever
- Rupture of membranes before term
- Decreased fetal movement
- Difficulty breathing or chest pain
- Unilateral swelling, pain, or redness of dependent extremity
  Rule out pregnancy if patient reports the following:
- Amenorrhea or irregular menses
- Fatigue or dizziness
- Nausea or vomiting
- Urinary frequency
- Breast tingling or tenderness
- Unprotected sexual intercourse

Etiology

Pregnancy occurs as a result of the union of an ovum and sperm with subsequent implantation and development of an embryo in the uterus or in some cases outside of the uterine cavity.

Incidence

Approximately 1 million adolescent pregnancies occur in the United States each year.

Risk Factors

- Sexual intercourse with inconsistent or no use of birth control
- Sexual abuse

Differential Diagnosis (Table 40-10)

Intrauterine pregnancy is a pregnancy that has appropriately implanted within the uterus. *Ectopic pregnancy* is a pregnancy in which the ovum implants outside the uterus, most commonly in a fallopian tube. *Molar pregnancy* is a pregnancy in which the ovum develops into a mole instead of an embryo. *Multiple gestation pregnancy* is a pregnancy in which more than one fetus is present in the uterus.

Management

Treatments and medications. If the patient plans to continue the pregnancy, the practitioner may prescribe prenatal vitamins with 0.4 to 0.8 mg of folic acid by mouth every day and ferrous sulfate 325 mg by mouth every day. Advise the patient to consult with an obstetrician or gynecologist before taking any OTC or prescription medication, and consult with an obstetrician or gynecologist regarding continuation of any current medications.

Counseling and prevention

- Counsel the adolescent regarding options:

  Therapeutic abortion—Depending on the state, this option may be available with or without parental, guardian, or legal consent. Depending on gestational age, the cost and availability of the procedure vary from state to state. If the patient elects termination, assist in arranging the procedure (including financial, legal, and emotional aspects) and appropriate follow-up care.

Table 40-10 Differential Diagnosis: Pregnancy

CRITERIA	INTRAUTERINE PREGNANCY	ECTOPIC PREGNANCY*	MOLAR PREGNANCY*	MULTIPLE GESTATION*
ICD-9 code	656.40	633.9	631.0	633.9
Subjective Data				
Pertinent history	Last menstrual period; onset of symptoms of pregnancy	Onset of symptoms of pregnancy and previous history of ectopic, pelvic inflammatory disease, or intrauterine device use	Onset of symptoms of pregnancy	Onset of symptoms of pregnancy
Presenting symptoms	Nausea, vomiting, breast tenderness, fatigue	May complain of lower abdominal pain, vaginal bleeding or spotting, dizziness, or referred shoulder pain	May complain of excessive nausea or vomiting and dark-colored vaginal bleeding or spotting	May complain of excessive nausea or vomiting
Objective Data *Physical examination*				
Fetal heart tone (by doptone)	Audible by about 12 weeks	Not audible in most cases before potential rupture	Not present	May hear more than one heart
Bimanual/pelvic examination	Size consistent with dates	Size may be consistent with dates; mass may be palpable in adnexae; blood may be present in vagina; pain may be elicited with adnexal palpation	Size may be greater than dates in first trimester; size may be less than dates after first trimester; dark blood may be present in vagina	Size greater than dates
Laboratory data	Positive HCG; quantitative HCG doubles about every 48°	Positive HCG; quantitative HCG rises less than 66% every 48°	Positive HCG; quantitative HCG may be abnormally elevated	Positive HCG; quantitative HCG may be higher than normal

*Refer immediately to a physician.

Continuation of pregnancy, including keeping the child or adoption—If the patient elects to continue the pregnancy, educate her about the importance of early and consistent prenatal care. If considering adoption, refer for counseling with a reputable agency. For the adolescent who elects to continue the pregnancy, the practitioner may perform initial prenatal evaluation (Box 40-2) and do appropriate initial prenatal teaching or refer the patient to a nurse midwife, obstetrician, or gynecologist to discuss the normal physical and emotional changes associated with pregnancy.

- Instruct the patient regarding general hygiene and activity. The adolescent may continue any exercise that is done regularly, but it is important to pay attention to changes in the center of gravity and balance as the pregnancy increases in size to avoid injury.
- Recommend walking for prevention of thromboembolic problems and constipation.
- Advise that bathing may continue as usual unless the membranes rupture.
- Advise that sexual activity may continue as usual unless there is rupture of the membranes, vaginal bleeding, placenta previa, or low-lying placenta. Advise the use of safe sex practices as appropriate.
- Counsel the patient regarding maternal and fetal safety: review and screen for domestic violence, use of seatbelts, alcohol, tobacco, illicit drugs, and prescription or OTC drugs, and avoidance of cat feces and raw or undercooked meats.
- Discuss the normal physical and emotional changes associated with pregnancy.
- Review common pregnancy-related discomforts (Table 40-11).
- Instruct the adolescent regarding danger signs in pregnancy (see the Alert box). Advise her to report signs immediately. Inform her how to contact the appropriate practitioner or facility during off-hours.

Follow-up. Provide follow-up care as outlined in Box 40-2.

Consultations and referrals. Promptly refer to an obstetrician or gynecologist any patient with the following preexisting medical conditions: cardiac disease, diabetes mellitus, asthma, hypertension, renal disease or recurrent UTIs, cancer, thyroid disease, liver disease, seizure disorder, anemias or hemoglobinopathies, severe varicosities or thromboembolic problems, lupus erythematosus, HIV infection, and acquired immune deficiency syndrome (AIDS).

Box 40-2 Guide to Antepartal Management

Gestational Age: 0-12 Weeks

Essential data

Diagnosis and dating of pregnancy

Subjective data

Date and normalcy of last menstrual period (LMP)

Signs and symptoms of early pregnancy—amenorrhea, nausea, vomiting, fatigue, urinary frequency, breast tingling or tenderness, date of positive pregnancy test

Obtain complete patient health history and family health history including current living conditions, enrollment in school or work, and financial resources, and assess for substance use, high-risk behaviors, domestic or partner abuse, and partner and parental involvement and support for pregnancy.

Objective data

At initial visist or soon thereafter, perform complete physical examination; pregnancy test (if not previously documented); weight gain or loss; blood pressure; urine dipstick for presence of glucose, protein, and ketones

Breast changes: increased size, more erectile nipples, pigmentation changes, Montgomery tubercles on areola, prominent venous pattern

Uterine changes: Goodell sign (softening of the cervix) at approximately 6 weeks; Hegar sign (softening and compressibility of the uterine isthmus) at approximately 6 weeks; and Chadwick sign (bluish color of cervix) at approximately 6 weeks. Increasing size: 6-8 weeks = small lemon; 8-10 weeks = medium orange; 10-12 weeks = approaching grapefruit size

At initial visit or soon thereafter, perform routine screening for sexually transmitted infection or vaginitis, urinary tract infection and cervical cancer including: gonorrhea, chlamydisis, candidosis, bacterial vaginosis, urine culture, Pap smear

Prenatal blood work: CBC/Hct/Hgb; VDRL or RPR; random glucose; sickle cell screen; rubella antibody screen; G6PD screen; HBsAg; blood typing, Rh factor and antibody screen; HIV antibody (with appropriate counseling, consent and confidentiality)

Ultrasound results as available

Obtain data related to specific patient complaints, discomforts, and danger signs if present (see Alert box)

Management

Options counseling (see Counseling and Prevention)

Initiate or reinforce diet counseling; refer for appropriate nutrition counseling or food supplementation services (e.g., WIC)

Initiate or reinforce vitamin and iron therapy (see Treatments and Medications)

Counsel about common discomforts of pregnancy and relief measures (see Table 40-11)

May order ultrasound for determining gestational age if size/dates discrepancy or unsure LMP.

Consult with a physician regarding any significant medical history, family history, findings on physical examination, or abnormal lab results.

Return visit in 4 weeks for routine prenatal check

Advise patient to report danger signs immediately (see Alert box)

Counsel about emotional changes related to pregnancy including ambivalence, disbelief or denial, emotional lability, or panic at being in uncontrollable situation.

Gestational Age: 12-20 Weeks

Essential data

Dating of pregnancy

Subjective data

Same as for weeks 0-12 as necessary

Assess for resolution of nausea, vomiting, and fatigue

Assess for additional discomforts related to pregnancy

Assess for fetal quickening

Objective data

Weight loss or gain: should gain 4-5 lb by week 20

Blood pressure

Urine dipstick for glucose, protein, and ketones if nausea, vomiting, and weight loss persists

Breast changes: colostrum may be present by 16 weeks

Uterine changes: 12 weeks—palpable as abdominal organ; 16 weeks—halfway between symphysis pubis and umbilicus; 18 weeks—three-fourths of way up from symphysis pubis to umbilicus; 20 weeks—at umbilicus or 20 cm above the symphysis pubis

Fetal heart tone audible by doptone at ∼ 12 weeks; by fetoscope at ∼ 20 weeks

Obtain data related to specific patient complaints, discomforts, and danger signs

Management

Same as for weeks 0-12

Offer triple marker test to screen for increased risk of neural tube defects and Down syndrome between 15-18 weeks

May order routine ultrasound for fetal survey around 16-18 weeks

Have patient return for weekly check of fetal heart if not present by 12-13 weeks by doptone; order ultrasound if not detectable by 14 weeks; have patient return for weekly check of fetal heart if not present by week 20 with fetoscope; if not detectable by 22 weeks, order ultrasound

Request patient report if quickening not noted by 20 weeks

Report any danger signs

Discuss emotional changes including greater acceptance of pregnancy; relief or excitement at presence of quickening; increased introspection

Gestational Age: 20-28 Weeks

Essential data

Dating of pregnancy

Subjective data

Same as for weeks 0-20

Assess for fetal movement, including patterns of movement

Box 40-2 Guide to Antepartal Management—cont'd

Objective data

Weight: should gain approximately 1 lb per week

Blood pressure

Urine dipstick for presence of glucose, protein

Uterine changes: height of uterus corresponds roughly to week of gestation in centimeters (e.g., 24 weeks = 24 cm)

Fetal heart tones clearly audible with doptone or fetoscope

Fetal lie and fetal parts palpable at 26-28 weeks; fetal movements detectable by examination

Obtain data related to specific patient complaints, discomforts, and danger signs

Management

Same as above

Routine screening for gestational diabetes between weeks 24-28 with 1 hour glucose load (50 g glucose); if abnormal result, patient follows a 3-day carbohydrate loading diet, followed by a 3-hour glucose tolerance test (100 g)

Routine administration of RhoGAM to Rh negative patients at 28 weeks following screening to rule out sensitization

Review danger signs, particularly signs of premature labor

Emotional changes: patient may begin having more thoughts and dreams about baby as a person; if sex is known, may call baby by name; begin thinking about and planning for labor

Return visit every 3-4 weeks from weeks 20-28

Gestational Age: 28-36 Weeks

Essential data

Dating of pregnancy

Subjective data

Same as for weeks 0-28

Assess for quality of fetal movement

Objective data

Weight: normal gain continues at about 1 lb per week

Blood pressure: may note slight drop in diastolic

Hematocrit: normal physiologic drop at this point in pregnancy due to expanded blood volume, but should not exceed 10%

Uterus continues to grow at rate of about 1 cm per week above symphysis pubis

Fetal presentation/parts easily palpable; fetal tones easily auscultated with normal rate 120-160 beats/minute

Obtain data related to specific patient complaints, discomforts, and danger signs

Management

Same as for weeks 0-28

Repeat hematocrit around week 28; prescribe ferrous sulfate treatment up to 325 mg three times a day if laboratory values are consistent with iron deficiency anemia

Refer for childbirth preparation classes as appropriate

Review signs of labor, when to go to hospital

Teach daily fetal movement count: client counts fetal movements one time each day after eating; if fetus moves less than 10 times in 2 hours to notify practitioner or hospital

Report danger signs

Emotional changes include increasing concern regarding labor, possible fear, and increasing thought and dreams about the baby

Return visit every 2 weeks for routine check from 28-36 weeks gestation

Gestational Age: 36-42 Weeks

Essential data

Dating of pregnancy

Subjective data

As for weeks 0-36

Assess for quality of fetal movement, particularly after 40 weeks

Assess for impending labor, including presence of "lightening," mucous plug, "blood show," contractions, and rupture of membranes

Objective data

Weight: patient may have slight weight loss (2-3 lb) before onset of labor

Blood pressure

Urine dipstick for glucose protein

Digital pelvic examination may reveal progressive changes in cervix including softening, movement from posterior to anterior, dilatation and effacement; fetal engagement and descent may occur

Uterine fundal height measurement may continue to increase 1 cm per week, but may also stay at same height due to descent of fetus

Fetal presentation and parts easily palpable; fetal heart tones easily auscultated

Obtain data related to specific patient complaints, possible labor/rupture of membranes, and danger signs

Management

Same as for weeks 0-36

Review signs and symptoms of labor, true vs false labor and daily fetal movement count

If fetus presents in breech, notify consulting obstetrician; arrange for external version as appropriate

Repeat VDRL/RPR; cervical cultures for gonorrhea and chlamydia, anogenital cultures for GABHS; and hematocrit at 35-36 weeks

Counsel regarding discomforts of late pregnancy

Emotional changes may include boredom with pregnancy, eagerness or fear of labor, and difficulty sleeping

Review danger signs

Return visit every week; after 40 weeks, perform biweekly nonstress test and biophysical profile. Schedule induction for 42 weeks if spontaneous delivery has not occurred

Table 40-11 Common Pregnancy-Related Complaints

PROBLEM	ETIOLOGY	CLINICAL MANIFESTATIONS	MANAGEMENT

Nausea and vomiting	Increased levels of estrogen and HCG; occasionally psychogenic if persistent or severe	Most severe in first trimester
		Usually occurs at same time(s) each day; not always in morning
		May take form of intolerance to certain foods or odors
		Can cause weight loss or failure to gain
			Medications:
			  Vitamin B$_6$ 25-50 mg orally three or four times a day, not to exceed 20 mg
			  Emetrol 15-30 ml orally on arising and every 3 hours as needed.
			  If there is no relief, consult.
			Counseling:
			  Explain the physiologic basis and probable duration
			  Avoid high-protein and fatty foods, an empty stomach, and specific foods which cause nausea
			  Increase carbohydrate intake and keep food in stomach (toast or dry cereal before arising; Coke or Coke syrup)
			Referral to physician:
			  If it persists beyond 14 weeks.
			  If severe enough to cause weight loss, dehydration or ketosis.

Heartburn	Hormonal relaxation of cardiac sphincter; reflux of gastric contents into esophagus; later in pregnancy may be caused by pressure on stomach from enlarging uterus	Sharp epigastric pain sometimes radiating to back
		May be related by specific foods or occur at specific times
		Differentiate from gallbladder disease
			Medication:
			  Give Maalox, 30 ml 1 hour after eating as needed.
			  Do not give antacids containing sodium bicarbonate (e.g., Rolaids).
			  Recommend avoiding spicy or fatty foods, lying down after meals, and allowing stomach to become empty.
			  Recommend drinking milk and eating small frequent meals.

Round ligament pain	Stretching and contraction of uterine round ligaments, which insert into inguinal canal and top of labia majora	Sharp, pulling twinge in inguinal area, radiating down into labia
		Exaggerated by activities such as walking or turning in bed
			Medications:
			  Give acetaminophen, 325 mg (one or two tablets) orally every 4 hours as needed.
			  Do not take aspirin or ibuprofen.
			Counseling:
			  Explain the physiologic basis.
			  Decrease activities which initiate or exacerbate the problem.
			  Stop activity when the pain occurs, and flex the hip on the affected side.
			  Apply local heat or take warm baths.

Constipation	Relaxation of large intestine because of hormonal effects; increased water absorption; exacerbated by oral iron intake, poor dietary intake of fluids and roughage, inadequate exercise	Hard, difficult-to-pass stools
		Must be differentiated from mere change in bowel habits
			Medications:
			  Milk of magnesia, 30 ml at bedtime
			  Colace, 100 mg at bedtime
			  Fermalox perhaps a less constipating form of oral iron but is expensive
			Counseling:
			  Explain the physiologic basis.
			  Increase exercise.
			  Increase fluid intake and dietary roughage.
			  Establish a relaxed, regular toilet routine.

Modified from Daniels, L.K. (1981). Pregnancy and labor. In Fox, J.A. (Ed.) Primary health care of the young. New York: McGraw-Hill.

Undescended Testes (Cryptorchidism)

MARGARET A. McCABE

Alert

Consult with or refer to a physician for the following:
- Unable to palpate either testicle in scrotum or inguinal canal
- Testicle that does not descend into the scrotum by 1 year of age

Etiology

The cause of this condition is congenital interference with the normal descent of the testicles into the scrotal sac.

Incidence

- Approximately 3% to 5% of cases occur in well male newborns, while 15% of cases are bilateral. Anorchism is present in 5% of cases
- About 20% of cases occur in males born prematurely
- About 80% of cases resolve by 1 year of age

Table 40-11 Common Pregnancy-Related Complaints—cont'd

PROBLEM	ETIOLOGY	CLINICAL MANIFESTATIONS	MANAGEMENT

Low backache	Muscle fatigue from accentuated lordosis of pregnancy; exacerbated by poor posture and poor body mechanics when bending or lifting; accentuated by wearing high-heeled or platform shoes	Dragging backache in lumbosacral area
		Frequency more severe in multiparas with poor abdominal muscle tone or who lift child or other heavy objects
		Differentiate from pyelonephritis and labor
			Medications:
			  Give acetaminophen, 325 mg every 4 hours as needed.
			  Do not take aspirin or ibuprofen in third trimester of pregnancy.
			Counseling:
			  Explain the physiologic basis.
			  Show patient how to use the legs for leverage when bending to pick up something.
			  Rest one foot on a stool or box when standing for long periods (ironing).
			  Teach pelvic rock.

Sciatica	Pressure on sciatic nerve from increased mobility of sacroiliac joint caused by hormonal effect on connective tissue	Sharp shooting pain down posterior area of thigh frequently initiated or exaggerated by exercise (e.g., walking, vacuuming)	Medications:
			  Acetaminophen, 325 mg (one or two tablets) every 4 hours as needed
			Counseling:
			  Explain the physiologic basis.
			  Avoid activities which initiate or exaggerate the problem.
			  Apply heat locally or take warm baths.
			  Remember that a maternity girdle will immobilize the pelvic joints but is expensive.

Dependent edema	Mechanical obstruction of venous return by enlarging uterus	Usually increases as day goes on rather than being present in morning upon awakening
		May occur after long periods of standing or in hot weather
		Usually in lower extremeties but can occur in hands
		Must be differentiated from more severe, generalized edema of preeclampsia
			Medications:
			  None. DO NOT GIVE DIURETICS IN PREGNANCY. DO NOT RESTRICT SODIUM.
			Counseling:
			  Explain the physiologic basis.
			  Have the patient rest on left side, flat in bed, at least 2 hours per day.
			  Maintain a diet high in protein.
			  Increase fluid intake to 2-3 L daily.
			  Elevate legs when sitting.
			  Report danger signs of preeclampsia.

Vaginal discharge	Normal leukorrhea of pregnancy because of increased vascularization and mucosal proliferation from hormonal effects	Profuse, white, cream discharge
		Nonirritating and non-odorous
		Must be differentiated from infections (e.g., candidaiasis, trichomoniasis, bacterial infections) (see Vulvovaginal Symptoms in this chapter)
			Medications:
			  See Vulvovaginal Symptoms in this chapter for treatment of specific infections.
			Counseling:
			  Explain the physiologic basis.
			  Keep perineal area clean and dry; expose it to the air.
			  Wear cotton underwear.
			  Avoid nylon underwear, pantyhose, tight pants, douching, feminine hygiene products, and water softeners in the bath water.

Risk Factors

- History of prematurity
- Presence of hydrocele or inguinal hernia
- Positive family history

Differential Diagnosis (Table 40-12)

Anorchism (anorchia) is the complete absence of testes. The scrotal sac appears smaller and softer than normal. This may be a result of a chromosomal anomaly.

Retractile testes is a physiologic variation of normal that results from an overactive cremasteric reflex. It is often bilateral. The incidence decreases with age as testes enlarge and the cremasteric reflex decreases. On examination the testes can be palpated in the inguinal canal and brought down into the scrotum.

True undescended testis is indicated when the testicle is not palpable in the scrotal sac. The testicle may be in the inguinal canal or in an intraabdominal location.

Management

Anorchism

Treatments and medications. The treatment depends on the underlying disorder.

Counseling and prevention

- Explain to the parents the cause for concern and the need for specialist referral.
- Reassure the parents and answer their questions honestly and thoroughly.
- Provide emotional support.

Table 40-12 Differential Diagnosis: Undescended Testicles

CRITERIA	ANORCHIA*	RETRACTILE TESTES	TRUE UNDESCENDED TESTIS
ICD-9 code	752.8	752.52	752.51
Subjective Data			
Age	Usually detected at birth or very shortly after	Usually detected at birth or very shortly after	Usually detected at birth or very shortly after
History	No report of seeing testicles in scrotum	May report seeing testicles in scrotum at times	History of prematurity; positive family history; no report of seeing testicles in scrotum
Description of problem	Report scrotal sac small; no visual evidence of testicles	Report testes not always in scrotum	Report no visual evidence of testes in scrotum
Objective Data *Physical examination*			
Genitalia	Small, soft scrotum; no testicles palpated in scrotum or inguinal canal	Testicles may be observed in scrotum; may be palpated in scrotum or in inguinal canal Examining child in cross-leg sitting or squatting may be helpful	Testicles not palpated in scrotum; may be palpated in inguinal canal
Laboratory data	Chromosomal analysis	None	Ultrasound of pelvis to locate testicle Laproscopy

*Refer to a pediatric urologist.

Follow-up
- Provide follow-up care at routine well-child care visits.
- Maintain communication with specialists regarding the plan of care.

Consultations and referrals. Refer the child to a urologist or an endocrinologist.

Retractile testes
Treatments and medications. None are necessary.
Counseling and prevention
- Explain the cremasteric reflex to the parents to enhance their understanding of the situation.
- Request that the parents observe the scrotum during dressing or bathing to identify the presence of the testicle.

Follow-up. Monitor testicular descent with observation and palpation at routine well-child visits.

Consultations and referrals. None are necessary.

True undescended testis
Treatments and medications. Examination under anesthesia may be done initially, followed by laparoscopy. Surgery or orchidopexy may be performed between 1 and 3 years of age. The effectiveness of hormonal therapy in true undescended testicle is controversial.

Counseling and prevention
- Explain to the parents that the testes usually descend within the first year of life.
- Request that the parents observe the scrotum during dressing or bathing to identify the presence of the testicle.
- If surgical treatment is necessary, explain the surgical plan (i.e., a simple procedure, short-stay surgery).
- Reinforce the importance of follow-up care after the procedure.
- Explain that monthly testicular examinations after puberty are important because of slightly increased risk of tumor.

Follow-up. Provide follow-up care through observation and palpation at routine well-child visits during the first 1 to 3 years of life.

Consultations and referrals. Refer the child to a urologist if the testes do not descend into the scrotum by 1 year of age.

Vulvovaginal Symptoms

MARGARET A. McCABE

Alert

Consult with or refer to a physician for the following:
- Unclear diagnosis
- Symptoms that are resistant to appropriate therapy
- Suspicion of sexual or physical abuse

Etiology

In prepubescent girls the vulvar skin is susceptible to irritation and trauma because of poor hygiene, the proximity of the vagina and anus, the lack of protective hair and labial fat pads, and the lack of estrogenization. A child or adolescent may acquire a vulvitis, a primary vulvitis with a secondary vaginitis, or a primary vaginitis with a secondary vulvitis. Contamination of the vulva or vaginal flora causing localized irritation or infection may be caused by respiratory pathogens, enteric pathogens, STDs, pinworms, a foreign body, polyps or tumors, systemic illness, vulvar skin disease, or trauma.

Incidence

- Nonspecific vulvovaginitis accounts for 25% to 75% of vulvovaginitis.
- Bacterial vaginosis occurs in 33% to 37% of women at STD clinics and in 4% to 15% of college students.

Risk Factors

- Positive past history of STD or vulvovaginitis
- Family or individual history of sexual abuse

- Sexual activity (risk increases when sex is unprotected or with multiple partners)
- Recent behavioral changes
- Poor hygiene
- Frequent bubble baths or use of hygiene products
- Wearing tight pants, pantyhose, or synthetic fibers
- Recent antibiotic therapy
- Recent systemic illness
- Chronic illness, including diabetes
- Masturbation
- Obesity

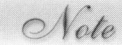

Child molestation always needs to be ruled out when one is assessing a child in this diagnostic category.

Differential Diagnosis

Vulvar or vaginal irritation may occur at any age and may be attributable to any number of causes (Table 40-13).

Nonspecific vulvovaginitis is localized irritation of the vulva and vagina caused by a variety of organisms.

Physiologic leukorrhea is an increased amount of thin white discharge.

Pinworms are parasites infesting the perianal region, causing localized irritation.

Abrasion is an open area caused by trauma.

Foreign body (an object in a body orifice) in the vagina can cause vulvovaginal symptoms.

Chemical irritation is localized atopy caused by the use of soaps, perfumes, cleaning products on clothing, or personal hygiene products.

Gonorrhea is an STD caused by *N. gonorrhoeae* bacteria. Presenting symptoms include dysuria, frequency, abdominal pain, and mucopurulent vaginal discharge.

Chlamydiosis is an STD caused by *C. trachomatis* bacteria. Presenting symptoms include dysuria, frequency, abdominal pain, and mucopurulent vaginal discharge.

Trichomoniasis is an STD caused by the *T. vaginalis* protozoon. Females may be asymptomatic or complain of pruritic vaginal discharge.

Pelvic inflammatory disease is an inflammation of the pelvic organs. Sexually transmitted organisms are implicated in most cases. Typical presentation includes lower abdominal pain including adnexal tenderness, fever, vaginal discharge, and cervical motion tenderness.

Bacterial vaginosis is a bacterial infection of the vagina that shows a profuse white, gray, or yellow discharge with a fishy odor.

Candidiasis, an infection caused by an overgrowth of *C. albicans*, is characterized by a thick, cheesy vaginal discharge with intense pruritus.

Management

Vulvovaginal symptoms in prepubescence
Nonspecific vulvovaginitis
Treatments and medications
- Prescribe broad-spectrum antibiotics, such as amoxicillin 20 mg/kg per day in three divided doses for 10 to 14 days or amoxicillin clavulanate (Augmentin) 20 mg/kg

per day based on the amoxicillin component in three divided doses for 10 to 14 days, or a cephalosporin (e.g., cephalexin, cefaclor) for 10 to 14 days.
- For persistent signs and symptoms, prescribe an estrogen cream at bedtime for 2 to 3 weeks, followed by every other day for 2 weeks.
- For pruritus, prescribe hydroxyzine hydrochloride (Atarax) 2 mg/kg per day in four divided doses or diphenhydramine hydrochloride 5 mg/kg per day in four divided doses.
- Recommend sitz baths for comfort.
- Suggest antibacterial cream at night.
- Suggest the patient or parents try A&D ointment, Vaseline, or Desitin to protect vulvar skin.

Counseling and prevention
- Educate the parents and child regarding the treatment plan and medication schedules.
- Instruct in good perineal hygiene, daily bathing, and handwashing. Good handwashing is especially important during a time of systemic illness.
- Recommend that the child wear cotton, loose-fitting underwear.
- Instruct the child not to use bubble bath or perfumed hygiene products.
- Suggest that the child should avoid tight-fitting pants, hose, or sleeper pajamas, especially those made of synthetic fibers.

Follow-up. If the child has been treated for a nonspecific vulvovaginitis, provide follow-up care by telephone or office visit after completion of the antibiotic course.

Consultations and referrals. Refer the child to a physician if symptoms are unresponsive to treatment.

Physiologic leukorrhea
Treatments and medications. Provide symptomatic relief measures to relieve patient discomfort, such as daily baths, cotton underwear, loose-fitting pants (suggest that no tight hose or sleepers be worn), and application of Desitin, A&D, or Vaseline on the irritated area.

Counseling and prevention
- Inform the parents and child that the condition usually resolves in 2 to 3 weeks.
- Instruct the parents and child in the importance of good perineal hygiene and daily bathing.
- Explain to the parents that some young girls do experience vaginal discharge. It will resolve, and following the recommended treatments aids in the child's comfort.

Follow-up. Provide follow-up care as needed.

Consultations and referrals. None is necessary.

Pinworms. See Perianal Itch and Pain in Chapter 35 and Parasitic Diseases in Chapter 44.

Treatments and medications
- Prescribe mebendazole 100 mg in one dose, to be repeated in 2 weeks.
- Remember that other family members may need to be treated.

Counseling and prevention
- Instruct the parents and child on the need for good hygiene. This includes bathing daily, good perineal hygiene, changing underwear daily, changing pajamas daily, and washing bedsheets weekly.
- Stress the importance of washing hands before eating and after bathroom use.

Table 40-13 Differential Diagnosis: Vaginal Symptoms—Prepubescence and Adolescence

CRITERIA	NONSPECIFIC VULVOVAGINITIS	PHYSIOLOGIC LEUKORRHEA	PINWORMS	ABRASION	FOREIGN BODY	CHEMICAL IRRITATION
ICD-9 code	616.10	623.5	127.4	959.1	939.2	623.9
Subjective Data						
Age	Any	Often newborn period; onset prepuberty	Any	Any	Any	Any
History: past and present	Exposure to respiratory pathogens, enteric pathogens; systemic illness	Possible past history, tends to have a cyclic pattern	Recent family history	Recent history of trauma; reports wearing tight-fitting pants, hose, or sleeper pajamas	Past history of foreign body in any orifice; retained tampon in adolescent	Reports use of bubble bath; use of new hygiene product; wears tight clothing
Description of problem and associated symptoms	Painful urination; vulvar and vaginal itching, burning, discharge, bleeding	Localized irritation; vulvar and vaginal itching or burning	Perineal itching, intensity may increase at night	Perineal discomfort, including burning and itching; possible bleeding	Painful urination; discharge; foul odor	Possible painful urination; possible itching
Objective Data						
Physical examination						
Temperature	Normal	Normal	Normal	Normal	Normal	Normal
General appearance	Appears normal	Appears normal	Appears normal	Appears normal	Appears normal	Appears normal
External genitalia	Vulvar and vaginal erythema or excoriation	Possible mild irritation	Adult pinworms visualized around anus at night; possible erythema, lesions from scratching	Localized edema, erythema; excoriation; abraded area; bruising	Localized erythema; foul odor; palpate mass through rectal wall; visualize foreign body	Erythema; excoriation
Internal genitalia (adolescence)	Appears normal	Appears normal	Appears normal	Appears normal	Appears normal; may visualize foreign body	Appears normal
Vaginal discharge	Minimal, mucoid	Copious creamy white	None	Blood stained	Purulent or bloody	None to minimal
Laboratory data	Normal urinalysis; normal wet prep; negative cultures	Normal urinalysis; normal wet prep; negative cultures	Normal urinalysis; pinworm eggs observed under microscope "tape test" (tape to rectal area at night and then put to glass slide)	Urinalysis normal or positive red blood cells	Urinalysis normal	Urinalysis normal, possibly a few red blood cells

GONORRHEA 098.0	CHLAMYDIOSIS 099.53	TRICHOMONIOSIS 131.0	CANDIDIASIS 112.9	BACTERIAL VAGINOSIS—*GARDNERELLA VAGINALIS*	PELVIC INFLAMMATORY DISEASE 614.9
Any	Any	Any	Any	Any	Any
Sexual contact, possibly unknown	Sexual contact, possibly unknown	Sexual contact, possibly unknown	Recent history of antibiotic or corticosteroid use	May or may not be related to sexual contact	Sexual contact; previous episode of PID; multiple sexual partners
Vaginal or urethral discharge; dysuria, frequency; labial tenderness; eye infection in newborn; urethritis in males; proctitis; pharyngitis; females often asymptomatic	Vaginal or urethral discharge; abdominal pain; dysuria, frequency; eye infection or pneumonia in newborn; urethritis in males; urethral syndrome in females	Copious discharge, painful urination, frequency; vulvar/vaginal itching; lower abdominal discomfort; postcoital bleeding	Painful urination; vulvar or vaginal itching; discharge; onset after menses or midcycle; increased symptoms postcoitally	Irregular, prolonged menses; abdominal pain	Onset following menses; lower abdominal pain; fever; vaginal discharge; irregular vaginal bleeding
Normal. Signs of infection in other mucomembranous regions, eye, throat, rectum	Normal. Conjunctivitis in infants; suprapubic tenderness; right upper quadrant tenderness in older children	Normal. Excoriated upper thighs	Normal. May affect oral mucosa	Normal. Appears normal	Normal to elevated. Lower abdominal tenderness
Rarely erythema, tenderness	Appears normal	Vulvar erythema, excoriation	Erythema and hyperemia of vulva; papulopustular perineal dermatitis; linear perineal fissures or excoriations	Possible erythema	May visualize external lesion due to HSV or HPV
Cervical discharge	Cervical tenderness; friable cervix; cervical hypertrophy; cervical discharge	Vaginal walls and cervix may have erythematous, granular appearance; cervical discharge	Erythema of mucosa	Discharge adherent to vaginal walls	Purulent cervical discharge; cervical motion tenderness; adnexal tenderness
Mucopurulent	Mucopurulent in females; white, clear, or mucopurulent in males	Frothy yellow-green, foul odor	Thick white discharge; no odor	Profuse gray, white, or yellow homogenous discharge, strong fishy odor	Minimal to moderate, may be purulent
Gonococcus culture positive; also collect *Chlamydia* culture; Gram stain positive for gram-negative diplococci; serologic RPR negative	*Chlamydia* culture positive; serologic rapid plasma reagin (RPR)	Wet prep positive—trichomonads; pH > 4.5	Wet prep positive hyphae, pseudohyphae, spores; pH > 4.5	Wet prep positive clue cells; positive "whiff" on KOH; pH > 4.5	Elevated white blood cell count and sedimentation rate; serologic RPR negative; collect *Chlamydia* culture and gonococcus culture

Follow-up. The practitioner may recheck the tape test with a microscope if symptoms continue after treatment.

Consultations and referrals. None are indicated.

Abrasion

Treatments and medications. Suggest an antibacterial cream (e.g., mupirocin, bacitracin) at bedtime and sitz baths for comfort and hygiene.

Counseling and prevention

- Instruct the parents and child on the need for good hygiene. This includes washing the area daily with soap and water and attempting to keep the abrasion and surrounding area clean.
- Educate the patient to use caution when engaging in activities with a risk of abrasion (e.g., bicycling).

Follow-up. Children treated for trauma need to be followed based on the severity of the injury.

Consultations and referrals. Refer the child to a physician if the trauma is extensive or requires sutures.

Foreign body

Treatments and medications

- Remove the foreign body. Inspect all body orifices (e.g., nose, ears) for additional foreign bodies.
- Irrigate with warm water.
- If there are signs or symptoms of infection, use a broad-spectrum antibiotic such as amoxicillin 20 mg/kg per day in three divided doses for 10 to 14 days or amoxicillin clavulanate (Augmentin) 20 mg/kg per day based on the amoxicillin component in three divided doses for 10 to 14 days, or a cephalosporin (e.g., cephalexin, cefaclor) for 10 to 14 days.

Counseling and prevention. Discuss the possible cause of the behavior with the parents.

Follow-up. No follow-up care is needed unless the child is treated for an infection.

Consultations and referrals

- Refer the child to a physician if unable to remove the object.
- Refer the child to a mental health professional if this is a recurrent event or behavioral problem.

Chemical irritation

Treatments and medications

- Advise the parents and child to identify and avoid the irritant.
- If the irritation is moderate to severe, apply 1% hydrocortisone cream or ointment each morning and night to decrease irritation until the symptoms are resolved.
- Recommend sitz baths for comfort.

Counseling and prevention. Instruct the parents and child on the need for good hygiene. This includes daily bathing, cotton underwear to decrease irritation, and loose-fitting pants.

Follow-up. The child may be followed up with by telephone for mild irritation and with an office visit for moderate to severe irritation.

Consultations and referrals. Refer the child to a physician if the source of the irritation cannot be verified.

Gonorrhea. See Sexual Abuse in Chapter 47.

Treatments and medications. Prescribe ceftriaxone 125 mg intramuscularly in one dose or spectinomycin 40 mg/kg intramuscularly in one dose, up to 2 g. Children who weigh more than 45 kg are treated with the adult regimen and doses.

Counseling and prevention

- Be sure that the parents understand the treatment regimen and medication schedule.
- Educate the parents to aid them in understanding that the transmission of gonorrhea is by sexual contact.

- Inform the parents about the process of reporting sexual abuse in their state of residence.
- Reassure the parents that the intent is to protect the child and help the perpetrator to modify or stop his or her actions.
- Encourage the parents to answer children's questions related to the illness factually and honestly.
- Discuss the implications for HIV screening.
- Discuss the benefits of human services, social work, and psychology referral.

Follow-up. Children who respond to treatment do not need a repeat culture. The practitioner may decide a follow-up visit is necessary for social considerations.

Consultations and referrals

- Report suspected child abuse to the appropriate agency. Children whose case involves suspected child abuse should be followed closely by both medical and social services professionals.
- Refer the parents and child to community support groups.
- Refer the child for HIV assessment.

Chlamydiosis

Treatments and medications. Prescribe erythromycin 50 mg/kg per day orally in four divided doses for 10 days, up to 500 mg per dose. For children 8 years of age and older, doxycycline 100 mg orally two times a day for 7 days may be prescribed.

Counseling and prevention. See the preceding discussion of Gonorrhea.

Follow-up. See the preceding discussion of Gonorrhea.

Consultations and referrals. See the preceding discussion of Gonorrhea.

Trichomoniasis. See Sexual Abuse in Chapter 47.

Treatments and medications. Prescribe metronidazole 125 mg (15 mg/kg per day) three times a day for 7 to 10 days.

Counseling and prevention. See the earlier discussion of Gonorrhea.

Follow-up. See the earlier discussion of Gonorrhea.

Consultations and referrals. See the earlier discussion of Gonorrhea.

Candidiasis

Treatments and medications. Apply topical nystatin, miconazole, or clotrimazole cream to the affected area for approximately 7 days. Suggest that the parents and child may need to apply the cream in the vagina in a moderate to severe case, giving one applicator of miconazole cream at bedtime for 7 nights or one vaginal suppository at bedtime for 3 nights or one applicator of clotrimazole cream in the vagina at bedtime for 7 to 14 nights.

Counseling and prevention

- Explain the treatment regimen to the parents.
- Educate the parents to aid them in understanding that candidiasis is not usually sexually transmitted.
- Encourage the parents to answer children's questions related to the illness factually and honestly.

Follow-up. Once the cause is determined, the child may be seen at routine well-child intervals for age. Schedule a return visit if symptoms recur.

Consultations and referrals. None are indicated unless the problem is recurrent or resistant to therapy, in which case consultation may be appropriate.

Vaginal discharge in adolescence

Nonspecific vulvovaginitis

Treatments and medications

- Prescribe broad-spectrum antibiotics, such as amoxicillin 250 mg three times a day for 10 to 14 days or amoxicillin clavulanate (Augmentin) 250 mg based on the amoxicillin component three times a day for 10 to 14 days, or a cephalosporin (e.g., cephalexin, cefadroxil) for 10 to 14 days.

- For persistent signs and symptoms, prescribe an estrogen cream at bedtime for 2 to 3 weeks, followed by every other day for 2 weeks.
- For pruritus, prescribe hydroxyzine hydrochloride (Atarax) 25 mg four times a day or diphenhydramine hydrochloride (Benadryl) 25 to 50 mg four times a day.
- Recommend sitz baths for comfort.
- Suggest antibacterial cream at night.

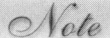

Adolescents have the right to confidentiality in health-care issues related to sexuality. Parents may be informed of treatment and included in counseling if desired by the adolescent.

***

Counseling and prevention
- Educate the adolescent regarding the treatment plan and medication schedules.
- Instruct the adolescent in good perineal hygiene, daily bathing, and hand washing. Good hand washing is especially important during a time of systemic illness.
- Recommend that the patient wear cotton, loose-fitting underwear.
- Instruct the adolescent not to use bubble bath or perfumed hygiene products.
- Suggest the patient wear no tight-fitting pants, hose, or sleeper pajamas, especially those made of synthetic fibers.

Follow-up. If the patient has been treated for a nonspecific vulvovaginitis, follow-up care by telephone or office visit should occur after completion of the antibiotic course.

Consultations and referrals. Refer the patient to a physician if symptoms are unresponsive to treatment.

Physiologic leukorrhea

Treatments and medications. Suggest symptomatic measures to relieve patient discomfort such as daily bathing, cotton underwear, loose-fitting pants (suggest that no tight hose or sleepers be worn), and apply Desitin to the irritated area.

Counseling and prevention
- Advise the patient that the condition usually resolves in 2 to 3 weeks.
- Instruct the adolescent on the importance of good perineal hygiene and daily bathing.
- Reassure the patient and explain that this problem will resolve and that the recommended treatments will aid in comfort.

Follow-up. Provide follow-up care as needed.

Consultations and referrals. None are necessary.

Pinworms. See Perianal Itch and Pain in Chapter 35 and Parasitic Diseases in Chapter 44.

Treatments and medications
- Prescribe mebendazole 100 mg in one dose, to be repeated in 2 weeks.
- Remember that other family members may need to be treated.

Counseling and prevention
- Instruct the adolescent on the need for good hygiene. This includes bathing daily, good perineal hygiene, changing underwear daily, changing pajamas daily, and washing bedsheets weekly.

- Stress the importance of washing hands before eating and after bathroom use.

Follow-up. The practitioner may recheck the tape test with the microscope if symptoms continue after treatment.

Consultations and referrals. None are indicated.

Abrasion

Treatments and medications
- Suggest an antibacterial cream (e.g., mupirocin, bacitracin) at bedtime.
- Recommend sitz baths for comfort and hygiene.

Counseling and prevention
- Instruct the adolescent in the need for good hygiene. This includes washing the area daily with soap and water and attempting to keep the abrasion and surrounding area clean.
- Educate the patient to use caution when engaging in activities with a risk of abrasion (e.g., bicycling).

Follow-up. Adolescents treated for trauma need to be followed based on the severity of the injury.

Consultations and referrals. Refer the patient to a physician if the trauma is extensive or requires sutures.

Foreign body

Treatments and medications
- Remove the foreign body. Inspect all body orifices for foreign bodies.
- Irrigate with warm water.
- If there are signs or symptoms of infection, use a broad-spectrum antibiotic such as amoxicillin 250 mg three times a day for 10 to 14 days or amoxicillin clavulanate (Augmentin) 250 mg based on the amoxicillin component three times a day for 10 to 14 days, or a cephalosporin (e.g., cephalexin, cefadroxil) for 10 to 14 days.

Counseling and prevention
- Discuss the possible cause of the behavior with the patient.
- Instruct the patient on the treatment plan.

Follow-up. No follow-up care is needed unless the adolescent is treated for an infection.

Consultations and referrals
- Refer the adolescent to a physician if unable to remove the object.
- Refer the patient to a mental health professional if this is a recurrent event and there is concern that it is a behavioral problem.

Chemical irritation

Treatments and medications
- Instruct the adolescent to identify and avoid the irritant.
- If the irritation is moderate to severe, have the patient try 1% hydrocortisone cream or ointment each morning and night to decrease irritation until the symptoms are resolved.
- Recommend sitz baths for comfort.

Counseling and prevention. Instruct the adolescent on the need for good hygiene. This includes daily bathing, cotton underwear to decrease irritation, and loose-fitting pants.

Follow-up. The patient may be followed up by telephone for mild irritation and with an office visit for moderate to severe irritation.

Consultations and referrals. Refer the adolescent to a physician if the source of the irritation cannot be verified.

Gonorrhea

Treatments and medications
- Prescribe one of the following in addition to azithromycin 1 g orally in one dose:
  Ceftriaxone 125 mg intramuscularly in one dose
  Cefixime 400 mg orally in one dose

Ciprofloxacin 500 mg orally in one dose
Ofloxacin 400 mg orally in one dose

Counseling and prevention

- Be sure that the patient understands the treatment regimen and medication schedule.
- Educate the patient in understanding that the transmission of gonorrhea is by sexual contact.
- Encourage proper and consistent condom use.
- Refer the partner for evaluation and counseling even if asymptomatic.
- If sexual abuse is suspected, inform the patient and parents about the process of reporting sexual abuse in their state of residence (see Sexual Abuse in Chapter 47).
- Reassure the patient and parents that the intent is to protect the adolescent and help the perpetrator to modify or stop his or her actions.
- Encourage the parents and adolescent to have open communication related to sexuality.
- Discuss the implications for HIV screening.
- Discuss the benefits of human services, social work, and psychology referral.

Follow-up

- Remember that patients who are symptom free after treatment do not need a follow-up culture.
- Schedule a return visit if symptoms recur.
- Recommend annual gynecologic examinations with Pap smears.

Consultations and referrals

- Report suspected sexual abuse to the appropriate agency.
- Remember that an adolescent whose case involves suspected child abuse should be followed closely by both medical and social service professionals.
- Refer the parents and adolescent to community support groups.
- Refer the adolescent for HIV assessment.

Chlamydiosis

Treatments and medications. Prescribe doxycycline 100 mg orally two times a day for 7 days or azithromycin (Zithromax) 1 g orally in one dose.

Counseling and prevention. See the earlier discussion of Gonorrhea.

Follow-up. See the earlier discussion of Gonorrhea.

Consultations and referrals. See the earlier discussion of Gonorrhea.

Trichomoniasis

Treatments and medications. Prescribe metronidazole 2 g orally in one dose or metronidazole 500 mg orally two times a day for 3 to 7 days.

Counseling and prevention. See the earlier discussion of Gonorrhea.

Follow-up. See the earlier discussion of Gonorrhea.

Consultations and referrals. See the earlier discussion of Gonorrhea.

Pelvic inflammatory disease

Treatments and medications. Refer to a physician for possible hospital admission

Counseling and prevention. See the earlier discussion of Gonorrhea.

Follow-up. See the earlier discussion of Gonorrhea.

Consultations and referrals. See the earlier discussion of Gonorrhea.

Candidiasis

Treatments and medications

- Prescribe one of the following:
  Butoconazole 2% cream (OTC) 5 g intravaginally for 3 days
  Clotrimazole 1% cream (OTC) 5 g intravaginally for 7 to 14 days
  Clotrimazole one 500 mg vaginal tablet
  Miconazole 200 mg vaginal suppository one time per day for 3 days
  Tioconazole 6.5% ointment 5 g intravaginally once
  Terconazole 0.8% cream 5 g intravaginally for 3 days
  Terconazole 80 mg vaginal suppository once a day for 3 days
  Fluconazole 150 mg orally in one dose.
- Recommend sitz baths for relief of irritation.
- Remember that recurrences require close assessment of risk factors.
- Recommend cotton underwear.
- Have the patient discontinue using perfumed vaginal hygiene products.

Counseling and prevention

- Treatment of the sexual partner is not usually required.
- Recommend abstinence or proper condom use until symptoms resolve.
- Educate the patient on the importance of practicing safe sex.
- Encourage good perineal hygiene.

Follow-up. A return visit is not required if the medication is used properly and symptoms subside. If the patient is at risk for noncompliance, a return visit is recommended in 1 to 2 weeks.

Consultations and referrals. None is indicated.

Bacterial vaginosis (Gardnerella vaginalis)

Treatments and medications

- Recommend symptomatic therapy: sitz baths, cotton underwear, loose-fitting pants.
- For nonpregnant adolescents prescribe metronidazole 500 mg orally two times a day for 7 days or clindamycin cream 2% 5 g intravaginally at bedtime for 7 days.
- For pregnant adolescents prescribe metronidazole 250 mg 3 times a day for 7 days or clindamycin 300 mg orally two times a day for 7 days.

Counseling and prevention

- Treat contacts only if there are recurrent symptoms.
- Educate the patient that this can be related to sexual contact but is not always sexually transmitted.
- Encourage good perineal hygiene.
- Instruct the patient on the treatment plan and medications.

Follow-up. See the earlier discussion of Gonorrhea.

Consultations and referrals. None are indicated.

Resources

Websites

The American College of Obstetricians and Gynecologists (www.acog.org)

The Alan Guttmacher Institute (www.agi-usa.org)

The Association of Reproductive Health Professionals (www.arhp.org)

Center for Young Women's Health, Children's Hospital, Boston (www.youngwomenshealth.org)

The Centers for Disease Control and Prevention (www.cdc.gov)

The Cochrane Collaboration (www.cochrane.org)

Double Sunrise (www.doublesunrise.com)

Medscape Women's Health (www.WomensHealth.medscape.com)

Museum of Menstruation and Women's Health (www.mum.org)

The National Guideline Clearinghouse (www.guideline.gov)

National Women's Health Advocacy Group (www.womenshealth-network.org)

The National Women's Health Information Center (www.4women.gov)

Ob-Gyn Net (www.obgyn.net)

The World Health Organization Reproductive Health Program (www.who.int/reproductive-health)

Bibliography

Baker, A. (1995). *Abortion and options counseling: A comprehensive reference.* Granite City, IL: Hope Clinic.

Bobak, I. & Jensen, M. (1993). *Maternity and gynecologic care: The nurse and the family*, St. Louis: Mosby.

Briggs, G.G, Freeman, R., & Yaffe, S.J. (1998). *Drugs in pregnancy and lactation: A reference guide to fetal and neonatal risk* (5th ed.). Baltimore: Williams & Wilkins.

Centers for Disease Control and Prevention. (1998). Sexually transmitted diseases treatment guidelines. *Morbidity and Mortality Weekly Report* (No. RR-1), 47.

Emans, S.J.H., Laufer, M.R., & Goldstein, D.P. (1998). *Pediatric and adolescent gynecology* (4th ed.). Philadelphia: Lippincott-Raven.

Hatcher, R., Robert, A., & Trussell, J. (1998). *Contraceptive technology* (17th ed.). New York: Ardent Media.

Henshaw, S.K. (1999). *US teenage pregnancy statistics with comparative statistics for women aged 20-24.* New York: Alan Guttmacher Institute.

Hillard, P.A. (1995). Abnormal uterine bleeding in adolescents, *Contemporary Nurse Practitioner, 1*(5), 21-28.

Hoekelman, R., Adam, H.M., Nelson, N.M., Weitzman, M.L., & Wilson, M.H. (2001). *Primary pediatric care* (4th ed.). St. Louis: Mosby.

Johnson, K. (2000). *The Harriet Lane handbook* (15th ed.). St. Louis: Mosby.

Lemcke, R. (1995). *Primary care of women.* Norwalk, CT: Appleton & Lange.

Scott, J., DiSaia, P.J., Hammond, C., & Spellacy, W. (1999). *Danforth's obstetrics and gynecology* (8th ed.). Philadelphia: Lippincott, Williams & Wilkins.

Shulman, L.P. (2000). Clinical trial results with MPA/E2C. *Journal of Reproductive Medicine, 45*(10 suppl.), 873-877.

Star, W.L., et al. (1999). *Ambulatory obstetrics: protocols for nurse practitioners/nurse midwives* (3rd ed.). San Francisco: University of California, Santa Barbara, School of Nursing.

Stewart, F.H., Harper, C.C., Ellertson, C.E., et al. (2001). Clinical breast and pelvic examination requirements for hormonal contraception: Current practice vs. evidence. *Journal of the American Medical Association, 287*(17), 2232-2239.

U.S. Preventive Services Task Force. (1996). *Guide to clinical preventive services* (2nd ed.). Baltimore: Williams & Wilkins.

Varney, H. (1997). *Varney's midwifery* (3rd ed.). Sudbury, MA: Jones & Bartlett.

Youngkin, E.Q. & Davis, M.S. (Eds.). (1998). *Women's health: primary care clinical guide.* Stamford, CT: Appleton & Lange.

Chapter 41 *Respiratory System*

Jennifer Piersma D'Auria

Breathing Difficulty, Stridor, and Wheezing, p. 645
Cough, p. 653
Nasal Bleeding (Epistaxis), p. 656
Nasal Congestion and Obstruction, p. 659
Sore Throat (Pharyngitis), p. 664
Voice Changes, p. 667

Risk Factors

- Neonate, infant, or young child (age-related differences in structure and function)
- Low–birth-weight (LBW) or premature infant
- Disease involving the airway (with any history of ventilation support) (e.g., bronchopulmonary dysplasia [BPD], respiratory distress syndrome, transient tachypnea of the newborn, cystic fibrosis [CF])
- Systemic disorders (e.g., immunosuppressed children, BPD, immotile cilia)
- Incomplete immunization status
- Emotional and physical stress
- Family or child history of asthma, CF, tuberculosis, or other pulmonary diseases
- Child history of recurrent respiratory problems
- Exposure to smoking or tobacco use
- Drug abuse (e.g., of cocaine, marijuana)
- Sudden infant death syndrome (SIDS) in a sibling
- Environmental hazards, including exposure to chemicals, animals, dust, asbestos, and other pulmonary irritants
- Environmental exposure to respiratory infections, influenza, or tuberculosis
- Obesity
- Congenital malformations of the airway (e.g., choanal atresia, cleft palate, tracheoesophageal fistula)

Health Promotion

Prevention of Infections

- Maintain general health and ensure balanced nutrition and adequate rest.
- Wash hands carefully.
- Dispose of respiratory secretions properly.
- Cover nose and mouth with a tissue when coughing and sneezing.
- Avoid exposure to pathogens as much as possible.
- Keep all immunizations up to date, including pertussis, influenza, and pneumococcal vaccines for high-risk groups.

Promotion of Respiratory Effort

Use a warm or cool mist humidifier for symptomatic relief of respiratory discomfort. Steam humidifiers are generally not recommended for safety reasons. Run a shower of hot water with the bathroom door closed to produce steam quickly. Have the child sit in the steamy bathroom for at least 10 minutes. (If upset or fearful, the child should be cuddled closely.) Have the parents and child notice whether cool or warm mist works more effectively to promote respiratory ease.

Positioning for Maximum Lung Expansion

- Avoid constricting clothes or blankets.
- Remember that the American Academy of Pediatrics (AAP) recommends that the prone position be avoided for healthy infants. Infants should be placed in the supine or side-lying position when put to bed during the first 6 months of life.
- During acute respiratory episodes, keep in mind that an older child may be put into a semiupright position supported by two pillows. For an infant, put a small blanket under the crib mattress to elevate it, or place the infant in a side position.

Maintenance of an Effective Airway

- Remember that saline nose drops may be used in infants (including infants less than 6 months of age). They may be purchased at a store or prepared at home (¼ teaspoon of table salt to 8 oz of warm tap water). If home preparation is recommended, provide the parents with written instructions and a demonstration of how to prepare saline nose drops.
- Use gentle suction with a nasal bulb syringe to clear nasal passages for infants. Teach parents to compress the bulb syringe before inserting it into the naris or both nares and then to release it slowly to remove nasal secretions to decrease irritation to the nasal mucosa.
- Consider topical decongestants for older children (over 6 years of age) with supervision. Use one bottle of topical nasal medication for each child. Do not administer topical preparations for more than 3 to 5 days to avoid rhinitis medicamentosa (rebound congestion). Nasal medications should be used sparingly in older infants (6 months of age or older) and in children under 6 years of age. If nasal congestion is severe, decongestant or vasoconstrictive nose drops may be helpful before feeding and at bedtime to promote nutrition and rest in younger age groups. Nasal decongestants also may be helpful for opening nasal passages during the first few days of using nasal cromolyn or intranasal corticosteroids.
- Keep in mind that the anticholinergic drying effects of first-generation antihistamines (e.g., chlorpheniramine, diphenhydramine, triprolidine) may provide relief from symptoms (e.g., runny nose, postnasal drip) associated with the common cold. In addition, the sedative effect of these first-generation antihistamines may prove helpful at night to quiet a nonproductive, irritative cough. They are not recommended for infants younger than 6 months and should be used sparingly in children from 6 months to

6 years of age. Recent nonsedative antihistamines (e.g., terfenadine, astemizole) lack anticholinergic drying effects and therefore do not help to diminish symptoms caused by the common cold. These newer antihistamines are an acceptable alternative for children with allergic rhinitis who cannot tolerate the sedative side effects of classic antihistamines. They have long half-lives and are prescribed for once or twice a day.

- Remember that oral decongestants may provide symptomatic relief from nasal stuffiness and congestion from the common cold. They are frequently used in combination with antihistamines. Oral decongestants and antihistamine-decongestant combination preparations are not recommended for infants younger than 6 months and should be used sparingly in children from 6 months to 6 years of age.

- Use antiinflammatory nasal sprays to possibly provide further relief for children with allergic and respiratory problems. Nasal cromolyn sodium is a safe drug with few side effects. It is prescribed three to six times a day, which may limit adherence. Nasal topical steroids are generally used for children whose allergic symptoms cannot be controlled by avoidance, antihistamines, or nasal cromolyn. They will take effect within 3 to 5 days, with a peak effect by 2 weeks. Side effects are minimal. Both nasal cromolyn and nasal topical steroids are best used as preventives but will provide relief during an illness. Shorts courses or bursts of oral steroids (e.g., prednisone) are generally reserved for severe cases that are not responsive to the previously described therapies.

- Keep in mind that the most commonly used antitussives include demulcents such as lollipops, honey, and throat lozenges. These local measures are safe and useful for coughs related to upper respiratory infections (URIs) or pharyngitis. Cough suppressants (centrally acting antitussives) should be used rarely in children. Dextromethorphan is the most frequently found nonopioid antitussive in over-the-counter (OTC) preparations. These preparations may contain a high percentage of alcohol and opioid ingredients that have a sedative effect. They may be used to control cough at bedtime to promote sleep in children over 3 years of age. They should be kept out of the reach of children. Antihistamines may also be classified as antitussives because of their sedative effect; however, they also have a drying effect on respiratory secretions. It is important to encourage parents to call before using cough medications in very young children. Parents should be counseled about the importance of cough as a protective reflex and the importance of treating the underlying disorder rather than the symptom.

- Remember that water is the most commonly prescribed expectorant, both orally and by inhalation. Cough expectorants, except for water, are rarely used in children. These drugs thin respiratory secretions and promote the flow of respiratory fluid so that the child can expectorate the mucus. Guaifenesin is the most commonly used expectorant in OTC preparations. It reduces the thickness of sputum but does not necessarily reduce the amount of coughing. Iodides were once popular in expectorants. The AAP Committee on Drugs recommends that iodides not be used in children.

- Counsel the child and the parents about the common behavioral side effects of OTC preparations used to treat minor respiratory illness, such as irritability, excess stimu-

lation, and insomnia with sympathomimetics; sedation with antihistamines, expectorants, and cough suppressants; and gastrointestinal (GI) upset with expectorants and cough suppressants.

- Encourage the child to avoid exposure to smoke. Assess factors that influence the child's or adolescent's desire to initiate smoking. Encourage parents who smoke to alter their behavior.

General Support Measures

- Encourage rest as needed.
- Use acetaminophen for mild fever, discomfort, and irritability associated with respiratory tract infections. Aspirin is contraindicated because of the association of influenza virus with the risk of developing Reye syndrome.
- Apply warm or cold compresses to sinuses.
- Promote hydration and nutrition appropriate for the age of the child. Increase fluid intake (especially of clear fluids, including Jell-O [gelatin dessert], popsicles, and iced drinks) to promote comfort and liquefy secretions to prevent dehydration, and to increase calorie intake during brief periods of anorexia.
- Suggest older children use warm salt water gargles, lozenges, and sour candies to alleviate throat discomfort.

Promotion of Parent and Child Competence in Well-Child and Illness Care

- Educate the parents about age-related differences in the respiratory system, especially for infants and very young children.
- Teach the parents what to look for (e.g., respiratory distress, dehydration, noticeable irritability), when to call the office, and what strategies to use at home when caring for a child with a respiratory problem.
- Use age-appropriate explanations and strategies to teach the child self-care with respect to respiratory health and illness.
- Help the parents and child recognize the influence of stress on respiratory problems.
- Promote discussion on environmental control to reduce precipitating factors.

Additional Areas for Anticipatory Guidance

- Discourage substance abuse and encourage adult and peer relationships with positive role-modeling.
- Promote parental and child understanding of age-appropriate safety concerns, including discussion of falls, suffocation, aspiration, accidents, and sports injuries.

Subjective Data

- Demographics, including age, gender, race, and socioeconomic status
- Reason for the visit and description of the problem (seek perceptions of the parents and child)
- Onset of symptoms (related to age and suspected cause)
- Course of the illness, including acute, recurrent, chronic, or progressive (getting better or worse)
- Precipitating factors, including feeding, allergy, acute or chronic infection, exercise, trauma, chronic irritation, foreign body, emotional stress, and exposure to infectious, chemical, or environmental irritants (e.g., fumes, smoke, weather changes, dust)
- Relieving factors (e.g., medications, positional changes)

- Current medications and treatments, including how they are diluted and administered, current prescription and OTC drugs, the purpose of their use, side effects, the response of the child, and when last administered
- Associated signs and symptoms, including fever, poor weight gain, anorexia, nasal discharge, sneezing, nosebleeds, sore throat, hoarseness, cough (worse at night or during the day), wheezing, stridor, shortness of breath or difficulty breathing, chest pain, difficulty swallowing or feeding, watery eyes, ear or tooth pain, drooling, vomiting, sweating, abdominal pain, irritability, rash, and chills
- Child's health habits, including eating or feeding behavior, relationship to feeding or difficulty feeding (for infants), and decreased appetite; changes in sleep patterns, activity level, or personality or temperament; school-related factors, including achievement, peer pressure, and number of absences from school; and medications, including difficulties with adherence
- Response to home management of respiratory problems
- Previous episodes of similar symptoms and the treatment methods
- Immunizations, including diphtheria, pertussis, tuberculin skin testing, *Haemophilus influenzae* type B, and pneumococcal vaccines (if indicated)
- Past health history, including hospitalizations or operations, infectious diseases, chronic illnesses: (if there is a history of allergies, describe extent of involvement, type of symptoms, and treatment methods), and past or recurrent problems related to the respiratory system, including the type, frequency, and treatments (e.g., BPD, asthma, croup, bronchitis, pneumonia, tuberculosis, sinusitis, number of colds or respiratory infections or otitis media in the previous 6 to 12 months, nasal polyps, foreign-body aspiration or insertion, cardiac disease)
- Birth history
- Feeding history (for neonates and infants)
- Date of last chest examination (or radiograph)
- Family health history, including:

  Present state of health of family members, including recent illness or infectious disease in the previous 2 weeks and any history of chronic illness in other family members (list age of onset)

  Level of family stress (child's and parents' perceptions), including method of coping with stress, perception of coping abilities, stability of the marriage, any recent moves, parent and sibling relationships, and any changes in jobs or unemployment

  Family history of disorders related to the respiratory system, including hematologic disorders, cardiopulmonary diseases, epistaxis, allergies, asthma, eczema, hay fever, allergic rhinitis, sinusitis, drug sensitivities, tuberculosis, obesity, and cystic fibrosis

  Experience with respiratory illness and home management
- Social history, including:

  Environmental screen, including location and condition of residence, occupation (including type of job), crowding, cleanliness, infectious disease, and chemical or environmental irritants (including pets)

  Exposure level, including number of settings the child spends time in (e.g., day care, preschool, elementary school, camp, high school, other)

  Economic factors, including family income sufficient for food, clothing, shelter, and health care treatment (including medications)

Exposure to smoking (e.g., Does the child smoke or chew tobacco? Do other family members or friends smoke?)

Child stress level, including friendship patterns; changes in intimate or peer relationships; sports or other competitive outlets; changes in schools; and transitions to elementary, middle, or high school

Objective Data

Physical Examination

A complete physical examination is generally indicated for all infants and children with significant upper or lower respiratory signs and symptoms. All procedures are explained to the child and the parents before being performed. The examiner is advised to evaluate the heart and lungs early in the examination of the infant and young child before crying and agitation occur. The examination should include:

- *Measurements*—Measure height and weight percentiles and vital signs.
- *General appearance*—Evaluate responsiveness (e.g., through play, smiling) to examiner and environment, as well as facial expression, posture, and body position.
- *Skin and lymph*—Inspect for color, edema, rash, lesions, and sweating; palpate to assess skin turgor; inspect nails for color; assess capillary refill in the fingernails; check for clubbing; and inspect and palpate the location and size of any lymphadenopathy.
- *Neck*—Palpate for position of the trachea, thyroid size, and masses.
- *Eyes*—Inspect eyes for swelling, tearing, discharge, or redness.
- *Ears*—Inspect color, integrity, position, and landmarks of tympanic membrane. Use pneumatic otoscopy to determine mobility.
- *Nose*—Inspect externally for deformity, swelling, and flaring of nostrils; assess character (e.g., unilateral or bilateral, thin, watery, bloody, purulent, foul smelling) and amount of discharge; palpate external nose for tenderness, deformities, swelling, and patency; perform direct inspection of internal mucosa and turbinates with otoscope handle with a nasal speculum (use a pen or flashlight to assess infants and toddlers); and inspect for moistness, color, lesions, polyps, drainage, foreign body, and inflammation of internal nasal mucosa.
- *Sinuses*—Inspect skin surfaces over and adjacent to the four paranasal sinuses, and assess location of pain (if any) to palpation and percussion of frontal and maxillary sinuses (for children under 8 years of age, the frontal sinuses are too small to palpate).
- *Mouth and throat*—Inspect for mouth breathing (make sure to test each nostril for patency), excessive pooling of saliva, and color and lesions of lips and oral mucosae; inspect tonsils for position, size, color, and exudates; inspect posterior pharynx for color, swelling, drainage; and notice quality of voice or cry; quality and character of cough, if present; and any breath odors.
- *Heart*—Palpate and auscultate for point of maximal impulse, and assess first and second heart sounds and the presence of any abnormal heart sounds (if an abnormal heart sound is present, find the location where it is heard best and note intensity, pitch, quality, and timing in the cardiac cycle).
- *Chest and lungs*

  Inspect chest configuration for size, shape, symmetry, and movement.

Assess type of respiratory movement (abdominal or diaphragmatic breathing in infants and young children, mixed thoracic and abdominal breathing in those from 5 to 7 years of age, and thoracic breathing in those from 7 to 8 years of age).

Assess respirations for rate, rhythm (in infants and children, rate and rhythm may be irregular), depth, quality, and character, and note inspiration-to-expiration (I:E) ratio.

If respiratory distress is observed, find the position of greatest ease of breathing and note other indications of respiratory distress, especially flaring of the nares, grunting, head bobbing, and stridor.

Palpate for symmetric chest expansion and tactile or vocal fremitus.

Auscultate and compare breath sounds from side to side for intensity, pitch, quality, and duration during inspiration and expiration.

Remember that percussion is less useful for evaluation of the respiratory system in smaller children and infants; the chest should be resonant to percussion, and any other sound indicates a pathologic condition.

- *Abdomen*—Inspect, percuss, and palpate abdomen for pain and organomegaly.
- *Neurologic*—For level of consciousness, observe irritability, restlessness, or confusion; examine for meningeal signs.

Diagnostic Procedures and Laboratory Tests

Diagnostic tests are dictated by the age of the child, the history, and the physical examination findings. They include:

- *Chest radiograph examination*—In general, an examination is indicated only to rule out a foreign body (inspiratory and forced expiratory) or infectious process (anteroposterior and lateral views).
- *Throat culture (if epiglottitis is ruled out)*—Current data indicate that rapid strep tests (RSTs) may be specific (90% to 96%) but lack sensitivity (76% to 87%). It is recommended that two swabs be obtained in a child who is suspected of having a streptococcal infection. If the RST is negative, a culture can then be done. When one is performing a throat swab, it is important to make contact with only the tonsils and the posterior aspect of the pharynx. Proper swabbing of exudates can greatly increase the chance of finding group A β-hemolytic streptococci (GABHS).
- *Blood cell and differential counts*—With respect to the respiratory system, a complete blood cell (CBC) count or white blood cell (WBC) count with or without a differential may be ordered as part of an evaluation of an infection (or of the course of an infection). A child's total WBC count and the total number of neutrophils (or number of immature and mature neutrophils) increase in response to tissue damage related to an infectious process. The release of increased numbers of neutrophils may occur during a severe bacterial infection and is called a "shift to the left." This term refers to the fact that neutrophils are generally reported in the first column on the left of a differential count and now occupy a higher proportion of the total population of WBCs. The number of eosinophils will increase in number and migrate to sites of an allergic reaction. (See Laboratory Tests in the Appendix.)
- *Pulmonary function tests*
  Peak expiratory flow rate (PEFR)—The peak expiratory flow meter or minometer is used to measure peak expiratory flow (in children at least 4 to 5 years of age).

PEFR may be used in numerous ways. It is a useful tool for measuring the severity of obstruction in an acute respiratory attack. (Less than a range of 30% to 50% of predicted baseline value or a child's personal baseline value indicates severe obstruction.) It also may be used to monitor a child's response to treatment during an acute attack or response to chronic treatments. It also may help the child and family monitor the daily course of a pulmonary disorder, thereby facilitating earlier treatment or showing the need for treatment changes.

Spirometer—Used for older children (5 to 7 years of age), the child is asked to take in a slow, full inhalation, hold it briefly, and then suddenly blow out as much air as possible over at least 3 seconds. The tracing that results shows the forced vital capacity (FVC) and the forced expiratory volume in the first second of exhalation (FEV_1). Diseases that obstruct airflow decrease the FEV_1 more than the FVC. An FEV_1/FVC ratio of greater than 0.85 in children is interpreted as normal airflow.

- *Sinus radiograph examination*—A sinus radiograph examination is rarely indicated. Consult with the physician before ordering. If it is ordered, a Waters' projection (maxillary sinuses) is usually sufficient.
- *Lateral neck radiograph examination*—This examination is indicated to rule out upper respiratory obstruction.
- *Tuberculin skin testing*—See Chapter 13.
- *Pulse oximetry*—Pulse oximetry may be used in the assessment and management of patients with respiratory problems. It is a fast and reliable way to continuously monitor arterial oxygen saturation noninvasively. Pulse oximetry measures light absorption by transillumination of the skin. The principle behind this method is that oxygenated hemoglobin absorbs red light at certain wavelengths. Measurement during a systolic pulse allows estimation of arterial oxygen saturation. Values as low as 80% oxygen saturation may be reliably measured with this method. Certain conditions reduce the reliability of oxygen saturation values such as hyperbilirubinemia, poor perfusion, and severe anemia.

Breathing Difficulty, Stridor, and Wheezing

Alert

Consult with or refer to a physician for the following:
- Respiratory rate of 60 breaths per minute or higher with respiratory distress
- Suspicion of foreign-body aspiration
- Persistent wheezing after therapy
- Infant with dyspnea and expiratory grunt
- Excessive drooling
- Dyspnea with muffled voice
- Stridor at rest (expiratory only, or both inspiratory and expiratory)
- Chronic stridor
- Signs of respiratory failure
- Infant less than 3 months of age
- Premature infant less than 6 months of age with a history of apnea
- Infant with chronic cardiopulmonary disease
- Anxious parents or parents with no access to a phone or transportation in case the child worsens rapidly

Etiology

Dyspnea, or difficulty in breathing, stridor, and wheezing are signs and symptoms of upper or lower respiratory disease in children. (See also Asthma in Chapter 45.) It is critical for the practitioner to determine whether the above symptoms are greatest during inspiration or expiration. This determination will help the practitioner localize the anatomic site of obstruction and develop a differential diagnosis. Increased inspiratory effort is suggestive of disease in the upper airway, whereas increased expiratory effort is suggestive of disease in the smaller airways or lower respiratory tract.

Upper airway problems generally interfere with air entry by variable obstruction of the airway. Stridor is the presenting "sound" with upper airway disease. It is generally described as a crowing or coarse sound and is usually heard during inspiration. Inspiratory stridor should direct the practitioner to consider common disorders above or below the glottis, such as croup, epiglottitis, laryngitis, and bacterial tracheitis. Stridor may occur on expiration or on both inspiration and expiration and is indicative of more significant obstruction. Expiratory wheezing is a high-pitched musical sound caused by partial airway obstruction. It is commonly associated with disorders of the lower respiratory tract that cause inflammation, infection, or bronchoconstriction. Pneumonia and asthma are the two most common clinical conditions associated with wheezing.

Psychogenic factors such as pain, fear, and hyperventilation syndrome are also associated with breathing difficulties in children.

Incidence

- Breathing difficulties are more frequent in infants and very young children because of developmental differences in the structure and function of the respiratory tract.
- They are more frequent during fall and early winter, since many disorders of the upper airway are viral in origin.
- Foreign-body aspiration is more common in children 6 months to 4 years of age.
- Children exposed to tobacco smoke have an increased incidence of lower respiratory infections and symptoms such as recurrent wheezing.
- Children with chronic cardiac, respiratory, congenital, or acquired immunodeficiency disorders (e.g., allergies, prematurity, BPD, congenital heart disease, cystic fibrosis, sickle cell, acquired immune deficiency syndrome [AIDS]) have an increased incidence of respiratory symptoms.

Risk Factors

- History of pulmonary disorders of the newborn (e.g., idiopathic apnea of infancy, respiratory distress syndrome, transient tachypnea)
- Neonates (including very-low–birth-weight [VLBW] infants), infants, and very young children because of age-related differences in structure and function of the respiratory tract
- Exposure to respiratory irritants or pathogens (e.g., tobacco smoke, air pollution, day care environment, house dust mites)
- Maternal infection during pregnancy (e.g., cytomegalovirus [CMV], *Chlamydia,* herpes simplex virus, rubella togavirus)
- Maternal chronic illness during pregnancy (e.g., diabetes, asthma)

- Maternal drug use during pregnancy (including smoking) or during labor and delivery
- Chronic cardiac, respiratory, congenital, or acquired immune deficiency problems (e.g., allergies, prematurity, BPD, CF, sickle cell, AIDS)
- History of recurrent aspiration or ventilation
- History of recurrent pulmonary infections
- History of apnea or hospitalization for pneumonia
- Family history of genetic diseases that affect the lung, atopy (e.g., asthma, eczema, hay fever), recent infectious diseases, apnea, or sudden infant death syndrome (SIDS)
- Incomplete immunization status
- Recent travel or exposure to pets, which potentially increase the possibility of unusual pathogens
- Anxious parents or parents with no access to a phone or transportation in case the child worsens rapidly

Differential Diagnosis

When attempting to develop a differential diagnosis, one must be critical in determining if the parents and child are using the same terminology for stridor and wheezing as the practitioner. Be prepared to imitate sounds for the parents or the child or ask them to imitate the sounds they are trying to describe to you (or during a telephone contact, ask the parents to put the phone by the child's nose and chest so you can hear the sound). During telephone or office contacts, always ask the parents or the child if the child is having trouble getting air in (inspiration) or out (expiration). Respiratory difficulty is an anxiety-producing situation for parents and children. Regardless of the severity of the illness, carefully assess the home environment and the parents' level of skill and comfort in caring for the ill child. Always ask parents if they have access to transportation or a telephone.

Acute stridor and upper airway obstruction (Table 41-1). *Viral croup (acute laryngotracheobronchitis)* is an acute inflammatory disease of the larynx and subglottic area. It is most often caused by parainfluenza virus serotypes. The predominant signs of upper airway obstruction in viral croup include a barking cough and inspiratory stridor.

Acute spasmodic laryngitis (spasmodic croup) is believed to be associated with a mild URI with an allergic component. It develops rapidly after exposure to a precipitating factor, occurs chiefly at night, and may recur. Clinically, physical signs and symptoms associated with spasmodic croup are generally very difficult to differentiate from those of viral croup. Therefore only viral croup is included in Table 41-1.

Epiglottitis is a medical emergency. It is usually caused by *H. influenzae* type B. Inflammation and swelling of the supraglottic structures may progress to complete airway obstruction. The practitioner in pediatric primary care must be aware of the diagnostic work-up associated with epiglottitis for immediate referral to a physician or hospital. The introduction of the *H. influenzae* conjugate vaccine has resulted in a dramatic decline in the incidence of this disease.

Lower airway involvement (Table 41-2). Acute bronchitis refers to inflammation of the trachea and bronchi and is generally caused by viral infections, such as adenovirus, influenza viruses, and respiratory syncytial virus (RSV). *Mycoplasma pneumoniae* is a common bacterial cause of acute bronchitis in children over 6 years of age. Acute bronchitis is generally a benign disease with few complications.

Acute pneumonia is acute inflammation of the lung and is classified according to the infecting agent. The causes of

Table 41-1 Differential Diagnosis: Viral Croup and Epiglottitis*

CRITERIA	VIRAL CROUP	EPIGLOTTITIS*
ICD-9 code	464.4	464.30
Subjective Data		
Age	6 months to 3 years	2 to 6 years
Season	Late fall and early winter	Any
Diurnal pattern	Worse at night	Throughout the day
Onset	Gradual and progressive; ask about the duration of symptoms	Sudden and progressive
Does your child look sicker than usual?	Variable; if severe, will appear gravely ill	Yes, gravely ill appearance
Preceding illness	Viral infection	Usually none
Fever	Low grade or absent	Moderate to high fever
Drooling	No	Yes
Voice quality	Hoarse	Muffled
Sore throat	No	Yes
Difficulty swallowing	No	Pronounced
Cough	Barking	None
Respiratory distress	Variable intensity of distress	Typically, inspiratory retractions and cyanosis
Stridor	Inspiratory (and/or expiratory)	Inspiratory
Past medical history	May have prior episodes of reactive airway disease, allergy, asthma	
Immunization status	Note any gaps in immunization schedule	Note any gaps in immunization schedule
Family coping and resources	Reliability of the caregiver; past experience with acute illness in children; access to telephone and transportation; distance from medical care	
Objective Data		
Physical examination		
Vital signs; especially respiratory rate	Mild fever or afebrile; respiratory rate mild to moderate increase (rate <40-50/minute)	High fever, rapid pulse and respirations
General appearance	Variable, depends on severity of obstruction; usually nontoxic, in sitting position, with restlessness and irritability	Toxic, agitated, restless, in sitting position leaning forward ("sniffing position")
Observe for signs of dehydration	Dry mucous membranes, poor tear production, decreased skin turgor, lethargy, sunken anterior fontanel	Dry mucous membranes, poor tear production, decreased skin turgor, lethargy
Cough	Harsh, barking	None
Voice quality	Hoarseness	Muffled
Ear, nose, and throat	Mild infection of nasopharynx, mild edema of mucous membranes	Pharynx beefy red, drooling Do not attempt to visualize epiglottis
Stridor	Inspiratory stridor with activity or at rest (increased severity)	Inspiratory
Respiratory status	Variable intensity; rate usually not more than 50/minute; labored with supraclavicular and intercostal retractions; may have wheezing and rhonchi on expiration; prolonged inspiratory phase	Severe respiratory distress
Laboratory tests		
Chest radiographs Lateral neck radiographs	May consider; generally not needed	May consider; generally not needed

*Immediate referral to a physician.

pneumonia in children are age related and depend on the season of the year. During the neonatal period, infants may have pneumonia caused by pathogens acquired from infection of the maternal genital tract. GABHS, *Escherichia coli,* and *Staphylococcus aureus* are common organisms causing newborn pneumonia. Chlamydial pneumonia is caused by *Chlamydia trachomatis* and occurs in infants 2 to 12 weeks of age. Respiratory syncytial virus (RSV) is the most common viral cause of pneumonia in infants 2 years of age and younger. It occurs in epidemics during the winter and early spring. Other uncommon causes of bacterial pneumonia in infants and young children may include CMV and *Pneumocystis carinii.*

Table 41-2 Differential Diagnosis: Lower Airway Disorders

CRITERIA	ACUTE BRONCHITIS	ACUTE BRONCHIOLITIS	ACUTE PNEUMONIA	BRONCHIAL ASTHMA
ICD-9 code	466.0	466.19	486.	493.9
Subjective Data				
Age	Young children because of viral etiology; M. pneumoniae common cause in school-age children and adolescents	Generally < 24 months; range of occurrence: 3 months to 3 years (RSV most common etiologic agent in this age group)	All ages; C. trachomatis etiologic agent in infants < 3 months; viral etiology more common in children 3 months to 4-5 years; M. pneumoniae in children > 5 years; RSV more common in infants 2 years of age and under	Majority present before 7 years of age
Season	Usually winter months	Common during late winter, early spring	Common during winter	Depends on precipitating or aggravating factors
Onset	Acute	Abrupt onset of wheezing and dyspnea; very young infants and premature infants may present with apnea, lethargy, few respiratory symptoms	Viral and mycoplasmal: Insidious; bacterial: Abrupt onset of fever and respiratory distress	May be insidious and prolonged or acute
Recent illness or precipitating factors	May have preceding URI	Rhinitis, cough, coryza for 1-2 days	Viral: URI signs and symptoms; then wheezing, increased respiratory rate, and intercostal retractions; or anyone in the family with recent infectious disease	Precipitating or aggravating factors may include allergy, infection, environmental changes (e.g., humidity, dust, temperature), exercise, emotional factors
Fever	Low-grade or absent	Low-grade or absent	Viral, mild to moderate; bacterial, high fever with chills	If concurrent infection
Associated signs and symptoms	Dry, nonproductive cough, worse at night; cough may become productive and accompanied by gagging or vomiting; chest pain in older children; complains of headache, myalgia, anorexia, and lethargy if attributable to M. pneumoniae or influenza viruses	Hacking cough; decreased appetite or difficulty feeding or sleeping; very young infants and premature infants may present with apnea, few respiratory signs or symptoms	Viral: dry hacking nonproductive cough, hoarseness, mild tachypnea, abdominal distension; bacterial: productive cough, respiratory distress, chest or abdominal pain; decreased appetite, difficulty taking fluids or sleeping	Mild to moderate respiratory distress, coughing, wheezing, tightness in chest; cough may be paroxysmal with vomiting; decreased appetite or difficulty taking fluids or sleeping
Family medical history	May have history of CF, immune disorders, asthma, other significant cardiopulmonary disease, smoking	May have history of CF; allergic reactions to foods, airborne allergens or insect stings; asthma, other cardiopulmonary disease, immune disorders	May have history of CF, sickle cell, immune disorders, AIDS, CMV, congenital heart disease, tuberculosis; atopy (asthma, eczema, hay fever)	May have history of asthma, allergic rhinitis, hay fever, chronic cough, eczema, atopic dermatitis
Child's past medical history	See Family Medical History; may have history of LBW, BPD, hospitalization, other episodes of bronchitis, recurrent aspiration, foreign-body aspiration, tobacco or marijuana smoking	See Family Medical History; allergy or atopy, foreign-body aspiration, congenital heart disease with congestive heart failure, BPD	See Family Medical History; LBW infant with hospitalization, previous hospitalization for pneumonia, immune disorders, recent case of measles, tuberculosis, any recent choking	See Family Medical History; may have history of chronic bronchitis, bronchiolitis, pneumonia, exposure to passive smoking

Recent exposures	Anyone in family with recent infectious illness (e.g., croup, URI; exposure to passive smoke or smoking; other precipitating factors associated with allergy or asthma)	Anyone in family with recent infectious illness (e.g., influenza, croup, URI)	Anyone in family with recent infectious illness; recent travel or exposure to pets episodes (foreign-body aspiration)	See Recent Illness for precipitating or aggravating factors
Immunization status	May have gaps in immunization schedule			
Family coping and resources	Reliability of the caregiver; past experience with acute illness in children; access to telephone and transportation and distance from medical care			
Objective Data *Physical examination*				
Vital signs	Fever generally low-grade or absent	Fever low-grade or absent, increased respiratory rate and heart rate	Depends on etiology: mild to pronounced fever, increased respiratory rate and heart rate	May have fever, depending on cause of attack; determine respiratory rate, heart rate, and blood pressure as baseline for comparison after treatment initiated
Growth percentiles	Note if height and weight are age-appropriate and if growth channels are being maintained			
General appearance	Nontoxic	Depends on severity; usually, signs of respiratory distress: shallow, rapid respirations; may have nasal flaring, cyanosis, retractions Note activity level and responsiveness	Variable—depends on etiology, age of child, and severity of disease Inspect at rest for dyspnea, grunting on expiration, respiratory rate > 50/minute, flaring of nostrils, intercostal and subcostal retractions (without stridor) Note activity level and responsiveness	Posture: May have rounded shoulders because of hyperinflation, anxious appearance, irritable; may have audible wheezing without stethoscope
Skin	—	May have pallor, cyanosis; poor capillary refill; signs and symptoms of dehydration: saliva, tears, skin turgor, dryness	May have pallor, cyanosis; poor capillary refill; signs or symptoms of dehydration: saliva, tears, skin turgor, dryness	May have pallor, sweating, cyanosis (if severe), poor capillary refill
Head, eye, ear, nose, and throat	Rhinitis usually present Dry, harsh cough	May have other concomitant foci of infection (e.g., otitis media, bacterial pneumonia)	May have other concomitant foci of infection (e.g. otitis media, sinusitis, meningitis)	Rhinorrhea and other signs of respiratory infection or allergy (e.g., allergic shiners, nasal crease, gaping facies)
Chest and lungs	High-pitched expiratory rhonchi, may also have inspiratory rhonchi that clear with coughing	Note abdominal respiratory movement; if paradoxical, immediate referral; symmetric expiratory wheezing or grunting; hyperresonant to percussion; prolonged expiratory phase, may have crackles (or rales)	May have normal auscultatory findings with pneumonia; may have decreased breath sounds with dullness to percussion, localized diminished breath sounds, tubular breath sounds, fine rales; older child may present with friction rub	Prolonged expiration with expiratory wheezes; may have inspiratory wheezes; may have greatly diminished air movement without wheezing; use of accessory muscles of respiration; intercostal retractions; hyperresonant to percussion
Cardiac	—	Tachycardia	Older child may have chest pain	Apex of heart and point of maximal impulse may be displaced
Abdomen	Liver and spleen may be palpable (because of hyperinflation of the lungs)	Abdominal distension or discomfort; liver and spleen may be palpable	Abdominal distension or discomfort	Abdominal distension or enlarged liver

Continued

Table 41-2 Differential Diagnosis: Lower Airway Disorders—cont'd

CRITERIA	ACUTE BRONCHITIS	ACUTE BRONCHIOLITIS	ACUTE PNEUMONIA	BRONCHIAL ASTHMA
Laboratory tests				
Chest radiographs	After consultation, usually not needed (films may be normal or show a mild increase in bronchovascular markings); inspiratory and expiratory chest radiographs if respiratory distress, wheezing, or cough of new onset in high-risk age group (6 months to 3 years) or history of choking episode	After consultation, usually not needed (films generally show hyperinflation with mild interstitial infiltrates)	Not needed in mild cases (films usually show perihilar streaking, increased interstitial markings, patchy bronchopneumonia; lobar consolidation may occur)	Not usually needed Inspiratory and expiratory chest radiographic if respiratory distress, wheezing, or cough of new onset in high-risk age group (6 months to 3 years) or history of choking episode
WBC count	Normal or slightly elevated, not usually needed	Normal, not usually needed	$> 15,000{-}20,000$ cells/mm^3 (usually not elevated with mycoplasmal or chlamydial pneumonia; C. trachomatis may have moderate eosinophilia)	Not usually needed
Other	—	Nasal and peripheral eosinophilia		PEFR $> 70\%$ of predicted or personal baseline value: Mild obstruction 50%-70% of baseline value: Moderate obstruction $< 50\%$ of baseline value: Severe obstruction Sputum: If necessary, culture and microscopic examination (Gram stain and Wright stain)

M. pneumoniae and GABHS are the most common causes of pneumonia in children older than 5 years of age. Although bacterial pneumonia is uncommon after the newborn period, *H. influenzae* type B and *Streptococcus pneumoniae* are frequently the offending organisms. *Chlamydia pneumoniae* is a newly identified agent recognized as second to *M. pneumoniae* as a cause for pneumonia in adolescents.

Acute bronchiolitis refers to a generalized inflammation of the small bronchi and bronchioles. Infectious agents generally associated with bronchiolitis are viruses, especially RSV. It is commonly seen in children under 2 years of age. Criteria for the diagnosis of bronchiolitis include a child 2 years of age or younger, a first episode of wheezing, and associated signs and symptoms of a viral respiratory infection (e.g., fever, cough, dyspnea, rhinitis) that are not the result of atopy or pneumonia. Infrequently *M. pneumoniae* may be associated with acute bronchiolitis in school-age children.

Bronchial asthma (see also Chapter 45) is the most common chronic lung disease in children. It is characterized by recurrent and reversible airway obstruction, inflammation, and hyperresponsiveness. A variety of stimuli may trigger an asthma attack. These stimuli include infections, exercise, airborne antigens (e.g., animal dander, molds, dust, house dust mites, food), environmental irritants (e.g., passive smoke, pollution), weather changes, and emotional factors. Morbidity and mortality rates have risen dramatically in the past three decades. It is noteworthy that underrecognition and undertreatment have been responsible for a high percentage of deaths from asthma.

Management

Viral and spasmodic croup. The first decision is whether the child should be managed at home, should be seen in the office, or requires hospitalization. An increasing respiratory rate is the best clinical measure of the degree of hypoxemia in children with croup. Other clinical signs of obstruction include the severity of stridor (especially stridor at rest) and the presence of retractions. Dehydration and fatigue are two additional clinical signs that affect the practitioner's management decisions. The majority of children with croup are treated at home. The following plan may be adapted for telephone contact or office visit. Children with a severe attack must be immediately referred to a physician for such treatment options as oxygen, racemic epinephrine, corticosteroid therapy, and hospitalization.

Treatments and medications
- Keep the child calm and quiet. (Have the parents hold the child.)
- Encourage clear fluids.
- Increase environmental humidity. Use a cool-mist humidifier for next 4 or 5 nights. If the child's breathing is still noisy, have the child sit in a steamy bathroom (by running hot water in the shower or bath) for 10 to 15 minutes.
- Watch the child for signs and symptoms of increased respiratory distress. Parents can monitor respiratory rate.
- Administer acetaminophen 10 to 15 mg/kg every 4 to 6 hours for fever or irritability. (Do not exceed five doses in 24 hours.)
- Do not use any medications that may depress the respiratory center (or make the child "sleepy") and mask anxiety and restlessness (e.g., antihistamines, cough syrups with codeine).

- Consider a dose of steroids (administered intramuscularly or orally) if indicated.
- Consider monitoring oxygen saturation if equipment is available in the office.

Counseling and prevention
- Acknowledge that respiratory illness can be very frightening and an anxiety-producing event for parents.
- Teach the parents about the signs and symptoms of respiratory distress, including rapid respiratory rate, increased agitation or fatigue, retractions, stridor at rest, turning blue, excessive drooling, and nasal flaring.
- Educate the parents and child about the cause and normal course of viral croup (e.g., 3 or 4 days, symptoms generally worse at night, URI signs and symptoms may persist longer).
- Educate the parents about the importance of humidity, fluids, close observation (e.g., a parent needing to sleep in the child's room), and no exposure to passive smoke.
- Acknowledge that although the spread of infection cannot be prevented, parents should keep the child home until fever is gone or for about 3 days into the illness.
- Review temperature control measures for the infant or young child.

Follow-up
- If parents make telephone contact, call back in 20 minutes to assess the child's response to treatment measures and to determine the level of parental anxiety.
- Schedule a return visit if there is no improvement in 48 hours or no response to treatment measures.
- If this is a case of moderate croup, first-time experience with croup, or heightened parental anxiety, call in 12 to 24 hours.
- Have the patient and parents return immediately or go to nearest emergency room if there are signs or symptoms of increased respiratory distress or stridor at rest.

Consultations and referrals. Immediately refer the child to a physician in the following situations:
- The child is under 1 year of age.
- The child develops stridor at rest or develops other signs or symptoms of increased respiratory distress.
- Signs or symptoms of epiglottitis (e.g., severe respiratory distress, toxicity, drooling, sore throat or difficulty swallowing, extreme agitation or exhaustion) occur.
- The caregiver is unreliable, has no readily accessible means of transportation, or lives far away from medical care.

Acute bronchitis

Treatments and medications
- Perform a tuberculin skin test if the child has had none in past year or the child has had exposure to tuberculosis.
- Increase fluid intake.
- Use throat lozenges or suck hard candy as needed.
- Increase environmental humidity.
- Avoid environmental irritants (e.g., fumes, tobacco smoke).
- Administer acetaminophen 10 to 15 mg/kg every 4 to 6 hours for fever or irritability. (Do not exceed five doses in 24 hours.)
- Avoid the use of cough suppressants in young children.
- Remember that antibiotics therapy may be indicated if the WBC count is elevated or there is purulent sputum.

Counseling and prevention
- Stress to the parents and child the importance of rest, fluids, and patience in the treatment of acute cough.

- Explain to the parents and child that the use of aspirin with an influenza viral infection is associated with Reye syndrome and should be avoided.
- Keep in mind that influenza virus vaccine is recommended for children over 6 months of age who have chronic cardiac or respiratory disorders or immunosuppression.

Follow-up

- Schedule a return visit if there is no improvement in 7 to 10 days.
- If there is a history of cardiopulmonary disease, schedule a return visit in 2 to 3 days.
- Have the patient and parents return immediately if there are signs or symptoms of respiratory distress.

Consultations and referrals. Refer the child to a physician if the following occur:

- Signs and symptoms of respiratory distress appear
- Symptoms last more than 3 weeks
- Foreign-body aspiration is suspected

Acute bronchiolitis

Treatments and medications

- Ensure rest or quiet activity, and place the child in a position of comfort.
- Increase fluid intake (small, frequent amounts).
- Increase environmental humidity.
- Clear secretions as needed: (1) with bulb syringe or (2) with percussion and postural drainage, especially before feedings and sleep.
- Avoid environmental irritants (e.g., fumes, tobacco smoke).
- Administer acetaminophen 10 to 15 mg/kg every 4 to 6 hours for fever or irritability. (Do not exceed five doses in 24 hours.)
- Administer antibiotics if secondary infection is present.

Counseling and prevention

- Acknowledge that respiratory illness can be a very frightening and anxiety-producing event for parents.
- Forewarn the parents that the child may be more tired than usual and may need to drink smaller amounts of fluid more frequently during the acute stage.
- Instruct the parents in percussion and postural drainage to clear secretions, especially before feedings.
- Discuss signs and symptoms of increased respiratory distress (e.g., increasing irritability, anxiety, turning blue, nasal flaring, wheezing, lethargy).
- Explain that antibiotics and other medications are usually not necessary.
- Discuss other supportive measures (e.g., temperature-control strategies, positioning of a small infant, maintenance of body warmth).
- Advise careful handwashing and protection of other siblings from droplet transmission.

Follow-up

- Call in 24 hours to evaluate response to supportive treatment and parental anxiety.
- Schedule a return visit in 48 hours if the temperature remains elevated or there is a poor response to supportive treatment.
- Schedule a return visit in 7 days if the child continues to be symptomatic.

Consultations and referrals. Refer the child to a physician in the following situations:

- Infant is less than 3 months of age
- Apneic episode occurs

- Respiratory rate is 60 per minute or greater with respiratory distress
- Child feeds poorly or shows signs or symptoms of dehydration
- Child is a premature infant younger than 6 months or has a history of apnea
- Infant has chronic cardiopulmonary disease, such as congenital heart disease or BPD
- Infant has congenital or acquired immune deficiency
- Caregiver is unreliable, has no readily accessible means of transportation, or lives far away from medical care
- Recurring episodes of bronchiolitis

Pneumonia

Treatments and medications

- Increase fluid intake.
- Ensure rest or quiet activity.
- Increase environmental humidity.
- Administer acetaminophen 10 to 15 mg/kg every 4 to 6 hours for fever or irritability. (Do not exceed five doses in 24 hours.)
- Avoid cough suppressants (and other cough medications) in children.
- Administer antibiotics as needed for the etiologic agent, and consult a physician.

Counseling and prevention

- Acknowledge that respiratory illness can be a very frightening and anxiety-producing event for parents.
- Forewarn the parents that the child may be more tired than usual and may need to drink smaller amounts of fluid more frequently during the acute stage.
- Instruct the parents in percussion and postural drainage to clear secretions, especially before feedings.
- Discuss signs and symptoms of increased respiratory distress (e.g., increasing irritability, anxiety, turning blue, nasal flaring, wheezing, lethargy).
- Discuss other supportive measures (e.g., temperature-control strategies, positioning of a small infant, maintenance of body warmth).
- Advise careful handwashing and protection of other siblings from droplet transmission.

Follow-up

- Schedule telephone contacts, home visits, or clinic visits until the patient is afebrile and there are no signs of respiratory distress.
- Schedule a return visit in 48 hours if there is no improvement.
- Recheck in 14 to 21 days.

Consultations and referrals. Refer the child to a physician in the following situations:

- Child less than 6 months of age who appears toxic
- Respiratory distress or cyanosis develops
- Child who feeds poorly or is unable to keep fluids down (or medications)
- Child with an underlying chronic illness (such as sickle cell, cancer, immune disorder)
- Caregiver is unreliable, has no readily accessible means of transportation, or lives far away from medical care
- Failure to improve in 48 hours
- Symptoms that fail to resolve in 3 weeks

Bronchial asthma (acute exacerbations). Treatment of acute exacerbations is based on the severity classification of the episode. Acute episodes are classified as mild, moderate, and severe. (For a complete discussion of asthma, see Asthma in Chapter 45.)

Treatments and medications

- Keep the child calm and quiet.
- For treatment at home (National Heart, Lung, and Blood Institute [NHLBI], 1997), have the child or parents check the PEF and provide initial therapy with a short-acting inhaled beta-agonist, 2 to 4 puffs from a metered-dose inhaler (MDI) up to three times every 20 minutes for a total of three doses, or a single treatment by nebulizer.
    1. If there is a good response (PEF greater than 80% of personal best or the predicted baseline value; no wheezing or shortness of breath with a response to the beta-agonist sustained for 4 hours), continue the beta-agonist every 3 to 4 hours for 24 to 48 hours. If the child is taking inhaled corticosteroids, double the dose for 7 to 10 days.
    2. If there is an incomplete response (PEF between 50% and 80% of personal best or predicted baseline value, or persistent wheezing and shortness of breath recurring within 4 hours of therapy), continue the beta-agonist (may be given by nebulizer), add oral corticosteroids, and contact the child's health care provider immediately for further instructions.
    3. If there is a poor response (PEF less than 50% with marked wheezing and shortness of breath) or noticeable distress, repeat the beta-agonist immediately and send child to the emergency department. If distress is severe, call 911.
- For treatment in the office (or emergency department) (which should include physician consultation):
    1. If PEFR is over 50%, provide initial treatment with a short-acting inhaled beta-agonist (e.g., albuterol) or by nebulizer, with up to three doses in the first hour. Check PEF after each treatment.
        a. If PEF is greater than 90% of the child's personal baseline or the predicted baseline value, stop treatments, observe for 1 hour, and repeat assessment.
        b. Give oxygen to maintain oxygen saturation greater than 90%.
        c. Provide oral steroids if there is a poor response to therapy or if the patient has recently been taking oral steroids,
    2. If the initial PEF is under 50% (severe exacerbation), refer immediately to a physician.
- For continued management of asthma exacerbations, refer to office or emergency department protocols or the guidelines of the NHLBI (1997). Puch clear fluids and avoid know precipitating factors or search for new ones across all settings the child is in (e.g., home, school, day care).

Counseling and prevention

- Provide further education to alleviate parental anxiety or overprotection or heightened anxiety in the child.
- Review the individualized home regimen with the child and the parents. Stress the importance of determining the child's PEF baseline value and promptly administering bronchodilators (if not following a daily regimen) at the first onset of signs or symptoms of a respiratory infection or bronchospasm before wheezing occurs.
- Assess and periodically promote the child's participation in self-management of asthma at home and school.

- Periodically review the purpose, dose, frequency, and side effects of medications.
- Review and reevaluate the child's readiness for new techniques for dispensing medications: nebulizer machine for infants and very young children; MDI with a spacer for children over 3 years of age.
- Set up periodic conferences to facilitate brainstorming with the child and the parents about possible solutions to problems encountered.

Follow-up

- Call immediately if recurrence of signs or symptoms of respiratory distress (or PEF is less than 70% of personal or predicted baseline value) or if chest pain or fever develops.
- Make telephone contact in 24 hours.
- Schedule a return visit in 1 to 2 weeks.

Consultations and referrals. Refer the child to a physician in the following situations:

- Child fails to respond to initial treatment
- Child does not improve or symptoms recur in 24 hours
- History of hospitalization for respiratory failure
- Concurrent infection occurs
- Caregiver is unreliable, has no readily accessible means of transportation, or lives far away from medical care

Cough

Alert

Consult with or refer to a physician for the following:
- Sudden onset of coughing, wheezing, or respiratory distress
- Purulent or blood-tinged sputum
- Limited chest expansion
- Chronic cough (3 weeks or longer)

Etiology

Coughing is a host defense mechanism to dislodge foreign matter or clear secretions from the respiratory tract. It is one of the most common respiratory symptoms in pediatric primary care. The most general way to characterize a cough is by duration, that is, as acute or chronic (3 weeks or longer). Across all age groups, the majority of coughs are acute and caused by mild to moderate cases of viral or bacterial URIs and allergy (e.g., rhinitis, asthma). The most common causes of chronic or persistent cough in children are infections, allergy, irritants (e.g., exposure to passive smoke, dry air), aspiration, and habit cough (from psychogenic factors). Congenital abnormalities and genetic disorders are less common causes of persistent cough in children.

Incidence

- Coughing is often associated with the common cold and other common URIs in children of all ages.
- Foreign-body aspiration occurs more frequently in toddlers and preschoolers.
- Coughing is common in children with allergic rhinitis and asthma.

Risk Factors

- URIs in children of all ages
- Allergic rhinitis

- Family history of asthma, allergic rhinitis, smoking, tuberculosis, cystic fibrosis, and other pulmonary disease or cardiac diseases
- Environmental exposure to passive smoke, chemical inhalants, tuberculosis or other pathogens, and travel

- History of foreign-body aspiration
- Immunocompromised children (e.g., premature infants, children with sickle cell or treated with steroids)
- History of immunodeficiency disorders, cardiac disease, or pulmonary disease (especially BPD)

Table 41-3 Subjective Findings that Suggest Respiratory Disease in Children with Recurrent Cough

SUBJECTIVE FINDINGS	MAY SUGGEST
Age of Onset	
Newborn or infancy	Congenital malformations (e.g., tracheoesophageal fistula, vascular ring, GER, congenital heart disease with congestive heart failure), perinatal infections (e.g., rubella, CMV, chlamydia, influenza, parainfluenza virus, RSV, pertussis), asthma, cystic fibrosis, AIDS
Preschool	Foreign-body aspiration, asthma, allergic rhinitis, bronchitis, infections (e.g., sinusitis), CF, AIDS, immune deficiency disorders, bronchiectasis, GER, congestive heart failure
School-age	Cigarette smoking, *M. pneumoniae*, sinusitis, postnasal drip, asthma, habit cough, CF
Characteristics of Cough	
Staccato	Pertussis, chlamydia
Barking	Viral croup, epiglottitis
Throat clearing	Allergy, chronic postnasal drip
Dry	Low humidity, allergy
Moist	Pneumonia, asthma
Honking or unusual	Habit or psychogenic
Paroxysms	Pertussis, chlamydia, asthma
Nocturnal	Asthma, postnasal drip, URI, GER, sinusitis
Absent during sleep	Psychogenic factors
Early morning	Allergy, smoking, sinusitis, CF
Seasonal	Allergy
Nonproductive	Viral rhinitis, allergic rhinitis, asthma, foreign-body aspiration
Productive:	
Clear or mucoid	Asthma, allergic rhinitis, smoking
Purulent	CF, bronchiectasis, pneumonia
Blood streaked	Tuberculosis, diphtheria, nasopharyngeal irritation, pneumonia
Malodorous	Sinusitis
Associated Findings	
Feedings	Congenital malformations, congenital heart disease, pneumonia, aspiration
Exercise	Asthma
Cold air	Asthma, vasomotor rhinitis, allergic rhinitis
Wheezing	Asthma, bronchiolitis, foreign-body aspiration
Stridor or voice change	Croup, epiglottitis, foreign-body aspiration
Drooling	Epiglottitis
Hemoptysis	Pneumonia (group A streptococci, tuberculosis), pertussis, CF, bronchiectasis
Conjunctivitis	Measles, chlamydia in newborns
Postnatal drip	Sinusitis, allergy
Cyanosis	Foreign body aspiration, bronchiolitis, asthma
Stopped breathing	Recurrent apnea
Failure to thrive	CF, congestive heart failure
Abnormal stools	CF
Exposure to Environmental Irritants	Tobacco or marijuana smoking, chemical inhalants
Exposure to Infection	Tuberculosis or other pathogens while traveling or in day care, school, home, and so on
Positive Family History	Asthma, allergic rhinitis, smoking, tuberculosis, CF, and other pulmonary or cardiac diseases
Stressful Family Interrelationships	Poor supervision that might increase possibility of aspiration or cough tics, or prolonged respiratory illness
Gaps in Immunization Status	Diphtheria, pertussis, measles, *H. influenzae*
Recurrent Respiratory Disorders	CF, asthma, immunodeficiency, BPD, congenital heart disease, bronchiectasis, foreign-body aspiration

- Incomplete immunization status (e.g., pertussis)
- Maternal infection with CMV or *Chlamydia*
- Increased family or child stress
- Anxious parents or parents with no access to telephone or transportation in case the child worsens rapidly

Differential Diagnosis

Subjective data. The majority of coughs during childhood are acute and self-limited. Recurrent or chronic cough in children demands a more thorough evaluation. Certain subjective findings related to a recurrent cough may assist the practitioner in developing a differential diagnosis (Table 41-3).

Objective data. For the majority of acute coughs, the physical examination findings will reveal an underlying upper or lower respiratory infection or allergic rhinitis. When a cough becomes recurrent or chronic, the practitioner must attempt to determine if it is related to acute, unrelated episodes of respiratory infection and irritation or related to more significant pulmonary disease. A complete physical examination must be performed. Table 41-4 outlines critical items to look for during the physical examination. It is noteworthy that a normal physical examination does not rule out the possibility of significant pulmonary disease.

Laboratory tests. Generally no laboratory tests are necessary if the cough is associated with common upper or lower respiratory infection or allergic rhinitis. For unexplained or recurrent cough associated with systemic disease, the practitioner may consider further diagnostic studies, such as tuberculin skin test, chest radiograph examination, sweat chloride determination, CBC, sputum culture and Gram stain, or spirometry.

Management

Management must be focused on determining the cause of the cough and formulating a treatment plan for that condition. In addition, the degree of illness and the complications of a specific condition will influence the therapeutic options for cough suppression.

Acute cough related to upper and lower respiratory infections (mild to moderate illness)
Treatments and medications
- Use a cool mist humidifier.
- Push fluids. (Warm liquids may help to relax the airway and loosen mucus.)
- Suggest throat lozenges or hard candy (for older children).
- Give 1 teaspoon of equal parts of honey (or corn syrup) and lemon juice every 10 minutes. (Do not give honey to infants under 1 year of age.)
- Avoid exposure to smoking and other respiratory irritants.
- Raise the head of the child's bed by placing a rolled blanket under the mattress; with an older child, two pillows may be used to elevate the head.
- Keep in mind the following general cough remedies (after determining the cough is not caused by bronchospasm):
  Expectorants increase the removal of secretions from airways; common expectorants include water and glyceryl guaiacolate that thin sputum. OTC expectorants are rarely used in children.
  Antitussives suppress coughing. *Demulcents* include water, throat lozenges, cough drops, and lollipops (for older children), a teaspoon of equal parts of honey or corn syrup (do not use honey in children under 1 year of age) and lemon juice, and topical anesthetics. Their duration of efficacy is limited, they are quickly washed away, and there is danger of overuse. *Centrally acting antitussives* include narcotic and nonnarcotic agents (usually only at night to promote sleep for the child and parents); codeine and hydrocodone are the most commonly used with children. The nonnarcotic drug dextromethorphan is the most commonly prescribed though its efficacy is unproved. *Antihistamines* may be used because of their sedative effect and their drying effect on the respiratory tree.
Counseling and prevention
- Explain the protective and self-limited role of cough in the disease process.

Table 41-4 Critical Physical Examination Items to Look for in the Child with Recurrent Cough

EXAMINATION ITEMS	WHAT TO LOOK FOR
Vital signs	Fever, tachycardia, tachypnea Use age-specific norms; count respirations and heart rate for 1 full minute
Growth percentiles	Abnormal patterns in length, weight, head circumference; poor growth
General appearance	Nutritional status, mental status changes, decreased activity, poor responsiveness to examiner or caregiver, leaning forward or sitting up, anxious facial expression, restlessness
Skin and lymph	Cyanosis, pallor, dehydration, capillary refill, clubbing, adenopathy
Ear, nose, mouth, and throat	Otoscopy to assess tympanic membranes; nasal flaring, purulent rhinorrhea, drooling, difficulty swallowing, sound of cough, characteristics of sputum, odor of sputum or breath, hoarseness, stridor; evidence of allergic facies, mouth breathing, nasal crease, allergic shiners, allergic salute, inflamed or boggy turbinates, masses; exudates of pharynx and tonsils
Chest and lungs	Increased respiratory rate: $\geq$ 60/minute in infant under 2 months; $\geq$ 50/minute in infant 2-12 months, $\geq$ 40/minute in child over 12 months; other signs of distress or dyspnea including tachypnea, head bobbing, nasal flaring, use of accessory muscles, grunting, wheezing, stridor at rest; poor air exchange; pattern of respiration, increased anteroposterior diameter; prolonged expiration; apnea; crackles (fine, medium, or coarse), or decreased breath sounds
Cardiac	Dysrhythmias, murmurs
Abdomen	Enlarged liver

- Discuss the therapeutic purpose of cough remedies (especially that water is the best expectorant for secretions of the upper airway) and advise the parents to stay with simple remedies.
- Use prescription or OTC cough agents sparingly and only in cases of severe symptoms or disruption of sleep; only use agents with one or two ingredients aimed at the most troublesome symptoms.
- Advise parents to keep cough medications out of the reach of children because they contain a high percentage of alcohol and may contain medications that have a sedative effect.
- Counsel the child and parents about the common behavioral side effects of ingredients in OTC medications, such as irritability, excess stimulation, and insomnia with sympathomimetics; sedation with antihistamines, expectorants, and cough suppressants; GI upset with expectorants and cough suppressants.
- Counsel about handwashing, covering the mouth with tissue, and avoiding exposure to others.
- Emphasize the need for proper sleep, a nutritious diet, and avoidance of stress.

Follow-up

- Have the parents call immediately if there is difficulty breathing, croup, wheezing, shortness of breath, blood in sputum, chest pain, or increased child or parental anxiety.
- Have the parents call if cough persists for more than 10 to 14 days or if the child develops a fever that lasts over 72 hours.

Consultations and referrals. Usually none are necessary. Refer if there are any signs or symptoms of complications associated with a specific condition.

Nasal Bleeding (Epistaxis)

Alert

> Consult with or refer to a physician for the following:
> - Profuse or persistent epistaxis (nasal bleeding that lasts over 30 minutes or will not clot with compression)
> - Physical findings of spontaneous bleeding at multiple sites
> - Suspicion of nasal fracture or neoplasm
> - Presence of nasal foreign body (unilateral purulent discharge)
> - Signs and symptoms associated with malignancy (such as hepatosplenomegaly, petechiae)
> - Current use or history of bleeding disorders or tendencies
> - Anatomic or vasculature abnormalities of the nose (e.g., polyps, telangiectasis, varicosities, deviated septum, perforated septum)
> - Decreased hematocrit secondary to epistaxis
> - Hypertension associated with epistaxis

Etiology

Epistaxis, or nasal bleeding, occurs frequently in childhood. The majority of cases of epistaxis originate in the nasal septum (Kiesselbach's area). Posterior epistaxis is more severe in nature and uncommon in children. The most common causes of anterior epistaxis in children are local irritation to the nasal mucosa, including nasal trauma, infections, allergic rhinitis, and topical nasal medications. Uncommon local causes of epistaxis include anatomic abnormalities (e.g., choanal atresia, septal deviation), nasal foreign bodies, and neoplasms. Juvenile angiofibroma is a benign tumor of the nose that may occur in male adolescents; it commonly appears as recurrent unilateral epistaxis with a nasopharyngeal mass. The sign of a nasal foreign body is usually unilateral purulent nasal discharge. The discharge may be foul smelling and streaked with blood.

Although systemic causes of epistaxis are infrequent during childhood, it is important for the practitioner to be familiar with them, especially in cases of recurrent epistaxis or when there are additional signs and symptoms of disease found in the history or physical examination. Factor XI deficiency (hemophilia C) and von Willebrand disease are the most common inherited bleeding disorders that cause epistaxis in children. Hereditary hemorrhagic telangiectasia is an autosomal dominant blood vessel disease that may appear during adolescence with severe epistaxis. Children with systemic diseases such as leukemia and lymphoma or who are undergoing chemotherapy have associated episodes of epistaxis caused by thrombocytopenia. Medications such as aspirin, ibuprofen, and anticoagulants may cause coagulopathies associated with epistaxis. Cocaine and other drugs abused by inhalation may contribute to recurrent epistaxis by causing nasal irritation or perforation and nasal bleeding. Hypertension is a rare cause of epistaxis in children.

Incidence

- From birth to 5 years of age, 30% of children have an episode of epistaxis.
- From 6 to 10 years of age, 56% of children have at least one nosebleed. Several isolated nosebleeds are common in childhood, rare during the neonatal period and infancy, and less common during adolescence.
- Epistaxis rarely occurs during infancy and after puberty.
- The incidence is higher during winter months because of a greater prevalence of URIs and low humidity.
- It is more common in boys than in girls.
- Less than 5% of children with recurrent epistaxis have a coagulation defect.

Risk Factors

- Use of forceps during delivery
- Allergies and allergic rhinitis
- Recurrent URIs with rhinitis
- Family history of bleeding disorders or tendencies
- Client history of bleeding disorders or tendencies
- Immunocompromised state (e.g., leukemia, lymphomas, chemotherapy, radiotherapy)
- Chronic use of topical nasal drugs (e.g., phenylephrine hydrochloride, cocaine)
- Anatomic or vascular abnormality of the nose
- Participation in sports
- Childhood from 2 to 10 years of age

Differential Diagnosis

Subjective data. See Table 41-5. Minor episodes of epistaxis are common during childhood. The majority of nosebleeds in childhood are mild and self-limited and are managed by the parents and child at home or by telephone care. When nosebleeds become recurrent or are difficult to handle, the child must be seen in the office.

Table 41-5   Differential Diagnosis: Epistaxis

CRITERIA	NASAL TRAUMA	INFECTIONS	ALLERGIC RHINITIS	MEDICATIONS
ICD-9 code	959.09	473.9	477.9	995.2; 784.7
Subjective Data				
Age	Nose picking and blunt trauma (including use of forceps during delivery) are the most common causes of epistaxis in childhood; foreign bodies common in early childhood	Infections common during early and middle childhood	Generally 2 to 4 years of age	All ages; adolescents may seek care for signs of nasal bleeding associated with drug abuse
Onset	Generally acute, sudden; intermittent or gradual onset may occur with foreign-body insertion; persistent bleeding that becomes more serous over time may suggest cerebral spinal fluid rhinorrhea if history of facial or nasal trauma	Associated with local or systemic infections; known to be associated with *Streptococcus*; may occur with some rare infectious diseases such as tuberculosis, diphtheria, pertussis, and syphilis; gradual if caused by medication overuse	May be acute, gradual, or chronic	Generally gradual
Circumstances	Nasal or facial injury; repeated nose picking, rubbing, blowing, sneezing; insertion of foreign body; exposure to dry environment (especially during winter months)	Signs or symptoms of URI or other infection 1 week before the episode	May be seasonal (suspect airborne pollens) or perennial (usually worse in winter because of heating systems, wool clothing, low humidity, and other allergens)	Use of OTC antihistamine or decongestant nasal sprays or oral drying agents; long-term use of topical antiallergic nasal sprays and drying agents for management of allergy; recent ingestion of aspirin, ibuprofen; drug abuse or sniffing
Location of bleeding	Generally anterior (out through the nose) and unilateral; if bilateral, suspect a posterior bleeding site or severe craniofacial trauma	Generally anterior	Generally anterior	Generally anterior
Length of bleeding time and response to compression	Generally bleeding does not last longer than 30 minutes or stops spontaneously or after compression for 10 minutes	Generally bleeding does not last longer than a few minutes or stops spontaneously or after compression a brief amount of time (10 minutes or less)	Generally bleeding does not last longer than a few minutes or stops spontaneously or after compression a brief amount of time (10 minutes or less)	Generally bleeding does not last longer than a few minutes or stops spontaneously or after compression a brief amount of time (10 minutes or less)
Related symptoms	If intermittent nasal obstruction, suspect foreign body; if unilateral mucopurulent discharge with bleeding or halitosis, suspect foreign body	Dependent on the infection involved; frequently have excoriated nares, coughing or sneezing, rhinorrhea associated with the episode; may have facial pain or headaches if sinusitis	Nasal stuffiness, watery and thin rhinorrhea, itching, sneezing, mouth breathing, snoring, allergic salute; chronic nasal obstruction with lower airway symptoms	Intermittent nasal obstruction or stuffiness; weight loss, conjunctivitis; psychosocial problems
Past medical history	May have had recent surgery or foreign-body insertion; history of deviated septum	Recent viral or bacterial infection; may have past history of chronic infection of nasopharynx with β-hemolytic streptococci	Allergies, allergic rhinitis; recurrent URIs, serous otitis media	Allergies, allergic rhinitis; infection; drug abuse, psychosocial problems; history of malignancy, chemotherapeutic agents, radiotherapy
Family history	No family history of bleeding disorders or tendencies	No family history of bleeding disorders or tendencies	May have family history of allergy, bleeding disorders, cystic fibrosis, polyps	May have family history of allergy, allergic rhinitis, aspirin idiosyncrasy, drug abuse

Continued

Table 41-5   Differential Diagnosis: Epistaxis—cont'd

CRITERIA	NASAL TRAUMA	INFECTIONS	ALLERGIC RHINITIS	MEDICATIONS
Subjective Data—cont'd				
Past episodes of epistaxis and response to treatment	Responds immediately to treatment	Associated with infection and responded immediately to treatment for nasal bleeding or eradication of the infectious agent	Associated with allergies or concurrent infection (e.g., sinusitis) that responded immediately to treatment	May or may not have had previous episodes of epistaxis, dependent on causative factor

Objective data. An extensive physical examination is not necessary in the majority of cases of mild epistaxis. A more comprehensive physical examination is conducted in cases of recurrent epistaxis. The practitioner should focus on determining the source of the bleeding and noting any evidence of underlying illness. The child's and the parents' level of apprehension about these episodes also should be assessed. If there are underlying factors (e.g., allergic rhinitis, medication) contributing to epistaxis, they also must be dealt with after the acute episode has been managed.

Blood pressure and vital signs are usually normal. The child should be observed for such behaviors as picking, rubbing, and blowing the nose, with notation of any evidence of apprehension or anxiety. Bleeding should stop spontaneously and not last more than 30 minutes, or more than 10 minutes with compression of the front part of the nose. The bleeding site is visualized in the anterior aspect of the nasal septum (Kiesselbach's area); the site of an active bleed is reddened, and a clot or crust is evident.

If there was blunt trauma, check that there is no ecchymosis, swelling, malalignment, or crepitus of the nose; that visual acuity is within normal limits for the age; that the sense of smell is intact; and that no cerebrospinal fluid leaks through the nose.

In performing a thorough nose, mouth, and throat examination, keep the following in mind:
- The child may have an excoriated area with crusted mucus, more often on the side of the dominant hand. A nasal crease, clear nasal discharge, and inflamed boggy mucosae are suggestive of allergic rhinitis.
- Dry mucous membranes are suggestive of trauma or medication as a cause of epistaxis.
- Enlarged red tonsils with or without exudate are suggestive of infection.
- Sinus tenderness and mucopurulent postnasal drip are suggestive of sinusitis.
- No evidence of masses of the oropharynx or nasopharynx should be seen.
- There should be no persistent mouth breathing as the result of nasal obstruction.

In performing a thorough examination of the skin and mucous membranes, there should be no evidence of a coagulopathy (e.g., bruising, petechiae, telangiectasia, spontaneous bleeding at other sites), and no lymphadenopathy or hepatosplenomegaly is present.

No laboratory tests are indicated if there is no family history of bleeding disorders and compression stopped the episode. If the history or observation indicates significant bleeding, the hematocrit should be determined.

Management
Telephone care of minor episodic epistaxis
Treatments and medications
- Keep the child and the parents calm.
- Have the child sit up and lean forward (to avoid swallowing blood).
- Provide reassurance for the parents and child.
- Instruct the parents or the child to pinch the nose over the bleeding site for a full 10 minutes (using a clock or timer).
- If bleeding continues, change the position of compression and pinch the nose for another full 10 minutes.

Counseling and prevention. Have the parents call if bleeding worsens or is persistent or if the parents' or the child's apprehension about the episode increases.

Follow-up. Schedule follow-up care as needed for recurrent episodes.

Consultations and referrals. Refer to a physician for the following:
- Bleeding lasting longer than 30 minutes or bleeding that cannot be controlled by compression (a situation requiring immediate referral)
- Recurrent bleeding from the same nostril
- Persistent bleeding occurring after trauma (because posterior bleeding usually cannot be controlled by the above measures)

Office care of recurrent epistaxis
Treatments and medications
- Keep the child and the parents calm.
- Give the child a basin and a towel to protect clothing.
- Place the child in a sitting position with the head tilted forward.
- Instruct the child to breathe through the mouth.
- Apply firm, constant pressure with the thumb and forefinger to both sides of the nose for 5 minutes, then 10 minutes, for a total of 15 minutes.
- Repeat the procedure if bleeding persists for longer than 10 to 15 minutes and change the position of compression.
- Encourage daily application of petrolatum or antibiotic ointment for 5 days after the nosebleed and then weekly for 1 month, resuming if nosebleeds recur. (Encourage the child to do this with parental supervision.)
- Initiate environmental control measures if an allergen or history of allergies is suspected.
- If epistaxis is caused by irritation from medication, stop or change the offending medications or refer the child to a specialist for treatment management.

Counseling and prevention
- Demonstrate to the child and parents the correct method of compression to stop nosebleeds.

- Encourage humidification of the home or the child's room, especially at night and during winter months.
- Educate the parents and child and reassure them about the causes of nosebleeds and the minimal blood loss associated with these episodes.
- Discourage picking of the nose.
- Encourage the use of petrolatum whenever nasal irritation is evident to the child or parents.
- If the child has swallowed a significant amount of blood, educate the parents and child about the possibility of hematemesis and black, tarry stools.
- If an underlying allergy or allergic rhinitis is suspected, counsel the parents and child regarding environmental control measures.

Follow-up. Schedule a return visit if nosebleeds recur frequently, become prolonged or profuse, or are difficult to control.

Consultations and referrals. Refer to a physician or an ear, nose, and throat specialist for the following:

- Described treatment does not stop the bleeding episode (noting that posterior bleeding usually cannot be controlled by these measures)
- Recurrent bleeding from the same nostril
- Family history of bleeding disorders
- Physical findings of systemic bleeding or malignancy
- Cause of epistaxis is complex (e.g., nasal foreign body, hereditary hemorrhagic telangiectasia, drug abuse)
- Unidentified cause of recurrent epistaxis

Nasal Congestion and Obstruction

Alert

Consult with or refer to a physician for the following:
- Nasal obstruction in a newborn
- History of head trauma followed by clear, watery nasal discharge
- Signs or symptoms of respiratory distress: nasal flaring, retractions, cyanosis, or tachypnea
- Suspicion of intranasal foreign body (unilateral purulent nasal discharge)
- Parent or child with history of substance abuse by inhalation

Etiology

The majority of cases of nasal rhinitis or obstruction during childhood are caused by inflammatory processes. These inflammatory processes are the result of viral or bacterial pathogens. Specific pathogens for the clinical entities reviewed in this section are covered in the discussion of differential diagnosis. Common clinical problems associated with nasal congestion or obstruction include viral rhinitis, allergic rhinitis, vasomotor sinusitis, and acute sinusitis. Acquired causes of nasal obstruction include rhinitis medicamentosa, adenoidal hypertrophy, foreign body, nasal polyps, trauma, and hormonal rhinitis (e.g., pregnancy, menses, hypothyroidism). Uncommon causes include congenital problems such as choanal atresia and neoplasms.

Incidence

- The common cold is the most frequent infection of humans.
- There is a higher incidence of the common cold in children under 5 years of age; young children may have 6 to 12 colds a year.
- Minor epidemics of the common cold occur during winter months. (Incidence is also higher in the fall and early spring. The peak month is September, coinciding with the return to school.)
- About 50% of cases of ethmoiditis occur between 1 and 5 years of age; maxillary sinusitis is seen after 1 year of age, and frontal sinusitis is seen at approximately 10 years of age.
- Approximately 5% of healthy children with a URI develop sinusitis.
- Allergic rhinitis is seen at 2 to 4 years of age and affects 10% of the population.
- Nasal foreign-body insertion is most common in toddlers and preschoolers.

Risk Factors

- Structural abnormalities (e.g., cleft palate, septal deviation, polyps, choanal atresia)
- Systemic disorder (e.g., cystic fibrosis, immune disorders, immotile cilia)
- Local insult (e.g., nasofacial trauma, swimming, diving, rhinitis medicamentosa)
- Allergic rhinitis
- Family history of nasal or sinus problems, allergic rhinitis, or allergies
- Neonate or young child (age-related differences in anatomy and physiology)
- Exposure to infectious groups of people (e.g., at day care, family, school)
- Incomplete immunization status
- Exposure to passive smoke
- History of substance abuse by inhalation (e.g., cocaine, glue, marijuana) by the parents or child or adolescent
- Adenotonsillar hypertrophy (peak incidence, 3 to 6 years of age)
- Predisposing conditions (e.g., pregnancy, menses, hypothyroidism)

Differential Diagnosis

Acute viral rhinitis, or the common cold, may be caused by well over 100 different viruses. The most common viruses associated with the common cold in children include rhinovirus, parainfluenza virus, RSV, and coronavirus. The most critical diagnostic clues include its classic mode of presentation and epidemiologic characteristics (Table 41-6).

Allergic rhinitis is the most common atopic disease in childhood. Nasal obstruction, rhinorrhea, and pruritus are classic signs and symptoms of this disease. It may be seasonal, perennial, or episodic. Seasonal allergic rhinitis, or hay fever, is caused by exposure to wind-borne pollens. Major pollen groups in the temperate zones are trees (late winter, early spring), grasses (spring to early summer), weeds (late summer, early fall), and mold spores (summer and fall). Perennial allergic rhinitis is generally a more significant problem during the winter months because of greater exposure to dust allergens, dust mites, and animal dander in the home. Symptoms associated with seasonal allergic rhinitis are generally more severe than those of perennial allergic rhinitis and are the result of airborne pollens. The most common complications of allergic rhinitis include serous otitis media, chronic sinusitis, increased frequency of respiratory infections, abnormal facial development, and drowsiness from antihistamine therapy.

Table 41-6   Differential Diagnosis: Nasal Congestion/Obstruction

CRITERIA	ACUTE VIRAL RHINITIS	ALLERGIC RHINITIS	VASOMOTOR RHINITIS	RHINITIS MEDICAMENTOSA	ACUTE SINUSITIS
ICD-9 code	472.0	477.9	477.9	472.0	461.2
Subjective Data					
Onset or duration	Sudden	Seasonal, after 2 years of age; perennial, before 2 years of age; (also may be a combination)	Most common in older children and adolescents; perennial episodes begin suddenly and go away suddenly	Onset with URI or acute exacerbation of allergic rhinitis	Recent illness: cold or allergic rhinitis
Fever	Low-grade or none in older children; infants may have more significant fever up to 105.1° F (40.6° C)	None	None		Low-grade fever up to 100.5° F (38.9° C)
Nasal symptoms	Stuffiness; profuse, thin discharge, intermittent and worse in morning; sneezing (if purulent for more than 7 to 10 days, see Acute Sinusitis)	Stuffiness; bilateral, thin, watery rhinorrhea, sneezing, intense itching or rubbing	Varying intensity of nasal stuffiness and clear or mucoid rhinorrhea	Varying intensity of nasal stuffiness and congestion; ask child specifically about frequency of use of OTC and topical nasal sprays	Mucopurulent nasal discharge; persistent postnasal drip
Cough	Mild nonproductive cough; mild sore throat; watery, red eyes	May have nonproductive cough (throat-clearing sound)	—	—	Choking cough (especially at night) or daytime cough longer than 7-10 days
Other symptoms	Malaise, decreased appetite, watery red eyes, mild irritability	Sore or scratchy throat; itchy, watery eyes; scratchy throat, palatal itching Epistaxis, nose picking, sniffing; lid and periorbital edema, allergic shiners; fatigue, irritability, anorexia	Occasionally sneezing, profuse rhinorrhea, moderate to pronounced congestion, no allergic eye symptoms	If overuse, may produce other systematic vascular symptoms, including increased blood pressure, central nervous system (CNS) stimulation	Headache (worse in morning and evening); intermittent periorbital edema; facial tenderness Swelling in the morning, anorexia, malaise, toothache, halitosis, epistaxis in children susceptible to them, facial tenderness (rare)

Exposure	To infection: Sick family members or others in child's environment (e.g., school, day care)	To environment: Seasonal frequently because of pollens; perennial because of animal dander, dust mites, mold, ingested allergens in rare cases	To environment: Temperature changes, air pollutants, tobacco smoke, perfumes, other nonspecific factors	To medication: Prolonged use of vasoconstrictor nose drops for more than 3-5 days, causing rebound reaction and secondary nasal congestion	
Child or family history	May have associated allergies, pattern of recurrent colds; other family member with similar illness	Hay fever, chronic nasal or sinus disease, asthma, eczema, allergies	No child or family history of allergy or coincidental	May have associated allergies, chronic nasal or sinus disease, asthma	Frequently allergic rhinitis or allergy; may have chronic nasal or sinus disease (e.g., septal deviation, cleft palate, polyps), asthma, eczema, CF, head injury
Objective Data *Physical examination*					
Vital signs	May have low-grade fever (temperature may be elevated in infants)	Afebrile	—	If long-term abuse, may be hypertensive	Usually low-grade fever
Eye	Mild inflammation of conjunctivae	Conjunctival edema and irritation, allergic shiners	No eye signs or other manifestations of atopy	May have manifestations of related atopy	May have periorbital edema
Ear, nose, mouth, and throat	Erythematous tympanic membranes, especially in infants; red, swollen nasal mucosa; thin and clear nasal discharge (first 2-3 days, then may become thick and mucopurulent); mild erythema of tonsils and posterior pharynx	Clear or mucoid rhinorrhea; edematous turbinates, frequently pale and boggy; dry, hacking cough; allergic facies (perennial): mouth breathing, nasal crease, malocclusion, high-arched palate, allergic salute; may have serous otitis media, associated hearing loss	Clear or mucoid rhinorrhea; moderate edema; may have mucus visible in posterior pharynx; no allergic facies or coincidental	Mucous membranes pale and edematous, obstruct airflow	Yellow, mucopurulent nasal discharge; swollen, injected nasal mucosa; tenderness or swelling over affected sinus(es); failure of frontal or maxillary sinuses to transilluminate in older children (rarely used)
Neurologic				If long-term abuse, may have signs of CNS stimulation	Normal gait, negative Brudzinski and Kernig signs
Laboratory tests	None usually	None usually; if necessary, nasal smear may be positive for eosinophils (more than 10% of the cells seen); on the differential WBC count, eosinophil count of > 5%; note that nasal eosinophilia may be absent if using antihistamines or between attacks	None usually; if done, nasal smear generally negative for eosinophils (in rare instances, may have eosinophilia)	None	Nasopharyngeal cultures not useful—results poorly correlated with cultures obtained by aspiration of sinus(es); radiographs not usually needed in uncomplicated cases

Vasomotor rhinitis is a category of chronic or intermittent nasal disease that is most commonly seen in older children and adolescents. It is a nonallergic form of rhinitis that is manifested by varying degrees of nasal obstruction accompanied by watery rhinorrhea and postnasal drip. It does not respond to environmental control or medication. There is no family history of allergy, and the nasal smear and skin tests (if done) are negative. It may be triggered by environmental changes such as temperature, humidity, or air pollution (especially smoke).

Rhinitis medicamentosa refers to rebound nasal congestion, most commonly the result of prolonged use of OTC topical nasal decongestant medications. It is important to specifically ask children and their parents about the use of topical nasal medications because they may not consider it important in their history.

Acute sinusitis (less than 30 days in duration) is a common complication of the common cold or allergic rhinitis. Common bacteria that cause sinusitis include *S. pneumoniae, H. influenzae, Moraxella catarrhalis,* and β-hemolytic streptococci. The onset of acute sinusitis may be gradual or sudden. With gradual onset, nasal congestion and discharge persists for 10 days or more without improvement. With sudden onset, high fever and periorbital inflammation or severe pain may be the signs or symptoms given. The most common serious complications of sinusitis include orbital cellulitis and intracranial infection (subdural empyema).

Management

Acute viral rhinitis

Treatments and medications

- Increase fluid intake (of fluid with calories, but avoid caffeinated products).
- Administer acetaminophen 10 to 15 mg/kg every 4 to 6 hours for fever or irritability during the first few days. (Do not exceed five doses in 24 hours.) Make sure you know whether child will be given drops, elixir, or tablets.
- To clear nasal secretions in infants, gently aspirate nasal secretions with a nasal bulb syringe as needed before feedings and sleep. For older children, encourage gentle nose blowing with tissues.
- For nasal stuffiness or discharge in children under 6 years of age, use normal saline nose drops (¼ teaspoon of table salt in 8 oz of warm tap water), 2 to 3 drops 15 to 20 minutes before eating or sleeping. If nasal blockage is severe (e.g., causing difficulty with feeding, interrupting sleep), the following may be considered:

    Decongestant nose drops or sprays (to be used sparingly with children under 6 years of age) may be prescribed. For children 6 months to 2 years of age, give 0.125% phenylephrine hydrochloride nose drops every 2 to 3 hours for up to 3 days. For children 2 to 6 years of age, give pediatric strength, long-acting nose drops (xylometazoline or oxymetazoline 0.05%) twice daily for up to 3 days. In children over 6 years of age, use adult-strength, long-acting drops every 12 hours as needed for up to 3 days

    Oral decongestants and antihistamine medications are not recommended in infants under 6 months of age and should be used sparingly in children under 6 years of age. Common ingredients in OTC products are pseudoephedrine hydrochloride and triprolidine hydrochloride plus pseudoephedrine. Dosages must be calculated

for the age or weight of the infant or child. Long-acting or sustained-release products are not recommended in children under 7 years of age. Use the lowest dose possible to achieve the desired relief.

- Use a cool mist humidifier (ultrasonic preferred) for 3 to 5 days.
- Limit exposure to others, if possible.
- Teach good handwashing.
- Encourage bed rest if there is a high fever.
- Apply petrolatum to nares if excoriated.

Counseling and prevention

- Discuss the normal course of the common cold (e.g., symptoms may last 10 to 14 days, fever is generally low grade and lasts less than 3 days, symptoms peak on days 3 to 5).
- Demonstrate the use of a thermometer and a nasal bulb syringe, as well as administration of nose drops and oral medications in infants and young children.
- Avoid OTC oral decongestants and antihistamines with infants and young children; increasing oral fluids is more helpful.
- If OTC oral medications are used or recommended, counsel the parents and child as follows:

    Common behavioral side effects of OTC preparations used to treat minor respiratory illness include irritability, excess stimulation, and insomnia with sympathomimetics; sedation with antihistamines, expectorants, and cough suppressants; and GI upset with expectorants and cough suppressants.

    Decongestants such as pseudoephedrine should not be administered at bedtime or later than 5:00 or 6:00 PM because of possible side effects of excess stimulation or insomnia.

    OTC "all-in-one" cold preparations should be avoided. Use single-ingredient preparations aimed at the most troublesome symptom.

- Use topical nasal medications only if there is severe blockage and for very brief periods of time as the result of rebound congestion. The practitioner may consider alternating administration of nasal medication; for example, use only in left nostril for first dose and in right nostril for second dose.
- Discuss the importance of cleaning the humidifier after a minor illness episode or every 3 days because of the buildup of molds in the humidifier that are being sprayed into the air.
- Educate the parents on the signs and symptoms of complications (especially if the child is an infant or toddler).
- Explain to the parents and child that the use of aspirin with an influenza viral infection is associated with Reye syndrome; therefore aspirin should not be given.
- Counsel about the prevention of colds (e.g., proper handwashing, avoiding exposure to others with colds, proper sleep, nutritious diet, avoidance of stress).
- Discuss feeding strategies for the breastfed infant to maintain the mother's milk supply in the event of a minor illness.

Follow-up. Call or schedule a return visit immediately if there are signs or symptoms of respiratory distress; if nasal discharge becomes thick, purulent, malodorous, or bloody; if fever persists more than 3 days; or if symptoms fail to resolve in 10 days.

Consultations and referrals. Usually none are necessary.

Allergic rhinitis. See Allergies in Chapter 43.

Treatments and medications

- Identify and avoid known or suspected antigen or antigens. If seasonal, have the patient avoid being outdoors during the early morning or late evening hours and use an air conditioner with an electrostatic filter to eliminate pollen. If perennial, focus on the child's room in the home and promote the use of dust control measures, such as keeping the room clean, avoiding the use of drapes and floor coverings, keeping windows and doors closed, removing pets, avoiding stuffed toys, avoiding damp places, and using an air conditioner.
- Prescribe an antihistamine or antihistamine-decongestant combination appropriate for the child's age; long-acting or sustained-release products are not recommended in children under 7 years of age. Use the lowest dose possible to achieve the desired relief.
- If nasal blockage is severe and for brief periods of time, consider sympathomimetic nose sprays for an acute episode only. They are not recommended for prolonged use (more than 3 or 4 days) because of worsening of symptoms with rebound congestion.
- Possibly use beclomethasone nasal spray 1 to 2 sprays to each nostril twice a day for acute seasonal problems.
- Possibly administer cromolyn sodium nasal solution 1 spray to each nostril three to four times a day for long-term therapy for seasonal problems.

Counseling and prevention

- Educate the parents and child about the cause of symptoms to promote adherence with treatment.
- Advise the parents that allergic rhinitis is a chronic problem that will "come and go" but that the symptoms can be controlled.
- Educate the parents about environmental control strategies for the atopic child.
- Discuss the side effects of oral medication, especially sedation, nervousness, tachycardia, dryness of the mouth or nasal mucosa, and constipation.
- Discuss the side effects of nasal medication (e.g., location irritation, stinging, nosebleeds). Discuss rebound congestion and the need to use nasal decongestants for only 3 or 4 days and only when there is complete obstruction. Consider alternating administration of nasal medication; for example, use in the left nostril for the first dose and in the right nostril for the next dose.
- Educate the parents and child about the need for continuous therapy with medication rather than sporadic use.
- Counsel the parents and child that use of cromolyn nasal solution must be initiated before exposure to allergens and continued until the end of pollen season. Advise that once cromolyn helps to control symptoms, the child may discontinue or decrease dosages of oral antihistamines or decongestants.
- Discuss indications for further allergy work-up.

Follow-up

- Call or schedule a return visit in 10 to 14 days for evaluation of the child's response to the treatment plan.
- Schedule a return visit if the symptoms are worse or unable to be controlled with the treatment measures.

Consultations and referrals. Refer the child to a physician in the following situations:

- Symptoms persist after 4 weeks of antihistamines, are perennial, or worsen each year

- Parents or the child request skin testing because symptoms are interfering with lifestyle
- Recurrent serous otitis media affecting hearing, speech, and language
- Recurrent or chronic sinusitis
- Nasal polyps present (suspicion of cystic fibrosis)
- Dental malocclusion problems develop from maxillary changes associated with chronic nasal obstruction

Vasomotor rhinitis

Treatments and medications. Generally the response is inconsistent (ranging from poor to fair) to drug therapy such as oral decongestants, antihistamines, or corticosteroids.

Counseling and prevention

- Discuss the possible causes of vasomotor rhinitis.
- Emphasize the nonallergic basis of this disorder and the inconsistent response the child may have to drug therapy.
- Avoid environmental triggers or seek to identify the irritant that precipitates attacks.

Follow-up. None is indicated.

Consultations and referrals. None are indicated.

Rhinitis medicamentosa

Treatments and medications

- Discontinue topical nasal decongestant sprays or drops.
- Let the child's history and physical findings guide further treatment or medication.

Counseling and prevention

- Educate the child and the family about the physiologic mechanism involved with rebound congestion.
- Discuss the addicting aspects of this class of medication.
- Advise the child and the family to avoid this class of medication or use only for 3 to 5 days as directed during the acute phase of an allergic attack or URI.

Follow-up. None is indicated.

Consultations and referrals. Refer the child to a physician in the following situation:

Cocaine abuse is suspected.

Acute sinusitis (bacterial)

Treatments and medications

- Administer antibiotics for 10 to 14 days for an acute episode, and continue 7 more days if the child is not totally asymptomatic or is responding slowly to therapy by end of the course of antibiotics. The course of therapy may be continued for up to 21 days for acute sinusitis
- Keep in mind the following first-line drugs:

  For the drug of choice for initial therapy of uncomplicated sinusitis, use amoxicillin 40 to 60 mg/kg per day in two divided doses for 10 to 14 days in uncomplicated cases in children who have not been on recent antimicrobial therapy.

  If the child is allergic to penicillin, use trimethoprim-sulfamethoxazole 8/40 mg/kg per day (8 mg of trimethoprim per 40 mg of sulfamethoxazole) in two divided doses, or erythromycin-sulfisoxazole 50/150 mg/kg per day (50 mg of erythromycin per 150 mg of sulfisoxazole), in three or four divided doses.

  If a β-lactamase-positive pathogen is suspected, use high-dose amoxicillin-clavulanate in two divided doses, or use trimethoprim sulfamethoxazole, a third-generation cephalosporin, a newer macrolide, or erythromycin-sulfisoxazole.

- Despite limited research investigating the effectiveness of decongestants and antihistamines in the treatment of acute sinusitis, keep in mind that a short course of decongestants to promote drainage of the sinuses until antibiotics take effect may be commonly recommended by some practitioners. The following may be considered:

Nose drops or spray for 3 to 4 days (see the treatment of Acute Viral Rhinitis)

An oral decongestant such as pseudoephedrine hydrochloride (not recommended in children less than 6 months of age)

An oral antihistamine-decongestant combination if the child has allergies or allergic rhinitis

- Consider administration of nasal steroids, such as beclomethasone dipropionate 1 spray to each naris twice a day. (Do not use for more than 4 weeks.)
- Administer acetaminophen 10 to 15 mg/kg every 4 to 6 hours during first few days for irritability, malaise, and fever. (Do not exceed five doses in 24 hours.)
- Increase fluid intake.
- Humidify the air in the child's room, especially at night.
- Keep the child's head elevated when lying down.
- Use warm compresses applied to the involved sinus or sinuses, steam inhalation, or periodic warm showers for an older child or adolescent to relieve pressure.
Counseling and prevention
- Demonstrate nasal hygiene, including the use of a nasal bulb syringe, the administration of nose drops, the disposal of nasal secretions, and gentle blowing of the nose to remove secretions.
- Instruct the child and the parents regarding medication, including the actions of medications, their side effects, the importance of continuous administration, and how to take or give medications (see the discussion of Acute Rhinitis).
- Instruct about the signs or symptoms of complications, which may indicate central nervous system (CNS) involvement (e.g., difficulty with balance, clumsiness, increased irritability, change in mental status, lethargy).
- If it is indicated, encourage cessation of smoking by the child or the parents.
Follow-up
- Call or schedule a return visit if there is no improvement in 48 hours (which may indicate a resistant organism or a complication).
- Call or schedule a return visit if symptoms are not completely resolved by the end of the antibiotic course.
Consultations and referrals. Refer the child to a physician in the following situations:
- Symptoms have not significantly improved in 1 week or disappeared in 2 or 3 weeks
- No response to treatment measures in 4 to 6 weeks
- Indication of complications

Sore Throat (Pharyngitis)

Alert

Consult with or refer to a physician for the following:
- Acute respiratory distress
- Drooling or difficulty swallowing
- Physical findings associated with rheumatic fever
- Adenotonsillar hypertrophy that causes upper airway obstruction
- Severe abdominal pain in the left upper quadrant (spleen)
- Membranous pharyngitis (especially if immunization status is incomplete)

Etiology

Pharyngitis, or "sore throat," refers to an inflammation of the tonsils or pharynx (tonsillitis and pharyngotonsillitis). However, it is important to keep in mind that a sore throat may occur without the presence of pharyngitis. Pharyngitis may be divided into two categories. The first category is pharyngitis that is associated with nasal discharge. Nasopharyngitis is more common in children younger than 2 years of age and is commonly caused by adenoviruses and influenza and parainfluenza viruses. Other viral pathogens include enteroviruses, Epstein-Barr virus, CMV, and herpes simplex virus. The second category is pharyngitis (including tonsillitis and pharyngotonsillitis) without nasal symptoms. GABHS are the most common cause of bacterial pharyngitis in children over 5 years of age. In adolescents, other causes include *M. pneumoniae,* gonococcus, and *Arcanobacterium haemolyticum.* Less common causes of pharyngitis include *Corynebacterium diphtheriae,* group C or G streptococci, *Francisella tularensis* (tularemia), and *Toxoplasma gondii.*

Although this section focuses on acute pharyngitis and tonsillitis, recurrent pharyngitis may occur in children and adolescents. The causes of noninfectious recurrent pharyngitis may include mouth breathing (such as secondary to nasal obstruction), postnasal drip, and school phobia.

Incidence

- The majority of cases of acute pharyngitis are attributable to viruses.
- Nasopharyngitis occurs most commonly in younger children (2 years of age or less).
- Pharyngitis occurs in 85% of patients with infectious mononucleosis.
- *M. pneumoniae* is a common cause of sore throat in adolescents and young adults.

Risk Factors

- Exposure to a streptococcal infection
- Carrier state if a family member or the child has a history of rheumatic fever, glomerulonephritis, or frequent streptococcal infections
- Recurrent streptococcal infections (documented)
- Children over 3 years of age
- Incomplete immunization status (e.g., for diphtheria)

Differential Diagnosis

Children may have a range of symptoms associated with pharyngitis. The cause cannot be determined by physical findings alone (Table 41-7). Age, environment, season of the year, and immune status will be important diagnostic considerations when seeking to identify the etiologic agent. Viral pharyngitis is more common in children under 2 years of age, and GABHS are most common in children 6 years of age and older.

A throat culture is indicated in children with fever, sore throat, anterior cervical lymphadenopathy, tonsillar exudate, or red throat. Two swabs should be obtained from the tonsils or pharynx. A rapid strep test (RST) should be obtained with the first swab. If the test is positive, treatment is initiated and a culture is not needed; the second swab can be thrown away. A negative RST should be confirmed with a routine throat culture for GABHS. In general, no further laboratory testing is indicated.

Several diagnostic generalizations may be helpful for establishing the cause of *viral pharyngitis.* Over 90% of cases of acute pharyngitis in children are attributable to viral pathogens. Acute viral pharyngitis is more common in children up to 5 years of

Table 41-7 Pharyngotonsillitis: Diagnostic Signs and Symptoms

| | GROUP A STREPTOCOCCI | | | |
	INFANT	SCHOOL-AGE	ADULT	VIRAL
Onset	Gradual	Sudden	Sudden	Gradual
Chief Complaint	Anorexia, rhinitis, listlessness	Sore throat	Sore throat	Sore throat, cough, hoarseness, rhinitis, conjunctivitis
Diagnostic Findings				
Sore throat	+	+++	+++	+++
Tonsillar erythema	+	+++	+++	++
Tonsillar exudate	+	++	+++	+
Palatal petechiae	+	+++	+++	+
Adenitis	+++	+++	+++	++
Excoriated nares	+++	+	+	+
Conjunctivitis	+	+	+	+++
Cough	+	+	+	+++
Congestion	+	+	+	+++
Hoarseness	+	+	+	+++
Fever	Low-grade	High	High	Rare or low-grade
Abdominal pain	+	++	+	+
Headache	+	++	++	+
Vomiting	+	++	++	+
Scarlatiniform rash	+	+++	+++	+
Streptococcal contact	+++	+++	+++	+
Ancillary Data				
Positive streptococcal culture	+++	++	+++	+
Elevated white blood cell count	++	++	+++	+

From Barkin, R.M., & Rosen, D. (1999). Emergency pediatrics: A guide to ambulatory care. St. Louis: Mosby.
+, Present.

age. The presence of a mild cough, rhinitis, or hoarseness and the absence of fever (or low-grade fever), tonsillopharyngeal erythema or exudates, and cervical lymphadenitis are supportive of a viral cause. Typically these signs and symptoms are general and do not direct the practitioner to a specific agent. However, there are several types of viral pharyngitis that have distinctive characteristics that allow the practitioner to identify the particular viral agent. These include infectious mononucleosis, pharyngoconjunctival fever (adenovirus), hand-foot-mouth disease, and herpangina (Table 41-8).

Group A β–hemolytic streptococcal pharyngitis is the most common cause of bacterial pharyngitis in children over 5 years of age. Fever is more commonly associated with GABHS. Usually infants and very young children with streptococcal infection have excoriated nares and appear listless but have no history of a common cold. In school-age children with a sore throat caused by streptococci infection, the practitioner should be alert for the triad of associated symptoms: headache, vomiting, and abdominal pain. Complications of GABHS infections include acute rheumatic fever and acute glomerulonephritis.

Management
Viral pharyngitis
Treatments and medications
- Administer acetaminophen 10 to 15 mg/kg as frequently as every 4 to 6 hours for fever or discomfort. (Do not exceed five doses in 24 hours.)
- Recommend warm saline gargles, lozenges, or sucking of hard candy for throat discomfort in older children and adolescents.
- Push fluids (but avoid carbonated drinks and citrus juices).

Counseling and prevention
- Inform the parents and child about the culture results and provide reassurance as needed.
- Educate the parents about the normal course of pharyngitis caused by a virus.
- Remember that the child may follow a normal diet as tolerated. Consider a soft diet for 2 days if swelling of tonsils or throat makes swallowing difficult.
- Avoid anesthetic throat sprays or lozenges.
- Suggest infection control measures, including good handwashing, proper disposal of respiratory secretions, and avoidance of unnecessary exposures.

Follow-up. None is indicated.
Consultations and referrals. None are indicated.

Group A β-hemolytic streptococcal pharyngitis
Treatments and medications.
- Administer potassium penicillin V at 50 mg/kg (up to 500 mg) two times a day for 10 days. This is the drug recommended by the American Heart Association. (It should be noted that penicillin V does not taste good. To enhance compliance, consider prescribing amoxicillin or a cephalosporin that tastes better.)
- Remember that other antibiotic options include the following: If the patient is at increased risk for rheumatic fever or has difficulty with compliance, administer benzathine penicillin G (Bicillin) intramuscularly one time. If the child weighs less than 27 kg, give 600,000 U of benzathine; if more than 27 kg, 1.2 million U. Observe the child in the office for 20 to 30 minutes after the injection.

Table 41-8   Differential Diagnosis: Viral Causes of Sore Throat with Distinctive Characteristics*

	INFECTIOUS MONONUCLEOSIS	HERPANGINA	HAND-FOOT-MOUTH DISEASE	PHARYNGOCONJUNCTIVAL FEVER
Subjective Data				
Age	Usually teenagers	Any	Any	Primarily children
Onset	Gradual	Acute	Acute, often in summertime epidemics	Acute, summer epidemics common (usually associated with public swimming facilities or local outbreaks in schools, camps, and so on)
Duration	1-4 weeks	4-7 days	1 week	1 week
Oral symptoms	Dysphagia	Dysphagia, sore throat	Pain in oral area	Sore throat
Associated exanthem	Yes	Yes	Yes	Yes
Associated symptoms	Fatigue, fever	Younger children: Fever, anorexia; Older children: sore throat, headache, myalgia; mild vomiting and diarrhea may occur	Mild fever, sore throat, malaise; may have diarrhea, pruritus, burning lesions	Fever, sore throat, eye exudates; may have headache, malaise, achiness, anorexia, mild to severe dysphagia
Objective Data				
Physical examination				
Vital signs	Fever	Fever	Fever	Fever
Lymphadenopathy	Generalized, cervical adenopathy, usually anterior and posterior cervical nodes are firm and mildly tender	Cervical adenopathy	May have cervical adenopathy	Cervical adenitis
Skin	Maculopapular or scarlatina rash in 5% of patients; universal if previous treatment with ampicillin or penicillin	None	Vesicles that do not ulcerate on palms, soles, interdigital areas, often with a linear configuration	May have flushed appearance of the face
Eye	May have eyelid edema	None	None	Conjunctivitis, both bulbar and palpebral involved; may be unilateral and then progress to bilateral
Mouth	Soft palate petechiae may be present	Sometimes vesicles and ulcers on soft palate and uvula	Vesicles that erode, leaving ulcers on tongue and oral mucosae	None
ENT	Injected pharynx with exudates	Vesicles and ulcers linearly arranged on anterior tonsillar pillars	None	Pharyngitis; may have exudative pharyngotonsillitis; may also have evidence of nasal stuffiness, epistaxis
Abdomen	Hepatomegaly in 30% of patients; spenomegaly in 50%-75% of patients	None	None	None
Laboratory data	Ebstein-Barr virus (EBV) serology	None	None	None

For viral pharyngitis, see Table 41-7.

If the patient has poor compliance, possibly prescribe amoxicillin 750 mg once daily for 10 days; this may be prescribed in children older than 3 years of age (Berman, Johnson, Chan, & Kelley, 2001).

- If the patient is allergic to penicillin, consider the following regimens:
  Erythromycin estolate 20 to 40 mg/kg per day in two to three divided doses for 10 days. (Erythromycin estolate causes less GI upset and is preferred by the American Heart Association).
  Cefadroxil 30 mg/kg per day once daily for 10 days.
  Do not prescribe if patient has a history of penicillin anaphylaxis.
- Administer acetaminophen 10 to 15 mg/kg as frequently as every 4 to 6 hours for fever or discomfort. (Do not exceed five doses in 24 hours.) Consider administering

ibuprofen if the child is very uncomfortable or has a high temperature. (See Chapter 44.)

- Recommend warm salt-water gargles, lozenges, or sucking hard candy for throat discomfort in older children and adolescents.
- Push fluids (but avoid carbonated or citrus juices).
  Counseling and prevention
- Remind the child and parents that any oral antibiotic must be taken for the full course.
- Teach infection control measures, including good hand-washing, proper disposal of respiratory secretions, and avoidance of unnecessary exposures.
- Isolate the child from others until medication has been taken for 24 hours.
- Suggest the child may return to school if afebrile and medication has been taken for 24 hours.
- Remember that family members who are symptomatic should have throat cultures performed.
  Follow-up
- Have the parents call immediately if the child has excessive drooling, difficulty swallowing, or enlarged lymph nodes.
- Have the parents call if the child has not improved in 48 to 72 hours.
- Have the parents call immediately if the child has an adverse reaction or reactions to medications or the child cannot keep the medication down.
- Have the parents call in 7 to 14 days if the child complains of malaise, headache, fever, dark urine, edema, decreased urinary output, or migratory joint pains.
- Take follow-up throat cultures of a child or a family member (or other close contact) who has a history of rheumatic fever or glomerulonephritis, if there is a history of frequent GABHS, if there is a community outbreak of GABHS, or if tonsillectomy is being considered because of chronic GABHS.
  Consultations and referrals. Refer the child to a physician for the following:
- Unresponsive cervical adenitis
- Signs and symptoms of peritonsillar abscess, retropharyngeal abscess; rheumatic fever, or glomerulonephritis
- Membranous pharyngitis (suspect diphtheria)
- Prolonged course with no improvement over 7 days

Voice Changes

Alert

Consult with or refer to a physician for the following:
- Progressive or persistent hoarseness lasting longer than 2 to 3 weeks.
- Signs of respiratory distress or obstruction accompanied by hoarseness
- Stridor associated with hoarseness
- History of foreign-body aspiration
- History of blunt trauma to the larynx
- Growth failure (height)
- Congenital hoarseness
- Painful hoarseness
- Chronic chest congestion and recurrent pneumonia
- Family history of hereditary type of laryngeal edema

Etiology

A change in voice quality is generally caused by dysfunction of the vocal cords. During the newborn period, laryngeal injuries may result from birth trauma (such as recurrent laryngeal nerve injury during a breech delivery), complications from intubation, or congenital anomalies (e.g., laryngeal web, laryngeal cysts, laryngeal cleft). The most common causes of acute voice changes in infants, children, and adolescents are viral URI, allergy, and voice trauma. Chronic voice abuse may lead to the development of vocal cord nodules in school-age children. Juvenile laryngeal papillomatosis is a common benign laryngeal tumor in children under 7 years of age. Common signs of juvenile laryngeal papillomatosis are hoarseness or stridor, aphonia or voice change, and respiratory compromise. Uncommon causes of hoarseness in children include hypothyroidism, exposure to toxins (e.g., smoke, lead, mercury), and vocal cord polyps. Rare causes of hoarseness or a change in voice quality include chromosomal abnormalities, neurologic disorders, congenital abnormalities, and diphtheria.

Incidence

- The prevalence of chronic hoarseness ranges from 5% to 20% in school-age children.
- Statistics on the prevalence of acute hoarseness are not known; however, approximately 90% of the cases of acute hoarseness are caused by viral infections of the upper respiratory tract.

Risk Factors

- Infants and children predisposed to acquired laryngeal paralysis as the result of birth trauma (specifically face presentation), neck or thoracic surgery, or CNS disease
- Acute infection of the respiratory tract
- History of gastroesophageal reflux (GER), allergy, chronic sinusitis, intubation, foreign-body aspiration, immunocompromise, maternal and congenital syphilis, or CNS disorder
- Environmental exposure to smoke, lead, mercury, chemotherapy, or irradiation
- School-age children and adolescents at risk for voice abuse from loud shouting and yelling
- Children 2 to 7 years of age at risk for juvenile laryngeal papillomatosis (which may also occur in newborns)
- Children entering puberty, especially males (i.e., pubertal voice changes)
- Incomplete immunization status (e.g., for diphtheria)
- Smoking

Differential Diagnosis

Subjective and objective data for determining a differential of acute episodes of a change in voice quality are presented in Table 41-9.

Acute laryngitis is commonly related to *respiratory tract infections* caused by adenoviruses and influenza A and parainfluenza type 1 viruses. Impaired nasal respiration and postnasal drip are the two most common precipitating factors of hoarseness as the result of an infectious inflammatory disease. Hoarseness is one of the hallmark symptoms of viral croup; a muffled voice is characteristic of severe tonsillitis and epiglottitis. However, in general, it is other signs and symptoms of respiratory distress or infection that precipitate an office visit and assist in determining a differential diagnosis. Other sections in this chapter discuss subjective data, objective data, and

Table 41-9 Differential Diagnosis: Common Causes of Acute Laryngitis in Children (464.0)

CRITERIA	RESPIRATORY TRACT INFECTION	ALLERGY	EXCESSIVE USE OF VOICE
ICD-9 code	519.8	477.9	784.40
Subjective Data			
Age	Variable, depends on the etiologic agent	Variable	≥ 4 years; most common in school-age children and adolescents
Onset	Follows associated signs and symptoms below	Sudden or gradual	Sudden
Associated signs and symptoms	Rhinorrhea, cough, nasal congestion, postnasal drip, sore throat, mouth breathing; may have fever, difficulty breathing	May have sore throat, difficulty swallowing	May have other allergic manifestations such as nasal congestion, sneezing, rhinorrhea; may have itchy, red eyes, palatal and throat itching, headaches, fatigue, malaise, nasal speech, snoring, epistaxis, and poor school performance
Precipitating factors	—	May be able to identify specific allergen; may include allergy to pollen, molds, animal dander, chemical fumes, smoke, or change in weather; may use inhaled steroids for asthma without a spacer device	School or social event with vigorous shouting, yelling, singing, and cheering
Child's health history	Exposure to infection	Allergic laryngeal disease; recurrent respiratory infections associated with hoarseness, enlarged tonsils or adenoids; otitis media, asthma, allergic rhinitis, chronic sinusitis	
Objective Data			
Physical examination			
Vital signs	Variable	Normal for age	Normal for age
General appearance	Variable, depends on child's age, etiologic agent, and level of involvement	Appears well, in no respiratory distress	Appears well, in no respiratory distress
Upper respiratory findings	Yes	Pale, bluish, boggy nasal mucosa, enlarged nasal turbinates, clear rhinorrhea; may have allergic facies (e.g., allergic shiners, mouth breathing, extra wrinkles below the lower eyelids), nasal salute; tonsils may be enlarged without exudates, postnasal drip; may have evidence of middle ear effusion	Possible sore throat on swallowing
Voice quality	Hoarse	Whispering or hoarseness upon phonation; may have to interrupt speech to clear throat or swallow mucus; may have difficulty swallowing	Hoarse
Breathing difficulties	Variable; depends on child's age, etiologic agent, and level of involvement	Variable; may have signs of increased respiratory effort	No

laboratory tests for respiratory disorders that may be associated with voice changes, especially viral croup and epiglottitis.

Children with documented *allergies,* especially allergic rhinitis or chronic sinusitis, may be more prone to develop acute episodes of hoarseness as the result of vocal cord edema and inflammation. Postnasal drip and mouth breathing may further contribute to the development of hoarseness or acute laryngitis during an allergic episode. In addition, long-term use of inhaled steroids without a spacer may occasionally precipitate hoarseness.

One of the most common causes of acute laryngitis or hoarseness in school-age children and adolescents is *excessive use of voice,* or vocal abuse as the result of excessive shouting and yelling at school or social events.

Management

Acute upper respiratory infection. Other sections in this chapter discuss the management of clinical entities associated with voice changes, especially viral croup and epiglottitis.

Allergy. Other sections in this chapter discuss the management of clinical entities associated with allergy (e.g., asthma, allergic rhinitis, sinusitis). See also Allergies in Chapter 43 and Asthma in Chapter 45.

Excessive use of voice

Treatments and medications

- Instruct the child to rest the voice by whispering or speaking softly.
- Increase environmental humidity, especially at night.
- Recommend throat lozenges and sucking hard candy for older children and adolescents.
- Increase fluid intake.

Counseling and prevention

- Explain the cause of hoarseness or laryngitis to the parents and child and stress the importance of voice rest.
- Discuss the role of supportive measures such as fluids and humidity.
- Educate the parents and child about the signs and symptoms of respiratory distress or infection.

Follow-up. None is indicated. The child should return immediately if there are increasing signs and symptoms of respiratory distress or infection.

Consultations and referrals. Refer the child to a physician or ear, nose, and throat specialist for the following:

- Signs and symptoms of airway obstruction
- Hoarseness progresses or lasts longer than 7 to 14 days
- Congenital hoarseness
- Painful hoarseness

Resources

Websites

American Academy of Pediatrics (www.aap.org)

Asthma Management Model System (www.nhlbisupport.com/asthma/educenter.html)

Virtual Hospital (University of Iowa), Multimedia Textbook: *Electric Airway* (www.vh.org/Providers/Textbooks/ElectricAirway/ElectricAirway.html)

Bibliography

Barkin, R.M. & Rosen, P. (Eds.). (1999). *Emergency pediatrics: A guide to ambulatory care* (5th ed.). St. Louis: Mosby.

Berman, S., Johnson, C., Chan, K., & Kelley, P. (2001). Ear, nose, and throat. In Hay, W.W., Hayward, A.R., Levin, M.J., & Sondheimer, J.M. (Eds.). *Current pediatric diagnosis and treatment* (15th ed.). New York: McGraw-Hill.

Darville, T. & Yamauchi, T. (1998). Respiratory syncytial virus. *Pediatrics in Review, 19*(2), 55-61.

Dershewitz, R.A. (Ed.). (1999). *Ambulatory pediatric care.* Philadelphia: J.B. Lippincott.

Lan, A.J. & Colford, J.M. (2000). The impact of dosing frequency on the efficacy of 10-day penicillin or amoxicillin therapy for streptococcal tonsillopharyngitis: A meta-analysis, *Pediatrics, 105*(2), e19.

National Heart, Lung, and Blood Institute. (1997). *Expert Panel report 2: Guidelines for the diagnosis and management of asthma.* Washington, DC: National Institutes of Health.

Pichichero, M.E. (1998). Group A beta-hemolytic streptococcal infections. *Pediatrics in Review, 19*(9), 291-302.

Tunnessen, W.W. (Ed.). (1999). *Signs and symptoms in pediatrics* (3rd ed.). Philadelphia: J.B. Lippincott.

Wald, E. (1999). Paranasal sinusitis. In McMillan, J.A., DeAngelis, C.D., Feigin, R.D., & Warshaw, J.B. (Eds.). *Oski's pediatrics: Principles and practice* (3rd ed.). Philadelphia: Lippincott, Williams & Wilkins.

Chapter 42 *Urinary System*

Mikel Gray & Fern Campbell

Abdominal Mass, p. 675
Bladder and Urethral Anomalies, p. 676
Blood in the Urine (Hematuria), p. 677
Diurnal Incontinence and Altered Patterns of Urine
    Elimination, p. 679
Nocturnal Enuresis, p. 684
Painful Urination, p. 686
Protein in the Urine (Proteinuria), p. 690

Risk Factors

Prenatal

- Maternal diabetes (risk for urogenital sinus or cloacal defect)
- Young maternal age during pregnancy (risk for bladder exstrophy but not epispadias)
- Older maternal age during pregnancy (risk for hypospadias)
- Multiparity (risk for exstrophy or epispadias defect)

Other

- Family history of congenital renal or urinary system defects, neurologic system defects, gastrointestinal (GI) tract defects (including imperforate anus), or hypertension
- Previous history of recurring, afebrile urinary tract infections (UTIs) or febrile infections
- Recent urologic instrumentation (e.g., catheterization, endoscopy)
- Indwelling catheter
- Interrupted or incomplete toilet training
- Recent emotional crisis or distress
- Urinary retention
- Trauma to the genitalia, flank, lower abdomen, or pelvis
- Recent streptococcal infection
- Constipation
- Stool incontinence
- Uncircumcised male
- Immunosuppression
- Diabetes
- Increased sexual activity

Health Promotion

Prevention of Infections

- Wash hands after toileting and before eating.
- Maintain adequate fluid intake (30 ml/kg per day).
- Maintain adequate hygiene of the perineal area and teach girls to wash from front to back.
- Avoid the use of urethral irritants, including bubble baths.
- Suggest showers rather than baths for girls with recurring UTIs.
- Avoid excessive intake of bladder irritants (e.g., caffeine, carbonated beverages, aspartame).
- Prevent constipation by maintaining adequate fluid and fiber intake in the diet.

- Provide additional counseling for sexually active adolescent girls:
  Urinate before and immediately after intercourse.
  Practice safe sex using barrier devices against transmission of sexually transmitted diseases (STDs).
  Avoid feminine deodorants, douches, and sprays.
  Seek immediate care for unusual vaginal discharge.

Subjective Data

- Complete history on initial visit (for other visits, the history should be adapted based on the presenting complaint)
- Demographics, including age, gender, and race
- Chief complaint and description of problem, including:
  Time and nature of onset (e.g., acute, gradual, after specific incident)
  Change in characteristics of urine, including color, concentration, odor, and presence of blood or sediment
  Blood noted on underclothing
  Associated symptoms, including changes in frequency of diurnal urination, nocturia, urgency to urinate, urinary leakage, dysuria, lower abdominal pain, flank or back pain, fever or chills, malaise, joint pain, anal itching, urethral or vaginal discharge, skin lesions or rashes, and polydipsia
- Toilet training, including age at toilet training, methods used in training, age at completion, and differentiation among primary enuresis, diurnal incontinence, or nocturnal enuresis, and secondary urinary incontinence
- Past medical history, including:
  Previous UTIs, including association with fever and results of testing
  Renal disease, including presenting problems, medical diagnosis, and treatments
  History of insertion of foreign bodies into body orifices, particularly with a mentally retarded child.
  Previous streptococcal infection.
  Diabetes
  Hospitalizations, including the reason for hospitalization, age of child, and treatments or surgery
  Injuries or illnesses, including infectious or trauma-induced illnesses, neurologic or urologic conditions, seizure disorders, undiagnosed febrile illness (particularly gastroenteritis), blood dyscrasias, sickle cell anemia, and diabetes mellitus
  Patterns and habits, including diurnal and nocturnal patterns of urine elimination, patterns of urine loss (if present), sleep patterns, patterns of sexual activity, and use of contraception
- Dietary history, including fluid intake (volume and choice of beverage), recent changes in diet or increase in intake of bladder irritants, and intake of dietary fiber sources

- Developmental history, including major milestones of motor and cognitive development as well as development of bladder control.
- Social history, including interpersonal relationships with parents, teachers, siblings, schoolmates, and others in the community
- School performance
- Family history, including urinary or renal anomalies, chronic or recurrent renal or urinary system disorders including calculi, polycystic renal disease, familial glomerulonephritis, UTIs, pinworms, varicella, scabies, blood diseases, enuresis, vesicoureteral reflux (particularly among siblings), congenital neurologic or GI defects, diabetes, and hypertension

Objective Data

Physical Examination

A complete physical examination should be performed on any child under 4 years of age, or if child is being seen for the first time. For older children, the examination should include the following procedures:

- Plot height and weight on an appropriate growth chart.
- Measure temperature, pulse, and blood pressure (supine and upright).
- Assess general appearance and nutritional status.
- Inspect skin for rashes, color, turgor, dryness, hematoma, and edema (of the eyes, hands, and lower extremities).
- Inspect ears for malformation.
- Auscultate heart for murmurs.
- Auscultate lungs for crackles and rhonchi.
- Assess abdomen for masses, and perform a bimanual examination of both kidneys in a smaller or thin child.
- Evaluate flanks for hematoma or ecchymoses; test for costovertebral-angle tenderness.
- Inspect external genitalia of both genders; assess perineal skin for rashes or altered integrity of skin; evaluate penis, testes, and epididymis in boys; inspect for urethral discharge; and perform complete digital rectal examination on older adolescents with signs or symptoms of prostatitis.
- Palpate lymph nodes.
- Observe joint mobility.

- Perform a complete neurologic examination for mental status, sensory and motor function (including perineal and perianal sensations), tone of anal sphincter, and bulbocavernosus reflux.
- Observe the act of voiding (when indicated) for quality of stream, intermittency, postvoid dribbling, pain with urination, and excessive hesitancy.

Diagnostic Procedures and Laboratory Tests

- *Urinalysis*—Dipstick analysis is used to assess for evidence of UTIs (e.g., nitrites, white blood cells [WBCs]), polyuria (e.g., low specific gravity with diabetes intoxication, glucosuria with diabetes mellitus), or evidence of renal disease causing polyuria (e.g., proteinuria, red blood cells [RBCs]) (Table 42-1). A microscopic analysis is indicated when dipstick results raise the suspicion of UTI. The urine is observed under high power for the presence of bacteria and WBCs. A urine culture and sensitivity test are indicated only when urinalysis raises the suspicion of infection.
- *Urine culture and sensitivity test*—A clean-catch, midstream specimen is typically adequate. However, repeated testing may be necessary because of contamination. Invasive methods of urine collection provide more accurate results. Catheterization with an appropriate-sized catheter (6 to 8 French) is preferred to larger-size catheters. Suprapubic aspiration of urine is the most reliable and most invasive method to collect urine for culture; it is rarely indicated in the evaluation of enuresis. A urine culture is used to identify the concentration and type of bacteria in the urine. Sensitivity testing determines the antimicrobial activity that various antibiotics exert against a specific strain of bacteria.
- *Calcium-to-creatinine ratio*—The calcium and creatinine concentrations of a random urine sample are obtained, and the ratio of urine calcium to urine creatinine is calculated. A calcium-to-creatinine ratio greater than 0.18 indicates hypercalciuria, a condition associated with hematuria that is caused by an unknown mechanism.
- *Twenty-four-hour urine study for calcium level*—The urine is saved over a 24-hour period for analysis of total calcium level. Consult the laboratory for directions for completing a 24-hour urine study. The 24-hour urine study for calcium is completed when the calcium-to-creatinine ratio is greater

Table 42-1 Components of the Dipstick Urinalysis and Their Significance

TEST	NORMAL	SIGNIFICANT FINDINGS
pH	5-7	> 8 Indicates alkaline urine
White blood cell count	< 3-4 HPF	> 3-4: Possible UTI
Red blood cell count	< 1-2 HPF	> 5: Possible UTI, underlying renal disease
Color	Clear to yellow	Dark yellow, turbid urine with debris near bottom of container may indicate pus (pyuria); clear with polyuria; bright red with fresh blood; darker red with old blood
Nitrate/nitrite	Negative	Positive with bacteriuria
Glucose oxidase	Negative	Positive with bacteriuria, diabetes mellitus
Bacteria	Negative	May indicate urinary tract infection
Protein	Negative	Fixed or persistent finding may indicate underlying renal disease
Specific gravity	1.010-1.025	Lower values (< 1.010) seen with diabetes insipidus and glomerulonephritis with renal tubular damage and inability to concentrate urine; higher values with diabetes mellitus, dehydration

From Fischbach, F.T. (1980). A manual of laboratory diagnostic tests. Philadelphia: J.B. Lippincott; Gray, M. (1992). Genitourinary disorders. St Louis: Mosby; Wilson, D. (1995). Nurse Practitioner, 20(11), 59-60, 68-74.
HPF, *High-power field.*

than 0.18. The 24-hour urine calcium level should be less than 4 mg/kg per day.

- *Complete blood cell count*—A complete blood cell (CBC) count is used to evaluate for evidence of postinfectious nephritis.
- *Serum antinuclear antibody study*—A serum antinuclear antibody (ANA) study is used to rule out the presence of systemic lupus erythematosus.

- *Ultrasonography of kidneys and bladder*—Ultrasonography images the anatomy of the upper and lower urinary tracts. It is particularly useful in the detection of hydronephrosis, significant ureteral dilatation, and solid or cystic structures in the kidney. It is used to image urinary calculi in conjunction with a plain abdominal film (kidneys and upper bladder). Ultrasonography of the bladder is used to determine postvoid residual urine

Voiding record for   **Name:**_____

Please record with a √ mark each time you leak, or don't make it to the bathroom before becoming wet.

For 2 days before starting your medicine, record all episodes of leakage

After you have been on the medicine 3 to 4 weeks, again record the number of times that you have leakage

Time	Day 1	Day 2		Time	Day 1	Day 2
8 A				8 A		
9 A				9 A		
10 A				10 A		
11 A				11 A		
12 P				12 P		
1 P				1 P		
2 P				2 P		
3 P				3 P		
4 P				4 P		
5 P				5 P		
6 P				6 P		
7 P				7 P		
8 P				8 P		
9 P				9 P		
10 P				10 P		
11 P				11 P		
M'nite				M'nite		
1 A				1 A		
2 A				2 A		
3 A				3 A		
4 A				4 A		
5 A				5 A		
6 A				6 A		
7 A				7 A		

Fig. 42-1 Example of a voiding record.

volumes and to determine the thickness of the bladder wall in obstructive conditions or the neuropathic bladder. Scrotal ultrasonography with Doppler blood flow measurement is used to differentiate epididymitis or epididymoorchitis from torsion of the testis and to image solid versus cystic or fluid testicular masses.

• *Bladder record and log*—This is a written record of time of urination, time and circumstances of incontinent episodes, volume voided, and type and volume of fluid intake. The log may contain one or all of these components and should be kept for 1 to 7 days (Fig. 42-1). The bladder log is an optional component of the routine evaluation of diurnal voiding dysfunction in children. It is used to evaluate patterns of urine elimination, functional bladder capacity, fluid intake, patterns of urine loss, and factors that provoke urinary incontinence.

Voiding Diary

Date	Time	Volume Voided	Volume Catheterized

Fig. 42-1 cont'd

- *Postvoiding urinary residual volume*—This is a measurement of urine left in the bladder after micturition. The postvoiding urinary residual volume (PVR) may be measured by catheterization immediately after urination (requiring invasive insertion of catheter) or by ultrasonic imaging of the bladder. A residual volume greater than 25% of the total bladder capacity (voided volume plus urinary residual volume) is generally considered significant for urinary retention. The PVR is an optional component in the routine evaluation of diurnal voiding dysfunction but an essential component when urinary retention is suspected or when incontinence is complicated by UTI.
- *Voiding cystourethrogram*—Radiographic imaging of the lower urinary tract requires catheterization and multiple radiographic images. The voiding cystourethrogram (VCUG) is used to determine the presence of vesicoureteral reflux and its grade. A radionuclide cystogram is substituted in children with severe allergies to contrast materials (as compared with allergy to intravenous infusion only).
- *Intravenous pyelogram and urogram*—Intravenous pyelogram and urogram (IVP/IVU) are serial radiographic images of the kidneys, ureters, and bladder after intravenous injection of an iodine-based contrast or nonionic contrast material. Radiographs are typically taken at 1 minute and 5 minutes and after compression of the abdomen over the kidneys. Tomography may be used to visualize structures at specific depths within the kidneys. A postvoiding image may be obtained.
- *Radionuclide renal scan*—This scan provides serial images of the kidneys, ureters, or bladder after intravenous injection of a radionuclide material. The diethylenetriaminepentaacetic acid (DTPA) radionuclide is used to determine obstruction of the upper urinary tracts and provide an esti-

mation of differential renal function (relative contributions of right versus left kidney function to total glomerular filtration rate [GFR]). The dimercaptosuccinic acid (DMSA) radionuclide provides a more accurate evaluation of differential renal function and the presence and severity of renal scarring among children with a history of pyelonephritis. However, it cannot be used to evaluate obstruction. The technetium 99m–mercaptoacetyltriglycine (MAG_3) radionuclide combines some of the advantages of DMSA and DTPA.

- *Urodynamic testing*—Urodynamics is a set of tests designed to measure the function of the bladder. Urodynamic evaluation is not indicated in the routine evaluation of diurnal incontinence or voiding dysfunction in children. Testing is indicated for children with complex voiding dysfunction, urinary incontinence of unknown origin, urinary retention, voiding dysfunction complicated by recurring or febrile UTI, vesicoureteral reflux, hydroureteronephrosis, or compromised renal function (Table 42-2).
- *Uroflowmetry*—Graphic representation of urinary flow, or uroflowmetry, is a noninvasive screening study. The patient is asked to urinate into a container that is placed on a flow transducer, which measures urinary flow in milliliters per second. The uroflow is indicated when urinary retention (bladder outlet obstruction or deficient detrusor contraction strength) is suspected. This screening test diagnoses abnormal urination patterns, but it does not differentiate obstruction from deficient detrusor contraction strength.
- *Cystometrogram*—A cystometrogram (CMG) is a graphic representation of bladder pressure as a function of volume. The bladder is catheterized, and a rectal tube is inserted to measure abdominal pressures. Intravesical (bladder) pressures and abdominal pressures are measured

Table 42-2 Indications for Urodynamic Testing and Significant Findings

CONDITION	INDICATIONS	SIGNIFICANT FINDINGS
Urge incontinence (unstable bladder of childhood)	Urine loss unresolved despite routine treatment	Persistent, unstable (hyperactive) detrusor contractions despite treatment, or previously undetected incontinence type (stress or extraurethral)
	Incontinence complicated by urinary retention, recurrent UTIs, single febrile UTI, vesicoureteric reflux	Unstable (hyperactive) detrusor contractions with detrusor sphincter dyssynergia (causes urinary retention and turbulence of urinary outflow, predisposing the bladder to bacterial colonization), or poor, deficient detrusor contraction strength with high urinary residual volume (videourodynamic testing preferred)
	Neurogenic bladder with urge or reflex incontinence	Detrusor sphincter dyssynergia with spinal lesions; deficient detrusor contraction strength with lower spinal disorders
Urinary retention	All cases	Bladder outlet obstruction with high detrusor contraction pressure and low peak and mean flow on voiding pressure study; obstruction predisposes the urinary system to urinary tract infections, vesicoureteric reflux, ureterohydronephrosis, and compromised renal function (videourodynamic testing preferred)
		Deficient detrusor contraction strength increases the risk of urinary tract infections
Stress urinary incontinence	All cases	Urine loss provoked by abdominal straining: An abdominal leak point pressure test is used to determine the severity; when caused by intrinsic sphincter deficiency (ISD), may indicate neurogenic bladder dysfunction and is managed differently than is urethral hypermobility (the most common cause of stress incontinence in adult women) (videourodynamic testing required to differentiate ISD from urethral hypermobility)

From Bauer, S.B., Retik, A.B., Colodny, A.H., et al. (1980). Urologic Clinics of North America, 7(2), 321-336; Gray, M. (1992). Genitourinary disorders. St Louis: Mosby.

directly, and detrusor pressure is calculated by subtraction of abdominal pressure from intravesical pressure. The filling CMG is used to determine the bladder's capacity and the compliance of the bladder wall during filling and to determine the cause of urinary incontinence. Unstable detrusor contractions occur with urge incontinence. Stress urinary incontinence is diagnosed by an abdominal leak-point pressure test.

- *Sphincter electromyogram*—Sphincter electromyogram (EMG) is a graphic representation of the pelvic muscle during bladder filling and micturition. The sphincter EMG is completed with a CMG or uroflowmetry (uncommon). Surface or needle electrodes are placed at the perianal and periurethral area, and kinesiology (gross muscle activity) of the pelvic floor is recorded.
- *Voiding pressure study*—This is a graphic representation of uroflowmetry and CMG during micturition. The child is asked to urinate after a filling CMG. The sphincter EMG also may be measured during the voiding pressure study.
- *Videourodynamic study*—This is a combination of urodynamic pressure, EMG, and uroflowmetry tracings with fluoroscopic imaging of the lower urinary tract. Videourodynamic testing combines physiologic measurements with a dynamic morphologic study of lower urinary tract function during bladder filling and micturition.
- *Serum creatinine and blood urea nitrogen levels*—For evaluation of renal insufficiency (the practitioner should refer to the local laboratory testing service for age-adjusted, normal-value ranges), indigo carmine dye is injected. Intravenous injection of it is used to determine the presence of ectopic ureter in girls (with the vagina stained purple).
- *Methylene blue test*—This is an intravesical infusion of methylene blue substance. The vagina stains blue with vesicovaginal fistula.

Abdominal Mass

Alert

Refer to a physician any child with an abdominal mass.

Etiology

Multiple factors can produce an abdominal mass (hydronephrosis). Obstruction of the ureteropelvic junction is common among infants and children, though ureteral strictures and the megaureter (a congenital dilatation of the ureter with stenosis at the ureterovesical junction) also may occur. The cause of multicystic kidney disease is unclear. The kidneys are dysplastic, possibly related to a vascular anomaly during embryogenesis.

The precise mechanism by which Wilms' tumor occurs is unknown, but some insight into its pathogenesis and origins or causes have been gained. Wilms' tumor assumes at least two forms, heritable and nonheritable malignancies. Heritable forms of Wilms' tumor account for approximately 15% to 20% of all reported cases. Wilms' tumor is associated with other anomalies. These relationships remain unclear, but children with these defects should be closely monitored for the presence of Wilms' tumor. The anomalies include aniridia, cryptorchidism, congenital renal anomalies, and cardiac anomalies as well as Beckwith-Wiedemann, Drash, and Perlman syndromes. The predisposition for Wilms' tumor is also associated with neurofibromatosis.

Little is known about the origin of neuroblastoma, partly because of the rarity of this tumor. The malignancy arises from the cells of the neural crest that develop into the sympathetic ganglia and the adrenal glands. A genetic predisposition toward neuroblastoma may exist.

The causes of urinary retention are bladder outlet obstruction and deficient detrusor contraction strength. See the discussion of Urinary Retention in this chapter.

Incidence

- The majority of abdominal masses are benign.
- Approximately half of abdominal masses in neonates arise from the kidneys.
- The majority of abdominal masses among neonates arise from hydronephrosis or multicystic kidney disorder.
- In one study, solid tumors accounted for slightly less than 2% of all masses among a combined data group of 115 neonates.
- The incidence of Wilms' tumor is 1 in 7.8 million children.
- Wilms' tumor becomes evident as an abdominal mass in over 90% of children.
- About 10% of Wilms' tumors are bilateral, affecting both kidneys and frequently creating bilateral abdominal masses.
- The incidence of neuroblastoma is 1 in 10 million live births.
- Neuroblastoma is the most common extracranial malignant tumor of infancy and early childhood, with 50% of all cases detected by the second year of life and 75% diagnosed by 4 years of age.

Risk Factors

- Polycystic or multicystic kidney disease
- Congenital urinary system defect

Differential Diagnosis

The majority of abdominal masses in infants arise from the kidneys, the retroperitoneal space, and the female genital tract. Initial assessment is accompanied by prompt referral to a physician for definitive diagnosis and management. A urinalysis should be completed on children who have an abdominal mass. Hematuria noted on dipstick analysis in infants may indicate renal vein thrombosis or, rarely, a urinary system tumor. Among children the coexistence of an abdominal mass and hematuria raises a greater suspicion of a tumor in the urinary system. Abdominal ultrasonography may be ordered in consultation with the physician to determine the presence of hydronephrosis, a solid tumor within the abdomen, or urinary retention with an enlarged bladder.

Management

Treatments and medications. All abdominal masses are referred for urgent evaluation and treatment. An abdominal ultrasonogram may be obtained to initially characterize the location of the mass and to differentiate cystic from solid masses or urinary retention with an overdistended bladder.

Counseling and prevention

- Reassure parents that many abdominal masses do not necessarily represent a malignancy but that a prompt evaluation and treatment are essential. Early detection is critical.

- Remember that routine screening has been advocated for neuroblastoma. A vanillylmandelic acid (VMA) spot urine test is inexpensive (less than $1) but has limited accuracy (i.e., limited sensitivity and specificity). High-performance liquid chromatography for urine VMA is more expensive (approximately $6), but it has a higher sensitivity and specificity. Widespread adoption for these screening tests in the United States is likely to occur if the test is proved cost-effective.

Follow-up. Follow-up care is determined in consultation with the consulting physician.

Consultations and referrals. Provide immediate referral to a physician for any child with an abdominal mass.

Bladder and Urethral Anomalies

Alert

Consult with or refer to a physician any case of bladder or urethral anomaly

Etiology

The most common anomalies of the lower urinary tract include hypospadias, exstrophy and epispadias anomalies, and prune-belly syndrome. Urine system anomalies often occur together. Other defects of the penis and bladder, such as penile or bladder duplication or agenesis, are extremely rare, occurring in only one in several million births.

The cause of hypospadias is unknown. The defect shows a familial predisposition, though no clear genetic factors for the condition have been identified. Hypospadias may occur as the result of an abnormal response to genital development, which is mediated partially by human chorionic gonadotropin.

Classic bladder exstrophy with epispadias and cloacal anomalies represents a spectrum of defects that occur with abnormal cloacal development. These defects affect the urinary system (classic exstrophy-epispadias complex), the GI system (imperforate anus), or both anorectal and urogenital sinus organs (cloacal anomalies). The mechanisms that produce this abnormal development of the cloacal membrane development are not known.

The cause of prune-belly syndrome is unknown. The condition may represent a chromosomal mutation, though the mechanism or location of such a defect has not been identified. Some postulate that the urologic and anterior wall defects of the syndrome are caused by obstruction of the posterior area of the urethra during embryonic development or that the condition represents the sequelae of prostatic dysgenesis and fetal ascites.

Incidence

- The urinary system is the most common site of congenital defects.
- The incidence of hypospadias varies among regions, ranging from as few as 0.26 per 1000 live births in Mexico to 8.2 per 1000 live births in Minnesota.
- The incidence of bladder exstrophy is approximately 3.3 per 100,000 live births.
- The risk of bladder exstrophy in a child with a parent who has the defect is 1 in 70 live births, a risk is 500 times greater than that faced by the general population.

- The incidence of prune-belly syndrome has been estimated to be 1 in 35,000 to 1 in 50,000 live births.
- As many as 20% of children with prune-belly syndrome die during infancy as a result of complications related to pulmonary hypoplasia.
- Cloacal anomalies are very rare, occurring in approximately 1 in 200,000 live births.

Risk Factors

- Sibling with a urinary system defect (particular risk for hypospadias, exstrophy or epispadias anomaly, prune-belly syndrome, and urogenital sinus defect)
- Family history of urinary system defects
- Turner syndrome (risk for prune-belly syndrome)

Differential Diagnosis

Evaluation of bladder and urethral anomalies should be completed in close consultation with a pediatric urologist. Prompt referral of the patient with a newly diagnosed anomaly is necessary. An abdominal ultrasonogram may be performed to identify the position, size, and architecture of the kidneys. In children with prune-belly syndrome, an exstrophy-epispadias anomaly, and urogenital anomalies, a voiding cystourethrogram may be performed to rule out vesicoureteral reflux and the presence of a fistulous tract. This study is typically obtained after referral to a pediatric surgeon and a pediatric urologist.

Signs of *hypospadias* include a ventral location of the urethral meatus in boys (as compared with the normal location at the distal end of the glans penis), incomplete formation of the foreskin, and possible ventral chordee (fibrous band causing "bend" during erection).

Classic *exstrophy* includes a wide separation of the symphysis pubis, externalization of the bladder with the midline red bladder mucosa open and draining urine, a shortened distance between the umbilicus and anus, and anterior displacement of anal sphincter. In boys, it may also include markedly short penile length with an anterior chordee, urethra is splayed open to the level of the bladder outlet, and bifid scrotum with retractile cryptorchid testes. In girls, it may include a shortened vaginal vault; short urethra open to level of bladder outlet, bifid clitoris, and a wide margin between labia.

Signs of *cloacal (urogenital sinus plus anorectal) anomalies* include abdominal distention, a single perineal opening with absent vagina and anal opening, or a hooded appearance to a single phalliclike opening, giving the appearance of an intersex state.

Symptoms of *prune-belly syndrome* include an absence of abdominal musculature with a prunelike appearance of the belly, or a scrotum with the absence of testes (cryptorchidism).

Management

Treatments and medications. Congenital urologic defects are initially managed by prompt referral to a pediatric urologist or another appropriate specialist. In most cases a single or staged surgical repair is combined with ongoing monitoring of the urinary system. In many instance, in particular, cloacal anomalies or the prune-belly syndrome, several specialists may follow the child throughout her or his lifetime.

Counseling and prevention

- Teach the parents about the defect and reassure them that treatment is available.
- Advise strict adherence with perineal hygiene for children with a urogenital sinus defect or an exstrophy-epispadias anomaly.

- Teach the parents to recognize the symptoms of UTI, and advise them to seek prompt care if these symptoms occur.
- Teach the parents of a child with prune-belly syndrome the symptoms of UTI and of pneumonia, because pulmonary hypoplasia associated with prune belly may increase the risk of these conditions.
- Teach the parents of a child with prune-belly syndrome to protect the child's abdominal area from pressure and to avoid constrictive clothing.
- Provide support and counseling for families of the child with a bladder or urethral anomaly.

Follow-up. Follow-up evaluation is typically handled by both the primary care practitioner (PCP) and the consulting pediatric urologist. Routine evaluation of the urine with a urinalysis and culture if indicated is justified whenever the child with exstrophy, cloacal defect, or prune-belly syndrome is seen by the practitioner. The blood pressure also should be checked regularly, and growth patterns assessed to detect potential changes in renal function. This surveillance is integrated with well-child care visits whenever possible.

Consultations and referrals. Immediate referral to a pediatric urologist or pediatric surgeon (urogenital defects) is indicated for any child with a defect of the bladder or urethra. Refer parents for genetic counseling if they are considering having additional children.

Blood in the Urine (Hematuria)

Alert

Consult with or refer to a physician for the following:
- Persistent hematuria of unclear origin
- Hematuria associated with hypercalciuria (elevated calcium-to-creatinine ratio or elevated 24-hour calcium level)
- Hematuria with suspected underlying renal disease (e.g., peripheral edema, hypertension, weight loss or failure to thrive [FTT], proteinuria)
- Hematuria with a febrile UTI
- Hematuria related to trauma (including insertion of a foreign body into the bladder, blunt or penetrating trauma to the flank or lower abdomen, and pelvic trauma)
- Vaginal bleeding from suspected sexual abuse (which may initially be perceived by the family as hematuria)

Etiology

Hematuria arises from several processes. UTI may produce hematuria, and it frequently occurs in cyclophosphamide cystitis. Disorders of the renal parenchyma frequently produce hematuria (Box 42-1). These conditions may be acquired or congenital, and the mechanisms by which they produce hematuria are sometimes unclear. Benign hematuria may occur after physical exertion, such as long-distance running or contact sports. The condition resolves over time though the risk of recurrence is significant.

Several familial conditions are associated with hematuria. Hypercalciuria may represent a familial or an acquired disorder that occasionally causes hematuria by means of an unclear mechanism. Familial benign hematuria occurs in at least one parent and the child. Several familial conditions may cause hematuria, including familial nephritis, either associated with deafness (Alport syndrome) or as an isolated finding. Polycys-

Box 42-1 Renal Disorders Associated with Hematuria

Congenital Conditions

Hypercalciuria
Benign familial hematuria
Structural defects of the urinary system
Benign recurrent hematuria
Hereditary nephritis

Acquired Conditions

Poststreptococcal glomerulonephritis
Postadenoviral glomerulonephritis
Perineal irritation
Coagulation disorders

Systemic Conditions

Hemolytic-uremic syndrome
Systemic lupus erythematosus
Polyarteritis nodosa
Necrotizing vasculitis
Goodpasture syndrome

Renal Trauma (from Blunt or Penetrating Insults)

Contusion
Minor laceration
Major laceration
Vascular injury

tic kidneys (autosomal recessive or dominant) often cause hematuria. In this case blood in the urine may arise after minor abdominal or flank trauma or as a result of spontaneous bleeding into a cyst.

Poststreptococcal glomerulonephritis usually follows a streptococcal pharyngitis or impetigo, causing edema, hypertension, and acutely impaired renal function. Other forms of glomerulonephritis can cause hematurias, and nephritis is frequently associated with blood in the urine on gross or microscopic examination. Disorders of the renal parenchyma, including nephritis, glomerulonephritis, and polycystic kidneys, may be associated with acute renal insufficiency or failure.

Urinary calculi frequently cause hematuria, particularly when they move through relatively narrow areas of the ureter, including the ureteropelvic junction, near the sacroiliac vessels, or at the ureterovesical junction.

Blunt or penetrating renal trauma is associated with hematuria, and significant or life-threatening bleeding can occur. Blunt insult to the abdomen or flank can cause a superficial bruise and an underlying renal contusion, with hematuria on gross or microscopic examination that resolves over time. More significant renal trauma, either lacerations or avulsion of the vascular pedicle, is associated with gross hematuria and potentially life-threatening blood loss in some cases.

The presence of spots of blood in the undergarments of boys, associated with dysuria, is often interpreted by parents as "blood in the urine." In this case, however, the source of bleeding is the urethra, and the condition is called *urethrorrhagia*. The condition is caused by a benign urethral lesion, and symptoms may recur for as long as 10 years.

Incidence

- UTI is the most common cause of hematuria among school-age children.
- Although tumors represent a significant cause of hematuria among adults, urinary tract malignancies account for less than 1% of all cases of hematuria among schoolchildren.

Risk Factors

- UTI
- Genitourinary (GU) trauma
- Renal disease
- Family history of benign familial hematuria
- Polycystic kidney disease in the family (autosomal dominant or recessive)
- Recent streptococcal infection
- History of urinary calculi
- Suspected renal vein thrombosis
- History of urinary system tumor

Differential Diagnosis (Table 42-3)

The initial step in the evaluation of blood in the urine is to determine whether the blood in a voided specimen is coming from the urinary tract. A midstream urine specimen is typically adequate, but a catheterized urine specimen is necessary if vaginal or rectal bleeding is suspected as the source of blood in a voided specimen. A dipstick urinalysis is performed to determine the presence of blood in the urine. A microscopic analysis also may be evaluated to confirm the diagnosis. The dipstick is further analyzed for the presence of nitrites and WBCs, and pyuria, bacteriuria, and casts are sought through microscopic analysis. If the urine specimen is suspected of infection, a culture and sensitivity test are completed, and the UTI is eradicated.

If urinalysis fails to reveal evidence of infection, a calcium-to-creatinine ratio is obtained. A ratio greater than 0.18 raises the suspicion of hypercalciuria, and this diagnosis can be confirmed or excluded by a 24-hour urine test for calcium level. The 24-hour urine calcium level should be less than 4 mg/kg per day. After infection and hypercalciuria have been excluded as the cause of hematuria, the parents' urine also may be subjected to urinalysis to rule out the presence of benign familial hematuria. If familial hematuria is not present, a CBC count is obtained to evaluate for evidence of postinfectious nephritis, and a serum ANA study is done to rule out the presence of systemic lupus erythematosus.

If these evaluations are negative or if renal disease is suspected as a possible source for the hematuria, the patient should be referred to a pediatric nephrologist. Cases of hematuria associated with a congenital defect of the urinary system are referred to a pediatric urologist.

Management

Treatments and medications. The appropriate management of hematuria relies on accurate diagnosis. Because hematuria commonly occurs among children without a serious underlying cause, the routine referral of every patient with hematuria to a specialist cannot be justified. In addition, even in the hands of a pediatric urologist or nephrologist, an unequivocal diagnosis of the cause of hematuria cannot be obtained in every case. Nonetheless, the practitioner can evaluate the child with blood in the urine, exclude significant underlying causes of hematuria, and manage the condition or refer the patient to a specialist for further testing and treatment.

An afebrile UTI can be managed by the practitioner (see Painful Urination in this chapter). Urethrorrhagia can also be managed by the practitioner. There is no clearly defined treatment for this condition. A urethral culture may be performed to determine the presence of a urethritis, though chlamydial (nongonococcal) urethritis will not yield positive results. If urethritis is suspected, a course of antimicrobial therapy may be prescribed, followed by a 30-day course of low-dose, suppressive antibiotics.

Counseling and prevention

- Reassure anxious parents that hematuria in a child is rarely associated with urinary system cancer. Emphasize the importance of testing for the child with hematuria. Explain the purpose of each examination and the significance of all negative as well as positive findings.
- Reassure the family of a boy with urethrorrhagia that the condition is benign and will resolve over time. Advise the family that recurrent bloody spotting of the undergarments and dysuria may occur and that the condition may persist

Table 42-3 Differential Diagnosis: Blood in the Urine

CRITERIA	URINARY TRACT INFECTION	BENIGN FAMILIAL HEMATURIA	HYPERCALCIURIA*	RENAL DISEASE*
ICD-9 code	599.0	599.7	275.40	593.9
Subjective Data				
Dysuria	Present	Absent	Uncommon	May be present
Fever	May be present	Absent	Absent	May be present
Frequency of urination/urgency	Present	Absent	Mild symptoms	May be present
Objective Data				
Laboratory data				
Urinalysis (dipstick findings other than hematuria)	Nitrites, white blood cells	None	Cloudy urine may be noted	Proteinuria with glomerulonephritis or other renal disease
Microscopic urinalysis (other than hematuria)	Pyuria, bacteriuria	No specific findings	Significant crystalluria	RBC and WBC casts, hyaline casts, granular casts

*Refer to a pediatric nephrologist.

for as long as 10 years without adverse consequences for the child.

Follow-up. Hematuria associated with UTI should be followed up after appropriate therapy (usually 7 to 14 days). A repeat urinalysis for resolution of signs of infection and resolution of hematuria is necessary, and additional evaluation of the hematuria is indicated if this condition is not resolved after successful treatment of the UTI.

Children with idiopathic hematuria should be assessed every year for evidence of compromised renal function, including blood pressure measurement, plotting of growth and development, and urinalysis for proteinuria. Referral to a pediatric nephrologist or urologist is indicated when any signs of compromised renal function are detected.

Children with urethrorrhagia should be reassessed annually or sooner if symptoms of the condition recur.

Consultations and referrals. Refer to a pediatric urologist if the symptoms associated with urethrorrhagia are recurrent or severe. In this case a retrograde urethrogram will be performed, and a diverticulum of the fossa navicularis, Cowper's gland cyst, or urethral polyp may be noted and resected. Refer to a pediatric nephrologist or urologist any child with hematuria and confirmed hypercalciuria; hematuria associated with proteinuria, hypertension, peripheral edema, or serum studies suggestive of compromised renal function; hematuria associated with recent abdominal or flank trauma; suspected urinary calculus; or recurrent or persistent hematuria when a cause cannot be determined.

Diurnal Incontinence and Altered Patterns of Urine Elimination

Alert

Consult with or refer to a pediatric urologist for the following:
- Voiding dysfunction not responsive to appropriate intervention
- Voiding dysfunction associated with recurrent UTIs or a single, febrile UTI
- Voiding dysfunction complicated by vesicoureteral reflux
- Voiding dysfunction associated with a neurologic condition
- Suspected Hinman syndrome
- Voiding dysfunction caused by urinary retention of unclear origin

Etiology

Several conditions are associated with diurnal urinary incontinence or other voiding dysfunction in children. The cause of voiding dysfunction among children is only partly understood.

Urge incontinence (or unstable bladder of childhood) is the occurrence of urine loss associated with a precipitous urge to urinate. The cardinal symptoms of urge incontinence among children are diurnal urinary frequency (voiding more than every 2 hours), urgency to urinate, urge incontinence (urine loss unless the urge to urinate is heeded immediately), and nocturnal enuresis. Among older children and adolescents nocturia may replace enuresis in this quadrangle of symptoms. The origin of urge incontinence in childhood is not clear. Urge incontinence in the "neurologically normal" child may be divided into two categories. In certain children, bladder control is never gained, and urge incontinence persists, despite attempts at toilet training. In others, urge incontinence occurs af-

ter a period of diurnal and nocturnal continence. When one is evaluating diurnal urge incontinence, it is important to exclude clinically significant, organic causes of unstable (hyperactive) detrusor contractions.

Neurologic disorders are known to cause urge incontinence with detrusor hyperreflexia or hyperactive contractions of the detrusor. These lesions may affect the brain, such as hydrocephalus caused by an Arnold-Chiari deformity or a brain tumor, or the suprasacral segments of the spine. Lesions of the sacral spine, such as the majority of myelomeningocele defects, affect the sacral spinal segments, causing detrusor areflexia (absence of detrusor contractions). Bladder outlet obstruction and irritative disorders of the lower urinary tract also have the potential to produce unstable detrusor contractions.

The origin of detrusor contractions among children without apparent neurologic conditions, obstruction, or inflammation of the lower urinary tract is not known. Subtle neurologic defects, a maturational lag, or developmental delay has been postulated to produce this condition.

Hinman syndrome, an uncommon voiding dysfunction, is a result of behavioral or psychologic disorders that are reflected in bladder dysfunction. The symptoms of Hinman syndrome are initially similar to those of urge incontinence. However, these children also have urinary retention and febrile UTIs as the syndrome progresses. In later stages persons with Hinman syndrome may have signs and symptoms of renal failure. The origin of Hinman syndrome remains unknown. It has been attributed to persistence of the "transitional phase of toilet training," when the child uses the sphincter to postpone voiding rather than suppressing contraction of the detrusor. It has also been attributed to a persistence of the normal response to unstable detrusor contractions. Psychologic factors, including personality and family dysfunction, and sexual abuse have also been associated with the Hinman syndrome.

Stress urinary incontinence is the leakage of urine associated with physical exertion (stress) in the absence of a detrusor contraction. Unlike in adult women, stress urinary incontinence in children is usually attributed to intrinsic sphincter deficiency. Neuropathic lesions affecting the sacral spinal segments, such as those produced by lumbosacral myelodysplasia, cause weakness of the muscular elements of the urethral sphincter and stress results in urinary incontinence. Iatrogenic damage to the sphincter from surgery of the pelvis or surgery also produces intrinsic sphincter deficiency in some children. Stress urinary incontinence is also associated with certain urologic system defects such as the exstrophy-epispadias complex.

Extraurethral (total) urinary incontinence is the continuous loss of urine from a source other than the urethra. Among children, extraurethral incontinence is typically caused by ureteral ectopia. In girls an ectopic urethra may drain urine into the vaginal vault. This condition produces a continuous, watery vaginal discharge superimposed on an otherwise normal voiding pattern. Extraurethral urinary incontinence also occurs among children with the exstrophy epispadias complex and those with cloacal deformities. This condition persists until these complex, significant defects can be surgically repaired.

In children of both genders, fistulas occasionally produce extraurethral urine loss. These fistulas may be the product of a congenital defect, such as an imperforate anus or a cloacal defect, or they may occur as a complication of a reconstructive surgery for hypospadias or epispadias.

Urinary retention is the condition that occurs when micturition fails to completely evacuate urine from the bladder vesicle.

Two conditions, bladder outlet obstruction and deficient detrusor contraction strength, cause urinary retention. Among children bladder outlet obstruction is typically caused by congenital or functional conditions. Urethral valves, polyps, or bladder neck contracture cause an anatomic obstruction of the bladder outlet. Functional causes of bladder outlet obstruction include detrusor sphincter dyssynergia sometimes associated with the unstable bladder of childhood and always associated with the Hinman syndrome. Rarely, tumors of the urethra or pelvic organs cause obstruction of the bladder outlet. As a result, the bladder contracts at high voiding pressures, predisposing the urinary system to ureterohydronephrosis, vesicoureteral reflux with febrile UTIs, and compromised renal function.

Deficient detrusor contraction strength causes urinary retention because the detrusor is unable to exert enough force to keep the bladder outlet open long enough to empty urine from the vesicle. Among children, deficient detrusor contraction strength is typically caused by neuropathic lesions of the sacral spinal cord or myogenic diseases affecting smooth muscle contractility. In other cases metabolic disorders, such as heavy-metal poisoning or diabetes mellitus, may be associated with poor detrusor contractility. Deficient detrusor contraction strength also may be produced by transient conditions including ingestion of antispasmodic or anticholinergic medications, certain antidepressants or antipsychotics, and illicit drugs including tetrahydrocannabinol of the *Cannabis* plant.

Incidence

- Urge incontinence is the prevalent type of incontinence among children.
- The prevalence of diurnal incontinence is approximately equal for boys and girls up to 14 years of age; after this time, girls are more likely than boys to have urine loss.
- The prevalence of diurnal urinary incontinence and nocturnal enuresis (combined) is approximately 15% in children 4 years of age. In one study, diurnal incontinence alone and combined daytime and nighttime urinary leakage occurred in approximately 10% of a group of 242 healthy schoolchildren.

Risk Factors

- Neurologic system defect
- GU system defects (particularly epispadias, exstrophy, and persistent cloacal anomalies)
- UTI
- Encopresis or fecal impaction

Differential Diagnosis

Diurnal voiding dysfunction can be divided into two categories. Transient incontinence in children is typically caused by inflammation (typically infection) of the lower urinary tract or by polyuria from diabetes mellitus, diabetes insipidus, or underlying renal disease. Established, or chronic, voiding dysfunction is either idiopathic or caused by an identifiable underlying condition that is managed along with the symptoms of urinary incontinence or urinary retention (Table 42-4).

Transient urinary incontinence is diagnosed by a focused history, careful physical examination, and urinalysis, with or without urine culture and sensitivity testing. Urinary infection is suspected when dipstick analysis reveals nitrites and WBCs and when microscopic urinalysis shows bacteriuria and pyuria. Underlying renal disease is suspected when urinalysis demonstrates hematuria and the history and physical examination demonstrate hypertension, changes in growth patterns, or other signs of renal parenchyma conditions (refer to Blood in the Urine in this chapter). UTI is a common cause of transient urinary leakage among children, but diabetes or renal disorders rarely become evident with incontinence as the primary symptom.

Established or chronic incontinence is diagnosed when causes of transient incontinence have been excluded or when management of these conditions does not cause relief from the symptoms of urine loss. For example, a child with diurnal urge incontinence may have bacteriuria, suggestive of UTI as the cause of the incontinence. Eradication of the bacteriuria may or may not relieve symptoms of urge incontinence. When established urge incontinence is suspected, the practitioner must identify the type of incontinence to determine appropriate treatment (Table 42-5). Urge incontinence is characterized by a history of urgency, frequency, diurnal urge incontinence, and enuresis or nocturia. When presented with a sudden urge to urinate, the child frequently squats or places a heel in the perineum in an attempt to arrest urine loss. These symptoms may be evaluated by history and physical examination, or they may be assessed after one checks a bladder log that the child and family are asked to keep. The bladder log is a written record of the pattern of urination, volume voided, fluid intake, occurrence of urine loss, and precipitating factors. The child with urge incontinence must be evaluated for urinary retention and for a history of recurring afebrile UTI or febrile UTIs. If these conditions occur, imaging of the urinary system (typically comprising a renal-and-bladder ultrasonogram, plus a videourodynamic evaluation or voiding cystourethrogram) and consulta-

Table 42-4 Differential Diagnosis: Transient Versus Established Urinary Incontinence

CRITERIA	TRANSIENT	ESTABLISHED
ICD-9 code	788.30	788.30
Subjective Data		
Onset of symptoms	Acute	Gradual, or child never masters bladder control despite toilet training
Objective Data		
Urinalysis	Nitrites and WBCs on dipstick analysis; bacteriuria and pyuria on microscopic examination; glucosuria or low specific gravity with diabetes	Negative or persistence of symptoms after eradication of UTI absent glucosuria or low specific gravity; concentrated urine with higher specific gravity frequently seen if child is attempting to manage urine loss by reducing fluid intake
Urine culture and sensitivity test	Positive	Negative or symptoms of urine loss persist after UTI is eradicated

tion with or referral to a pediatric urologist are warranted. If the child has a history of urge incontinence, recurring UTIs, and abnormal upper urinary tract imaging studies or an abnormal videourodynamic test with pseudodyssynergia, Hinman syndrome should be suspected and the child should be promptly referred to a pediatric urologist.

Stress incontinence is diagnosed when urine loss is associated with physical exertion in the absence of a precipitous urgency to urinate. One can elicit the sign of stress urinary incontinence during the physical examination by asking the child to bear down or cough while the urethral meatus is visualized. The passage of urine in the absence of a sudden urge to void determines the presence of stress incontinence. Because stress incontinence is typically caused by intrinsic sphincter deficiency and usually associated with a neurologic disorder or a structural defect of the urinary system, a pediatric urologist is consulted or a referral is obtained.

Extraurethral incontinence is diagnosed when continuous urine loss is not associated with a precipitous desire to urinate or with physical exertion. Parents frequently report "continuous dampness or leakage" in a child with urge or stress incontinence. To differentiate these conditions, it is necessary to phrase questions very specifically. The practitioner may ask the parents whether their child may be dry for at least 30 minutes to 1 hour. Likewise, the symptom of squatting or placing the heel in the perineum is associated with urge incontinence rather than with extraurethral incontinence though parents and the child may describe this condition as being "continuously wet." Vaginal secretions also may be confused with extraurethral incontinence among girls. A simple phenazopyridine-pad test may be used to differentiate these conditions. The child is provided with an absorbent pad to absorb vaginal secretions or urinary leakage after phenazopyridine is administered. The parents are instructed to place the bag in a sealed plastic bag and bring it to the practitioner within 24 hours. Since phenazopyridine causes a characteristic orange discoloration of the urine, incontinence can be easily differentiated from vaginal discharge, which does not produce this characteristic stain on the pad.

Management

Urge incontinence

Treatments and medications. Specific dietary recommendations are designed to reduce the irritative properties of urine and related incontinence. The following measures also may reduce the risk of UTI and urinary retention associated with dehydration and constipation.

- *Avoid dehydration*—Many families and children reduce fluid intake in an attempt to alleviate urine loss. However, instead of reducing urine incontinence, fluid restriction

Table 42-5 Differential Diagnosis: Incontinence Types

CRITERIA	URGE	STRESS	EXTRAURETHRAL*	URINARY RETENTION*
ICD-9 code	788.31	788.32	599.9	788.20
Subjective Data				
Frequency of urination	Positive	May be absent	Absent	Frequency may be greater during sleep as opposed to waking hours
Urgency to urinate	Positive	Absent	Absent	May be positive
Precipitating factor for urine loss	Sudden desire to urinate	Physical exertion	No identifiable cause	May be associated with urgency or physical exertion
Nocturnal enuresis	Positive	Urine loss alleviated during night	Unaffected by time of day	Not applicable
Objective Data				
Physical examination				
Neurologic examination	Normal or signs of neurologic condition	Signs of neurologic or urologic defect common	Normal or signs of urologic defect	Normal or signs of neurologic condition or urologic defect
Laboratory data				
Bladder log	Diurnal frequency, reduced functional bladder capacity, urine loss associated with urge to urinate	Diurnal frequency may be normal; urine loss associated with physical activity	Persistent urine loss with otherwise normal pattern or urine elimination, or massive urine loss without identifiable patterns of urine elimination	Frequent urine elimination
Postvoid residual volume determination (by catheterization or ultrasonography)	Normal or elevated with learned dyssynergia; residual volume may be greater than voided volume with Hinman syndrome	Normal unless associated with urinary retention	Normal	Elevated (> 25% of total bladder capacity)

*Refer to a pediatric urologist.

that is sufficient to produce even mild dehydration concentrates the urine, increasing its irritability to the bladder and its potential to promote unstable detrusor contractions and sensory urgency. Recommend that the incontinent child receive the recommended dietary allowance (RDA) for fluids (30 ml/kg of body weight per day).

- *Reduce the intake of bladder irritants*—Certain foods and beverages may produce bladder irritation or serve as natural diuretics. These substances may be eliminated or reduced to alleviate urine loss. Because bladder irritants have different effects in different persons, they should be reduced or eliminated one at a time to determine their effect on voiding dysfunction. Common bladder irritants include caffeine, coffee, tea, aspartame, carbonated beverages, alcohol, and cigarette smoke.
- *Avoid constipation and regulate bowel elimination patterns*—Constipation may predispose the bladder to urinary retention, and it has been associated with an increased risk of UTI. A combination of adequate fluid intake and dietary fiber is used to manage and prevent constipation in most children (see Constipation in Chapter 35). Constipation or encopresis may also be aggressively managed by a combination of initial evacuation of the rectum and colon, followed by regular use of a stool softener and dietary modifications ensuring adequate fluid and fiber intake and regular bowel movements with soft formed stool. (See Constipation in Chapter 35.)

Specific behavioral methods can also be used to manage urinary incontinence in selected children. Prompted or timed voiding is feasible for most children. However, other behavioral methods require the patient to isolate and contract the pelvic muscles. Application of these techniques implies that the child is old enough to identify and tighten the pelvic muscles and that she or he has sufficient perineal sensations to identify proprioceptive and exteroceptive stimuli including bladder fullness, urgency to urinate, and a pelvic versus abdominal versus thigh muscle contraction.

- *Prompted, or timed, voiding*—The child with urge incontinence should be placed on a prompted, or timed, voiding schedule, whether or not medications are being used to manage unstable detrusor contractions. Timed voiding should apply both to home and during school, and a letter should be written to the school-age child's teachers explaining the nature of the voiding dysfunction and the rationale for prompted voiding. A schedule of 2 to 3 hours is typically instituted for urge incontinence.
- *Quick-flick contractions for episode of urgency*—The child with unstable detrusor contractions (urge incontinence) can be taught to isolate and contract the pelvic muscles in response to an episode of precipitous urgency. The child is taught to complete either a "quick-flick" contraction (maximal strength contraction for a period of 2 to 4 seconds) or a sustained contraction (lasting 6 to 10 seconds). The child should repeatedly contract the pelvic muscles until the contraction and precipitous urgency subsides and then proceed to the bathroom immediately.
- *Pelvic muscle relaxation*—Behavioral training techniques also may be used for the child with unstable bladder contractions and detrusor sphincter dyssynergia. The child is taught to isolate and contract the pelvic muscles. However, rather than being taught graded exercises designed to improve maximal strength and endurance, the child is taught progressive relaxation exercises. Once this maneu-

ver is mastered, it is practiced with urination to prevent obstruction and urinary retention associated with dyssynergia of the detrusor and sphincter muscles.

The management of urinary incontinence and altered patterns of urinary elimination may also require use of medications:

- *Oxybutynin chloride (Ditropan)*—The dosage is 2.5 to 5 mg (for children 5 years of age and older) two or three times per day (not to exceed 15 mg in 24 hours) for a 6-month trial and then ongoing. Safety in children younger than 5 years of age has not been established. An antispasmodic, this drug is used to increase small-bladder capacity. Side effects include drowsiness, mydriasis, dizziness, dry mouth, urinary retention, and constipation. It is available in liquid form. Advise the child and family that dry mouth is likely to occur and that adequate fluid intake and chewing sugar-free gum reduce this symptom. Mild blurring of vision is a frequent side effect during initial therapy, and reading small print may be difficult. If the vision is significantly blurred, the medication is discontinued or the dosage adjusted. Oxybutynin requires 5 to 7 days for maximum effectiveness; as-needed dosing is not recommended. Heat intolerance characterized by flushing and fever related to exertion or a hot climate may occur. The dosage of anticholinergics-antispasmodics frequently requires readjustment during summer months. Constipation may be significant. Increased fluid and fiber are recommended as preventive measures.
- *Propantheline bromide*—The child dosage is 0.5 mg/kg twice a day. The adult dosage is 7.5 to 15 mg two to four times a day for a 6-month trial and then ongoing. An anticholinergic, this drug is used to inhibit unstable detrusor contractions. For side effects, see oxybutynin. Propantheline reaches maximum effectiveness after 1 to 3 days of use; refer to oxybutynin for other considerations.
- *Hyoscyamine sulfate*—The dosage is 0.03 to 0.1mg/kg two to four times a day for a 6-month trial and then ongoing. An antispasmodic, this drug is used to inhibit unstable detrusor contractions. The side effects are similar to those for oxybutynin. It is available in liquid (sublingual), tablet, and sustained-release forms. The side effect of dry mouth is typically less noticeable than with propantheline or oxybutynin.
- *Imipramine hydrochloride*—The dosage is 25 mg 1 hour before bedtime and may increase to 50 mg in children less than 12 years of age and 75 mg in children greater than 12 years of age for a 6-month trial and then ongoing. Medication should be decreased slowly over 6 to 8 weeks once improvement is seen. With its combination anticholinergic and α-sympathomimetic effects, this drug is used to treat urge incontinence or mixed urge and stress urinary incontinence. Side effects include dryness of mouth, blurred vision, restlessness, sleep disturbance, mood swings, and hypertension. Refer to oxybutynin for considerations related to anticholinergic-antispasmodic effects. α-Sympathomimetic effect may contribute to side effects such as restlessness, difficulty with sleep, and high blood pressure. Do not exceed the dosage prescribed. Keep this and all medications out of reach of children. There is danger of toxicity if the drug is ingested by other children or if the prescribed dosage is exceeded.

Altered skin integrity and rashes are frequent complications of urinary incontinence. Children with severe stress urinary incontinence and extraurethral urinary leakage are at particular risk, just as those with double urinary and fecal incontinence. A preventive skin care program is begun for any child with severe urinary leakage and for those with altered skin integrity at the time of presentation.

- Clean the skin thoroughly with soap and water or an incontinence cleanser at least daily.
- Avoid excessive use of soap and drying cleansers. Rinse skin with water when changing containment devices or use an incontinence cleanser; use soap or cleanser when necessary.
- Prescribe an ointment to act as a moisture barrier or a skin barrier when urine loss is severe or when altered skin integrity is observed.
- Prescribe an over-the-counter (OTC) or prescription product for candidal rash (red maculopapular rash with satellite lesions) as indicated. When urine loss is severe, recommend a powder form. Advise the family to spread the powder lightly over the affected area and to avoid applying large volumes, which promote moisture retention.
- Thoroughly dry the skin daily; use a hair dryer set at the lowest or cool setting to promote complete drying of the perineal skin.

Counseling and prevention

- Counsel the family that the condition frequently improves with age.
- Teach the family to recognize common skin complications associated with urinary leakage, including ammonia dermatitis and candidal rash. Review instruction concerning a preventive skin program, and emphasize the importance of regular cleansing and drying of skin exposed to continuous urinary leakage.
- Review medications, including dosages and side effects. Reinforce the relationship between behavioral management of urine loss and pharmacotherapy. Keep all medications out of the reach of children.
- Teach the family to recognize the signs and symptoms of UTI; include the importance of obtaining a urinalysis and urine culture when evaluating any fever of unclear origin.

Follow-up

- Schedule a return visit after institution of therapy. Oxybutynin, propantheline, and hyoscyamine require several days to 1 week to be effective, and an evaluation of the efficacy of the medication requires at least 1 week of ongoing therapy.
- Schedule a return visit every 3 to 6 months as indicated. Children frequently have resistance to the effects of a particular medication, requiring substitution of a similar drug. In addition, changes in weather may alter the child's susceptibility to the side effect of flushing as a response to heat, and the dosage of the antispasmodic medication may need to be adjusted accordingly.
- Schedule a return visit whenever symptoms of UTI occur, or when the child has a fever.

Consultations and referrals

- Refer to a physician any child with infection that is unresponsive to appropriate treatment; recurrent UTIs or a single febrile UTI; reflux; neurologic condition; suspected Hinman syndrome; or urinary retention of unclear origin.
- Keep in mind that letters concerning scheduled toileting are frequently required to assist the child with diurnal urge incontinence to maintain a timed voiding schedule while in school. The nature of the condition, medications, and required voiding schedule with a rationale are typically forwarded to teachers and to the principal of the school.

Stress urinary incontinence

Treatments and medications. Because stress urinary incontinence among children is usually attributed to intrinsic sphincter deficiency caused by a neuropathic condition or congenital anomaly, referral to a pediatric urologist is usually indicated. Occasionally an adolescent girl has pelvic floor relaxation with urethral hypermobility that may be managed with behavioral or pharmacologic therapy.

Pelvic muscle (Kegel) exercises may be effective for an adolescent girl who has stress urinary incontinence. The patient is taught to identify and contract the pelvic muscles, and a graded exercise program designed to improve strength and endurance is completed. However, although pelvic muscle exercises have been shown to be effective in the treatment of stress urinary incontinence caused by urethral hypermobility, the efficacy of this program among patients with intrinsic sphincter deficiency and among children has not been documented.

Medications may be used to provide temporary relief from mild to moderate stress urinary incontinence. An α-adrenergic agonist such as pseudoephedrine or ephedrine may be administered for transient relief of stress incontinence. Pseudoephedrine is typically administered in an oral dosage of 15 to 60 mg every 6 hours, or every 12 hours if a sustained-release preparation is used. The medication should not be administered at night because insomnia is a common side effect and because the occurrence of mild to moderate stress urinary incontinence is not significant during sleep.

Counseling and prevention

- Teach the family to recognize common skin complications associated with urinary leakage, including ammonia dermatitis and candidal rash. Review instructions concerning a preventive skin program, and emphasize the importance of regular cleansing and drying of skin that is exposed to continuous urinary leakage.
- Encourage the patient to remain on a regimen of pelvic muscle exercises for the entire course of prescribed treatment. The effectiveness of this exercise program, like any fitness regimen, is improved when exercises are repeated over time.
- Review medications, including dosages and side effects. Reinforce the relationship between behavioral management of urine loss and pharmacotherapy.
- Teach the family to recognize the signs and symptoms of UTI, including the importance of obtaining a urinalysis and urine culture when evaluating any fever of unclear origin.

Follow-up. Schedule a return visit for the adolescent on a pelvic muscle exercise program every 1 to 2 weeks during the initial month of therapy and every 2 weeks for 3 months. After completion of an initial program, he or she should be prescribed a maintenance program involving exercises 3 or 4 days each week and followed as needed. Immediate visits are indicated if symptoms of a UTI occur.

Consultations and referrals. Refer to continence nurse specialist patients with stress urinary incontinence without evidence of a neurologic condition or urologic anomalies.

Extraurethral incontinence

Treatments and medications. This condition is caused by fistula or ectopia; both are surgical issues. The practitioner's primary management is focused on identification of the incontinence type and referral to a pediatric urologist.

Counseling and prevention. Before referral and definitive management of extraurethral incontinence, teach the child and family skin care and provide education concerning an adequate containment device. The containment device may be a pad or an incontinence brief, depending on the volume of urine loss. The pad or brief should contain superabsorbents to maximize containment and keep moisture away from the skin (refer to discussion of skin care in Management of Urge Incontinence).

Follow-up. Follow-up care is scheduled in consultation with the pediatric urologist. Schedule a return visit if symptoms of a UTI occur or if perineal rashes are observed.

Consultations and referrals. See the Alert box.

Urinary retention

Treatments and medications. Because urinary retention is typically associated with neuropathic conditions or a congenital urologic anomaly, practitioner management generally focuses on identification of the condition with referral to a pediatric urologist.

Clean, self-intermittent catheterization may be used to manage urinary retention. The decision to prescribe intermittent catheterization for a child is made in consultation with a pediatric urologist. The child or family are taught a clean technique of catheter insertion, and catheterization is scheduled every 3 to 6 hours. Nighttime catheterization is avoided whenever feasible though this strategy may be necessary for infants or in other special cases. The catheter may be cleaned by use of soap and water and stored in a dry, clean container before reuse. Microwave "sterilization" in the home is occasionally recommended for intermittent catheters. Each catheter is cleansed with soap and rinsed with water. The catheters are then placed in the microwave, along with a container containing at least 8 ounces of water. The water serves as a heat bath, and the catheters are exposed to the heat and radiation of the microwave for a period of 1 minute per catheter.

An indwelling catheter is rarely used to manage urinary retention. The decision to insert an indwelling catheter is made in consultation with the pediatric urologist. The catheter should be constructed of silicone or a lubricious coating and used with a bedside drainage bag and a leg bag as indicated. The indwelling catheter is used as a "last resource" for the management of urinary retention. It is not an appropriate management program for urinary incontinence.

Counseling and prevention. Teach the child and family the signs and symptoms of a UTI and how to obtain a urine specimen when the child has a fever of unclear origin (see Painful Urination in this chapter).

Follow-up. Follow-up care should be scheduled in consultation with the pediatric urologist.

Consultations and referrals. Referral to a pediatric nephrologist is indicated if urinary retention is associated with compromised renal function.

Nocturnal Enuresis

Alert

Consult with or refer to a physician for the following:
- Evaluation of enuresis demonstrating polyuria consistent with diabetes mellitus, diabetes insipidus, or possible underlying renal disorder
- Adverse reaction to pharmacotherapy
  Consult with or refer to a pediatric urologist for the following:
- Urogenital anomaly noted on the physical examination or during ultrasound of the kidneys or bladder
- UTI in a boy of any age, or recurrent UTIs in preadolescent girls
- UTI associated with enuresis that is resistant to antibiotic therapy
- Secondary nocturnal enuresis occurring with diurnal urinary incontinence in a child with previously normal continence

Etiology

The exact cause of primary monosymptomatic nocturnal enuresis is unknown. In the absence of infection or structural defects several theories have been proposed (Kelalis et al, 1992). There may be delayed maturation of the central nervous system (CNS), causing incomplete control of the detrusor reflex during sleep. This theory is supported by the spontaneous remission of enuresis with maturation and the observation that the majority of enuretic children have adequate urinary control during waking hours as well as adequate control of bowel function. This pattern of mastery of continence closely reflects the normal pattern of toilet training, in which bowel control and diurnal bladder control precede nocturnal continence.

Enuresis may occur as a developmental delay. Children who have enuresis are frequently delayed in the mastery of other developmental milestones when compared with nonenuretic children. Sleep patterns have been associated with enuresis, though sleep studies with electroencephalogram tracings on enuretics failed to correlate bedwetting with any particular stage of sleep.

Inappropriate secretions of antidiuretic hormone during sleep also have been postulated as a cause of enuresis. According to this theory, the secretion of antidiuretic hormone, which normally peaks during sleep, is depressed. As a result, the bladder must deal with an abnormally large volume of urine and responds by uncontrolled micturition.

Primary enuresis is known to follow a familial pattern, and this observation has been used to support several theories, including the maturational lag and developmental delay theories. The significance of the familial pattern of enuresis, however, remains unclear.

Secondary enuresis has been associated with emotional distress such as that caused by divorce, a death in the family, or the birth of a sibling. In addition, primary and secondary enuresis has been postulated to arise from psychologic causes. However, no serious psychologic disorders have been associated with enuresis, and the relationship between emotional distress and the predisposition to bedwetting remains unclear.

Food allergies have been blamed for primary and secondary enuresis. Nonetheless, only anecdotal evidence exists of this relationship.

Incidence

- About 5 to 7 million children in the United States have nocturnal enuresis.
- Boys are affected twice as often as girls.
- Bedwetting occurs in 20% of 5-year-olds.
- About 5% of children have enuresis at 10 years of age; approximately 1% have enuresis at 15 years of age.
- About 45% to 50% of children with UTI have nocturnal enuresis.
- About 25% of children attaining initial nocturnal continence by 12 years of age become enuretic for approximately 2.5 years.
- Familial history is significant. One parent being enuretic results in a 44% occurrence rate in offspring, while both parents being enuretic results in a 77% occurrence rate in offspring.

Risk Factors

- Interrupted or incomplete toilet training (anecdotal evidence only)
- Emotional distress or recent emotional crisis

- Family history of enuresis
- UTI (secondary enuresis is uncommon)
- Delayed developmental milestones

Differential Diagnosis (Table 42-6)

Enuresis is the uncontrolled discharge of urine; *nocturnal enuresis* is the uncontrolled discharge of urine during sleep. These terms are often used synonymously. The evaluation of enuresis requires differentiation of monosymptomatic enuresis from bedwetting associated with voiding dysfunction or another underlying disorder. Monosymptomatic enuresis is separated into two categories. Primary enuresis occurs when a child continues to wet the bed after successful toilet training. Secondary enuresis occurs when a child has a recurrence of bedwetting after a period of diurnal and nocturnal continence. Diurnal incontinence is frequently associated with enuresis, but that condition is clinically different from primary or secondary monosymptomatic enuresis.

When enuresis exists as a single finding, evaluation of the condition is postponed until 6 to 7 years of age whenever possible. If the child is less than 6 years of age and the parents demand immediate evaluation, an initial assessment to exclude UTI or polyuria is completed. A low specific gravity on urinalysis warrants further evaluation only when associated with other signs of diabetes (such as polyuria during the day and at night, polydipsia and excessive thirst, and weight loss) or underlying renal disease (such as hypertension, changes in growth patterns, and weight loss). An ultrasonogram is not necessary, but this noninvasive test may be completed both to allay the anxiety of parents and to exclude the possibility of underlying structural defects of the urinary system.

Management

Treatments and medications. Treatment for nocturnal enuresis is deferred until the child reaches 6 years of age unless the family is insistent on a more aggressive course or the child exhibits signs of serious psychologic distress caused by the enuresis. Behavioral treatments recommended for every enuretic child include decreased fluid intake in the evening (limited to sips after dinner) and teaching the child to urinate immediately before sleep. Bladder irritants in the diet (including caffeine, aspartame, and carbonated beverages) should be avoided, particularly before sleep. A chart or reward system provides positive reinforcement for dry nights and allows the child to have greater control over the condition. The child should be taught to assume responsibility for successful (dry) nights, but no punishment should be applied to nights that enuresis occurs.

Table 42-6 Differential Diagnosis: Nocturnal Enuresis

CRITERIA	PRIMARY	SECONDARY	UNDERLYING RENAL DISORDER*
ICD-9 code	307.6	307.6	593.9
Subjective Data			
Onset of bedwetting	Persistent since before toilet training	Acute onset after previous period of nocturnal continence	Acute onset after previous period of nocturnal continence
Associated symptoms			
Dysuria (pain on urination)	Absent	Observed when secondary enuresis related to symptomatic UTI	Absent
Hematuria	Absent	Rarely observed with symptomatic UTI	Sometimes observed with specific renal parenchyma disorders (refer to Blood in the Urine in this chapter)
Objective Data			
Physical examination			
General findings	Usually normal	Usually normal	May note hypotension, hypertension, edema, and skin rash; may find signs of other infection
Laboratory data			
Nitrites and WBCs on dipstick urinalysis; bacteriuria, pyuria on microscopic urinalysis	Absent	Rarely observed when UTI is associated with enuresis	Absent
Positive urine culture	Rarely positive with underlying urinary tract infection	Rarely positive with underlying UTI	Absent
Red blood cells and hematuria on urinalysis	Absent	Rarely with symptomatic UTI	Sometimes observed with specific renal parenchyma disorders (refer to Blood in the Urine in this chapter)
Structural defect on ultrasonography	Rarely positive	Rarely positive	May be positive (refer to Blood in the Urine [Hematuria] in this chapter)
Diurnal urinary frequency (voids more often than every 2 hours)	Frequently positive	Frequently positive	Positive with early-stage renal insufficiency

Alarm therapy is the most successful treatment strategy for enuresis, and its effect lasts longer than other therapies, including drugs. This type of therapy requires commitment from the child and the parents. An alarm system is sewn into pajamas (preferably) or attached to a pad in the bed. The alarm sounds when wetting is detected. The child must then get out of bed, change his or her clothing, and empty the bladder before returning to bed. This process is repeated each time the alarm sounds. In one study alarm therapy remained effective among 63% and 56% of children at 6 and 12 months after discontinuation of treatment respectively. In contrast, 36% and 16% of children receiving treatment with imipramine and 68% and 10% of those whose cases were managed by desmopressin acetate remained continent at 6 and 12 months respectively.

Two medications are used to manage enuresis. The primary pharmacologic effect of imipramine is unclear. It is known to exert an antispasmodic effect and a CNS effect similar to an α-adrenergic agonist and to influence sleep patterns; it may influence antidiuretic hormone secretion. Desmopressin acetate diminishes the volume of urine created by the kidneys during sleep. It has several potential advantages over imipramine therapy, including its rapid onset of action.

- *Imipramine hydrochloride (Tofranil)*—The dosage is 25 mg 1 hour before bedtime; this may be increased to 50 mg in children younger than 12 years of age and 75 mg in children older than 12 years of age. Medication should be decreased slowly over 6 to 8 weeks once improvement is seen. It is about 40% to 60% effective. Side effects include dryness of mouth, blurred vision, sleep disturbance, and mood swings. The mechanism of action is unclear; it may reduce bedwetting by altering sleep patterns and through anticholinergic effects.
- *Desmopressin acetate (DDAVP)*—Children older than 6 years of age should initially receive 20 mg at bedtime (10 mg [1 squirt] per nostril) for 2 weeks. The dosage may be increased by 10 mg (1 squirt) each nostril per week to maximum of 40 mg. Use should be discontinued if no improvement is seen at maximum dosage. The drug has approximately a 70% success rate, but there may be a relapse after discontinuance. Advantage for short-term success (e.g., sleepovers, camping trips). Side effects include headache, rhinitis, nasal congestion, flushing, and fluid retention or water intoxication.

Alternative therapies may be used in selected children with enuresis, though there is only anecdotal evidence for their efficacy. Hypnotherapy and dietary therapy aimed at identifying and eliminating allergens from foods are the most common alternative therapies used for enuresis.

Counseling and prevention

- Educate the parents and the child regarding the origins of enuresis; include a discussion of proper, consistent toilet training at the appropriate age of readiness for the child.
- Explain the usual age at which nocturnal continence can be expected and when nocturnal enuresis therapy is most likely to be successful (6 years or older). Advise parents that nocturnal enuresis typically resolves between 6 and 10 years of age but that a small number of adults (0.5% to 1%) have occasional episodes of bedwetting.
- Explain the rationale for beginning with noninvasive, preventive methods such as restricting nighttime fluid intake. Discuss available treatment options with the child and parents. Emphasize the potential advantages and disadvantages of each treatment to allow informed consent.

- If alarm therapy is used, advise the parents that commitment to consistent therapy is required for long-term success. Discuss the need to be patient with therapy, and support parental support and encouragement for the child. Instruct the parents to give praise for continence, but emphasize that punishment or ridicule should be avoided when they are coping with incontinent episodes.
- If medications are prescribed, provide oral and written instructions on proper administration. When prescribing imipramine chloride, advise the parents not to exceed the dosage prescribed and to notify their PCP if urinary retention occurs. Instruct the parents to apply sunscreen to their child to prevent photosensitivity. Keep this and all medications out of reach of children; there is a significant danger of toxicity if ingested by other children or if prescribed dosage is exceeded.
- When prescribing desmopressin acetate, instruct the parents in proper technique for intranasal administration. Advise them that retention of water with edema of the feet and hands, lethargy, and behavioral changes should be reported promptly.

Follow-up. Schedule a return visit in 2 weeks to evaluate the efficacy of therapy and every month thereafter until the condition is resolved or there is a determination of a need for additional treatment.

Consultations and referrals

- Refer the child to a psychologist or psychiatrist if enuresis is associated with significant psychologic distress.
- Refer to the Alert box for additional indications for referral.

Painful Urination

Alert

Consult with or refer to a physician for the following:
- Child under 2 years of age
- Elevated blood pressure
- Febrile UTI (for which the practitioner should obtain a culture and sensitivity and initiate empiric treatment pending culture results)
- Costovertebral angle tenderness and complaints of flank pain
- Evidence of sexual abuse or trauma
  Consult with or refer to a pediatric urologist for the following:
- Ureterohydronephrosis of vesicoureteral reflux noted on ultrasound or voiding cystourethrography
- Suspicion of foreign body in the urinary tract
- Boy or prepubertal girl with a recurrent UTI, or a child having first documented UTI when imaging studies are unobtainable
- Hematuria persisting following resolution of infection

Etiology

The origin of UTI is unclear. Two primary factors are believed to determine the likelihood that a certain child will have bacteriuria or a symptomatic UTI. The majority of UTIs are caused by a group of gram-negative bacterial pathogens. *Escherichia coli* is the most common causative organism in children and in adults. Other causative organisms include *Klebsiella, Enterobacter, Proteus,* and *Pseudomonas* species. Gram-positive pathogens also have the potential to infect the urinary tract; *Staphylococcus* and *Enterococcus* species are most common.

Several host factors have an influence on the person's risk of UTI. The most common route of entry of pathogens in the urinary system is ascension through the urethra. Because girls have a shorter, straighter urethra as compared with boys, they are more prone to UTIs. In addition, sexual activity increases the risk of UTI, probably as a result of mechanical factors. In addition to systemic immune mechanisms, several inherent factors in the urinary system also act to inhibit bacterial growth and reproduction. A thin mucopolysaccharide layer in the bladder inhibits the adherence of pathogens to the bladder wall, rendering them free to be flushed from the system during urination.

The urine contains inhibitory factors. The osmolality of the urine influences bacterial growth and reproduction. A urine with increased osmolality and high urea concentrations is bacteriostatic, and a dilute urine also may be bacteriostatic. An acidic pH inhibits the growth of certain pathogens, and a specific glycoprotein, the Tamm-Horsfall protein, which is secreted by the ascending loop of Henle, produces a urinary "slime" that inhibits bacterial adherence.

In contrast to the host defense mechanisms, the bacteria have certain pathogenic factors that may bypass or limit the effectiveness of the host defense mechanisms. These include fimbriae, which act as anchors, or pili, which assist bacteria to adhere to the bladder wall, despite micturition. Certain bacteria also secrete toxic substances that interfere with host defense mechanisms. The K antigen interferes with lysis of the bacteria after invasion of WBCs and macrophages. Hemolysin is a cytotoxic substance that interferes with the actions of WBCs, and other bacteria become resistant to complement activation by unknown mechanisms.

Certain conditions render the child more susceptible to bacteriuria and symptomatic UTIs. Incomplete evacuation of the bladder (urinary retention) increases the susceptibility to UTI, since the child is unable to evacuate bacteria and toxic substances from the urinary system during micturition. Unstable detrusor contractions and detrusor sphincter dyssynergia also increase the risk of infection because they create turbulence of urine during voiding or episodes of incontinence. This turbulence may assist ascension of bacteria from the distal to proximal ends of the urethra and bladder. Calculi or foreign bodies in the urinary tract also increase the risk of UTI because they serve as a safe harbor for bacteria to grow and multiply, even in the presence of antimicrobial therapy.

Constipation may predispose the child to urinary infections. The precise mechanism of this relationship remains unclear. Obstruction of the bladder in the presence of a large mass of hardened stool in the rectum has been postulated but never proved. It seems more likely that constipation predisposes the child to poor detrusor contractility. As a result, bladder evacuation is compromised, and the risk of infection is increased. The possible role of an increased community of local pathogens caused by bacterial overgrowth within the retained stool mass has not been explored.

Other conditions that may produce painful urination include urethritis, or inflammation of the urethra. Nongonococcal (nonspecific) urethritis is common among sexually active adolescents but rare among children. *Chlamydia* and *Ureaplasma* organisms are the most common pathogens in nongonococcal urethritis, accounting for 50% to 60% of all cases. GU trauma may produce painful urination, particularly when the penis, urethra, or bladder is directly injured. Voiding dysfunction that causes detrusor sphincter dyssynergia occasionally produces painful urination because of elevated voiding pressures.

Incidence

- In the first 6 months of life, boys are more prone to UTIs than girls.
- After infancy, girls are more prone to UTI than boys.
- About 40% of children with UTI are asymptomatic.
- Approximately 3% to 5% of girls will have at least one UTI before puberty.
- Asymptomatic bacteriuria is more common than symptomatic UTI.
- The incidence of UTI increases in adolescence, especially with sexual activity.

Risk Factors

- Urinary system defects
- Previous UTI
- Vesicoureteral reflux
- Recent urologic instrumentation
- Intermittent catheterization or indwelling catheter
- Constipation
- Voiding dysfunction associated with urinary retention
- Urinary calculi
- Foreign body in the urinary system
- Bubble baths (anecdotal evidence only)
- Diabetes

Differential Diagnosis (Table 42-7)

Cystitis, or infection of the lower urinary tract (bladder), is characterized by dysuria, frequency, cloudy, odorous urine, and urgency to urinate. Suprapubic or lower abdominal discomfort are commonly noted in older children and adolescents but not in younger children. A febrile UTI creates symptoms of a lower UTI along with flank pain and a fever of 101° F or more. Nausea and vomiting may be present and may precipitate dehydration. If pyelonephritis has progressed to urosepsis, the child may have episodes of chills and changes in mental status.

All suspected UTIs are evaluated by urinalysis, and most children should undergo urine culture and sensitivity testing to identify the causative organism and antimicrobial sensitivities. Additional diagnostic testing is indicated for special populations.

Indications for urinalysis, urine culture and sensitivity testing, and upper urinary tract imaging (typically renal and bladder ultrasonography and voiding cystourethrogram) include:

- Infants and toddlers under 2 years of age
- All boys, regardless of age
- Preadolescent girls after second afebrile UTI
- Children with congenital anomalies
- All complicated UTIs (i.e., those with fever or hematuria)
- All persistent UTIs (i.e., persistence of bacteriuria, despite pharmacotherapy)

Indications for urinalysis only, followed by empiric therapy, include:

- Uncomplicated UTIs in sexually active adolescent girls
- Initial uncomplicated UTI in prepubertal girls

The symptoms of a UTI are particularly vague in a younger child or an infant. Dysuria and lower abdominal or suprapubic pain are reported only in a minority of younger children with documented UTIs. Among older children the classic cluster of symptoms—dysuria, suprapubic or lower abdominal discomfort, frequency of urination, and urgency to urinate—occur.

Table 42-7 Differential Diagnosis: Pain on Urination

CRITERIA	LOWER URINARY TRACT INFECTION	PYELONEPHRITIS*	GASTROENTERITIS	URETHRITIS	PINWORMS
ICD-9 code	595.0	590.80	558.9	597.80	127.4
Subjective Data					
Pain on urination	Dysuria among older children and adolescents; frequently absent among younger children or infants	Dysuria among older children and adolescents; frequently absent among younger children or infants	Absent dysuria	Continuous urethral pain exacerbated by urination	Anal and perineal itching, absent dysuria
Associated symptoms					
Lower abdominal or suprapubic discomfort	Vague or absent in younger child or infant, typically observed in older child or adolescent, pain is alleviated by urination and aggravated by postponing micturition	Similar to lower UTI but flank pain and costovertebral angle tenderness and pain noted in older child or adolescent	Cramping abdominal discomfort, pain is not aggravated or alleviated by urination or bladder filling	Typically absent	Absent
Fever	Low-grade or absent fever (100° F or less)	High-grade fever (100° F or above)	Fever usually mild (100° F or less)	Absent fever	Absent fever
Urethral discharge	Absent	Absent	Absent	Purulent discharge with gonococcal urethritis; clear discharge with nongonococcal urethritis	Absent
Nocturia or diurnal urge incontinence	May be present with child after toilet training or in adolescent	May be present with child after toilet training or in adolescent	Absent	Absent	Absent
Objective Data **Laboratory data**					
Urinalysis	Dipstick: Positive for nitrites, WBCs; microscopic analysis: Bacteriuria and pyuria	Dipstick: Positive for nitrites, WBCs; microscopic analysis: Bacteriuria and pyuria	Negative	Initial 10 to 15 ml of early morning stream contains WBCs; midstream urine negative for nitrites or white blood cells	Negative
Urine culture and sensitivity testing	Positive for bacteria	Positive for bacteria	Negative	Midstream urine negative for bacteria	Negative
Urethral swab	Negative	Negative	Negative	Positive for gonococcus; negative for bacteria with nongonococcal urethritis	Negative

From Gray, M. (1993). Nursing assessment and diagnosis of urinary function. In Broadwell, D.B., Parrish, R.C., & Saunders, R.C. (Eds.). Child health nursing. Philadelphia: J.B. Lippincott.
*Consult with or refer to a pediatric urologist.

Nocturia may occur in adolescents, but younger children often have an acute recurrence of nocturnal enuresis with or without diurnal urge incontinence. Pyelonephritis also may precipitate relatively few signs among younger children and infants. Some infants have a low-grade fever, despite significant infection of the upper urinary tract, and others have seizures or other atypical responses.

Because *pyelonephritis* produces such a vague complex of symptoms in the younger child or infant, it is often misdiagnosed as gastroenteritis. Gastroenteritis is an infection of the GI tract. Overgrowth of a bacteria or viral pathogen produces the characteristic symptoms of lower abdominal pain or cramping, mild fever, nausea and vomiting, and diarrhea. A urinalysis is negative and must be performed any time a child has a fever of unclear origin.

Urethritis is characterized by urethral burning that is relatively continuous and exacerbated by urination. The undergarments may be spotted with blood or a serous or purulent discharge, and the child may complain of discomfort and itching in the perineal area.

Painful urination related to trauma is characterized by a recent history of trauma to the genitalia, lower abdomen, or pelvic area.

Management

Urinary tract infection

Treatments and medications. The role of "forcing fluids" for a urinary infection remains controversial. Dehydration should be avoided because it increases the irritative symptoms associated with UTI and the risk for urgency or urge incontinence. Copious fluid intake probably should be avoided, since it dilutes the concentration of urea, Tamm-Horsfall protein, and other glycoproteins in the urine, possibly reducing the body's natural defenses against infection. In addition, dilute urine has a lower concentration of any prescribed antimicrobial drug, which may reduce its effectiveness against bacteria in the urine. Children with a UTI should be encouraged to drink the RDA of fluids, which is 30 ml/kg of body weight per day.

Reduce or eliminate the intake of bladder irritants, including caffeine, carbonated beverages, aspartame, alcoholic beverages, and some spicy foods.

The discomfort associated with a UTI may be severe. Ensuring an adequate fluid intake alleviates the irritative effects of concentrated urine. In addition, a warm sitz bath or warm shower may alleviate the lower abdominal or suprapubic discomfort and lower back pain associated with a UTI. The bath water should come above the child's waist, and it should not contain any perfumes or detergents (e.g., bubble bath).

Symptomatic UTI requires the administration of antimicrobials. In certain situations antimicrobials are chosen empirically. In other situations an empiric antimicrobial is administered for 1 or 2 days, but the final choice is dictated by the results of a sensitivity panel. The choice of antimicrobial agent is influenced by multiple considerations. These include the cost of the drug, the route and frequency of administration, the age of the child, and the practitioner's preferences for and familiarity with certain agents. Generally a twice-a-day dosage schedule is preferred to medications that are given three or four times daily. Oral medications are preferred whenever possible. Parenteral medications are required for resistant strains of bacteria. Intravenous medications are administered for the child with a febrile UTI who is unable to tolerate oral intake

and when the UTI is deemed to be severe or when urosepsis is suspected.

The duration of therapy varies according to the severity of the infection and the presence of complicating factors. For first-time, uncomplicated UTIs in adolescent girls, a 3- to 5-day course of therapy is adequate. However, for complicated UTIs, including those associated with a fever, hematuria, or pathogens with multiple antimicrobial resistance, a 7- to 10-day course is required. Longer courses of treatment also should be given to children with vesicoureteral reflux, voiding dysfunction, or other factors that reduce their resistance to bacteriuria.

The following medications are commonly prescribed for the treatment of UTI:

- *Trimethoprim-sulfamethoxazole (TMP-SMX) (Bactrim)*— The dosage is 7.5 to 8 mg/kg TMP with 37.5 to 40 mg/kg SMX every 12 hours for 3 to 7 days. Side effects include headache, nausea, and vomiting. Additional considerations are that it is available in liquid and tablet forms, is relatively inexpensive, may cause severe allergic reactions, and may cause vaginitis in adolescent girls.
- *Amoxicillin*—The dosage for a child weighing 6 kg is 25 to 50 mg every 8 hours for 3 to 7 days. For a child weighing 6 to 8 kg, the dosage is 50 to 100 mg every 8 hours for 3 to 7 days. For a child weighing 8 to 20 kg, the dosage is 6.7 to 13.3 mg/kg every 8 hours for 3 to 7 days. Side effects include rash, nausea, vomiting, and diarrhea. Additional considerations are that it is available in liquid and capsule forms, is inexpensive, and may cause vaginitis in adolescent girls.
- *Nitrofurantoin (Macrodantin)*—This drug may be given to children greater than 1 month of age. The regular dosage is 5 to 7 mg/kg per day in four divided doses every 6 hours, or 1 capsule of Macrobid every 12 hours for 3 days if needed for pain. Side effects include nausea, vomiting, diarrhea, dizziness, and headache. Additional considerations are that it is moderately expensive and not available in liquid form (but capsule may be opened and powder mixed in a small amount of food for administration). The medicine should be given with milk or food to prevent nausea or vomiting. It may intensify peripheral neuropathies with long-term administration; transient pneumonitis-like syndrome may occur; and this medication is not first choice for persons with compromised pulmonary function.
- *Cephalexin (Keflex)*—This drug is not given to children less than 1 month of age. The regular dosage is 50 to 100 mg/kg per day in four doses for 3 to 7 days. Side effects include nausea, vomiting, headache, weakness, fever, chills, and a rare occurrence of pseudomembranous colitis. Additional considerations are that it is relatively inexpensive and requires frequent administration. Children with sensitivity to penicillins may have increased risk for hypersensitivity to cephalexin.
- *Ciprofloxacin (Cipro)*—The dosage is 250 to 500 mg by mouth every 12 hours. Side effects include headache, fatigue, dizziness, diarrhea, photosensitivity, and nephrotoxicity (rare). Additional considerations are that it is relatively expensive, frequently effective against *Pseudomonas aeruginosa,* affects collagen deposition, and should not be administered to children under 16 years of age. (Consult a physician or pharmacist for advice concerning administration in adolescents.)

In addition to antimicrobials, antipyretics may be administered for fever. Acetaminophen is commonly preferred as an antipyretic, since aspirin has been associated with Reye syndrome when administered to treat viral influenza.

Urinary analgesics may be given to relieve the discomfort associated with UTI. Phenazopyridine is administered at 12 mg/kg per day every 6 hours. The medication provides an analgesic and anesthetic effect on the bladder by means of unclear mechanisms. Possible side effects of phenazopyridine include thrombocytopenia, agranulocytosis (uncommon), nausea or vomiting, and diarrhea. Phenazopyridine is available only in a tablet form; it causes the urine to assume a deep orange or reddish yellow appearance, and the urine may stain clothing. The medication is typically administered over a 2- to 3-day period until the antimicrobial has a chance to alleviate the discomfort of UTI by eradicating the majority of urinary tract pathogens.

Combination agents are available to manage UTI-related pain. Typically they contain atropine or another anticholinergic, methylene blue, phenyl salicylate, or benzoic acid. Refer to a standard drug reference for specific dosages. These medications are designed to provide urinary analgesia. Potential adverse effects include anticholinergic actions such as dry mouth, blurred vision, and heat intolerance and analgesic actions such as hematuria and bloody stools. Examples of combination agents include Atrosept, Dolsed, Hexalol, Uridon, Urised, Uriseptic, Uritab, and Uro-Ves.

Counseling and prevention. See Urethritis.

Follow-up

- Repeat the urine culture if there is no improvement in 72 hours or the patient remains symptomatic.
- Perform urinalysis at every visit or every 3 to 6 months for 2 years.

Consultations and referrals. See the Alert box.

Urethritis

Treatments and medications. Gonococcal urethritis is managed according to guidelines promulgated by the Centers for Disease Control and Prevention (CDC). Typically, 75,000 to 100,000 U of aqueous procaine penicillin G per kg of body weight is administered four times a day by intramuscular injection. Alternatives for treatment include amoxicillin 50 mg/kg orally divided four times a day for 7 to 10 days. Children over 8 years of age who are allergic to penicillin may be given tetracycline 25 mg/kg as an initial oral dose, followed by 40 to 60 mg/kg divided three or four times a day for 7 days. Among younger children, ceftriaxone 125 mg in a one-time intramuscular dose may be given. The practitioner should refer to CDC guidelines for the most current information concerning the management of gonococcal urethritis. Nongonococcal urethritis is managed by a 10- to 14-day oral course of tetracycline, erythromycin, or sulfonamide. When *Trichomonas vaginalis* is suspected, metronidazole is prescribed.

GU trauma is managed by referral to a pediatric urologist. Voiding dysfunction associated with painful urination also may be managed by referral to a physician. Refer to Diurnal Incontinence and Altered Patterns of Urine Elimination in this chapter for a description of the management of voiding dysfunction in children.

Counseling and prevention

- Discuss proper cleaning and wiping of the perineum with the parents and child, if age-appropriate. Stress need to use a front-to-back method to avoid fecal contamination of the urethral orifice. If the child is male, teach proper cleaning of the penis with special emphasis on retraction and replacement of foreskin on an uncircumcised boy.

- Caution parents regarding use of urethral irritants (e.g., bubble bath). Encourage the child to maintain an adequate fluid intake. If attempting to toilet train, advise parents to postpone training until infection is resolved.
- Educate parents regarding proper administration of any prescribed medication. Caution parents to keep medications out of the reach of children. Advise parents to notify practitioner if symptoms of UTI persist after 72 hours, if side effects of medications are noted, or if symptoms worsen.
- Educate the sexually active adolescent with gonococcal urethritis about safer sex practices, including the use of a condom barrier to protect against STDs (see also Vulvovaginal Symptoms, Penile Discharge, and Genital Lesions in Chapter 40).

Follow-up. A return visit is indicated if symptoms of UTI are not completely resolved or if side effects of medication occur. A follow-up appointment should be scheduled when urinary incontinence or related voiding dysfunction is not resolved, despite treatment of the UTI. A repeat urinalysis is obtained, and a urine culture is repeated if indicated. If these test results are negative, an evaluation of voiding dysfunction is begun. If vesicoureteral reflux or structural abnormality of the urinary system is discovered, the child is evaluated by a pediatric urologist and receives follow-up care from both the urologist and the PCP. A follow-up urethral culture is obtained after treatment of gonococcal or nongonococcal urethritis. This follow-up is particularly important when one is employing empiric treatment of a nonspecific urethral infection.

Consultations and referrals. See the Alert box.

Protein in the Urine (Proteinuria)

Alert

Consult with or refer to a physician for the following:
- Persistent, asymptomatic proteinuria
- Creatinine-to-protein ratio in the nephrotic range (greater than 1.0)
- Evidence of compromised renal function (e.g., hypertension, peripheral edema, altered growth patterns)
- History of febrile urinary infections with vesicoureteral reflux
- Systemic disease (e.g., diabetes mellitus, hepatitis B)
- Immunosuppressive condition (e.g., acquired immune deficiency syndrome [AIDS])

Etiology

Proteinuria can signal the presence of significant underlying renal disease, or it can be a benign response to stress or a prolonged time in the upright position. Positional or stress proteinuria may be transient, recurrent, or fixed. Nonetheless, the protein-to-creatinine ratio remains low, and kidney function remains unaffected. Stress-induced proteinuria occurs after vigorous exercise. Positional proteinuria occurs as an exaggerated response to an upright position. The mechanisms that cause positional or stress-induced proteinuria are unknown.

Several renal disorders may produce proteinuria. Reflux nephropathy can lead to proteinuria. (In this case significant cortical damage has occurred, and evidence of compromised renal function [including significant hypertension] should be sought.) Acute tubulointerstitial nephritis can produce nephrotic-range proteinuria. Tubulointerstitial nephritis is caused by infection, a drug reaction (to antimicrobials, diuretics, or nonsteroidal antiinflammatory drugs [NSAIDS]), or the inflammation produced by sarcoidosis. Primary renal disease also may produce proteinuria. Nephrotic syndrome, membranous glomerulopathy, congenital nephrotic syndrome, and intrinsic acute renal failure cause significant proteinuria.

Incidence

- Proteinuria is found in approximately 11% of randomly screened school-age children and is persistent in 2.5%.
- Orthostatic proteinuria usually occurs in children over 8 years of age.

Risk Factors

- Recent physical stress (e.g., fever, acute illness, vigorous physical exertion)
- History of renal disease

Differential Diagnosis

No symptoms are directly attributable to the presence of protein in the urine though many of the underlying causes of proteinuria result in various symptoms. Proteinuria is typically detected on a routine dipstick analysis of the urine. Proteinuria is clinically categorized according to its frequency of presentation and by its underlying cause (Table 42-8).

Transient orthostatic proteinuria occurs after intense physical exertion, an acute illness, or a fever. In a small portion of children, proteinuria is found to be present when a urine sample is collected later in the day but absent in specimens collected early in the morning. The term "postural proteinuria" has been used to describe this condition.

Stress-induced proteinuria is typically seen in healthy adolescents. Protein is typically detected in the urine for a transient period after physical stress. Vigorous physical exercise, an acute illness, or a febrile episode is a common precipitating factor. Proteinuria resolves spontaneously without intervention.

In contrast to the orthostatic and stress-induced types, *nephrotic-range persistent,* or *fixed, proteinuria* is detectable on urinalysis, regardless of the time of day or the presence of recent physical stress. In contrast to orthostatic or stress-induced proteinuria, the ratio of protein to creatinine in the urine is greater than 2.0. Persistent proteinuria is distinguished from orthostatic or transient proteinuria because it may represent a serious underlying renal disorder. Urinalysis typically reveals additional signs of renal disease, including hematuria, RBC casts, WBC casts, or granular casts. Compromised renal function with peripheral edema, altered growth patterns, and hypertension may coexist with proteinuria. The child with nephrotic-level proteinuria should be referred to the physician promptly.

Management

Treatments and medications

- When stress-induced proteinuria is suspected, urinalysis is repeated to determine persistence of the findings. If proteinuria is absent from subsequent urinalysis and there are no other findings suggestive of underlying renal disease, no further evaluation or management is indicated.
- When proteinuria below the nephrotic range is found on urinalysis specimens obtained later during the day but

Table 42-8 Differential Diagnosis: Protein in the Urine

CRITERIA	POSTURAL PROTEINURIA	STRESS-INDUCED PROTEINURIA	NEPHROTIC-RANGE PROTEINURIA*
ICD-9 code	593.6	593.6	791.0
Subjective Data			
Associated symptoms	None	None	Edema; appears swollen to parents; possible fever, oliguria, abdominal pain, and respiratory difficulty (shortness of breath)
Onset of symptoms	Typically older than 8 years of age	Usually in adolescents	Any age
Relevant history	Negative for recent physical stress	Recent acute illness, febrile illness, vigorous physical exertion	Possible recent infection (usually upper respiratory tract); recurrent UTIs; systemic disease (e.g., systemic lupus erythematosus); chronic disease such as hepatitis B or diabetes mellitus
Objective Data			
Physical examination	Normal	Normal	Findings may include fever; peripheral and central edema (periorbital edema); hypertension or hypotension; dullness to percussion at lung bases (large pleural effusions); ascites; signs of infection (e.g., pneumonia, peritonitis, otitis media, skin rashes)
Laboratory data			
Protein-to-creatinine ratio (measured in mg)	> 0.3 but < 2.0	> 0.3 but < 2.0	> 2.0
Microscopic urinalysis	Negative	Negative	Hyaline casts, RBC and WBC casts, and granular casts

*Refer to a pediatric nephrologist.

with first specimens being free of protein and there are no additional signs of underlying renal disease, no further evaluation is indicated.

- When asymptomatic proteinuria persists or when the creatinine-to-protein ratio is in the nephrotic range, prompt referral to a pediatric urologist or pediatric nephrologist is indicated.

Counseling and prevention

- Emphasize the importance of follow-up observation for the child who has persistent or nephrotic-range proteinuria. Explain that a lack of symptoms may not necessarily indicate absence of a treatable but significant underlying renal disorder.
- Explain the cause of transient, stress-induced proteinuria or orthostatic proteinuria, and reassure the child and family that the condition does not represent a serious underlying condition.

Follow-up. Obtain subsequent urinalysis for protein in the child with a history of proteinuria. Evaluate growth patterns, check for peripheral edema, and measure blood pressure and serum creatinine and blood urea nitrogen levels in the child with a history of proteinuria and significant underlying renal disease.

Consultations and referrals. Refer to a physician when persistent, nephrotic-range proteinuria is detected, when proteinuria below the nephrotic range persists without explanation, or when there is evidence of progressive deterioration of renal function.

Resources

Websites

Keep Kids Healthy (www.keepkidshealthy.com/welcome/conditions/hematuria.html)

National Institute of Diabetes and Digestive and Kidney Diseases (www.niddk.nih.gov)

National Kidney Foundation (www.kidney.org/patients/bedwet.cfm)

Your Family Doctor (familydoctor.org/handouts/329.html)

Bibliography

Abrams, P., Khoury S., & Wein, A. (Eds.). (1999). *Incontinence: 1st International Consultation on Incontinence.* Plymbridge, UK: Plymouth.

Baird, P.A. & McDonald, E.C. (1981). An epidemiologic study of congenital malformations of the anterior wall in more than half a million consecutive live births. *American Journal of Human Genetics, 33,* 470.

Bauer, S.B. (1992). Neurogenic vesical dysfunction in children. In Walsh, P.C., Retick, A.B., Stamey, T.A., et al. (Eds.). *Campbell's urology* (6th ed.). Philadelphia: W.B. Saunders.

Bauer, S.B., Retik, A.B., Colodny, A.H., et al. (1980). Symposium on pediatric urology: The unstable bladder of childhood. *Urologic Clinics of North America, 7*(2), 321-336.

Bobson, W.L. & Leung, A.K. (2000). Secondary nocturnal enuresis. *Clinical Pediatrics, 39*(7).

Burstein, J.D. & Furlit, C.F. (1985). Anterior urethra. In Kelalis, P.P., King, L.R., & Belman, A.B. (Eds.). *Clinical pediatric urology* (2nd ed.). Philadelphia: W.B. Saunders.

De Paepe, H., et al. (2000). Pelvic-floor therapy and toilet training in young children with dysfunctional voiding and obstipation. *BJU Inernational, 85*(7), 889-893.

Diven, S.C., et al. (2000). A practical primary care approach to hematuria in children. *Pediatric Nephrology, 14*(1):65-72.

Escribano, J., et al. (1999). Symptomatology and development of urolithiasis in children with frequency-dysuria syndrome associated with hypercalciuria. *CMJ, 40,* 80-84.

Fischbach, F.T. (2000). *A manual of laboratory and diagnostic tests.* (6th ed.). Philadelphia: J.B. Lippincott.

Gearhart, J.P. (1999). Bladder exstrophy: Staged reconstruction. *Current Opinion in Urology, 9*(6), 499-506.

Gillenwater, J.Y., Grayhack, J.T., Howards, S.S., et al. (Eds.). (1996). *Adult and pediatric urology* (3rd ed.). St Louis: Mosby.

Glazener C.M. & Evans, J.H. (2000). *Desmopressin for nocturnal enuresis in children.* Cochrane Database of Systematic Reviews.

Goessl, C., et al. (2000). Efficacy and tolerability of tolterodine in children with detrusor hyperreflexia. *Urology, 55*(3), 414-418.

Gray, M. (1996). Atraumatic urethral catheterization in children. *Pediatric Nursing, 22*(4), 306-311.

Gray, M. (1993a). Nursing assessment and diagnosis of urinary function. In Broadwell, D.B, Parrish, R.S., & Saunders, R.C. (Eds.). *Child health nursing.* Philadelphia: J.B. Lippincott.

Gray, M. (1993b). *Sphincter re-education for pediatric voiding dysfunction complicated by dyssynergia* (Continence for All Conference: A Global Perspective). London: Association for Continence Advice.

Hendren, W.H. (1992). Cloacal malformations. In Walsh, P. C., Retick, A. B., Stamey, T.A., et al. (Eds.). *Campbell's urology* (6th ed.). Philadelphia: W.B. Saunders.

Hinman, F. (1986). Non-neurogenic neurogenic bladder (the Hinman syndrome): 15 years later, *The Journal of Urology, 136*(10), 769-777.

Kaplan, G.W. & Brock, W.A. (1982). Idiopathic urethrorrhagia in boys. *Journal of Urology, 128,* 1001-1003.

Kelalis, P.P., King, L.R., & Belman, A.B. (Eds.). (1992). *Clinical pediatric urology* (3rd ed.). Philadelphia: W.B. Saunders.

Klein, N.J. (2001). Management of primary nocturnal enuresis. *Urologic Nursing, 21*(2), 71-82.

Lancaster, P.A.L. (1987). Epidemiology of bladder exstrophy: A communication from the International Clearinghouses for Birth Defects monitoring system. *Teratology, 36,* 221.

Leung, A.K. & Robson, W.L. (2000). Evaluating the child with proteinuria. *Journal of the Royal Society of Health, 120*(1), 16-22.

Loening-Baucke, V. (1998). Toilet tales: Stool toileting refusal, encopresis, and fecal incontinence. *Journal of Wound, Ostomy, & Continence Nursing, 25*(6), 304-313.

Loghman-Adham M. (1998). Evaluating proteinuria in children. *American Family Physician.* Available online at www.aafp.org/afp/981001ap/loghman.html.

Mattsson, S. (1994). Urinary incontinence and nocturia in health schoolchildren. *Acta Pediatrica, 83*(9), 950-954.

Meorman, P., Fryns, J., Goddeeris, P., et al. Pathogenesis of the prune belly syndrome: A functional urethral obstruction caused by prostatic hypoplasia. *Pediatrics, 73,* 470, 1984.

Monda, J.M. & Hussman, D.A. (1995). Primary nocturnal enuresis: A comparison among observation, imipramine, desmopressin acetate and bed-wetting alarm systems. *Journal of Urology, 154,* 745-748.

Nishi, M., Miyake, H., Takeda, T., et al. (1987). Mass screening for neuroblastoma in Sapporo City, Japan. *American Journal of Pediatric Hematology and Oncology, 14,* 327-331.

Pagon, R.A., Smith, D.W., & Shepard, T.H. (1979). Urethral obstruction malformation complex: A cause of abdominal muscle deficiency and the "prune belly." *Journal of Pediatrics, 94,* 900.

Ritchey, M.L. & Andrassy, R.J. (1996). Pediatric urologic oncology. In Gillenwater, J.Y. (Ed.). *Adult and pediatric oncology.* St. Louis: Mosby.

Roberts, J.A. (1990). Is routine circumcision indicated in the newborn? An affirmative view. *The Journal of Family Practice, 31*(2), 185-196.

Rogers, J. (1991). Pass the cranberry juice. *Nursing Times, 87*(48), 36-37.

Sengler, J. & Minnaire, P. (1995). Epidemiology and psychosocial consequences of urinary incontinence. *Revue de Praticien, 45*(3), 281-285.

Shapiro, E., Lepor, H., & Jeffs, R.D. (1984). The inheritance of classical bladder exstrophy. *Journal of Urology, 132,* 308.

Shaw, K.N. & Gorelick, M.H. (1999). Urinary tract infection in the pediatric patient. *Pediatric Clinics of North America, 46*(6), 11-24.

Thompson, R.S. (1990). Routine circumcision in the newborn: An opposing view. *The Journal of Family Practice, 31*(2), 189-196.

Tobias, N.E. (2000). Management of nocturnal enuresis. *Nursing Clinics of North America, 35*(1), 37-60.

Verco, P.W., Khor, B.H., Barbary, J., et al. (1986). Ectopic vesicae in utero. *Australasian Radiology, 30,* 117-120.

Wein, A.J., Malloy, T.R., Shofer, F., et al. (1980). The effects of bethanechol chloride on urodynamic parameters in normal women and in women with significant residual urine volumes. *Journal of Urology, 124,* 397-399.

Wilson, D. (1995). Assessing and managing the febrile child. *Nurse Practitioner, 20*(11), 59-60, 68-74.

Woodard, J.R. & Gosalbez, R. (1992). Neonatal and perinatal emergencies. In Walsh, P.C., Retick, A.B., Stamey, T.A., et al. (Eds.). *Campbell's urology* (6th ed.). Philadelphia: W.B. Saunders.

Woodard, J.R. & Parrott, T.S. (1976). Urologic surgery in the neonate. *Journal of Urology, 116,* 506.

Chapter 43 *Nonspecific Complaints or Problems*

Allergies, p. 694
Failure to Thrive, p. 699
Fever, p. 704
Irritability, p. 710
Lymphadenopathy, p. 714
Obesity, p. 718

Allergies

LINDA GILMAN

Alert

Consult with or refer to an allergist or physician for the following:

- Signs and symptoms of anaphylaxis, including lightheadedness or syncope, flushing or pallor, paresthesias, generalized pruritus, urticaria, vomiting and diarrhea, palpitations, tachycardia, pulmonary edema, bronchial asthma (severe), and vascular collapse
- Signs and symptoms of angioedema, characterized by swelling of the tongue, pharynx, larynx, trachea, joints, hands, feet, and lips
- Systemic symptoms
- Symptoms unresponsive to appropriate treatment
- Perennial symptoms
- Chronic infections

Etiology

Allergic reactions are caused by a hypersensitivity of the body's immune system to an allergen, resulting in tissue inflammation. If there is a genetic predisposition to atopy and the child is exposed to an allergen, antigen-specific immunoglobulin E (IgE) molecules are produced. These molecules bind to mast cells in the respiratory tract. Once the child becomes sensitized in this manner, the same antigen will cause an immediate type 1 hypersensitivity reaction with release of mast cell mediators such as histamine, prostaglandin, and leukotrienes, as well as the synthesis of cell-interactive compounds called *cytokines.* Gell and Coombs (1968) classify four different types of allergic reactions based on the physiologic processes in which they occur.

Type I reactions are atopic, or hypersensitivity, reactions. These are IgE-mediated and encompass anaphylaxis, allergic rhinitis, urticaria, and allergic asthma. Type I reactions can be classified as immediate, typically occurring within 30 minutes of antigen exposure, or late onset, occurring within 2 to 12 hours. Immediate hypersensitivity reactions are caused by the release of histamines from a mast cell, or basophil, to which two specific IgE molecules have attached, when exposed to an antigen. The release of histamine causes an immediate inflammatory process. The delayed or late-onset reaction is mediated by leukotrienes, primarily causing infiltration of tissues with neutrophils, eosinophils, and fibrin. A later phase releases macrophages and fibro-

blasts into surrounding tissues, causing cellular destruction. Aspirin and nonsteroidal antiinflammatory drugs (NSAIDs) do not involve the IgE antibody. These drugs use the prostaglandin pathway. When urticaria and angioedema do occur as a result of the sensitivity of aspirin or NSAIDs, it is usually seen with chronic urticaria and in older patients.

Type II reactions are caused by the activation of the complement system, particularly the protein fragments C3a and C5a. When activated by antigens, they trigger the release of mediators from mast cells and basophils, causing cell damage and destruction (e.g., Rh and ABO hemolytic disease of the newborn).

Type III reactions are antigen-antibody reactions affecting the vascular endothelium and brought about by direct stimulation of mast cells and basophils by various foreign agents (e.g., serum sickness).

Type IV reactions involve T-cell–mediated hypersensitivity of a delayed type (e.g., contact dermatitis).

Incidence

- Allergies affect about 20% of the total U.S. population.
- Allergic rhinitis is the most common of all allergic disorders, affecting about 15% of the pediatric population. It is more common in boys.
- Asthma occurs in 10% of children and is the most common chronic illness in childhood.
- Food allergy accounts for 95% of food sensitivity problems seen in clinical settings. Less than 5% of these are true allergic disorders.
- About 10% of children have atopic dermatitis (eczema), and the prevalence has been increasing over the past few decades.
- Allergies have a strong genetic predisposition. A high incidence of allergies occurs within family members, including the triad of eczema, asthma, and allergic rhinitis.
- Climate affects allergies. There is an increased incidence of mold-related reactions in warm, moist environments all year round; dust allergies in dry, hot areas; and pollen allergies in areas of trees and weeds (especially ragweed and grasses).
- Housing affects allergies. Cockroach allergies are prevalent in inner city dwellings, and mold allergies are common in basement apartments. Dust mite and animal dander allergies are more common but less dramatic than sensitivity reactions. Many people are sensitive to various chemicals that are used within the home and chemicals from local industry.
- Penicillin is the most common cause of anaphylaxis, with one reaction per 10,000 administrations.

Risk Factors

- Family or child history of anaphylaxis, allergies, eczema, asthma, or urticaria

- Previous history of food intolerance (e.g., cow's milk sensitivity)
- Residing in geographic areas with high levels of air pollution or naturally occurring respiratory irritants (e.g., pollen, mold spores)
- Exposure to allergens in the home (e.g., dust, dust mites, pet danders, tobacco smoke, household chemicals, feather bedding, cockroaches, formaldehyde [and formalin], other agents used in construction materials)

Differential Diagnosis

Any child who is suspected of having an allergic disease or complains of allergic symptoms requires a comprehensive history and physical examination.

Anaphylaxis is a pediatric emergency (see Airway Obstruction in Chapter 48). Acute respiratory distress is caused by a reexposure to a sensitizing antigen in a hypersensitive person. The reaction can range from mild distress to severe, life-threatening anaphylaxis with respiratory distress and cardiovascular collapse. Common causes of anaphylaxis include penicillin (especially injected), foods (commonly eggs, fish, milk, peanuts, shellfish, soybeans, and tree nuts), foreign serum, inhaled pollen, insect stings (especially by bees, hornets, and wasps), diagnostic agents (iodine), and local anesthetics.

Allergic rhinitis and *conjunctivitis* combined make a set of symptoms including clear rhinorrhea, nasal congestion, pruritus, and sneezing (often paroxysmal). Ocular symptoms such as watery, itchy eyes frequently accompany nasal symptoms and a grainy appearance to the conjunctivae. A stringy, mucoid discharge is often found in the conjunctival sac. Other, associated symptoms include itching of the throat and ears, snoring, sleep disturbance, dry sore throat (especially in the morning), irritability, dry cough (usually exacerbated in the early part of the night), and headache or facial pain with tenderness of sinus areas. Allergic rhinitis and conjunctivitis are IgE-mediated immediate hypersensitive reactions to airborne allergens.

Common causative allergens include dust, mold, pollen, mites, animal danders, and seasonal allergens such as grass and trees in spring and ragweed and mold in late summer and fall.

Food allergies can also produce allergic rhinitis; however, only a small percentage of cases are IgE-mediated and associated with histamine release (causing an immediate reaction). Most cases of rhinitis caused by food allergies are produced by a delayed hypersensitivity, making diagnosis more difficult. Detection is primarily made by history, elimination, and rechallenge. Dairy allergy is frequently associated with chronic nasal congestion. The patient commonly has watery, itchy eyes; injected sclerae; and conjunctivae with cobblestone appearance and mucoid discharge. Bluish purple circles under the eyes ("allergic shiners") and double creases under the lower eyelids (Dennie Morgan folds) are often seen. Sneezing is often paroxysmal, and nasal secretions may be clear or mucoid. Turbinates tend to be pale and edematous. The older child with allergic rhinitis often has a crease across the bridge of the nose ("allergic salute") from chronic rubbing with the palm of the hand and various facial grimaces secondary to intense nasal itching. Tonsils and the posterior area of the pharynx may be erythematous as a result of irritation from postnasal secretions. These secretions are also responsible for the frequent attempt to clear the throat and the dry to mildly wet cough often seen with allergies.

Atopic dermatitis, also known as *eczema,* is a skin response to an ingested substance to which the child has developed IgE antibodies. The pathogenesis of this condition is not clearly understood, nor is the role of the immune defect. Common foods typically involved are milk, legumes (including peanuts and soybeans), wheat, and corn. Citrus and tomatoes can cause flushing and erythema but rarely are associated with a more extensive dermatitis. Direct skin contact with allergens such as dust and animal dander can also produce dermatologic symptoms. Diagnosis is usually not difficult, because atopic dermatitis usually follows a pattern:

- *Acute phase*—An exacerbation involving erythema, vesiculation, edema, and excoriation resulting from intense pruritus
- *Chronic phase*—Involvement of scaling, lichenification, and changes in the pigmentation of the skin

The expression of atopic dermatitis also changes with the life cycle:

- *Infantile phase*—The onset is in the first 6 months of life and involves the scalp, cheeks, forehead, trunk, and extensor surfaces, with sparing of nasolabial folds and diaper area. Lesions are typically crusting and oozing.
- *Childhood phase (4 years of age to puberty)*—This mainly involves the flexor surfaces of extremities, neck, ankles, wrists, and posterior area of thighs. Lesions are dry, papular, and intensely pruritic, and excoriations and infections from scratching are common.
- *Adult phase*—In the chronic form, as with the childhood form, antecubital and popliteal fossae are primarily affected, along with hands, feet, and neck. The skin becomes thickened and lichenified because of repetitive scratching. Although the condition is not clearly understood, the child with atopic dermatitis frequently has double creases under the lower eye lids (Dennie Morgan folds), creases and deep lines on the palms of the hands, and excessive skin dryness (xerosis).

Allergic contact dermatitis becomes evident with erythema and a papular rash that may progress to vesicles, bullae, and a more extensive denuding of the skin. This reaction is caused by a substance contacting the skin. It is intensely pruritic and may be immediate (IgE mediated) or a delayed hypersensitivity reaction of up to 2 weeks (T-cell mediated). Common causative allergens include fur, leather, formaldehyde, neomycin, *Toxicodendron* (formerly *Rhus*) oils (i.e., poison ivy, poison sumac, poison oak), nickel, topical anesthetics, shoe dyes or glue, and latex (especially in children with spina bifida). Photosensitive contact dermatitis requires sun exposure to elicit the allergic response. This is often seen with drugs such as tetracycline, sulfonamides, thiazides, and topical preparations such as coal tar. The diagnosis of photosensitive contact dermatitis is made when the rash develops in sun-exposed areas. Severe contact dermatitis can also involve other areas of the body not in contact with the offending substance (an "id" or "autoeczematous" reaction, as with poison ivy).

Allergic pulmonary disorders often refers to asthma (see Chapter 45). The child with asthma usually has wheezing and acute symptoms of cough and shortness of breath. These children may have a history of other atopic reactions. An allergic cough may be an early manifestation of a bronchospasm. The allergic cough is a persistent, irritating cough in an allergic individual. Upper respiratory tract symptoms, such as clear rhinorrhea, sneezing, and an allergic shiner, may accompany the cough.

Many food reactions termed *food allergies* are caused by factors other than immunologic (toxic or pharmacologic substances in the food or metabolic disorders). However, certain reactions to food and food substances are true food hypersensitivities. These fall into two groups:

- IgE-mediated reactions that produce anaphylaxis, acute angioedema of upper airway, and bronchospasm
- Nonanaphylactoid reactions, which are immunoglobulin G (IgG), immunoglobulin M (IgM), or T-cell mediated (the more common form of reaction)

Common food allergens in children include milk, soybeans, and wheat. Older children tend to be more allergic to fish, shellfish, and nuts. The expression of food allergies can include the following:

- Gastrointestinal (GI) tract disorders related to food hypersensitivity include swelling and pruritus of the oropharynx, nausea, abdominal pain and distension, bleeding, bloating, cramps, vomiting, diarrhea, steatorrhea, weight loss, failure to thrive (FTT), and ulcers.
- Respiratory problems include rhinoconjunctivitis, periocular erythema and pruritus, tearing, nasal congestion, rhinorrhea, sneezing, and wheezing.
- Cutaneous disorders include urticaria, angioedema, atopic dermatitis, and dermatitis herpetiformis (gluten-sensitive enteropathy).
- Systemic disorders include anaphylaxis.

Urticaria, or *hives,* is caused by vasodilatation and edema of the skin as a result of histamine being released from the dermal mast cells. The patient usually has an acute onset of intensely pruritic, erythematous, raised wheals in varying size with pale papular centers. The lesions may coalesce, and the rash blanches on pressure. (See Hives [Urticaria] in Chapter 37.)

Angioedema is an extension of urticaria into the lower dermis of the skin. Hereditary angioedema is a rare condition appearing as angioedema of the upper airway, face, and GI tract and is potentially life threatening.

Management

Anaphylaxis

Treatments and medications. Immediate referral should be made to an emergency facility and physician. Early recognition and prompt intervention are critical to the outcome. Epinephrine 1:1000 (0.01 ml/kg up to 0.3 ml) is the treatment of choice. All children at risk for anaphylaxis should have readily available autoinjectable epinephrine such as EpiPen Jr. (0.15 mg of 1:12000 epinephrine). Children weighing over 20 kg should use Epi Pen (0.3 mg of 1:1000 epinephrine). Give liquid or intramuscular diphenhydramine (1 mg/kg up to 50 mg) in addition to epinephrine. The patient should use an inhaled bron-

chodilator in addition to epinephrine for lower airway involvement. Corticosteroids are also useful for all episodes of significant anaphylaxis, either oral (2 mg/kg up to 60 mg) for mild cases or injectable for severe cases.

Counseling and prevention

- Advise parents of children with anaphylactoid reactions to carry an epinephrine autoinjector kit. Older children should carry their own kits. Instruct family and child in proper use of kit.
- Remind parents of children with drug allergies to alert pharmacists and health practitioners of their child's allergies each time a prescription is written or a vaccine is to be given.
- Instruct children with beesting allergies to avoid scented perfumes and cosmetics during warm months and avoid walking barefooted outdoors.
- Suggest the elimination of wasp and bee nests when possible near the child's home to decrease the incidence of beestings.
- Educate parents of children with shellfish allergies to prohibit diagnostic testing using contrast dyes containing iodine.
- Instruct children at risk for anaphylaxis to wear an identification bracelet such as Medic Alert.
- Remind parents to carefully scrutinize food labels for known allergens and prepare alternative foods when necessary.

Follow-up. Follow-up care is determined by a physician. Children with systemic reactions (e.g., urticaria, urethema, pruritus, angioedema) to insect stings should have skin testing for venom-specific IgE antibodies. Testing can be done as soon as 1 week after the child was stung. A radioallergosorbent test (RAST), which measures serum IgE antibodies, is not advised because of the high incidence of false-negative results.

Consultations and referrals. Provide immediate referral to an emergency facility or physician.

Allergic rhinitis. See Nasal Congestion and Obstruction in Chapter 41.

Treatments and medications. See Tables 43-1 to 43-3. Orally administered antihistamines are effective first-line drugs in the management of mild to moderate allergic symptoms such as rhinitis, sneezing, itchy eyes, and itchy nose. Children should be started on antihistamines just before onset of the allergy season and kept on them until the season is over.

Orally administered antihistamines for management of acute exacerbations have a main side effect of sedation (e.g., over-the-counter [OTC] preparations including brompheniramine

Table 43-1 First-Generation Antihistamines

ANTIHISTAMINE	H₁ BLOCKADE	SEDATION	ANTICHOLINERGIC EFFECTS	DOSE
Ethanolamines (diphenydramine [Benadryl])	+++	++	++	12.5-25 mg every 6-8 hours
Alkylamines (chlorpheniramine [Chlor-Trimeton])	+++	+	++	12 years and older: 4 mg every 4-6 hours
Piperazines (hydroxyzine [Atarax])	+++	++	++	2 mg/kg per day divided every 4-6 hours
Piperadines (Azatadine)	+++	++	++	12 years and older: 1-2 mg twice a day
Ethylenediamine (Tripelennamine)	+++	++	++	5 mg/kg per day in 4-6 divided doses

Data from Sharma, P. (2001). Chronic Allergies. In Green-Hernandez, C., et al. (Eds.). Primary care pediatrics. Philadelphia: J.B. Lippincott.
+ indicates the specificity of the drug's ability to have H₁ blockade, the amount of the drug's sedative effect, and the amount of the drug's anticholinergic effects.

[Dimetapp Allergy], chlorpheniramine [PediaCare Allergy, Chlor-Trimeton], clemastine fumarate [Tavist], diphenhydramine [Benadryl]). For more severe symptoms not controlled by OTC drugs, prescription antihistamines are available (e.g., promethazine hydrochloride [Phenergan], hydroxyzine [Atarax], cyproheptadine [Periactin]).

Nonsedating allergy preparations are currently available for children 12 years of age and older (e.g., loratadine [Claritin], cetirizine [Zyrtec], and fexofenadine [Allegra]).

Sympathomimetics (e.g., pseudoephedrine, phenylpropanolamine) should be used alone or in combination with an antihistamine if nasal congestion is present (e.g., phenylpropanolamine HCL and brompheniramine maleate [Dimetapp], phenylpropanolamine HCL and chlorpheniramine maleate [Triaminic allergy]). For more severe symptoms, preparations are available by prescription (e.g., Rynatan, Phenergan VC).

For management of allergy symptoms associated with coughing, a combination antihistamine, decongestant, and cough suppressant may be used (e.g., dextromethorphan 10 mg, pseudoephedrine HCL 30 mg, brompheniramine maleate 2 mg, and alcohol at 0.95% [Dimetane DX]).

Intranasal, short-term oral corticosteroids for acute exacerbations are potent antiinflammatory agents that decrease the population of inflammatory cells in the nasal mucosa and reduce the level of mediators of the allergen and cytokines. Corticosteroids may be used topically. The lowest dose possible is used to decrease the potency for short-term treatment to avoid systemic effects.

Nasal cromolyn (e.g., cromolyn sodium [Nasalcrom], triamcinolone nasal inhaler [Nasacort]), a mast cell stabilizer, is useful for perennial rhinitis and mild to moderate allergic rhinitis. Nasal cromolyn must be used three or four times per day to be effective. Azelastine (Astelin Nasal Spray) is an alternative for children 12 years of age and older at a dosage of 1.1 mg/day (2 sprays per nostril twice a day).

Nasal decongestant sprays may be effective for short-term use. Limit use to 3 days to avoid dependence resulting from the rebound effect on the nasal mucosa.

Immunotherapy should be considered when symptoms tend to be chronic rather than seasonal, when medical therapy provides suboptimal relief, or when the allergic condition is complicated by recurrent infections such as sinusitis, pharyngitis, and otitis media.

For allergic conjunctivitis, the following preparations may be used either alone or in combinations with the previously mentioned medications: ophthalmic cromolyn sodium (Opticrom); NSAIDs, such as ketorolac-tromethamine ophthalmic (Acular); phenylephrine HCL ophthalmic; and tetrahydrozoline HCL (Visine). Olopatidine HCL (Patanol 0.1 %) ophthalmic solution may be used for a dual-action ocular allergy that inhibits mast cell–mediator release and possesses antihistamine activity. Patanol is indicated for temporary relief of itching of the eyes as a result of allergic response; it is effective for up to 8 hours and should be administered as 2 drops in each effected eye. The individual should not use if wearing contact lenses.

Identifiable household allergens should be removed whenever possible. Air purifiers may be of some value, especially when used in the area where the child sleeps.

Counseling and prevention

- Instruct the parents and child on avoidance of known and suspected allergens.
- Educate on home-setting modifications as follows:

  Control dust particles and dust mites through frequent vacuuming and covering of the mattress.

  Remove from the child's sleeping area carpeting, toys, draperies, and other objects that attract dust.

Table 43-2 First-Generation Antihistamines

ANTIHISTAMINE	H₁ BLOCKADE	SEDATION	ANTICHOLINERGIC EFFECTS	DOSE
Fexofenadine (Allegra)*	+++	−	−	12 years and older: 60 mg twice a day orally
Loratadine (Claritin)	+++	−	−	6 years and older: 5-10 mg/day orally
Cetirizine (Zyrtec)	++++	−	−	2 years and older: 5-10 mg/day orally
Azelastine (Astelin)	+++	+	−	12 years and older: 2 sprays each nostril twice a day as needed

From Sharma, P. (2001). Chronic allergies. In Green-Hernandez, C., et al. (Eds.). Primary care pediatrics. Philadelphia: J.B. Lippincott.
*Application for approval for use in children 3 years of age and older is before the Food and Drug Administration.
+ indicates effects. − indicates no effects.

Table 43-3 Intranasal Corticosteroids

MEDICATION	DOSAGE PER ACTUATION (μg)	FORMULATION	DOSAGE
Beclomethasone (Vanceril, Beconase)	42/84	AQ/MDI	6 years and older: 1-2 sprays in each nostril twice a day
Budesonide (Rhinocort)	32	MDI	6 years and older: 2 sprays in each nostril per day (not for use with nonallergic rhinitis)
Flunisolide (Nasarel)	25	AQ	2 sprays in each nostril per day
Fluticasone (Flonase)	50	AQ	2 sprays in each nostril per day
Mometasone (Nasonex)	50	AQ	2 sprays in each nostril per day
Triamcinolone (Azmacort)	55	AQ/MDI	2 sprays in each nostril per day

From Sharma, P. (2001). Chronic allergies. In Green-Hernandez, C., et al. (Eds.). Primary care pediatrics. Philadelphia: J.B. Lippincott.
AQ, Aqueous; MDI, metered-dose inhaler.

Avoid feather and down bedding.

Use air-purification systems, especially deionizing machines.

Use nonaerosol, non–fragrance-containing cleaners.

Cease tobacco use.

Frequently bathe pets, or remove them if necessary.

Use dehumidifiers for mold allergies, and use light in darkened areas such as closets to reduce mold growth.

- Suggest avoidance of outdoor activities during days of high levels of allergens.
- Discuss with parents the side effects of medications, such as drowsiness with antihistamines and irritability with decongestants.

Follow-up. Follow-up care is based on the following factors:

- Age of the child
- Severity of symptoms
- Frequency of recurrence
- Seasonal versus perennial
- Parents' or child's ability to adhere to treatment

Consultations and referrals

- Refer to an allergist for testing or immunotherapy if symptoms persist, despite treatment, or if there are frequent related infections (e.g., otitis media, tonsillitis, sinusitis).
- Refer to an otolaryngologist if persistent middle-ear effusion, chronic sinusitis, or chronic throat infections are present.
- Refer to a pulmonologist if there is persistent cough or frequent lower respiratory tract infections.

Atopic dermatitis. See also Rash in Chapter 37.

Treatments and medications

- Remove or avoid any identifiable allergen when possible.
- Prescribe antihistamines to provide relief from itching during exacerbations. Hydroxyzine (Atarax) 2 mg/kg per day is preferred, while diphenhydramine (Benadryl) 5 mg/kg per day or cyproheptadine (Periactin) 0.25 mg/kg per day may be used. Alternating antihistamines every 2 weeks can be of benefit in controlling chronic symptoms.
- With topical corticosteroids, use the lowest dose possible for short-term treatment of inflammation to avoid systemic side effects. Apply two or three times a day for 2 weeks. Apply corticosteroids before use of a moisturizer. The form of a topical preparation affects the rate of absorption, therefore affecting potency (i.e., lotions are usually low in potency but creams, ointments, and emollients are high in potency). (See Table 43-1.)
- Possibly prescribe oral corticosteroids for 1 week for acute exacerbations.
- Keep in mind that bathing is controversial among dermatologists. Frequency is based on individual response and may range from daily to two times per week. The patient should lightly pat self dry and coat the skin with moisturizing agents (e.g., Lubriderm, Eucerin). Aquaphor is helpful for areas of thickened, scaly skin. Alpha-Keri bath oil added to bath water helps retain moisture.
- Advise the wearing of cotton, loose-fitting clothes and avoidance of wool and synthetics.
- For soap, advise the use of nondrying cleansing lotions (e.g., Dove) and avoidance of soap entirely for severe cases. Use a nonsoap skin cleanser (e.g., Cetaphil).
- Advise liberal use of moisturizing agents (e.g., Eucerin, Curel, Sensitive Skin, Lubriderm, Aquaphor).
- Advise the use of alpha-hydroxy acid (Lac Hydrin), applied twice daily to retain skin moisture and decrease skin thickness in cases of chronic dermatitis.
- Possibly use psoralen ultraviolet-A range in severe cases.

- For herbal therapy, suggest evening primrose oil (Etamol).
- Possibly prescribe antimicrobial treatment (e.g., cefadroxil monohydrate [Duricef]) for secondary skin infections.

Counseling and prevention

- Advise humidifying the household during winter months.
- Provide supportive care for the parents and child because of the discomfort, disfigurement, and chronicity of this condition.
- Advise expectant mothers who have a strong family history of allergies to eat a varied diet before and during the time of breastfeeding to avoid sensitizing the infant with large quantities of a specific food.
- Promote hypoallergenic homes by educating parents about the most common household offenders and techniques to control them.
- Stress the importance of maintaining skin integrity.
- Instruct on need to lubricate dry skin through daily bathing (controversial) and use of moisturizing cleansing agents (Cetaphil for severe cases). Alpha-Keri bath oil adheres water to the skin. Advise the patient to pat dry and apply a moisturizing lotion (e.g., Eucerin) to slightly damp skin.
- Advise wearing cotton clothing to avoid irritation from wool and synthetics.
- Keep nails clean and short.
- Inspect skin and provide prompt antimicrobial treatment of secondary infections.
- Apply ointments such as Aquaphor Healing Ointment to areas of skin thickening and scaling. Use corticosteroid creams sparingly and only for acute exacerbations.
- Educate parents regarding the proper use of prescribed medications and their potential side effects.
- Instruct parents to seek early detection and treatment of any illness, which tends to exacerbate skin conditions.
- Attempt to determine and avoid the underlying allergen. Any infant with allergic dermatitis should have a trial of a dairy-free diet. Mothers of infants who are breastfed should eliminate dairy products from their diet for a trial period.

Follow-up. Follow-up care is based on the same criteria as for Allergic Rhinitis. Because atopic dermatitis is resistant, a strict follow-up schedule (i.e., every 2 weeks initially) is important to assess response to treatment.

Consultations and referrals

- Refer to a dermatologist for skin conditions not responding to treatment and for frequent or severe secondary bacterial infections.
- Refer to an allergist to determine underlying allergies.

Allergic pulmonary disorders. See Asthma in Chapter 45.

Allergic contact dermatitis

Treatments and medications. If allergic contact dermatitis is localized, use topical corticosteroids (see Table 37-1) to relieve pruritus and inflammation. More extensive reactions may require several days of oral antihistamines. Severe cases can also be treated with oral corticosteroids such as prednisone in a tapering course of 1 to 2 weeks. Milder cases may be managed with OTC creams, baking soda, or colloidal oatmeal baths (e.g., Aveeno).

Counseling and prevention

- Recommend the removal of offending plants from child's environment where possible.
- Teach the parents and child to identify and avoid offending plants (e.g., poison ivy, remembering the phrase "If the leaves are three, let them be").

- Suggest wearing long pants during hiking.
- Instruct that if contact with a suspect plant occurs, the exposed area should be washed immediately with soap and water to decrease the reaction.
- Instruct on prescribed medications and relief measures.
- Advise that the condition is self-limited.
- For other types of allergic contact dermatitis, keep in mind that prevention primarily consists in identifying the irritating substance and future avoidance.

Follow-up. Follow-up care is necessary only for severe cases or if secondary bacterial infection develops from scratching.

Consultations and referrals. Refer to a physician or dermatologist for severe cases and those patients not responding to treatment.

Food allergies

Treatments and medications. Strict avoidance of allergy-causing substances is the only proved treatment for food allergies. Rechallenge timing is based on the age of onset, foods involved, and nature of the allergic reaction. A change of infant formula, first to soybean suspension ("soy milk"; 50% of children allergic to cow's milk are also soybean sensitive) and then to protein hydrolysate formula (e.g., Alimentum, Nutramigen) may be needed (see also Infantile Colic in Chapter 35). Breast-feeding in most cases is best for infants with suspected food hypersensitivity or with a strong family history of allergies. However, in some cases, if allergic symptoms persist in breast-fed infants, mothers must eliminate suspected foods from their diets (e.g., dairy products, peanuts, nuts, eggs).

Oral antihistamines (e.g., diphenhydramine) are the drugs of choice for treatment of mild allergic symptoms from food ingestion. For more severe reactions epinephrine is the drug of choice (see Anaphylaxis).

Counseling and prevention

- Advise introducing in infants new solid foods no sooner than 3 to 5 days apart to assess tolerance.
- Counsel parents that one third of children with food sensitivity lose the immediate reaction response after 1 year of strict food avoidance. (Reactions to peanuts, nuts, and fish tend to be long term.)
- Teach parents (and older children) to read food labels. For example, a child with a milk allergy needs to avoid ingredients containing milk or milk solids, butter, casein, caseinate, whey, lactalbumin, and cheese.
- Advise all caregivers, school personnel, and other contacts of the child's food sensitivity and special diet. Children with severe reactions should wear an identification bracelet such as Medic Alert.
- Provide information and support to parents and child through information sources such as the Food Allergy Network.

Follow-up

- Schedule a return visit in 2 weeks after the institution of a food-restricted diet.
- If symptoms improve, continue the restriction and discuss a plan for rechallenge with the parents.

Consultations and referrals

- Refer to an allergist if symptoms persist despite an elimination diet.
- Refer to a dermatologist if dermatologic symptoms persist after institution of an elimination diet.
- Refer to a gastroenterologist if GI tract symptoms persist, for confirmation of celiac disease or other malabsorption diseases, or for protracted vomiting or diarrhea.

Urticaria. See Hives (Urticaria) in Chapter 37.

Failure to Thrive

KATHLEEN KENNEY

Alert

Consult with or refer to a physician for the following:
- Infants who appear septic or lethargic
- Signs and symptoms of shock or impending shock
- Infants or children who continue to have unexplained weight loss despite appropriate treatment
- Suspected cardiac, renal, pulmonary, or other life-threatening organic causes for poor weight gain
- Signs or symptoms of pyloric stenosis: projectile vomiting; palpable, sausage-shaped mass; no weight gain or minimal weight gain
- Signs or symptoms of intussusception (e.g., "currant jelly" stools, lethargy, poor sign turgor)
- Signs or symptoms of child abuse

Etiology

FTT, or growth deficiency, is described as inadequate weight gain based on the standard growth charts of the National Centers for Health Statistics (NCHS). FTT is most commonly divided into two categories: organic and nonorganic. Organic causes of FTT include disease processes and congenital or genetic disorders (e.g., cardiac, metabolic, central nervous system [CNS], pulmonary, GI tract, immunologic disorders) that result in inhibition or alteration of enzyme or hormone secretion, digestion, absorption, or transport of nutrients to tissues.

Nonorganic FTT refers to psychosocial causes of growth failure that may come from many sources within the child's environment. Nonorganic FTT can be subdivided into the following subcategories:
- Accidental FTT includes children who receive inadequate nutrition as a result of a mistake or lack of understanding (e.g., improper preparation of formula).
- Neglectful FTT results from parents who are overwhelmed with psychologic issues, financial burdens, or other psychosocial issues.
- Deliberate FTT is a result of child abuse and deliberate food withholding.

Family dysfunction, child abuse, financial burdens, and the emotional status of parents are only a few of the psychosocial issues that may cause an infant or child to fall below the appropriate growth curve.

Incidence

- Nonorganic FTT occurs in approximately 50% of the cases of FTT. Organic causes encompass about 25% of the children with FTT. The remaining 25% of cases are a result of combined causes (organic and nonorganic).
- Diagnosis is usually made during infancy and early childhood but may occur throughout childhood.
- Children from economically deprived areas are more likely than those from affluent areas to have nonorganic FTT.
- Children with nonorganic FTT have a higher incidence of poor adaptive family relationships and family dysfunction.
- Overall the incidence of nonorganic FTT is greater than that of organic FTT.
- Leading causes of organic FTT are cardiac, neurologic, and GI disorders, as well as cystic fibrosis.

Risk Factors

Nonorganic failure to thrive
- Inadequate caloric intake
- Low socioeconomic status
- Family dysfunction
- Stress
- Child abuse or neglect
- Lack of knowledge or teaching
- Insufficient lactation
- Cultural beliefs
- Psychosocial issues
- Emotional deprivation and depression
- Food withholding
- Maternal-infant dysfunction
- Maternal drug use
- Mechanical problems (e.g., cleft palate)
- Maternal or paternal psychiatric disorder
- Colic
- "Difficult feeder"
- Inexperienced or impatient child caregiver
- Incorrect preparation of formula
- Normal variant (e.g., "slightness")

Organic failure to thrive
- Acute infection or sepsis
- Chronic disorders (e.g., CNS, pulmonary, cardiac, metabolic, endocrine, GI tract disorders)
- Malignancy
- Chronic infection (e.g., tuberculosis [TB], acquired immune deficiency syndrome [AIDS])
- Genetic or chromosomal disorders
- Prematurity
- Lead poisoning

Differential Diagnosis

FTT is a sign, not a specific diagnosis. It is a term that is used to identify children whose weight and growth pattern consistently falls below the 3rd to 5th percentiles for age or whose weight drops below significant percentiles. FTT generally refers to inadequate weight gain or weight loss because this may be the only sign in early FTT. The causes of FTT are either insufficient provision of nutrients or inability to retain sufficient nutrients to grow. After 18 to 24 months of age, changes in growth trajectories are rarely physiologic in nature. Weight changes are the most common initial findings in children with FTT. Head circumference and height and length ratios tend to be altered with long-standing FTT, and most children are diagnosed before this stage. Early intervention in children with FTT is essential because altered neurologic development is possible from prolonged nutritional deficiency. Plotting the height, weight, and head circumference on the age-appropriate growth chart allows for simple observation of the child's growth pattern. Children with a gradual decline (i.e., they may not yet be below the 5th percentile but have a constant decline) or those who fall below the 5th percentile over a consistent period should be evaluated for FTT. Evaluation of any child with symptoms of FTT or poor weight gain should include assessing the following four dimensions of the child and family: medical, nutritional, developmental or behavioral, and psychosocial. Any child with signs of pathologic causes for FTT should be referred to the appropriate physician or specialist for evaluation and management with consultation. Once pathologic causes have been ruled out, the practitioner should continue with the appropriate management of nonorganic FTT. Certain children may always be below the 5th percentile yet be paralleling their "normal" curve. These children may not have FTT but may have short stature, prematurity, or endocrine disorders.

Nonorganic FTT is the most common cause of inadequate weight gain. It results from psychologic, cultural, or financial issues and has no pathophysiologic cause. Most of the diagnostic clues become evident with an in-depth history and physical examination.

Organic FTT is poor, insufficient weight gain or weight loss as a result of ongoing physiologic conditions such as CNS abnormalities, congenital heart defects, pulmonary disorders, GI tract disorders (e.g., pyloric stenosis, intussusception, malabsorption), endocrine disorders, mechanical difficulties (e.g., cleft lip or palate), or genetic disorders. Symptoms related to the specific organic cause often declare themselves during the assessment process. Laboratory tests and other testing used to diagnose organic FTT are included in Table 43-4. Children with suspected organic FTT should be referred to a physician.

The practitioner must keep in mind that there may be overlapping of the causes and origins of FTT.

Management

Nonorganic failure to thrive

Treatments and medications

Nutritional management

- Determine the average weight for the child. Using an appropriate growth chart, note the weight at the 50th percentile for a child of the same age. This is the goal weight. Using this goal weight, determine the amount of calories required in a 24-hour period to maintain proper growth and development by using Table 43-5.
- Develop with the parents a plan to achieve appropriate caloric intake within 1 week. To increase caloric intake per oz of formula, use 2 fewer oz of water when mixing the formula. By means of this method of formula preparation, the child receives 24 calories per oz (instead of 20 calories per oz). Parents may also purchase formula of higher caloric content.
- If the child is over 4 months of age, add cereal to the diet. Review preparation with the parents and teach basic feeding techniques.

Hospitalization

- Hospitalization depends on an assessment of the home environment, safety, and parents' level of concern for the child's welfare.
- Hospitalization in the presence of psychologic issues may increase the child's anxiety level, promote separation issues, and ultimately result in behavior such as withdrawal, anorexia, or impaired parent-child relationships.
- Children with accidental FTT often do not require hospitalization and can be easily managed at home.
- Neglectful FTT does not automatically require hospitalization of the child. If the home environment is considered safe and parental interest is present, the child may be managed at home.
- Foster care placement is sometimes necessary.
- Hospitalization is required if there is child abuse or endangerment, continued weight loss even with reporting of adequate calories, or suspicion of underlying organic disease.

Counseling and prevention

- Encourage parents to attend parenting classes (and provide them with referrals).
- Help parents in identifying stressful issues or concerns.
- Reassure parents regarding the child's ability to overcome stresses and achieve adequate nutrition.

Table 43-4 Differential Diagnosis: Organic and Nonorganic Failure to Thrive

CRITERIA	NONORGANIC	ORGANIC*
ICD-9 code	783.41	783.41
Subjective Data		
Age of onset	Usually in infancy but can be diagnosed throughout childhood	Any age
Prenatal history	May be history of no prenatal care, maternal drug use or psychiatric disorder, unwanted pregnancy, or unplanned pregnancy	May be history of genetic defect detected in utero, maternal illness or infection before delivery, alcohol or drug use, HIV
Birth history	May have positive toxicology screen, history of prematurity	May be history of abnormalities detected in utero, birth trauma, premature birth, meconium-stained amniotic fluid
Developmental history	May be normal but with prolonged nutritional deprivations; many have some developmental delays	May see developmental delays with many CNS disorders
Immunizations	May not be up to date on immunizations because of poor parental compliance	May not be up to date, resulting in infectious process (e.g. measles)
Family history	Possible history of family dysfunction, financial burdens, social problems, abuse, psychiatric disorders, or cultural issues	Possible genetic or congenital disorders
Social history	New parents may verbalize lack of experience or knowledge of appropriate feeding patterns or formula preparation	Parental anxieties related to an ongoing organic process can result in parents decreasing feeds or fear of feeding
	Parental psychiatric disorders may result in improper or lack of feeding or neglectful behavior	Mechanical problems such as "cleft palate" may result in increased parental anxiety pertaining to feeds or avoidance of feeding
	Conflict between parents or grandparents concerning child care and nutrition	
	Financial concerns or issues may not allow provision of food to infant or child	
	Parents may be distracted by other concerns (e.g., financial, illness, death in family, sibling needs)	
Nutritional history	Parents report that infant has disinterest in feeding, withdrawn behavior, poor concentration during feeds, poor suck	Parental complaints of poor or inappropriate suck, tachypnea with feeds, diaphoresis with feeds, mechanical difficulty (e.g., cleft palate), lethargy with feeds, colicky behavior
	Parents describe improper preparation of formula, use of supplementary juices or water for formula	Possible history of pica may lead to lead poisoning
Associated symptoms		
Vomiting	May be present, but not enough to cause weight loss	May be new onset: Infectious/viral illness
		May have projectile or nonprojectile: Pyloric stenosis vs. reflux
		Gagging or poor gag reflex: CNS disorder
Diarrhea	Not causative factor	May be present
Objective Data		
Physical examination		
Parent-child interactions	Poor parent-child interaction observed; withdrawn child, no eye contact with people	Appropriate parent-child interactions
Appearance	May be small; apathetic	May be lethargic, with altered mental status and irritability
	May be lethargic, altered mental status	
Signs of abuse	Unexplained bruises, scars; poor hygiene	Not present
Dysmorphic features	None	Possible with genetic defects (e.g., cleft palate or lip, Down syndrome)
Weight	Consistently falls below 5th percentile on growth chart	Child plots below 5th percentile on growth chart
	Decrease of two or more percentiles along growth chart	May be gradual weight loss or poor weight gain
Height	May fall within normal range; may be below 5th percentile with long-term FTT	May be below 5th percentile for age with "short stature," dwarfism, prematurity
Head circumference	Inappropriate head circumference ratios with long-standing FTT	Inappropriate head circumference with CNS abnormalities (hydrocephalus); genetic deformities (craniosynostosis)

*Refer to a physician.

Continued

Table 43-4 Differential Diagnosis: Organic and Nonorganic Failure to Thrive—cont'd

CRITERIA	NONORGANIC	ORGANIC*
Vital signs		
Temperature	Normal	Fever may be present with infectious processes
Heart rate	Normal or elevated depending on degree of nutritional anemia and dehydration	May be elevated with congenital heart defects, pulmonary compromise, CNS abnormalities or infection
Respiratory rate	Normal	May have tachypnea at rest or with feeds
Head, eyes, ears, nose, and throat	Normal	Cleft palate; poor gag reflex; signs of infection
Heart	Normal	Possible bradycardia, tachycardia, murmur, altered blood pressure, poor pulses, altered oxygen saturation
Lungs	Normal	Possible tachypnea, retractions, nasal flaring, rales, wheezing
Abdomen	Normal	Possible palpable pyloric ring, palpable mass, abdominal distension, "currant jelly" stools, organomegaly
CNS	Normal	Possible altered mental status, poor gag reflex, hypotonia, lethargy, poor suck, abnormal cranial reflexes
Developmental testing	May be altered with long-standing FTT from chronic nutritional deficiencies	May be altered because of CNS defects, abnormalities
Laboratory data		
CBC	Hematocrit and hemoglobin may be low from nutritional anemia Mean corpuscular volume may be low from iron deficiency or lead poisoning	May have high WBC count because of infection or low count because of malignancy or viral infection May have low hematocrit and hemoglobin related to anemia from infection, malignancy, chronic disease
Electrolytes	Usually within normal range	Based on organic cause, electrolytes may be normal or abnormal; specific organic cause affects result
Urinalysis	Specific gravity may be elevated because of dehydration	May have leukocytes and bacteria with infection May have protein, glucose in urine with metabolic, endocrine disorders
Other tests†		
X-rays	To check bone age or child abuse	May be used to rule out pneumonia, pyloric stenosis, mass, congenital heart or lung disease
Computed tomography scans	None needed	May be used to rule out CNS disorders, mass
Ultrasonograms	Not needed	Used to rule out pyloric stenosis, cardiac defects, renal disorders, CNS disorders

*Refer to a physician.
†Other laboratory tests may be necessary with organic FTT, so consult a physician.

Table 43-5 Caloric Requirements

AGE (MONTHS)	AVERAGE CALORIC INTAKE (PER 24 HOURS)
0 to 6	110 calories/kg
6 to 12	105 calories/kg
12 to 24	100 calories/kg

- Teach the mother proper breastfeeding techniques.
- Discuss with parents the normal caloric requirements for the child.
- Develop a goal for adequate caloric intake and plan to achieve this in an appropriate period (see Table 43-5).
- Teach basic feeding techniques. Review burping, positioning and timing of feeds, and methods of formula preparation to increase caloric content of formula.

- Instruct parents not to let infants go longer than 4 to 6 hours between feeds. If an infant sleeps through feeding, instruct parents to wake the infant if it has been longer than 6 hours since the last bottle.
- Encourage parents to feed the infant in a quiet area to decrease distractions to the infant and parents.
- Teach parents of toddlers with disinterest in eating to have specific mealtimes scheduled in a controlled atmosphere without distractions (e.g., television, toys).
- Discuss cultural beliefs pertaining to nutrition and attempt to incorporate them into the feeding plan. Discuss cultural beliefs that may be harmful in an open-ended, nonthreatening manner.
- Promote regular checkups and routine pediatric health care in an attempt to avoid inadequate nutrition, recognize early symptoms of FTT, and identify potential issues that may result in inadequate caloric intake, stress, or anxiety.
- Provide teaching booklets on feeding and nutrition to parents and families.

Table 43-6   Synopsis of the Practitioner's Role in Management of Organic Failure to Thrive

POSSIBLE CAUSES	CONSULTATION/REFERRAL	COUNSELING/PREVENTION	FOLLOW-UP
Mechanical problems or congenital abnormalities (e.g., cleft palate)	Refer to a surgeon	Use special nipples Teach proper feeding techniques Instruct on chin-lifting to help improve suck Reassure parents about fears or concerns with the infant's feeding and appearance	Once surgery is complete, continue with routine pediatric follow-up
Infection or sepsis	Refer to a physician	Inform parents of the diagnosis and explain the referral and treatment process Provide support and reassurance to parents	Once child has been discharged, continue with routine pediatric follow-up
Central nervous system disorders	Refer to a neurologist	Provide reassurance and support to parents as needed Act as a support system and liaison with the neurologist to help parents in understanding the diagnosis and treatment	Continue with regular pediatric follow-up
Reflux	Consult a physician	Teach parents proper positioning of the child at a 45-degree angle for 1 hour before meals and 1 hour after meals Demonstrate proper burping techniques and positioning for sleeping at an angle for reflux precautions Reassure parents that this is often a self-limited disorder that improves with age Answer any questions parents may have	Continue with routine pediatric follow-up
Pyloric stenosis	Refer to a surgeon	Explain to parents the diagnosis and need for referral Reassure parents and answer any questions they may have	Once surgical correction has been completed and child is discharged, continue with normal pediatric care and follow-up
Cardiac, pulmonary, and metabolic disorders	Refer to an appropriate specialist	Explain to parents the diagnosis and need for follow-up	Continue with normal pediatric follow-up

Follow-up

- Schedule weekly visits to check weight, height, head circumference, and physical assessment until weight has reached the 5th percentile. Each visit should include food diary and ongoing assessment of parental concerns, issues, or anxieties.
- Schedule monthly visits until adequate weight gain has been achieved and maintained for at least 3 consecutive months.
- Continue routine pediatric follow-up care throughout childhood with continued assessment for regression of weight.

Consultations and referrals

- Consult a social worker for financial, housing, support, and insurance issues.
- Refer parents to support groups or new parenting groups.
- Refer mothers with breastfeeding difficulties to a breastfeeding consultant at the hospital or to the La Leche League.

- Refer to an appropriate agency if child abuse is suspected. Inform the parents and discuss with them the reasons for reporting findings and concerns.
- Provide references on available support services for abusers and encourage parents to seek help.
- Refer parents to the Women, Infants, and Children (WIC) Program for aid in providing formula, as well as the Medicaid office for insurance and reimbursement.
- Consult a nutritionist for any child with special nutritional needs to aid in developing a feeding plan to achieve adequate daily caloric intake.
- Refer to a physician any child who, with adequate nutritional intake, continues to have weight loss.
- Refer to a mental health professional any parents or families with psychologic or psychiatric disorders, recurrent drug abuse, or family dysfunction.

Organic failure to thrive. Refer to a physician (and see also Table 43-6).

Fever

JENNIFER PIERSMA D'AURIA

Alert

Consult with or refer to a physician for the following:
- Any child appearing toxic or very ill
- Any infant under 2 to 3 months of age
- Any child with a temperature greater than 100.4° F (38° C) or less than 97° F (36° C) during the first 2 to 3 months of life
- Any child between 3 and 24 months of age with a temperature of 105° F (40° C) or higher
- Fever associated with chills, abnormal vital signs, difficulty breathing, excessive drooling, and difficulty swallowing
- Fever associated with seizure; meningeal signs; or non-blanching rash, petechiae, or purpura
- Altered mental status (e.g., lethargic, disoriented, inconsolable)
- Clinical signs of dehydration
- History of underlying disease, especially neurologic disease, seizures, cardiopulmonary compromise, and immunodeficiency
- Prolonged fever (temperature greater than 100.4° F [38° C]) for more than 7 to 10 days
- Febrile episodes that cannot be confirmed though parents believe they exist
- Anxious or unreliable caregivers with no access to telephone or transportation in case the child's condition worsens rapidly

Etiology

For purposes here, *fever* is defined as an elevation in the set-point temperature of the body as a result of a pathologic stimulus. Body temperature is regulated by the hypothalamus. Although the set-point temperature may vary among individuals, many experts define a fever by a rectal temperature greater than 100.4° F (38° C), oral temperature greater than 99.5° F (37.5° C), axillary temperature greater than 99.0° F (37.2° C), or ear (tympanic) temperature greater than 100.4° F (38° C) (rectal mode) or 99.5° F (37.5° C) (oral mode). (A practitioner should remember that tympanic temperatures are not reliable in infants under 6 months of age.) During the first 2 months of life, any departure from normal body temperature, including hypothermia, may indicate serious illness. In addition, children with chronic illnesses, especially those who are immunocompromised, may not generate a febrile reaction with serious infection.

Incidence

- Acute episodes of fever accounts for approximately 15% of outpatient clinic visits and 20% of emergency room visits.
- Fever is commonly associated with viral and bacterial infections of the respiratory and GI tracts. Complaint of fever is most common during the first few years of life.
- Occurrence of fever is uncommon and infrequent during the first 3 months of life.
- There is an increase in occurrence of fever from November to March in children 3 to 36 months of age (often from respiratory and GI viral pathogens).
- Up to 40% of febrile episodes occur in July through September (often from enteroviruses).
- About 5% to 20% of children under 5 years of age have fever without source (FWS). The peak incidence of FWS occurs in children 6 to 24 months of age.

- Infection is most common cause of fever of unknown origin (FUO) in children under 6 years of age. Collagen-vascular disorders [CVDs] appear more commonly in children over 6 years of age.

Risk Factors

- Children from 6 to 24 months of age (at greatest risk for occult bacteremia if they have a temperature of 103° F [39.5° C] without an apparent source of infection)
- History of underlying disease, especially cardiopulmonary compromise or immunologic impairment (e.g., congestive heart failure, cardiac infections, asplenia, cancer chemotherapy, cystic fibrosis, asthma, sickle cell anemia, human immunodeficiency virus [HIV] infection)
- History of prolonged stay or complicated course in the nursery, or maternal infection during pregnancy
- Infants under 2 months of age treated for unexplained hyperbilirubinemia, or previous treatment with antimicrobial agents
- Children from 3 moths to 3 years of age with a temperature greater than 104° F (40° C)
- Incomplete immunization status
- History of recent immunization (e.g., diphtheria, pertussis, and tetanus [DPT] vaccine in the preceding 24 to 48 hours; measles, mumps, and rubella [MMR] vaccine 7 to 10 days before onset of fever)
- History of previous bacteremic illness
- Environmental exposure (e.g., day care, ill family member, recent travel) to *Haemophilus influenzae, Neisseria meningitidis, Streptococcus pneumoniae,* or *Salmonella.*
- Anxious or unreliable caregiver with no access to telephone or transportation in case the child's condition worsens rapidly

Differential Diagnosis

A careful history and physical examination identifies the cause of fever in the majority of children. The history and physical examination should focus on the age of the child, severity of the illness, height of fever, parents' or caregiver's report of child's behavior or symptoms, immunocompromised states, epidemiologic factors, evidence of dehydration, source of infection, and ability of the parents to participate in the child's care. Many settings have protocols or established algorithms for evaluation of febrile infants and very young children.

Fevers in children are generally categorized by their duration and whether a cause for the fever can be determined. Clinical knowledge of physical findings and the epidemiology of common diagnostic entities associated with acute fever in children generally guide the practitioner to a correct diagnosis. An important aspect of determining a differential diagnosis for a child with fever is to determine if a fever is really present. The parent's level of understanding about fever and ability to read a thermometer, as well as the possibility of a factitious fever, must be carefully weighed during the diagnostic process.

Most acute episodes of *fever related to an apparent source* in children range in temperature from 101° to 104° F (38.3° to 40° C) and last only 2 or 3 days. Localized infections of the upper respiratory tract (e.g., common cold, otitis media, sinusitis), lower respiratory tract (e.g., pneumonia, bronchiolitis), GI tract (e.g., viral and bacterial gastroenteritis), and urinary tract are the most common causes of an acute fever of short duration. Other less common causes include musculoskeletal infections, bacteremia, and meningitis. Nonfocal causes include varicella and roseola. Frequently, few or no laboratory investigations are necessary because the history and physical examination reveal an apparent cause for the infection and age and temperature risk factors are not present.

Unexplained episodes of *fever without source* that persist for less than 7 days are commonly encountered in children under 5 years of age. Many cases of FWS resolve on their own or are attributable to minor acute infectious diseases that are later determined to be either localized or nonlocalized (e.g., chickenpox). In these cases laboratory testing may be necessary to uncover "silent" foci of infection, such as a urinary tract infection (UTI) or pneumonia. Rare causes of FWS include heat illness, drug reaction, or allergic disorders.

Research indicates that although most children with FWS do not have bacteremia, approximately 50% of children with occult bacteremia have FWS. The majority of cases of occult bacteremia are attributable to *S. pneumoniae*. Children at high risk for occult bacteremia include children under 2 years of age, those who have a temperature greater than 103° F (39.4° C), those who appear ill (or toxic), those who have an abnormal white blood cell (WBC) count (less than 5000 cells/mm³ or greater than 15,000 cells/mm³), immunologic impairment, or history of exposure to *H. influenzae* or *N. meningitidis*.

Different criteria exist among practitioners for defining *fever of unknown origin*. Lorin and Feigin (1999) define FUO as a fever that continues for 8 or more days in a child who appears well and in whom a careful history, physical examination, and initial laboratory screening have failed to determine a diagnosis for the prolonged fever. Others define FUO as a prolonged fever that continues more than 7 to 10 days (McCarthy, 1998).

The majority of cases of FUO resolve on their own without a diagnosis. Viral and bacterial infections are the leading cause of FUO in children under 6 years of age. Rheumatologic disorders and rarely malignancies are the other two commonly identified causes of FUO in children.

Criteria for evaluation (subjective and objective data) of a child with an acute fever caused by a localized infection are contrasted with those for a child with FUO in Table 43-7. The diagnostic evaluation of a child with FWS falls somewhere between these two categories.

Management

The practitioner must consider the child's age, significant historical (including epidemiologic factors and exposures) and objective factors (e.g., observational variables, severity of the illness, evidence of dehydration, ability of the parents to participate in the child's care) including laboratory findings in deciding whether the management plan should include home care, a sepsis evaluation, antibiotic therapy, or hospitalization. Again the practitioner should refer to any algorithms or protocols that exist in the practice setting. However, the practitioner's clinical judgment of the child's health state supersedes any decision-making guides that are used in the practice setting.

Acute fever
Treatments and medications
- Provide reassurance and parent support.
- Push fluids with calories (e.g., no diet sodas) and a light diet. Avoid caffeinated drinks.
- Advise keeping the patient lightly dressed (i.e., no bundling).
- Advise both rest and activity as needed.

- For infection control, advise the patient to wash hands carefully, dispose of respiratory secretions properly, cover the nose and mouth with tissue if coughing or sneezing, and avoid exposing others.
- If the parents are observing the child at home, instruct them to check at regular intervals for changes in mental status or behavior; evidence of rashes, bruising, or bleeding under the skin; respiratory difficulty; decreasing urinary output; dry mouth; no tears; and abdominal pain.
- For fever resulting from a localized infection, prescribe antibiotics aimed at the cause. Infants less than 1 month of age or infants who appear seriously ill (toxic) or are predisposed to serious bacterial infection caused by an underlying disease should be hospitalized and receive intravenous antibiotic therapy.
- If antipyretics (Table 43-8) are needed for an acute illness, keep in mind that they are needed primarily during the first 24 hours of the illness course. Aspirin is contraindicated in children and adolescents with fever because of the association of aspirin with Reye syndrome.
  In children greater than 2 months of age antipyretics are usually recommended for temperatures greater than 102° to 103° F (39° to 39.4° C) or if the child is uncomfortable. Children with a history of febrile seizures, underlying chronic disease, or immune disorder may need earlier or more aggressive antipyretic schedules. Neither clinical improvement nor defervescence after antipyretic administration is a useful indicator for differentiating serious from less serious illness in children.
  The drug of choice is acetaminophen 10 to 15 mg/kg per dose every 4 to 6 hours (up to five doses in 24 hours). Acetaminophen is contraindicated in neonates and young infants because its elimination half-life is prolonged. Do not use it if a child is dehydrated (because it is eliminated primarily by hepatic metabolism).
  An alternative therapeutic option is ibuprofen. The smallest effective dose should be used, and it is contraindicated in the last 3 months of pregnancy. In children between 6 months and 12 years of age with a temperature less than 102.5° F (39.2° C), give 5 mg/kg per dose every 6 to 8 hours. If the temperature is 102.5° F (39.2° C) or higher, give 10 mg/kg per dose every 6 to 8 hours. Do not exceed a maximum daily dose of 40 mg/kg per day. In children 12 years of age and older, give 1 tablet (200 mg) every 6 to 8 hours. If fever does not respond to 1 tablet, dosage may be increased to 2 tablets. Do not exceed 6 tablets in 24 hours.
  Alternating acetaminophen and ibuprofen is not recommended. It does not increase fever reduction and may lead to dosage errors and accidental poisoning. If children need longer coverage, they may do better with ibuprofen since it has a longer-lasting effect than acetaminophen.
- Sponging is unnecessary in the majority of febrile episodes but must be used with antipyretic therapy. If sponging is recommended, tell the parents to use lukewarm water (85° to 90° F) and to stop sponging if shivering occurs. Sponging with alcohol or ice water is contraindicated.
  Counseling and prevention
- Acknowledge that fever is an anxiety-provoking event. Inform the child and parents that fever tells a person that body defenses are working correctly and assure parents

Table 43-7   Differential Diagnosis: Fever

CRITERIA	ACUTE FEVER CAUSED BY A LOCALIZED INFECTION	FEVER OF UNKNOWN ORIGIN
ICD-9 code	780.6 (136.9)	780.6
Subjective Data		
Age	Children younger than 2 years of age are at highest risk for occult bacteremia; incidence of some diagnostic entities commonly associated with fever are age-specific (e.g., incidence of otitis media peaks from 6 to 18 months of age).	Consider separate interview with older children and adolescents to get their perception of the illness. Age determines the probability of certain entities and urgency of a work-up; infectious disease most common cause of fever of unknown origin in children younger than 6 years of age.
Gender and ethnicity	Gender and ethnicity may affect the diagnostic process (e.g., boys, Native Americans, Eskimos, and children from developing countries have a higher incidence of severe ear infections).	Gender may affect the diagnostic process (e.g., autoimmune disease is more common in girls; certain immune deficiencies are more common in boys; pelvic inflammatory disease in adolescent girls).
Fever patterns	Majority of fevers are less than 2 to 3 days in duration (FWS may persist for up to 7 days); pattern may suggest origin. Height, duration, and response of fever to antipyretics are generally not helpful in determining the severity of an illness.	Prolonged fever for at least 8 days; pattern (e.g., spiking, sustained, relapsing, recurrent) may provide clues for determining the origin.
Temperature measurement	Technique for taking temperature, type of measurement device, person responsible for taking and reading thermometer; time(s) of day temperature is taken, activity level.	Documentation of fever (may have daily record); technique for taking temperature, type of measurement device, person responsible for taking and reading thermometer; time(s) of day temperature is taken, activity level.
Associated symptoms	May have diarrhea, abdominal pain, vomiting, eye discharge, coughing, respiratory symptoms, rashes, behavioral changes (e.g., irritability, lethargy), decreased urine output. Note that a neonate or very young infant may have very few symptoms other than fever, irritability, and poor feeding.	In addition to symptoms for Acute Fever, search for weight loss, failure to grow, fatigue, malaise, anorexia, eye discharge, abdominal pain, cough, headache, chest pain, dyspnea, edema, dysuria, fever occurring with joint pain or rash; also onset of menses and sexual activity.
Activity patterns	Any age: May have decreased appetite, decreased activity level, alterations in sleeping.	Any age: May have sudden or progressive alterations in sleeping, eating, playing or other activities of daily living; if school-aged or adolescent, include missed school days, peer relationships, sexual activity, drug experimentation.
Exposures	May have other family members who are ill, ill contacts in other settings (e.g., day care, school).	Investigate more thoroughly for animal exposure (cats, dogs, rats, birds, turtles); travel history to regions of the United States or other countries with endemic diseases such as malaria, hepatitis, tuberculosis, histoplasmosis, coccidioidomycosis; wooded areas (Lyme disease, Rocky Mountain spotted fever, mosquito bites, tick).
Immunizations	Recent diphtheria, pertussis, tetanus, measles, mumps, rubella (fevers more likely in children younger than 2 years of age); date and results of last TB test.	Results of last TB test.
Hospitalizations or chronic illnesses	Prior hospitalizations; serious infections (sepsis, meningitis); recurrent bacterial infections; asplenia, immunologic disorders (e.g., HIV, sickle cell); neurologic disease, cardiopulmonary compromise.	In addition to those for Acute Fever, carefully screen for unrelated recurrent illnesses with fever; recent surgical procedure, transfusion of blood; any history of near-fatal or significant illness in child or other family member.
Medication	May be receiving medications or drugs they are sensitive to or may have had toxic ingestions (e.g., salicylates, amphetamine, tricyclic antidepressants).	May be receiving medications or drugs they are sensitive to or may have had toxic ingestions (e.g., salicylates, amphetamines, tricyclic antidepressants).
Family health history	May have history of febrile seizures in other family members.	May have immune disorder, inflammatory bowel disease, tuberculosis, neurologic disease, cardiopulmonary compromise; any family member with history of near-fatal or significant illness or drug abuse; exposure to AIDS.

Table 43-7 Differential Diagnosis: Fever—cont'd

CRITERIA	ACUTE FEVER CAUSED BY A LOCALIZED INFECTION	FEVER OF UNKNOWN ORIGIN
Dietary history	See Activity Patterns	May have consumed raw meat, game meat, raw fish, unpasteurized milk; history of pica, imported cheese.
Home treatment	May have given child antibiotics and antipyretics (use of antibiotics may alter culture results, and use of antipyretics may make it difficult to assess presence of serious illness); note dose of medications and response to treatment.	May have taken or been given antibiotics and antipyretics; note dose of medications and response to treatment.
Family coping and resources	Determine what concerns the child and parent have about the fever; determine whether they have been able to manage episode and obtain follow-up care; whether they have accessibility to phone, transportation, thermometer, distance from health care facility.	Determine what concerns the child and parent have about the fever; consider possibility of misinterpretation of several unrelated illnesses with fever; ask about family stress or parental fear of significant or serious illness; determine whether they have accessibility to phone, transportation, thermometer, distance from health care facility.
Objective Data		
Physical examination	A focused but careful examination should be performed.	A complete physical examination should be performed. The following areas should be emphasized: Keep in mind that the three most common causes of FUO are infectious disease, autoimmune disease, and malignancy.
General appearance	Use YALE observation scales (see Table 44-5) or other approach for evaluating febrile child: Document alertness, activity level or motor ability, interactional style, quality of cry or voice, degree of irritability, consolability, state of hydration, color.	Note affect of both parent and child, interactional style between parent and child and with examiner; note activity level if febrile (see YALE observation scales)
Vital signs (temperature, pulse, respirations, blood pressure)	Variable; note temperature; very young child (younger than 2 years of age) with temperature more than 40° C (104° F) has greater chance of bacteremia; note if pulse (P) or respirations (R) are elevated in proportion to temperature or if P and R more than 2 standard deviations above norm for age; note presence of hypertension or hypotension.	Variable; document if fever is present; note if pulse or respiration is elevated in proportion to temperature; note presence of hypertension or hypotension.
Height and weight	Maintaining growth percentiles	May have weight loss, FTT
Skin and lymph	Cyanosis, pallor, peripheral perfusion, hydration, skin turgor, rashes, petechiae, purpura, enlarged or tender regional lymph nodes.	Note if rash is present with fever event; generalized or regional adenopathy; pallor, petechiae, purpura, hydration, perfusion.
Head, eyes, ears, nose, throat	Note characteristics of anterior fontanel; purulent rhinorrhea, injection of pharynx, exudate on tonsils, mouth ulcers, Koplik spots, barking cough, excessive salivation or drooling; nasal flaring; bulging, red or immobile tympanic membranes; sinus tenderness.	In addition to those for Acute Fever, carefully observe evidence of conjunctivitis, papilledema; palpate sinuses and mastoid area for tenderness; examine teeth and gums for cavities, abscesses.
Cardiorespiratory	Note presence of murmurs; breathing difficulty, retractions, wheezing, diminished breath sounds, stridor.	Note heart murmurs, chest pain, wheezing.
Abdomen	Note characteristics of bowel sounds, tenderness, distension, rigidity, enlarged spleen, enlarged or tender liver.	Note characteristics of bowel sounds, tenderness, distension, rigidity, organomegaly.
Genitourinary tract and rectum	Note inflamed meatal area, suprapubic tenderness, costovertebral tenderness, tenderness or enlargement of testes, circumcised or uncircumcised.	In addition to items for Acute Fever, consider rectal examination, test stools for occult blood loss (guaiac test); pelvic examination in adolescent girl for inflammation of cervix, areas of localized tenderness.
Musculoskeletal	Note gait, joint swelling, rashes, erythema, bony tenderness.	Note gait, joint swelling or restricted range of motion, rashes; bony tenderness, muscle soreness, pain.
Neurologic	Note changes in mental status, irritability, nuchal rigidity; presence of meningeal signs (may not be present in children under 12 to 18 months of age with meningitis).	Note changes in mental status, deep tendon reflexes, cerebellar function, cranial nerves, other items as indicated.

Continued

Table 43-7   Differential Diagnosis: Fever—cont'd

CRITERIA	ACUTE FEVER CAUSED BY A LOCALIZED INFECTION	FEVER OF UNKNOWN ORIGIN
Laboratory tests	Generally none if there is a localized focus of infection, the child appears well, and age and temperature risk factors are not present. Overall, the younger and more toxic or ill-appearing the febrile child is, the stronger are the indications for laboratory investigation. This is true with or without abnormal findings on the history and physical examination. The two most common screening tests include a CBC count with differential count and erythrocyte sedimentation rate. In general, a WBC count of < 5000 cells/mm³ or ≥ 15,000 cells/mm³ and an erythrocyte sedimentation rate of ≥ 30 mm/hour indicates that a febrile child may be at risk for bacteremia. Other tests may include urinalysis, urine culture, stool for WBC counts, chest radiograph (only if there is suspicion of pneumonia); blood culture or lumbar puncture (if child appears seriously ill or other high-risk factors are present).	Consult or refer to physician. Laboratory testing is individualized for the age and situation of the child. If no clues are present, initial screening tests may include CBC count with differential, blood urea nitrogen, creatinine, hepatic enzymes, alkaline phosphatase, ESR, urinalysis, urine culture, tuberculin skin testing, chest radiograph, Epstein-Barr virus serologic study, HIV antibody (if risk factors present).

Table 43-8   Antipyretics

BRAND	DOSE OF FEVER MEDICINE							
	0-3 MO	**4-11 MO**	**12-23 MO**	**2-3 YR**	**4-5 YR**	**6-8 YR**	**9-10 YR**	**11-12 YR**
Acetaminophen drops (80 mg/0.8 ml)	0.4 ml	0.8 ml	1.2 ml	1.6 ml	2.4 ml			
Acetaminophen elixir (160 mg/tsp)		½ tsp	¾ tsp	1 tsp	1½ tsp	2 tsp	2½ tsp	
Chewable tablet acetaminophen or aspirin (80 mg)			1½	2	3	4	5	6
Junior swallowable tablet (160 mg)				1	1½	2	2½	3
Adult tablet acetaminophen or aspirin (325 mg)						1	1	1½
Ibuprofen suspension (100 mg/5 ml)	½ tsp	¾ tsp	1 tsp	1¼ tsp	1¾ tsp	2 tsp		
Ibuprofen capsule (200 mg)						1	1½	2

From Barkin, R.M. & Rosen, P. (1999). Emergency pediatrics: A guide to ambulatory care (5th ed.). St. Louis: Mosby.

that high temperatures resulting from infection do not cause brain damage. Take extra time for counseling with parents who have had minimal experience with minor illness in children or who care for a child with a history of febrile convulsions.

- Remind parents that observation of the child's appearance or behavior is the key to managing children with fevers, not noting the height of the fever.
- Teach parents, especially parents with a child with a FWS, to assess the child at regular intervals for changes in mental status or behavior; evidence of rashes, bruising, or bleeding under the skin; respiratory difficulty; decreasing urinary output; dry mouth; no tears; and abdominal pain.

- Demonstrate or review the proper method for taking a body temperature in a young child to reduce injury and emotional trauma (e.g., rectal temperature for children under 5 years of age).
- Review infection control measures (since most infections associated with fever are contagious). Teach good hand-washing technique. Advise parents to keep the child away from others, especially pregnant women and others with immune problems.
- Instruct parents to avoid OTC combination medications, especially those that contain aspirin, when managing a child with fever. Advise parents and children to not use aspirin with chickenpox or

influenza because of the association of aspirin and Reye syndrome.

- Demonstrate or review written materials for administration of antipyretics and the correct dosage for parents of younger children and for older children who manage their own care.
- Instruct parents to not give antipyretics to infants under 6 months of age without consultation with a health care provider.
- Teach parents to offer young children fluids. Older children should drink extra fluids to replace body fluids lost because of sweating. Remind parents to not force fluids but to encourage small, frequent amounts of iced drinks, popsicles, and gelatin. Advise them to avoid diet products and caffeinated products.

Follow-up

- Keep in mind that follow-up care depends on the age of the child, degree of fever, subjective and objective findings, and origin or cause.
- Schedule a return visit in a few hours if the temperature remains greater than 103° F (39.5° C) in a child under 2 years of age, if fever persists for more than 2 to 3 days, or if the condition worsens.
- Advise parents to call immediately or return promptly if vomiting and diarrhea associated with a febrile episode persist for more than 12 hours.
- Make telephone contact within 12 to 24 hours with any parents or caregivers who are anxious or have minimal experience monitoring children with fever at home.
- Consider telephone contact in 24 hours or reexamine in the office any infant or very young child with significant fever or underlying chronic disorder or disorders.

Consultations and referrals. Consult with or refer to a physician for the following:

- All febrile infants under 2 to 3 months of age
- All children who are ill-appearing or toxic
- Children with altered mental status, extreme irritability, meningeal signs, petechiae, purpura, excessive drooling and difficulty swallowing, respiratory distress, or dehydration
- Any fever that persists beyond 7 days (especially an FUO)
- Children with a predisposing illness or significant exposure, immune deficiency, underlying chronic illness, or history of febrile seizures
- Parents or caregivers who are unable to reliably participate in the child's care or have no access to transportation or telephone for close contact

Fever without source

Treatments and medications. See Acute Fever. Hospitalization may be necessary for all toxic-appearing infants and children for intravenous antibiotic therapy after a full laboratory investigation (i.e., septic evaluation) (e.g., complete blood cell [CBC] with differential count, erythrocyte sedimentation rate [ESR], urinalysis, blood cultures, urine culture, cerebrospinal fluid [CSF] culture).

In infants less than 3 months of age, management may range from hospitalization with a full sepsis evaluation to close surveillance if there is a low risk for serious bacterial infection (Box 43-1) and caregivers are observant and reliable with access to transportation and telephone.

It is generally recommended that:

- Infants less than 1 month of age be hospitalized for intravenous antibiotic therapy pending culture results.
- Febrile infants less than 3 months of age receive a full sepsis evaluation and initial course of antibiotic therapy

---

Box 43-1 Low-Risk Rochester Criteria

Well-appearing infant, with normal vital signs and good hydration and perfusion
Healthy infant:
- Term (greater than or equal to 37 weeks of gestation)
- No antibiotic therapy (antenatal or postnatal)
- No unexplained hyperbilirubinemia
- No underlying illness
- No previous hospitalizations; discharged with the mother as a newborn
- No focal infection (e.g., of skin, soft tissue, bones and joints)
- Good social situation
Laboratory criteria:
- WBC count of 5000 to 15,000 cells/mm³
- Band form count less than or equal to 1500 cells/mm³
- Normal urinalysis (less than 5 WBC/HPF)
- Normal stool (less than 5 WBC/HPF, if done)

From Barkin, R.M. & Rose, P. (1999). Emergency pediatrics: A guide to ambulatory care *(5th ed.). St. Louis: Mosby.*
HPF, *High-power field.*

---

pending culture results. If indicated, a stool culture and chest radiograph should be obtained. In some situations, depending on age of the infant, height of the fever, and clinical appearance, hospitalization and a full sepsis evaluation may not be necessary. However, in these situations, caregivers must be observant and reliable and have easy access to transportation and telephone for close follow-up study.

- The history, physical examination findings, and clinical appearance of febrile children 3 months to 3 years of age guide decisions about doing a lumbar puncture or chest radiograph as part of the sepsis evaluation. Whether the child is hospitalized depends on the clinical appearance, ability to take fluids and medications orally, and reliability of the caregivers to observe and maintain close follow-up.
- Antibiotic therapy may be indicated if: (1) the temperature is 102.2° F (39° C) or higher, or (2) the temperature is 102.2° F (39° C) or higher and the WBC count is greater than 15,000 cells/mm³. (Perform a urinalysis and culture before prescribing antibiotics to the child, especially if the child is a male less than 6 months of age or female less than 2 years of age.)

Counseling and prevention. See Acute Fever.

Follow-up

- See Acute Fever.
- Provide close observation and telephone contact in 6 to 12 hours, especially if the patient is a child less than 2 years of age (a high-risk age group for occult bacteremia).
- Monitor laboratory results and update parents on the findings.

Consultation and referrals. Consult with or refer to a physician for the following:

- All children who are ill-appearing or toxic
- Children with altered mental status, extreme irritability, meningeal signs, petechiae, purpura, excessive drooling and difficulty in swallowing, or respiratory distress
- All febrile infants under 2 to 3 months of age or child with a predisposing illness or significant exposure, immune deficiency, underlying chronic illness, or history of febrile seizures
- Children with clinical symptoms or signs of dehydration

- Parents or caregivers who are unable to reliably participate in the child's care or have no access to transportation or telephone for close contact

Fever of unknown origin

Treatments and medications

- See Acute Fever.
- Provide close observation and daily recordings of morning and afternoon and evening temperatures for at least 1 week (rectal temperatures are preferred in infants and young children; tympanic temperatures are unreliable).

Counseling and prevention

- See Acute Fever.
- Provide parent and child reassurance and support as needed as a result of uncertainty over the meaning of fevers.
- Inform the parents and child that most FUOs go away on their own in 6 weeks or less, so the evaluation process will be staged to avoid unnecessary costs and invasive procedures.

Follow-up

- Schedule a return visit to the clinic in 1 week to discuss the final results of initial laboratory evaluation, obtain an update on the child's status, and discuss additional testing.
- Continue interim histories and physical examinations as indicated.

  Consultation and referrals. Consult with or refer to a physician for the following:

- Additional studies indicated (consult to discuss selection)

- Inpatient observation indicated
- Weight loss or decreased activity during febrile episodes
- FTT
- Unconfirmed febrile episodes when parents believe they exist
- Underlying child, parent, or family psychopathology
- Laboratory evaluation indicative of serious infectious disease, autoimmune disease, or malignancy

Irritability

NANCY E. ALFIERI

Alert

Consult with or refer to a physician for the following:

- Signs and symptoms of increased intracranial pressure (e.g., full, tense fontanelle; disorientation; sluggish pupillary reaction; vomiting)
- Irritability in infants less than 3 months of age (with or without fever), or in infants of any age with FUO that is associated with vomiting, headache, or seizures
- Recent history of head trauma
- Recent history of viral illness and concurrent aspirin use
- Infants with cyanosis
- Hyperthermia or hypothermia
- Dehydration

Table 43-9   Acute Causes of Irritability

INFANT/TODDLER	PRESCHOOL AND SCHOOL-AGE CHILDREN	ADOLESCENTS
Cardiovascular	**Cardiac**	**Infection**
Congenital heart disease*	Myocarditis*	Meningitis*
Paroxysmal atrial tachycardia*	Pericarditis*	Osteomyelitis
Child Abuse	**Infection**	**Intoxication**
Shaken-baby syndrome*	Minor acute infections	Illicit drug use*
	Osteomyelitis	Medications*
Hypothermia or Hyperthemia	Otitis externa (swimmer's ear)	Carbon monoxide poisoning*
	Reye syndrome	
Infection		**Infection**
Encephalitis*	**Inflammatory Disease**	Minor acute infections
Kawasaki's disease*	Toxic synovitis	
Meningitis*		**Trauma**
Otitis media	**Trauma**	Fractures, sprains, and dislocations
Acute sinusitis	Fractures, sprains, and dislocations	
		Miscellaneous
Trauma	**Miscellaneous**	Asthma*
Subdural hematoma*	Asthma*	Dental caries and abscesses
Acute blood loss*	Dental caries and abscesses	Malignancy*
Foreign body*	Insect bites	Migraine headaches
Fracture, sprains, and dislocations	Malignancy*	
Tourniquet (digit or penis)	Migraine headaches	
Corneal abrasion	Sunburn	
Miscellaneous		
Asthma*		
DPT vaccination reaction		
Incarcerated hernia		
Insect bites		
Intussusception*		
Malignancy*		
Parasites (e.g., lice, scabies, tics, worms)		
Sunburn		

Denotes life-threatening causes of irritability.

Etiology

Irritability is a behavioral symptom that may be described by parents as irritable, cranky, fussy, agitated, oversensitive, touchy, testy, colicky, short-tempered, or constantly crying. Although irritability is a nonspecific symptom and may be evident alone, it frequently appears with other contributing factors. Irritability may be the initial sign of an acute, life-threatening illness, a chronic systemic illness, or maturational stress such as teething (Tables 43-9 and 43-10).

Incidence

- Irritability may accompany most pediatric illnesses.

- The most common sign of irritability is acute infections and fever.

Risk Factors

- History of head trauma
- History of child abuse
- Congenital heart disease
- Pica
- History of maternal alcohol or illicit drug use
- Depression
- Allergies
- Feeding difficulties

Table 43-10   Causes of Chronic or Recurrent Irritability

INFANT/TODDLER	PRESCHOOL AND SCHOOL-AGE CHILDREN	ADOLESCENTS
Allergies Food or food formula and environmental contact dermatitis eczema	**Allergies** Environmental	**Allergies** Environmental
Child Abuse* (Physical, Sexual, or Emotional)	**Child Abuse* (Physical, Sexual or Emotional)**	**Child Abuse* (Physical, Sexual or Emotional)**
Child Neglect*	**Developmental Disorders** ADHD Autism Developmental delay	**Endocrine** Hormone disturbances Hyperthyroidism Premenstrual syndrome
Developmental Disorders ADHD Autism Developmental delay Speech delay	**Endocrine** Hyperthyroidism	**Hematologic Disorders** Leukemia* Sickle cell disease*
Hematologic Leukemia* Sickle cell disease*	**Inflammatory Disease** Juvenile rheumatoid arthritis Lyme disease	**Infection** HIV* Mononucleosis
Intoxication Lead and other heavy metals Medications	**Psychiatric** Depression or mania Family stress or discord Maternal depression Mood disorders Post–traumatic stress syndrome	**Intoxication** Illicit drug use* Medications
Metabolic Disorders Urea cycle disorders* Hypoglycemia* Hyponatremia or hypernatremia* Hypocalcemia or hypercalcemia* Phenylketonuria*	**Neurologic** Migraine headaches Seizures	**Psychiatric** Depression or mania Family stress or discord Maternal depression Mood disorders Post–traumatic stress syndrome (PTSS)
Neonatal Drug-Withdrawal Syndrome	**Miscellaneous** Asthma* Degenerative diseases Dietary deficits Fetal alcohol syndrome Malignancy	**Neurologic** Migraine headache seizures
Nutritional Disturbances Iron-deficiency anemia Malnutrition		**Miscellaneous** Asthma* Dietary deficits Malignancy
Miscellaneous Asthma* Colic Constipation Deafness (unrecognized) Family stress or discord GER Malignancy* Motion sickness Parental anxiety Teething Vision impairment		

*Denotes life-threatening causes of irritability.

Table 43-11 Irritability: Diagnostic Considerations

CONDITION	DIAGNOSTIC FINDINGS	COMMENTS
Infections		
Minor acute infections		
Upper respiratory tract infections	Rhinorrhea, cough, variable fever, decreased activity, nontoxic	Irritability decreases with antipyretic therapy; must rule out other abnormality; see Nasal Congestion in Chapter 41
Otitis media	Rhinorrhea, fever, ear pain	Irritability usually decreases with antipyretic therapy and local therapy (eardrops) if needed; see Ear Pain in Chapter 34
Urinary tract infection	Fever, dysuria, frequency, burning	Irritability decreases in 24 hours with appropriate antibiotics; see Painful Urination in Chapter 42
Other		
Meningitis and encephalitis	Fever, anorexia, changed mental status, lethargy, variable stiff neck, headache	Important infection to consider in irritable child; may exist even in presence of other infection such as otitis media
Osteomyelitis	Bone pain, redness	Orthopedic consultation
Kawasaki's disease	Fever, reddened conjunctivae, rash, chapped and cracked lips, stomatitis, elevated ESR	Extreme irritability may be the most pronounced sign; treatment within the first 10 days of illness is crucial to preventing coronary artery vascularities and formation of an aneurysm
Colic	Episodic, intense, persistent crying in an otherwise healthy child; usually occurs in late afternoon or evening	Usually begins at 2 to 3 weeks of age and continues until 10 to 12 weeks; must be certain no abnormality exists; advise soothing, rhythmic activities (rocking, wind-up swing), avoiding stimulants (e.g., coffee, tea, cola) if breastfeeding, and minimizing daytime sleeping; soy or hydrolyzed casein formula may be transiently beneficial; make sure that mother gets adequate sleep and is handling stress; diagnosis of exclusion; see Infantile Colic in Chapter 35
Teething	Irritated, swollen gum; does not cause high fevers, significant diarrhea, or diaper rash	Advise teething ring, wet washcloth to chew on; rubbing gums with small amount of Scotch (or other liquor) or proprietary products; avoiding salty foods; see Chapter 16
Intrapsychic		
Parental anxiety	Insecure, anxious parents; overly responsive, irritable well child	Unstable or changing home environment, inconsistent parenting; attempt to support parents
Intoxication		
Ephedrine, phenobarbital, aminophylline, amphetamines	In therapeutic or high dose may cause irritability as either a primary or paradoxic effect	May try different form of drug or substitute
Lead	Weakness, weight loss, vomiting, headache, abdominal pain, seizures, increased intracranial pressure	Dimercaprol, EDTA (Ethylenediaminetetraacetic acid); see Lead Poisoning in Chapter 47

Modified from Barkin, R. Rosen, P. (1999). Emergency pediatrics: A guide to ambulatory care (5th ed.). St. Louis: Mosby.

- Chronic otitis media
- Constipation
- Aspirin use
- Malnutrition
- History of chronic disease
- Chronic pain
- Fatigue
- Hearing loss
- Developmental delays

Differential Diagnosis

The differential diagnosis should be guided by the child's age and an analysis of the symptoms. A detailed history should be obtained, and attention should be given to patterns of irritability, alleviating factors, and course over time. Assessment should be made of psychosocial parent-child interactions and the parents' response to the child's irritability. Perform a thorough physical examination to identify the pattern of irritability, contributing factors, and physical findings. Attempt to console

Table 43-11 Irritability: Diagnostic Considerations—cont'd

CONDITION	DIAGNOSTIC FINDINGS	COMMENTS
Narcotics withdrawal in newborn	Yawning, sneezing, jitteriness, tremor, constant movement, seizures, vomiting, dehydration, collapse	Symptoms begin in first 48 hours but may be delayed; support child: phenobarbital 5 mg/kg per 24 hours every 8 hours intramuscularly or orally with slow tapering over 1 to 3 weeks; see Chapter 28
Trauma		
Foreign body, fracture, or tourniquet (hair around digit)	Local tenderness, swelling, often following injury; thread or cloth around digit or penis	Splinter or other foreign body, hairline fracture; contusion; tourniquet around digit or penis
Subdural hematoma	History of head trauma; progressively impaired mental status; vomiting, headache, seizures.	May be acute or chronic; requires recognition, computerized tomography scan; neurosurgical consultation; see Head Injury in Chapter 48
Epidural hematoma		
Corneal abrasion	May not have history; patch; fluorescein positive; see Eye Trauma in Chapter 34	
Deficiency		
Iron-deficiency anemia	Pallor, learning deficit, anorexic, poor diet, microcytic, hypochromic anemia	Peaks at 9 and 18 months of age; diet insufficient; elemental iron 5 mg/kg per 24 hours every 8 hours orally; see Anemia in Chapter 36.
Malnutrition	Wasted, distended abdomen	May be caused by neglect or poverty
Endocrine and Metabolic		
Hyponatremia or hypernatremia	Dehydration, edema, seizures, intracranial bleeding	Multiple causes
Hypocalcemia	Tetany, seizure, diarrhea	Multiple causes
Hypercalcemia	Abdominal pain, polyuria, nephrocalcinosis, constipation, pancreatitis	Multiple causes
Hypoglycemia	Sweating, tachycardia, weakness, tachypnea, anxiety, tremor; cerebral dysfunction	Multiple causes; dextrose 0.5 to 1.0 g/kg per dose intravenously
Diabetes insipidus	Polydipsia, thirst, constipation, dehydration, collapse	May be hyponatremic; urine specific gravity less than 1.006; inability to concentrate urine on fluid restriction; see Diabetes Mellitus in Chapter 46
Cardiovascular		
Congenital heart disease	Cyanosis, other cardiac findings	Usually cyanotic
Congenital heart failure	Tachypnea, tachycardia, rales, pulmonary edema	Cardiac and noncardiogenic
Paroxysmal atrial tachycardia	Heart rate greater than 180 beats per minute; restless, variably cyanotic, variable congestive heart failure	Irritability if prolonged; see Chapter 32
Miscellaneous		
Incarcerated hernia or intussusception	Specific abdominal findings	Surgical consultation; may be more common cause than expected; see Hernias and Abdominal Pain in Chapter 35
DPT reaction	Immunization within 48 hours	Analgesia; see Chapter 13

the child to rule out any other significant disorders. In puzzling cases, serial examinations and laboratory investigation may be necessary. Identify all children with life-threatening illnesses and immediately refer them to a physician or an emergency room as appropriate.

Management

Treatments and medications. Treatments and medications are determined by the diagnosis (Table 43-11).

Counseling and prevention
- Instruct and demonstrate for parents the methods of consoling the child.
- Address parental anxiety and coping skills that may be aggravating the child's emotional state.
- Evaluate the level of irritability and appropriateness of the response.

Follow-up. Per the diagnosis, follow-up by telephone for reassurance as needed.

Consultations and referrals

- Refer to a physician for all life-threatening illnesses (see the Alert box) and for the initial presentation of chronic systemic illness.
- Refer to Child Protective Services when abuse or neglect is suspected.
- Refer parents to appropriate support groups or counseling for children with chronic illnesses.

Lymphadenopathy

KATHLEEN KENNEY

Alert

Consult or refer to a physician for the following:
- Regional lymphadenopathy lasting longer than 3 weeks without an identified source
- Lymphadenopathy in the presence of an FUO
- Generalized lymphadenopathy lasting longer than 3 weeks
- Enlargement of supraclavicular, epitrochlear, mediastinal, or abdominal nodes
- Suspicion of malignancy
- Suspicion of underlying autoimmune disorder
- Lymphadenopathy in the presence of immunosuppression
- Nodes that increase in size or number or are of rubbery consistency

Etiology

Children normally have lymphadenopathy, or enlarged lymph nodes, because of a steady increase in lymphoid tissue after birth and during early childhood in response to environmental antigens. Lymphoid tissue growth peaks between 8 and 12 years of age. Children commonly have easily palpable nodes, especially in the head and neck region. Lymph node enlargement is considered pathologic in children when nodes are larger than 1 cm in size, with certain exceptions. Generally, epitrochlear nodes greater than 0.5 cm are considered abnormal, and inguinal nodes measuring up to 1.5 cm may be normal. Supraclavicular nodes of any size are worrisome and are cause for further investigation. Occipital nodes are almost always associated with scalp infections and epitrochlear nodes in children are often associated with cat-scratch disease. Lymphadenopathy can be divided into two categories, regional or generalized. Regional lymphadenopathy refers to enlargement of nodes within the same drainage region. Generalized lymphadenopathy is enlargement of two or more noncontiguous areas.

The origin of nodal enlargement is most often related to an ongoing infectious process in the area that drains into the node. Cervical, axillary, and inguinal nodes are easily palpable in children, and enlargement in these areas often represents a transient response to local infections or viruses. Causes of regional lymphadenopathy include viral upper respiratory tract illnesses, adenovirus infection, cytomegalovirus (CMV) infection, and local bacterial infections (e.g., pharyngitis, cat-scratch disease, otitis media). Causes other than infectious include Kawasaki's disease, histiocytosis, sarcoidosis, and lymphomas. Generalized lymphadenopathy manifests as invasion of numerous nodes throughout the body. It is usually the result of more serious infectious processes, antigen reaction, immunosuppression, or malignancy.

Incidence

- About 45% of children and 34% of neonates have palpable head and neck nodes.
- Infection is the most common cause of lymphadenopathy in children, viral more than bacterial.
- Generalized lymphadenopathy has a higher incidence of more serious disorders and malignancies.
- The incidence of Hodgkin's disease increases in the teenage years.
- Atypical mycobacterial infection has a higher incidence in children between 1 and 6 years of age.
- Cervical adenopathy is the primary sign in 80% to 90% of children with Hodgkin's disease.

Risk Factors

- Exposure to illness or recent illness
- Recent travel
- Inadequate immunizations
- Recent immunizations with DPT vaccine
- Exposure to TB
- History of drug ingestion
- Cat exposure, thorn scratch, or rat bite
- Trauma to area
- Hepatosplenomegaly
- Ingestion of undercooked raw meat
- Rash
- Blood transfusion
- Suspected immunodeficiency (e.g., HIV)
- Systemic disorder (e.g., juvenile arthritis, systemic lupus erythematosus, rheumatic fever, storage disease [rare])

Differential Diagnosis

When one is evaluating enlarged nodes of any kind in infants, children, and adolescents, a good acronym to aid in making the differential diagnosis is ALL AGES. This acronym identifies essential components to consider when one is evaluating the child:

- **A** (age)—Recognize that young children often have palpable or enlarged nodes.
- **L** (location)—Identify and recognize common and uncommon areas for enlarged nodes in children.
- **L** (length of time present)—Prolonged lymphadenopathy may represent a more invasive process than a short-term disease.
- **A** (associated signs and symptoms)—Fever, upper respiratory infection, sore throat, cough, and night sweats, for example, may aid in identifying the origin of the enlarged nodes.
- **G** (generalized)—Generalized lymphadenopathy is more consistent with pathologic causes or systemic involvement.
- **E** (extranodal associations)—Common symptoms are associated with specific nodes (as with occipital nodes and scalp disease).
- **S** (splenomegaly and fever)—Consider viral and bacterial causes. (See also Table 43-12.)

With *localized lymphadenopathy,* infection may be caused by numerous viral or bacterial sources related to common organisms found in the area of drainage into the specific node. The specific diagnosis relates to signs and clinical manifestations. Viral upper respiratory tract infections are the causative factor in the majority of cases of regional lymph node enlargement. Common bacterial pathogens resulting in localized

Table 43-12   Differential Diagnosis: Lymphadenopathy

CRITERIA	INFECTION	AUTOIMMUNE DISORDERS/ HYPERSENSITIVITY REACTIONS	MALIGNANCIES*
ICD-9 code	683.	279.4/995.3	239.8
Subjective Data			
Age of onset	Any age	Any age	Any age
Onset	Usually see rapid enlargement of nodes	May see slow or gradual enlargement of nodes	Usually slow increase in node size is documented
Past medical history	May be history of exposure to infectious process	May be history of gradual progression of symptoms or other episodes of acute exacerbation	May be history of frequent illnesses or progression of symptoms
Family history	May be history of family member with infection or TB	May be family history of autoimmune disorder	Not contributory
Immunization status	May report inadequate immunizations; consider MMR	Recent immunization with DPT	Not contributory
Medications	Not contributory	May be history of recent use of drugs such as phenytoin (serum sickness)	Not contributory
Social history	Possible increased risk factors for exposure to infectious processes (e.g., TB)	Not contributory	Not contributory
Contributory history			
Cat exposure	May be history of recent scratch or bite	Not contributory	Not contributory
Blood transfusion	May report history of transfusion; consider: hepatitis, HIV	Not contributory	Not contributory
Travel	May report recent travel	Not contributory	Not contributory
Sexual exposure	May report episodes of unprotected sexual activity	Not comtributory	Not contributory
Associated symptoms			
Fever	Usually present	May be present in some CVDs	May have prolonged, unexplained fever; may have history of low-grade fevers or night-time fevers
Chills	Often present, prominent in bacteremia or sepsis	Rare	May be present
Malaise	May be present	May be present	Common
Pallor	May be present	Rare	Common presenting symptom, especially with anemia or leukemia
Weight loss	Not significant with short-term, acute illness; may be present with prolonged infection (e.g., as HIV, TB)	Not contributory	Common
Easy bruising	Present in ITP	Not contributory	Seen in leukemia
Epistaxis	Present with sinus infections	Not contributory	May be present in leukemia
Rash	Present in many viral exanthems (e.g., measles, roseola, enterovirus); may be present in some bacterial infections (e.g., scarlet fever)	Can be present with some CVDs (e.g., juvenile arthritis, systemic lupus erythematosus)	Not contributory
Arthralgia	Viral illness may present with generalized arthralgia; bacterial viral infections of specific joints may present with pain to affected joint	Present with many CVDs (e.g., juvenile arthritis, systemic lupus erythematosus, rheumatic disorders)	May be present in leukemia
Generalized pruritus	Possible (e.g., varicella, scarlet fever)	Reported in drug hypersensitivity and serum sickness	May be present (Hodgkin's disease)
Bone pain	Reported in osteomyelitis, septic joints	Usually complain of generalized bone pain vs. specific bone pain	Highly suggestive of hematologic malignancy (leukemia, neuroblastoma)
Cough	Often present with pneumonia, TB, fungal infections	Present in lymph node syndrome	May be present

*Refer to a physician.

Continued

Table 43-12   Differential Diagnosis: Lymphadenopathy—cont'd

CRITERIA	INFECTION	AUTOIMMUNE DISORDERS/ HYPERSENSITIVITY REACTIONS	MALIGNANCIES*
Objective Data			
Physical examination			
Temperature	Usually elevated	Normal or possibly elevated	May be elevated for prolonged periods, during nighttime; or may be normal
Skin			
Petechiae	Occasional (e.g., meningitis, ITP)	None	Present with many malignancies: leukemia
Pallor	May be present	Not contributory	May have mild or severe pallor
Rash	Present in many infectious and viral processes	Present in many CVDs and hypersensitivity reactions	Usually not present
Lymph nodes			
Location	Isolated to area of infectious process	Usually generalized with most CVDs	Isolated or generalized
Size	1 to 3 cm; Usually normal or in response to transient illness	Usually see enlargement greater than 2.5 cm	May have many slightly enlarged nodes or nodes greater than 2.5 cm
Mobility	Fully mobile	Normal mobility	Fixed and matted adjacent to structures
Consistency	Soft, shotty nodes with transient illness; fluctuence may be present with adenitis	Usually normal consistency	Usually have hard, rubbery characteristics
Overlying skin	May be warm, erythematous, fluctuant	Not affected	Not affected
Head, eyes, ears, nose, and throat	Usually have findings of infectious process in area of nodal enlargement (e.g., tonsilar enlargement, exudate on palate show cervical lymphadenopathy; tympanic membranes bulging, dull, nonmobile, erythematous show preauricular, cervical, or postauricular lymphadenopathy)	Usually within normal limits	Mass may be present
Heart and lungs	Possible (e.g., crackles, rhonchi, tachypnea, tachycardia)	May have murmur with rheumatic disorders	May have absent breath sounds, murmur related to mass or obstruction
Abdomen	May be signs of ongoing infectious process (e.g., right lower quadrant tenderness, diffuse abdominal pain)	Usually not contributory	Mass may be palpable
Genitourinary tract	Possible signs of ongoing infection: Pelvic pain, vaginal discharge, cervical motion tenderness, testicular enlargement	Usually not contributory	Mass may be palpable
Extremities	May have swelling of certain infected joints or extremities with ongoing infectious processes	May have swelling, pain, stiffness of specific or generalized joints or extremities	May palpate mass along extremity
Laboratory data			
CBC count with differential count	Elevated WBC count with a leftward shift	Often normal	May have elevation or suppression of WBC count, may have profound anemia, may see neutropenia
Erythrocyte sedimentation rate	Elevated with many infectious processes	Elevated	Can be normal or elevated
Monospot	Positive with mononucleosis	Negative	Negative
Throat culture	May be positive for β-hemolytic streptococcal or streptococcal group A infection	May have positive culture for streptococcal infection (rheumatic fever)	Negative
Blood culture	Positive with bacterial sepsis and bacteremia	Negative	Negative

Table 43-12   Differential Diagnosis: Lymphadenopathy—cont'd

CRITERIA	INFECTION	AUTOIMMUNE DISORDERS/ HYPERSENSITIVITY REACTIONS	MALIGNANCIES*
Stool culture	Positive for bacteria with infectious diarrhea	Negative	Negative
Viral culture	May be positive for certain viral entities	Negative	Negative
Toxoplasmosis	May be positive	Negative	Negative
Venereal Disease Research Laboratory test	May be positive (may have false-positive result with hepatitis, mononucleosis, TB, malaria, varicella, measles, Lyme disease, CVDs, narcotic use)	Negative	Negative
Purified protein derivative	May be positive with TB	Negative	Negative
Gonorrhea culture or Chlamydia culture	May be positive	Negative	Negative
Epstein-Barr virus titers	May be positive	Negative	Negative
Rheumatoid factor	Negative	May be positive with many CVDs	Negative
Antinuclear antibodies	Negative	May be positive with most CVDs	Negative
Anti-streptolysin	May be positive with active strep infection	Positive in many CVDs (e.g., juvenile arthritis)	Negative

ITP, Idiopathic thrombocytopenia.

lymphadenopathy include *Staphylococcus* and *Streptococcus* organisms and nontypable *H. influenzae*.

Lymphadenitis is a primary infection of an isolated node. The cause of adenitis is frequently bacterial; the most common organisms include staphylococcal, streptococcal, *H. influenzae*, and anaerobes. Other origins include TB and atypical mycobacteriosis (atypical TB).

Malignancies including Hodgkin's disease, non-Hodgkin's lymphoma, and other lymphomas (e.g., mediastinal lymphoma), neuroblastoma, and rhabdomyosarcoma may become evident on clinical examination as regional lymph node enlargement. Nodes that become evident with or without fever, have a rubbery characteristic, and continue for longer than 2 weeks should be evaluated by a physician to rule out malignancy.

Autoimmune disorders or hypersensitivity reactions may become evident as regional lymphadenopathy. Disorders such as systemic lupus erythematosus, juvenile arthritis, rheumatic fever, and serum sickness should be included in the differential diagnosis with appropriate signs. Children with these suspected diagnoses should be referred to a physician.

Generalized lymphadenopathy usually represents more significant disease processes. When the appearance is generalized lymphadenopathy accompanied by fever, possible classifications of infection include varicella, mumps, measles, CMV infection, rubella, mononucleosis, enterovirus infection, toxoplasmosis, and immunodeficiency. Each specific diagnosis depends on the clinical signs or symptoms, including laboratory data. Other diagnoses that must be entertained with generalized lymphadenopathy with fever include AIDS and Kawasaki's disease. All children with generalized lymph node enlargement should be referred to a physician for further work-up and management.

Generalized lymphadenopathy with low-grade or no fever may represent hypersensitivity reactions (e.g., serum sickness, CVDs, neoplasm [such as leukemia]).

Management

Localized lymphadenopathy. Indications for biopsy (refer to a physician) include the following (biopsy after 1 to 2 months of observation):

- Age greater than 10 years
- FUO, weight loss, or hepatosplenomegaly
- Mass fixed to skin or underlying structures
- Skin ulceration
- Supraclavicular location
- Increased size greater than 3 cm and firmness of mass
- No regression after more than 6 weeks of observation

Lymphadenitis

Treatments and medications

- Treat the suspected causative agent. Most commonly isolated are *Staphylococcus* and *Streptococcus* organisms and *H. influenzae*.
- Prescribe cephalexin 40 mg/kg per day in four divided doses for 10 days, amoxicillin-clavulanic acid (Augmentin) 40 mg/kg per day in three divided doses for 10 days, or erythromycin 30 to 50 mg/kg per day in four divided doses for 10 days. (Instruct parents that medication may cause gastric upset.)
- For fever and pain, prescribe acetaminophen 10 to 15 mg/kg per dose every 4 hours for fever or pain (up to five doses in 24 hours) (contraindicated in neonates and young infants) or ibuprofen suspension (100 mg/5 ml) 5 to 10 mg/kg per dose every 6 hours for fever or pain for children older than 6 months of age.

Counseling and prevention

- Teach parents medication dosing, timing, and administration techniques.
- Educate parents on the use of warm soaks on affected nodes three or four times a day.
- Educate parents on the importance of observing for signs of increased swelling, high fevers, difficulty swallowing or

breathing, and continued fevers after 3 full days of antibiotic therapy.

- Inform parents of the need to seek immediate medical attention for difficulty breathing or swallowing.
- Discuss with parents the need for a return visit if there are signs of dehydration (e.g., absent tears in infants and toddlers), for poor urine output, or if lethargy develops.
Follow-up
- Schedule a return visit after 24 to 48 hours of antibiotic therapy to assess for regression of nodes, decreased erythema, decrease in fever, and improvement of child's clinical status.
- If lymphadenitis is improved, schedule a visit after antibiotic therapy is completed.

Consultations and referrals. Refer to a physician if a child is dehydrated or has difficulty breathing or swallowing (refer for admission), if lymphadenitis persists after appropriate treatment with proper antibiotics, or if lymphadenitis recurs.

Regional lymphadenopathy
Treatments and medications
- Prescribe appropriate antibiotics related to the specific infection.
- Prescribe acetaminophen 10 to 15 mg/kg per dose every 4 hours for fever (temperature of 101° F [38.3° C] or more) (not to exceed five doses in a 24-hour period) or ibuprofen suspension 10 mg/kg per dose every 6 hours for fever or pain in children over 6 months of age.
Counseling and prevention
- Educate parents on proper dosing and administration of antibiotics.
- Discuss with parents the diagnosis and expected recovery time.
- Review with parents the need to use acetaminophen or ibuprofen with active high fevers as prescribed to avoid high fever spikes and seizures.
- Instruct parents to provide clear liquids, juices, water, and soda to child in small, frequent amounts to avoid dehydration.
- Reassure parents that refusal of solid food is common during times of illness and will resolve when child feels better.
- Discuss with parents the issues of viral illnesses and clinical manifestations.
- Review with parents the signs of a worsening condition and the need for a return visit.
- Reassure parents regarding any concerns or anxieties they may have.
Follow-up
- Schedule a return visit or call within 48 to 72 hours of antibiotic initiation.
- Schedule a return visit in 24 hours if hydration is of concern.
Consultations and referrals
- Refer to a physician if a child continues with fever or significant lymphadenopathy after appropriate treatment has been completed; for suspected systemic infection, immunodeficiency, or other organic diseases; or if there is no sign of improvement or worsening of lymphadenitis after a course of antibiotics is begun.
- Immediately refer cases of generalized lymphadenopathy with or without fever to a physician for further work-up and evaluation.

- Refer children with suspected autoimmune disorders or hypersensitivity reactions to a physician for work-up and management.
- If malignancy is suspected, immediately refer to a physician for further evaluation and management.

Obesity

ELIZABETH F. GUNHUS

Alert

Consult with or refer to a physician for the following:
- Suspected endocrine disorders with associated subnormal linear growth or delayed bone age
- Obesity that becomes evident after prolonged corticosteroid therapy
- Obese children with associated developmental delay or hypogonadism
- Cases of depression or psychologic illness

Etiology

Obesity is the most prevalent nutritional disorder affecting children in the United States. Obesity is the condition of excessive body adipose tissue. There are various defining criteria for obesity. Most commonly the definition includes a weight-to-height comparison in which the weight exceeds 120% of the standard ideal body weight. A body mass index (kilogram per meter squared) exceeding the 95th percentile for age and sex is also diagnostic for obesity. Obesity is also evident when the triceps skinfold measurement is greater than or equal to the 85th percentile on standardized charts of triceps measurements. In many individuals the presence of excessive adipose tissue is clearly evident during the physical examination. The conditions of obesity and excessive body weight frequently occur together. Overweight is a state of weighing more than average for height or body build. This excess of weight does not always coexist with an excess of fat tissue and therefore is not definitive in the diagnosis of obesity. Obesity clearly arises when an individual's dietary caloric intake is greatly in excess of his or her caloric or energy expenditure. Therefore obesity results from excessive dietary intake or inadequate energy expenditure, or a combination of the two. Although rare, endocrine and metabolic disorders can also cause obesity.

Incidence

- The incidence of childhood obesity has increased an estimated 30% over the past 25 years.
- Nearly 15% of American children are affected to some degree by childhood obesity.
- Obesity occurs across all segments of the population, though the prevalence increases in urban and lower socioeconomic populations.

Risk Factors

- Child or adolescent spending a great deal of waking time involved in sedentary activities
- Excessive television watching and video game activity
- Changes in lifestyle (such as increased dependence on automobiles, contributing to decline in activity)
- Inadequate physical activity

- Patterns of "gorge" eating, with a large amount of calories ingested at one meal
- History of parental obesity
- Children without consistent adult supervision, including latchkey children
- Boredom and inaccessibility to recreational activities

Differential Diagnosis (Table 43-13)

A thorough history and physical examination are critical in developing an individualized treatment plan for a child afflicted with obesity. The history should include details regarding the child's dietary intake and physical output. For this purpose it is often useful for the practitioner to request a food-and-exercise diary from the child and family. A diary covering at least 3 days provides some insight into the life-style habits of the patient. The food diary should include all foods and drinks consumed during the period, with a detailed account of preparation styles and quantities. In older patients the diary could also include the child's mood or emotion that triggered the eating, such as anger or sadness. It is important to review the food diary for patterns of binge eating or repeated overeating. The exercise diary should include activities that required physical exertion but also track the amount of time spent in sedentary activities, such as watching television. Identify any use of prescription or nonprescription medications, dietary supplements, or weight-loss programs.

A psychologic and social assessment of the child and family may help to identify any emotional or social factors contributing to the child's obesity. Key elements that should be identified in this assessment include details of the child's daily life, such as time spent with primary caregivers and the amount of supervision. Also address afterschool and weekend childcare and supervision. Assess the value the family places on food and mealtimes. In addition, determine where the child eats meals and who prepares these meals. A latchkey child, who spends a great deal of time without direct parental supervision, may be at an increased risk for excessive eating. The potential increases when unsupervised children are restricted from participating in physical activities outside of the home for lack of adult supervision.

The physical examination should involve all body systems. Plot height and weight on a standardized growth curve as a method of monitoring growth patterns for an individual child. Assess the body fat stores of all overweight children. An easy, indirect method of doing this is by using a caliper measurement of the skinfold thickness of subcutaneous fat stores in the triceps and subscapular areas. The practitioner should be attentive to the possible physical complications associated with obesity, including constipation issues and orthopedic difficulties. Obese children may have breast enlargement as a result of adipose stores. Excess adipose tissue in the suprapubic area may also cause the male genitalia to appear falsely small. Include an accurate blood pressure reading. Screening laboratory studies should include a complete blood count, serum glucose, fasting cholesterol, and urinalysis as appropriate.

A physical examination alone can frequently rule out the majority of the endocrine and metabolic causes of obesity. Such disorders are relatively rare in children of average stature, normal mental development, and no unusual phenotypic characteristics. If there are any suspicions of such disorders causing the child's obesity, the appropriate evaluation and referral should then be initiated.

Metabolic causes of obesity are generally rare but should be considered when one is assessing an obese child. Prader-Willi syndrome is the most common metabolic cause of obesity in children. Individuals with this syndrome generally exhibit hypotonia, feeding difficulties, and FTT in infancy. Facial features may include almond-shaped eyes and a triangular mouth. Hyperphagia and obesity are later developments. Other associated findings include developmental delay, hypogonadism, and short stature.

Hypothyroidism is a deficiency in the secretion of thyroid hormones. Either congenital or acquired, it is among the most common endocrine disorders of childhood. Clinical appearance of an affected child may include a subnormal linear growth rate, increased weight gain, and delayed bone age. Other symptoms include dry skin, constipation, and fatigue. Diagnosis is made through a simple thyroid function test. Treatment with exogenous thyroxine is effective at low cost and has a low risk of adverse side effects (see Thyroid Disorders in Chapter 33).

Table 43-13   Differential Diagnosis: Obesity (Requiring Physician Referral)

CRITERIA	PRADER-WILLI SYNDROME	HYPOTHYROIDISM	GROWTH HORMONE DEFICIENCY	CUSHING SYNDROME
ICD-9 code	759.81	244.9	253.3	255.0
Subjective Data				
Cause	Metabolic disorder	Endocrine disorder	Endocrine disorder	Endocrine disorder, prolonged corticosteroid therapy
Clinical presentation	Infants: Hypotonia, feeding difficulties, FTT; older children: Hyperphagia	Subnormal linear growth, weight gain, delayed bone age	Subnormal linear growth, short stature, delayed bone age	Truncal obesity, fat pads on neck and back, "moon" face
Associated signs and symptoms	Developmental delay, hypogonadism, short stature	Constipation, fatigue, dry skin	None	None
Objective Data				
Laboratory data	None	Thyroid profile	Growth hormone profile	Cortisol levels

Growth hormone deficiency results from a diminished or deficient pituitary function. Causes of the deficiency may have idiopathic, organic, or genetic origins. The clinical appearance generally includes short stature, poor linear growth rate, delayed bone age, and obesity. In addition, fasting hypoglycemia and hypogonadism may be detected in boys (see Chapter 33).

Cushing syndrome results from an excess of circulating free cortisol in the body. Cortisol is a glucocorticoid secreted by the adrenal cortex. Although there are various origins, Cushing syndrome in children is generally a result of prolonged or excessive corticosteroid therapy. Manifestations of Cushing syndrome generally include truncal obesity, fat pads on the neck and back, and rounded "moon-shaped" face. Any suspected or diagnosed endocrine disorder should be referred to a pediatrician or a pediatric endocrine specialist.

Patterns of repeated obesity within various families are suggestive of genetic predispositions to various body shapes and sizes. It is also possible that various genetic factors influence the metabolic rate and function within members of the same family. It is clear that children with obese parents have a much greater propensity toward obesity than children with parents of normal weight and body size have. Lifetime risk for obesity increases by 40% if one parent is obese and by 80% if both parents are obese. In contrast, approximately 5% of children born to nonobese parents will have obesity. Although genetic factors clearly contribute to the condition of obesity, it is sometimes difficult to separate a hereditary influence from the many environmental factors involved in the development of obesity.

Environmental factors play a major role in influencing much of a child's lifestyle. Most cases of childhood obesity are a direct result of excessive dietary intake or inadequate physical activity, or a combination of the two. Children live in an environment where their food intake is strongly affected by a variety of outside influences. These include both positive and negative influences from family and peers. Many advertising campaigns strongly target children to direct their food choices, usually steering them toward foods that are high in caloric and fat content. In general, young children have very little control over their meal selections, food purchases, or food preparations. As children mature, the balance gradually shifts, and a split develops between the child and family over dietary control.

In most cultures there is a great value placed on food, not only for its nutritional significance, but also for the role it plays in social occasions and celebrations. When food is symbolically a comfort or reward, it can often lead to excessive dietary intake. Eating becomes a response to anxiety, depression, and even boredom. Personal difficulties or instability of the family structure may have a negative effect on a child's self-esteem, increasing the desire for excessive eating and therefore the risk of pediatric obesity. The social life of an obese child or adolescent may also suffer. This can often be reflected in a negative body image, social isolation, and feelings of rejection and depression. All such influences may again cause the child to use food as a comfort measure.

Inadequate physical activity is also a contributing factor to the condition of obesity. Some children may be inactive as a result of illness or physical handicaps. A smaller energy expenditure through diminished physical activity must clearly be balanced by a commensurate dietary intake, or the dietary excess will lead to the condition of obesity. Chronic conditions such as asthma result in intolerance for physical exertion. This lack of physical activity, which results in weight gain, serves only to increase such exercise intolerance and exacerbates the initial health concern. The technologic advances of modern society have led to a more sedentary life-style, where cars are the main form of transportation and television is a major source of recreation. Video games and computer activities have increased the volume of sedentary activities for American children. Such changes in the American lifestyle have increased the risk factors for childhood obesity throughout the population.

Management

Treatments and medications

- Remember that clinical goals should focus on the treatment of already obese individuals and on prevention strategies directed at those at highest risk for obesity.
- Aim for dietary balance between caloric intake and energy expenditure.
- Implement dietary suggestions that help to maintain current weight without increasing body fat stores. As the child continues to grow in height, a healthier equilibrium will be achieved.
- Seek out support groups for obese adolescents.
- Be aware that energy needs are affected by additional influences, especially fever and illness.
- Keep in mind that a treatment team for an obese child should include the family, child, and pediatric provider. Additional support from nutritional and mental health services is often beneficial.
- Maintain a diet log book that includes date, time, quantity, and type of food eaten. For older children it should include emotion and activity at the time of eating.
- Implement an exercise program to increase caloric expenditure. Begin with activities such as walking or swimming. Initial activities may start with 20 to 30 minutes of physical activity three times weekly and gradually increase as the child's endurance increases. This can be accomplished if worked into child's routine activities, such as walking rather than riding to a friend's house. Activity programs should be medically safe and involve exercise that is enjoyable, convenient, and realistic.

Counseling and prevention

- Remember that early identification of children at high risk for obesity allows for a focus on preventive strategies.
- Educate families that obesity is often a multigenerational problem and encourage all family members to adopt a lifestyle that includes a healthy diet and adequate physical activity.
- Offer tips to reduce caloric intake:
  Decrease quantity of food purchased and serve smaller portions.
  Make low-fat, reduced-calorie substitutions when possible (e.g., 1% milk in place of whole milk).
  Sever associations between external stimuli and eating, especially with television watching. Suggest that foods be eaten only while the child is sitting at the table, not at the refrigerator or while watching television.
  Make dietary allowances to incorporate favorite foods or satisfying substitutes.
  Remember that snacks of complex carbohydrates are often more satisfying than those containing simple sugars.
  Encourage children of all ages and weights to express feeling of satiety, and encourage parents to acknowledge a child's perception of feeling full.
  Instruct parents that children should not be forced to "clean their plates" when not hungry.

- Provide reinforcement and encouragement for all accomplishments. Focus on short-term goals of weight management or increased physical activity.
- Advise parents that nutritional patterns that begin early in life are often perpetuated throughout a lifetime. Counsel parents to initiate healthful eating habits for young children (see Chapter 15).
- Recommend that parents avoid use of food as a comfort or reward.
- Inform the child and parents that weight-management programs require extended periods of time and extensive effort from all individuals involved.
- Reinforce to the parents and child the concept that dietary changes are sought to prevent long-term health complications for the child. Esthetic changes are not the primary goal.
- Find ways to make child's exercise more enjoyable.
- Encourage family members to begin an activity program with the child.
- Suggest to the parents and child that organized, noncompetitive activities with other children of the same age group may make increased activity more appealing.
- Remind parents that dietary and lifestyle examples set by important adult figures often have a great influence on children.

Follow-up. Visits should be scheduled every 2 weeks initially with the dietary changes. Visits may then be scheduled monthly to assess progress and provide positive encouragement and support.

Consultations and referrals
- Refer to a physician all children with suspected endocrine disorders or suspected metaolic disorders.
- Refer obese adolescent females with menstrual irregularities, severe acne, and hirsutism to gynecologic assessment for polycystic ovarian syndrome.
- Provide nutritional consultation or referral for evaluation and development of an individualized diet with attention to providing a supply of adequate vitamins and nutrients for the growing child.
- Consult with a mental health professional for coexistent depression or self-esteem difficulties.
- Refer morbidly obese children with a weight greater than 200% of ideal weight to a pediatric weight loss specialist for a weight-reduction regimen.

Resources

Organizations
National Information Center for Children and Youth with Disabilities (NICHCY) (which can provide a list of national resources for children with a wide variety of diseases and disorders, PO Box 1492, Washington, DC 20013-1492; (800) 695-0285 or (202) 884-8200; e-mail at nichcy@aed.org; www.nichcy.org

Websites
American Academy of Ophtalmology (www.eyenet.org)
American Optometric Association (www.aoanet.org)
Centers for Disease Control and Prevention (www.cdc.gov)
Family Practice Notebook: Failure to Thrive Management (*www.fpnotebook.com/PED50.htm*)
A Guide for Parents: Television and your Child (www.vh.org/patients/IHB/Peds/General/TVChildren.html)
Joint Program in Nuclear Medicine Findings: Fevers and Cervical Lymphadenopathy (brighamrad.harvard.edu/Cases/jpnm/hcache/1010/findings.html)

Journal of the American Academy of Ophtalmology (www.aao.org)
Library of the National Society of Medicine's *Journal of Family Medicine* (www.ccspublishing.com/j_fammed.htm)
National Center for Education in Maternal and Child Health: Childhood Nutrition (www.ncemch.org/RefDes/kpchildnutr.html)
National Institute of Diabetes and Digestive and Kidney Diseases (www.niddk.nih.gov)
National Library of Medicine (www.nlm.nih.gov/medlineplus)
National Society for Medicine Online Medical Diagnosis: Enlarged Lymph Node and Lymphadenopathy (www.medical-library.org/journals/mddx/lymphadeno/1_lymphadenopathy.htm)
National Society of Medicine Online Medical Diagnosis: Failure to Thrive (www.medical-library.org/journals/mddx/failure_to_thrive/1_failure_to_thrive.htm)
North American Association for the Study of Obesity's *Obesity Research Journal* (www.naaso.org)
U.S. Food and Drug Administration (www.fda.gov)

Bibliography

Abelson, M. (1998). Evaluation of olopatidine, a new ophtalmic antiallergic agent with dual activity, using a conjunctival allergen challenge model. *Annals of Allergy, Asthma, and Immunology, 81*(3), 211-218.

Anderson, R.E, Crespo, C.J, Bartlett, S.J, Cheskin, L.J, & Pratts, M. (1998). Relationship of physical activity and television watching with body weight and level of fatness among children: Results from the third national health and nutrition examination survey. *Journal of the American Medical Association, 279,* 938-942.

Baraff, L.J. (1993). Management of infants and children 3-36 months of age with fever without source. *Pediatric Annals, 22,* 497-504.

Baughcum, A.E, Burklow, K.A, Deeks, C.M, Powers, S.W, & Whitaker, R.C. (1998). Maternal feeding practices and childhood obesity. *Archives of Pediatric and Adolescent Medicine, 152,* 1010-1014

Barkin, R.M. & Rosen, P. (Eds.). (1999). *Emergency pediatrics: A guide to ambulatory care* (5th ed.). St. Louis: Mosby.

Behrman, R.E., Kliegman, R.M., & Jenson, H.B. (Eds.). (2000). *Nelson textbook of pediatrics* (16th ed.). Philadelphia: W.B. Saunders.

Bray, G.A. (1998). *Contemporary diagnosis and management of obesity.* Newton, PA: Handbooks in Healthcare.

Buckley, R. (1998). Allergic eye disease: A clinical challenge. *Clinical and Experimental Allergy, 28*(Suppl), 39-42.

Chesney, P.J. (1994). Cervical adenopathy. *Pediatrics in Review, 15*(7), 276-284.

Dietz, W. (1999). Childhood obesity. In McMillan, J., DeAngelis, C.D., Feigin, R.D., & Warshaw, J.B. (Eds.). *Oski's pediatric principles and practices* (3rd ed.). Philadelphia: Lippincott, Williams & Wilkins.

Ehrmann, W. G. (2000). Obesity. In Hoekelman, R.A., Adam, H.A., Nelson, N.M., Weitzman, M.L., & Wilson, M.H. (Eds.). *Pediatric primary care* (4th ed.). St. Louis: Mosby.

Epstein, L.H, Paluch, R.A, Gordy, C.C, & Dorn, J. (2000). Decreasing sedentary behaviors in treating pediatric obesity. *Archives of Pediatric and Adolescent Medicine, 154,* 220-226.

Erickson, S.J., Robinson, T.N., Haydel, K.F., & Killen, J.D. (2000). Are overweight children unhappy? *Archives of Pediatric and Adolescent Medicine, 154,* 931-935.

Gahagan, S. & Holmes, R. (1998). A stepwise approach to evaluation of undernutrition and failure to thrive. *Pediatric Clinics of North America, 45*(1), 169-187.

Gell, P. & Coombs, R. (1968). *Clinical aspects of immunology* (2nd ed.). Philadelphia: F.A. Davis.

Gortmaker, S.L, Peterson, K., Wiecha, J., et al. (1999). Reducing obesity via a school-based interdisciplinary intervention among youth. *Archives of Pediatric and Adolescent Medicine, 153,* 409-418.

Habermann, T. (2000, July). Lymphadenopathy. *Mayo Clinic Proceedings, 75*(7), 723-732.

Hamme, L.D. (1997). Obesity. In Schwartz, M.W., Curry, T., Sargent, A.J., Blum, N.J., & Fein, J.A. (Eds.). *Pediatric primary care: A problem oriented approach.* St. Louis: Mosby.

Jaskiewicz, J.A. & McCarthy, C.A. (1993). Evaluation and management of the febrile infant 60 days of age or younger. *Pediatric Annals, 22,* 477-483.

Kline, M.W. & Lorin, M.I. (1999). Fever without source. In McMillan, J., DeAngelis, C.D., Feigin, R.D. & Warshaw, J.B. (Eds.). *Oski's pediatric principles and practices* (3rd ed.). Philadelphia: Lippincott, Williams & Wilkins.

Margileth, A.M. (1995). Lymphadenopathy: When to diagnose and treat. *Contemporary Pediatrics, 12*(2), 71-91.

McCarthy, P.L. (1998). Fever. *Pediatrics in Review, 19*(12), 401-408.

Myers, M.D, Raynor, H.A, & Epstein, L.H. (1998). Predictors of child psychological changes during family-based treatment for obesity. *Archives of Pediatric and Adolescent Medicine, 152,* 855-861.

Robinson, T.N. (1999). Reducing children's television viewing to prevent obesity. *Journal of the American Medical Association, 282,* 1561-1567.

Schwartz, D. (2000). Failure to thrive: An old nemesis in a new millennium. *Pediatrics in Review, 21*(8), 257-264.

Chapter 44 *Infectious Diseases*

Nancy E. Kline

Diphtheria, p. 723
Fungal Infections (Superficial), p. 724
Influenza, p. 727
Lyme Disease, p. 728
Meningitis, p. 730
Mumps, p. 731
Parasitic Diseases, p. 731
Pertussis (Whooping Cough), p. 735
Poliovirus Infections, p. 737
Reye Syndrome, p. 738
Roseola, p. 738
Rubella (German Measles), p. 739
Rubeola (Measles), p. 740
Scabies, p. 741
Tetanus, p. 742
Tuberculosis, p. 743
Varicella–Zoster Virus, p. 745
Viral Hepatitis, p. 746

Diphtheria

Alert

Consult with or refer to a physician for the following:
- Signs of epiglottis (e.g., anxious, toxic-appearing child with a high fever, respiratory distress, stridor, and drooling)
- Signs of respiratory distress (e.g., wheezing, crackles, or rhonchi; nasal flaring; retractions; cyanosis)

Etiology

Corynebacterium diphtheriae is the bacterial agent that causes the illness known as *diphtheria*. The bacteria are present in discharges from the nose, eye, throat, and skin lesions and are transmitted by close personal contact with a patient or carrier. Diphtheria is classified into several groups: respiratory, tonsillar or pharyngeal, laryngeal, laryngotracheal, conjunctival, skin, and genital. Individuals with untreated disease are contagious for about 2 weeks; those who receive antibiotic therapy are contagious for less than 4 days. The incubation period is 2 to 5 days.

Incidence

- Diphtheria is usually prevalent in the fall and winter months, although outbreaks can occur during the summer in warmer climates.
- The illness is common in crowded conditions and lower socioeconomic groups

Risk Factors

- Failure to appropriately immunize against *C. diphtheriae*
- Contact with an infected individual or carrier (persons who have been immunized may become infected)

Differential Diagnosis

The following diagnoses must be considered and ruled out when making the diagnosis of diphtheria (see Chapter 41):

- *Upper respiratory tract infection*—This is a viral illness characterized by rhinorrhea, sneezing, cough, congestion, and mild fever, usually lasting 7 to 10 days.
- *Streptococcal pharyngitis*—This is a bacterial illness characterized by high fever, erythema, and purulent material on the tonsils.
- *Laryngotracheitis (croup)*—This is a viral illness characterized by a cough similar to that of a "barking seal," possibly accompanied by fever.
- *Epiglottitis*—This is a bacterial, life-threatening infection of the supraglottic areas characterized by a sudden onset of respiratory distress, high fever, and drooling. These children appear anxious and quite ill.
- *Infectious mononucleosis*—This is an acute infection of the lymphoid tissue characterized by fever, lymphadenitis, rash, splenomegaly, and pharyngitis.
- *Diphtheria*—Refer to Table 44-1.

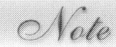

Note

The signs and symptoms of diphtheria depend on the site of the infection and the immunization status of the individual.

Management

Treatments and medications

- A diagnosis of suspected diphtheria infection must be confirmed by culture. Special culture medium is required for culture; therefore the laboratory needs to be notified when specimens will be obtained.
- Equine serum diphtheria antitoxin (DAT) is given to neutralize circulating antitoxin in a patient with confirmed diphtheria infection. DAT can cause anaphylactic and serum sickness reactions. Therefore skin testing is required before administration of the full dose. A patient requiring DAT therapy must be in a hospital and under the care of staff that are able to manage emergency complications and anaphylaxis.
- Treatment of diphtheria also includes antibiotic therapy with intravenous penicillin in a dose of 50,000 to 100,000 U/kg divided into four daily doses. Patients that are sensitive to penicillin can receive erythromycin 40 mg/kg per day (maximum of 2 g/day). The remainder of the treatment is primarily supportive.

Table 44-1 Classification of Diphtheria

CRITERIA	NASAL DIPHTHERIA*	TONSILLAR AND PHARYNGEAL DIPHTHERIA*	LARYNGEAL DIPHTHERIA*	CUTANEOUS, VAGINAL, CONJUNCTIVAL, AND AURAL DIPHTHERIA*
ICD-9 code	032.2	032.1	0.32.3	032.85
Subjective Data				
Exposure	Exposure to an individual with active diphtheria infection	Exposure to an individual with active diphtheria infection	Exposure to an individual with active diphtheria infection	Exposure to an individual with active diphtheria infection
Associated findings	May report recent upper respiratory tract symptoms (cough, rhinorrhea); red, brown nasal discharge, which progresses to purulent discharge	May report low-grade fever, sore throat, malaise, anorexia	May report noisy breathing, hoarseness, dry cough	May report lesions on the skin or conjunctivae, ear pain, or a draining ear
Immunization history	Inadequate against diphtheria	Inadequate against diphtheria	Inadequate against diphtheria	Inadequate against diphtheria
Objective Data				
Physical examination	Mucopurulent rhinorrhea: May have foul odor, excoriated nares and upper lip, white membrane on nasal septae	Low-grade fever, white or gray membrane over the posterior pharynx and tonsils (bleeds when disturbed), enlarged cervical lymph nodes, edema in the soft tissues of the neck, difficulty swallowing, unilateral or bilateral paralysis of the palate, stupor, coma (rare)	Extension of the white membrane down past the pharynx, noisy breathing, stridor, hoarseness, dry cough, retractions, airway obstruction	Ulcerative, sharply demarcated lesions on the skin, vulva, or lining of the vagina; reddened, edematous conjunctivae; corneal erosions, otitis externa with purulent discharge (which may have a foul odor)

*Immediate referral to a physician.

- Patients may need encouragement to eat and drink because anorexia is a problem. Intravenous fluid therapy is an alternative.
- Cardiac, neurologic, and respiratory complications are common and require close monitoring.
- Patients with cutaneous diphtheria need to have the wound cleaned thoroughly with soap and water and have contact isolation implemented. These patients may also require antimicrobial therapy.
- As immunity does not develop following the active disease state, a patient must be immunized with diphtheria toxoid following the illness.

Counseling and prevention
- Educate parents on the benefits of immunizations.
- Remember that the incidence of diphtheria has declined dramatically with the advent of the diphtheria vaccine. Since the mid-1980s, only 24 cases of respiratory diphtheria were reported in the United States. However, with limited access to health care for some segments of the population, it would not be surprising to see periodic outbreaks of the disease.
- Keep in mind that currently, 97% of children entering school have had at least three diphtheria immunizations. However, it is estimated that 50% of Americans over the age of 60 years lack sufficient protection against the disease. Practitioners must take advantage of updating immunization boosters in both pediatric and adult populations.

- Instruct parents regarding the use of contact isolation to prevent spread of the disease, and give specific instruction regarding medication administration. Individuals are contagious for 4 days after antibiotic therapy is initiated.

Follow-up. Patients who have had diphtheria infection require periodic follow-up care until they have returned to their normal state of health. A multidisciplinary team may be required if there are cardiac or neurologic sequelae.

Consultations and referrals
- Provide immediate referral to a physician for any individual suspected of having diphtheria.
- Report all cases of diphtheria to the health department.
- Contact the school nurse or day-care center.

Fungal Infections (Superficial)

Alert

Consult with or refer to a physician for the following:
- High fever
- Petechiae
- Purpura
- Progressively worsening oral candidal infection
- Anorexia
- Dehydration

Etiology

Candida albicans is the most common species of the genus *Candida* that causes superficial infection in children (i.e., candidiasis). It is present in the intestinal tract, vagina, and mucous membranes of normal hosts. Newborn infants can acquire the organism in utero, during delivery, or postnatally. Most infections are endogenous.

Tinea capitus is a fungal infection of the scalp occurring most often in children between the ages of 2 and 10 years. Often transmission occurs after a break in the skin and subsequent personal contact with an infected individual or fomite (e.g., combs, brushes). Transmission can occur as long as fungal spores are present on examination with Wood's lamp fluorescence.

Tinea corporis (ringworm) is a fungal infection of the skin that occurs worldwide and is transmitted by direct contact with infected persons, animals, or fomites. Transmission occurs as long as fungal spores are present.

Tinea cruris is a fungal infection of the skin on the groin and upper thighs that occurs most often with increased moisture, tight clothes, and obesity. Transmission can also occur following direct or indirect person-to-person contact.

Tinea pedis is a fungal infection that occurs on the skin of the feet and toes. Infection occurs after contact with fungi in swimming pools, showers, or locker rooms, or with infected skin scales.

Tinea versicolor is a superficial fungal infection caused by *Malassezia furfur* via personal contact during scaling. Tinea versicolor occurs worldwide.

Incidence

- Candidal infection is a common cause of diaper dermatitis, vaginitis, and thrush in normal, healthy infants and children.
- With candidal infection, children with human immunodeficiency virus (HIV) infection or who are immunosuppressed (e.g., through diabetes mellitus, cancer chemotherapy, daily corticosteroids) are unusually susceptible to infection.
- Tinea capitus is not often seen in infants or adolescents.
- Tinea corporis (ringworm) is a common superficial fungal infection worldwide.
- Tinea cruris occurs most often in adolescent boys and young adult men.
- Tinea cruris often occurs along with tinea pedis.
- Tinea pedis occurs in adolescents and young adults but not often in young children.
- Tinea versicolor is most often seen in adolescents and young adults but occasionally in infants as well.

Risk Factors

- Candidal infection (previous antibiotic therapy, immunosuppression)
- Tinea infection (contact with fungal spores through direct person-to-person contact or fomites)

Differential Diagnosis (Table 44-2)

Common superficial fungal infections and other disorders which must be considered in the differential diagnosis of each are included below.

Cutaneous candidal infection

- *Diaper dermatitis*—Irritation of the skin in contact with a diaper. See Diaper Rash in Chapter 37.

Mucosal candidal infection. Oropharyngeal infection may be mistaken for curds of milk or formula.

Tinea capitus

- *Seborrheic dermatitis*—An increase in sebaceous secretions, causing increased oil production, erythematous patches, and scaling.
- *Psoriasis*—A chronic skin disorder characterized by erythematous papules that coalesce to form plaques. New lesions tend to appear at sites of trauma. If left untreated, a silvery white scale develops.
- *Alopecia areata*—Hair loss in well-defined patches on the scalp. Causes include seborrheic dermatitis, drugs, irradiation, and systemic illnesses.
- *Impetigo*—Bacterial skin disease characterized by isolated pustules that rupture and become crusted.
- *Lupus erythematosus*—Rheumatologic disorder causing a facial form of seborrhea that appears as elevated, erythematous patches with scales.

Tinea corporis (ringworm)

- *Tinea incognita*—Appearance of skin lesions following application of topical corticosteroids. It resolves spontaneously after application ceases.

Tinea cruris

- *Seborrheic dermatitis*—An increase in sebaceous secretions, causing increased oil production, erythematous patches, and scaling.
- *Psoriasis*—A chronic skin disorder characterized by erythematous papules that coalesce to form plaques. New lesions tend to appear at sites of trauma. If left untreated, a silvery white scale develops.
- *Allergic dermatitis*—Inflammation of the skin (because of an allergy) characterized by erythema, pruritus, and various lesions.
- *Intertrigo*—A superficial dermatitis found in skin folds.

Tinea pedis

- *Eczema*—An acute or chronic inflammation of the skin that causes erythema, papules, vesicles, scales, scabs, and crusts (alone or in combination).
- *Allergic dermatitis*—Inflammation of the skin (due to an allergy) characterized by erythema, pruritus, and various lesions.

Tinea versicolor

- *Seborrheic dermatitis*—An increase in sebaceous secretions, causing increased oil production, erythematous patches, and scaling.
- *Pityriasis alba*—A skin disease with decreased melanin that causes patches of round or oval macular lesions with fine scales. It is often seen on the faces of children. The patches usually disappear spontaneously.
- *Pityriasis rosea*—An inflammatory skin disease characterized by rosy macular lesions with fine scales and a clearing center on the back and ribs. The lesions usually disappear spontaneously after 2 to 10 weeks.
- *Vitiligo*—An acquired skin condition characterized by white patches surrounded by normally pigmented areas. It is more common in tropical areas and in darker-skinned individuals. The cause is not known.

Management

Candidal infection

Treatments and medications. For cutaneous infection, the treatment is application of an antifungal cream (e.g., clotrimazole [Lotrimin], nystatin [Mycostatin]) with each diaper change.

Table 44-2 Differential Diagnosis: Fungal Infections (Superficial)

CRITERIA	CANDIDAL INFECTION	TINEA CORPORIS/ TINEA CAPITIS	RINGWORM	TINEA CRURIS	TINEA PEDIS	TINEA VERSICOLOR
ICD-9 code	112.9	110.5/110.0	110.5	110.3	110.4	111.0
Subjective Data						
Description of problem (appearance)	Cutaneous: parents report diaper rash, baby cries when diaper is wet with urine; mucosal: white spots in mouth, poor feeding	Parents or patient reports red rash on scalp, swelling, pustules, vesicles, itching, hair loss	Parents or patient reports circular rash, itching	Parents or patient reports red rash in the groin area, excessive itching	Parents or patient reports red rash on the feet and toes; itching	Parents or patient reports areas of fine scaling in oval lesions; itching
Objective Data						
Physical examination						
Inspection of lesions	Cutaneous: vivid, red diaper dermatitis that involves the intertriginous folds; mucosal: White, curd-like plaques on a red base; weight loss, signs of dehydration	Red, scaly scalp with short broken hairs and alopecia; pustules, vesicles, presence of a kerion	Pruritic, circular lesion with slightly raised borders and clearing center; well demarcated	Well-demarcated, scaly lesion on the upper thighs and groin; bilaterally symmetric; secondary infection may be present	Scaly, vesicular, or pustular lesions on the feet and toes; secondary infection may be present	Multiple scaly patches over the upper trunk and arms; areas fail to tan in the summer
Laboratory data		Wood's lamp for fluorescence of lesions or scrapings and microscopic visualization (diagnostic)	Wood's lamp for fluorescence of lesions or scrapings and microscopic visualization (diagnostic)	Wood's lamp for fluorescence of lesions or scrapings and microscopic visualization (diagnostic)	Wood's lamp for fluorescence of lesions or scrapings and microscopic visualization (diagnostic)	Wood's lamp for fluorescence of lesions or scrapings and microscopic visualization (diagnostic)

For an oral mucosal infection (oral), the treatment is nystatin suspension (100,000 U/ml) orally four times a day for 14 days in a dose of 2 ml for infants and 4 to 6 ml for children and adolescents, or clotrimazole troches 10 mg, with one troche dissolved slowly five times a day for 14 days. If an infant is being breastfed, examine and treat the mother for candidiasis of breast.

Counseling and prevention
- Instruct parents that completion of therapy is important. Many parents are tempted to cease therapy as soon as lesions disappear. Advise parents that lesions commonly recur if therapy is not adequate.
- Instruct parents on the proper administration of medication. Apply suspension directly to the oral mucosa with a finger or cotton application. Good handwashing is important to prevent transmission to caregivers.
- If an infant is bottle-fed, instruct parents to boil nipples and pacifiers.

Follow-up. Infants and children with oral candidiasis may require a return visit in 2 weeks to ensure that the condition is improving and they are able to eat and drink normally.

Consultations and referrals. Consult with a physician if children require oral antifungal therapy for persistent cutaneous fungal infection. Immediate attention by a physician is warranted if the infant or child is severely dehydrated or has evidence of a more serious cutaneous condition (see the Alert box).

Tinea capitus

Treatments and medications. The treatment is griseofulvin 10 to 20 mg/kg per day divided two times a day for 4 to 8 weeks. Ketoconazole 3 to 4 mg/kg per day may be substituted if griseofulvin is not tolerated, but ketoconazole has more side effects.

Counseling and prevention
- Instruct the parents and child that completion of therapy is important. Many parents are tempted to cease therapy as soon as lesions disappear. Advise that lesions commonly recur if therapy is not adequate.
- Advise that contact with individuals with active tinea infections often causes others to become infected.
- Instruct the parents and child that good handwashing, thorough cleaning of bathrooms and personal effects, and avoidance of sharing bath towels may slow transmission of the fungi.
- Instruct parents that persisting fungal infections, despite adequate treatment, may require oral antifungal therapy.

Follow-up. Children who are taking oral griseofulvin should have liver enzymes monitored monthly because the medication can cause liver damage.

Consultations and referrals
- Provide immediate referral to a physician for all infants and children with severe dehydration or evidence of a more serious cutaneous condition (see the Alert box).
- Consult with a physician if a child requires oral antifungal therapy for persistent cutaneous fungal infection.

Tinea corporis (ringworm), tinea cruris, tinea pedis, and tinea versicolor

Treatments and medications. The treatment is topical application of miconazole, tolnaftate, or clotrimazole twice daily for 4 weeks, or ketoconazole, oxiconazole, or sulconazole once daily for 4 weeks.

Counseling and prevention
- Instruct the parents and child that completion of therapy is important. Many parents are tempted to cease therapy as

soon as the lesions disappear. Advise parents that lesions commonly recur if therapy is not adequate.
- Inform the parents and child that contact with individuals with active tinea infections often causes others to become infected.
- Instruct that good handwashing, thorough cleaning of bathrooms and personal effects, and avoidance of sharing bath towels may slow the transmission of the fungi.

Follow-up. Schedule a return visit if the condition persists despite adequate treatment because these children may require oral antifungal therapy.

Consultations and referrals
- Provide immediate referral to a physician for all infants and children with severe dehydration or evidence of a more serious cutaneous condition (see the Alert box).
- Consult with a physician if a child requires oral antifungal therapy for persistent cutaneous fungal infection; an underlying immunosuppressive disorder may be present.

Influenza

Alert

Consult with or refer to a physician for the following:
- Meningeal signs and symptoms (e.g., lethargy, anorexia, irritability, stiff neck, vomiting, Kernig's or Brudzinski's sign, severe headache)
- Signs of dehydration (e.g., poor skin turgor, dry lips, sticky mucous membranes, sunken fontanel)
- Signs of respiratory distress (e.g., nasal flaring, retractions, wheezing, crackles, rhonchi, cyanosis, stridor)
- Anxious child with a high fever, respiratory distress, stridor, and drooling

Etiology

Epidemic disease is caused by types A and B influenza virus. It is spread by person-to-person, direct contact, large airborne droplets, or articles contaminated with nasopharyngeal secretions. During an influenza outbreak, school-age children are most frequently infected; they in turn infect their siblings and parents in the home. Epidemics occur when the circulating strain is not the same as strains in the recent past. Influenza is highly contagious, and patients are most infectious in the 24 hours before symptoms are evident. Contagiousness lasts for 7 days in older children and adults but may persist for a longer period in younger children. The incubation period is 1 to 3 days.

Incidence

- In normal, healthy children influenza rates are estimated at 10% to 40% each year.
- Influenza season is typically from mid-October through mid-February.

Risk Factors

- School-age child
- Institutionalized populations
- Household contact with an infected person (usually a school-age child)
- No annual influenza vaccination

Differential Diagnosis

Refer to Table 44-3.

Management

Treatments and medications

- Nasopharyngeal cultures, if obtained, should be done within the first 72 hours of illness because the viral load is greatest during this time.
- Diagnosis is usually made based on the clinical signs and available prevalence data.
- Treatment in a normally healthy child is primarily supportive. Bed rest may be necessary because fatigue is common. Acetaminophen or ibuprofen may be used for fever and myalgias; however, aspirin should be avoided because of the relation between aspirin use and Reye syndrome.
- The parents may need to encourage the child to maintain adequate hydration and nutrition because many times anorexia is a problem.
- Antiviral therapy should be considered for patients with severe disease or underlying conditions (e.g., HIV infection, cystic fibrosis, cardiac dysfunction, asthma, receipt of immunosuppressive therapy) that may cause them to have an increased risk for complications.
- Amantadine (Symmetrel), an antiviral, diminishes the severity of influenza A but is not effective in the treatment of influenza B. It is currently the only antiviral agent used in children for treatment of influenza. The dosage is 5 mg/kg in one or two divided doses for 7 days or until symptoms have subsided. Total daily dosage for children 1 to 9 years of age is 150 mg; for children 10 years of age and older, it is 200 mg. Rimantadine is an antiviral agent that can be used for prophylaxis in an attempt to prevent infection in exposed children. The dose of rimantadine is the same as that for amantadine. These agents are not approved by the Food and Drug Administration (FDA) for use in children less than 1 year of age.

Counseling and prevention. Annual influenza vaccination is safe and carries minimal side effects. The composition of the vaccine is changed periodically in anticipation of the expected prevalent strains. Vaccination is recommended for children 6 months of age and older who have a disease or condition (e.g.,

HIV infection, cystic fibrosis, cardiac dysfunction, asthma, receipt of immunosuppressive therapy) that predisposes them to complications from influenza infection. Vaccine-naïve children less than 9 years of age require two doses of vaccine 1 month apart to achieve an adequate antibody response. Children who have primary or secondary immune deficiency should be vaccinated but may not have an optimal response. The household contacts of these children should be vaccinated to assist in preventing influenza transmission. Educate parents regarding the fact that the vaccine only protects against certain strains of the virus and is not 100% effective in preventing influenza. Protection in healthy subjects is 70% to 80%.

Follow-up. Uncomplicated influenza infection does not require follow-up care. Children with chronic illnesses or those who are immunosuppressed should be observed until they have returned to their normal state of health.

Consultations and referrals. Refer to a physician any normal, healthy children who require antiviral treatment for severe influenza infection. Children with chronic illnesses and immunosuppression may be followed in conjunction with a physician because they may require hospitalization.

Lyme Disease

Alert

Consult with or refer to a physician for the following:
- Meningeal signs and symptoms (e.g., lethargy, anorexia, irritability, stiff neck, vomiting, Kernig's or Brudzinski's sign, severe headache)
- Cranial nerve palsies
- Peripheral neuropathy

Etiology

Lyme disease is caused by a spirochete, *Borrelia burgdorferi*. It is most often transmitted via the deer tick; however, there is recent evidence to suggest that there are other vectors that aid the transmission of Lyme disease (e.g., rodents). The disease is clustered in three geographic areas of the United States. These

Table 44-3 Differential Diagnosis: Influenza

CRITERIA	INFLUENZA	UPPER RESPIRATORY TRACT INFECTION	MENINGITIS*
ICD-9 code	487.1	465.9	322.9
Subjective Data			
Present history	Classmates sent home with flulike illness (e.g., fever, chills, malaise, headache, myalgia, sore throat, cough, abdominal pain, nausea, vomiting, anorexia)	Sneezing, cough, congestion, mild fever	Lethargy, irritability, vomiting, stiff neck, anorexia
Objective Data			
Physical examination	Fever, with or without chills, malaise, rhinorrhea, cough, abnormal breath sounds (e.g., wheezing, crackles, rhonchi), dehydration, weight loss	Rhinorrhea, cough, mild fever	Lethargy, high fever, irritability, stiff neck, weight loss, Kernig or Brudzinski sign

*Immediate referral to a physician.

include the Northeast, from Massachusetts to Maryland; the Midwest, primarily Wisconsin and Minnesota; and California. Lyme disease has also been reported in other countries. The incubation period from a tick bite to the appearance of erythema migrans is 3 to 32 days.

Incidence

- All ages and both sexes may be affected.
- Most cases occur in June and July.

Risk Factors

- Recent tick bite, especially in highly endemic areas

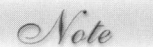

The patient may have late signs, including joint involvement, cardiac abnormalities, cranial nerve findings, and meningeal symptoms, without ever having early symptoms or erythema chronicum migrans.

Differential Diagnosis

Refer to Table 44-4.

Management

Treatments and medications. If the diagnosis is not made clinically during the early stages or if erythema chronicum migrans was never present, serologic tests are available for diagnostic purposes. Immunoglobulin M (IgM)–specific antibody titer peaks between 3 to 6 weeks after infection. Immunoglobulin G (IgG)–specific antibody titer peaks weeks to months later. An indirect fluorescent antibody test and enzyme-linked immunosorbent assay (ELISA) are available, but both false-negative and false-positive test results occur with each.

For children eight years of age or older, doxycycline (100 mg orally twice a day for 14 to 21 days) should be given at the time of the appearance of the annular rash. For all ages of children, amoxicillin (25 to 50 mg/kg orally twice a day for 14 to 21 days) may be given. If the child is allergic to penicillin, erythromycin or cefuroxime may be substituted. Early antibiotic therapy should prevent the later stages of the disease.

A child with early disease should be reevaluated after a 14-day course of antibiotic therapy because relapses are common and the antibiotic therapy may need to be continued or changed. If the disease is not identified until late signs and symptoms have developed, treatment may vary. Children with isolated seventh-nerve palsy (and normal cerebrospinal fluid [CSF] findings), mild carditis, or arthritis can be treated with the same antibiotics as recommended for early disease. More advanced cardiac disease, persistent arthritis, and extensive neurologic involvement should be treated with intravenous ceftriaxone or penicillin G.

Counseling and prevention. In 1998, a Lyme disease vaccine was licensed for use by the FDA for persons 15 to 70 years of age. The vaccine should be used in conjunction with personal protective measures for persons in geographic areas of moderate to high risk whose activities cause them to be exposed frequently to vector ticks. The vaccine is not recommended for persons who reside, work, or recreate in high-risk areas who do not have prolonged or frequent exposure to infected ticks.

A practitioner should also:
- Instruct on identification of the deer tick.
- Encourage compliance with antibiotic therapy because relapse of Lyme disease is common and requires retreatment.

Table 44-4 Differential Diagnosis: Lyme Disease

CRITERIA	LYME DISEASE	INFLUENZA	TINEA CORPORIS
ICD-9 code	088.81	487.1	110.5
Subjective Data			
Rash	Erythematous annular rash; development of secondary rash, malar rash or urticaria	No rash	Erythematous, circular lesion
Associated symptoms	History of a tick bite, malaise, conjunctivitis, headache, fever, arthralgias, mild neck stiffness	Fever, chills, body aches, headache, and malaise	Itching
Objective Data			
Physical examination			
Inspection of skin	Erythema chronicum migrans: Begins as a red papule at site of tick bite and expands to form large annular rash with central clearing, secondary annular lesions, malar rash	No rash	Well-circumscribed, circular lesion with slightly raised borders and a clearing center
Associated findings	Urticaria, fever, cranial nerve palsies (e.g., Bell palsy), nonsymmetric arthritis in large joints	Coryza, cough, and cold	None
Laboratory data	Positive ELISA; confirm with Western blot		Wood's lamp, fluorescence of lesions

- Instruct that prompt removal of ticks from the skin and use of tick repellant decreases the incidence of Lyme disease. In areas where Lyme disease is prevalent, long pants and long-sleeved shirts with pants tucked into the socks prevent deer tick bites. Heavily wooded areas should be avoided.
- Instruct parents to carefully examine children for ticks after the children play outdoors.

Follow-up. Children receiving oral antibiotic treatment for early-stage disease should be evaluated at 14 days to determine disease status and the need to continue or change antibiotic therapy. Other children who have progressed to late-stage disease require follow-up care until they have resumed their previous state of health, and they may require follow-up with specialty services (e.g., cardiology, rheumatology, neurology, ophthalmology).

Consultations and referrals

- Consult with a physician if a child has suspected Lyme disease.
- Provide immediate referral to a physician if the child exhibits cardiac or central nervous system (CNS) involvement (see the Alert box).

Meningitis

Alert

Consult with or refer to a physician or emergency center for the following:
- Signs of meningitis (e.g., irritability, fever, lethargy, nuchal rigidity, confusion, severe headache)
- Fever or low body temperature in an infant younger than 2 months of age

Etiology

Bacterial meningitis in children 2 months to 12 years of age is usually caused by *Streptococcus pneumoniae* or *Neisseria meningitidis*. Infection with *Haemophilus influenzae* type B may occur at any age but is most common before the age of 4 years. With the widespread use of the conjugate vaccine against *H. influenzae*, the incidence of meningitis as a result of this organism has decreased significantly. Meningitis associated with ventriculoperitoneal shunts is most often due to *Staphylococcus epidermidis*, while meningitis in children with an open neural tube defect may be due to *Streptococcus aureus* or enteric bacteria. Children who are immunosuppressed with T-cell defects are susceptible to cryptococcal and *Listeria monocytogenes* infections of the CNS. Aseptic meningitis, an acute inflammation of the meninges, is most often caused by a virus. Enterovirus, coxsackievirus, and echoviruses type 4, 6, 9 and 11 are the most common types. St. Louis and California encephalitis are the most commonly implicated arboviruses that cause aseptic meningitis. Other etiologic viral agents such as HIV, varicella, Epstein-Barr virus (EBV), measles, mumps, rubella, polio, rabies, influenza, and parainfluenza can cause aseptic meningitis. *Mycoplasma, Chlamydia,* fungi, protozoa and parasites can also cause CNS infection leading to aseptic meningitis. The incubation period is variable depending on the causative organism or virus, but it is usually in the range of 1 to 10 days.

Incidence

- Infection occurs throughout childhood and adulthood.
- Bacterial meningitis occurs more frequently during winter and spring, in more males than females, and most often between 2 months and 2 years of age.

Risk Factors

- Close exposure to individuals infected with *N. meningitidis*
- Failure to immunize against measles, mumps, and rubella
- Failure to immunize against *H. influenzae* type B
- Varicella infection
- Exposure to mosquitoes, ticks, or sandflies carrying St. Louis or California encephalitis
- Recent upper respiratory infection
- Penetrating head trauma
- Ventriculoperitoneal shunt
- Day-care attendance

Differential Diagnosis

Manifestations of bacterial meningitis may be preceded by several days of upper respiratory tract symptoms. Rapid onset of meningeal symptoms (in less than 1 day) is common with *S. pneumoniae* or *N. meningitidis*, whereas 2 to 3 days may elapse before symptoms occur in patients with *H. influenzae* type B infection. In young infants (younger than 2 months of age), meningeal symptoms may be vague and nonspecific, including irritability, restlessness and poor feeding. Fever or low body temperature usually is present. Older infants and children may exhibit fever, headache, irritability, nausea, vomiting, anorexia, nuchal rigidity, lethargy, diplopia and photophobia. Seizures and coma may occur. On physical examination, patients may demonstrate Kernig's and Brudzinski's signs, lethargy, bulging fontanel, ptosis, focal neurologic signs, petechiae, purpura, papilledema, anisocoria, bradycardia with hypertension, and apnea. Lumbar puncture should be performed on any child who suspected of having meningitis, except when signs (other than a bulging fontanel) of increased intracranial pressure are present. Skin infection at the site of the lumbar puncture, suspicion of a mass lesion, and extreme clinical instability are also reasons to not perform a spinal tap. Following lumbar puncture, CSF should be sent to the laboratory for cell count, glucose, protein, and Gram stain and culture. If fungi, viruses, or other agents are suspected cultures should also be sent for these.

Management

Treatments and medications. Treatment of bacterial meningitis is directed at decreasing the damage to the CNS caused by the inflammatory response; administration of antibiotics as determined by the CSF culture results; and maintenance of systemic and cerebral perfusion. Supportive therapy is directed at reversing shock and treatment of disseminated intravascular coagulation (DIC), inappropriate antidiuretic hormone secretion, seizures, increased intracranial pressure, apnea, dysrhythmias, and coma. Aseptic viral meningitis is usually a benign, self-limited disease. Hospitalization is necessary for young infants and children because of the possibility of bacterial meningitis. Treatment of supportive for viral meningitis, except in cases of herpes simplex virus (HSV), varicella, and herpes zoster, which is treated with acyclovir. Lyme disease is treated with high-dose parenteral ceftriaxone. Headache, which may be severe in all cases of aseptic meningitis, should be treatment with nonsteroidal antiinflammatory drugs (NSAIDS) or narcotics.

Counseling and prevention.

- Chemoprophylaxis with rifampin for family contacts of patients with *N. meningitidis* is recommended.
- Meningococcal vaccine is recommended for at-risk individuals (e.g., those with sickle cell disease, institutionalized persons).
- Routine immunization against *H. influenzae* is recommended for all infants.

Follow-up. Follow-up care for uncomplicated aseptic meningitis is not needed. Children who develop neurologic, cardiac, renal, hematologic, audiologic or other organ system sequelae should be treated by a specialist as recommended.

Consultations and referrals. Consult a physician or send the child to an emergency center immediately if meningitis is suspected

Mumps

Alert

Consult with or refer to a physician for the following:
- Signs of meningitis (e.g., lethargy, anorexia, irritability, stiff neck, Kernig's or Brudzinski's sign, severe headache)
- Signs of an acute condition of the abdomen (e.g., persistent vomiting, pain, tenderness)
- Testicular pain or scrotal swelling

Etiology

Humans are the only known host of mumps, which is caused by a virus spread by direct contact. The incubation period is between 12 and 25 days after exposure. The individual is contagious for as many as 7 days before and as long as 9 days after the onset of symptoms. Mumps infection in adults can be severe.

Incidence

- Infection occurs throughout childhood and rarely during adulthood.
- Mumps infection is more common in late winter and throughout spring.

Risk Factors

- Exposure to infected individuals
- Failure to immunize against the mumps virus

Differential Diagnosis

Submandibular lymphadenitis causes enlarged, erythematous, tender, warm lymph nodes. It may be associated with tonsillitis, dental abscess, or infection.

Preauricular lymphadenitis causes enlarged, erythematous, tender, warm lymph nodes. It may be associated with infection or inflammation of the conjunctivae or eyelids.

Salivary duct obstruction causes swelling and tenderness at the parotid gland.

Epididymitis is an inflammation of the epididymis that causes unilateral scrotal swelling, erythema, and tenderness. Bacterial organisms or viruses are the primary causes.

Mumps is caused by a virus in an unimmunized child. The child may complain of malaise, decreased appetite and activity, pain when chewing, swelling of salivary glands (which may not occur in all cases), scrotal swelling, and pain. The physical examination may reveal a child who appears listless, swelling and tenderness of the salivary glands (may not occur in all cases), scrotal swelling, testicular pain on palpation, abdominal pain on palpation, meningeal signs (15% of all cases), arthralgias (rare), and audiologic impairment (rare).

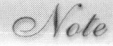
Note

The mumps virus can invade any tissue of the body; therefore one must be aware of symptoms involving the meninges, brain, kidney, testicles, epididymis, pancreas, and ovaries.

Management

Treatments and medications. There is no antiviral therapy available to treat mumps infection. The care is primarily supportive. Acetaminophen may be used to control fever or pain. If salivary gland swelling is present, warm compresses may provide some relief. Pain associated with mastication may be diminished if a soft or liquid diet is provided. Isolation of the hospitalized child is necessary until the swelling and other symptoms have resolved.

Counseling and prevention

- Instruct the parents and child that any food which increases salivary flow (e.g., citrus fruits, spicy foods, candies) should be avoided because this causes pain.
- Instruct parents that a child with an active infection should refrain from attending day care or school until all symptoms have subsided because the period of contagion may persist for as long as 9 days.
- Instruct parents on the benefits of immunizations and advise that their child should be immunized against mumps virus according to the standard immunization schedule.
- Advise that family members exposed to mumps who are not immunized and have not had the virus should be observed for signs and symptoms.

Follow-up. Follow-up care for uncomplicated mumps infection is not required. Children who require physician referral for meningeal, renal, testicular, scrotal, audiologic, or abdominal involvement should be observed until they return to their normal state of health. Specialists (e.g., renal, genitourinary, neurology) may need to follow the child on a long-term basis if various organ systems were involved.

Consultations and referrals

- Consult a physician if mumps is suspected.
- Refer to an emergency center immediately if the child exhibits involvement of various organ systems (see Alert box).
- Report all cases of mumps infection to the health department.
- Notify day-care workers or the school nurse when a case of mumps is diagnosed.

Parasitic Diseases

Alert

Consult with or refer to a physician for the following:
- Signs of dehydration (e.g., poor skin turgor, dry lips, sticky mucous membranes, sunken fontanel)
- Signs of acute condition of the abdomen (e.g., persistent vomiting, pain, tenderness)

Giardiasis and Cryptosporidiosis

Etiology

Giardiasis is caused by a protozoan, and humans are infected by fecal contamination of the water supply. Most infections occur after ingestion of infected food or water, and infection is limited to the intestine or biliary tract. Person-to-person contact has been responsible for transmission of giardiasis in day-care centers. The incubation period is 1 to 4 weeks. *Cryptosporidium* is a protozoan found in numerous hosts, including birds, mammals, reptiles, and humans that causes cryptosporidiosis. Person-to-person transmission occurs, as does transmission from animals to humans and humans to animals. The parasite is not affected by chlorine and can pass through water filters. Contaminated water is also a source of infection. The incubation period is 2 to 14 days.

Incidence

- Depending on the geographic location, serial surveys of stool samples in the United States have shown prevalence rates of 1% to 20% for *Giardia*.
- Most community-wide epidemics of giardiasis are related to contaminated water supplies.
- Giardiasis is the most common intestinal protozoal infection in children in the United States and in most areas worldwide.
- *Cryptosporidium* organisms are a common cause of diarrheal illness in the United States and abroad.

Risk Factors

- Contact with children in day-care centers (especially in areas where children are not toilet trained) or institutions for the mentally retarded

Table 44-5 Differential Diagnosis: Giardiasis and Cryptosporidiosis

CRITERIA	GIARDIASIS	CRYPTOSPORIDIOSIS
ICD-9 code	007.1	007.4
Subjective Data		
History	May be asymptomatic; recent foreign travel, foul-smelling diarrhea or soft stool (may be intermittent), flatulence, poor appetite	Recent foreign travel; low-grade fever; frequent, watery diarrhea; abdominal pain; poor appetite
Objective Data		
Physical examination	Abdominal distension, weight loss, anemia, failure to thrive	Abdominal pain, weight loss, poor skin turgor, sticky mucous membranes
Laboratory data	Stool for ova and parasites positive for *Giardia* organisms	Stool for ova and parasites positive for *Cryptosporidium* organisms; electrolyte imbalance

- Ingestion of unprocessed, contaminated water
- For giardiasis, recent travel to an endemic area
- For giardiasis, patients having cystic fibrosis
- For cryptosporidiosis, persons who routinely handle animals in zoos or in the wild

Differential Diagnosis

Because giardiasis and cryptosporidiosis cause many of the signs and symptoms of diarrheal illness, the differential diagnosis includes all illnesses that cause diarrhea and abdominal pain (Table 44-5). The definitive diagnosis is made when diagnostic tests are obtained and the protozoa are identified (see Treatments and Medications, as well as Diarrhea in Chapter 35).

Management

Treatments and medications. *Giardia* and *Cryptosporidium* organisms are detectable in stool specimens sent for microscopic examination for ova and parasites. Three different stool specimens obtained on different days should be sent to detect infection. Patients with suspected parasitic disease should be placed on enteric precautions. Treatment for these diarrheal diseases includes the measures listed in Box 44-1.

Counseling and prevention

- Warn individuals who are traveling to foreign countries about the potential risks associated with unfiltered and untreated drinking water.
- Instruct parents that children who are infected should refrain from attending day-care facilities until their symptoms have resolved.
- Instruct parents on the signs and symptoms of dehydration.
- Instruct parents on prescribed medications.
- Instruct parents that these protozoans are spread in families by fecal-oral transfer of cysts from the feces of an infected person. Persons are contagious until approximately 2 days after antibiotic therapy has been started.
- Advise parents and caregivers to wash their hands thoroughly after each diaper change.

Follow-up. Children who require hospitalization for dehydration should have a follow-up visit after discharge to ensure weight gain and a return to their previous state of health. Two negative stool cultures should be obtained to determine resolution of the infection.

Box 44-1 Treatments for Giardiasis and Cryptosporidiosis

Giardiasis

Quinacrine hydrochloride (Atabrine) 6 mg/kg per day in three divided doses for 7 days

Furazolidone (Furoxone) 5 to 8 mg/kg per day in four divided doses (maximum of 400 mg/24 hours; child must be older than 1 month of age; only stable suspension)

Metronidazole (Flagyl) 3 to 50 mg/kg per day in three divided doses for 5 to 10 days

Cryptosporidiosis

Supportive care (e.g., intravenous fluids, correction of electrolyte abnormalities)

No specific antibiotic therapy

Consultations and referrals

- Refer to a physician for any child who is severely dehydrated (see the Alert box).
- Notify the day-care center or school nurse when giardiasis or cryptosporidiosis is diagnosed.
- Report to the local health department (as required).

Cysticercosis

Alert

> Consult with or refer to a physician for the following:
> - Signs of retinal detachment (e.g., visual changes, blindness, pain)
> - Signs of acute condition of the abdomen (e.g., persistent vomiting, pain, tenderness)
> - Signs of increased intracranial pressure (e.g., vomiting, headache, dizziness, cranial nerve deficits, visual changes)

Etiology

Cysticercosis (tapeworm infection) is caused by intestinal infestation of several different parasites (of the genus *Cysticercus*). Although most parasites are endemic to countries other than the United States, some infections are acquired here; however, the majority are imported. Beef or pork tapeworm can be transmitted by ingesting undercooked beef or pork.

Incidence

- Cysticercosis is widespread in countries where human feces are used as fertilizer or where disposal of feces is not regulated (e.g., areas of Africa, Central and South America, Europe, Asia).

Risk Factors

- Ingestion of raw or undercooked beef or pork
- Improper disposal of human feces
- Travel to endemic areas

Differential Diagnosis

Tapeworm infestation results in space-occupying lesions in the eyes, muscles, viscera, and brain; therefore conditions that produce symptoms associated with space-occupying lesions must be considered. In the eyes, tapeworm infestation may cause retinal detachment, resulting in visual changes, blindness, and pain. In the muscles, these lesions produce pain and vascular and lymphatic compromise similar to the symptoms associated with soft tissue masses or tumors. In the viscera, space-occupying lesions produce pain and intestinal obstruction that may mimic symptoms of an acute condition of the abdomen (e.g., appendicitis, ileus). In the brain, symptoms associated with increased intracranial pressure are observed, including vomiting, headache, visual changes, and dizziness. These symptoms are also associated with neoplastic disease, arteriovenous (AV) malformations, and brain abscess. The history may reveal recent travel to endemic areas, and segments of tapeworm (proglottids) may be noticed in the child's stool by parents. Associated symptoms may include abdominal pain, diarrhea, increased appetite, headache, visual changes, and muscular pain.

The physical examination may reveal abdominal pain and tenderness on palpation, weight loss (regardless of increased appetite), cranial nerve deficits, gait instability, soft tissue mass, retinal detachment, and blindness. Laboratory data will indicate ova or proglottids in feces or on the perianal skin. (Use the tape method as described in Enterobiasis [Pinworm Infestation].)

Management

Treatments and medications

- Stool examination for evidence of ova or proglottids is necessary.
- Serologic tests are available through the Centers for Disease Control and Prevention (CDC).
- Praziquantel and albendazole, broad-spectrum anthelmintics, have become the treatments of choice for cysticercosis.
- Patients with neurocysticercosis require hospitalization for observation of neurologic status.

Counseling and prevention. Instruct parents that contact with human waste is necessary for transmission of tapeworm. It is also important to cook all pork and beef thoroughly to prevent transmission of the encased parasites.

Follow-up. Periodic diagnostic imaging (computed tomography [CT] scan or magnetic resonance imaging [MRI] scan) is required for patients with ocular, muscular, visceral, or intracranial involvement. Office visits should be scheduled following the scans to discuss the results and perform a physical examination. Children with tapeworm infestation may require follow-up care by a multidisciplinary team, depending on which organ systems are involved.

Consultations and referrals

- Provide immediate referral to a physician for any child with signs of retinal detachment, intestinal obstruction, or increased intracranial pressure (see the Alert box).
- Refer patients with suspected tapeworm infection to a physician for treatment.

Ascariasis

Alert

> Consult with or refer to a physician for the following:
> - Signs of respiratory distress (e.g., wheezing, crackles or rhonchi, nasal flaring, retractions, cyanosis)
> - Signs of an acute condition of the abdomen (e.g., persistent vomiting, pain, tenderness)

Etiology

Ascaris lumbricoides is a roundworm that infects humans and causes ascariasis. The adult worm lives in the intestines, and the female lays 200,000 eggs per day. The eggs are excreted in the stool and require incubation in the soil for 2 to 3 weeks to become infectious. Infection occurs after ingestion of the eggs.

Incidence

- Ascaris is common in areas where human feces are used as fertilizer or where there is poor sanitation. It is more prevalent in tropical areas.
- *A. lumbricoides* is the most common parasitic worm in humans worldwide.
- In the United States, *A. lumbricoides* is second only to pinworms as most common parasitic worm.

Risk Factors

- Improper disposal of human feces
- Travel to endemic areas

Differential Diagnosis

Refer to Table 44-6.

Management

Treatments and medications. Visual identification of worms in emesis or at the anus, or stool specimens for ova and parasites, confirm infestation with ascaris, although suspected infection should be treated without laboratory confirmation. Anthelmintics (e.g., albendazole, mebendazole [Vermox], levamisole, pyrantel pamoate [Antiminth]) are given to eradicate the infestation.

Treatment of intestinal obstruction is primarily supportive because it commonly resolves without surgical intervention. Nasogastric suction, fluid and electrolyte management, and close observation are appropriate measures. If the patient's condition worsens, surgical correction may be required.

Counseling and prevention

- Instruct parents that sanitary disposal of feces is necessary to prevent transmission. Special attention should be paid to disposal of diapers from infected infants.
- Dispel myths regarding the source of infection (e.g., nocturnal grinding of teeth, sleeping in a knee-chest position).

Follow-up. Stool specimens for ova and parasites examined 3 to 4 weeks after therapy may be helpful in determining whether infection has resolved. Uncomplicated ascariasis does not require further follow-up care. Children with respiratory or intestinal complications may need periodic follow-up until they have attained their previous state of health.

Consultations and referrals

- Provide immediate referral to a physician for any child with signs of respiratory distress or intestinal obstruction (see the Alert box).
- Notify day-care workers or the school nurse when ascariasis is diagnosed.

Hookworm Disease

Alert

Consult with or refer to a physician for the following:
- Severe anemia
- Signs of respiratory distress (e.g., wheezing, crackles or rhonchi, nasal flaring, retractions, cyanosis)
- Signs of acute condition of the abdomen (e.g., persistent vomiting, pain, tenderness

Etiology

Hookworm disease is caused by infestation with one of two different worms, *Ancylostoma duodenale* and *Necator americanus*. These worms can be found worldwide. Larvae can remain infective in damp soil for several weeks (though for a shorter period in dry areas). The larvae penetrate skin in contact with contaminated soil (primarily the soles of the feet) or are ingested through the digestive system.

Incidence

- Hookworm disease is primarily found in Europe, the Mediterranean, Asia, South America, sub-Saharan Africa, the Western Hemisphere, and many Pacific islands.
- It is more common in deprived areas where shoes are not commonly worn.

Risk Factors

- Improper disposal of human feces, which may cause soil contamination
- Walking barefoot in high-risk areas
- Travel to endemic areas

Table 44-6 Differential Diagnosis: *Ascaris*

CRITERIA	ASCARIS	PNEUMONIA	ACUTE APPENDICITIS*
ICD-9 code	127.0	486.	540.9
Subjective Data			
History	Recent travel to endemic areas; may be asymptomatic; abdominal pain; cough; fever; vomiting: may be bilious; worms seen in emesis (common) or expelled from the anus (rare)	Fever, cough, wheezing, abdominal pain, decreased appetite, malaise	Fever, severe abdominal pain, malaise, vomiting, constipation
Objective data			
Physical examination	May be asymptomatic; fever; adventitious breath sounds (e.g., wheezing, crackles, rhonchi); abdominal tenderness and rigidity; jaundice	Fever, cough, wheezing, respiratory distress, weight loss	Fever, abdominal rigidity, and tenderness (usually right upper quadrant), abdominal guarding
Laboratory data	Eosinophilia; stool specimen for ova and parasites confirms infestation with *Ascaris*	Chest radiograph reveals infiltration	Elevated white blood cell count

*Immediate referral to a physician.

Differential Diagnosis

The diagnosis may include iron-deficiency anemia, which is an abnormally low hemoglobin level caused by nutritional iron deficit, or pneumonia, a viral or bacterial infection of the lungs characterized by fever, cough, wheezing, and respiratory distress. The history may reveal recent travel to endemic areas. The patient may be asymptomatic, or associated symptoms may include intense pruritus (usually soles of feet and between toes), abdominal pain and tenderness, and cough.

The physical examination may be unremarkable, or the patient may show weight loss. There may be adventitious breath sounds (e.g., wheezing, crackles, rhonchi) during auscultation in heavily infected individuals. Laboratory data may indicate hypochromic, microcytic anemia; eosinophilia; guaiac-positive stool; and hookworm eggs (identified on microscopic examination of stool specimen).

Management

Treatments and medications. Examination of stool specimens under the microscope reveals hookworm eggs. Adult worms are rarely seen. Pyrantel pamoate 11 mg/kg (maximum dose of 1 g) daily for 3 days or mebendazole 100 mg twice a day for 3 days is the treatment of choice. Treatment may be repeated if necessary. Iron supplementation or blood transfusion in severe cases may be required to correct the associated anemia.

Counseling and prevention
- Instruct parents that sanitary disposal of feces is necessary to prevent transmission.
- Recommend wearing shoes in high-risk areas to prevent infection with hookworm, but this may not be possible in economically deprived areas.
- Provide caregivers with explicit instructions regarding administration of medications.

Follow-up. Hemoglobin or hematocrit should be monitored until the associated anemia has resolved. Otherwise, follow-up care of uncomplicated hookworm infection is not required.

Consultations and referrals. Provide immediate referral to a physician for children with severe anemia or respiratory distress (see the Alert box).

Enterobiasis (Pinworm Infestation)

Etiology

Enterobiasis, or pinworm infestation, is caused by a nematode, *Enterobius vermicularis*. It is distributed worldwide and has no gender predilection. Female nematodes deposit eggs on the perianal skin, and autoinfection, as well as transmission from another infected individual, is common.

Incidence

- There is no seasonal variation in incidence.
- Preschool and school-age children are most often infected and often transmit infection to other family members.

Risk Factors

- Children in day-care settings and schools
- Household or institutional contacts with an infected child

Differential Diagnosis

The clinical presentation of pinworm infestation is distinctively different from other parasitic infections and therefore limits the differential diagnosis to conditions that cause intense itching in the perianal or vaginal area. (See Chapter 35, Perianal Itch and Pain, and Chapter 40, Vulvovaginal Symptoms.) Vaginal candidiasis is a monilial infection involving the vagina, which causes erythema, white discharge, and intense pruritus. Hemorrhoids are varicose veins located in the rectum or anus, causing burning and itching.

In regard to enterobiasis, the history may reveal intense itching (primarily around the anus, less often around the vulva) and vaginal discharge. Findings on physical examination may include an excoriated anal area and purulent vaginal discharge (which may be bloody).

Management

Treatments and medications. The most effective method of obtaining pinworm eggs for diagnosis is to apply a piece of transparent tape to the perianal skin at bedtime. The tape is removed the next morning before washing and subsequently examined under a microscope to identify pinworm ova. The treatment of choice is mebendazole 100 mg (regardless of weight), treatment to be repeated in 2 weeks. An alternative treatment is a single dose of pyrantel pamoate 11 mg/kg (maximum dose of 1 g). If infestation persists, reevaluate for possible retreatment. Use of these drugs should be limited in children less than 2 years of age, and all household contacts should be treated as well.

Counseling and prevention
- Instruct parents that there are no specific cleansing measures to be employed in the treatment of pinworm infection.
- Inform parents that pinworm infection is not a reflection of personal hygiene and that they should not feel guilty.
- Give explicit medication instruction to caregivers.
- Advise parents that because of the high infectivity, recurrence is common.

Follow-up. Usually none is indicated.

Consultations and referrals. Consult a physician if the infection does not respond to treatment or if a secondary skin infection arises from intense scratching.

Pertussis (Whooping Cough)

Alert

Consult with or refer to a physician for the following:
- Infants younger than 6 months of age with suspected pertussis infection, because these patients require hospitalization most frequently and have the highest mortality
- Respiratory distress or cyanosis
- Decreased oral intake resulting in dehydration

Etiology

Pertussis is caused by infection with *Bordetella pertussis*. Humans are the only known hosts of pertussis, and infection occurs following person-to-person contact via aerosolized droplets from the respiratory tract. Infants and children frequently acquire the illness from an infected adolescent or adult. The incubation period is 6 to 20 days. Infectivity is highest in the catarrhal stage.

Incidence

- The incidence of pertussis has decreased since the advent of pertussis vaccine in the 1940s.
- About 35% of cases occur in infants less than 6 months of age, and these children have the highest mortality.
- Periodic outbreaks occur.

Risk Factors

- Failure to appropriately immunize an infant or child against pertussis
- Direct person-to-person contact with an infected individual

Differential Diagnosis

Refer to Table 44-7, and see Cough in Chapter 41.

Management

Treatments and medications. Erythromycin is the antimicrobial agent of choice, and therapy should be started as soon as the diagnosis of pertussis is suspected (40 to 50 mg/kg divided four times a day for 14 days [maximum dosage of 2 g/day]). If therapy is started in the catarrhal phase, it is likely that the course of illness will not progress to the paroxysmal phase. Once the infant or child has reached the paroxysmal phase, erythromycin primarily prevents the spread of illness.

Hospitalized children should remain in isolation until they have received 5 days of erythromycin. Children who are managed on an outpatient basis should refrain from attending day care or school until they have had 5 days of erythromycin therapy.

Supportive treatment may be required for infants and children who are unable to tolerate oral intake because of the persistent coughing episodes. These children may require hospitalization for hydration. During the paroxysmal coughing episodes hypoxemia is common. Infants and children who are hospitalized may benefit from supplemental oxygen. Some children require intensive care management for severe cases of pertussis.

Counseling and prevention

- Instruct parents that pertussis is very easily transmitted because infection occurs following person-to-person contact via aerosolized droplets from the respiratory tract. The period of highest infectivity is during the catarrhal stage.
- It is important to stress the benefit of pertussis immunization with parents. Acellular pertussis vaccines are now used in combination with diphtheria and tetanus toxoids (DTaP), and do not cause the same complications as are associated with the whole-cell pertussis vaccine (see Chapter 13).
- For infants and children who contract pertussis and are not hospitalized, teach parents the signs of complications (e.g., respiratory failure, dehydration) so that they are prepared to seek emergency medical attention.

Follow-up. Children managed on an outpatient basis should have one follow-up visit after the period of contagiousness has

Table 44-7 Differential Diagnosis: Pertussis

CRITERIA	PERTUSSIS*	CROUP	UPPER RESPIRATORY TRACT INFECTION	PNEUMONIA
ICD-9 code	033.9	464.4	465.9	486.
Subjective Data				
Fever	Usually no fever	No fever or mild fever	No fever	Fever
Description of cough	Mild upper respiratory tract infection symptoms with cough for approximately 2 weeks (catarrhal stage); severe coughing episodes in the paroxysmal stage	"Barking cough"	Dry cough	Cough with acute onset
Associated symptoms	Vomiting, decreased oral intake; parents report that sucking from a bottle precipitates a coughing episode; poor feeding		Rhinorrhea, sneezing	Coryza, hoarseness
Immunization history	Inadequate or unvaccinated for pertussis	Usually current	Usually current	Usually current
Objective Data				
Physical examination				
Fever	No fever	No fever or mild fever	No fever	Fever
Cough	Paroxysmal coughing episodes associated with an inspiratory whoop	"Barking" cough	Dry cough	Wet cough
Associated findings	Face becomes red with coughing and then cyanotic; seizure activity		Rhinorrhea, sneezing	Wheezing, crackle; respiratory distress and respiratory failure may develop
Laboratory data				Chest radiograph indicates infiltrate

*Refer to a physician.

passed. Those who are hospitalized should be observed until they have reached their previous state of health. Infants and children who have lost weight with the illness should have periodic weight checks to ensure appropriate weight gain in the convalescent period.

Consultations and referrals
- Provide immediate referral to a physician for infants 6 months of age or younger (see the Alert box).
- Refer to a physician any infant or child under 5 years of age who is suspected of having a pertussis infection.
- Report all cases of pertussis infection to the health department.
- Notify day-care workers or the school nurse when a case of pertussis is diagnosed.

Poliovirus Infections

Alert

Consult with or refer to a physician for the following:
- Meningeal signs and symptoms (e.g., lethargy, anorexia, irritability, stiff neck, vomiting, Kernig's or Brudzinski's sign, severe headache)
- Signs of paralysis (e.g., weakness, decreased deep tendon reflexes, intense muscle pain, urinary incontinence, respiratory difficulty)

Etiology

Polioviruses are types of enteroviruses. Poliovirus infections occur in humans and are transmitted by the fecal-oral or (possibly) respiratory route. When a susceptible person comes into contact with a poliovirus, one of three responses occur: (1) nonspecific febrile illness (most frequent), (2) aseptic meningitis (nonparalytic poliomyelitis), or (3) paralytic poliomyelitis (least frequent). Paralytic poliomyelitis is the only type that is clinically identifiable as a poliovirus and accounts for 1% to 2% of infections during epidemics. The incubation period to onset of paralysis is 4 to 21 days. The greatest communicability occurs directly before and after onset of symptoms. The virus persists in the throat for about 1 week but may be excreted in the stool for weeks to months after the infection. Mild cases may involve only one side, and once the fever subsides, no further paralysis is likely to develop.

Incidence

- Infection with poliovirus occurs more often in infants and young children.
- Infection occurs more commonly in conditions of poor hygiene.
- Currently, poliovirus infection is very rare in the United States. The most recent outbreak occurred in 1979 in a group of individuals who refused immunization.
- Live oral poliovirus vaccine (OPV) has been associated with paralytic disease. The incidence is one case per 7.8 million doses of OPV distributed. The greatest risk of paralysis occurs with the first dose of OPV.

Risk Factors

- Failure to appropriately immunize against poliovirus
- Infection via the fecal-oral route in immunocompromised patients

Differential Diagnosis

Refer to Table 44-8.

Management
Poliomyelitis
Treatments and medications. Treatment of poliovirus infection is primarily supportive. Acetaminophen or ibuprofen may be used to treat fever. If paralysis ensues, respiratory support may be necessary. Physical therapy may be required to manage the deficits associated with weakness or paralysis.

Counseling and prevention. Immunization according to recommended guidelines is paramount in preventing poliovirus infection. The American Academy of Pediatrics (AAP) recommends the use of an all inactivated poliovirus vaccine (IPV) schedule for routine immunization of children in the United States (see Chapter 13).

It is very important to limit contact between immunosuppressed children and persons recently vaccinated with OPV, because the fecal-oral route of transmission can result in paralytic poliovirus infection. Children who are due for immunization and reside in the same household with immunocompromised individuals (e.g., those with HIV or severe combined immune deficiency, persons receiving cancer chemotherapy or prolonged corticosteroid therapy) should receive IPV according to the AAP guidelines and avoid the risk of exposing others to poliovirus.

Follow-up. Children who have paralytic poliovirus require close follow-up care by a multidisciplinary team to prevent further complications.

Consultations and referrals
- Provide immediate referral to a physician for any child suspected of having poliovirus infection.
- Report cases of poliovirus to the health department.
- Contact the school nurse or day-care center.

Table 44-8 Differential Diagnosis: Poliomyelitis

CRITERIA	POLIOMYELITIS*	MENINGITIS*
ICD-9 code	045.90	322.9
Subjective Data		
Immunization history	History of inadequate polio immunization or recent immunization	Up to date
Associated symptoms	Fever, muscle weakness, anxiety, urinary incontinence, headache, stiff neck	Lethargy, irritability, vomiting, stiff neck, anorexia
Objective Data		
Physical examination	Fever, Kernig or Brudzinski sign, decreased superficial or deep tendon reflexes, progressive weakness, respiratory difficulty (e.g., increased respiratory rate, inability to speak without frequent pauses)	Lethargy, irritability, stiff neck, weight loss, Kernig or Brudzinski sign

Immediate referral to a physician.

Reye Syndrome

Alert

Consult with or refer to a physician for the following:
- Signs of meningitis or encephalitis (e.g., full, tense or bulging fontanelle; lethargy, anorexia, irritability, high-pitched cry; stiff neck, Kernig's or Brudzinski's sign, severe headache.
- Any suspected case of Reye Syndrome (e.g., symptoms of protracted vomiting; confusion, combative behavior, agitation, stupor, coma), which must be referred to an emergency center immediately.

Etiology

Reye syndrome is characterized by encephalopathy and the noninflammatory fatty infiltration of the liver and kidney. Development of Reye syndrome has been associated with epidemics of influenza A or B and varicella. Administration of aspirin in conjunction with one of these viral illnesses predisposes a patient to this condition.

Incidence

- This condition occurs most commonly in school-age children
- The incidence of Reye Syndrome has decreased dramatically as aspirin-containing products are avoided in children with influenza, viral illness, or varicella

Risk Factors

- Taking aspirin and aspirin-containing products during a case of viral illness

Differential Diagnosis

Clinical manifestations of Reye syndrome begin with intractable vomiting during or immediately following recovery from an upper respiratory tract infection. Over a period of several hours to a more than a day, the child becomes confused, combative, agitated, stuporous, and eventually comatose. In addition to the altered level of consciousness (LOC), physical findings include dilated pupils, hyperactive deep tendon reflexes, and respiratory changes. The liver is normal in size or may be moderately enlarged. Jaundice is not present. Serum transaminase and ammonia levels are elevated, and the prothrombin time may be prolonged. Hypoglycemia and acidosis may also be present. CSF examination is normal. Definitive diagnosis of Reye syndrome is made by liver biopsy. Children and infants under 2 years of age should also be evaluated for inborn errors of metabolism.

Management

Treatments and medications. Treatment of Reye syndrome is supportive and includes intravenous hydration to prevent hypoglycemia and dehydration, central venous pressure monitoring, intracranial pressure monitoring and treatment of increased intracranial pressure as needed (with mannitol and hyperventilation), frequent assessment of laboratory parameters, and administration of vitamin K or fresh frozen plasma to improve clotting ability.

Counseling and prevention. The prognosis of Reye syndrome correlates with the depth and length of the comatose state. Death is usually due to increased intracranial pressure and not liver failure. Prevention is possible by avoiding aspirin or aspirin-containing products during viral illnesses.

Follow-up. Children who develop neurologic sequelae should be followed by a specialist as recommended.

Consultation and referrals. Consult a physician, or send the child to an emergency center immediately if Reye syndrome is suspected.

Roseola

Alert

Consult with or refer to a physician for the following:
- Signs of meningitis or encephalitis (e.g., full, tense, or bulging fontanel; lethargy, anorexia, irritability, high-pitched cry; stiff neck, Kernig's or Brudzinski's sign, severe headache)
- Febrile seizures

Etiology

Roseola (exanthem subitum, or sixth disease) is caused by human herpesvirus 6. The mode of transmission is not known, and the incubation period is estimated to be 5 to 15 days. The infected individual is thought to be contagious during the febrile period before the appearance of the rash.

Incidence

- This is a common, acute, febrile illness in infants and toddlers.
- This most commonly occurs in children 6 to 24 months of age.
- Infection after 4 years of age is rare.
- Most cases occur in the spring or summer months.

Risk Factors

- Exposure to infected individuals
- Day-care settings

Differential Diagnosis

Roseola is an acute viral infection (Table 44-9). It occurs in children 6 months to 3 years of age. There is an acute onset of fever with a temperature of up to 105° F (40.6°C), which can last up to 8 days (average duration is 4 days). Fever abruptly disappears with the onset of a pink, maculopapular rash (over 10% to 29% of the body) that begins on the trunk and spreading to the face, neck, and extremities. The lesions are nonpruritic and discrete and disappear in 1 to 2 days. There is no desquamation.

Scarlet fever, or *scarlatina*, is an acute infectious disease usually caused by a circulating toxin produced by group A β-hemolytic streptococcus (GABHS). This is rare in children under 2 years of age, with the highest incidence in those from 6 to 12 years of age. Usually there is an acute onset of fever, pharyngitis, and headache. On physical examination a "strawberry tongue" and red pharynx may be noted. A rash appears within 48 hours after infection and appears as diffuse pin-size eruptions on an erythematous base. It blanches with pressure, has a "sandpaper" texture, and desquamates in 1 to 2 weeks. Complete resolution takes approximately 3 weeks. The rash appears on the neck, axilla, and inguinal areas before quickly becoming generalized. The patient may appear flushed and have circumoral pallor. Throat culture will be positive for GABHS.

Rubella is caused by an ribonucleic acid (RNA) virus. History reveals a lack of or inadequate rubella immunization. Postauricular and occipital lymphadenopathy is common. Rash and fever usually appear together. The rash is mild and maculopapular, rapidly spreads from the face to the extremities, and resolves by the fourth day. (See Rash in Chapter 37.)

Table 44-9 Differential Diagnosis: Roseola

CRITERIA	ROSEOLA	SCARLET FEVER	RUBELLA
ICD-9 code	057.8	034.1	056.9
Subjective Data			
Age	6 to 24 months	Any	Any
Fever	Abrupt onset of high fever (temperature of 102° F to 105° F) lasting about 7 days	Fever present	Mild fever
Rash	Parents report that appearance of the rash follows defervescence	Parents or child report pruritic rash, which occurs with fever	Parents or child reports rash occurring with fever
Associated symptoms	Usually playful with normal appetite	Listless; sore throat	Listless
Objective Data			
Physical examination			
Fever	High fever precedes rash	Moderate fever	Mild fever
Rash	Erythematous, maculopapular rash	Pinpoint pruritic rash	Maculopapular rash
Associated signs	Child does not usually appear toxic	Listless; erythematous throat with enlarged tonsils	Listless; postauricular and suboccipital lymphadenitis
Laboratory data		Throat culture positive for GABHS	Rubella titer: Inadequate antibodies

Management

Treatments and medications. Diagnostic tests to confirm the diagnosis of roseola are not commercially available, and there is no specific management or treatment. Acetaminophen or ibuprofen may be used to control the associated fever. Isolation of the child is not necessary.

Counseling and prevention

- Instruct parents that roseola is a normal, acute childhood illness and that the period of contagion is during the febrile stage before the onset of the rash.
- Reassure parents that the fever and rash will resolve spontaneously.
- Instruct parents to call or return if the child worsens.
- Instruct parents on fever control.

Follow-up. No specific follow-up is necessary unless the child exhibits associated febrile seizures.

Consultations and referrals

- Refer to a physician immediately any child with signs of meningeal involvement or febrile seizures.
- Notify day-care personnel regarding the diagnosis.

Rubella (German Measles)

Alert

Consult with or refer to a physician for the following:
- Severe headache
- Inconsolable
- Lethargy
- Bulging fontanel
- High fever
- Purpura
- High-pitched cry
- Stiff neck
- Anorexia
- Persistent vomiting
- Photophobia
- Pregnancy

Etiology

Rubella virus is classified as a rubivirus and is transmitted postnatally via contact from nasopharyngeal secretions. Most cases occur in late winter to early spring, although the risk of contracting the disease has declined dramatically since the advent of the rubella vaccine. Before vaccine development, most cases of rubella occurred in children. However, in the postvaccine era the majority of cases have occurred in unvaccinated adolescents and young adults. The incubation period ranges from 14 to 21 days. The period of contagion is thought to be 1 to 2 days before appearance of the rash and 5 to 7 days afterwards. Fetal infection with rubella virus usually results in the death of the fetus or development of a syndrome of congenital anomalies (congenital rubella).

Incidence

- The incidence of rubella infection has declined by more than 99% since the prevaccine era.
- Rubella infection is extremely uncommon, although serologic surveys show that 10% to 20% of young adults are susceptible to the virus.

Risk Factors

- Failure to immunize against rubella virus
- Exposure of susceptible postpubertal girls or women who are pregnant

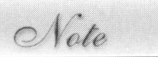

Note

Children who were not identified as having congenital rubella at birth may be noted to have features of the disorder in later childhood or at time of school entry.

Differential Diagnosis

The differential diagnosis of postnatally acquired rubella includes all erythematous, maculopapular rashes (Table 44-10). (See also Rash in Chapter 37.)

Table 44-10 Differential Diagnosis: Postnatal or Congenital Rubella

CRITERIA	POSTNATAL RUBELLA	CONGENITAL RUBELLA*
ICD-9 code	647.50	771.0
Subjective Data		
Exposure and immunization history	Known exposure to rubella in an unimmunized host	Known exposure to rubella in an unimmunized pregnant female
Associated findings	Parents or child report that rash begins on the face and spreads rapidly over the entire body within 24 hours; rash begins to fade on day 2 and is nearly resolved by day 3; minimal fever; transient polyarthralgia (more common in females, adolescents, young adults); malaise, decreased appetite	
Objective Data		
Physical examination	Erythematous, maculopapular, discrete rash; suboccipital and postauricular lymphadenopathy; minimal fever; transient polyarthralgia; thrombocytopenia (rare); purpura (rare); meningeal signs (rare)	Congenital anomalies including cataracts, glaucoma, patent ductus arteriosus, atrial or ventricular septal defects, sensorineural deafness, neurologic deficits and mental retardation, failure to thrive, organomegaly, thrombocytopenia, jaundice, purpura ("blueberry muffin" skin lesions), thyroid disorders, insulin-dependent diabetes

*Refer to a physician.

Toxoplasma infection, infectious mononucleosis, and enteroviral illnesses all cause suboccipital and posterior auricular lymphadenopathy.

Management

Postnatal rubella

Treatments and medications. Confirmation of infection by serologic testing may be helpful in identifying a patient with postnatal infection. Rubella virus is also isolated through nasopharyngeal or throat swabs, urine, and CSF. The diagnosis of congenital rubella infection is difficult after the child has reached the age of 1 year because these studies are no longer diagnostic.

Management of uncomplicated rubella infection is primarily supportive, with the focus on bed rest, fever control, and pain management. Acetaminophen and ibuprofen may be used for fever and arthralgias. Children who contract postnatal rubella infection should be isolated for 7 days after the appearance of the rash. Children with congenital rubella may shed the virus until they are over 1 year of age unless urine and nasopharyngeal cultures are negative before that time.

Counseling and prevention. Children who are known to be infected, either postnatally or with congenital rubella, should avoid contact with susceptible persons, including women of childbearing age. Instruct parents of these children about the potential risk of exposing pregnant women to their infected child. Individuals are contagious 1 to 2 days before onset of the rash and 5 to 7 days thereafter.

Rubella virus vaccine protects 98% of those immunized. The vaccination is given in conjunction with the recommended two-dose measles vaccine at ages 12 to 15 months and 4 to 6 years. The incidence of rubella infection in adolescents and women of childbearing age is primarily due to deficient immunization. A history of clinical infection is unreliable and should not be considered as evidence of immunity.

Follow-up. Follow-up care for uncomplicated rubella infection is not indicated. Children who have required treatment for thrombocytopenic purpura or rubella encephalitis should be observed until platelet counts normalize and the children have returned to their previous state of health.

Consultations and referrals

- Provide immediate referral to a physician for any child exhibiting encephalopathy or meningeal signs and symptoms (see the Alert box).
- Remember that an exposed, susceptible pregnant woman must be referred for obstetric management, because she will require a determination of rubella antibody.
- Keep in mind that children with congenital rubella infection and subsequent development of chronic neurologic, audiologic, cardiac, or developmental problems are best managed by a multidisciplinary team approach.
- Report all cases of rubella infection to the health department.
- Notify day-care workers or the school nurse when a case of rubella is diagnosed.

Rubeola (Measles)

Alert

Consult with or refer to a physician for the following:
- Respiratory distress
- Croup
- Severe headache
- Lethargy
- Persistent vomiting
- Anorexia
- Confusion
- Dehydration
- Full, tense, or bulging fontanel

Etiology

Rubeola (measles) is a viral disease of humans transmitted by direct contact. In recent years the incidence of measles has increased because of failure to immunize preschool children, as well as outbreaks in adolescents and young adults who were vaccinated appropriately at the time but did not receive the second vaccine according to current guidelines. Infected individuals are contagious from 3 to 5 days before the appearance of the rash to 4 days after the appearance of the rash. Symptoms including fever, cough, malaise, coryza, and conjunctivitis, and Koplik's spots are present before the rash appears. The incubation period is between 8 and 12 days from exposure to onset of symptoms.

Incidence

- Since the development of the measles vaccine, there has been a 95% reduction in the reported incidence of measles.
- Winter and spring are the seasons of peak incidence in individuals who are unvaccinated.

Risk Factors

- Exposure to an infected individual
- Failure to appropriately immunize against the measles virus

Differential Diagnosis

Differential diagnosis includes all diseases in which a maculopapular, erythematous rash occurs (see Rash in Chapter 37). However, the appearance of a brown, intense rash following cough, coryza, and conjunctivitis should set measles apart from the other exanthems.

Rubeola, or *9-day measles,* is characterized by acute onset of fever, coryza, cough, and conjunctivitis, as well as a confluent, erythematous, brownish maculopapular rash that develops 3 to 4 days after the initial symptoms and progresses in a caudal direction. Malaise and anorexia may be present. Immunization status is inadequate for measles. The physical examination may reveal fever, coryza, cough, and conjunctivitis; presence of Koplik spots on the buccal mucosa before the appearance of the rash; confluent, maculopapular exanthem generalized over body; otitis media; and crackles or rhonchi (clinical or radiographic evidence of pneumonia). To determine the diagnosis, laboratory data should show measles-specific IgM antibody.

Management

Treatments and medications. There is no specific treatment available for the measles virus, although IgG can be given to prevent or modify the course of disease if given within 6 days of exposure (dose of 0.25 ml/kg intramuscularly; maximum of 15 ml). Supportive care measures are necessary. Bed rest and adequate hydration are important. Acetaminophen or ibuprofen may be used to control fever, while cough may be managed with antitussive agents and a cool-mist vaporizer. Antibiotics are not necessary unless a secondary bacterial infection ensues.

Otitis media is the most common complication of measles infection and may be treated with the same antibiotics as for standard otitis media. If the patient is hospitalized, respiratory isolation is necessary for 4 days following the onset of the rash to prevent exposure of other susceptible individuals.

Counseling and prevention. Measles vaccine protects 95% of those immunized. By 12 years of age, children should have received two doses of live measles vaccine. Parents must be educated regarding the importance of measles vaccination. A history of clinical measles infection is unreliable, so unless there is documented physician- or practitioner-diagnosed measles, laboratory evidence of measles immunity, or documented immunization, one cannot presume that immunity is present.

Instruct parents that individuals are contagious until 4 days after the rash appeared.

Follow-up. Follow-up care for uncomplicated measles is not necessary. Children who have been treated for pneumonia or otitis media or required hospitalization for associated complications should have follow-up visits until they have returned to their normal state of health.

Consultations and referrals

- Immediately refer any child with meningeal signs, respiratory distress, or dehydration to the nearest emergency center.
- Refer all cases of rubeola infection to the health department.
- Notify day-care workers or the school nurse when a case of rubeola is diagnosed.

Scabies

Alert

Consult with or refer to a physician for the following:
- Infants
- Pregnant girls or women

Etiology

Scabies is caused by a mite, *Sarcoptes scabiei,* that affects humans. Transmission occurs by close personal contact with an infected individual or with infected clothing or linens. Scabies is very contagious because there are a large number of mites in the exfoliating skin. The incubation period in persons without previous exposure is 4 to 6 weeks. In those with previous exposure, symptoms develop in 1 to 4 days.

Incidence

- Scabies occurs worldwide in 15- to 30-year cycles.
- Scabies affects persons of all socioeconomic levels without regard to age, gender, or personal hygiene.

Risk Factors

- Close personal contact with an infected individual

Differential Diagnosis

A diagnosis of dermatitis should be considered when making a diagnosis of scabies (Table 44-11). Dermatitis is inflammation of the skin characterized by erythema, pruritus, and various skin lesions.

Management

Treatments and medications. Effective management involves treating the entire household at one time, because untreated family members may cause reinfection. The treatment of choice is 5% permethrin (Elimite). For many years the treatment of choice was application of lindane lotion (1%). However, there is concern regarding the potential for neurotoxicity if absorption is increased. High levels of lindane occur in infants with decreased body fat and in individuals with areas of broken skin. Lindane lotion cannot be used in pregnant or nursing women and should be used in others with great caution.

Table 44-12 summarizes agents used in the treatment of scabies. Oral medications may be required to control itching. These include hydroxyzine hydrochloride (Atarax) 0.6 mg/kg per dose every 6 hours or diphenhydramine (Benadryl) 5 mg/kg per day

divided every 6 hours (maximum dosages of 150 mg/24 hours in children weighing less than 9 kg (20 lbs), and 300 mg/24 hours in children weighing greater than 9 kg).

Counseling and prevention

- Instruct that avoidance of infected individuals is the only way to prevent contracting the mite.
- Emphasize that scabies can infect persons of any socioeconomic group, age, or gender, regardless of the state of personal hygiene.
- Inform parents and caregivers that scabies is very contagious and transmission occurs through close personal contact with an infected individual.
- Instruct parents that all bedding and clothing must be washed in hot water and dried in a dryer on the hot cycle. Nonwashable items should be stored in sealed plastic bags for 4 days. Mites cannot survive longer than 4 days without skin contact.
- Instruct on the importance of treating all household members.
- Inform parents that the child should not return to day care or school until treatment is completed.
- Instruct parents to observe for signs and symptoms of secondary infections and call if they develop.

Follow-up. Follow-up care for uncomplicated scabies infection is not indicated. If an infant or child is treated for a secondary bacterial infection, follow-up care may be necessary.

Consultations and referrals

- Refer to a physician any infants and pregnant girls or women.
- Notify day-care personnel or the school nurse regarding diagnosed cases of scabies.

Tetanus

Alert

Consult with or refer to a physician for the following:
- Generalized muscle spasms
- Muscle rigidity

Etiology

Clostridium tetani produces an endotoxin that binds to the CNS structures. It is present in animal and human intestines and throughout the environment. Tetanus is not transmitted by

Table 44-11 Differential Diagnosis: Scabies

CRITERIA	SCABIES
ICD-9 code	133.0
Subjective Data	
Less than 2 years of age	Parents report itching; may precede appearance of the rash by several weeks; presence of a vesicular rash most commonly on the head, neck, palms, and soles
2 Years of age and older	Parents or child report intense itching; may precede appearance of the rash by several weeks; presence of a papular rash most commonly between the fingers, flexor aspects of the wrists, extensor surfaces of the elbows, axillary folds, belt line, thighs, navel, penis, nipples, abdomen, other aspects of feet, and lower part of the buttocks
Objective Data	
Less than 2 years of age	Observe intense itching; presence of a vesicular rash most commonly on the head, neck, palms, and soles; secondary infection may be present if scratching the lesions has caused skin breakdown
2 Years of age and older	Observe intense itching; presence of a papular rash most commonly between the fingers, flexor aspects of the wrists, extensor surfaces of the elbows, axillary folds, belt line, thighs, navel, penis, nipples, abdomen, other aspects of feet, and lower part of the buttocks; secondary infection may be present if scratching the lesions has caused skin breakdown

Table 44-12 Selected Scabicidal Agents

AGENT	APPLICATION	COMMENTS
Permethrin 5% (Elimite)	Apply to dry skin from the chin down to the toes; in babies, apply to the scalp and forehead as well; leave on for 8 to 12 hours before washing	Treatment of choice
Lindane 1% (Kwell, Scabene)	Apply to dry skin from the chin down to the toes (cannot be used in infants under 2 years of age); keep in mind the CDC recommends use of other scabicides for children under 10 years of age; leave on for 8 to 12 hours before washing	Potential for neurotoxicity if misused
Crotamiton 10% (Eurax)	Apply from the chin down to the toes; reapply at 24 hours; wash off at 72 hours	Least effective; does have antipruritic effect

person-to-person contact but through wounds in the skin, where the organism multiplies and toxin is released. Neonatal tetanus is common in countries where women do not routinely receive tetanus immunizations. The incubation period is 3 to 21 days; in neonates, it is 5 to 14 days.

Incidence

- Tetanus occurs throughout the world.
- The disease is more common in warmer climates and months.
- With the advent of vaccination in the United States, the incidence of the disease has dramatically decreased.

Risk Factors

- Failure to immunize against tetanus
- Deep or contaminated wounds

Differential Diagnosis

Refer to Table 44-13.

Management

Treatments and medications. Although there is a culture available to confirm tetanus infection, the diagnosis is usually made on the basis of clinical findings. Tetanus immune globulin is given as soon as possible to prevent circulating tetanus toxin from binding to CNS sites, but additional treatment is primarily supportive. Respiratory support may be required because the muscle spasms may interfere with adequate ventilation. Medications to treat muscle spasms (e.g., diazepam) are of primary importance. Intravenous fluid therapy is also necessary because the patient is not usually able to maintain adequate oral hydration. Infection with tetanus does not result in immunity from future infection; therefore the patient should be immunized in the convalescent period to prevent reinfection.

Counseling and prevention

- Encourage parents to maintain current tetanus immunization on all persons in the household.
- Educate the parents regarding required medications and dosing (Table 44-14).

Follow-up. Children who have had active tetanus infection require follow-up care until they have achieved their previous state of health or, if neurologic sequelae are present, for an extended period.

Consultations and referrals

- Provide immediate referral to a physician and emergency center for any suspected case of tetanus (see the Alert box).
- Remember that cases of tetanus must be reported to the health department.
- Contact the school nurse or day-care center.

Tuberculosis

Alert

> Consult with or refer to a physician for the following:
> - Signs of meningeal irritation
> - HIV-positive child with a positive tuberculosis (TB) test result

Etiology

TB is caused by *Mycobacterium tuberculosis* in the United States. Transmission to children is usually via droplet inhalation from an adult infected with pulmonary TB. Adults with active infection are contagious until 2 to 4 weeks after starting therapy. Children with TB do not transmit infection very often because the pulmonary lesions are much smaller and cough is rare or not present. The incubation period from infection to the development of a positive TB skin test is 2 to 10 weeks.

Incidence

- Since 1987, the number of cases of TB in children under 15 years of age has increased by almost 40%.
- Of children in the United States, infants and adolescents are at greatest risk of developing TB.
- Currently the highest rates of infection are among minorities.

Risk Factors

- Recent TB skin test conversion
- Close contact with an adult with pulmonary TB

Table 44-13 Differential Diagnosis: Tetanus

CRITERIA	TETANUS*	MUSCLE SPASMS
ICD-9 code	037.	728.85
Subjective Data		
Present history	History of a wound or laceration, incomplete tetanus immunization series, painful muscle spasms occurring gradually over several days	Painful muscle spasms, may be associated with recent injury, immunization status current
Objective Data		
Physical examination	Muscle spasms, may be aggravated by stimuli (e.g., noise, sudden movement), muscle rigidity, increased oral secretions, respiratory distress	Muscles tense, no respiratory involvement

Immediate referral to a physician.

Table 44-14 Tetanus Vaccination Recommendations for Wounds

IMMUNIZATION STATUS	CLEAN OR MINOR WOUND	CONTAMINATED OR DEEP WOUND
Three or more previous tetanus immunizations	Requires immunization if last dose > 10 years earlier	Requires immunization if last dose > 5 years earlier
Unknown tetanus immunization history	Immunize; does not require tetanus immune globulin	Immunize; requires tetanus immune globulin

Table 44-15 Differential Diagnosis: Tuberculosis

CRITERIA	TUBERCULOSIS	LYMPHADENITIS	MENINGITIS*	ERYTHEMA NODOSUM
ICD-9 code	011.90	289.3	322.9	695.2
Subjective Data				
Fever	No fever	Mild fever	High fever	No fever
Associated symptoms	Usually none	Painful lymph nodes	Lethargy, irritability, vomiting	Painful nodules on legs
Exposure	Known exposure to an adult with pulmonary tuberculosis	None known	Possible	
Objective Data *Physical examination*				
Associated findings	Usually asymptomatic; positive tuberculosis skin test defined as an area 10 mm or greater of induration at 48 or 72 hours; an area of 5 mm or greater in a high-risk child (see Risk Factors) should be treated as suspect; painless, enlarged lymph nodes; meningeal signs (rare), erythema nodosum, vesicular conjunctivitis	Swollen, tender lymph nodes; may have fever	High fever, lethargy, irritability; full, tense, or bulging fontanel, high-pitched cry, stiff neck, Kernig or Brudzinski sign	Erythematous, tender nodules on legs

*Immediate referral to a physician.

Table 44-16 Antituberculosis Drugs in Children

DRUG (DOSE)	ADVERSE EFFECTS
Isoniazid (10 to 15 mg/kg per day in two divided doses; maximum of 300 mg/24 hours)	Hepatotoxicity, peripheral neuritis, hypersensitivity; when used in a dosage exceeding 10 mg/kg per day in combination with rifampin, may cause increased incidence of hepatotoxic effects
Rifampin (10 to 20 mg/kg per day in two divided doses)	Red urine and tears, stains contact lenses, flulike reactions, hepatotoxicity
Pyrazinamide (20 to 40 mg/kg per day in two divided doses; maximum of 2 g/24 hours)	Hepatotoxicity, hyperuricemia
Ethambutol (15 to 25 mg/kg per day once daily)	Optic neuritis (reversible), decreased red-green color discrimination

- HIV infection or other immune deficiencies
- Diabetes mellitus
- Renal disease
- Malnutrition
- Poverty and overcrowding
- Immunosuppressive therapy (e.g., cancer chemotherapy, daily corticosteroid therapy)

Differential Diagnosis

Infants and children with TB are usually asymptomatic. Table 44-15 identifies possible conditions that may mimic some of the occasional symptoms found in children with TB.

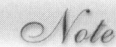

Note

About 10% to 20% of children with TB do not test positive when given a skin test, so a negative TB skin test result does not exclude the diagnosis of TB. If infection is suspected, consult with a physician.

Management

Treatments and medications. After confirmation of a positive TB test or suspected clinical infection, anti-TB therapy should be started (Table 44-16). Children with TB infection without disease may be given a single-agent therapy, whereas children with primary pulmonary TB or extrapulmonary disease should be treated with two or more agents. If two agents are used in the treatment of pulmonary TB, the duration of treatment is 12 months, whereas the use of three agents reduces the treatment to 6 months. Noncompliance is less of a problem if the duration of therapy is shorter.

Counseling and prevention

- Explain to the parents and child that compliance with the treatment regimen is necessary to obtain a cure.
- Explain to parents the importance of completing entire course of therapy.
- Instruct parents that transmission from the child to another individual is extremely uncommon because children do not produce sputum and aerosolization of the bacillus is not likely. However, parents should limit contact with susceptible individuals (e.g., immunocompromised persons, diabetics). (See Risk Factors.)
- Inform parents that children who are receiving anti-TB drugs may have some adverse reactions (see Table 44-16).

Follow-up. Follow-up care should continue throughout the duration of the treatment to encourage compliance and monitor for side effects. Patients may need to be observed by a public health nurse or visiting nurse to encourage compliance with the treatment regimen.

Table 44-17 Differential Diagnosis: Varicella

CRITERIA	CHICKENPOX (VARICELLA)	HERPES ZOSTER	BULLOUS IMPETIGO
ICD-9 code	052.9	053.9	684.
Subjective Data			
Fever	Fever present	No fever	No fever
Rash	Appearance of vesicular rash, usually initially on trunk	Appearance of grouped vesicular lesions	Appearance of grouped vesicular lesions
Associated symptoms	Pruritus, poor appetite, malaise, arthralgia	Pain and pruritus	Pruritus
Immunization history	No varivax	History of chickenpox	Adequate immunization
Objective Data			
Physical examination			
Rash	Generalized, vesicular, pruritic rash	Vesicular lesions lie along a sensory dermatome	Discrete or grouped vesicles on an erythematous base
Fever	Fever present	Afebrile	Afebrile
Associated findings	Listlessness, purulent fluid in vesicles, arthralgias, hepatomegaly (rare), meningeal symptoms (rare)	Usually none	Usually none
Laboratory data	Thrombocytopenia (rare), elevated liver enzyme levels (rare)	Usually none	None

Consultations and referrals

- Provide immediate referral to a physician for any child with meningeal signs and symptoms.
- Consult with or refer to a physician for all cases of TB.
- Refer to a physician any children who have vesicular conjunctivitis, elevated liver enzyme levels, or other adverse reactions to therapy.
- Notify day-care workers or the school nurse when a case of TB is diagnosed.
- Report all cases of TB to the health department.
- Refer to a visiting nurse service if there are problems complying with treatment.

Varicella-Zoster Virus

Alert

Consult with or refer to a physician for the following:
- Signs of meningeal irritation (e.g., lethargy, irritability; full, tense, or bulging fontanel; high-pitched cry, stiff neck, Kernig's or Brudzinski's sign)
- Signs of respiratory compromise (e.g., nasal flaring, retractions, wheezing, crackles, rhonchi)
- Patient who is immunosuppressed (e.g., a child who is HIV, a child who is receiving chemotherapy or daily corticosteroids)
- Lesions on the eyelids or eyes
- Signs of dehydration
- Signs of Reye syndrome (e.g., lethargy, persistent vomiting, disorientation, confusion, seizures)

Etiology

Varicella-zoster virus (VZV) is a herpesvirus, and primary infection results in chickenpox. Following the primary infection, the virus remains in the body in the latent form, and reactivation results in herpes zoster, or shingles. Humans are the only host of this virus, which is highly contagious. Person-to-person spread occurs by direct contact with the varicella or zoster lesions or by airborne droplet infection. The incubation period is between 10 and 21 days. The infected individual is contagious for 24 to 48 hours before the outbreak of the lesions and until the lesions have crusted over. Following varicella infection, the patient has lifelong immunity.

Incidence

- Varicella is the most common rash illness of childhood. An estimated 3 million cases occur yearly.
- Most reported cases occur in children between 5 and 10 years of age.
- Most varicella infections occur during late winter and early spring.

Risk Factors

- Inadequate or no immunization against varicella
- Primary infection with varicella occurs in susceptible individuals after direct contact with a person with chickenpox or herpes zoster infection
- Day-care and classroom settings
- Infected household contacts

Differential Diagnosis

Refer to Table 44-17. (See also Rash in Chapter 37.)

Management

Treatments and medications. Oral acyclovir has been shown to be of benefit in reducing the duration of new lesion formation and the total number of lesions when given at a dose of 20 mg/kg four times a day. (The adult dose is 800 mg four times a day.) The treatment is most beneficial if started within 24 hours of onset of the rash.

Other than the use of acyclovir, the treatment of VZV is primarily supportive. Acetaminophen may be used to control fever; however, the use of aspirin should be avoided because of the association between aspirin and Reye syndrome. Intravenous hydration may be required if the patient has chickenpox lesions on the oral mucosa and oral intake is decreased. Pruritus may be controlled with diphenhydramine. Secondary infection may develop following scratching of the lesions. Oral antibiotic therapy with dicloxacillin 40 mg/kg per day in three divided doses or cephalexin (Keflex) 25 to 50 mg/kg per day in four divided doses may be initiated.

Counseling and prevention. Instruct parents of infected children about the potential risk of exposing susceptible pregnant women to their infected child, because fetal infection may occur. Children with chickenpox or zoster should be isolated from the time of appearance of the lesions until all lesions have crusted over.

The live-attenuated varicella vaccine is now commercially available in the United States. Vaccine efficacy during clinical trials in the United States was approximately 86%. Instruct parents of the importance of their child receiving this vaccine.

Parents should be taught the signs and symptoms of complicated varicella infection (e.g., meningeal signs, respiratory distress, dehydration, ocular involvement) in order for them to seek appropriate emergency medical care.

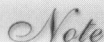

Any infant, child, or adolescent who is immunosuppressed (e.g., has HIV, is receiving chemotherapy agents or daily systemic corticosteroids) and contracts primary varicella or herpes zoster infection must be referred to a physician immediately.

Follow-up. Follow-up care for uncomplicated varicella infection is not indicated. For a child hospitalized with varicella encephalitis or pneumonia, follow-up care should continue until the child has reached their previous state of health. If a child had anorexia, periodic weight checks are necessary until appropriate weight gain is established. If there was ocular involvement, the child needs follow-up care by an ophthalmologist.

Consultations and referrals
- Provide immediate referral to a physician for any child with meningeal symptoms, signs of Reye syndrome, severe dehydration, respiratory compromise, ocular involvement, or thrombocytopenia
- Notify day-care workers or the school nurse when a case of varicella is diagnosed.

Viral Hepatitis

Alert

Consult with or refer to a physician for the following:
- Vomiting with dehydration
- Jaundice
- Irritability
- High fevers
- Severe headache
- Combative behavior

Etiology

Viral hepatitis is identified as hepatitis A virus (HAV), hepatitis B virus (HBV), hepatitis C virus (HCV), hepatitis D virus (HDV) or non-A, non-B hepatitis. It is important to determine which type of hepatitis is present, both for diagnosis and treatment and for determining appropriate measures to prevent spread of the virus. HAV is spread by the fecal-oral route and may be transmitted by contaminated water or food (e.g., shellfish). In the United States, young adults are infected most often. In developing countries, children age 10 years or younger are primarily infected. No seasonal variation has been noted, and the incubation period is 15 to 50 days. The infection is spread primarily during the incubation period.

HBV is spread by sexual activity and through contaminated blood or body fluids containing blood. HBV is not transmitted through contaminated water or food or by the fecal-oral route, and the virus can result in chronic infection. The incubation period is 45 to 160 days. Infants of mothers who are carriers or have active infection are at high risk for contracting the virus before birth.

HCV is spread by contact with infected blood or blood products, but not by blood transfusion. Person-to-person spread of the virus is not well understood. Those who are infected are at risk for chronic infection. The incubation period is 7 to 9 weeks.

Incidence

- HAV is the most common cause of hepatitis in children ages 5 to 15 years.
- In children, HBV infection is most common in HBV-endemic areas, children in custodial care facilities, those receiving blood products, and those undergoing hemodialysis.
- Infection with HCV in children under the age of 15 years is not common.

Risk Factors

Hepatitis A
- Poor hygiene or inadequate handwashing
- Exposure to infected household contacts, infected caregivers, or other children in day-care settings

Hepatitis B
- Exposure to infected blood or blood products
- Intravenous drug use
- Poor hygiene
- Active or chronic infection in women of childbearing age
- Multiple sex partners
- Diagnosis of a sexually transmitted disease (STD)
- No immunization or incomplete immunization series for hepatitis B

Hepatitis C
- Intravenous drug use
- Frequent exposure to blood products (e.g., by health care workers)

Differential Diagnosis

Refer to Table 44-18.

Management

Treatments and medications. Serologic tests for viral hepatitis include:

Hepatitis A
- Hepatitis A antibody (anti-HAV) IgM indicates recent infection.
- Anti-HAV IgG indicates past infection.

Hepatitis B
- Hepatitis B surface antigen (HBsAg) indicates acute infection or chronic infection.
- IgM anti-HBc indicates acute or recent HBV infection.

Table 44-18 Differential Diagnosis: Hepatitis

CRITERIA	INFECTIOUS MONONUCLEOSIS	REYE SYNDROME*	HEPATITIS A	HEPATITIS B	HEPATITIS C
ICD-9 code	075.	331.81	070.10	070.30	070.51
Subjective Data					
Associated symptoms	Fatigue, fever	Fatigue, encephalopathy, history of recent viral infection or varicella	Fever, jaundice, nausea, vomiting, anorexia, malaise, may be asymptomatic	Jaundice, nausea, anorexia, malaise, arthralgias, rash; may be asymptomatic	Jaundice, malaise; may be asymptomatic
Objective Data					
Physical examination					
Associated findings	Enlarged lymph nodes, pharyngitis, splenomegaly	Confusion, combative, hepatic failure	Fever, jaundice, weight loss	Jaundice, weight loss, macular rash, hepatomegaly	Jaundice, malaise
Laboratory data	Elevated liver enzymes, bilirubin, SGOT, SGPT, alkaline phosphatase	Indicates hepatic failure, ammonia level elevated	Elevated bilirubin level	Elevated bilirubin level	Elevated bilirubin level

*Immediate referral to a physician.
SGOT, *Serum glutamate oxaloacetate transaminase;* SGPT, *serum glutamate pyruvate transaminase.*

- Antibody to hepatis B core antigen (Anti-HBc) indicates past infection.
- Anti–hepatitis Be antibody (anti-HBe) indicates HBsAg carriers with a low risk of infectiousness.
- Hepatis B e antigen (HBeAg) indicates carriers at increased risk of transmitting infection
- Antibody to hepatitis B surface antigen (Anti-HBs) indicates past infection and determines immunity after vaccination.
  Hepatitis C
- Elevated hepatitis C antibody (anti-HVC) indicates acute or past infection but does not always indicate persistent infection.
  Other treatment considerations include:
- Keep in mind that treatment of uncomplicated viral hepatitis is usually supportive.
- Remember that bed rest is important because fatigue is common.
- Keep in mind that many patients are anorexic and need encouragement to eat and take fluids.
- Avoid medications that are metabolized by the liver (e.g., acetaminophen, sedatives, tranquilizers).
- Keep in mind that α-interferon injections may be used to treat persons with chronic HBV and HCV infections.

Counseling and prevention
- Keep in mind that immune globulin is highly effective in preventing HAV and HBV virus following exposure. In HAV-exposed persons (e.g., household contacts, those at day-care centers, sexual partners), immune globulin should be given within 2 weeks of exposure in a single dose.
- Instruct the parents and child on the disease process and treatment.
- Instruct the family on the prevention of spread (see Etiology).
- Educate parents on importance of hepatitis B vaccine (HepB). A combination vaccine for hepatitis B and *H. influenzae* type B is available for use at 2, 4, and 12 to 15 months of age (Merck and Company, Inc., West Point, PA).
- Keep in mind that newborn infants exposed to HBV should receive hepatitis B immune globulin (HBIG) as soon as possible after birth or within the first 12 hours of life. The HBV vaccine should also be given before hospital discharge and repeated at 1 month and 6 months of age.
- Advise that children exposed to infected household contacts or infected blood or body fluids should receive HBIG within 1 to 2 weeks.

Follow-up. Children with viral hepatitis should be monitored until their liver enzyme levels have normalized and they have returned to their previous state of health.

Consultations and referrals
- Remember that any child exhibiting encephalopathy, ascites, elevated ammonia levels, or abnormal coagulation times requires immediate referral to an emergency center (see Alert box).
- Notify day-care workers or the school nurse when a case of hepatitis is diagnosed.
- Report to the health department.

Resources

Websites
American Academy of Pediatrics (www.aap.org)
American Lyme Disease Foundation, Inc. (www.aldf.com)
Centers for Disease Control and Prevention (CDC) (www.cdc.gov)
Infectious Diseases in Children (www.slackinc.com/child/idc/idchome.htm)
National Center for Infectious Diseases (www.cdc.gov/ncidod)
Preventable Diseases (www.merck.com/disease/preventable)

Bibliography

American Academy of Pediatrics (2000). *2000 Red book: Report of the Committee of Infectious Diseases* (25th ed.). Elk Grove Village, IL: American Academy of Pediatrics.
American Academy of Pediatrics, Committee on Infectious Diseases (2000). Prevention of Lyme Disease. *Pediatrics, 105*, 142-147.
Centers for Disease Control and Prevention (2000). Prevention of varicella: Update recommendations of the Advisory Committee on Immunization Practices (ACIP). *Morbidity and Mortality Weekly Report, 48*(RR-6), 1-5.

Centers for Disease Control and Prevention (2000). Recommended childhood immunization schedule—United States, 2000. *Morbidity and Mortality Weekly Report, 49*(2), 35-38.

Feder, H.M. Jr. (2000). Lyme disease vaccine: good for dogs, adults, and children? *Pediatrics, 105,* 1333-1334.

Feigin, R.D. & Cherry, J.D. (Eds.). (1998). *Textbook of pediatric infectious diseases* (4th ed.). Philadelphia: W.B. Saunders.

Lesko, S.M. & Mitchell A.A. (1999). The safety of acetaminophen and ibuprofen among children younger than two years old. *Pediatrics, 104,* e39.

Mandell, G.L. & Wilfert, C.M. (Eds.). (1999). *Pediatric infectious diseases.* Philadelphia: Current Medicine.

Prior, M.J., Nelson, E.B., & Temple, A.R. (2000). Pediatric ibuprofen use increases while incidence of Reye's syndrome continues to decline. *Clinical Pediatrics, 39,* 245-247.

Wadsworth, L. (1999). Polio immunization: dealing with new recommendations and helping parents understand the changes. *Journal of Pediatric Health Care, 13,* S21-30.

Ward, M.R. (1997). Reye's syndrome: an update. *Nurse Practitioner, 22*(12), 45-46, 49-50, 52-53.

Section 4
Families with Children Requiring Long-Term Management

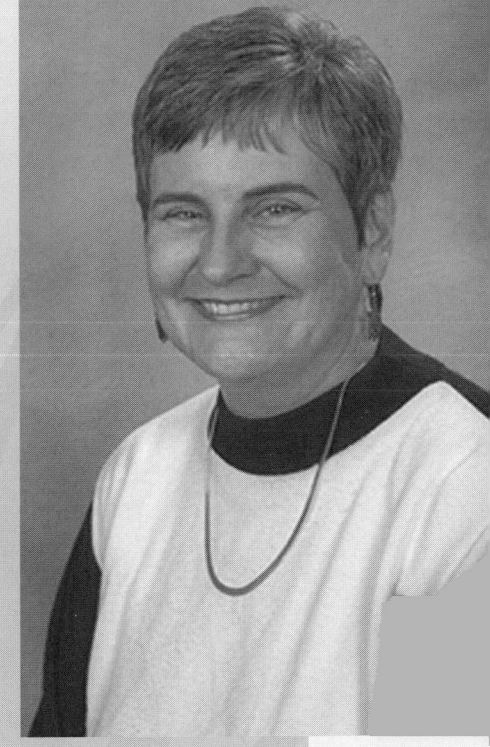

*F*or most readers, Dr. Marie Scott Brown needs no introduction. She has been a leader and inspiration to pediatric nurse practitioners (PNPs) for over 35 years. Dr. Brown was one of the first to complete the PNP certification program at the University of Colorado at Boulder. Since that time she has had a distinguished career as a scholar, educator, author, researcher, anthropologist, and clinician. The following is a brief review of a few of the many accomplishments Dr. Brown has achieved during her long and distinguished career.

Dr. Brown's original texts (co-authored with Dr. Mary Murphy), *Pediatric Physical Diagnosis for Nurses* and *Ambulatory Pediatrics for Nurses*, were the first books written by PNPs for PNPs that documented clinical skills in history-taking, physical assessment, diagnosis, and management. Since then she has authored 5 more books, 13 book chapters, and nearly 100 articles in professional and lay publications. Additionally, she has authored 24 audio-visual productions and 11 computer-assisted instructional programs. Dr. Brown is also a much sought-after speaker on topics related to research, theory, and practice about childbirth, children, families, and crosscultural approaches, and she has presented more than 30 papers internationally and 61 papers nationally.

Dr. Brown is currently a Professor of Nursing at the School of Nursing Oregon Health Sciences University in Portland, Oregon (first appointed in 1980). She maintains a clinical practice in pediatrics and has done so throughout her career. In 1994, she returned to school and completed in 1996 a Post-Master's Certificate in Nurse Midwifery/Women's Health Care. Since then she has also practiced as a nurse midwife in the Midwifery Service at Oregon Health Sciences University. Dr. Brown received her MA and PhD degrees in Anthropology from the University of Colorado at Boulder, where she also completed a two-year post-doctorate in Nursing and Anthropology. Her nursing education began at Marquette University in Milwaukee, Wisconsin, where she earned a BSN, and it continued at the University of Colorado in Denver, where she completed her MSN.

Dr. Brown has held numerous professional appointments. Before her current appointment, she spent several years at the University of Colorado School of Nursing in the Graduate Parent-Child Program in positions such as Co-Director of a federal research grant, "Facilitation, Preparation and Use of Expanded-Role Nurse Practitioners," and Director of the Robert Wood Johnson Fellowship Program.

Dr. Brown's expertise and interest in anthropology and culture have taken her around the world where she has been able to combine her clinical expertise while working in such countries as Mexico, Vietnam, China, Russia, and the Philippines, as well as parts of Africa. Most recently (in 2002), she was awarded a Fullbright Scholarship to study and work in Botswana.

Jane A. Fox

Chapter 45 *Diseases and Problems*

Anorexia and Bulimia, p. 751
Asthma, p. 757
Cystic Fibrosis, p. 770
Diabetes Mellitus, p. 778
Hemophilia and Bleeding Disorders, p. 787
Human Immunodeficiency Virus and Acquired Immune
   Deficiency Syndrome, p. 796
Neoplastic Disease, p. 815
Rheumatic Fever, p. 826
Sickle Cell Anemia, p. 829

Anorexia and Bulimia

MARY E. MUSCARI

Alert

Immediate hospitalization is required for children and adolescents with:
- Acute suicidal ideation
- Cardiac dysrhythmias
- Cardiomyopathy
- Severe dehydration, electrolyte disturbance, and metabolic crises
- Acute pancreatic failure

Anorexia nervosa (AN) is characterized by the persistent quest for thinness. Characteristics include refusal to maintain body weight at or above a minimally normal weight for height and age (or failure to make expected weight gain during a period of growth); intense fear of gaining weight or becoming fat, even when underweight; disturbance in the way in which one's body weight or shape is experienced; and, in postmenarchal females, amenorrhea for at least three consecutive menstrual cycles.

Anorectics believe that they are obese even when extremely emaciated. This body-image disturbance can range from mild distortion to severe delusion, and it is not related to the degree of weight loss. The adolescents may be concerned with their entire body, or they may focus on specific body areas such as the abdomen, thighs, and buttocks. The basis of body-image distortion lies in the feelings of ineffectiveness, evoking a sense of helplessness and passivity manifested as difficulty in mastering bodily functions.

The American Psychiatric Association (APA) specifies two types of AN. The first is the restrictive type in which the person has not regularly engaged in bingeing or purging behaviors during the current episode of anorexia. The second is the binge-eating, purging type in which the person regularly engages in either bingeing or purging during the anorexia period.

Bulimia nervosa (BN) signifies the chaotic eating patterns that characterize the disorder. These patterns include recurrent episodes of binge eating (eating a larger than average amount of food in a discrete period of time, with a feeling of lack of control over eating during these episodes), repeated compensatory mechanisms to prevent weight gain (e.g., self-induced vomiting, laxative or diuretic abuse, use of other medications [such as ipecac], fasting, excessive exercise), binge eating and compensatory mechanisms such that both occur on average at least twice a week for 3 months, and self-evaluation unduly influenced by body shape and weight.

Bulimia typically begins with the discovery that self-induced vomiting and laxative abuse may be used for weight control. Bingeing subsequently develops, possibly as a result of the physiologic changes of dieting, and a vicious cycle begins. The bingeing episodes are usually secretive and primarily involve the ingestion of carbohydrate-rich, easily digested foods in amounts that may range from 5000 to 20,000 kcal per episode. Binge episodes may be associated with feelings of anxiety, depression, boredom, or loneliness or with an unpleasant event. Binges may be planned and may occur at any time; however they usually occur in the late afternoon or evening. Binge eating may become very expensive, with the individual spending or stealing large amounts of money to support the "habit."

In bulimic adolescents an intense, covert preoccupation with food develops and progressively interferes with educational, vocational, or social activities. Shame follows bingeing, and they are usually quite distressed by their symptoms. They are also at risk for impulsive behaviors such as substance abuse, shoplifting, and promiscuity, increasing their chances for chemical dependency and sexually transmitted diseases (STDs), including acquired immune deficiency syndrome (AIDS).

The APA specifies two types of bulimia. The first is the purging type during which the person regularly engages in purgative activities. The second is the nonpurging type, during which the person uses other inappropriate compensatory mechanisms such as fasting or excessive exercise. The latter may be missed because many health care professionals are not aware of its existence.

Etiology

Numerous theories addressing the causes and origins of eating disorders have been developed. It is now generally accepted that eating disorders are multifactorial in origin and that no one element is responsible. Twin studies have suggested a genetic component, since a female is 10 to 20 times more likely to have an eating disorder if she has a sibling with the disease. Family dysfunction increases the likelihood for eating disorders, as it does with other psychiatric disorders. Patients with eating disorders may have family histories of eating disorders, affective disorders, and substance abuse. A past history of sexual abuse has also been elicited in many patients with eating disorders. Cultural factors must be considered because eating disorders are primarily seen in Western and industrialized countries where thinness is the ideal.

Incidence

- Approximately 1% of all teenage and college-age women suffer from AN.
- Approximately 5% to 8% of all teen-age and college-age women suffer from BN.
- The male-to-female ratio ranges from 1:6 to 1:10.
- Eating disorders are more prevalent among young Caucasian females under 25 years of age from middle to upper social classes in Western culture.
- The majority of eating disorders develop somewhere between 12 and 18 years of age, but if untreated or treated unsuccessfully, the disorder may persist into adulthood.

Risk Factors

- Maladaptive early eating patterns (may increase the likelihood of later problems)
- Incidence of sexual abuse
- Body dissatisfaction before or during puberty
- Family history of eating disorders, affective disorders, or substance abuse
- Adolescents considering careers in which thinness is required (e.g., acting, modeling, dancing, wrestling, gymnastics).

Differential Diagnosis

All adolescents should be screened for eating disorders during routine physical assessments and when episodic illnesses come to medical attention in a manner that is suggestive of anorexia or bulimia as part of the differential diagnosis (e.g., gastritis, menstrual irregularities, weight loss). Box 45-1 lists the criteria to consider when one is assessing for an eating disorder.

Subjective Data

If anorexia or bulimia is suspected, a complete history should be obtained with careful attention to the following:

- *Weight history*—Include the frequency of weighing, premorbid weight, menstrual threshold, and a detailed history of fluctuations. Graphing is exceptionally helpful when looking for patterns that may be associated with specific stressors. Assess the amount of stress associated with weight by observing nonverbal and verbal communication during the interview and the actual weighing. Question adolescents about their ideal weight and their perception of their total body appearance as well as specific body parts. Because they may have difficulty in verbalizing these perceptions, it may be useful to have them draw pictures of themselves and their families.
- *Dieting history*—Determine the onset of dieting behaviors, what prompted them, and whether there was a source of outside encouragement, as well as what types of diets were used and their frequency and duration. This aids in determining impulsiveness and overall health factors related to malnutrition. It is helpful to determine whether adolescents diet alone or with others. High school and

---

Box 45-1 The Eating Disorder Pocket Assessment Guide

Subjective Assessment

Solicit a weight history.
Ask about ideal weight and perception of body appearance.
Determine the onset of dieting behaviors.
Establish what types of diets were used, as well as their frequency and duration.
Determine if the adolescent diets alone or with others.
Establish when binge eating began and the precipitating circumstances.
Elicit the types of purgative behaviors used.
Ask the adolescent how he or she obtains laxatives.
Question the adolescent about other substance use.
Question the type, frequency, and duration of exercise.
Assess sexual activity and sexuality.
Assess activities.
Assess social interactions.
Assess for depression and suicide ideation.
Elicit the systems review.
Obtain a comprehensive family psychiatric history.

Objective Assessment

Measurements—Weight: Decreased or fluctuating; blood pressure: Low, orthostatic hypotension; Pulse: Low, bradycardia; Temperature: Low, hypothermia
General appearance—Hyperactive; listless or lethargic
Integumentary system—Dry, desquamated, yellow; lack of acne; dullness or loss of scalp hair; lanugo; brittle nails; signs of dehydration
Head, eyes, ears, nose, and throat—Tiny conjunctival hemorrhages, hypertrophied salivary glands, dental enamel erosion, caries, and adenopathy

Heart—Bradycardia and ejection click (mitral valve prolapse)
Breast—Decreased adipose tissue
Abdomen—Concave, left lower quadrant mass
Genitourinary system—Pubic hair loss and history of amenorrhea or oligomenorrhea
Musculoskeletal system—Muscle wasting, Russell's sign, and lower extremity edema
Neurologic system—Possible abnormalities in mental status examination

Differential Diagnoses

Depression, schizophrenia, substance abuse, inflammatory bowel disorder, pancreatitis, peptic ulcer disease, hypothalamic tumors, frontal lobe tumors, seizure disorders, diabetes mellitus, and effects of medications (e.g., neuroleptics, lithium preparations, tricyclic antidepressants, opiates, corticosteroids, oral contraceptives)
The critical key factor that differentiates anorexia and bulimia from other disorders is body-image disturbance.

Diagnostic Studies

Complete blood cell count—Usually normal
Thyroid function tests—Triiodothyronine (T_3) and thyroxine (T_4) low with anorexia
Erythrocyte sedimentation rate—Low with malnutrition
Electrolytes—Abnormal, related to purgative methods
Creatine phosphokinase—Elevated with ipecac use
Drug screens—For laxatives and illicit drugs
Reproductive hormones—Low with weight loss
Electroencephalogram—May have dysrhythmia

From Mary E. Muscari, 1997, 2001.

college students may have difficulty with treatment if their peers are actively involved in dieting or eating-disorder behaviors.

- *Bingeing and purging history*—Establish when binge eating began, the precipitating circumstances, and whether fluctuations in symptoms correlate with recurrent life events. Assess the daily and weekly frequency of bingeing, type and amount of foods used, time of day, and feelings of lack of control over binges. Purging behavior assessment begins with eliciting the types of purgative behaviors used. Onset, frequency, time of day, and precipitating factors should be established, as well as the method of self-induced vomiting. Some adolescents use instruments (e.g., fingers, spoons) to stimulate the gag reflex, others "water-load," and some have "advanced" to where they no longer need stimulation. Those who have lost their gag reflex after persistent self-induced vomiting are at risk for aspiration. Some adolescents may resort to the use of ipecac, which causes cardiac, gastrointestinal (GI) tract, and neuromuscular toxicity. Stimulant laxatives are preferred because of their rapid action, and many adolescents consume high amounts. Ask adolescents how they obtain laxatives, since many resort to stealing because of expense or embarrassment. Over-the-counter (OTC) diuretics are usually used; however, prescription diuretics may be stolen from family members or requested for premenstrual syndrome. Enema and synthetic thyroid abuse are rare, but the possibility should be questioned. Screen adolescents for drug and alcohol use or abuse; boys and men should be questioned about anabolic steroid use.
- *Exercise history*—Question about the type, frequency, and duration of exercise and the possibility of compulsiveness. Establish the latter by asking adolescents what would happen if they did not exercise at their specified time or for their specified amount. In general, bulimic adolescents engage in exercise much less frequently than their anorectic counterparts; however, both groups must be assessed.
- *Sexual history*—Sexual and sexuality problems may arise in adolescents with eating disorders. Empathetically discuss sexual issues and assess each adolescent on an individual basis, strongly considering developmental level and experience. Assess sexual experience, the consequences of intrapersonal and interpersonal factors, the adolescent's affective range when discussing sex, and whether the adolescent is receiving secondary gain relating to sex and sexuality from the eating disorder. Assess whether bingeing with purging has become a substitute for sexual activity.
- *Activities and goals*—Assess present activities and goals; specific vocations have been suggested to be risk factors for the development of eating disorders. AN and BN may also severely interfere with school, vocational, and social activities. School and vocational skills may be hindered because of physiologic effects or psychosocial preoccupations, or they may be falsely enhanced because of feelings of perfectionism. Leisure activities may no longer exist because of disorder-related preoccupations or depression, creating even greater stress. Although adolescents with bulimia are usually more social than their anorectic counterparts, they tend to be more superficial in their relationships. Many feel distanced and self-conscious and may have difficulty expressing and asserting themselves. Assess social interactions and social skills.
- *Substance use or abuse*—Assess for use or abuse of nicotine, alcohol, diet pills, and prescription and illicit drugs. Substance abuse is associated more with bulimia, but it is necessary to assess anorectics as well. Assessment should include the amount, frequency, and circumstances of substance use, keeping in mind the fact that substance use may take place in "bingelike" patterns.
- *Psychosocial history*—Assess for depression because depression may be associated with anorexia and may either precede or follow bulimic behaviors. Ask adolescents directly about suicidal thoughts, including when these thoughts occurred and a full account of the plan, if one exists. An acutely suicidal adolescent requires immediate referral for evaluation and probable psychiatric admission. Major depressive disorder and dysthymic disorder have been observed in numerous anorectic patients. Obsessive-compulsive disorder has also been reported in a significant number. Personality problems found in bulimics include impulsiveness (e.g., shoplifting, promiscuity), poor self-esteem, and cognitive distortions. Adolescents may have accompanying personality disorders that significantly affect their recovery. Borderline, avoidant, histrionic, dependent, and obsessive-compulsive personality disorders are the ones typically observed.
- *Sleep history*—Assess sleep patterns and observe for sleep disturbances, a starvation-related symptom. There is often a decrease in the amount of sleep, including fragmented sleep and early morning awakening.
- *Review of systems*—Ask about eating disorder-related symptoms such as cold intolerance, fatigue, dry skin, hair loss, irregular menses, fluid and electrolyte imbalance, GI tract problems (e.g., constipation), lethargy, and dental problems. There have been incidences of eating disorders in adolescents with medical disorders such as diabetes mellitus and cystic fibrosis (CF), necessitating careful screening of these patients.
- *Comprehensive family psychiatric history*—Include the quality of relationships and communication styles. Investigate other family issues, including physical and sexual abuse, how family decisions are made, what the patient likes or dislikes about the family, who provides emotional support, how anger is expressed, discipline, and family roles.

Objective Data

A thorough physical examination should be performed with careful attention to the following (also see Box 45-1):

Physiologic signs and symptoms

Anorexia. The physiologic manifestations in AN result from starvation. These starvation-related symptoms may be clinically important as one of a series of perpetuators to the illness. Cognitive changes may include impaired concentration, increased indecisiveness, and loss of general interests. There is social withdrawal, and interests become restricted to food and food-related areas. Irritability, anxiety, and mood lability are common. Depression is frequently observed, and the predominant affect may be apathy.

Reduced gastric emptying is common and may be responsible for feelings of bloating, dyspepsia, and early satiety. Other symptoms include amenorrhea, hypotension, bradycardia, reduced body temperature, insensitivity to pain, loss of scalp hair, and development of lanugo.

Amenorrhea is one of the earlier manifestations observed in AN. It is associated with a reversion of gonadotropin secretion to the prepubertal pattern. Low levels of plasma luteinizing hormone (LH) and follicle-stimulating hormone (FSH) are accompanied by a profound estrogen deficiency. This decrease in estrogen may be responsible for the development of osteoporosis, which is common in anorexia.

Other endocrine abnormalities may be observed. Some patients have difficulty concentrating their urine in response to water deprivation, possibly because of defective osmoregulation of the secretion of vasopressin. A small number of patients have vasopressin responses consistent with partial diabetes insipidus. Many patients exhibit abnormal thermoregulatory responses when exposed to hot and cold as well as a lack of shivering. All of these responses are controlled by mechanisms that are most likely hypothalamic and that are probably the result of starvation.

Despite their extremely low weights, anorectics are likely to exhibit hypothyroidlike symptoms. These include constipation, cold intolerance, hypotension, bradycardia, slow relaxation of reflexes, hypercarotenemia, and dry skin and hair. Serum levels of thyroxine and triiodothyronine are lower than normal.

GI tract manifestations are common. There are delayed gastric emptying and decreased intestinal mobility, which lead to the complaints of bloating, abdominal pain, and constipation. An increase in hepatic enzymes may signify fatty infiltrates of the liver. Other changes observed in AN include thinning of the left cardiac ventricle and decreased cardiac chamber size: anorectics literally "eat their hearts out." These changes are associated with decreased blood pressure and decreased cardiac output. Dysrhythmias are also common, particularly when there is electrolyte imbalance. Renal changes generally reflect dehydration.

Bulimia. Physiologic signs and complications are chiefly associated with purgative behaviors such as self-induced vomiting and laxative and diuretic abuse. These behaviors frequently prove to be the most physically damaging, demonstrating that bulimia can be associated with significant life-endangering medical complications.

Physical signs associated with bulimia are few and are not seen in all patients. The first is evidence of skin changes on the dorsum of the hand that vary from abrasions to scarring (Russell's sign), which is possibly related to using the hand to stimulate the gag reflex. The second is hypertrophy of the salivary glands, associated with high carbohydrate intake. The third is the presence of dental erosion, a pattern associated with an acid bath to the back of the mouth.

Complications range from discomfort to life-threatening problems. The adolescent may have headaches, fatigue, muscle cramps, polydipsia, polyuria, and irregular menses. Vomiting may result in esophageal perforation; binge eating may cause gastric dilatation or rupture. Laxative abuse may be associated with laxative dependency, profound constipation, cathartic colon, steatorrhea, protein-losing gastroenteropathy, and GI tract bleeding. Dehydration may relate to vomiting, excessive exercise, and diuretic and laxative abuse, creating significant electrolyte abnormalities that include hypochloremia, hypokalemia, and hyponatremia.

Cardiovascular problems may also develop. Abuse of ipecac (used to stimulate vomiting) has highly toxic effects, causing irreversible myocardial damage and diffuse myositis resulting from emetine toxicity.

Psychologic signs fand symptoms. Adolescents with eating disorders exhibit several cognitive distortions. Thinking is concrete and dichotomous with a superstitious quality, causing them to see many things in an all-or-none or black-or-white fashion ("If I eat one cookie, I'll be a total failure, so I may as well eat the whole box"). Other distorted beliefs include a morbid fear of fatness, dissatisfaction with body shape, and the intense belief that strict control over body weight or thinness is necessary for happiness and well-being.

Behavior is motivated by a fear of fatness and all that this implies, as well as cognitive self-reinforcement. Dietary restraint is often fueled by its own induction of gratification and sense of control. Gastric emptiness is identified with virtue and mastery, fullness with weakness and lack of self-discipline.

Feelings of disgust for their bodies may lead to sexual problems in adolescents. They may fear exposing their bodies, becoming pregnant, losing control, expressing intimate feelings, or being rejected. Many may have a history of sexual abuse, an extremely significant factor in sexual problems.

They may also have complications such as substance abuse, depression, suicidal ideation or attempts, impulsivity, posttrauma symptoms, and self-destructive and self-mutilating behaviors. Families may also be undergoing psychosocial problems (divorce) or psychopathologic disorders (affective disorders). Families may also consciously or unconsciously reinforce eating-disordered behavior and sabotage treatment.

Physical examination. A comprehensive examination is essential. Begin with a mental status examination. Observe general appearance, cognitive functioning, affect, judgment, reality orientation, and ability to think abstractly. Notice signs of depression, anxiety, obsessional thoughts, and self-abusive behaviors (e.g., cutting). A thorough psychosocial history and mental status examination aid in ruling out other possible psychiatric differential diagnoses. Obtain temperature, pulse, and blood pressure; these are decreased with eating disorders.

Early physical signs of anorexia are minimal; the adolescent has a decreased weight, probable amenorrhea, hyperactivity, and sleep disturbance. The adolescent may also have constipation. Once signs of starvation are present, anorexia has more noticeable features than bulimia. Vital signs may reveal hypotension, bradycardia, and hypothermia. Hyperactivity may be replaced with lethargy and fatigue. The skin is dry, desquamated, and yellow (carotenemia); there is dullness and loss of scalp hair and the development of lanugo over the body (compensatory response for loss of the shivering ability to maintain body heat). Decreased androgen levels result in a lack of acne. Gastric slowing results in abdominal discomfort, bloating after eating, and constipation. The adolescent may also exhibit lower-extremity edema and polyuria.

There is usually little physical evidence of bulimia; however, observe for the three cardinal signs mentioned earlier: skin changes on the dorsum of the hand, hypertrophied salivary glands, and dental erosion. Assess for signs of complications of bulimia such as dehydration, edema, electrolyte imbalance, acidosis, and alkalosis. Adolescents with bulimia may have regular menses; however, some have amenorrhea (with low-weight bulimia) or irregular menses (with normal-weight bulimia). A pelvic examination is usually indicated to rule out other diseases, and a pregnancy test is warranted if the adolescent is sexually active.

The differential diagnosis should include the possibility of comorbid problems and alternative disorders. Comorbid problems have already been discussed and include other psychiatric diagnoses such as depression, substance abuse, and personality disorders. Alternative diagnoses include depression, schizophrenia, substance abuse, inflammatory bowel disorder, pancreatitis, peptic ulcer disease, hypothalamic tumors, frontal lobe tumors, seizure disorders, diabetes mellitus, and the effects of medications (e.g., tricyclic antidepressants, neuroleptics, lithium preparations, opiates, corticosteroids, oral contraceptives). The key factor that differentiates anorexia and bulimia from other disorders is body-image disturbance.

Diagnostic procedures and laboratory tests

- Complete blood cell (CBC) count (usually normal in eating disorders)
- Serum electrolyte levels (results depend on severity of dehydration and mechanism of purging), glucose level, and renal, liver, and thyroid function tests (triiodothyronine and thyroxine levels are usually low in anorexia)
- Electrocardiogram with a rhythm strip (patients with AN have significantly lower heart rates, longer QRS intervals, shorter mean QTc and lesser QTc dispersion, whereas patients with BN have slightly longer mean QTc dispersion)
- Urine and stool samples to detect diuretic and laxative abuse
- Possible erythrocyte sedimentation rate (ESR) to rule out inflammatory processes
- Estrogen or testosterone levels when indicated (adolescents with chronic amenorrhea and a low estrogen level may need to be estrogenized to decrease the risk for later osteoporosis)
- Follow-up laboratory tests, depending on the patient's status

Management

Treatments and medications. Once the diagnosis has been established, it is necessary to develop a treatment plan. Establish the necessity of psychotherapy and the adolescent's and family's commitment to treatment. Collaborate with the mental health professional and nutritionist (if available) to prevent manipulation and allow for continuity of care in a nonconfusing manner. Consistency is critical. A realistic, comprehensive plan helps to minimize treatment-related problems such as resistance and noncompliance.

Physiologic management is primarily targeted toward nutritional restoration and maintenance and the prevention and treatment of complications. The intensity, frequency, and duration of intervention depend on the severity of the disorder. However, it is highly recommended that some form of physiologic management exist while the adolescent is in psychotherapy.

The primary goal of nutritional therapy is to assist the adolescent in learning how to eat a well-balanced diet. A nutritional consultation and follow-up evaluation are recommended. Instruct adolescents to develop and use a daily log or diary for self-monitoring. Logs add structure, a workable reality to the disorder, and the ability to follow self-progress. The log may be used in psychotherapy; therefore it should be written in a manner that may be shared with both providers without burdening the patient.

Underweight adolescents should gain approximately 2 pounds per week. Rapid weight gain can lead to congestive heart failure (CHF) and thus should be avoided. The underweight patient should be started on a regimen of approximately 1500 calories per day divided into three meals and two snacks, with the emphasis on portions, not calories. Using a diabetic food exchange can accomplish this. The amount of calories can be gradually increased to 2000 calories, and up to 3000 calories as needed.

Decreasing or stopping purging, especially laxative abuse, produces fluid retention, constipation, and bloating and may result in the adolescent requesting a diet. This should be discouraged with sensitivity to the fact that the adolescent's metabolism has slowed somewhat. The target calorie level should be adjusted for this lowered metabolic rate. The estimated decrease for bulimia is 10% to 15%. About 5% is possible for milder cases, whereas up to 35% may be needed for more severe cases. Again, even though a calorie-based regimen is used, portion control (using three meals and two snacks per day) should be taught to reduce calorie counting. The adolescent needs a significant amount of support to deal with the weight fluctuations.

Proper nutrition can be better initiated and maintained by use of cognitive-behavioral techniques and effective patient teaching. Cognitive-behavioral techniques are especially useful for a variety of distortions in bulimia. The first method is stimulus control to alter the environment by removing factors that induce bingeing. These alterations include not engaging in other activities while eating, restricting eating to one room, and ridding the house of binge food. A second method is substituting alternative behaviors such as exercise, hot baths, crafts, brushing the teeth, or taking walks to occupy free time. There are also the palliative techniques of distraction (e.g., going for a walk immediately after eating) and parroting (e.g., "I can handle this without binge eating"). When adolescents feel stressed and consider bingeing, they can use decatastrophizing to challenge arbitrary consequences by asking themselves, "What is the worst thing that could happen if...?" Visualization techniques assist in developing mental images of handling the binge-purge situation when it arises.

Relaxation techniques may reduce anxiety, thus possibly reducing bingeing. A telephone support network, preferably made up of other adolescents with bulimia, allows for verbalization to avoid negative behaviors.

A written contract is helpful for enhancing compliance and for reinforcing reality. The contract should be typed, and clear, concise, concrete terminology should be used so that a patient may fully understand what is expected of them, leaving little room for manipulation resulting from "loopholes." Goals should be realistic, measurable, and time-framed. Contracts should be for short-term periods from a few days to a month to minimize anxiety and feelings of hopelessness. Both the practitioner and patient should sign them. If the mental health professional is also using the contract approach, the practitioner and mental health professional must work together to assess the feasibility for the patient. The decision may be to use a combined contract signed by all three parties, two separate contracts, or alternating contracts. The combined contract has the advantage of being more holistic while demonstrating the cohesiveness of the practitioner and mental health professional as a treatment team whose primary goal is the well-being of the patient.

As noted, there are numerous disorder-related physical complications that must be assessed and managed. Management of complications is the same as for any adolescent with those specific problems. Depending on the severity, the adolescent may require physician consultation or may need to be hospitalized medically for a brief period until the problem can be corrected. If the problem does not warrant hospitalization, the adolescent should be followed up very closely in the outpatient setting.

Additional recommendations include a dental referral and the use of baking soda wash to counteract acidity after vomiting, use of a multivitamin and mineral supplement (1000 mg of calcium carbonate [1500 mg when amenorrheic]), and consideration of estrogenization in patients with amenorrhea for 6 months or more. Antidepressant medications have been found to help decrease the symptoms of depression and the frequency of bingeing in patients with bulimia. They may also be of help in medically stable anorectics. However, because of the possibility of comorbid diagnoses and the potential side effects of psychotropics, it is strongly suggested that patients be referred to either a psychiatric nurse practitioner (NP) or a psychiatrist for medication therapy.

Physical management is more difficult than it appears. Assessments and interventions are not complicated; however, an adolescent's psychologic status may allow for the perpetuation of physical symptoms if the underlying psychologic issues are left unaddressed.

The psychologic problems associated with AN and BN affect both the adolescent and the family; therefore psychiatric referral is crucial. The practitioner and therapist, along with the nutritionist, need to work as a team right from the beginning. Role clarification prevents confusion and reduces manipulation, since the adolescent may play one care provider against another. Some aspects of care, such as self-esteem development, nutritional teaching, and cognitive-behavioral training, overlap. However, this is beneficial when care is provided in a manner that reinforces these important issues. After the initial "team meeting" (typically by telephone), team members should be in contact with each other at regular intervals. Team members should obtain written consent from the adolescent and parents (or guardian) allowing for confidential release of information between them.

A critical role in caring for adolescents with eating disorders is assisting them and their families in initiating and maintaining treatment. Often it is the NP who makes the diagnosis and who assists the adolescent and family in the decision to accept assistance. The practitioner must present the need for treatment in a positive manner. It is very important to engage the patient's family. Lack of support from the family may endanger compliance, and the family may try to sabotage treatment, especially when the adolescent is improving, to keep their own problems hidden and maintain the facade of the good family.

Family members need to verbalize their own frustrations, and they should be allowed to do so without feeling blamed for the disorder. Family members should also be included in the treatment plan without breaching confidentiality or affecting the adolescent's independence. Teaching the family about the disorder and its effect on them assists in alliance development.

A significant amount of shame, denial, and lack of insight are associated with bulimia. Development and maintenance of a therapeutic alliance are difficult at best and require continuous effort. Not all adolescents are ready to relinquish a disorder that has become their identity. Some adolescents deny their disorder outright, while others refuse treatment or feign compliance and never return. The practitioner must accept this reality and analyze it when it happens, not personalize it.

Counseling and prevention. Educate regarding proper nutrition. Despite their preoccupation with food, most eating-disordered adolescents have little nutritional knowledge; therefore they need to learn basic nutrition. Adolescents are still growing and should be informed of their nutritional growth requirements. When appropriate, they should also be taught that food deprivation may lead to bingeing and that adherence to a regular meal plan significantly decreases binge eating. The adolescent should learn to recognize the precipitating factors that may result in bingeing—loneliness, tension, anger, guilt, boredom, and depression—and how to use cognitive-behavioral techniques to control bingeing when precipitating factors occur. It may also be helpful to assist adolescents in calculating the actual cost of binge eating and discuss using the saved money to purchase nonfood rewards.

Teach about the devastating consequences of purging and its ineffectiveness as a weight-loss method. Purging may be used to prevent weight gain or relieve guilt associated with bingeing, or it may be used as a release mechanism for negative emotions such as anger. In patients who have been sexually abused, purging may serve as a mechanism for ridding themselves of the traumatic experience. Vomiting and diarrhea may give a sense of existence to the patient with a borderline personality disorder. The weight loss that results from purging is minimal and affects only a small amount of calorie absorption.

Address the self-esteem deficit. Eating-disordered adolescents frequently demonstrate low self-esteem with feelings of inadequacy, helplessness, ineffectiveness, guilt, and self-doubt. Many rely on the opinions of others, overaccommodate other's needs, and ignore their own needs to gain approval, which lowers their self-esteem and makes them particularly vulnerable. The first intervention in fostering self-esteem is the development of effective communication skills. Although better taught in group settings, communication skills may be initiated on a one-to-one basis. Assist adolescents in discovering their needs and how to verbalize them. Mind reading should be actively discouraged, and the adolescent should learn to become an active listener, a difficult task for a patient who is egocentric. Discuss nonverbal communications and the messages that they give as well as mixed messages from conflicting verbal and nonverbal messages. Role playing and audiovisual taping are very useful. A nonthreatening topic can be chosen for discussion from a newspaper, a magazine, or a television show to teach that mutual understanding does not necessarily mean mutual agreement. This can later be expanded to more intensive issues such as family concerns and peer-related issues. Other methods that foster self-esteem include identifying areas of competence and providing an adolescent with positive reinforcement; encouraging self-appraisal and ownership of accomplishments and positive risks taken; exploring areas of self-nurturing with the goal of developing guilt-free, nurturing self-care using nonfood rewards; encouraging self-expression through writing, art, music, and the like; and using family work to enhance positioning in the family.

Discuss sexuality. There will be adolescents who have had no experience, pleasurable experiences, or traumatic experiences. There will be adolescents who are heterosexual, homosexual, or bisexual. For some, bingeing may be a substitute for sex. Anorectics may have little interest in sex; bulimics may be promiscuous. Discuss anatomy and physiology and the changes that occur in the presence of bulimia. Give information about identified sexual problems, and offer suggestions in better meeting the adolescent's needs, including recognizing and labeling feelings. Discuss sexuality, since the adolescent may have concerns and difficulties about becoming a woman or becoming a man. Exploration of roles and sociocultural expectations in relation to sexuality further enhances its development.

Help adolescents with goal-setting. All-or-none thinking leads to unattainable notions concerning success and contentment. Eating-disordered adolescents tend to set unrealistic and unattainable goals, thereby reinforcing a negative self-evaluation and further diminishing self-esteem. Goal-setting should focus on realistic short-term goals and should include specific desired outcomes, necessary conditions, outcome achievement time frame, and level of accepted outcome performance. These allow the adolescent to develop an understanding of realistic and attainable goals. For example, the goal may be as follows: "Immediately upon awakening, (name) will begin to follow her or his meal plan for that day, and continue to do so every day for 1 week." This gives the specific desired outcome (following the meal plan), needed conditions (immediately upon awakening), outcome achievement time (every day for 1 week), and minimum accepted performance of outcome (commitment). Eventually adolescents will be able to develop their own meal plans. Initially, just facing the idea of eating on a regular basis is a difficult goal.

Assist adolescents in developing healthful coping mechanisms. Eating-disordered adolescents use food and negative eating behaviors as maladaptive coping mechanisms. Therefore they must learn how to adapt by using effective direct and indirect coping mechanisms. Adolescents must first learn to differentiate solvable problems from unsolvable ones. This begins by teaching the principles of problem-solving and then encouraging an adolescent to consistently practice these skills and apply them to day-to-day situations. To enhance these skills, the NP can have the adolescent practice on a relatively nonthreatening issue, such as choosing an article of clothing. Later, more complex issues such as choosing a food item may be used.

Help adolescents learn alternatives for problems that cannot be solved. First, they should develop some behaviors that may be substituted for bingeing and purging when stressed by nonsolvable problems. These may include writing poetry, reasonable exercise, calling a friend, dancing, or listening to music. Second, they should be taught relaxation techniques and stress management. Adolescents may also be taught time management using a daily calendar with time set aside for self-nurturing and the unexpected. Third, discuss the advantages of a healthful lifestyle, including proper nutrition, exercise, and adequate rest and sleep.

Follow-up. Eating disorders are chronic disorders that result in recovery, not cure. Therefore patients need to be observed for a significant time, usually years. In the initial phases of the illness many children and adolescents may need to be followed up weekly or more frequently to be monitored for possible complications. Patients requiring significant outpatient follow-up care over time may require in-patient treatment. Most patients do not require such close monitoring, and each should be assessed individually.

A specific history must be obtained at the onset of each visit, including questioning about fatigue, weakness, fainting, loss of concentration, evidence of malnutrition or fluid deprivation, confusion, polyuria, polydipsia, muscle cramping, constipation, steatorrhea, chest pain, bloating, abdominal pain, dental hypersensitivity, and edema. Routinely monitor logs to ascertain intake, frequency of binge-purge episodes, and exercise.

Orthostatic vital signs and an accurate weight should be monitored at each visit. Adolescents should be carefully weighed after voiding. Some patients may "hold in their urine" or drink copious amounts of water (tanking) to artificially raise their weights. These practices are more common in anorexia but may also be observed in the low-weight adolescent with bulimia. The physical examination should be comprehensive, focusing on specific problems that relate to purgative methods.

Laboratory evaluation is necessary whenever signs and symptoms of complications arise. Electrolyte levels must be monitored when deficits are suspected. An increased amylase level may assist in the detection of vomiting in a patient who denies the same. Urine and stool specimens may also be collected to check for laxative and diuretic abuse, and urine and serum specimens may be sent to detect substance abuse. Urine tests for specific gravity assist in assessing hydration status; however, be aware that some patients dilute their urine with water to alter the results. Fresh stools and urine should be collected to prevent substitutions.

Every visit should be supportive. The chronic nature of these disorders leads to significant frustration for all family members and the patient.

Consultations and referrals

- Consult with or refer to a mental health professional and a nutritionist who have experience treating children with eating disorders.
- Refer to a dentist for evaluation and treatment of dental problems secondary to starvation and purging.

Refer adolescents to a support network of other adolescents with eating disorders.

Resources

Websites

American Anorexia-Bulimia Association (www.aabainc.org)
Anorexia Nervosa and Related Eating Disorders, Inc. (www.anred.com)
Eating Disorders Awareness and Prevention Inc. (www.edap.org)
Eating Disorders Foundation of Canada (www.eating-disorders.org/edfoc.htm)
National Association of Anorexia Nervosa and Associated Disorders (ANAD) (www.anad.org)

Asthma

MARIJO RATCLIFFE

Alert

Consult with or refer to a physician for the following:
- Past history of intensive care unit (ICU) hospitalization, intubation, or respiratory arrest
- Multiple emergency room visits or hospitalizations
- Steroid dependence (e.g., oral corticosteroids)
- Poor response to usual therapy, or therapy associated with significant side effects
- Child younger than 3 years of age with moderate or persistent asthma (Table 45-1)
- Failure to perceive symptoms or severity, or detection of a poor clinical response to treatment
- Associated complicating conditions (e.g., severe rhinitis or sinusitis, nasal polyps, gastroesophageal reflux [GER], aspiration, pneumonia, pneumothorax)
- Additional diagnostic work-up indicated (e.g., skin testing, pulmonary function testing, exercise testing)
- Additional therapy indicated (e.g., immunotherapy)
- Suicidal ideation, depression, or a severely dysfunctional family

Asthma is a chronic disease that occurs in all age groups, resulting in reversible airflow obstruction within the large and small airways. The major pathologic processes that contribute

Table 45-1 Asthma Severity Classification

ASTHMA SEVERITY CLASSIFICATION	INTERMITTENT	MILD PERSISTENT	MODERATE PERSISTENT	SEVERE PERSISTENT
Symptoms	Less than two times per week; brief exacerbations (few hours to few days); normal between exacerbations	More than two times per week; exacerbations affect activity	Daily exacerbations; affect day and night activities	Continuous, frequent exacerbations; limited physical activities
Nighttime symptoms	Less than two times per month	More than two times per month	One or more times per week	Frequent
Lung function (PEFR or FEV$_1$)	≥ 80% predicted; variability < 20%; can be normal values	≥ 80% predicted; variability 20% to 30%	> 60% and < 80% predicted; variability > 30%	≤ 60% predicted; variability > 30%
Medications needed for control	Intermittent rescue* medication; may need oral steroid for exacerbations	For infants and children, daily controller medication (cromolyn or low dose of inhaled corticosteroid); consider leukotriene modifier medication; need rescue* medication for exacerbations	For infants and children, daily controller medication (low to medium dose of an inhaled corticosteroid); add long-acting bronchodilator if appropriate; consider leukotriene modifier medication; need rescue* medications for exacerbations	For infants and children, daily controller medication (high dose of an inhaled corticosteroid); may also need systemic corticosteroids every day or every other day; add long-acting bronchodilators if appropriate; consider leukotriene modifier medication; need rescue* medication for exacerbations

Modified from Pediatric asthma: Promoting best practice. (1999). Milwaukee, WI: American Academy of Allergy, Asthma and Immunology, Inc.
Short-acting bronchodilator or oral prednisone.
FEV$_1$, Forced expiratory volume in 1 second; PEFR, peak expiratory flow rate.

to airflow obstruction are inflammation with mucosal edema, bronchospasm from smooth muscle contraction, and mucus production. Although chronic, the disease is reported to have intermittent exacerbations and symptoms. Although a greater understanding of the predominance of inflammation in the pathology of asthma has developed over the last 15 years, the origin of asthma remains incompletely understood. Despite research regarding the underlying pathophysiology, which has improved our understanding and led to refined treatment modalities, the prevalence, morbidity, and mortality associated with asthma have continued to increase in children at a time when these are declining in many other childhood illnesses.

The needs of a chronically ill child can be felt throughout the family. Families must deal with uncertainty regarding exacerbations, fears for their child with respiratory distress, loss of parental work time, and the special care needs of a child with asthma. Those needs can include unexpected, more frequent and additional medical appointments, locating and properly using equipment to monitor asthma and administer medications, and ensuring the safety and care of their child within all the environments that the child spends time in during the day.

Asthma is responsible for more school absences and hospital visits than any other chronic childhood disease. Asthma continues to seriously affect family life and productivity in terms of health care costs and the significant burden to families. In 1994 the total direct and indirect cost of asthma in the United States was estimated to be $10.7 billion, an increase of 54.1% since 1985. Direct costs included hospitalizations, which

decreased because of shorter length of stay rather than less admissions, emergency room visits, physician visits, and prescribed medications, which increased 10.1% over the last 10 years; indirect costs were attributable primarily to parental loss of work time and school absences. Despite the increase in the prevalence of asthma, estimated costs per person with asthma decreased 3.4% during this same time period. National efforts targeting specific asthma outcomes and resource utilization combined with a reduction in hospital length of stay may be responsible for this overall reduction in asthma costs.

Two factors contributing to the increased mortality and morbidity of asthma in children are underdiagnosis and inappropriate treatment. To be effective and reduce costs, asthma treatment must be family centered and combine a variety of components, both pharmacologic and nonpharmacologic.

Etiology

Asthma is the result of a complex, multicellular reaction in the airways in which many types of cells are involved, primarily mast cells, eosinophils, and T lymphocytes. Airway inflammation, airway hyperresponsiveness, and bronchoconstriction, resulting in airflow obstruction, which by definition is at least partially reversible, characterize asthma.

Airway inflammation with hyperreactivity is the common denominator in all children with asthma. Regardless of whether a child has intermittent, mild, moderate, or severe persistent asthma (see Table 45-1), evidence of inflammation in airway tissue has been documented through analysis of bronchoalveolar lavage fluid obtained from a child's airways. Inflammation is present in all children with or without the presence of symptoms.

The inflammatory process is begun when immunoglobulin E (IgE) binds to high-affinity receptors on the surface of resident mast cells, epithelial cells, and circulating basophils and low-affinity receptors on lymphocytes, eosinophils, platelets, and resident macrophages. When an allergen-trigger interacts with these IgE receptors, activation of the cell and the release of preformed as well as newly generated mediators occurs. Mast cell degranulation releases histamine, leukotrienes, and cytokines, which cause bronchoconstriction of smooth muscle. Inflammatory cells (i.e., eosinophils, lymphocytes, neutrophils, basophils) are recruited to the airways and activated releasing cytokines, superoxides, enzymes, and other bronchoconstrictors. The cumulative action of these mediators causes an increase in airway responsiveness, bronchospasm, epithelial cell sloughing, mucus production, and edema. Airway repair and remodeling occurs subsequent to the inflammation.

Mast cells contribute to inflammation by releasing preformed mediators such as histamine, peroxidase, and neutral proteases and form molecules such as superoxide, cytokines (e.g., interleukin 4 [IL-4], IL-5, interferon-γ), and platelet-activating factor, all of which play a role in allergic inflammation. Eosinophils are the principal effector cell of injury to the airway. They are recruited into the lung from the epithelium through actions of the T-cell cytokines and degranulate to release damaging chemical mediators. Through the interaction of these cells with the epithelium, adhesion proteins release oxidants and proteases, which degrade the basement membrane and interstitial matrix molecules. Macrophages contribute to airway injury through the release of cytokines, lipid mediators, and lysosomal enzymes and function as antigen-presenting cells that further stimulate T-lymphocyte proliferation and cytokine production. Basophils release preformed mediators such as histamine and cytokines while increasing in number 24 hours and longer after the allergen has occurred. Their actions seem to provide a basis for the chronicity of inflammation and symptoms in the late-phase asthma response. T lymphocytes also provide stimulation to activate and continue the chronic and persistent inflammatory processes and regulate airway repair processes.

The result of this persistent damage of epithelial cell sloughing, cell injury, mucus production, and edema causes the characteristic bronchospasm, airway hyperresponsiveness, and chronicity of symptoms seen in children with asthma. Ensuing remodeling of the airway, which can ultimately change the structure and function of the wall, can have a significant effect on future pulmonary function.

A balance between the subpopulation of T-lymphocyte cells and helper T cells (Th-1 or Th-2) may influence the expression or suppression of asthma and allergic disease. Current evidence indicates that the presence or absence of an allergic response may be attributable to a directing influence toward a predominant Th-1 or Th-2 cytokine expression response to environmental stimuli. If a Th-2 response with cytokines such as IL-4 prevails along with a diminished production of interferon-γ, allergic inflammation is likely. But if the Th-1 pathway is influenced with the release of IL-12, a protective effect against the generation of the allergic response occurs. Newborn cord blood indicates a predisposition toward a Th-2 phenotype caused by an imbalance of Th-2 and Th-1 cells from the placenta. The initial influence on the release of these cytokines is

---

Box 45-2 Factors that May Affect Balance between Th-1 and Th-2 Cytokine Responses in Early Life*

Influences that May Promote Th-1 Environment

Older siblings
Child-care setting in early life
Rural environment
Certain bacterial and viral infections

Influences that May Promote the Th-2 Environment

Minimal to no infection exposure
Frequent antibiotic use
Urban environment
Sensitization to house dust mites, cockroaches, and allergens

Adapted from Busse, W.W. & Lemanske, R.F. (2001). New England Journal of Medicine, 344, 350-362.
Factors that may cause an imbalance in the Th-1 and Th-2 cytokine response may increase the likelihood of developing allergic disease (Th-2) or reduce the likelihood of allergy (Th-1).

---

believed to be a bacterial infection of the airways, leading to the expression of the "hygiene hypothesis" as a possible determinant of asthma development. If a neonate under 6 months is exposed to infectious microbes or develops a respiratory infection, it is hypothesized the neonate will be directed to the Th-1 pathway and not develop the allergic sensitization pattern. Furthermore, lack of early exposure to these microbial infections or frequent use of antibiotics may predispose the infant to the development of IgE-mediated response to allergens. In support of this hypothesis, it has been reported that asthma is less frequent in children who attend day care or have older siblings or live on farms with endotoxin exposure. To reduce the risk of asthma, a suggestion has been made to provide some kind of "exposure" to the infants at risk for allergy (parents with history of allergy or asthma) to stimuli that would lead to an increased Th-1 mediated response at a critical time in the development of their immune system (Box 45-2).

Generalized alterations in the immune response of children early in life may play a significant role in the development of asthma and perhaps even lead to strategies for its prevention. Asthma development seems to be a multifactorial process influenced by the genetic makeup of an individual, the effect on his or her immune system, and the timing of occurrences of respiratory infections and environmental exposures.

Most children with asthma have a specific IgE antibody response when exposed to specific allergic triggers, which leads to their asthma symptoms. However, their airways may also be affected by neural control mechanisms located in the airway, which regulate inflammatory processes and airway caliber. Within the airways there is an extensive network of nerve fibers, and they contain neurotransmitters capable of producing the characteristic features of asthma exacerbations. With vagal stimulation, the parasympathetic nervous system causes airway constriction, and sympathetic adrenergic stimulation causes dilatation. In asthma, these systems may not function or respond appropriately. There is interest in the neurotransmitters from the nonadrenergic noncholinergic neural pathways and the effect they may have on the neural control of airway caliber.

Early- and late-phase asthma response. An acute asthma exacerbation is superimposed on a child with varying degrees of chronic airway inflammation. Therefore early and aggressive treatment is necessary to reduce the severity of the exacerbation as well as the duration. During the early airway response phase to an inhaled trigger, bronchospasm occurs within minutes as the child's airways react to the allergen that binds with a specific IgE surface on a mast cell, causing mast cell degranulation. This response can spontaneously remit in some children, but most need treatment and respond to a bronchodilator such as a β_2-adrenergic receptor agonist. During the late-phase response, which may occur from 4 to 6 hours later, the bronchospastic response is still present, but the inflammatory response predominates. This perpetual inflammation may contribute to the long-term airway hyperresponsiveness, which may persist for weeks to months after an exacerbation. The process can be further aggravated by allergic as well as nonallergic or irritant stimuli such as smoke, mucus, strong odors, and cold air. Therefore treatment is based on reducing the inflammatory response with antiinflammatory agents and bronchodilators to minimize airway constriction.

Incidence

- Asthma is the most common chronic disease of childhood affecting approximately 4.4 million children in the United States.
- Asthma occurs in all races and in all age groups but more severely affects children and low-income and minority populations.
- National survey data from 1960 to 1995 (from the National Center for Health Statistics) revealed that the number of people with asthma had more than doubled in the previous 15 years.
- The most rapid increase in new cases of asthma occurs in children less than 5 years of age, with over 160% percent increase between 1980 and 1994. Approximately 5 million children under 18 years of age have asthma, and there are 1.3 million cases in children under 5 years of age.
- Although wheezing in the first few years of life is common, many children experience a resolution of these symptoms by early school age. After 5 years of age, the overall incidence of wheezing in childhood is relatively low but associated with persistent symptoms into adulthood if continuing from an earlier age or initiated at this age.
- Asthma is more prevalent in boys than in girls until approximately 18 years of age.
- Asthma is a leading cause of school absenteeism, leading to over 10 million missed school days annually (three times more days for children without asthma).
- Hospitalization rates for children increased in children under 4 years of age between 1979 and 1994 and remained steady in other age groups, averaging approximately 164,000 per year.
- Emergency room visits averaged approximately 570,000 annually and decreased as age increased, but the overall rate remained stable between 1992 and 1995.
- Deaths caused by asthma have increased nationally over the last 15 years and remain highest for African Americans and older adults.
- African Americans are slightly more likely to have asthma than Caucasians, but African Americans and Hispanics are more likely to die from it, which is possibly related more to socioeconomic status than to ethnicity.

Risk Factors

Predisposing factors
- Atopy
- Gender (male until approximately 18 years)
- One or more parents with asthma, allergies

Contributing factors
- Small airway size
- Small size at birth (less than 2500 g)
- Diet (i.e., food allergy)
- Smoking, including perinatal and passive exposure

Exacerbating triggers and factors
- Respiratory infections
- Allergens
- Weather, including high humidity, cold air, weather changes
- Smoking, both active and passive
- Strong odors
- GER
- Allergic rhinitis and sinusitis
- Sensitivity to selected medications and sulfites
- Dysfunctional family situation
- Restricted access to medical care

Differential Diagnosis

Beginning in the newborn period, cough and wheezing may indicate other conditions (Box 45-3) and common pediatric illnesses (see Chapter 41).

Respiratory syncytial virus (RSV) is a ubiquitous respiratory virus that can cause bronchiolitis and injure the upper or lower respiratory system, causing wheezing and coughing in all age groups. Because of its universality, RSV usually infects all children by 2 years of age and may lead to wheezing and

---

Box 45-3 Differential Diagnosis: Cough and Wheeze*

Usual Respiratory Causes

Asthma (493.91)
Infection (465.9)
Foreign-body aspiration (934.9)
Cystic fibrosis (493.91)

Unusual Respiratory Causes

Bronchopulmonary dysplasia (770.7)
Pulmonary structural abnormalities (770.8)
Laryngotracheal malacia (519.1)
Tracheoesophageal fistula (530.84)
Bronchiectasis (494.0)
Vocal cord dysfunction (478.5)
Primary ciliary dyskinesia (781.3)
Allergic bronchopulmonary aspergillosis (117.3)
Functional cough (306.1)

Possible Cardiovascular Causes

Congenital heart defects (746.9)
Vascular rings or slings (747.21)

Possible Gastrointestinal Causes

Gastroesophageal reflux or aspiration (530.81)
Foreign body in the esophagus (935.1)

See also Chapter 41.

airway obstruction with subsequent viral illnesses for several years.

Foreign-body aspiration should be considered in any baby around 1 year of age or older if monophonic wheezing and diminished breath sounds are present and confined to one lung region. The history may or may not be congruent with aspiration (sudden onset of cough or choking).

Cystic fibrosis (see Cystic Fibrosis later in this chapter) should be considered in a child with chronic or recurring respiratory tract or GI tract symptoms. Chronic pulmonary infections and sinusitis are frequently part of the illness resulting in asthma-like symptoms of wheezing, shortness of breath, and an obstructive respiratory disease pattern. Pancreatic insufficiency and GI tract symptoms of meconium ileus at birth, steatorrhea, and malabsorption are associated with CF but may not be present in a small proportion of children. The sweat test to determine the diagnosis for CF should be done in a laboratory that performs the test frequently because of the numerous technical problems associated with it. Genetic testing for CF is done at specific laboratories throughout the country.

Subjective Data

History is the most important aspect of diagnosis. Consider a diagnosis of asthma with the following:
- Persistent or recurrent cough or wheeze with the following: prolonged viral respiratory tract infections; disturbed sleep at night; physical activity; history of atopy, allergic rhinitis, prematurity, or recurrent pneumonia or bronchitis; vomiting associated with coughing; respiratory symptoms associated with exposure to allergens or irritants; frequent school or day-care absences; crying, laughing, or shouting; or parental history of cough only, especially at night or with strenuous activity and no wheeze (cough-variant asthma)
- Parental description of a decrease in child's quality of life (including activity, playfulness, sleep patterns, and appetite that are disturbed because of cough or wheeze)
- Family history of asthma or atopy
- Parent reports that child complains of or exhibits the following:
  Chest tightness, pain, or shortness of breath
  Restlessness or anxiousness with cough, wheeze, or shortness of breath
  Persistent cough (at nighttime, during the day, or with activity)

Preference for upright position rather than lying down to sleep
Abdominal pain or "tummy ache" with cough or wheeze (resulting from abdominal muscles contracting on expiration and coughing)

Objective Data

Physical examination. During an asthma exacerbation, the practitioner may observe the following physical findings of respiratory distress caused by asthma:
- Tachycardia, tachypnea, increasing expiratory phase, coughing, or wheezing
- Increased anteroposterior diameter of the chest wall
- Grunting respirations
- On auscultation, multiphonic wheezes, initially on expiration; as episode worsens, inspiratory wheezes and rhonchi; if poor air movement, possible inaudible breath sounds (a very ominous sign of significant distress)
- Accessory muscle use (e.g., nasal flaring, sternocleidomastoid, scalene, abdominal muscle use)
- Possible intercostal and subcostal retractions
- Child stopping for breaths between words
- Pallor or cyanosis
- Increased anteroposterior (AP) diameter of chest wall
- Preference for upright position
- Altered level of consciousness associated with previous symptoms

In a child with asthma not currently having an exacerbation, the following physical findings may be observed:
- Increased AP diameter of chest wall
- Mild prolonged expiratory phase
- Evidence of allergy or atopy (e.g., skin dryness, eczema, dark circles under eyes, pale, bluish nasal turbinates)

Diagnostic procedures and laboratory tests. See Table 45-2.

Primary Care Issues and Implications

Growth and development. Asthma is a disease that may wax and wane throughout a child's life; therefore it is important to reassess the treatment plan every 3 to 6 months with child and family. Allow the child to "grow" into responsibilities and participate in treatment decisions as skills and knowledge increase. Assist the family in placing reasonable expectations on the child and to support the child's efforts.

The child's growth potential should not be affected because of asthma, though some research has indicated that puberty may be

Table 45-2 Laboratory Evaluation for Exacerbations

LABORATORY STUDIES	EVALUATION	COMMENTS	FOLLOW-UP
Assessment of airway obstruction* Spirometry Peak Flow Rate	FEV₁, FEF 25% to 75%, FVC, PEFR	Evaluate and compare with best previous values either with spirometer or peak flowmeter; need baseline spirometry periodically	Reevaluate after bronchodilator and oxygen administered; should normalize
Oxygenation	Oxygen saturation	To determine severity of exacerbation, have oxygen or oximeter available	
Radiography	Chest radiograph	If there is concern for pneumothorax, pneumomediastinum, or pneumonia; rule out other causes of wheezing if the diagnosis is uncertain; may or may not see hyperinflation	Follow-up film as needed

*For normal values, see Table 45-5.
FEF, *Forced expiratory flow;* FEV₁, *forced expiratory volume in 1 second;* FVC, *forced vital capacity;* PEFR, *peak expiratory flow rate.*

delayed. Frequent exacerbations may lead to a slowing of growth velocity, but catch-up growth should occur with stabilization.

Inhaled corticosteroids in prepubertal children are of concern if greater than the prescribed dose is taken and a spacer is not used. The swallowed portion of the inhaled medication is related to the increasing proportion that is absorbed into the circulation. To minimize this absorption and increase the amount of medication that reaches the lungs, it is recommended that a large volume spacer is used and, when the child is old enough, rinsing their mouth with water after use. Research conducted over 9 years in children evaluating growth suppression and inhaled corticosteroid use indicated transient growth-velocity suppression in the first year of treatment, with subsequent attainment of predicted adult height.

If the practitioner notices growth delay, consideration should also be given to other physiologic, nutritional, and social factors as well. Referral for evaluation may be needed.

Exercise. Practitioners should assist the child and family in determining the type of physical activities that the child is capable of, wants to do, and is comfortable in performing.

Exercise-induced asthma is believed to occur secondary to the evaporation of water from the airway cells leading to a release of inflammatory mediators causing smooth muscle contraction. This prevents the water loss and subsequent bronchoconstriction; children with asthma may need instruction in preexercise asthma treatment (with a β-agonist, cromolyn sodium, or nedocromil sodium) or the use of controller drugs such as inhaled corticosteroids or montelukast (Table 45-3). Adequate fluid intake and a cooling-down period are also advised. In addition, the current belief is that warming up with submaximal exercise to increase bronchial blood flow and water delivery to airways may decrease symptoms. Children with asthma may find more success in activities that are not prolonged or can be intermittent, such as swimming, bicycling, walking, baseball, volleyball, and soccer.

Nutrition and diet. Although not common, food allergies are suspected by many parents as a cause for asthma in children and may play a role in a child's symptoms. Rather than the needless restriction of a child's diet, a child may benefit from a referral to a local dietitian or from skin testing. In addition, skin testing may answer further questions the parents may have regarding allergens in the environment and strategies for environmental prevention.

Children with asthma may have severe exacerbations when ingesting sulfites, which have been banned by the Food and Drug Administration (FDA) for use in fresh foods. Sulfites may still be present in processed potatoes, shrimp, dried fruits, molasses, nonfrozen lemon and lime juices, beer, and wine, as well as in labeled bulk preparations of fruits and vegetables.

Parenting and sleep issues. Some of the medications and methods of administration of asthma treatment have the potential to cause child-parent conflicts. β-Agonists and oral corticosteroids may have a side effect of wakefulness and increased activity, and a child may be required to sit still for a 5- to 10-minute nebulizer treatment three or four times a day. These can be difficult for parents to accept if they are not forewarned.

Assist the parents by providing practical suggestions to facilitate asthma care (e.g., adjust the timing of doses with bedtime in mind, give the early morning or late night treatment while the child is asleep, read a book together, have markers and coloring books for treatment times, place the child in a high chair or watch a video during treatments). Currently, the use of spacers with face masks and metered-dose inhalers (MDIs) can significantly abbreviate the time required for medication administration. Most medications do come in MDI form and offer an alternative delivery method to nebulized drugs.

Immunizations and vaccines. Children over 6 months of age with chronic asthma should receive the flu vaccine in the fall if the child is not allergic to eggs or chicken. For children between 6 months and 3 years of age, the first split virus dose is given in two halves separated by a month and then in one dose annually thereafter. For children 3 to 8 years of age with no previous flu vaccine or influenza illness, the split virus vaccine should also be given in two doses a month apart and annually thereafter. Children 9 to 12 years of age can receive one dose of the split virus each year. A single dose of the whole virus is recommended annually for children over 12 years of age. It is also recommended that family members and practitioners who care for chronically ill children receive the vaccine.

A routine immunization schedule should not be precluded unless the child is following an oral regimen of corticosteroids. If illness prevents routine immunization, immunizations should be rescheduled as soon as possible.

Management

Treatments and medications. The goals of asthma treatment are described in Box 45-4.

Pharmacologic treatment. The understanding of chronic airway inflammation has led to the current treatment approaches rec-

Table 45-3 Medication Guidelines for Outpatient Management of Acute Asthma

	INHALED β-AGONISTS (ALBUTEROL)	CORTICOSTEROIDS (PREDNISONE)
Home usage	MDI: Two inhalations through a spacer with 2 to 3 minutes between inhalations; may repeat every 4 to 6 hours; nebulizer: 0.25-0.5 ml (1.25-2.5 mg) or 0.15-0.25 mg/kg of 0.5% solution in 2 to 3 ml of saline; may repeat every 4 to 6 hours	Oral: 2 mg/kg per day divided every 12 hours for 3 to 5 days and then discontinued
Side effects	Jitteriness, headache, tachycardia, nausea, wakefulness	In the short-term, increased appetite, activity, mood changes
Comments	May be combined with an antiinflammatory treatment if not effective or needed more often than every 4 to 6 hours	May be in liquid or tablet form; may be given with favorite food or beverage to minimize the bitter taste; emphasize the reason for prescribing and the importance of taking only as prescribed; if minimal or no improvement 6 to 12 hours after starting, refer for further treatment; new formulations are available with a better taste

ommended by the National Heart, Lung, and Blood Institute consensus panel regarding the management of acute and chronic asthma. The American Academy of Allergy, Asthma and Immunology published refinement of these guidelines for children in 1999. Children with asthma should have a prescribed asthma management plan (AMP) (Box 45-5) to consult at home (or in any environment that they spend time in) when the exacerbation begins as well as for routine care and monitoring of their asthma. Table 45-3 illustrates a common approach to home management of an acute exacerbation.

Asthma drugs currently fall into two major categories: (1) quick-relief "rescue" medications, and (2) long-term "controller" medications. Asthma drugs used for acute and chronic management are listed in Table 45-4.

Controller drugs attempt to "control" symptoms by modifying the underlying process of asthma with antiinflammatory agents, long-term bronchodilators, and leukotriene modulators. Controller medications for children are used long term to keep persistent asthma under control. Antiinflammatory medications may control symptoms by interrupting the inflammatory process and prophylactically suppressing future inflammation within the airways.

The long-acting bronchodilators act to relax airway smooth muscle, thereby preventing or reversing bronchoconstriction, but have a longer onset and mode of action than the "rescue" bronchodilators. Rescue drugs are short-acting medications that improve or relieve airflow limitation in a lesser period of time; they are not prescribed for antiinflammatory or hyperresponsiveness purposes.

Studies have shown that long-term antiinflammatory treatment improves lung function, reduces hyperresponsiveness, and controls symptoms more effectively than bronchodilators alone. It is postulated that these medications may prevent or minimize airway remodeling. When used concomitantly, long-acting bronchodilators and antiinflammatory medications may address the needs of children with moderate to severe persistent asthma and are superior to the single use of one or the other. The combination allows them to participate more fully in daily activities while reducing exercise and nighttime symptoms.

Rescue medications, most commonly albuterol or levalbuterol, are the bronchodilators used for rapid relief of symptoms. Ipratropium bromide (an anticholinergic) is an adjunct treatment to be considered if albuterol or levalbuterol is ineffective or bronchorrhea is a problem.

Assessing severity. The National Asthma Education Panel of the National Heart, Lung, and Blood Institute has developed an asthma-severity classification (see Table 45-1). This classification should be made before treatment. No single test precisely categorizes patients; however, an attempt has been made to combine symptoms and lung function to clarify treatment strategies. Although the asthma severity classification is variable and will require reevaluation, it is a good starting point for systematically evaluating a child's treatment needs.

Children with mild asthma and intermittent symptoms may require an occasional β-agonist treatment with exercise or allergen exposure or multiple asthma medications with an acute respiratory infection. This may entail use of a β-agonist and an antiinflammatory, such as a short burst of corticosteroids. Even a child with mild intermittent asthma is capable of having a severe exacerbation.

In general, use of nebulized albuterol or an MDI preparation provides faster bronchodilatation with fewer side effects than an oral preparation. In children with intermittent asthma, an oral preparation may be of occasional use, though most parents complain of the disruptive side effects of wakefulness and hyperactivity.

Children with mild to moderate persistent asthma symptoms need more treatment to avoid compromising their quality of life, maximizing cardiopulmonary reserve and, one would hope, prevent chronic airway hyperreactivity and remodeling. Many children become accustomed to low-grade, chronic symptoms and adjust their activity to these or simply accept their symptoms as part of their life. Parents and practitioners can inadvertently promote this unless they are aware of the possibility and frequently evaluate the child.

Medications such as inhaled corticosteroids, leukotriene modulators, cromolyn, nedocromil, or long-acting bronchodilators are needed for persistent symptoms, with home monitoring to control symptoms. Short-term bronchodilators

---

Box 45-4 Goals of Asthma Treatment

Minimize or eliminate asthma symptoms and maintain normal activities, including participation in sports and exercise, school and day-care attendance, and sleeping through the night.

Maintain as near a normal pulmonary function as possible.

Minimize airway hyperreactivity.

Minimize the adverse effects of medications.

Prevent further asthma exacerbations and symptoms.

Box 45-5 Minimal Content for Asthma Management Plan

A. *Identification information*—Name, address, date of birth, parent's name, phone, asthma care provider, and hospital

B. *Medications*—Dose, frequency, duration, and purpose (e.g., for exacerbation, for daily maintenance and exercise)

C. *PEFR*—Personal best of the child if followed with:
- Green Zone—Able to do usual activities, no symptoms of asthma episode, PEFR 80% to 100% of child's best (indicating no changes needed in medications)
- Yellow Zone—Increased asthma symptoms, usual activities limited, PEFR 50% to 80% of child's best (indicating need for addition of "rescue" medications and other action)
- Red Zone—Significant asthma symptoms, usual activities severely limited, asthma symptoms return less than 4 hours after use of "rescue" medication, PEFR less than 50% of child's best (indicating possible need for oral steroid dose and requiring contact with parents or asthma care provider)

D. *Early warning signs*—Physical symptoms and what to do when they occur (e.g., check PEFR if appropriate, increase short-acting β-agonist to every 4 hours, start oral corticosteroid burst at prescribed dose, call providers to notify of change in status)

E. *When to call providers for help*—If previous measures not effective, medications needed more often than every 4 hours, respiratory distress increases, or PEFR decreases or does not change

(Call 911 when there is a blue color to the lips or fingernails or extreme respiratory distress!)

Table 45-4 Asthma Medications Currently Available for Chronic and Acute Asthma Management in Children

Controller Medications

	DOSAGE FORM	LOW DOSE	MEDIUM DOSE	HIGH DOSE
Beclomethasone dipropionate (Beclovent, Vanceril, Vanceril-DS)	MDI: 42 μg/puff 84 μg/puff	2-8 puffs/ day 1-4 puffs/day	8-16 puffs/day 4-8 puffs/day	> 16 puffs/day > 8 puffs/day
Budesonide (Budesonide Turbuhaler, Budesonide Respules)	DPI: 200 μg/puff 0.25 mg/2 ml and 0.5 mg/2 ml	1 puff/day Not established (maximum recommended dose is 0.5 mg/day)	1-2 puffs/day Not established (maximum recommended dose is 1 mg/day)	> 2 puffs per day Not established (maximum recommended dose is 1 mg/day)
Flunisolide (AeroBid, AeroBid-M)	MDI: 250 μg/puff	2-3 puffs/day	4-5 puffs/day	> 5 puffs/day
Fluticasone propionate (Flovent)	MDI: 44 μg/puff 110 μg/puff 220 μg/puff	2-4 puffs/day — —	4-10 puffs/day 2-4 puffs/day —	> 10 puffs/day > 4 puffs/day > 2 puffs/day
	DPI: 50 μg/puff 100 μg/puff 250 μg/puff	2-4 puffs/day — —	4-10 puffs/day 2-4 puffs/day —	> 10 puffs/day > 4 puffs/day > 2 puffs/day
Triamcinolone (Azmacort)	MDI: 100 μg/puff	4-8 puffs/day	8-12 puffs/day	> 12 puffs/day

Systemic corticosteroids

Prednisone (Pediapred) — Chronic use is 0.5-2 mg/kg, divided twice a day or every other day; in severe cases dosage may differ. Long-term use may lead to hypertension, weight gain, hirsutism, diabetes, cataracts, glaucoma, osteoporosis, gastric bleeding, growth suppression caused by HPA suppression, peptic ulcers, acne, edema, skin atrophy. Emphasize the reason for prescribing and necessity of only giving as prescribed. Attempt to taper off to a minimal dose from every day to every other day, and then discontinue or wean to inhaled steroids if possible. Use with caution in children with TB, parasitic infections, diabetes, depression, peptic ulcers, and glaucoma. Caution regarding exposure to varicella and varicella immunization; instruct to parents to call if patient is exposed; discontinue steroids if possible; consider acyclovir

Nonsteroidal antiinflammatory drugs

Cromolyn sodium (Intal) — Inhalation by nebulizer: 20 mg three or four times/day; inhalation by MDI: 2 puffs three or four times/day (800 μg/puff); NSAIDs inhibit early- and late-response phase; needs routine use for effectiveness; initial trial may take 3 to 4 weeks to determine efficacy; has minimal to no side effects

Nedocromil sodium (Tilade) — Inhalation by MDI: 2 puffs 3 or 4 times/day (1.75 μg/puff); may reduce to twice a day based on response; needs routine use for effectiveness; use with spacer to minimize bad taste, clinical trials still ongoing in children; has minimal to no side effects

Long-acting inhaled β-agonists

Salmeterol (Serevent) — Inhalation by MDI: 2 puffs twice a day (25 μg/puff); not to be used for acute exacerbations; this form of bronchodilator is used as a controller, not a "rescue" drug; short-acting β-agonists are needed for acute problems; helpful for controlling nocturnal and exercise-induced symptoms; side effects may include tachycardia, jitteriness, headache, wakefulness, and increased activity

Formoterol (Foradil Aerolizer) — Inhalation by DPI: 2 puffs twice a day (12 μg/capsule) for a child older than 12 years of age; not to be used for acute exacerbations; this form of bronchodilator is used as a controller, not a "rescue" drug; short-acting β-agonists are needed for acute problems; helpful for controlling nocturnal and exercise-induced symptoms; may be used 15 seconds before exercise; side effects similar to those of other β-agonists

Table 45-4 Asthma Medications Currently Available for Chronic and Acute Asthma Management in Children—cont'd

Combination inhaled corticosteroid and long-acting β-agonists

Fluticasone/Salmeterol (Advair Diskus)	Inhalation by DPI: 1 puff twice a day for a child older than 12 years of age; variable dosages: 100 μg/50 μg, 250 μg/50 μg, 500 μg/50 μg; dosage based on child's current asthma therapy; see package insert or *Physician's Desk Reference* for initial and maximum dosage; side effects include pharyngitis, sinusitis, hoarseness, oral candidiasis, and headaches

Sustained-release bronchodilators

Theophylline (Slo-Bid)	Many forms available; age-dependent dosages; usually given every 12 hours; may need every 8 hours in some children; 6 to 9 years of age: 24 mg/kg per day; 9 to 12 years of age: 20 mg/day; 12 to 16 years of age: 18 mg/day; not used frequently with the advent of short- and long-acting β-agonists; appropriate dosing and monitoring of serum levels to maintain between 5 and 15 μg/ml is essential because of the significant side effects of tachycardia, dysrhythmias, headaches, nausea and vomiting, seizures, and even death; can be useful with nocturnal symptoms; conditions known to alter metabolism include febrile illness, pregnancy, lover disease, and CHF; medications such as cimetidine, erythromycin, ciprofloxacin, oral contraceptives, and propanolol can increase clearance; medications that can decrease clearance are rifampin and phenytoin; adverse effects do not necessarily occur according to serum levels; start with lower serum levels to evaluate therapeutic effect

Leukotriene modifiers

Montelukast (Singulair)	Tablet 10 mg, chewable tablet 4 mg or 5 mg; children 2 to 5 years of age: 4 mg once a day at night; children 6 to 14 years of age: 5 mg once a day at night; children older than 14 years of age: 10 mg once a day at night; may be helpful in exercise-induced asthma; side effects include headache, dizziness, drowsiness, and fatigue

"Rescue" Medications

Short-acting β-agonists

Albuterol (Ventolin, Proventil)	Inhalation/nebulizer 0.5% solution (5 mg/ml); children less than 12 years of age: 0.15-0.25 mg/kg per dose every 4 to 6 hours (maximum dose not to exceed 12 to 24 mg/day); children older than 12 years of age: 2.5 to 4 mg/dose every 4 to 6 hours (maximum dose not to exceed 32 mg/day); inhalation by MDI 90 μg/ puff: 1-2 puffs every 4 to 6 hours as needed; inhalation by Rotacaps 200 μg/capsule: children: 200-400 μg every 4 to 6 hours; possible side effects include jitteriness, tachycardia, increased activity and wakefulness, nausea, and headache; use spacer with MDI
Levalbuterol (Xopenex)	Inhalation/nebulizer solution 0.63 mg/3 ml or 1.25 mg/3 ml: children 2 to 11 years of age: Limited data (see package insert); children older than 12 years of age: 0.63 mg three times a day every 6 to 8 hours (may be increased to 1.25 mg three times a day (0.63 mg of levalbuterol comparable to 2.5 mg of albuterol); significantly fewer side effects than albuterol

Anticholinergics

Ipratropium bromide (Atrovent)	Inhalation by MDI 18 μg/puff; children younger than 12 years of age: 1 or 2 puffs every 6 to 8 hours; children older than 12 years: 2 to 4 puffs every 6 hours (maximum dose of 12 puffs every 24 hours); safety and efficacy not established in children younger than 12 years of age; not for use with initial treatment of bronchospasm; slower onset of action (30 to 60 minutes); used as an alternative or adjunct bronchodilator for those with increased secretions; possible side effects include dryness in the mouth and a bad taste

Systemic corticosteroids

Prednisone (Prelone, Pediapred, Orapred)	Acute "burst": 2 mg/kg per day once a day or divided twice a day for 3 to 5 days only; side effects may include mood changes and increased appetite and activity; for long-term side effects, see the listing for prednisone under Controller Medications

are still needed for exacerbations. Additionally, early and aggressive short-term oral glucocorticoids for acute exacerbations may also be needed.

Severe persistent asthma symptoms require multiple daily asthma medications. These include antiinflammatory medications and long-acting bronchodilators for daily use, leukotriene modulators, rescue medications (short-acting bronchodilators) with exacerbations, and use of oral corticosteroids on a continuous or every-other-day basis. Methotrexate, intravenously administered immunoglobulin, and cyclophosphamide are occasionally used in a small subpopulation of severe asthmatics as a corticosteroid-sparing therapy when corticosteroid side effects persist or progress.

Counseling and prevention

Nonpharmacologic treatment. Prevention is a key aspect of asthma management, with reduction or avoidance of allergens and monitoring and early treatment of symptoms accomplished in the home setting.

Asthma management plan. An asthma management plan (see Box 45-5) is required for all children with asthma. The practitioner formulates the plan with the family based on the needs and capabilities of the child and family. It provides clear instruction on how to proceed on a daily basis for those children with persistent symptoms on controller medications and when an exacerbation occurs. This shared home management approach among the child, family, and practitioners can reduce exacerbations in number, duration, and severity. An asthma management plan should be physically available on site and understood in all settings for the child (e.g., home, school, day care, grandma's house).

Box 45-6 Metered-Dose Inhaler Techniques

Metered-Dose Inhaler with Spacer

Stand or sit upright and remove gum or anything else from mouth.
Shake MDI for 3 seconds.
Insert MDI into spacer.
Exhale maximal amount.
Seal lips around the mouthpiece of the spacer.
Press down on the canister of the MDI to fill the spacer with medication.
Take a slow deep breath in and hold it for a slow count to 10.
Release breath and wait 2 to 3 minutes.
Repeat the procedure.
Rinse out mouth with water if using an inhaled corticosteroid to prevent thrush.

Metered-Dose Inhaler without Spacer

Stand or sit upright and remove gum or anything else from mouth.
Shake metered-dose inhaler for 3 seconds.
Exhale maximal amount of air.
Place MDI two fingerbreadths in front of mouth and pointing toward the back of the throat.
With the MDI in this position, open mouth and start to take a slow deep breath while pressing down on the canister of the MDI.
Hold breath for a slow count of 10 seconds.
Release breath and wait 2 to 3 minutes.
Repeat the procedure.
Rinse out mouth with water if using an inhaled corticosteroid to prevent thrush.

Metered-Dose Inhaler with Face Mask (for Infants and Young Children)

Stand or sit upright (if possible) and remove gum or anything else from mouth.
Shake MDI for 3 seconds.
Insert the MDI into the spacer.
Explain to the child that a mask will be put over the nose and mouth but that her or she will be able to breathe normally.
While keeping a good seal on the mask around the child's mouth and nose, press down on the canister once to release the medicine.
Hold the mask in place while child takes six normal breaths.
Wait 1 to 2 minutes and repeat the procedure.
Wipe the skin around the child's mouth and face with a wet cloth if using a spacer and mask with an inhaled corticosteroid to prevent fungal infection.

Appropriate use of asthma medications. Because there are now long- and short-acting bronchodilators, inhaled antiinflammatory corticosteroids, inhaled antiinflammatory nonsteroidal medications, combination medications and leukotriene modulators, many children and families can become confused or misinformed regarding the proper use of medications. It becomes important to reiterate the use and purpose of the medications while emphasizing the fact that these are not "addictive" drugs, nor do they cause a "weakening" of the respiratory system with continued use.

An increase in treatment is necessary as the severity or frequency of symptoms increases. Before stepping up treatment, assess the following:

- The child and family's understanding and use of the medications.
- Proper technique in using equipment to administer the drug. (Although use of an MDI with a spacer is preferable, there may be instances when a spacer is not available. Both techniques are described in Box 45-6.)
- Appropriate timing for medications.

Peak expiratory flow rate monitoring. A child over 4 or 5 years of age can be taught to perform peak-flow monitoring. Assess the child's demonstration of technique at intervals to verify continued accuracy and performance. Peak expiratory flow rate (PEFR) can be especially useful for children who do not perceive their asthma symptoms or airflow limitation well.

Ideally the child would monitor the PEFR in the morning to evaluate changes over time. If decreases are documented, an increase in daily controller medications should be considered along with a review of other asthma symptoms. Once a personal best PEFR has been established when the child is well and asymptomatic, the values can be placed in the green, yellow, and red zones for future reference. (Box 45-7 provides PEFR technique and zones). Remember that the child's personal best PEFR will change as the child grows in height.

During an exacerbation the decision to increase or decrease treatment can be correlated with the PEFR, symptoms, and history. The PEFR should never be the sole rationale to change treatment, because, unlike spirometry, it is a very effort-dependent maneuver and measures predominantly larger airway obstruction. Therefore, even if the PEFR is within normal limits, other symptoms or history should not be ignored.

Environment. Avoidance of allergens and other asthma triggers as identified by the history or diagnostic work-up is an important part of the plan to control asthma exacerbations (see Chapters 41 and 43). Not all children with asthma have allergies, although allergies are more common in children over 5 years of age. Allergens such as pollens, grasses, house dust mites, pet dander from warm-blooded animals, molds, and cockroaches are the most common allergy triggers for children with allergies.

Box 45-7 Peak Expiratory Flow Rate Monitoring Technique

Stand up and set the arrow on the device to 0.
Remove gum or anything else in the mouth.
Breathe in deeply.
Seal lips around the mouthpiece
Blow as hard and fast as possible.
Write down the number at the arrow.
Repeat the procedure.
Record the best of three attempts.

Immunotherapy, if available, is an option for children with diagnosed allergies if medications do not control the problem and avoidance is not possible. In many children irritants such as cigarette smoke, wood-burning smoke, strong odors, or poor air quality also trigger asthma. Passive smoking exposure is an irritant to the child's airways whether it occurred when the child was present or hours before. Once identified, avoidance of these triggers should be emphasized. Adverse indoor environments require modifications whenever possible. If this is not possible, consistent use of asthma medications will be necessary. Not all families can intervene in their homes to the same degree. Therefore a reasonable environmental modification approach can be discussed with the family based on the child's needs and family finances. Listed in Box 45-8 are common problems and solutions that can be explored with the family.

Education. Asthma education provided for the families by the practitioner and a shared management approach to treatment have become an effective treatment modality for children with asthma. It is not unrealistic to envision asthma education becoming a standard of care similar to that found with diabetes education.

Parents need asthma education to begin as soon as the diagnosis is made and need a year of intermittent education and assistance before they start to feel a level of comfort in managing their child's asthma at home. Over that year, the content of the education program must be comprehensive, and the lines of communication must be open so that skills, understanding, and trust develop over time.

Asthma education for a family can be approached in the following ways. Initially the family must know and understand enough to safely care for the child at home. This assumes a basic knowledge of symptom recognition, the purpose and use of medications and equipment, and when to call for further medical assistance. Subsequent visits or educational sessions can be organized to include formal education time or health care follow-up visits that incorporate educational components. Whichever way the educational component is addressed, it is useful to have a "master" content of curriculum (Box 45-9) to ensure that all aspects of care are included.

Individualizing the asthma education and plan to the child and family is a strength of this approach that also lays the groundwork for a cooperative, shared management approach. Both the practitioner and family must understand the overall plan for care and how this will become part of the child's and family's daily life for their mutual goal to be achieved. As parents accept more responsibility for care decisions, an interactive partnership is formed with the practitioner, with each partner having distinct as well as complementary responsibilities. Communication and compliance are enhanced as the parents learn to make crucial observations and judgments in a variety of circumstances and obtain reinforcing feedback from the practitioner. It is a powerful advantage for the child to have the practitioner know and understand the skills of the parents and the parents feel that the practitioner trusts and listens to them as well. Evaluation studies of families participating in asthma education programs have demonstrated appropriate decision-making during home treatment of their children with asthma.

Follow-up

Pulmonary function. After an asthma exacerbation, it may take 4 to 6 weeks for the child's airways to return to baseline value, assuming that there have been no intercurrent infections or problems. In some children this process may take even longer.

Parents must be aware of the need to treat symptoms early and aggressively, should they recur, because the child's air-

---

Box 45-8 Environmental Modifications

Bedroom (First Priority)

Encase mattress, box spring, and pillow in zippered plastic.
Remove clutter, vacuum or dust weekly with the child out of the room.
Remove carpets if possible or use synthetic, easily washable rugs.
Use dacron fiber pillows, not down or animal feathers.
Wash bedding weekly in 130° F water to kill dust mites.
Machine wash stuffed toys frequently or remove them from the room.
Remove curtains or use shades.
Keep the closet door closed.
Remove pets and house plants.
Reduce humidity to less than 50%.
Use filters (even cheesecloth) on air ducts.
Avoid vaporizers.

Home

For the heating system, change the furnace filter monthly, have the duct system professionally vacuumed annually, and dust electric baseboard heaters monthly.
Vent the clothes dryer outside.
Place a vapor barrier in crawl spaces to reduce mold.
Prevent mold accumulation with bleach (diluted 1 part bleach to 3 parts water) or use a commercial product.
Have only minimal house plants.
Vacuum rugs and damp mop other floors when the child is not present.
Keep pets out of the house or at least off upholstered furniture and carpets.
Allow no smoking anywhere in the house, car, or any closed environment.
Use a wood stove or fireplace if it is the only source of heat.
Remove carpets laid on cement if possible.

Box 45-9 Essential Components for an Asthma Education Program

Perceptions and personal feelings about asthma and prescribed medications
Goals of the child and family
Definition of asthma and its related basic anatomy, physiology, and pathophysiology
Asthma triggers and how to avoid them
Signs and symptoms of exacerbations, as well as early and late warning signs
Medication, equipment, and indications for the use of each
Home monitoring
Asthma management plan, with instructions on when to call the care provider
Environmental modifications if indicated
Consideration of the family's individual needs

---

ways may be increasingly hyperresponsive during this time. It is important to have a written asthma care plan that supports this recovery time and follow-up visits and phone calls to track the child's progress. Without an adequate understanding, parents may make treatment decisions that are not appropriate.

Children with asthma who are old enough to perform pulmonary function tests (usually over 6 years of age) should have follow-up assessment routinely to evaluate treatment effectiveness, in addition to PEFR monitoring. Rather than categorically stating a frequency, it makes much more sense to determine the need based on the severity of the disease. At minimum, a child with mild asthma should have pulmonary function reevaluated yearly. Children with persistent disease that is in good control may benefit from evaluations of spirometry (Table 45-5) two to four times per year in addition to PEFR monitoring at home. However, a child with daily symptoms that are under poor control may need spirometry as often as weekly or monthly. Monitoring of PEFR at home is a useful tool between formal evaluations, but it is not considered adequate as the only measurement of lung function.

Plan of care. Routine assessment of all the aspects of the plan of care, understanding of medication purpose and use, and appropriate use of equipment such as a spacer, MDI, and nebulizer should be routine every 3 to 6 months. Children's capabilities, the school, and the family's home situation can change, and unless carefully scrutinized, the asthma plan may become inadequate to the current situation. Because most children have an average of eight viral upper respiratory tract infections a year and these are the most frequent triggers for a young child's asthma, it is essential to maintain a proactive plan during the viral infection season. The fall is the time when school-age children return to classes and may be a natural time to review the plan of care, ensure that the school has the appropriate paperwork for emergency and routine asthma needs, and evaluate pulmonary function.

If a patient's condition has been stable for 3 months or longer, a decrease in maintenance therapy may be considered unless there are other concerns. This step down in treatment is just as important as is the step up when symptoms intensify. Children and families benefit from an evaluation to determine

Table 45-5 Pulmonary Function Norms

HEIGHT		FVC (L)				
cm	INCHES	BOYS	GIRLS	FEV$_1$ (L)	PEFR (L/MINUTE)	FEF 25% TO 75% (L/SECOND)
100	39.4	1.00	1.00	0.70	100	0.9
102	40.2	1.03	1.00	0.75	110	0.99
104	40.9	1.08	1.07	0.82	120	1.08
106	41.7	1.14	1.10	0.89	130	1.16
108	42.5	1.19	1.19	0.97	140	1.25
110	43.3	1.27	1.24	1.01	150	1.34
112	44.1	1.32	1.30	1.10	160	1.43
114	44.9	1.40	1.36	1.17	174	1.51
116	45.7	1.47	1.41	1.23	185	1.60
118	46.5	1.52	1.49	1.30	195	1.69
120	47.2	1.60	1.55	1.39	204	1.78
122	48.0	1.69	1.62	1.45	215	1.86
124	48.8	1.75	1.70	1.53	226	1.95
126	49.6	1.82	1.77	1.59	236	2.04
128	50.4	1.90	1.84	1.67	247	2.12
130	51.2	1.99	1.90	1.72	256	2.21
132	52.0	2.07	2.00	1.80	267	2.30
134	52.8	2.15	2.06	1.89	278	2.39
136	53.5	2.24	2.15	1.98	289	2.47
138	54.3	2.35	2.24	2.06	299	2.56
140	55.1	2.40	2.32	2.11	310	2.65
142	55.9	2.50	2.40	2.20	320	2.74
144	56.7	2.60	2.50	2.30	330	2.82
146	57.5	2.70	2.59	2.39	340	2.91
148	58.3	2.79	2.68	2.48	351	3.00
150	59.1	2.88	2.78	2.57	362	3.09
152	59.8	2.97	2.88	2.66	373	3.17
154	60.6	3.09	2.98	2.75	384	3.26
156	61.4	3.20	3.09	2.88	394	3.35
158	62.2	3.30	3.18	2.98	404	3.44
160	63.0	3.40	3.27	3.06	415	3.52
162	63.8	3.52	3.40	3.18	425	3.61
164	64.6	3.64	3.50	3.29	436	3.70
166	65.4	3.78	3.60	3.40	446	3.78
168	66.1	3.90	3.72	3.50	457	3.87
170	66.9	4.00	3.83	3.65	467	3.96
172	67.7	4.20	3.83	3.80	477	4.05
174	68.5	4.20	3.83	3.80	488	4.13
176	69.3	4.20	3.83	3.80	498	4.22

Modified from Polgar, G. & Promadhar, V. (1971). Pulmonary function testing in children: Techniques and standards. Philadelphia: W.B. Saunders.
FEF, *Forced expiratory flow;* FEV$_1$; *forced expiratory volume in 1 second;* FVC, *forced vital capacity;* PEFR, *peak expiratory flow rate.*

the least amount of medication required keeping the child's pulmonary status as close to normal as possible and maintaining normal activities without symptoms.

Once control is established, routine follow-up visits should be based on the severity of asthma and the family's level of understanding and skill in caring for the child. Intervals may be from 1 to 6 months. Children with persistent asthma benefit from consultations with an asthma specialist one to four times or more per year, depending on their level of asthma control, response to therapy, family functioning, and so on.

Consultations and referrals. See the Alert box. Any child with asthma who is unresponsive to usual treatment, is hospitalized, or has frequent emergency room visits may benefit from consultation with a physician.

Future research and treatments. With ongoing research, asthma management is continuing to undergo changes, making it imperative that the practitioner stay updated and keep the families within their practice informed of changes.

Future developments in asthma therapy will be directed toward antiinflammatory mechanisms with more specificity of action and prevention strategies. Selective inhibitors, which would relax airway smooth muscle and enhance the current β-agonist effect, are being explored, and leukotriene and cytokine antag-

onists and inhibitors may be available. Since IgE plays a major role in the pathogenesis of allergy, the development of a human monoclonal antibody, referred to as anti-IgE, is being explored as a possible treatment for managing asthma and allergic disease. The introduction, timing, and nature of microbial or viral exposures is being explored with the possibility of using "probiotics" through the GI tract or vaccines as a source of protecting children against an allergic response by enhancing the development of the Th-1 type of cytokine response.

Strategic plans are being developed and implemented by the Department of Health and Human Services to establish and address priorities for asthma care. These priorities include determining the cause of asthma, reducing the burden of care for all those with asthma but especially the disproportionate burden in minority populations and those living in poverty and improving surveillance systems of the disease with the assessment of the effectiveness of asthma programs. Until the genetic cause of asthma and the maturation of the immunologic response is further elucidated, molecular biologic research will continue to involve investigation of drugs and cellular interactions that seem to affect related genes and the mechanisms of asthma.

Table 45-6 displays special considerations for children with asthma.

Table 45-6 Special Considerations for Children with Asthma

PROBLEM	CLINICAL MANIFESTATIONS	TREATMENT	COMMENTS
Exercise-induced bronchospasm	Cough with or shortly after exercise, PEFR down from preexercise levels	Pretreatment before exercise: (1) Short-acting bronchodilator 10 seconds before activity, (2) long-acting bronchodilator every day, (3) cromolyn sodium 15 seconds before or nedocromil 30 seconds before activity, and (4) consideration of leukotriene modulator or montelukast daily	Reassure children that they can participate in sports and inform them that many Olympic athletes have asthma; pretreatment with an inhaled β-agonist gives rapid bronchodilatation but children with daily or frequent activities may find long-term controller medications more convenient; may need referral for exercise testing if therapy not effective; notify coaches or teachers of pretreatment needs and update the asthma management plan at school
Gastroesophageal reflux	Recurrent cough with or without symptoms of pain after eating; nonspecific vomiting, regurgitation; may exacerbate asthma episode with increased secretions and wheezing; may have chronic aspiration	Treatment with H_2-blocker; small, frequent feedings; remaining upright for 1 hour after eating	Theophylline preparations may relax lower esophageal sphincter and may interact with H_2-blocker (cimetidine), causing decreased clearance of theophylline
Sinusitis	Upper respiratory tract congestion, yellowish-green drainage, foul breath, cough for more than 10 days	Antibiotic therapy for 3 weeks; may also treat with inhaled nasal steroids to promote drainage	Consider if child not responding to asthma therapy
Aspirin or NSAID sensitivity	Symptoms of asthma exacerbation	Treat as any exacerbation and discontinue aspirin or NSAID	Counsel families to avoid these drugs; more commonly seen in adults, but approximately 12% to 28% of children may have aspirin sensitivity with possible crossover to NSAIDs
Allergic rhinitis	Nasal itching, sneezing, rhinorrhea, epistaxis, and congestion; allergic conjunctivitis is a common comorbidity	Antihistamines, nasal steroids, environmental modifications to reduce or avoid allergens, decongestants	May often exacerbate asthma or coexist with it

Resources

Cystic Fibrosis

SUSANNE MEGHDADPOUR

Alert

> Patients with symptoms consistent with a diagnosis of CF must be referred to a CF center for diagnosis and evaluation. Patients with known CF should be referred to a primary physician and the appropriate CF center if the following conditions exist:
> - Pulmonary exacerbation with significantly increased cough refractory to oral antibiotics or, if in combination with shortness of breath, to loss of energy or weight loss
> - Pneumothorax
> - Hemoptysis
> - First onset of or recurrent rectal prolapse
> - Constipation refractory to OTC enemas or laxatives
> - Hematemesis

CF is the most commonly inherited lethal disease among the white population. It is an autosomally recessive disorder affecting the exocrine glands and secretions, particularly of the respiratory, GI, and reproductive systems. In most instances viscous secretions obstruct ducts and airways and lead to pulmonary infections, pancreatic insufficiency, intestinal malabsorption, azoospermia, and long-term cirrhosis of the liver. The salivary and sweat glands excrete abnormal amounts of sodium chloride. Although many presentations have been noted, the most common include diarrhea or constipation (or both), difficulty gaining weight, and recurrent respiratory infections (Table 45-7).

Etiology

A significant breakthrough occurred in 1989, when it was discovered that the basic genetic mutation in CF is caused by a gene on the long arm of chromosome 7 and is responsible for a chloride regulator in cells, also known as the *cystic fibrosis transmembrane conductance regulator* (CFTR). The mutation, caused by the alteration of some essential amino acids in a long chain of deoxyribonucleic acid (DNA), causes abnormal chloride conductance by epithelial cells on mucosal surfaces. The most common mutation of the gene is the DF508 (deletion of phenylalanine at the 508 position on the protein). However, more than 700 mutations that result in CF have been identified. The prevalence of mutations of CFTR vary among different populations. Whereas the DF508 deletion explains about 50% of the disease among persons of northern European ancestry, the most common mutation in Ashkenazi Jews is W1282x. The effects of the disease are seen in organ systems where cells expressing the gene are found. Researchers are working on trying to correlate certain mutations with various degrees of pancreatic insufficiency as well as severity of pulmonary disease. This would allow some ability to predict health outcome for children diagnosed with CF

Incidence

It is estimated that the incidence of CF is as follows:
- 1 in 4250 live Caucasian births
- 1 in 8035 live Native American births

Table 45-7 Abnormalities of Various Organ Systems in Cystic Fibrosis

ORGAN SYSTEMS	SYMPTOMS TO NOTE	PATHOLOGIC PROCESSESS
Sinuses and nose	Discolored nasal secretions; positive cultures of *S. aureus, P. aeruginosa,* or *H. influenzae* bacteria; nasal polyps	Infection, viscous secretions obstructing the sinuses
Lungs	Cough, airway reactivity, cystic changes on chest radiograph, atelectasis, bronchopneumonia, air trapping, pneumothoraces,* hemoptysis,* sputum culture positive for *S. aureus, H. influenzae,* and *P. aeruginosa* bacteria, digital clubbing	Obstruction of the airways, viscous secretions, chronic infection
Intestines, pancreas	Meconium obstruction in neonates, rectal prolapse, malabsorption (particularly fat and fat-soluble vitamins, especially A, E, and K†), diarrhea, FTT, distal intestinal obstruction (observed as constipation), intussusception, diabetes	Intestinal obstruction with large, bulky stool; pancreatic duct obstruction, abnormality of epithelial cells at mucosal surface
Liver	Neonatal jaundice, cirrhosis,* portal hypertension,* esophageal varices,* hematemesis (related to varices),* splenomegaly	Obstruction, fibrosis
Sweat and salivary glands	Abnormal sweat chloride with salty taste to skin, heat prostration, tendency toward metabolic alkalosis	Presumed to be caused by chloride-channel abnormality
Reproductive organs	Reduced fertility in females, absence of the vas deferens or azoospermia in males	Obstruction, viscous mucus in cervical canal

From Bye, M.R., Ewig, J.M., & Quitell, L.M. (1994). Lung, 172,251-270; Murphy, T.M. & Rosenstein, B.J. (1995). Cystic fibrosis lung disease: Approaching the 21st century. Chicago: University of Chicago, Pritzker School of Medicine.
*Usually appears in the advanced stages of the disease.
†Note that vitamin deficiencies themselves have other signs and symptoms.

- 1 in 15,540 live African-American births
- 1 in 60,250 live Asian-American births
- 1 in 11,070 live Hispanic or Latino births

Risk Factors

Because CF is a recessive disorder requiring the transmission of two affected chromosomes, the risk factor is having parents who either are carriers or have the disease. For a child to have CF, both parents must pass a CF gene onto their offspring. Carriers are symptom free. The most common situation involves parents with unknown carrier status. With each pregnancy they have a 1-in-4 chance of having a child with CF, a 1-in-4 chance of having an unaffected child, and a 1-in-2 chance of having a child who is also a carrier.

Subjective Data

When obtaining a history of a child who is suspected of having CF, begin by asking the parents or caregiver to speak open-endedly about the child's early infancy and childhood. Explore the following areas (refer also to Table 45-7):

Review of systems

- *Skin*—Note any history of profuse sweating or comments that the child tasted salty when kissed. Abnormal amounts of sodium and chloride are excreted by the sweat glands, leading to excessive sweating and a "salty taste" on the skin.
- *Head, eyes, ears, nose, and throat*—Note any history of recurrent otitis media; incidence of sinusitis in older children; and nasal polyps or significant nasal congestion. The cellular defect discussed results in abnormalities of the epithelial lining of the sinuses.
- *Lungs*—Review any history of "chest colds" or "asthma"; required hospitalization, treatments, and results; any wet or dry cough; history of sputum production and amount; and the child's exercise tolerance during formal physical education and at play. The excess production of tenacious mucus observed in CF provides a medium for chronic bronchitis and pulmonary infections. About 30% of children with CF also have airway reactivity or asthma. Most children with CF who cough have a wet-sounding cough. The cough may not be responsive to broad-spectrum antibiotics. Worsening lung disease, shortness of breath, cough, and airway obstruction are often observed first as an inability to "keep up" with peers.
- *GI tract*—Note any history of diarrhea, constipation, malodorous stools, steatorrhea, or rectal prolapse. Have the patient describe his or her appetite, and ask for 2- to 3-day dietary recall. Note any difficulty gaining weight. Pancreatic insufficiency causes malabsorption, especially of fats, leading to failure to thrive (FTT). Large, foul-smelling stools and a layer of grease in the toilet bowl are commonly mentioned in the history. The insufficiency of pancreatic enzymes can lead children to eat continually without weight gain.
- *Other*—The symptoms listed here, if related to CF, will most likely come in combination with other GI or respiratory symptoms:
  History of excess urination or thirst, especially in combination with weight loss
  Mucosal excoriation
  Vision abnormalities (may be related to vitamin A deficiency)
  Excessive bleeding or abnormal blood cell counts (Vitamin K deficit can cause decreased prothrombin production)

  Gait or hand-eye discoordination (may be associated with vitamin E deficit)
  Glucose intolerance is observed in 30% to 60% of patients, usually with progression of disease or in adolescence
  In children, ketonuria and ketoacidosis (not usually present)

Objective Data

Physical examination

- *Height and weight*—Height and weight should be recorded on a growth chart at each visit. Compare past weights (percentage) with current weight. Plot weight for height on a growth chart. A child with CF is often but not always at the lower end of the growth curve. Often weight for height is out of proportion. The older the child is at diagnosis, the more remarkable the growth abnormalities usually are. However, 8% to 10% of new diagnoses are made in late school age or early adolescence because there are children who grow well enough to stay on normal growth curves until they reach adolescence when the typical growth spurts do not occur.
- *Respiratory rate*—The respiratory rate is a simple measure that provides important information for children about their respiratory effort (Box 45-10). Younger children especially make use of accessory muscles when their work of breathing increases. The way a child is breathing should also be observed. Count the respiratory rate and observe accessory muscle use, with the child remaining in his or her mother's lap before beginning the physical examination to keep him or her calm. A child with an elevated respiratory rate or using accessory muscles to breathe has an increased respiratory effort and may have pulmonary obstruction or restriction.
- *Heart rate and blood pressure*—Measurements in children with CF should be normal.
- *Head, eyes, ears, nose, and throat*—There should not be any abnormal skull structure in CF. However, an infant may have bulging fontanels and edema because of hypoproteinemia. This should correct itself once the protein deficiency is addressed. Assess the child who has required frequent courses of corticosteroids for posterior retinal cataracts. Check nasal passages for bogginess and congestion. Check for nasal polyps. Nasal polyps are evident not just in CF but also in children with allergies. They are predominantly seen in adolescents and to a lesser degree in school-age children.
- *Neck*—The examination should be normal. There may be lymphadenopathy related to upper respiratory tract infection of the sinuses or oropharynx.
- *Chest*—If the child coughs, the practitioner should assess the quality of the cough and, when possible, the sputum. Cough, when present, is usually wet sounding and productive in children with CF. Young children do not

---

Box 45-10 Normal Respiratory Rates for Children (Breaths per Minute)

Neonate—30 to 60
Infant to child 2 years old—20 to 35
Child 2 to 6 years old—20 to 30
Child 6 to 10 years old—18 to 26
Child 10 to 18 years old—15 to 24

expectorate, but the child who does most often produces yellow-tinged sputum. Sputum color changing from pale yellow to green is evidence of increasing bronchiectasis and infection. Assess lung sounds for crackles and wheezes. Many children with CF have few crackles. However, when the presence of a productive cough signals infection or as airway obstruction progresses from smaller to larger airways, more crackles and wheezes are audible.

Measure the inspiration-to-exhalation time (inhalation-to-exhalation ratio [I:E ratio]). The normal I:E ratio is about 1:2. As expired air is forced to move past obstructed airways, exhalation requires more time, thereby increasing the I:E ratio to 1:3 or 1:4. Initially this may be abnormal in a child with CF.

Measure the anteroposterior (AP) and lateral diameters ratio. Measurement of the AP and lateral diameters of the chest can be made with calipers or a tape measure. The ratio of the AP to lateral diameter of the thorax should not exceed 0.8. As obstructive airway disease and air trapping become more pronounced and the chest more barrel shaped, this ratio (or thoracic index) approaches 1.

- *Heart*—Heart sounds should be normal. In severe or late-stage disease, when bronchopulmonary obstruction leads to hypoxemia and pulmonary vascular constriction, right ventricular hypertrophy may be present.
- *Abdomen*—The practitioner should assess bowel sounds and check for masses and any enlargement of the liver or spleen. The constipation common in CF is usually a distal intestinal obstruction, with stool often palpable in the region of the cecum or the ileocecal valve. In young children this is sometimes preceded by a history of rectal prolapse. In about 16% of infants with CF, meconium ileus is present at birth. Enlargement of the liver or spleen is usually not present until advanced stages of CF. At times, the liver may not be enlarged, but its lower margin may be palpable. This may be the result of hyperinflation of the lungs pushing the diaphragm and the liver downward.
- *Genitourinary system*—Examination of the genitourinary (GU) system in boys and girls indicates abnormalities. Hydroceles and undescended testicles are respectively 4 and 15 times more common in boys with CF. The vas deferens is atrophied or obstructed more than 90% of the time. This is consistent with obstruction of the epididymis and seminal vesicles. The testes are generally normal, and the prostate is not affected. Sexual function is normal. Girls have few clinically assessable abnormalities of reproductive organs. There is significant mucus accumulation in the cervical canal. The vaginal canal, fallopian tubes, and ovaries are normal. Sexual function is normal. Onset of puberty and development of secondary sexual characteristics are often delayed.
- *Skin and extremities*—The practitioner should assess for excessive sweating. Children with CF usually sweat profusely and can become dehydrated easily, especially in hot weather and with intensive exercise. Also assess for digital clubbing. Digital nail-bed clubbing correlates with increasing pulmonary bronchiectasis.

Diagnostic procedures and laboratory tests

- *Chest radiograph*—Look for indications of air trapping and hyperinflation, increased perihilar airway markings, small cyst-shaped obstructions on cross-section of airway, atelec-tasis, and bronchopneumonia. Chest radiographic findings may not be present in very young children with CF. The first findings are usually air trapping and hyperinflation, often first observed in the apices.
- *Pulmonary function test*—Note any flow and volume parameter abnormality. An increased ratio of residual volume to total lung capacity (RV:TLC) greater than 30% is abnormal. Parameters may be normal while children are younger and when pulmonary disease is minimal. Small airway flow is usually the first measure to become abnormal. Forced expiratory volume drop is a sensitive indicator of acute infections. Rising RV:TLC points to increased hyperinflation.
- *Abdominal radiograph*—Note any constipated stool in the ileocecal region or a general pattern of large amounts of stool and gas in the bowel. Abdominal radiographs are needed only to confirm the presence of severe constipation or of bowel obstruction.
- *Sputum culture*—Look for the presence of *Haemophilus influenzae, Staphylococcus aureus,* and *Pseudomonas aeruginosa,* especially mucoid *Pseudomonas* organisms. This must be a broad-spectrum culture, not one simply done for β-hemolytic streptococci. Very young children with CF appear to be initially colonized with *S. aureus* and *H. influenzae.* Usually colonization with *P. aeruginosa* comes later. However, bronchoscopy findings have shown *Pseudomonas* organisms in infants as young as 2 months of age. Mucoid *Pseudomonas* organisms are a strain of *P. aeruginosa* seen almost exclusively in CF.
- *Sweat test*—Keep in mind that sweat chloride values in excess of 60 mEq/L are considered positive for CF; a value less than 40 mEq/L is normal; and 40 to 60 mEq/L is considered borderline. This test is based on the sweat gland duct abnormality. Increased amounts of sodium chloride are excreted in sweat because there is a reabsorption abnormality on the cellular level. Pilocarpine iontophoresis (or a sweat test) must be performed by technicians with standardized techniques and equipment, preferably at a CF center, to minimize false-positive and false-negative results. False-positive results may be attributable to malnutrition, celiac disease, untreated adrenal insufficiency, ectodermal dysplasia, nephrogenic diabetes insipidus, hypothyroidism, mucopolysaccharidoses, glucose-6-phosphate dehydrogenase deficiency, type 1 glycogen storage disease, fucosidosis, atopic dermatitis, or Klinefelter syndrome. False-negative results may be attributable to edema or hypoproteinemia.

    The sweat test is performed by stimulation of the sweat glands with application of pilocarpine to the skin surface of the arm or leg and application of electrical stimulation. The sweat is collected and analyzed for chloride content. If borderline results are obtained, the diagnosis must be confirmed by genetic testing or clinical findings. In some CF centers measurement of voltage across nasal epithelium can be made. This is increased in persons with CF and can help confirm an unclear diagnosis.
- *Genetic testing*—Families with a child suspected of having CF (or with a positive sweat test) can have genetic testing performed. Direct DNA analysis is performed for the DF508 gene. If it is not found, linkage analysis can be performed to look for specific DNA markers, which are linked with CF gene. As was previously noted, genetic analysis cannot yet identify 100% of individuals with CF.

Box 45-11 Confirmation of a Diagnosis of Cystic Fibrosis*

- Postive sweat iontophoresis test result, or
- Genetic testing positive for CF, and
- Clinical data of pulmonary disease consistent with CF, or
- Clinical findings of pancreatic insufficiency

It is important that more than one component be present.

Thus the sweat test remains a vital diagnostic tool. Prenatal testing is now also available, especially for high-risk families. If the testing result is positive and the mother chooses to continue her pregnancy, a sweat test is subsequently performed to confirm the diagnosis (Box 45-11.)

Primary Care Issues and Implications

Although care of the CF patient is directed by the protocols of the CF center, there are primary-care and well-child concerns that apply to these children as they do to all other children. The primary care practitioner (PCP) being attuned to these needs becomes particularly important for a child with a chronic illness.

Immunizations. The child should be given all the usual immunizations, including *H. influenzae* type B (Hib) vaccine. Children with CF also need an annual injection of influenza vaccine. The heptavalent pneumococcal conjugate vaccine is indicated for infants only. The 23-valent pneumococcal polysaccharide vaccine is recommended for those over 65 years of age or if other risk factors for invasive pneumococcal infection are present.

Growth and development. Cognitive and physical development should follow usual parameters in children with CF, except in the area of sexual characteristics (see Sexuality). Emotionally, it is important to remember that these children deal with issues of morbidity and death, particularly their own, much sooner than other children do. In addition, emotional development often has a great deal to do with what hopes and expectations parents have had for their children and how they have communicated expectations to them.

Use the same growth curves as those used for other children to track growth of children with CF. Gaining weight and height is difficult for children with CF. Their growth may track along the lower percentiles, but all efforts should be made to maximize growth. Inadequate growth has been correlated with increased morbidity and mortality. Weight should be calculated as a percentage of ideal weight for height. Plot the height and actual weight on a growth chart. If the weight is not on the same percentile as height, calculate what the weight would be if the same percentile had been achieved. Calculate Actual Weight divided by Ideal Weight for Height × 100. Children whose growth drops below 85% to 89% of ideal weight for height are considered underweight, and close attention must be paid to their dietary intake and use of enzymes.

Nutrition. Children with CF require the same foods that other children do, but with special emphasis on increasing calories. Use basal metabolic rates as guidelines. Caloric needs may be as high as 120% to 150% of the Recommended Dietary Allowance (RDA) for age and sex. Periodic diet histories can point out areas of deficiency. Remember that fats are the most calorie-dense foods. They should play a large role in the diet of a child with CF and not be restricted as they might otherwise be. Food, especially fat, intake should never be decreased if malabsorption occurs. Instead, pancreatic enzymes must be optimized. Children with diabetes who have CF need to have liberal access to all foods except pure sugars. Insulin must be adjusted accordingly.

Peer pressure sometimes instigates noncompliance. Adolescents, especially, dislike feeling different. Preadolescent and adolescent girls with CF can become extremely thin and anorectic, simply by reducing or eliminating their use of enzymes. They are often reinforced for being thin by peers. Careful monitoring of weight and enzyme use is critical at this time.

Exercise. Exercise is encouraged. It provides a method for airway clearance and improvement of pulmonary reserve as well as contributing positively to a child's self-esteem. Aerobic exercise should be entered into with an exercise program that permits gradual increase in aerobic work load. Swimming is particularly advantageous, since it allows for aerobic exercise in a moist environment, which decreases concerns of electrolyte loss in sweat. Weight training is often enjoyed by boys who have a difficult time with being smaller than their peers and have to work hard to maintain their weight. A program of gradual training should be used. CF should not be used as a reason to avoid physical education (see School Concerns).

Discipline. Parents need to recognize that children with CF require discipline in the same manner that all children do. These children should have timeouts, withholding of privileges, and so forth used the way they are used with all other children. This is sometimes difficult, and parents may require support.

Food and food intake can become an arena of contention for parents of children with CF at all ages. Although food should not become a battleground or an area in which the child learns that he or she can manipulate parents, withholding food should never be used as a method of discipline.

School concerns. Both parents and school personnel are often concerned when a child begins school. A parent-teacher conference at the beginning of the school year should be encouraged. Clarification of the following items may be helpful to all involved:

- Children with CF, though they have a cough, are not usually contagious.
- These children should be encouraged to cough, to aid in mucus clearance. Special arrangements may need to be made so that this is not disruptive to the rest of the class.
- Children with CF have a greater-than-usual need to access restroom facilities. They need to feel that this is all right and not be embarrassed about asking to leave a class.

Nutrition is vitally important, and snacks should be accessible. Medications, including bronchodilators and pancreatic enzymes, must be able to be given. The health care practitioner must outline the medication needs. The school must identify someone who will be responsible for helping the child get his or her medication. If the child is not permitted to keep enzymes, they especially should be readily accessible to decrease both the amount of time needed to take them and the child's sense of being different.

Physical education is usually encouraged. Most children with CF can usually tell when they need to stop and "take a break." The pulmonologist at the CF center should help determine a child's exercise capacity. This is especially important if a child has more advanced disease and might become hypoxemic. Exercise should not be withheld, despite its sometimes precipitating coughing.

In extremely hot weather, fluids should be available, and sodium replacement may be needed.

Sexuality. Development of secondary sexual characteristics and puberty are sometimes delayed in CF. Adolescents need to be assured that they will develop normally, even if a little later. Boys with CF need to be reminded that, although the reproductive system in CF is involved, if they are sexually active, they are not protected from STDs. Many adolescent boys begin to explore the issues of male sterility in CF and may want to know definitively if they are sterile. Referral to a knowledgeable urologist is appropriate. Girls need to be reminded that, if sexually active, they are not only at risk for STDs but can also become pregnant. Pregnancy is often associated with exacerbation of illness.

Family concerns. Besides issues of discipline and general care, families of children with CF undergo significant stress and benefit from support in the following areas:

- Emotional concerns are greater. Even when a child is doing relatively well (medically), the family is always contending with the fear that their child may die.
- Financial costs can be enormous. The need to consider finances often ties parents to jobs for fear of insurance loss. Losing a job because of time away as a result of a child's medical concerns is not uncommon. Many OTC medications and other treatments are not covered by even the best insurance plans.
- Siblings often feel either guilty about not being sick or being left out because they receive less attention from their parents, or both. Parents may recognize this as a problem.

Specific screening. Ongoing measurements of growth including height, weight, triceps skinfold measurements, and midarm muscle circumference. Annual laboratory blood work includes a CBC count, electrolyte levels, prothrombin and partial thromboplastin times, liver function tests, and vitamins A and E levels. A chest radiograph is needed at least annually. Sputum cultures are often needed multiple times throughout the year. Decide with the CF center what testing should be done locally versus at the center. (See Table 45-8 for CF complications that may require screening.)

Management

Pulmonary disease and its complications contribute to 90% of the deaths in CF. Treatment is directed at controlling pulmonary obstruction and infection. The main focus for GI tract management is addressing pancreatic dysfunction and GI tract malabsorption. Measure achievement of success by maintaining pulmonary function testing results as close to normal as possible, avoiding bronchial obstruction with mucus and secretions, minimizing infection, and maintaining growth in height and weight. Management includes use of medications and treatments, parent and patient education to encourage adherence to an agreed-upon regimen, and appropriate consultation and referral.

Treatments and medications

Antibiotics. Antibiotics may be given orally, intravenously, or by aerosol. Some CF centers use long-term suppressive treatment with chronic antibiotics; others treat for specific organisms for specific periods of time. The organisms targeted are *H. influenzae* and *S. aureus* in young children and with initial exacerbation of disease. The PCP usually must begin treatment for mild infections. If left untreated in a child with CF, these illnesses can progress and worsen quickly.

Oral antibiotics used to treat *H. influenzae* and *S. aureus* (and dosage) are as follows:

- Dicloxacillin 40 to 100 mg/kg per 24 hours, divided every 6 hours
- Amoxicillin with clavulanic acid 40 to 80 mg/kg per 24 hours, divided every 8 to 12 hours
- Cephalexin 40 mg/kg per 24 hours, divided every 6 to 12 hours
- Cefaclor 40 mg/kg per 24 hours, divided every 8 hours
- Clarithromycin 15 mg/kg per 24 hours, divided every 12 hours

If *P. aeruginosa* is believed to be contributing to the exacerbation or the patient's respiratory condition worsens, the oral antibiotic ciprofloxacin may be prescribed. This drug has been associated with rapid development of drug-resistant organisms. Therefore it should be used judiciously. The dosage is 20 to 30 mg/kg per 24 hours, divided every 12 hours. (All of the previously listed antibiotics should be used for a 2- to 3-week period.)

To treat *P. aeruginosa,* tobramycin is now available for delivery by aerosol in the form of TOBI. It is given at 300 mg twice each day. Colistimethate sodium (Coly-Mycin) is also sometimes used in aerosolized form. There is currently no aerosol-specific formulation of the drug. Therefore the intravenous formulation must be diluted with a minimum of 2.5 ml of diluent to ensure that the size of the aerosol particle is small enough to allow adequate deposition in the lower airway. A compressor nebulizer is used to deliver both medications.

Intravenous antibiotics. Because intravenous antibiotic therapy is frequently started in the hospital but continued at home, the practitioner may be in contact with a child receiving home intravenous therapy. These intravenous regimens are generally regulated through the CF center. However, it should be known that these children are generally receiving a combination of aminoglycosides and β-lactams for treatment of *P. aeruginosa* and *S. aureus.* It is not uncommon for aminoglycoside dosages to be significantly higher than usual to achieve drug levels in obstructed airways and because drug clearance in CF patients is very rapid. Peak and trough levels must be measured.

Bronchial dilatation and control of airway inflammation. Medications are used both to dilate the bronchial airways (usually β-agonists) and decrease the hyperreactivity and inflammation observed in many patients with CF. This is done in an attempt to ease mucus clearance. Some studies have found that β-agonists may cause airway irritability and be contraindicated in some CF patients. Most of these medications are delivered by a compressor nebulizer or an MDI. MDIs are more commonly used with older children, and a spacer must also be used to aid in deposition of particulate matter. Young children using a nebulizer may need to use a face mask instead of a mouthpiece. Commonly used β-agonists include the following:

- Albuterol sulfate 2.5 mg added to a diluent of 2.5 ml of saline in a nebulizer every 4 to 6 hours, or 2 puffs by MDI every 4 to 6 hours
- Bitolterol mesylate 2.5 mg added to a diluent of 2 ml of saline in a nebulizer every 12 hours, or 2 puffs by MDI every 8 to 12 hours
- Serevent (a longer-acting β-agonist available as an MDI or in powder form in a disk dispenser), 2 puffs of the MDI or 1 click of the dispenser every 12 hours

Antiinflammatory medications. These drugs are used to control and provide preventive effect for children with significant airway inflammation and hyperreactivity. All must be used regu-

Table 45-8 Complications of Cystic Fibrosis

COMPLICATION	SIGNS AND SYMPTOMS	PHYSICAL ASSESSMENT	LABORATORY FINDINGS	MANAGEMENT
Allergic bronchopulmonary aspergillosis (airway reactivity to the presence of the mold *Aspergillis fumigatus* in the airways)	Cough secondary to airway reactivity; often refractory to usual treatment	Nonspecific	Chest radiograph may show fluffy infiltrates; positive skin test for *A. fumigatus*; elevated *Aspergillus*-specific serum immune globulin E	Directed at decreasing airway reactivity; long course of oral and inhaled corticosteroids tapered over a number of weeks
Sinusitis	Nasal congestion; discolored nasal secretions; frontal headaches	Tenderness of maxillary sinus region; decreased sinus transillumination	Sinus radiograph and sinus CT with evidence of sinusitis; may be chronic in CF	Nasal corticosteroids every 12 to 24 hours; antibiotics directed at *S. aureus* and *H. influenzae* for 4 to 6 weeks
Hemoptysis (related to enlarged bronchial arteries and progressing infection)	More than 100 ml of blood per day for 3 to 7 days or more than 240 ml in 24 hours is considered significant	Nonspecific; check for decreased breath sounds	Chest radiograph may indicate changes associated with exacerbation of disease	If child is able to detect site of bleeding, keep affected lung in dependent position, treat infection; may require arterial embolization
Pneumothorax	Chest pain, respiratory distress, tachypnea, dyspnea, pallor	Decreased breath sounds, vocal fremitus	Layering of air on decubitus chest radiograph; distorted lung and heart borders	Provide supplemental oxygen; may need chest tube placement
Distal intestinal obstruction syndrome	Abdominal pain, history of constipation	Stool palpable in ileocecal region on abdominal examination	Abdominal radiograph indicates stool obstructing bowel	"Soap suds" enemas; large volume of polyethylene glycol solution (Golytely) by mouth or nasogastric tube
Rectal prolapse	Protrusion of intestinal mucosa from anus; associated with malabsorption or constipation; usually seen in younger patients	Visualization of prolapse	None needed	Reduce with gentle pressure, child in knee-chest position or bent over a chair
GER (related to reduced tone of gastroesophageal reflux; exacerbated by cough)	Midabdominal or midsternal pain; usually present after food intake, when prone; emesis with cough	Nonspecific except for history	None usually needed; if severe, may require a gastric pH probe study; evaluation of gastric emptying	Medical treatment with metoclopramide and histamine$_2$ channel blockers; raise head of bed; avoid lying down immediately after eating
Hematemesis (bleeding caused by gastric or esophageal varices)	GI tract bleeding	Observation of bleeding; reduced hematocrit; history of gastroesophageal varices	Monitor hematocrit; once stable, if varices not known, evaluation will be required	Replacement of blood loss; may need surgical management of varices
Diabetes	Weight loss, increased incidence of infection	Weight loss; infection refractory to treatment	Elevated fasting serum glucose level; proteinuria and glucosuria	Insulin; can moderate diet but avoid decreasing calories

larly to gain the desired effect. Nonsteroidal preparations include the following:

- Cromolyn sodium 20 mg/2 ml vial aerosolized every 6 to 8 hours, or 2 puffs by MDI every 6 to 8 hours (must be used three or four times a day)
- Nedocromil sodium 2 puffs every 12 hours by MDI (not yet available in the United States for use in a nebulizer)

Inhaled corticosteroids (none available for use with a nebulizer) include:

- Beclomethasone 2 puffs every 8 to 12 hours by MDI
- Triamcinolone (Azmacort) 2 to 4 puffs every 8 to 12 hours by MDI
- Flunisolide (AeroBid) 2 to 4 puffs every 8 to 12 hours by MDI
- Flovent (available in three concentrations of 44, 110, and 220 μg) 2 puffs every 12 hours
- Pulmicort 2 puffs once or twice a day, or 0.25 or 0.5 mg nebulized every 12 hours.

Oral corticosteroids are used when hyperreactivity and cough cannot be controlled with nonsteroidal agents or with inhaled steroidal preparations. "Bursts" over 5-days of 1 to 2 mg/kg per day, given either every 12 or every 24 hours, are used.

Mechanical clearance. After bronchodilatation, various techniques are used to clear the airways. The oldest technique involves placing the child in prone positions at an angle for postural drainage. Percussion and vibration are then provided by use of cupped hands or a mechanical percussor-vibrator. Although relatively simple, this technique is time consuming, difficult for persons with arthritis or joint abnormalities to perform for long periods, requires an available "therapist" (parent, sibling, friend), and is especially difficult for families with more than one child with CF. Newer techniques have been developed, including the following:

- Positive expiratory pressure mask
- High-frequency oscillation by means of a fitted vest
- Autogenic drainage techniques
- Flutter device, which employs oscillations of expiratory pressure to encourage movement of mucus

Mucolytics. Various mucolytic agents such as guaifenesin have been used over the years with very limited benefit. Dornase alfa (Pulmozyme), a recombinant human deoxyribonuclease, is an enzyme that has been shown to reduce the adhesive, viscous quality of CF sputum and to enhance mucus clearance. No longer experimental, it is now used particularly with patients with advancing but not acute exacerbation of lung disease. The dosage is 2.5 mg aerosolized (from a nebulizer) once or twice a day.

Enzyme replacement. The child's degree of malabsorption is usually determined at the time of diagnosis. If the child is determined to have pancreatic insufficiency, enzyme replacement is needed. Most enzyme preparations now available are enzyme-coated microspheres. Granules or powders are still available but can cause excoriation of the mouth and perianal region. Once the upper limit of enzyme dosage has been reached, the addition of a histamine$_2$-blocker can enhance effectiveness. Recommended pancreatic enzyme dosages are shown in Box 45-12.

Vitamin supplementation. Fat malabsorption also results in malabsorption of fat-soluble vitamins, especially vitamins A, E, and K. Vitamin D is usually replenished by adequate exposure to sunlight. Vitamins A and E levels can be obtained. Prothrombin time can be measured to assess adequate vitamin K absorption. Vitamin supplementation should be accomplished

---

Box 45-12 Recommended Pancreatic Enzyme Dosages

- *Infants*—Begin with 2000 to 4000 IU lipase per 120 ml of food. Remove the microspheres from the capsule and feed with foods such as mashed bananas or applesauce.
- *Children younger than 4 years of age*—Begin with 1000 IU lipase per kg per meal.
- *Children older than 4 years of age*—Begin with 500 IU per kg per meal.

The goal is not to exceed 2500 IU lipase per meal. Enzyme adjustments in all children are made in accordance with stool frequency and consistency.

---

with water-miscible preparations. Vitamin preparations in liquid and tablet form are now available that target specifically the fat-soluble vitamins and should be used for general vitamin supplementation, even if deficiency does not appear to be present.

More recent and emerging therapies. Many new therapies are being tried at various CF centers in the country. None currently available represents a cure, but all attempt to ameliorate the morbidity of CF and to improve life quality and life expectancy.

- *Lung transplant*—No longer considered experimental, bilateral lung transplant can now be offered to both pediatric and adult patients (based on stringent selection criteria) in the United States at a large number of CF centers.
- *Nonsteroidal antiinflammatory drugs*—Nonsteroidal antiinflammatory drugs (NSAIDs), particularly ibuprofen, were investigated for many years. They are now being used by some CF centers in an effort to reduce inflammation, reduce adhesiveness of neutrophils, and suppress elastase activity, which seems to promote lung injury.
- *Gene therapy*—Gene therapy remains under investigation. Efforts are directed at correcting CFTR dysfunction by an attempt to transfer normal CFTR gene into CF epithelial cells using a variety of vectors.

Other therapies under investigation represent an attempt to alter defective chloride-transport mechanisms and alter the regulation of mutated CFTR.

Complications. Secondary complications that occur in CF and may require specific evaluation and management are noted in Table 45-8.

Counseling and prevention. Teaching families and patients begins at diagnosis and is ongoing. It involves providing new information and reiterating old information. These discussions are most often begun at the CF center and should be reinforced by the PCP:

- Explain anticipated testing. The sweat test, though not painful, may be uncomfortable. The results should be available on the same day testing is done. Review the results, and discuss what CF is. Note the variability of the disease and the inability to anticipate an outcome based on the sweat test results. Grandparents should be included in this discussion.
- Review genetic information. Emphasize the need not to "blame" any member or side of the family for the inheritance of the CF gene. Recall that both parents must carry the gene and that in most cases neither parent has any way of knowing he or she is a carrier.

- Review the management outlined by the CF center team. Clarify that you will continue as the PCP and will be involved not only in the child's CF care but especially in the routine pediatric care that any child needs.
- Assist the family in considering how they will accommodate the need for medications, aerosol treatments, chest physical therapy, increased visits for care, and so forth into their lives.
- Review the potential effect on the family and on siblings.
- Discuss the financial implications.
- For school-age children, discuss who at the school should be informed and how.
- Provide all children age-appropriate information about their disease.
- Involve school-age and older children in decisions regarding alterations to their routines, discussing their disease with peers, and the like, as much as is possible.
- Review medications and side effects that the family should either know about or notify someone about, as follows:
  Antibiotics—These may cause nausea or lead to allergic response of hives or airway reactivity, which should be reported immediately. They may also interact or interfere with other medications.
  Bronchodilators—When first started, these can cause "jittery" feelings, which should resolve. They may also cause tachycardia, which is not usually cause for alarm.
  Antiinflammatory aerosolized medications and inhaled corticosteroids—These should be used on a regular basis and considered preventive (i.e., not useful if used only during exacerbation). If aerosolized medications are being delivered by a nebulizer, appropriate cleaning of the equipment is important. If the patient is using an MDI, the spacer should be checked for defects and the family taught how to detect when the inhaler is empty.
  Oral corticosteroids—When used persistently over long periods (years), these can cause growth retardation. Long-term use has also been associated with posterior retinal cataracts, necessitating regular eye examinations. Occasionally glucose intolerance develops. Some patients also develop a cushingoid appearance, which can be distressing. Studies do indicate that in CF, the benefits outweigh the risks.
  Enzymes—These have few side effects. Dosages or concentrations greater than 2500 U/kg per meal should be used only under the express direction of a pediatric pulmonologist. High-concentration enzyme doses have been associated with GI tract obstruction.
- Review techniques determined by the physical or respiratory therapist to be most effective for an individual patient. Airway clearance techniques must be performed regularly.
- Encourage and discuss options for aerobic activity or weight training.
- If airway clearance is to be accomplished by manual chest percussion and drainage, help the family determine who will do it and who will give that person a break!
- Reinforce the need for large caloric intake. Sources of calories should come from all food groups.
- Explain that times of rapid growth (e.g., puberty) and times of decreased appetite (pulmonary exacerbations) are also times of increased caloric need that parents must anticipate.
- Advise that fats should not be restricted because they are a prime source of calories. This can lead to the child with CF requiring a diet different from that of the rest of the

family. Help parents, especially mothers, determine how to accommodate this.
- Discuss peer pressure and how this can affect a child's nutrition.
- Keep in mind that a child who does not gain weight appropriately may need oral supplements. These are available either commercially or through the use of recipes (usually available from CF centers) to prepare high-calorie puddings and milkshakes. Help parents determine how to best address this need.
- Discuss both with the parents and the child issues of peers and peer relationships, school, and siblings.
- Assist families in helping children identify themselves as more important than their disease.
- Remember that excelling either academically, athletically, or in a hobby is helpful in development of self-esteem. Parents need to be encouraged to allow their children to explore interests and to see life as more than a series of medications, treatments, and hospitalizations.
- Help teenagers learn to make good decisions. Discussions and roleplaying are helpful.
- If it is determined that an adolescent is not going to continue formal education beyond high school, discuss jobs and life options.
- As a child's CF progresses, consider issues of morbidity (e.g., whether and how to continue an education, changes in family life, need for changes in the child's routines).
- Remember that despite advances in the care of children with CF, death continues to come prematurely. Parents of children who have had ongoing deterioration in their health status and in whom death is a possibility need to discuss issues of death and dying. Children often think about these issues before their parents do. It is important for a child to feel confident in discussing them and in asking questions. Such thoughts often occur even when death is not expected, such as at times of pulmonary exacerbation, but it is not uncommon for a child to feel as though he or she needs to spare his or her parents the pain of considering death, even when the child wants and needs to talk about it.

Follow-up. Follow-up care of the child with CF needs to be a joint venture between the primary care practice and the CF center. Well-child care, common childhood illnesses, monitoring growth and nutrition, and early-onset respiratory and GI tract illnesses should be able to be managed by the local practitioner.

Severe exacerbations or treatment failure should be managed by or in consultation with the CF center. In addition, in accordance with the Cystic Fibrosis Foundation guidelines, all children with CF should be seen at a CF center quarterly for medical assessment, monitoring of pulmonary function, and evaluation of status by the nutritionist, respiratory or physical therapist, nurse, and social worker specialized in the care of children with CF.

A child with CF benefits most from the support and availability of both the PCP and the specialist team.

Consultations and referrals. Consultations and referrals are recommended as follows:

Initial diagnosis. Consultation and referral to the appropriate CF center are needed for the following:
- Diagnosis
- Initial management plan
- Recommendations regarding a child's particular nutritional needs

- Airway clearance plan
- Family and child psychosocial assessment by the social worker or psychologist
- Genetics counseling

Ongoing physical needs

- *Medical treatment*—Care must be taken with any failure of oral antibiotics, uncontrollable airway reactivity; side effects of medications necessitating treatment change; inability to regulate enzymes; or indications of the complications noted in Table 45-8. Refer to the physician at the CF center or to the appropriate specialist.
- *Nutrition*—Children who drop below 85% of ideal weight for height should be referred to the nutritionist and physician.
- *Airway clearance*—Children who for medical, family change, or financial reasons cannot continue their previously established airway clearance routine should be referred to the physical or respiratory therapist for reevaluation and development of a new routine.

Ongoing developmental and psychologic needs

- Children with ongoing school issues (e.g., absenteeism, inability to keep up with class work, inability to physically keep up with friends) may need evaluation by a school psychologist.
- Teenage boys who are interested in exploring issues of fertility need to be referred to a knowledgeable urologist.
- Teenage girls should receive routine gynecologic care. If this is not done in the primary care setting, referral should be made to a gynecologist.
- Pregnant adolescents choosing to continue their pregnancy must be referred to an obstetrician familiar with the care of teenagers with chronic diseases.
- Parents of any child with CF who may not have had genetics counseling at diagnosis should be referred to a counselor if they are considering having another child.

Resources

Most CF centers develop teaching materials for families within their own centers, emphasizing their guidelines for care. Frequently these materials are available to other providers as well. In addition, numerous pamphlets are published by pharmaceutical and home care companies with interests in CF. These materials are endorsed to varied degrees by different centers. The local CF center should be contacted for a list of recommended resources.

Organizations

(In addition to patient resources, some pharmaceutical companies have care assistance programs to help with the cost of medications.)

Axcan Scandipharm, 22 Inverness Center Parkway, Birmingham, AL 35242; (800) 950-8085

Cystic Fibrosis Foundation, 6931 Arlington Road, Bethesda, MD 20814; (800) FIGHT CF

Genentech, Inc., 460 Point San Bruno Boulevard., South San Francisco, CA 94080; (415) 225-1000

McNeil Pharmaceutical Co., #1000 Route 202, PO Box 300, Raritan, NJ 08869; (908) 218-6000

Solvay Pharmaceutical Co., 901 Sawyer Road., Marietta, GA 30063; (800) 241-1643

Publications

Croal, D.A (1994). *CF and your tomorrow*. Madison, WI: University of Wisconsin, The Cystic Fibrosis Family Education Program.

Cunningham, J.C., & Taussig, L.M. (1999). *An introduction to CF for patients and families* (2nd ed.). Bethesda, MD: Cystic Fibrosis Foundation and Ortho-McNeil Pharmaceutical.

Orenstein, D. (1997). *Cystic fibrosis: A guide for patient and family* (2nd ed.). New York: Raven.

Hopkins, K. (1998). *Understanding cystic fibrosis*. Jackson, MS: University Press of Mississippi.

Smith, S.T. (1996). *Big pats or little pats?* Buffalo, NY: Western New York Cystic Fibrosis Center and McNeil Pharmaceutical.

Smith, S.T. (1994). *CF and me*. Buffalo, NY: Western New York Cystic Fibrosis Center and McNeil Pharmaceutical.

Websites

Association of Adults with Cystic Fibrosis (www.iacffa.com)
Canadian Cystic Fibrosis Foundation (www.ccff.ca)
Cystic Fibrosis Foundation (www.cff.org)
Cystic Fibrosis Library (www.HealingWell.com/library/cysticfibrosis)
The Dreamsurfer Network (www.dreamsurfer.org)
HealthBoards.com (www.healthboards.com)
MyCysticFibrosis.com (www.mycysticfibrosis.com)
Everyday Warriors (www.everydaywarriors.com)

Diabetes Mellitus

JOHN C. KIRCHGESSNER

Alert

Consult with or refer to a physician for the following:
- Hyperglycemia (blood glucose greater than 250 mg/dl)
- Nausea and vomiting
- Arterial pH less than 7.35, or venous pH less than 7.30
- Serum bicarbonate level less than 15 mEq/L
- Carbon dioxide less than 16 mEq/L
- Ketone bodies in the urine (ketonuria) or elevated serum ketone levels greater than mg/dl (ketonemia)
- Severe hypoglycemia (blood glucose level less than 50 mg/dl) that has not responded promptly to glucagon
- Semiconscious, unconscious, or comatose state
- Seizures

Diabetes mellitus is the most common endocrine disorder in childhood. In the past, type I diabetes was the most common form of diabetes in children, and only approximately 1% to 2% were diagnosed with type II, or nonimmune-mediated, diabetes. However, over the past decade there has been a rapid increase in the incidence of type II diabetes in children 10 years of age older. Some experts are fearful of an emerging epidemic of type II diabetes in the pediatric population. This increase in type II diabetes in the pediatric population also coincides with the increase in overweight and obese youth, and obesity has been identified as a risk factor for the development of type II diabetes in the adult population. Most diagnoses of type I diabetes occur either during the early school-age years or during the prepubertal and pubertal years; type II diabetes is generally diagnosed in the prepubertal and pubertal year. Although diabetes is relatively easily controlled, management of this disorder encompasses all aspects of a child's and family's life. Pediatric endocrinologists play a major role in assisting patients and their families in managing diabetes. However, these children have all the common pediatric health care problems their peers without diabetes do, and it is not unusual for pediatric health care practitioners to encounter the child with diabetes. For this reason it is essential for those in pediatric primary care to clearly understand the disorder, its management, and how common health care problems can affect diabetes and its management.

Etiology

Diabetes mellitus is a disorder of carbohydrate metabolism resulting from the decrease in insulin production or inadequate utilization of insulin. The potential to develop type I diabetes is influenced by three major factors: human leukocyte antigens, the environment, and immunologic processes. Type I diabetes, also known as *juvenile-onset* or *insulin-dependent diabetes mellitus,* is an autoimmune disease in which islet cell antibodies lead to the destruction of the pancreatic beta cells and eventually to a relative lack of insulin. When approximately 90% destruction of the beta cells occurs, clinical manifestations of the disorder become apparent, including hyperglycemia, ketonuria, and acidosis. Type II diabetes, also known as *adult-onset diabetes,* or *nonimmune-mediated diabetes,* is clearly the result of an entirely different disease process from type I diabetes. The development of hyperglycemia in type II diabetes occurs as a result of any one cause or a combination of the following causes: decreased insulin production, insulin resistance, hepatic glucose production, or reduced glucose uptake by target tissue.

Incidence

- Approximately 798,000 people are diagnosed each year with diabetes.
- Of all people diagnosed with diabetes, 5% to 10% have type I, while type II diabetes accounts for approximately 90% to 95% of all diagnosed diabetes.
- Approximately 0.16% of all people under 20 years of age have diabetes.
- About 1 in 600 school-age children develops type I diabetes mellitus.
- The majority of children diagnosed with type I diabetes are diagnosed either during the early school-age years or in adolescence, with incidence increasing as the age of the child increases.
- Type II diabetes is increasing at an alarming rate among children older than 10 years of age.
- Asian, Hispanic, African-American, and Native American children are at greater risk of developing type II diabetes than their peers of western European descent.

Risk Factors

- Family history of type I or type II diabetes mellitus
- Being American Indian, Hispanics, or African Americans (all of these groups have a greater risk of developing type II diabetes than Caucasian individuals. On the other hand, the development of type I diabetes is lower in African-American, Mexican-American, and Asian-American populations)
- Obesity (more than 20% over ideal body weight)
- Past medical history of pancreatitis, hemochromatosis, pancreatectomy, Cushing syndrome, acromegaly, CF, congenital rubella syndrome, Down syndrome, and hyperlipidemia
- Medications, including glucocorticoids, furosemide, and thiazides

Subjective Data

The following information should be obtained on the initial visit:
- Age, sex, and race
- Reason for the visit and history of present illness, including:
  Onset and duration—In type I diabetes the onset of symptoms may be relatively acute, with rapid progression and deterioration in the child.

Presence of the "polytriad" of polyuria, polydipsia, and polyphagia—Other, more subtle symptoms may be enuresis in a previously toilet-trained older child, lethargy, irritability, and a decrease in school performance. The onset of type II diabetes is often more insidious and may not manifest as dramatically as type I diabetes.

Associated symptoms—This includes weight loss (related to the relative lack of insulin and resulting catabolism), obesity (often one of the symptoms with type II diabetes), abdominal pain, nausea and vomiting (often seen in diabetic ketoacidosis), growth failure (relative lack of insulin also causes a deceleration in linear growth), and fatigue (related to the inability of the body's cells to properly metabolize glucose for energy, resulting in a chronic fatigue state). Associated symptoms related to type II diabetes may include blurred vision, nocturia, hyperpigmented skin patches in intertriginous areas (acanthosis nigricans), and recurrent vaginitis.

- Past medical history, including:
  Recent viral illnesses—Coxsackievirus B and rubella and mumps viruses are believed to have a role in the development of type I diabetes and the autoimmune process.

  Any chronic illnesses—Endocrine disorders, CF, congenital rubella syndrome, and Down syndrome are related to the increased likelihood of diabetes mellitus.

  Eating disorders—Although eating disorders may not contribute directly to the onset of diabetes, a history of eating disorders may influence the approach to management or the management of the diabetes itself.

  Growth and development—Growth and development may be delayed by undiagnosed hyperglycemia or poor glycemic control. Generally parents or caregivers first notice a loss of weight or lack of weight gain followed by failure to grow taller.

  Menstrual history—Menarche, amenorrhea, oligomenorrhea (menstrual cycle onset and frequency can be affected by undiagnosed hyperglycemia or poorly controlled blood glucose in an already diagnosed individual). Amenorrhea in a child suspected of having type II diabetes may be the result of polycystic ovarian syndrome; often associated with obesity and insulin resistance.

  History of impaired glucose tolerance or hypoglycemia—Some children are given the diagnosis of either impaired glucose tolerance or hypoglycemia months to years before the diagnosis of diabetes.

  Hospitalizations or major acute illnesses

  Childhood illnesses—This includes chickenpox and mumps.

- Family history, which, because of the genetic nature of diabetes and its long-term implications, should include inquiries about some of the following chronic illnesses: autoimmune diseases (e.g., lupus erythematosus, pernicious anemia, rheumatoid arthritis, thyroid dysfunction, Addison disease), hypoglycemia, types I and type II diabetes, endocrine disorders, cardiovascular disease, renal disease, and hyperlipidemia The family's ethnic background should also be explored. Individuals whose genetic traits include Asian, Hispanic, American Indian, and African-American backgrounds are at greater risk for developing type II diabetes.

- Psychosocial history, including child and family stressors, child and family coping styles, primary caregivers, and level and quality of child care

- School, including grade, performance (if blood glucose levels are poorly controlled, performance often declines), and schedule and activities (to assist in identifying times throughout the day in which hypoglycemia may occur as a result of late meals or increased activity)
- Recreation and activities, including type, time of day, and duration
- Family economic resources (although the economic status does not have a direct effect on the development of diabetes, the economic resources available to the child and family may influence the plan of management and which support services are used)
- Lifestyle and cultural factors that may influence the plan of management (e.g., ethnic and religious practices, habits).
- Current health status:
  Diet history—Use a 24-hour recall, 3-day diary, or food group frequency to determine the following: eating patterns, weight history, nutritional status, use of vitamin and mineral supplements, food intolerances, likes and dislikes, food allergies, use of food assistance programs (e.g., the Women, Infants, and Children [WIC] program, food stamps), past nutrition education, whether the family is interested in seeing a dietitian, number of

meals and snacks, types of snacks, how is food prepared and who prepares it, and how often the family eats outside the home.

Exercise history (including recess and physical education for school-age children and adolescents)—This includes frequency, intensity, timing, and type (aerobic exercise is preferred over isometric exercise).

Medications—Prescription medications such as thiazides, glucocorticoids, furosemide, estrogen-containing products, β-blockers, and nicotinic acid may cause the elevation of blood glucose levels, whereas oral hypoglycemic agents, insulin, and β-blockers can cause hypoglycemia.

Substance abuse—This includes tobacco, alcohol, and illicit drugs.

Allergies

Immunization status

A comprehensive health history, including a complete review of systems, is essential if the diagnosis of diabetes mellitus is suspected. However, a complete health history is not necessary at each interim visit. Box 45-13 shows examples of health histories for quarterly interim and annual visits. The history that is included in a quarterly visit is generally focused on

---

Box 45-13   Diabetes History

Quarterly Diabetes History

Insulin

Type: humulin, Novolin, Pure Pork, other
Dosage: For each injection of the day
Most recent dosage change: Date and amount
Timing of injections
Who is preparing and administering injections: Caregivers, child, other

Blood glucose monitoring

Product: Accucheck; One-Touch; Glucometer, other
Blood glucose patterns: Obtained from client's blood glucose diary
Who is performing blood glucose monitoring: Caregivers, child, other

Exercise or activity

Type
Time of day
Length/duration
Frequency

Severe hypoglycemia since last visit

Severe hypoglycemia is defined as hypoglycemia resulting in semiconscious or unconsciousness; requiring the use of glucagon or emergency services

Diet

Total number of carbohydrates
Number of calories, if applicable
Number of meals and snacks
Timing of meals and snacks
Current medications

Intercurrent illnesses

Particularly those that affected blood glucose, caused the production of ketones, or required medical intervention

Other issues

School: Grade, performance, activities
Lifestyle changes
Compliance: Wears Medic-Alert identification, carries rapid glucose
Tobacco and alcohol use

Annual Diabetes History

Include all items from the quarterly diabetes history, in addition to the review of systems below:
General: Fatigue; weight loss or gain
Skin: Rash, color changes, hair changes, thickening
Head: Headache
Eyes: Glasses, blurred vision, double vision, pain, date of last ophthalmology examination
Ears: Decreased hearing; pain
Nose: Bleeding; decreased sense of smell
Mouth: Gingival hypertrophy or bleeding, sore tongue, dental problems, hoarseness, date of last dental examination
Neck: Stiffness, pain, thyroid enlargement
Breasts: Pain, lumps, discharge
Respiratory: Cough, chest pain, wheezing
Cardiac: Chest pain, edema, palpitations, cyanosis, murmur
Hematologic: Easy bruising, easy bleeding, lymph node enlargement
Gastrointestinal tract: Anorexia, nausea, vomiting, bloody stools, constipation, diarrhea, jaundice
Genitourinary system: Dysuria, urgency, frequency, incontinence, hematuria, urinary tract infections, enuresis
Menstrual: menarche; last menstrual period, type of flow, dysmenorrhea, amenorrhea, gravida, para, abortions
Musculoskeletal: pain; cramps; joints: pain, stiffness, swelling
Neurologic: Seizures, dizziness, numbness, tremor, incoordination
Psychiatric: Nervousness, depression, insomnia, suicidal thoughts, behavior changes
Endocrine: Heat or cold intolerance; change in hair texture, distribution
Habits: Tobacco; alcohol; drugs

the diabetes. The history that is obtained at an annual visit, however, should include all of the diabetes management history and a general review of systems. Children with chronic illnesses should be encouraged to seek routine health maintenance from their PCP. The review of systems may assist the specialist in identifying additional health care problems or areas of concern.

Objective Data

Physical examination. See Table 45-9.
Diagnostic procedures and laboratory tests. See Table 45-10.

Primary Care Implications and Issues

Growth and development. At each continuing care visit, obtain both height and weight and plot measurements on an appropriate growth chart. Perform Tanner staging yearly to assess sexual maturation. If changes have occurred in physical growth, namely deceleration or no growth, explore the reasons with careful attention paid to glycemic control.

Vision. Remember that each continuing care visit should include inquiry into any changes in sight or problems involving the eyes and a funduscopic examination; assess visual acuity at least once a year.

Diet, exercise, and diabetes education. Keep in mind that each continuing-care visit should include assessment of diet and nutritional status; assessment of activity level; and frequent review of diabetes management. Developmental issues related to diabetes management include driving safety, drinking and diabetes, leaving home, and going to college.

Immunizations. Note that children with diabetes should receive all the routine immunizations that any other child would receive. Recommend a flu shot each year. Children with diabetes are at risk for hyperglycemia and ketosis if they become infected with the influenza virus.

Safety. Note that this includes issues of increased activity and hypoglycemia prevention. Planned activity is ideal, preferably after a meal, with blood glucose monitoring before and after exercise. Extended periods of increased activity may also require glucose monitoring during the activity. Snacks before, during, and after exercise may be necessary to prevent hypoglycemia. If exercise is planned, reduce the insulin dose accordingly.

Driving with diabetes. Advise the patient to monitor blood glucose level before driving and to wear diabetes identification in the form of a bracelet, necklace, or wallet card. Always have the patient carry a source of "quick" sugar (e.g., glucose tablets, regular soda) in the vehicle and eat before beginning to drive if a mealtime or snack time is near; advise not wait to get to the destination. The patient should never skip a meal or snack while driving. If hypoglycemic symptoms occur or are suspected while driving, the patient should pull the vehicle over to the side of the road and turn off the engine. Hypoglycemia can distort judgment and slow response time, so advise the patient to treat the hypoglycemia appropriately and not resume driving until all symptoms have subsided. If driving on long trips, the patient should be certain to carry plenty of snack foods or a small meal.

Sexuality. Note that birth control methods appropriate for the patient with diabetes include barrier methods and oral contraceptives (with routine screening for risk factors). Ideally all pregnancies should be planned; there is a strong correlation between optimal blood glucose control (both before conception and during pregnancy) and successful, healthy pregnancies.

Substance use and abuse

Alcohol. Because of alcohol's suppression of hepatic gluconeogenesis, remember that severe hypoglycemia can occur if blood glucose levels drop after alcohol has been consumed, and hypoglycemia can persist for up to 12 hours after alcohol consumption. Alcohol use should occur only after consultation with a health care provider, and blood glucose should be under optimal control. A patient should limit the intake of alcohol. Alcohol should never be consumed on an empty stomach, so the patient should drink alcohol with a meal. He or she should also avoid alcoholic beverages that contain high concentrations of sugar (e.g., sweet wines, cordials).

Tobacco. Note that risk factors for cancer, heart disease, and chronic lung disease that apply to the general population also apply to the patient with diabetes who uses tobacco, and diabetes in and of itself is a risk factor for cardiovascular disease. Therefore tobacco use, particularly smoking, is contraindicated. Smoking cessation is strongly encouraged, and nicotine patches and nicotine gum can be safely prescribed for a patient with diabetes.

Drugs. Remember that all illicit drugs have deleterious effects on diabetes control and management, including altered perception and judgment, hyperglycemia, hypoglycemia, masking of hypoglycemic symptoms, and altered eating patterns (with decreased appetite leading to hypoglycemia and increased appetite leading to hyperglycemia).

Management

Management of both type I and type II diabetes in a pediatric patient is multifaceted and multidisciplinary. The overall goals should include maintaining normal growth and development of the child, optimal glycemic control, prevention of future complications, and empowerment of the patient and family. As with any child diagnosed with a chronic illness, both the child and the family become patients. Maintaining the daily blood glucose level at as near to normal a level as possible involves balancing food intake, exercise, and medication.

Treatments and medications

Nutrition. Nutrition management should ideally be prescribed and monitored by a registered dietitian. The goals of nutrition therapy include, but are not limited to, euglycemia and the prevention of hyperglycemia and hypoglycemia; the attainment of normal growth and development through adequate caloric intake; maintenance of lipid levels at levels that are appropriate for the pediatric patient; maintenance of optimal health; and prevention of obesity.

Determining caloric requirements

- *Infancy to prepuberty*—Begin with 1000 calories and add a minimum of 100 calories for each year of life, up to a minimum of 2000 calories by 11 years of age.
- *Adolescence*—At 12 to 15 years of age, add 100 calories per year for girls and 200 calories per year for boys. At 15 to 20 years of age, the number of calories is influenced greatly by the activity level of the individual. Approximately 30 kcal/kg is used for young women, with the number of calories increased to accommodate increased activity levels. Young men who have a relatively sedentary lifestyle can be maintained on approximately 30 kcal/kg. Young men with average to very active physical lifestyles require approximately 40 to 50 kcal/kg per day.

Nutrition plans. Before deciding which plan is best for the patient, it is important to consider the age of the patient, the sophistication of the patient and family, and which system fits

Table 45-9 Objective Data for Diabetes Mellitus: Physical Examination

COMPONENTS OF PHYSICAL EXAMINATION	ANTICIPATED PHYSICAL FINDINGS
Vital Signs*	
Respirations	Tachypnea or Kussmaul respirations if client is in ketoacidosis.
Blood pressure (orthostatic measurements in adolescence)	In older adolescents and young adults, potential for autonomic neuropathy and orthostatic hypotension. Orthostatic hypotension may also be the result of severe hyperglycemia and dehydration. Hypertension can also be found in older adolescents and young adults.
Height and Weight*	
Recorded on appropriate growth chart for gender and age	If diabetes is poorly controlled, particularly with ketosis, weight loss may result. Prolonged periods of poorly controlled blood glucose can cause a deceleration in linear growth. Obesity has also been associated with insulin resistance.
Integumentary System	
Skin*: Moisture; texture; turgor; lesions; injection sites; fingerstick sites; intertriginous areas Nails: Color; debris; shape	Dry, rough skin with poor turgor may occur with chronic or severe hyperglycemia. Integumentary signs of dehydration are to be expected with diabetic ketoacidosis. General observation for lesions showing signs of poor healing, infection, and ulceration. All insulin injection sites must be inspected and palpated for hypertrophy. All fingerstick sites must be inspected for signs of infection. Other less common skin lesions and conditions are intertriginous candidal infections, necrobiosis lipoidica diabeticorum, and acanthosis nigricans.
Hair: Pattern; texture	Dry, course, brittle hair, reflecting changes that occur with hypothyroidism or poor nutrition status.
Head, Eyes, Ears, Nose, and Throat	
Eyes*: Acuity; funduscopic examination	Decreased acuity and blurred vision are common problems found with prolonged hyperglycemia. Retinal vascular changes (hemorrhages, background retinopathy, proliferative retinopathy) may be found in late adolescence and young adults with diabetes of 5 years or greater duration; those with hypertension or nephropathy may be at an increased risk for retinopathy.
Ears: External auditory canals	Chronic drug-resistant otitis externa may be found in clients with long-standing hyperglycemia.
Mouth: Breath; mucosa; moisture; gingivae	Oral assessments may reveal dry buccal mucosa with sweet "fruity-like" breath if hyperglycemia and ketosis are occurring. Gingival hypertrophy, bleeding gums, and other signs of periodontal disease may be present if poor oral hygiene and chronic hyperglycemia are problematic.
Thyroid*: Hypertrophy	Approximately 30% of clients with diabetes also develop hypothyroidism. Hypertrophy of the thyroid may be present; true goiters are rare.
Respiratory System	
Pattern: Tachypnea; Kussmaul	Tachypnea and Kussmaul respirations may be present with severe ketosis.
Cardiovascular and Peripheral Vascular System	
Heart and extremities*: Color; temperature; pulses; complete hand, finger, and foot examination	Extremities should be assessed for changes in color (pallor, rubor) and decreased temperature indicating a compromised vascular system. Decrease in lower extremity pulses may be noted in clients with chronic vascular changes.
Abdomen	
Bowel sounds	Decreased bowel sounds may be present if client is ketotic.
Tenderness	Abdominal tenderness may be present if client is ketotic.
Organomegaly*	Hepatomegaly has been found in clients with chronic hyperglycemia.
Genitourinary System	
Tanner staging	Delayed growth and maturation may occur with poorly controlled blood glucose.
Vaginal examination	Vulvovaginitis may be a problem resulting from candidal infection.
Costovertebral angle tenderness	
Neuromuscular System	
Deep tendon reflexes,* proprioception,* vibratory sensation, pain or light touch, gait; heel walking	Peripheral paresthesias may be present in newly diagnosed clients; if the presentation has been subacute and hyperglycemia has been present for an extended period, these generally resolve spontaneously with improved glycemic control. Older adolescents and young adults (< 5 years with diagnosis) may have peripheral neuropathy changes such as hyporeflexia; reduced proprioception of great toes; reduced vibratory sensation; reduced pain and light touch sensation, and poorly coordinated heel walking. Remember, most peripheral neuropathy begins in lower extremities and later develops in upper extremities. Also, peripheral neuropathy develops distally and progresses proximally.

Table 45-10 Laboratory Data for Diabetes Mellitus

LABORATORY TESTS	NORMAL VALUES
Fasting plasma glucose level	1 week to 16 years: 60 to 105 mg/dl; >16 years: 70 to 115 mg/dl
Random plasma glucose level (may be used if patient is undiagnosed and symptomatic)	1 week to 16 years: 60 to 105 mg/dl; >16 years: 70 to 115 mg/dl
Oral glucose tolerance test	Rarely used in diagnosis; if needed, refer to a physician
Glycosylated hemoglobin: Should be performed with initial workup; however, the glycohemoglobin may not be solely diagnostic of diabetes; a glycosylated hemoglobin test should be performed at least every 3 months if the patient is insulin treated	3.9% to 7.7% of total hemoglobin (values may vary depending on method used by individual laboratory)
Fasting lipid profile: A lipid profile should be obtained on all children older than 2 years of age and only after control of blood glucose has occurred. If values are at the normal upper limits, the lipid profile must be repeated. If values are within normal limits, lipid levels should be assessed every 5 years.	Normal upper-limit values for cholesterol, triglycerides, high-density lipoprotein, low-density lipoprotein, and very-low-density lipoprotein depend on age and gender
Serum creatinine: In children with proteinuria	Infant: 0.2 to 0.4 mg/dl Child: 0.3 to 0.7 mg/dl Adolescent: 0.5 to 1 mg/dl
Urinalysis	Glucose: Negative Ketones: Negative Protein: Dipstick negative Albumin
24-hour or overnight urine collection: In postpubertal patients with diabetes more than 5 years in duration. If abnormal albumin or protein excretion is present, serum creatinine or blood urea nitrogen level must be measured in addition to glomerular filtration rates.	4 to 16 years 3.35 to 15.3 mg/24 hours
Thyroid function tests: Triiodothyronine, thyroid-stimulating hormone, thyroxine	***Triiodothyronine (ng/dl)*** 1 to 3 days of age: 89-405 1 week of age: 91-300 1 to 12 months of age: 85-250 Prepubertal children: 119-218 Pubertal children and adults: 55-170 ***Thyroid-stimulating hormone (μU/ml)*** 1 to 30 days of age: Boys, 0.52-16; girls, 0.72-13.1 1 month to 5 years of age: Boys, 0.53-7.1; girls, 0.46-8.1 6 to 18 years of age: Boys, 0.37-6; girls, 0.36-5.8 ***Thyroxine (μg/dl)*** 1 to 2 days of age: 11.4-25.5 (147-328 nmol/L) 3 to 4 days of age: 9.8-25.2 (126-324 nmol/L) 1 to 6 years of age: 5-15.2 (64-196 nmol/L) 11 to 13 years of age: 4-13 (51-167 nmol/L) >18 years of age: 4.7-11 (60-142 nmol/L)

best into the patient's or family's lifestyle. There are various nutrition plans that can be used to ensure that the patient is receiving adequate calories and nutrition. Each system is designed to allow the patient to achieve the nutrition goals outlined earlier. Currently the most common system used by most nutritionists and health care providers is carbohydrate counting. Carbohydrate counting assures that the child receives adequate caloric intake while offering the child and family ease in management of their nutrition.

After determining the caloric requirements and current food intake, a practitioner can design meal plans by dividing daily food intake into meals and snacks. All meal plans must accommodate the individual's eating habits, activity level, and insulin regimen. It is most important to synchronize food intake with the peak action of insulin and activity.

- *Children less than 6 years of age*—Three meals and three snacks a day. Generally children in this age group cannot go for longer than 4 hours without eating. Snacks are usually in the midmorning, midafternoon, and before bed.
- *Children older than 6 years of age*—Three meals and two snacks a day. The meal plan generally includes three meals and midafternoon and bedtime snacks.

Nutrition education should be comprehensive and ongoing, with frequent evaluation by the NP and a registered dietitian.

Exercise. Exercise and aerobic activity have been proved to reduce the risk of cardiovascular disease in the overall population.

For individuals with diabetes, who by virtue of the illness are at a greater risk for macrovascular disease, aerobic activity has an even greater importance. Therefore children with diabetes should be encouraged to participate in regular aerobic activity. Benefits include cardiovascular health, improved glucose tolerance, increased insulin sensitivity, reduced hyperinsulinemia, and reduced body fat and weight.

The following precautions should be kept in mind:

- *Hypoglycemia prevention*—The practitioner should help plan the exercise (ideally 60 to 90 minutes after a meal) and decrease the insulin dose. Advise the patient to consume additional snacks (snacks containing complex carbohydrates, protein, and fat). Older children and adolescents participating in strenuous or lengthy organized sports may require snacks before and during the period of exercise. Monitor blood glucose levels before and after exercise.
- *Prevention of post-exercise, late-onset hypoglycemia*—This form of hypoglycemia can actually occur up to 12 hours after exercise has ceased. Prevention includes monitoring blood glucose levels closely, adjusting the food intake (i.e., eating complex carbohydrates and protein-rich foods), adjusting insulin, and avoiding strenuous exercise in the evening and before going to bed.
- *Exercising with elevated blood glucose levels*—Prevention includes avoiding strenuous exercise when blood glucose level is greater than 240 mg/dl or ketonuria is present.

Medications. Insulin is the only medication used to treat type I diabetes because oral hypoglycemic agents have no use in the treatment of type I diabetes. Insulin is responsible for utilization of glucose, protein synthesis, fat storage, and glycogen storage.

- *Precautions*—Lipodystrophies (hypertrophy and atrophy) affect absorption and efficacy of insulin. Hypertrophy is related to poor injection-site rotation, and the incidence increases with the use of beef-derived insulin. Atrophy is an immune response to the frequent injection of one site with beef-derived insulin.
- *Prevention*—Rotation of insulin injection sites and avoiding the hypertrophied site; use of human or purified pork insulin; injection into and around atrophied sites with human or purified pork insulin may help already damaged tissue return to normal.
- *Determination of the initial insulin dosage*—Considerations are age, weight, development, and metabolic state. Younger children have a higher sensitivity to regular insulin and are less likely to recognize hypoglycemic symptoms, while older school-age children and adolescents have larger insulin requirements as a result of the hyperglycemic and insulin-resistant effect of growth and development hormones.

The acceptable starting dose is based on the formula 0.5 to 1.0 U/kg per day. Younger children require approximately 0.5 U/kg per day, while adolescents may require 1.5 U/kg per day. After the daily requirement of insulin is determined, with the assumption that most children will be started on a "split-mixed" dosage (i.e., two injections per day of intermediate-acting and fast-acting insulin), the dosage is divided as shown in Box 45-14.

- *Injections*—Split-mixed injection schedule is usually two injections per day of intermediate-acting and fast-acting insulin. Three- and four-injection schedules may prove effective for some older children, adolescents, and young

---

Box 45-14   Initial Insulin Dose Determination

Formula:	0.5 to 1.0 U/kg per day ($^2/_3$ total dose in morning, $^1/_3$ total dose in evening)
Morning dose:	NPH/Lente = $^2/_3$; Regular = $^1/_3$
Evening dose:	NPH/Lente = $^1/_2$; Regular = $^1/_2$

Example: In a 16-year-old, 60-kg boy with newly diagnosed type I diabetes, the initial dosage (using 1.0 U/kg per day) would be determined as follows:

Daily requirement:	1.0 × 60.0 kg = 60 U/day
Morning dose:	$^2/_3$ of daily requirement = 40 U
	NPH/Lente = $^2/_3$ of total morning dose = 27 U
	Regular = $^1/_3$ of total morning dose = 13 U
Evening dose:	$^1/_3$ of daily requirement = 20 U
	NPH/Lente = $^1/_2$ of total evening dose = 10 U
	Regular = $^1/_2$ of total evening dose = 10 U

---

adults, but decreased compliance becomes an issue as the number of injections per day is increased. These schedules are usually initiated to improve fasting blood glucose control or to accommodate individual life-styles.

- *Adjustment of initial insulin doses*—Based on blood glucose patterns, use a conservative approach when you are making insulin increases. Increase insulin only 1 to 2 U at a time, and adjust only one insulin dose at a time. Dosage increases should be made only every 2 or 3 days. If hypoglycemia is the problem and insulin doses need to be adjusted, decreasing insulin can be done more aggressively. For mild hypoglycemia, decreasing the insulin by 1 to 2 U should be adequate. For severe hypoglycemia, decreasing all insulin doses by 10% for the next 48 hours may be necessary. If after 48 hours no further hypoglycemia has occurred, small increases can be made as necessary. Monitor blood glucose patterns closely during insulin adjustment and explore the reasons why the blood glucose levels are not in the target range (e.g., food, activity, illness, stress) before making insulin adjustments.

Insulin and insulin administration is changing at a rapid pace with new preparations and methods being developed all the time. Currently, multiple injection schedules using Ultralente, Regular, and Humalog insulin are being used successfully by some children. Insulin analogs are also being used. Many older children are also using insulin pumps, which provide a continuous subcutaneous infusion of insulin and allow children greater flexibility in the daily management of their diabetes. Inhaled insulin is currently being studied as a potential method of insulin delivery in the future.

In regard to oral hypoglycemic agents, the management of type II diabetes in the pediatric population begins with lifestyle changes, most importantly diet and exercise. However, as in the adult population, diet and exercise alone cannot attain euglycemia, and medications must be considered. Although insulin is the only agent approved by the FDA to manage diabetes in children, it is known to cause an increase adiposity, which further contributes to insulin resistance. The etiology and pathophysiology of type II diabetes in children appear to be similar to that of type II diabetes in adults; therefore many pediatric en-

Box 45-15 Determining the Glucagon Dosage

Infant—Approximately 0.25 mg
Child younger than 5 years—0.5 mg
School-age child or adolescent—1 mg

docrinologists assume that oral glucose-lowering agents will be effective in children. Those agents that have been used with relative success in the pediatric population are the biguanides and sulfonylureas. It is strongly recommended that PCPs collaborate closely with a pediatric endocrinologist before prescribing any oral hypoglycemic agents for a child or adolescent.

All patients treated with insulin should have glucagon available to them at all times.

- *Indications*—Inability to swallow without risk of aspiration, or uncooperative or combative behavior resulting from hypoglycemia.
- *Administration and dosage*—Administered subcutaneously or intramuscularly, with doses based on approximate age. Box 45-15 lists dosages for glucagon.
- *Considerations*—The child should begin to awaken 15 to 20 minutes after administration. Once the child is awake and can safely swallow, juice, milk, or glucose tablets should be given, followed by a snack containing complex carbohydrate and protein. A possible side effect of glucagon is nausea, so lay the child on his or her side after administration of insulin to prevent aspiration if vomiting should occur before consciousness is regained. Careful monitoring of blood glucose level should occur for the next 12 to 24 hours because the risk for another episode of severe hypoglycemia is greatest during this time.

Counseling and prevention

- Remember that goals should be developmentally appropriate. Topics that must be included during initial education include nutrition, exercise, insulin (including timing, storage, injections), blood glucose monitoring, hypoglycemia, and glucagon usage. Other topics that must be discussed during the first several weeks after diagnosis are sick-day rules, insulin adjustment, foot care, safety, driving, and traveling with diabetes.
- Because of the volume and intensity of the material, frequently review all teaching topics.
- Provide the child and parents with material for review, including in the areas of pathophysiology (basic pathophysiology), explanations of type I and type II diabetes, and the causes of diabetes.
- Give monitoring instructions to the child and parents. Blood glucose monitoring is the preferred method of monitoring glucose levels. It should be done three or four times a day, with one 3:00 AM glucose check a minimum of once a week. More frequent monitoring should be provided during times of illness, increased stress, or increased exercise and activity. Hands should be washed with soap and water before a fingerstick is performed. Alcohol may be used to cleanse the individual finger; however, alcohol has been shown to cause drying of the skin, and this may be of concern for those individuals who have dry skin in general. Fingersticks should be performed on the sides of the finger, with avoidance of fingertips and unnecessary discomfort. Lancets should then be disposed of in a puncture-resistant container to prevent injury to others.

With electronic blood glucose monitors, the choice of a product should be based on the family income, child's developmental level, child's ability to use a blood glucose monitor accurately, child's ability to obtain a large-enough blood sample, and manufacturer provision of a toll-free customer service number.

Successful blood glucose monitoring depends on the size of the blood sample; timing of test being accurate and according to manufacturer specifications; cleanliness of the monitor; and age and condition of the reagent strips. Instruct patients to periodically bring their monitors and supplies to clinic visits so that their technique and the monitor itself can be assessed for cleanliness and accuracy.

Urine testing for glucose level has little value in the management plan of type I diabetes and should not be encouraged. Urine testing for ketones may be done. Test the urine for ketones any time blood glucose levels are greater than 240 mg/dl, as well as during times of illness. The selection of ketone test strips should be based on cost, accuracy, ease of performance, and ease of interpretation.

- Demonstrate and instruct on insulin administration. Insulin should be refrigerated between 36° and 46° F, not frozen, and removed from the refrigerator a few minutes before administering. Cold insulin may be uncomfortable when injected. Insulin may be stored at room temperature (59° to 68° F) provided that the vial will be used within a month. Direct exposure to sunlight and heat should be avoided, and encourage patients and families to write the date the vial was opened on the vial itself.

When drawing up and preparing split-mixed insulin injections, Humalog and regular insulin should always be drawn into the syringe before the intermediate-acting or long-acting insulins. Insulin is administered into the subcutaneous tissue. To ensure subcutaneous injection, the skin should be pinched and the syringe needle angled at 90 degrees. To prevent intramuscular injections in thin individuals or young children, angling the syringe at 45 degrees may be necessary. Do not massage the injection site. Aspiration of the syringe after the needle is placed is not necessary. Insulin injection sites should be rotated on a regular basis. Suggest that patients use regions for several days before rotating to the next region. Regions or sites are (in order of decreasing insulin absorption rates) the abdomen, arms, legs, and buttocks.

- When a child is sick, advise that blood glucose monitoring and urine testing for ketones should be increased to every 4 to 6 hours around the clock.
- Advise that insulin must be taken even if anorexia, nausea, or vomiting is a problem. Intermediate-acting and long-acting insulin may not require adjustment of the routine dose. However, regular insulin must be available and adjusted to accommodate hyperglycemia and ketonuria. Supplemental doses of regular insulin are usually required every 4 to 6 hours if hyperglycemia and ketonuria are present.
- Instruct that orally administered fluids should be increased to prevent dehydration, especially if ketosis, hyperglycemia, or fever is present.
- If nausea and vomiting occur and solid foods are not tolerated, possibly convert the meal plan to clear liquids or more palatable foods while still maintaining the daily

caloric requirement and preventing hypoglycemia. Examples of such foods are regular colas, ginger ale, juices, regular Jell-O, pudding, broth, and Popsicles.

- Advise that a physician should be contacted for the following: treatment of precipitating infection or illness; assistance with insulin dosage adjustments; blood glucose levels that remain greater than 240 or less than 80 mg/dl despite following the guidelines for illness; presence of ketones; nausea and vomiting, with an inability to tolerate oral fluids; persistent diarrhea (five times per day or lasting longer than 24 hours); changes in mental status; and labored respirations or dyspnea.
- Instruct the parents and child about hypoglycemia:

Causes—Insulin excess, decrease in or lack of food intake, increased exercise and activity, and alcohol consumption

Symptoms:

Mild—Pallor, palpitations, diaphoresis, shakiness, hunger, and fatigue

Moderate—Confusion, poor concentration, irritability, poor coordination, blurred vision, slurred speech, and fatigue

Severe—Disorientation, combative behavior, loss of consciousness, seizures, and inability to be aroused

Treatment—Treatment should be as rapid as possible. Determine if the person can swallow safely: If aspiration is not a threat, oral treatment is usually appropriate (severe hypoglycemia can be treated with a glucose gel placed between the cheek and gums); if aspiration is a concern, alternative parenteral routes are necessary, such as glucagon injections or intravenous dextrose. Whenever hypoglycemic symptoms are experienced, a blood glucose level should be obtained; if blood glucose monitoring is not possible, the child should be taught to treat the hypoglycemia based on the symptoms being experienced. Determining what to eat and how much depends on how soon the next meal is and the guidelines in Box 45-16. Monitor blood glucose levels for the next several hours. If severe hypoglycemia has occurred, the health care practitioner or diabetes manager should be notified.

Prevention

- Routine blood glucose monitoring before, during, and after increased activity, with a minimum of one 3:00 AM blood glucose test once a week
- Knowledge regarding causes, signs, and symptoms of hypoglycemia
- Knowledge regarding appropriate treatment of hypoglycemia
  Timing of meals and snacks
  Education of family, friends, teachers, and significant others regarding the identification and treatment of hypoglycemia
  Wearing proper diabetes identification (e.g., necklaces, bracelets, wallet cards)
  Adjustment of insulin to accommodate increased activity.

Follow-up. Follow-up care should be provided 1 to 2 weeks after the initial diagnosis, then 4 weeks after the initial diagnosis, and then every 3 months. Telephone follow-up should be provided as necessary for insulin adjustment. Laboratory follow-up includes:

- Glycosylated hemoglobin test every 3 months
- Screening for microalbuminuria yearly in postpubertal adolescents with type I diabetes or in children with diabetes for more than 5 years; for those children with type II diabetes, screening for microalbuminuria beginning at the time of diagnosis and then annually

---

Box 45-16 Guidelines for Management of Hypoglycemia

Mild Hypoglycemia

Treat with 10 to 15 g of carbohydrate (e.g., three glucose tablets, five Lifesavers, 4 oz of orange juice, 8 oz of milk, 4 to 6 oz of regular soda, 2 tbsp of raisins, commercial glucose gel).

If after 15 minutes the symptoms have not subsided, another 10 to 15 g of carbohydrate can be taken.

Moderate Hypoglycemia

Treat with 15 to 30 g of carbohydrate.

After 10 to 15 minutes, if the next meal is not imminent, additional, more complex food must be eaten and include a complex carbohydrate and protein. If the next meal is within the next 15 to 20 minutes, this should suffice.

Severe Hypoglycemia

Glucagon should be administered for severe hypoglycemia using the dosages discussed earlier.

It is imperative that after administration of glucagon the person be monitored closely, and observed for regaining of consciousness, vomiting, and seizures. It is recommended that after the glucagon is administered the person be positioned lying on his or her side to prevent aspiration should vomiting occur.

After consciousness is regained, a liquid source of 10 to 15 g of carbohydrate should be provided.

After all nausea has subsided, a small snack should be eaten or the next meal provided.

- Thyroid function tests yearly
- Lipid profile annually unless there is low risk

Consultations and referrals

- All children over 10 years of age or who have had a diagnosis for 3 to 5 years should have an annual dilated funduscopic examination.
- A child should be referred to podiatry for common problems such as ingrown toenails, warts, and fungal infections.
- Dental health maintenance and hygiene should be encouraged with routine dental visits.
- Referral to or consultation with a pediatric endocrinologist should be considered for the following: every child with diabetes, especially at onset or diagnosis and if blood glucose management is recalcitrant despite following developmentally appropriate diabetes management standards; diabetic ketoacidosis; and any changes in growth and development have occurred.
- Ideally each child and family should be referred to a dietitian at the time of diagnosis, with periodic follow-up assessments to ensure adequate caloric intake and dietary management. If a registered dietitian is not readily available, consultation provides support and assistance to the health care provider and diabetes manager.
- For some families it may be necessary to consult social services regarding financial concerns of family adjustment and coping. Child psychology can also be an excellent resource for child and family adjustment problems related to chronic illness.
- Both school nurses and public health nurses can be assets to any management team when you are dealing with children and chronic illness. Both school nurses and public health

nurses can follow up the child and family in the community and assist in diabetes education and management.

Resources

Organizations

American Association of Diabetes Educators, 100 West Monroe Street, Suite 400, Chicago, IL 60603; (312) 424-2426; www.aadenet.org

American Diabetes Association (ADA), 1701 North Beauregard Street, Alexandria, VA 22311; (800) DIABETES; www.diabetes.org

Diabetes Trust Fund, 48 Medical Park East Drive, Suite 154, Birmingham, Alabama 35235; (800) 577-1383; www.diabetestrustfund.org

Juvenile Diabetes Foundation, 120 Wall Street, New York, NY 10005; (212) 785-9595; www.jdf.org

Hemophilia and Bleeding Disorders

JACQUELINE G. IOLI

Alert

Refer to a physician for any known hemophiliac with the following:

- Any actual or suspected head, spine, or back injury
- Flank or abdominal injury or pain (rule out iliopsoas and hip joint bleeds)
- Neck, mouth, tongue, or pharyngeal injury or bleeding
- Evidence of circulatory or neurovascular compromise (compartment syndrome) in an extremity
- No clinical improvement in bleeding after factor product administration (usually two doses)
- Recurrent bleeding into the same joint
  Also refer for any infant or child with the following:
- Family history of a bleeding problem
- Any recurrent or unexplained bleeding
- Palpable bruises on the trunk, abdomen, or back

Because inherited bleeding disorders affect 1% to 3% of the general population, virtually all PCPs encounter such children in their practices. There are three hemophilia syndromes: hemophilia A, or factor VIII deficiency (classic hemophilia), hemophilia B, or factor IX deficiency (Christmas disease), and hemophilia C, or factor XI deficiency, this last being characterized by mucocutaneous bleeding and clinically similar to von Willebrand's disease (vWD) (which has a much less severe course than the name would indicate).

In factor VIII and factor IX deficiencies, bleeding typically occurs deep in muscles, soft tissues, or joints. This bleeding is not immediate but occurs characteristically several hours after injury (a "stopping and starting" pattern). This delay reflects the failure of the deficient clotting factor to contribute to the formation of a firm fibrin clot. Instead, a soft, mushy mass that is prone to rebleeding is formed. In contrast, superficial cuts and scrapes usually do not pose a bleeding problem because other hemostatic phases, namely, platelet aggregation, tissue pressure, and vasoconstriction, may be sufficient to stop any bleeding. Female carriers of factor VIII or factor IX deficiency can have bleeding symptoms similar to those in vWD.

vWD (hereditary pseudohemophilia) can be coinherited with platelet function abnormalities or factor XII deficiency. There are three common forms of vWD; types I and II are the most common forms and are characterized by a mild course with mucocutaneous bleeding; type III is quite rare and clini-

cally indistinguishable from severe hemophilia since there is no detectable serum von Willebrand's factor (vWF).

Platelet function defects (PFDs) form a varied group of disorders in which the platelets respond poorly to normal triggers of aggregation (e.g., epinephrine, adenosine, diphosphate, or collagen). PFDs are often with vWD and have a clinically indistinguishable course from vWD.

Factor XII deficiency, often coinherited with vWD or PFD, causes no alterations in bleeding by itself but paradoxically prolongs the activated partial thromboplastin time (aPTT).

Etiology

Hemophilia A and B are transmitted as X-linked recessive genetic traits, passed on through the X or female chromosome, and so males are almost exclusively affected. Approximately one third of all new cases of hemophilia are the result of spontaneous genetic mutations.

Female carriers of factor VIII and factor IX may be symptomatic because of the Lyon hypothesis. It is commonly accepted that both X chromosomes in a cell do not operate at the same time and a "shutting-down" process occurs with half of the X chromosomes. Because this is a random event, unique to each person, some females may "turn off" a larger percentage of the "normal" X chromosomes, leaving less of the normal factor VIII chromosomes "working" to make factor VIII. Hemophilia C is inherited in an autosomal recessive manner; thus both girls and boys are affected, and a symptomatic child is usually homozygous for the disorder (inheriting two abnormal genes, one from each parent). The level of factor XI and prolongation of the aPTT correlates poorly with the amount of bleeding experienced.

Types I and II vWD are autosomal dominant disorders (males and females equally affected, with the child inheriting one affected gene); the affected gene is located on chromosome 12. Type III vWD, the most severe form, occurs when a child inherits two affected vWD genes. Spontaneous genetic mutations resulting in vWD occur as well. Only 1% of vWD patients have type III vWD where there is absence of vWF and ristocetin cofactor (no protein and thus no function).

vWD is a disorder of the vWF protein the role of which in hemostasis is to act as a stabilizing carrier protein for the factor VIII molecule. It is also necessary for the formation of a secure platelet plug, a component of platelet aggregation. When vascular injury occurs, vWF acts as an adhesive bridge, linking circulating platelets to the site of injury at the blood vessel wall. vWD results either from deficiencies in the amount of vWF present or from structural abnormalities in the protein itself. In the most common form of vWD, type I, the total amount of vWF is decreased. Further, vWF circulates in small, medium and large clusters of the vWF antigen. About 80% of vWD patients have type I vWD in which multimers of all sizes are present but in decreased quantity, as is the total amount of vWF. Factor VIII may also be mildly decreased (with fewer carrier molecules for factor VIII leading to stable factor VIII). Ristocetin cofactor is a measure of the function of the vWF antigen, and this too may be decreased in type I vWD. Just under 20% of patients have one of the two subtypes of type II vWD; type IIA is characterized by absence of the medium and largest vWF multimers; and type IIB is characterized by the largest multimers and hyperfunction of the vWF, which can cause excessive binding of platelets and may appear with thrombocytopenia. The hemophilia treatment center (HTC) needs to determine subtype to determine appropriate therapy. Mucocutaneous bleeding is characteristic of vWD, and so profuse nosebleeds and excessive bleeding from lesions or sites in the mouth are common. Bruising, particularly those out of proportion to injury with hard centers, can occur. Other examples of bleeding include prolonged bleeding from skin cuts, excessive menstruation, or menorrhagia, and postoperative bleeding or unexplained swelling. Because of the wide clinical heterogeneity of vWD with some affected persons having very few symptoms and others much more, many persons with vWD are undiagnosed.

Incidence

- Hemophilia A occurs in approximately 1 per 10,000 live male births. There are an estimated 20,000 affected individuals in the United States.
- Hemophilia B occurs in approximately 1 per 25,000 live male births. There are an estimated 4500 affected individuals in the United States.
- Hemophilia C affects approximately 1% to 3% of Ashkenazi Jews (Jews of Eastern European descent). Other groups are also affected.
- vWD affects between 1% and 3% of the general population. A more precise incidence is not known because symptoms are generally mild. A high incidence has been observed in certain geographic areas, such as the Åland Islands (Ahvenanmaa) of Finland, Sweden, Israel, and Iran.
- Both hemophilia A and B and vWD occur in all the world's populations.
- Life expectancy for hemophilia A and B is near normal with appropriate medical care and the absence of HIV and hepatitis C infection.
- Life expectancy for vWD is normal.

Risk Factors

- Family members with bleeding disorders
- Women related through the maternal line to an individual with hemophilia (i.e., sisters, aunts, nieces of an affected male)

Subjective Data

The bleeding history is perhaps the single most sensitive test for inherited bleeding disorders. Special attention should be paid to hemostatic challenges (e.g., surgeries, menses) in children especially; there is simply not enough time for many children to have been so challenged. Any child with a suspected or known bleeding disorder should have a complete history taken including a careful review of systems. Special emphasis should be placed on the following areas:

Family history. Absence of a positive family history does not rule out presence of a bleeding disorder. Obtain a bleeding history of the patient and all first-degree relatives of both biologic parents (e.g., the child's parents, aunts and uncles, grandparents). This three-generation pedigree is quite useful. Signs and symptoms of vWD are often mild or accepted as the "family norm" and unreported for medical evaluation.

History of bruising or bleeding episodes. Bruising in infants and toddlers is less common (outside of tibial bruising), and evaluation needs to focus on the nature of the hemostatic challenge. Note the nature of any bruising or bleeding, the site or sites of bruising or bleeding, and when the bruising or bleeding episode occurred (e.g., rough play, spontaneous occurrence). Did the child awaken from sleep with a nosebleed? Do the nosebleeds occur more in cold weather? Note the length of the bleeding episode, how the bleeding was finally stopped, and the effect of bruising or bleeding on the child's activities (Table 45-11). Do bruises have hard centers? Does the child or anyone in the family have menorrhagia (heavy menses defined as greater than six to eight saturated pads per day)? A history of iron-deficiency anemia or blood transfusions? A history of bleeding or unusual swelling after dental work or surgery (especially circumcision and tonsillectomy)? Was there bleeding after umbilical cord exfoliation?

Past medical history. This includes abnormal presurgical laboratory study results such as a prolonged aPTT or bleeding time.

Current medications. This includes medication use by an infant or child or the presence in the household of agents with known antiplatelet effects such as acetylsalicylic acid (including bismuth subsalicylate [Pepto-Bismol]), NSAIDs, and warfarin (Coumadin).

Allergy history. Allergic rhinitis, breathing dry air without adequate humidification, and mechanical trauma from nose picking may contribute to nasal bleeding.

History for follow-up visits. This section of the history (for an individual with a known bleeding disorder) should include the history of bleeding episodes, their frequency, the sites involved, the treatment, and the patient's response.

Table 45-11 Age-related Patterns of Bleeding: Hemophilia A and B

AGE	EVENT	DESCRIPTION
< 1 month	Birth process	Intracranial hemorrhage, cephalohematomas
	Invasive procedures	Circumcision, intramuscular injection, heel stick, venipuncture
> 1 month	Spontaneous bleeding leading to bruising and hematoma formation; characteristic appearance: Hematoma is raised, known as "palpable purpura"	
1 month to 1 year	Occurrence unrelated to any identifiable precipitating event	Unusual sites such as back, abdomen, trunk, or under the arms (from picking infant up); suspicion of child abuse may prompt diagnostic evaluation
	Crawling, cruising, pulling to stand; teething, immunizations	Superficial hematomas on extensor surfaces
1 to 3 years	Ambulation with normally anticipated falls and bumps of a toddler	Oral bleeding from frenulum tears, intramuscular bleeds; soft tissue: Especially in scrotum and gluteal region; CNS bleeding
3 to 5 years	Increasing motor skills (e.g., climbing, running, jumping)	Joint bleeds evident
5 to 12 years	Physical activities	Groin, hip bleeds evident
> 12 years	Physical activities	Denial; risk-taking; behaviors may contribute to occurrence of bleeding episodes; hematuria

Menstrual history. The menstrual history for female patients should include the age at menarche, number of days of flow, and number of saturated pads per day (six to eight or less is normal). Cycle-to-cycle variability in flow volume is common. Is school or sleep disrupted by menorrhagia? Is there dysmenorrhea? What treatment has been tried? (Many NSAIDs can worsen menorrhagia.)

Developmental history. This area includes gross motor achievements in infants, toddlers, and preschool-age children.

School history. This includes any time lost from school that is related to bleeding episodes.

Physical activities. This includes sports, exercise, physically related behaviors for school-age children and adolescents. Assess for activities that invite accidents or trauma, with resulting bleeding.

Psychosocial history. This area includes family coping and adaptation, finances, support groups. Also, is sleep disrupted because of pain or bleeding?

Objective Data

Physical examination. The initial visit and complete physical examination for know or suspected bleeding disorders (see Table 45-11) includes the following:

- Describe the exact location of bruising or bleeding.
- Carefully evaluate the skin for telangiectasia (which may be associated with bleeding disorders) and for elasticity (excessive elasticity may be a sign of a connective tissue disorder such as Ehlers-Danlos or Marfan syndrome, both of which are associated with PFDs).
- Assess the joints for hypermobility (common with connective tissues disorders that are associated with PFDs).
- For bruises, observe for appearance, size, and number.
- For bleeding, observe for evidence of fresh bleeding or oozing, the presence of any clot and its nature, and any abnormal laboratory data (Table 45-12). If it is a known

Table 45-12 Laboratory Assessment for Bleeding Disorders

LABORATORY TEST	PURPOSE	RESULTS	INTERPRETATION	COMMENTS
Complete blood cell count	Screen	Normal*	Expected finding	Findings that may be consistent with vWD: Decreased hemoglobin, hematocrit from profuse, recurrent nosebleeds, excessive menstrual bleeding; thrombocytopenia
Prothrombin time	Screen	Normal	Expected finding in hemophilia A, B and vWD	
Activated partial thromboplastin time	Screen	Prolonged	Prolonged correlates with factor activity <30% finding in hemophilia A, B and vWD	Requires further evaluation: Hematologist referral, assay of factor level, vWF functional activity (see below)
Factor VIII level (coagulant activity)	Diagnostic	Decreased	Hemophilia A, vWD, carrier states for each	Activity expressed as a percentage; normal range from 50% to 150% depending on laboratory values
Factor IX level (coagulant activity)	Diagnostic	Decreased	Hemophilia B, carrier state	Activity expressed as a percentage; normal from 50% to 150% depending on laboratory values; low levels in infancy normal secondary to immature liver synthesis of factor IX; repeat assays may be needed to determine exact baseline value
vWF antigen	Diagnostic	See Comment 1	Level of circulating vWF	Hematologist interpretation necessary, since exact diagnosis required for accurate treatment
vWF functional activity* (also known as ristocetin cofactor [RCoF])	Diagnostic	See Comment 2	Measures binding agglutination of vWF to platelets in presence of ristocetin	Repeat testing not unusual, since vWF is increased in certain disease states and under stressful conditions such as pregnancy or venipuncture
Ristocetin-induced platelet aggregation to low-dose ristocetin (RIPA-LD)*	Diagnostic	See Comment 3	Measures binding and ability of binding to induce platelet aggregation in presence of small amounts of ristocetin	1. Useful in factor VIII carrier state determination: Usual 1:1 relationship between vWF antigen and factor VIII is decreased in carrier state
Multimer analysis	Diagnostic	See Comment 4	Assesses structure of vWF using immunoelectrophoresis test available only in specialized reference laboratory	2. vWF:RCoF decreased in type 1, most common type of vWD; decreased in carrier state
				3. Increased level indicates a structural problem in vWF, causing hyperplatelet aggregation and thrombocytopenia
				4. Multimer analysis useful in diagnosing types of vWD where bleeding results from abnormal structure of vWF

DNA analysis for genetic mutations causing hemophilia A and B is useful for carrier state determination and prenatal diagnosis. Latter accomplished by chorionic villus sampling at 9 to 11 weeks of gestation or by amniocentesis at 12 to 15 weeks of gestation. At birth, confirmation of diagnosis from cord blood samples taken from infant's side, since factors VIII, IX do not cross placenta. DNA analysis is of limited use in diagnosis of vWD. Bleeding time may or may not be ordered, since results can be variable and depend on the technique of the individual performing test.
*Should be done at an HTC.

bleeding disorder, it is usually not necessary to repeat documented diagnostic laboratory studies.

Interval and follow-up visits. Physical examination should include the following, keeping in mind that any deviation from baseline values can result from bleeding episodes:

- *Neurologic system*—Assess for weakness, motor or sensory impairments in the extremities, or asymmetries. New-onset

seizures or severe headache are sometimes caused by intracranial bleeding, and new-onset neck stiffness or loss of limb may be a sign of spinal epidural hematoma.

- *Development*—Look for any loss of previously attained motor or cognitive skills.
- *Musculoskeletal system*—Assess the range of flexion, extension, and rotation at the elbows, knees, and ankles (the

Table 45-13 Hemophilia and Bleeding Disorders: Specific Issues and Concerns

ISSUE	AGE TO DISCUSS	COUNSELING	OTHER
Parental responses of guilt, anger, fear	Time of diagnosis, ongoing	Responses reemerge with each developmental stage	Inherited nature, unpredictability of bleeding events, potential for life-threatening bleeding unique to this chronic illness; ask about support systems; reactions of other family members (partner, siblings, grandparents), friends to illness
Safety	Infancy, ongoing	Expect physical activity of infant and young child to cause bleeding; reassurance of available treatment and medical care; should parental effort focus on ensuring safe environment rather than restricting activity; at older ages, avoid activities that would cause injury to any child	Inform parents about after-hours care; establish plan for office or emergency department care for infusions; check for Medic Alert bracelet, necklace, or information pinned to infant; discuss car seat, seat belt use, and for older children, use of protective equipment such as helmet for biking; Read labels of over-the-counter medications to avoid use of aspirin, nonsteroidal antiinflammatory drugs
Discipline	Infancy, ongoing	Goal: Balance between overprotection and extreme permissiveness	Assess parental attitude, usual methods of discipline and how they were disciplined as children; introduce alternative strategies such as contracts, time-outs if needed; threatening child with infusion for misbehavior is not appropriate
Out-of-home care	All ages	Interaction with children outside home contributes to development	Assess parent's comfort with play groups, babysitters, and so on; assist parent in discussing bleeding disorder with others; if leaving child with others, instructions about signs, symptoms of bleeding; actions to take if bleeding occurs
School	Preschool-age and older	Peer relationships; school work, performance	Inform school personnel about bleeding disorder and signs, symptoms of bleeding; action to take if bleeding occurs at school; sports participation; school visit by hemophilia treatment center nurse, educator may be helpful
Sports, exercise	School-age, adolescence	No contact sports such as football, hockey	Exercise and sports that strengthen all muscles for joint stability and increase joint flexibility are best, such as swimming, golf; assess child's sports interests and recognize peer pressure to perform certain sports; consider introducing role models for other sports
Sexuality	Birth, adolescence	Circumcision, actual inheritance	May be delayed until diagnosis confirmed; inheritance, carrier testing for relatives addressed by hemophilia treatment center genetic counselor
		Safer sex: Condom use, sexually transmitted diseases such as human immunodeficiency virus, hepatitis B	Reproductive concerns, especially if human immunodeficiency virus positive; other issues: Intimacy, disclosing information about bleeding disorder or HIV status
Adjustment to chronic illness	School-age, adolescence	Child's, adolescent's perspective of bleeding disorder	Includes information related to school performance, peer relationships, sibling relationships, activities, knowledge of bleeding disorder, participation in treatment; in addition, for adolescent: Career or education plans after high school
Menstruation in carrier females and vWD	School-age	Anticipatory guidance	Teach that six to eight pads per day is normal. Heavier bleeding should prompt consultation with HTC to consider use of Stimate and Amicar; dysmenorrhea managed with COX-2 inhibitors (e.g., Celebrex, Vioxx) if acetaminophen does not relieve pain

most frequent sites of joint bleeding). Comparison with the HTC assessment may be helpful in evaluating the extent of acute joint bleeding. The measurement of joint circumference may be helpful in following the course of resolution of a joint bleed.

Diagnostic procedures and laboratory tests. See Table 45-12. Generally performed as part of a comprehensive hemophilia visit are the following, though frequency of assessment depends on the HTC protocol and signs and symptoms of the patient:

- *Performed at least yearly*—CBC count, inhibitor screen, liver enzyme studies, and CD4 cell counts on those persons known to have human immunodeficiency virus (HIV)
- *Performed approximately every 2 to 3 years*—Assays for hepatitis A, B, and C (despite completion of hepatitis B vaccination, negative seroconversion can occur, so presence of protective antibody against hepatitis B should be monitored), with an HIV screen only if risk factors are present

Primary Care Implications and Issues

Refer any child with a known or suspected bleeding disorder to the HTC. Provision of well-child care should follow current American Academy of Pediatrics (AAP) recommendations for regular assessments, physical examination, and routine screening. Special attention should be paid to the following:

- *Immunizations*—Remember that hepatitis A vaccine is recommended for children with hemophilia or clotting factor–dependent vWD over 2 years of age.
- *Growth*—Monitor weight and height at every visit. Growth rates exceeding normal, especially for weight, add stress to joints. Nutritional assessment may be necessary.
- *Dental care*—Advise that the first dental visit should be during the toddler years. Dental care is usually available at the HTC but may also be provided by a local dentist after consultation and with observance of the HTC's recommendations for circum-procedure hemostasis with factor or aminocaproic acid.

Issues and concerns that are typically addressed in the primary care setting should take into account the diagnosis of hemophilia (Table 45-13). Also, episodes of acute illness should be evaluated with bleeding as a possible origin. Examples are shown in Box 45-17.

Management

Management requires a comprehensive approach facilitated by the HTC. Baseline levels of either factor VIII or factor IX coagulant activity can provide a rough guideline to the expected frequency and type of bleeding in hemophilia A and B (Table 45-14).

Treatments and medications

- Bleeding episodes should be treated by supplying the missing or deficient clotting factor in sufficient amounts to achieve coagulation or hemostasis. Factor replacement products for hemophilia A and B and vWD are described in Table 45-15.
- Currently used virus-inactivation methods for human plasma–derived factor replacement products are considered effective against HIV and hepatitis B and C only, while hepatitis A and parvovirus cannot be inactivated.
- Cryoprecipitate and fresh frozen plasma are no longer standard treatments of hemophilia or vWD.
- HTC protocols should be followed for usual replacement therapy. These protocols specify the most appropriate replacement therapy product for the child (see Box 45-15) and a dosage according to the site of bleeding and the child's weight.
- As needed, a bolus dose may be provided according to most common dosing schedule. It is initiated at the first sign of bleeding with the aim of preventing complications from uncontrolled bleeding. Repeat the bolus dose based on the half-life of the factor product (i.e., half-life of factor VIII product, 12 hours; half-life of factor IX product, 18 to 24 hours). Prophylaxis dosing refers to the routine scheduling of factor replacement product infusions two or three times a week with the goal of preventing bleeding. It is useful in children with severe hemophilia.
- Interventions are implemented according to the magnitude or severity of the bleeding episode (e.g., calling the HTC for known or suspected head injuries).
- Desmopressin (synthetic vasopressin, or DDAVP) causes release of factor VIII and vWF from the endothelial stores. DDAVP is prescribed by the HTC for children with vWD or mild factor VIII (factor VIII greater than 5%) after a test dose is given and an adequate response is documented. The intranasal form, Stimate, can also be used and is a convenient and fairly low-risk alternative to intravenous DDAVP or intravenous clotting factor.
- Antifibrinolytic medications (epsilon-aminocaproic acid and tranexamic acid) are considered adjunctive hemostatic agents. They prevent clot dissolution from fibrinolysis,

---

Box 45-17 Evaluation of Acute Illness as Related to Hemophilia

Blood in the urine—UTI versus spontaneous bleeding
Abdominal and groin pain—Hip joint, retroperitoneal, and iliopsoas bleeds verse acute surgical problem (e.g., appendicitis, inguinal hernia)
Headache and vomiting—CNS bleed versus viral illness

Table 45-14 Baseline Levels in Hemophilia A and B

BASELINE LEVEL: FACTOR VIII OR FACTOR IX	CLASSIFICATION OF SEVERITY	FREQUENCY AND TYPE OF BLEEDING
< 1%	Severe	Frequency of bleeding ranges from weekly to several episodes per month; spontaneous bleeding common; life-threatening bleeds may occur; hemorrhage with trauma or surgery
1% to 5%	Moderate	Frequency variable; spontaneous bleeding less common; hemorrhage with trauma or surgery
> 5%	Mild	Spontaneous hemorrhage rare; hemorrhage only with significant trauma or surgery

Table 45-15 Common Treatment Options for Children with Inherited Bleeding Disorders

PRODUCT	INDICATIONS	DOSAGE	ADMINISTRATION
Recombinant factor 8 (F VIII)	Moderate and severe bleeding in F VIII deficiency	1 unit of F VIII per kg raises F VIII level 2%	10 ml/minute intravenous push % correction × kg × 0.5 = U to be infused May be given at home safely after caregivers are trained in home infusion by the HTC May be stored in home refrigerator
Factor 8 and vWF	Severe bleeding in vWD	50 units/kg every 24 hours	See package insert for specific dosing and consider dosing based on activity of vWF (100 units/kg/ 24 hours) May be stored in a home refrigerator
Activated factor complex	Moderate and severe bleeding in F VIII deficiency with inhibitors	50 to 75 units/kg	See package insert for specific infusion rates May not be given at the same time with aminocaproic acid Associated with allergic reactions Large doses (over 100 units/kg) are associated with disseminated intravascular coagulation, so monitor PT
Recombinant factor 9 (F IX)	F IX deficiency with moderate and severe bleeding	0.5 to 1 units/kg raises F IX level 1%	Higher risk of allergic reactions than rF VIII. May be stored in a home refrigerator
Recombinant rf VIIa	F VIII or F IX deficiency with inhibitor possible use in other bleeding disorders	45 to 90 μg/kg per dose	Half-life of rF VIIa is 2.5 hours In hemophilia requires every 2-3 hour dosing May be stored in a home refrigerator
DDAVP intravenous or intranasal (Stimate)	Mild bleeding in mild F VIII deficiency and von Willebrand's and platelet function defect	Intravenous: 0.3 μg/kg/dose of Stimate Intranasal: 1 spray (150 μg) < 50 kg; 2 sprays (300 μg) > 50 kg body weight	Intravenous form is given in 25 to 50 NSS over 20 to 30 minutes. Intravenous form has reports of tachyphylaxis and hyponatremic seizures in patients with tenuous fluid balance. Never give intravenous form intranasally. Do not give low-dose (generic) intranasal DDAVP (10-15 μg/spray) in lieu of Stimate. Stimate may be given only after a test dose in the HTC documents efficacy.
Aminocaproic acid (Amicar)	Bleeding disorders with mucous membrane bleeding or as an adjunctive in special situations	100 mg/kg/dose orally once daily for 5 days (maximum dose of 24 g/day) Suspension: 250 mg/ml as 480 ml bottle Tablets: 500 mg	May not be given with Autoplex or Feiba. Syrup is easier than tablets for most children and adults to take because of the large number of very large tablets required to achieve dosage. Stabilizes clots in mouth and nose bleeds; there must be a clot already for the product to be optimally effective (usually DDAVP, Stimate, or a dose of factor). Store Stimate in the home refrigerator to prolong shelf-life.

particularly in the mouth but also in the nose, throat, and endometrium.

- Pain medications such as acetaminophen and (with physician consultation) codeine and narcotic analgesics are preferred to relieve pain associated with bleeding episodes. Aspirin-containing medications and NSAIDs are contraindicated because of their potential inhibiting effect on platelet function. However, the newer COX-2 inhibitors (celecoxib [Celebrex] and rofecoxib [Vioxx]) do not have antiplatelet effects and are safe to use in the bleeding disorders population. Insurance precertification is often required but is fairly easy to obtain once the carrier is aware of the diagnosis of a bleeding disorder.

- Bed rest and use of ice, compression, or Ace wraps are helpful.
- Physical therapy consultation for splinting or crutches may be necessary.
- Invasive procedures require hematologist consultation and factor replacement before or after the procedure. These include lumbar puncture, arterial blood gas samples, dental extractions or dental work when regional anesthetic agents are injected, lacerations that require suturing, and femoral or jugular venipuncture.
- Routine procedures include immunizations. Immunizations should be given by the route they are designed to be given through. Intramuscular injections rarely cause bleed-

ing even in hemophiliacs. Furthermore, muscle bleeds are far easier to treat than immunization-preventable illnesses such as pertussis or polio. Avoid giving immunizations by the subcutaneous route unless the immunization is designed to be given subcutaneously because there are no data to support efficacy by the nonstandard route. Children with vWD may have immunizations without any special precautions. For hemophiliacs, take the following simple precautions:

Give all immunizations in the vastus lateralis muscle of the thigh regardless of age. Avoid the deltoid and gluteus muscles. There are few nerves in the thigh that could be affected in the rare event of postimmunization bleeding or swelling.

Ask the family to assist with direct pressure to the injection site for about 15 minutes after the immunization.

Apply a small ice bag (a glove is fine, and use gauze to protect the skin) for another 15 minutes

Instruct the family to report any unusual swelling to the HTC.

- Complications of therapy include:

Allergic reactions to factor replacement products (VIII or IX)—Occurrence is during an infusion or up to 1 to 2 hours later. Signs and symptoms include hives, itching, chills, nausea, redness, or stinging at infusion site. Treatment is intravenous or oral administration of diphenhydramine before infusion.

Inhibitors—Antibodies may form as an immune response to a foreign protein (i.e., the infused factor VIII or IX replacement product). These inhibitory antibodies inactivate the replacement product and are clinically associated with failure of bleeding episodes to respond to appropriate replacement therapy. Inhibitor development is a serious and, depending on the inhibitor level and clinical situation (e.g., surgery), potentially fatal complication. Inhibitors can develop at any age and after thousands of factor replacements. However, the following features in their development have been observed: More likely to occur during childhood and after relatively few factor product exposure days (days on which a patient receives one or more factor product doses), higher incidence in severe hemophilia A, and may be more common with the use of recombinant factor products.

Infection—The transmission of bloodborne infectious disease such as HIV and viral hepatitis B, C, and D has been associated with the use of factor replacement products derived from human plasma in the past and continues to be a significant health burden. Since the mid-1980s, transmission of these viruses has been significantly reduced, if not entirely eliminated, because of improved donor screening practices, vigorous virus-inactivation methods, and administration of the hepatitis B vaccine. Long-term consequences of chronic hepatitis infections include cirrhosis and hepatocellular carcinoma.

Counseling and prevention

- Provide general teaching to the parents and child related to bleeding disorders, beginning at the time of diagnosis.
- Address early the parents' or child's misconception or fear that the individual with a bleeding disorder will "bleed to death." Teach that bleeding is "long and slow," not "hard and fast." Teach that the lifespan is normal for patients with vWD and near normal for patients with hemophilia (with proper medical care).
- Recommend Medic Alert bracelets (for children under 8 years of age) or necklaces (for children over 8 years of age).
- Take into account patterns of bleeding for anticipatory guidance to ensure appropriate parental interventions.
- Use developmentally appropriate explanations to facilitate the outcome of self-care.
- Teach the parents and child possible signs and symptoms related to the site of bleeding and the recommended treatment for bleeding episodes. The parents and child should be knowledgeable about the complications of bleeding, especially the long-term consequences of musculoskeletal and central nervous system (CNS) bleeding. (Table 45-16 provides clinically relevant information.)
- Instruct the parents and child about the administration of replacement product. A home health care infusion company is needed for a supply of factor replacement product at home. Replacement product is not available from local pharmacy, and a hospital may not have in stock the specific type prescribed because of its high cost and infrequent use. Always use the product prescribed.
- Instruct the parents and child that factor replacement product should be stored in the refrigerator at home. A cooler and freezer pack should be available to transport the product for travel out of the immediate home area.
- Review with the family the ordering of sufficient supplies of replacement product based on the child's past and anticipated factor replacement needs. Practice reading expiration dates.
- Discuss home infusion by parents, with later self-infusion by child. Demonstrate the procedure, with a return demonstration by the parents and child. Venipuncture by parents generally occurs around 4 years of age, with the child performing it by about 12 years of age. Developmentally appropriate child participation in administration should be encouraged. Instruct parents and child on the following:

Vein selection, use of tourniquet, possible use of analgesic cream to numb skin before venipuncture, and application of pressure for 5 to 10 minutes after venipuncture

Reconstitution of factor product and use of a filter needle to withdraw reconstituted factor product

Universal precautions when reconstituting and withdrawing factor product and during venipuncture

Appropriate disposal of sharps and material contaminated with blood

- Document bleeding episodes, factor replacement product given, and responses.
- Stress the importance of communication with the HTC for assistance with bleeds that do not respond to usual replacement therapy; accidents or trauma; bleeds into potentially dangerous sites such as head, mouth, retropharyngeal or retroperitoneal areas; recurrent bleeds into the same joint; or any other question or concern. The HTC is available by phone 24 hours a day.
- Discuss access to a local medical provider or emergency department for assistance with venipuncture, administration of replacement, and emergency care of bleeding episodes. Develop and review an emergency plan.

Table 45-16 Sites of Bleeding

SITE	SIGNS AND SYMPTOMS	COMPLICATIONS	TREATMENT
Joints			
Most common clinical problem in hemophilia A, B; knees, elbows, ankles most frequently affected; then hip, wrist, shoulder	Complains of "funny feeling" or tingling, warmth in joint Heat, swelling Pain Limitation of movement Very young child refuses to walk or use extremity	Increased chance of rebleeding in same joint (known as "target joint") Chronic pain Inflammation Long term: joint deformity, crippling arthritis	Factor replacement per hemophiliac treatment center guidelines Repeat dose sometimes necessary Pain medication as needed Physical therapy consultation depending on bleed

1. Radiograph not diagnostic for acute episode of joint bleeding; more likely to show chronic bony changes from repeated joint bleeds.
2. Hip joint bleed clinically significant: May result in aseptic necrosis of femoral head because of increased intraarticular pressure:
   Signs or symptoms: Limited abduction, adduction, paresthesias below inguinal ligament.
   Ultrasonogram to confirm clinical observation.
   Consult hematologist.
   Hospitalization usually necessary with follow-up physical therapy plan for rehabilitation.

SITE	SIGNS AND SYMPTOMS	COMPLICATIONS	TREATMENT
Soft Tissue and Muscle			
Common sites of muscle bleeds: thigh, calf, forearm, iliopsoas*	Early: Aching, swelling Cutaneous warmth Pain Limitation of movement Discoloration	Muscle wasting Scarring, fibrosis Contracture Neurovascular damage (i.e., compartment syndrome) caused by pressure from bleeding into confined spaces such as wrist, hand, forearm, tibial areas, plantar surface of foot Pseudocyst formation	Factor replacement per hemophiliac treatment center guidelines Consult hematologist whenever clinically significant bleeding such as deep muscle or internal bleeding, compartment syndrome is suspected Application of ice and observation may be all that is needed for some superficial soft-tissue hematomas that are limited in size (and depending on their location)

Clinically significant bleeding may occur in the soft tissues or muscles.
Pharyngeal or retropharyngeal bleeding may occur from trauma or after infection. Airway obstruction is possible.
Signs and symptoms: Drooling, inability to swallow.
Radiograph to confirm.
Hospitalization usually necessary.
Evidence of neurovascular damage.
Bleeding into the thigh or iliopsoas-retroperitoneal area: Anemia or massive blood loss is possible depending on the extent of bleeding.
Sign and symptoms of iliopsoas-retroperitoneal bleeding: Abdominal, inguinal, or hip area pain, limited hip extension, numbness from femoral nerve compression.
Differential diagnosis of iliopsoas-retroperitoneal bleeding includes hip joint bleed, groin muscle pull, gastroenteritis, acute surgical condition of abdomen.
Radiograph, ultrasonogram to confirm presence of hematoma.
Hospitalization and physical therapy plan for rehabilitation.

SITE	SIGNS AND SYMPTOMS	COMPLICATIONS	TREATMENT
Central Nervous System			
CNS	Head, neck, or spinal injury; headache, blurred vision, vomiting, change in pupil size or response to light Weakness in extremities Change in speech, behavior Drowsiness, loss of consciousness	Brain damage Related motor deficits, paralysis	Prompt replacement per hemophiliac treatment center guidelines Consult hematologist Watch closely for signs of increased intracranial pressure Hospitalization likely

CNS bleeding is a life-threatening medical emergency.
History of trauma not always present.
Presence or absence of "goose-eggs," bruises, lacerations on head is not reliable indicator of injury or extent of possible internal bleeding.
Replacement therapy should be given *before* any diagnostic evaluation is started.

Iliopsoas refers to a combination of the iliacus muscle, which originates in the iliac fossa and inserts into the greater trochanter, and the psoas muscle with its thoracolumbar vertebral origin and insertion at the lesser trochanter.

Continued

Table 45-16 Sites of Bleeding—cont'd

SITE	SIGNS AND SYMPTOMS	COMPLICATIONS	TREATMENT
Unexplained headache lasting 4 hours or more may be a symptom of intracranial bleeding.			
Oral areas	Bleeding from frenulum tear, tongue, lip, or other mucosal areas in mouth Nausea, vomiting Choking	Anemia Airway obstruction Severe blood loss	Instruct patient to avoid swallowing blood Antifibrinolytic medications Replacement if bleeding persists Consult hematologist if bleeding is severe Consider dental consult or other surgical assessment, depending on extent of injury Hospitalization for intravenous hydration if oral intake interferes with clot formation

Emergency measures may be necessary to keep the airway open or replace significant blood loss.
Hospitalization for intravenous hydration may be considered if oral intake interferes with clot formation.

Before any dental procedure, consult a hematologist; antifibrinolytic medication alone or in combination with factor replacement or desmopressin may be necessary.

SITE	SIGNS AND SYMPTOMS	COMPLICATIONS	TREATMENT
Nose (common problem in vWD)	Mild: < 10 minutes Severe: Prolonged or recurrent	Same as oral areas if bleeding severe	Pressure bilaterally over soft tissue of nares: Have child sit with head bent slightly forward to prevent aspiration or swallowing of blood If bleeding persists, consult hematologist Replacement necessary if bleeding severe Ear, nose, throat consultation may be useful in some cases Other measures include ample indoor humidification; topical intranasal moisturizing agent; salt pork gently inserted in the nares to produce vasoconstriction, prevent rebleeding
Abdomen and Pelvis			
Urinary tract	Blood in urine Flank pain	Chronic kidney damage (rare)	Consult hematologist Bed rest, increased fluid intake usually prescribed; factor replacement possible Do not use antifibrinolytic medication (may cause clot formation in renal vasculature) Although spontaneous hematuria of unknown origin occurs in hemophiliacs, further medical evaluation may be necessary to rule out other causes (e.g., UTI)
GI tract	Abdominal pain Vomiting blood Bloody or tarry stools Hypotension Weakness	Anemia Severe blood loss	Consult hematologist Replacement therapy and aggressive diagnostic evaluation to determine source of bleeding are necessary Hospitalization is possible

- Review the complications of treatment, including allergic reactions, inhibitor development, and infectious diseases.
- Teach the parents and child not to use aspirin and NSAIDs.
- Review safety precautions with the parents and child.
- Stress to parents the importance of genetic counseling, especially if future pregnancies are desired. Explain that the risk of a child inheriting a bleeding disorder is determined both by parental carrier status (the potential to carry the genetic trait) and by the bleeding disorder's pattern of genetic transmission.
- Stress involvement in noncontact sports for all children with inherited bleeding disorders. Swimming, golf, walking, and biking are excellent choices. There is no substitute for careful adult supervision during all sports whether formal team sports or informal "pick-up" games in the neighborhood.

Follow-up. A routine HTC visit is scheduled every 3 to 12 months depending on the age of the child and severity of the bleeding disorder. Follow-up care after a bleeding episode includes daily telephone contact or office visits until the bleeding episode is resolved. If the family is receiving home therapy, telephone or office consultation should be provided for the following: bleeds that do not respond to usual replacement or require more than two treatments; recurrent bleeds into the same joint; injury to the head, neck, or spine; bleeding into potentially dangerous sites such as mouth, retropharyngeal or retroperitoneal areas, or hip; and neurovascular or circulatory changes accompanying bleeding episodes.

Consultations and referrals

- Remember that any child with a bleeding disorder such as hemophilia or vWD should be managed at an HTC. Many health care personnel are available through such a center to assist in care, both at the center and through community outreach and referrals. These health care professionals include hematologists, dentists, social workers, physical therapists, genetic counselors, orthopedic surgeons, educators, nurses, psychologists, and nutritionists.
- Provide information about the National Hemophilia Foundation (NHF) to families.
- Keep in mind that family stress is common and usually related to the unpredictability of bleeding episodes, compliance with treatment regimens, and the high cost of replacement therapy. Family-to-family support may be possible through the HTC and state chapters of the NHF.
- Obtain a travel letter that describes the child's diagnosis, treatment guidelines for factor replacement, and instructions for contacting the child's hematologist whenever the child or the family travels some distance from the HTC.
- Notify the school nurse.
- Refer for genetic counseling at an HTC.
- Refer to a home health care infusion company.

Resources

Organizations
National Hemophilia Foundation; (800) 42HANDI;
www.hemophilia.org
Websites
Shemophilia (www.shemophilia.org/resources/index.html)
World Federation of Hemophilia (www.wfh.org)
AllAboutBleeding (www.allaboutbleeding.com)

Human Immunodeficiency Virus and Acquired Immune Deficiency Syndrome

KATHLEEN A. SHEA & SUSAN M. HEFFERNAN

Alert

Consult with or refer to a pediatric HIV and AIDS specialist for any of the following:
- Child or adolescent diagnosed with HIV
- Signs of *Pneumocystis carinii* pneumonia (e.g., fever, cough, tachypnea, dyspnea)
- Child with fever
- Pain
- Disease progression (e.g., growth failure, neurodevelopmental decline, decrease in CD4+ T-cell count, increasing HIV ribonucleic acid [RNA] copy number)

In the United States, at the end of 1999, there were approximately 317,000 persons living with AIDS. This increased prevalence reflects increases in survival of persons diagnosed with AIDS because of improved treatments. Pediatric AIDS changed dramatically in the late 1990s as a result of the steep decline in perinatally acquired AIDS. The implementation of AIDS Clinical Trials 076 and of the Public Health Service Guidelines (Zidovudine administered during pregnancy and labor and to the newborn) has significantly reduced the incidence of babies born with HIV infection (Fig. 45-1), and improved treatment modalities have delayed the onset of AIDS-defining illnesses in children (Fig. 45-2).

The management of HIV-infected infants, children, and adolescents is rapidly changing and increasingly complex. It should be directed by a specialist in pediatric AIDS, and when that is not possible, experts should be consulted regularly. Effective management requires a multidisciplinary approach including physicians, nurses, social workers, psychologists, nutritionists, outreach workers, and pharmacists.

Etiology

HIV and its sequela AIDS affect infants, children, adolescents, and adults. The disease is characterized by profound immunosuppression and results in susceptibility to opportunistic infection and neoplasms.

HIV is an RNA retrovirus in the lentivirus family. Lentiviruses are often characterized as producing neurodegeneration and are often fatal. The HIV enters the human host cell and transcribes its RNA into DNA fueled by the viral enzyme reverse transcriptase. This proviral DNA can integrate into the human cellular DNA. The virus targets CD41 T lymphocytes, resulting in a reduction of the number of circulating T cells and noticeable cytopathologic features. HIV is transmitted through blood and body fluids and is detectable in blood, semen, vaginal and cervical secretions, amniotic fluid, breast milk, alveolar fluid, saliva, tears, throat swabs, and cerebrospinal fluid. Replication of the virus depends on viral and host factors. Viral mutations may lead to variants with more cytopathicity. High levels of circulating HIV correlate with decreasing numbers of CD41 T cells, and both correlate with clinical disease progression. Factors associated with maternal fetal transmission of HIV include low CD41 T cell count, high viral load, prolonged rupture of membranes, and intrapartum exposure to blood.

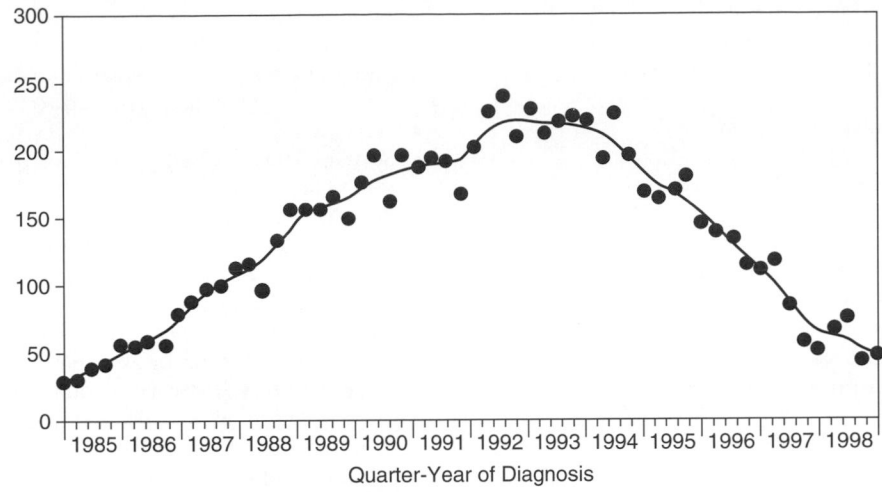

Fig. 45-1 Perinatally acquired AIDS (1985 through 1998, United States). (From Centers for Disease Control and Prevention [1999]. *HIV/AIDS Surveillance Report, 11*[No. 2], 1.)

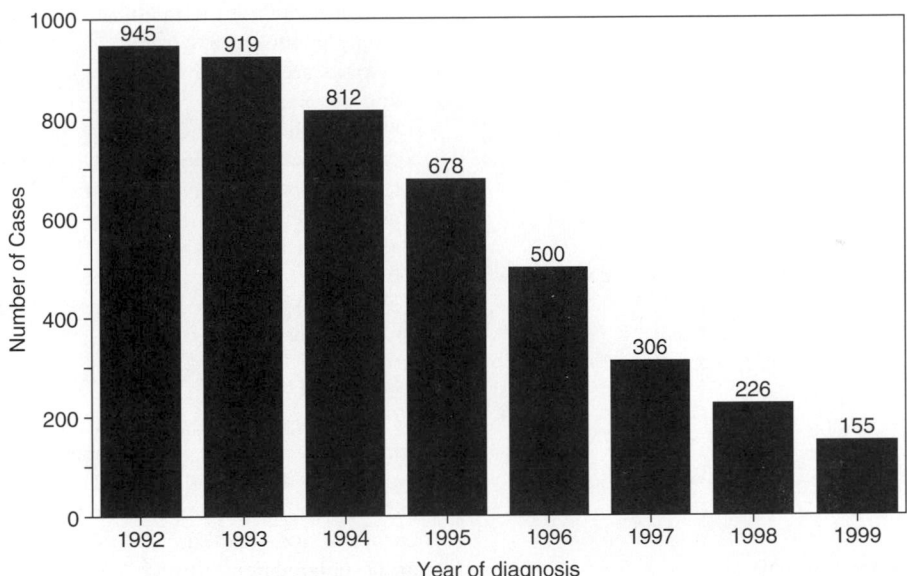

Fig. 45-2 Estimated pediatric AIDS incidence, by year of diagnosis (1992 through 1999, United States). (From Centers for Disease Control and Prevention (2000). *HIV/AIDS Surveillance Report, 12*[No. 1].)

The pathogenesis of HIV disease in children differs from that of adults. Children have a shorter latency period, with 80% of children being symptomatic by 2 years of age. Lower viral burdens are found in asymptomatic and mildly symptomatic children, whereas those with severe disease may have a high viral burden similar to that of adults. Children with perinatally acquired HIV infection have higher viral burdens than those whose transmission was through transfusions after 3 months of life. An infant's immature immune system may make them particularly vulnerable hosts.

Incidence

- There were approximately 4300 persons under 19 years of age living with AIDS at the end of 1999. The majority of pediatric cases are from perinatal exposure. African Americans and Hispanics continue to be disproportionately rep-

resented. Approximately two thirds of the children with AIDS reside in seven states: Florida, New York, California, Illinois, New Jersey, Texas, and Pennsylvania. The majority of these patients reside in metropolitan areas with populations over 500,000.

- The prevalence of persons living with HIV but not diagnosed with AIDS is uncertain because not all states conduct HIV case surveillance. According to data from 34 states, there were 2063 children under 13 years of age and 5263 adolescents 13 to 19 years of age reported through June 2000.

- Exposure category (pediatric):
Hemophilia or coagulation disorder: 3%
Mother with or at risk for HIV infection: 91%
Receipt of blood transfusion, blood components, or tissue: 4%
Risk not reported or identified: 2%

- Exposure category (adolescent males):
  Men who have sex with men: 34%
  Injecting drug use: 6%
  Men who have sex with men and inject drugs: 5%
  Hemophilia or coagulation disorder: 5%
  Heterosexual contact: 4%
  Receipt of blood transfusion, blood components, or
    tissue: 4%
  Risk not identified: 13%
- Exposure category (adolescent females):
  Injecting drug use: 14%
  Hemophilia or coagulation disorder: 1%
  Heterosexual contact: 52%
  Receipt of blood transfusion, blood component or
    tissue: 6%
  Risk not identified: 28%
- Race:
  African American, not Hispanic: 59%
  Hispanic: 23%
  Caucasian, not Hispanic: 17%
  Asian and Pacific Islander: 0.5%
  Native American and Alaska Native: 0.3%

Risk Factors

- Intravenous drug use
- Use of crack cocaine
- Homosexuality
- Multiple sex partners
- Unprotected sexual intercourse
- History of STDs
- Transfusion recipient before 1985
- Sexual partner of intravenous drug user, bisexual, or HIV-infected person
- Infant born to mother with HIV infection
- Infant born to a mother with risk factors for HIV
- Hemophilia

Subjective Data

A complete history should be obtained with special attention to the following:

Initial visit

- Did the mother receive prenatal care?
- Has the mother been tested for HIV? If so, did she receive the results?
- Does the mother have risk factors for HIV, such as a history of intravenous drug or crack cocaine use; a sexual partner who is an intravenous drug user, bisexual, or an HIV-positive male; being a transfusion recipient before 1985; a history of STDs; or inadequate or no prenatal care?
- Is there a history of any of the following: sexual abuse; fever (persistent and unexplained); opportunistic infections; STDs; recurrent bacterial infections; FTT; encephalopathy; interstitial lung disease; cardiomyopathy; chronic diarrhea; recurrent vaginitis (candidal); thrombocytopenia; tuberculosis (TB); severe, prolonged, or recurrent gastroenteritis; bronchiolitis; or fungal mucocutaneous or skin infection?
  The mother should also be asked about the following:
- Past history, including illnesses, hospitalizations, sources of care, medications, immunizations, and allergies
- Social history, including living situation, emotional supports, finances, peer relationships, education, occupation, legal status (emancipation), and legal problems

Adolescents should be questioned on:

- Substance use, including alcohol, tobacco, marijuana, cocaine, crack cocaine, opiates, anabolic steroids, and other drugs (including type and route)
- Menstrual history
- Sexual history, including gender of partner, age at initiation of sexual intercourse, number of sexual partners, types of sexual experience (e.g., oral, anal, vaginal intercourse), any sexual partner at risk for HIV, contraceptive history and current practices, use of condoms, pregnancy history, and STDs
- Mental health status, including general mood, depression, and suicidal ideation or attempts.

Interval history. Information on the following topics should be obtained at the initial visit and at each visit:

- Diet, including food intake, calorie count as indicated, use of nutritional supplements, loss of appetite, vomiting, and difficulty swallowing
- Elimination, including bowel patterns and any history of diarrhea
- Development, including milestone attainment, loss of milestones, school performance, and school absences
- Social, including the death of family members, any ill family members, foster care, disclosure of diagnosis, respite care, care for caregiver, and family coping patterns and problems
- Medication, including what has been prescribed and what child is actually taking (check dosages, frequency, ability to obtain medications [e.g., through insurance], difficulty getting the child to take many medications, and the use of alternative therapies)
- Problems, including any illnesses since the last visit or any recurrent symptoms (e.g., cough, fever, night sweats, pain, fatigue, social issues)

Objective Data

Physical examination. A complete physical examination should be performed on all infants, children, and adolescents suspected of having HIV or AIDS. Physical findings may include generalized lymphadenopathy, hepatosplenomegaly, neurodevelopmental deficits, FTT, recurrent otitis media, parotid enlargement, thrush, and rash.

Diagnostic procedures and laboratory tests. In addition to a positive HIV culture or positive HIV polymerase chain reaction (PCR), laboratory findings may include lymphopenia, anemia, thrombocytopenia, increased quantitative immunoglobulin, inverted CD4-to-CD8 ratio, decreased percentage of CD4 cells, and increased percentage of CD8 cells. (See HIV Testing later in this chapter.)

Most Commonly Reported AIDS Indicator Diseases

- Pneumocystis carinii *pneumonia*—Airborne organism, resembling a protozoan, that in immunosuppressed individuals causes pneumonitis characterized by abrupt onset of fever, cough, tachypnea, and dyspnea.
- *Lymphoid interstitial pneumonitis*—Chronic lymphocytic infiltration of the lungs characterized by an initially asymptomatic period that may progress to tachypnea, cough, wheezing, and hypoxemia. It is accompanied by lymphoid proliferation at other sites such as generalized lymphadenopathy, hepatosplenomegaly, and parotid enlargement.
- *Recurrent bacterial infections*—Two or more bacteriologically documented systemic infections such as bacteremia,

pneumonia, meningitis, osteomyelitis, septic arthritis, or abscess of body cavity or internal organ.

- *HIV wasting syndrome*—Diagnosed in the absence of a concurrent illness other than HIV infection that could explain the following findings: (1) persistent weight loss greater than 10% of baseline, or (2) downward crossing of at least two of the following percentile lines on the weight-for-age chart in a child older than 1 year of age, or (3) greater than 5th percentile on weight-for-height chart on two consecutive measurements more than 30 days apart, plus (4) chronic diarrhea (i.e., at least two stools per day for more than 30 days), or (5) documented fever for 30 days (intermittent or constant).

- *Candida esophagitis*—Inflammation of the esophagus caused by *Candida albicans*. Patients may have symptoms such as substernal pain, dysphagia, odynophagia, weight loss, or vomiting, or they may be asymptomatic. It may occur with or without oropharyngeal candidiasis.

- *HIV encephalopathy*—Severe form of developmental delay manifested by progressive deterioration in cognitive, motor, language, and adaptive function with loss of previously acquired milestones.

- *Cytomegalovirus (CMV) disease*—A herpesvirus that in immunocompromised hosts may cause chorioretinitis, esophagitis, pneumonitis, hepatitis, colitis, encephalitis.

- *Pulmonary candidiasis*—A less common manifestation of candidiasis resulting in laryngitis or epiglottitis.

- Mycobacterium avium–*intracellulare complex infection*—Non-TB, or atypical, mycobacteria resulting in disseminated infection characterized by weight loss, fever, night sweats, malaise, anemia, and neutropenia. It may result in chronic diarrhea, abdominal pain, colitis, malabsorption. CD41 T-cell counts lower than 100 cells/mm³ are primary risk factor.

- *Cryptosporidiosis*—Parasitic GI disease associated with high-volume, watery diarrhea; anorexia; and weight loss. Stools often contain mucus, but not blood or leukocytes. Persistent disease is more likely in patients with low CD41 T-cell counts.

- *Herpes simplex disease*—In immunocompromised hosts, may result in oral and genital mucocutaneous lesions, retinitis, esophagitis, encephalitis, chorioretinitis, hepatitis, and pneumonitis.

HIV Testing

HIV DNA PCR is the preferred virologic method for diagnosing HIV infection in infancy because the test is highly sensitive and specific and available and results can be obtained within 24 hours. HIV culture has similar sensitivity to DNA PCR but is more expensive, is not readily available, and requires 2 to 4 weeks to obtain results.

Most HIV-infected infants can be identified by 1 month of age, and virtually all can be identified by 6 months of age. Viral diagnostic testing should be performed at 48 hours, 1 to 2 months, and 3 to 6 months of age. A positive result should be confirmed by a second sample as soon as possible. HIV is diagnosed by two positive HIV virologic tests performed on separate blood samples. HIV can be excluded among children with two or more negative virologic tests, two of which are performed after 1 month of age and one of those being after 4 months of age.

For children over 18 months of age antibody testing is recommended. Enzyme immunoassays (EIAs) are used for HIV antibody testing. Western blot or immunofluorescent antibody tests should be used for confirmation. A positive antibody test in a child over 18 months of age is usually indicative of infection.

Table 45-17 lists the Centers for Disease Control and Prevention (CDC) current surveillance definitions for AIDS in adolescents. Box 45-18 lists the CDC clinical categories for children under 13 years of age who are HIV infected. Table 45-18 lists the CDC immunologic categories based on CD4+ lymphocyte counts and percentages; Table 45-19 lists the CDC classification system based on immunologic and clinical categories.

Early identification of HIV-infected infants begins with early identification of HIV-infected women. Universal HIV counseling and voluntary testing are recommended as the standard of care for pregnant women. Early identification of HIV-infected

---

Table 45-17 Revised Case Definition of AIDS-Defining Conditions for Adults and Adolescents 13 Years of Age and Older

Candidiasis of bronchi, trachea, or lungs	Lymphoma, immunoblastic (or equivalent term)
Candidiasis, esophageal	Lymphoma, primary or brain
Cervical cancer, invasive	*Mycobacterium avium* complex or *Mycobacterium kansasii*,
Coccidioidomycosis, disseminated or extrapulmonary	disseminated or extrapulmonary
Cryptococcosis, extrapulmonary	*Mycobacterium tuberculosis*, any site, pulmonary or extrapulmonary
Cryptosporidiosis, chronic intestinal (> 1-month duration)	*Mycobacterium*, other species or unidentified species, disseminated
Cytomegalovirus disease (other than liver, spleen, or nodes)	or extrapulmonary
Cytomegalovirus retinitis (with loss of vision)	*Pneumocystis carinii* pneumonia
Encephalopathy, HIV related	Pneumonia, recurrent
Herpes simplex, with chronic uclers (> 1-month duration), or	Progressive multifocal leukoencephalopathy
bronchitis, pneumonitis, or esophagitis	*Salmonella* septicemia, recurrent
Histoplasmosis, disseminated or extrapulmonary	Toxoplasmosis of brain
Isosporiasis, chronic intestinal (> 1-month duration)	Wasting syndrome because of HIV
Kaposi sarcoma	CD4+ T lymphocyte count less than 200 μL, or CD4+ percentage
Lymphoma, Burkitt (or equivalent term)	less than 15%

Centers for Disease Control and Prevention. (1992). 1993 revised classification system for HIV infection and expanded case surveillance definition of AIDS among adolescents and adults. Morbidity and Mortality Weekly Report, 41(RR-17), 1-19.

Box 45-18 Clinical Categories for Children with Human Immunodeficiency Virus (HIV) Infection

Category N: Not symptomatic

Children who have no signs or symptoms that are considered to be the result of HIV infection or who have only one of the conditions listed in category A.

Category A: Mildly symptomatic

Children with two or more of the conditions listed below but none of the conditions listed in categories B and C:

Lymphadenopathy ($\geq$ 0.5 cm at more than two sites; bilateral at one site)

Hepatomegaly

Splenomegaly

Dermatitis

Parotitis

Recurrent or persistent upper respiratory tract infection, sinusitis, or otitis media

Category B: Moderately symptomatic

Children who have symptomatic conditions other than those listed for category A or C that are attributed to HIV infection. Examples of conditions in clinical category B include, but are not limited to, the following:

Anemia (< 8 g/dl), neutropenia (< 1000 cells/mm³), or thrombocytopenia (< 100,000 cells/mm³) persisting $\geq$ 30 days

Bacterial meningitis, pneumonia, or sepsis (single episode)

Candidiasis, oropharyngeal (thrush), persisting (for more than 2 months) in children > 8 months of age

Cardiomyopathy

CMV infection, with onset before 1 month of age

Diarrhea, recurrent or chronic

Hepatitis

Herpes simplex virus (HSV) stomatitis, recurrent (more than two episodes within 1 year)

HSV bronchitis, pneumonitis, or esophagitis with onset before 1 month of age

Herpes zoster (shingles) involving at least two distinct episodes or more than one dermatome

Leiomyosarcoma

Lymphoid interstitial pneumonia or pulmonary lymphoid hyperplasia complex

Nephropathy

Nocardiosis

Persistent fever (lasting > 1 month)

Toxoplasmosis, onset before 1 month of age

Varicella, disseminated (complicated chickenpox)

Category C: Severely symptomatic

Serious bacterial infections, multiple or recurrent (i.e., any combination of at least two culture-confirmed infections within a 2-year period), of the following types: Septicemia, pneumonia, meningitis, bone or joint infection, or abscess of an internal organ or body cavity (excluding otitis media, superficial skin or mucosal abscesses, and indwelling catheter–related infections):

Candidiasis, esophageal or pulmonary (bronchi, trachea, lungs)

Coccidioidomycosis, disseminated (at site other than or in addition to lungs or cervical or hilar lymph nodes)

Cryptococcosis, extrapulmonary

Cryptosporidiosis or Iaosporiasis with diarrhea persisting > 1 month

Cytomegalovirus disease with onset of symptoms at age > 1 month of age (at a site other than liver, spleen, or lymph nodes)

Encephalopathy (at least one of the following progressive findings present for at least 2 months in the absence of a concurrent illness other than HIV infection that could explain the findings):

Failure to attain or loss of developmental milestones or loss of intellectual ability, verified by standard developmental scale or neuropsychologic tests.

Impaired brain growth or acquired microcephaly demonstrated by head circumference measurements or brain atrophy demonstrated by CT or MRI (serial imaging is required for children < 2 years of age).

Acquired symmetric motor deficit manifested by two or more of the following: Paresis, pathologic reflexes, ataxia, and gait disturbance.

Herpes simplex virus infection causing a mucocutaneous ulcer that persists for > 1 month; or bronchitis, pneumonitis, or esophagitis for any duration affecting a child > 1 month of age

Histoplasmosis, disseminated (at a site other than or in addition to lungs or cervical or hilar lymph nodes)

Kaposi sarcoma

Lymphoma, primary, in brain

Lymphoma, small, noncleaved cell (Burkitt) or immunoblastic or large cell lymphoma of B-cell or unknown immunologic phenotype

Mycobacterium tuberculosis, disseminated or extrapulmonary

Mycobacterium, other species or unidentified species, disseminated (at site other than or in addition to lungs, skin, or cervical or hilar lymph nodes)

Mycobacterium avium–intracellulare complex or *Mycobacterium kansasii*, disseminated (at site other than or in addition to lungs, skin, or cervical or hilar lymph nodes)

Pneumocystis carinii pneumonia

Progressive multifocal leukoencephalopathy

Salmonella (nontyphoid) septicemia, recurrent

Toxoplasmosis of the brain with onset at > 1 month of age

Wasting syndrome in the absence of a concurrent illness other than HIV infection that could explain the following findings:

Persistent weight loss > 10% of baseline, or

Downward crossing of at least two of the following percentile lines on the weight-for-age chart (e.g., 95th, 75th, 50th, 25th, 5th) in a child $\geq$ 1 year of age, or

Less than 5th percentile on weight-for-height chart on two consecutive measurements taken $\geq$ 30 days apart, plus chronic diarrhea (i.e., at least two loose stools per day for $\geq$ 30 days) or documented fever (for $\geq$ 30 days, intermittent or constant)

From Centers for Disease Control and Prevention (1994). Morbidity and Mortality Weekly Report, 43, 6-8.

Table 45-18 Immunologic Categories Based on Age-specific CD41 T-lymphocyte Counts and Percentage of Total Lymphocytes

	AGE OF CHILD					
	YOUNGER THAN 12 MONTHS		1 TO 5 YEARS		6 YEARS AND OLDER	
IMMUNOLOGIC CATEGORY	CELLS/mm³	(%)	CELLS/mm³	(%)	CELLS/mm³	(%)
1. No evidence of suppression	≥1500	(≥25)	≥1000	(≥25)	≥500	(≥25)
2. Evidence of moderate suppression	750 to 1499	(15 to 24)	500 to 999	(15 to 24)	200 to 499	(15 to 24)
3. Severe suppression	<750	(<15)	<500	(<15)	<200	(<15)

From Centers for Disease Control and Prevention (1994). Morbidity and Mortality Weekly Report, 43(RR-12), 4.

Table 45-19 Pediatric HIV Classification*

	CLINICAL CATEGORIES			
IMMUNOLOGIC CATEGORIES	N: NO SIGNS OR SYMPTOMS	A: MILD SIGNS AND SYMPTOMS	B: MODERATE SIGNS AND SYMPTOMS†	C: SEVERE SIGNS AND SYMPTOMS†
1. No evidence of suppression	N1	A1	B1	C1
2. Evidence of moderate suppression	N2	A2	B2	C2
3. Severe suppression	N3	A3	B3	C3

Children whose HIV infection status is not confirmed are classified by using the above grid with a letter E (for perinatally exposed) placed before the appropriate classification code (e.g., EN2).
†Both category C and lymphoid interstitial pneumonitis in category B are reportable to state and local health departments as acquired immunodeficiency syndrome.
From Centers for Disease Control and Prevention (1994). Morbidity and Mortality Weekly Report, 43, 12.

women enables these women to receive appropriate care for their own health, antiretroviral therapy to prevent perinatal transmission, proper counseling against breastfeeding for HIV-infected mothers living in the United States (where safe breast milk substitutes are available), proper prevention of PCP in HIV-exposed infants, and early treatment of HIV-infected infants when indicated.

Primary Care Issues and Implications

Growth

- Plot growth measurements of height, weight, and head circumference every 1 to 3 months depending on age and symptom status.
- Assess growth velocity every 3 months; if it is less than the 3rd percentile for age, refer to a pediatric GI tract or endocrine specialist.
- Note that FTT occurs in 20% to 80% of children with HIV and is usually caused by GI tract abnormalities leading to malabsorption and malnutrition. It may be related to an HIV-induced hypermetabolic state.
- Remember that adolescents may have delayed pubertal onset because of delayed hypothalamic pituitary-gonadal axis maturation, which may affect self-esteem.

Development. Symptomatic HIV-infected children may have developmental delays of varying degrees that are manifested by neurologic and neuropsychologic impairments in the cognitive, motor, and behavioral areas. Evidence indicates that the CNS may be directly infected with HIV. Genetic and environmental factors also play a major part.

HIV-associated progressive encephalopathy is the most severe form of delay, manifested by progressive deterioration in cognitive, motor, language, and adaptive function with loss of previously acquired milestones. Encephalopathy with a less severe course is more common, with children experiencing a gain of few or no further skills over time, decreasing intelligence quotient scores, lack of acquisition of new milestones, and slower gain of milestones.

Children should have neurodevelopmental testing on a regular basis as a measure of disease progression and also a measure of treatment efficacy. Testing should be done when children are well and afebrile; should not be done after painful or stressful procedures.

Counsel parents regarding normal growth and development and the child's individual needs, and refer to early intervention program as indicated.

Immunizations. HIV-infected children should be immunized with routine inactivated vaccines (e.g., diphtheria-tetanus-pertussis [DTaP] vaccine, inactivated polio vaccine [IPV], Hib vaccine, hepatitis B vaccine) following the recommended schedule for uninfected children. Influenza vaccine is recommended annually. Pneumococcal vaccine is recommended based on age and vaccine-specific recommendations. Children with HIV may have an impaired response to Prevnar, and Prevnar does not replace the use of Pneumovax 23 in children over 24 months of age.

Measles, mumps, and rubella (MMR) vaccine should be given to HIV-infected children at 12 months unless they are severely immunocompromised. (See Box 45-18 and Table 45-18.) A second dose may be given 1 month after the first to induce seroconversion as early as possible.

Varicella vaccine should be considered in HIV-infected children in CDC classes N1 and A1 (no or mild signs or symptoms of disease; see Box 45-18 and Table 45-18) after the risks and benefits are considered.

Hepatitis A vaccine is recommended for children living in areas with known consistently elevated hepatitis A rates and for persons with chronic liver disease.

HIV-infected children may not respond appropriately to vaccines and are considered susceptible to vaccine-preventable diseases if exposed. Passive immunoprophylaxis with immunoglobulin is recommended for measles, tetanus and varicella exposure regardless of immunization status.

Screening and monitoring. The schedule and frequency of monitoring is determined by the patient's degree of HIV-related complications, with highly symptomatic patients requiring more frequent evaluations. Generally the following are recommended:

- Medical history initially, with an interval history at each subsequent visit
- Physical examination initially and each subsequent visit, with close attention to standard growth curves
- Neurodevelopmental evaluation initially and then annually

Laboratory evaluation

- HIV RNA plasma viral load initially and then every 3 to 4 months
- CD4 and CD8 lymphocyte counts and percentages initially and then every 3 to 4 months
- Quantitative serum immunoglobulins initially
- CBC count initially and then every 1 to 3 months as indicated
- Serum electrolytes initially and then every 6 months or as indicated
- Liver function tests initially and then every 2 to 6 months as indicated
- Hepatitis B, hepatitis C, infectious mononucleosis (Epstein-Barr virus [EBV]), cytomegalic inclusion disease (CMV), and toxoplasmosis testing initially
- Chest radiograph initially and then annually
- Electrocardiogram (ECG) and echocardiogram initially and then annually
- TB testing initially and then annually
- Routine preventive care and anticipatory guidance as indicated at each visit

Safety

- Provide basic age-appropriate injury-prevention counseling.
- Because an immunosuppressed child may be at risk for infection, ask the school to inform the family of outbreaks (e.g., of varicella, salmonellosis).
- Teach universal precautions to family members.
- Instruct the family on the need for safe and proper storage of medications.

Discipline

- Parents may be reluctant to discipline because of terminal illness.
- Family life may be disorganized and disrupted by drug use, illness, hospitalization, and death.
- Emphasize consistency and limit-setting as hallmarks of discipline with the intent to provide stability for children.
- Referral may be made to a social worker or psychotherapist as appropriate.

School

- Children should be encouraged to attend school regularly as their health permits.
- Participation in activities should not be limited.
- No case of HIV transmission in schools has been reported.
- HIV status should not be disclosed without consent of parents or guardian, as well as the child when age-appropriate.
- School staff (e.g., teacher, nurse, medical advisor) should be informed if both the child and parents consent.

Adolescence. Teenagers have a higher female-to-male ratio of HIV infection. Heterosexual contact is the most common risk factor for teenage girls, while homosexual contact as a risk factor is more common with teenage boys. Discuss issues of confidentiality. Adolescents who choose not to disclose an HIV diagnosis to their families should be encouraged to inform a supportive adult. Additional problems may include homelessness, pregnancy, parenting, and substance abuse.

Sexuality

- Instruct HIV-infected adolescents regarding the possibility of infecting a partner through oral, anal, or vaginal sex.
- Discuss notification of sexual partners.
- Instruct regarding the use of condoms with spermicide containing nonoxynol-9.
- Advise adolescent girls of childbearing age of the risk of maternal-fetal transmission.
- Counsel regarding birth control options.
- Advise uninfected adolescents of how HIV is and is not transmitted.
- Instruct uninfected adolescents regarding prevention, including abstinence or delaying intercourse, use of condoms, and avoiding injectable drug use and needle sharing.

Nutrition. Nutritional manifestations of HIV disease are eventually seen in most HIV-infected children. The cycle of immune deficiency, enteric infections, malabsorption, and malnutrition contributes to clinical deterioration. Collaboration with GI tract and nutritional specialists is recommended for this complex problem. Assess nutritional status and observe for signs of growth failure at every visit, with special attention to the following:

- Elicit history of dietary intake, refusal to eat, vomiting, diarrhea, dysphagia, interval illness.
- Record anthropomorphic measurements including height, weight, and head circumference. Plot on standardized growth charts, and monitor closely for signs of growth failure.
- Calculate growth velocity every 3 to 6 months.
- Calculate the caloric needs of children (100 kcal/kg for the first 10 kg of body weight, 50 kcal/kg for the second 10 kg of body weight, and 20 kcal/kg for each kg over 20 kg of body weight).
- Provide nutritional counseling or referral to a nutritional specialist.
- Evaluate common GI tract symptoms such as diarrhea, dysphagia, and abdominal pain in collaboration with a gastroenterologist.
- Provide nutritional supplementation in consultation with GI tract and nutritional specialists.
- Remember that oral interventions for supplementation include the addition of high-calorie foods and formulas such as Pediasure, Advera, and Peptamen.
- Include age-appropriate and ethnically appropriate foods when possible.
- When caloric needs cannot be met orally, consider enteral supplementation. These supplements include nasogastric feedings and placement of gastrostomy tube. Many children can be given nighttime supplements, which allows for normal feedings during the day. Total parenteral feedings are reserved for children with severe weight loss unresponsive to gastrostomy feedings and children with pancreatitis.

Psychosocial issues. Families affected by HIV disease are often isolated and may have suffered from the great effect of poverty and drug abuse. The additional burdens encountered by these families are often overwhelming. PCPs should be aware of issues confronting these families, such as receipt of a diagnosis of terminal illness, fear of disclosing the diagnosis to family and friends, depression, fear of disclosing the diagnosis to the child and school, cost and stress of administering medications, frequent clinic appointments, death, and permanency planning for children affected by parental death. Families affected by HIV should be assigned a consistent social worker who can know them and their needs and work with mental health community agencies.

Pain. See Chapter 7. Children and adolescents with HIV disease experience pain. Pain may be related to infectious complications, procedures, medications, and HIV itself. Perception of pain may be influenced by cultural background, social experiences, previous experiences with pain, and drug abuse. Pain management in the primary care setting begins with preventing pain associated with procedures (e.g., use of eutectic mixture of local anesthetics [EMLA] cream before routine blood drawing). It is important that children be adequately medicated for pain control.

Management

Treatments and medications

Reduction of perinatal HIV transmission. The implementation of AIDS Clinical Trials Group study 076 has resulted in a nationwide 66% reduction of perinatal AIDS since 1993. Zidovudine is administered to HIV-infected pregnant women orally beginning at 14 to 34 weeks of gestation, intravenously during labor, and orally to newborns for the first 6 weeks of life (Table 45-20). Treatment guidelines for HIV-infected pregnant women are the same as those for nonpregnant women, and pregnant women may receive combination therapy for treatment of their own disease. Long-term follow-up care of infants exposed to antiretroviral drugs while in utero is recommended.

Prophylaxis against Pneumocystis carinii pneumonia. Pneumocystis carinii pneumonia is the most common opportunistic infection in children who have AIDS. Among children with perinatally acquired HIV, infants 3 to 6 months of age are at greatest risk. Prophylaxis should begin at 4 to 6 weeks of age for infants born to HIV-infected women regardless of their CD41 T-cell count. For HIV-infected children over 1 year of age, the decision whether to begin or continue prophylaxis is based on CD41 T-cell count and symptoms. For HIV-infected adolescents, *Pneumocystis carinii* pneumonia prophylaxis should be started when the CD41 T-cell count is less than or equal to 200 cells/mm³. Table 45-21 provides specific recommendations based on age and HIV infection status.

The recommended chemoprophylaxis for children and adolescents is TMP-SMX. When starting a regimen of TMP-SMX, obtain a CBC count, differential count, and platelet count. Repeat monthly while prophylaxis is being received (Table 45-22).

Routine immunoglobulin intravenous (IGIV) therapy in combination with antiretroviral therapy is recommended for the following:

- Hypogammaglobulinemia (IgG less than 250 mg/dl)
- Recurrent, serious, bacterial infections (two or more infections such as bacteremia, meningitis, or pneumonia in a 1-year period)
- Children who fail to form antibodies to common antigens
- Treatment of parvovirus B19 infections
- Treatment of thrombocytopenia
- A single dose for children exposed to measles (the dose of IGIV is 400 mg/kg per dose every 4 weeks or once after measles exposure)

Table 45-21 Recommendations for Pneumocystis carinii Pneumonia Prophylaxis for HIV-Exposed Infants and Children by Age and HIV Infection Status

AGE AND HIV INFECTION STATUS	PCP PROPHYLAXIS
Birth to 4-6 weeks, HIV exposed	No prophylaxis
4-6 weeks to 4 months, HIV exposed	Prophylaxis
4-12 months	
HIV-infected or indeterminate	Prophylaxis
HIV infection excluded	No prophylaxis
1-5 years, HIV infected	Prophylaxis if CD4+ T lymphocyte count is < 500 μl or < 15%
> 5 years, HIV infected	Prophylaxis if CD4+ T-lymphocyte count is < 200 μl or percentage is < 15%

From Centers for Disease Control and Prevention. (1999). USPHS/IDSA guidelines for the prevention of opportunistic infection in persons with human immunodeficiency virus. MMWR Morbidity and Mortality Weekly Report, 48(RR-10), 1-59, 61-66.

Table 45-20 Zidovudine Regimen for the Reduction of Perinatal Transmission of HIV

TIME	ROUTE	DOSAGE
During pregnancy, beginning anytime after 14 weeks of gestation	Oral	200 mg three times a day or 300 mg two times a day
During labor and delivery	Intravenous	2 mg/kg during the first hour and then 1 mg/kg per hour until delivery
Newborn baby, beginning 8 to 12 hours after birth until 6 weeks of age	Oral	2 mg/kg four times per day

From Centers for Disease Control and Prevention (1998). Public Health Service Task Force recommendations for the use of antiretroviral drugs in pregnant women infected with HIV-1 for maternal health and for reducing perinatal HIV-1 transmission in the United States. Morbidity and Mortality Weekly Report, 47(RR-2), 1-30.

Table 45-22 Drug Regimens for *Pneumocystis carnii* Pneumonia Prophylaxis for Children 4 Weeks of Age or Older

RECOMMENDED REGIMEN	ACCEPTABLE ALTERNATIVE TRIMETHOPRIM-SULFAMETHOXAZOLE DOSAGE SCHEDULE	ALTERNATIVE REGIMENS IF TRIMETHOPRIM-SULFAMETHOXAZOLE IS NOT TOLERATED
• Trimethoprim-sulfamethoxazole, 150 mg/m² per day of trimethoprim with 750 mg/m² per day of sulfamethoxazole administered orally in divided doses twice a day three times per week on consecutive days (e.g., Monday, Tuesday, Wednesday)	• 150 mg/m² per day of trimethoprim with 750 mg/m² per day of sulfamethoxazole administered orally as a single daily dose three times per week on consecutive days • 150 mg/m² per day of trimethoprim with 750 mg/m² per day sulfamethoxazole administered orally in divided doses twice a day and administered 7 days per week. • 150 mg/m² per day of trimethoprim with 750 mg/m² per day sulfamethoxazole administered orally in divided doses twice a day and administered three times a week on alternate days (e.g., Monday, Wednesday, Friday)	• Dapsone (children > 1 month of age), 2 mg/kg (maximum of 100 mg) administered orally once a day, or 4 mg/kg (maximum of 200 mg orally ever week) • Aerosolized pentamidine (children > 5 years of age), 300 mg administered via Respirgard II inhaler monthly • Atovaquone (children 1-3 months of age and > 24 months of age), 30 mg/kg orally once a day; children 4-24 months of age, 45 mg/kg orally once a day

From Centers for Disease Control and Prevention. (1999). USPHS/IDSA guidelines for the prevention of opportunistic infections, in persons with human immunodeficiency virus. Morbidity and Mortality Weekly Report, 48(RR-10), 1-59, 61-66.

Table 45-23 Indications for Initiation for Antiretroviral Therapy in Children with HIV Infection

Clinical symptoms associated with HIV infection (i.e., clinical categories A, B, or C [see Box 45-18])

Evidence of immune suppression, indicated by CD4+ T-lymphocyte absolute number or percentage, (that is, immune category 2 or 3 [see Table 45-18])

Age younger than 12 months regardless of clinical, immunologic, or virologic status

For asymptomatic children older than 1 year of age with normal immune status, two options can be considered:

PREFERRED APPROACH	ALTERNATIVE APPROACH
Initiate therapy regardless of age or symptom status	Defer treatment in situation in which the risk for clinical disease progression is low and other factors (e.g., concern for the durability of response, safety, adherence) favor postponing treatment. In such cases, the health care provider should regularly monitor virologic, immunologic, and clinical status. Factors to be considered in deciding to initiate therapy include the following: • High or increasing HIV RNA copy number • Rapidly declining CD4+ T-lymphocyte number or percentage to values approaching those indicative of moderate immune suppression (i.e., immune category 2 [see Table 45-18]). • Development of clinical symptoms.

From Centers for Disease Control and Prevention. (1998). Guidelines for the use of antiretroviral agents in pediatric HIV infection. Morbidity and Mortality Weekly Report, 47(RR-4). Updated as a living document on Jan. 7, 2000 at www.hivatis.org

Antiretroviral therapy. Treatment guidelines for antiretroviral use in pediatric patients are rapidly evolving, and methods for monitoring response to treatments are increasingly complex. Whenever possible, delivery of care should be directed by experts in the care of children with HIV infection. Enrollment of HIV-infected children in clinical trials should be encouraged when available (see Resources).

Antiretroviral therapy is recommended for most children (Table 45-23). The decision to start therapy is based on virologic, immunologic, and clinical criteria. Clinical trials have demonstrated superior outcomes with combination therapy as opposed to monotherapy (Table 45-24). Strict adherence to drug regimens is vital to enhance viral suppression and prevent emergence of drug resistance. The family, caregivers, and child should be assessed for their capacity to adhere to strict regimens and a multidisciplinary team should be available for support and ongoing monitoring.

Guidelines for antiretroviral therapy for adolescents are the same as those for adults. Currently, treatment is recommended to all patients with acute HIV syndrome, those within 6 months of HIV seroconversion, and all patients with symptomatic HIV infection. Treatment of asymptomatic patients requires analysis of real and potential risks and benefits. (For the current guidelines, go to www.HIVATIS.org.)

Table 45-24 Recommended Antiretroviral Regimens for Initial Therapy for HIV Infection in Children

STRONGLY RECOMMENDED	RECOMMENDED AS AN ALTERNATIVE	ONLY IN SPECIAL CIRCUMSTANCES	NOT RECOMMENDED
Clinical trial evidence of clinical benefit or sustained suppression of HIV replication in adults and children • One highly active protease inhibitor, plus two nucleoside analog reverse trascriptase inhibitors (NRTIs). Preferred protease inhibitor for infants and children who cannot swallow pills or capsules is nelfinavir or ritonavir. Alternative for children who can swallow pills or capsules: Indinavir. • Recommended dual NRTI combinations: The most data on use in children are available for the combinations of zidovudine (ZDV) and dideoxyinosine (ddi) and for ZDV and lamivudine (3TC). More limited data are available for the combinations of stavudine (d4T) and ddi, d4T, and 3TC, and ZDV and zalcitabine (ddC). • Alternative for children who can swallow capsules: Efavirenz (Sustiva), plus 2 NRTIs (see above) or efavirenz (Sustiva), plus nelfinavir and 1 NRTI.	Clinical trial evidence of suppression of HIV replication, but (1) durability may be less in adults or children than with strongly recommended regimens, (2) the durability of suppression is not yet defined, or (3) evidence of efficacy may not outweigh potential adverse consequences (e.g., toxicity, drug interaction, cost). • Nevirapine and two NRTIs • Abacavir in combination with ZDV and 3TC	Clinical trial evidence (1) of limited benefit for patients, or (2) data are inconclusive but may be reasonably offered in special circumstances. • Two NRTIs • Amprenavir in combination with 2 NRTIs or abacavir	Evidence against use (1) because of overlapping toxicity or (2) because use may be virologically undesirable. • Any monotherapy • d4T and ZDV • ddC and ddi • ddC and d4T • ddC and 3TC

From Centers for Disease Control and Prevention (1998). Guidelines for the use of antiretroviral agents in pediatric HIV infection. Morbidity and Mortality Weekly Report, 47(RR-4). Updated as a living document on Jan. 7, 2000 at www.hivatis.org

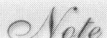

Note

With adolescents, medications for treating HIV and opportunistic infections should be dosed based on Tanner staging of puberty and not specific age. Adolescents in early puberty (Tanner I and II) should be dosed under pediatric guidelines, whereas those in late puberty should be dosed by adult guidelines. Those in the midst of a growth spurt (Tanner III females and Tanner IV males) should be closely monitored for medication efficacy and toxicity when the practitioner chooses adult or pediatric guidelines.

The goals of therapy are to reduce viral load to undetectable levels, preserve immune function, and prevent disease progression. Criteria for changing therapy are disease progression (virologic: increasing HIV RNA levels; immunologic: decreasing CD4+ T-lymphocyte count or clinical symptoms), toxic effects or intolerance of drugs, or data suggestive of a superior regimen (Table 45-25). Table 45-26 provides a list of antiretroviral drugs, doses, side effects, and interactions.

Counseling and prevention

• Explain and provide information to the parents, caregivers, and child or adolescent about HIV infection:

HIV causes AIDS.

HIV cannot be cured, but there are treatments that may prevent disease progression and secondary infections.

The HIV virus attaches to a type of white blood cell (WBC) (called CD41 T cells, helper T cells, T helpers, or T4s) that helps the body fight against infection. This results in a decreased number of T cells and T cells that are less effective against fighting infection.

As the virus spreads, more CD41 T cells are destroyed, and the body loses its ability to fight against infection.

• Explain to the parents, caregivers, child, or adolescent how HIV can be spread (e.g., through sexual intercourse [oral, anal, and vaginal sex]; by sharing needles for intravenous drug use; from mother to infant while the fetus is growing in utero, during delivery, or through breast milk; through transfused blood [from before 1985] contaminated with HIV).

Table 45-25 Considerations for Changing Antiretroviral Therapy for HIV-Infected Children

VIROLOGIC CONSIDERATIONS	IMMUNOLOGIC CONSIDERATIONS	CLINICAL CONSIDERATION
• Less than a minimally acceptable virologic response after 8 to 12 weeks of therapy. For children receiving therapy with two nucleoside analog reverse transcriptase inhibitors (NRTIs) and a protease inhibitor, such a response is defined as a onefold (1.0 log^{10}) decrease from baseline HIV RNA levels. For children who are receiving less potent therapy (e.g., dual NRTI combinations), an insufficient response is defined as a less than fivefold (0.7 log^{10}) decrease in HIV RNA levels from baseline value. • HIV RNA not suppressed to undetectable levels after 4 to 6 months of antiretroviral therapy • Repeated detection of HIV RNA in children who initially responded to antiretroviral therapy with undetectable levels • A reproducible increase in HIV RNA copy number among children who have had a substantial HIV RNA response but still have low levels of detectable HIV RNA. Such an increase would warrant change in therapy if, after initiation of the therapeutic regimen, a greater than threefold (0.5 log^{10}) increase in copy number for children ≥ 2 years of age and greater than fivefold (0.7 log^{10}) increase for children < 2 years of age is observed.	• Change in immunologic classification (see Table 45-19) • For children with CD4+ T-lymphocyte percentages of < 15% (i.e., those in immune category 3), a persistent decline of five percentiles or more in CD4+ cell percentage (e.g., from 15% to 10%) • A rapid and substantial decrease in absolute CD4+ T-lymphocyte count (e.g., a > 30% decline in < 6 months)	• Progressive neurodevelopmental deterioration • Growth failure as persistent decline in weight and growth velocity despite adequate nutritional support and without other explanation • Disease progression defined as advancement from one pediatric clinical category to another (i.e., from clinical category A to clinical category B).

From Centers for Disease Control and Prevention (1998). Guidelines for the use of antiretroviral agents in pediatric HIV infection. Morbidity and Mortality Weekly Report, 47(RR-4). Updated as a living document on Dec. 14, 2001 at www.hivatis.org

• Explain that HIV is not spread by hugging or kissing people; using the same toilet, tub, or shower; sharing eating utensils; or coughing or sneezing.

• Teach about good nutrition and advise the parents, caregivers, and child that nutrition plays important role in maintaining general health. Children are more likely to have symptomatic illness if poorly nourished. Encourage a well-balanced diet and instruct the family to inform the PCP of any decreased appetite, difficulty eating, and pain with swallowing. Explain the need for supplementation when appropriate.

• Instruct parents, caregivers, child, or adolescent about infection control, including proper handwashing before food preparation, after toileting and diaper changes, and before medication administration, as well as the avoidance of raw eggs, meats, and fish, which should be thoroughly cooked.

• Remember that children with HIV should not change cat litter.

• Advise parents to notify the PCP if the child has been exposed to chickenpox or measles so child may receive preventive treatment.

• Explain the importance of immunizations and use of inactivated instead of live polio vaccine.

• Teach universal precautions to family members and caregivers:

Avoid direct contact with blood.

Do not share personal items such as razors, toothbrushes, pierced earrings.

Keep open sores covered.

Use latex gloves or other barrier when caring for child with bleeding.

For minor cuts, clean with soap and water, apply povidone-iodine, and cover.

For blood spills, wipe with a paper towel, wash the area with soap and water, and rinse with a 1:10 bleach water solution.

For disposable waste soiled with blood, wrap in a newspaper or in plastic bag with a tie, then discard in a plastic-lined, covered trash can.

For blood-stained clothing, rinse in cold water or hydrogen peroxide and wash as usual.

Recommend proper handwashing after contact with urine, vomitus, nasal secretions, oral secretions, stool, tears, and dirty diapers.

Text continued on page 815

Table 45-26 Characteristics of Antiretroviral Drugs: Nucleoside Analog Reverse Transcriptase Inhibitors

DRUG (ABBREVIATION)/ TRADE NAME	DOSAGE	MAJOR TOXIC EFFECTS	DRUG INTERACTIONS	SPECIAL INSTRUCTIONS
Abacavir (formerly 1592U89) (ABC)/ Ziagen *Preparations:* Pediatric oral solution: 20 mg/ml Tablets: 300 mg	*Neonatal:* not approved for infants younger than 3 months of age. For infants between 1 and 3 months of age, a dosage of 8 mg/kg of body weight twice daily is under study. *Pediatric and adolescent:* 8 mg/kg of body weight twice daily; maximum dosage 300 mg twice daily *Adult:* 300 mg twice daily	*Most frequent:* Nausea, vomiting, headache, fever, rash, anorexia, and fatigue. *Unusual (more severe):* Approximately 5% of adults and children develop a potentially fatal hypersensitivity reaction. Symptoms include fever, fatigue, malaise, nausea, vomiting, diarrhea, and abdominal pain. Physical findings include lymphadenopathy, ulceration of mucous membranes, and maculopapular or urticarial skin rash. A hypersensitivity reaction can occur without a rash. Laboratory abnormalities include elevated liver function test results, elevated creatine phosphokinase and creatinine levels, and lymphopenia. This reaction generally occurs in the first 6 weeks of therapy. For patients suspected of having a hypersensitivity reaction, ABC should be stopped and not restarted since hypotension and death have occurred on rechallenge.	No significant interactions between ABC, zidovudine (ADV), and lamivudine (3TC). Abacavir does not inhibit and is not metabolized by hepatic cytochrome P-450 enzymes. Thus, it should not cause changes in drug levels or clearance of agents metabolized through these pathways, such as protease inhibitors and NNRTIs.	
Didanosine (ddI)/ Videx *Preparations:* Pediatric powder for oral solution (must be mixed with antacid): 10 mg/ml Chewable tablets with buffers: 25, 50, 100, and 150 mg Buffered powder for oral solution: 100, 167, and 250 mg	*Usual pediatric:* in combination with other antiretrovirals: 90 mg/m² every 12 hours *Pediatric range:* 90 to 150 mg/m² every 12 hours (May need higher dosage for patients with central nervous system disease.) *Neonatal (<90 days of age):* based on pharmacokinetic data from PACTG 239: 50 mg/m² every 12 hours	*Most frequent:* diarrhea, abdominal pain, nausea, vomiting *Unusual (more severe):* peripheral neuropathy (dose-related), electrolyte abnormalities, hyperuricemia *Uncommon:* pancreatitis (dose related) seems less common in children than adults; increased liver enzyme levels, retinal depigmentation (asymptomatic, reported with pediatric administration)	Possible decrease in absorption of ketoconazole, itraconazole, tetracycline; administer at least 2 hours before or 2 hours after ddI. Ciprofloxacin absorption significantly decreased (chelation of drug by antacid); administer 2 hours before or 6 hours after ddI. Concomitant administration of ddI and delavirdine may decrease the absorption of these drugs; separate dosing by at least 2 hours. Ganciclovir may increase the AUC and peak levels of ddI and predispose to toxic effects. Administration with protease inhibitors: indinavir should be administered at least 1 hour apart from ddI on an empty stomach. Ritonavir should be administered at least 2.5 hours apart from ddI.	ddI formulation contains buffering agents or antacids. Food decreases absorption; administer ddI on an empty stomach (1 hour before or 2 hours after meal). Further evaluation in children regarding administration with meals is under study. For oral solution: shake well, and keep refrigerated; admixture stable for 30 days.

Adolescent dosing by Tanner Stage: Adolescents in early puberty (Tanner I–II) should be dosed using pediatric schedules, whereas those in late puberty (Tanner stage V) should be dosed using adult schedules. Youth who are in the midst of their growth spurt (Tanner III females and Tanner IV males) should be closely monitored for medication efficacy and toxic effects when choosing adult or pediatric dosing guidelines. NNRTI indicates nonnucleoside reverse transcriptase inhibitor; AUD, area under the curve; D₅W, dextrose 5% in water; TMP-SMX, trimethoprim-sulfamethoxazole.

Continued

Table 45-26 Characteristics of Antiretroviral Drugs: Nucleoside Analog Reverse Transcriptase Inhibitors—cont'd

DRUG (ABBREVIATION)/ TRADE NAME	DOSAGE	MAJOR TOXIC EFFECTS	DRUG INTERACTIONS	SPECIAL INSTRUCTIONS
Didanosine (ddI)/ Videx—cont'd	*Adolescent and adult:* weight, >60 kg: 200 mg twice daily; weight, <60 kg: 125 mg twice daily			
Lamivudine (3TC)/ Epivir *Preparations:* Solution: 10 mg/ml Tablets: 150 mg	*Pediatric:* 4 mg/kg every 12 hours *Neonatal (<30 days of age):* under study in clinical trials: 2 mg/kg every 12 hours *Adolescent and adult:* 150 mg twice daily	*Most frequent:* headache, fatigue, nausea, diarrhea, skin rash, abdominal pain *Unusual (more severe):* pancreatitis (primarily seen in children with advanced HIV infection receiving multiple other medications), decreased neutrophil count, increased liver enzyme levels	TMP-SMX increases 3TC blood levels (possibly competes for renal tubular secretion); unknown significance. When used with ZDV may prevent emergency of resistance, and for ZDV-resistant virus, revision to phenotypic ZDV sensitivity may be observed.	Can be administered with food. For oral solution: Store at room temperature. Decrease dosage for patients with impaired renal function.
Stavudine (d4T)/Zerit *Preparations:* Solution: 1 mg/ml Capsules: 15, 20, 30, and 40 mg	*Pediatric:* 1 mg/kg every 12 hours (up to weight of 30 kg) *Neonatal:* under evaluation in PACTG 332 *Adolescent and adult:* weight, >60 kg: 40 mg twice daily; weight, 30-60 kg: 30 mg twice daily	*Most frequent:* headache, GI disturbances, skin rashes *Uncommon (more severe):* peripheral neuropathy, pancreatitis *Other:* increased liver enzyme levels	Drugs that decrease renal function could decrease clearance. Should not be administered in combination with ZDV (poor antiretroviral effect).	Can be administered with food. Decrease dosage for patients with renal impairment. For oral solution: shake well and keep refrigerated; solution stable for 30 days.
Zalcitabine (ddC)/ Hivid *Preparations:* Syrup: mg/ml (investigational) Tables: 0.375 mg and 0.75 mg	*Usual pediatric:* 0.01 mg/kg every 8 hours *Pediatric range:* 0.005 to 0.01 mg/kg every 8 hours *Neonatal:* Unknown *Adolescent and adult:* 0.75 mg three times a day	*Most frequent:* headache, malaise *Unusual (more severe):* peripheral neuropathy, pancreatitis, hepatic toxic effects, skin rashes, oral ulcers, esophageal ulcers, hematologic toxic effects	Cimetidine, amphotericin, foscarnet, and aminoglycosides may decrease renal clearance of zalcitabine. Antacids decrease absorption. Concomitant use with ddI is not recommended because of the increased risk of peripheral neuropathy. Intravenous pentamidine increases the risk of pancreatitis (do not use concurrently).	Administer on an empty stomach (1 hour before or 2 hours after a meal). Decrease dosage in patients with impaired renal function.
Zidovudine (ZDV, AZT)/Retrovir *Preparations:* Syrup: 10 mg/ml syrup Capsules: 100 mg Tablets: 300 mg Concentrate for injection/for IV infusion: 10 mg/ml	*Usual pediatric:* Oral: 160 mg/m² every 8 hours IV (intermittent infusion): 1-2 mg/kg every 4 hours IV (continuous infusion): 20 mg/m² per hour *Pediatric range:* 90 mg/m² to 180 mg/m² every	*Most frequent:* hematologic toxic effects, including granulocytopenia and anemia, headache *Unusual:* myopathy, myositis, hepatic toxic effects	Increased toxic effects may be observed with concomitant administration of the following drugs (therefore more intensive monitoring for toxic effects may be warranted): ganciclovir, interferon, TMP-SMX, acyclovir. The following drugs may increase ZDV concentration (and therefore potential toxic effects): probenecid, atovaquone, methadone, valproic acid. Decreased renal clearance may be observed with coadministration of	Can be administered with food (though the manufacturer recommends administration 30 minutes before or 1 hour after a meal). Decrease dosage for patients with severe renal impairment.

Table 45-26 Characteristics of Antiretroviral Drugs: Nucleoside Analog Reverse Transcriptase Inhibitors—cont'd

DRUG (ABBREVIATION)/ TRADE NAME	DOSAGE	MAJOR TOXIC EFFECTS	DRUG INTERACTIONS	SPECIAL INSTRUCTIONS
Zidovudine (ZDV, AZT)/Retrovir—cont'd	6-8 hours *Neonatal:* Oral: 2 mg/kg every 6 hours IV: 1.5 mg/kg every 6 hours *Premature infants:* (Standard neonatal dose may be excessive for premature infants Under study in PACTG 331:1.5 mg/kg every 12 hours from birth to 2 weeks of age; then increase to 2 mg/kg every 8 hours after 2 weeks of age *Adolescent and adult:* 200 mg three times daily or 300 mg twice daily		cimitidine (may be significant in patients with renal impairment). Fluconazole interferes with metabolism and clearance of ZDV (increases ZDV AUC). ZDV metabolism may be increased with coadministration of rifampin and rifabutin; clarithromycin decreases concentrations of ZDV probably by interfering with absorption (administer 4 hours apart). Ribavirin decreases the intracellular phosphorylation of ZDV (conversion to active metabolite). Phenytoin concentrations may increase or decrease., Should not be administered in combination with stavudine (poor antiretroviral effect).	Significant granulocytopenia or anemia may necessitate interruption of therapy until marrow recovery is observed; use of erythropoietin or reduced ZDV dosage may be necessary for some patients. Reduced dosage may be indicated for patients with significant hepatic dysfunction. Infuse loading doses and IV doses over 1 hour. Dilute with D_5W to concentration of ≤ 4 mg/mL. For IV solution: refrigerated diluted solution stable for 24 hours. Some experts use a dosage of 180 mg/m^2 every 12 hours when used in combination with other antiretroviral compounds, but data on this dosing in children are limited.
Delavirdine (DLV)/ Rescriptor *Preparations:* Tablets: 100 mg	*Pediatric:* Unknown *Neonatal:* Unknown *Adolescent and adult:* 400 mg three times daily	*Most frequent:* headache, fatigue, gastrointestinal complaints, rash (may be severe).	Metabolized in part by hepatic cytochrome P-450 3A; potential for multiple drug interactions. Before administration, the patient's medication profile should be reviewed carefully for potential drug interactions. Not recommended for concurrent use (DLV decreases the drug's metabolism, resulting in increased drug levels): antihistamines (astemizole, terfenadine); sedative-	Can be administered with food. Should be taken 1 hour before or 1 hour after ddl or antacids. Tablets can be dissolved in water and the resulting dispersion taken promptly.

Note: Drugs metabolized by the hepatic cytochrome P-450 3A (CYP 3A) enzyme system have the potential for significant interactions with multiple drugs, some of which may be life-threatening. These interactions are outlined in detail in the guidelines for use of antiretroviral agents in HIV-infected adults and adolescents (Centers for Disease Control and Prevention [1998]. Report of the NIH Panel to Define Principles of Therapy of HIV infection and guidelines for the use of antiretroviral agents in HIV-infected adults and adolescents. Morbidity and Mortality Weekly Report, 47[RR-5], 1–82) and in prescribing information available from the drug companies. These interactions will not be reiterated in this document, and the health care professional should review those documents for detailed information. Before therapy with these drugs is initiated, the patient's medication profile should be reviewed carefully for potential drug interactions.

Continued

Table 45-26 Characteristics of Antiretroviral Drugs: Nucleoside Analog Reverse Transcriptase Inhibitors—cont'd

DRUG (ABBREVIATION)/ TRADE NAME	DOSAGE	MAJOR TOXIC EFFECTS	DRUG INTERACTIONS	SPECIAL INSTRUCTIONS
Delavirdine (DLV)/ Rescriptor—cont'd			hypnotics (alprazolam, midazolam, triazolam); calcium channel blockers (nifedipine); ergot alkaloid derivatives; amphetamines; cisapride, warfarin; rifabutin or rifampin (also increase clearance of DLV); anticonvulsants (phenytoin, carbamazepine, phenobarbital; also increase clearance of DLV). Decreased absorption of delavirdine if given with antacids, histamine$_2$-receptor antagonists. Increased trough concentrations of delavirdine if given with ketoconazole, fluoxetine (increases trough by ~50%); increased levels of both drugs if delavirdine given with clarithromycin. DLV also increases levels of dapsone, quinidine. Administration with protease inhibitors: decreases metabolism of saquinavir and indinavir, resulting in a significant increase in saquinavir and indinavir concentrations and a slight decrease in DLV concentrations.	
Efavirenz (formerly DMP 266)/Sustiva *Preparations:* Capsules: 50, 100, and 200 mg	*Pediatric:* Administered once daily. Body weight 10 to <15 kg: 200 mg; 15 to <20 kg: 250 mg; 20 to <25 kg: 300 mg; 25 to <32.5 kg: 350 mg; 2.5 to <40 kg: 400 mg; ≥40 kg: 600 mg. Currently no data are available on the appropriate dosage for children younger than 3 years of age. *Adolescent and adult:* 600 mg once daily	*Most frequent:* Skin rash, central nervous system (somnolence, insomnia, abnormal dreams, confusion, abnormal thinking, impaired concentration, amnesia, agitation, depersonalization, hallucinations, euphoria), primarily reported in adults; increased aminotransferase levels, teratogenic in primates (use in pregnancy should be avoided, and women of childbearing potential should undergo pregnancy testing before starting therapy).	Mixed inducer/inhibitor of cytochrome P-450 3A4 enzymes; concentrations of concomitant drugs can be increased or decreased depending on specific enzyme pathway involved. Not recommended for concurrent use; antihistamines (astemizole or terfenadine), sedative-hypnotics (midazolam or triazolam), cisapride, or ergot alkaloid derivatives. Drug interactions requiring careful monitoring if coadministered: warfarin levels potentially increased; while of uncertain clinical significance, a reliable method of barrier contraception should be used in addition to oral contraceptives. Enzyme inducers such as rifampin, rifabutin, phenobarbital, and phenytoin may decrease efavirenz concentrations; clinical significance unknown. Efavirenz is highly plasma-protein bound and has the potential for	Efavirenz can be taken with and without food. The relative bioavailability of efavirenz was increased by 50% (range 11%-128%) after a high-fat meal (1070 kcal, 82 g of fat, 62% of calories from fat). Because there is no information on safety of efavirenz in dosages higher than recommended, administration with a high-fat meal should be avoided because of the potential

Adolescent dosing by Tanner Stage: Adolescents in early puberty (Tanner I–II) should be dosed using pediatric schedules, whereas those in late puberty (Tanner stage V) should be dosed using adult schedules. Youth who are in the midst of their growth spurt (Tanner III females and Tanner IV males) should be closely monitored for medication efficacy and toxic effects when choosing adult or pediatric dosing guidelines. NNRTI indicates nonnucleoside reverse transcriptase inhibitor; AUD, area under the curve; D$_5$W, dextrose 5% in water; TMP-SMX, trimethoprim-sulfamethoxazole.

Note: Drugs metabolized by the hepatic cytochrome P-450 3A (CYP 3A) enzyme system have the potential for significant interactions with multiple drugs, some of which may be life-threatening. These interactions are outlined in detail in the guidelines for use of antiretroviral agents in HIV-infected adults and adolescents (Centers for Disease Control and Prevention [1998]. Report of the NIH Panel to Define Principles of Therapy of HIV infection and guidelines for the use of antiretroviral agents in HIV-infected adults and adolescents. Morbidity and Mortality Weekly Report 47[RR-5], 1–82) and in prescribing information available from the drug companies. These interactions will not be reiterated in this document, and the health care professional should review those documents for detailed information. Before therapy with these drugs is initiated, the patient's medication profile should be reviewed carefully for potential drug interactions.

Table 45-26 Characteristics of Antiretroviral Drugs: Nucleoside Analog Reverse Transcriptase Inhibitors—cont'd

DRUG (ABBREVIATION)/ TRADE NAME	DOSAGE	MAJOR TOXIC EFFECTS	DRUG INTERACTIONS	SPECIAL INSTRUCTIONS
Efavirenz (formerly DMP 266)/Sustiva— cont'd			drug interactions with other highly protein-bound drugs (eg, pheno-barbital, phenytoin). Clarithromycin levels are decreased, whereas the levels of its metabolite are increased; alternatives to clar-ithromycin, such as azithromycin, should be considered. Other macrolide antibiotics have not been studied in combination with efavirenz. Administration with protease inhibitors: coadministration decreases levels of saquinavir (AUC decreased by 50%) and indinavir (AUC decreased by 31%). Coadmin-istration of saquinavir as a sole protease inhibitor is not recom-mended; indinavir dose should be increased if given with efavirenz (for adults, from 800 mg to 1000 mg every 8 hours). Coadministration increases levels of both ritonavir and efavirenz (AUC increased by 20% for both) and is associated with a higher frequency of adverse clinical and laboratory findings; monitoring of liver enzyme levels is recommended if coadministered. Coadministration increases levels of nelfinavir (AUC increased by 20%), but no dose adjustment is needed.	for increased absorption. Capsules may be opened and added to liquids or foods, but efavirenz has a peppery taste; grape jelly has been used to dis-guise the taste. Bedtime dosing is recommended; particularly during the first 2 to 4 weeks of therapy, to improve tolera-bility of central nervous system side effects.
Nevirapine (NVP)/ Viramune *Preparations:* Suspension: 10 mg/mL (investigational) Tablets: 200 mg	*Pediatric:* 120 to 200 mg/m² every 12 hours Note: start therapy with 120 mg/m² given once daily for 14 days. Increase to full dose adminis-tered every 12 hours if no rash or other unto-ward effects. *Neonatal (through 3 months of age):* under study in PACTG 356: 5 mg/kg once daily for 14 days, fol-lowed by 120 mg/m² every 12 hours for 14 days, followed by 200 mg/m² every 12 hours. *Adolescent and*	*Most frequent:* skin rash (some severe), sedative effect, headache, diarrhea, nausea *Unusual:* elevated liver enzyme levels, rarely hepatitis	Induces hepatic cytochrome P-450 3A; autoinduction of metabolism occurs in 2 to 4 weeks with a 1.5 to 2 times increase in clearance. Potential for multiple drug interactions. Before administration, the patient's medication profile should be reviewed carefully for potential drug interactions. Drugs having suspected interactions should be used only with careful monitoring: rifampin and rifabutin; oral contraceptives (alternative or additional methods of birth control should be used if coadministering with hormonal methods of birth control); sedative-hypnotics (tria-zolam, midazolam); oral anticoagu-lants; digoxin; phenytoin; theophylline. Administration with protease inhibitors: decreases indinavir and saquinavir concentrations signifi-cantly; may also decrease ritonavir concentration. Not known if increased doses of protease	Can be adminis-tered with food. May be adminis-tered concur-rently with ddI. For investigational suspension: Must be shaken well; store at room temperature.

Continued

Table 45-26 Characteristics of Antiretroviral Drugs: Nucleoside Analog Reverse Transcriptase Inhibitors—cont'd

DRUG (ABBREVIATION)/ TRADE NAME	DOSAGE	MAJOR TOXIC EFFECTS	DRUG INTERACTIONS	SPECIAL INSTRUCTIONS
Nevirapine (NVP)/ Viramune—cont'd	*adult:* 200 mg every 12 hours. Note: start therapy at half dose for the first 14 days. Increase to full dose if no rash or other untoward effects.		inhibitors are needed.	
Indinavir/Crixivan *Preparations:* Capsules: 200 and 400 mg	*Pediatric:* under study in clinical trials: 350-500 mg/m² every 8 hours *Neonatal:* unknown Because of adverse effect of hyperbilirubinemia, should not be given to neonates until further information available *Adolescent and adult:* 800 mg every 8 hours	*Most frequent:* nausea, abdominal pain, headache, asymptomatic hyperbilirubinemia (10%) *Unusual (more severe):* nephrolithiasis (4%) *Rare:* spontaneous bleeding episodes in patients with hemophilia; hyperglycemia; diabetes mellitus	Cytochrome P-450 3A4 responsible for metabolism. Potential for multiple drug interactions. Before administration, the patient's medication profile should be reviewed carefully for potential drug interactions. Not recommended for concurrent use (indinavir decreases the drug's metabolism, resulting in increased drug levels): antihistamines (astemizole, terfenadine); disapride; ergot alkaloid derivatives; sedative-hypnotics (triazolam, midazolam); rifampin (greatly reduces indinavir levels). Rifabutin concentrations are increased, and a dose reduction of rifabutin to half the usual daily dose is recommended. Ketoconazole and itraconazole cause an increase in indinavir concentrations (consider reduction of adolescent and adult indinavir dosage to 600 mg every 8 hours). Clarithromycin coadministration increases serum concentration of both drugs. Nevirapine coadministration may decrease indinavir serum concentration. Administration with other protease inhibitors: ritonavir decreases the metabolism of indinavir and results in greatly increased indinavir concentrations.	Administer on an empty stomach 1 hour before or 2 hours after a meal (or can take with a light meal). Adequate hydration required to minimize risk of nephrolithiasis. If coadministered with ddl, give at least 1 hour apart on an empty stomach. Grapefruit juice decreases serum levels of indinavir (by about 26%). Decrease dosage for patients with cirrhosis. Capsules are sensitive to moisture and should be stored in original container with desiccant.

Adolescent dosing by Tanner Stage: Adolescents in early puberty (Tanner I–II) should be dosed using pediatric schedules, whereas those in late puberty (Tanner stage V) should be dosed using adult schedules. Youth who are in the midst of their growth spurt (Tanner III females and Tanner IV males) should be closely monitored for medication efficacy and toxic effects when choosing adult or pediatric dosing guidelines. NNRTI indicates nonnucleoside reverse transcriptase inhibitor; AUD, area under the curve; D₅W, dextrose 5% in water; TMP-SMX, trimethoprim-sulfamethoxazole.

Note: Drugs metabolized by the hepatic cytochrome P-450 3A (CYP 3A) enzyme system have the potential for significant interactions with multiple drugs, some of which may be life-threatening. These interactions are outlined in detail in the guidelines for use of antiretroviral agents in HIV-infected adults and adolescents (Centers for Disease Control and Prevention [1998]. Report of the NIH Panel to Define Principles of Therapy of HIV infection and guidelines for the use of antiretroviral agents in HIV-infected adults and adolescents. Morbidity and Mortality Weekly Report 47[RR-5], 1–82) and in prescribing information available from the drug companies. These interactions will not be reiterated in this document, and the health care professional should review those documents for detailed information. Before therapy with these drugs is initiated, the patient's medication profile should be reviewed carefully for potential drug interactions.

Table 45-26 Characteristics of Antiretroviral Drugs: Nucleoside Analog Reverse Transcriptase Inhibitors—cont'd

DRUG (ABBREVIATION)/ TRADE NAME	DOSAGE	MAJOR TOXIC EFFECTS	DRUG INTERACTIONS	SPECIAL INSTRUCTIONS
Nelfinavir/Viracept *Preparations:* Powder for oral suspension: 50 mg per one level scoop (200 mg per one level teaspoon) Tablets: 250 mg tablet	*Pediatric:* 30 mg/kg three times a day *Neonatal:* Under study in PACTG 353: 10 mg/kg three times a day (Note: no preliminary data available, investigational) *Adolescent and adult:* 75 mg three times a day	*Most frequent:* diarrhea *Less common:* asthenia, abdominal pain, rash *Rare:* hyperglycemia and diabetes mellitus	Nelfinavir is in part metabolized by cytochrome P-450 3A4. Potential for multiple drug interactions. Before administration, the patient's medication profile should be reviewed carefully for potential drug interactions. Not recommended for concurrent use (nelfinavir decreases the drug's metabolism, resulting in increased drug levels): antihistamine (astemizole, terfenadine); cisapride; ergot alkaloid derivatives; sedative-hypnotics (triazolam, midazolam); rifampin (greatly reduces nelfinavir levels). Rifabutin causes less decline in nelfinavir concentrations; if coadministered with nelvinavir, rifabutin should be reduced to one half the usual dose. Oral contraceptives: estradiol levels are reduced by nelfinavir, and alternative or additional methods of birth control should be used if coadministering with hormonal methods of birth control. Administration with other protease inhibitors: nelfinavir increases levels of saquinavir and indinavir.	Administer with meal or light snack. For oral solution: powder may be mixed with water, milk, pudding, ice cream, or formula (for up to 6 hours). Do not mix with acidic food or juice because of resulting poor taste. Do not add water to bottles of oral powder; a special scoop is provided with oral powder for measuring. Tablets readily dissolve in water and produce a dispersion that can be mixed with milk, chocolate milk; tablets also can be crushed and administered with pudding.
Ritonavir/Norvir *Preparations:* Oral solution: 80 mg/mL Capsules: 100 mg	*Pediatric:* 400 mg/m² every 12 hours To minimize nausea and vomiting, initiate therapy at 250 mg/m² every 12 hours and increase stepwise to full dose over 5 days as tolerated. *Pediatric range:* 350 to 400 mg/m² every 12 hours *Neonatal:* under study in PACTG 354 (single-dose pharmacokinetics) *Adolescent and adult:* 600 mg every 12 hours	*Most frequent:* nausea, vomiting, diarrhea, headache, abdominal pain, anorexia *Less common:* circumoral paresthesias, increased liver enzyme levels *Rare:* spontaneous bleeding episodes in patients with hemophilia; pancreatitis; increased triglycerides and cholesterol levels; hyperglycemia; and diabetes mellitus	Ritonavir is metabolized extensively in the liver by the cytochrome P-450 enzyme 3A (CYP3A). Potential for multiple drug interactions. Before administration, the patient's medication profile should be reviewed carefully for potential drug interactions. Not recommended for concurrent use: analgesics (meperidine, piroxicam, propoxyphene); antihistamines (astemizole, terfenadine); certain cardiac drugs (amiodarone, bepridil, encainide, flecainide, propafenone, quinidine); ergot alkaloid derivatives; cisapride; sedative hypnotics (clorazepate, diazepam, estazolam, flurazepam, midazolam, triazolam, zolpidem); certain psychotropic drugs (bupropion, clozapine); rifabutin. Oral contraceptives: estradiol levels are reduced by ritonavir, and alternative or additional methods of birth control should be used if one is coadministering with hormonal methods of birth control.	Administration with food increases absorption. If administered with ddl, should be administered 2.5 hours apart. Oral capsules must be kept refrigerated. For oral solution: must be kept refrigerated and stored in original container; can be kept at room temperature if used within 30 days. To minimize nausea, therapy should be initiated at a low dose and increased to full dose over 5 days as tolerated. Techniques to

Continued

Table 45-26 Characteristics of Antiretroviral Drugs: Nucleoside Analog Reverse Transcriptase Inhibitors—cont'd

DRUG (ABBREVIATION)/ TRADE NAME	DOSAGE	MAJOR TOXIC EFFECTS	DRUG INTERACTIONS	SPECIAL INSTRUCTIONS
Ritonavir/Norvir— cont'd			Ritonavir decreases levels of sulfamethoxazole; theophylline (levels should be monitored, and dosage may need to be increased); zidovudine. Ritonavir increases levels of clarithromycin (dosage adjustment may be necessary for patients with impaired renal function); desipramine; warfarin (monitoring of anticoagulant effect necessary). Ritonavir may increase or decrease digoxin levels (monitoring of levels is recommended). Drugs that increase CYP3A activity, such as carbamazepine, dexamethasone, phenobarbital, and phenytoin (anticonvulsant levels should be monitored as ritonavir can affect the metabolism of these drugs as well), can lead to increased clearance and therefore lower levels of ritonavir. Administration with other protease inhibitors: decreases the metabolism of indinavir and saquinavir and results in greatly increased concentrations of these drugs.	increase tolerance by children: Mixing oral solution with milk, chocolate milk, vanilla or chocolate pudding, or ice cream; dulling the taste buds before administration by chewing ice, giving Popsicles or spoonfuls of partially frozen orange or grape juice concentrates; coating the mouth by giving peanut butter to eat before the dose. Administration of strong-tasting foods, such as maple syrup or cheese or strong-flavored chewing gum immediately after dose.
Saquinavir/Fortovase **Preparations:** Soft gel capsules: 200 mg	*Pediatric:* under study in clinical trials: 50 mg/kg three times a day *Neonatal:* Unknown *Adolescent and adult:* 1200 mg three times a day	*Most frequent:* diarrhea, abdominal discomfort, headache, and nausea *Rare:* spontaneous bleeding episodes in patients with hemophilia; hyperglycemia; diabetes mellitus	Saquinavir is metabolized by the cytochrome P-450 3A system in the liver, and there are numerous potential drug interactions. Before administration, the patient's medication profile should be reviewed carefully for potential drug interactions. Not recommended for concurrent use (saquinavir decreases the drug's metabolism, resulting in increased drug levels): antihistamines (astemizole, terfenadine); cisapride; ergot alkaloid derivaties; rifampin and rifabutin (decrease saquinavir levels by 80% and 40% respectively). Saquinavir levels are decreased by carbamazepine, dexamethasone, phenobarbital, and phenytoin. Saquinavir levels are increased by DLV, ketoconazole. Saquinavir may increase levels of calcium channel blockers, dapsone, quinidine, triazolam. Administration with other protease inhibitors: coadministration of ritonavir decreases the metabolism of saquinavir and results in greatly increased saquinavir concentrations.	Administer within 2 hours of a full meal to increase absorption. Concurrent administration of grapefruit juice increases saquinavir concentration. Sun exposure can cause photosensitivity reactions; sunscreen or protective clothing is recommended.

- Discuss disclosing the HIV diagnosis to others.
- Encourage the adolescent to inform sexual partners of his or her HIV status. Offer support as needed.
- Assess the family's or adolescent's knowledge and attitudes about illness and feelings regarding disclosure.
- Assess the child's developmental and cognitive level and understanding of illness causation.
- Try to find out what child or adolescent really wants to know.
- Answer questions honestly and use correct terms for describing illness (e.g., virus, germs).
- Present disclosure as a process over time, with opportunities for expansion and clarification at later times.
- Encourage parents to respect the child's or adolescent's right to privacy.
- Encourage the family or adolescent to inform medical staff when using emergency departments and other medical settings where he or she is not known.
- Inform the family that the school does not need to know the child's diagnosis because HIV is not spread through casual contact. If parents choose to disclose to the school, encourage discussion with the child's teacher, school nurse, and principal.
- Educate regarding prevention of HIV and AIDS transmission.
- Advise abstinence or delay of sexual intercourse.
- Encourage HIV testing.
- Advise the use of latex condoms with nonoxynol-9 when having vaginal or anal sex with male penetration. Advise the use a barrier such as dental dam or nonmicrowavable plastic wrap during oral sex.
- Advise not to share needles or at least to wash needles in a 1:10 bleach-water solution if drug use is continuing.
- If the patient is HIV infected, advise not to breastfeed or donate blood or organs; to use condoms to prevent HIV transmission to an uninfected partner; and to use birth control such as Norplant, the pill, or tubal ligation to prevent unplanned pregnancy.
- Instruct parents, caregiver, child, or adolescent on all prescribed medications.

Follow-up. HIV-infected and exposed children and adolescents need frequent follow-up visits with the PCP every 1 to 3 months depending on the disease state and symptoms. Children and adolescents may also require frequent appointments with specialists; when possible, schedule appointments on the same day to facilitate compliance and limit school absences.

Consultations and referrals

- Remember that HIV-infected children and adolescents should be evaluated by a specialist in HIV every 3 to 6 months. Most major urban medical centers have specialty services dedicated to comprehensive care for these families.
- Consult with physician specialists as indicated (e.g., gastroenterologist, cardiologist, pulmonary specialist, ophthalmologist).
- Keep in mind that all families should be referred to and followed up regularly by a social worker knowledgeable about HIV.
- Contact state and local health departments regarding HIV and AIDS reporting requirements.
- Possible provide the school nurse and other school personnel regular updates on the child's status (only with parent's, guardian's, or adolescent's permission).
- Refer to an early intervention program if appropriate.

Resources

Websites

AIDS Clinical Trials Information Service (www.ACTIS.org)

AIDS Education Global Information System (AEGIS) (www.aegis.com)

The Association of Nurses in AIDS Care (www.anacnet.org)

Camp Sunburst (www.sunburstprojects.org/camp.html)

Centers for Disease Control and Prevention, National Center for HIV, STD, and TB Prevention, Divisions of HIV/AIDS Prevention (www.cdc.gov/hiv/dhap.htm)

HIV/AIDS Treatment Information Service (www.hivatis.org)

Joint United Nations Programme on HIV/AIDS (www.unaids.org)

National AIDS Treatment Advocacy Project (www.NATAP.org)

The National Pediatric and Family HIV Resource Center (www.pedhivaids.org)

New York State Department of Health AIDS Institute Online (www.hivguidelines.org)

The Pediatric AIDS Foundation (www.pedaids.org)

Neoplastic Disease

SUSAN DULCZAK & MARILYN J. HOCKENBERRY

Alert

Any child suspected of having a malignancy should be immediately referred to a physician. A child with a diagnosis of cancer should be managed at a pediatric cancer center.

Signs and symptoms of neoplastic disease include:

- *Pain*—Pain may be generalized or present at a specific location. For example, pain and swelling at the tumor site may be the initial presentation in a child with a bone tumor. Generalized bone aches and difficulty walking can be a symptom of leukemia.
- *Fever*—Although fever is a frequent occurrence during childhood, many children with cancer come to medical attention with unexplained persistent fever as an initial symptom.
- *Anemia*—Cancer such as leukemia or lymphoma invades the bone marrow, causing a decrease in the production of red blood cells (RBCs). Many children have anemia at diagnosis.
- *Increased bruising*—Cancers that invade the bone marrow cause a decreased production of platelets, increasing a child's susceptibility to bleeding.
- *Abdominal mass*—An abdominal mass is a common presentation of Wilms' tumor and neuroblastoma and B-cell lymphoma.
- *Lymphadenopathy*—Enlarged painless lymph nodes, prolonged fever, and weight loss are serious symptoms that may indicate a malignancy.
- *White pupillary reflex*—The presence of a white reflection from a child's pupil is the classic sign of retinoblastoma, a tumor of the eye.
- *Frequent headaches, often associated with vomiting*—Children with brain tumors may have frequent headaches and vomiting depending on the location of the brain tumor.
- *Excessive, rapid weight loss*—A history of recent weight loss in the presence of other symptoms may be a sign of serious illness such as cancer.

Etiology

Childhood cancer, once a uniformly fatal disease, is now a highly curable illness. As more children survive cancer, the primary care practitioner becomes more responsible for managing the effects of the disease and treatment. For this reason it is essential that the practitioner become knowledgeable about cancer in children.

The cause of childhood cancer is unknown. Some childhood tumors may demonstrate patterns of inheritance that indicate a probably genetic basis for the development of cancer. Children with certain types of chromosomal abnormalities have an increased incidence of cancer. For example, children with Down syndrome have 15 times a greater chance of developing leukemia than other children. Factors associated with adult onset of cancer cannot be directly linked to the development of cancer in children. These factors include environmental agents such as carcinogens, drugs, and certain foods.

Incidence

- More than 12,400 people younger than 20 years of age are diagnosed with cancer each year in the United States.
- Over 70% of these children survive the disease if treated properly; nonetheless, they pose a significant challenge to a health care provider in the primary care setting.
- Cancer is the leading cause of death from disease in children 3 to 15 years of age and the second-leading cause of death overall, with injuries being the primary cause of death in this age group.
- The most common type of cancer found in children is leukemia (Table 45-27).
- Brain tumors are the second most common childhood cancer, while lymphomas are the third.
- Boys are slightly more affected than girls, though this depends on the type of tumor.

Risk Factors

- Genetic alterations
- Immunodeficiency syndromes
- Late effects of treatment (e.g., secondary malignancies related to treatment)
- Radiation
- Chromosome abnormalities

Subjective Data

The following data should be obtained from a child who arrives at the primary care setting when the diagnosis of cancer is suspected. When there is evidence to indicate a malignancy,

Table 45-27 Childhood Cancer Incidence: Age Adjusted (All Races, Both Sexes; 1975-1995)

SITE	PERCENTAGE OF TOTAL	RATE PER 1,000,000 CHILDREN
Leukemia	25	37
Brain and nervous system	17	25
Lymphoma	16	24
Kidney	4	6
Soft tissue	7	11
Bone	6	9
Eye	2	3
Liver	1	2
All other	22	32
All sites	100	149

the child and family should be referred to a pediatric cancer center to complete the diagnostic evaluation and begin treatment. The role of the PCP is to identify possible signs and symptoms associated with cancer and to facilitate a timely transfer to a pediatric cancer center.

A complete history should be obtained with careful attention to the following:

- History of present illness, including onset of symptoms, severity and duration, and alleviating or potentiating factors
- History of previous illnesses, including communicable diseases, infections, previous hospitalizations or surgeries, exposure to blood products, and immunization status
- Family history, including previous family members with cancer (including type, treatment, and outcome), present health status of family members, and construction of a complete a family genogram (see Chapter 5)
- Growth, including a review of a growth chart for all children and a head circumference chart for children under 3 years of age
- Developmental history, including milestones obtained and recent regression in any milestones
- Psychosocial history, including any family concerns and problems

The review of systems should include:

- Skin, including any history of bruising or bleeding, lesions, or sores
- Head, eyes, ears, nose, and throat, including any history of infection, proptosis, pupil discoloration, or eye muscle weakness
- Heart, including any history of murmur or thrill, dyspnea, shortness of breath, cyanosis, edema
- Respiratory system (lungs), including any history of infection, cough, wheezing, or shortness of breath
- GI system (abdomen), including any history of abdominal swelling, pain, mass, change in bowel or bladder patterns, nausea, and vomiting
- Musculoskeletal system, including any history of weakness in extremities, limited range of motion (ROM), tenderness or swelling, and joint pain
- Neurologic system, including altered consciousness, mood changes, decreased sensations, abnormal reflexes, and abnormal cerebellar functions
- Lymphatic system, including any history of enlarged lymph nodes or frequent infections
- Hematologic system, including any history of bruising, nosebleeds or gum bleeding, paleness, fatigue, blood or tar-colored stools, and hematuria

Objective Data

A complete physical examination should be performed. Any of the following findings require careful investigation:

- General, including orientation, state of health, and abnormal vital signs
- Skin, including petechiae or ecchymosis, lesions or sores, presence of blood from gums or nasal bleeding, color of skin, and number and size of any café-au-lait spots
- Head, eyes, ears, nose, and throat, including evidence of infection, proptosis, pupil discoloration, extraocular muscles not intact, limited peripheral vision, and nystagmus
- Heart, including murmurs or thrills and peripheral pulses
- Lungs, including evidence of infection, crackles (rales) or rhonchi, decreased breath sounds, and chest asymmetry
- Abdomen, including hepatosplenomegaly, mass, decreased bowel sounds, striae, and ascites

- Musculoskeletal system, including altered ROM, tenderness or swelling, joint pain, effusion, and limpness
- Neurologic system, including altered consciousness, cranial nerve deficits, decreased sensations, abnormal reflexes, abnormal cerebellar functions, and unstable gait
- Lymphatic system, including enlarged lymph nodes.

Differential Diagnosis

Table 45-28 discusses common childhood cancers that may be seen initially in a primary care setting. It is important for the practitioner in the primary care setting to have an understanding of the various types of childhood cancers to facilitate early detection of the disease. Although many of the diagnostic tests are not ordered by the practitioner, it is important to have an understanding of how the diagnosis of cancer is established. Table 45-29 reviews specific clinical manifestations and assessment of brain tumors in children. Table 45-30 reviews signs and symptoms related to the site of the tumor.

Primary Care Issues and Implications

A child diagnosed with cancer poses many concerns for the practitioner in primary care. Cancer and its treatment can alter the child's growth and development, diet and nutrition, and sleep patterns. Issues relating to discipline can be of great concern to the family and must be addressed. Table 45-31 lists the major primary care concerns for a child with cancer.

Management

Any child with cancer should be managed at a pediatric cancer center. The PCP should be involved in the care of a child receiving treatment for cancer when the child returns to the home community. Table 45-32 reviews the types of treatment used for each type of childhood cancer and the common side effects. The most common side effects of cancer therapy are related to bone marrow suppression. This can lead to infection, bleeding, and anemia. Each of these symptoms is discussed in the following section.

Common side effects of cancer treatment and management

Fever
- *Risk factors*—Infection, dehydration, systemic chemotherapy, bone marrow transplantation, blood cell counts with an absolute neutrophil count (ANC) less than 1000 cells/mm³
- *Signs and symptoms*—Fever over 100.4° F (38° C), malaise, possible infection (e.g., at needle puncture sites, mucosal ulcerations, abrasions, or skin tears, intravascular catheter site)

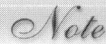
Note

Children with neutropenia may be unable to produce an inflammatory response to infection, and the usual symptoms of an infection may be absent.
- *Prevention*—Filgrastim (Neupogen), a growth factor that increases production of WBCs, is used to decrease the duration of neutropenia. Use of Neupogen is protocol specific.
- *Treatment*—For children with an ANC less than 1000 cells/mm³, the following measures should be taken as soon as possible: blood cultures from central venous lines or peripheral source; Culture of throat, urine, lesions, and catheter exit site as appropriate; chest radiograph; broad-spectrum intravenous antibiotics

Varicella-zoster virus infection (chickenpox or shingles). This is potentially life-threatening for an immunocompromised child.
- *Risk factors*—Immunosuppression, children who have never had chickenpox or varicella vaccine
- *Signs and symptoms*—Rash, fever, pain and tingling along a dermatome, vesicular lesions

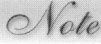
Note

Children receiving chemotherapy who have a direct varicella exposure should receive varicella-zoster immunoglobulin 125 U/10 kg (maximum of 625 U) intramuscularly within 96 hours of the exposure. Children who develop varicella while receiving chemotherapy should be treated with intravenous acyclovir. Reactions in the form of zoster or shingles can occur in immunosuppressed children; these children should be treated with intravenous acyclovir.

Pneumocystis carinii pneumonia
- *Risk factors*—Immunosuppression
- *Signs and symptoms*—Shortness of breath, dyspnea, fever, oxygen saturation less than 95%
- *Prevention*—Children receiving chemotherapy are given prophylactic treatment with TMP-SMX 150 mg/kg twice a day for 3 consecutive days a week during treatment for cancer. For children who cannot tolerate TMP-SMX, dapsone 2 mg/kg orally daily or aerosolized pentamidine at a dose of 300 mg administered monthly are options. Preventive treatment for *Pneumocystis carinii* pneumonia continues throughout the course of cancer therapy and continues after completion of chemotherapy according to protocol.
- *Treatment*—Children with symptoms of *Pneumocystis carinii* pneumonia should be transferred immediately to a pediatric cancer center. Diagnosis usually is confirmed by bronchoalveolar lavage, and TMP-SMX, oxygen, and corticosteroids are started.

Anemia. Children receiving therapy for cancer can develop anemia, so CBC count should be closely monitored.
- *Signs and symptoms*—See Anemia in Chapter 36; also pallor, headache, dizziness, shortness of breath, fatigue, possible tachycardia
- *Management*—Children are treated symptomatically. Packed RBC transfusions are not given unless the hemoglobin falls below 7 to 8 g/dl, except when the child is symptomatic. Epoetin (Epogen), which stimulates bone marrow production of RBCs, is being studied for use in children.

Bleeding. Children receiving therapy for cancer are at risk for bleeding when the platelet count falls below 100,000 cells/mm³. They are at risk for spontaneous hemorrhage when the platelet count falls below 20,000 cells/mm³.

Note

Advise parents and child to avoid rectal temperature measurements, contact sports, eating or chewing sharp food items, use of hard toothbrushes, dental flossing, razors, and aspirin-containing products.

- *Management*—Remember that prevention is essential. If nosebleeds occur, teach parents and the child to stop the

Text continued on page 824

Table 45-28 Common Childhood Cancers

TYPE	INCIDENCE	SIGNS AND SYMPTOMS	SUBJECTIVE DATA (HISTORY)
Leukemia: Most common type of childhood malignancy	Peak incidence 4 years of age 2500 to 3000 children diagnosed each year with acute lympho-cytic leukemia 4 per 100,000 children under 15 years of age	Fever, easy bruisability, pallor and lethargy, recurrent infections, hepatosplenomegaly, bone pain and arthralgias	Complete history as discussed earlier in this chapter; carefully assess for the presence of signs and symptoms previously mentioned and the date of onset
Brain tumors: Most common histologic types: astrocytoma, medullablastoma, and ependymoma	• Second most common child-hood malignancy and most common solid tumor • Approximately 1500 cases of brain tumors diagnosed each year in the United States • 3 per 100,000 children under age of 15	Depend on location of brain tumor (see Table 45-29)	Complete history
Neuroblastoma: Tumor of the sympathetic nervous system	Accounts for approximately 50% of malignant tumors in neonates 50% occur by 2 years of age 1.2 per 100,000 children under 15 years of age	Weight loss, anorexia, fatigue; diarrhea and vomiting; fever; hypertension; proptosis or orbital ecchymosis; paralysis if there is spinal compression; hepatomegaly; bone pain; lym-phadenopathy; paresis; presence of abdominal mass	Complete history
Non-Hodgkin lymphoma	• Accounts for approximately 6% of all childhood cancers • Peak age 5 to 15 years • Increased incidence in chil-dren with immunodeficiency syndromes • 4.6 per million	Depends on the location of the lymphoma; painless enlarged lymph nodes, fever; weight loss, lethargy, night sweats, malaise, pain, GI bleeding, intussuscep-tion, palpable mass, obstructive jaundice Head and neck: Lymphodenopathy, jaw swelling, nasal obstruction, snoring, rhinorrhea, cranial nerve palsy Mediastinum: Superior vena cava syndrome with distorted neck veins, edema of head and neck, and dyspnea CNS: Height and age, vomiting, irritability, papilladema	Complete history; focus on the duration of symptoms and the possibility of previous infectious disease exposures

CT, *Computed tomography;* HMA, *homovanillylmandelic acid;* LDH, *lactate dehydrogenase;* MRI, *magnetic resonance imaging,* TSH, *thyroid-stimulating hormone*

OBJECTIVE DATA (EXAMINATION)	DIAGNOSTIC TESTS	DIFFERENTIAL DIAGNOSIS	TREATMENT
Complete physical examination; assess for: Evidence of infection, lymphadenopathy, petechiae or ecchymosis, hepatospleno-megaly, testicular enlargement, bone tenderness	Complete blood cell count; reticu-locyte count; renal and liver chemistries, LDH, uric acid; coagulation profile, fibrinogen, fibrin split products; urinalysis; chest radiograph, bone marrow aspiration or biopsy; spinal fluid examination	Infection; juvenile rheumatoid arthritis; infectious mononucle-osis; idiopathic thrombocy-topenic purpura; aplastic anemia; other malignancy	Chemotherapy with or without CNS radiation therapy
Complete neurologic examination. Infratentorial tumors: Unsteady gait, nystagmus, slow or altered speech, cranial nerve weakness, hemiparesis; brainstem tumors: Nerve palsies, facial weakness, hearing loss, dysarthria or dys-phagia, altered sensations, spastic hemiparesis; midline tumors: Paralysis of upward gaze, impaired light reaction, loss of convergence, nystagmus, visual impairment, visual field cuts, precocious puberty; cere-bral tumors: lethargy, hemipare-sis, seizures	CT scan of the brain with and without contrast; MRI of the brain and spinal cord as indi-cated; endocrine evaluation; complete blood cell count; liver and renal chemistry assays	Hydrocephalus in the young infant; encephalitis; abscess; hematoma; pseudotumor; optic neuritis; hemangioma; failure to thrive; arteriovenous malforma-tion; metabolic disorder; Guil-lain-Barré syndrome; venous sinus thrombosis	Surgical resection, radiotherapy, and chemotherapy may be used, depending on type of brain tumor
Complete examination; carefully assess for lymphadenopathy, petechiae or ecchymosis, hepatomegaly, mass in the abdomen, blood pressure, orbital proptosis or ecchymosis, skin lesions ("blueberry muffin")	Complete blood cell count; liver enzymes, coagulation profiles; urinalysis and spot urine test for catecholamines (VMA and HVA); 50 ml spot urine sample for cat-echolamines; bone marrow aspi-ration and biopsy; CT scan or MRI of primary site; chest radio-graph; skeletal survey and bone scan; ultrasonogram of the abdomen and pelvis	Other malignancy; systemic infec-tions; osteomyelitis; juvenile rheumatoid arthritis; inflamma-tory bowel disease; cystic or storage disease	Surgical resection, radiotherapy, chemotherapy, depending on the stage of the disease. Children with poor prognosis may benefit from intensive chemotherapy followed by autologous bone marrow transplant
Complete physical examination; carefully assess for lym-phadenopathy; abdominal mass; hepatomegaly; petechiae and ecchymosis; altered respirations, shortness of breath	Complete blood cell count; reticu-locyte count; liver and renal chemistry assays, LDH, uric acid tests; coagulation profile, fi-brinogen, fibrin split products; urinalysis; chest radiograph; CT scan of the involved area; abdominal ultrasonogram to include liver, spleen, kidneys, abdomen, and pelvis; gallium scan; tuberculosis skin test; bone marrow aspiration or biopsy; spinal fluid examination	Infection; other malignancy	Chemotherapy with or without radiotherapy

Continued

Table 45-28   Common Childhood Cancers—cont'd

TYPE	INCIDENCE	SIGNS AND SYMPTOMS	SUBJECTIVE DATA (HISTORY)
Hodgkin disease	• Accounts for approximately 5% of all childhood cancers • The incidence in males is less than in females • The incidence is bimodal • With a peak at 15 to 36 years of age then again > 50 years of age • The incidence is rare in children > 5 years of age • < 1 per 100,000 children (adolescents)	Painless enlarged lymph node(s); fever; weight loss; lethargy, malaise; night sweats	Complete history; focus on the duration of symptoms and the possibility of previous infectious disease exposures
Wilms' tumor: Tumor of the kidney	Accounts for approximately 5 to 6% of all childhood cancers < 1 per 100,000 under 15 years of age 80% occur before 5 years of age Bilateral kidney involvement is seen in 5% to 10% of patients Hereditary form: Autosomal dominance inheritance	Abdominal mass; hypertension; hematuria; (rare) fever, dyspnea, anemia, diarrhea, pain	Complete history; focus on the duration of symptoms; mass usually detected by family
Rhabdomyosarcoma: Tumor of striated muscle tissue	5% to 8% of all cases of childhood cancer Primary sites include the head and neck, genitourinary system, and extremities < 1 per 100,000 under 15 years of age	Related to the site of the tumor (see Table 45-30)	Perform a complete history; focus on the location of the symptoms
Bone tumors: Osteosarcoma	Most common bone tumor Peak incidence for osteosarcoma is during the rapid bone growth period: 15 years of age for boys and 14 years of age for girls < 1 per 100,000 children	Osteosarcoma: Pain, swelling, limping, constant tenderness. Most commonly involves the long bones	Complete history
Ewing's sarcoma	Peak incidence for Ewing's is during the second decade of life Most frequently occurs in bone but may also arise from soft tissue (extraosseous Ewing) < 1 per 100,000 children younger than 15 years of age	Ewing sarcoma: Intermittent pain, palpable mass, pathologic fractures are common	

CT, *Computed tomography;* HMA, *homovanillylmandelic acid;* LDH, *lactate dehydrogenase;* MRI, *magnetic resonance imaging,* TSH, *thyroid-stimulating hormone*

OBJECTIVE DATA (EXAMINATION)	DIAGNOSTIC TESTS	DIFFERENTIAL DIAGNOSIS	TREATMENT
Complete examination; carefully assess for: Lymphadenopathy (firm, nontender, rubbery, and mobile)	CBC count; sedimentation rate; copper values; liver and renal chemistry assays, alkaline phosphate; TSH, T_4; coagulation profile; urinalysis; chest radiograph; CT scan of the chest, abdomen, and pelvis; tuberculosis skin test; bone marrow aspiration or biopsy; nodal biopsy; staging laparotomy may be performed if the findings would significantly alter staging and therapy; spinal fluid examination	Infectious mononucleosis; atypical mycobacterial infections; toxoplasmosis; reactive hyperplasia	Therapy may include radiotherapy, chemotherapy, or both
Complete physical examination; carefully assess for the following in a child being evaluated for Wilms' tumor: Abdominal mass. Children with the hereditary form of Wilms' tumor can have the following anomalies: Aniridia, hemihypertrophy, sexual ambiguity, genitourinary or renal abnormalities, microcephaly, Beckwith-Widemann syndrome	CBC count; reticulocyte count; liver and renal chemistries; urinalysis; chest radiograph; abdominal radiograph; abdominal ultrasonogram; chest and abdominal CT scans; cytogenetic analysis	Multicystic kidney; neuroblastoma; hematoma; renal carbuncles	Surgery is performed to remove the affected kidney; therapy may include radiotherapy, chemotherapy, or both
Perform a complete physical examination	CBC count; reticulocyte count; liver and renal chemistry assays; urinalysis; chest radiograph; chest and abdominal CT scans; CT scan of the primary location; bone scan, skeletal survey; bone marrow aspiration or biopsy, surgical biopsy of tumor	Other malignancy	Therapy may include radiotherapy, chemotherapy, or both
Complete physical examination; carefully assess for: Tenderness at site of tumor; swelling; decreased range of motion	CBC count; liver and renal chemistry assays; urinalysis; chest radiograph; plain film of the involved area; chest CT scan; CT scan and MRI of the primary lesion; bone scan, skeletal survey, biopsy	Osteomyelitis; benign tumor; other malignancy	For osteogenic sarcoma: Chemotherapy/surgical resection and reconstruction of the limb; Ewing sarcoma: Chemotherapy with the use of radiation therapy and surgery based on tumor location and response to chemotherapy

Table 45-29 Clinical Manifestations and Assessment of Brain Tumors

SIGNS AND SYMPTOMS	ASSESSMENT
Headache	
Recurrent and progressive in frontal or occipital areas	Relieved after vomiting
Usually dull and throbbing	Record description of pain, location, severity, and duration
Worse on arising, less during day	Use pain rating scale to assess severity of pain
Intensified by lowering head and straining, such as during bowel movement, coughing, sneezing	Note changes in relation to time of day and activity
	Observe changes in behavior in infants (persistent irritability, crying, head rolling)
Vomiting	
With or without nausea or feeding	Record time, amount, and relationship to feeding, nausea, and activity
Progressively more projectile	
More severe in morning	
Relieved by moving about and changing position	
Neuromuscular Changes	
Incoordination or clumsiness	Test muscle strength, gait, coordination, and reflexes
Loss of balance (use of wide-based stance, falling, tripping, banging into objects)	
Poor fine-motor control	
Weakness	
Hyporeflexia or hyperreflexia	
Positive Babinski's sign	
Spasticity	
Paralysis	
Behavioral Changes	
Irritability	Observe behavior regularly
Decreased appetite	Compare observations with parental reports of normal behavioral patterns
Change in school performance	Monitor growth and food intake
FTT	Monitor activity and sleep
Fatigue (frequent naps)	
Lethargy	
Coma	
Bizarre behavior (staring, automatic movements)	
Cranial Neuropathy	
Cranial nerve involvement varies according to tumor location	Assess cranial nerves, especially nerves VII (facial), IX (glossopharyngeal), X (vagus), V (trigeminal, sensory roots), and VI (abducens)
Most common signs: head tilt, visual defects (nystagmus, diplopia, strabismus, episodic "graying out" of vision, visual field defects), absent gag reflex	Assess visual acuity, binocularity, and peripheral vision
Vital Signs Disturbances	
Decreased pulse and respirations	Measure vital signs frequently
Increased blood pressure	Monitor pulse and respirations for 1 full minute
Decreased pulse pressure	Record pulse pressure (difference between systolic and diastolic blood pressure)
Hypothermia or hyperthermia	
Other Signs	
Seizures	Record seizure activity
Cranial enlargement*	Measure head circumference daily (infant and young child)
Tense, bulging fontanel at rest*	Perform funduscopic examination if skilled in procedure
Nuchal ridigity	
Papilledema (edema of optic nerve)	

From Wong, D. (1999). Nursing care of infants and children *(6th ed.)*. St Louis: Mosby.
*Present only in infants and young children.

Table 45-30 Relationship between Site of Tumor and Symptoms

SITE OF PRESENTATION	ASSOCIATED SYMPTOMS
Head and Neck	
Orbit	Pain, swelling, ptosis, visual disturbances, and changes in cranial nerves II, III, IV, VI
External auditory canal	Earache, ear drainage, hearing loss unilaterally, poor visualization of tympanic membrane with suspected foreign object (tumor)
Surface muscle	Swelling, mass not associated with injury, cranial nerve deficits, enlarged firm cervical lymph nodes
Nasopharyngeal	Chronic sinusitis, purulent or clear nasal discharge, chronic unilateral otitis media, dizziness, headaches, mastication or feeding difficulty, epistaxis
Central nervous system	Headaches, vision changes, cranial nerve change, gross motor changes, paralysis, pain or numbness, behavioral changes
Trunk	
Chest wall	Swelling, asymmetry, distended veins, pleural inflammation; usually asymptomatic until mass very large; respiratory distress
Retroperitoneal, pelvis, perineum	Flank or back pain, renal obstruction, constipation, hematuria (rare), hypertension
	Changes in gait, pain, decreased use of limb, enlarged lymph node proximal to lesion, enlarging mass
Extremities	
Bladder, urinary tract, prostate	Urinary obstruction, hematuria, dysuria, progressive regression in toilet training, urinary tract infection
Vagina	Vaginal bleeding, vaginal drainage, protruding mass

Table 45-31 Primary Care Concerns for Children Receiving Treatment for Cancer

CONCERN OR ISSUE	INTERVENTION
Immunizations	Children receiving immunosuppressive therapy should not receive live virus vaccinations
	Live MMR vaccine should be administered to household contacts; these viruses are not transmissible after vaccination
	Diphtheria-pertussis-tetanus, Hib, pneumococcal vaccines, and hepatitis B vaccines can be administered safely to the child receiving therapy for cancer
	Live varicella zoster vaccine should be given to siblings and household contacts. The vaccine virus is occasionally trasmitted; it is safer than contracting mild virus
	Children who received chemotherapy or radiation therapy should not receive live vaccinations until at least 6 months after the completion of therapy
Nutrition	Frequent assessment of nutritional status and nutrition consultation
	Plot height and weight every month during treatment
	Small, frequent feedings
	Encourage high-calorie diet and well-balanced nutrition
	Offer supplements as indicated
Vision and hearing screening	Continue routine screening as designated for age
	Periodic hearing testing for children receiving aminoglycosides or cisplatin
Dental screening	Teach parents and child to be meticulous in oral hygiene practices
	Continue routine checkups with approval from oncology team
	Obtain CBC count with differential before dental appointment
	Premedication before dental procedures may be indicated
Sleep	Encourage frequent rest periods throughout the day
	Teach parents that children may have difficulty sleeping through the night
Safety	Observe blood cell counts to determine restrictions that may need to be made in the child's activities (e.g., low platelet count means no contact sports)
	Teach usual safety practices according to development stage or age of the child
School	Contact cancer center social worker or nurse to determine information sent to the school
	Assess child's progress in school
	Assist with obtaining teacher for homebound when needed (if cancer center personnel have not pursued it)
Discipline	Encourage parents to maintain discipline
	Stress importance of the child's continued responsibilities in the family
	Discuss other means of discipline than spanking
Activity	Encourage the child to live as normal and active a life as possible
	Physical therapy consultation

Table 45-32   Effects of Treatment for Childhood Cancer

TREATMENT	ACUTE SIDE EFFECTS
Surgery	Change in function (i.e., of an organ or limb)
Chemotherapy	Myelosuppression (infection, bleeding, anemia)
	Nausea and vomiting
	Alopecia
	Mucositis or stomatitis
	Corticosteroid effects
	Cardiomyopathy (anthracyclines)
	Leukoencephalopathy (methotrexate)
	Nephrotoxicity
	Neuropathy (vinca alkaloids)
	Ototoxicity (cisplatin, carboplatin)
	Cystitis (cyclophosphamide)
	Allergic reactions (L-asparaginase, bleomycin)
	Pancreatitis (L-asparaginase)
	Pneumonitis (methotrexate, BCNU, bleomycin)
	Syndrome of inappropriate secretion of antidiuretic hormone (vincristine, cyclophosphamide)
Radiation therapy	Skin and mucosal inflammation
	Tissue edema and inflammation
	Pneumonitis
	Nausea and vomiting
	Enteritis
	Myelosuppression
	Alopecia
	Somnolence
	Leukoencephalopathy

Major organ dysfunction can occur, depending on the treatment for cancer, extent of disease, and age of the child at diagnosis. Careful evaluation of the child's growth and development is essential, since endocrine abnormalities and CNS toxicities can occur as a result of treatment. It is important for all children to continue to be monitored at the pediatric cancer center.

Counseling and prevention. Explain to the parents and child the pathophysiology of the disease, including the following areas:

- Basic concepts related to the development of childhood cancer
- Diagnosis and prognosis
- Diagnostic tests and implications of the results as they relate to treatment
- Misconceptions associated with cancer and recommended treatment
- Remission and relapse
- Differences between stable disease, progressive disease, and recurrent disease

Explain to the parents and child the treatment for the disease, including the following areas:

- Specific forms of therapy (e.g., chemotherapy, radiation therapy, surgery, bone marrow transplantation)
- Experimental therapy and research protocol therapy
- Informed consent
- Patient rights as a subject in a research study
- How to read a treatment "road map"
- The various phases of chemotherapy
- Specific chemotherapy agents being given
- How radiation therapy is given
- Side effects of radiation therapy
- The need for surgery and the risks

Explain to the parents and child the general side effects of treatment, including the following areas:

- Nausea and vomiting related to treatment
- Decreased appetite, with encouragement and support for good nutrition
- GI tract symptoms of constipation or diarrhea related to treatment (e.g., change in bowel habits, constipation after vincristine [VCR], diarrhea).
- Mouth care during treatment
- Hair loss occurring during treatment
- Prevention of sun exposure during treatment and the need to use sunscreen (because several drugs increase sun sensitivity)
- Signs and symptoms related to decreased hemoglobin during treatment (e.g., tiredness, paleness)
- Children sometimes needing more rest and increased sleep when blood cell counts are low
- Specific side effects related to the child's treatment protocol

Explain to the parents and child precautions after chemotherapy, including the following areas:

- Proper handwashing
- Use of gloves when handling diapers, stool, vomitus, or urine

Explain to the parent and child the risk of infection, including the following areas:

- Bone marrow suppression
- Symptoms of infection that are the result of a low WBC count
- When to report fever (temperature greater than 100.4° F [38° C])

nosebleed by having the child sit upright and pinch the nostril together for at least 10 minutes without releasing. If bleeding persists in any child with low platelet counts, the child needs a platelet transfusion.

Mucositis. Mucositis can occur as a side effect of numerous chemotherapy agents and radiotherapy.

- *Risk factors*—Chemotherapy: methotrexate, doxorubicin hydrochloride (Adriamycin); radiotherapy (head and neck region); bone marrow transplantation; neutropenia
- *Signs and symptoms*—Oral lesions, erythema, swelling, fever
- *Management*—Maintain adequate oral hygiene; assess for fever, and implement appropriate evaluation for patients with neutropenia. Advise diligent mouth care as suggested by the pediatric oncology center.

Children with indwelling catheters. Many children with prolonged or intensive treatment protocols require long-term venous access. Access devices are classified as external catheters such as the Hickman or Broviac, or indwelling catheters such as the Infusaport or Port-A-Cath. NPs in primary care settings need to be aware of the care for these catheters. Each center will provide guidelines for care of the central venous catheter.

Children who have completed therapy. NPs in the primary care setting may provide care for survivors of childhood cancer. Table 45-33 discusses specific clinical signs and symptoms related to the particular treatment for cancer.

Table 45-33 Late Effects of Cancer Treatment

SYSTEMIC EFFECTS AND CLINICAL MANIFESTATIONS	ASSOCIATED MODE OF TREATMENT
Central Nervous	
Leukoencephalopathy (syndrome ranging from lethargy, dementia, and seizures to quadriplegia and death)	Methotrexate, CNS irradiation, or both
Mineralizing microangiopathy (headaches, focal seizures, incoordination, gate abnormalities)	Methotrexate, CNS irradiation, or both
Peripheral neuropathy (footdrop, incoordination)	Vincristine
Cognitive deficits (intelligence, nonlanguage skills)	Intrathecal chemotherapy, cranial irradiation (especially before 3 years of age), or both
Cardiovascular	
Cardiomyopathy (tachycardia, tachypnea, dyspnea, shortness of breath, edema, palpitations)	Anthracyclines (doxorubicin and daunorubicin), irradiation to heart, or both High-dose cyclophosphamide
Pericardial damage (pleural effusion, cardiomegaly)	Mediastinal irradiation
Respiratory	
Pneumonitis (dyspnea, nonproductive cough, fever)	Lung irradiation; alkylating agents; possibly bleomycin, vinblastine, cisplatin
Pulmonary fibrosis (dyspnea, restrictive ventilation, decreased exercise tolerance)	
Gastrointestinal	
Chronic enteritis (colic, abdominal pain, vomiting, diarrhea, obstipation, bleeding)	Abdominal irradiation, methotrexate, cytosine arabinoside
Hepatic fibrosis (jaundice, hepatomegaly)	Methotrexate, 6-mercaptopurine
Urinary	
Hemorrhagic cystitis (chronic microscopic hematuria to gross hemorrhage)	Cyclophosphamide; ifosfamide irradiation, especially with radiomimetic chemotherapeutic agents (e.g., doxorubicin, daunorubicin)
Bladder fibrosis (decreased bladder capacity, ureteral reflux)	
Tubular necrosis (decreased creatinine clearance)	Cisplatin
Endocrine	
Growth retardation (abnormal growth velocity)	Irradiation to the thyroid, pituitary gland, testes, ovaries
Thyroid dysfunction	
Gonadal dysfunction	
Reproductive	
Possible gonadal damage: Both sexes (amenorrhea, decreased sperm counts, increased follicle-stimulating and luteinizing hormones, decreased testosterone or estrogen)	Alkylating agents Irradiation to the pituitary gland, testes, ovaries
Skeletal	
Linear growth retardation (short stature)	Irradiation, long-term corticosteroids
Spinal deformities, scoliosis, kyphosis, asymmetric growth, pathologic fractures	Irradiation
Immune	
Asplenia (overwhelming infection, fever)	Splenectomy (Hodgkin's disease)
Sensory Organs	
Cataracts (opacity over pupil)	Cranial irradiation, high-dose corticosteroids
Hearing (decreased hearing associated with high-frequency loss)	Cisplatin
Additional Effects	
Dental problems	
Increased caries, periodontal disease, hypoplastic teeth, hypodontia (delayed or absent tooth development)	Irradiation to maxilla and mandible
Second malignancies	
Bone and soft-tissue tumors	Irradiation, alkylating agents, epipodophyllotoxins
Leukemia	
Nonlymphocytic leukemia	

Modified from Wong, D. (1999). Nursing care of infants and children. (6th ed.). St Louis: Mosby.

- Ways to prevent infection (e.g., proper handwashing, good hygiene, minimization of exposures)
- The proper way to take a temperature
- Avoidance of the use of a rectal thermometer
- Varicella exposure and when to call
- Chickenpox exposure and the need to report it immediately
- Live immunizations not being given to the patient during treatment, but all appropriate immunizations being given to siblings and other household members (see Chapter 13)

Explain to the parents and child the risk of bleeding, including the following areas:

- Signs and symptoms of decreased platelet counts (e.g., increased bruising, nosebleeds, headaches, abdominal pain, tarry stools, hematuria)
- The proper way to stop a nosebleed
- Precautions to take when the platelet count is low (e.g., soft toothbrush, no flossing, prevent head injury, obtain blood cell counts before dental care)
- Avoidance of aspirin- or ibuprofen-containing medications.

Discuss with the parents and child the need for laboratory work, including the following areas:

- Blood cell function (e.g., of WBCs, RBCs, platelets)
- Normal blood cell values
- Specific signs and symptoms of low blood cell counts
- Calculation of the ANC
- Concerns related to a low ANC count
- Specific laboratory tests related to the child's disease or treatment

Explain to the parents and child diagnostic tests, including the following areas:

- Tests to be performed
- Risks involved
- Strategies to decrease discomfort associated with the tests
- Preparation to be done before the tests (e.g., nothing-by-mouth status, topical anesthesia, conscious sedation)
- Time and location of the tests in the outpatient setting

Explain to the parents and child the need for venous access, including the following areas:

- Need for a venous access device
- The procedure and what the catheter looks like
- Proper care of the venous access device
- How to obtain proper supplies for care of the line
- Signs of infection and who to call if these signs develop
- Removal of the catheter and care for the catheter site after completion of therapy

Explain to the parents and child changes in activities, including the following areas:

- Returning to school or homebound education
- Information the staff can provide to the school
- Accessing services in the school district
- Importance for the child to remain in school and participate in activities as much as possible
- Specific restrictions necessary when the blood cell counts are low (e.g., stay away from crowds, remain home from school for an ANC less than 500 cells/mm³)
- Activity limitations related to the child's disease or treatment

Explain to the parents and child the effect of the diagnosis on the family, including the following areas:

- Need to evaluate existing support systems
- Available community resources
- Financial needs and potential resources
- Applications for financial assistance

- Support services
- Need to involve siblings
- Maintaining consistency in disciplining all children
- Child care concerns and possible solutions
- Working with employer
- Support groups offered for families with cancer

Follow-up. Children with cancer are followed closely by the cancer center. Any concerns that may develop when a child is being seen in a primary care setting should be immediately conveyed to the pediatric oncology center.

Consultations and referrals. Children receiving treatment for cancer are followed up by a pediatric oncologist or NP. Problems encountered in the primary care setting should be immediately referred to the cancer center. Most childhood cancer centers provide consultation to the child's school at diagnosis and continue to follow the child's school progress during treatment and once therapy has been discontinued. Oncology social workers are usually assigned to each child and family and are available for assistance when the primary care practitioner encounters problems in the home environment. The intensity of treatment causes alterations in the child's nutritional status, requiring dietary consultation early in therapy. Most childhood cancer centers have nutritionists who follow up children with cancer closely during each return visit to the hospital or clinic.

Resources

Organizations

American Cancer Society, 90 Park Ave., New York, NY 10016; (800) ACS-2345

Cancer Information Service, NCI, Building 31, National Institutes of Health, Bethesda, MD 20892

Candlelighters Childhood Cancer Foundation, Inc., 2025 I Street NW, Suite 1011, Washington, DC 20006

Leukemia Society of America, 800 Second Avenue, New York, NY 10017

National Childhood Cancer Foundation; (800) 458-6223; www.nccf.org/index.htm

Websites

Association of Pediatric Oncology Nurses (www.apon.org)

CancerSource.com (www.cancersource.com)

Candlelighters Childhood Cancer Family Alliance (www.candle.org)

Last Acts (www.lastacts.org)

The Leukemia & Lymphoma Society (www.leukemia.org)

Oncology Nursing Society (www.ons.org)

Rheumatic Fever

KATHLEEN KENNEY

Alert

Consult with or refer to a physician for the following:
- Family history of rheumatic fever
- Recent history of group A β-hemolytic streptococcus (GABHS) infection in the presence of the Jones criteria
- History of untreated GABHS infection or poor compliance with medication regimen
- Presence of two major symptoms and one minor symptom from the Jones criteria

Rheumatic fever (RF) is an inflammatory connective tissue disorder that results as a delayed response to the sequela of GABHS infection. This response primarily involves the heart, blood vessels, joints, CNS, and subcutaneous tissue. The discovery of the role of GABHS in the development of RF combined with the introduction of antibiotic therapy led to the ability to prevent RF. During the 1960s and 1970s in the United States there was a significant decline in the number of reported cases of rheumatic fever. In the 1980s a sudden steady increase in the number of reported cases of RF was seen across the United States. Studies thus far have been able to identify the reason for this resurgence. More recently there appears to be a decrease in the reported cases possibly because of better recognition and treatment of streptococcal pharyngitis.

The diagnosis of RF does not rely on one specific symptom or blood test but rather on many criteria (known as the *Jones criteria*) (Table 45-34) and evidence of a recent streptococcal infection (e.g., pharyngitis, impetigo). The clinical manifestations may vary; therefore it is important to use the Jones criteria to diagnose RF. According to these criteria the patient must have two of the major criteria and one of the minor criteria, or one of the major criteria and two of the minor. The guidelines also state that documentation of a recent streptococcal infec-tion is now a requirement for the diagnosis. Streptococcal infection can be documented by means of culture, rapid antigen, or antibody rise or elevation.

Etiology

The origin of RF is related to GABHS infection. The mechanism that causes the development of the manifestations of RF is poorly understood. There are several hypotheses. The most popular is that there is an abnormal immune response by the human host to some component of the group A streptococcus. This response results in the development of antibodies that may lead to the immunologic damage that occurs and is seen in the clinical manifestations. The only clinical manifestation that results in chronic changes is those immunologic responses that occur in the heart (most commonly as valvular changes and insufficiency). It is not understood why certain people are more susceptible to the development of RF than others. Because of the inability to predict a certain population's risk for developing RF, it is imperative to identify streptococcal infections through appropriate diagnostic tests (e.g., rapid strept, strept agar, ASO titers) and appropriately document and treat them to avoid the development of further complications.

Table 45-34 Jones Criteria

CRITERIA	CLINICAL MANIFESTATIONS
Major Criteria	
Carditis	Murmurs of valvular insufficiency
	May see dysrhythmia (usually first-degree heart block)
	May see signs of CHF
	Occurs in 40% to 80% of patients with rheumatic fever
Polyarthritis	Most confusing of major criteria
	Leads to many errors in diagnosis
	Joints exquisitely tender, warm, red, and swollen
	Pain is migratory, affecting several different joints, especially the elbows, knees, ankles, and wrists
	Does not need to be symmetric
	Does not cause chronic joint disease
Sydenham chorea	Occurs in 15% of cases
	Is a late manifestation that may be very subtle in onset
	Careful history is required
	May present as a complaint of clumsiness
	Best sign is change in handwriting
	May include emotional lability
	May affect all four extremities or be unilateral, with jerky movements of extremities
	Usually disappears within 6 months
Erythema marginatum	Occurs in less than 10% of cases
	Rash is nonspecific pink macules seen on the trunk and proximal parts of limbs
	Late in the development of the rash there is blanching in the middle of the lesions
	Rash is nonpruritic and worsens with application of heat
Subcutaneous nodules	Occurs in 2% to 10% of the patients
	Most commonly seen in patients with severe carditis
	Nodules pea-sized, firm, nontender, with no inflammation
	Seen on the extensor surface of joints: knees, elbow, and spine
Minor Criteria	
Fever	Usually no higher than 102° F
Arthralgia	Discomfort in joints without the pain, redness, and warmth seen in polyarthritis
Elevated acute-phase reactants (ESR, C-reactive protein)	These tests are ways to identify an acute inflammatory process (may be seen with many other inflammatory processes)
Prolonged P-R interval on electrocardiogram	Nonspecific finding that can occur with many other processes; therefore must use other criteria

Incidence

- The peak incidence is at greater than 3 years of age (with a range of 5 to 15 years of age)
- It is rare under 4 years of age
- It is more common in families with previous history of RF
- There is a higher incidence in lower socioeconomic settings
- It is more common in winter and spring

Risk Factors

- Presence of rheumatic fever in another family member
- Documented previous GABHS infection with inappropriate
- Low socioeconomic setting

Subjective Data

A thorough history should be completed on a child suspected of having RF, with careful attention to the following:

- *Description of the problem*—The most common complaint with RF is joint symptoms. Ask if one or several joints are affected. There is often complaint of the pain migrating from one joint to another joint. Clarify the pain as to the severity based on the child's ability to perceive pain. The joint pain of RF is usually severe (e.g., any inflammation affecting the lower extremities may cause the child to be unable to walk). Joint pain that the child states is relieved with rubbing is not indicative of RF. The child may have complaints of chest pain and abdominal pain, as well as a history of recent nosebleeds. Children with choreiform movements can be easily overlooked in their mildest forms as a result of the condition being misdiagnosed as a behavioral problem, emotional distress, or clumsiness.
- *Past history*—There may be recent history of sore throat, upper respiratory infection, or abdominal pain within the previous 4 weeks. The neurologic complaints that may accompany RF include a recent history of emotional lability, change in behavior, difficulties in school, or a change in handwriting. Complaints of jerky, involuntary movements by the child are highly suggestive of Sydenham's chorea, which is seen with RF.

Objective Data

Physical examination. Any child with possible RF requires a complete physical examination with careful attention paid to the clinical manifestations described in the Jones criteria:

- *Heart*—Auscultation for murmurs should be performed. Cardiac findings include murmurs consistent with valvular insufficiency or possible cardiac rubs.
- *Musculoskeletal system*—The findings of polyarthritis include joints that are swollen, red, warm, and exquisitely tender to palpation. Palpation of extensor surfaces may lead to identification of subcutaneous nodules. These nodules are pea sized, firm, and nontender, with no inflammation.
- *Skin*—Inspection occasionally allows for the visualization of an erythematous rash over the trunk and proximal part of the limbs (only in 10% of cases). This rash may be further identified through the application of heat, which causes a worsening of the rash.
- *Neurologic system*—Findings include choreiform movements, emotional lability, and possible irritability.

Diagnostic procedures and laboratory tests. There is no specific test to diagnose RF, but several tests help in confirming the final diagnosis. The most commonly used is the anti-streptolysin titer, which documents the presence of previous GABHS infection (modestly elevated is 320 Todd units in children). There may also be previous documentation of a positive throat culture for GABHS within the preceding weeks. The ESR and the C-reactive protein may be elevated, reflecting an ongoing inflammatory process. A CBC count may reveal an elevated WBC count as a result of an ongoing bacterial infection. An electrocardiogram may demonstrate heart block or other dysrhythmias.

Primary Care Issues and Implications

- *Growth and development*—The neurologic component of RF may include emotional lability, involuntary movements, and poor fine-point hand control. Reassure parents that these are temporary occurrences and will resolve with time, leading to no permanent neurologic damage.
- *Immunizations*—AAP guidelines for routine immunizations should be followed.
- *Safety*—Remind parents that while children are actively suffering from Sydenham's chorea, dangerous activities such as climbing a ladder, playing on monkey bars, or driving a car (for adolescents) must be avoided because there is increased risk for injury. The joint pain and inflammation caused by the polyarthritis of RF necessitates decreased exercise and an awareness by playmates and siblings to avoid injuring the child's area of pain and swelling.
- *Discipline*—The practitioner should discuss the effect of emotional lability on the child's behavior (see Discipline in Chapter 19).
- *Sexuality*—Issues are the same as for other children.
- *Nutrition*—There are no specific restrictions or recommendations for nutritional management of children with RF.

Management

Treatments and medications. Treatment is directed at prevention of RF, treatment of the GABHS infection which caused the RF, treatment of the symptoms and inflammatory responses, and other supportive therapy including management of subsequent CHF and secondary prevention of recurrences of RF, as follows:

- *Prevention of sequelae of GABHS infection*—Culture and treat all suspected (initially) and diagnosed GABHS infections with penicillin V potassium 25 to 50 mg/kg per day divided every 6 hours for 10 days or (if the patient is allergic to penicillin) erythromycin 40 mg/kg per day divided into four doses for 10 days.
- *Acute rheumatic fever*—Provide hospital admission with the following treatment: aspirin 100 mg/kg per day divided every 6 hours, plus oral penicillin (see above for doses) for 10 days or penicillin G benzathine injection intramuscularly (children weighing less than 27 kg should receive 600,000 U; children weighing more than 27 kg should receive 1.2 million U)
- *Carditis or CHF*—Determine treatment by consultation with a cardiologist or pediatrician.
- *Prevention of recurrences of RF (maintenance after initial diagnosis):*
  Penicillin G benzathine 1.2 million U intramuscular every 4 weeks, or

Penicillin potassium 250 mg orally two times a day, or (if allergic to penicillin)

Erythromycin 250 mg orally two times a day

Also, sulfadiazine 500 mg daily for patients weighing less than 27 kg, with 1 g daily for patients weighing more than 27 kg

- *Duration of prophylaxis (American Heart Association [AHA] recommendations)*—Rheumatic fever without carditis should be treated for 5 years or until 21 years of age. Rheumatic fever with carditis but no residual disease after episode should be treated for 10 years or until adulthood. Rheumatic fever with residual heart disease should be treated for at least 10 years after the last episode of rheumatic fever.

Counseling and prevention

- Instruct parents on the need for prompt and appropriate treatment of sore throat and fevers.
- Educate the parents and child on the disease process and treatment regimen.
- Teach the parents and child importance of continued antibiotic prophylaxis to avoid recurrence of RF.
- Educate the family on the effect that the disease has had on the child's heart and the need for continued monitoring with a cardiologist.
- Inform families with a history of RF of the higher incidence and need to be more aware of possible GABHS infections.
- Educate families on importance of completing course of antibiotics when GABHS infection is identified.
- Advise parents on the need for added prophylaxis for dental and other invasive procedures.

Follow-up. Provide follow-up care per the physician or specialist.

Consultations and referrals. Refer to physician or cardiologist.

Resources

Websites

HeartCenterOnline for Patients (www.heartcenteronline.com/ myheartdr/Articles_about_the_heart/Heart-Threatening_ Illnesses.html)

Sickle Cell Disease

JACQUELINE G. IOLI & MIRIAM GILDAY

Alert

Refer to a physician any child with known sickle cell disease (SCD) and:

- Seizures, unilateral weakness, slurred speech, or altered level of consciousness (possible stroke)
- Bilateral pulmonary auscultatory abnormalities, especially crackles, chest pain, and pulse oximetry less than 95% (possible acute chest syndrome)
- Fever over 101.5° F (38.6° C), even if the source can be identified (possible sepsis, with a minimum of one dose of parental antibiotics needed)
- Palpable spleen in the context of sudden onset, abdominal pain, fever, paleness, or jaundice (possible acute splenic sequestration crisis [ASSC])
- Moderate to severe pain that does not respond to first-line analgesics (i.e., standard doses of acetaminophen alone or with codeine and ibuprofen)
- Signs of urinary tract infection (UTI) (e.g., pyuria, dysuria, flank pain, hematuria [possible pyelonephritis or sepsis])

SCD is a group of autosomal recessive genetic disorders characterized by the production of hemoglobin S, hemolytic anemia, and acute and chronic tissue damage secondary to the blockage of blood flow by abnormally shaped RBCs. The most common four sickling disorders are described in Table 45-35. Life span is predicted to be in the mid-40s for persons with sickle cell anemia (SS) and sickle β^0-thalassemia and near normal for persons with sickle "C" disease (SC) and sickle β^+-thalassemia. Each type of SCD is characterized by wide clinical heterogeneity between individuals within that group. As a group, persons with SS and sickle β^0-thalassemia are generally more symptomatic, and as a group, persons with SC and sickle β^+-thalassemia are generally less symptomatic. (However, individual cases will vary.)

Etiology

The most common hemoglobin, hemoglobin A (for Adult), is made up of two α-globin chains and two β-globin chains.

Table 45-35 Differences between the Most Common Types of Sickle Cell Disease

DISEASE	GENOTYPE	INCIDENCE	CLINICAL SEVERITY	USUAL Hgb (g/dl)	USUAL PERCENTAGE OF RETICULOCYTES	USUAL Hgb ELECTROPHORES
Sickle cell anemia	SS	1 in 375 African-American live births	Usually severe	6-10	5-20	> 90% Hgb S; possibly some Hgb F
Sickle "C" disease	SC	1 in 835 African-American live births	Mild to moderate	10-15	5-10	50% Hgb C 50% Hgb S
Sickle β^0-thalassemia	Sickle and thalassemia	1 in 1667 African-American live births	Severe to moderate	6-10	5-20	> 80% Hgb S; < 3.5% Hgb A_2; possibly some Hgb F
Sickle β^+-thalassemia			Mild to moderate	9-12	5-10	> 60 Hgb S; > 3.5% Hgb A_2; 20% Hgb A; possibly some Hgb F

Sickle hemoglobin (Hgb S, for Sickle) has two normal α-globin chains, but on the β-globin chain there is a substitution of valine for glutamic acid at the sixth position. Persons with sickle trait are carriers and not clinically affected (for a more detailed description of sickle trait, see Chapter 36).

The shape of the RBC changes to a C or sickle shape. This causes blood-flow blockage to various areas of the body with effects to all body systems. RBCs change shape because Hgb S molecules polymerize easily. When hemoglobin S is polymerized, the RBC becomes elongated and rigid. Exposure to low oxygen states, dehydration or hyperosmolarity, or high or low temperatures creates conditions that enhance polymerization and thus sickling. Cells can change shape from sickle to normal (biconcave disk) several times before they are permanently damaged and hemolyze. Further, sickled cells "stick" to each other easily because of altered electrical charge. The sickled cells irritate the endothelium of the blood vessels, especially in high flow areas like the brain, which leads to narrowing of vessels in these areas because of scarring and accumulation of fibrin and platelets. Thus obstruction occurs more easily in areas of narrowed vessels. All body tissues are at risk for damage as a consequence of the vascular obstruction from sickled RBCs. Body tissues with the lowest oxygen tension are at highest risk for damage (e.g., kidney, eye).

Incidence

- The sickling disorders are the most common hemoglobinopathies worldwide.
- Sickle trait and SCD are most common in malaria-prone areas such as Africa, the Mediterranean, Asia, and western India. (In some areas, 25% of the population has the sickle trait.) Also affected are people of the Caribbean and of South and Central America.
- About 50,000 people in the United States are affected with SCD.

Risk Factors

- Two parents with the trait (25% risk of having a child with SCD with every pregnancy)
- Persons with SCD who have children with a partner with the trait (50% risk of having a child with SCD; all of their children will have the trait)
- African, Mediterranean, Hispanic, Caribbean, or South American descent

Subjective Data

Initially, a complete history should be obtained, including a careful review of systems on any child with a known or suspected hemoglobinopathy, with special emphasis on family history. Absence of a positive family history of sickle trait or other unusual hemoglobin traits does not rule out the presence of SCD because many adults are unaware of their trait status or had poor quality counseling. Also be sure to cover the following areas:

- *History of pain episodes*—Keep in mind that there is no clinical or laboratory test to "confirm" a painful episode! (See Chapter 7.) Pain exists when and where the patient says it does. Is there a usual site or sites? What usually helps pain (i.e., pharmacologic or nonpharmacologic means, or both)? What worsens pain (e.g., heat, cold, exercise, distraction)?

- *History of other sickle-related problems:*
  Life-threatening complications of SCD, including cerebrovascular accident (CVA or stroke), ASSC, aplastic crisis, acute chest syndrome (ACS), or pneumonia, infections (Table 45-36)
  Disabling complications of SCD (Table 45-37), including hand-foot syndrome (most common in infants and toddlers; most frequent initial complication of SCD), priapism, leg ulcers, avascular necrosis of the hips or shoulders, and sickle retinopathy
- *Past medical history*—Ask in particular about reactive airway disease.
- *Allergy history*—Remember that itching related to opioid analgesics is a known side effect and is not necessarily an allergy.
- *Current medications*—Keep in mind that children under 5 years of age with known SCD should be taking prophylactic penicillin. Does the family commonly keep any pain medications on hand just in case? How often are these medications used? Does the child take folic acid?
- *History of follow-up visits in a child with known SCD*—Has the child been seen at an SCD center? When was the last visit?
- *Immunization history*
- *Developmental history*—Ask about toilet training and common developmental milestones, such as speech and gross and fine motor skills (e.g., dressing, feeding, walking, development of hand preference).
- *School history*—Note days lost because of illness; grades; and general performance.
- *Physical activities*—Is there dyspnea with normal activity? Easy fatigability?
- *Sleep*—Does pain interfere with sleep? Does the child snore?
- *Nutrition history*—What is the child's food intake in general? How much milk per day? Does the child complain of epigastric pain after eating fatty foods? Does the child experience constipation with use of opioid analgesics?
- *Psychosocial history*—With whom does the child live? What do siblings or other family members know about SCD? How does the family adapt to the stress of sickle pain episodes and related hospitalizations? What family supports exist, and who are they? Is there insurance coverage? Is there a need to refer to social work for assistance with referral to community resources for housing, transportation, financial and utility bill assistance?
- *Family history*

Objective Data

Physical examination. The initial visit for known or suspected SCD includes a complete physical examination. Assess for the following:

- *Head, eyes, ears, nose, and throat*—Presence of frontal bossing or upper mandibular hypertrophy (secondary to extramedullary hematopoiesis), scleral icterus (usually not an indicator of liver disease; merely an indication of hemolysis typical of SCD), and tonsillar hypertrophy
- *Neurologic system*—Symmetric facial expressions, use of and strength in extremities, clonus, and developmental delays
- *Cardiac system*—Presence of murmur with an appropriate description (e.g., grade I to IV systolic ejection murmur)

Table 45-36 Life-Threatening Complications of Sickle Cell Disease

COMPLICATION	PATHOPHYSIOLOGY AND INCIDENCE	SIGNS AND SYMPTOMS	PREVENTION AND MANAGEMENT
Cerebrovascular accident (CVA)	Sickled cells block circulation to brain, most commonly the carotid, anterior, and middle cerebral arteries (areas of high blood flow) 6% to 10% of SCD patients are affected; median age is 7 years, with a 67% recurrence rate in untreated patients	Aphasia Hemiplegia or hemiparesis Seizures Cranial nerve palsies Coma	Monitor for unilateral weakness in an extremity whether or not it is painful Refer to SCD center for risk assessment with transcranial Doppler screening Refer to SCD center for suspected CVA. Immediate treatment: exchange transfusion. Long-term prevention of future CVAs with chronic transfusion program (usually monthly).
Acute chest syndrome (ACS)	Sickled cells block microcirculation to lungs, resulting in ventilation-perfusion mismatching Over time, repeated episodes cause chronic restrictive lung disease with pulmonary hypertension and cor pulmonale Significant cause of mortality and morbidity in all age groups	Decreased pulse oximetry Fever Pleuritic chest pain (in older children and adults) Tachypnea (in younger children) Pulmonary infiltrates on chest radiograph	Children with SCD are also at the same risk for reactive airways disease as other children, complicating care. To establish baseline value, monitor pulse oximetry on every SCD patient at every well-child visit. Refer to SCD center because it is difficult to distinguish both clinically and radiographically from bacterial and viral pneumonia; consequently, suspected ACS is treated exactly as pneumonia.
Acute splenic sequestration crisis (ASSC)	Usually occurring in young children 6 months to 4 years of age; sickled cells block venous outflow circulation of the spleen; blood enters spleen but cannot leave (platelets and WBCs may also become trapped) Up to 25% of circulating blood volume can be sequestered in the spleen, causing profound anemia, shock, pallor, and a greatly enlarged spleen with abdominal distension in as little as a few hours Most children autosplenectomize by about 2 or 3 years of age after a series of smaller, less life-threatening infarcts	Enlarged spleen Paleness Lethargy Abdominal pain Dropping hemoglobin and platelet count, with possible drop in WBC	Palpate spleen to check for enlargement; it may be as far down as the pelvis. Refer to SCD center or nearest emergency department. Remember than uncrossmatched blood may be required to treat profound shock. Large amounts of crystalloid fluids are not indicated because they can cause hemodilution, but blood pressure may need to be initially supported with fluids.

- *Pulmonary system*—Baseline pulse oximetry on all visits with careful auscultation of all fields, observing for presence of crackles or coarse breath sounds
- *Abdomen*—Palpation for spleen and inspection for the presence of cholecystectomy or splenectomy scars
- *GU system*—Tanner staging
- *Musculoskeletal system*—ROM of shoulders and hips

Interval and follow-up visits should be performed with observation of the areas just listed and notations made as to deviation from patient's baseline values.

Diagnostic procedures and laboratory tests. A complete blood cell (CBC) count with reticulocyte count should be performed every 6 months to 1 year to monitor baseline status. Each person with SCD has a baseline value that is normal for them. Most persons with SCD have an elevated reticulocyte count (above 5%), while lower values indicate an aplastic crisis. Some persons with SC and sickle β^+-thalassemia have near-normal hemoglobin levels and thus their reticulocyte counts would be expected to be near normal; these patients are the exception to the generalization. Infection and pain can cause the hemoglobin to drop below baseline value. A falling hemoglobin combined with thrombocytopenia indicates splenic sequestration whether or not the spleen is palpable. This finding necessitates referral to a SCD center.

Hemoglobin electrophoresis should be done in infancy to confirm the diagnosis of SCD after a positive newborn screening test. If an infant has had prenatal diagnosis with amniocentesis, the newborn screening test may serve as the confirmatory testing. There is no role for a sickle prep or sickle dex test in the care of children with SCD. The sickle prep does not detect the presence of unusual hemoglobin traits states such as hemoglobin C trait or β-thalassemia trait. To monitor the proportions of fetal hemoglobin (hemoglobin F), the hemoglobin electrophoresis should be repeated every 2 to 3 years thereafter, with care being taken not to draw if it has been less than 3 months since a blood transfusion. Because it does not sickle, hemoglobin F often has an ameliorating effect on the clinical course in SCD.

Table 45-37 Disabling Problems in Sickle Cell Disease

COMPLICATION	PATHOPHYSIOLOGY	SIGNS AND SYMPTOMS	MANAGEMENT
Sickle retinopathy	Sickled cells block the central retinal artery resulting in proliferative sickle retinopathy (PSR), vitreous hemorrhage, and retinal detachment. The biochemical and metabolic conditions in the aqueous humor favor RBC sickling, which plugs the outflow pathways and causes increased intraocular pressure. Moderate elevation of intraocular pressure in eyes of people with SCD can produce permanent visual deterioration.	Any change in visual acuity.	Refer to ophthamology for general examination with detailed retinal examination. Avoid referral to optometrists who cannot perform the details of retinal examination required.
Anemia	Sickled cells have decreased oxygen-carrying capacity Chronic hemolytic anemia and decreased oxygen-carrying capacity result in increased cardiac output (50% above normal at rest to meet tissue needs for oxygen) and occasionally left ventricular enlargement (from increased stroke volume) and systolic flow murmur.	Exercise capacity can be reduced as much as 50% to 75% of that of nonaffected children. Flow murmur is common, especially in persons with low baseline hemoglobin (< 9 g).	Encourage children to have activity as tolerated allowing rest periods as needed. Gym restriction should be individualized; some children need no restrictions. Some children who have more limited energy reserves may benefit from saving their energy for other activities besides physical education.
Sickle nephropathy	The relatively hypoxic and hyperosmolar conditions in the kidney favor sickling.	In the first decasde of life, this results in a loss of urine concentrating ability and increased total urine output (with enuresis in some cases), but total kidney function is normal. Serum creatinine is below normal because of increased glomerular filtration from cardiac output. In the second and third decades of life chronic sickling can result in impairment of kidney function. Creatinine rises to "normal" levels, indicating worsening of kidney function. Serum albumin fall, and proteinuria is common.	Monitor serum creatinine and urinalysis. Counsel parents that enuresis is the result of SCD, not the child's fault. Help parents develop strategies to cope. Continue to encourage fluids; dehydration causes hyperosmolarity and further sickling. Refer to nephrology for rising creatinine with proteinuria. Transplant may be indicated and patients with SCD are good transplant candidates.
Cholelithiasis	RBC hemolysis increases bilirubin production, resulting in gallstones, composed of desiccated bile and in 60% of cases calcium bilirubin. Gallstones occur in 14% of children under 10 years, 30% of adolescents and 75% of adults by 30 years of age.	Common symptoms include nausea, vomiting, and RUQ pain or diffuse abdominal pain.	Refer for surgical evaluation in consultation with SCD center. Treatment is elective cholecystectomy.

Table 45-37 Disabling Problems in Sickle Cell Disease—cont'd

COMPLICATION	PATHOPHYSIOLOGY	SIGNS AND SYMPTOMS	MANAGEMENT
Avascular necrosis of femoral head	Sickled cells block the circulation to bones resulting in avascular necrosis and subsequent collapse of the femoral head. Similar pathophysiologic problems can occur in the shoulder.	Limitation in range of motion Pain with weight-bearing in the hip or referred pain to back or leg. Venous stasis ulcers.	Rest, no weightbearing. NSAIDs. Surgical decompression. Total joint replacement is only an option after skeletal maturity is achieved to avoid leg-length discrepancy.
Leg ulcers	Sickling increases in distal areas of the body, which have relatively lower oxygen tension and temperature. Leg ulcers occur because of circulatory insufficiency, most commonly around the ankles and in males more often than females. Risk increases in the late teens into adulthood. Persons with low baseline hemoglobin (< 7 g/dl) are at higher risk.		Refer to SCD center for wound care. Skin grafting, Unna's boot, hyperbaric oxygen therapy, and transfusions may all be used to promote healing.
Infection	Spleen is the primary site of immune response in the child under 2 or 3 years of age. Sickled cells block circulation to spleen, causing small infarcted areas resulting in functional asplenia. SCD patients have impaired opsonization (surrounding and engulfing foreign bacteria) and reduced antibody synthesis in response to intravenous antigens, which causes a life-long vulnerability to infection (serum antibody response to killed and live vaccines is normal). Children from 6 months to 3 years with SCD are 400 times more likely to become infected by *S. pneumoniae* and 2 times more likely to become infected by *H. influenzae.*	Fever, usually, but not exclusively over 101.5° F.	Monitor and treat signs of sepsis or shock. Fever 101.5° F in the child with SCD is an emergency requiring sepsis work-up (blood, urine cultures, possible CSF culture by spinal tap, stool culture if diarrhea is present). However, fever below 101.5° F may be a sign of early sepsis; observation over 2 or 3 hours often demonstrates a rising temperature, the hallmark of sepsis. Remind parents to avoid antipyretics because these may mask fever. Refer to SCD center or emergency department for IV administration of antibiotics to children with suspected sepsis that are effective against *H. influenzae* and *S. pneumoniae;* usually cefuroxime, or ampicillin sulbactam (Unasyn). *Antibiotic administration should not be delayed even to obtain cultures.* An alternative to hospitalization is observation in the emergency department with homecare and outpatient follow-up visits. This is appropriate in children with SCD over 2 to 3 years of age who are febrile yet who look well and have remained stable in the emergency department for 6 to 8 hours after blood cultures are obtained and one IV dose of antibiotics is received. Further, the family must be reliable in giving oral antibiotics and revisiting the PCP or SCD center the following day. Cultures should be checked at this visit along with a careful PE
Aplastic crisis	Parvovirus B19 (fifth disease) causes brief (about 1 to 2 weeks) aplastic crisis (no production of RBCs) in normal persons. In persons with chronic hemolytic anemia, a profound (Hgb = 2) anemia, and reticulocytopenia (low reticulocyte count, new blood cell count) can occur during even brief periods of RBC aplasia. Anemia may be so severe that congestive heart failure results.	Paleness Lethargy Pallor	Obtain CBC with reticulocyte count. A low reticulocyte count is unusual in SCD patients, who should have an elevated reticulocyte count to compensate for chronic hemolytic anemia. A normal reticulocyte count in a SCD patient with flu-like symptoms may be an early sign of aplastic crisis. Refer to SCD center or closest emergency department for management with packed RBCs. Avoid large volumes of fluid because cardiac failure from hemodilution can occur.

A chemistry screen should be performed at least yearly with urinalysis. Pay careful attention to the serum creatinine and urine protein. Children with SCD should have low creatinine; a normal creatinine may be a sign of early kidney disease. Likewise, elevation of urinary protein may also herald early kidney disease. Both a "normal" creatinine (above 0.9) and presence of urinary protein should prompt consultation with the SCD center or pediatric nephrologist and with assessment of 24-hour urine for creatinine and protein as a first-line evaluation. Liver function should be normal in SCD. However, an elevated GGT could indicate biliary tract obstruction or be a sign of hemolysis.

Common medical problems with SCD include:

- Potentially life-threatening complications (see Table 45-36).
- Potentially disabling complications (see Table 45-37).
- Pain (Table 45-38). The diagnosis of vaso-occlusive crisis (VOC, also known as *pain crisis*) is made based on

history; it is ultimately a diagnosis of exclusion. Sickled cells can block circulation to any bone, muscle, or organ in the body. Decreased circulation causes a vicious cycle of ischemia and pain and further sickling. Recall that there is no clinical or laboratory test to "confirm" a painful episode. VOC has a waxing and waning quality and may last for hours to days or weeks. Fever may accompany VOC; however, sepsis should be assumed until proved otherwise by blood culture and clinical improvement of the patient. Pain may occur as infrequently as once every few years and not require hospital admission (in about one third of patients) or as often as twice or more per month, requiring hospital admission. Failure to rule out all other potential causes of pain can result in inappropriate treatment. For example, headaches may result from sinusitis, tension, migraines, or meningitis. Abdominal pain (see Abdominal Pain in Chapter 35) may be caused by gall-

Table 45-38 Common Pain States Associated with Sickle-Cell Disease

PAIN STATES	CLINICAL SIGNS AND SYMPTOMS	SIGNS AND UNDERLYING CAUSE	SPECIAL FEATURES OR CONSIDERATIONS
Acute painful event	Sudden onset Pain in any and all parts of body	Vaso-occlusion Endothelial damage Inflammation	Unpredicatable, recurrent Great variability All ages
Acute hand-foot syndrome (dactylitis)	Painful dorsal swelling of hands and feet	Symmetrical infarcts of metacarpal and metatarsal bones because of obstruction of developing blood vessels	More common in childhood Often first manifestation of disease (occuring as early as 6 months of age)
Acute inflammation of joints	Painful swollen joints	Vaso-occlusion or injury Inflammation Infected joints	May accompany dactylitis Acute flare-ups as isolated events May involve disease of endothelium
Acute chest syndrome	Chest pain, particularly rib and substernal area Chest pain posteriorly (upper back) Fever, tachypnea, or hypoxia	Pulmonary infiltrates May be associated with infarction or infection Unilateral pain (splinting from atelectasis)	May require exchange transfusion and can be fatal Common cause of mortality in children and adults
Splenic sequestration	Left upper-quadrant pain Noticeable pallor Sudden decrease in hemoglobin concentration Enlarged spleen	Blood trapped in the spleen	Can be catastrophic in young children, with possibility of circulatory collapse Insidious onset in adults Occurs in older children and adults with HbSC and sickle β-thalassemia
Intrahepatic sickling or hepatic sequestration	Right upper-quadrant pain Sudden decrease in hemoglobin Enlarged liver	Blood pooling in the liver	Occurs more commonly in adults
Abdominal and intraabdominal pain	Jaundice	Cholelithiasis Splenic infarction	Can be intial manifestation of acute chest syndrome
Priapism	Painful erection	Sickling in sinusoids of penis	May last for a few hours (acute and brief) to days (acute and prolonged) or may be chronic or stuttering (intermittent)
Avascular necrosis of femur or humerus	Prolonged, constant bone pain Shoulder pain Knee pain Hip pain	Associated with bone infarction, sickle arthritis	Physical therapy may be useful for reducing pain and maintaining function
Chronic-neuorpathic pain	Pain in back Spontaneous Lancinating	Older adults: Disk disease, infections Collapsed vertebrae Iron-overload neuropathy	Often not considered in sickle-cell disease

From American Pain Society. (1999). Glenview, IL.

stones, appendicitis, renal stones, cystitis, or tubal pregnancy. VOC may be precipitated by hypoxia, infection, fever, acidosis, dehydration, exposure to extreme cold, anxiety, depression, and physical exhaustion. Often no precipitating event can be found.

Primary Care Issues and Implications

- *Well-child visits with the PCP*—Children with SCD should see the PCP at standard intervals for routine well-child care and, especially, immunizations.
- *Dental care*—Routine dental care is most important for children with SCD because of their susceptibility to infection. There is no contraindication to nitrous oxide (in fact, this decreases sickling) or local anesthetics, including those with epinephrine. The use of prophylactic antibiotics is controversial and should be decided in consultation with the SCD center.
- *Sexuality*—Adolescents with SCD usually have normal fertility and normal sexuality. Sexual development may lag behind by a year or more. This can be worrisome to both children and parents. Reassurance should be given that sexual development will proceed normally, even if it starts later than expected.
- *Menstruation*—Teens with SCD are quite able to distinguish sickle-related pain from dysmenorrhea and usually report that the latter as less painful. Menorrhagia is quite uncommon and should be evaluated in consultation with an adolescent medicine specialist and the SCD center, the staff of which can evaluate for a concomitant bleeding problem.
- *Immunizations*—These children require the same immunizations as other children, as outlined by the AAP. Of particular importance is Prevnar, the 7-valent (heptavalent) conjugated pneumococcal vaccine (PCV7), because children with SCD are especially vulnerable to pneumococcal infections as a result of their decreased splenic function. Since Prevnar is standard for all infants, older children should be considered for immunization in consultation with the SCD center. Additionally, in SCD, children should receive the 23-valent polysaccharide pneumococcal vaccine at 2 years of age and every 5 years thereafter. This provides broader, if somewhat less effective protection against pneumococcal infections. If splenectomy is planned, children should receive a dose of meningococcal vaccine, in addition to the above, at least 2 weeks preoperatively. Care should be taken to assess whether older children have had a dose of Hib vaccine after 18 months of age.
- *Nutrition*—A well-balanced diet is important to support normal growth and development and to meet the increased demands of the disease. However, parents should be cautioned not to place too many demands around this issue. The child with SCD will go through the same appetite fluctuation and picky eating habits as other children. Nutritional needs are best met by offering a variety of foods and allowing the child to choose what and how much he or she will eat. Because hydration is particularly important for children with SCD, noncaffeinated beverages that the child enjoys should be readily available and encouraged. A children's chewable multiple vitamin tablet can help provide for minimum dietary needs. However, high doses of supplemental iron should be avoided because iron overload can result, especially if intermittent or routine blood transfusions are required. If iron deficiency is suspected, testing should be done to document this (total iron binding capacity [TIBC], serum iron, and ferritin; see Chapter 36) before therapy is begun (one and two α-globin gene deletions are common in children with SCD, and these can cause mild microcytosis, which can mimic the microcytosis seen in iron deficiency). If a child's weight and height fall below the 5th percentile for age, or if the child crosses percentiles downward on the growth curve, a dietary supplement such as Pediasure or Resource can be given.

- *Safety*—Children with SCD have normal coagulation. Standard age-appropriate safety precautions are adequate.
- *Sleep*—Since children with SCD are usually anemic, enlarged tonsils with snoring can cause large drops in pulse-oximetry during sleep. Question the family about snoring at each visit, especially if tonsils are large, and refer snorers with SCD to the SCD center for evaluation for tonsillectomy.
- *Discipline*—During infancy, distraction is often the only way to manage unwanted behavior. Physical discipline is inappropriate for all children, while excellent supervision is important for all children at all ages. The importance of age-appropriate and consistent discipline among all the children at home, including age-appropriate chores, and encouragement of age-appropriate independence in self-care should be stressed. Children with SCD are more similar to their siblings in terms of their need for discipline than they are different. Parenting a child with a chronic illness and walking the fine line between unnecessary restriction and fostering independence is a topic for discussion at every clinic visit.
- *Exercise*—Exercise tolerance is highly individual, but participation in group activity is critical to self-esteem. Children with SCD should be encouraged to participate in activities to their level of tolerance and allowed to rest when tired or out of breath.
- *School issues*—Excellent education is a foundation for success in adult life. Encourage daily reading and participation in learning experiences within the family. Communication with school staff is critical to the child's success at school. School staff need to be aware of the child's need for hydration, access to bathroom facilities, pain management during the school day, decreased activity tolerance (with possible needs for gymnasium exemption and an elevator pass), and transportation. The school nurse needs to be aware of the need to report to the SCD center any fever over 101.5° F, chest pain, abdominal pain, or signs of stroke. Investigate the availability of intermittent homebound instruction for chronically ill children; at the very least, at the beginning of every school year, establish a makeup plan for school work missed because of illness.
- *Growth*—Children with SCD, especially SS, may be shorter and weigh less than other children their age as a result of the increased caloric requirements of heightened RBC production.
- Development
  Infants—As with many chronic illnesses, parents experience the "death" of their "perfect child." Generally, SCD does not interrupt normal developmental milestones in infancy.
  Toddlers and preschoolers—Parents must be encouraged to use positive reinforcement rather than punitive

disciplinary methods and to encourage their children to develop a sense of independence and competence despite their illness. Children with SCD may not tolerate play outside in very cold weather. Likewise, they may not tolerate swimming in cool water. Parents must learn how their individual child responds to these stressors and plan activities accordingly. Children with SCD toilet train at similar ages to their siblings without SCD. However, enuresis is a common problem, even after achievement of nighttime dryness at 2 to 4 years of age, because of sickle cell–related kidney changes causing hyposthenuria and blunting of the normal diurnal variation in urine output. New or refractory enuresis is quite distressing to families. Table 45-37 provides a discussion of potentially disabling problems.

School-age children—Parents may experience denial, anger (e.g., toward the child, health care staff, each other, teachers, siblings), fear, and helplessness. These are typical responses to grief and loss in the initial stages but, over time, they may lead to chronic sorrow. School performance is often unaffected unless absences are frequent. Growth delay may cause decreased feelings of self-worth. Because of decreased exercise tolerance, children with SCD may not be able to keep up with peers (and should be allowed to rest when tired), and because of growth delay, children with SCD may be smaller and shorter than peers. As a result of frequent absences from school, children with SCD may fall behind, resulting in illiteracy and feelings of inadequacy in school. Other school problems may result if school staff do not understand that children with SCD must be allowed to drink water during the school day and allowed frequent access to the bathroom.

Adolescents—Some adolescents deny their SCD and exhibit "testing" behavior by refusing to seek anticipatory or preventive medical care. Delay in achieving secondary sex characteristics may affect self-esteem. Scleral icterus, in the face of normal liver function studies, can be a troubling cosmetic problem.

Management

Life-threatening or suspected life-threatening complications should be managed by referral to an SCD center (see Tables 45-36 and 45-37). Further, the patient and the NP must have a working relationship with an SCD center, which can provide as-needed guidance in the evaluation and treatment of complications and act as a resource for prevention of complications. Both excellent medical care and excellent patient and family education are critical to the lifetime success of affected individuals.

Treatments and medications

Antibiotic prophylaxis. Twice-daily penicillin for children from 2 months to 5 years of age (longer if history of documented pneumococcal sepsis) reduces this risk to that of the normal populations. Prophylactic penicillin does not reduce bacterial nasopharyngeal colonization, but it does prevent bacteremia and tissue invasion even in the face of continued nasopharyngeal carriage or reexposure. Liquid penicillin must be refrigerated for no more than 2 weeks, after which it loses potency. Dosages are Pen VK 125 mg twice a day for children 2 months to 3 years of age and Pen VK 250 mg twice a day for children 3 to 5 years of age

In coordination with the SCD center, erythromycin may be substituted for children with documented penicillin allergies.

Amoxicillin 250-mg chewable tablets may be also substituted for Pen VK 250 mg and has the advantage of not requiring refrigeration.

Folic acid. Although it is reasonable to give 1 mg of folic acid daily to children with hemolytic anemias like SCD to assist with formation of new RBCs, there is no conclusive documentation that this practice improves outcome. Certainly this practice is not harmful and may be undertaken by motivated families. The tablet may be crushed and mixed with applesauce in younger children or simply chewed by older children.

Hydroxyurea. A form of chemotherapy, hydroxyurea (HU) allows the bone marrow to make more fetal hemoglobin, which does not sickle. Adults with two or more VOC episodes per year are good candidates for HU therapy, and, of these, about two thirds to three fourths find the drug clinically beneficial in reducing VOC. Patients must be reliable about taking medication and coming in for visits for monitoring of serum chemistry, urinalysis, and CBC as directed by the SCD center. Children with frequent pain may also be good candidates and should be referred to the SCD center for initiation of HU therapy. Growth should be carefully monitored while the child is receiving HU therapy. However, most adolescents and adults tend to gain weight, possibly from feeling better. Expect mean cell volume (MCV) to rise (over 100 fl) initially and hemoglobin to rise after 3 months of therapy. The clinical benefit (in contrast to the hematologic response) may take 3 or more months to become evident. Folic acid supplementation is indicated when HU therapy is being followed. In coordination with SCD center, Actigall can be given for cosmetic reasons if a patient is bothered by frequent scleral icterus.

Pain. Pain is now the fifth vital sign. Assess pain with age-appropriate scales. Nonpharmacologic management of mild to moderate pain at home involves rest, oral fluids, application of heat, warm compresses, massage (if tolerated), age-appropriate distractions (e.g., pacifier, games, music, television, relaxation techniques), and any other supportive measures the child and family find helpful. However, the cornerstone of pain management is the stepwise use of pharmacologic agents.

1. Mild pain in SCD can be treated with acetaminophen (at 10 to 15 mg/kg per dose every 4 hours) or an NSAID such as ibuprofen (at 10 mg/kg per dose every 6 hours). These agents may be alternated or used together. Parents should be cautioned to measure temperature before giving either acetaminophen or ibuprofen so that fever is not masked. NSAIDs should be used with caution in children with renal impairment and always administered with food to prevent gastric irritation.

2. A weak opioid such as codeine may be added to acetaminophen and ibuprofen (1 to 2 mg/kg per dose of codeine).

3. Acetaminophen or NSAIDs may be given with a potent opioid such as morphine, often in long-acting formulation to improve patient's day-to-day function by preventing the peaks and valleys in analgesia common with the short-acting opioids. The SCD center should be involved in the treatment of pain that is unresponsive to steps 1 and 2. The most common drug given with VOC is intravenous morphine, given slow intravenous push or dripped over 10 to 20 minutes.

Common side effects of this regimen include severe itching, which can be managed with Benadryl (diphenhydramine), and constipation, which can be managed by the usual means (e.g., stool softeners, laxatives). Analgesia must be balanced against side effects (e.g., sedation, nausea, pruritus). During acute pain, administer analgesics around the clock with appropriate frequency (based on the drug's pharmacology and route of administration). Drugs such as NSAIDs and acetaminophen have dosage ceilings, meaning higher doses do not produce additional relief. However, opioids often need to be titrated to higher than common doses to produce relief in SCD patients. SCD patients metabolize drugs faster and more efficiently than non-SCD patients because of their anemia and resulting increased cardiac output, which causes an increased glomerular filtration rate (GFR) in the kidneys and increased hepatic blood flow and hepatic clearance.

Counseling and prevention

- Refer to an SCD center for initial disease education, which includes SCD pathophysiology, inheritance, and management. Good communication is essential between the center staff and NP so that the family receives consistent information and appropriate reinforcement from the NP about SCD. Most states in the United States routinely screen all newborns for hemoglobinopathies, including SCD, to facilitate early referral to an SCD center for education and treatment with twice-daily penicillin (greatly reducing mortality and morbidity from pneumococcal disease, which can affect infants as young as 4 months of age). Many persons at risk do not know their hemoglobin trait status, particularly those of ethnic groups in whom the sickle trait is less prevalent.

- At visits to both the SCD center and the PCP, remember that children should be taught about SCD and their own care needs as they grow in age-appropriate language and content.

- Teach teenagers the pathophysiology and rational for management of SCD in anticipation of taking on responsibility for their health care as adults.

- Keep in mind the importance of penicillin administration in children with SCD under 5 years of age cannot be overstated. Parents must be warned to refill medications regularly and not to allow prescriptions to lapse.

- Teach parents of children with SS or sickle β^0-thalassemia under 7 years of age the spleen palpation technique. The family should be instructed to palpate the abdomen daily (in the context of morning or evening care to be helpful) as a baseline test and more often if the child is ill or complaining of abdominal pain. Alterations in baseline values should be reported to the SCD center immediately or the child brought to the nearest emergency room. With SS and sickle β^0-thalassemia, after 7 years of age the risk of ASSC drops significantly and daily palpation is no longer necessary. However, children with SC or sickle β^+-thalassemia have a risk of an enlarged spleen even into adolescence. Although this is not usually life-threatening, alterations should be reported to the SCD center.

- Avoid using ibuprofen and acetaminophen for fever. All fever, regardless of source, needs to be reported to the SCD center. Parents should check OTC cold medications carefully because some contain acetaminophen or ibuprofen, which could mask the presence of fever.

- Encourage extra fluid intake. Parents should be taught about the risks of dehydration (which enhances sickling) and high urine output (because of changes in the kidneys) in SCD, which necessitate extra fluid intake.

- Avoid temperature extremes. Temperature extremes can enhance sickling and lead to vasoocclusive episodes.

Swimming may be well tolerated in a heated pool, particularly if the child changes to dry clothing immediately afterward. In winter, layered clothing is best.

- Regarding out-of-home care, remember that group day care is not specifically contraindicated. However, children in group day care tend to have more frequent febrile illnesses, which could result in more frequent hospitalizations for the child with SCD. In general, a small setting may result in fewer exposures to infection. Parents should be cautioned to keep immunizations up to date. Caregivers need to be educated by the parents about general issues in SCD, including reporting suspected fever, pain symptoms, paleness, or any other unusual finding immediately to the parents.

- Encourage healthy psychosocial development. Teach the family to view the child as a healthy person with a chronic medical problem rather than as a sick child. Children with chronic illnesses are vulnerable to being viewed as weak, helpless, or inadequate, and such a view fosters helplessness and poor self-esteem. The role of "sick child" is disabling and can become a refuge used to avoid coping with difficulties in school, at home, and among peers. Children should be encouraged to think of SCD as one facet of their lives but not their whole identity.

- Encourage positive coping with illness. Encourage families to develop a plan to manage home responsibilities (including the needs of siblings) during a child's hospitalization. Parents should be encouraged to keep a bag packed (just as is advised for prenatal care) for themselves and for their child in case hospitalization is required. Teach parents that although VOC is often called a "crisis," the medical definition is simply "sudden onset"; parents often assume crisis means "life-threatening."

- Discuss age-appropriate discipline.

- Advise that SCD patients should avoid travel in unpressurized aircraft above 10,000 feet and to mountainous areas above 10,000 feet. (Normal individuals may experience altitude sickness in these circumstances; thus the risk of sickling is increased). Standard pressurized aircraft present no difficulty to SCD patients.

- Keep in mind that both parents of children with SCD and adolescents with SCD should receive genetic counseling to fully appreciate their risk of having children with SCD.

- Address exercise.

- Address school issues.

Follow-up

- Routine care at a SCD Center should occur at diagnosis and every 3 to 12 months thereafter depending on the child's clinical course.

- Follow-up care for hospitalizations can occur with the NP or at the SCD center, depending on the specific reason for hospitalization.

- Afebrile children with painful episodes can be managed at home with oral medications under telephone guidance by the SCD center or NP.

Consultations and referrals

- Remember that annual eye examinations by an experienced ophthalmologist are needed beginning at 10 years of age. Hyphema, or acute loss of vision from hemorrhage in the anterior chamber, in SCD and sickle trait is an ophthalmologic emergency requiring immediate intervention by an ophthalmologist because of the risk of developing elevated intraocular pressure, even if only small amounts of blood are present.

- Refer children with hypertension, proteinuria, or creatinine at "normal" levels (over 0.8 mg/dl).
- Refer for poor school performance, lagging developmental milestones, or history of stroke. Neuropsychologic testing can form the baseline for monitoring neurologic change and the foundation for intervention in the school setting.
- Refer for surgery any children with cholelithiasis or poor venous access who may require infusion port placement.
- Keep in mind that children with SCD who will undergo general anesthesia require a consultation with the SCD center for perioperative planning. To prevent sickling complications postoperatively, children with SCD need to have a hemoglobin greater than 10 g/dl on the day of their procedure (even if this would require a blood transfusion) and prophylactic intravenous hydration for a few hours preoperatively. If baseline hemoglobin is greater than 10 g/dl, transfusion may not be necessary. The timing of transfusion and monitoring for iron overload requires coordination with the SCD center.
- Refer to the local chapter of the National Association for Sickle Cell Disease for family support and community advocacy.

Resources

Websites
American Academy of Pediatrics Policy Statement on Health Supervision for Children with Sickle Cell Disease and their Families (www.aap.org/policy/01564.html)

American Pain Society (www.ampainsoc.org)

City of Hope Pain Resource Center, Nursing Research and Education (www.mayday.coh.org/_private/frbanner_new.htm)

International Association of Sickle Cell Nurses and Physician Assistants (IASCNAPA): (www.emory.edu/PEDS/SICKLE/parnpage.htm)

Joint Center for Sickle Cell Disease and Thalassemia (www.sickle.bwh.harvard.edu/menu_sickle.html)

National Heart, Lung and Blood Institute: Sickle Cell Disease (www.nhlbi.nih.gov/health/prof/blood/sickle/sick-mt.htm)

Sickle Cell Advocates for Research and Empowerment, Inc. (www.defiers.com)

Sickle Cell Disease Association of America (www.sicklecelldisease.org)

The Sickle Cell Information Center at the Georgia Comprehensive Sickle Cell Center at Grady Health System (www.emory.edu/PEDS/SICKLE/)

Texas Department of Health-Sickle Cell Disease (www.tdh.state.tx.us/newborn/sickle.htm)

Bibliography

Agertoft, L. & Pederson, S. (2000). Effect of long-term treatment with inhaled budesonide on adult height in children with asthma. *New England Journal of Medicine, 343,* 1064-1069.

AIDS Institute, New York State Department of Health (1995; updated 1997). *Criteria for the care of children and adolescents with HIV infection.* New York: New York State Department of Health.

American Academy of Pediatrics (2000). Human immunodeficiency virus infection. In Pickering, L.K. (Ed.). *2000 Red book: Report of the Committee on Infectious Diseases* (25th ed.). Elk Grove Village, IL: American Academy of Pediatrics.

American Academy of Pediatrics (2000). Type 2 diabetes in children and adolescents. *Pediatrics, 105*(3), 671-680.

American Academy of Pediatrics (1999). *Pediatric human immunodeficiency virus (HIV) infection: A compendium of AAP guidelines on pediatric HIV infection.* Elk Grove Village, IL: American Academy of Pediatrics.

American Academy of Pediatrics (1996). Health supervision for children with sickle cell diseases and their families. *Pediatrics, 98*(3), 467-472.

American Diabetes Association (2000). Consensus statement: Type 2 diabetes in children and adolescents. *Diabetes Care, 23*(3), 381-397.

American Diabetes Association. (2001). Standards of medical care for patients with diabetes mellitus. *Diabetes Care, 24*(Suppl 1).

American Diabetes Association (1999). Epidemiology of diabetes interventions and complications (EDIC): Design, implementation, and preliminary results of a long-term follow-up of the Diabetes Control and Complications Trial cohort. *Diabetes Care, 22*(1), 99-111.

American Diabetes Association (1999). Screening for type 2 diabetes. *Diabetes Care, 22*(1S), 20S-23S.

American Pain Society (1999). *Guidelines for the management of acute and chronic pain in sickle cell disease.* Glenview, IL: American Pain Society.

Anderson, S.D. & Daviskas, E. (2000). The mechanism of exercise-induced asthma is.... *Journal of Allergy Clinical Immunology, 106,* 453-459.

Armstrong, D.S., Grimwood, K., Carlin, J.B., et al. (1997). Lower airway inflammation in infants and young children with cystic fibrosis. *American Journal of Respiratory and Critical Care Medicine, 156,* 1197-1204.

Ball, T.M., Castro-Rodríguez, J.A., Griffith, K.A., Holberg, C.J., Martínez, F.D., &

Wright, A.L. (2000). Siblings, day-care attendance, and the risk of asthma and wheezing during childhood. *New England Journal of Medicine, 343,* 538-543.

Barnes, P.J. (2000). New directions in allergic diseases: Mechanism-based anti-inflammatory therapies. *Journal of Allergy and Clinical Immunology, 106,* 5-16.

Beyer, J.E., Simmons, L.E., Woods, G.M., & Woods, P.M. (1999). A chronology of pain and comfort in children with sickle cell disease. *Archives of Pediatric and Adolescent Medicine, 153,* 913-920.

Boat, T.M. (2000). Cystic fibrosis. In Behrman, R.E., Kliegman, R.M., & Jenson, H.B. (Eds.). *Nelson textbook of pediatrics* (16th ed.). New York: W.B. Saunders.

Bousquet, J., Jeffrey, P.K., Busse, W., Johnson, M., & Vignola, A.M. (2000). Asthma. *American Journal or Respiratory and Critical Care Medicine, 161,* 1720-1745.

Busse, W.W. & Lemanske, R.F. (2001). Advances in immunology: Asthma. *New England Journal of Medicine, 344,* 350-362.

Centers for Disease Control and Prevention. (2000). *Diabetes projects: Children and diabetes.* Available online at www.cdc.gov/diabetes/projects/cda2.htm.

Centers for Disease Control and Prevention (1999). *HIV/AIDS Surveillance Report, 11*(2); 12(1).

Centers for Disease Control and Prevention (1998). Guidelines for the use of antiretroviral agents in pediatric HIV infection. *Morbidity and Mortality Weekly Report, 47*(RR-4), 1-43.

Centers for Disease Control and Prevention (1998). *National diabetes fact sheet 1998.* Available online at www.cdc.gov/diabetes/pubs/facts98.htr.

Centers for Disease Control and Prevention (199?). *HIV/AIDS Surveillance Supplemental Report, 7*(1).

Cystic Fibrosis Foundation (2000, August). *Patient registry annual data report 1999.* Bethesda, MD: Cystic Fibrosis Foundation.

Department of Health and Human Services (2000). *Action against asthma.* Washington, DC: Office of Science Policy.

Dershewitz, R. (1999). *Ambulatory pediatric care* (3rd ed.). Philadelphia: Lippincott-Raven.

Di Sant'Agnese, P.A. & Hubbard, V.S. (1984). The gastrointestinal tract. In Taussig, L.M. (Ed.). *Cystic fibrosis*. New York: Thieme-Stratton.

DiMichele, D. & Neufeld, E.J. (1998). Hemophilia: A new approach to an old disease. *Hematology/Oncology Clinics of North America, 12*(6), 1315-1344.

Ewenstein, B.M. (1997). Von Willebrand's disease. *Annual Review of Medicine, 48,* 525-542.

FitzSimmons, S.C., Burkhart, G.A., Borowitz, D., et al. (1997). High dose pancreatic enzyme supplements and fibrosing colonopathy in children with cystic fibrosis. *New England Journal of Medicine, 336,* 1283-1289.

Gibson, L. E., & Cooke, R. E. (1959). A test for concentrations of electrolytes in sweat in cystic fibrosis of the pancrease utilizing pilocarpine iontophoresis. *Pediatrics, 23,* 545-549.

Gonsalves, M.Y. (2000). Coordinating care for patients with type 2 diabetes. *Patient Care for the Nurse Practitioner, 3*(9), 15-17, 21-22, 25-26, 31-34.

Grant, E.N., Lyttle, C.S., & Weiss, K.B. (2000). The relation of socioeconomic factors and racial/ethnic differences in US asthma mortality. *American Journal of Public Health, 90,* 1923-1925.

Graumlic, S.E., Powers, S.W., Byars, K.C., Schwarber, L.A., Mitchell, M.J., & Kalinyak, K.A. (2001). Multidimensional assessment of pain in pediatric sickle cell disease. *Journal of Pediatric Psychology, 26*(4), 203-214.

Grothaus, K. (1998). Eating disorders and adolescents: An overview of maladaptive behavior. *Journal of Child and Adolescent Psychiatric Nursing, 11*(4), 146-150.

Harley, J.R. (1997). Disorders of coagulation misdiagnosed as nonaccidental bruising. *Pediatric Emergency Care, 13*(5), 347-349.

Hockenberry-Eaton, M.J. (Ed.). (1998). *Essentials of pediatric oncology nursing: A core curriculum.* Glenview, IL: Association of Pediatric Oncology Nurses.

Holt, P.G. & Sly, P.D. (2000). Prevention of adult asthma by early intervention during childhood: Potential value of new generation immunomodulatory drugs. *Thorax, 55,* 700-703.

Hubbard, V.S. (1985). Gastrointestinal complications in cystic fibrosis. *Seminars in Respiratory Medicine, 6*(4), 299-306.

Kerem, B.S., Rommens, J.M., Buchannan, J.A., et al. (1989). Identification of the cystic fibrosis gene: Genetic analysis. *Science, 245,* 1073-1080.

Klinehart, D., Orto, C., Gioia, K., & Hannan, M. (1997). Von Willebrand disease: A nursing Perspective. *Journal of Obstetric Gynecologic and Neonatal Nursing, 26*(3), 271-276.

Knowles, M.R. & Noone, P. (1994). Evaluation of the patient with borderline sweat test results. *Pediatric Pulmonology, 10*(Suppl), 141-142.

Langenderfer, B. (1998). Alternatives to percussion and postural drainage. *Journal of Cardiopulmonary Rehabilitation, 18,* 283-289

Linet, M.S., Ries, L.A., Smith, M.A., Tarone, R.E., & Devesa, S.S. (1999, June). Cancer surveillance series: Recent trends in childhood cancer incidence and mortality in the United States. *Journal of the National Cancer Institute, 91*(12), 1051-1058.

Lusher, J.M. (1996). Screening and diagnosis of coagulation disorders. *American Journal of Obstetrics and Gynecology, 175*(3), 778-783.

Mannino, D.M., Homa, D.M., Pertowski, C.A., et al. (1998). Surveillance for asthma—United States, 1960-1995. *Morbidity Mortality Weekly Report, 47*(SS-1), 1-28.

Marshall, B.C. & Samuelson, W.M. (1998). Basic therapies in cystic fibrosis: Does standard therapy work? *Clinics in Chest Medicine, 19,* 487-504.

Martínez, F.D. (1999). Maturation of immune responses at the beginning of asthma. *Journal of Allergy and Clinical Immunology, 103,* 355-361.

Martínez, F.D., Stern, D.A., Wright, A.L., Taussig, L.M., & Halonen, M. (1998). Differential immune responses to acute lower respiratory illness in early life and subsequent development of persistent wheezing and asthma. *Journal of Allergy and Clinical Immunology, 102,* 915-920.

Miller, S.T., Sleeper, LA., Pegelow, C.H., et al. (2000). Prediction of adverse outcomes in children with sickle cell disease. *New England Journal of Medicine, 342*(2), 83-89.

Murphy, T.M. & Rosenstein, B.J. (1995, October). *Cystic fibrosis lung disease: Approaching the 21st century.* Chicago: University of Chicago, Pritzker School of Medicine.

Muscari, M. (1998). Screening for eating disorders. *American Journal of Nursing, 98*(11), 18-19.

Muscari, M. (1998). Walking a thin line: Managing adolescents with anorexia and bulimia. *American Journal of Maternal Child Nursing, 23*(3), 130-141.

National Asthma Education Program Expert Panel (1997). *Expert panel report II: Guidelines for the diagnosis and management of asthma* (NIH Pub. No. 97-4051). Bethesda, MD: US Department of Health and Human Services, National Heart, Lung and Blood Institute.

Panagiotopoulos, C., McCrindle, B., Hick, K., & Katzman, D. (2000). Electrocardiographic findings in adolescents with eating disorders. *Pediatrics, 105*(5), 100-103.

Pediatric Asthma Committee (1999). *Pediatric asthma: Promoting best practice: Guide for managing asthma in children.* Rochester, NY: American Academy of Allergy Asthma & Immunology, Academic Services Consortium.

Pickering, L. (Ed.). (2000). *2000 Red book: Report of the Committee on Infectious Diseases.* Elk Grove Village, IL: American Academy of Pediatrics.

Pizzo, P. & Poplack, D. (Eds.). (1997). *Principles and practice of pediatric oncology* (3rd ed.). Philadelphia: J.B. Lippincott.

Pizzo, P.A. (1998). *Pediatric AIDS: The challenge of HIV infection in infants, children and adolescents* (3rd ed.). Baltimore: Williams & Wilkins.

Quinn, C.T. & Buchanan, G.R. (1999). The acute chest syndrome of sickle cell disease. *Journal of Pediatrics, 135*(4), 416-422.

Quittner, A.L. (1998). Measurement of quality of life in cystic fibrosis. *Current Opinions in Pulmonary Medicine, 4,* 326-331.

Robinson, M.R. (1999). There is no shame in pain: Coping and functional ability in adolescents with sickle cell disease. *Journal of Black Psychology, 25*(3), 336-355.

Rodgers, G.M. (1999). Overview of platelet physiology and laboratory evaluation of platelet function. *Clinical Obstetrics and Gynecology, 42*(2), 349-359.

Rommens, J.M., Ianuzzi, M.C., Kerem, B.S., et al. (1989). Identification of the cystic fibrosis gene: Chromosome walking and jumping. *Science, 245,* 1059-1065.

Rosenbloom, A.L., Joe, J.R., Young, R.S., & Winter, W.E. (1999). Emerging epidemic of type 2 diabetes in youth. *Diabetes Care, 22*(2), 345-354.

Rosenstein, B.J. & Langbaum, T.S. (1984). Diagnosis. In Taussig, L.M. (Ed.). *Cystic fibrosis.* New York, NY: Thieme-Stratton.

Rubin, B.K. (1999). Emerging therapies for cystic fibrosis lung disease. *Chest, 115,* 1120-1127.

Schidlow, D.V. (1999). *A continuing medical education program on cystic fibrosis, from theory to practice.* Philadelphia: Hahneman School of Medicine.

Soucie, J. M., Nuss, R., Evatt, B., et al. (2000, July 15). Mortality among males with hemophilia: Relations with source of medical care. *Blood, 96*(2), 437-442.

Steiner, H. & Lock, J. (1998). Anorexia nervosa and bulimia nervosa: A review of the past 10 years. *Journal of the American Academy of Child and Adolescent Psychiatry, 37*(4), 352-359.

Strollerman, G.H. (1997, March). Rheumatic fever, *The Lancet, 349*(9056), 935-942.

Taub, L.F. (1998). The ADA's clinical practice recommendations in action. *American Journal of Nursing, 98*(10), 16B-16C, 16F.

Taussig, L.M. (1984). Cystic fibrosis: An overview. In Taussig, L.M. (Ed.). *Cystic fibrosis*. New York: Thieme-Stratton.

Thomas, V.J., Gruen, R., & Shu, S. (2001). Cognitive-behavioral therapy for the management of sickle cell disease pain: Identification and assessment of costs. *Ethnicity and Health, 6*(1), 59-67.

Venkateswaran, L., Wilimas, J.A., Jones, D.J., & Nuss, R. (1998). Mild hemophilia in children: Prevalence, complications, and treatment. *Journal of Pediatric Hematology/Oncology, 20*(1), 32-35.

Vichinsky, E.P., Styles, L.A., Colangelo, L.H., Wright, E.C., Castro, O., Nickerson, B., & the Cooperative Study of Sickle Cell Disease (1997). Acute chest syndrome in sickle cell disease: clinical presentation and course. *Blood, 89*(5), 1787-1792.

Welsh, M., Tsui, L.C., Boat, T.E., & Beaudet, A.L. (1995) Cystic fibrosis. In Scriver, C.R., Beaudet, A.L., & Valle, D. (Eds.). *The metabolic basis of inherited disease* (3rd ed.) (vol. 3). New York: McGraw-Hill.

Weiss, K.B., Sullivan, S.D., & Lyttle, C.S. (2000). Trends in the cost of illness for asthma in the United States, 1985-1994. *Journal of Allergy and Clinical Immunology, 106,* 493-499.

Wethers, D.L. (2000). Sickle cell disease in childhood: Part I. Laboratory diagnosis, pathophysiology and health maintenance. Part II. Diagnosis and treatment of major complications and recent advances in treatment. *American Family Physician, 62*(5), 1013-1020, 1027-1028; 62(6), 1309-1014.

Wierenga, K.J.J., Hambleton, I.R., & Lewis, N.A. (2001). Survival estimates for patients with homozygous sickle-cell disease in Jamaica: A clinic-based population study. *Lancet, 357,* 680-683.

Wong, D.C., Hockenbery-Eaton, M.J., Winkelstein, M., & Wilson, D. (Eds.). (2000). *Nursing care of infants and children* (6th ed.). St. Louis: Mosby.

Chapter 46 *Developmental Difficulties*

Autism, p. 841
Cerebral Palsy, p. 844
Down Syndrome, p. 850
Duchenne and Becker Muscular Dystrophy, p. 856
Learning Difficulties, p. 862
Mental Retardation, p. 867
Spina Bifida, p. 869

Autism

STEPHANIE BONNEY

Alert

Consult with or refer to a physician for the following:
- *In infants*—Poor eye contact, lack of social interest or imitation, history suggestive of infantile spasms, slowed head growth.
- *In toddlers*—Loss of previously acquired words and hand skills; self-abusive or self-stimulatory behaviors, evidence of neurocutaneous syndromes, decreased or increased response to sensory input.
- *In preschoolers or school-age children*—Loss of previously acquired language, failure to use language for communication, lack of peer interactions and imaginative play.

In 1943 Leo Kanner described a group of children with extreme language disorder, extreme social isolation, and unusual responses to their environment believed to be secondary to emotional disturbance. Since that time, *autism* has become recognized as a developmental difficulty that has an underlying biologic basis. Manifestations of the disorder range from mild expression characterized by fairly subtle deviations that may be overlooked in the young child to severe impairment of function that is readily apparent. Although there may be variations in degree, three types of behavioral deviations are shared by all individuals with autism: (1) a qualitative impairment of reciprocal social interaction, (2) a qualitative impairment in the development of language and communication, and (3) a restricted range of activities and interests. The *Diagnostic and Statistical Manual of Mental Disorders, fourth edition* (DSM-IV) criteria also require that the onset is before 3 years of age. It is critical that the disorder be recognized early because there is some evidence that early intervention may make a significant difference in outcome. By 18 months of age, most parents have some concern about social language development. Diagnosis, however, is frequently not made until after 3 years of age, especially in children with milder forms of the disorder. The primary care practitioner's (PCP's) recognition of a qualitative impairment in social interaction may be the key to early identification of autism and pervasive developmental disorder (PDD).

Etiology

The cause of autism is unknown. It is clear, however, that in at least some cases there is a genetic component, with a 3% risk of recurrence in siblings of autistic children. In addition, autism may be associated with several genetic disorders, including fragile X syndrome, Rett syndrome, Williams syndrome, Möbius syndrome, tuberous sclerosis, untreated phenylketonuria (PKU), and possibly neurofibromatosis. Although prenatal problems are often reported for children who develop autism, there is no evidence that there is any causal relationship. Imaging studies, electrophysiologic studies, brain tissue, and neurochemical studies frequently show abnormalities, but no clear pattern is specifically associated with autism and PDD.

Incidence

- Autism and PDD occur in approximately 5 to 15 births per 10,000.
- An apparent increase in the number of children affected is probably the result of changing definitions of autism. Some authorities report even higher rates when the mildest cases along the spectrum are included.
- Autism is more common in boys than girls. A ratio of 3:1 to 4:1 is generally reported, but this may be even higher at the milder end of the spectrum.

Risk Factors

- Family history of autism, language deficits, psychiatric conditions such as mood disorders, and certain patterns of personality characteristics
- Prenatal factors such as prematurity, dysmaturity, bleeding in pregnancy, toxemia, maternal accidents, viral infections or exposure, and poor vigor in the neonatal period
- Encephalitis

Subjective Data

A complete history should be taken on any child suspected of having autism, with careful attention paid to the following areas:

General
- Pregnancy or birth complications (see Risk Factors)
- Newborn complications (nonspecific)
- Developmental and behavioral history

Infants. Parents may report the following:
- Infant is difficult to console or prefers self-calming activities (e.g., rocking)
- Lack of social responsiveness (i.e., eye contact, facial responsiveness, social smile)
- Failure to cuddle
- Nonspecific "mama" and "dada," with or without acquisition of two or three single words followed by a plateau in language development
- Failure to respond to name and acting as though he or she is deaf

- Failure to imitate sounds
- Failure to respond to a command, with or without a gesture
- Lack of separation anxiety, or excessive distress at separation from primary caregiver
- Failure to engage in gesture games (e.g., patty-cake, peekaboo)

Toddlers. Parents may report the following:

- Loss of fine motor skill (which may indicate a degenerative disorder)
- Lack of interest in toys, or a restricted range of interests
- Fascination with a single object such as piece of string or other small object
- Lack of pretend play or social play
- Lack of gestures, pointing, and so on
- Use of people as objects, and taking of an adult's hand to manipulate an object
- Failure to engage in joint attention (i.e., does not draw another's attention to an activity or object)
- Delayed onset of expressive language or failure to use words for communication
- Persistent use of immediate echolalia (repetition of words or phrases just heard) or delayed echolalia (use of "pat phrases" or repetition of parts of advertising jingles)
- Unusual responses to sensory stimulation (e.g., may be unresponsive to pain or may be tactilely defensive and resistant to body contact; may seek out certain sensory experiences by turning in circles or smelling things; may be unresponsive to sound or hypersensitive to noise; may show unusual attention to visual details, such as identification of logos or early recognition of letters or numbers)
- Exceptional adherence to routines or rituals
- Difficulty with transitions

Preschoolers (3 to 6 years of age). Parents may report the following:

- Speech and language delay and deviant patterns of speech
- Persistent pronoun reversal or referral to self in third person
- Unusual rhythm or intonation, speaking in singsong fashion or monotone, whispering, speaking too loudly, or sounding stilted
- Failure to initiate communication
- Failure to engage in turn-taking in conversation
- Poor language comprehension
- Carrying-on of conversations with self or reenacting of favorite video presentations (with themes repetitive and lacking original thought or imagination)
- Lack of symbolic play
- Average or precocious development in skills involving rote memory (e.g., counting without having number concepts or reading words without comprehension)
- Social withdrawal or persistence in parallel play instead of interactive play, and seeking of solitude
- Gaze avoidance
- Lack of empathy or responsiveness
- Inability to interpret others' facial expressions or tone of voice
- Perseverance on a certain topic or object of interest
- Repetitive movements such as hand flapping, rocking, and twirling

School-age children. Only atypical, mildly impaired children or those who were misdiagnosed earlier are likely to appear for diagnosis at this age. A spurt in language development may occur around 5 years of age. This phenomenon or a good response to intervention may cause the original diagnosis of autism or PDD to be questioned at this time. Although functional communication and social skills may improve, qualitative impairments remain. These children are frequently described as "aloof." Language and early academic skills may appear normal; however, there is a discrepancy between rote, memory-based skills and those requiring abstract thinking. There are also deficits in pragmatic and conversational skills. Such a child may be interested in friends but is viewed as "different" by peers. Interests are limited and may "specialize" in one area. The child may also display subtle repetitive behaviors or mannerisms.

Other things to include in the history of a child this age include any illnesses and injuries (e.g., encephalitis, head injury, seizures); a review of systems, including hearing and notation of any atypical seizures; and any family history of PDD or autism, speech delay or language deficits, mood disorders, mental retardation (MR), and individuals with mild degrees of impairment of social relatedness.

Objective Data

Physical examination. A complete physical examination should be performed with special attention to the following areas:

- *Hearing evaluation*—Be sure to include the brainstem auditory evoked response (BAER) test if behavioral audiometry is not definitive.
- *General appearance*—Note whether the child has dysmorphic features suggestive of a syndrome. (Generally, autistic children do not have dysmorphic features and are attractive, healthy-appearing youngsters.)
- *Skin*—Observe for signs of neurocutaneous disorders.
- *Neurologic system*—Rule out focal abnormalities.
- *Developmental assessment*—Keep in mind that verbal and social skills are more delayed than nonverbal problem-solving skills. Autistic children are difficult to test because they often have their "own agenda" and do not respond to the test structure. Informal assessment or having a parent present tasks may be helpful. Start with nonverbal activities. The assessment may be limited to history.
- *Behavioral assessment*—Remember that behavioral assessment requires the examiner to attempt to engage the child in interactive play (e.g., for an infant or toddler, rolling the ball, having "tea," talking on the telephone). Attempt to engage the preschooler in play with dolls or "little people" and the verbal child in conversation about various topics. Observing the child play in the waiting room may be a useful part of the assessment. Again, it may be very useful to encourage a parent to engage the child in an interactive game while the examiner observes. Several diagnostic tools are available to assist in diagnosing autism, but their usefulness in the primary care setting is limited by the need for specialized training and by time constraints.

Diagnostic procedures and laboratory tests. Perform laboratory tests as indicated. The practitioner should have a low threshold for obtaining an electroencephalogram (EEG). EEG abnormalities are present in 40% to 60% of children with autism. The most common abnormalities are diffuse or focal spikes or slowing and paroxysmal spike-and-wave activity. Clinical seizures occur in about 25% of cases. Seizures often start in childhood, but another peak is associated with puberty.

Magnetic resonance imaging (MRI) and other imaging studies often show nonspecific abnormalities but are not indicated as part of a routine evaluation. Deoxyribonucleic acid (DNA) testing for fragile X syndrome should be conducted. Chromosome studies may be considered for any child with dysmorphic features, and BAER testing should be performed if behavioral audiologic assessment is inconclusive.

Differential Diagnosis

Other conditions to consider in the differential diagnosis of PDDs depend somewhat on the child's age and overall developmental level. For those children probably manifesting autism, the category most applicable becomes the diagnostic issue. Although there are not clear lines of division, the DSM-IV criteria are most commonly used in making the diagnosis.

Also called *Kanner syndrome, early infantile autism,* or *childhood autism, autistic disorder* requires greatly impaired and disordered, not merely delayed, development in social interaction, communication, activities, and interests. A careful history usually reveals abnormalities were present by 24 months of age or earlier, but they must be manifest by 3 years of age. Most individuals with autism are also mentally retarded.

Pervasive developmental disorder not otherwise specified includes *atypical autism.* This term is used when the individual has severe impairments in the development of reciprocal social interaction, communication, or stereotypical behavior but does not meet the criteria for autistic disorder. The degree of socialization and relatedness is most often used to differentiate them. Some social interest and empathy are exhibited.

Social interaction, activities, and interests are affected in *Asperger syndrome,* but there are no significant delays in language or cognitive development. Individuals do not meet the criteria for schizophrenia.

Often children with severe *mental retardation without autism* exhibit stereotyped behaviors, emotional lability, and self-stimulatory behaviors. An additional diagnosis of autism is not indicated unless social interaction and communication are more impaired than would be expected for the child's developmental level.

When semantic and pragmatic language difficulties are severe enough to impair communication and social interaction, some authorities place *developmental language disorder* at the mildest end on the continuum of autism. The presence of echolalia, rote reciting of phrases and other auditory patterns, and reversal of pronouns may determine the decision.

Some children with *attention deficit hyperactivity disorder* (ADHD) may be rigid and overly focused at times. On the other hand, children with autism may be hyperactive and have a short attention span. These characteristics may be difficult to sort out in some children.

Nonverbal learning disorders may include difficulties with social perception and interaction but are distinguished by the overall cognitive profile and relative lack of language disability.

Emotional disturbances such as anxiety disorder, schizotypal and personality disorders, and thought disorders are distinguished from autism by the history of developmental disorder, with symptoms present in early childhood.

Only females have been diagnosed with *Rett syndrome.* Defining characteristics include deceleration of head growth, loss of previously acquired hand skills, and subsequent development of stereotyped hand movements.

Childhood disintegrative disorder is a clinically significant loss of previously acquired skills occurring after 2 years and before 10 years of age. This disorder is usually associated with severe MR.

In *Landau-Kleffner syndrome* (*acquired epileptic aphasia* in children), the onset of language problems is usually between 3 and 7 years of age. Some children exhibit psychotic behavior. The language problems may start abruptly or be insidious in nature. Clinical seizures are rare and often nocturnal. EEG abnormalities may not always be present or may occur only during sleep.

Primary Care Issues and Implications

- *Growth and development*—Physical growth is unaffected. Cognitive, language, social, and emotional development are always affected to some degree.
- *Nutrition*—Tactile sensitivity and resistance to change often make it difficult to maintain a well-balanced diet. This may result in inadequate nutrition, though growth is rarely affected.
- *Immunizations*—The regular schedule for immunizations should be followed.
- *Safety*—Behavioral characteristics and developmental delays require provision of a safe play area and increased supervision.
- *Discipline*—Children with autism are extremely difficult to manage behaviorally. Almost all parents need to periodically consult with behavioral therapists familiar with their child's special needs in this area.
- *Sexuality*—Language and developmentally delayed children are particularly vulnerable to sexual abuse. Self-stimulation in the form of masturbation may become an issue. Adolescents and young adults who have higher functioning may experience distress secondary to interpersonal skill deficits in developing intimate relationships.
- *Exercise*—There are no restrictions except those related to seizure activity. Regular safe physical activity may require planning and creative use of resources.

Management

Treatments and medications. The practitioner may provide family advocacy and case management services, especially during the initial diagnostic evaluation and determination of educational placement. Educational programming and behavioral training are the most important aspects of management.

Positive reinforcement and education are most effective in promoting growth in functional skills and shaping other behaviors. An autism specialist may be helpful in developing an individual behavior management program.

The role of medications in managing symptoms is limited. A variety of medications have had some success in selected cases. Stimulants, tricyclic antidepressants, anxiolytics, β-adrenergic receptor blockers, neuroleptics, serotonin reuptake inhibitors, dopamine receptor blockers, clozapine, risperidone, and others have been used. None of these treatments has had consistently positive effects across large groups of autistic children. Recommendations for a specific medication trials are best left to a developmental pediatrician, child psychiatrist, or neurologist experienced in the management of autistic children.

Counseling and prevention

- Provide parents and family support, especially around the initial evaluation and diagnosis. It is important to ask parents what they believe might have caused the problem to try to alleviate inappropriate feelings of guilt.
- Educate parents about the diagnostic continuum of PDDs because this is often confusing for families.

- Provide information about the special education process and services (Box 46-1). Autistic disorder is a specific disability category under the Individuals with Disabilities Education Act. Before 3 years of age, home-based early intervention programs are offered by many communities under Part H of the Education of the Handicapped Amendments.
- Discuss the issue of unconventional therapies. Facilitated communication is an alternative communication modality in which a trained "facilitator" supports the arm of the autistic child to type messages on a keyboard. Studies have demonstrated that the facilitator, though unintentionally, is the source of the communication. Use of this technique should be considered experimental. Auditory integration training is a series of lessons in which the child listens to music with specific frequencies filtered out. This also should be considered an experimental treatment.
- Review the importance of adequate nutrition. Counsel parents on creative ways to improve intake by offering a variety of foods that are acceptable and by behavior modification techniques (e.g., offering a preferred food immediately after a less desirable one). A child may have a preference for specific foods only.
- Consider the need for a multivitamin supplementation.
- Instruct parents in ways to create a safe play area. A Dutch door on a room designated as a playroom is one such option. Increased supervision and vigilance are needed as the result of general delays, lack of comprehension of danger, and frequent lack of response to the caregiver's tone of voice.
- Discuss discipline. Positive reinforcement is usually more effective than aversive action; however, finding reinforcers that motivate the autistic child is often difficult. Help parents explore the options.
- Address sexuality issues. Assess vulnerability to abuse and guide parents in appropriate prevention. Older, higher-functioning individuals may benefit from counseling regarding sexuality.
- Stress the importance of exercise. Discuss opportunities available for special needs children in the community.
- Monitor growth and level of development to provide individualized counseling throughout childhood and adolescence.

Follow-up. Perform a routine follow-up evaluation for well-child care. Reevaluation for special education is required at least every 3 years.

Consultations and referrals. Consult with the child's teacher and the school nurse regarding school programs and resources, and also refer the child to:

- A developmental pediatric interdisciplinary clinic for initial evaluation and diagnosis
- A developmental pediatrician, neurologist, or child psychiatrist for medication recommendations when indicated
- A pediatric neurologist for evaluation of possible seizures
- The child study team in the public school or a local early intervention program to explore eligibility for special education services

Refer the parents to the Autism Society of America or a local autism resource center for parental support and information.

Resources

Organizations

Autism Research Institute, 4182 Adams Avenue, San Diego, CA 92116; (619) 281-7165

Autism Society of America, 7910 Woodmont Avenue, Suite 650, Bethesda, MD 20814; (800) 3AUTISM; www.autism-society.org

Publications

The Autism handbook. (2000). London: National Autistic Society.

Box 46-1 The Special Education Process

Referral

The child is referred to the principal, guidance counselor, or special education coordinator by the parent, teacher, other school personnel, or health care provider.

Child Study Committee Meeting

The committee reviews the referral information and the student's school performance within 10 working days. The committee may then recommend the following:

- Consultations with a specialist, teachers, or other individuals working with the child
- Strategies that have not yet been tried in the classroom
- Formal evaluation (requires parent permission)

Formal assessment must be completed within 65 working days:

- Educational
- Medical (vision screen; hearing screen)
- Sociocultural
- Psychologic
- Classroom observation
- May include speech and language therapy and occupational or physical therapy

Eligibility Committee Meeting

Parents are invited to participate. The committee meets to determine if the student is eligible for special services.

Individualized Educational Plan

The committee, including the parents, must meet and complete the IEP within 30 calendar days of eligibility. The parents must sign the IEP before special education services can begin. The IEP must be reviewed and evaluated at least once each school year.

Reevaluation must be done at least every 3 years to determine progress and ongoing eligibility.

Cerebral Palsy

STEPHANIE BONNEY

Alert

Consult with or refer to a physician for the following:

Newborns

- Lethargy and irritability
- Weak, high-pitched cry
- Little interest in surroundings
- Asymmetric movements
- Feeding problems (e.g., poor suck, tongue thrust, tonic bite)
- Unusual posturing (may be floppy or hypertonic)

Older Infants

- Failure to attain motor milestones (e.g., sitting, crawling, walking)
- Poor head control

- Persistence of primitive reflexes (e.g., asymmetric tonic neck reflex, grasp, plantar, crossed extension, tonic labyrinthine reflexes)
- Asymmetry or exaggeration of primitive reflexes
- Abnormal muscle tone (e.g., hypotonia, hypertonia)
- Posturing, scissoring of the legs, plantar flexing of the feet, or opisthotonos (arching of the back with head and heels bent backwards)
- Facial grimacing or writhing movements that are not seen when the child is as rest
- Hand dominance before 1 year of age
- Microcephaly
- Fisting of hands after 3 months of age

Cerebral palsy (CP) is defined as a static, nonprogressive disorder of movement and posture caused by an injury to the central nervous system (CNS) occurring during the period of early brain development. Brain injury may occur during pre-natal development, in the perinatal period, or postnatally during the first 3 to 5 years of life.

Although the brain lesion is static, its manifestations can change over the first few years of life because of maturation of the impaired neurologic system and its expression in neuro-motor development. Any child suspected of or diagnosed with CP should be referred to a multidisciplinary team for further evaluation.

Etiology

CP can be attributed to a variety of causes occurring during the period of early brain development. Prenatal causes include drug exposures; intrauterine infections such as cytomegalic in-clusion disease (by cytomegalovirus [CMV]) and toxoplasmo-sis; maternal hypertension; placenta previa or abruptio placen-tae; and congenital brain malformations. Perinatal causes include birth trauma, hypoxia, preeclampsia, low birth weight (LBW), prematurity, postmaturity, fetal distress, and sepsis. Postnatal events associated with CP include meningitis, en-cephalitis, kernicterus, and traumatic brain injury, including that caused by child abuse.

There is a strong correlation between the development of CP and prematurity. In fact, the risk of CP increases as the birth weight decreases. In 25% to 40% of the children diagnosed with CP, the cause is unknown.

Incidence

- CP occurs in approximately 1 to 3 live births per 1000.
- The recent higher incidence of spastic diplegia is a result of the increased survival of children born prematurely.
- The recent decrease in the incidence of extrapyramidal CP is the result of the prevention of kernicterus.

Risk Factors

- Prematurity
- LBW infants
- Fetal distress
- Neonatal seizures
- Intracranial hemorrhage
- Birth asphyxia
- Birth trauma
- Intrauterine CMV
- Viruses or bacteria that infect the CNS (e.g., meningitis, encephalitis)
- Apgar scores of 3 or less at 20 minutes

- Precipitous or prolonged labor
- Kernicterus
- Meconium staining
- Acquired brain injury in children less than 3 years of age

Differential Diagnosis

Because there is no specific diagnostic test that allows one to make a firm diagnosis of CP, a thorough history is necessary to exclude closely resembling disorders. CP is a nonprogressive disorder, which also distinguishes it from the following:

- *Neurodegenerative disorders*, where there is a loss of pre-viously existing cognitive, motor, and fine motor skills
- *Mental retardation*, where delays exist in both motor and cognitive development
- *Neuromuscular disorders*, where weakness, muscle atrophy, and decreased deep tendon reflexes may exist

There is no specific diagnostic test for CP. Diagnosis may be made after a detailed history and comprehensive evaluation. Computed tomography (CT) scan of the brain may be useful in establishing the cause of CP. MRI may also help determine when the insult to the brain occurred (e.g., during prenatal de-velopment, perinatal period, postnatally).

Classification of cerebral palsy (Table 46-1). *Spastic cere-bral palsy,* the most common type of CP, implies involvement of the pyramidal tracts. In this type of CP, there is increased tone in the extremities with a characteristic clasp-knife quality as well as increased deep tendon reflexes. These characteris-tics persist even during relaxed periods of sleep and do not seem to be affected by stress or emotional change. Spastic CP is further defined by the areas of the body involved. Quadri-plegia refers to involvement of all four extremities. Spastic diplegia implies more extensive involvement in the lower ex-tremities, with mild involvement of the upper extremities. Hemiplegia refers to involvement of one side of the body only.

The other main category of CP is *extrapyramidal cerebral palsy,* referring to those tracts outside of the pyramidal system, most commonly the basal ganglia and the cerebellum. Ex-trapyramidal CP is subclassified by the quality of the muscle tone or movements. One common tone pattern in this type of CP is rigid, or "lead pipe." Rigid, or dystonic, limbs are typically difficult to put through range of motion (ROM) exercise, partic-ularly when the child is stressed or emotionally upset. Other manifestations of this type of CP include athetosis (slow writhing movements) and chorea (abrupt, involuntary movements).

Ataxic cerebral palsy is a much less common form of ex-trapyramidal CP manifested by a broad-based gait, truncal titu-bation (staggering gait), and dysmetria (inability to carry out a learned motor skill).

Often there is a mixed picture *(mixed cerebral palsy),* with the clinical examination revealing characteristics of both spas-tic and extrapyramidal involvement. This type of CP is often the result of extensive brain injury; therefore other develop-mental difficulties are often associated with the mixed subtype.

Primary Care Issues and Implications

- *Nutrition*—Failure to thrive (FTT) is often seen in children with CP. Causes may include oral motor deficits such as hypotonia, weak suck, poor coordination of swallowing mechanisms, exaggerated tongue thrust, hyperactive gag reflex, and tonic bite reflex, and inadequate access to food because of either inappropriate feeding techniques or lack of family resources. Suggest to parents the addition of food supplements to increase caloric density (Box 46-2).

Table 46-1 Types of Cerebral Palsy

CRITERIA	SPASTIC QUADRIPLEGIA	SPASTIC HEMIPLEGIA	SPASTIC DIPLEGIA	EXTRAPYRAMIDAL	ATAXIC	MIXED
Subjective Data						
Tone	Infant floppy in early months; difficulty holding infant, very rigid or stiff; difficulty changing diaper because of scissoring of legs	Child keeps one hand fisted while other remains open	Difficulty changing diaper because of scissoring of legs	Arching of back; rigidity in extremities; slow, writhing movements	Head bobbing	May include items listed under subjective data for extrapyramidal, ataxic, hemiplegic, diplegic, or quadriplegic cerebral palsy
History	Congenital malformations of the brain; intrauterine viral infections	History of traumatic brain injury	Prematurity	Kernicterus	Ataxic cerebral palsy in family members	
Feeding	Poor suck, difficulty feeding infant; difficulty handling oral secretions			Increased drooling; swallowing difficulties; tongue thrust		
Other findings	Delay in attaining developmental motor milestones, (e.g., holding up head, sitting, crawling, walking); irritability or excessive sleeping; weak cry			Involuntary movements; often abrupt; unusual facial movements, not seen when sleeping	Difficulty with balance; cognitive delays	
Objective Data						
Tone	Hypotonia in first few months of life (hypertonicity and spasticity may be evident by 1 year of age); scissoring of legs caused by tight abductors; those with spastic quadriplegia seldom walk; upper and lower extremities are affected	Increased upper extremity involvement on the affected side; posturing, fisting of the hand on the affected side; toe walking on affected side; heel cord tightening on the affected side	Increased spasticity in legs; scissoring of legs caused by tight abductors; toe walking caused by tight heel cords; upper extremities may be mildly involved	Opisthotonos; choreoathetoid movements; hypotonia in infancy followed by variable tone and athetoid movements later; upper extremities more involved than lower extremities; lead-pipe rigidity in extremities		May exhibit symptoms associated with spastic, diplegic, hemiplegic, extrapyramidal, and ataxic cerebral palsy

Neurologic	Sustained ankle clonus; nystagmus, strabismus; persistence of primitive reflexes; asymmetric tonic neck reflex, Moro reflex, tonic labyrinthine reflex, positive support; positive Babinski reflex; microcephaly	Asymmetric deep tendon reflexes, increased reflexes on the affected side; high risk for seizures, particularly focal seizures; asymmetry noted in parachute response and lateral propping; sensory deficits (e.g., astereognosis; visual field deficits)	Bilateral ankle clonus	In kernicterus: Paralysis of upward gaze, sensorineural hearing loss, tooth enamel dysplasia	Unbalanced, wide-based gait; tremor; dysmetria
Cognitive involvement	MR likelihood increases with the severity of cerebral palsy; fine motor difficulties	Decreased incidence of MR but occurrence of learning disorders, particularly in the area of perceptual difficulties			
Other	Oral motor dysfunction; contractures; dislocation of hip; scoliosis	Scoliosis		Facial grimacing (not noted when sleeping)	Associated cognitive difficulties

---

Box 46-2 Food Supplements to Increase Caloric Density

Fortified milk—Add dry milk powder (20 calories per tbsp) to whole milk to increase calories and protein.

Double-strength milk—Combine 1 qt milk and 1 cup powdered milk. This can then be added to cooked foods (e.g., mashed potatoes, cream soups), milkshakes, and other recipes that call for milk or water. Milk may also be fortified using commerical milk drinks such as Instant Breakfast or Alba.

Fat supplements—Add extra butter or margarine to foods that are offered, especially pureed ones. Add extra mayonnaise to meat salads and salad dressings.

Snacks—Snacks may include cheese and crackers, peanut butter and crackers, whole-milk yogurt, and other high-calorie items.

- *Immunizations*—In general, all immunizations should be administered according to the regular schedule.
- *Growth and development*—Growth and development are often affected, depending on the type of CP and the specific motor limitations. Routine screening tools such as the Denver II may not be adequate to assess developmental abilities (see Consultations and Referrals).
- *Seizures*—Seizure activity is present in approximately one third of children with CP, more commonly in those with spastic hemiplegia or quadriplegia. Treatment should follow the same guidelines as for other children with seizure disorders.
- *Elimination*—Constipation is often present and may be exacerbated by lack of mobility, inadequate fiber and fluid in the diet, and abnormal muscle tone affecting peristalsis. Impaction may also be present. (See Management for specific interventions.) Urinary tract infections (UTIs) are more common in children with CP because of inadequate fluid intake, more frequent constipation, and abnormal voiding patterns. Management should follow standard guidelines. The practitioner should be alert to urine with a strong odor, as well as fever with no identifiable cause.
- *Drooling*—Drooling is often present and may cause the following problems: social isolation for the school-age child, skin excoriation, wet clothing requiring frequent changes, foul odor, and discomfort. It may interfere with learning activities if a child drools on the worktable or adaptive equipment. (See Management for specific interventions.)
- *Orthopedic issues*—Increased muscle tone may cause discomfort and difficulty with daily care activities such as bathing, dressing, and positioning. Unbalanced muscle tone may also lead to such problems as hip dislocation (unilateral or bilateral), scoliosis, and contractures. Increased tone and limited mobility may lead to shortening of muscles and permanent contractures. Orthotic devices such as splints and braces are often used to prevent contractures and to provide stability at specific joints. (See Management for specific interventions.)
- *Communication*—Speech motor problems are the result of the inability to organize the muscles to produce clear speech. These problems include dysarthria (difficult speech because of impairment of the tongue and other speech-related muscles) and apraxia (difficulty with the motor-planning component of speech). Receptive language–processing disorders are related to cognitive impairments in affected children. (See Consultations and Referrals.)
- *Sensory deficits*—Visual impairment is present in approximately 50% of children with CP. Deficits include refractive errors, strabismus, nystagmus, and amblyopia. Premature infants may have problems related to retinopathy of prematurity. Vision screening should be performed by an ophthalmologist if there is any concern regarding visual deficit. Hearing deficit is also common, present in approximately 10% of children with CP, particularly those with a history of prenatal or postnatal CNS infection. Hearing screening should be performed by an audiologist because many children with CP are not able to participate in routine audiograms.
- *Cognitive impairments and educational needs*—Approximately two thirds of children with CP have some degree of cognitive impairment, ranging from mild learning difficulty (LD) to severe MR. Children with CP should be closely monitored for signs of developmental delay and learning difficulties. Referral to early intervention programs should be made in infancy. (See Learning Difficulties later in this chapter for a more in-depth discussion of educational resources for the handicapped child.)
- *Sexuality*—Sexuality and other issues of adolescence such as independent living and vocational training need to be addressed in an individualized fashion. Adaptations based on individual physical limitations can be developed. Counseling should be provided as needed.
- *Safety*—Children with CP may be at higher risk of injury depending on their physical abilities. Children with ataxic or extrapyramidal CP are more likely to have frequent falls. Care should be taken when one is evaluating a child for adaptive equipment such as walkers or motorized wheelchairs because such a child may not have appropriate judgment ability to handle these devices safely.

Management

Treatments and medications. Treat constipation as follows:

- *Diet*—The initial mode of intervention is diet. Increase fluids and increase dietary fiber by introducing fruits, vegetables, whole grains, and legumes. (Cultural preferences may limit the success of this approach.) Many formulas come in a high-fiber version (e.g., Pediasure with fiber, Ensure with fiber).
- *Stool softeners*—Docusate sodium (Colace) is the most commonly prescribed stool softener. It is available as a 20 mg/5 ml syrup. The recommended dose is 10 to 40 mg daily if the child is younger than 3 years of age; 20 to 60 mg daily if the child is 3 to 6 years of age; 40 to 150 mg daily if the child is 6 to 12 years; and 50 to 500 mg if the child is over 12 years of age.
- *Laxatives*—Senokot comes in liquid form (218 mg/5 ml). The dose varies with the size of the child. Start with ½ tsp one or two times daily and titrate to a successful regimen. The maximum dose is 1 tsp two times a day for children. For Milk of Magnesia, the dose varies with the size of the child. Start with ½ to 1 tsp one or two times daily and titrate up to a successful regimen. Monitor for diarrhea. Instruct the family to work with the medication to find the dose and schedule that works best for their child.

- *Impaction*—The first step is to clean out the bowels. This should be accomplished by daily enemas (Fleet or Pediatric Fleet) until the return is clear. Follow-up treatment should be a combination of stool softeners and laxatives for at least 1 month. The regimen can be slowly withdrawn based on the response of the child.
- *Regular bowel regimen*—Once a successful program has been developed, it should be used on a regular basis.

For drooling, treatment can be accomplished with glycopyrrolate 0.04 to 0.1 mg three to six times daily. The maximum adult dose is 1 to 2 mg/dose up to three times a day. The most common side effects include decreased secretions, exacerbation of constipation, decreased urine output, drowsiness, decreased sweating, and overheating in the summer. Surgical interventions are available but should be considered only after other interventions have failed.

For management of increased tone:

- Baclofen is classified as a CNS inhibitor and skeletal muscle relaxant. Start at 5 mg (½ of a 10-mg tablet) three times a day and increase to a maximum of 60 mg/day. Side effects include drowsiness, nausea, constipation, and urinary frequency.
- Dantrolene may be started at 0.5 mg/kg per dose twice a day, increasing gradually to a maximum of 3 mg/kg per dose two to four times a day (up to 400 mg daily). Dantrolene is also a muscle relaxant but works by inhibiting muscle contraction directly. Common side effects include drowsiness, nausea, increased drooling, and weakness. Children who depend on their high tone to sit or stand erect may become less functional when taking this medication, even though their tone becomes more normal. It may also cause liver damage, and so liver function must be monitored closely.
- An intrathecal baclofen pump may be implanted when oral medications have failed to adequately control spasticity. Side effects are the same as for oral baclofen. Studies have shown this method to be effective in dealing with severe spasticity.
- Botulinum toxin injections along with physical therapy have been shown to reduce spasticity.
- A neurosurgical procedure called a "selective dorsal rhizotomy" can be performed to help manage increased tone in children with spastic diplegia.

Equipment needs are common in the child with CP. Specific equipment prescriptions are usually determined by consultation with an orthopedist as well as a physical and occupational therapist. Ankle-foot orthoses (AFOs) prevent shortening of the heel cord. They usually consist of a molded plastic splint that can fit inside the shoe. This device keeps the foot in flexion, allowing the child to sit in a more stable position and stand with a flat foot. Hand splints help to keep the wrist in a flexion position, preventing contracture of this joint. Thumb splints prevent the thumb from becoming contracted and losing function of the hand. Wheelchairs and other ambulation devices are also often necessary. Depending on the type and severity of CP, many children have limited ambulation skills and require assistive devices to move about the community and school. Special adaptive strollers and wheelchairs are available to maximize stability in sitting and promote good posture; these chairs are also flexible to allow easy use and transportation.

Counseling and prevention. Routine preventive monitoring should be performed in the following areas to prevent secondary complications:

- Monitor nutritional status for FTT or increased weight gain, particularly in a tube-fed child.
- Review with parents elimination patterns and any prescribed management program, particularly bowel regimens.
- Monitor for progression of orthopedic anomalies (e.g., worsening contractures, hip subluxation, scoliosis).
- Determine whether the patient is receiving appropriate therapeutic and educational services.
- Ensure that medical needs (e.g., medications, feedings) are being provided properly in the school or day-care setting. Counseling may be indicated for the following areas:
- Ensure that the family is enrolled in the appropriate supplemental programs, such as the Women, Infants, and Children (WIC) program; Early and Periodic Screening Diagnosis and Treatment (EPSDT) program; and any other state block grant programs that support specialized medical care for children with handicaps.
- Provide referrals for appropriate financial resources for the family (e.g., to Aid to Families with Dependent Children [AFDC], Supplemental Security Income [SSI].)
- Offer emotional and psychologic support to both the individual child or adolescent and the family in dealing with a child with special needs.
- Identify respite or community resources to assist the family in caring for their child.
- Instruct parents that the child with CP should have well-child visits based on the routine recommended schedule for all children.

Follow-up. Follow-up contact with specialists (e.g., orthopedist, developmental pediatrician, occupational therapist, physical therapist, speech and language pathologist) should occur on a regular basis. A young child (infant to preschool age) should be seen every 6 months if there are no intervening concerns. Once the child reaches school age, a yearly follow-up visit is adequate because it is likely that the school will identify any more immediate concerns and make the appropriate referrals.

Consultations and referrals. Any child showing symptoms listed in the Alert box or the Risk Factors section should be referred to a neurodevelopmental pediatrician or a child neurologist for initial comprehensive evaluation and diagnostic work-up as well as for periodic follow-up monitoring for progress.

Referral for comprehensive feeding assessment by a speech and language pathologist may be indicated and should include evaluation of oral motor skills and the best type of diet (e.g., pureed foods, thickened liquids). Refer for dietary assessment by a registered dietitian to determine appropriate caloric needs. Supplement recommendations can be made accordingly (see Box 46-2). Multidisciplinary input may be required to determine whether a feeding tube is necessary to supplement oral intake.

Social work evaluation may be helpful in determining if the family is participating in appropriate supplemental programs such as WIC and EPSDT.

Communication deficits can be managed with the assistance of a speech and language pathologist. An occupational therapist may be required to assist with modification of communication equipment. Augmentative communications systems are extremely helpful for children in developing functional communication. Systems may be as simple as a picture board with two or four pictures or as sophisticated as a programmable computerized system with a voice modulator that can "talk" for the child. Children with CP should be referred to a qualified speech and language pathologist for evaluation of communication deficits and recommendations for therapy and augmentative systems.

A social worker can be very helpful to the family of a child with CP. Specific areas to be addressed include accepting and adjusting to having a child with a disability, financial strain, availability of respite services and community support systems, and issues of adjustment for the child. Issues of independence and other matters for the adolescent can also be addressed.

Resources

Organizations

American Academy of Cerebral Palsy and Developmental Medicine (AACPDM), 6300 North River Road, Suite 727, Rosemont IL 60018; (847) 698-1635; www.aacpdm.org

United Cerebral Palsy Association, Inc., 1660 L Street NW, Suite 700, Washington, DC 20036; (800) 776-0414; www.ucpa.org

United States Cerebral Palsy Athletic Association, 25 West Independence Way, Kingston, RI 02881; (401) 792-7130; www.uscpa.org

Publications

Exceptional Parent Available from the Psych-Ed Corp, 209 Harvard Street, Suite 303, Brookline MA 02146-5005; (800) 247-8080.

Geralis, E. (1998). *Children with cerebral palsy: A parent's guide.* Rockville, MD: Woodbine House.

Down Syndrome

STEPHANIE BONNEY

Alert

A child with Down syndrome should be followed by a multidisciplinary team for coordination and management. The following issues also frequently occur in association with Down syndrome and should be referred to a physician:

* *Congenital heart disease*—Complete atrioventricular (AV) canal, ventricular septal defect, tetralogy of Fallot, mitral valve prolapse (adolescence through adulthood)
* *Gastrointestinal (GI) problems*—Hypotonia causing poor oral intake, duodenal obstruction or atresia, Hirschsprung's disease (first year of life), gastroesophageal reflux (GER), imperforate anus (at birth), FTT (which may develop within the first year of life)
* *Musculoskeletal problems*—Cervical spine (atlantoaxial instability), hip clicks, hypotonia.
* *Genitourinary (GU) conditions*—Urinary anomalies (e.g., hypospadias, undescended testes, underdeveloped testicles)
* *Other*—Congenital cataracts, abnormal newborn screening for thyroid

Down syndrome is a condition associated with a recognizable phenotype, limited intellectual capacity because of extra chromosome-21 material, and a predisposition to certain medical conditions. Down syndrome (trisomy 21) is the single most common cause of MR.

Etiology

Down syndrome is an autosomal chromosomal disorder; with karyotyping, it is divided into three areas: (1) nondisjunction of the chromosome 21, which is an uneven division of the chromosomes because of failure of separation and migration during cell division, (2) translocation, in which extra chromosomal pieces occur in 3% to 4% of individuals, and (3) mo-

Box 46-3 Clinical Signs of Down Syndrome during the Neonatal Period

Hypotonia or floppy posture
Flat face (i.e., low nasal bridge and small nose)
Small and dysplastic auricle of the ear
Poor or absent Moro reflex
Brachycephalic skull (seen in normal infants also)
Upward-slanting palpebral fissures (i.e., eye openings slant upward)
Epicanthic folds (i.e., skin folds in the inner corners of the eyes)
Brushfield spots
Maxillary underdevelopment
Tongue protrusion (often prominent)
Clinodactyly
Gap between the first and second toes
Redundant skin at the base of the neck
Simian crease

saicism, in which some cells have normal chromosomes and some have 47, with the extra being chromosome 21.

During the neonatal period, many clinical signs can be identified that help with making the diagnosis. The literature has identified over 300 signs and symptoms in the spectrum. No infant has all the signs, and no one single sign is characteristic of Down syndrome. The most common signs in the neonatal period are listed in Box 46-3. Box 46-4 addresses all the common findings in Down syndrome.

Morbidity is highest during the first year of life for a child with Down syndrome. Cardiac anomalies are responsible for almost 60% of the deaths, with respiratory infections following in frequency. Down syndrome can be diagnosed in three ways:

1. Ultrasonography is not the most accurate method; however, it is used to measure the length of fetal extremities and raise a level of suspicion for Down syndrome.

2. Triple screen measures three different substances in the mother's bloodstream and detects about 60% of pregnancies in which the baby has Down syndrome. These substances are decreased α-fetaprotein (AFP), increased human chorionic gonadotropin (HCG), and decreased unconjugated estriol (uE_s). Factors such as twins and gestational age can affect the interpretation of this particular battery of tests.

3. For chromosomal testing, amniocentesis is done at 16 to 18 weeks of gestation. Test results take 2 to 3 weeks, but results can be obtained by rapid chromosome analysis in 3 to 5 days. Chorionic villus sampling (CVS) can be performed at 10 to 12 weeks of gestation. Test results take 1 to 2 weeks, and results can be obtained by rapid chromosome analysis in 3 to 5 days.

Incidence

Down syndrome occurs in the following:
* All cultures
* All ethnic groups
* All socioeconomic levels
* All geographic regions
* Approximately 1 per 1000 live births
* Through trisomy 21 in 95% of cases
* More boys than girls (by a small number)

Box 46-4 Common Findings in Down Syndrome

Skull

Flat occipital area
Brachycephaly
Hypoplasia of midfacial bones
Reduced interorbital distance
Underdeveloped maxilla
Obtuse mandibular angle
False fontanel
Separated sagittal suture

Eyes

Oblique narrow palpebral fissures
Epicanthic folds
Brushfield spots
Strabismus
Nystagmus
Myopia
Hypoplasia of the iris

Ears

Small, shortened ears
Low and oblique implantation
Overlapping helices
Prominent antihelix
Absent or attached earlobes
Narrow ear canals
External auditory meatus
Structural aberrations of the ossicles
Stenotic external auditory meatus

Nose

Hypoplastic
Flat nasal bridge
Anteverted, narrow nares
Deviated nasal septum

Mouth

Prominent, thickened and fissured lips
Corners of the mouth turned downward
High-arched, narrow palate
Shortened palatal length
Protruding enlarged tongue
Papillary hypertrophy (early preschool)
Fissured tongue (later school years)
Periodontal disease
Partial anodontia
Microdontia
Abnormally aligned teeth
Anterior open bite
Mouth held open

Neck

Short broad neck
Loose skin at nape

Chest

Shortened rib cage
Twelfth-rib anomalies
Pectus excavatum or carinatum
Congenital heart disease

Abdomen

Distended and enlarged abdomen
Diastasis recti
Umbilical hernia

Muscle Tone and Musculature

Hyperflexibility
Muscular hypotonia
Generalized weakness

Integument

Skin appears large for the skeleton
Dry and rough
Fine, poorly pigmented hair

Extremities

Short extremities
Partial or complete syndactyly
Clinodactyly
Brachyclinodactyly

Upper

Short, broad hands
Single palmar transverse crease
Incurved short fifth finger
Abnormal dermatoglyphics

Lower

Short and stubby feet
Gap between first and second toes
Plantar crease between first and second toe
Second and third toes grouped in a forklike position
Radial deviation of the third to the fifth toe

Physical Growth and Development

Short stature
Increased weight in later life

Other Findings Seen in Newborns

Enlarged anterior fontanel
Delayed closing of sutures and fontanels
Open sagittal suture
Nasal bone not ossified, underdeveloped
Reduced birth weight

From Jackson, P.L. & Vessey, J.A. (2000). Primary care of the child with a chronic condition (3rd ed.). St Louis: Mosby.

Risk Factors

- Advanced maternal age
- Advanced paternal age (20% to 30% increased risk)
- Down syndrome in immediate family or sibling's family

Subjective Data

An infant or child who is suspected of or diagnosed with Down syndrome requires a complete history on the initial visit. On subsequent visits, special attention should be given to the following:

- Parental concerns
- Perinatal history, including any prenatal diagnosis (how and when)
- Pregnancy, including history, laboratory tests, prenatal care, medications, and knowledge of Down syndrome, if known by testing
- Labor and delivery, including where, length of time, weight and height, Apgar scores, length of time in nursery, and problems at birth
- Feeding history, including breast or bottle, solids, any difficulty with sucking, length of time feeding, easily tiring, frequent interruptions, vomiting, spitting up or choking, and weight gain or loss
- Elimination, including toilet-training age, problems with stooling (hard or soft), urinating well, and a good urine stream
- Sleep patterns, including snoring with apnea, sleeping through the night, unusual sleeping positions, and the reappearance of napping in older children
- Growth and development, including approximate ages as to when infant or child first accomplished the following: smiled, responded to sound, followed to midline, rolled over, transferred objects, sat unsupported, cruised, pulled to stand, walked alone, fed self, said "dada" or "mama," put two words together, and used sentences as examples of development
- Immunizations, including names and dates administered
- Any current or past problems, including:
  Respiratory problems (e.g., breathing difficulty or breath-holding, snoring, gagging, choking, respiratory infections, sinusitis)
  Ear problems (e.g., ear infections, discharge)
  GI problems (e.g., vomiting, persistent diarrhea, constipation, weight gain or loss)
  Eye problems (e.g., discharge, crusting, tearing)
  GU problems (e.g., on Pap smear or gynecologic examination [for adolescents])
  Neurologic problems (e.g., seizures [including what type and medication used], headaches, changes in neurologic status [such as weakness in one arm, clumsiness, or loss of established motor skills])
  Psychosocial problems (e.g., in sibling relationships or friendships; problems such as distractibility, hyperactivity, and falling asleep in the classroom)
- Screening, including hearing (when, type, and results), vision (when, type, and results), and dental (last examination)
- Educational history, including name of school, grade, type of educational program (e.g., special education, mainstreaming, inclusion), and performance and function

Objective Data

Physical examination. Areas of pertinent interest include the following:

- *Height and weight*—Plotted on Down syndrome chart; head circumference also plotted (microcephaly in 20% of cases)
- *Vital signs*—Includes blood pressure screening
- *Eyes*—Red reflex; if absent, immediate referral to an ophthalmologist; observation for nystagmus, blepharitis, tearing, discharge, and crusting
- *Ears*—Narrowness of opening, visualization of tympanic membrane, and cerumen impaction because of the smallness of the ear canals and hypomobility of tympanic membranes
- *Nares*—Size and mucous membranes
- *Mouth*—Inspection of tongue, oral cavity, teeth, gums, and tonsillar size
- *Heart*—Auscultation for irregular heart rate and cardiac murmur
- *Skin*—Notation of dryness around elbows, knees, hands, and so on; nailbeds and mouth for any cyanosis; areas of alopecia; and inspection of genital area, buttocks, and thighs for folliculitis (usually around school age and adolescence)
- *Musculoskeletal system*—Hypotonia of infants, head control, and oral motor control; checking of spine for abnormal subluxation of the atlantoaxial vertebrae, scoliosis, knee dislocation and foot deformity, slipped femoral epiphysis, hip click or dislocation, joint tenderness
- *GU system*—Pelvic examination and Papanicolaou (Pap) smear at approximately 18 years of age; also a check for early or late puberty (Tanner staging)
- *Developmental screening*—Denver II and Rapid Developmental Screening Checklist; screening for speech and language (Table 46-2 provides developmental milestones for children with Down syndrome.)

Diagnostic procedures and laboratory tests

- Complete blood cell (CBC) count yearly
- Chromosomal karyotype (with appropriate referral if not done in the nursery)

Table 46-2 Developmental Milestones and Skills in Children with Down Syndrome

	AVERAGE (MONTHS)	RANGE (MONTHS)
Milestone		
Smiling	2	1½ to 3
Rolling over	6	2 to 12
Sitting	9	6 to 18
Crawling	11	7 to 21
Creeping	13	8 to 25
Standing	10	10 to 32
Walking	20	12 to 45
Talking, words	14	9 to 30
Talking, sentences	24	18 to 46
Skill		
Eating		
Finger-feeding	12	8 to 28
Using spoon and fork	20	12 to 40
Toilet training		
Bladder	48	20 to 95
Bowel	42	28 to 90
Dressing		
Undressing	40	29 to 72
Putting clothes on	58	38 to 98

From Pueschel, S.M. (1999). The child with Down syndrome. In Levine, M.D., et al. (Eds.). Developmental behavioral pediatrics. (3rd ed.). Philadelphia: W.B. Saunders.

- Brainstem auditory evoked response (BAER) at birth to 3 months of age
- Tympanometry at 12 months of age and annually
- Thyroid function test (thyroid-stimulating hormone [TSH]) at birth and at 6 months and then yearly (as the child ages, there is an increased [40%] risk of hypothyroidism)
- Cervical spine radiographic examination from a lateral view, as well as with head flexed and extended, at approximately 3 to 5 years of age and as needed to rule out atlantoaxial instability, which can be asymptomatic and present in 20% of the population with Down syndrome
- Possible hip and scoliosis radiographic examination
- Echocardiogram during first 2 to 4 weeks of life and again during adolescence if there is evidence of valvular disease on clinical examination, because of the possibility of mitral valve prolapse
- Ultrasound examination, which can be performed in lieu of a gynecologic examination (if the adolescent is unable to cooperate for the gynecologic examination, sedation may be required)

Box 46-5 is an example of a preventive medical checklist to be used for patients with Down syndrome.

Primary Care Issues and Implications

- *Growth and development*—Plot height and weight on a Down syndrome graph. These children have a tendency to gain weight. Refer to an early intervention program because of global delays. Infants and children may be taught language using the total communication approach, which includes signing as well as spoken language. (See also Nutrition and Diet.)
- *Immunizations*—Use the same immunization schedule as for other children, except for immunosuppressed children, who should not receive live viral vaccines. Influenza vaccine is given yearly.
- *Safety*—Keep harmful materials such as poisons out of reach. Advise parents to "childproof" the kitchen and keep electrical outlets covered. Avoid the use of a pillow with these infants because of hypotonia. These children are prone to joint injuries because of laxity of the joints. Infants in car seats need to be properly aligned because of hypotonia.
- *Screenings*—Conduct a BAER test at birth to 3 months of age. Tympanometry is performed at 12 months and annually as the result of shifting hearing loss (over 60% of these children have hearing loss). Vision screening should be done at each visit because of the high risk of myopia, astigmatism, and cataracts. A dental examination should be performed before 2 years of age because of malocclusion and small pointed teeth, with 6-month follow-up visits.
- *Nutrition*—Keep in mind that breastfeeding may cause frustration and difficulty because of low muscle tone. Recommend a high-fiber diet with fluids. Plot growth measurements on Down syndrome graphs and compare with standard graphs. If the child is below the 3rd percentile or is falling off the expected percentile, consider congenital heart disease, endocrine disorders (thyroid or pituitary), or nutritional factors. Weight can be a problem because of hypotonia, undiagnosed hypothyroidism, and retardation of growth resulting in short stature. Review caloric intake and monitor weight. Children with Down syndrome require fewer calories than other children of the same age.
- *Elimination*—Discuss constipation, which can be attributable to lack of variety in the diet secondary to hypotonia

of the oral cavity and a tendency toward oral defensiveness. The following may also contribute or cause constipation: hypothyroidism, delay in achieving upright posture, decreased gross motor mobility, lack of exercise, low-fiber diet, lack of fluids, and Hirschsprung's disease. Toilet training often may be delayed or may take longer to achieve.

- *Exercise*—Encourage the child to enroll in Special Olympics, a community program, or a physical fitness program for weight control and social participation. A child who has atlantoaxial instability needs to avoid contact sports, somersaults, diving, the butterfly stroke (when swimming), handstands, and certain warming-up exercises.
- *School*—Discuss the need for finding the least restrictive school environment. Assist the family in becoming an advocate for the child in the individualized education program (IEP).
- *Sexuality*—Note that males may have some delays in the secondary sex characteristics. However, by late adolescence they will complete sexual maturity. Girls who start menses before 10 years of age or beyond 18 years of age need referral to a gynecologist. Problems related to menses, such as hygiene problems, irregular or heavy bleeding, pain or dysmenorrhea, premenstrual behavior problems, seizures during menses, or cessation of menses, need further medical evaluation. Preexamination counseling and education is helpful before the first gynecologic examination. Discuss or review the risks of oral contraceptives with the family. About 5% to 15% of women (including adolescents) who have more severe levels of MR may have severe premenstrual symptoms such as self-destructive behavior, increased seizure activity, hyperactivity, or increased irritability or angry outbursts because of their inability to verbalize feelings. Those with Down syndrome are capable of having children, and so discussion is necessary regarding contraception and appropriate sexual behavior. Discussion at an early age regarding appropriate private and public behaviors, such as group security, silence about last names and phone numbers, avoidance of strangers, and appropriate socialization (even with family members) is important.

Management

Treatments and medication. There are no specific treatments for Down syndrome. Medications are dependent on the particular illness or body system involved.

- A multivitamin may be considered if oral intake is limited or if heart disease or failure is present.
- Known hypersensitivity to cholinergic drugs (e.g., atropine) is possible.
- A thyroid supplement is often needed. This population is at greater risk for developing problems with thyroid gland function.
- Antibiotics may be prescribed for short-term and prophylactic use for frequent ear infections, sinusitis, and cardiac problems.
- Antihistamines may be prescribed to decrease both fluid in the middle ear and nasal congestion.
- Cardiac medications are often indicated in the early years because of congenital heart disease and again in the later years for mitral valve prolapse.
- Psychotropic medications may be prescribed during adolescence for behavioral problems.

Box 46-5 Health Care Guidelines for Individuals with Down Syndrome

Infant (Birth to 12 months)

History

Prenatal diagnosis of Down syndrome
Subjective assessment of hearing
Feeding and caloric intake
Stooling pattern and constipation
Review parental concerns
Respiratory and other infections

Physical Examination

Irregular heart rate
Heart murmur
Cataracts (must see red reflex)
Intact hearing; otoscopic exam
Fontanels
Neurologic examination
Musculoskeletal examination
Visualize tympanic membranes

Laboratory and consultations

Chromosomal karyotype
Thyroid function test (TSH and T_4) at birth and at 6 months
Results of state-mandated screening
Echocardiogram
Cardiology (even in the absence of a murmur)
Genetic counseling
Feeding specialist (lactation nurse or occupational therapist)
Brainstorm Auditory Evoked Response (BAER) Test (birth to 3 months); auditory testing birth and at 6 months
Ear, nose, and throat examination (by 3 months)
Ophthalmology examination (by 6 months of age)

Developmental

Discuss early intervention and refer to a local program
Developmental evaluation (by 3 months)

Recommendations

Parent (family) support
Reinforce the need for subacute bacterial endocarditis (SBE) prophylaxis in susceptible children with cardiac disease
Enrollment with Supplemental Security Income (SSI) and Medical Assistance, depending on income
Consider a will, trust, and custody arrangements
Continue SBE prophylaxis for children with cardiac defects

Childhood (1 to 12 years)

History

Review parental concerns
Ear, nose, and throat problems
Constipation
Review educational program
Monitor for behavior problems
Review current level of functioning
Sleep problems (snoring or obstructive sleep apnea)
Review audiologic and thyroid function tests
Review ophthalmology and dental care

Physical examination

General childhood examination
Neurologic examination regarding atlantoaxial instability
Brief vulvar examination for girls

HEALTH CARE GUIDELINES FOR INDIVIDUALS WITH DOWN SYNDROME (Down Syndrome Preventive Medical Checklist) is published in *Down Syndrome Quarterly* (Vol 4, Number 3, Sept, 1999) and is reprinted with permission of the Editor. The **Health Care Guidelines** also may be accessed and downloaded via the Internet from the *Down Syndrome Quarterly* HomePage at: www.denison.edu/dsq/health99.shtml. Information concerning publication policy or subscriptions may be obtained by contacting Dr. Samuel J. Thios, editor. Denison University, Granville, OH 43023 (email: Thios@Denison.edu)

Data from Cohen, W.I. (1999). Down syndrome preventive medical checklist. Down Syndrome Quarterly, 4(3), 1. Available online at www.denison.edu/dsq/health99.shtml.
*Recommendations for screening asymptomatic individuals with Down syndrome.

- Creams and antibiotics for dry skin, folliculitis, and other staphylococcal infections as a result of immunologic deficiency are often needed.
- Stool softeners and volume expanders may be used if constipation becomes a problem.

Counseling and prevention

- Provide literature and information on Down syndrome to the family.
- Discuss the feeding patterns of infants and children. Observe for poor feeding, failure to retain feeding, or not stooling (which can indicate a bowel obstruction in the infant).
- Discuss developmental concerns. Delays are noted in all areas. Social and emotional development is the least affected. Language and motor skills will show a greater delay (see Table 46-2).
- Advise the family to keep a notebook to record appointments, tests, studies, provider's telephone numbers, hospitalizations, and other significant information.

- Help the family to anticipate sibling issues, such as concern, misconceptions, disappointment, guilt, sadness, and feelings of helplessness.
- Advise that feeding difficulties can indicate cardiac problems, low muscle tone, or a GI problem. Some possible feeding difficulties are poor suck, tongue thrust, vomiting or reflux, delay in eye-hand coordination, delay in grasp for finger feeding, delay in holding utensils or cup, weak bite, immature chewing patterns, poor weight gain, oral defensiveness with textures, fatigue, cyanosis, and physical anomalies such as a small oral cavity and underdevelopment of the midface.
- Discuss the signs and symptoms of hypothyroidism, such as decreased stamina, intolerance to hot or cold, slowing of learning or development, increasing weight, and constipation.
- Discuss the signs and symptoms of atlantoaxial instability, which is a subluxation of the upper spine vertebrae as a result of joint laxity. Signs and symptoms in the 1% to 2%

Box 46-5 Health Care Guidelines for Individuals with Down Syndrome—cont'd

Laboratory and consultations

TSH (annually)

Auditory testing (every 6 months until 13 years of age)

Cervical spine radiographic examination, lateral view in flexion, extension, and neutral (at 3 to 5 years and as needed) to rule out atlantoaxial instability

Ophthalmology examination every year

Dental examination at 2 years of age with 6 month follow-up visits

Echocardiogram by a pediatric cardiologist if not done previously

Celiac disease screening (between 2 and 3 years of age)

Developmental

Enrollment in developmental or educational program

Complete annual educational assessments

Evaluation by a speech and language pathologist

Consider referral for augmentative communication device

Recommendations

Twice-daily teeth brushing

Total caloric intake below recommended dietary allowance for children of similar age and height

Well-balanced, high-fiber diet and healthful eating patterns

Regular exercise program

Respite care

Recreational programs

Continue speech therapy and physical therapy

Begin to acquire good self-care, grooming, dressing, and housekeeping skills, as well as money-handling skills

Reinforce the need for SBE prophylaxis in susceptible children with cardiac disease

Adolescence (12 to 18 years)

History

Review interval medical history questioning specifically about the possibility of obstructive airway disease and sleep apnea

Behavior problems

Vision and hearing problems

Address sexuality issues

Physical examination

General physical examination; gynecologic examination if sexually active only

Monitor for obesity by plotting for height and weight

Neurologic examination regarding atlantoaxial instability

Laboratory and consultations

TSH (annually)

Auditory testing every year

Ophthalmologic evaluation every year

Cervical spine radiographic examination, lateral view in flexion, extension, and neutral as needed

Echocardiography if evidence of valvular disease on clinical examination

Adolescent medicine consultation for sexuality issues

Dental examination twice yearly

Developmental

Continue speech and language therapy

Psychoeducational evaluations annually as part of IEP

Health, abuse prevention, and sex education

Smoking, drug, and alcohol education

Recommendations

Functional transition planning (16 years of age)

Discuss plan for future living arrangements, such as community living arrangements

Update will, trust, and custody arrangements

Encourage social and recreational programs with friends

Register to vote and for the Selective Service at 18 years of age

Refine good self-care, grooming, dressing, and housekeeping skills, as well as refining money and banking skills

Enrollment with SSI and Medical Assistance, depending on income

Dietary and exercise recommendations

Reinforce the need for SBE prophylaxis in susceptible individuals with cardiac disease

---

of the population affected are persistent neck pain, loss of established motor skills, loss of bowel and bladder control, increasing clumsiness, weakness of arms, changes in sensation in the hands and feet, gait changes, torticollis, sudden preference for sitting, dyspnea, and increased muscle tone in legs.

- Inform parents that children with Down syndrome are at greater risk for developing diabetes; pernicious anemia; certain skin conditions such as alopecia, vitiligo, folliculitis, and seborrheic dermatitis; respiratory infections; scoliosis; and leukemia, which can strike 1 in 1000 children with Down syndrome.
- Discuss the importance of learning self-help skills to foster independence.
- Discuss behavioral issues, such as oral defensiveness, obstinacy, low frustration level, hyperactivity, short attention span, and self-stimulating behavior, as well as discipline, all of which should be looked at from the standpoint of the child's developmental age and assessed for possible causes.

- Teach parents the importance of the following: annual hearing tests because of shifting hearing loss, which can affect speech development; vision testing every year because children with Down syndrome often need to wear glasses at an early age; and dental screening beginning at 2 years of age, with 6-month follow-up visits.
- Alert the family to certain surgical procedures requiring general anesthesia (e.g., myringotomy, tonsillectomy, adenoidectomy, hernia repair) that need special precautions if C1-C2 dislocation is present.
- Instruct parents in common symptoms associated with Down syndrome, including snoring with obstructive sleep apnea from chronic upper respiratory infections; obesity; increased amounts of saliva (drooling); and hypotonia.
- Discuss the need for brushing the teeth twice daily because of high tendency for periodontal disease.
- Instruct parents that subacute bacterial endocarditis (SBE) prophylaxis needs to be started in children with cardiac

problems when surgery, dental work, or other invasive procedures are to be done.

- Discuss nutritional intake because older children with Down syndrome tend to gain weight easily; they require fewer calories than other children the same age.
- Discuss the possibility of neurologic changes (e.g., persistent neck pain, loss of bowel and bladder control, changes in sensation).
- Address psychosocial issues.
- Assist the family in coordination of services. Many providers will be involved in care, and many tests will be required.
- Assist the family in finding resources for financial aid.
- Discuss the availability of respite hours and care.
- Assist the family in finding a sibling group and a parent support group or parent-to-parent network.
- Discuss health, abuse prevention, sex education, smoking, alcohol, and drugs with the teenager and family.
- Discuss vocational programming and setting up leisure-time activities with the adolescent and family.
- Discuss encouraging independence in daily living activities, such as housekeeping skills, money management, good hygiene measures, cooking, travel skills, coping with emergencies, and food selection and preparation.
- Discuss future planning for guardianship, SSI, community living environments, trusts, and estate planning.
- Encourage the child to enroll in Special Olympics, a community program, or a physical fitness program for social participation and weight control.
- Discuss health issues when appropriate.
- Teach breast self-examination and testicular self-examination, taking into account the developmental level of the individual.
- Prepare the adolescent for gynecologic examination by discussion and demonstration of materials and pictures.
- Discuss obtaining medical care with a PCP as the adolescent moves into young adulthood.

Follow-up. Provide follow-up care as needed for well-child care.

Consultations and referrals. The following referrals may be indicated:

- A pediatric cardiologist at birth
- A pediatric ear, nose, and throat (ENT) specialist for evaluation of the oral pharyngeal cavity
- An audiologist for an initial hearing consultation and yearly evaluation
- A speech and language therapist for consultation and evaluation
- An early intervention program (birth to 3 years) for evaluation of developmental level and intervention modalities, physical and occupational therapy, speech and language, and special education issues, with referral to other services as needed
- An augmentative communication specialist (only as indicated by lack of speech development) and an assistive technology specialist for evaluation (if warranted)
- An ophthalmologist at birth and 1 year of age and follow on a yearly basis
- A dentist for checkups beginning at or before 2 years of age
- A nutritionist for advice on formula adjustments, weight problems, and nutritional intake

Refer the parents to a genetic counselor because of the increased incidence of Down syndrome in subsequent pregnancies. Other providers who can be used for referrals are a pediatric surgeon, an endocrinologist, a neurologist, a gynecologist, a pediatric gastroenterologist, and a social worker.

Resources

Organizations

The Arc of the United States, 1010 Wayne Avenue, Suite 650, Silver Springs, MD 20910; (310) 565-3842; www.thearc.org

Association for Children with Down's Syndrome, 4 Fern Place, Plainview, NY 11803; (516) 933-4700; www.acds.org

National Down Syndrome Society, 666 Broadway, New York, NY 10012; (800)221-4602; www.ndss.org

Duchenne and Becker Muscular Dystrophy

CAROLYN D. FARRELL & CHRISTINA TROUT

Alert

Consult with or refer to a physician for the following:
- Respiratory difficulty (e.g., paroxysmal nocturnal dyspnea, recurrent upper respiratory infections)
- Cardiac irregularities (e.g., signs of cardiomyopathy; supraventricular tachycardia [SVT])
- Delay or loss of motor capabilities
- Bowel obstruction
- Urinary frequency, urgency, or incontinence
- Scoliosis

Duchenne muscular dystrophy (DMD) is a genetically determined form of muscular dystrophy that affects 1 in 3500 males. The disease process demonstrates initial involvement with skeletal muscle of the proximal extremities, first evident in the lower extremities. The disorder is progressive and eventually involves muscles of the upper extremities, chest wall, and heart. Ultimately the cause of death in these individuals is attributable to respiratory or cardiac complications. A clinically milder variation involving a mutation in the same gene results in the phenotype (physical and clinical manifestations of a disorder) known as *Becker muscular dystrophy* (BMD). Box 46-6 lists common manifesting signs and symptoms of DMD.

Etiology

DMD and BMD are X-linked recessive genetic disorders caused by a mutation within the dystrophin gene. This is an extremely large gene (with more than 2 million base pairs) coding for the assembly of about 3685 amino acids to form the

---

Box 46-6   Signs and Symptoms Consistent with a Diagnosis of Duchenne Muscular Dystrophy*

History of "clumsiness"; tendency to trip and fall easily
Tendency to push off one's own upper legs (i.e., Gower maneuver) or use nearby furniture to get up from a prone or seated position
Large, "muscular-looking" calves
History of delayed motor development
Inability to keep up with peers when running

Average age of diagnosis is 3 to 5 years.

dystrophin protein, which is critical to the structure and functioning of the muscle cell membrane. Dystrophin quantitatively accounts for only a small percentage of total muscle protein but has greater representation in the membrane cytoskeleton, especially in skeletal and cardiac muscle. Disruptions in the gene result in absence, significant reduction, or altered structure and function of the dystrophin protein. Mutations within the DMD gene, generally DNA deletions of varying sizes, are detectable in about 70% of affected males. These mutations are distinct from one family to another.

Consistent with X-linked recessive disorders, DMD more typically affects males, since, in contrast to females, they have only one copy of the X chromosome and therefore all genes that are located on that chromosome. Inheritance of the DMD (or BMD) gene in a family is transmitted through and by (typically) unaffected female carriers. However, approximately one third of DMD (or BMD) cases are a result of a new or sporadic mutation in that individual's dystrophin gene. Although females are not typically affected with DMD, this diagnosis should not be excluded simply because the presenting symptomatic individual is a female. (In some cases, manifesting females have been misdiagnosed as having limb-girdle muscular dystrophy.)

The clinically milder disorder termed BMD is associated with a similar distribution of muscle weakness as that of DMD, but the age of onset may be later and the progression slower than that of DMD. Genetically both of these disorders are caused by mutations within the dystrophin gene, but the nature of the mutations differs.

Incidence

- DMD affects 1 in 3500 males.
- One third of all DMD cases are caused by new mutations.
- About 1 in 1750 females are carriers.
- Approximately 60% of female carriers will have elevated serum muscle enzymes (creatine kinase); however, a normal creatine kinase level does not rule out carrier status.
- Carrier females may exhibit manifestations of this disorder from muscle fatigue, mild weakness, or enlarged calves to a milder symptomatic dystrophy involving the limb-girdle muscle regions.

Risk Factors

- Positive family history of Duchenne, Becker, or "limb-girdle" muscular dystrophy
- Male gender
  Risks associated with DMD or BMD
- Respiratory insufficiency
- Cardiac muscle, function, or conduction involvement
- Scoliosis
- MR or impairment (30% of cases), or subnormal intellectual capacity

Subjective Data

Any child who has a history of "clumsiness" or a tendency to trip and fall easily should be considered at risk for DMD. This common presenting history frequently occurs at a developmental stage when a young male, typically 2 to 3 years of age, is beginning to run and become very active. It can easily be explained away by the normal childhood tendency to try to do too much too quickly. This will truly be the case in the majority of situations, but unfortunately dismissal without further evaluation delays diagnosis and intervention in an affected child, causes additional parental anguish and frustration, and results in a delay in advising parents of potential risk to future children. BMD is usually compatible with continuation of ambulation into adult life, which is a useful clinical criterion. (Males with BMD may report a history of wheelchair dependency after an accidental injury, such as a fall.) Those who remain ambulatory into adolescence and adulthood may show symptoms of cardiomyopathy (such as dyspnea upon exertion). If DMD or BMD is suspected, obtain a comprehensive history with careful attention to three areas:

- *Family history*—Obtain a complete three-generation pedigree, inquiring specifically about any history of DMD or BMD, about male siblings or maternal uncles with muscular dystrophy or weakness, and generally about all siblings, parents, aunts, uncles, or grandparents concerning any history of muscle disorders or weakness. If the family history is positive, obtain copies of medical records of the affected individuals, if possible. The age of onset and distribution of body involvement of muscle problems may provide clues in assessing this diagnosis. Furthermore, it is sometimes helpful to ask the child's mother if she has any personal history of muscle weakness or cramping and assess if she has large calves, because carrier females may exhibit these features.
- *Developmental history* (Table 46-3)—Review the intellectual and motor development of the symptomatic child and the age at which the child achieved motor milestones. Normal childhood milestones of sitting up and raising the head while prone are achieved. Once the child is ambulating, peculiarities in gait are observed. Although these gait abnormalities may be attributed to the novice walker, these findings persist and become more exaggerated. Other presenting descriptions include a floppy infant, reluctance to walk, delayed walking, walking on toes, difficulty getting up, and difficulty in crawling. Parents report the gait to be "waddling," "swaying," "like a crab," "like a duck," "as if he had a stone in his shoe," and "like a penguin." Parents may comment that their son has "well-muscled" calves with complaints of cramping, especially after exercise. Assess intellectual status (such as verbal ability, play activity). Talk with the child and ask questions. Inquire of the parents about speech, reading, and school abilities. The intellectual history and development are generally normal. However, there may be speech delay or inappropriate level of comprehension since about 30% of affected males are mentally impaired.
- *Medical history*—No other classic presenting signs (see the Alert box) or history raises suspicion of this diagnosis. However, a small percentage of males initially are evaluated for GI complaints related to DMD, and liver enzyme abnormalities are often detected. Thus, in the absence of determining a metabolic cause for such a presenting problem, consider the diagnosis of DMD (or BMD) and explore family and developmental histories.

Objective Data

Physical examination. Any child suspected of having DMD requires a thorough physical examination with careful assessment. The practitioner should do the following:

- Obtain routine measurements of height, weight, and head circumference and plot them on an appropriate growth charts. Although not a common feature, some affected males will be small for age.

Table 46-3 Developmental Status of Those Affected with DMD/BMD

MILESTONES	DEVELOPMENT (AGE)*	GAIT AND POSTURE
Holds head up when prone	Normal	
Sits up	Normal	
Initial walking, parents report clumsiness with frequent falling	Normal	Slightly waddling, heel slapping
Parents report abnormality in walking	May be delayed (2-3 years of age)	Wide-based with feet externally rotated, heels slightly off the ground
Parents report inability to keep up with peers	Climbing stairs difficult (taken one at a time); difficulty getting up from a prone position; running never well achieved; cannot hop; difficulty riding bicycle, if even achieved (4 to 6 years of age)	Waddling with associated hyperlordosis

*May be older with BMD.

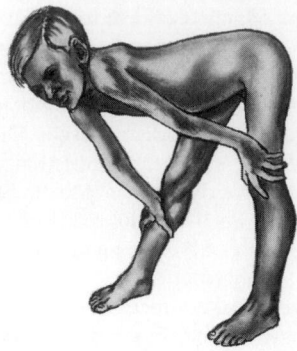

Fig. 46-1 Gower sign. (From Wong, D.L. [1999]. *Nursing care of infants and children* [6th ed.]. St. Louis: Mosby.)

- Assess vital signs, including pulse, respirations, and blood pressure.
- Auscultate heart sounds.
- Percuss the chest and auscultate lung sounds.
- Assess for calf hypertrophy, a reflection of enlarged, hypertrophied muscle cells and replacement of normal tissue with fat and fibrous tissue; it is almost invariably present in these young affected males. The calves may feel rubbery or tough on palpation.
- Assess for muscle strength and reflexes; proximal muscle strength is diminished, and ankle reflexes may be depressed. Weakness of the proximal area of the lower extremities is evidenced by the presence of the Gower maneuver (use of the hands to "climb up oneself" by progressively positioning the hands up the lower extremities to assist in pushing into a standing position) (Fig. 46-1). A simple method to evaluate for presence of this sign is to place the child on the floor with no nearby furniture and ask the child to get up; affected males will resort to a form of Gower maneuver or may move to an adjacent piece of furniture for assistance. To assess muscle strength it also may be helpful to have the child lie on the examination table with legs outstretched and ask the child to raise a leg from the hip while posing some pressure on the upper thigh in opposition to the leg lift.
- Observe for an enlarged tongue and a wide mandibular and maxillary arch with separation of the front teeth, which is present in some cases.

Diagnostic procedures and laboratory tests. If the diagnosis of DMD or BMD is suspected, the initial testing should include measurement of creatine kinase (CK) levels in the blood. The level of this muscle enzyme will invariably be greatly elevated in affected males. (Values are typically greater than 10,000 IU; normal values range between 20 and 320 IU, depending on the laboratory.) Although CK values can be elevated in other disorders affecting muscle, DMD (BMD) is one of the few disorders (excepting myasthenia gravis) causing levels to be elevated to that extent. Upon confirmation of elevated CK consistent with DMD, the following tests are options for confirmation of the diagnosis and may be ordered by the neurologist and neuromuscular clinic team:

- Genetic testing may be used as a first-line approach in confirming the diagnosis rather than immediately proceeding to a muscle biopsy (consult with a genetics expert). This testing specifically refers to DNA analysis of the DMD (BMD) gene. DNA testing uses white blood cells (WBCs) obtained from a blood specimen. The DNA is extracted, amplified, and then analyzed for deletions or duplications within the most commonly mutated regions of this extremely large gene. (Note that mutations cannot be corrected; they are present in each cell.) The rationales for a decision to proceed with DNA testing instead of a muscle biopsy are that: (1) the identification of a mutation within the dystrophin gene confirms the diagnosis without the invasive procedure of a muscle biopsy, (2) the genotype (precise DNA mutation) may provide clues as to the potential phenotype (physical manifestations of DMD versus BMD), and (3) knowledge of the specific DNA mutation provides the basis for assessing other female relatives at carrier risk in the family (e.g., child's mother, sister, maternal aunt), and (4) allowance is given for the option of prenatal testing if desired. With current technology, genetic mutations are not identifiable in approximately 30% of affected males.
- Muscle biopsy was routinely performed in the past but is no longer needed for diagnostic purposes if a DNA mutation is identified in the affected individual. However, a biopsy may be helpful for information about severity and for case management. Histologically the muscle tissue demonstrates a dysmorphic appearance, meaning that there is evidence of regenerating muscle cells as well as degenerating cells undergoing phagocytosis. Other findings include the infiltration of the necrotic area with fat and fibrous tissue.

- Immunofluorescent antibody staining for dystropin can determine the absence or presence and distribution of dysmorphin associated with the cell membrane.
- With biochemical assay of the dystrophin protein, a western blot technique is used to assess the amount and quality of dysmorphin in the muscle tissue. This analysis is useful in distinguishing DMD from BMD because the level of reduction and degree of abnormalities in dysmorphin are directly related to the clinical severity. DMD is associated with absent or extremely low levels of dystrophin protein but to a lesser extent than DMD. Female carriers may also demonstrate alterations in the dystrophin protein and levels.

Primary Care Issues and Implications

Growth and development

- Remember that there is normal growth in most cases. Rare cases may be associated with FTT or growth retardation.
- Remember that intellectual development is normal in most cases, while cognitive impairment in occurs in about 30% of cases. Intelligence quotient may be (IQ) 1 standard deviation below normal.
- Keep in mind that motor milestones are normal to delayed in first year, with slowed progression, reduction, or loss of motor abilities evident by 2 to 3 years of age. (See Exercise.)

Immunizations

- Follow recommended American Academy of Pediatrics (AAP) guidelines.
- Administer annual influenza shots to avoid potential pulmonary compromise.
- Consider the risk for immunosuppression in males treated with corticosteroids.

Exercise. To address progressive muscle weakness, deterioration, loss of function, and contractures, encourage the following:

- Maintain normal functioning as long as possible.
- Encourage overall range-of-motion (ROM) exercises for all joints to maintain optimal mobility and prevent the weakness associated with nonuse.

Note

Muscles should not be exercised to the point of exhaustion; overexercise or inappropriate increase in stress to muscles does not increase strength as with normal muscle but instead may contribute to muscle damage.

- Encourage heel-cord stretching exercises daily to address problems with ankle dorsiflexion that result in toe walking because of hip-girdle region weakness and tightening of iliotibial bands.
- Encourage calf muscle–stretching exercises daily.
- See additional information in the Management section.

Diet and nutrition

- Keep in mind that no special diet or dietary restrictions are necessary.
- Advise maintenance of a well-balanced diet.
- Remember that caloric intake needs to be adjusted because energy needs decrease with decreased activity.

Safety

- Keep in mind that the child is at risk for injury and poor body mechanics and alignment. The distribution of weakness affects balance, mobility, gait, and strength.

- Assist the child and family in understanding the mechanics of altered balance and muscle strength as it affects gait and so on.
- Remember that "foot drop" increases the risk of tripping and falling. Assess for AFOs, braces, and a wheelchair as needed.
- After loss of ambulation, promote upper body alignment and a properly fitted wheelchair.
- When lifting for transfers is anticipated, teach proper body mechanics to parents or caregivers, or consider mechanical lifts and devices.
- See Chapter 14.

Discipline

- Advise that parents should follow same discipline practices as with other children. (See Discipline in Chapter 19.)
- Remember that some boys with DMD have difficulty remembering and understanding a series of verbal instructions; such difficulty may inadvertently lead to conflict.

Sexuality

- Remember that the majority of these children are normal in intellectual and sexual development.
- Note that by puberty, many males with DMD are in leg braces or wheelchairs.
- Remember that psychosocial implications are posed by progressive physical limitations and altered identity.
- Advise that these children need peer support and help with positive self-image and confidence because social isolation is common.
- See Chapter 17.

Screening. Upon confirmation of the diagnosis, the child with DMD should have a cardiac and respiratory evaluation. The child will need to be evaluated regularly by a physician specializing in physiatry or rehabilitation medicine, or by a member of the neuromuscular team to: (1) determine the child's current capabilities, (2) make recommendations for appropriate exercise and maintenance or enhancement of capabilities, (3) make recommendations for supportive orthotics, as needed, and (4) provide an ongoing assessment of the spine. Scoliosis develops as the muscle weakness progresses, which can compromise pulmonary function and body alignment.

Management

The diagnostic, medical, genetic, individual, psychosocial, interpersonal, and family needs and considerations associated with the diagnosis of DMD are best addressed through an interdisciplinary team approach. The needs are complex, ongoing, and not discrete. A team of dedicated professionals working in concert with the child and family assures optimal care and the ability to address needs as they arise and demonstrates commitment to the value of the individual and family.

Treatments and medications. Because there is no cure at this time for DMD, the treatment and management of the child are essentially symptomatic and are aimed at prevention and support (Table 46-4). Exercises to maintain strength and mobility and eventually the use of AFOs, bracing, spinal support measures, and a wheelchair are all employed as the needs arise.

Drug therapy. Studies have demonstrated that administration of steroids, specifically prednisone or deflazacort (Calcort), is associated with improved muscle strength and function. Steroids may delay the progression of muscle weakness thus prolonging the child's ability to ambulate by up to 2 years of age. This treatment has side effects that include osteoporosis,

Table 46-4 Physical Complications Associated with DMD

PHYSICAL FINDING OR COMPLICATION (APPROXIMATE AGE)	MANAGEMENT
Tight iliotibial bands and Achilles tendons (3-6 years of age)	Active and passive stretching daily
Hip, knee, and ankle contractures (3-6 years of age)	Active and passive ROM
Prominent toe-walking (6-10 years of age)	Orthopedic consultation; AFOs; possibly surgery
Spinal curvature (10-16 years of age)	Orthopedic consultation; proper positioning; possibly surgery
Equinovarus deformity of feet (10-16 years of age)	Supportive boots; proper positioning to maintain ankles at 90 degrees
Declining forced vital capacity (12-18 years of age)	Regular pulmonary exercise by blow bottles, spirometry, singing, swimming; special attention to respiratory illness with prompt antibiotic coverage
Pressure sores of elbows, buttocks, ankles (12-18 years of age)	Preventive measures (e.g., position changes, massage, prompt intervention) Refer for physical and orthotic therapy for proper padding and cushioning to distribute weight
Constipation (12-18 years of age)	Design individual bowel regimen; assure adequate hydration (maintain urine specific gravity of 1.010); diet inclusive of fruits, roughage, and bulk; active and passive ROM
Forced vital capacity of 1 L with report of morning headache, disrupted sleep, daytime drowsiness, or mental confusion	Arrange overnight oximetry and capnography monitoring anticipating need for mechanical assistance

emotional lability, immune suppression, and weight gain. If weight gain is not managed, it may in and of itself diminish ambulatory ability. Steroids have a limited effect, and the side effects eventually outweigh the potential benefits. Deflazacort (Calcort) is a drug similar to prednisone, possibly with fewer side effects, but it is not approved by the Food and Drug Administration (FDA) in the United States. There are also reports of improvement related to dietary supplementation with creatine, but research is needed to substantiate this.

Scoliosis surgery. The development of truncal weakness leads to lumbar lordosis and scoliosis. The scoliosis is not halted by orthotic bracing. Surgical straightening can improve pulmonary ventilation and may improve positioning for comfort later in the disease process.

Respiratory therapy. Muscles that aid in breathing are also affected by muscular dystrophy, thus eventually leading to respiratory insufficiency. Measures to prevent early complications such as pneumonia include use of an incentive spirometer or other breathing exercises. Chronic hypoventilation is an inevitable and life-threatening situation. The patient and family are faced with options such as hospice and palliative care or mechanical ventilation (e.g., bilevel positive airway pressure [BiPAP], tracheostomy). The treatment options may extend life but also alter quality of life. Extensive counseling is recommended in making these life-altering decisions. Not only do the decisions affect longevity and quality of life for the patient, but also affect the quality of life for caregivers. Respite care is essential for the parents and caregivers to maintain personal well-being and relationships with other family members and community.

Gene therapy. The current research focus in potential treatment for DMD is on gene therapy. The approach would involve the synthesis of the dystrophin gene and incorporation into a vector (e.g., an attenuated virus) capable of transfecting (penetrating and getting the gene into the cell) human muscle cells while not disturbing that or other genes. The goal is that the incorporated gene would then prompt the deficient human cells to produce the gene product and continue to make the gene. The practical limitation will be the problem of getting the gene to the target tissue and having the gene be effectively incorporated to produce the necessary product, in addition to the difficulty of finding a vector that will accommodate an extensive gene. The body's immune response to the gene product, in this case the protein dystrophin, may also be a barrier to successful treatment.

Counseling and prevention (Table 46-5)

- Address parental concerns and questions. Most children with DMD are of normal intelligence and have the same needs as all normal children. Yet their physical prognosis is that of progressive decline. Therefore they are thrust into an environment where they must have regular examinations, testing, and contact with health care providers beyond that of the average child. In the early stages of this diagnosis, neither they nor their parents know what to expect. Encourage them to verbalize their concerns and questions. Parents often request guidance in talking with the children about the advancement of symptoms.

- Provide basic genetic information about the disorder. It is important that the family understand that DMD is a genetically determined condition and that they could be at risk to have future affected children. This information should be balanced, however, with an understanding that how the family deals with this concern may affect the self-image of the affected child. Also, DMD (BMD) can be a sporadic occurrence in some families. The diagnosis of a genetically determined disorder tends to engender guilt in some persons or families; thus information needs to be conveyed in a nonthreatening and nonaccusatory fashion. (See also Chapter 5.)

- Proactively anticipate, explore, and educate about reproductive concerns and options, risks to future children, and prenatal testing considerations.

- Educate families about newborn testing or screening for DMD. Serum CK levels can be tested as early as 24 hours after delivery. (Screening programs have been started in some hospitals using blood from a heel stick applied to filter paper to screen for elevated CK or the most common DNA deletions in the DMD gene.)

Table 46-5 Counseling and Interventions: DMD and BMD

CARE CONCERN	RECOMMENDATION
Initial diagnosis: Parental shock and denial, need for education and knowledge about expectations	Teach about disease course and preventive measures. Encourage participation in health care decisions, management, and support groups. Follow-up by telephone after diagnosis or subsequent visits. • Refer to the MDA, which can provide supportive services, materials, and so on. • Inform family of local support group.
Appropriate physical and occupational therapy: School-age or preschool, as function indicates	• Make referrals to agencies or schools as physical examination indicates (e.g., tightening of heel cords, restriction of ROM). • Contact school system concerning needed accommodations (e.g., modification in physical education activity, getting to second-floor classes).
Home accommodation to mechanical aids, implemented as needed	Provide referral to vendors and agencies who assist in adapting home environment to mechanical devices.
Teacher, counselor, and therapist knowledge deficit concerning disease	Facilitate meeting of involved educators and care providers to inform and educate about the disease, its process, and expectations.
Family or caregiver involvement in care delivery: Problems associated with total responsibility, limitations in ability to provide care	Refer to a visiting nurse service or other appropriate community agency.
Patient need for control: Desire for independence	Respect individual concerns regarding aspects of care. Assist in facilitating choices in care and life aspirations (e.g., living arrangements, caregivers, school).
Carrier risk for mother, sisters (or maternal aunts) of affected males; risk to future grandchildren	• Provide referral for genetic consultation. • Recognize critical importance of DNA analysis of affected for potential future analysis of female relatives, if desired. If testing is not desired at present, offer and facilitate option of DNA banking (storage of genetic material from the affected person). Consult with a genetics specialist.
Medical and supportive care, equipment; financial burden	• Arrange for social work consultation as needed. • Facilitate registration with MDA.
Respiratory decline: progressive through end stage of disease	• Monitor lung capacity and pulmonary function at regular visits, increasing frequency as needed. • Educate and inform patient and family concerning ventilatory support options. Encourage further discussion with rehabilitation medicine specialist or physiatrist.
Grief and end-of-life issues	• Address parental needs: Encourage sharing of feelings (e.g., fear, guilt, anger, hopelessness); recognize need for private time but inability to leave child; resolution of relationship with child; difficulty in decision about DNA testing, if not previously done, since it equates with finality of situation. • Address needs of person with DMD (BMD): encourage sharing of feelings (e.g., fear, anger, hopelessness, loneliness); assist in facing issue of death; facilitate communication with family and friends; promote physical comforts. • Address feelings of siblings and friends (e.g., guilt, fear, resentment). • Promote awareness of future family needs and orientation. • See Chapter 23.

• Help families understand the benefits, risks and limitations of diagnostics, treatment, management, and genetic testing facets of DMD or BMD, such as steroid therapy, muscle biopsy versus DNA analysis for affected males, and meaning to potential female carriers.
• Provide appropriate referrals.

Follow-up. Initially, after the diagnosis is confirmed, an otherwise healthy child can be followed by the PCP for well-child care, together with regular evaluations every 6 months to 1 year by the neuromuscular diseases professional team. These follow-up visits must increase in frequency as the disorder progresses or as the child is enrolled in treatment regimens (e.g., prednisone therapy).

Consultations and referrals
• Refer the child and family for genetic consultation and counseling.

• Refer parents to professional and community resources (e.g., the Muscular Dystrophy Association [MDA], local support groups, and so on. (See Resources at the end of this section.)
• Consult with specialists, including a neurologist, genetic counselor or geneticist, and rehabilitation medicine physician, to guide diagnostic testing and evaluations to effect a smooth, effective, and minimally stressful approach. Consultation before the diagnosis may avert unnecessary or suboptimal evaluations.
• With parent or child permission, inform the school nurse and the child's teacher of the child's special needs.
• Facilitate integrated care management with other health care providers (e.g., physical and occupational therapists) and social workers.

Resources

Also see Resources in Chapter 5

Organizations

Genetic Alliance; (800) 336-GENE; www.geneticalliance.org

International Society of Nurses in Genetics; (603) 643-5706; nursing.creighton.edu/isong

Muscular Dystrophy Association (MDA), 3300 East Sunrise Drive, Tucson, AZ 85718-3208; (520) 529-2000; www.mdausa.org

The Parent Project for Muscular Dystrophy Research, PO Box 5324; Department 1092, Cincinnati, OH 45201; (800) 714-KIDS

Publications

Hyde, S. (1996). *Duchenne muscular dystrophy: A parent's guide to physiotherapy in the home.* Muscular Dystrophy Group of Great Britain and Northern Ireland, 7-11 Prescott Place, London SW46BS; 071-720-8055.

Emery, A. (1994). *Muscular dystrophy: The facts.* New York: Oxford University Press.

Learning Difficulties

STEPHANIE BONNEY

Alert

Consult with or refer to a physician for the following:
- Delay of 6 months or more in attainment of developmental milestones
- Loss of developmental skills
- Microcephaly or macrocephaly
- Dysmorphic features
- Aberrant sexual development or growth, or significant change in the rate of growth
- Focal neurologic deficits or seizures
- Vision or hearing deficits
- In the school-age child, any of the above in addition to the following:
  Motor or vocal tics
  Significant decrease in tested cognitive abilities or loss of previously mastered academic skills
  Change in neurologic examination (e.g., increased prominence of "soft" neurologic signs)
  Thyromegaly and abnormal thyroid function tests
  Severe headaches of unclear cause
  Evidence of clinical depression
- In the adolescent, any of the above in addition to evidence of substance abuse

LDs impair an individual's ability to perceive, integrate, store, retrieve, or produce information. These difficulties cannot be attributed to motor or sensory deficits, MR, cultural, environmental, or emotional causes. They may, however, coexist with other disabilities. Such deficits usually result in significant discrepancies on tests of cognitive ability and academic achievement in reading, math, or written language. Socialization skills also may be impaired.

These disorders of function are neurologic in origin and static in nature; their manifestation changes across the lifespan because of the maturation of the CNS and environmental demands. Symptoms suggestive of the presence of neural system abnormalities may appear in the preschool years, but a diagnosis of LD is usually not made until the child has been exposed to academic instruction.

Etiology

LDs can be attributed to a variety of causes. Heredity is implicated when similar learning problems are reported in other family members. Genetic studies indicate an autosomal dominant inheritance pattern with 90% penetrance. Certain genetic conditions such as fragile X syndrome or Prader-Willi syndrome are also associated with LDs or MR. Other possible causes include intrauterine exposure to tobacco, alcohol, drugs, perinatal infections, birth trauma, head injuries, nutritional deprivation, and exposure to toxins. The same factors or events that can cause CP or MR may also result in LDs. Most often a specific cause cannot be identified.

Incidence

- In the United States, special education services are provided to 2.8 million children for LDs.
- Of children in public school special education, 52% have LDs.
- Basic deficits in language and reading occur in 85% to 90% of school-age children with LDs.

Risk Factors

- Family history of learning problems
- Genetic syndrome
- Prenatal exposure to alcohol, tobacco, or other drugs
- Prenatal infection or poor nutrition
- Toxemia or pregnancy
- Gestational diabetes
- Fetal distress
- Prematurity
- Precipitous or prolonged labor
- Birth trauma
- Small for gestational age (SGA)
- Acquired brain injury

Subjective Data

A complete history should be obtained with careful attention to the following areas:

- Prenatal and birth history, including pregnancy or birth complications (see Risk Factors); inadequate prenatal care; prenatal exposure to alcohol, tobacco, or other drugs; poor maternal weight gain; gestational diabetes; toxemia; preeclampsia; prematurity; labor of less than 3 hours or more than 30 hours; and fetal distress
- Neonatal history, including low Apgar scores (less than 7), small or large for gestational age, congenital or perinatal infection, respiratory distress, and jaundice of a significant degree (requiring prolonged phototherapy or transfusion)
- Infant characteristics, including temperament, sleep, and feeding pattern
- Developmental history, including language, social adaptation, and motor skills
- Current development, including school history (e.g., grade, retentions, subject strengths or weaknesses, homework, learning style, organizational skills, tutoring, special services), school performance (information obtained directly from the teacher), extracurricular activities, interests, hobbies, friends, level of independence, and chores assigned
- Past medical history, including recurrent otitis, meningitis, seizures, iron deficiency anemia, allergies, chronic illness (e.g., cancer, sickle cell disease, asthma), or psychiatric disorders
- Review of systems, including somatic complaints, hearing or vision problems, seizures or tics, medications, substance abuse (e.g., of inhalants, tobacco, alcohol, other drugs), eating patterns and nutrition, and sleep patterns

- Accidents or ingestions, including acquired brain injury or concussion and lead poisoning
- Behavior and affect, including school performance and behavior (information obtained directly from the teacher and parents), frustration tolerance, response style, motivation, fears and worries, perfectionistic or compulsive behaviors, habits, attention, activity level, anxiety, sadness, anger, sleep pattern, interpersonal style, and peer interactions (assessed using standardized child behavior checklists such as the Achenbach Child Behavior Checklist or Conner's Questionnaire)
- Family and social history, including speech delays, school underachievement, LDs, congenital defects, MR, ADHD, tic disorder, PDD or autism, mental health problems and substance abuse, independent functioning level of adults in the family, and recent changes in the family (e.g., births, deaths, divorce, moves)

Objective Data

Physical examination. A complete physical examination should be performed with special attention to the following:

- *Growth pattern*—Measure height, weight, and head circumference, and plot on a growth chart.
- *Vision and hearing screen*
- *General appearance*—Observe minor congenital anomalies (e.g., epicanthal folds, hypertelorism, high-vaulted palate, low-set ears, fifth finger curved toward other fingers, single transverse palmar crease). Assess skin for signs of neurocutaneous disorders (e.g., more than eight café-au-lait spots, axillary freckling, ash-leaf depigmented areas). Inspect genitalia for premature or aberrant development.
- *Neurologic assessment*—Perform a complete examination, including cranial nerves and peripheral examination, to rule out focal signs or ataxia. Conduct a neuromaturational assessment to identify subtle neurologic signs suggestive of an immature or inefficient nervous system, often associated with LDs or ADHD. These "soft signs" are frequently seen in preschoolers and may be insignificant; they are expected to fade out by 7 to 8 years of age. Examples include general motor clumsiness secondary to qualitative impairment in performance of a variety of motor activities (e.g., skipping, tandem gait, alternate hopping, ball skills). Motor overflow results from failure to isolate the muscle groups needed to perform the task. Synkinesia (mirroring), in which one side of the body mimics an activity being carried out by the contralateral side, may be observed during sequential finger opposition or rapid repetitive alternating movements. Dysdiadochokinesia is difficulty performing rapid repetitive alternating movements. During sequential pronation and supination of the hands, the child fails to suppress movement in the proximal muscle groups. Associated movements include facial posturing or movements during fine motor activities or hiking of the shoulder during paper-and-pencil tasks.
- *Developmental assessment*—Few developmental screening tests are available for use with the school-age child or adolescent. The practitioner usually relies on developmental charts (see Appendix A) to screen for developmental dysfunction. However, it is important that the practitioner engage the child in some form of direct assessment. Human figure drawing tests, Gesell figures, and the Peabody Picture Vocabulary Test provide a sampling of a child's skill and style. It may also be useful, if the practitioner is interested in establishing a more active role in the

---

> **Box 46-7 Common Psychoeducational and Language Tests Used by Psychologists and Educational Specialists to Diagnose Learning Difficulties**
>
> Wechsler Intelligence Scale for Children III (WISC-III) yields full scale, verbal, and performance IQs in children 6 to 12 years of age.
> Woodcock-Johnson Psycho-Educational Battery measures verbal ability, reasoning, perceptual speed, achievement, memory, knowledge, and interests.
> Key Math Diagnostic Arithmetic Test measures skills and applications.
> Beery Visual Motor Integration Test (VMI) assesses visual processing, attention to detail, visual motor integration, motor planning, and dexterity.
> Peabody Picture Vocabulary Test assesses receptive vocabulary.
> Test of Language Development (TOLD) measures receptive and expressive language skills. Composite scores may be derived in syntax, semantics, speaking, listening, and total spoken language.
> Standford-Binet Intelligence Scale, fourth edition.

assessment of learning problems, to become trained in the use of a neurodevelopmental tool such as the Pediatric Early Elementary Examination (Levine, 1999).

- *Behavioral assessment*—Throughout the assessment, behavior and style should be observed. Observe whether the response varies according to the type of task. Reactions include:
  Confidence versus performance anxiety or the need for excessive reassurance
  Cooperation versus noncompliance
  Pleasant versus oppositional or avoidant
  Enthusiastic versus disengaged
  Communicative versus excessively quiet
  Reflective versus impulsive
  Focused versus distractible
  Persistent versus having a low frustration tolerance
  Consistent versus erratic
  Happy versus sad, anxious, or irritable
  Quick response versus slow response
- *Psychoeducational and language tests*—These tests are done by psychologists and educators (Box 46-7).

Diagnostic procedures and laboratory tests. Perform complete laboratory tests as indicated:

- If there is a family history of LDs, autistic traits, or MR on the maternal side, obtain DNA testing for fragile X. Some authorities recommend fragile X testing on all individuals diagnosed with LDs.
- In the presence of dysmorphic features or growth aberrations and low cognitive functioning, obtain chromosomes for karyotype.
- If there is evidence of clinical seizures, including absence seizures induced during examination with hyperventilation, obtain an EEG.
- In the case of decreased rate of linear growth, dry skin and hair, thyromegaly, increased heart rate, or decline in school performance, obtain thyroid function tests.
- If there are focal neurologic abnormalities or a change in neurologic functioning, consider head-imaging studies.

- If there is a history or observation of problems with attention or behavior, determine whether the child meets the criteria for ADHD.

Classification of Learning Difficulties

LDs may be language-based, caused by perceptual handicaps, or mixed. Although there are many subtypes of LDs, each manifesting a particular cluster of deficits, there is currently no widely accepted nosology. However, it is helpful to be familiar with the following frequently used terms:

- *Dyslexia*—Impaired ability to use language, manifested by difficulty in reading, spelling, writing, or speaking fluently
- *Dysgraphia*—Difficulty producing legible handwriting with age-appropriate speed

- *Dyspraxia*—Difficulty performing or sequencing fine motor acts, as well as impaired motor planning
- *Dysnomia*—Difficulty in remembering names or recalling words to use in a given context
- *Dyscalculia*—Difficulty in understanding or using mathematical symbols or functions

Differential Diagnosis

Uneven development is the most consistent finding in individuals with *learning difficulties*. Inconsistencies may be noted between or within areas of development.

Borderline and *mild mental retardation* are characterized by global developmental delays with no significant strengths or weaknesses identified, except in gross motor functioning,

Table 46-6 Developmental Domains

PRESCHOOL	SCHOOL-AGE	ADOLESCENCE
Language		
Learning new vocabulary	Phonologic awareness	Abstract language
Articulation	Discriminating among sounds	Use of figurative speech
Auditory comprehension	Reading comprehension	Written language fluency
Following directions	Story writing	
Expressing wants or needs using mature syntax	Difficulty following complex oral or written instructions	
Motor and Visual Motor		
Manipulating objects	Controlled fine motor function (e.g., pencil control, handwriting)	Performance of complex motor patterns
Balance		
Fine motor coordination	Visual motor integration, (e.g., copying)	
Coloring, drawing	Letter and number reversals and word inversions	
Cutting with scissors		
Social		
Peer interaction	Appreciate perspective of others	Intimacy in friendships
Frustration tolerance	Formation of close friendships	Small group membership
Behavioral control		
Participation in groups		
Sharing		
Cognitive		
Cause and effect	Application of rules	Analysis and integration of information
1:1 correspondence	Use of logic	
Number concepts	Abstract concepts	
Concepts of place and attribute	Conscious problem solving	
Self-Help		
Eating and dressing	Independence in personal hygiene	Increase in independence
	Beginning independence in neighborhood and community	
Attention		
Self-regulation	Sustained listening	Increase in use of active working memory
Delaying of gratification	Concentration	
Sustaining a response	Filtering ambient noise	
Listening	Self-monitoring	
Planfulness	Organization	
Academics		
Letter and number recognition	Mastery of reading, including word recognition and comprehension at grade level	Same as school-age
Simple addition	Mastery of math calculations and concepts at grade level	
	Mastery of written language at grade level	
	Discrepancies between standardized school testing and academic performance	

which may be age appropriate. Attainment of developmental milestones is often delayed.

The performance of children with *attention deficit hyperactivity disorder* during limited periods is age-appropriate. Tested academic achievement is usually age-appropriate, though school performance is usually poor. Distractibility, impulsivity, and deterioration of attention over time are the prominent characteristics of ADHD. Hyperactivity may or may not be present.

With *sociocultural disturbance,* the family history reveals significant loss or trauma, basic needs that have not been consistently met, or family expectations that are inconsistent with the demands of the educational system.

Children with *emotional and behavioral disturbances* show evidence of significant levels of anxiety, depression, inadequate coping strategies, behavioral patterns, or other psychiatric disorders that interfere with school performance. Children may be brought for evaluation because of failure to meet developmental or academic expectations in any of the developmental domains (Table 46-6).

Primary Care Issues and Implications

- *Nutrition*—It is especially important that children with learning problems have good nutrition so that their ability to benefit from their educational program is maximized.
- *Immunizations*—Immunizations should be given according to the regular schedule.
- *Safety*—Children with LDs may be more immature and lack the judgment of their age-mates, placing them at greater risk for injury. They may require more supervision and guidance than their peers.
- *Discipline*—Immaturity and difficulty in reading social cues place learning-disabled children at greater risk for inappro-

priate behavior. They may have less understanding of consequences and be at increased risk for abuse.

- *Sexuality*—Immaturity, lack of awareness of social cues, and increased risk of low self-esteem place these children at higher risk of abuse or inappropriate sexual behavior. For young adults, deficits in coordination may have a negative effect on sexual functioning.
- *Exercise*—Poor coordination, visual perceptual problems, and problems with laterality and kinesthetic sense may reduce general physical competence. These children may be subjected to ridicule from peers and thus may avoid participating in both "sandlot" and organized games and sports. Others with language-based disabilities may be competent physically but prevented from participation because of homework demands or grades.
- *Growth and development*—Physical development is unaffected. Cognitive, social, and emotional development is always affected to some degree. As many as 50% of children with LDs also have attention deficit disorders.

Management

Treatments and medications. Treatment is primarily through appropriate educational programming. Attention deficits may require pharmacotherapy (Box 46-8).

Counseling and prevention

- Reassure the parents if there is no indication of a specific identifiable medical cause. It is important to ask the parents what they think might have caused the problem in order to identify and try to alleviate inappropriate feelings of guilt.
- Educate the parents about the special education process, services, and parental rights (Box 46-9). If possible,

Box 46-8 Medications for Attention Deficit Hyperactivity Disorder

Ritalin (methylphenidate)	It is approved by the FDA to treat ADHD in children 6 years of age and above; it is also used for children 3 to 5 years of age. It is safe and effective for 75% or more of children with ADHD.
Dosage schedule	The usual effective dose is between 0.3 and 1 mg/kg per day administered two to three times per day for a daily maximum of 2.0 mg/kg or 60 mg per day. Few side effects are experienced at 1 mg/kg per day. Start with a low dose and gradually titrate up. During the trial period, obtain standardized teacher questionnaires weekly to monitor response. The timing of each dose should be individualized in order to obtain the best overall response.
Dose forms	Tablets: 5 mg, 10 mg, 20 mg Sustained-release tablets (Ritalin SR 20). Note that the onset of action is less predictable and may release only 6 to 8 mg over 6 to 8 hours.
Dexedrine (dextroamphetamine)	It is FDA approved to treat ADHD in children 3 years of age and older. It may be more effective than Ritalin in younger children.
Dosage schedule	The usual starting dose is between 2.5 mg and 5 mg/day titrated weekly for a maximum dose of 40 mg/kg per day. Obtain teacher questionnaires weekly to monitor response.
Dose forms	Tablets: 5 mg, 10 mg Sustained release spansules: 5 mg, 10 mg, 15 mg. Note that these are more predictable and better absorbed than Ritalin SR.
Adderall	It is FDA approved to treat ADHD in children 3 years and older.
Dosage schedule	The usual dose is 2.5 to 5 mg/day, titrated weekly to a maximum dose of 40 mg/day.
Dose forms	Tablets: 5 mg, 10 mg, 20 mg, 30 mg
Catapres (clonidine)	It is not FDA approved for treatment of ADHD. It may be useful for children who cannot take stimulants, or it may be used in conjunction with stimulants. It may be particularly useful in targeting low frustration tolerance and disinhibition. It is not recommended for children with cardiovascular disease or history of depression. Caution family not to stop medication suddenly.
Dosage schedule	The initial dose is 0.05 mg at bedtime. Begin gradual (every 3 to 7 days) titration by 0.05 mg. Maximum dose should not exceed 0.3 to 0.4 mg/day divided three to four times. Monitor BP and heart rate.
Dose forms	Tablets: 0.1 mg, 0.2 mg, 0.3 mg

Box 46-9 The Special Education Process

Referral

The child is referred to the principal, guidance counselor, or special education coordinator by the parent, teacher, other school personnel or health care provider.

Child Study Committee Meeting

The committee reviews the referral information and the student's school performance within 10 working days. The committee may then recommend the following:

- Consultations with a specialist, teachers, or other individuals working with the child
- Strategies that have not yet been tried in the classroom
- Formal evaluation (requires parent permission)

Formal Assessment

Must be completed within 65 working days:

- Educational
- Medical (e.g., vision screen, hearing screen)
- Sociocultural
- Psychologic
- Classroom observation
- May include speech and language, as well as occupational or physical therapy

Eligibility Committee Meeting

Parents are invited to participate when the committee meets to determine if the student is eligible for special services.

Individualized Education Plan

The committee, including the parents, must meet and complete the IEP within 30 calendar days of eligibility. The parents must sign the IEP before special education services can begin. The IEP must be reviewed and evaluated at least once each school year. Reevaluation must be done at least every 3 years to determine progress and ongoing eligibility.

logic age and specific areas of development. Consistency is of even greater importance.

- Explore sexuality issues with the parents and child. Assess vulnerability, and guide parents in appropriate prevention. Talk with the older adolescent about the possible effect of his or her difficulties on sexual functioning. Assess the need for fragile X testing in females if it has not already been done.
- Stress the importance of exercise. Counsel the parents regarding alternative activities for those with poor coordination. Swimming, dancing, karate, horseback riding, running, track, or body-building may build self-esteem and enhance coordination. Counsel the parents about the need to balance the child's educational needs with social, leisure, and self-esteem–building activities.
- Counsel the parents regarding growth and development and the need to monitor development so that individualized counseling can be provided when needed. Anticipatory guidance is especially important.

Follow-up. Reevaluation for special education is required at least every 3 years. Individual children may need earlier reevaluation depending on age, severity of difficulty, and overall progress. It is the school's responsibility to do the psychologic, social, and educational components. The practitioner completes the medical component for the triennial and interval well-child examinations.

Consultations and referrals

- Remember that the following referrals may be indicated. Refer the child to or for:

  The school child study team or developmental clinic for further evaluation if development is uneven or school performance is poor

  An ophthalmologist if the vision screen is abnormal

  Full audiometric testing if there is an abnormal hearing screen or behaviors suggestive of problems with auditory comprehension (consider auditory processing testing)

  Comprehensive speech and language evaluation for language difficulties with or without articulation problems

  A neurologist for evaluation of abnormal EEG or head-imaging studies

  A geneticist for counseling if the karyotype or DNA result is positive for fragile X

- Consider referral to a child psychiatrist for medication evaluation if there are complex emotional or behavioral issues.
- Consult with the child's teacher and the school nurse regarding school programs and resources. Advocate for the child as needed.
- Consider occupational, physical, or recreational therapy if evaluation of motor coordination is poor.

  Refer the parents to LD organizations such as the National Center for Learning Disabilities (NCLD) or the Learning Disabilities Association of America (LDA) for parent education and support.

alleviate fears about the child being stigmatized. Offer suggestions about how to handle such fears on the part of their child.

- Educate the parents about controversial therapies (e.g., sensory integration therapy may improve coordination but does not affect learning).
- Remember that megavitamins and mineral supplements are not useful and may be harmful. Optometric vision training concentrates on a program of eye exercises to improve the ability of the eyes to move smoothly and focus together. Studies are few and have problems with methodology.
- Counsel the parents on the importance of good nutrition. Emphasize the need to provide a breakfast that is high in protein. Assess overall nutrition and suggest a multivitamin course if appropriate.
- Counsel the parents on accident prevention and safety. Help them understand the need for additional supervision while fostering increased independence. Some activities such as driving may require specialized instruction or a delay in attainment. Monitor the use of helmets and seatbelts.
- Counsel parents on discipline. Help them learn appropriate expectations given the discrepancies between chrono-

Resources

Organizations

Learning Disabilities Association of America (LDA), 4156 Library Road, Pittsburgh, PA 15234; (412) 341-1515; www.ldanatl.org

National Center for Learning Disabilities (NCLD), 381 Park Avenue South, Suite 1420, New York, NY 10016; (212) 545-7510; www.ncld.org

Publications
Silver, L.B. (1998). *The misunderstood child: A guide for parents of children with learning disabilities* (3rd ed.). New York: McGraw-Hill.

Mental Retardation

STEPHANIE BONNEY

Alert

Consult with or refer to a physician for the following:
- Delay in attainment of developmental skills
- Failure to progress beyond a certain stage of development
- Loss of previously attained developmental milestones
- Delayed language development
- School failure
- Microcephaly
- Physical features commonly seen in syndromes associated with MR:
  Upward slanting eyes, epicanthal folds, and simian creases (Down syndrome)
  Short stature (Prader-Willi syndrome, Williams syndrome)
  Enlarged pinnas and macroorchidism (fragile X syndrome)
  Café-au-lait spots (neurofibromatosis)
  Hypopigmented spots, adenoma sebaceum and shagreen patches (tuberous sclerosis)
  Microcephaly, phocomelia (absence of the proximal portion of a limb), and synophrys (condition in which the two eyebrows grow together) (Cornelia de Lange syndrome)

MR refers to significantly subaverage general intellectual functioning existing concurrently with deficits in adaptive behavior, all manifested during the early developmental period.

All three components—subaverage intellectual functioning, adaptive deficit, and onset before 18 years of age—must be present to meet the criteria for this diagnosis. Intellectual functioning is determined by use of standardized psychometric testing (Box 46-10). Adaptive functioning refers to socialization skills, skills of daily living, and the ability to get along in the community. The age of onset must be considered because cognitive impairment during the early developmental years has an influence on the individual different from what impairment has during adulthood.

Etiology

The causes of MR are varied (Box 46-11). In approximately 30% to 40% of cases a direct cause cannot be identified. Of note is that the more severe the degree of retardation, the more likely an organic cause can be identified.

Incidence

- Of the general population, 6.2 to 7.5 million people have MR.
- Approximately 85% of all persons with MR fall into the mild range.

Risk Factors

- Poor prenatal care
- Genetic defects
- Microcephaly
- Premature birth
- Birth trauma with associated hypoxic-ischemic episode
- Congenital infections
- Prenatal exposure to toxins

Box 46-10   Diagnostic Studies

Routine Screening for the Child with Developmental Delays of Unknown Etiology

Chromosome karyotyping
DNA studies for fragile X
Urine and plasma amino acids
Urine metabolic screen

Additional Tests (Depending on Clinical Presentation)

Urine organic acids
Ammonia level
Serum pyruvate and lactate
Screen for mucopolysaccharoidosis
Long-chain fatty acids
EEG
Head imaging (MRI or CT scan)

Psychologic Tests

Stanford-Binet Intelligence Scale (fourth edition)
Bayley Scales of Infant Development
Wechsler Scales: Wechsler Preschool and Primary Scale of Intelligence (WPPSI-R) (3 to 7 years of age); Wechsler Intelligence Scale for Children (WISC-III) (6 to 16 years of age); Wechsler Adult Intelligence Scale (WAIS) (16 years of age and older)

Box 46-11 Causes of Mental Retardation

Chromosomal anomalies (e.g., fragile X syndrome, Down syndrome)
CNS malformations
Metabolic disorders, including inborn errors of metabolism (e.g., phenylketonuria, homocystinuria, maple syrup urine disease, galactosemia, Lesch-Nyhan syndrome)
Neurocutaneous syndromes (e.g., neurofibromatosis, tuberous sclerosis)
Intrauterine infections (e.g., toxoplasmosis, rubella, CMV, HSV, HIV)
Maternal exposure to drugs or toxins (e.g., cocaine, alcohol, Dilantin, over-the-counter [OTC] medications)
Hypothyroidism
Lead poisoning
CNS infection during the developmental period (e.g., herpes, meningitis, encephalitis)
CNS trauma
Diseases (e.g., meningitis, encephalitis)

- Meningitis and encephalitis
- Metabolic disorders
- Thyroid disease
- Family history
- Inadequate or lack of immunizations

Subjective Data

Any child suspected of being mentally retarded must have a comprehensive history completed with special attention to the following areas:
- Prenatal history, including lack of prenatal care, exposure to viral infections (e.g., rubella; toxoplasmosis; cytomegalic

inclusion disease [from HIV]; herpes simplex virus [HSV]); maternal exposure to drugs, alcohol, anticonvulsants, and STDs

- Perinatal history, including birth asphyxia, trauma, and neonatal seizures
- Postnatal history, including prematurity, LBW, infantile spasms, and metabolic disorders
- Past medical and family history, including Down syndrome, fragile X syndrome, autism, CP, metabolic diseases, Prader-Willi syndrome, neurocutaneous syndromes, hypothyroidism, trauma, diseases (e.g., meningitis, encephalitis), and elevated lead levels
- Developmental history (reported by the parents), including:
  Birth to 2 years of age—Failure to achieve developmental milestones at the appropriate age, decreased interest in surroundings, and feeding difficulties (e.g., inadequate suck)
  2 to 6 years of age—Speech delays, abnormal behaviors (e.g., perseveration, self-stimulation)
  Older than 6 years of age—School failure, distractibility, short attention span, difficulty following directions

Objective Data

Physical examination. A complete physical examination should be performed with careful assessment of development. Global developmental delays are often observered, with language and cognitive abilities often being more affected than gross motor skills. Other possible findings include hypotonia; macrocephaly or microcephaly; and other dysmorphic features that may be associated with MR, including upward slanting eyes, epicanthal folds, and single transverse palmar creases (signs of Down syndrome); short stature and obesity (Prader-Willi syndrome); enlarged pinnas and macroorchidism (fragile X syndrome); café-au-lait spots (neurofibromatosis); and thin upper lip, short palpebral tissues, maxillary hypoplasia, and smooth philtrum (fetal alcohol syndrome) (see Fetal Alcohol Syndrome in Chapter 47).

Diagnostic procedures and laboratory tests. Box 46-10 lists the appropriate diagnostic studies for MR.

Differential Diagnosis

The child with MR displays primary delays in cognitive and language skills, though there also may be some motor delays. This distinguishes MR from CP, in which motor deficits are more significant than cognitive deficits (Box 46-12).

The child with a communication disorder (e.g., an autism spectrum disorder) displays more severe deficits in language skills, with higher abilities in motor and nonverbal problem-solving tasks.

Evidence of regression, change in neurologic examination results, or slowing or arrest in the rate of development may indicate a neurodegenerative disorder.

Work-up of the child with developmental delays of unknown cause must include a comprehensive history, including family history, and a complete physical examination (looking particularly for dysmorphic features).

Primary Care Issues and Implications

The practitioner can provide comprehensive primary care for a mentally retarded child and much-needed anticipatory guidance for the parents. The following issues should be addressed as they relate to caring for a child with MR.

- *Growth and development*—Development is affected, though the degree of retardation varies. Expectations regarding

---

Box 46-12 Classification of Mental Retardation

Mild

May have third- to sixth-grade level skills
Able to follow social norms
Able to develop vocational skills
Capable of self-maintenance

Moderate

More delayed skills, with simple communication skills and self-care abilities
May be able to perform simple skills under sheltered conditions
May be capable of self-maintenance, or may require a supervised residential setting

Severe

Limited communication skills
Usually ambulatory
Able to follow simple routines
Needs assistance with self-care
Needs close supervision

Profound

Has significant delays
Dependent for self-care
Needs constant supervision

Adaped from the President's Panel on Mental Retardation. (1985). Mental retardation: A national plan for a national problem. Washington, DC: Chart Book, US Department of Health, Education, and Welfare.

---

development should be tailored according to the mental age rather than the chronologic age of a child with MR.
- *Immunizations*—All immunizations should be administered according to the regular schedule.
- *Safety*—Children with MR often lack judgment and have no fear of danger. They require close supervision, especially in new environments.
- *Discipline*—Discipline should be consistent and appropriate for mental age. Rules and expectations should be explained simply and concretely. These children may not understand rationales for rules and expectations but usually respond to simple cause-and-effect behavior management (e.g., time-out). Positive reinforcement is also an effective behavior management tool.
- *Sexuality*—Parents need to explain sexuality issues (e.g., menstruation, reproduction) simply, using mental age as a gauge for the amount of detail presented. Role modeling appropriate social behaviors is often helpful. Parents need to be vigilant and protective of these children because they may become targets of sexual abuse or exploitation.
- *Nutrition*—Optimal nutrition is important in aiding learning.
- *Exercise*—Children with MR should be encouraged to participate in exercise as tolerated.

Management

Treatments and medications. Any child believed to be mentally retarded should be thoroughly evaluated by an interdisciplinary team. This team should consist of a developmental pediatrician or practitioner, a psychologist, an educational specialist, and a social worker. In addition, speech, occupa-

Table 46-7 Federal Legislation for Education of Children with Disabilities

PUBLIC LAW	DATE	TITLE	DESCRIPTION
94-142	1975	Education for All Handicapped Children Act	Mandated free appropriate public education for school-aged children with developmental disabilities
94-142	1975	Preschool Incentive Program	Funded states to develop services for children 3 to 5 years of age
99-457	1986	Preschool Incentive Program amended	Funded services to children younger than 3 years of age
101-476	1990	Individuals with Disabilities Education Act, Infants and Toddlers with Disabilities Program	Extended services to children up to 3 years of age by 1993
102-119	1991	Individuals with Disabilities Education Act	Funding for children up to 5 years of age
103-227	1994	Goals 2000: Educate America Act	Eight national educational goals for all children
105-17	1997	Individuals with Disabilities Educatiton Act Amendments	Continued services to disabled children

Data from National Center for Learning Disabilities. Available online at www.ncld.org/advocacy/fedlaws.cfm.

tional, and physical therapists may be helpful in providing additional information to support the diagnosis of MR.

The treatment of MR primary involves ensuring that the child receives appropriate educational services and associated therapies (e.g., speech, occupational, physical, recreational therapies) if needed.

The practitioner should be knowledgeable regarding community and educational opportunities available to persons with MR, thereby being able to serve as a parent and patient advocate as needed. Knowledge of federal laws (Table 46-7) is helpful when explaining the rights of persons with disabilities to parents.

Counseling and prevention

- Offer emotional support to parents in helping them deal with a mentally retarded child. Many parents may experience anger, denial, and guilt before finally accepting the diagnosis of MR.
- If MR is attributable to a genetic or a known etiologic disorder, advise parents to seek genetic counseling.
- Stress the importance of good prenatal care. In addition, a thorough immunization update should be performed before conception.
- Educate the parents regarding the ill effects drugs and alcohol have on the developing fetus.
- Remember that screening for metabolic diseases should be performed in the newborn period (after 24 hours of age) and as needed.
- Educate parents regarding childhood safety (e.g., use of seat belts, bike helmets). (See Chapter 14.)

Follow-up. Follow the routine guidelines for well-child care unless associated disorders exist that require more frequent monitoring.

Consultations and referrals. Refer the child to:

- An interdisciplinary team that includes a developmental pediatrician or practitioner, a psychologist, and an educational specialist for an initial evaluation and diagnosis
- An audiologist for a hearing evaluation
- A physical or occupational therapist if gross or fine motor delays exist
- A speech therapist if speech delays exist
- An educational specialist to ensure that the child receives appropriate, individualized education (e.g., early infant stimulation programs, Head Start, preschools for children with special needs)

Refer adolescent females to a gynecologist experienced in dealing with women with disabilities if self-care during menses

is problematic. Medroxyprogesterone acetone (Depo-Provera) therapy may be warranted in this situation.

Resources

Organizations

The Arc of the United States, 1010 Wayne Avenue, Suite 650, Silver Springs, MD 20910; (301) 565-3842; www.thearc.org

The Council for Exceptional Children, 1110 North Glebe Road, Suite 300, Arlington, VA 22201; (800) CEC-SPED; www.cecsped.org

National Child Care Information Center, 243 Church Street NW, Vienna, VA 22180; (800) 716-2242; www.nccic.org

Spina Bifida

STEPHANIE BONNEY

Alert

A child with spina bifida should be followed by a multidisciplinary team for coordination and management. Refer to a physician in the following situations:
- Spina bifida occulta suspected
- Dimple or hair tuft on lower area of spine
- Child diagnosed with spina bifida who has one or more of the following:
  Increasing head circumference
  Sleep apnea
  Subtle or sudden change in bladder function
  Seizures
  Vomiting (other than that caused by GI problems)
  Fever of unknown cause
  Allergic reaction (cause unknown)
  See Tables 46-8 and 46-9 and Box 46-13 for a more comprehensive list of signs and symptoms of spina bifida

This neural tube defect (NTD) occurs within the first 28 days of gestation and is present at birth. However, it is not completely static, and significant changes in neurologic function affecting mobility and continence can occur throughout childhood and adolescence. The type of defect, its level on the spinal cord, and central problems such as hydrocephalus, Arnold-Chiari malformation, and agenesis of the corpus callosum can be present and affect the extent of the disability associated with spina bifida. It can range from minor foot imbalance to full paraplegia with global delay.

Table 46-8 Signs and Symptoms of Hydrocephalus Shunt Malfunction or Infection

INFANT	TODDLER	SCHOOL-AGE CHILD
Fussiness or irritability	Headaches	Headaches or stiff neck
Vomiting	Crankiness or irritability	Irritability
Full or bulging fontanel	Vomiting	Vomiting
Increase in head size	Crossing of eyes	School problems
Change in eating habits	Lethargy	Learning difficulties
Lethargy	Sleepiness	Difficulty with balance or coordination
Sleepiness	Visual blurring	Crossing eyes or difficulty raising eyes
Sunset eyes	Seizures	Lethargy
Seizures	Swelling along shunt	Sleepiness
Swelling along shunt	Decrease in sensory or motor functions	Visual blurring
		Seizures
		Swelling along shunt
		Personality changes
		Decrease in sensory or motor functions
		Upper extremity tremors

Table 46-9 Signs and Symptoms of Arnold-Chiari Malformation*

NEWBORN/INFANT	CHILD/ADOLESCENT
Diffculty swallowing or hands	Stiffness or spasticity of the arms
Weak or poor cry	Loss of feeling in the hands or arms
Sleep apnea at any age	Hiccups
Inspiratory wheeze	Gagging or choking
Diminished gag reflex	
Possible facial weakness	
Stridor	
Aspiration	

Main cause of hydrocephalus in 80% of children.

Box 46-13 Signs and Symptoms of Tethered Cord

Tethered cord is attachment of the cord to a bony or fixed structure or, in the case of a lipomeningocele, adherence of the cord to a fatty tumor, which may particularly cause problems during the child's periods of rapid growth.

Signs and Symptoms

Deterioration of gait
Increased lumbar lordosis or flexion of the knees
Regression in the lower extremities as demonstrated by a rapid
   increase in orthopedic deformity or a loss of previous motor
   or sensory status
Change or increase in deep tendon reflexes
Weakness and atrophy
Back or lower extremity pain or paresthesia
Change in previously achieved bowel and bladder function
Spasticity in the back or lower extremities

Etiology

The cause of spina bifida is multifactorial.

Incidence

- In the United States, the incidence of spina bifida is 1 out of 1000 live births.
- Fewer affected infants are born than in past because of folic acid therapy.

Risk Factors

- Positive family history or other child born with NTD
- One of the partners having an NTD (risk increase to 4% to 5%)
- Maternal history of valproate sodium, alcohol, or aminopterin (an anti-folic acid) use, as well as diabetes mellitus
- Folic acid deficiency
- Maternal hyperthermia in early pregnancy (treated with hot tubs or saunas) and fever from infection

Subjective Data

A complete history should be gathered on any child with spina bifida, including a complete family and birth history on the initial visit. On subsequent visits, carefully explore the following areas:

- Parental concerns
- Prenatal history, including prenatal care, types of diagnostic studies done (e.g., ultrasound examinations) and results, medications taken, folic-acid tablets or vitamins with folic acid, any problems with pregnancy (especially in the first trimester), maternal serum AFP screening, and genetic counseling
- Birth history, including hours of labor, type of delivery, length, weight, head circumference, Apgar scores, length of stay in neonatal intensive care unit (NICU) or transfer to another hospital, and length of hospitalization of mother or infant
- Past medical history, including surgeries, diagnostic tests, and past illnesses (e.g., UTIs, unexplained fevers)

- Immunization history, including names and dates
- Nutritional history, including dietary intake, fiber and fluids, and difficulty with any of these
- Allergy history, including allergies to latex, medications, or foods
- Current medications, including anticholinergics, antibiotics, anticonvulsants, and medications to regulate stool
- Elimination history, including normal stool pattern (as controlled by diet, suppository, stool softeners, or other means); bladder program, which may include clean intermittent catheterization (CIC); how many times per day; dryness between catheterizations; self-catheterization or need for assistance; urethral or abdominal opening; and voiding on own
- Screening, including hearing (e.g., type, dates, results; developmental type, dates, results), school readiness, and psychologic testing (e.g., type, dates, results)
- Therapies, including physical, occupational, speech and language, and others
- Educational history, including name of school, grade, type of educational program, performance and function, academic difficulties, social behavior, and peers
- Social history, including involvement with community agencies such as WIC, SSI, Early Intervention, community programs, department of social services, school district, committee on preschool special education, committee on special education, friends, sports activities, extracurricular activities, or others
- Family history, including chronic or genetic diseases, seizures or other neurologic diseases, bowel or bladder difficulties, musculoskeletal problems, and developmental delays
- Review of systems, including head (e.g., shunt problems [see Table 46-8]); eyes (e.g., history of esotropia, sunset eyes, nystagmus, vision screening [including when and results]); GI system (e.g., gagging, choking, sleep apnea, vomiting when feeding, reflux; musculoskeletal); infant or child being able to move upper and lower extremities; orthotics and type (e.g., AFOs, wheelchair, scoliosis jacket); neurologic system (e.g., seizures, type and medication); and integumentary system (e.g., reddened areas, abrasions, ulcers, swelling, warmth over bony prominences)
- Habits, including sleeping (note any stridor, "snoring noises," or episodes of hypoxia)

Objective Data

Physical examination. A complete physical examination should be performed with special attention to the following. Height, weight, and head circumference should be measured and plotted on a growth chart). Vital signs, including blood pressure, should be taken. Also, special attention should be paid to the following areas:

- *Head*—Examine the fontanels for bulging, suture line (younger than 18 months of age); examine the shunt for physical signs of swelling at or near the valve or along the shunt line and for redness at the site of the shunt.
- *Eyes*—Examine the eyes for extraocular movements (EOMs), strabismus, and esotropia, and the retina for papilledema.
- *Musculoskeletal system*—Assess for strength in the upper and lower extremities, spasticity, fine motor coordination, inflammation of joints, changes in the spine, gibbus formation, contractures of the lower extremities, subluxation of the hip, congenital displaced hips, feet, or legs turning in or out, gait, scoliosis, positioning, and type of activity.
- *Neurologic system*—Elicit reflexes of the lower extremities, especially to sensations of touch, pain, and movement, and observe eye-hand coordination.
- *Integumentary system*—Observe for reddened or excoriated areas over bony prominences and swelling, ulcers, or abrasions. Feel for excess warmth in any area, particularly where braces or splints are touching the skin.
- *GU system*—Palpate for undescended testes. Observe for hypospadias, urinary stream irritation around urethral opening, and Tanner stages.
- *GI system*—Observe for anal wink and tone; inspect stomas for color, ulcerations, and sediment.

Diagnostic procedures and laboratory tests. Perform urinalysis, urine culture, CBC count, and electrolytes, including blood urea nitrogen (BUN), creatinine, and anticonvulsant levels (if appropriate). The protocol for studies is determined by the spina bifida team and may include ultrasound examination of the kidneys and bladder; voiding cystourethrography (VCUG); urodynamics; radiographic examination of the spine, hips, knees, feet, and shunt series; MRI or CT scan of the head and spine; and EEG.

Differential Diagnosis

The four types of lesions discussed here may include hydrocephalus, Chiari malformation (see Table 46-9), and tethered cord involvement (see Box 46-13).

Spina bifida occulta is the most common type of lesion. There is a defective fusion of a vertebral arch in the lumbosacral area but no protrusion, and it may be marked only by a dimple in the skin or a tuft of hair. Often it is diagnosed on a routine back radiograph. It may affect the gait in a progressive way, or a change may occur in bowel or bladder function.

A skin-covered fatty tumor, *lipomeningocele* encompasses neural tissue and can protrude from an unfused area in the lumbosacral area of the spine. It can affect lower extremity musculoskeletal function and bowel and bladder control.

Meningocele is a protrusion of the sac that contains meninges and cerebrospinal fluid and can be found in any level of the spinal cord. After surgical repair only minor sensory and motor deficits are present.

A protrusion of the sac that contains meninges, cerebrospinal fluid, spinal cord, and spinal nerves, *myelomeningocele* can occur at any level of the spinal cord. It is usually associated with hydrocephalus, Arnold-Chiari malformation, and tethered cord involvement. Surgical intervention is needed, but it does not heal the defect. There is significant impairment, depending on where the defect lies (midthoracic, midlumbar, or sacral area), which determines the extent of the physical disability.

Primary Care Issues and Implications

- *Growth and development*—Plot the patient's height, weight, and head circumference on a chart. Observe any discrepancies, particularly in the head size, and note on the weight and height graph whether jacket or braces are included. Use arm-span measurement to approximate height if the child is unable to stand. Routine developmental screening, particularly in the areas of gross and fine motor development and speech and language, is important.
- *Immunizations*—All immunizations should be administered according to the same schedule as other children.

However, because of frequent hospitalizations and surgeries, the immunizations may be delayed. Practitioners need to carefully assess status.

- *Integumentary issues*—The integumentary system requires special attention because sensation in the lower extremities is often diminished or absent; the child cannot feel hot water, friction burns, sunburn, scratches, or ulcers.
- *Safety*—Accessible environments need to be constructed if the child is in a wheelchair, wearing long leg braces, or has gross motor difficulties.
- *School*—Discuss with the parents school progress and learning problems. Shunt revisions caused by infections can affect cognitive skills. Difficulties may first appear in middle school as words take on increased difficulty.
- *Bladder management*—Assess the bladder program. Determine if the child is voiding spontaneously or with CIC. A child with a neurogenic bladder has little or no sensation of bladder fullness. Other problems may include poor or large bladder capacity, no awareness of urine passing through the urethra, no ability to stop urinary flow or poor stream, and constant dribbling. It is not recommended to treat asymptomatic positive urine cultures in persons with neurogenic bladder who use CIC. Asymptomatic bacteriuria is frequently found in patients using CIC without typical UTI symptoms.
- *Bowel management*—Bowel management is the most difficult and challenging task because of the time commitment, the patience required, and the cultural connotation that elimination elicits. Regulating the stool consistency and predictable evacuation is the goal to avoid constipation. Severe constipation can cause UTIs, shunt malfunction, stomach distension (resulting in loss of appetite), nausea or vomiting, and respiratory difficulties. Chronic constipation can occur early in life and may delay the success of a bowel program. Children can develop nasal fatigue and not be able to smell when they have an accident.
- *Latex allergy*—All individuals with spinal bifida have the potential for an allergy to latex (natural rubber products). Starting in the nursery, instruct the parents or caregiver to make the environment latex-safe. Some common signs of latex allergy are swelling of the lips (particularly when blowing up a balloon), unexplained rash on the hands or face, and wheezing or difficulty breathing. Box 46-14 provides a comprehensive list of items containing latex.

Management

Treatments and medications

Bowel management. Bulk-forming agents result in increased peristalsis and motility and help to regulate stool consistency. The bowel must be thoroughly cleaned out before these medications are taken to avoid impaction of fecal material in the intestine. Increase fluid intake when the medication is taken (eight 8-oz glasses of fluid per day). The following are examples of possible agents:

- *Metamucil*—Give 1 rounded tsp stirred into an 8-oz glass of water or juice one to three times a day.
- *Malt soup extract (Maltsupex)*—Give children 1 or 2 tbsp in 8 oz of liquid once or twice daily. Take with cereal, milk, or a preferred beverage. Give bottle-fed infants (over 1 month of age) 1 to 2 tbsp in the day's total formula or 1 or 2 tsp in a single feeding to correct constipation. Give the breastfed infant 1 or 2 tsp in 2 to 4 oz of water or fruit juice once or twice daily. It has a gentle laxative action and promotes soft, easily passed stool.

Lubricants help soften stool and lubricate the large intestine, making it easier for stool to pass through the bowel. Prolonged use (over 6 months) of mineral oil can cause a deficiency of fat-soluble vitamins A, D, E, and K and may cause soiling accidents. Contraindications are a weak swallow reflex, exaggerated gag, and problems with vomiting, which may lead to aspiration pneumonia.

Stimulants to ease stool through the colon and rectum should be used only when other methods have failed because they may cause cramping. They should not be used on a long-term basis. It is important to take 6 to 8 oz of liquid when taking a laxative. A laxative takes effect in to 12 hours. Possible agents include:

- *Bisacodyl (Dulcolax)*—This comes in tablets (5 mg) or rectal suppositories (10 mg). Children 12 years and older can take 1 to 3 tablets in a single dose, while those 6 to 12 years of age can receive 1 tablet daily. Advise not to chew or crush the tablet. For suppositories, children 12 years and older can take 1 suppository daily, while those younger than 12 years can receive $\frac{1}{2}$ of a suppository daily
- *Magnesium citrate*—This comes in a 12-ounce bottle: Adults (12 years and older) may be given $\frac{1}{2}$ to 1 full bottle divided into two doses, while children (6 to 12 years of age) should receive $\frac{1}{3}$ to $\frac{1}{2}$ bottle. The dosage for children less than 6 years of age is 4 ml/kg given two times a day. A full glass of liquid must be taken with each dosage. Do not exceed the daily dose. A bowel movement should occur in $\frac{1}{2}$ to 6 hours.

Stool softeners increase the amount of water absorbed into the stool as it moves through the intestine, producing a softer stool. Long-term use is not recommended because of its effect on the lining of the bowel. Drink plenty of fluids and follow a diet rich in fiber. Do not use oral medication if constipation is present.

Supplied in capsules, tablets, and oral solution, idocusate sodium (Colace) acts within 24 to 48 hours. Give adolescents 50 to 500 mg daily; children 6 to 12 years of age 40 to 150 mg daily; children 3 to 6 years of age 20 to 60 mg daily; and infants and children younger than 3 years of age 10 to 40 mg daily.

A natural bowel stimulant, senna (Senokot) is best given at bedtime. It takes 6 to 8 hours to act. The resulting stools may look yellow to yellow-green. The drug may cause cramps. It is available in a syrup (218 mg/5 ml). Adolescents may be given 2 to 3 tsp of syrup daily; children older than 5 years of age should be given 1 or 2 tsp of syrup daily; and children younger than 5 years of age can receive $\frac{1}{2}$ to 1 tsp of syrup daily.

Lactulose (Cephulac) is available in syrup form (10 g/15 ml). Give older children and adolescents 40 to 90 ml/day divided three or four times a day. Give infants 2.5 to 10 ml/day divided three or four times a day.

Various enemas are another treatment that can be used to help regulate bowel movements. Two additional bowel interventions include biofeedback and appendicostomy.

Bladder management. CIC is prescribed by the urologist and dependent on urologic studies. The frequency is usually three or four times a day during waking hours. This is a clean procedure with a nonlatex catheter. It can be performed by a family member, and eventually the child when the child is able to follow directions and has good eye-hand coordination. Review the procedure for CIC at the time of the visit. Ditropan relaxes smooth muscle of the bladder, while its contraindications are megacolon and hypersensitivity to the drug. Possible side

Box 46-14 Latex Occurrence

FREQUENTLY CONTAIN LATEX	EXAMPLES OF LATEX-SAFE ALTERNATIVES OR BARRIERS

Latex in the Hospital Environment

FREQUENTLY CONTAIN LATEX	EXAMPLES OF LATEX-SAFE ALTERNATIVES OR BARRIERS
Adhesives, skin (Smith & Nephew)	Mastisol (Ferndale)
Anesthesia circuits, bags, oxygen masks	Neoprene (Anesthesia Associates, Ohmeda adult), *some* Vital Signs
Band-Aids	Active Strip (3M), Curad Flexible Neon, Readi-Bandages
Blood pressure cuff, tubing (J & J)	Cleen Cuff (Vital Signs), nylon (*some* Trimline)
Bulb syringe	*Selected* Davol, Medline, Rusch, Premium, Baxter
Casts: Delta-Lite Podiatry, Orthoflex (J & J)	Scotchcast soft, Delta-Lites, *recent* Conformable (J & J), Caraglas Ultraliners (Gore)
Catheters (condom)	Clear Advantage (Mentor), ProSys NL (ConvaTec), *selected* Coloplast, Rochester, PolyTech (Hollister)
Catheters (indwelling and systems, UDS)	*Some* Am BioMed, Argyle, Bard, Cook, Dale, Kendall, Lifetech, Mentor, Rochester
Catheters (cardiac, vascular, pulmonary)	Rusch, Vitaid. Adapters & plug (Addto)
Catheters (straight, coudé)	*Some* World Medical, Am BioMed,
Catheters (feeding)	Mentor, RobNel (Sherwood), Coloplast, *selected* Bard, Rusch catheters
	Accumark feeding catheter (Sims Portex)
CPR manikins and medical training aids	*Most* Laerdal products
Dressings: Dyna-flex, butterfly closures (J & J), BDF Elastoplast, Action Wrap, Coban (3M), Lyofoam (Acme), Spandage (Medi-tech)	Duoderm (Squibb), Reston foam (3M), Opsite, Venigard, Comfeel (Coloplast), Xeroform (Sherwood), PinCare (Hollister), Bioclusive, Montgomery strap (J & J), Webril, Kendall, Metalline, Selopor, Opraflex (Lohmann), Centurion brief, *some* Airstrips

Latex in package only: Steri-Strip wound closure system (J & J), Tegaderm, Tegasorb, Active Strips (3M), Nu-Derm (J & J), Curad

FREQUENTLY CONTAIN LATEX	EXAMPLES OF LATEX-SAFE ALTERNATIVES OR BARRIERS
Ear plugs	Grainger
Elastic wrap: ACE, Esmarch, Zimmer, Dyna-Flex, Elastikon (J & J)	E-Cotton, CEB elastic (coNco), Champ (Carolon), Adban Adhesive, X-Mark (Avcor), Co-Flex, PowerFlex (Andover), Comprilan (Jobst), Esmark (DeRoyal, NHP)
Electrode bulbs, pads, grounding	*Some* Baxter, Dantec EMG, Conmed, ValleyLab, Vermont Med, Staodyn, Neotrode
Endotracheal tubes, airways	*Selected* Berman, Mallinckrodt, Polamedco, Portex, Rusch, Sheridan, Shiley
Enemas	BabyLax, *some* Adult (Fleet), Theravac, Bowel Manot Tube (MIC), Pharmaseal set (Baxter), cone irrigation set (Convatec), silicone retention cuff tip (Lafayette), all Fleet, Ready-To-Use
G-tubes, buttons	Silicone (Bard, Flexiflo, MIC, Rusch, Stomate)
Gloves: sterile, clean, surgical, orthodontic	Allergard (J & J), Dermaprene (Ansell), N-Dex (Best), Safeskin Nitrile, Neolon, SensiCare*, Tru-touch (Maxxim), Nitrex, Tactyl 1, 2 (SmartPractice), Duraprene (Allegiance Healthcare), Elastyren (Hermal, Center Labs), Boston Medical, Masel, Neotech
Incentive deep-breathing exerciser	Voldyne 5000 (Sherwood David & Geck), Triflo II
IV access (e.g., injection ports, Y-sites, bags, pumps, Buretrol ports, PRN adapters, needleless systems)	Cover Y-sites and bag ports—do not puncture. Use stopcocks for medications
	Polymer injection caps and Safsite (Braun), Abbot systems, Walrus, Gemini (IMED), *selected* Baxter (InterLink), Braun burettes, Statlock, Ready Med, ConMed, Clave, Alaris, Hudson, *selected* Sims, IV boards (Avcor), Terumo; pumps: Mach II, ADS 100, Clic-Open
Operating room and infection control (e.g., masks, hats, shoe covers)	*Some* by Kimberly Clark, TECNOL; OR and sterile packs (CML, DeRoyal) twill ties
Medication vial stoppers	*Some* AmRegent, Astra, Bedford Labs, Fujisawa, Gensia, Glaxo, Lilly, Roche
Miscellaneous items	Soft-grip fabric clamp covers (Scanlan), Precision Dynamics I.D. bracelets
Penrose drains	Jackson-Pratt, Zimmer Hemovac
Pulse oximeters, thermometer probes	Nonin oximeters, *selected* Nellcor sensors, Diatec probe covers

Modified from Spina Bifida Association of America (2001). Washington, DC. Updated in Spring, 2001.
This list is offered as a guideline to individuals, families, and professionals by the Latex Committee of the Nursing Council, Spina Bifida Association of America, and is updated twice a year. It is very difficult to obtain full and accurate information on the latex content of products, which may vary between companies and product series. PLEASE NOTE: The companies offering "alternatives" often also make many latex products. Checking with suppliers before use with latex-allergic individuals is strongly recommended. The information in this list is constantly changing as manufacturers improve their products and as we learn more about latex allergy. For the most current version of this list, visit the SBAA website at www.sbaa.org or send an SASE with $0.34 postage to Spina Bifida Association of America, 4590 MacArthur Blvd NW, Suite 250, Washington, DC 20017-4226, (800)-621-3141. (For the Latex Allergy Information packet, which includes a current bibliography, guidelines for writing policies and procedures, and recommendations to avoid latex reactions, please send $5.00.)

Continued

Box 46-14 Latex Occurrence—cont'd

FREQUENTLY CONTAIN LATEX	EXAMPLES OF LATEX-SAFE ALTERNATIVES OR BARRIERS
Reflex hammers	Cover with plastic bag
Respirators	Advantage (MSA), HEPA-Tech (Uvex), PFR 95 (Tecnol), 3M 1860
Resuscitators, manual	*Certain* Ambu, Armstrong, Laerdal, Puriton Bennett, Vital Blue, Respironics, Rusch
Spacer (for MDIs)	ACE spacer (Center Labs), OptiHaler (HealthScan)
Stethoscope tubing	PVC (*some* Littman) cover with ScopeCoat or latex-free stockinette (Albahealth)
Suction tubing	PVC (Davol, Laerdal, Mallinckrodt, Superior, Yankauer, Medline, Ballard)
Syringes, disposable	Terumo Medical, Abbott PCA, Abboject, Norm-Ject (Air-Tite), EpiPen, *selected* BD syringes, AdvantaJet (Activa)
Tapes: pink, Waterproof (3M), Zonas, Moleskin, cloth, Waterproof (J & J), adhesive felt (Acme)	Dermicel (J & J), Durapore, Microfoam, Micropore, Transpore (3M)
Tonopen disposable covers (glaucoma tester)	Cath-Strip (Genetic Labs), Ice Tape (P.O. Pak), All-Felt (Universal Foot Care)
Tourniquets	Children's Medical, Grafco, VelcroPedic, X-Tourn straps (Avcor), Free-Band (KLP)
Theraband (also strip, tube), other OT supplies	REP Bands and Cords (OPTP), Exercise putty (Rolyan)
Tubing, sheeting	Plastic tubing: Tygon LR-40 (Norton), thread, sheets (JPS Elastomerics)
Vascular stockings (Jobst)	Compriform Custom (Jobst)

Latex in the Home and Community

Art supplies (e.g., paints, glue, erasers, fabric paints)	Elmers (School Glue, Glue-All, GluColors, Carpenters Wood Glue, SnoDrift paste), FaberCastel erasers, Crayola (except stamps, erasers), Liquitex paints, DickBlick, Play-Doh
	Tempera and acrylic paints and soap erasers, Play-Doh
Balloons	Mylar balloons, self-sealing *Myloons*
Balls: Koosh balls, tennis balls, bowling balls	PVC (Hedstrom Sports Ball), Nerf Foam Balls
Carpet backing, gym floor, basement sealant	Provide barrier—cloth or mat
Chewing gum	Trident (Warner-Lambert), Wrigley gums
Clothes: appliqué on T-shirts, elastic on socks, underwear, sneakers, sandals	Cloth-covered elastic, neoprene (Decent Exposures, Nolatex Industries), Buster Brown elastic-free socks (Vermont Country Store)
Condoms, contraceptive sponges, diaphragm	Polyurethane (Avanti), female condom (Reality), Trojan Supra Condom
Crutches: tips, axillary pads, hand grips	Cover with cloth, tape
Dental dams, cups, bands, root canal material, orthodontic rubber bands	PURO/M27 intraoral elastics (Midwest Orthodontic), wire springs, sealant (Delton) Dams (Meer Dental, Hygenic Corp), John O Butler, Earloop masks (Richmond)
Diapers, incontinence pads, rubber pants	Huggies, First Quality, Gold Seal, Tranquility, Always, *some* Attends, Drypers diapers (not training pants), Confidence (Paper-Pak), Pampers, Luvs
Feeding nipples	Silicone, vinyl (*selected* Gerber, Evenflo, MAM, Ross, Mead Johnson)
Food handled with latex gloves	Synthetic gloves for food handling
Associated allergies are reported to banana, avocado, chestnut, kiwi, and other fruits	
Handles on racquets, tools	Vinyl, leather handles, or cover with cloth or tape
Infant toothbrush-massager	Soft bristle brush or cloth, Gerber/NUK
Kitchen cleaning gloves	PVC MYPLEX (Magla), cotton liners (Allerderm)
Miscellaneous items	Some medical stickers by MediBadge, UAL, Cushie Tushie Potty Seat
Newsprint, ads, coupons, lottery scratch tickets	
Pacifiers	Soothies (Children's Med Ventures), *selected* Binky, Gerber, Infa, Kip, MAM
Rubber bands, bungee cords	Plasti bands
Toys (e.g., Stretch Armstrong, old Barbies)	Jurassic Park figures (Kenner), 1993 Barbie, Disney dolls (Mattel), many toys by Fisher Price, Little Tikes, Playschool, Discovery, Trolls (Norfin), Silly-Putty
Water toys and equipment: (e.g., beach thongs, masks, bathing suits, caps, scuba gear, goggles)	PVC, plastic, nylon, Suits Me Swimwear
Wheelchair cushions, tires	Jay, ROHO cushions, Use leather gloves, Sof Care bed/chair cushions (Gaymar)
Zippered plastic storage bags	Waxed paper, plain plastic bags, Ziploc bags

Modified from Spina Bifida Association of America (2001). Washington, DC. Updated in Spring, 2001.

effects are constipation and decreased sweating. In tablet form, give children older than 5 years of age 5 mg two to three times a day. In syrup form, give children older than 5 years of age 1 tsp (5 mg) two to three times a day.

Other medications used for patients with neurogenic bladder are propantheline bromide, pseudoephedrine hydrochloride, phenylephrine hydrochloride, bethanechol chloride, and tricyclic antidepressants. The side effects are dry mouth, blurred vision, drowsiness, dizziness, weakness, nervousness, rapid heart rate, headache, skin flushing, and constipation. The risks are heat exhaustion in very warm conditions and sensitivity to the sun (creating a need to use sun block).

Mobility and positioning. Alterations in the structure and alignment of the bones, muscles, and joints can lead to varying degrees of impairment of mobility in these children. The level of the lesion usually determines what type of equipment is needed. Discuss positioning, which can involve the supine, side-lying, prone, floor-sitting, and standing positions. A child who is unable to ambulate or needs to use braces and crutches may use a wheelchair to conserve energy. Goals to be maintained for these children are to maximize function and learning, to maintain ROM, and to prevent contractures. Orthotics are frequently used to support or help to correct a misalignment. The most commonly used orthotics are AFO, knee-ankle-foot orthosis, hip-knee-ankle-foot orthosis, reciprocating gait orthosis, and thoracolumbosacral orthosis.

Antibiotics. Antibiotics are used for the treatment of UTIs.

Anticonvulsants. If warranted, anticonvulsants are used for seizures.

Counseling and prevention
- Provide information to all women of childbearing age regarding the use of folic acid to reduce the risks of having a child with NTDs.
- Stress to parents the importance of well-child care and the need for immunizations.
- Provide the family information regarding spina bifida.
- Assist the family in finding resources for financial assistance.
- Teach and reinforce the importance of knowing the signs and symptoms of hydrocephalus, shunt malfunction and infection, Arnold-Chiari malformation, and tethered cord (see Tables 46-8 and 46-9 and Box 46-13).
- Review with the parents and child the bowel and bladder program, if appropriate.
- Teach the parents and child the signs and symptoms of a UTI (e.g., fever, abdominal or flank pain, nausea and vomiting, change in color or odor of urine, lack of appetite).
- Provide current information regarding latex allergy to the family, child, caregivers, and school or community personnel (Box 46-14). Inform the parents and child about the need to wear a Medic-Alert bracelet or tag for latex allergy. Provide information describing the symptoms of allergic reactions to latex. Instruct the parents to report a reaction to the practitioner.
- Have the parents encourage the child toward independence in the areas of diet, bathing, dressing, toileting, skin care, and safety.
- Suggest that the child or adolescent participate in sports, physical activity, recreational activities, and adaptive physical education programs.
- Provide age-appropriate information regarding sexuality and sexual development.
- Prepare families for early pubertal changes (earlier than 8 years of age), which can be normal in the spina bifida population.

- Alert families to the possibility of LDs and the resources available.
- Review safety issues with parents, including the use of caution when transferring the child in and out of the wheelchair, locking the brakes, and using the transfer board; turning on hot water (i.e., check the water temperature); and when around radiators or anything that is hot and could touch the skin.
- Discuss with the parents and child the importance of good nutrition, including eight 8-oz glasses of fluid a day (e.g., noncaffeinated, low-sugar drinks, water), which are needed to avoid constipation and maintain diluted urine. A diet high in fiber should be maintained while avoiding milk, chocolate, greasy foods (pizza), corn, corn syrup, and spicy foods.
- Teach the parents and child the importance of good skin care.
- Advise the parents and child to check the skin daily, observing for any abrasions, scratches, reddened or excoriated areas, especially where the orthotics touch the skin. The use of a mirror may be helpful.
- Discuss skin protection and the need for sun block because of decreased feeling in the lower extremities and sun sensitivity caused by the drug oxybutynin chloride (Ditropan).
- Suggest wearing socks under AFOs to help prevent pressure areas.
- Advise keeping the skin moist. Use lotion on the skin immediately after bathing.
- Suggest using soaps that do not change skin pH (e.g., Neutrogena, Basis, Aveeno).
- Advise the avoidance of Mercurochrome, a blow dryer, peroxide, alcohol, and povidone-iodine (Betadine) for cleaning or drying a wound.
- Advise parents to report any skin breakdowns immediately.
- Discuss with the parents and adolescent ways to facilitate independence. Encourage the adolescent to meet other individuals with disabilities and participate in group projects. Suggest that the parents offer the child or adolescent opportunities away from home (e.g., camps, games for the physically challenged, Special Olympics).
- Encourage participation in the development of IEPs at school.
- Discuss transition planning, independent-living centers, skill-building seminars, vocational-rehabilitation services, college programs, and group homes.
- Discuss the Americans with Disabilities Act and the effect it has on the family.
- Assist in finding a family practitioner, internist, nurse practitioner, or gynecologist, if appropriate, as the young adult state nears.

Follow-up. Follow-up care is determined by the spina bifida team and also provided as needed for well-child care.

Consultations and referrals. A child with spina bifida should be referred to and managed by a spina bifida team (which may consist of a neurosurgeon, neurologist, orthopedist, urologist, pediatrician, psychiatrist, nurse, social worker, and therapists). The child should also be referred to:
- An ophthalmologist for yearly eye examinations as a result of the high incidence of strabismus in children with hydrocephalus
- An orthopedist who specializes in spine surgery to evaluate for scoliosis and corrective interventions, if necessary

- A physical therapist if orthotics are used or needed
- A nutritionist to discuss and plan with the family and child a diet and weight-control program, particularly if the child uses a wheelchair as the primary mode of ambulation
- An endocrinologist if there are signs of precocious puberty
- An assistive or augmentative program when there is a question of eye-hand coordination or learning difficulties in school
- An early intervention program for the services of a physical therapist or occupational therapist, special education, and speech and language
- A service coordinator to facilitate multiple services and assist the family in meeting the complex health care needs of the child
- A neuropsychologist for testing if academic and learning problems are identified by the parents and teacher
  In addition:
- Refer the parents to a parent-to-parent group or parents support group.
- Refer the family to social services for identification of additional resources, including financial ones.
- Refer the family for genetic counseling to help answer any concerns regarding future pregnancies.

Resources

Organizations

Centers for Independent Living, National Council on Independent Living, 1916 Wilson Boulevard, Suite 209, Arlington, VA 22201; www.ncil.org

March of Dimes Birth Defects Foundation, 1275 Mamaroneck Avenue, White Plains, NY 10605; (888) MODIMES; www.modimes.org

Spina Bifida Association of America, 4590 MacArthur Boulevard NW, Suite 250, Washington, DC 20007-4226; (202) 944-3285 or (800) 621-3141; www.sbaa.org

Websites

For Parents

American Association of People with Disabilities (www.aapd.com)

Association for Children and Adults with Learning Disabilities (www.acldonline.org)

Disability Network, Inc. (www.disabilitynetwork.com)

Down Syndrome for New Parents (www.downsyn.com)

KidNeeds.com (www.kidneeds.com)

KidPower (www.kid-power.com)

National Birth Defects Prevention Network (www.nbdpn.org)

World Association of Persons with Disabilities (www.wapd.org)

For Professionals

Internet Resources for Special Children (www.irsc.org)

Cerebralpalsy.com (www.cerebralpalsy.com)

Chapel Hill Area Local Unit (an autism resource) (www.autism-info.com)

Council for Exceptional Children (www.cec.sped.org)

Down Syndrome Information Network (www.down-syndrome.net)

Bibliography

Agerter, D.C. & Rassmussen, N.H. (2000). Diagnosing and treating ADHD in children. *Minnesota Medicine, 83*(6), 51-54.

Barron-Cohen, S. (2000). Is Asperger syndrome/high-functioning autism necessarily a disability? *Developmental Psychopathology, 12*(3), 489-500.

Bennett, F.C. (1999, July). Diagnosing cerebral palsy—the earlier the better. *Contemporary Pediatrics, 16,* 7.

Brent, R.L., Oakley, G.P., & Mattison, D.R. (2000). The unnecessary epidemic of folic acid: Preventable spina bifida and anencephaly. *Pediatrics, 106*(4), 825-827.

Cartwright, C. (2000). Primary tethered cord syndrome: Diagnosis and treatment of an insidious defect. *Journal of Neuroscience Nursing, 32*(4), 210-215.

Cate, S. (1999). Multiple marker screening for Down syndrome—Whom should we screen? *Journal of the American Board of Family Practice, 12*(5), 367-374.

Daily, D.K., Ardinger, H.H., & Holmes, G.E. (2000). Identification and evaluation of mental retardation. *American Family Physician, 61*(4), 1059-1067, 1070.

Dworkin, P.H. & Glascoe, F.P. (1997, April). Early detection of developmental delays: How do you measure up? *Contemporary Pediatrics, 14*(4), 158-168.

Elias, E.R. & Hobbs, N. (1998, April). Spina bifida: Sorting out the complexities of care. *Contemporary Pediatrics, 15*(4) 156-171.

Engsberg, J.R., Olree, K.S., Ross, S.A., & Park, T.S. (1998). Spasticity and strength changes as a function of selective dorsal rhizotomy. *Journal of Neurosurgery, 88*(6), 1020-1026.

Fehlings, D., Rang, M., Glazier, J., & Steele, C. (2000). An evaluation of botulinum-A toxin injections to improve upper extremity function in children with hemiplegic cerebral palsy. *Journal of Pediatrics, 137*(3), 331-337.

Fletcher, J.M., Shaywitz, S.E., & Shaywitz, B.A. (1999). Comorbidity of learning and attention disorders: Separate but equal. *Pediatric Clinics of North America, 46*(5), 885-897.

Gottesman, R.L. & Kelly, M.S. (2000, November). Helping children with learning disabilities toward a brighter adulthood. *Contemporary Pediatrics, 17*(11), 42-61.

Klinger, L.G. & Renner, P. (2000). Performance based measures in autism: Implications for diagnosis, early detection, and identification of cognitive profiles. *Journal of Clinical Child Psychology, 29*(4), 479-492.

Newberger, D.S. (2000). Down syndrome: Prenatal risk assessment and diagnosis. *American Family Physician, 62*(4), 825-832, 837-838.

Northrup, H. & Volcik, K.A. (2000). Spina bifida and other neural tube defects. *Current Problems in Pediatrics, 30*(10), 313-332.

Pastore, E., Marion, B., Calzolari, A., Digilio, M.C., Giannotti, A., & Turchetta, A. (2000). Clinical and cardiorespiratory assessment in children with Down syndrome without congenital heart disease. *Archives of Pediatric Adolescent Medicine, 154*(4), 408-410.

Phillips, D.M., Longlett, S.K., Mulrine, C., Kruse, J., & Kewney, R. (1999). School problems and the family physician. *American Family Physician, 59*(10), 2816-2824.

Potenza, M.N. (1997). New findings on the causes and treatment of autism. *Medscape Mental Health, 2*(8).

Rapin, I. (1997). Autism. *The New England Journal of Medicine, 337*(2), 97-104.

Rawiciki, B. (1999). Treatment of cerebral origin spasticity with continuous intrathecal baclofen delivered via an implantable pump: Long-term follow-up review of 18 patients. *Journal of Neurosurgery, 91*(5), 733-736.

Saenz, R.B. (1999). Primary care of infants and young children with Down syndrome. *American Family Physician, 59*(2), 381-390, 392, 395-396.

Smith, T. (1997). Sexual differences in pervasive developmental disorders. *Medscape Mental Health, 2*(6).

Sventz, M.V., Ireland, M., & Blum, R. (2000). Adolescents with learning disabilities: Risk and protective factors associated with emotional well-being: Findings from the national longitudinal study of adolescent health. *Journal of Adolescent Health, 27*(5), 340-348.

Szepfalusi, Z., Seidl, R., Bernert, G., Dietrich, W., Spitzauer, S., & Urbanek, R. (1999). Latex sensitization in spina bifida appears disease-associated. *The Journal of Pediatrics, 134*(3), 344-348.

Wolraich, M.L. (2000, October 28). *Attention deficit hyperactivity disorder: Current diagnosis and treatment.* American Academy of Pediatrics Annual Meeting. American Academy of Pediatrics.

Chapter 47 *Social Disorders*

Barbara A. Elliott & Christie Sandra Ehle Erickson

Fetal Alcohol Syndrome and Alcohol-Related Neurologic Disorder, p. 877
Lead Poisoning (Plumbism), p. 879
Physical Abuse and Neglect, p. 882
Poverty and Homelessness, p. 884
Sexual Abuse, Incest, and Rape, p. 886
Substance Abuse, p. 889

Fetal Alcohol Syndrome and Alcohol-Related Neurologic Disorder

Alert

Consult with or refer to a physician when signs and symptoms of fetal alcohol syndrome (FAS) and alcohol-related neurologic disorder (ARND) occur:
- Prenatal and postnatal growth retardation
- Central nervous system (CNS) dysfunction, including intellectual, neurologic, and behavioral symptoms
- Facial dysmorphology (of eyes, maxilla, nose, and mouth)
- Maternal history of alcohol use or abuse

FAS and ARND have profound, lifelong effects on children and their families. Although they cannot be cured, FAS and ARND can be prevented.

Specific physical and behavioral attributes are associated with FAS and ARND. Practitioners need to know these characteristics so that they can be a part of the diagnostic effort, provide relevant services, and make appropriate referrals for children and families.

Etiology

FAS and ARND are the fetal consequences of a mother's drinking of alcohol during pregnancy, which exposes the fetus to toxic levels of alcohol. FAS is a severe condition with obvious physical defects and changes in the central nervous system (CNS), including retardation. ARND is milder, with fewer abnormalities, but with significant CNS changes that may not be obvious until the child is older.

How exposure to alcohol during pregnancy produces FAS and ARND is still unclear. The brain develops throughout the pregnancy, and drinking alcohol at any time during gestation can be harmful. Chronic use or binge drinking causes the most CNS damage to the fetus.

Diagnosis of a child with ARND is often missed. These children are often only mildly affected, with low-to-average intelligence, subtle lags in development, and facial attributes that look abnormal only to experienced observers.

Incidence

- The incidence of FAS has increased sixfold in the last 15 years.
- FAS and ARND is found in all races and socioeconomic groups.
- Approximately 20 children per 10,000 are born with FAS. ARND occurs more frequently than FAS.
- Indigenous American populations have the highest incidence.
- The effects of FAS and ARND persist throughout life.
- One of six women of childbearing age habitually or occasionally drinks enough to harm an unborn child.
- The Centers for Disease Control and Prevention (CDC) report that pregnant women are drinking more now than they were 5 years ago.
- Children with FAS and ARND are at increased risk of neglect and physical abuse.
- A significant proportion of those with mental retardation and learning disabilities are believed to have FAS or ARND.

Risk Factors

- Gestational history of maternal alcohol abuse (including binge drinking)
- Foster or adopted child
- Neglected child

Subjective Data

Any child suspected of having FAS and ARND requires a comprehensive history. There are no definitive tests for FAS and ARND. Instead, diagnosis is based on a combination of evidence. FAS and ARND are often misdiagnosed as attention deficit hyperactivity disorder (ADHD) (Table 47-1). There are four diagnostic categories for FAS and ARND:
- Growth retardation, including low birth weight (LBW), failure to thrive (FTT), being short and thin for age, and reduced head circumference
- CNS involvement, including developmental delay, intellectual impairment, poor motor control, attention deficits, hyperactivity, and muscle weakness
- Facial dysmorphology, including an underdeveloped groove in the upper lip, thin upper lip, flat midface, short or upturned nose, low nasal bridge, ear anomalies, short palpebral fissures, epicanthal folds, and micrognathia (small chin and jaw)
- Maternal history of alcohol use during pregnancy

Findings at birth
- LBW (below the 10th percentile)
- Below-normal length
- Smaller-than-normal occipitofrontal circumference

Findings in infants
- Irritability and overreaction to sounds
- Excessive crying

Table 47-1 Distinguishing Characteristics of Attention Deficit Hyperactivity Disorder and Fetal Alcohol Syndrome/Alcohol-Related Neurologic Disorder

ADHD	FAS/ARND
Has trouble focusing and sustaining focus	Can focus and sustain focus
When focus is attained, can learn to problem-solve	Has trouble learning presented material
Can shift focus when necessary	Has difficulty shifting focus
May act impulsively and not think things through	May act impulsively
When things go wrong, able to process, understand, and problem-solve	When things go wrong, unable or slow to process, problem-solve, or take responsibility for actions

From DeVries, J. (1997). Imagine the possibilities: A new study documents the difference between ADHD and FAS. FAS Times, Summer, 1–5. Reprinted with permission of J. DeVries, FAS Family Resource Institute.

- Poor sleep patterns
- Poor muscle tone
- FTT
- Problematic attachment to a parent or parents
- Seizure disorders or congenital defects (e.g., physical anomalies, sensory deficits, developmental or behavioral problems)

Findings in young children
- Attention-span deficits
- Clumsiness and hyperactivity
- Lack of bonding
- Little caution with strangers
- Problems with phobias, tantrums, and emotional instability
- Gregarious and affectionate nature

Findings in school-age children
- Peak academic functioning in grades 6 to 8
- Average intelligence quotient (IQ) of 70 to 90
- No connection between actions and consequences
- Frequent arithmetic and language deficits
- Interpersonal naïveté
- Increasingly susceptible to victimization
- Impulsive actions

Findings in adolescents. The most typical characteristics of FAS and ARND are behavioral, summarized as follows:
- "Poor judgment" (i.e., inattentive, impulsive, repeats mistakes, no consideration of consequences)
- Carelessness with possessions and money
- Need for immediate gratification
- Poor use of time
- Plateaued reasoning and judgment abilities
- Inappropriate sexual behaviors (as victim or perpetrator)
- Risk of alcohol abuse

Objective Data
A complete physical examination should be done on any child with suspected FAS or ARND. Physical examination and objec-tive findings associated with FAS and ARND in infancy are as follows (listed in order of common occurrence; a * indicates a finding that is less observable with increasing age):
- Diminished IQ
- Microcephaly
- Underdeveloped or absent groove in upper lip*
- Posteriorly displaced jaw*
- Prenatal or postnatal growth deficiency
- Teeth anomalies
- Thin or wide lips*
- Hyperactivity
- Eye ptosis
- Strabismus
- Slanting eyes
- Epicanthal folds*
- Abnormal hair or head shape
- Hypertonia
- Finger anomalies
- Short, flat nose with a high nasal tip*
- Malformed ears or hearing deficits
- Unusually creased palms
- Back, neck, and spine defects
- Midface hypoplasia*
- Small stature

Primary Care Issues and Implications
- *Early discovery*—Early case-finding is important because ample nutrition, health care, and nurturance may prevent the damage that can occur with neglect.
- *Short parentage*—The average child with FAS and ARND stays with the birth mother less than 4 years and is at increased risk of neglect and child abuse.
- *Guilt consequence*—Birth mothers who learn the diagnosis is a consequence of their own drinking suffer tremendous guilt. Support, addiction treatment, and counseling can be important.
- *Growth and development*—Often FAS and ARND are evident only in the delays observed in these areas. Growth retardation, intellectual and motor delays, attention deficits, and muscular weaknesses can be diagnostic. Careful monitoring of a child's development can indicate where and when additional interventions might be helpful.
- *Nutrition*—Careful and appropriate nutrition can allay further retardation in growth and development.
- *Sleep*—Sleep disorders are common among children with attention disorders and hyperactivity.
- *Exercise*—Guided exercise and coordination efforts can help develop a child's limited motor and muscular potential to its greatest advantage. Exercise also can be a productive use of the child's energy to avoid some of the consequences of hyperactivity.
- *Sexuality*—As a child with FAS and ARND matures, his or her impassivity and poor judgment can become obvious in sexuality. Education about sexual development, birth control, and sexually transmitted diseases (STDs) is needed.
- *School*—Appropriate school placements, classroom settings, and educational goals depend on the extent of the disabilities. Evaluate the child's potential and opportunities carefully, working with the school and parents or guardian appropriately.

Management

The major roles for practitioners in FAS and ARND are prevention, case-finding, anticipatory guidance, and case management.

Treatments and medications. There is no cure for FAS and ARND; however, drugs can be used to control behaviors such as hyperactivity and aggression. Refer the child to a provider expert in managing the care of children with FAS and ARND.

Counseling and prevention. FAS and ARND are completely preventable. Educate and warn young women about the effects of alcohol on their unborn children. Counseling families with a child who has FAS and ARND should include the following:

In infancy and early childhood
- Alcohol intervention with parents
- Education regarding the physical and psychosocial needs of the child
- Careful monitoring of the child's health and development
- Safe, stable, structured home
- Discipline, use of rewards for good behavior, and redirection
- Avoidance of overstimulation
- Respite care opportunities for the parents or caregiver
- Referral to early childhood, special education services

In childhood
- Stable, safe, structured home or residence
- Careful monitoring of the child's health and development
- Appropriate education and skills development for the child
- Realistic parental expectations and goals
- Support groups for parents or caregiver
- Discipline focused on immediate, clear, and concrete consequences and rewards, with intervention before a behavior escalates
- Respite care for the parents or caregiver

In adolescence
- Education about sexual development, birth control, and protection from sexually transmitted diseases (STDs)
- Residential planning (for a safe, stable, structured environment)
- Vocational training and placement
- Support groups for the parents or caregiver
- Respite care for the parents or caregiver
- Teaching of healthy choices

Follow-up. As needed, remain in contact with the family or caregivers to provide anticipatory guidance and counseling, case management, and counseling with other pregnancies. Remain in contact with the child to provide evaluation of health and development, primary health care, referrals, and case management.

Consultations and referrals
- Refer the child to physicians, home services, school nurses, social workers, and others with expertise in FAS and ARND.
- Refer the caregivers to support groups, respite care, and counseling.
- Provide case management for these children and their families.
- Refer families with infants and young children with FAS and ARND to early intervention programs.

Resources

Organizations

National Organization on Fetal Alcohol Syndrome (NOFAS), 216 G Street NE, Washington, DC 20002; (202) 785-4585; e-mail address: information@nofas.org; www.nofas.org

Publications

Dorris, M. (1989). *The broken cord.* New York: Harper & Row.

Lead Poisoning (Plumbism)

Alert

Consult with or refer to a physician for the following:
- Capillary blood lead screening levels over 45 μg/dl (an inpatient emergency)
- Screening levels over 20 μg/dl, which should involve referral for full medical evaluation as well as educational, nutritional, and environmental interventions

Lead poisoning is a major environmental public health problem of children in the United States. It occurs in every geographic area and social stratum, but poor inner-city minority children are most often affected.

Lead interferes with the development and functioning of essentially all body organs and systems. At high levels, lead causes coma, convulsions, and death. Although the outward signs may be subtle, lead poisoning also causes mental retardation, impaired growth, hearing loss, and behavioral problems. Intervention for potential lead toxicity are needed whenever a child's blood lead level (BLL) is 10 μg/dl or higher.

Screening, education, and prevention of lead poisoning are routine practice for practitioners. Familiarity with treatment responses when lead-screening tests are positive and coordination of care and long-term follow-up evaluation for children with higher lead levels is important.

Etiology

For lead poisoning to occur, lead needs to get into a child's body. The usual source of exposure to lead is decomposing lead-based paint in the child's home. The primary pathway is lead-contaminated dust and soil, but lead may also be in air, water, or food. It is ingested, often by normal hand-to-mouth activities of the children.

There is increasing evidence that lead, even in small amounts, can cause harmful and long-lasting effects. A high level of lead in the body has long been known to have life-threatening consequences; now it is known that even low amounts of lead exposure in young children interfere with the development and functioning of all body organs and systems.

Lead is persistent in the body; once it is absorbed, it takes more than 20 years for half of a given dose to be naturally removed by the body. Small amounts of lead can cause effects that endure long after the exposure.

Practitioners need to remain well informed regarding recommendations for the reduction and elimination of this completely preventable childhood illness. The lowest acceptable BLL concentration is now less than 10 μg/dl; levels over 20 μg/dl call for environmental, educational, and medical intervention. At a level of 45 μg/dl and above, chelation therapy is indicated. Chelation therapy, which is done through referral to a physician, may also be introduced at a level below 45 μg/dl.

Incidence

- Even low levels of lead exposure can cause CNS damage, hearing impairments, and growth deficits.

- It is estimated that 890,000 United States children have BLLs greater than 10 μg/dl.
- Children absorb more than 50% of the lead they ingest.
- If calcium or iron deficiency exists, even more lead is absorbed through the gastrointestinal (GI) tract.
- High concentrations of lead exist in paints that were made before 1950.
- Children are also at risk of being born with lead poisoning when their mothers have elevated BLLs.
- The amount of lead ingested by U.S. children is dropping because of improvements in understanding and treating lead poisoning and because of the ban on the use of lead-based paint.
- Some populations are more heavily exposed than others. Poor children, African-American children, and children living in housing built before 1946 are at greater risk.
- African-American children are affected six times more often than Caucasian children.

Risk Factors

- Living in poverty
- Living in older, poorly maintained housing
- Siblings or playmates with high lead levels
- Location of home or child care near heavily traveled roadways
- Housing painted (especially) before 1950
- Minority race
- Inner city residence
- Pica
- Warm weather (e.g., more outdoor activities, windows open)
- Home built before 1978 that is being remodeled

Subjective Data

Any infant or child at high risk for elevated lead levels requires a comprehensive history. There are subjective screening questions to ask every child's parents when a child is being screened with the capillary blood screening test. These questions, which are recommended by the CDC, are found in Chapter 12.

When the lead screen level is over 10 μg/dl, assess the child's general health, behavior, and appearance, with attention paid to:
- General health
- Condition of living and day-care environment
- Developmental status and behavioral concerns
- Social service needs
- Family's knowledge of exposure-limiting measures
- Nutritional habits
- Siblings' lead status
- Parental occupation

When the blood lead level is over 20 μg/dl, further documentation of the child's behavior and appearance should be made as part of the referral, with special attention to the following:
- Listlessness
- Loss of appetite
- Irritability
- Behavioral changes
- School problems
- Developmental or growth delays

Objective Data

Physical examination. When the BLL is greater than 10 μg/dl:
- Perform a complete physical examination.
- Record the current weight and any change.
- If the blood lead level is above 20 μg/dl, check for pallor.
- Perform a careful neurologic examination, observing especially for any incoordination, balance problems, hearing loss, listlessness, irritability, or seizures.
- Evaluate for delayed development using the Denver II.
- Measure venous lead levels (Table 47-2).
- Evaluate for anemia, because anemia is often the manifesting condition) (see Anemia in Chapter 36).

Diagnostic procedures and laboratory tests. Screening tests are done on capillary blood. Follow-up diagnostic evaluations are done using venous blood, following the recommendations based on the screening BLLs (see Table 47-2). There are two

Table 47-2 Follow-Up for Capillary Blood Lead Levels

BLOOD LEAD LEVEL (μg/dl)	INTERVENTION
Less than 10	Not considered poisoned
10-14	Perform diagnostic tests on venous blood every 3 months; provide family lead education; refer for social services if necessary
15-19	Perform diagnostic tests on venous blood every 2 months; provide family lead education; refer to social services if necessary; if blood lead levels persist or worsen, proceed according to actions for blood lead levels 20-44
20-44	Perform diagnostic tests on venous blood within 48 hours, with follow-up testing in 1 to 2 months, then every 3 months; provide coordination of care (case management) or services, including cnvironmental intervention, medical evaluation, educational and nutritional intervention, and possible pharmacologic treatment
45-69	Perform diagnostic tests on venous blood with 24 hours, and carefully monitor after that; within 48 hours, begin coordination of care (case management) or clinical management, including environmental intervention, medical intervention, educational and nutritional intervention, and chelation therapy
Over 70	Perform diagnostic tests on venous blood as a diagnostic emergency; hospitalize child and immediately begin coordination of care (case management) or clinical management with chelation therapy and full medical, environmental, and educational interventions

Modified from Centers for Disease Control and Prevention. (1997). Screening young children for lead poisoning: Guidance for state and local public health officials. Atlanta: Centers for Disease Control and Prevention.

approaches to screening, depending on the local public health recommendations. Some settings recommend universal screening of all children; children are to be screened when they are between 12 and 24 months of age, or between 36 and 72 months of age if they have not been previously screened. Other settings recommend that only high-risk children be screened (see Risk Factors). In these settings, only children having one or more of the criteria are to be screened between 12 and 24 months of age, or between 36 and 72 months of age if not previously done.

Primary Care Issues and Implications

Identifying children with elevated blood lead levels is a priority to prevent CNS damage. When several children are identified with BLLs greater than 10 μg/dl, community-wide interventions are needed Lead poisoning is a multifaceted environmental problem with no simple solutions. Primary care practitioners (PCPs), lawmakers, the legal system, public health officials, homeowners, housing officials, educators, and families must work together to address the challenge.

For an affected child, the practitioner must address the following areas:

- *Growth and development*—Careful assessment is indicated at each visit. Especially monitor CNS development, hearing, and growth, watching for deficits.
- *Nutrition*—The child may report no desire to eat, constipation, and stomach cramps. It is vitally important to maintain a low-fat diet with high iron, vitamin C, and calcium intake. Educate the child and family about regular meals.
- *Sleep*—The child may report trouble sleeping.
- *Exercise*—The effects of higher lead levels are often evident in problems with coordination, balance, strength, and lack of energy. Encourage activity, and work with occupational and physical therapists, as appropriate.
- *School*—Concentration, behavior, and learning problems are associated with higher lead levels. Assess the child carefully and refer for further work-up as appropriate.

Management

Well-child care is through universal screening or targeted screening for high-risk children. Screen at 12 to 15 months of age, or between 36 and 72 months of age if not previously screened. Follow-up diagnostic tests using venous blood and referrals depend on community and family-specific risk and previous BLLs (see Table 47-2).

Treatments and medications. When an elevated BLL is documented:

- Removal from lead exposure is the primary treatment.
- Chelation treatment is indicated when blood lead levels are high (over 40 μg/dl) and is performed with the participation of a physician.
- Referral should be made to a lead clinic or specialized team for treatments.
- Both outpatient and inpatient chelation should be made available. (A confirmed lead-safe environment is necessary for outpatient treatment.)

Counseling and prevention. For primary prevention:

- Educate parents about lead poisoning (e.g., pathways of exposure, age of house paint, community risks).
- When several children are identified with elevated levels, keep in mind that community intervention is needed.
- Have brochures about lead exposure in waiting areas.
- Empower families to reduce lead exposure in their environments.

When elevated lead levels have been documented, counsel as follows:

- Review the protective measures for families found in Box 47-1.
- Educate parents specifically about the child's exposures and how to reduce them.
- Counsel supportively yet clearly about the housing health risk. (A housing crisis is often precipitated for the family.)
- Report elevated BLLs to the local health department as required.
- Work with the public health department and social services to reduce exposures.

Box 47-1 Protective Measures for Families Dealing With Household Lead

1. Place furniture or other objects in front of large peeling paint areas until more permanent steps can be taken.
2. Cover smaller peeling areas with sticky-backed paper.
3. Damp-dust and mop all hard surfaces of the household, such as floors, moldings, window frames, and door frames with a high (5% to 8%)–phosphate cleaner about twice a week to decrease the amount of lead dust in the environment.
   - Trisodium phosphate contains over 5% phosphates and is usually available in local hardware stores.
   - Other cleaners and some automatic dishwasher detergents contain 5% or more phosphates (read the label carefully).
   - Dry sweeping and vacuuming actually spread the dust further.
4. Pick up and remove loose paint chips with a disposable rag or paper towel saturated with a high-phosphate cleaning solution and dispose in a manner that will not spread the lead further.
5. Never sand, scrape, or burn lead paint off surfaces; this puts large amounts of lead dust or fumes into the air.
6. Be certain the decomposing paint is removed or encapsulated in a safe manner, preferably by a certified lead abatement specialist. All young children and pregnant women should be out of the house during this work and should not return until a thorough high-phosphate clean-up has been done.
7. Provide a diet high in calcium and iron for the children; consider a daily vitamin with an iron supplement.
8. Wash and dry children's hands and faces frequently, especially before eating or after playing outside.
9. Keep toys, pacifiers, and other frequently mouthed objects clean and dry.
10. Be certain all young children in the home are tested for lead.
11. Be prepared to relocate if lead hazards cannot be abated in a timely manner.
12. Use only cold tap water for cooking (warm water causes lead to leach from the solder), and run tap water 2 to 3 minutes in the morning to flush the pipes before using them.

Modified from Centers for Disease Control and Prevention. (1997). Screening young children for lead poisoning: Guidance for state and local public health officials. Atlanta: Centers for Disease Control and Prevention.

- Counsel the family to maintain nutrition with regular meals that include plenty of iron (e.g., fortified cereals, legumes, spinach, raisins), vitamin C, and calcium (e.g., milk, cheese, cooked greens).

Follow-up. For children with elevated BLLs:

- Follow the recommendations for follow-up care listed in Table 47-2.
- Refer the child for appropriate medical and environmental interventions.
- Counsel the family regarding nutritional needs.
- Observe the child's growth and development carefully.
- Work carefully with other agencies to serve the child's needs, possibly coordinating services.

After chelation therapy:

- Discharge only to a confirmed lead-safe environment.
- Coordinate care and services from many agencies to serve the child's and family's needs (or participate in care if another is coordinating services).
- Follow BLLs carefully. Reductions in levels should occur within a few months, but multiple chelations may be needed.

Consultations and referrals

- Notify the public health department as directed for the given setting.
- Know the community and region's resources for referrals.
- Refer the child to a lead clinic or physician when the screening BLL is 20 μg/dl or greater.
- Contact social services and housing assistance when the BLL is 20 μg/dl or greater.
- Work with agencies and schools to provide assessments and services to children with elevated BLLs.

Resources

Organizations

Lead Poisoning Prevention Branch, Division of Environmental Hazards and Health Effects, National Center for Environmental Health, 1600 Clifton Road, Mailstop E 25, Atlanta, GA 30333; (404) 639-2510

Websites

Centers for Disease Control and Prevention (CDC) Childhood Lead Poisoning Prevention Program (www.cdc.gov/nceh/lead/lead.htm)
The Coalition to End Lead Poisoning (www.leadsafe.org)
National Safety Council's Environmental Health Center's Lead Poisoning Prevention Outreach Program (www.nsc.org/ehc/lead.htm)

Physical Abuse and Neglect

Alert

Consult with or refer to a physician and report to the local authorities any child suspected of having been or reported to have been physically abused or neglected.

Practitioners are mandated reporters in all states for all types of abuse of children, including physical, emotional, sexual, and neglect. When abuse is suspected (i.e., when it comes to mind as a part of the differential diagnosis), contact the appropriate local authorities. This process usually involves a oral report followed within a few days by a written report. It is imperative to know the reporting requirements in the practice setting.

A child with physical injuries needs to have the injuries treated and have a full assessment for child abuse. A referral to a practitioner who is experienced in these assessments is appropriate. However, the most common symptoms of child abuse are behavioral changes rather than physical findings.

Etiology

Child maltreatment has been recognized for generations, but it was not defined as a health issue until the early 1960s. Child abuse is a symptom of family abnormalities with complex, multigenerational causes and particular family dynamics.

Treatment needs to be focused on several levels: the injuries and consequences suffered by the child, the family and parenting dysfunction, any (individual) parental pathologic condition, and related community circumstances. Prevention is also focused at the individual, family, and community levels.

Child abuse can be inflicted by anyone responsible for caring for children, and it occurs in all types of families and settings. There is more child abuse and neglect reported in minority families with lower incomes, but that does not mean that more abuse occurs there; it occurs in all settings. It is unfortunate to miss children living in danger by assuming that majority culture, middle-class children are not abused. Children of all ages are physically abused and neglected, though infants and young children are at greatest risk for life-threatening injury.

Incidence

- An estimated 5000 children die each year as a result of child abuse; three times that number suffer permanent brain damage from abuse.
- Every year more than 2.8 million cases of child abuse and neglect are reported.
- Approximately one third of the reported child abuse and neglect cases are substantiated each year. Of substantiated cases, 60% of the children are neglected and 25% are physically abused. (The others were sexually abused; see Sexual Abuse, Incest, and Rape, later in this chapter.)
- Infants and young children are at the greatest risk for life-threatening injuries from abuse.
- In children under 3 years of age, 25% of fractures and 10% to 15% trauma are inflicted on them.
- African Americans and American Indians have the highest rates of victimization; Asians and Pacific Islanders have the lowest rates.
- More women than men are perpetrators of physical abuse and neglect of children.

Risk Factors

For parents (to abuse)

- Dysfunctional attachment in a new mother
- Unrealistic expectations of child development
- Overconcern or underconcern about injury
- Refusal of appropriate hospitalization
- Alcohol or drug addiction
- Other types of violence in the home
- Social isolation
- High levels of stress
- Abused as children

For children (to be abused)

- Premature birth
- Poor self-concept
- Habit disorders
- Chronically ill
- Handicap or disability
- High-need infant
- Difficult pregnancy or birth

Subjective Data

A comprehensive history must be completed on any child suspected of having been physically abused or neglected. It is important to approach the family in a nonjudgmental manner and to be an advocate for both the child and the family. The task of an interview is to gather data that guides the physical examination and laboratory study and builds a relationship with the parents and child. Interview questions need to be worded in a nonleading way. Parents should be interviewed separately when possible. It is important to remember that more than half of the women whose children are abused are themselves victims of domestic violence.

When a referral for a full assessment is made, it is important to include the presence of any of the following behavioral indicators (with the appropriate risk factors and any observed pattern) in the medical record of repeated trauma in the documentation:

- Fearful of adults
- Depressed
- Too accepting of painful procedures
- Inconsolable
- Seeking constant reassurance
- Aggressive or withdrawn
- Frightened of parent or parents
- Overanxious to please
- Evasive when asked about injuries
- Experiencing a sleep disorder

Subjective data that may indicate child neglect includes the following:

- Inadequate immunizations
- No medical care
- Unsafe environment
- Little supervision
- Abandonment

Objective Data

The physical examination of a suspected victim of physical abuse should be thorough and conducted in an unhurried way. The examination begins with a developmentally appropriate approach. Do not simply focus on an obvious injury; it is important that the entire body be examined (so all of the child's clothes need to be taken off for the examination). Photographs of obvious physical injuries should be taken and drawings on a body sketch should be done as part of the documentation.

Physical examination. An examination should be performed on the following areas:

- *Head*—Common injuries (in both infants and older children) include those on the scalp skin, in the mouth, and on the neck and face. They also include retinal hemorrhages (from "shaken baby syndrome" or "shaken impact syndrome"); if eye trauma is suspected, refer to an ophthalmologist.
- *Chest, abdomen, and genitals*—Common injuries are to the upper, middle, and lower back and across the buttocks. Organ injury is possible even without external abdominal bruising (from "shaken baby syndrome"). There may also be current or past genital bruising, discharge, or other signs of injury (because physical and sexual abuse often found together).
- *Extremities*—There may be injuries to the arms and legs (including the palms and soles).

Suspicious findings related to physical abuse may include:

- Bruises and welts on soft tissue (in different stages of healing)
- Burns (e.g., cigarette burns, scald injury)
- FTT
- Fractures (multiple and in different stages of healing)
- Genital injury or infection
- Hemorrhage (e.g., retinal, intraabdominal, renal)
- Lacerations and abrasions (multiple and neglected)
- Neurologic injuries (e.g., brain hematomas, coma)
- Optic injuries (e.g., retinal injuries, black eyes)

Suspicious findings related to neglect may include:

- Poor hygiene
- Inappropriate clothing for the current weather
- Extreme diaper rash
- Lack of routine health care
- Lack of continuity of health care

Diagnostic procedures and laboratory tests. Radiographic surveys of part or all of the child's body may be indicated when broken bones are suspected. The practitioner doing the full assessment can order this survey.

Primary Care Issues and Implications

The practitioner's primary concern is ensuring the child's safety. There are many modes of injury, and abuse needs to be kept in mind when a child has an unusual pattern of manifesting symptoms. The practitioner's role in cases of child physical abuse and neglect includes aiding prevention through anticipatory guidance, identifying and addressing of risk factors, reporting suspicions to proper authorities, assessing and documenting findings, referring appropriately, and supporting children and families when community and court interventions occur through long-term follow-up study.

Reporting to and intervention by the authorities raises an ethical dilemma for mandated reporters because the family unit is inevitably changed by the report, and major dislocations and economic consequences can result. Remaining a care provider and advocate for the patient and family is important when the family (or a portion of it) is willing to remain a part of the practice.

Other issues involve the following areas:

- *Growth and development*—Physical abuse is traumatic and destructive to a child's well-being. It can interfere with normal developmental progression and age-appropriate tasks. Assess the child's development carefully after abuse has occurred and refer appropriately.
- *Sleep*—Children who have been abused commonly experience sleep disturbances, ranging from nightmares and needing to sleep with a protector or in a safe place to night terrors and insomnia. Have a professional who is an expert in healing after abuse evaluate the sleep disturbances and manage any problems.
- *School*—Physical abuse can predispose a child to respond to frustration with bullying, conflict, or violence. Relationships at school should be discussed frequently, and nonviolent conflict resolution skills taught. Work with and refer to the schools and other professionals appropriately.

Management

When there are suspicious physical findings, they need to be discussed with the child and family. It is also important to discuss the mandatory reporting laws with the child and family to prepare them for the involvement of social services or law enforcement agencies. It is helpful to present the investigative agency as a partner in understanding what has happened, stopping the abuse, and looking after the child's best interest.

The PCP's charted record can provide important evidence about the abuse of a child. The child abuse expert who receives the referral for the work-up also uses it in guiding that assessment. If court action becomes necessary, the charted documentation from all settings becomes a part of the proceedings. Document the following carefully and objectively:

- Medical and relevant social history
- Statements made by the child and the parents or guardian
- Child and family behaviors
- Detailed description of the injuries
- Laboratory data
- Pictures or drawings of the injuries

Treatments and medications. Treatment should be planned to help any injuries heal and avoid permanent physical impairment (when possible). The greatest overall damage is to the child as a developing being, whether the abuse is physical, emotional, or neglect. Counseling the abused child, working with dysfunctional families, and treating post–traumatic stress disorders needs to be done by skilled providers.

Counseling and prevention

Prenatal care

- Watch for maternal neglect or physical abuse of a pregnancy or fetus (through addictions).
- Discuss the mother's past and current experience with violence. Inquire if she feels safe with her partner and in her environment.
- Advocate for the infant's well-being.
- Identify any increased risk for violence and refer appropriately.

Well-child care

- Explain the need for routine well-child visits.
- Educate about child development and identify realistic behavior expectations.
- Discuss changing safety concerns.
- Investigate child care options and discuss how to choose safe child care.
- Talk about parenting and discipline issues.
- Model nonviolence in the office.
- Discuss the mother's experience with violence.
- Review other risk factors.
- Identify any increased risk for violence and refer appropriately.

Counseling and support for the family after abuse has occurred

- Clearly place responsibility for the abuse. (The child did not cause or deserve it.)
- Inquire about and support ongoing therapies and interventions.
- Provide anticipatory guidance for the child's development, including expected and appropriate child behaviors, child's skill development, and developmental milestones.
- Teach parenting skills, emphasizing age-appropriate communication, safety, and nonviolent discipline.
- Continue discussing the child's recovery from previous abuse, emphasizing emotional, behavioral, and physical consequences. Discuss these topics over time and with each new milestone.
- Support the parents' recovery from the abuse with discussion and appropriate referrals.

Counseling and support for the child after abuse has occurred

- Clearly place responsibility for the abuse. (The child did not cause or deserve it.)
- Inquire about and support work with other therapists.
- Educate the child regarding physical, social, and emotional development.

- Assess the child for post–traumatic stress problems, depression, and anxiety, and refer appropriately.
- Educate the child regarding nonviolent conflict-resolution skills.

Follow-up

- Carefully follow the child's health, development, and safety.
- Support parental, family, and child involvement in counseling.
- Coordinate or participate in multidisciplinary and multiagency interventions.
- Perform routine well-child care.

Consultations and referrals

- Refer disclosed or suspected cases to a multidisciplinary team for full assessment of potential abuse, which should be done by providers who are experts in interviewing children and evaluating for inflicted injuries.
- Refer to a physician when abuse has resulted in injuries (depending on the nature, location, and severity of the injuries).
- Refer high-risk cases to social services and school support services for assessment of the needs of the child and family, protection of the child, coordination of counseling, and other services the family may need (e.g., homemaker services, parent aide programs, respite care, alcohol and substance abuse programs, foster homes, Parents Anonymous).
- Refer high-risk families to community parenting groups for support and skills training, mentor mothers, and individual and family counseling.
- Refer dysfunctional families and those with post–traumatic stress disorders to a mental health professional.

Resources

Organizations

National Child Abuse Hotline (Child Help USA); (800) 422-4453; www.childhelpusa.org

Parents Anonymous, Inc., 675 W Foothill Boulevard., Suite 220, Claremont, CA 91711; (909) 621-6184; e-mail parentsanon@msn.com; www.parentsananymous-natl.org

National Clearinghouse on Child Abuse and Neglect Information, 330 C Street SW, Washington, DC 20447; 1-800-394-3366; http://www.calib.com/nccanch

National Foundation for Abused and Neglected Children, PO Box 608134, Chicago, IL 60660; e-mail nfanc@hotmail.com; www.gangfreekids.org

Websites

Child Abuse Prevention Network (www.child-abuse.com)

Poverty and Homelessness

Alert

Refer the child to another physician, agency, or provider for the following:

- Needs beyond the capacity of the current site or scope of the current provider's practice (providing transportation for the child and family when possible)
- Child diagnosed with or at high risk for human immunodeficiency virus (HIV) and acquired immune deficiency syndrome (AIDS)
- Child with an unstable chronic disease

Health problems faced by homeless children are similar to those faced by all impoverished children and their families. They are in special need of continuity in disease prevention and health promotion services because of the adverse settings in which they live. The profile of illnesses they experience (distribution, cause, and severity) varies to some degree based on the physical environment, level of access to health care, and range of social and emotional stressors they face.

There are barriers to receiving health care that homeless and impoverished families particularly encounter; these include finding or accessing a provider, waiting for and during appointments, meeting the costs of health care (for both office visits and prescribed treatments), overcoming cultural barriers, and obtaining transportation to and from appointments. These barriers need to be addressed.

Etiology

Poverty and homelessness are caused by a variety of circumstances, including lack of affordable, low-cost housing; unemployment; low wages; family violence and dysfunction; mental and physical illness; and inadequate public assistance. These circumstances, alone or in combination, can result in the continuum of impoverishment for families. In recent years, poverty has become a gender issue as well, with women becoming impoverished at increasing rates. It should be noted that homeless women with children are not as likely to have mental illness or substance-abuse issues when compared to individual homeless women or men.

Incidence

- There are approximately 2 million homeless persons every day in the United States.
- Families with children make up more than one third of the homeless population.
- Women and children are the fastest growing subgroup of the homeless population.
- Children represent 25% of the homeless population.
- Every night, 100,000 children go to sleep homeless.
- Government support for low-income housing has been cut by 80% in the last decade.
- Nearly 10% of Americans are malnourished, and almost two thirds of them are part of family units.

Risk Factors

- Single parenthood
- State of residence (some states have better governmental assistance programs)
- Parental unemployment or low wages
- Few community and family support systems
- Family violence
- Parental substance abuse
- Parental mental illness
- Lack of available, low-cost housing
- Racial or ethnic minority

Subjective Data

A complete history should be obtained with careful attention to the areas described here. The listed conditions are each a consequence of the environments in which the children and adolescents live, the lack of opportunities to buy or prepare food, and the family priority to provide food and shelter before health care. Health care for these children involves attending to the specific health concerns they have when they are seen. Important questions to ask during history-taking include any family member's psychiatric problems, substance abuse, and sources of social support.

Impoverished and homeless children and adolescents have a particular profile of illnesses and diseases that result from their circumstances. Among them are the following that need to be explored:
- Alcohol and chemical abuse
- Dental concerns
- Fewer immunizations
- Foot problems
- Frostbite
- Hearing loss from middle ear infections
- Increased risk of lead poisoning
- Increased susceptibility to infections and communicable diseases
- Injuries (especially from violence)
- Obesity, anemia, and nutritional deficiencies
- Parasites
- Physical or psychologic delays in development
- Skin disorders (from poor hygiene and infestations of parasites)
- Tuberculosis (TB)

In addition, among adolescents, the following problems should be explored:
- Alcohol and chemical abuse
- Hepatitis C
- HIV
- Mental illness issues
- Pregnancy and contraception issues
- STDs

Objective Data

A complete physical examination should be done, with special sensitivity to respiratory, ear, and skin conditions and developmental delay, neglect, and inflicted injuries. The practitioner should follow child and teen checkup guidelines or the American Academy of Pediatrics' health maintenance schedule for examinations, immunizations, growth and development, and so on.

Primary Care Issues and Implications

The following are the goals of practitioners who care for homeless and impoverished children and adolescents:

General
- Assess the need for health care and other services.
- Plan and coordinate the needed services.
- Provide skilled services.
- Monitor to ensure multiple service needs are met (possible case management role).
- Advocate for the child and family.
- When the health issues are acute, as when a child has an infection or asthma in a shelter, provide immediate attention and referral.
- When the need is for preventive, diagnostic, and treatment services, provide the services, working to prevent the serious, long-term health consequences associated with being homeless or impoverished (e.g., hearing loss, dentition problems, malnutrition, obstetric issues).

Growth and development
- Assess anthropometric measurements carefully at every visit, measuring height and weight. Assess development using appropriate developmental screening tool (Denver II).
- Note placement on the malnutrition continuum, including anemia, weight loss, slowing of growth in body mass, loss

of muscle and tissue mass, slowing of growth in height, and arrest of growth.
- Provide anticipatory guidance and refer as needed.

Immunizations
- Assess the child's immunization status at every visit.
- Give all appropriate immunizations (e.g., influenza vaccine, pneumococcal vaccine, Mantoux test) whenever possible, including at appointments for minor illness.
- Limit barriers to immunizations (e.g., lack of evening and weekend hours, requiring prescheduled appointments).

Nutrition
- Use a food-frequency questionnaire to carefully assess what is being eaten and the sources of food.
- Relate nutrition to growth and development.
- Counsel the child and parents regarding diet, obesity, and malnutrition.
- Set mutually acceptable realistic nutrition goals with the parents.
- Refer the family to appropriate community resources (e.g., Women, Infants, and Children [WIC] program, children's nutrition programs, emergency food shelves, soup kitchens).

Sleep
- Assess sleep patterns, habits, routines, and arrangements carefully.
- Advise the family of resources.
- Provide guidance on managing sleep problems.
- Refer the family when possible.

Exercise
- Assess the child's activity levels and strength.
- Provide guidance.

Sexuality
- Assess appropriately.
- Educate the child and parents about STDs (including HIV and AIDS), safe sex, birth control, and sexual violence.

School
- Assess carefully if the child attends school (including when, where, and why or why not).
- Advise the parents about resources.
- Refer the family when possible.

Screening (age-appropriate)
- Screen for anemia; TB; lead toxicity; HIV and AIDS; STDs; hearing, vision, and dental problems; substance abuse; pregnancy; violence; and abuse.
- Treat appropriately.
- Refer when possible.

Management

It is important to set clear priorities when one is seeing homeless or impoverished children, perhaps in this order:
- Acutely ill children and those with unstable chronic conditions
- Pregnant adolescents without prenatal care
- Children needing immunizations
- Children needing checkups or well-child care
- Others

Treatments and medications
- Consider the living circumstances of the child and family. (For example, if a child has scabies, treatment may be impossible unless there is access to medication, laundry services to wash clothing, and bathing or water to complete the treatment regimen.)

- Consider the family's readiness and ability to follow through with the prescription. (For example, injected antibiotics may be manageable in circumstances where oral antibiotics that need refrigeration are not.)
- Arrange for a sponsor to help transport the child and parents to any referral site and help negotiate the system, if possible.
- Have medications and social and mental health services available on site.
- Offer opportunities for personal hygiene, some supplemental food, and basic essentials (e.g., diapers, tampons) on site if possible.

Counseling and prevention. Health care becomes a priority for these children and their families only after their basic needs (e.g., food, shelter) are met. Primary prevention of these health problems comes through public policy changes (e.g., related to housing, job training, adequate public assistance). Secondary and tertiary preventive efforts are needed for treatment of and education related to malnutrition, frostbite, STDs, trauma, and so on.

Follow-up. Provide follow-up services (when possible) when needed for well-child care or as indicated for other problems.

Consultations and referrals
- When possible, maintain continuity of care.
- Manage cases with the help of agencies and other professionals in the community (e.g., shelters, schools, social service agencies).
- Locate practitioner services where these families gather (e.g., a shelter or soup kitchen in an urban setting, a mobile service center in rural areas).
- Provide families with assisted referrals whenever possible.

Resources

Organizations

Health Care for the Homeless, Policy Research Associates, Inc., 262 Delaware Avenue, Delmar, NY 12054; (888) 439-3300, x. 246; e-mail address: wvcc@prainc.com; www.prainc.ocm

Interagency Council on the Homeless, 451 Seventh Street SW, Suite 7274, Washington, DC 20410; (202) 708-1480

National Health Care for the Homeless Council, PO Box 60427, Nashville, TN 37206-0427; (615) 226-2292; e-mail address: council@nhchc.org; www.nhchc.org

National Law Center on Homelessness and Poverty, 1411 K Street, NW, Suite 1400, Washington, DC 20005; (202) 638-2535; www.nlchp.org

Sexual Abuse, Incest, and Rape

Alert

Consult with or refer to a physician and report to the appropriate authorities any child who is suspected of having been sexually abused or discloses sexual abuse.

Practitioners are mandated reporters of sexual abuse (including rape) of children in all states. When it is suspected (i.e., when it comes to mind as a part of the differential diagnosis), contact with appropriate authorities in the jurisdiction must be made. This process usually involves an oral report followed within a few days by a written report. A practitioner should know the reporting requirements in the current practice setting.

Etiology

Sexual abuse and assault include any form of nonconsenting sexual activity. The legal definitions vary from state to state; however, most definitions include the use of power (or force when the abuse is defined as rape), sexual contact, and non-consent of the victim. Intrafamilial sexual abuse (incest) is defined as any form of sexual activity between a child and an immediate family member (e.g., parent, stepparent, sibling), extended family member (e.g., grandparent, uncle, aunt, cousin), or surrogate parent (i.e., adult whom the child perceives to be a member of the family unit). Extrafamilial sexual abuse is defined as any form of sexual contact between a non-family member and a child. In a majority of these cases, the adult is known to the child and has had access to the child as a friend, neighbor, or caregiver.

Central to the issue of child sexual abuse is the power differential between the abuser and the child. This power differential, combined with the child's trust of the known adult, results in damage to the child. The child is developmentally unable to understand or give informed consent to the sexual activities initiated by an older person, and refusal is simply not possible. Children are "groomed" or prepared over time to participate in sexual behavior. Rape is one form of sexual abuse, usually perpetrated by someone who is known to the victim as a nonfamily member.

Incest occurs in all social settings, with no relationship to parental education, income, or employment. It also occurs in all geographic locations and across all religious and ethnic backgrounds. Incest happens between generations of a family and within the immediate family unit, and it can continue over an extended period of time.

Incidence

Sexual abuse

- Conservative estimates approximate that there are 300,000 cases of child sexual abuse each year in the United States.
- The numbers of unreported incidents are greater than the reported ones because of the secrecy and shame that accompany child sexual abuse.
- The average age of onset of incest is 9 years of age for girls and 8 years of age for boys.
- Of the incest cases, 75% are father and daughter (including stepfathers, live-in boyfriends, or other men in the parental role).
- Most sexual abuse of children is perpetrated by male family members.

Sexual assault

- Before 18 years of age, one girl in four and one boy in eight (conservatively estimated) have nonconsensual sex, but only 6% of these incidents are reported to the authorities.
- About 80% of the victims know their abusers; two thirds of abusers are family members, and 80% are male perpetrators.

Risk Factors

- Living in a home where other family violence is ongoing
- Parental history of child sexual abuse
- Family portrayal that "everything is okay"
- Geographic and social isolation (i.e., a closed family system)
- Extreme mistrust of outsiders
- Family secrets (i.e., dysfunctional family communication)
- Enmeshment (i.e., unhealthy closeness among family members)
- Imbalance of parental power
- Child caring for parental needs (i.e., role reversal)
- Shame-based discipline
- Parental substance abuse

Subjective Data

A thorough, careful history must be obtained for any child suspected of having been sexually abused. Since most children have been threatened or specifically told to "keep the secret," practitioners must be alert to the possibility of sexual abuse even if it is denied. When a child does disclose a history of sexual abuse, it must be taken seriously and carefully evaluated.

History-taking is essential in making a diagnosis of child sexual abuse. Children should be interviewed about the abuse once (or as few times as possible) by trained and experienced interviewers. The interviewers will obtain taped or video documentation that can be used as admissible evidence in court.

When one is making the referral for the evaluation, presenting behavioral symptoms, even if they are nonspecific, should be noted and described. The most common symptoms of sexual abuse are often behavioral rather than physical findings; findings may include:

Preschool indicators

- Excessive crying
- Fretful or extreme agitation
- FTT
- Developmental regression
- Excessive fears
- Repetitive sex play beyond normal sexual exploration
- Excessive masturbation
- Sleep disturbances
- Toileting difficulties
- Excessive clinging, particularly to certain adults and in response to certain others

School-age indicators

- School problems, including school-related phobias
- Noticeable themes of violence in artwork or schoolwork
- Withdrawal from peers
- Age-inappropriate friendships
- Distorted body image and related problems
- Advanced sexual knowledge
- Excessive mood swings
- Extreme temper
- Depression and suicidal ideation or attempts
- Acting out behaviorally or verbally
- Secondary enuresis
- Overt sexual acting-out toward adults
- Sophisticated sexual play with younger children

Adolescence indicators

- Prevailing lack of trust
- Low self-esteem
- Running away
- Sleep disorders
- School problems, including changed performance and truancy
- Withdrawal and isolation from peers
- Drug or alcohol abuse
- Self-mutilation
- Multiple sexual contacts
- Clinical depression
- Suicide attempts

Objective Data

When a child needs to be examined for the possibility of sexual abuse, a referral to a skilled clinician is indicated because a careful, thorough physical examination must be completed. A child with physical injuries caused by sexual activity needs to be referred to a setting that is prepared to treat the injuries and to use an evidentiary kit (if sexual activity has reportedly occurred within the previous 48 hours) to gather evidence for court follow-up. When the referral is made, include documentation about the following objective issues if they are present:

- STDs
- Poor sphincter tone
- Abrasions or bruises of the external genitalia
- Pain or itching in genital area
- Pain on urination
- Pregnancy

Primary Care Issues and Implications

Practitioners are mandated to report suspicions or evidence of child sexual abuse to the authorities in their area, usually social services or law enforcement agencies. The obligation to report is when "there is reason to believe" that sexual abuse occurred. Informing the parents of the obligation to report can be handled with a clear statement: "When I see injuries, behaviors, and concerns of this type, I am obligated by law to report them to the authorities. They will be coming to interview you about them." Many parents, despite the neutrality and legal obligation of the practitioner, will then end their relationship with the practitioner.

Reporting and intervention by the authorities raises an ethical dilemma for practitioners and other mandated reporters because the family unit is inevitably changed with the report, and major dislocations and economic consequences can result. Remaining the care provider and advocate for the patient and family is important when the family (or a portion of it) is willing to stay a part of the practice.

The practitioner should also examine issues related to the following areas:

- *Growth and development*—Any sexual abuse that a child experiences is traumatic and destructive to the child's well-being. It interferes with normal developmental progression and age-appropriate tasks. Assess development carefully after abuse has occurred and refer appropriately. Such a profound breach of trust can affect the child's emotional and physical health for life. The degree of harm depends on several factors, including:

  Child's age (younger children are more vulnerable)
  Preexisting emotional health of the child and family members
  Type of assault (more force and bodily penetration increase the trauma)
  Duration of the abuse (repeated abuse causes more psychologic harm)
  Relationship to the offender (more destructive when the offender is someone the child knows and trusts)
  Reactions of others (negative reactions by family or professionals exacerbate the trauma)

- *Sleep*—The effects of sexual abuse can range from nightmares to suicide. Some sleep disturbances can be a normal part of the flashbacks that occur as part of the healing process. Others indicate underlying emotional difficulties. Evaluation by a professional expert in healing after sexual abuse is needed for clarification.

- *Sexuality*—Sexual abuse commonly affects the child's sexual growth and development. Depending on when and for how long the abuse occurred, the child may only know how to relate sexually to adults who are the gender of the perpetrator. There may be inappropriate sexual acting-out, masturbation, early sexual activity, promiscuity, or prostitution. Careful supervision of growth and development, appropriate conversation about the consequences of sexual abuse, and appropriate referrals for healing are indicated.

- *School*—Changes in performance and friendships at school can be consequences of sexual abuse. Dropping out of school and running away are not uncommon.

Management

The way a practitioner responds to suspicions or disclosures of child sexual abuse is critical to the child and to family healing. A supportive response from adults in the child's life decreases the devastation that can result from the abuse. The practitioner's charted record can provide important evidence about the abuse of a child. The child abuse expert who receives the referral for the work-up also uses it in guiding that assessment. If court action becomes necessary, charted documentation from all settings becomes a part of the proceedings. Document the following carefully and objectively:

- Medical and relevant social history
- Statements made by the child and the parents or guardian
- Child and family behaviors
- Detailed description of the injuries
- Laboratory data
- Pictures or drawings

Treatments and medications

- Treat any physical health needs (e.g., lacerations) and provide medications for infections.
- When sexual intercourse has occurred within the previous 48 hours, keep in mind that injuries need to be documented and evidence needs to be collected. Refer the child to a setting capable of doing this for the examination.

Counseling and prevention

Anticipatory guidance at the preschool examination

- Talk with parents about the risk.
- Investigate any parental history of sexual abuse and refer appropriately.
- Educate the child to tell an adult whom he or she trusts about any "touch" that makes them feel uncomfortable.
- Use the names of genitalia for "private parts" during a child's examination.
- Encourage the parents to use appropriate terminology in talking with children.

Anticipatory guidance at the preadolescent and adolescent examination

- Talk with the child about sexuality and sexual experiences.
- Educate the child or teenager about the risks of date rape (when developmentally appropriate).
- Offer assistance and further discussion as desired or needed.
- Also talk at this time about alcohol and drug use and their effect on decision-making and risk-taking.

Counseling parents at the time sexual abuse is disclosed or suspected

- Inform the parents about the reporting process and expected follow-up evaluation.
- Explain that you will not abandon them and that you will make appropriate referrals towards healing.
- Listen.
- Answer any questions.

Counseling parents over time

- Describe rape-trauma syndrome with its process of denial and anxiety, acute disorganization with depression, and gradual reorganization.
- Educate the parents about the child's developmental consequences and the healing process (including emotional, physical, and social aspects).
- Support parents as they experience their own therapy and treatment.
- Counsel parents regarding parenting skills; discipline; and management of specific stressors, safe living choices for family members, and self-esteem and development.
- Hold the offender accountable while maintaining a compassionate relationship.

Counseling a child or adolescent victim at the time sexual abuse is disclosed or suspected

- Inform them about the reporting process and expected follow-up evaluation (as is developmentally appropriate).
- Explain that you will not abandon them and that you will make appropriate referrals toward healing.
- Reassure the child and parents that any physical trauma will heal and that the child will return to normal physically.
- Answer any questions.

Counseling a child or adolescent victim over time

- Clearly hold the offender accountable (the child did not deserve or invite the abuse).
- Describe the healing process (rape-trauma syndrome also, as appropriate).
- Carefully monitor growth, health, development, and safety.
- Assess for post–traumatic stress disorder, depression, and anxiety disorders, and refer appropriately.
- Over time, discuss the effects of the abuse on health and development, as appropriate.

Follow-up

- Manage the health care needs of the child and family after suspicion or disclosure of child sexual abuse.
- Carefully monitor the growth, health, development, and safety of the child.
- Attend to emotional and psychologic trauma with counseling and psychiatric referrals. (See Counseling and Prevention.)
- Follow the rape-trauma healing process, with referrals for supportive counseling as appropriate.

Consultations and referrals

- Know the community resources.
- For diagnosis, refer to a capable, skilled team, agency, or person (perhaps in the emergency department at a hospital) to interview, examine, and obtain evidence from any potentially sexually abused child.
- Refer the child to skilled and trained interviewers who will obtain information in the least traumatic and most legally helpful way.
- Refer the parents and child to supportive counselors when the child is experiencing uncomplicated recovery from abuse.
- Refer a child with a complicated or pathologic recovery from abuse to psychiatrists and family therapists.

Resources

Organizations

National Child Abuse Hotline (Child Help USA); (800) 422-4453; www.childhelpusa.org

Parents Anonymous, Inc., 675 W Foothill Boulevard, Suite 220, Claremont, CA 91711; (909) 621-6184; e-mail address: parentsanon@msn.com; www.parentsananymous-natl.org

National Clearinghouse on Child Abuse and Neglect Information, 330 C Street SW, Washington, DC 20447; (800) 394-3366; www.calib.com/nccanch

National Foundation for Abused and Neglected Children, PO Box 608134, Chicago, IL 60660; e-mail address: nfanc@hotmail.com; www.gangfreekids.org

Websites

Child Abuse Prevention Network (www.child.cornell.edu)

Substance Abuse

> **°Alert**
>
> Consult with or refer to a physician for the following:
> - Coma, seizures, cardiac disturbances, or psychosis as a result of drug use
> - Use of highly dangerous drugs such as opiates, amphetamines, cocaine, barbiturates, and hallucinogens (refer for possible detoxification, drug treatment, psychologic testing, psychiatric evaluation, and intervention)
> - Behaviors indicating a potential danger to self or others
> - Pregnancy
> - Physical or sexual abuse (which must be reported)
> - Frequent use of alcohol, marijuana, and inhalants, especially by those suffering changes in their academic, social, or vocational progress (refer for evaluation, assessment, and intervention)

Etiology

Use, abuse, and addiction. Tobacco, alcohol, and other drugs are used, abused, and become sources of addiction for youths. Use of drugs, particularly alcohol or marijuana, as a recreational activity without obvious changes in behavior or performance is not regarded as a health issue by many children or adolescents and families. Abuse of chemicals occurs when a young person is actively seeking the chemical because of dependence. At this point, the young person may use often to produce "good feelings" and to escape reality; behaviors may also begin to change and schoolwork may slip. Addiction occurs when there is a pronounced preoccupation with the drug, loss of control over its use, and behaviors that focus on its acquisition (Table 47-3).

Alcohol and other substances. There are genetic and environmental factors that predispose a person to substance abuse and addiction. When the predisposition is combined with an introduction to the substance and an enabling setting, use begins and there is no encouragement to stop. Experimental use can progress to excessive use (abuse) and then to addiction. The use progresses through this sequence if taking the drug is seen as pleasurable or rewarding, the supportive system approves of the behavior, and no one in the environment observes that dependence is occurring. An enabling setting removes the negative consequences, and there is no reason to stop.

Tobacco. Most smokers adopt the cigarette habit during adolescence and follow this with a lifetime of cigarette consumption. Adverse health effects experienced by adolescents include a decrease in fitness, increased coughing and phlegm, more respiratory illnesses, more sick and hospital days, early development of artery disease, and a slower rate of lung growth. The younger the age at which a person begins smok-

Table 47-3 Drugs Commonly Used by Adolescents

DRUG	STREET NAMES	HOW USED	SIGNS AND SYMPTOMS OF OVERDOSE	WITHDRAWAL SYMPTOMS
Cocaine	Blow, Hard, Flake, Coke, Base, White Powder, Dome, Rock	Inhaled, injected, orally, smoked	Agitation, confusion, hallucinations, cardiac arrest, panic attacks, paranoia, convulsions	Irritability, sluggishness, prolonged period of sleep, depression, nausea
Ecstasy (methylenedioxy-methamphetamine [MDMA])	Rolls, Pills, Beans, X, XTC, Adam, Clarity	Swallowed, snorted, smoked, injected	Teeth grinding, scratching or rubbing skin, dizziness, loss of consciousness, eye twitching, panic attacks, muscle cramping, seizures, increased body temperature, increased heart rate, increased blood pressure, heart attack, stroke	Hangover symptoms, tired feeling, dullness of senses and mental process
GHB (gamma hydroxybutyratic acid)	Liquid E, Georgia Homeboy, Scoop, Grievous Bodily Harm, Liquid X, G, Easy Lay, Gamma 10, Salty Water	Inhaled, injected, swallowed	Dizziness, loss of consciousness, decreased heart rate, memory loss, nausea, vomiting, headache, passing out, respiratory depression, muscle fatigue, coma, death	Insomnia, anxiety, tremors, depression
Heroin	Smack, Junk, Bindles, Bags, Black Tar, Manteca, Horse, Bundles, Tar	Inhaled, smoked, injected, orally	Restlessness, constipation, droopy eyelids, slow breathing, depressed cough reflux, sweatiness, lethargic, slow heart rate, sedation, respiratory failure, death	Insomnia, hot and cold flashes, nausea, vomiting, weakness, abdominal cramps, diarrhea
Inhalants	Whippets, Ozone, Thrust, Poppers, Climax, Rush, Locker Room, Nitrous, Canisters	Inhaled through nose, fumes breathed into mouth	Acute: Double vision, headache, tinnitis, chest pain, anxiety, confusion, nausea Long-term: Tremors, weight loss, impaired respiratory system, lack of concentration, damage to CNS, cardiac arrest, irritation to nose and mouth, death	Hallucinations, headache, nausea, chills, tremors
Ketamine	Special K, K, Cat Valiums, K-Wave, Business Man's LSD	Inhaled, injected, swallowed, smoked	Tunnel vision, delirium, amnesia, depression, impaired motor function, high blood pressure, seizures, coma, potentially fatal respiratory problems	None documented
LSD (lysergic acid diethylamide)	Acid, Boomers, Yellow Sunshine, Double Dome, Sid, Stamps, A-Bombs, Paper, Dots, Blotter, Trips, Doses	Orally	Visual hallucinations, distortion of sizes and shapes, impaired judgement, increased body temperature, increased blood pressure, sweating, sleeplessness	Can have persistent psychosis and persisting perception disorders
Marijuana	Weed, Pot, J, Herb, Joint, Blunt, Kind Crippie	Smoked, orally	Paranoia, increased appetite, impaired coordination, altered perception, restlessness, anxiety attacks, panic attacks	Insomnia, decreased appetite, nausea, irritability, anxieties
Methamphetamine	Batu, Speed, Meth, Crack Meth, Go Fast, Crank, Glass, Ice Chalk, Fire, Crystal, Poor Man's Coke	Inhaled, injected, swallowed, smoked	Malnutrition, physical burnout, aggressive behavior, rapid weight loss, paranoia, memory loss, psychotic behaviors, cardiac and neurologic damage, seizure, stroke, death	Depression, nausea, severe craving for drugs, shaking, desire to sleep, loss of energy
Rohypnol (flunitrazepam)	Roofies, Ruphies, Forget-Me Pill, Dulcita, Wheel, R-2, Roach 2, Landing Gear, Mind Eraser	Swallowed, inhaled, injected, smoked, dissolved in drink	Slowed breathing, headaches, poor judgment, memory loss, drowsiness, confusion, hallucinations, decreased blood pressure, urinary retention, blackouts, coma, death	Headaches, tension, irritability, hallucinations, muscle aches, confusion, delirium, seizures

Data from Drug identification designer and club drugs quick reference guide *(1st ed.). (1999). Reprinted with permission of South-Western College Publishing, Mason, OH, a division of Thomson Learning; fax (800) 730-2215.*

ing, the greater is the risk for developing the numerous illnesses associated with smoking.

Incidence

Tobacco

- Tobacco use usually begins in early adolescence.
- Among adolescents, about the same number of females and males smoke cigarettes. More males than females use other forms of tobacco (e.g., cigars, pipes, smokeless tobacco).
- Minority adolescents smoke cigarettes at significantly lower rates than Caucasian adolescents.
- Approximately 40% of young people who try cigarettes become regular smokers.
- The average age that most try smoking is between 11 and 13 years, while the average age that most become daily smokers is 17 years.
- Children who begin smoking at an early age are more likely to develop more severe levels of nicotine addiction than those who start at a later age.
- More than one third of high-school youths smoke or use smokeless tobacco, and 25% of 17- and 18-year-olds smoke.
- Some children begin using smokeless tobacco before 6 years of age, and more than half of smokeless tobacco users begin by 13 years of age.
- Nicotine is generally the first drug used by young people who later use alcohol, marijuana, and harder drugs.

Alcohol and other drugs

- Substance abuse is now encountered in the elementary grades.
- With each advancing level in school, there is a progressive increase in the number of users, frequency of use, and variety of drugs used (except for inhalants and heroin).
- Reported use of drugs is higher for males (except for amphetamines).
- In the first half of the 1990s, drug use in teenagers dramatically increased; it then stabilized in the second half.
- Of adolescents who use drugs or alcohol, 16% meet the criteria for a diagnosis of dependence.
- Once addiction is evident in an adolescent, it can become highly chronic.
- Comorbidities among addicted adolescents are common, with depression the most common secondary diagnosis (in more than 50% of cases).
- Substance abuse during pregnancy is associated with increased rates of infant prematurity, anomalies, and death.
- Alcohol and other drug use are significant in all social strata and ethnic backgrounds.
- African-American adolescents report lower rates of drug use than other racial or ethnic groups, whereas Hispanic adolescents have the highest rates of use for cocaine, heroin, and steroids.
- Intoxication is a significant contributing factor in accidental deaths, homicides, and suicides.
- The leading cause of death in 15- to 24-year-olds is alcohol-related motor-vehicle accidents.

Risk Factors

For development of alcohol and other drug use in children

- Fetal exposure to alcohol or other drugs
- Alcohol or other drug abuse by parents, peers, or siblings

- Sexual or psychologic abuse
- Mental health problems
- Economically disadvantaged background
- Delinquency
- Physical disability or chronic pain

For development of alcohol and other drug use in adolescents

- Alcohol or other drug abuse by parents, peers, or siblings
- Low self-esteem
- Depression
- Poor relationship with parents
- Suicide attempts
- Lack of religious commitment
- Low academic performance and motivation
- Peer use of alcohol and other drugs
- Antisocial behavior

For development of tobacco use

- Peers who smoke
- Family members who smoke
- Rebelliousness
- Low academic performance and motivation
- External locus of control
- Low concern with the health consequences of smoking
- Low socioeconomic background
- Tobacco being accessible and available
- Tobacco use being perceived as normal and positive
- Lack of parental support and involvement

Subjective Data

Any child or adolescent suspected of substance abuse requires a comprehensive history.

Screening for tobacco, alcohol, and other drug use. As part of periodic health care with every grade-school-age or older child, examine these issues without parental pressure or presence:

- Review the extent of tobacco, alcohol, and other drug use of peers and family members.
- Investigate the child's or adolescent's attitudes toward use of tobacco, alcohol, and other drugs.
- Ask which specific drugs (including tobacco and alcohol) the child or adolescent has tried or is using.
- If the child or adolescent reports ongoing use (keeping in mind that use is often underreported), learn which drugs are in current use; the extent of the use; the settings in which the use occurs; and the amount of social, educational, and vocational disruption, if any, caused by the use.
- Keep in mind that an age-appropriate psychosocial history also is part of the screening history (see Risk Factors and Box 47-2).
- Refer to Box 47-3, which illustrates the RAFFT technique for screening children and adolescents for alcohol and drug use.

Assessment of alcohol and other drug use. This assessment is performed to determine whether a child with a positive screen needs a referral for full assessment and intervention.

- Use a compassionate, nonjudgmental attitude, without condemnation or alarm, to allow honesty.
- Interview the child or adolescent alone, investigating psychiatric issues and symptoms, family issues, and issues included among the risk factors.
- Interview the family, investigating the relationships and history of addictions in the family by developing a genogram (see Chapter 5).

Box 47-2 Smoking Cessation Strategies for Youths

1. Have the patient set a specific date to quit.
2. Write a contract with the patient.
3. Teach or provide the strategies and materials in A, B, or C below. (Utilizing more of these categories, possibly all three of them, is more effective.)
   A. Behavioral strategies (e.g., self-help materials, regular exercise, formal treatment program, social support)
   B. Nicotine-replacement strategies (e.g., nicotine gum, patch, spray, inhaler)
   C. Antidepressant strategies (e.g., bupropion)

Box 47-3 RAFFT

A relatively new screening instrument, RAFFT is particularly valuable because it focuses equally on alcohol and drug use. It was developed at Brown University for Project ADEPT.

- Do you drink or use drugs to *relax*, feel better about yourself, or fit in?
- Do you ever drink or use drugs while you are by yourself *(alone)*?
- Do you or any of your closest *friends* drink or use drugs?
- Does a close *family* member have a problem with alcohol or drug use?
- Have you ever gotten into *trouble* from drinking or drug use?

From Riggs, S.G. & Alario, A.J. (1989). Adolescent substance abuse. In Dube, C.E., et al. (Eds.). The project ADEPT curriculum for primary physician training, Providence, RI: Brown University. Reprinted with permission of the National Volunteer Training Center, Center for Substance Abuse.

- Determine whether a low, high, or problematic risk of abuse or addiction is present. (See Management later in this chapter.)

Objective Data

Physical examination. Objective data are documented as part of screening and assessment of alcohol and other drug use. There are few formal instruments for adolescent substance screening. Of these, the RAFFT and the Personal Experience Inventory (PEI) appear most suited to screening adolescents, addressing both alcohol and drug use and related behaviors in young people. The RAFFT is discussed in Box 47-3, while the PEI can be ordered by use of the address in the Resources section.

A thorough physical examination should be performed. Objective findings to observe and document include the following:

- Red eyes
- Extremely dilated or constricted pupils
- Evidence of intravenous use (e.g., tracks)
- Odors of alcohol or inhaled substances
- Emaciation
- Hyperexcitability
- Unexplained lethargy

Diagnostic procedures and laboratory tests

- Keep in mind that drug screening is appropriate in the following situations:

Patient has life-threatening symptoms (e.g., seizures, coma, cardiac rhythm disturbances)

Screening required for sports competition, school screenings, and preemployment evaluations, as well as after motor-vehicle accidents

An adolescent is pregnant

Drug abuse treatment is being monitored

- Consider issues of consent and confidentiality (see Consent to Laboratory Drug Screens).
- When ordering drug screens, talk with the laboratory to determine available, appropriate tests.
- Observe the gathering of the urine sample to avoid getting a contaminated specimen.
- Remember that screening is not helpful in making diagnoses.
- Keep in mind the following limitations:

A positive drug screen indicates recent drug use only. It does not indicate the pattern of use, level of impairment, or drug dependence.

A positive screen must be confirmed by a more reliable testing method to diagnose drug abuse.

False-positive screens result from antibody cross-reactions, while false-negative screens result from technologic shortcomings, pharmacokinetic characteristics, and intentional specimen tampering.

- Keep in mind the following issues related to consent to laboratory drug screens:

Use of laboratory drug screening tests raises legal, clinical, and ethical issues, including issues of confidentiality, mature minors, how to integrate the findings into the management of the adolescent and family care, and consent concerns.

Drug screening without patient approval is a legal invasion of privacy. Unless it is a medical emergency, involuntary screening should not be performed.

Voluntary screening of adolescents is discouraged. Those using are least likely to consent.

When a parent requests a drug screen or the practitioner is suspicious of substance abuse, allow the adolescent the right to refuse the screening test. Doing the test poses a threat to the adolescent-parent or practitioner-patient relationship.

Manage the underlying family dysfunction with counseling.

Maintain the previously established relationship with the adolescent.

When the screen is required as part of joining or continuing a sport or employment, keep in mind that the adolescent is providing prior consent to periodic testing; discuss this with the adolescent when the drug screen is first done.

If a screening is done, consider whether to share the results with parents or guardians. If the screening is ordered because of an acute medical condition, share the results so that the parents or guardians can be informed about the acute condition. Otherwise, do not inform the parents or guardian unless the adolescent agrees according to state laws (see Chapter 6).

Primary Care Issues and Implications

Mastery of the basic skills of screening, routine assessment, education, and referral for further assessment and treatment are essential practitioner skills. Further assessment and treatment should be done by health care professionals who are experienced and knowledgeable in the complexities of dealing with child or adolescent substance-abuse issues.

The PCP's assessment of alcohol and other drug use by children or adolescents should determine the level of risk for use that is occurring. With an assessment of low risk, primary prevention is indicated. With an assessment of high risk (moderate to heavy use of alcohol and experimentation with other drugs), appropriate intervention includes the following:

- Counseling and anticipatory guidance
- Careful follow-up evaluation
- Consideration of referral for assessment and counseling

When the assessment reveals active problematic use of alcohol and other drugs, the intervention focuses on the following:

- Treatment of medical and other complications
- Collection of an accurate, comprehensive data base
- Referral to a specialized facility for full assessment and treatment

Management

If an initial assessment indicates the likelihood of active alcohol or other drug abuse or dependence, decide whether medical intervention is indicated immediately or within a prescribed time. Practitioners from an evaluation or treatment facility should complete the detailed assessment. Know and be familiar with the referral resources in the local community, including inpatient and outpatient care and private and public resources, as well as their availability and costs.

Treatments and medications

- The use of medications (e.g., Antabuse, methadone) to directly treat alcohol and other drug abuses should be managed by physicians and groups providing specialized services.
- Nicotine addiction can be addressed with the use of nicotine replacement therapy, which allows gradual withdrawal. Combine this therapy with referral to a smoking cessation program or counseling interventions (see Box 47-2).

Counseling and prevention. Box 47-4 lists primary factors that can prove very effective in protecting children and adolescents against drug and alcohol use. Substance use is pervasive, extending across all regions, levels of population density, and economic and ethnic groups, so prevention efforts must be broadly aimed. They also must reach children in elementary schools and be continuous through high school.

At well-child visits during elementary school, encourage parents to begin discussions at home about tobacco, drug, and alcohol use, to share their values, and to model appropriate behaviors. Also, inform parents who smoke that their children are much more likely to smoke than children from homes whose parents are free of tobacco. Smoking parents who work on quitting smoking not only improve their own but also their children's immediate and future health.

Use of drugs, particularly alcohol or marijuana, as a recreational activity without significant disruption of behavior or performance is not often regarded by children or adolescents or their families as a health issue. Practitioners may need to offer counseling regarding the associated risks (even though no counseling has been requested). Recreational use, even at low frequencies and amounts, has a potential risk for causing serious problems, including future abuse and intentional or unintentional injury.

Box 47-4 Resiliency Factors against Drug and Alcohol Use

Relationship with a caring adult
Having the opportunity to contribute and be seen as a resource
Effectiveness in school and relationships
Positive outlook
Healthy expectations
Self-esteem and an internal locus of control
Self-discipline
Problem-solving and critical-thinking skills
Sense of humor

Tobacco products. Prevention efforts are concerned with increasing children's protective resiliency factors and decreasing their risk factors. The most effective tobacco-use prevention programs are community-wide combinations of education and public policy approaches. Steps in a primary prevention effort include:

- Screen and assess a patient's risks for starting tobacco use and follow-up at each opportunity.
- Establish trusting, supportive relationships with the child or adolescent.
- Discuss the deceptions in advertisements featuring young adults as smokers.
- Offer to speak about tobacco use in young people to parent and teacher groups.
- Work with schools to offer programs that teach the skills to resist tobacco use.
- Develop or support programs in the community to discourage tobacco use.

Alcohol and other drugs. For a low-risk child (primary prevention efforts), focus on education and strengthening positive coping strategies for the youth and family. Education includes information, the development of decision-making skills, values clarification, stress management, and refusal skills. Community efforts are essential in this process, and practitioners can participate in supporting effective prevention programs, which include the following:

- Recreation and fitness facilities for children or adolescents
- Parental commitment to nonalcoholic parties
- Active involvement of religious institutions
- Curtailment of media messages that glamorize substance use

For a high-risk child (secondary prevention), preventive contacts should include the following:

- Education about modifying behaviors
- Counseling about increasing resilience (see Box 47-4)
- Close contact and assessment to monitor changes in drug use
- Referrals for therapy or self-help groups as needed

Secondary prevention also involves working with the family and educating them about the risk factors. Counseling includes referrals to therapy or a self-help group and efforts to improve the quality of family interactions and decrease the enabling behaviors.

Know the referral sources available in the immediate geographic area so that appropriate and informed referrals can be made in a timely way. Support the child and family during this difficult time.

Follow-up

Tobacco products. Visits are important in assisting children or adolescents and families to stop using tobacco products. Box 47-2 describes the process of working with a child or adolescent who wants to stop using. Keep in mind that it may take a child several "practice" attempts at quitting smoking before one is successful.

Alcohol and other drugs. Follow-up care for children who have alcohol or other drug use issues is a matter of continuing health care and ongoing support, including the following steps:

- Follow health and development carefully.
- Maintain a relationship with the child or adolescent.
- Assess for changing use, abuse, or addiction patterns, and refer appropriately.
- Be supportive of ongoing therapies.
- Keep talking about the treatment, its use, and any associated morbidities.
- Accept relapses and encourage abstinence as part of the follow-up care.

Consultations and referrals

- Know the available resources, including the following information:
  Names of the agencies and their approaches to treatment
  Telephone numbers
  Names of contact persons at treatment facilities
  Costs
  Data that each agency needs for a referral from a practitioner
- Select a treatment program that requires family involvement and includes treatment of both the family and child.
- Explain to the child and family what they can expect.
- If there are no severe medical or psychiatric complications of the addiction, remember that the most cost-effective treatment may be an outpatient treatment program.

Resources

Organizations

Alcohol and Other Drugs: Al Anon, Alateen; (888) 425-2666; e-mail address: wso@al-anon.org; www.al-anon.org

Narcotics Anonymous, NA World Service, PO Box 9999, Van Nuys, CA 91409; (818) 773-9999; www.na.org

National Clearinghouse for Alcohol and Drug Information (NCADI), a service of the Substance Abuse and Mental Health Services Administration (SAMHSA); (800) 487-4890; www.health.org

Office on Smoking and Health, Department of Health and Human Services, 200 Independence Avenue SW, Washington, DC 20201; (877) 696-6775; www.dhhs.gov/topics/smoking.html

Personal Experience Inventory (PEI), Western Psychological Services, 12301 Wilshire Boulevard, Los Angeles, CA 90025; (310) 478-2061

Stop Teenage Addiction to Tobacco (STAT), Northeastern University, 360 Huntington Avenue, 241 Cushing Hall, Boston, MA 02115; (617) 373-7826; e-mail address: info@stat.org

Bibliography

American Medical Association. (1993). *Diagnostic and treatment guidelines on child physical abuse and neglect.* Chicago: American Medical Association.

Applebaum, M.G. (1995). Fetal alcohol syndrome: Diagnosis, management, and prevention. *Nurse Practitioner, 20*(10), 24-36.

Centers for Disease Control and Prevention. (1991). *Preventing lead poisoning in young children.* Atlanta: Centers for Disease Control and Prevention.

Centers for Disease Control and Prevention. (1997). *Screening young children for lead poisoning: Guidance for state and local public health officials.* Atlanta: Centers for Disease Control and Prevention.

Healton, C., Messeri, P., Reynolds, J., et al. (2000). Tobacco use among middle and high school students—U.S., 1999. *Morbidity and Mortality Weekly Review, 49*(3), 49-53.

Norton, D. & Ridenour, N. (1995). Homeless women and children: The challenge of health promotion. *Nurse Practitioner Forum, 6*(1), 29-33.

Perkins, S.W. (1999). *Drug identification: Designer and club drugs.* Carollton, TX: Alliance Press.

Riggs, S.G. & Alario, A.J. (1989). Adolescent substance abuse. In Dube, C.E., et al. (Eds.). *The project ADEPT curriculum for primary physician training.* Providence, RI: Brown University.

Rogers, P.D., Spears, S.R., & Ozbek, I. (1995) .The assessment of the identified substance-abusing adolescent. *Pediatric Clinics of North America, 42*(2), 351-370.

U.S. Department of Health and Human Services. (2000). *Child maltreatment 1998: Reports from the states to the National Child Abuse And Neglect Data System.* Washington, DC: US Government Printing Office.

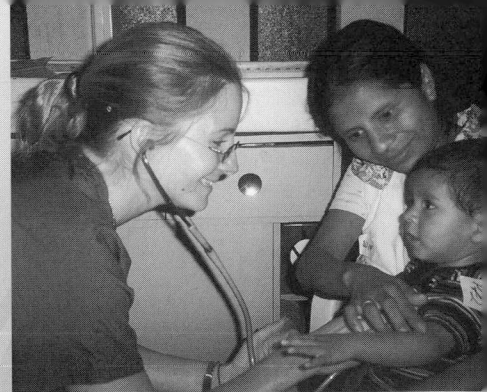

Section 5

Emergencies and Preparation for Hospitalization

As a pediatric nurse practitioner (PNP), performing a physical examination on a 2½-year-old child, even under the best of circumstances, can be quite strenuous. Performing that same exam as a student NP in a third-world country with little knowledge of the culture and language is another obstacle altogether. Add the extreme heat to the crowded and dirty environment and performing that physical exam on the most well-behaved child becomes nearly impossible.

But what NP doesn't enjoy a challenge? Twice, as a student and then again as a practicing PNP, I participated in a medical mission to Nueva Santa Rosa, a small village in Guatemala. As a student, I anticipated and prepared for the trip by reading about diseases and common illnesses indigenous to that area of the world. I also attempted to learn some important Spanish phrases. Yet nothing could have prepared me for the frustrations I would feel on that first trip. Imagine trying to teach a poor, uneducated mother who speaks a different language that overdressing her 2-month-old infant when it is 85° outside is unhealthy. Simultaneously, imagine losing your light because the sun is setting, a line of patients with no end in sight, and a dirty, emaciated dog who has found a new home under your feet.

As a student, the expectations I had for providing care for these families far exceeded the eventual reality, which inevitably led to complete frustration. I felt obligated to work quickly to see every patient who had traveled all day in the heat to receive care. I became frustrated with myself when I did not know what to do. And worst of all, I was unable to communicate with my patients and wasn't even noticing their little faces and smiles.

Returning home after that first trip to Guatemala, I felt different. I felt a deeper appreciation and renewed outlook on my profession, my colleagues, my family, and the patients for whom I cared. At first, I honestly thought that the trip would be a "once in a lifetime" experience.

However, it was only a few months after returning home that I began thinking about the next trip.

A full year later, I went on my second medical mission. Within that year I had graduated and was now practicing as a PNP. My clinical skills were improved and I was more prepared for the emotional effects of caring for the families in Guatemala. I did not become as impatient when I was unsure what to do, because I realized that sometimes even those with 10 years more experience than myself were unsure too! I also took my time with every patient, particularly in regard to health teaching. It is wonderful to be able to treat scabies with the proper medication, but it does not do an inflicted young infant any good if his mother is unable to protect him from reoccurrence.

Following the second trip, I came to appreciate the confusion and obstacles of caring for those who have a different language, culture, and educational background, and I recognized that you could never teach enough. This is true when caring for any 5-year-old child with an ear infection, whether the child lives in Nueva Santa Rosa or New York City.

Missionary work in countries like Guatemala is not only interesting and educational, but also rewarding and uplifting. As an inexperienced new graduate, possibly one having a hard time finding a first job, you are guaranteed experience and then some if you spend some time, even a week, caring for families in a third-world country. Or, if you have been practicing for years and are feeling bored, unchallenged or unappreciated, spending time caring for those who are so desperately in need of expert skills and knowledge will certainly be re-energizing. Donating time and skills to empower people with knowledge and to provide health services to those who are severely underprivileged is more gratifying than one could ever imagine.

Jenny Zethner

Chapter 48 *Managing Pediatric Emergencies in a Primary Care Setting*

Jane A. Fox

Acute Foreign–Body Aspiration (Choking), p. 897
Acute Hemorrhage, p. 898
Acute Respiratory Arrest, p. 898
Airway Obstruction, p. 899
Burn Injury, p. 900
Coma and Loss of Consciousness, p. 901
Frostbite, p. 902
Head Injury, p. 903
Hyperthermia, p. 904
Near Drowning, p. 904
Orthopedic Fractures, p. 906
Shock, p. 906

A medical emergency is any situation that requires immediate medical attention to preserve life or limb. Primary care providers (PCPs) encounter emergencies through direct presentation in the clinic and through telephone triage. The PCP is responsible for recognizing an actual or potential emergency situation, providing initial stabilization, and facilitating transport to an emergency care setting for further management. Proficiency with basic life support is essential; ideally PCPs are also equipped with advanced life-support skills.

This chapter focuses on emergencies that may appear in a primary care setting. For emergencies requiring cardiopulmonary resuscitation (CPR), the practitioner is concurrently referred to the American Heart Association's (AHA's) guidelines for basic and advanced life support for both adults and children. Emergency situations that do not require immediate resuscitation but warrant immediate management to preserve life or limb are also presented. The practitioner should provide families, as a part of well-child care anticipatory guidance, information on recognizing emergencies, immediate intervention, and how to access emergency services, such as 911 and the local poison information center. Parents and caregivers should be encouraged to learn CPR and to enroll in a first-aid course.

Acute Foreign-Body Aspiration (Choking)

Alert

The following are cardinal signs of complete airway obstruction:
- Inability to speak, cough, or make sounds
- Clutching at throat (a universal sign)
- Acute cyanosis

A choking individual requires immediate maneuvers to remove the aspirated foreign body to prevent a full pulmonary or cardiopulmonary arrest. Foreign-body aspiration causes more than 200 deaths per year in children under 5 years of age. The most common causes of choking include food (e.g., hot dogs, nuts, seeds), coins, small toys, and small objects.

Assessment

Acute airway obstruction findings may include cyanosis, apnea, stridor, wheezing, cough, and inability to speak. Facial petechiae may be seen as a result of increased intrathoracic pressure. Laryngotracheal foreign bodies produce acute obstruction, and round objects are more likely to completely block the airway. Bronchial foreign bodies cause a less acute clinical course. Patients develop air trapping, wheezing, cyanosis, muffled voice, and cough. Immediate intervention is needed if airway is totally obstructed, while if there is partial obstruction, the practitioner may order arterial blood gases (ABGs) or oximetry and chest radiographs (inspiratory and expiratory).

Management

If the individual is unable to speak, cough, or make sounds, the AHA's guidelines are implemented immediately. These interventions include the following steps:
- *Infants under 1 year of age*—Four back blows, four chest thrusts, and repetition of four back blows and four chest thrusts until choking is resolved

- *Children 1 year of age and older*—Five manual abdominal thrusts (Heimlich maneuver), which can be repeated as indicated

If the individual has aspirated foreign material into the airway but is able to speak or cough, no intervention is warranted other than supportive care and reassurance. If dyspnea does not easily resolve, transport emergently for further evaluation and management.

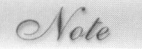

Do not sweep the mouth of an infant or child because the foreign material may be forced even farther into the airway.

Acute Hemorrhage

Alert

The following are warning signs of impending shock from acute bleeding:
- Low blood pressure
- Tachycardia
- Poor capillary refill
- Decreased skin temperature
- Altered mental status
- Decreased urinary output

Acute hemorrhage (internal or external) becomes significant when 20% of the circulating blood volume is lost. Continued uncontrolled bleeding can lead to shock (hypovolemic) and death within a matter of minutes because of impaired blood flow to the skin, muscles, and major organs. Recognition of blood loss and emergency bleeding control is essential to preventing loss of life or limb.

Assessment
- Pallor
- Weak and thready pulse
- Hypotension
- Thirst
- Restlessness
- Shock
- Pain over an affected area (e.g., a fracture)
- Signs of acute internal bleeding (e.g., frank blood in the urine or stool; pink, foamy blood in the emesis; frank blood in emesis; severe vaginal bleeding; black tarry stools)

Management
For external hemorrhage, use:
- Direct pressure
- Elevation of the affected area
- Pressure over the artery proximal to any bleeding not controlled with direct pressure
- Splinting of the fracture to prevent further injury
- Tourniquet application (when a combination of all listed methods is not sufficient to control the bleeding)

For suspected internal hemorrhage, the emergency management is similar to the emergency management of shock (see Shock).

Acute Respiratory Arrest

Alert

The following are warning signs of impending respiratory arrest:
- Respiratory rate greater than 60 beats per minute
- Bradycardia (which is considered a prearrest state)
- Tachycardia, indicated by a heart rate greater than 180 beats per minute for children under 5 years of age or a heart rate greater than 150 beats per minute for children over 5 years of age
- Signs of respiratory distress
- Cyanosis
- Failure to recognize parents
- Change in level of consciousness (LOC)
- Seizure
- Fever with petechiae

Acute respiratory arrest requires immediate airway management and artificial breathing to avert full cardiopulmonary arrest. Emergency life-support techniques and concurrent transfer to an emergency medical facility are essential to achieving the best possible outcome for the person suffering respiratory or cardiopulmonary arrest. Refer to the AHA's guidelines for basic and advanced life-support techniques.

Primary care practitioners (PCPs) are more likely to encounter an emergency situation in which respiratory arrest is pending. Recognition of warning signs (see the Alert box), initial rapid cardiopulmonary assessment, evaluation of potential causes (Box 48-1), and early stabilizing interventions concurrent with transfer to an emergency medical facility can prevent an actual respiratory arrest.

Assessment

Data is gathered emergently and concurrently with stabilization. Rapid cardiopulmonary assessment includes the following:
- Airway patency
- Breathing, including rate, air entry (e.g., chest rise, breath sounds, stridor, wheezing), pattern (e.g., retractions, grunting), and color
- Circulation, including heart rate, blood pressure, peripheral pulses, skin perfusion (e.g., capillary refill, temperature, color, mottling), and cerebral perfusion (e.g.,

Box 48-1 Potential Causes of Respiratory Arrest

Pulmonary:
- Upper airway causes: Foreign-body aspiration, croup epiglottis
- Lower airway causes: Asthma, bronchiolitis, pneumonia, foreign-body aspiration
- Other: Drowning, bronchopulmonary dysplasia, respiratory distress syndrome

Cardiovascular: Congenital heart disease, septic shock, sever dehydration, pericarditis, myocarditis, congestive heart failure

Central nervous system: Hydrocephalus, shunt failure, meningitis, seizure, tumor, head trauma

Other: Sudden infant death syndrome (SIDS), multiple trauma, poisoning, botulism, anaphylaxis

recognition of parents, response to pain, muscle tone, pupil size)
- Emergency history
- Previous medical history
- Current medications
- Possible ingestants
- History of recent illness
- Known trauma
- Allergies
- Initial treatment already provided

Management

Management of acute respiratory arrest includes airway stabilization and management and artificial breathing techniques. Supportive oxygen is given if available. Immediate transfer to an emergency care setting is essential for further stabilization, evaluation, and management. Refer to the AHA's basic and advanced life-support algorithms for management.

Airway Obstruction

Impending respiratory arrest can be the result of either upper or lower airway obstruction. Causes of upper airway obstruc-

tion include foreign-body aspiration (as previously discussed), croup, and epiglottitis. Lower airway obstruction can be caused by asthma, bronchiolitis, pneumonia, and foreign-body aspiration.

Assessment

See Table 48-1 for differential diagnosis and management.
   History
- Previous medical history
- Onset, duration, and character of symptoms
- Possibility of foreign-body aspiration
- Presence of upper respiratory infection (URI) symptoms
- Fever
- Medications and treatments given at home and time elapsed before seeking care
- Immunization record (suspect pertussis in an unimmunized child)

Physical examination and findings. In addition to the rapid cardiopulmonary assessment (as described in Acute Respiratory Arrest), assess for the following:
- Inspiratory or expiratory stridor
- Retractions (e.g., suprasternal, supraclavicular, intercostal, subcostal)

Table 48-1 Differential Diagnosis and Management: Airway Obstruction (519.8)

DIAGNOSIS	CRITERIA	MANAGEMENT
Croup (see Chapter 41)	Viral illness (generally influenza virus) edema around vocal cords Most common under 3 years of age Occurs in late fall and early winter Onset over 1 to 2 days Low-grade fever Barklike cough Inspiratory stridor present URI symptoms present	Administer oxygen. Administer racemic epinephrine by aerosol. Hydrate. Rule out epiglottitis with lateral neck radiograph.
Epiglottitis (see Chapter 41)	Bacterial infection of epiglottis (Incomplete or no immunization for *H. influenzae* type B (generally caused by *H. influenzae* type B) Life-threatening airway obstruction can occur Most common 2 to 6 years of age Onset over a few hours High fever Cough absent Inspiratory stridor present URI symptoms variable Drooling present Tripod sitting position	Allow parents to remain with child. Administer oxygen. Prepare for emergency airway management. Avoid invasive procedures. Do not perform oral examination. Immediately transfer to an emergency facility.
Asthma (see Chapter 49)	Caused by allergies or infection Age over 1 year Dyspnea Wheezing present Prolonged expiratory phase Possible fever	Administer oxygen. Administer inhaled (nebulized) bronchodilators. Control fever. Transfer to a medical facility if severe or unresolved.
Bronchiolitis (see Chapter 41)	Age under 1 year Usually caused by respiratory syncytial virus Hoarseness and cough present Gradual onset of respiratory distress Possible apnea spells in infants	Administer oxygen. Administer nebulized bronchodilators. Transfer to medical facility.
Pneumonia (see Chapter 41)	All ages Viral etiology: Gradual onset of cough, fever, and tachypnea Bacterial etiology: Abrupt onset of fever, chills, tachypnea, and chest pain	Consult with a physician. Provide supportive care. Provide penicillin and supportive care.

- Pallor or cyanosis
- Lethargy or agitation
- Posture (tripod position)
- Nasal flaring
- Drooling

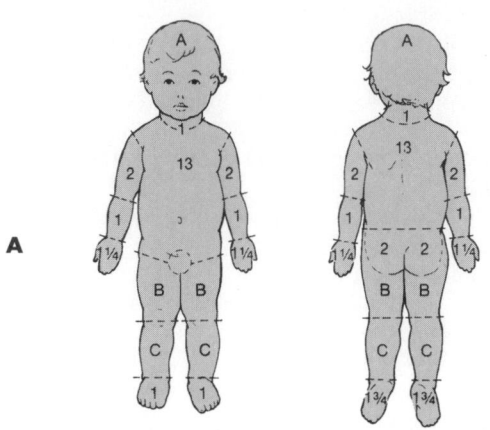

A

RELATIVE PERCENTAGES OF AREAS AFFECTED BY GROWTH

AREA	BIRTH	AGE 1 YR	AGE 5 YR
A = ½ of head	9½	8½	6½
B = ½ of one thigh	2¾	3¼	4
C = ½ of one leg	2½	2½	2¾

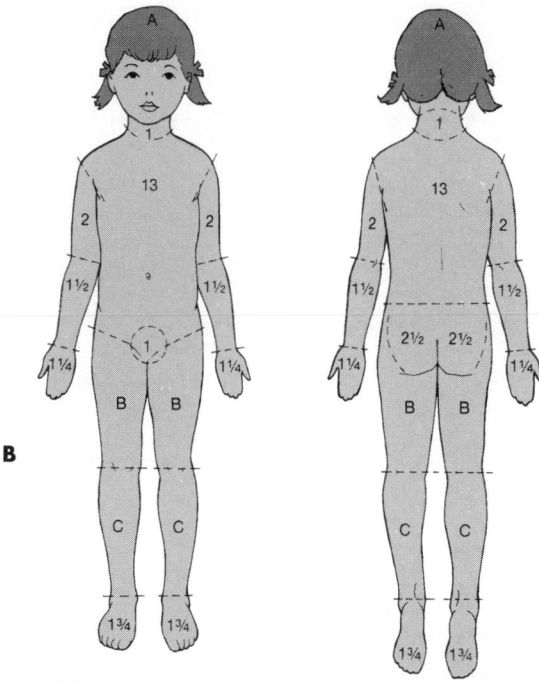

B

RELATIVE PERCENTAGES OF AREAS AFFECTED BY GROWTH

AREA	AGE 10 YR	AGE 15 YR	ADULT
A = ½ of head	5½	4½	3½
B = ½ of one thigh	4½	4½	4¾
C = ½ of one leg	3	3¼	3½

Fig. 48-1 Estimation of distribution of burns in children. **A,** Children from birth to 5 years of age. **B,** Older children. (From Wong, D.L. [1999]. *Whaley and Wong's nursing care of infants and children* [6th ed.]. St. Louis: Mosby.)

Management

- See Acute Foreign-Body Aspiration (Choking).
- For patients who are unconscious or cannot breathe, speak, cough, or cry, use back blows with chest thrusts (for those less than 1 year of age) and abdominal thrusts (for those 1 year of age and older).

Burn Injury

Alert

The following are severe burns requiring emergent referral to a medical facility:

- Full-thickness (third- and fourth-degree) burns
- Partial-thickness (first- and second-degree) burns
- Children with preexisting medical problems that could complicate management
- Children with associated trauma in which the burn injury poses the most risk
- Inadequate care in the home environment for wound care
- Suspected child abuse
- Burns involving the face or perineum
- Electrical burns
- Burns involving smoke inhalation
- Circumferential burns

A burn is a thermal injury to the skin. Burn injury is the fourth leading cause of accidental death in children 5 to 14 years of age, with an incidence of 1.9% in boys and 1.5% in girls (per 100,000 children). The degree and severity of a burn injury is dependent upon the type of burn (e.g., electrical, flame, liquid, chemical, radiation); the duration of exposure to the burning agent; the area injured, including the percentage of body surface area or burn surface area (BSA), also referred to as total body surface area (TBSA) and any injury to vital anatomy; the presence of associated injuries (e.g., trauma, smoke inhalation); and the individual's premorbid condition.

Assessment

History

- Mechanism and history of the burn injury, including type of exposure, duration of skin contact with the burning agent, and the elapsed time from injury to seeking treatment
- Possibility of smoke inhalation
- Chemical burns, including chemical name and concentration
- Tetanus status
- Previous medical history, including any cardiac valve disease or recent streptococcal infection

Physical examination and findings

- General appearance, including any evidence of distress
- Vital signs
- Area of the burn, calculating the BSA involved (Fig. 48-1) and using the following percentages as guides:

Infants—Arms, 9%; legs, 13% (increasing to 18% by 15 years of age); anterior trunk, 13% (increasing to 18% by 5 years of age); posterior trunk, 18%; head, 18% (decreasing 1% per year until 9 years of age); perineum, 1%

Adolescents 15 years and over (using the "rule of nines")—Arms, 9%; legs, 18%; anterior trunk, 18%; posterior trunk, 18%; head, 9%; perineum, 1%

- Distribution of burn
- Depth of classification of burn injury (Box 48-2)
- Severity of the burn, determined by the depth of the burn
- Sensation in the burn area
- Complete pulmonary examination
- Other system examinations based on the location and extent of the burn
- Old burns, including assessment for infection

Diagnosis and classification of burns. Minor burns cover less than 10% of the BSA and involve less than 2% full-thickness injury (see Box 48-2). Severe burns require emergent referral to a medical facility (see the Alert box).

A diagnosis of physical abuse or child neglect (see Chapter 47) is indicated by the following:

- Unexplained burns
- Burns to the palms, soles, back, buttocks, or genitalia
- Burn patterns resembling a cigar or cigarette, electric burner, or iron
- A burn distribution resembling a rope burn around the neck, body, or extremities

Management

- For initial first aid, provide immediate removal of the causative factor, lavage with cool water or normal saline, immediate removal of clothing involved, and extended lavage for burns involving chemical agents.
- For first-degree burns, clean with a mild detergent and water or saline. Apply a topical anesthetic (e.g., benzocaine) three or four times a day as needed.
- For second-degree burns, cleanse the area with a mild detergent or povidone-iodine solution (e.g., Betadine) and then with sterile saline. Débride the area of loose skin. Do not unroof blisters from the palms or soles. Apply 1% silver sulfadiazine (Silvadene) cream to the area and dress with a closed sterile dressing; use nonadherent gauze and a bulky dressing to absorb wound drainage.
- Remember that application of cold water soaks (not ice packs) may offer some pain relief for first- and second-degree burns.
- Administer tetanus toxoid if indicated.
- Orally administer penicillin 50,000 to 100,000 U/kg per day in three divided doses for 5 days if there is a history of valvular heart disease or concomitant streptococcal infection.
- Provide pain management (see Chapter 7).
- Teach the parents and child to keep the area clean and dry, increase fluid intake, elevate the affected areas, maintain range of motion (ROM) in the affected joints, and schedule a return visit if signs or symptoms of infection occur.
- Have the patient or parents schedule a return visit in 24 to 48 hours for an infection check and dressing change, and teach the child or family to clean and change the dressing every day thereafter
- Have the patient return in 1 week to evaluate the healing process. Observe for complications.

Coma and Loss of Consciousness

Alert

Coma or loss of consciousness warrants emergency transport to a medical facility.

Assessment

Although the causes of coma are widely varied (Box 48-3), the initial assessment and management is the same until transport to a medical facility is achieved. The depth of coma or LOC is best initially determined by use of the Glasgow Coma Scale (Table 48-2). Obtain a careful history from family members or caregivers. Perform a physical examination, including a complete neurologic examination. In addition, measure initial vital signs and assess and manage the airway, breathing, and circulation.

Box 48-2 Burn Severity Grading System

Superficial (First-Degree) Burns

Pain is predominant symptom
No skin loss
Heals without scarring in 5 to 10 days

Partial-Thickness (Second-Degree) Burns

Involves the upper layer of the epidermis
Tender
Erythematous
Blisters and weeping skin
Painful
Heals in about 2 weeks with variable amounts of scarring

Full-Thickness (Third-Degree) Burns

Involves entire skin to subcutaneous level
Absent sensation in area of injury
Often severe pain in areas at the periphery (where superficial and partial-thickness burns may occur)
Skin charred or white, with a dry, leathery appearance
Requires grafting to close

Fourth-Degree Burns

Also a full-thickness injury
Involves underlying structures (e.g., muscles, fasciae, bone)

Box 48-3 Causes of Coma

Uncontrolled diabetes mellitus
Hypoglycemia
Postictal state
Electrolyte imbalance
CNS infection
Head injury
Cerebrovascular accident
Reye syndrome
Shock
Asphyxia
Drug or poison ingestion
Renal failure
Addison's disease

Table 48-2 Pediatric Modification of Glasgow Coma Scale (GCS) by Age of Patient*

GLASGOW COMA SCORE	PEDIATRIC MODIFICATION		
Eye Opening			
≥ 1 year	**0-1 year**		
4 Spontaneously	4 Spontaneously		
3 To verbal command	3 To shout		
2 To pain	2 To pain		
1 No response	1 No response		
Best Motor Response			
≥ 1 year	**0-1 year**		
6 Obeys			
5 Localizes pain	5 Localizes pain		
4 Flexion withdrawal	4 Flexion withdrawal		
3 Flexion abnormal (decorticate)	3 Flexion abnormal (decorticate)		
2 Extension (decerebrate)	2 Extension (decerebrate)		
1 No response	1 No response		
Best Verbal Response			
> 5 years	**0-2 years**		**2-5 years**
5 Oriented and converses	5 Cries appropriately, smiles, coos		5 Appropriate words and phrases
4 Disoriented and converses	4 Cries		4 Inappropriate words
3 Inappropriate words	3 Inappropriate crying or screaming		3 Cries or screams
2 Incomprehensible sounds	2 Grunts		2 Grunts
1 No response	1 No response		1 No response

From Barkin R.M. & Rosen, P. (1999). Emergency pediatrics: A guide to ambulatory care (5th ed.). St Louis: Mosby.
*Score is the sum of the individual scores from eye opening, best verbal response, and best motor response, using age-specific criteria. GCS of 13 to 15 indicates mild head injury, GCS of 9 to 12 indicates moderate head injury, and GCS less than 8 indicates severe head injury.

Management

- Maintain safety.
- Stabilize airway and provide oxygen.
- Position to prevent aspiration of vomitus.
- Provide a glucagon injection for diabetic individuals (see Chapter 45).

Frostbite

Alert

Referral to a medical facility is indicated if a child has:
- Hypothermia (e.g., a core temperature 95° F [35° C] or less)
- Third- or fourth-degree frostbite
- A preexisting medical condition that may cause complications

Frostbite injury occurs from freezing of tissue. Exposed areas are most likely to suffer frostbite, especially the earlobes, nose, cheeks, hands, and feet. The affected part becomes numb, hard, and blue. Although light frostnip is easily treated and poses no adverse sequelae, deep frostbite can threaten loss of limb or life.

Assessment

- Early signs of frostbite, including shivering, decreased flexibility, aching or numbness, and low body temperature

Box 48-4 Classification of Frost Injury

First-degree (frostnip)—Erythema, edema, no blistering, and minimal tissue damage
Second-degree—Bulla and blister formation
Third-degree—Full skin-thickness necrosis without loss of the body part
Fourth-degree—Complete necrosis with gangrene and loss of the body part

- Progressive signs, including drowsiness; apathy; loss of consciousness; cold, cyanotic, mottled skin; and hard, inflexible skin and muscle
- Degree of frost injury (Box 48-4)

Management

For frostnip:
- Rewarm with warm hand.
- Blow through cupped hands.
- Rewarm in armpit.
For deep frostbite:
- Rapidly rewarm with warm water.
- Loosen clothing.
- Do not rub the frostbitten part (to prevent further tissue damage).
- Do not use direct or ambient heat to rewarm.

- Elevate the affected part.
- Have the affected person drink warm beverages.

Head Injury

Alert

Emergency transfer to a medical facility is indicated when the following occur with a head injury:
- Loss of consciousness
- Persistent vomiting
- Unequal pupil size
- Change in LOC (e.g., increased lethargy, somnolence)
- Change in neuromotor function (e.g., weakness in an extremity, change in gait)
- Seizure
- Drainage of blood or fluid from nose or ears
- Severe headache

Head injuries occur commonly and follow etiologic patterns according to age group. For all ages, falls are the most common cause of head injury. In infants, child abuse is also a cause. Preschool and school-age children more commonly experience head injuries related to automobile accidents. For adolescents, sports-related head injury or assault contribute to head injuries. PCPs must recognize severe head injuries and begin emergency interventions. The practitioner differentiates the severity of the head injury and determines appropriate care and home monitoring tactics.

Head injury is classified according to the level of injury and the subsequent effect on neurologic status. Box 48-5 classifies the types of head injuries, and Box 48-6 describes the severity of head injuries.

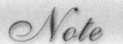

Note

For the child who is unconscious, neurologic evaluation is deferred until assessment and management of airway, breathing, and circulation are achieved.

Assessment

History
- Age
- Mechanism of injury, including event, force of impact, and direction of forces
- Behavior and LOC since the injury
- Previous medical conditions, medications, and allergies

Physical examination and findings
- Airway, breathing, and circulation
- Vital signs
- Results of Glasgow Coma Scale (see Table 48-2)
- Neurologic examination, including pupil size and reaction to light; LOC and orientation (a useful mnemonic is AVPU [alert, responds to verbal stimulus, responds to painful stimulus; unresponsive]); neurosensory and neuromotor function, including symmetry; cranial nerve assessment; gait assessment; coordination; and reflexes
- Presence of hemotympanum, cerebrospinal fluid (CSF), or rhinorrhea

---

Box 48-5 Types of Head Injury

Concussion

Transient loss of consciousness
Amnesia of the event
No structural brain damage

Contusion

Structural damage to brain tissue (e.g., hemorrhage, edema)
Presence of a neurologic defect
Possible seizures

Intracranial Hemorrhage

Accumulation of blood within the cranium
Acute or latent occurrence
Epidural: Rapid deterioration of neurologic status within hours of the injury
Subdural: Chronic or acute depending on the onset and progression of the neurologic defect

---

Box 48-6 Severity of Head Injury

Mild

Positive injury to the head
No loss of consciousness
No vomiting
Absence of a neurologic defect
Possible mild headache

Moderate

Head injury with positive transient loss of consciousness
Decreased LOC after the injury
Possible vomiting after the injury

Severe

Persistent loss of consciousness
Persistent vomiting
Seizure
Irregular respirations
Pallor
Possible CSF drainage from the external ear canal (possible basilar skull fracture)

- Presence of palpable or visible cranial injuries (e.g., lacerations, hematomas, depressed cranium)
- Battle sign or raccoon eyes
- Presence of fontanels

Management

Emergency transfer to a medical facility is indicated for severe head injury or for individuals with persistent change in sensorium. Management of individuals with a mild head injury rests strictly on advising the parents to monitor for signs and symptoms that warrant immediate emergency care. The child should be kept quiet and on a clear liquid diet for 24 to 48 hours after a mild head injury. Headache pain is treated with aceta-minophen. Narcotics should be avoided. If it is a recent trauma, application of an ice pack may reduce swelling. Finally, evaluation of the child's arousability, sensorium, and basic neurologic status should be done every 1 to 2 hours for the first 24 hours. Parents should be advised to monitor the following and to seek emergency care if signs of a deteriorating neurologic status develop:

- Decreased LOC
- Agitation
- Seizures
- Persistent, forceful vomiting
- Unequal pupils
- Weakness or loss of use of an extremity
- Slurred speech
- Blurry vision
- Severe unrelenting headache

Hyperthermia

Alert

Individuals with the following should be transferred to an emergency facility:
- Signs and symptoms of heat stroke
- Burns
- Chronic disease causing a decreased ability to sweat (e.g., cystic fibrosis)
- Ingestion of medications that may impair normal sweating

Individuals exposed to environmental heat without appropriate acclimatization, fluids, or equipment are subject to various heat-related illnesses (Table 48-3). Most of these illnesses are preventable. Young children, athletes, and the chronically ill are at increased risk. Heat stroke is a life-threatening accumulation of body heat and concurrent disturbance of the sweating mechanism. Excessive and unrelenting body heat results in generalized cellular damage to the central nervous system (CNS), liver, kidneys, and blood-clotting mechanisms.

Assessment
History
- Cause of overheating
- Duration of overheating
- Initial measures taken
- Preexisting health conditions
- Current medications
- Known allergies
Physical examination and findings
- Temperature greater than 104.6° F (40.5° C)
- Profuse sweating or absent sweating with hot and dry skin
- Convulsions (in 60% of cases)
- Delirium to coma
- Incontinence
- Hypotension
- Tachycardia
- Shock
- Oliguria
- Vomiting
- Diarrhea
- Headache

- Dizziness
- Abdominal pain

Management
- Remove all of the patient's clothing.
- Apply or immerse the patient in cool water until temperature is lowered to 102.2° F (39° C).
- Apply ice packs to the groin, axilla, and neck areas. Fan the patient. (This can be done immediately at the scene.)
- Prevent shivering.
- Administer oxygen.
- Treat shock.
- Massage the extremities to maintain peripheral circulation.

Near Drowning

Alert

Emergency management of the drowning victim includes:
- Immediate and persistent CPR
- Evacuation of vomitus from airway
- Correction of hypothermia
- Emergency cricothyrotomy if laryngospasm persists

Drowning is the second most common cause of accidental death in children, and the third most common cause of death from all causes in children between 1 and 13 years of age. Toddlers and teenage boys are the two groups most at risk. Drowning causes death by suffocation after submersion in liquid. Survival past 24 hours after a submersion episode is called *near drowning.*

Drowning is defined as death within 24 hours of a submersion incident. The drowning process includes aspiration of liquid, creation of an alveolar-arterial oxygen difference, decreased lung compliance, and resulting hypoxemia. Continued hypoxemia and persistent changes in alveolar function lead to damage to vital organs. Although the mechanisms of lung injury differ based on whether a drowning episode occurred in saltwater or freshwater, the result is the same, as are the emergency interventions. The outcome is dependent on the drowning victim's age and preexisting health, water temperature, duration of submersion, and presence of resuscitation attempts immediately after submersion.

Assessment
- Rapid cardiopulmonary assessment (see Acute Respiratory Arrest in this chapter)
- Age
- Submersion event, including the type of water, duration of submersion, and any initial resuscitative attempts
- Potential for associated trauma (e.g., cervical spine injury)
- LOC
- Response to painful stimulation

Management
The near-drowning victim who is awake and alert and has signs of minimal injury requires a complete physical examination and a baseline chest radiographic examination. The near-drowning victim who is unconscious but has normal respirations, normal pupillary responses, and purposeful response to pain stimulation is treated with airway management, supportive oxygen, rewarming, and immediate transfer to an emergency facility. The

Table 48-3 Environmental Heat Illnesses: Clinical Presentation

CONDITION	PREDISPOSING CAUSE	CENTRAL NERVOUS SYSTEM	SKIN	MUSCLE CRAMPS	THIRST	RECTAL TEMPERATURE	BLOOD PRESSURE	PULSE	MANAGEMENT
Heat cramps	Muscle work, sodium depletion, drinking large quantities of water	WNL	Sweating	Severe	WNL	<104° F (40° C)	WNL	WNL	Replacement of salt
Heat exhaustion	Heat exposure without access to water or with replacement of sweat loss with water only	Fatigue, weakness, headache, anxiety	Sweating	Variable	Variable	<104° F (40° C)	Tends to be low	Tends to be low	Replacement of salt or water
Heat stroke	Heat exposure, potassium and sodium depletion, impaired sweating, increased heat production	Headache, listlessness, confusion, seizure, psychosis, coma	Hot, dry	Variable	Abnormal	>104° F (40° C)	Abnormal (high or low)	Elevated	Cooling and support

From Barkin, R.M., & Rosen, P. (1999). Emergency pediatrics: A guide to ambulatory care. (5th ed.). St. Louis: Mosby.
WNL, Within normal limits.

near-drowning victim who is comatose with impaired respirations, abnormal response to pain, or impaired cardiovascular function also requires CPR and ventilatory support.

Orthopedic Fractures

Alert

Extra caution is required if the following fractures are suspected:
- Vertebral fracture (possible spinal cord injury)
- Basilar skull fracture (suspect a hemorrhage into the middle ear, as seen behind the tympanic membrane)
- Parietal fracture (possible middle meningeal artery laceration [epidural hemorrhage])
- Rib fracture (possible underlying lung injury or hemothorax)

Fractures can be defined as any break in the continuity of bone or cartilage. They are described in terms of the anatomic location on the bone, the fracture pattern, and how the fracture fragments relate to each other. Epiphyseal fractures are described in Fig. 48-2. The risk of growth disturbance increases from a type 1 fracture to a type 5 fracture.

Assessment

History
- Age
- Cause of injury
- Mechanism of injury, including the child's position before and after the injury and the direction of traumatic forces
- Source of pain or tenderness
- Hearing or feeling a "snap" at the time of injury
- Time of last food and water intake
- Any first aid already performed
- Past medical history, including activity level, medications, and allergies
- History of previous trauma

Physical examination and findings
- Airway, breathing, circulation, and LOC
- Vital signs and signs of possible shock

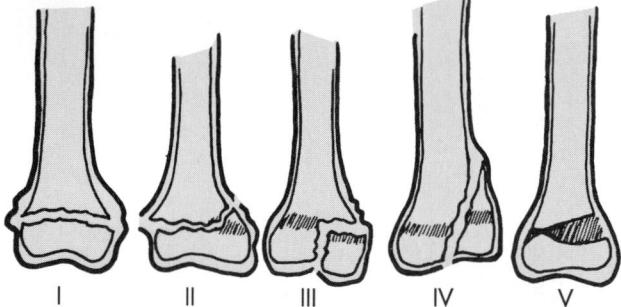

Fig. 48-2 Types of epiphyseal injuries in order of increasing risk. Injuries are classified as follows: *type I*, separation or slip of growth plate without fracture of the bone; *type II*, separation of the growth plate and breaking off a section of metaphysis; *type III*, fracture of epiphysis extending through the joint surface; *type IV*, fracture of growth plate, epiphysis, and metaphysis, and *type V*, crushing injury of epiphysis (can be diagnosed only in retrospect). This classification of epiphyseal injuries was developed by orthopedists R.B. Salter and W.R. Harris. (First published in Salter, R.B. & Harris, W.R. [1963]. Injuries involving the physeal plate. *Journal of Bone and Joint Surgery, 45*[3], 587-622.)

- Injury assessment, including assessment for edema, erythema, ecchymoses, and obvious angulation; assessment for the 5 *P*s (pain, pallor, paralysis, paresthesia, and pulselessness); examination of deformities, including abnormal angulation, crookedness, and shortening, rotation; and assessment of any open wound over a bone, point tenderness at a suspected site of fracture, swelling, and discoloration of soft tissue (indicating hemorrhage)

Management
- Elevation above heart to decrease swelling or pain
- Cold or ice packs
- Limitation of activity
- Medications for pain relief (see Chapter 7)
- Nothing by mouth (NPO status)
- Emergency transfer to a medical facility if there are signs of hemodynamic instability (e.g., blood loss, shock) or open fractures; otherwise, urgent transfer to a medical facility

Shock

Alert

Any child or adolescent who is in shock should be immediately transferred to a medical facility

Shock is a metabolic crisis in which the body's organs and tissues experience an acute insufficiency of oxygen and metabolites because of inadequate blood perfusion. Uncorrected shock leads to irreversible organ and tissue damage and death. Shock is either hypovolemic (e.g., acute hemorrhage), cardiogenic (e.g., pump failure), or distributed (e.g., sepsis, anaphylaxis) in nature. Prompt recognition of a preshock or shock state, coupled with emergency interventions, is essential to preserving vital tissues, organs, and life.

Assessment
- Change in LOC (i.e., decreased mental alertness)
- Cool skin temperature with diaphoresis
- Sluggish capillary refill
- Abnormal vital signs (e.g., hypotension, tachycardia, tachypnea)
- Decreased urine output
- Hypothermia

Management

Initial management of a shock state, concurrent with emergency transfer to a proper medical facility, includes the following:
- Positioning in a recumbent, or Trendelenburg's, position
- Judicious administration of supportive oxygen
- Evaluation and early intervention of the cause of shock (e.g., control of hemorrhage, treatment for anaphylaxis)
- Intravenous fluid resuscitation with normal saline or lactated Ringer's solution (if available)

Resources

Websites
American Board of Emergency Medicine (www.abem.org)
The Completely Different Pedictric Emergency Medical Journal (pediatric-emergency.com)

Emergency Medical Services for Children (www.ems-c.org)

Emergency Medicine and Emergency Medical Services (Hardin, MD) (www.lib.uiowa.edu/hardin/md/emerg.html)

The Virtual ER (www.virtualer.com)

Bibliography

Adreoni, C.P., Tipsord-Klinkhammer, B., & Klinkhammer, B. (2000). *Quick reference for pediatric emergency nursing.* Philadelphia: W.B. Saunders.

American Academy of Pediatrics (2001). *Textbook of neonatal resuscitation* (4th ed.). Elk Groove, IL: American Academy of Pediatrics.

American Heart Association, International Liaison Committee on Resuscitation (2000). Guidelines 2000 for cardiopulmonary resuscitation and emergency cardiovascular care: An international consensus on science. *Circulation 2000, 102*(8, suppl), 1.

American Heart Association (1990). *Textbook of advanced cardiac life support.* Dallas: American Heart Association.

American Heart Association and American Academy of Pediatrics (1988). *Textbook of advanced pediatric life support.* Dallas: American Heart Association.

Barkin, R.M. (Ed.). (1997). *Pediatric emergency medicine* (2nd ed.). St. Louis: Mosby.

Barkin, R.M. & Rosen, P. (Eds.). (1999). *Emergency pediatrics: A guide to ambulatory care* (5th ed.). St. Louis: Mosby.

Bolte, R. (1999). Drowning: A preventable cause of death. *Contemporary Pediatrics, 16*(7), 94-115.

Conn, A.W, Edmonds, J.F., & Barker, G.A. (1979). Cerebral resuscitation in near-drowning. *Pediatric Clinics of North America, 26,* 691-701.

Curley, M. & Moloney-Harmon, P. (2001). *Critical care nursing of infants and children* (2nd ed.). Baltimore: W.B. Saunders.

Knapp, J.F. & Seidel, J.S. (Eds.). (2000). *Childhood emergencies in the office, hospital and community.* Elk Grove, IL: American Academy of Pediatrics.

Rogers, M. & Helfaer, C.D. (1998). *Textbook of pediatric intensive care* (3rd ed.). Baltimore: Williams & Wilkins.

Schuman, A.J. (2001). New guidelines for pediatric life support. *Contemporary Pediatrics, 18*(9), 39-53.

Selbst, S.M. & Korin, J.B. (2000). Malpractice and emergency care: Doing right by the patient—and yourself. *Contemporary Pediatrics, 17*(7), 88-106.

Smith, M.L. (2000). Pediatric burns: Management of thermal, electrical, and chemical burns and burn-like dermatologic conditions. *Pediatric Annals, 29*(6), 367-378.

Zuckerman, G.B. & Conway, E.E. (2000). Drowning and near drowning: A pediatric epidemic. *Pediatric Annals, 29*(6), 360-366.

Chapter 49 *Preparation for Painful Procedures, Hospitalization, and Surgery*

Theresa M. Eldridge

Helping Children and Families Cope with Hospitalization and Surgery

Hospitalization of children has changed drastically from the restricted visiting policies of one to two times a week in the 1950s to the current practices of rooming-in and liberal visiting policies. Hospitalization is very stressful for children and their families, with the potential for interrupting the developmental processes and causing negative behavior outcomes. Although current trends are for decreased lengths of stay and more outpatient procedures, many children are chronically ill and may have multiple hospitalizations. Additionally, more procedures and diagnostic tests are being done on an outpatient basis, often in the home or health care clinic. The practitioner can provide children and their families with information, support, skills, and strategies to help with effective coping and adjustment, to prevent undue anxiety, and to minimize adverse medical and behavioral outcomes. To accomplish this, it is essential that the practitioner establish a trusting, honest relationship with the family. Numerous factors influence how children perceive illness, hospitalization, and surgery:

- Age
- Developmental level of the child
- Anxiety level of the parents or caregiver
- Individual characteristics and temperament of the child
- Coping styles and skills
- Parent-child relationships
- Religion
- Previous experience with hospitalization, surgery, and procedures
- Ethnic and cultural beliefs
- Amount, quality, and type of preparation for hospitalization, surgery, and procedures

Hospitalization and surgery disrupt the child's normal routine, which can increase the child's vulnerability and decrease coping ability. Children between 6 months and 6 years are the most susceptible to distress following hospitalization because of their immature cognitive level and lack of coping skills. Factors that place a child at greater risk for negative outcomes following hospitalization or surgery are:

- Age between 6 months and 6 years or developmental delay
- Moderate hospital stay of 4 to 8 days
- Prolonged hospital stay (longer than 8 days)
- More serious illnesses or traumas, especially those resulting in pain or painful procedures

- Hospitalizations that necessitate isolation of the child from the family
- Parents who exhibit high anxiety or have poor coping skills
- Inadequate preparation of the child and family for hospitalization and surgery
- Individual characteristics of the child that adversely affect the child's ability to cope with stressful events (e.g., external locus of control, temperament characteristics found in the difficult or slow-to-warm-up child)
- Children who have had a previous or multiple previous hospital, surgical, or procedure experiences or who have had a negative health care experience(which could also have been at the doctor's or dentist's office)

Short hospital stays of 3 days or less cause less disruption for a child than moderate stays of 4 to 8 days when the child does not have adequate time to adjust to the hospital environment. Prolonged hospital stays longer than 7 to 8 days provide the child with time to adapt to the hospital environment but also increase the disruption of the child's daily routine and separation from parents and home. Children who are hospitalized or have surgery have many fears that increase their anxiety. Key issues and fears of hospitalized children are:

- Separation from loved ones
- Interruption in normal daily routine
- Fear of abandonment
- Unfamiliar environment and equipment
- Loss of self-identity
- Loss of autonomy
- Decreased mobility
- Frightening and painful procedures
- Thoughts that illness, hospitalization, or surgery are punishments for being "bad"
- Loss of control
- Mutilation and bodily injury
- Isolation from peers

Separation Anxiety

One of the major stresses for children 6 to 30 months of age is separation anxiety, also called *anaclitic depression*. A summary of the three phases of separation anxiety is located in Box 49-1. It is important to help parents understand and appropriately respond to the child exhibiting these behaviors. Although separation anxiety is primarily associated with young children, school-age children and adolescents also indicate fears about being away from their families and may demon-

Box 49-1 Phases of Separation Anxiety

Protest Phase

Infancy behaviors

Cries or screams loudly
Clings to parents
Displays inconsolable grief
Rejects and avoids contact with strangers

Toddler behaviors

Verbally attacks strangers (e.g., "Go away! I don't like you.")
Physically assaults strangers (e.g., kicks, bites, hits, pinches)
Attempts to escape and find parents
Attempts to physically force parents to stay
Possibly continues behavior for hours until physically exhausted
Possibly renews protest when a stranger approaches

Despair Phase

Generally stops crying
Becomes depressed, hopeless, or mournful
Becomes disinterested in playing and eating
Becomes withdrawn, sad, lonely, and isolated
Becomes uncommunicative
May regress to earlier behaviors (e.g., bedwetting, thumbsucking)
May continue behaviors an indeterminate amount of time and can become physically at risk because of a lack of eating and drinking

Detachment Phase

Appears to be adjusting but is actually resigned and not coping well
Shows increased interest in surroundings and playing
Interacts with and develops superficial relationships with strangers
Appears happy and content but is actually exhibiting a superficial adjustment to loss
Usually only shows detachment after a prolonged separation from parents

Box 49-2 Identifying Coping Styles of Children

Question 1—Which approach is most effective when your child is going to have a possibly painful procedure?
  a. To tell the child everything in detail
  b. To tell the child very little about the procedure before-hand
  c. To not tell the child until the procedure happens

Question 2—How does your child usually cope with medical procedures?
  a. Wants to know what will happen
  b. Becomes upset if procedures are discussed
  c. Pretends nothing special is happening
  d. Closes eyes while procedure is happening
  e. Likes to distract self
  f. Tells jokes

Question 3—How does your child react to pain or fear?
  a. May yell but will cooperate
  b. Totally "loses control"
  c. Calm, cooperative, even though fearful

Question 4—How does your child react to new situations or strangers?
  a. Fearful and rejecting of new experiences and people
  b. Actively seeks out new people and situations
  c. Accepting but not overly enthusiastic
  d. Warms up after some exposure

Question 5—How would you describe your child's mood, reaction to stimuli, predictability? (Children who are adaptable, positive in mood, less intense, less responsive to stimuli, more predictable in everyday behavior, approaching, approachable, and distractible adjust better to hospitalization than children who are not.)

strate feelings of loneliness, boredom, isolation, and depression. Older children, however, generally have better coping skills and tend to be less distressed.

Coping Styles

Children use a variety of coping patterns to adapt to and master stressful life experiences. Frequently used coping styles are aggression, regression, intellectualization, recapitulation, reversal, denial, and humor. Extreme forms of these coping styles can be detrimental, although there may be some temporary benefit. For example, a child might benefit from denial, such as a child who initially denies feelings of fear or anxiety about a cancerous tumor until a later time when the child feels more emotionally capable and stable. Regression is frequently seen in children after a hospitalization, severe illness, or surgery. Previously toilet-trained preschoolers may begin to have "accidents." Children of all ages may revert to temper tantrums, clinging, fearfulness, and other previously mastered behaviors. Teaching children and their families appropriate coping skills can minimize the negative effects of hospitalization. Questions to identify the individual coping styles of children are found in Box 49-2.

Coping Skills

Teaching children positive coping skills lessens anxiety, improves their cooperation, enhances physical recovery, and provides a sense of control for the child to develop mastery. Box 49-3 offers some of the cognitive-behavioral coping strategies that can be used to prepare children for hospitalization and other stressful procedures.

Assessment

Each child and family should be assessed before hospitalization or surgery to identify strengths and those at higher risk for distress. A general assessment should include the following:

- Family's understanding of child's illness or reason for surgery
- Family's coping styles
- Type and quality of family supports
- Family's cultural and socioeconomic background
- Primary language
- Educational and learning style of the parents
- The effect that hospitalization will have on family, siblings, job, child care, and so on
- Ability of parents to be available to stay with their child in the hospital

Box 49-3 Coping Interventions

Procedural and Sensory Information

Provide information to the child along with the sensations the child will experience (e.g., information about how a cast is cut off in two pieces; the child will feel vibrations, tingling, and warmth; seeing chalk dust fly and smelling chalk).

Filmed Modeling

Show children a film in which a child experiences and successfully adapts to a hospitalization or surgery. Many videos depict events that children encounter when hospitalized and stress explanations of hospital procedures and the feelings experienced.

Therapeutic Play

Use various play modalities such as puppets, dolls, and roleplaying to assess the child's knowledge and concerns about hospitalization and surgery. These tools also can be used to teach children about procedures and equipment. Dolls or anatomically correct pictures can be used to show children where their tonsils or appendix are located.

Coping Skills

Relaxation—Stretching then tensing muscles; using a cue word such as "calm"

Deep breathing—Abdominal or "belly" breathing with long expiration

Imagery—Imagining a positive scene with the smell, sounds, "pictures"

Comforting self-talk—"I will be better soon" (saying it out loud and then thinking it)

Distraction—Distracting children from the procedure by talking about something they are interested in or distracting young children with toys, music, stories, or having the child count the number of tiles on the floor

Reinforcement—Using positive reinforcement immediately after cooperative behavior (e.g., giving a sticker to a child who holds still for venipuncture)

Desensitization—Using a calming technique such as imagery or deep breathing to help the child develop a desensitization to fear about an approaching procedure such as an immunization (must be used over time)

Music—Playing music with a slow tempo at a low pitch and volume often promotes relaxation (allow the child to select the music if possible)

Biofeedback

Teach the child to recognize and manage the body's physiologic responses to stress.

Hypnosis

Use deep relaxation to help children control anxiety and pain (generally used for children who have multiple painful procedures [e.g., hemophiliacs]).

Specific information about the child that will help the practitioner identify potential needs for hospital and surgery preparation includes.

- Preferred name
- Past responses to new situations, strange people, and fearful things
- Previous experiences and reactions to hospitalizations, surgeries, testing, and health and dental care
- Experience with and response to pain
- Developmental level
- Daily routine, eating patterns (including likes and dislikes), and sleeping routine
- Self-care activities (e.g., dresses self, brushes teeth)
- School and preschool
- Language development, including special words used for *urination, bottle,* and so on
- Special routines, toys, blanket, and comfort items
- Individual temperament characteristics
- Perceptions about illness, surgery, and the reason for hospitalization
- Special needs

Preparation for Procedures, Hospitalization, and Surgery

Practitioners can improve a family's adaptation to their child's illness or surgery by advance preparation of the child and family whenever possible. Emergency admissions do not allow for much preparation, but baseline data about the child and family can be shared with hospital personnel and greatly improve the family's adjustment. It is also necessary for the practitioner to be familiar with the hospital policies and practices in the local community. Rooming-in, visiting hours, play and recreational facilities, child life programs, preparation programs, and information on medical and nursing staff can be discussed with families. Preparation guidelines based on the child's cognitive level and developmental issues are identified in Table 49-1.

Fear of the unknown and lack of understanding often contribute to a child's anxiety. Communication in a language that the parents and child understand is critical in helping families cope with their anxiety. Some words have different meanings and can be confusing to parents and children. Children tend to be concrete in their interpretation of words and not fully grasp acronyms (e.g., *ICU* being understood as "I see you," *IV* being understood as "ivy"). Children and parents should be asked if they know what nurses and doctors mean when they say these words. Some words may be helpful to some children and threatening to others. The practitioner must listen carefully and be sensitive to the family's understanding and response to language. Table 49-2 provides suggestions for communicating in language appropriate for children.

Hospitalization and surgery can be very traumatic for the parents and child but need not be an entirely negative experience. Careful preparation of family members can alleviate much of the fear and anxiety. Sudden illnesses or surgeries will not have the advance preparation that is desirable; however, positive interventions can still be helpful in adapting to the situation and upon the family's return home. The following are some general guidelines that the practitioner can use to assist parents and children:

- Prepare a child according to his or her age. An infant requires little preparation because of limited cognitive and language capabilities, but an infant does respond to the feelings of his or her parents. Preparation of the parents can alleviate the child's stress and increase comfort and relaxation, which is then communicated to the infant. Infants 1 to 2 years of age can be told about going to the hospital on the day of or evening before admission or

Table 49-1 Preparing the Family for Hospitalization, Surgery, and Procedures

DEVELOPMENTAL CHARACTERISTICS	RESPONSIBILITIES AND INTERVENTIONS
Infant: Developing Trust	
Attachment to parent	Encourage a parent to stay with hospitalized child and assist in child's care as much as possible (i.e., rooming-in).
	Encourage parents to assist and participate with procedures if allowed.
	If a parent is unable to be with infant, use security item (e.g., stuffed toy, blanket, pacifier).
	Meet child's needs promptly (e.g., feeding, diaper change, crying).
Stranger and separation anxiety	Encourage usual caregivers to participate with procedures or examination.
	Encourage consistent caregivers (e.g., primary nurse).
	Limit the number of strangers child is exposed to, especially at one time.
	Approach child in a slow, nonthreatening manner.
	Teach parents behavior responses of stranger anxiety and separation anxiety and appropriate responses.
Sensorimotor phase of development	Cuddle and hug child after examinations and procedures.
	Encourage parents to comfort child using sensory measures (e.g., stroking skin, talking softly, giving pacifier, using a tape recording of music).
	Use appropriate analgesics to control discomfort.
Increased muscle control	Expect older infants to resist, so restrain adequately.
	Keep harmful objects out of reach.
	Provide necessary restraints but allow for as much freedom as possible (e.g., intravenous line in foot, not hand).
Memory of past experiences	Recognize that older infants may associate objects or persons with previous experiences and may cry or resist.
	Keep frightening objects out of view.
	Perform painful procedures in another area, not in crib or bed.
	Use nonintrusive procedures whenever possible (e.g., tympanic temperature).
Imitation of gestures	Model desired behaviors (e.g., opening mouth).
Toddler: Developing Autonomy	
Egocentric	(Use approaches for Infant and the following.)
	Explain procedure in terms of what child will see, hear, smell, feel, and taste.
	Emphasize when certain behaviors are required (e.g., lying still).
	Tell child it is all right to yell, cry, or use other means to verbally express feelings.
	Follow toddler's usual routines as much as possible.
Negative behavior	Encourage parents to bring familiar objects from home (e.g., toys, books, clothes, pictures of family members and pets).
	Expect that child may resist or try to run away.
	Use a firm, direct approach.
	Ignore temper tantrums.
	Use distraction techniques.
	Restrain adequately.
	Explain to parents that regression is a result of separation and is often most evident in this age group.
	Support and encourage parents to use positive parenting practices and set limits.
	Teach parents to never threaten the child with abandonment or painful procedure (e.g., shot) if child is not cooperative or acts out.
Limited language skills	Communicate using behaviors.
	Use a few simple terms that are familiar to the child.
	Give one direction at a time (e.g., "Lie down" and then "Hold my hand").
	Use small replicas of equipment; allow child to handle equipment.
	Use therapeutic play, use doll (not child's favorite doll) to demonstrate experiences (e.g., mask anesthesia, blood pressure).
	Prepare parents separately to avoid child's misinterpreting words.
Limited concept of time	Prepare child shortly or immediately before procedure, surgery, or task.
	Use teaching sessions of 5 to 10 minutes.
	Have all needed equipment and materials available to avoid delays.
Striving for independence	Tell child when procedure, examination, or surgery is over.
	Explain procedures, situations, or events in terms child can understand (Table 49-2).
	Encourage and allow choices whenever possible, but realize child may continue to be resistant and negative.
	Encourage and allow child to participate in care and to help whenever possible (e.g., drink medicine from a cup, hold a dressing).
	Encourage and allow toddler to explore as much as possible within safety guidelines.
	Promote play activities in a play area with other children if possible.

Continued

Table 49-1 Preparing the Family for Hospitalization, Surgery, and Procedures—cont'd

DEVELOPMENTAL CHARACTERISTICS	RESPONSIBILITIES AND INTERVENTIONS
Preschooler: Developing Initiative and Preoperational Thought	
Egocentrism Separation	Explain reasons for hospitalization, surgery, or procedure in simple terms and how it relates to child (stress sensory aspects). Demonstrate use of equipment. Allow child to play with miniature or toy equipment (e.g., stethoscope). Encourage therapeutic play (e.g., doll play, drawings). Use neutral words to describe equipment, procedures (Table 49-2). Encourage play activities and interaction with peers if possible (e.g., playroom and play equipment in hospital, surgery admission area). Support parents in accepting regressive behaviors. Encourage child to discuss home and family. Promote acceptable coping behaviors.
Increased language skills	Use verbal exploration but continue to employ sensory techniques; avoid overestimating child's comprehension. Encourage child to verbalize feelings and ideas.
Concept of time and frustration tolerance still limited	Use techniques and approaches as for toddler but increase teaching time to 10 to 15 minutes; may divide information into more than one session. Encourage play, with doll, puppets, clay as teaching methods. Offer predictability and continue to promote usual routines (e.g., bedtime, eating, play) as much as possible.
Illness and hospitalization often viewed as punishment	Explain why child is hospitalized or needs surgery or procedure (e.g., "This surgery will make your throat feel better"). Ask child his or her thoughts about why he or she is being hospitalized or having surgery or procedure. State directly that the hospitalization, surgery, procedure, or medicine is not a form of punishment. Encourage parents not to use the threat of hospitalization or shot if child does not cooperate or comply.
Fear of bodily harm, intrusion, and castration; rich fantasy life and magical thinking	Explain anatomy in simple terms. Discuss the limits of treatment; inform child what body areas will and will not be touched; use appropriate body drawings and dolls to teach and show exactly where dressing, incision, and so on, will be. Use nonintrusive procedures whenever possible. Apply adhesive bandage over puncture site (child may believe all his blood will leak out, so children this age need adhesive bandages for even tiny scratches; body integrity is very important). Realize that procedures involving genitals promote anxiety. Allow child to wear underpants with gown. Explain unfamiliar situations and equipment, especially noises and lights; use sensory techniques for coping. Allow child opportunities to use appropriate coping techniques (Box 49-3). Keep equipment out of sight except when used or shown.
Striving for initiative	Allow as much mobility as possible; child needs gross motor play, and peer play. Involve child with care whenever possible. Give choices whenever possible but avoid excessive delays. Praise child for helping and cooperating; never shame child for uncooperative behavior.
School-Age Child: Developing Industry	
Increased language skills; interest in acquiring knowledge	Explain procedures using correct scientific and medical terminology; ask children their understanding. Explain reason for hospitalization, surgery, or procedure using simple diagrams of anatomy and physiology. Explain functioning and mechanism of equipment in concrete terms. Allow child to manipulate equipment; use doll or another person as model to practice using equipment (older school-age child may feel doll play is "childish"). Encourage the child to ask questions and express concerns and feelings.

Table 49-1 Preparing the Family for Hospitalization, Surgery, and Procedures—cont'd

DEVELOPMENTAL CHARACTERISTICS	RESPONSIBILITIES AND INTERVENTIONS
School-Age Child: Developing Industry—cont'd	
Improved concept of time	Plan for longer teaching sessions (20 minutes).
	Prepare in advance for hospitalization, surgery, or procedure.
Increased self-control	Gain child's cooperation.
	Tell child what is expected.
	Suggest ways of maintaining control (Box 49-3).
	Provide opportunities that promote mastery.
	Child still needs parents but can use other adults and peers to meet needs.
Striving for industry	Allow responsibility for simple tasks (e.g., collecting specimens).
	Include in decision making (e.g., preferred site for injection; older child can decide if mask or intravenous anesthesia induction).
	Encourage active participation (e.g., removing dressings, handling equipment, opening packages).
	Maintain rules and rituals.
Developing relationships with peers	Possibly prepare two or more children for hospitalization, surgery, or procedure and encourage child to help another child.
	Provide privacy from peers during procedures and examinations to maintain self-esteem.
	Provide opportunities for peer interaction without parents.
	Encourage parents to support significant peer relationships (child may or may not want parents rooming-in).
	Encourage continued schoolwork.
Adolescent: Developing Identity	
Increasingly capable of abstract thought and reasoning	Supplement explanations with reasons why procedure, hospitalization, or surgery is necessary.
	Explain long-term consequences of procedure, hospitalization, or surgery.
	Realize that adolescent may fear death, disability, disfigurement, or other potential risks.
	Encourage discussion of concerns, fears, options, and alternatives.
Conscious of appearance	Provide privacy.
	Discuss what to expect (e.g., scar, hair loss) and how to minimize it.
	Emphasize any physical benefits of surgery or procedure.
Concerned more with present than future	Realize that immediate effects of procedure, surgery, or hospitalization are more significant than future benefits.
Striving for independence	Involve in decision-making and planning (e.g., time, place, individuals present during procedure or hospitalization, clothing to wear).
	Impose as few restrictions as possible.
	Suggest methods of maintaining control (coping strategies).
	Accept regression to less positive methods of coping.
	Realize that adolescent may have difficulty accepting new authority figures and may resist complying with procedures and hospital routines.
	Encourage individuality and personalize hospital room, casts, and so forth.
Developing peer relationships and group identity	Use same interventions as for school-age child, but remember that peers assume greater significance.
	Provide individualized schooling and recreation if needed.
	Provide opportunities for maintaining peer relationships and activities.
	Encourage adolescent to talk with other adolescents who have had the same disease, surgery, or procedure.
	Recognize that adolescent is individuating from parents but still needs parental support.
	Support parents and adolescent in recognizing and coping with normal growth and development issues.

Table 49-2 Considerations in Choosing Language

WORDS AND PHRASES TO AVOID	ALTERNATIVES
Vitals, vital signs	See how warm your body is; see how fast and strongly your heart is beating; hug your arm.
Incision	Small opening (compare it to something familiar, such as size of little finger)
IV	Medicine that goes into your vein (tube/straw) in your arm/hand and helps you get better quicker
Flush IV	Help medicine work better by putting special water in
Stretcher	Bed on wheels
Urine, stool, BM	Child's usual term (e.g., "pee pee," "poop")
Dye	Special medicine in a tube that will help your practitioner see your [part of body] more clearly
NPO	Nothing to eat or drink; your tummy needs to be empty
Shot, bee sting, stick	Medicine under the skin
Pain	You may feel sore, achy, scratchy, tight, snug (use manageable terms); some children say they feel a warm feeling. After you take it, let me know how it feels to you.
Cut, fix	Make better
Deaden	Make numb or sleepy
Specimen	Sample
Take a picture (x-ray, CT scan, MRI)	A picture of the inside of you (describe what child will see, hear, feel and what the equipment is like)
Electrode	Sticky Band-Aids with a wet spot in the middle with small strings
Dressing change	Clean, new bandages
Gas, anesthesia, put to sleep	Give you medicine that will help you go into a deep sleep; you won't feel anything until the operation is over, and then the doctor will stop giving you the medicine so you can wake up; breathe special air through a mask
Tell your parents goodbye	Say "See you later" to parent
Good girl/boy	You did a good job of holding still.
You seem angry, sad, scared; That was hard for you	How was that for you? Was it the way you thought it would be? Is there something else we should tell people about this?
As long as . . . (as with duration of procedure)	For less time than it takes you to . . .
As big as . . . (as with size of incision or catheter)	Smaller than . . .
As much as . . .	Less than . . .

Box 49-4 Preparation of Siblings

Be honest.

Find out if the sibling would like to visit and respect the child's feelings (especially if the answer is "no").

Allow the child to participate in a hospital tour if desired.

Act out hospital experiences with puppets, dolls, and roleplaying.

Encourage the child to express feelings (e.g., anger, guilt, jealousy, worry, fear).

If a parent must be at the hospital away from a sibling, have the parent call daily if possible, write or tape-record letters or stories, or send home safe, unused items from the hospital (e.g., emesis basin, straws).

Have the hospitalized child and sibling draw pictures for each other and bring or send photos.

Encourage the sibling to bring something from home for the hospitalized child (if allowed).

- Always be honest with the child and siblings. Parents should talk to their child when they have some emotional control.

- Assess each child's knowledge and understanding of the situation before deciding what information to share with the child.

- Select the materials and method of preparation to match the child's cognitive level, experience, special circumstances, and interest.

- Involve the child and siblings in the preparations as much as possible (Box 49-4).

- Encourage discussion about the hospitalization and surgery by reading books to the child or having the child read or color. Also use the other intervention strategies already identified in Box 49-3.

- Explain to the parents the stages of separation and how to appropriately deal with the behaviors exhibited by the child.

- Encourage parents to hold children in a position of comfort during procedures such as lab draws and intravenous insertions whenever possible.

- Explain to the parents, child, and siblings what to expect in clear and simple terms.

- Discuss different options of how the child might effectively cope during hospitalization and with various procedures.

- Have the parents, child, and siblings attend a hospitalization and surgery preparation tour or program.

surgery; 2- to 3-year-olds can be prepared 2 to 3 days before surgery or hospitalization; 4- to 7-year-olds can receive preparation 4 to 7 days before admission; and children over 7 years of age can be involved in preparation and planning a few weeks before the admission or surgery.

- Discuss ways the parents can support their child before, during, and after procedures, hospitalization, and surgery.
- Allow a parent to stay with the child as much as possible at the hospital.
- Have the parents bring items from home to the hospital (e.g., the child's own clothes, pictures, security items).
- Explain to parents that the child may revert to previously mastered behaviors (e.g., thumbsucking, clinging, fear of being left alone, toileting regression).
- Remember that older children also need a great deal of support and reassurance.
- Be sure the hospital staff know special events and people in the child's life and specific routines and preferences of the child (nickname, preferences and patterns for eating, sleeping, etc.).
- Encourage parents to discuss with the staff their child's specific reactions to stress and pain and the coping behaviors generally used.
- Encourage the parents, child, and siblings to express their feelings and help them identify positive aspects of the hospitalization and surgery.
- Model appropriate behaviors. Children imitate their parents and health care personnel.
- Encourage parents never to leave without saying goodbye. Parents should not sneak away when the child is sleeping or preoccupied so the child will develop a sense of trust.
- Use language that is age-appropriate.
- Allow the child to play with medical equipment, and always practice possible procedures and promote effective coping behaviors.
- Encourage preparation of the child using sensory aspects of the experience (i.e., what will the child smell, hear, feel, see, taste).
- Adapt the preparation and care of the child based on individual needs (e.g., child is learning disabled, developmentally disabled, of a different culture).
- Consider the use of enteric mixture of local anesthetics (EMLA) cream to eliminate the pain of needles for local anesthesia and intravenous liquids.
- Do not force any information on a child if he or she clearly indicates not wanting to hear or experience it.

Special Considerations

Children with chronic illnesses often must deal with repeated hospitalizations and surgeries. In addition, they may use the disease as a means of dealing with other issues. The following are some of the issues that the practitioner may need to address in relation to children with chronic illnesses:

- *Seizure disorder*—Children may fear the loss of control. Children with seizures have a significant incidence of behavioral and emotional problems. (See Seizures, Breath-Holding Spells, and Syncope in Chapter 39.)
- *Diabetes*—Children may act out their anger at their parents and themselves by refusing to comply with dietary restrictions and the medical regimen. (See Diabetes Mellitus in Chapter 45.). Often, bulimia and anorexia nervosa may be a result of maladaptive coping. (See Anorexia and Bulimia in Chapter 45.)
- *Heart disease*—Children with heart disease who are asymptomatic may have difficulty in complying with restrictions because they do not feel "sick." (See Chapter 32.)
- *Renal disease*—Children may feel they are controlled by machines and have issues of independence and dependence. If the illness is severe, there may be anxiety about transplantation and rejection.
- *Gastrointestinal disorders*—Children may have a preoccupation with food and concerns about eating the "wrong" foods. Children with gastrointestinal (GI) disorders often have school phobia, depression, or chronic psychogenic abdominal pain.
- *Asthma*—Children may fear suffocation, drowning, or strangulation. Depression and suicide are of concern with this group of children. (See Asthma in Chapter 45.)
- *Cancer*—Children who are diagnosed before 3 years of age seem to adapt emotionally to their disease partly because they cannot cognitively comprehend the seriousness of their disease. Older children not only understand the ramifications of their illness but also have an understanding of death. In addition, older children who have significant sequelae (e.g., hair loss, loss of a limb or body function), experience significant reactions to their disease, affecting their self-concept. (See Neoplastic Disease in Chapter 45.)

All children may experience a negative reaction to illness, hospitalization, or surgery. Children with certain personality characteristics may respond with significant maladaptive traits. Children who are overly dependent, inhibited, and fearful may react by giving up, while overly independent children may exhibit risk-taking behaviors. Children who have chronic illnesses also have issues regarding loss of control, dependence, changes in self-concept, depression, and suicide. The practitioner can provide a thorough assessment of each child, address concerns, and provide appropriate interventions.

Conclusion

Teaching coping techniques to older children and using play therapy for younger children has been shown to significantly decrease the anxiety and stress experienced by the children. Minimizing the psychologic distress through preparation and adapting the hospital environment to decrease the disruption of a child's daily routine have also demonstrated positive outcomes. Providing for predictability in the hospital environment and allowing a child as much control as possible over situations such as dressing changes provides optimal adaptation to hospitalization or surgery. Providing continuity in the nursing staff and allowing for surrogate parents (i.e., "hospital grandmothers") who are consistent care providers also minimize the negative effects of hospitalization and surgery.

Resources

Publications

At the hospital coloring book, available from the Channing L. Bete Company, Inc, 200 State Road, South Deerfield, MA 01373-0200, (800) 628-7733; www.channing-bete.com.

Howe, J. (1998). *A night without stars.* New York: Atheneum Scholastic.

Howe, J. (1994). *The hospital book.* New York: William Morrow and Company.

Keene, N. & Prentice, R. (1999). *Your child in the hospital.* Sebastopol, CA: O'Reilly and Associates.

Landsdown, R. (1996). *Children in hospital: A guide for family and carers.* New York: Oxford University Press.

Melamed, B.G. & Siegel, L.J. (1975). Reduction of anxiety in children facing hospitalization and surgery by use of filmed modeling. *Journal of Consulting and Clinical Psychology, 43,* 511-521.

Miller, M. (1996). *Behind the scenes at the hospital.* Austin, TX, 1996, Steck-Vaughn.

Moe, B.A. (1976). *Pickles and prunes.* New York: McGraw-Hill.

Moses, A. (1998). *At the hospital.* Naperville, IL: The Child's World.

Rey, M. & Rey, H. (1966). *Curious George goes to the hospital.* New York: Houghton Mifflin.

Rogers, F. (1997). *Going to the hospital.* New York: Putnam Grosset.

Santesteban, A. (1997). *The complete guide to pediatric hot lines and resources* (2nd ed.). Bedford, TX: ABC Press.

Organizations

Association for the Care of Children's Health (ACCH), 19 Mantua Road, Mt. Royal, NJ 08061; (609) 224-1742; www.acch.org

Channing L. Bete Company, Inc., 200 State Road, South Deerfield, MA 01373-0200; (800) 628-7733; www.channing-bete.com

Film Ideas, 3710 Commercial Avenue, Suite 13, Northbrook, IL 60062; (800) 475-3456; www.filmideas.com

Maxishare, PO Box 2041, Milwaukee, WI 53201; (800) 444-7747; www.maxishare.com

Universal Health Communication, Inc., 1200 S Federal Highway, Suite 202, Boynton Beach, FL 33435; (800) 229-1842; www.universalhealthonline.com

Bibliography

Bar-Mor, G. (1997). Preparation of children for surgery and invasive procedures: milestones on the way to success. *Journal of Pediatric Nursing, 12,* 252-255.

Brewer, S.L. & Lambert, C.S. (1997). Preparing children for same day surgery: Innovative approaches. *Journal of Pediatric Nursing, 12,* 257-259.

Bricher, G. (2000). Children in the hospital: issues of power and vulnerability. *Pediatric Nursing, 26,* 277-282.

Carson. D.K., Council, J.R., & Gravely, J.E. (1991). Temperament and the family characteristics as predictors of children's reactions to hospitalization. *Developmental and Behavioral Pediatrics, 12,* 141-147.

Ferrari, L.R. (Ed.). (1999). *Anesthesia and pain management for the pediatrician.* Baltimore, MD: Johns Hopkins University Press.

Greenberg, L.A. (1991). Teaching children who are learning disabled about illness and hospitalization. *Maternal Child Nursing, 16,* 260-263.

LaMontagne. L.L. (2000). Children's coping with surgery: a process-oriented perspective. *Journal of Pediatric Nursing, 15,* 307-312.

LaMontagne, L.L. (1993). Bolstering personal control in child patients through coping interventions. *Pediatric Nursing, 19,* 235-237.

Lancaster, K.A. (1997). Care of the pediatric patient in ambulatory surgery. *Nursing Clinics of North America, 32,* 441-455.

Melnyk, B.M. (2000). Intervention studies involving parents of hospitalized young children: an analysis of the past and future recommendations. *Journal of Pediatric Nursing, 15,* 4-13.

Melamed, B.G. (1988). Helping children and families cope with hospitalization and outpatient medical treatment. *Feelings and the Medical Significance, 30,* 15-20, 1988.

Norred, C.L. (2000). Minimizing preoperative anxiety with alternative caring-healing therapies. *AORN Journal, 72,* 839-843.

Ott, M.J. (1996). Imagine the possibilities! Guided imagery with toddlers and preschoolers. *Pediatric Nursing, 22,* 34-38.

Wright, M.C. (1995). Behavioral effects of hospitalization in children. *Journal of Pediatric Child Health, 31,* 165-167.

Appendix A *Growth Charts and Developmental Screening Tools*

Jane A. Fox

This appendix includes reference charts and tools to assess physical growth, development, and language in the pediatric population. Charts to assess physical growth (e.g., weight, length, stature, head circumference) in girls and boys from birth to 20 years of age can be found here (Figs. A-1 through A-9). Maturational Assessment of Gestational Age (New Ballard Score) (Fig. A-10) and gestational age charts (Fig. A-11) have also been included, as have age-specific percentiles of blood pressure measurements for boys and girls from birth to 18 years of age (Figs. A-12 and A-13). Also included in this appendix are copies of the Denver II (Fig. A-14) and two tools used to assess language development, the Denver Articulation Screening Examination (for children 2 to 6 years of age) (Fig. A-15) and the Early Language Milestone Scale (for children from birth to 36 months of age) (Fig. A-16).

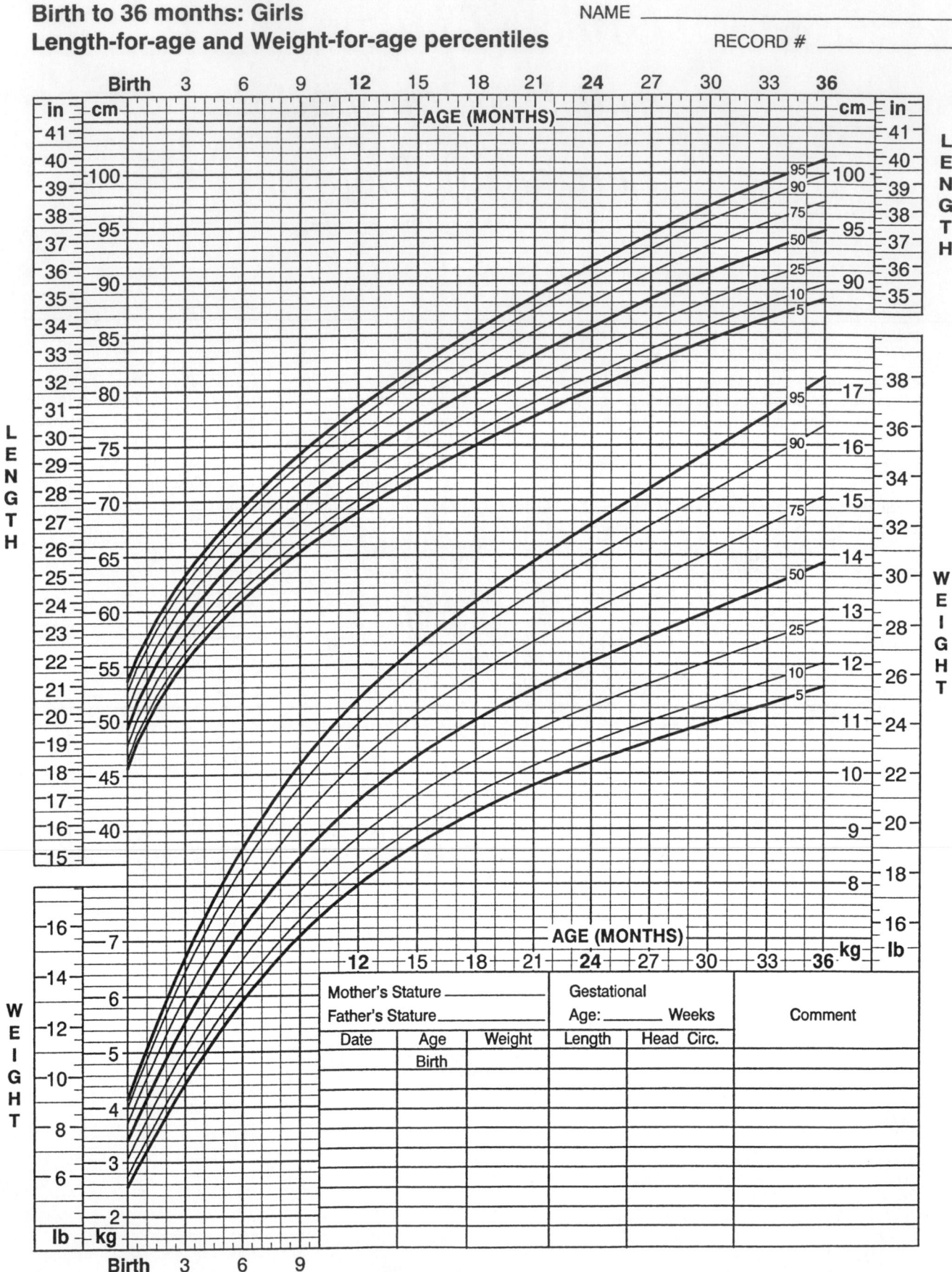

Fig. A–1 Length-for-age and weight-for-age percentiles for girls from birth to 36 months old.

Birth to 36 months: Girls
Head-circumference-for-age and
Weight-for-length percentiles

NAME _____

RECORD # _____

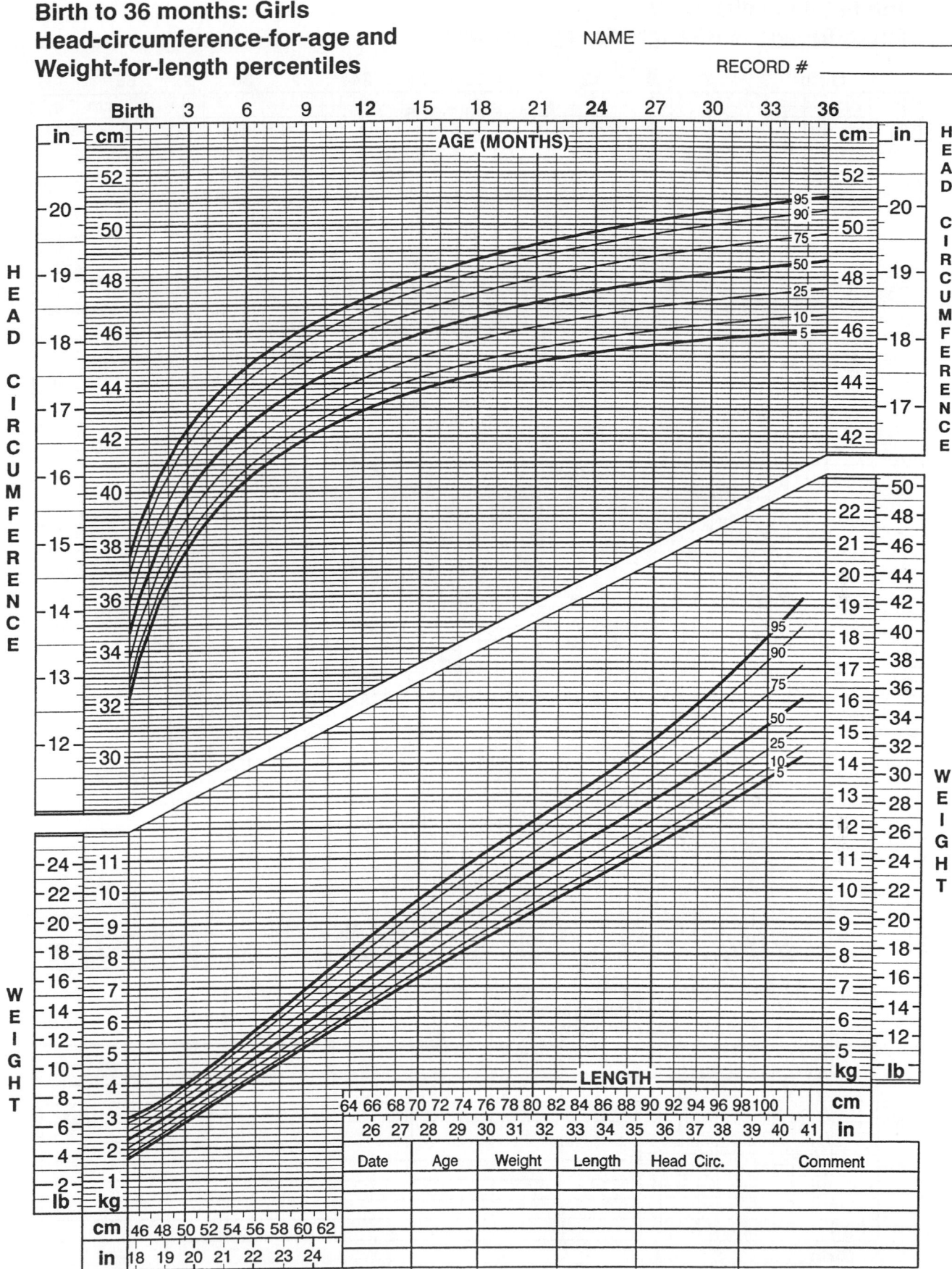

Fig. A-2 Head-circumference-for-age and weight-for-length percentiles for girls from birth to 36 months old.

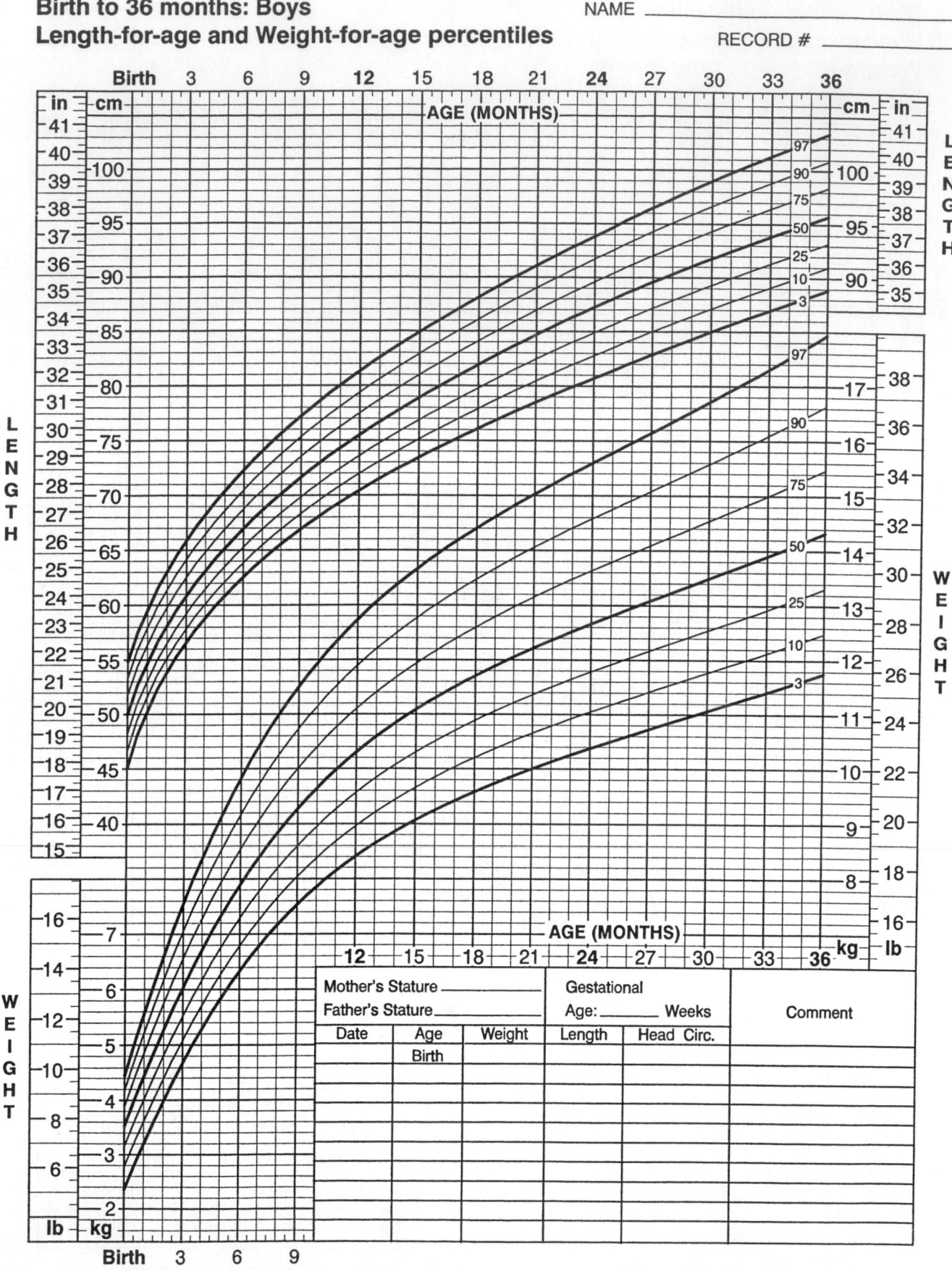

Birth to 36 months: Boys
Length-for-age and Weight-for-age percentiles

NAME _____

RECORD # _____

Fig. A-3 Length-for-age and weight-for-age percentiles for boys from birth to 36 months old.

Birth to 36 months: Boys
Head-circumference-for-age and
Weight-for-length percentiles

NAME _____

RECORD # _____

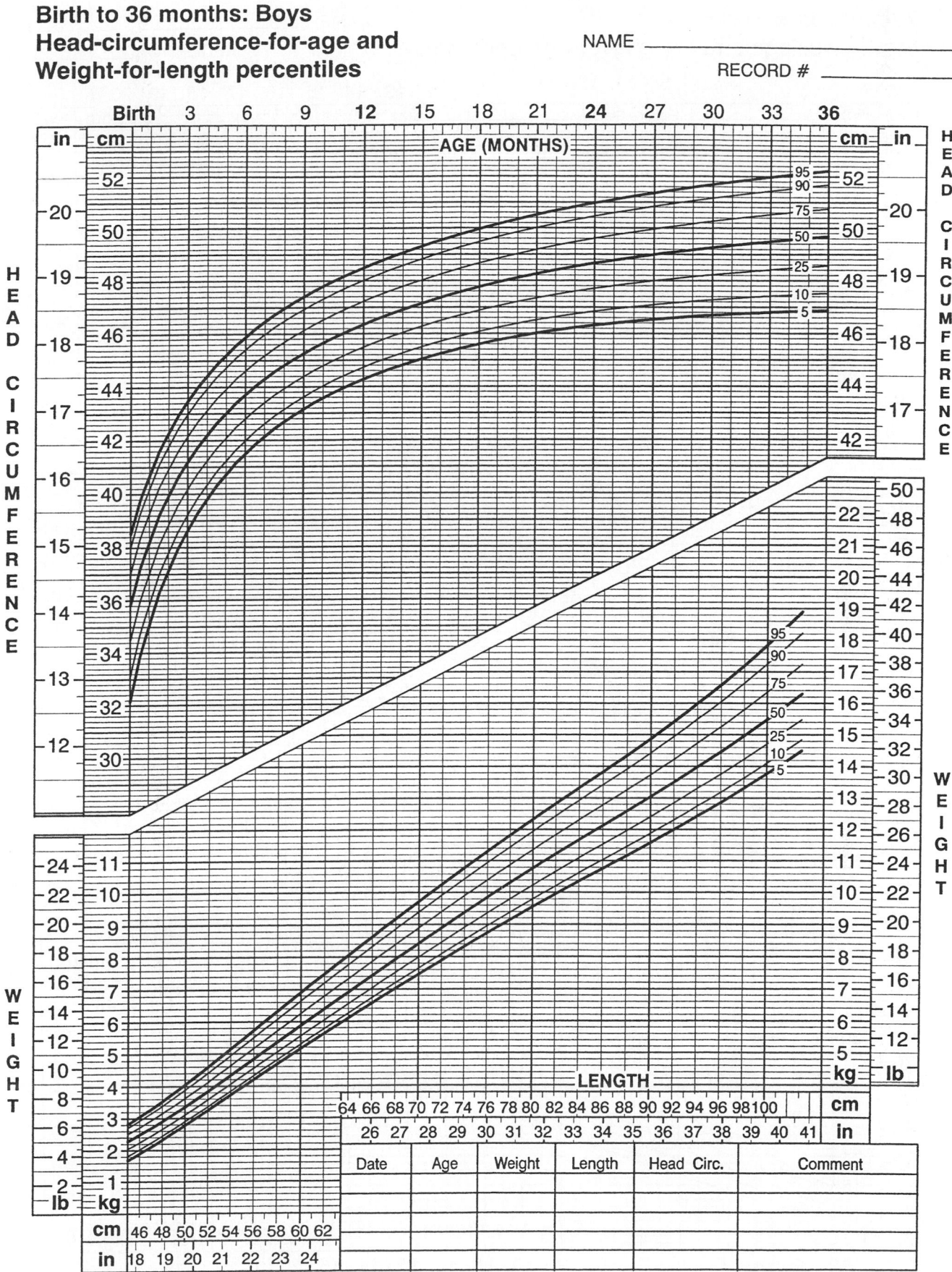

Fig. A–4 Head-circumference-for-age and weight-for-length percentiles for boys from birth to 36 months old.

2 to 20 years: Girls
Stature-for-age and Weight-for-age percentiles

NAME _____

RECORD # _____

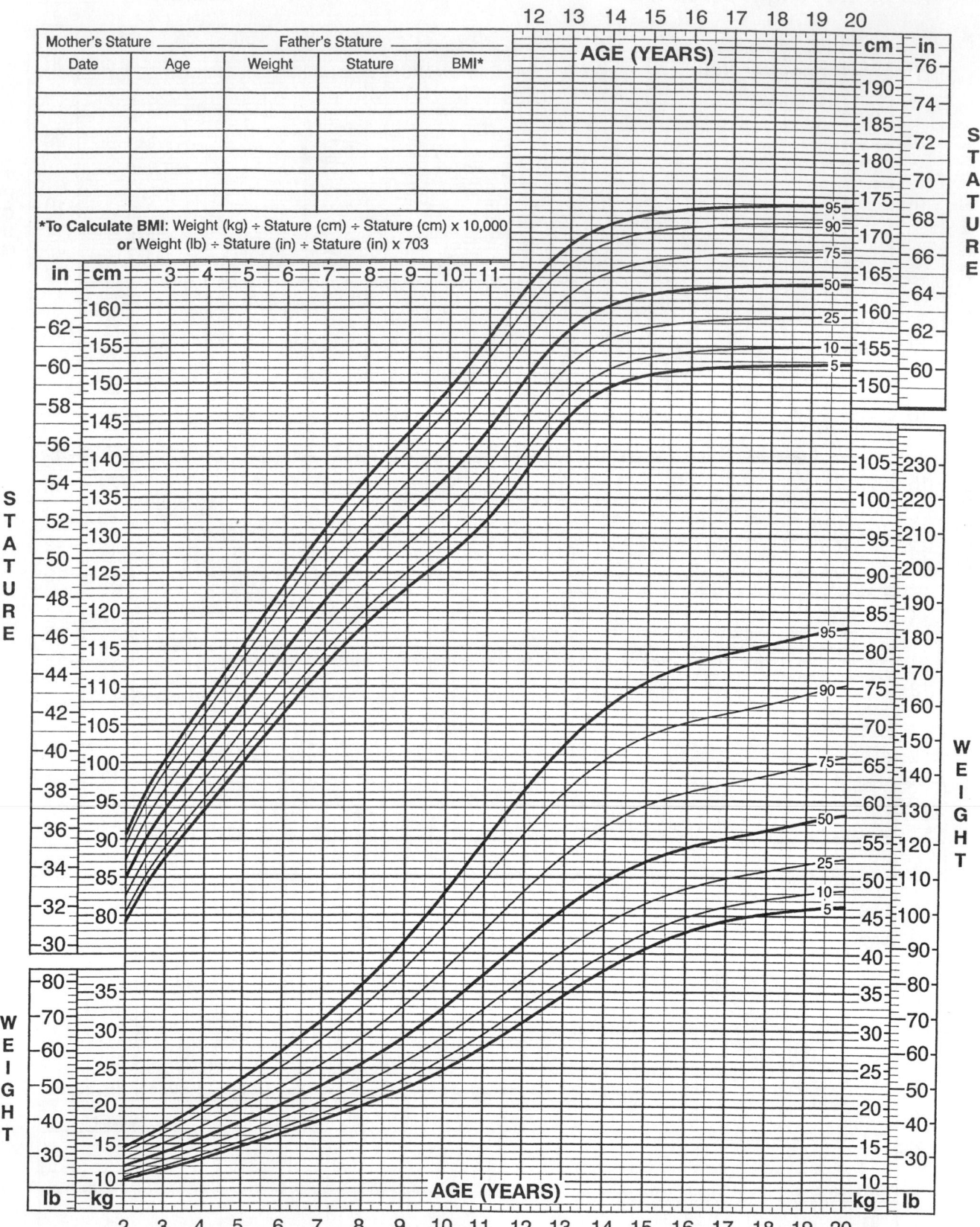

Fig. A-5 Stature-for-age and weight-for-age percentiles for girls from 2 to 20 years old.

NAME ______________________

RECORD # __________

Weight-for-stature percentiles: Girls

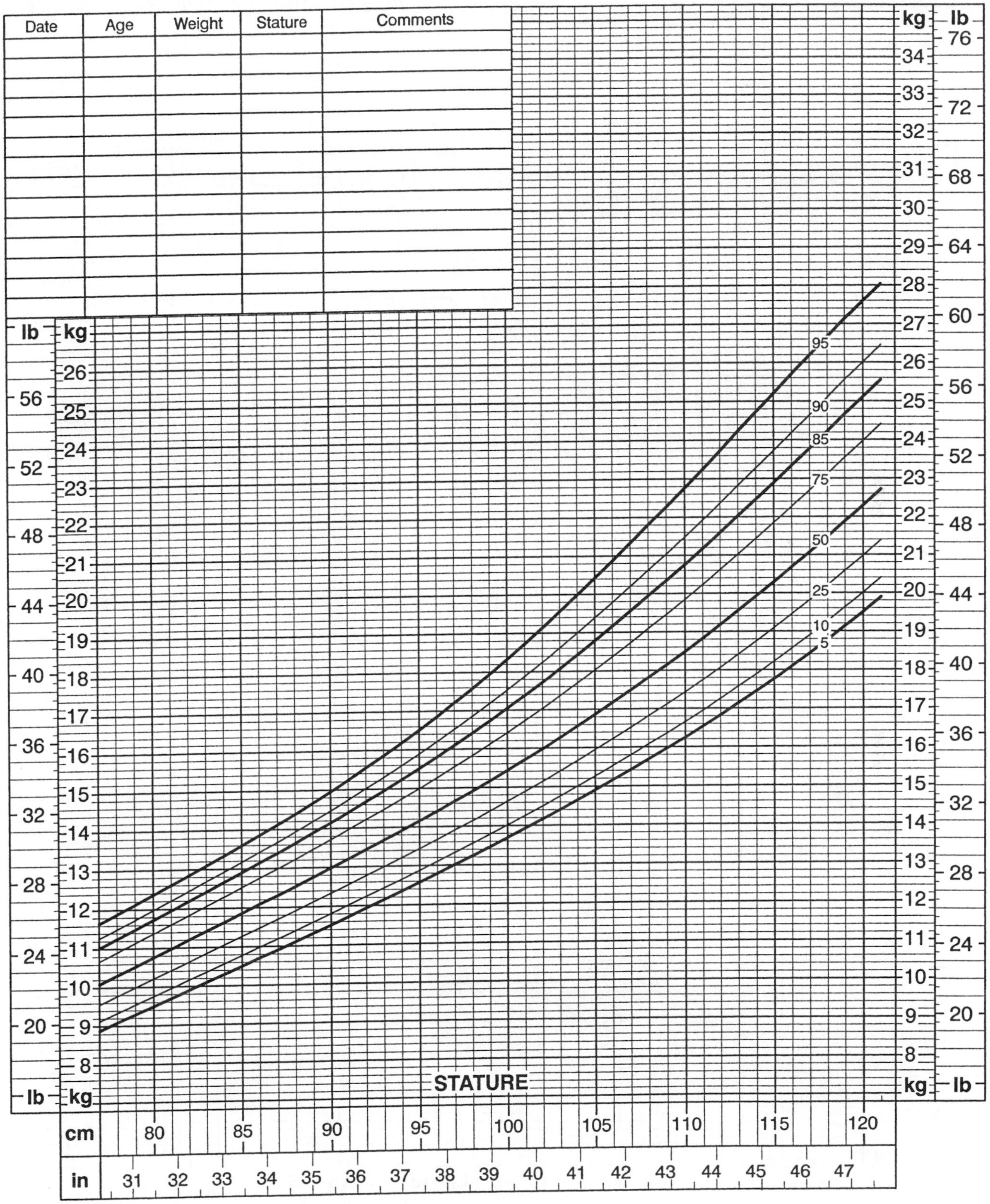

Fig. A-6 Weight-for-stature percentiles for girls.

2 to 20 years: Boys
Stature-for-age and Weight-for-age percentiles

NAME _____

RECORD # _____

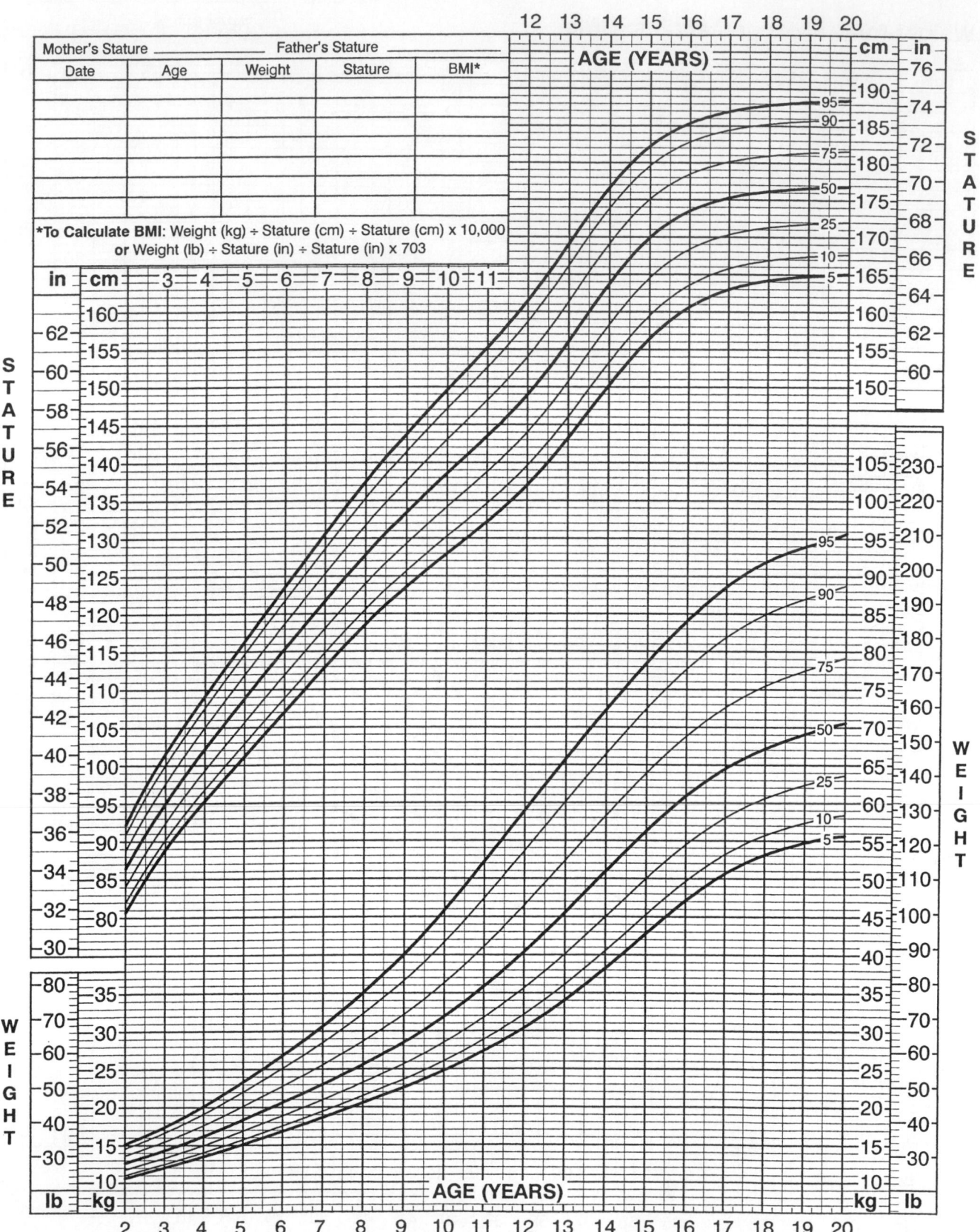

Fig. A-7 Stature-for-age and weight-for-age percentiles for boys from 2 to 20 years old.

Weight-for-stature percentiles: Boys

NAME _____

RECORD # _____

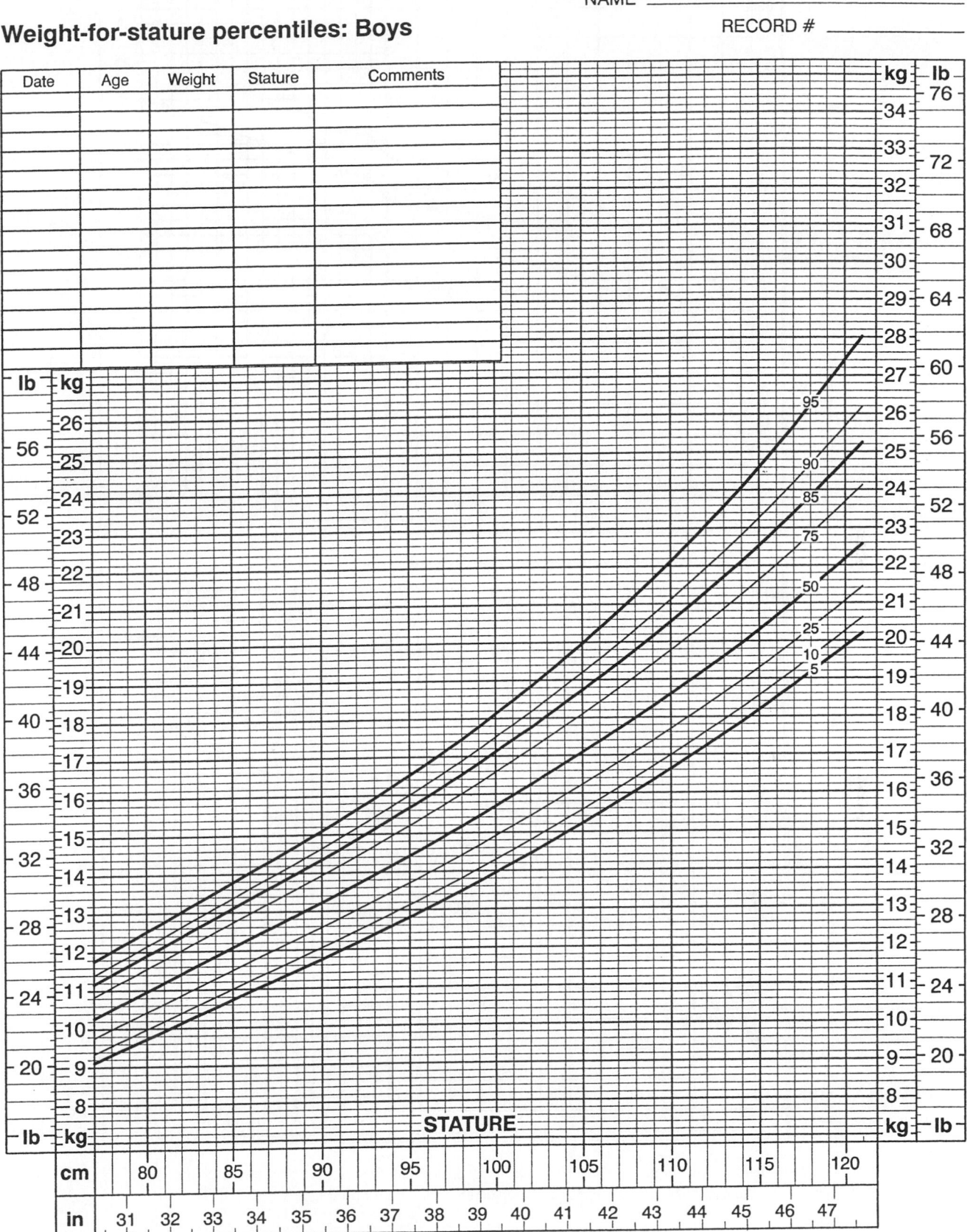

Fig. A-8 Weight-for-stature percentiles for boys.

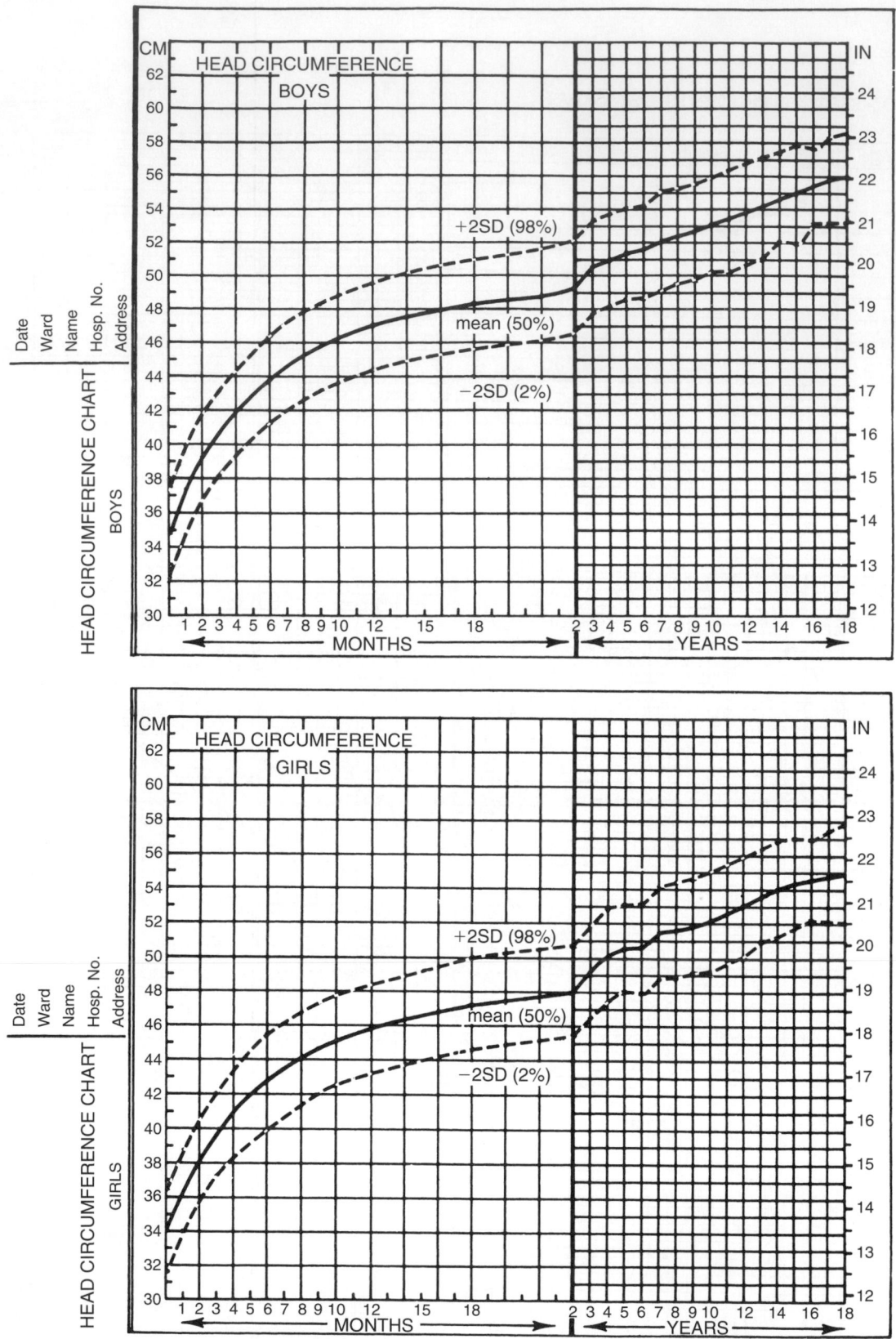

Fig. A-9 Head circumference charts. (From Nellhaus, G. [1968]. Composite international and interracial graphs. *Pediatrics, 41,* 106. University of Colorado Medical Center Printing Services.)

MATURATIONAL ASSESSMENT OF GESTATIONAL AGE (New Ballard Score)

NEUROMUSCULAR MATURITY

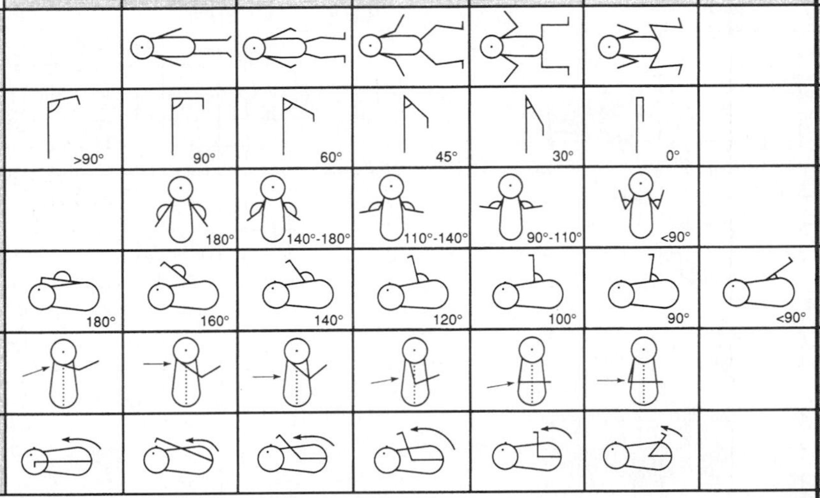

NEUROMUSCULAR MATURITY SIGN	SCORE							RECORD SCORE HERE
	-1	0	1	2	3	4	5	
POSTURE								
SQUARE WINDOW (Wrist)	>90°	90°	60°	45°	30°	0°		
ARM RECOIL		180°	140°-180°	110°-140°	90°-110°	<90°		
POPLITEAL ANGLE	180°	160°	140°	120°	100°	90°	<90°	
SCARF SIGN								
HEEL TO EAR								

TOTAL NEUROMUSCULAR MATURITY SCORE

PHYSICAL MATURITY

PHYSICAL MATURITY SIGN	SCORE							RECORD SCORE HERE
	-1	0	1	2	3	4	5	
SKIN	sticky friable transparent	gelatinous red translucent	smooth pink visible veins	superficial peeling &/or rash, few veins	cracking pale areas rare veins	parchment deep cracking no vessels	leathery cracked wrinkled	
LANUGO	none	sparse	abundant	thinning	bald areas	mostly bald		
PLANTAR SURFACE	heel-toe 40-50 mm:-1 <40 mm:-2	>50 mm no crease	faint red marks	anterior transverse crease only	creases ant. 2/3	creases over entire sole		
BREAST	imperceptible	barely perceptible	flat areola no bud	stippled areola 1-2 mm bud	raised areola 3-4 mm bud	full areola 5-10 mm bud		
EYE/EAR	lids fused loosely: -1 tightly: -2	lids open pinna flat stays folded	sl. curved pinna; soft; slow recoil	well-curved pinna; soft but ready recoil	formed & firm instant recoil	thick cartilage ear stiff		
GENITALS (Male)	scrotum flat, smooth	scrotum empty faint rugae	testes in upper canal rare rugae	testes descending few rugae	testes down good rugae	testes pendulous deep rugae		
GENITALS (Female)	clitoris prominent & labia flat	prominent clitoris & small labia minora	prominent clitoris & enlarging minora	majora & minora equally prominent	majora large minora small	majora cover clitoris & minora		

TOTAL PHYSICAL MATURITY SCORE

SCORE

Neuromuscular _____

Physical _____

Total _____

MATURITY RATING

score	weeks
-10	20
-5	22
0	24
5	26
10	28
15	30
20	32
25	34
30	36
35	38
40	40
45	42
50	44

GESTATIONAL AGE (weeks)

By dates _____

By ultrasound _____

By exam _____

Fig. A-10 Maturational Assessment of Gestational Age (New Ballard Score). (From Ballard, J.L., et al. [1991]. New Ballard Score, expanded to include extremely premature infants. *Journal of Pediatrics, 119,* 417-423. Reprinted with permission of Dr. Ballard and Mosby.)

CLASSIFICATION OF NEWBORNS (BOTH SEXES) BY INTRAUTERINE GROWTH AND GESTATIONAL AGE

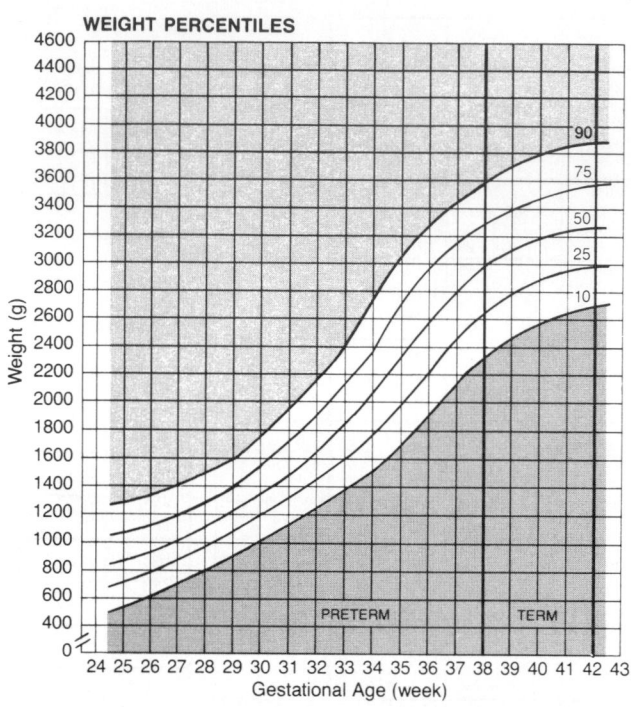

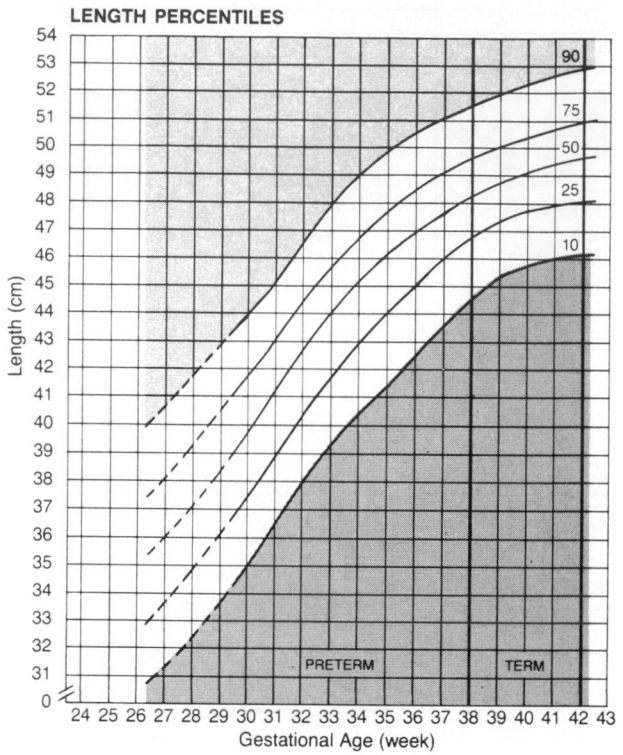

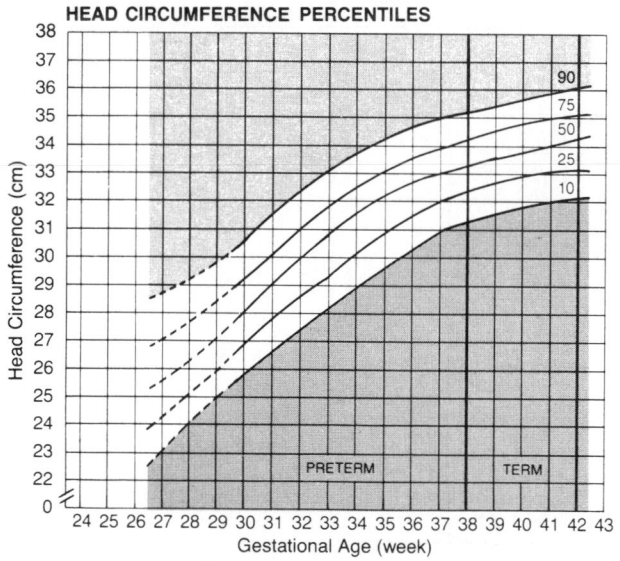

CLASSIFICATION OF INFANT*	Weight	Length	Head Circ.
Large for Gestational Age (LGA) (>90th percentile)			
Appropriate for Gestational Age (AGA) (10th to 90th percentile)			
Small for Gestational Age (SGA) (<10th percentile)			

*Place an "X" in the appropriate box (LGA, AGA or SGA) for weight, for length, and for head circumference.

Fig. A-11 Classification of newborns (both sexes) by intrauterine growth and gestational age. (From Battaglia, F.C. & Lubchenco, L.O. [1967]. A practical classification of newborn infants by weight and gestational age. *Journal of Pediatrics, 71,* 159-163; Lubchenco, L.O., Hansman, C., & Boyd, E. [1966]. Intrauterine growth in length and head circumference as estimated from live births at gestational ages from 26 to 42 weeks. *Pediatrics, 37,* 403-408.)

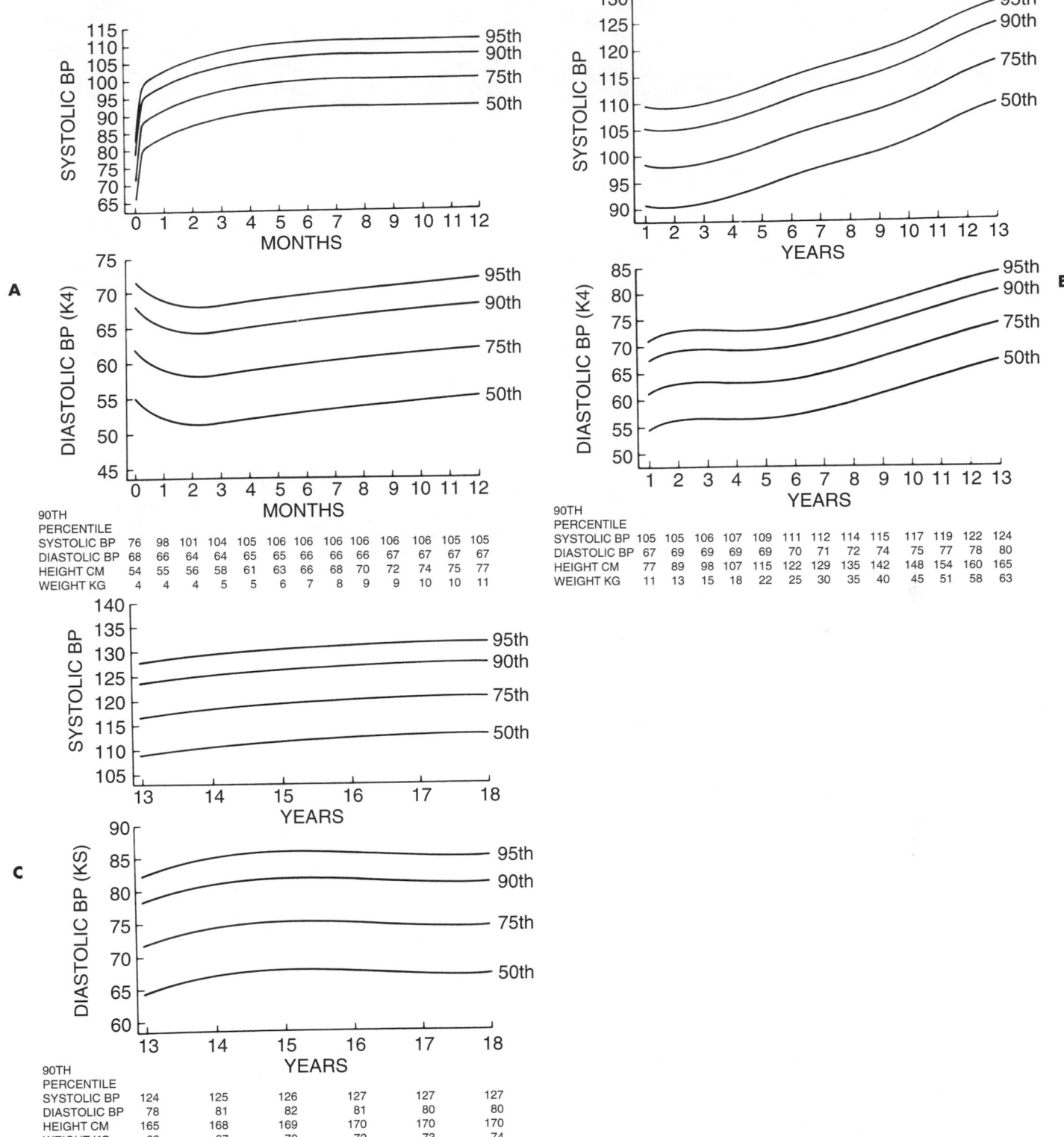

90TH PERCENTILE (Birth to 12 months)

SYSTOLIC BP	76	98	101	104	105	106	106	106	106	106	106	105	105
DIASTOLIC BP	68	66	64	64	65	65	66	66	66	67	67	67	67
HEIGHT CM	54	55	56	58	61	63	66	68	70	72	74	75	77
WEIGHT KG	4	4	4	5	5	6	7	8	9	9	10	10	11

90TH PERCENTILE (1 to 13 years)

SYSTOLIC BP	105	105	106	107	109	111	112	114	115	117	119	122	124
DIASTOLIC BP	67	69	69	69	69	70	71	72	74	75	77	78	80
HEIGHT CM	77	89	98	107	115	122	129	135	142	148	154	160	165
WEIGHT KG	11	13	15	18	22	25	30	35	40	45	51	58	63

90TH PERCENTILE (13 to 18 years)

SYSTOLIC BP	124	125	126	127	127	127
DIASTOLIC BP	78	81	82	81	80	80
HEIGHT CM	165	168	169	170	170	170
WEIGHT KG	63	67	70	72	73	74

Fig. A-12 Age-specific percentiles of blood pressure measurements in boys. **A,** Birth to 12 months of age; **B,** 1 to 13 years of age; **C,** 13 to 18 years of age. (Data from the Report of the Second Task Force on Blood Pressure Control in Children. [1987]. *Pediatrics, 79,* 1.)

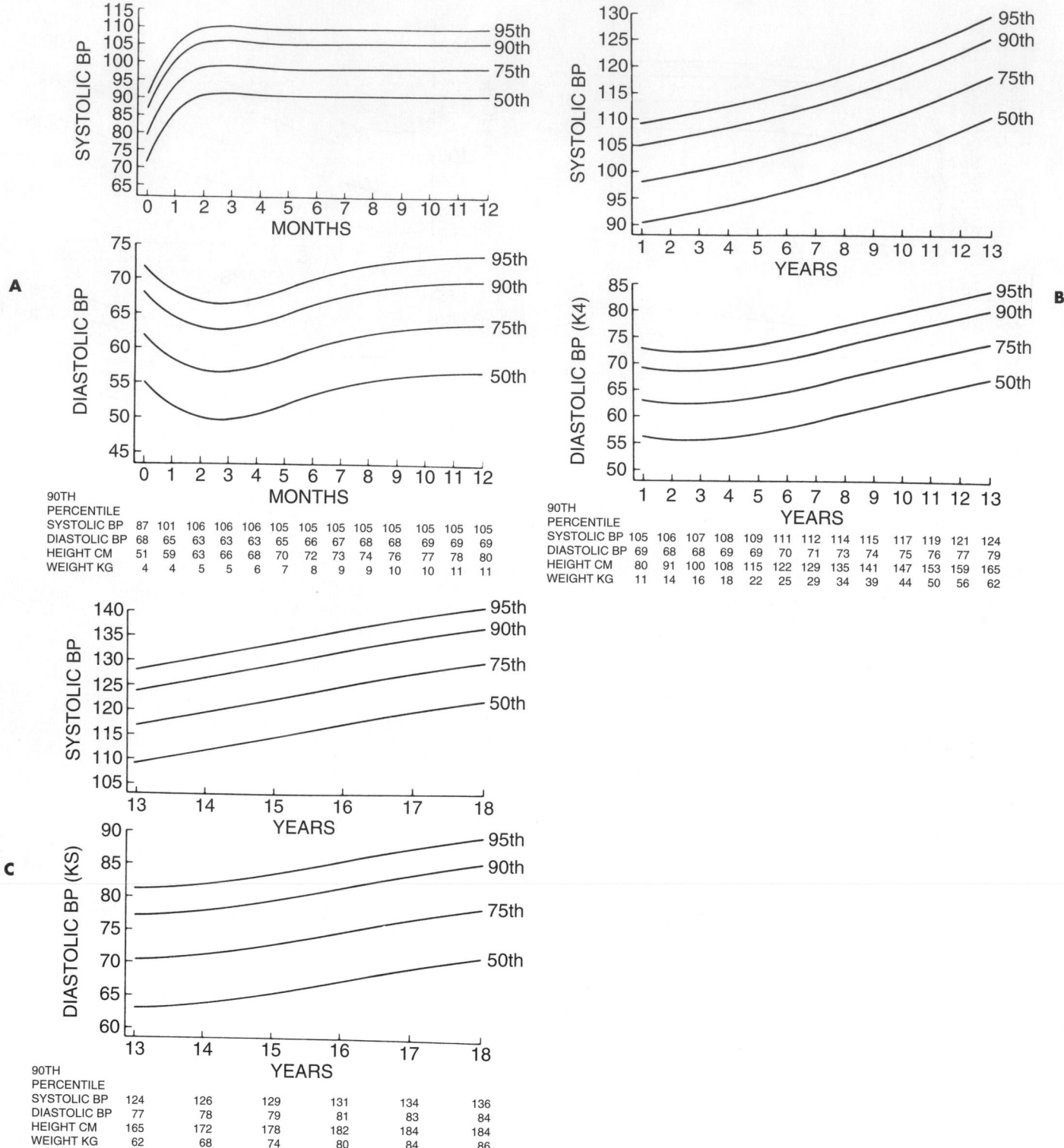

Fig. A-13 Age-specific percentiles of blood pressure measurements in girls. **A,** Birth to 12 months of age; **B,** 1 to 13 years of age; **C,** 13 to 18 years of age. (Data from the Report of the Second Task Force on Blood Pressure Control in Children. [1987]. *Pediatrics, 79,* 1.)

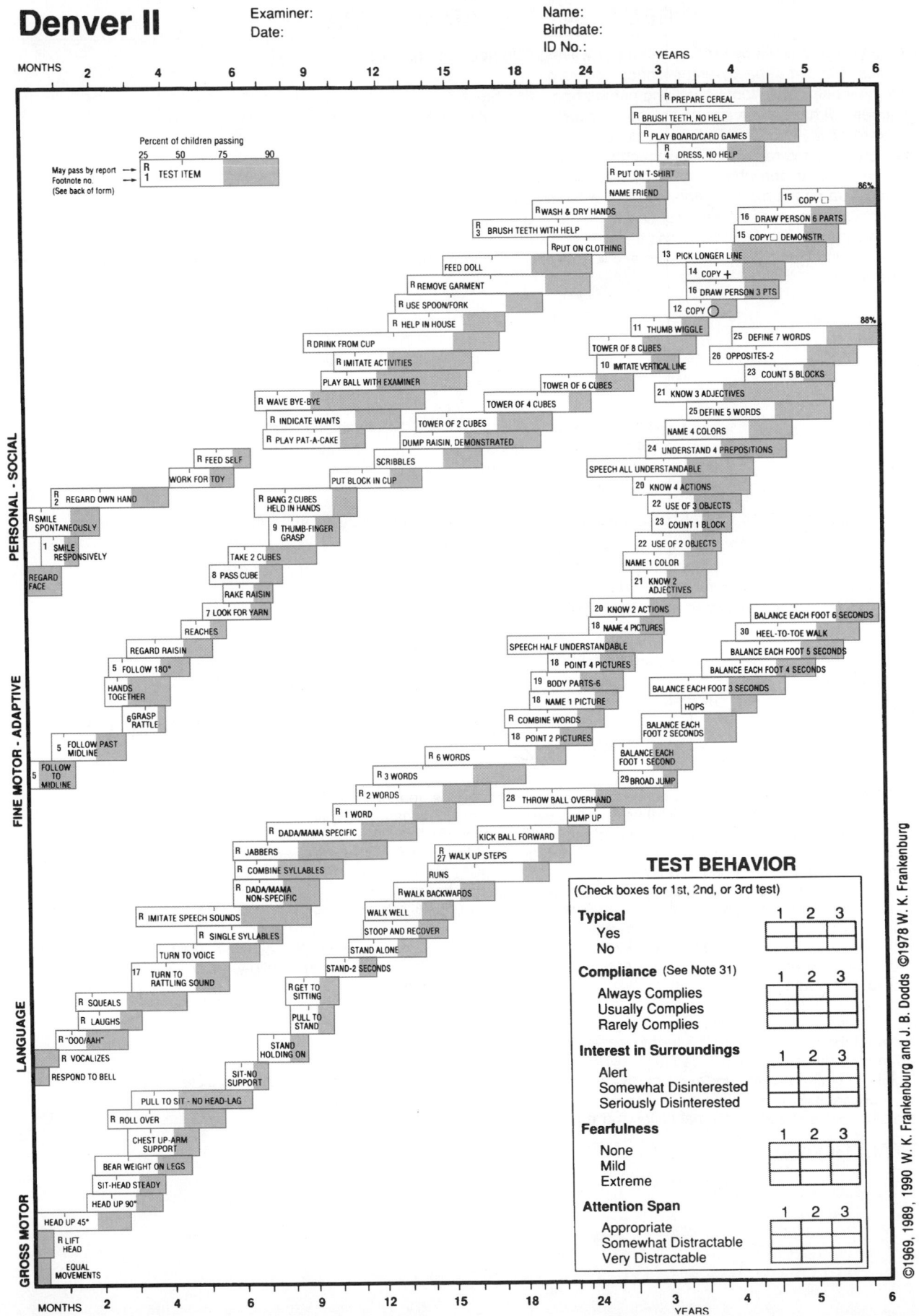

Fig. A-14 Denver II. (From Frankenburg , W.K. & Dodds, J.B. [1990].)

DIRECTIONS FOR ADMINISTRATION

1. Try to get child to smile by smiling, talking or waving. Do not touch him or her.
2. Child must stare at hand several seconds.
3. Parent may help guide toothbrush and put toothpaste on brush.
4. Child does not have to be able to tie shoes or button/zip in the back.
5. Move yarn slowly in an arc from one side to the other, about 8" above child's face.
6. Pass if child grasps rattle when it is touched to the backs or tips of fingers.
7. Pass if child tries to see where yarn went. Yarn should be dropped quickly from sight from tester's hand without arm movement.
8. Child must transfer cube from hand to hand without help of body, mouth, or table.
9. Pass if child picks up raisin with any part of thumb and finger.
10. Line can vary only 30 degrees or less from tester's line. |/
11. Make a fist with thumb pointing upward and wiggle only the thumb. Pass if child imitates and does not move any fingers other than the thumb.

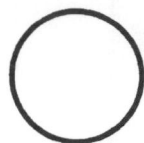   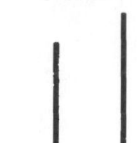   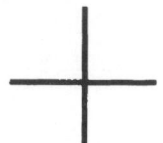   

12. Pass any enclosed form. Fail continuous round motions.

13. Which line is longer? (Not bigger.) Turn paper upside down and repeat. Pass 3 of 3 or 5 of 6.

14. Pass any lines crossing near midpoint.

15. Have child copy first. If failed, demonstrate.

When giving items 12, 14, and 15, do not name the forms. Do not demonstrate 12 and 14.

16. When scoring, each pair (2 arms, 2 legs, etc.) counts as one part.
17. Place one cube in cup and shake gently near child's ear, but out of sight. Repeat for other ear.
18. Point to picture and have child name it. (No credit is given for sounds only.)
    If less than 4 pictures are named correctly, have child point to picture as each is named by tester.

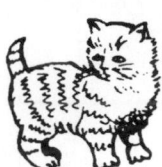   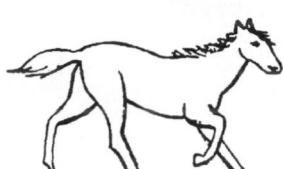   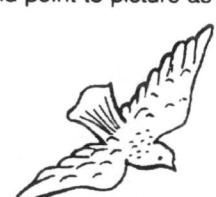   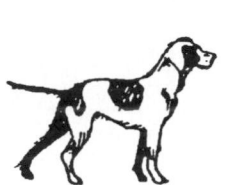   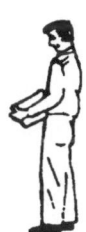

19. Using doll, tell child: Show me the nose, eyes, ears, mouth, hands, feet, tummy, hair. Pass 6 of 8.
20. Using pictures, ask child: Which one flies?... says meow?... talks?... barks?... gallops? Pass 2 of 5, 4 of 5.
21. Ask child: What do you do when you are cold?... tired?... hungry?   Pass 2 of 3, 3 of 3.
22. Ask child: What do you do with a cup? What is a chair used for? What is a pencil used for?
    Action words must be included in answers.
23. Pass if child correctly places <u>and</u> says how many blocks are on paper. (1, 5).
24. Tell child: Put block **on** table; **under** table; **in front of** me; **behind** me. Pass 4 of 4.
    (Do not help child by pointing, moving head or eyes.)
25. Ask child: What is a ball?... lake?... desk?... house?... banana?... curtain?... fence?... ceiling? Pass if defined in terms of use, shape, what it is made of, or general category (such as banana is fruit, not just yellow). Pass 5 of 8, 7 of 8.
26. Ask child: If a horse is big, a mouse is __? If fire is hot, ice is __? If the sun shines during the day, the moon shines during the __? Pass 2 of 3.
27. Child may use wall or rail only, not person. May not crawl.
28. Child must throw ball overhand 3 feet to within arm's reach of tester.
29. Child must perform standing broad jump over width of test sheet (8½ inches).
30. Tell child to walk forward, ⊂○⊂⊃⊂○⊃➤ heel within 1 inch of toe. Tester may demonstrate.
    Child must walk 4 consecutive steps.
31. In the second year, half of normal children are noncompliant.

OBSERVATIONS:

Fig. A-14, cont'd.

DENVER ARTICULATION SCREENING EXAMINATION (DASE)

Denver Articulation Screening Examination

NAME

HOSPITAL NO.

ADDRESS

(For children 2.5 to 6 years of age)

Instructions: Have child repeat each word after you. Circle the underlined sounds that he or she pronounces correctly. Total number of correct sounds is the raw score. Use charts below to score results.

Date: _____ Child's age: _____ Examiner: _____ Raw score: _____

Percentile: _____ Intelligibility: _____ Result: _____

1. <u>t</u>able	6. zip<u>per</u>	11. <u>s</u>ock	16. <u>wagon</u>	21. <u>leaf</u>
2. shi<u>rt</u>	7. <u>gr</u>apes	12. vac<u>uu</u>m	17. <u>gum</u>	22. <u>ca</u>r<u>r</u>ot
3. <u>d</u>oor	8. <u>fl</u>ag	13. <u>y</u>arn	18. <u>house</u>	
4. tru<u>nk</u>	9. <u>th</u>umb	14. <u>mother</u>	19. <u>pen</u>cil	
5. <u>j</u>umping	10. too<u>th</u>brush	15. <u>tw</u>inkle	20. fi<u>sh</u>	

Intelligibility (circle one):   1. Easy to understand   3. Not understandable
                               2. Understandable half of the time   4. Cannot evaluate

Comments:

Fig. A-15 Denver Articulation Screening Examination. (From Drumwright, A.F. & Frankenburg, W.K. [1971-1973].)

DENVER ARTICULATION SCREENING EXAMINATION (DASE)—cont'd

To score DASE words: Note raw score for child's performance. Match raw score line (extreme left of chart) with column representing child's age (to the closest *previous* age group). Where raw score line and age column meet denotes percentile rank of child's performance when compared with other children that age. Percentiles above heavy line are *abnormal*, below heavy line are *normal*.

Percentile Rank

Raw score	2.5 yr	3.0 yr	3.5 yr	4.0 yr	4.5 yr	5.0 yr	5.5 yr	6 yr
2	1							
3	2							
4	5							
5	9							
6	16							
7	23							
8	31	2						
9	37	4	1					
10	42	6	2					
11	48	7	4					
12	54	9	6	1	1			
13	58	12	9	2	3	1	1	
14	62	17	11	5	4	2	2	
15	68	23	15	9	5	3	2	
16	75	31	19	12	5	4	3	
17	79	38	25	15	6	6	4	
18	83	46	31	19	8	7	4	
19	86	51	38	24	10	9	5	1
20	89	58	45	30	12	11	7	3
21	92	65	52	36	15	15	9	4
22	94	72	58	43	18	19	12	5
23	96	77	63	50	22	24	15	7
24	97	82	70	58	29	29	20	15
25	99	87	78	66	36	34	26	17
26	99	91	84	75	46	43	34	24
27		94	89	82	57	54	44	34
28		96	94	88	70	68	59	47
29		98	98	94	84	84	77	68
30		100	100	100	100	100	100	100

To score intelligibility:

	NORMAL	ABNORMAL
2.5 years	Understandable half of the time or easy to understand	Easy to understand
3 years and older	Easy to understand	Understandable half of the time or easy to understand

Test result: 1. Normal on DASE and intelligibility = *normal*
2. Abnormal on DASE or intelligibility = *abnormal**

*If abnormal on initial screening, rescreen within 2 weeks. If abnormal again, child should be referred for complete speech evaluation.

Fig. A-15, cont'd.

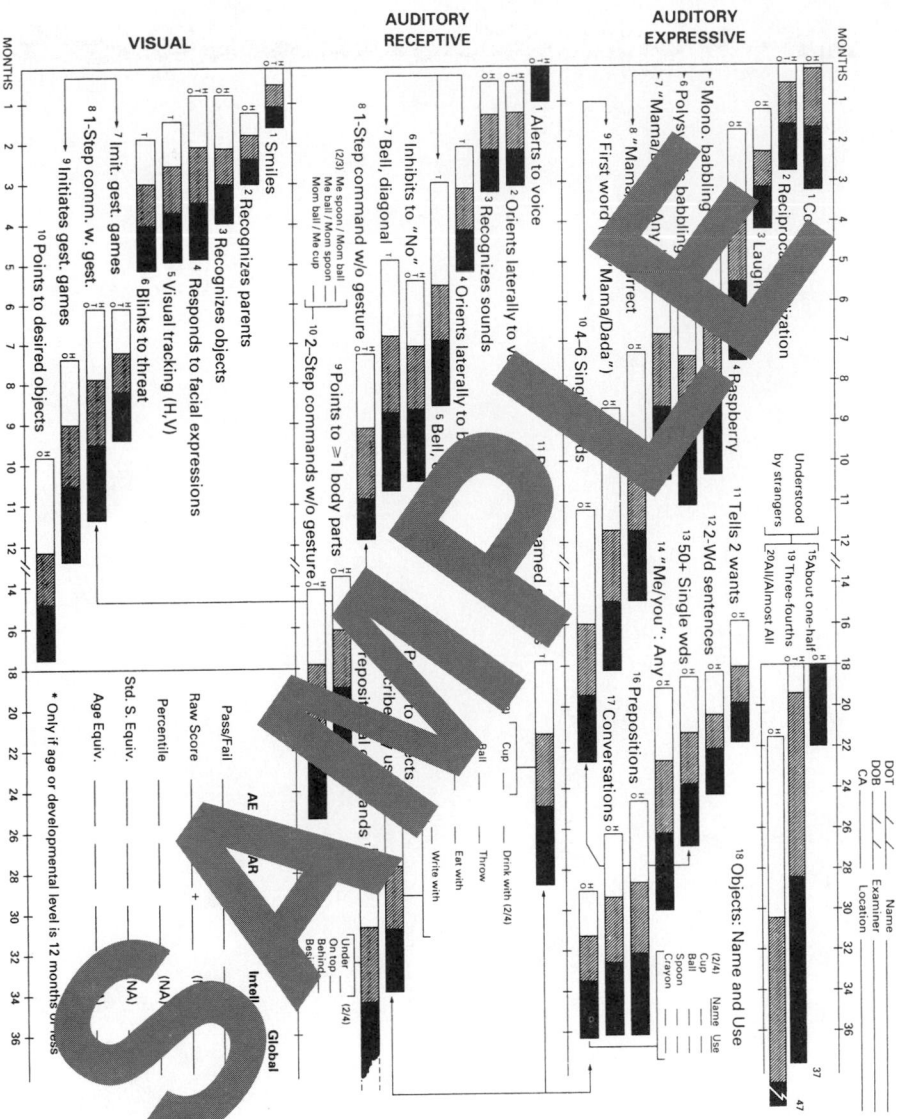

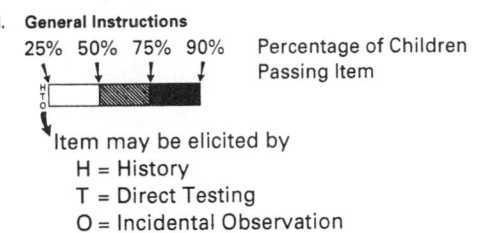

I. General Instructions

25% 50% 75% 90% Percentage of Children
Passing Item

Item may be elicited by
H = History
T = Direct Testing
O = Incidental Observation
• Always start with H, where allowed.
• Child passes item if passed by any of the
allowable means of elicitation for that item.
• Basal = 3 consecutive items passed (work down from age line).
• Ceiling = 3 consecutive items failed (work up from age line).

Fig. A-16 Early Language Milestone Scale. (Reprinted with permission from PRO-ED, Inc. Austin, TX.)

Appendix B Age-Appropriate Reference Charts for Well-Child Care Visits

Barbara Jones Deloian

The reference charts provided here (Tables B-1 through B-4) have been developed as guides for routine well-child care. Multiple references have been consulted regarding the timing of examinations, routine screening tests, immunizations, and anticipatory guidance. Age ranges rather than specific ages are given because of differences among the various agencies. Each clinical setting determines its own practices based on its community standards of care.

Anticipatory guidance must be approached based on the individual needs of a particular family and child. Topics have been included to demonstrate the variety of issues that may be covered at routine well-child visits. The specific ages for each topic vary because of the differing rates of development among children and the concerns of each family. A practitioner should refer to the respective chapters for further information about these anticipatory guidance topics.

Resources

Websites
American Academy of Pediatrics (www.aap.org)
Bright Futures (www.brightfutures.org)
Centers for Disease Control and Prevention Immunization Schedule (www.cdc/gov/recs/child-schedule.pdf)
National Guideline Clearinghouse (www.guidelines.gov)

Bibliography

American Academy of Pediatrics. (2000). *Recommendations for preventive pediatric health care: Policy statement*. Elk Grove Village, IL: Committee on Practice and Ambulatory Medicine.

Dixon, S. & Stein, M. (2000). *Encounters with children: Pediatric behavior and development*. St. Louis, Mosby.

Green, M. (Ed.) (2000). *Bright futures: Guidelines for health supervision of infants, children, and adolescents* (2nd ed.). Arlington, VA: National Center for Education in Maternal and Child Health.

Isaacs, S.L. & Knickman, J.R. (2001). *To improve health and health care 2001: The Robert Wood Johnson Foundation anthology*. San Francisco: Jossey-Bass.

Offit, P.A. & Bell L.M. (1999). *Vaccines: What every parent should know*. New York: IDG Books.

Pickering, L.K. (Ed.). (2000). *2000 Red book: Report of the Committee on Infectious Diseases* (25th ed.). Elk Grove Village, IL: American Academy of Pediatrics.

Table B-1 Newborns to 1-Year-Old Infants

ASSESSMENT AREA	PRENATAL COUNSELING	BIRTH	3 DAYS (<48-HOUR STAY)	2 WEEKS
History and physical examination	Prenatal and family history	X	X	X
Vital signs/BP if indicated		X	X	X
Growth: Ht, Wt, and HC		X/HC	Wt/HC	X/HC
Dental examination/referral				
Screening:				
Vision		Developmental screen	Developmental screen	Development screen
Hearing		Newborn screen		
Tests:				
Hereditary/metabolic/newborn screen and follow-up		As state requires	As state requires	As state requires
Hemoglobin/hematocrit				
Lead screening				
Sickle cell screening				
Urinalysis				
Tuberculin skin test				
Cholesterol				
Development/behavior/temperament assessment		Consider Brazelton	Consider Brazelton	Consider Brazelton
Anticipatory guidance:				
Nutrition/feeding/elimination	Type of feeding Circumcision	Hunger/satiation cues Elimination patterns	Volume, frequency, duration	Wt gain Feeding ease
Sleep/wake activities	Maternal sleep patterns	State modulation Back to sleep	Daily patterns, sleep location/position	Sleep routines Play activities
Safety/injury prevention	Car seat	Car seat/positioning Burns	Siblings	Multiple handlers protection
Health promotion/disease prevention	Immunizations	Well-child care Immunizations	Handwashing Skin care	Passive smoke Illness signs
Family/social interactions	Parental expectations	Family supports	Mother's rest, nutrition, pain management	Parent roles Establishing trust
Development/behavior/temperament counseling	Parent education programs and resources	Infant behaviors Consoling	Establishment of sleep/wake patterns	Irritability Consoling
Immunizations	See Chapter 13 or www.cdc.gov/nip/recs/child-schedule.pdf			

X: Recommended by major authorities.
At risk: Should be considered for children who are at risk for problems in these areas.
Anticipatory guidance activities may be relevant at different ages of a child. All are interchangeable and offer guidance about topics that may be discussed.

4 WEEKS AND 2 MONTHS	4 MONTHS	6 MONTHS	9 MONTHS	12 MONTHS
X	X	X	X	X
X	X	X	X	X
X/HC	X/HC	X/HC	X/HC	X/HC
		PE	PE	PE as needed
Developmental screen	Developmental screen	Developmental screen	Developmental screen	Developmental screen
Developmental screen	Developmental screen	Developmental screen	Developmental screen	Developmental screen
			X	X
			At risk	At risk
				At risk
			At risk	At risk
				At risk
Developmental screen	Developmental screen	Developmental screen	Developmental screen	Developmental screen
Return to work	Starting solids	Avoid bottle-propping	Self-feeding cup	Whole milk
Frequency		Pace feeding	Discontinue bottle	Table foods
Duration				Utensils
Sleeping through the night	Night time rituals	Regular bedtime	Night time waking	Night time rituals
Naps	Need pacifer	Naps		Reading
Rolling over				
Choking	CPR	Aspiration	Bottle caries	Toddler childproofing
Outings	Falls	Home safety/childproofing	Poisoning	
OTC drugs			Falls	
Immunizations	Allergies	Care of URIs	Care of teeth	Vitamins
Child care plans	Fever	Vomiting and diarrhea		Need for iron
	Immunizations	Immunizations		Immunizations
	Effects of child care			
		Consistency	Separation anxiety	Infant initiative
		Predictability		Weaning
		Infant imitation		
Head control	Grasping	Sitting up	Object permanence	Walking
Coordinated suck, swallow, and	Reading	Vocal games	Crawling	Discipline
breathing	Singing	High-chair readiness	Toys	Interactive games
	Security object			

Table B-2 Toddlers and Preschool Children

ASSESSMENT AREA	15 MONTHS	18 MONTHS
History and physical examination	X	X
Vital signs/BP if indicated	X	X
Growth: Ht, Wt, and HC	X/HC	X/HC
Dental examination/referral	As recommended by dentist/referral as needed	As recommended by dentist/referral as needed
Screening:		
Vision	Developmental screen	Developmental screen
Hearing	Developmental screen	Developmental screen
Tests:		
Hemoglobin/hematocrit	As needed if at risk	As needed if at risk
Lead screening		
Sickle cell screening	As needed if at risk	As needed if at risk
Urinalysis		
Tuberculin skin test	As needed if at risk	As needed if at risk
Cholesterol		
Development/behavior/temperament assessment	X	X
Anticipatory guidance:		
Nutrition/feeding	Self-feeding Picky eater	Vegetables and fruit Quantity of fruit juices
Sleep/wake activities	Day and night patterns and activities and naps	Playtime variety Daytime outings
Safety/injury prevention	Home childproofing Poisons	Supervised play First aid information
Health promotion/disease prevention	Dental care and bottle caries Immunizations	Immunizations Safety with animals
Family/social interactions	Tantrums	Family activities Power of praise
Development/behavior/temperament counseling	Initiation of play Stacking or container play Reading	Approach to toilet training Reading
Immunizations	See Chapter 13 or www.cdc.gov/nip/recs/child-schedule.pdf	

X: Recommended by major authorities.
At risk: Should be considered for children who are at risk for problems in these areas.
Anticipatory guidance activities may be relevant at different ages of a child. All are interchangeable and offer guidance about topics that may be discussed.

24 MONTHS	36 MONTHS	4 YEARS	5 YEARS
X	X	X	X
X	X/BP	X/BP	X/BP
X/HC	X/HC if needed	X	X
As recommended by dentist/ referral as needed	As recommended by dentist/ referral as needed	As recommended by dentist/ referral as needed	As recommended by dentist/ referral as needed
Developmental screen	X Re-screen if uncooperative within 6 months	X	X
Developmental screen	Developmental screen	X	X
As needed if at risk	As needed if at risk	As needed if at risk	As needed if at risk
At risk			
As needed if at risk	As needed if at risk	As needed if at risk	As needed if at risk
			X
As needed if at risk	As needed if at risk	As needed if at risk	As needed if at risk
As needed if at risk	As needed if at risk	As needed if at risk	As needed if at risk
X	X	X	X
Portions and choices	Food Pyramid	Food jags and preferences	Food selection
Caffeine and sugar	Snacks		
Attention span	Day care	Preschool	School preparation
Variety of activities	TV viewing and play	TV viewing and play	TV
	Crib to bed		Reading
			Outdoor play
Water safety	Swimming pools	Fire safety	Helmets
	Gun safety		
Passive smoke	Behavior management issues	Update immunizations	Update immunizations
Violence prevention			
Strangers	Parallel play	Imitative play	Family mealtime
Discipline and punishment			
Toilet training	Toilet-training progress	Chores	Hygiene
Masturbation	Reading	Self dressing	Home chores
Discipline	Drawing	Assistance with hygiene	Activities for success
	Puzzles		

Table B-3 School-Age Children and Preadolescents

ASSESSMENT AREA	6 YEARS	7 YEARS	8 YEARS
History and physical examination	X		X
Vital signs/BP if indicated	X/BP		X/BP
Growth: Ht and Wt	X		X
Dental examination/referral	As recommended by dentist, with referral as needed	As recommended by dentist, with referral as needed	As recommended by dentist, with referral as needed
Screening:			
Vision	X		X
Hearing	X		X
Tests:			
Hemoglobin/hematocrit			
Lead screening	At risk	At risk	At risk
Sickle cell screening	At risk	At risk	At risk
Urinalysis			
Tuberculin skin test	As needed if at risk	As needed if at risk	As needed if at risk
Cholesterol	As needed if at risk	As needed if at risk	As needed if at risk
Development/behavior/school assessment	X		X
Anticipatory guidance:			
Nutrition	Healthy lunches	Snacks and food choice	Junk food and sodas
Sleep/wake activities	TV time/sports	TV	Appropriate sleep and TV time
		Hobbies	
Safety/injury prevention	Helmets	Helmets with bicycles,	Sports protective equipment
	Protective equipment needs	skateboards, and skates	
Health promotion/disease prevention	Self care	Exercise	Healthy decisions
	Flossing	Bowel/bladder function	Unusual habits
			Energy level
Family/social interactions	Communication styles	Home responsibilities	Self-direction
	Ability to deal with frustration	Loss of family member	Moods and emotion
Development/behavior/temperament/ sexuality/counseling	School progress	School progress	School progress
	Favorite friend	One special wish	Favorite subject
Immunizations	See Chapter 13 or www.cdc.gov/nip/recs/child-schedule.pdf		

X: Recommended by major authorities.
At risk: Should be considered for children who are at risk for problems in these areas.
Anticipatory guidance activities may be relevant at different ages of a child. All are interchangeable and offer guidance about topics that may be discussed.

9 YEARS	10 YEARS	11 YEARS	12 YEARS
	X	X	X
	X/BP	X/BP	X/BP
	X		X
As recommended by dentist, with referral as needed	As recommended by dentist, with referral as needed	As recommended by dentist, with referral as needed	As recommended by dentist, with referral as needed
	X	History	X
	X	History	X
		Menstruating females	Menstruating females
At risk	At risk	At risk	At risk
At risk	At risk	At risk	At risk
As needed if at risk	As needed if at risk	As needed if at risk	As needed if at risk
As needed if at risk	As needed if at risk	As needed if at risk	As needed if at risk
	X	X	X
Fat/sugar	Food Pyramid	Weight	Diets
Peer activities	Clubs	Increasing need sleep	Sleep activities
TV and reading	Gangs		
Fire and gun safety	Violence prevention	Reduction of high risk behaviors	Importance of extracurricular activities
Problem solving	Behavior problems	Updated immunizations	Updated immunizations
Aches and pains	Bullying or peer abuse	Tobacco and alcohol	Drugs and alcohol
			Tobacco use
Family mealtimes	Family routines and schedules	Time management priorities	Peer pressure
Conflicts			
School progress	School progress	School progress	School progress
Homework	Study strategies	Body changes	Sexuality

Table B-4 Adolescents

ASSESSMENT AREA	12 YEARS	13 YEARS	14 YEARS
History and physical examination	X	X	X
Vital signs/BP if indicated	X/BP	X/BP	X/BP
Growth: Ht and Wt	X	X	X
Dental examination/referral			
Screening:			
Vision	History	History	History
Hearing	History	History	History
Tests:			
Hemoglobin/hematocrit	Menstruating females	Menstruating females	Menstruating females
Lead screening			
Sickle cell screening			
Urinalysis	Dipstick for sexually active teens	Dipstick for sexually active teens	Dipstick for sexually active teens
Tuberculin skin test	As needed if at risk	As needed if at risk	As needed if at risk
Cholesterol	As needed if at risk	As needed if at risk	As needed if at risk
Development/behavior/school assessment	X	X	X
Anticipatory guidance: HEADSS(N)			
Home/family	Parents relationships Siblings	Interactions with parents/ conflicts	Chores Discipline
Education/school	Progress Attendance	Performance	High school expectations
Activities	Friends Sleep patterns	Clubs Sports	Church Regular exercise
Drugs/health	Drugs/alcohol	Self-care BSE/TSE*	Self-care STDs
Sexuality/behavior	Masturbation Abstinence Sexuality	Sexuality concerns Healthy decisions	Abstinence Birth control Condoms
Suicide/abuse	Affect Depression	Emotions/moods Fears	Abuse Traumas
Nutrition	Appetite Weight gain	Diet fads Eating patterns	Food Pyramid Growth concerns
Immunizations	See Chapter 13 or www.cdc.gov/nip/recs/child-schedule.pdf		

X: Recommended by major authorities.
At risk: Should be considered for children who are at risk for problems in these areas.
Anticipatory guidance activities may be relevant at different ages of a child. All are interchangeable and offer guidance about topics that may be discussed.
BSE, breast self-examination; STD, sexually transmitted disease; TSE, testicular self-examination.

15 YEARS	16 YEARS	17 YEARS	18 YEARS
X	X	X	X
X/BP	X/BP	X/BP	X/BP
X	X	X	X
X	History	History	X
X	History	History	X
Menstruating females	Menstruating females	Menstruating females	Menstruating females
Dipstick for sexually active teens	Dipstick for sexually active teens	Dipstick for sexually active teens	Dipstick for sexually active teens
As needed if at risk	As needed if at risk	As needed if at risk	As needed if at risk
As needed if at risk	As needed if at risk	As needed if at risk	As needed if at risk
X	X	X	X
Driving privileges	Living arrangements	Best friends	Graduation plans
	Car		Living arrangements
Career plans	College	Homework	Career, college, or technical school
		Time management	
Reading	Music	Parties	Part-time job hours
TV	Sleep	Self-reliance	Finances
Sleep patterns	Jobs		
Self-care	Self-care	Self-care	Self-care
Seatbelts	Alcohol and tobacco	Date-rape drugs	OTC medications
Relationships	AIDS protection	STDs and AIDS	Pregnancy plans
Trust	Peer pressures	Protection	
Number of partners			
Violence	Suicide thoughts	Breakups	Date abuse
Bullying	Peer conflicts	Problem friendships	
Snacks	Fat, sugar, and caffeine	Anorexia and bulemia	Meal preparation
Weight concerns			

$\mathscr{A}$ppendix C *Laboratory Tests*

Kathleen Kenney

Laboratory tests are used in combination with the presenting subjective (history) and objective (physical examination) findings to arrive at an appropriate diagnosis and treatment plan. The table (Table C-1) in this appendix includes normal values for each test and common interpretations of the results. These interpretations are only a guideline to aid in proper diagnosis and treatment.

Bibliography

Bakerman, S. (1994). *ABCs of interpretive laboratory data* (3rd ed.). Myrtle Beach, SC: Interpretive Laboratory Data.

Barone, M. (2000). *The Harriet Lane handbook*. St. Louis: Mosby.

Pagana, K.D. & Pagana, T.J. (1998). *Manual of diagnostic and laboratory tests*. St. Louis: Mosby.

Table C-1 Normal Values and Interpretations of Laboratory Tests

TEST	NORMAL VALUE	INTERPRETATION
Complete Blood Cell (CBC) Count		
White blood cell (WBC) count	Newborn: 9000 to 30,000/mm³ 2-week-old: 5000 to 20,000/mm³ 1-year-old: 6,000 to 18,000/mm³ 2-year-old to adult: 5000 to 10,000/mm³	*Increased (leukocytosis):* First week of life and during adolescence; bacterial infection, acute hemorrhage, hemolysis, malignancy, intoxication, serum sickness, steroid therapy, trauma, stress *Decreased (leukopenia):* Viral infection, rickettsial infection, hypersplenia, primary bone marrow disorders (e.g., leukemia), myeloma, bone marrow suppression, drug-related (e.g., antibiotics, antihistamines, anticonvulsants, diuretics, analgesics), cyclic neutropenia
WBC differentials		
Neutrophils (total)	Child: 33% to 60% of WBCs Adult: 60% to 70% of WBCs Bands: Newborn: 1.6 to 2.3 1-month-old: 0.5 Child: 0.2	*Increased (neutrophilia):* Myelocytic leukemia, pregnancy, nausea and vomiting, strenuous physical exercise, parasitic infections, rickettsial infections, metabolic disturbances, trauma, inflammatory disorders (e.g., acute rheumatoid arthritis, rheumatic fever), hypersensitivity reactions *Decreased (neutropenia):* Bacterial infections (e.g., typhoid fever, hepatitis, infectious mononucleosis, measles, influenza, chickenpox), aplastic anemia, vitamin B_{12} deficiency, folic acid deficiency, bone marrow depressants, drug therapies
Eosinophils	1% to 4% of WBCs	*Increased:* Allergies, parasitic infections, tumors (e.g., Hodgkin's disease, lymphoma, brain tumors), Addison's disease, chronic skin infections, gastrointestinal (GI) diseases, certain drugs (e.g., phenothiazines, ampicillin, phenytoin) *Decreased:* Infectious mononucleosis and other acute infections, use of certain drugs (e.g., adrenocorticotropic hormone [ACTH], epinephrine, thyroxine, prostaglandin)
Basophils	0.5% to 1.0% of WBCs	*Increased:* Leukemia, polycythemia, Hodgkin's disease, allergy or inflammation, chronic hemolytic anemia, endocrine problems, infections (e.g., tuberculosis [TB], varicella), influenza *Decreased:* Allergic reactions, hyperthyroidism, prolonged steroid treatment
Monocytes	2% to 6% of WBCs	*Increased:* Recovery phase of acute infections, viral infections, subacute bacterial endocarditis (SBE), collagen diseases, leukemia, Hodgkin's disease, rickettsial infection, parasitic diseases: malaria, preleukemic states *Decreased:* Prednisone treatment, rheumatoid arthritis, hairy cell leukemia, human immunodeficiency virus (HIV) infection
Lymphocytes	Child: 31% to 57% of WBCs Adult: 20% to 40% of WBCs	*Increased:* Infection, mononucleosis, viral infections (e.g., mumps, measles, upper respiratory infections [URIs]), infectious hepatitis, leukemia, lymphoma, toxoplasmosis, ulcerative colitis, serum sickness, idiopathic thrombocytopenia *Decreased:* Hodgkin's disease, systemic lupus erythematosus (SLE), after administration of ACTH and cortisone, after burns or trauma, Cushing syndrome, HIV infection
Red blood cell (RBC) count	Birth 5 to $6.3 \times 10^6/\mu l$ 3 months: 3.8 to $5.2 \times 10^6/\mu l$ Infant: 3.5 to $5.9 \times 10^6/\mu l$ Child: 3.7 to $5.2 \times 10^6/\mu l$	*Increased:* Dehydration, acute poisoning, severe diarrhea, hemorrhage, vigorous exercise, high altitude *Decreased:* Blood loss, dietary insufficiency of iron, lead poisoning, Hodgkin's disease, leukemia, SLE, Addison's disease, rheumatic fever (RF), SBE
Hematocrit (Hct)	Newborn: 42% to 64% Child: 34% to 40% Male: 40% to 50% Female: 37% to 47%	*Increased:* Polycythemia, severe dehydration, erythrocytosis *Decreased:* Anemia, leukemia, hemorrhage, hyperthyroidism, cirrhosis

Continued

Table C-1 Normal Values and Interpretations of Laboratory Tests—cont'd

TEST	NORMAL VALUE	INTERPRETATION
Hemoglobin (Hgb)	Newborn: 14 to 20 g/dl Child: 12 to 14 g/dl Male: 13.5 to 17.5 g/dl Female: 12 to 26 g/dl	*Increased:* Intravascular hemolysis, dehydration, polycythemia *Decreased:* Anemia, iron deficiency anemia, sickle cell anemia, thalassemia, hemorrhage, hyperthyroidism
Reticulocyte count (Retic)	Infant: 2% to 5% of RBCs Child: 0.5% to 4% of RBCs Male: 0.5% to 1% of RBCs Female: 0.5% to 2.5% of RBCs	*Increased:* Hemorrhage or blood loss, increased RBC destruction, following iron therapy, hemolytic anemias *Decreased:* Iron deficiency anemia, aplastic anemia, chronic infection, radiation therapy, chronic disease state, more than 100 drugs
RBC indices		
Mean corpuscular volume (MCV)	1 to 3 days old: 95 to 120 μm^3 Infant or child: 70 to 95 μm^3 Male: 78 to 98 μm^3 Female: 78 to 102 μm^3	(Used to identify anemia) *Increased:* Folate deficiency, cobalamin deficiency, vitamin B_{12} deficiency, liver disease, hypothyroidism *Decreased:* Lead poisoning, disorders of iron metabolism (e.g., iron deficiency anemia, anemia of chronic disease), disorders of globin synthesis, hemolytic anemias (especially thalassemia minor)
Mean corpuscular Hgb concentration (MCHC)	31 to 37 Hgb/dl RBCs	*Increased:* Spherocytosis *Decreased:* Iron deficiency anemia, thalassemia minor, lead poisoning
Mean corpuscular hemoglobin (MCH)	26-34 pg	*Increased:* Macrocytosis *Decreased:* Microcytosis, iron deficiency, thalassemia, hypochromia, lead poisoning, sideroblastic anemia, anemia of chronic disease
Menser index (MCV/RBC)	Normal: 11 to 14 Abnormal: More than 14	*Less than 11:* Thalassemia minor *More than 14:* Lead poisoning, iron deficiency anemia of chronic disease

Platelet count	Premature: 100,000 to 300,000/mm³
	Newborn: 140,000 to 300,000/mm³
	Neonate: 150,000 to 300,000/mm³
	Infant: 200,000 to 475,000/mm³
	Child: 150,000 to 450,000/mm³
		Increased: Acute infections, malignancy, postsplenectomy, rheumatoid arthritis, trauma, TB, Kawasaki's disease
		Decreased: Idiopathic thrombocytopenia purpura (ITP), leukemia, viral infections, toxic effects of many drugs, HIV infection
		Decreased production:
		   Marrow suppression (aplastic anemia, radiation, chemotherapy, drugs
		   Marrow infiltration (leukemia)
		   Congenital
		Increased destruction:
		   Immunologic (ITP, leukemia, SLE)
		   Other causes of destruction (drugs, coagulopathies [hemolytic uremic syndrome (HUS), disseminated intravascular coagulation (DIC), septicemia])
		   Severe hemorrhage

Erythrocyte sedimentation rate (ESR)	Westergren: Child: 0 to 10 mm/hour Cutler: Child: 4 to 13 mm/hour Wintrobe: Child: 0 to 13 mm/hour	*Increased:* Acute bacterial infection, inflammatory process or disease, acute rheumatic fever, rheumatoid arthritis, collagen disease
Coagulation Tests		
Partial thromboplastin time (PTT) and activated partial thromboplastin time (APTT)	APTT: 30 to 40 seconds PTT 60 to 70 seconds (Varies between laboratories)	*Prolonged:* Defects of factors, I, II, V, VIII, IX, X, XI, and XII; vitamin K deficiency; liver disease; DIC; nephrotic syndrome
Prothrombin time (PT)	10 to 15 seconds	*Prolonged:* Biliary obstruction; prothrombin deficiency; heparin therapy; low fibrinogen levels; vitamin K deficiency; DIC; Coumadin ingestion; rat poison ingestion; deficiencies of factors I, II, V, VII, and XVII
Tourniquet test	Positive pressure test: Occasional (5 to 10) petechiae Negative pressure test: 1 to 2 petechiae or more	*Increased:* Petechiae formation in thrombocytopenia

Table C-1 Normal Values and Interpretations of Laboratory Tests—cont'd

TEST	NORMAL VALUE	INTERPRETATION
Bleeding time	Ivy method: 2 to 9.5 minutes (forearm) Duke method: Less than 8 minutes (earlobe)	*Prolongation of bleeding time*: Clotting factor deficiency (e.g., von Willebrand's disease, hepatic failure, DIC), specific factor deficiency (e.g., fibrinogen, V, VII, VIII, IX, X, XI, XII), drugs (e.g., aspirin, nonsteroidal antiinflammatory drugs [NSAIDs], high-dose penicillin and cephalosporins *Decreased:* Abnormality in plasma factors and fibrinogen, aplastic anemia
Glucose-6-phosphate dehydrogenase (G6PD)	5 to 15 U	*Decreased:* 13% of African-American males, 3% of African-American females, nonimmunologic hemolytic diseases of the newborn *Increased:* Pernicious anemia, ITP, hyperthyroidism
Blood Chemistries		
Calcium, total serum	Full-term infants: 7 to 12 mg/dl Children: 8 to 11 mg/dl Ionized calcium: Newborn: 4.2 to 5.58 mg/dl; less than 2 months old: 4.4 to 5.6 mg/dl	*Increased total calcium*: Hyperparathyroidism, excess intake of vitamin D, acute osteoporosis, idiopathic hypercalcemia of infancy, sarcoidosis *Increased ionized calcium*: Primary hyperparathyroidism, excessive intake of vitamin D, various malignancies *Decreased total calcium*: Hypoparathyroidism, malabsorption of vitamin D and calcium, renal disease, diarrhea, rickets (vitamin D deficiency), pancreatitis, pregnancy, respiratory alkalosis, diuretics *Decreased ionized calcium*: Hypoparathyroidism, pseudohypoparathyroidism, vitamin D deficiency, renal failure
Chloride (Cl⁻)	Newborn: 96 to 110 mmol/L Child: 98 to 106 mmol/L	*Increased:* Dehydration, Cushing syndrome, hyperventilation, anemia, diabetes insipidus, renal disease *Decreased*: Severe vomiting, severe diarrhea, pyloric obstruction, diabetic acidosis, fever, Addison's disease, burns
Magnesium (Mg)	Newborn: 1.5 to 2.3 mEq/L Child: 1.4-1.9 mEq/L Adult: 1.3-2.1 mEq/L	*Increased:* Renal dysfunction or failure, diabetic acidosis, hypothyroidism, Addison's disease, dehydration, use of antacids containing Mg, multiple magnesium sulfate enemas *Decreased:* Chronic diarrhea, hemodialysis, chronic renal disease, use of diuretics, malabsorption syndromes
Potassium (K⁺)	Newborn: 3.7 to 5.9 mEq/L Child: 3.4 to 4.7 mEq/L	*Increased:* Acidosis, renal failure, Addison's disease *Decreased (hypokalemia):* Diarrhea, vomiting, dehydration, pyloric obstruction, starvation, malabsorption, use of certain diuretics, chronic fear, antiinflammatory drugs
Sodium (Na⁺)	Newborn: 134-144 mEq/L Child: 138-144 mEq/L	*Increased:* Dehydration, Cushing disease, tracheobronchitis, diabetes insipidus, inadequate thirst, profuse sweating, vomiting or diarrhea *Decreased:* Vomiting, diarrhea, severe burns, pyloric obstruction, diabetic acidosis, Addison's disease, syndrome of inappropriate antidiuretic hormone (SIADH) (acute or chronic renal failure)
Glucose	Child: 60 to 100 mg/dl Full-term newborn: 20 to 90 mg/dl	*Increased:* Diabetes, Cushing's disease, acute stress *Decreased:* Overdosage of insulin, vomiting, dehydration, bacterial sepsis, glycogen storage disease
Blood urea nitrogen (BUN)	Child: 5 to 18 mg/dl	*Increased:* Kidney disease, urinary obstruction, renal dysfunction, shock, dehydration, GI hemorrhage, infection, diabetes, malignancies, Addison's disease *Decreased:* Liver failure, nephrotic syndrome, overhydration, pregnancy, malnutrition
Creatinine	Child: 0.3 to 0.7 mg/dl	*Increased:* Acute rheumatoid arthritis, systemic lupus erythematous, leukemia, burns

Continued

Table C-1 Normal Values and Interpretations of Laboratory Tests—cont'd

TEST	NORMAL VALUE	INTERPRETATION
Liver Function Tests		
Alkaline phosphatase (Alk Phos)	Less than 2 years: 85 to 235 ImU/ml 2 to 8 years: 65 to 210 ImU/ml 9 to 15 years: 60 to 300 ImU/ml 16 to 21 years: 30 to 200 ImU/ml Adult: 39 to 117 ImU/ml	*Increased:* Acute viral hepatitis, obstructive jaundice, cirrhosis, rickets, bone growth, healing fracture, hyperparathyroidism; osteomalacia, juvenile Paget disease *Decreased:* Hypothyroidism, hypoparathyroidism, malnutrition, pernicious anemia; scurvy, dwarfism, placental insufficiency
Bilirubin	Total: 0.2 to 1 mg/dl Conjugated: 0 to 0.2 mg/dl Indirect conjugated: 0.2 to 0.8 mg/dl Newborn: 1.5 to 12.0 mg/dl	*Increase in unconjugated:* Hemolytic anemias, hepatitis, lymphoma, hereditary glucuronyl transferase deficiency *Increased conjugated:* Acute and chronic hepatitis, biliary duct obstruction, cancer of the head of the pancreas, cirrhosis
Lactate dehydrogenase (LDH)	Newborn: 160 to 450 U/L Infant: 100 to 250 U/L Child: 60 to 170 U/L	*Increased:* Acute leukemia, hemolytic anemias, chronic hepatitis, sickle cell anemia, pernicious anemia, skeletal muscle necrosis, hepatic disease, infectious mononucleosis, shock and anoxia, seizure, pneumonia, cancer, alcoholism
Serum glutamic-oxaloacetic transaminase (SGOT)*	3 to 6 years: 15 to 50 (U/L) 6 to 12 years: 10 to 50 (U/L) Adult: 5 to 40 IU/L	*Increased:* Acute liver disease, musculoskeletal diseases, acute pancreatitis, acute fulminating hepatitis, post-trauma, generalized infectious shock, Reye syndrome *Decreased:* Pyridoxine deficiency, terminal stages of hepatic failure
Serum glutamate pyruvate transaminase (SGPT)†	5 to 35 IU/L	*Increased:* Same as for SGOT *Decreased:* Sam as for SGOT
Thyroid Function Tests		
Triiodothyronine (T$_3$)	Child: 100 to 240 ng/dl Adult: 120 to 200 ng/dl	*Increased:* Primary hyperthyroid states, acute thyroiditis *Decreased Levels:* Pituitary insufficiency, hepatic disease
Total thyroxine (T$_4$)	Child: 7 to 15 μg/dl Adult: 5 to 13 μg/dl	*Increased:* Hyperthyroidism, thyroxine administration, estrogen administration, pregnancy, thyrotoxicosis *Decreased Total T$_4$:* Hypothyroidism
Free thyroxine (FT$_4$)	0 to 4 days: 2 to 6 ng/dl 2 weeks to 20 years: 0.8 to 2 ng/dl	*Increased:* Hyperthyroidism, thyroxine administration *Decreased:* Hypothyroidism
Thyroid-stimulating hormone (TSH)	Newborn: 3 to 18 mU/L Adult: 0.5 to 10 mU/L	*Increased:* Primary hypothyroidism *Decreased:* Hyperthyroidism, secondary and tertiary hypothyroidism, dwarfism associated with decreased pituitary growth hormone
Mononucleosis screen	Monospot: Negative Heterophile: Negative titer: More than 1:56	Monospot aids in diagnosis of mononucleosis; usually negative in young children; titer of 1:56 is suspicious; titer of 1:224 or more is diagnostic of mononucleosis
Phenylalanine (blood) (phenylketonuria [PKU] test, Guthrie test)	Less than 2 mg/dl for samples collected between 12 and 48 hours after birth More than 4 mg/dl for samples collected after the third day of life	*Increased:* Greater than 15 mg/100 ml in PKU; greater than 4 mg/100 ml is positive
Glucose tolerance test (GTT) (oral)	Fasting blood sugar: Less than 115 mg/dl 90 minutes: Less than 200 mg/dl 2 hours: Less than 140 mg/dl 3 hours: Less than 125 mg/dl	*Increased:* Intestinal diseases, hypothyroidism, Addison's disease *Decreased:* Diabetes mellitus, hyperthyroidism, steroid effect, severe liver damage.
Total iron-binding capacity (TIBC)	Infant 100-400 μg/dl Child/adult: 240- 450 μg/dl	*Increased:* Iron deficiency anemia, pregnancy, oral contraceptives *Decreased:* Anemia of chronic diseases, sideroblastic anemia
Transferrin	240 to 480 mg/dl	*Increased:* Inadequate dietary iron, iron deficiency anemia due to hemorrhage, acute hepatitis, polycythemia, oral contraceptives *Decreased:* Pernicious anemia, thalassemia, sickle cell anemia, chronic infection, cancer, hepatic disease, uremia, rheumatoid arthritis, nephrotic syndrome, malnutrition

Previously called aspartate aminotransferase (AST).
†*Previously called alanine aminotransferase (ALT).*

Table C-1 Normal Values and Interpretations of Laboratory Tests—cont'd

TEST	NORMAL VALUE	INTERPRETATION
Serum iron	Infant: 100 to 250 μg/dl Child: 50 to 120 μg/dl	*Increased:* Hemosiderosis, iron poisoning, hemolytic anemia, estrogen therapy; hemochromatosis, transfusion, acute hepatitis *Decreased:* Iron deficiency, chronic diseases (e.g., SLE, rheumatoid arthritis, chronic infections), third trimester of pregnancy, severe physiologic stress (e.g., surgery, infections, myocardial infarction)
Antistreptolysin O titer (ASO)	Less than 166 Todd units	*Increased:* RF, rheumatoid arthritis, acute glomerulonephritis, streptococcal infection, collagen diseases
Antinuclear antibody test (ANA)	Negative: Less than 1:20 or less than 1:40 (in some laboratories)	Positive is titer of 1:10 or 1:20 (depending on the laboratory) *Positive:* SLE, lupoid hepatitis, scleroderma, rheumatoid arthritis, discoid lupus erythematosus, Sjögren syndrome, dermatomyositis, polyarteritis, rifampin ingestion
Sickle cell screen (Sickledex)	Negative	*Positive:* Sickle cell disease, sickle cell trait *False Positive:* Transfusion of sickling blood within 4 months of test, newborn
Venereal disease research laboratory (VDRL) test	Nonreactive	*Reaction:* Syphilis (confirm with fluorescent treponemal antibody absorption [FTA-ABS] test) *False Positive:* Hepatitis, mononucleosis, tuberculosis, malaria, varicella, measles, Lyme disease, collagen vascular diseases, narcotic use
Urinalysis		
Specific gravity	1.005 to 1.025	*Increased:* Diabetes mellitus, nephrosis, dehydration, glomerulonephritis *Decreased:* Diabetes insipidus, glomerulonephritis, pyelonephritis, severe renal damage
Color	Normal is yellow-straw colored	*Colorless:* Large fluid intake, chronic interstitial nephritis, untreated diabetes mellitus, alcohol ingestion, diuretic therapy *Orange:* Concentrated urine, restricted fluid intake, dehydration, fever *Brownish-yellow or greenish-yellow:* May indicate bilirubin, pseudomonal infection *Red or reddish-dark brown:* Hemoglobinuria (trauma) *Dark brown:* Melanotic tumor, Addison's disease *Blue or green:* Bilirubin (jaundice)
pH	Average range: 4.6 to 8	*Increased (alkaline):* Diabetes mellitus, glomerulonephritis, urinary tract infection, salicylate intoxication *Decreased (acidic):* Acidosis, diabetes insipidus, renal failure, diarrhea, dehydration
Blood	Negative	*Hematuria:* Lower urinary tract infection, SLE, polyarteritis nodosa, renal stones, glomerulonephritis, malignant hypertension, hemorrhagic cystitis (adenovirus)
Protein	Slight to none	*Positive:* Nephritis, nephrosis, teenagers, exercise, asymptomatic proteinuria, SLE, diabetes mellitus, renal calculi; toxemia, orthostatic proteinuria
Glucose	Up to 0.3 g/24 hours; dipstick negative	*Increased:* Diabetes mellitus, liver disease, other metabolic disorders, renal tubular disorders, central nervous system (CNS) disorders.
Ketones	Negative	*Positive:* Dehydration, fever, anorexia, diarrhea, fasting, starvation, prolonged vomiting, following anesthesia, poorly controlled diabetes
Bilirubin	Negative or 0.2 mg/dl	*Increased:* Hepatitis, liver disease, obstructive biliary tract disease
Urobilinogen	1-4 mg/24 hours	*Increased:* Excessive destruction of RBCs, hemolytic anemias, pernicious anemia, malaria, infectious hepatitis, pulmonary infarct, biliary disease, severe infection, infectious mononucleosis, cirrhosis, hemolytic jaundice or anemia

Continued

Table C-1 Normal Values and Interpretations of Laboratory Tests—cont'd

TEST	NORMAL VALUE	INTERPRETATION
Microscopic Examination of Urine		
RBCs	1-2 RBCs/high-power field (hpf)	*Increased:* Pyelonephritis, SLE, renal stones, cystitis, trauma, TB, hemophilia, polyarteritis nodosa, malignant hypertension
WBCs	0-4 WBCs/hpf	*Increased:* Infection of urinary tract, nephrosis, pyelonephritis, fever, TB
Epithelial cells	Occasional/hpf	*Increased:* Nephrosis, poisoning from heavy metals or other toxins, glomerulonephritis, acute tubular necrosis.
Hyaline casts	Occasional/hpf	*Increased:* Disorders of kidney tubules, hemorrhage or inflammatory disease, dehydration, nephritis, malignant hypertension
Granular casts	Occasional	*Increased:* Acute tubular necrosis, advanced glomerulonephritis, pyelonephritis, chronic lead poisoning
Urine culture and sensitivity	No growth	*Positive:* Skin contamination if bacterial count greater than 50,000 to 100,000 colonies/ml of a single urinary pathogen on clean catch; greater than 1000 colonies/ml of a single organism or catheterized specimen indicates active urinary tract infection
Feces Examination		
Blood	Negative	*Positive:* Ulcerative lesions of GI tract, bleeding hemorrhoids (false positive), nosebleed
Mucus	Negative	*Positive:* Ulcerative colitis, bacillary dysentery, ulcerating cancer of colon, acute diverticulitis
Fat	Less than 7 g/24 hours	*More than 7 g/24 hours:* Enteritis; pancreatic diseases; malabsorption syndrome; history of mineral oil, rectal suppository, or Metamucil ingestion; steatorrhea
WBCs	Few/hpf	*Increased:* Shigellosis, salmonellosis, invasive *Escherichia coli*, ulcerative colitis, typhoid, *Yersinia enterocolitica*, fissure, hemorrhoids, polyps, pseudomembranous colitis
Urobilinogen	125-250 Ehrlich units/24 hours	*Increased:* Hemolytic anemias *Decreased:* Complete biliary obstruction, severe liver disease, oral antibiotics
Ova and parasites	None	*Positive:* Parasitic infection
Examination of Cerebrospinal Fluid (CSF)		
Pressure	70-180 mm H_2O	*Increased:* Space-occupying lesion, cerebral hemorrhage, meningitis, pseudotumor cerebri, obstructed shunt
Appearance	Clear, colorless	*Yellow:* Bilirubinemia or jaundice, metastatic melanoma, meningitis *Bloody:* Traumatic tap, cerebral hemorrhage, subdural hematoma with contusion *Turbid:* Yeast, bacteria
Culture and smear	No growth Negative Gram stain No acid-fast bacilli	*Positive:* Bacterial meningitis, TB meningitis
Glucose	60 to 80 mg/dl	*Decreased:* Bacterial meningitis, TB meningitis, hypoglycemia, leukemia with meningeal spread *Increased:* Diabetes
Protein	15 to 45 mg/dl	*Increased:* Acute encephalomyelitis, bacterial meningitis, TB meningitis, acoustic neuroma
Total cell count	Infant: 0 to 20/mm³ Adult: 0 to 10/mm³	*Increased:* Bacterial meningitis, early viral meningitis, aseptic meningitis, cerebral abscess

Appendix D Radiologic Tests

Ericka K. Leibold Waidley

Many radiologic procedures, no matter how simple, are traumatic experiences for an unprepared child. Every child or adolescent has the right to know what to expect before being sent for radiographs. Summarized here are a few important facts that should be used as guidelines when planning a radiology preparation program:

- Effective preparation must be timely, well-organized, complete, and factual.
- Each child or adolescent should be assessed before the preparation to determine individual needs for knowledge, emotional support, and "after-care."
- Parental involvement during preparation and during the procedure, if allowed, offers the child trustworthy and reliable support before and after the radiographs. In working with adolescents, always give the patient the choice of desired level of parental involvement.
- Adequate time must be allotted during the preparation for questions from the child or adolescent and parents and answers to those questions, and after the procedure for the family to verbalize and work out feelings.

Table D-1 presents specific preparation considerations and techniques that may be used for radiologic procedures. Table D-2 describes the developmental needs of children of different ages in relation to such problems.

Resources

Websites

Virtual Hospital—Iowa Health Book, Pediatric Radiology (www.vh.org/Patients/IHB/PedsRad.html)
A Pediatric Radiology Digital Library (www.pediatricradiology.com)
University of North Carolina Department of Radiology (www.ibiblio.org/jksmith/UNC-Radiology-webserver/Pediatric.html)

Bibliography

Burton, E.M. (1999). *Essentials of pediatric radiology*. New York: Thieme Medical Publishers.

Cohen, M. & Burton, E.M. (1990). *Magnetic resonance imaging of children*. Philadelphia: B.C. Decker.

Donnelly, L.F. & Donnelly, L.F. (2001). *Fundamentals of pediatric radiology*. Philadelphia: W.B. Saunders.

Erikson, E. (1983). *Childhood and society*. New York: W.W. Norton.

Harned R.K. & Strain, J.D. (2001, April). MRI-compatible audio/visual system: impact on pediatric sedation. *Pediatric Radiology, 31*(4), 247-50.

Phillips, J. (1975). *The origins of intellect: Piaget's theory*. San Francisco: Freeman.

Rumack, C., Wilson, S., & Charboneau, J. (1991). *Diagnostic ultrasound*. St. Louis: Mosby.

Shady, K., Siegal, M.J., & Glazer, H.S. (1992). CT of focals: Pulmonary masses in childhood. *Radiographics, 12*(3), 505-514.

Waidley, E. (1977). Preparing children for radiology procedures. *Journal of the Association for the Care of Children in Hospitals, 6,* 6-11.

Table D-1 Common Pediatric Diagnostic Imaging Procedures

EXAMINATION	POSSIBLE PURPOSE AND/OR INDICATIONS	POSSIBLE PHYSICAL PREPARATION NEEDED*

Computed tomography (CT) scan—A computerized recording/picture of a slice or cross-section of a part of the body	Head scans to detect or rule out
	  Tumors
	  Blood clots
	  Enlarged ventricles
	  Abnormalities in nerves or muscles of the eye
	Body scans
	  To distinguish bone, tissue, fat, gas, fluid, and so on
	  To determine if a growth is solid or fluid filled
	  To determine if an organ's size and shape are normal
		Sedation
		  Infants and newborns < 1 month
		    Plan feeding close to time of examination.
		    Bundle in warm blanket.
		  Children (1 month to 5 years)
		    Remember they often require sedation to ensure immobility (intramuscular [IM] injection approximately 20 minutes before scanning procedure).
		Immobilization
		  Infants are wrapped securely in blankets and sandbags are used to hold positioning.
		  Older children (> 5 years) can often cooperate after verbal explanation and reassurance.
		  Intravenous (IV) contrast material may be used for vascular studies, especially in liver and kidneys.
		  If IV contrast material will be used, IV line should be in place.
		  Opacification of bowel may be needed for examinations of abdomen.
		  Contrast media are given orally or through nasogastric (NG) tube.
		  Contrast media may be mixed with fruit juice.
		  Time of oral contrast media depends on visualization needed (anywhere from 45-60 minutes before scan to 3-4 hours or night before).

Magnetic resonance imaging (MRI)—Produces two- or three-dimensional images without using x-rays	Can target specific atoms, "see" through bone, and clearly define soft tissue; can be a valuable tool for determining a diagnosis in the following:
	Brain and nervous system disorders
	  Multiple sclerosis
	  Tumors
	  Hydrocephalus
	  Diseases of brain and interior of spine
	Cardiovascular disease
	Cancer
	Organ diseases
	Musculoskeletal problems
		The elimination of patient motion is extremely important to good images.
		Sedation
		  It is required for all patients < 5 years and any age uncooperative child.
		  It may also be needed for any older child who experiences claustrophobia.
		  Infants may avoid sedation if a feeding is given immediately before procedure and infant is bundled securely.
		  Explain to parents that younger children will be sedated.
		Nothing by mouth (NPO); the minimal period of NPO is 4-8 hours (depending on patient's age).
		• Hospitals and outpatient facilities may have specific protocols for procedural (conscious) sedation.
		• A patient under conscious sedation has a depressed level of consciousness but retains the ability to independently and continuously maintain a patent airway and respond to physical stimulation and verbal commands.

Table D-1 Common Pediatric Diagnostic Imaging Procedures—cont'd

EXAMINATION	POSSIBLE PURPOSE AND/OR INDICATIONS	POSSIBLE PHYSICAL PREPARATION NEEDED*

		• The following are general guidelines for infants and children:
		Pre-procedure diet
		  Less than 2 years
		    NPO for milk and solids for 6 hours pre-procedure
		    NPO for clear liquids 2 hours pre-procedure
		  2 or more years
		    NPO for milk and solids for 8 hours pre-procedure
		    NPO for clear liquids for 4 hours pre-procedure

Ultrasound—The mainstay of pediatric diagnostic imaging because of the advent of real-time ultrasound, higher resolution scanners, and the competency of ultrasonographers	Head and neck
	  To help classify a lesion as inflammatory, neoplastic, congenital, traumatic or vascular
	  To follow the progression or regression of a lesion
	Chest
	  To identify pleural effusion
	  To guide thoracentesis procedures
	  To assess diaphragmatic paralysis to differentiate between cystic or solid intrathoracic mass
	  To evaluate diaphragmatic hernia
	  To detect underlying tumors as a cause of persistent pleural fluid
	  To assist in placement of endotracheal tube
	Abdomen
	  Doppler examination often limited to determination of the presence and direction of the flow within a vessel
	Kidney/adrenals
	  MRI—No contrast media required (using nonionizing radiation instead); has replaced the intravenous pyelogram (IVP) as the primary modality for the pediatric urinary tract
		Fluids
		  Child must have full bladder.
		    Offer fluids to child who is assessed as being able to "hold urine."
		    Infants < 3 months can be fed or given a pacifier during procedure.
		Sedation
		  Infant/toddlers 3 months to 3 years probably require sedation (usually given immediately before procedure).
		  Children > 3 years can watch TV or videos, play with toys, read books instead of sedation.
		
		Stomach must be fully distended with fluid.

Radiographic Examinations Abdomen	To detect any abnormalities (e.g., bowel obstruction) In newborn infants with imperforate anus, immediate preoperative films done to determine the lowest end of the colon that is patent as a guide for surgical intervention	None
Barium enema—The insertion of an enema tip (usually a soft rubber catheter) into the anal orifice	To visualize the large colon and detect any large-bowel obstruction; small-bowel follow-through (the visualization of the terminal ileum at the end of fluoroscopy) To diagnose chronic constipation or megacolon, acute abdominal conditions, ulcerative colitis, colonic bleeding, polyps, and so on.	Preparation varies with indications for examination. Check with physician for specific orders. Chronic constipation, megacolon, acute abdomen; preparation is needed. Ulcerative colitis Liquid diet for 12 hours; NPO after midnight prior to the examination

Continued

Table D-1 Common Pediatric Diagnostic Imaging Procedures—cont'd

EXAMINATION	POSSIBLE PURPOSE AND/OR INDICATIONS	POSSIBLE PHYSICAL PREPARATION NEEDED*

		Colonic bleeding
		  Liquid diet for 24 hours before examination
		  Laxative afternoon before examination
		  Saline or Fleet enema at bedtime and morning of examination
		Other indications
		  0-2 years
		    NPO for 3 hours before examination
		  2-6 years
		    Clear-liquid dinner, NPO for 4 hours before examination
		    One-half suppository at bedtime and one-half 3 hours before examination
		    If poor results: Fleet or normal saline enema
		  6-16 years
		    Clear liquid dinner; NPO after midnight before examination
		    One suppository afternoon before examination
		    One suppository morning of examination
		    If poor results: Fleet enema

Bone age series
  Birth to 2 years: hands, wrists, and knees
  2 years and older: hands and wrists
	To determine if child is at desired bone growth for chronologic age
	Evaluation of the "bone age" based on the appearance of the bones, the extent of bone formation in the epiphyses and round bones, and the extent to which the epiphyses have begun to unite with their shafts
		None

Cardiac catheterization—The introduction of a catheter under fluoroscopic control into the blood vessels or into the chambers of the heart	To obtain samples of blood from the chambers of the heart To monitor the functioning of the heart To obtain information for the diagnosis of congenital heart malformations, especially prior to cardiac surgery	Sedation is usually ordered—NPO after midnight before the examination.
Chest	To detect any anomalies of the chest, ribs, lungs, etc. To determine the true size of the heart To visualize lung or pleural areas where extreme densities or fluid is present (including horizontal fluid levels) To visualize foreign bodies in the tracheo-bronchial tree	No preparation is needed. Inform parents that smaller children often need to be immobilized (usually by placing child in or on type of apparatus that prevents movement, (e.g., "papoose board").

Intravenous pyelogram (IVP)—Also called excretory urography (ultrasound often used as first-choice diagnostic modality)	To visualize the collecting and transporting system of the urinary tract (e.g., the renal calyces, pelvises, and bladder); can roughly determine excretory capacity of the individual kidneys by appearance, time and concentration of the radiopaque dye as it is being excreted	Fluids and bowel preparation
		  0-1 years
		    Clear liquids in morning; NPO for 3 hr prior to examination
		  2-6 years
		    Clear liquids in morning; NPO for 4 hours before examination
		    One-half suppository at bedtime
		    One-half suppository in morning
		    If not effective: normal saline enema in morning

Table D-1 Common Pediatric Diagnostic Imaging Procedures—cont'd

EXAMINATION	POSSIBLE PURPOSE AND/OR INDICATIONS	POSSIBLE PHYSICAL PREPARATION NEEDED*
		6-16 years NPO after midnight prior to examination or clear-liquid breakfast then NPO One suppository at bedtime Suppository in morning If not effective, normal saline enema in morning

Surveys
  Skeletal survey
  Metastatic survey
  Joint or arthritic survey
	To detect the presence or extent of localized lesions
	To evaluate the degree of involvement of the skeleton in a generalized disease process
	Indications
	  Metastatic survey for neoplasms or chronic granuloma
	  Skeletal survey for leukemia and anemia, osteochondrodystrophy, mongolism, or multiple congenital defects
		None

Upper gastrointestinal series—Includes pharynx, esophagus, stomach, and duodenum	In neonates and young infants: for evaluation of esophageal atresia, difficulty with feeding, regurgitation, vomiting, abdominal distention
	In older infants or children: for evaluation of repeated pneumonias, aspiration, tracheoesophageal fistula; also for esophageal foreign bodies, vomiting, abdominal distention, failure to thrive, abdominal pain, diarrhea, and GI bleeding
		Fluids
		0-2 years
		  Clear liquids after 6 PM the night before examination; NPO for 3 hr before examination
		2-16 years
		  NPO after midnight before examination
		  No gum chewing on day of examination

Table D-2 Developmental Considerations in Relation to Radiologic Procedures

DEVELOPMENTAL CONSIDERATIONS	CHILD/ADOLESCENT AND PARENT PREPARATION

Infancy (Birth to 1 Year of Age)

During the first year, the infant is basically egocentric and is concerned with need satisfaction and physical safety. Separation from the mother (or caregiver) produces a form of primary anxiety that is behavioralized as increased tension (continued crying, frenzied movements, and rigid muscle tone). Because of this anxiety and the resulting movement, infants are usually placed on an immobilization board so that the x-ray procedure can be done successfully the first time (thus preventing further exposure to radiation and increased infant and parent anxiety due to repeated attempts to complete the procedure).

It is obvious that the infant cannot be emotionally prepared for the radiologic procedure, but it is important to inform and prepare the parents or significant caregiver. Research supports the theory that by lowering the mother's stress, the child's stress will be indirectly reduced. This suggests that by interacting with and preparing the mother for stressful events she will in turn interact with her child and lower the child's anxiety.

If the mother is adequately prepared for what will be happening to the infant during the procedure (e.g., the immobilization board, injection of sedation, etc.), and she feels able to cope with this, then she should be allowed to stay with the infant during the procedure (although many radiology departments do not allow this). For CT scans and MRI, an infant between 1 month and 1 year usually requires IM sedation. The parents need a full explanation regarding the effect of this sedation since many are fearful to have their infant "put to sleep."

One of the infant's main concerns for need satisfaction is food. For procedures that examine the digestive tract, the infant usually has to be NPO for a certain length of time (see Table D-1). It is extremely important to make every attempt with the radiology department to schedule these procedures between feeding times so that the infant does not have to go for an extended period of time without adequate nutrition. If this scheduling is not possible, then the physician should be consulted as to how long the child has to be NPO before the procedure for it to still be successful. This can range from 2 to 6 hr, depending on the age of the infant and the type of procedure.

Even if the mother or caregiver cannot accompany the infant, certain comfort measures should be considered. Most radiology departments, because of their location, are usually cold, therefore the infant should be well covered with blankets. Also, for older infants a pacifier can be used to satisfy the sucking needs if feedings have been withheld. The infant should be clean and have dry diapers applied before being sent to the radiology department so that further delays are prevented.

Toddlerhood (1 to 3½ Years of Age)

In this stage of development the utmost concern for the child is separation from the mother (or caregiver) because she is still the main component for need satisfaction. When separation occurs, the child may appear to miss the mother and doubt that she will return.

An important developmental task at this stage is muscle control of elimination and retention of urine and feces. It is difficult for the toddler to let go of this newly acquired control, which is sometimes necessary with several of the radiologic procedures and/or their preparation (MRI, CT, voiding cystourethrogram). With this increasing body independence, the body products become associated with sexual and aggressive behavior, and the toddler may feel a considerable loss when forced to give them up without control.

The toddler's major concerns with off-unit procedures are separation anxiety and permanent desertion by the mother. It may be important to a child in this age group to leave a note on the pillow to "tell Mommy where I am" or to encourage the parents, after adequate preparation, to accompany the child to the x-ray department and wait in the waiting room (if not allowed to stay with the child) until the procedure has been completed.

Imagination also begins to play an important part in the daily life of the older toddler, and each new effort is usually preceded by fantasy play. In stressful situations this can be hazardous because toddlers may perceive the radiologic procedure as threatening to their well-being and may fight to maintain self-integrity. Defenses that the toddler uses to cope with this anxiety are imitation, avoidance, denial, and increasing stubbornness.

Some toddlers may also have a fear of shots and doctors because they probably have had past experience with both. For MRIs and CTs, this age group usually requires IM sedation, which may increase their feelings of loss of control, activate their imagination, and intensify their fantasies.

Another common fear is that of strange and unfamiliar places and new people. Preparation that involves using pictures of the environment and strange equipment can help reduce some of these fears. Because the toddler has such a vivid imagination when left alone in stressful situations, the child should be told exactly what will and will not happen. An example of this is to tell the toddler that the x-ray equipment cannot move by itself (this has become increasingly more difficult to explain with computer-activated equipment), that it will not crush the child, or that even though it looks and sounds scary it does not hurt. Being honest and factual with the child usually results in success. Because of the attention span of this age group, it is usually best to prepare the child 1 to 3 hours before the procedure.

Table D-2 Developmental Considerations in Relation to Radiologic Procedures—cont'd

DEVELOPMENTAL CONSIDERATIONS	CHILD/ADOLESCENT AND PARENT PREPARATION

Preschool (3½ to 6½ Years of Age)

The preschool age is a tender time for hospitalization and diagnostic testing because of the child's limited vocabulary and ability to understand. The thinking process is still egocentric, and conclusions are based on intuitive and magical beliefs, e.g., on what the child wants to believe (preoperational thought).

During this stage, children are also trying to discover what kind of person they are going to be. The child is developing a conscience and a sense of autonomy, and there is an increasing interest in competence, prowess, and dominance. Toward the end of this stage is the Oedipal phase, when the child identifies with the parent of the opposite sex and turns away from the parent of the same sex. This phase can also involve a fear of castration by the parent of the same sex and can be projected to include fear of harm by a technologist who is the same sex as the child.

It is also during this stage of development that children begin to find pleasure in genital manipulation. They develop a sense of reward gratification and, at the same time, a sense of guilt associated with this activity. For example, one radiologic procedure, the IVP, can be done to determine if the kidneys, bladder, and urinary tract are functioning correctly. If the child is having an IVP and has been experimenting with masturbation, the guilt and shame can be overwhelming. Fortunately, as technology has improved, an ultrasound examination may now be the diagnostic modality used first.

The preschooler has a vivid imagination that allows fantasizing when left alone in an unfamiliar and threatening situation. Common fantasies of this age group are similar to those of the toddler: animation of the machinery with fears of mutilation and bodily harm and beliefs that the machine can "see inside the head" (thought invasion) and know what the child is thinking. The preschooler is also afraid of injections and IVs (which may be needed for sedation prior to MRIs and CTs). These procedures are especially stressful for children who may feel that they are being punished for bad behavior.

With this age group it is often beneficial to use drawings, dolls, or actual equipment (radiograph films, syringes, "play" radiograph tables, etc.) during the preparation to help increase the child's comprehension. When explaining an MRI or CT scan, do not explain the technology by using the analogy that "it can see inside the body." The preschooler is capable of understanding simple explanations of the body parts and should be shown what areas of the body the doctor needs to see. Explaining and showing children which parts will be examined helps them to cope with fears of mindreading, mutilation, and castration. This is an inquisitive age group, and all the child's questions need to be answered appropriately. Repeated reassurance and compliments on the child's ability to understand increase feelings of mastery and self-pride.

School-Age (6½ to 13 Years of Age)

The school-age child looks to peers or a special friend for support and encouragement. This is a time when secrets are kept and only confided to each other, thought processes become more organized (concrete operational thought), and a more stable self-identity begins to form. The most important task, however, is competence in school, and interruption from this can be devastating.

Latency occurs between 7 and 11 years with the sexual drive being controlled and repressed. In order to do this, the child may use several unconscious mechanisms: isolation, pseudo-compulsion, turning to the opposite (e.g., denying anger), and sublimation of wishes (channeling drives into acceptable outlets).

In this stage the child may still fear castration, and even death. An example of how this fear can be potentiated is when the technologist places a heavy rubber plate or "apron" over the child's genitals with an explanation that the x-ray machine may hurt these areas. It is better to offer an explanation that the doctor does not need to see these parts on the picture, and therefore they need to be covered.

Visual aids, equipment, and tours can be useful with this age group to increase their knowledge of health and the hospital system. It is helpful to instruct children in the medical terminology for body parts and procedures after you have learned their own words for them.

Many children need to know the sequence of events (including time of day, how they will be transported, who will be with them, strange or unusual smells or sounds, etc.), how it will feel (including a description of the coldness of the radiology table, positioning, lightness or darkness, and the sensations they might experience), and how long it will take. Telling the child what to expect provides time to rally forces and decide upon acceptable ways to cope. It is helpful to discuss with children ways they have coped with uncomfortable situations in the past. If the child is not able to think of any coping behaviors that have been successful, then the practitioner should offer some suggestions, e.g., counting to 10 until the injection is over, watching the minutes advance on a nearby clock, singing a favorite song or rhyme, or practicing the multiplication tables. The child can even be encouraged to practice the chosen strategy prior to the procedure in order to be able to remember it more easily.

Adolescence (13 to 18 Years of Age)

"Modern" teenagers have become much more sophisticated in their basic understanding of the world around them and in their expectations for respect and consideration. This age group has an adult level of cognition and fully developed deductive reasoning.

Adolescents are seeking to know more about themselves and their bodies. They are in the process of identifying their own,

It may be difficult for adolescents to express concerns in the presence of their parents. The professional needs to respect this need for privacy and work with the parents to understand this as a normal developmental need of teenagers. The teenager must be able to trust the professional caregiver team and rely on their confidentiality with any information discussed.

Continued

Table D-2 Developmental Considerations in Relation to Radiologic Procedures—cont'd

DEVELOPMENTAL CONSIDERATIONS

Adolescence (13 to 18 Years of Age)—cont'd

unique identity. Illness during this crucial developmental time can be just one cause of "identity confusion" and form fears of not "fitting in" with friends and peers.

The natural tendency for rebellion (seeking independence) at this stage typically causes strained relationships within the family unit. Commitment to the adolescent peer group and the process of seeking a new idealized self often discredit the parents (e.g., the recognition that adolescents do not want to become like "them") and are a consistent cause of concern for both adolescents and parents.

Adolescent patients may make assumptions about their diagnosis based on misinformation (often received from their peers) and/or misinterpretation of information they have heard. It is important to have teenage patients repeat back what they have heard and clarify any misconceptions. Complete honesty and factual information are essential for this age group.

CHILD/ADOLESCENT AND PARENT PREPARATION

The adolescent may be preoccupied with physical changes and having a body that is different from others. This may lead to fears about the potential outcomes/diagnosis that may result from the tests or procedures being performed. Castration anxiety may be exhibited through concerns about body size and shape, secondary sexual development, and hostility towards the opposite sex. Adolescents benefit greatly from consistency in staff, allowing them to develop a trusting relationship and build confidence.

When preparing adolescents for tests and/or procedures, it is important to determine the terminology that is used for body parts (e.g., clarification of "slang words") and function. Using tools such as anatomically descriptive body outlines or models can be helpful. It also builds trust if the practitioner recognizes, and compliments, teenagers on their knowledge level and understanding.

Preparation and teaching can usually be done in one session as long as adequate time is allocated for questions and answers. Often, written brochures and/or handouts can be given to the teenager to read, with time available to clarify the information or answer questions. If high-technology equipment (MRI, CT scan, ultrasound) is to be used, extra time immediately prior to the procedure should be scheduled. This allows the technician to show the equipment to the teenager, demonstrate how it works, and answer questions. Encouraging this interaction, and scheduling enough time for it, will assist the teenager in fully understanding the procedure and in generating some last-minute questions.

Appendix E *CPT and ICD-9 Codes*

Physicians' Current Procedural Terminology, known as CPT, is a list of descriptive terms and identifying codes for reporting medical, surgical, and diagnostic services (Table E-1). It provides communication among health care practitioners, patients, and third-party payers. Each procedure or service is identified by a five-digit code.

International Classification of Diseases (9th revision) Clinical Modification is commonly referred to as ICD-9. It is a numerical and alphabetical list of all available codes for diseases used by practitioners when writing a diagnosis or by a coder when preparing a claim for third-party reimbursement (Table E-2). Basic guidelines regarding the use of ICD-9 codes is defined by the Centers for Medicare and Medicaid Services (CMS) (formerly the Health Care Financing Administration [HCFA]).

For a list of new, revised, and invalid codes and subclassification of diseases, see the Resources given here.

Resources

Publications

CPT 2001 Physician's current terminology. (2001). Chicago: American Medical Association.

ICD-9CM (9th ed.) (vols. 1&2). (2000). New York: Medicode, Inc.

Table E-1 CPT Codes

SERVICE	CODE
Consultation	
Level 1	99241
Level 2	99242
Level 3	99243
Level 4	99244
Level 5	99245
Office Visit (New Patient)	
Level 1	99201
Level 2	99202
Level 3	99203
Level 4	99204
Level 5	99205
Office Visit (Established Patient)	
Level 1	99211
Level 2	99212
Level 3	99213
Level 4	99214
Level 5	99215
General Pediatrics	
Abscess drainage	10160
Aerosol treatment (initial)	94664
Aerosol treatment (subsequent)	94665
Arterial blood gas	36600
Arterial puncture	36600
Bladder catheterization	53670
Bone age (radiograph)	76020
Cardiopulmonary resuscitation (CPR)	92950
Cerumen removal	69210
Cervical mucus (penetration test)	89330
Cervical smear	88150
Chlamydia culture	87110
Culture preparation	99000
Diaphragm fitting	57170
Electrocardiogram	93010
Fungus culture (skin)	87101
Fungal wet mount	87220
Glucose tolerance test	82951
Gram stain	87205
Gram stain/Tzanck test	87207
Hearing (audiologic function test, tympanometry)	92567
Hearing evaluation	92506
Hematocrit	85014
Injection of medication (intramuscular, and specify)	90782
Injection of medication (intravenous, and specify)	90784
Intradermal skin prick test (specify number of tests)	95024
Introduction of catheter (vein)	36000
Intravenous infusion by MD (first hour)	90780
Intravenous infusion by MD (second through eighth hour, and specify number of hours)	90781
Kolt 3 wet prep	87220
Lead	83655
Lumbar puncture	62270
Nasogastric intubation	89130
Nebulizer treatment	94650
Norplant insertion	11975
Norplant removal	11976
Papanicolaou (Pap) smear	88150

Table E-1 CPT Codes—cont'd

SERVICE	CODE
Parasite smears	87177
Peak flow analysis	94160
Potassium hydroxide (KOH) preparation	87220
Pulse oximetry (single)	94760
Pulse oximetry (multiple)	94761
Purified protein derivative (PPD)	86580
Rapid strep test	87430
Rubella titer	86762
Skin biopsy (skin lesion)	11100
Spirometry	94010
Spirometry (prebronchodilator/postbronchodilator)	94060
Stool (occult blood test)	82270
Suprapubic bladder tap (by needle)	51010
Sweat test	82435
Throat culture	87081
Tine tuberculin test	86585
Tympanogram	92567
Urinalysis dip	81000
Urinalysis without microscopic examination	81002
Venipuncture	
For collection of specimens	36415
Under 3 years of age	36400
Over 3 years of age	36410
Wet mount/KOH preparation (for suspected vaginitis when doing pelvic examination)	87210
X-ray film (chest)	71010-71035
X-ray film (extremity)	73592

Developmental and Behavioral Pediatrics

SERVICE	CODE
Developmental test (per hour, and specify number of hours)	96111
Gesell Development Assessment	96111
Psychiatry evaluation (specify)	90885

Immunizations

SERVICE	CODE
Diphtheria-tetanus-acellular pertussis vaccine (DTaP)	90700
Diphtheria-tetanus-pertussis vaccine (DTP)	90701
Diphtheria and tetanus toxoids (DT)	90702
Tetanus toxoid	90703
Mumps virus vaccine (live)	90704
Measles virus vaccine (live attenuated)	90705
Rubella virus vaccine (live)	90706
Measles, mumps, and rubella virus (MMR) vaccine (live)	90707
Measles and rubella virus vaccine (live)	90708
Rubella and mumps virus vaccine (live)	90709
Measles, mumps, rubella, and varicella vaccine	90710
DTP and injectable poliomyelitis vaccine	90701
Poliovirus vaccine (live oral) (any type)	90712
Poliomyelitis vaccine	90713
Typhoid vaccine	90690
Varicella zoster virus (chickenpox) vaccine	90716
Tetanus and diphtheria toxoids adsorbed for adult use (Td)	90718
Diphtheria toxoid	90719
DTP and *Haemophilus influenzae* type B (HIB) vaccine	90720
Influenza virus vaccine	90657
Hepatitis B (under 1 year of age)	90744
Hepatitis B (over 1 year of age)	90745
HIB	90645

Other

Refer to CPT manual

Table E-2 ICD-9 Codes

DESCRIPTION	CODE
Abdominal pain (unspecified site)	789.00
ABO/RH incompatibility	773.0
Abortion (legal; elective and under medical supervision)	635.
Abortion (spontaneous)	634.
Abscess	682.9
Abuse (child neglect)	995.52
Accessory nipples or breast	757.6
Acne	706.1
Acne neonatorum	706.1
Acne vulgaris	706.1
Acquired cataract	366.9
Acquired immune deficiency syndrome (AIDS)	042.
Acute lymphoblastic leukemia (ALL)	204.00
Addison's disease	255.4
Adhesions (foreskin)	752.69
Adhesions (penis to scrotum [congenital])	752.69
Adhesions, vaginitis (congenital)	752.49
Adolescence growth	V21.2
Adrenal insufficiency	255.4
Airway obstruction	519.8
Alcohol dependence	303.9
Allergic bronchopulmonary aspergillosis	117.3
Allergic conjunctivitis	372.14
Allergic contact dermatitis	692.9
Allergic reaction	995.3
Allergy	995.3
Allergy (food; any, ingested)	693.1
Alopecia	704.00
Alopecia areata	704.01
Alopecia (congenital)	757.4
Amblyopia	368.00
Amebiasis	006.9
Amenorrhea	626.0
Anal fissure	565.0
Anemia (unspecified)	285.9
Anorchia	752.8
Anorexia	783.0
Anteversion femur (neck; congenital)	755.63
Antibiotic-associated diarrhea/colitis	960.
Aphthous ulcers	528.2
Aphthous ulcers (oral; recurrent)	528.2
Apnea	786.03
Apparent life-threatening event (ALTE)	786.09
Appendicitis	541.
Appendicitis (acute)	540.9
Arthritis	716.9
Ascaris	127.0
Asthma	493.9
Asthma without status asthmaticus	493.90
Ataxic (unspecified)	781.3
Atlantoaxial instability	723.9
Atopic dermatitis	691.8
Attention deficit disorder with hyperactivity	314.01
Attention deficit disorder with no hyperactivity	314.00
Autoimmune disorder	279.4
Backache/back pain	724.5
Back strain	847.9
Bacterial paronychia	681.9
Balanoposthitis	607.1
Behavior disorder or problem	312.9
Benign premature adrenarche	259.1

Table E-2 ICD-9 Codes—cont'd

DESCRIPTION	CODE
Benign premature thelarche	259.1
Bile acid pancreatic insufficiency	577.8
Birthmark	757.32
Bites (insect)	911.4
Black eye (ecchymosis)	921.0
Blepharitis	373.0
Blindness and low vision	369
Blindness of both eyes	369.00
Blount disease (tibia vara)	732.4
Blunt abdominal trauma	959.1
Body lice	132.1
Brachial plexus stretch	953.4
Breast asymmetry	757.6
Breast discharge	611.79
Breast infection	611.0
Breast mass	611.72
Breast tenderness	611.71
Breath-holding (child)	312.81
Breath-holding spells	786.9
Bronchiectasis	494.0
Bronchiolitis (acute)	466.1
Bronchitis	466.0
Bronchopulmonary dysplasia	770.7
Bulimia	307.51
Bullous impetigo diaper rash	684.
Burn	949.0
Café au lait spots	709.09
Calluses	700.00
Campylobacter	041.86
Candida albicans (monilial)	112.9
Candidal infection	112.9
Caput succedaneum	767.1
Carbuncle and furuncle	680
Cataract	366
Celiac disease	579.0
Cellulitis (specify site)	682.9
Cephalhematoma	761.1
Cerebral palsy	343.
Cerebral palsy (mixed)	343.8
Cerumen (impacted)	380.4
Cervical lymphadenitis	289.3
Cervical lymphadenopathy	785.9
Chalasia	530.51
Chalazion	373.2
Chancroid	099.0
Chemical burn (eye)	940.0
Chemical conjunctivitis	372.05
Chemical irritation	623.9
Chest pain	786.50
Chest pain (noncardiac)	786.59
Child abuse	995.50
Chlamydia and nongonococcal urethritis (NGU)-nonspecific urethritis (NSU)	099.41
Cholecystitis	575.1
Cholelithiasis	574.2
Chondromalacia patellae	717.7
Cleft lip	749.1
Cleft lip and cleft palate	749.2
Cleft palate	749.0
Colic/infantile irritability	789.0
Colitis	558.9
Coma	780.01

Continued

Table E-2 ICD-9 Codes—cont'd

DESCRIPTION	CODE
Common warts	078.10
Concussion (cerebral)	850.9
Condylomata acuminata	078.11
Congenital cataract	743.30
Congenital heart defect	746.9
Congenital heart disease (CHD)	746.9
Congenital hypothyroidism	243.
Congenital rubella	771.0
Conjunctivitis	372.30
Constipation	564.0
Constitutional delay of growth and development	783.40
Constitutional delay of growth and puberty	259.0
Contact dermatitis	692.9
Contact dermatitis and other eczema	692
Contraception	V25.9
Contraception counseling	V25.09
Contraceptive management (family planning advice)	V25.09
Contraceptive management (unspecified)	V25.9
Convulsions	780.3
Corneal abrasion	918.1
Corns	700.00
Coronary atherosclerosis	414.0
Costochondritis	733.6
Cough	786.2
Cow's milk allergy	693.1
Cow's milk intolerance	271.3
Coxsackievirus B	079.2
Craniopharyngioma	237.0
Craniosynostosis	756.0
Crohn's disease	555.9
Crohn's disease (regional, unspecified)	555.9
Croup	464.4
Cryptorchidism (undescended testicle)	752.5
Cryptosporidiosis	007.4
Cushing disease	255.0
Cutaneous, vaginal, conjunctival, and aural diphtheria	032.85
Cystic fibrosis	277.00
Cystic fibrosis without ileus	277.00
Cytomegalovirus (CMV)	078.5
Dacryocystitis	375.30
Dandruff	690.18
Dehydration	276.5
Delayed puberty	259.0
Dental caries	521.0
Depression, nonspecific	311.
Development (delayed)	783.4
Developmental dysplasia of the hip (congenital hip dislocation)	754.30
Diabetes (uncomplicated, type I)	250.01
Diabetes (uncomplicated, type II)	250.00
Diaper dermatitis	691.0
Diaper or napkin rash	691.0
Diarrhea	558.9
Diarrhea (acute)	787.91
Diarrhea as a result of poisoning	973.9
Diskitis	722.90
Displacement (intervertebral disk)	722.2
Down syndrome (trisomy 21)	758.0
Drug dependence	304.9
Duchenne-muscular dystrophy	
Dysmenorrhea	625.3
Ear discharge	388.60

Table E-2 ICD-9 Codes—cont'd

DESCRIPTION	CODE
Ear pain	388.70
Eating disorder (unspecified)	307.50
Ecchymosis	459.89
Ectopic pregnancy	633.9
Encephalitis	323.9
Encopresis	787.6
Enuresis (primary, secondary)	307.6
Enuresis (unspecified)	788.30
Ephelides (freckles)	709.09
Epiglottitis (acute)	464.30
Epilepsy	345.9
Epispadias (female)	753.8
Epispadias (male)	752.62
Epistaxis	784.7
Epstein-Barr virus (EBV)	075.
Equinovarus (acquired)	736.71
Equinovarus (congenital)	754.51
Erythema multiforme (Stevens-Johnson syndrome)	695.1
Erythema nodosum	695.2
Escherichia coli	041.4
Esophagitis	530.10
Esotropia	378.00
Exotropia	378.10
Extrapyramidal	343.8
Extraurethral	599.9
Eye deviations	378.87
Eye injury	921.9
Eyelid cellulitis	373.13
Eyelid infection	373.9
Eyelid injury	921.1
Failure to thrive (FTT)	783.41
Familial short stature	783.43
Fear of health-related procedures	300.29
Febrile seizure	780.31
Fecal impaction	560.39
Femoral hernia	553.00
Fetal alcohol syndrome (FAS)	760.71
Fever as a result of infection	780.6/136.9
Fever of unknown origin	780.6
Fibroadenoma	611.72
Fibroadenosis of breast	610.2
Fibroangioma (unspecified site)	210.7
Fibrocystic mass	610.1
Fifth disease (eruptive)	057.0
Filiform wart	078.10
Flat wart	078.10
Folate deficiency	281.2
Folic acid deficiency	281.2
Folliculitis	704.8
Food intolerance	579.8
Foot-and-mouth disease	078.4
Foreign body in anus/rectum	937.
Foreign body in or on cornea	930.0
Foreign body in ear	931.
Foreign body in esophagus	935.1
Foreign body in external eye	930.9
Foreign body in lung	934.9
Foreign body in vagina	939.2
Fracture	829.0
Fragile X syndrome	759.83
Frostbite	991.3

Continued

Table E-2 ICD-9 Codes—cont'd

DESCRIPTION	CODE
Functional cough	306.1
Fungal paronychia	681.9
Furuncle/abscess (face)	680.0
Furuncle/carbuncle	680.9
Glucose-6-phosphate dehydrogenase (G6PD) deficiency	282.2
Gastritis	535.5
Gastroenteritis (unspecified)	558.9
Gastroesophageal reflux	530.81
Gastrointestinal (GI) tract bleeding	578.9
Gender identity disorder of adolescent or adult life	302.85
General medical examination (other specified)	V70.8
Genital herpes simplex virus (HSV)	054.10
Genital wart	078.11
Genu valgum (acquired)	736.41
Genu valgum or varum	736.4
Genu varum (acquired)	736.42
Giardia lamblia infestation	007.1
Giardiasis	007.1
Gingivitis	523.1
Glioma	191.9
Glomerulonephritis	583.9
Glucose malabsorption	271.3
Gonadal failure	257.2
Gonorrhea	098.0
Gonorrhoeae	098.40
Granuloma (umbilicus of newborn)	771.4
Graves disease	242.0
Groin pull	848.8
Growing pains	781.99
Growth hormone deficiency	253.3
Gynecologic examination (annual Pap smear)	V72.3
Gynecomastia	611.1
Hand-foot-mouth disease	074.3
Hashimoto's disease	245.2
Head lice	132.0
Headache	784.0
Hearing loss	389.9
Heart murmur (functional/undiagnosed)	785.2
Heatstroke/sunstroke	992.0
Helicobacter pylori infection	041.86
Hemangioma	228.0
Hematuria	599.7
Hemophilia A	286.0
Hemorrhage	459.0
Hemorrhoids	455.6
Henoch-Schönlein purpura	287.0
Hepatitis	573.3
Hepatitis A	070.10
Hepatitis B	070.30
Hepatitis C	070.51
Hepatitis (viral)	070.9
Hereditary spherocytosis	282.0
Hernia of unspecified site	552.9
Herniated disc	722.2
Herpangina	074.0
Herpes (genital)	054.10
Herpes gingivostomatitis	054.2
Herpes simplex	054.43
Herpes zoster	053.9
Herpetic whitlow	054.6
Hip pointer	922.2

Table E-2 ICD-9 Codes—cont'd

DESCRIPTION	CODE
Hirschsprung's disease	751.3
Human immunodeficiency virus (HIV)	079.53
HIV counseling	V65.44
HIV disease	042.
HIV infection (asymptomatic)	V08.
Hordeolum externum	373.11
Hordeolum (sty)	373.11
Hydrocele	603.9
Hydrocephalus	331.4
Hydronephrosis	591.
Hypercalciuria	275.40
Hypercholesterolemia	272.0
Hyperlipidemia	272.4
Hyperphoria	378.40
Hypersensitivity reaction	995.3
Hypertension	401.9
Hypertension (essential)	401.9
Hypertension (secondary)	405.99
Hyperthyroidism	242.9
Hypertonia	779.8
Hypertriglyceridemia (essential)	272.1
Hypertrophy	611.1
Hypertropia	378.31
Hypoglycemia	251.2
Hyponatremia	276.1
Hypospadias	752.6
Hypothalamic/pituitary failure	253.
Hypothyroidism	244.9
Hypothyroidism (congenital)	243.
Idiopathic scoliosis	737.30
Idiopathic thrombocytopenic purpura	287.3
Impetigo	684.
Impetigo (bullous)	684.
Infantile autism (current or active)	299.00
Infantile colic	789.00
Infantile spasms	345.6
Infectious mononucleosis	075.
Influenza	487.1
Inguinal hernia (unilateral)	550.90
Injury (site unspecified)	959.9
Innocent murmur	785.2
Internal femoral torsion	736.89
Internal tibial torsion	736.89
Intrauterine pregnancy	656.40
Intussusception	560.0
Iron deficiency anemia	280.9
Irregular menstrual cycle	626.4
Irritable bowel syndrome	564.1
Jammed finger	959.5
Jaundice	782.4
Jaundice (physiologic)	774.6
Juvenile arthritis	714.30
Kawasaki's disease	446.1
Knee sprain	844.9
Kyphosis	737.1
Laceration (wound open)	879.8
Lactose intolerance	271.3
Langerhans cell histiocytosis	277.8
Laryngeal diphtheria	032.3
Laryngitis	464.0
Laryngotracheomalacia	519.1

Continued

Table E-2 ICD-9 Codes—cont'd

DESCRIPTION	CODE
Lead poisoning	984.9
Learning disability	315.2
Leg-length discrepancy	755.30
Legg-Calve'-Perthes' disease	732.1
Leukemia of unspecified cell type	208.91
Lice (head)	132.0
Limited exposure to sun	368.13
Little League elbow	718.82
Lyme disease	088.81
Lymphadenitis	289.3
Lymphadenopathy	785.6
Lymphoid leukemia	204.
Lymphoma (malignant)	202.8
Lymphosarcoma	200.10
Malabsorption syndrome	579.9
Malnutrition (calorie)	263.9
Meckel diverticulum	751.0
Melanoma (malignant)	172.8
Meningitis	322.9
Meniscal injury (knee)	959.7
Mental retardation (mild)	317.
Mental retardation (moderate)	318.0
Metatarsus adductus valgus	754.60
Metatarsus adductus varus	754.53
Miliaria	705.1
Miliaria rubra	705.1
Milk and soy protein intolerance	579.8
Milk intolerance	579.8
Molar pregnancy	631.
Molluscum contagiosum	078.0
Mongolian spots	757.33
Mononucleosis	075.
Mouth sores	528.9
Multiple gestation	633.9
Mumps	072.
Munchausen syndrome	301.51
Muscle spasms	728.85
Myocarditis	429.0
Nasal diphtheria	032.2
Nasal infection	473.9
Nasal trauma/injury	959.09
Nasolacrimal duct obstruction	375.56
Nausea	787.02
Nausea and vomiting	787.01
Necrotizing ulcerative gingivitis	101.
Neisseria gonorrhoeae	098.19
Neonatal conjunctivitis	771.6
Neonatal conjunctivitis and dacryocystitis	771.6
Nephrotic range proteinuria	791.0
Neurofibromatosis	237.70
Nevus	448.1
Nipple discharge	611.79
Nongonococcal urethritis	099.40
Normal fatigue	780.79
Nystagmus	379.50
Obesity (unspecified)	278.00
Observation for suspected condition	V71.8
Obstruction of GI biliary tract	576.2
Optic neuritis	377.30
Oral candidiasis (thrush)	112.0
Orbital cellulitis	376.01

Table E-2 ICD-9 Codes—cont'd

DESCRIPTION	CODE
Orbital fracture	802.8
Osgood-Schlatter disease	732.4
Osteochondritis dissecans of elbow	732.78
Osteochondritis dissecans of knee	732.78
Osteoma	213.9
Osteomyelitis	730.2
Otitis externa	380.10
Otitis media (acute)	382.00
Otitis media (chronic serous, simple)	381.01
Overfeeding	783.6
Pallor	782.61
Pancreatitis	577.0
Panic attack	300.01
Panner disease	732.3
Patellofemoral syndrome	719.46
Pathologic murmur	785.2
Pectus excavatum (congenital)	754.81
Pediculosis (crabs and lice; pubic)	132.2
Pelvic inflammatory disease (PID)	614.9
Penile trauma	607.9
Peptic ulcer disease	533.90
Perianal itch	698.0
Pericarditis	423.9
Personal history of exposure to lead	V15.86
Pertussis	033.9
Pes cavus	754.71
Pes cavus (acquired)	736.73
Pes planus (acquired)	734.
Pes planus (congenital)	754.61
Pharyngitis (acute)	462.
Phimosis (congenital)	605.
Photosensitive skin reaction	692.82
Phthirus pubis	132.2
Physiologic leukorrhea	623.5
Pica	307.52
Pinworms	127.4
Pityriasis rosea	696.3
Plantar warts	078.19
Pleural effusion	511.9
Pneumonia	486.
Poisoning (accidental; as below)	E850-E858
Poisoning (with drugs, medicinals, and biologic substances)	960-979
Poliomyelitis	045.90
Port-wine nevus or mark	757.32
Port-wine stain	757.32
Postnatal rubella	647.50
Postural proteinuria	593.6
Prader-Willi syndrome	759.81
Precocious puberty	259.1
Pregnancy	V22.2
Pregnancy examination or test	V72.34
Premature ventricular contractions (PVCs)	427.69
Prematurity	765.1
Prepubescent acne	706.1
Primary ciliary dyskinesia	781.3
Primary irritant dermatitis	692.9
Proteinuria	791.0
Pruritus ani	698.0
Pseudostrabismus	378.9
Pubic lice	132.2
Pulmonary structural abnormality	770.8

Continued

Table E-2 ICD-9 Codes—cont'd

DESCRIPTION	CODE
Puncture wound	879.8
Pyelonephritis	590.80
Pyloric stenosis (infantile)	750.5
Rape	E960.1
Rash or skin eruption (nonspecific)	782.1
Renal disease	593.9
Respiratory tract infection	519.8
Retractile testis	752.52
Reye syndrome	331.81
Rheumatic fever with heart involvement	391.
Rheumatic fever without heart involvement	390.
Rhinitis (allergic)	477.9
Rhinitis (viral acute)	472.0
Rickets	268.0
Rocky Mountain spotted fever	082.0
Roseola	057.8
Rotator cuff tear	840.4
Rotavirus	008.61
Rubella without mention of complication	056.9
Rubeola (measles)	055.9
Salmonella infection	003.29
Salpingitis	614.2
Scabies	133.0
Scarlet fever	034.1
Scoliosis (acquired)	737.30
Scoliosis (congenital)	754.2
Screening for cardiovascular disease	V81.2
Scrotal mass	608.89
Seborrheic dermatitis	690.
Seborrheic diaper dermatitis	690.12
Seizure	780.39
Separated shoulder	831.00
Sepsis (generalized)	038.9
Septic arthritis	711.0
Septicemia of a newborn	771.8
Sexual and physical abuse	V61.21
Sexual precocity	259.1
Shigella	004.9
Shock	785.50
Short stature (constitutional)	783.4
Shoulder dislocation	831.00
Sickle cell anemia	282.60
Sinusitis (acute)	461.9
Sinusitis (chronic)	473.9
Skeletal dysplasia	742.9
Sleep disturbance	780.50
Slipped upper femoral (nontraumatic) epiphysis	732.2
Snake bite	989.5
Spastic diplegia	343.0
Spastic hemiplegia	342.1
Spastic quadriplegia	343.2
Speech language disorder or speech delay	315.39
Spermatocele	608.1
Spermatocele (congenital)	752.8
Spina bifida	741.90
Spondylolisthesis	756.12
Spondylolysis (congenital)	756.11
Staphylococcus aureus	041.11
Status epilepticus	345.3
Stenosis (congenital)	713.65
Stenosis (infantile)	750.5

Table E-2 ICD-9 Codes—cont'd

DESCRIPTION	CODE
Stenosis (lacrimal duct)	375.52
Stiff neck (also see torticollis)	723.5
Stomatitis	528.0
Strabismus	378.9
Strain/sprain	848.9
Strep throat	034.0
Stress	308.9
Stridor	786.1
Sturge-Weber disease	759.6
Suicide attempt	E958.9
Sunburn	692.71
Superficial folliculitis	704.8
Syncope	780.2
Synovitis	727.00
Syphilis (acquired)	097.9
Systemic illness	783.43
Systemic juvenile rheumatoid arthritis	714.30
Systemic lupus erythematosus	710.0
Tantrum	312.10
Teething syndrome	520.7
Testicular torsion	608.2
Tetanus	037.
Thalassemia	282.4
Thrombocytopenia (infectious)	287.5
Tics	307.2
Tinea capitis	110.0
Tinea corporis	110.5
Tinea cruris	110.3
Tinea pedis	110.4
Tinea versicolor	111.0
Tonsillar and pharyngeal diphtheria	032.1
Tonsillitis (acute)	463.
Tonsillopharyngitis (streptococcal)	034.0
Torticollis	723.5
Tourette syndrome	307.23
Tracheoesophageal fistula	530.84
Trachomatis	076.1
Traction alopecia	704.09
Transient synovitis	727.00
Trauma-induced petechiae	772.6
Trichomonas	131.09
Trichotillomania	312.39
True undescended testis	752.21
Tuberculosis	011.9
Turner syndrome	758.6
Ulcerative colitis	556.9
Umbilical hernia with obstruction	552.1
Umbilical hernia with obstruction and gangrene	551.1
Umbilical hernia without mention of obstruction	553.1
Upper respiratory infection (acute)	465.9
Uremia	586.
Urethritis	597.80
Urinary incontinence (transient/established)	788.30
Urinary tract infection	599.0
Urinary tract infection (lower; cystitis)	595.0
Urinary tract infection (upper)	590.80
Urticaria	708.80
Vaginal abrasions	959.1
Vaginal bleeding	623.8
Vaginal discharge	623.5
Varicella	052.9

Continued

Table E-2 ICD-9 Codes—cont'd

DESCRIPTION	CODE
Varicocele (scrotal)	456.4
Vascular rings	747.21
Venereal disease (other)	099.9
Viral exanthem	057.9
Viral infection (unspecified)	079.99
Viral warts	078.1
Visual impairment	369.9
Vitamin B_{12} deficiency	266.2
Vitiligo	709.01
Vocal cord dysfunction	478.5
Vomiting	787.03
Vulvovaginitis	616.10
Warts (common)	078.10
Warts (plantar)	078.19
Warts (venereal)	078.19
Whooping cough	033.9
Wilms' tumor	189.0
Wrist fracture	814.00
Wrist sprain	842.00
Yersinia	027.9

Appendix F General Health, Pediatric, and Nurse Practitioner Internet Sites

Jane A. Fox

Search Engines

Alta Vista (altavista.com)
Excite (www.excite.com)
HotBot (www.hotbot.com)
Infoseek (www.infoseek.com)
Lycos (www.lycos.com)
Northern Light (northernlight.com)
Yahoo (www.yahoo.com)

Metasearch Engines

Metacrawler (www.metacrawler.com)
National Center for Biotechnology Information Literature Databases (www.ncbi.nlm.nih.gov:80/Literature/index.html)
National Library of Medicine Gateway (gateway.nlm.nih.gov/gw/Cmd)
Search (www.search.com)

Access to MEDLINE

Centre for Evidence-Based Medicine (cebm.jr2.ox.ac.uk/docs/otherebmgen.html)
CliniWeb (International) (www.ohsu.edu/cliniweb)
Cumulative Index to Nursing and Allied Health Literature (Cinahl) (subscription required) (www.cinahl.com)
Doctor's Guide—Global (requires registration) (www.docguide.com)
Hardin Meta Directory (www.lib.uiowa.edu/hardin/md) (www.lib.uiowa.edu/hardin/md/nurs.html)
Healthfinder—Consumer Guide to the Internet (www.healthfinder.gov)
HealthWeb (healthweb.org)
MDChoice (free subscription) (www.mdchoice.com)
MedWeb—Emory University (www.medweb.emory.edu/MedWeb)
National Library of Medicine Gateway (gateway.nlm.nih.gov/gw/Cmd)
NCBI Literature Databases (www.ncbi.nlm.nih.gov:80/Literature/index.html)
New York Academy of Medicine Evidence-Based Medicine Resource Center (www.ebmny.org)
ScHARR Netting the Evidence (www.sheffield.ac.uk/scharr/ir/netting)

Bookmarks

Mari Stoddard's Bookmarks (numerous medical links) (amber.medlib.arizona.edu:80/Bookmarks.html)
Medical Bookmarks (miscellaneous) (www.musc.edu/pa_program/medbkmrk.htm)

Clinical Practice Guidelines and Systematic Reviews

Agency for Healthcare Research and Quality National Guideline Clearinghouse (www.guidelines.gov)
American Medical Association Adolescent Health Resources (www.ama-assn.org/ama/pub/category/1981.html)

Bandolier (www.jr2.ox.ac.uk/bandolier)
Centers for Disease Control and Prevention Wonder Prevention Guidelines (wonder.cdc.gov/wonder/prevguid/prevguid.shtml)
Cochrane Database of Systemic Reviews (topics and abstracts free; complete clinical practice guidelines require paid membership) (cochrane.org)
Guidelines for Adolescent Preventive Services (www.ama-assn.org/ama/pub/category/1980.html)
Madigan Army Medical Center Referral (www.mamc.amedd.army.mil/Referral/index_rg.htm)
Medical Matrix (requires log-in) (www.medmatrix.org/_Spages/Practice_Guidelines.asp)
Medscape (www.medscape.com/Home/topics/pediatrics/pediatrics.html)
National Health System Center for Reviews and Dissemination, The University of York (www.york.ac.uk/inst/crd/list.htm)
National Center for Complimentary and Alternative Medicine, National Institutes of Health (altmed.od.nih.gov)
Norbert's Medical Links (www.geocities.com/HotSprings/2233/medical.html)
Primary Care Clinical Practice Guidelines—Pediatrics (medicine.ucsf.edu/resources/guidelines/guide15.html)
Sigma Theta Tau Online Journal (abstracts free; full texts require paid subscription) (www.stti.iupui.edu/library/ojksn/soj_content.html)
U.S. National Network of Libraries of Medicine Evaluation of Health and Medical Websites (nnlm.gov/healthinfoquest/help/eval.html)
Virtual Naval Hospital (www.vnh.org/Providers.html)

Organizations

American Academy of Nurse Practitioners (www.aanp.org)
American Academy of Pediatrics (www.aap.org)
American Academy of Physician Assistants (www.aapa.org)
American College of Nurse Practitioners (www.nurse.org/acnp)
American Nurses Association (www.nursingworld.org)
National Association of Pediatric Nurse Practitioners, Inc. (napnap.org/)

General Pediatric Sites

Clinical Pharmacology 2000 (free subscription) (www.cp.gsm.com/)
Harriett Lane WWW Links (162.129.72.40/poi/)
Medem—The Medical Library, American Academy of Pediatrics (www.medem.com/MedLB/bufferpage_aap.cfm)
NP Central (www.nurse.net/np/)
Nursing and Nurse Practitioner Sites (www.geocities.com/HotSprings/2350/)
Pediatric Database (PEDBASE) (www.icondata.com/health/pedbase/pedlynx.htm)

Pediatric Infectious Diseases (www.pedid.uthscsa.edu/)

PedInfo—Index of the Pediatric Internet (www.pedinfo.org)

PediatricLinx (requires free registration) (www.pediatriclinx.com/)

Points of Pediatric Interest (www.med.jhu.edu/peds/neonatology/link.html#Links)

University of California School of Nursing (nurseweb.ucsf.edu/www/arwwebpg.htm)

The Virtual Children's Hospital (www.vh.org/VCH/CommonProblems/CommonProblems.html)

The Virtual Nursing Center (www-sci.lib.uci.edu/HSG/Nursing.html)

Virtual PNP (home.earthlink.net/emgoodman/virtualpnp.htm)

Listservs

Npinfo (send message with subscribe npinfo first name last name) (majordomo@nurse.net)

Pedinfo (send message with subscribe first and last name) (pedinfo@u.washington.edu)

Bibliography

American Academy of Pediatrics. (1999). *Clinical practice guidelines of the American Academy of Pediatrics*. Elk Grove Village, IL: American Academy of Pediatrics.

Balas, E.A. (1999). From appropriate care to evidence-based medicine. *Pediatric Annals, 27*(9), 581-584.

Bennett, S.D. (1998). Pediatric resources on the web. *Clinical Excellence for Nurse Practitioners, 2*(3), 188-189.

Feldman, W. (2000). *Evidence-based pediatrics*. St. Louis: B.C. Decker.

Kibbe, D.C., et al. (1997). A guide to finding and evaluating best practices health care information on the Internet: The truth is out there? *Journal of Quality Improvement, 23*(12), 678-689.

McKibbon, A. (1999). *PDQ evidence-based principles and practice*. Hamilton, Ontario, Canada: B.C. Decker.

McSweeney, M., Spies, M., & Cann, C.J. (2001). Finding and evaluating clinical practice guidelines. *The Nurse Practitioner, 26*(9), 30-47.

Sackett, D.L., et al. (1997). *Evidence-based medicine: How to practice & teach EBM*. New York: Churchill-Livingstone.

Werk, L.N., Bauchner, H., & Chessare, J.B. (1999). Medicine for the millennium: Demystifying EBM. *Contemporary Pediatrics, 16*(12), 87-107.

Appendix G *Telephone Triage and Protocols*

Susan M. Watson

Role of the Practitioner in Telephone Management

- Triaging of phone calls
- Facilitation of access to health care for emergent and urgent conditions
- Advising parents on how to manage illness or injuries at home
- Anticipatory guidance
- Counseling
- Provision of emotional support and reassurance

Steps in the Management of Phone Calls

- Information gathering
  Develop rapport with the parents.
  Use effective communication and history-taking skills.
  Determine the caller's needs.
- Careful assessment and planning
  Determine the parents' reliability.
  Verify the family's resources.
  Ascertain the parents' ability to handle the illness or concern.
- Intervention (generally there are three dispositions)
  The child requires immediate or urgent evaluation by a health care provider.
  The child requires same-day evaluation or evaluation within 24 hours.
  The illness or injury can be managed at home.
- Evaluation
  Assess the parents' understanding and agreement with the plan of care. If necessary, ask the parents to repeat the information given.
  Instruct the parents to call back with changes in the child's condition. Inform the parents when to seek further medical attention. Provide noncompliance warnings to inform the parents of possible ramifications of not complying with the treatment plan; these warnings aid with appropriate care for the child and help protect the nurse.
  Order a follow-up phone call.

Benefits of Telephone Protocols

- Telephone protocols ensure that the advice given is consistent, precise, and accurate.
- Protocols help to determine which patients need to be seen, where and when they should be seen, and who should see them.
- Parents are not faced with differing opinions on how to manage illnesses at home or when to bring the child in for evaluation.
- Health care providers know what information has been shared with the parents.
- Telephone protocols may decrease the number of unnecessary office visits, which can provide more time to see truly ill patients.
- Health care costs may be decreased.

Documentation of an Illness-Related Telephone Call Using a Protocol System

- Date and time
- Child's name, date of birth, and gender
- Name of child's health care provider
- Name and relationship of the caller to the child
- Phone number and location of call
- Child's weight
- Any allergies
- Current medications
- Child's temperature (if applicable)
- History of the presenting problem, including signs and symptoms
  How long have they been occurring?
  Has the caller given medications or treatment?
  What is the child's activity level?
  Are other family members ill?
- Protocol used
  Working diagnosis
  Recommended disposition (where and when follow-up should occur)
  Advice given per protocol, including drug dosages
  Call-back advice
- Patient's or caller's intended action
  Agreement with plan
  Warning of medical consequence of noncompliance to the follow-up advice if condition worsens
- Any professional collaborations or referrals made
- Time call ended
- Nurse's signature

- Copies of all telephone interactions via telephone logsheets, audiotapes, or computerized entries to be put into the patient's permanent medical record

Legal Liability of the Telephone Triage Nurse

Telephone triage nurses can be held legally liable for the advice they give, and negligence is the most common reason for a lawsuit in medical malpractice. There are four components to be demonstrated in negligence:
1. The duty to meet the standard of care
2. A breach of the duty to meet the accepted and reasonable standard of care
3. The breach of duty causing foreseeable harm
4. The actual harm or injury that was incurred

There are no standards of practice established for telephone care. Therefore it is very important for telephone triage nurses to be familiar with the legal aspects of their practice. As professionals, nurses are accountable and autonomous. Accountability means the nurse must make conscientious use of protocols, document correctly, and adhere to quality assurance guidelines. Autonomy means using an independent judgement for each call and deciding to override the protocol if the situation requires it. Following these principles helps to defend against allegations of malpractice.

The three best ways to protect triage nurses from legal liability are:
1. Accurate documentation
2. Use of established pediatric protocols
3. Quality assurance measures such as good orientations and ongoing training, audit checks, and patient satisfaction surveys

Recommendations

1. Be an advocate for the child.
2. Include in the orientation:
   - Review of policy and procedures and written protocols
   - Training in triage and telephone assessment
   - Precepted call situations and initial actual calls
3. Become familiar with the medico-legal aspects of telephone triage nursing.
4. Obtain individual malpractice insurance.
5. Practice prudently within the confines of job description and collaborative practice agreement.

6. Remember that documentation is paramount. Practice risk management.
7. Use established protocols, and adapt and modify them to meet the needs of the office or institution. Update annually.
8. Document noncompliance warnings. The primary reason for lawsuits is delayed medical treatment.
9. Be autonomous and override the protocol or consult the covering physician when necessary.
10. Include in the quality assurance program:
    - Critiques of telephone logs
    - Audits of checklists
    - Reviews of parent satisfaction surveys
    - Analysis of data and necessary improvements
    - Continued education for practitioners

Resources

Publications
Baker, R. (1997). *Pediatric telephone advice* (2nd ed.). Philadelphia: Lippincott-Raven.
Schmitt, B. (2000). *Pediatric telephone protocols: Office version* (8th ed.). Elk Grove Village, IL: American Academy of Pediatrics.
Websites
Ars Medica (www.ramex.com)
Telephone Nurse Triage (www.psna.org/career/telehealth.htm)
TeleTriage Systems (www.teletriage.com)

Bibliography

Brown, J. (1994). *Telephone medicine.* Philadelphia: J.B. Lippincott.
Coleman, A. (1997). Where do I stand? Legal implications of telephone triage. *Journal of Clinical Nursing, 6*(3):227-231.
Osterhaus, J. (1995). Telephone protocols in pediatric ambulatory care. *Pediatric Nursing, 21*(4):315-355.
Princiotta, C. (1999). Telephone triage: Good business. *Advance for Nurse Practitioners, 7*(10):2.
Robinson, D., Anderson, M., & Erpenbeck, P. (1997). Telephone advice: New solutions for old problems. *The Nurse Practitioner, 22*(3):179-192.
Schman, A. (1998). Is there a pediatric call center in your future? *Contemporary Pediatrics, 15*(8):75-93.
Schmitt, B. (1998). Calls about sick children: A triage system for the office. *Contemporary Pediatrics, 15*(7):138-152.
Schmitt, B. (1998). Calls about sick children: A triage system for the office. *Contemporary Pediatrics, 15*(8):49-79.

Index

A

Abacavir, 807t
Abdomen
  bleeding disorder and, 795t
  cancer and, 816
  cystic fibrosis and, 772
  diabetes and, 782t
  Down syndrome and, 851b
  gastrointestinal disorder and, 410
  neuropsychiatric disorder and, 580
  in newborn assessment, 113t, 126t-127t
  physical abuse and, 883
  in physical examination, 101t
  of preterm infant, 324
  respiratory disorder and, 645
  sickle cell disease and, 831t
Abdominal mass, 675-676
Abdominal migraine, 588b
Abdominal pain
  differential diagnosis of, 413t-416t, 417-418
  etiology of, 412, 417
  incidence of, 417
  management of, 418-420
  risk factors for, 417
ABO incompatibility, 481t, 482
Abortion
  genetic evaluation and, 45
  therapeutic, 628
Abrasion, 525-526
  corneal, 396, 397t, 398
  vulvovaginal
    in adolescence, 639
    differential diagnosis of, 636t
    in prepubescence, 638
Abscess, 496-499, 498t
  of ear, 380t
  periungual, 526-528, 527t
Absence seizure, 600
Abstinence, sexual, 273t
Abuse
  behavior patterns causing, 130-131
  child, colic vs, 444
  physical, 882-884
  sexual, 886-889
    of foster child, 303
    in stepfamily, 333
    vaginal bleeding and, 623
  substance
    diabetes and, 781
    by parent, 283-286, 284b, 285b
Acceptance, unconditional and universal, 70
Accessory nerve, 105t
Accessory nipple, 616, 618t
Accident
  definition of, 186
  motor vehicle. See Motor vehicle accident
  patient history of, 88t
Accident-prone profile, 206t
Accommodation, visual, 375
Accommodative esotropia, 395

b, Box; f, figure; t, table.

Accountability, 71
Accutane, 502t, 504
Acetaminophen
  bleeding disorder and, 792
  fever and, 705, 708t
  lymphadenopathy and, 717
  pharyngitis and, 666
  rash and, 532
  recurrent headache and, 590t
  sickle cell disease and, 836
  sinusitis and, 664
Acetylcholinesterase, 53t
Achilles tendinitis, 205t
Achondroplasia, 48t
Acidosis, vomiting with, 454t
Acne, 499-504
  differential diagnosis of, 500, 501t-502t
  etiology of, 499
  incidence of, 499
  management of, 500, 503-504
  prevention of, 491
  risk factors for, 499-500
Acoustic nerve, 105t
Acoustic reflectometry, 376
Acquired immune deficiency syndrome,
    796-815. See also Human immuno-
    deficiency virus infection
Activity
  cancer and, 823t
  neonatal assessment of, 119t
  pain and, 74
Acute chest syndrome, 831t
Acyanotic heart disease, 346, 348
Acyclovir
  for genital herpes, 275t
  for varicella zoster, 745
Adapalene, 502t
Adderall
  learning disability and, 865t
  for tic, 610t
Addiction, 75, 889. See also Substance abuse
Addictive family, 283-286, 284b, 285b
Addison disease, 454t
Adhesion, foreskin, 627, 627t, 628
Adjunctive management for pain, 80t
Adjustment disorder, 585
Adolescent
  adopted, 292
  anemia screening of, 469b
  assault on, 195-196
  bell-clapper deformity in, 435
  blood in stool of, 463t
  burn injury of, 900
  causes of death of, 186t
  cerebral palsy in, 848
  contraception for, 270-272, 272b, 273t-274t
  death and grief and, 293
  depression in, 584-586, 585b
  developmental counseling about, 145t
  developmental domains of, 864t
  developmental milestones for, 139t
  diabetes and, 781
  diarrhea in, 432t

Adolescent—cont'd
  Down syndrome and, 855b
  drugs abused by, 890t
  eating disorder in, 751-757
  family affected by, 15
  fetal alcohol syndrome and, 877, 878
  genetic disorder in, 66
  growth and maturation of, 269
  herpes infection in, 620-621
  HIV infection in, 802
  homicide by, 195
  hospitalization of, 913t
  injury prevention for, 192t
  irritability in, 710t, 711t
  nutrition assessment of, 269, 271
  office visits by, 268-269, 269t
  oral care for, 222-223
  pain in, 76t, 80t
  as parent, 278
  parenting issues about, 276
  parenting tasks during, 21t
  piercing and tattooing in, 277
  pregnancy in, 277-278. See Pregnancy
  screening of, 270t
  sexual abuse of, 887
  sexuality and, 232t-233t
  sexually transmitted disease and, 272, 275-
    276, 275t
  sickle cell disease and, 835, 836
  skin infection in, 491
  vaginal discharge in, 638
  vomiting in, 456t
  vulvovaginal symptoms in, 634-640
Adoption, 287-292
  data about, 288-289
  incidence of, 288
  management of, 290-292
  primary care issues of, 289-290
  risk factors of, 288
  types of children, 287-288
  types of families, 287
Adrenal hyperplasia, 149t
Adrenarche, premature, 365t, 366
Adrenocorticotropic hormone, 363
Adult diphtheria tetanus vaccine, 158-159
Advanced practice nurse, 3
Adverse reaction to vaccine, 166t-168t,
    177, 182t
Advocacy, 70
Aerosol, 494
Affection, parental expression of, 26
Affinity, 22
African-American parent, 24t-25t
African culture, 39t
Age
  of assent, 69
  bleeding disorder and, 790t
  bone, 615
    endocrine disorder and, 362
  caloric requirements and, 702t
  of discretion, 69
  divorce and, 297
  gestational, 110, 630t

Age—cont'd
hemophilia and, 788t
Pneumocystis carinii pneumonia prophylaxis and, 803t
of preterm infant, 323b
stool changes and, 462t
topical corticosteroid and, 492
vomiting causes and, 456t
Agreement, collaboration, 5
AIDS, 796-815. *See also* Human immunodeficiency virus infection
Airway
asthma and, 758-759
breathing difficulty and, 645-653. *See also*
Breathing difficulty
cystic fibrosis and, 774, 776, 778
maintenance of, 642-643
obstruction of
in anaphylaxis, 695
as emergency, 899-900, 899t
stridor with, 646, 647t
Alarm therapy for enuresis, 686
Albuterol
asthma and, 765t
cystic fibrosis and, 774
Alcohol
abuse of, 889, 891
diabetes and, 781
fetal alcohol syndrome, 877-879, 878t
Alcohol-related neurologic disorder,
877-879, 878t
in adopted child, 288
Algorithm for pain, 77, 78f
Allergy, 694-699
anaphylaxis caused by, 695
asthma and, 766-767
to coagulation factor, 793
conjunctivitis with, 403, 405t, 407
dermatitis from, 532
atopic, 491, 695
contact, 514, 515t-516t, 517, 695
differential diagnosis of, 725
management of, 698
differential diagnosis of, 695-696
etiology of, 694
food, 426, 695
differential diagnosis of, 695-696
management of, 699
hives caused by, 520-521, 521t
incidence of, 694
laryngitis and, 668, 668t, 669
latex, 872, 873t-874t
management of, 696-699, 696t, 697t
milk
colic vs, 442t-443t, 444
management of, 446-447
milk or soybean protein, 431t, 433
pallor and, 484, 485t
patient history of, 88t
of preterm infant, 323
rhinitis with
asthma and, 769t
differential diagnosis of, 658t-659t,
659, 695
management of, 663, 696-697, 696t, 697t
nasal bleeding and, 657t
risk factors for, 694-695
Alliance, in family assessment, 18b
Alliance in family, 17

Allis sign, 547, 547f
Alopecia, 518-520, 519t, 725
Alpha-fetoprotein, 53t
Alpha-thalassemia, 471-472
Alport syndrome, 677
Ambiguous genitalia, 616
Amblyopia, 390-391, 390t, 392
Amebiasis, 428t, 431
Amenorrhea
androgen insensitivity syndrome and, 66
anorexia and, 753-754
differential diagnosis of, 623
management of, 623-624
American Academy of Pediatric Dentistry, 221
American Academy of Pediatrics
on fluoride, 221
on vaccine administration, 171t
American Dental Association, 221
American Nurses Credentialing Center, 3
American Psychiatric Association, 751
Aminocaproic acid, 792t
Amitriptyline, 590t
Amniocentesis
Down syndrome and, 850
for genetic screening, 53t
Amoxicillin
Lyme disease and, 729
middle ear infection and, 383-384
pharyngitis and, 666
sinusitis and, 663
urethritis and, 690
urinary tract infection and, 689
Amoxicillin clavulanate
cystic fibrosis and, 774
lymphadenopathy and, 717
sinusitis and, 663
vaginal foreign body and, 639
vulvovaginitis and, 635, 638-639
Amphetamine, 316t
Anal fissure
differential diagnosis of, 421t-422t, 423,
459, 459t
management of, 425, 461
Anal foreign body
differential diagnosis of, 459, 459t
management of, 462
Analgesic
bleeding disorder and, 792
for dysmenorrhea, 418
sickle cell disease and, 836-837
Anaphylaxis
differential diagnosis of, 695
etiology of, 694
management of, 696
Androgen insensitivity syndrome, 66
Anemia
cancer and, 817
differential diagnosis of, 472, 473t-475t,
476-478
etiology of, 471
incidence of, 471-472
irritability in, 713t
management of, 478-480
otitis media and, 384
pallor with, 484
pernicious, 476, 478
risk factors for, 472
sickle cell, 829-838, 832t. *See also* Sickle
cell disease

Anemia—cont'd
differential diagnosis of, 473t-475t,
476-477
genetics of, 49t
incidence of, 471
Angioedema, 696
Angiotensin-converting enzyme inhibitor, 357
Anglo-European/American culture, 24t-25t
Animal bite, 509t-510t, 511
Ankle, sports injury to, 549
Ankyloglossia, 227
Anomalous pulmonary venous return,
348, 349
Anomaly, 61t, 62t
Anorchism, 364, 633-634
Anorectal manometry, 412
Anorexia nervosa, 751-757
amenorrhea and, 622-623
assessment of, 752t
data on, 752-755
etiology of, 751
incidence of, 752
management of, 755-758
risk factors for, 752
Anovulation, 623
Antepartal management, 630b-631b
Anterior draw test, 549, 549f
Anterior leg pain syndrome, 204t
Anteversion, femoral, 566-567, 567t
Anthropometrics, 213
Antibiotic
acne and, 502t, 503
cystic fibrosis and, 774, 777
diphtheria and, 723
gastroenteritis and, 418
Lyme disease and, 729
otitis media and, 383-384
pharyngitis and, 665
pneumonia and, 418
sickle cell disease and, 836
urinary tract infection and, 689-690
Antibiotic-associated diarrhea, 426, 429t, 433
Antibiotic prophylaxis for dental procedures,
227, 227f
Antibody
antinuclear, 555
bleeding disorder and, 793
hepatitis, 746-747
HIV, 799-800
muscular dystrophy and, 859
Anticipatory guidance
for dental care, 223t
developmental assessment and, 139
for neuropsychiatric disorder, 576
prenatal, 84-85
for respiratory disorder, 643
sexual abuse and, 888
Anticonvulsant
serum levels of, 581
types of, 602t-603t
Antidepressant, 586
Antidiuretic hormone, 684
Antifibrinolytic drug, 791-792
Antigen
administration of, 170t
hepatitis, 746-747
human leukocyte, musculoskeletal disorder
and, 555
Antigen-antibody reaction, 694

Antihistamine
effects of, 642-643
first-generation, 696t
for rhinitis
allergic, 696-697, 696t
viral, 662
Antihypertensive agent, 357, 359t
Antiinflammatory drug
asthma and, 763
cystic fibrosis and, 774, 776, 777
nonsteroidal
for abnormal uterine bleeding, 624
asthma and, 769t
bleeding disorder and, 792
cystic fibrosis and, 776
for dysmenorrhea, 418, 625, 625t
sickle cell disease and, 836
Antiinflammatory nasal spray, 643
Antinuclear antibody test, 555
Antipyretic, 705, 708t
Antiretroviral therapy for HIV infection, 803t-813t, 804-805
Antitoxin, diphtheria, 723
Antitussive, 643, 655
Anus
neonatal assessment of, 128t
in physical examination, 102t
Anxiety
separation, 258-259, 259b, 908-909, 909b
stranger, 263-264
Aorta, coarctation of, 348-349
Aortic stenosis, 348, 349
Aphasia, acquired epileptic, 843
Aphthous ulcer, 447
differential diagnosis of, 449t
management of, 450
Aplastic crisis, 833t
Apophysitis of tibial tubercle, 205t
Appearance
neonatal assessment of, 119t
in physical examination, 95t
Appendicitis, 417
ascariasis vs, 734t
differential diagnosis of, 413t-415t
Apprehension test, patellar, 549
Arabic culture, marriage in, 40b
Arm. *See also* Extremity
in Down syndrome, 851b
of neonate, 128t-129t
Arnold-Chiari malformation, 870
Arrest, respiratory, 898-899, 898b
Arrhythmia, 345
Arterial blood gases, 342
Artery, transposition of, 349
Arthralgia, patellar-femoral, 205t
Arthritis
juvenile rheumatoid, 562, 563t-564t, 565-566
septic, 562, 563t-564t
sports-related, 204t
as vaccine adverse event, 169t
Ascariasis, 733-734, 734t
Ascites, 455t
Aseptic necrosis, 562
Asian culture
assessment of, 39t
newborn care in, 41b
parenting in, 24t-25t
postpartum practices in, 40b
symptoms in, 42b

Asperger syndrome, 842
Asperillosis, 775t
Aspiration
foreign body, 897-898
by infant, 188t, 189t
by preschool-aged child, 190t
strategies to prevent, 199
by toddler, 190t
joint, 555
Aspirin
asthma and, 769t
for fever, 708t
rheumatic fever and, 828
Assault, 195
Assessment
biochemical, 213
Calgary Family Assessment Model, 10-17
contraception, 272
cultural, 38, 39t, 40-42
developmental. *See* Developmental assessment
of drug-exposed infant, 318t
of foster child, 301-302
genetic
in adolescent, 66
in child, 65-66
in newborn or infant, 59-62
hearing, 375
of preterm infant, 324
of neonatal jaundice, 482
newborn, 107-135. *See also* Newborn assessment
nutritional, 208, 212-213
parenting, 30-31, 30b, 31b, 32b
of pregnancy, 278b
of school readiness, 235-245. *See also* School readiness
Asthma, 757-770
airway obstruction in, 899t
classification of, 758t
data on, 761, 761t
differential diagnosis of, 648t-650t, 760-761, 760t
etiology of, 758-760, 759b
exercise and, 762
growth and development in, 761-762
hospitalization for, 915
immunization and, 762
incidence of, 760
management of, 652-653, 762-770, 762t, 763b, 764t-765t, 766b, 767b, 768t, 769t
nutrition in, 762
risk factors for, 760
sleep and, 762
Asymmetry of breast, 616, 618t
Ataxic cerebral palsy, 845, 846t-847t
Atelolol, 359t
Athlete's foot, 725, 726t
Athletic activity, 544-545
amenorrhea and, 623
bleeding disorder and, 790t
injury from. *See* Sports injury
Atlantoaxial instability, 575, 575t
Down syndrome and, 853, 854-855
Atonic seizure, 600
Atopic dermatitis
differential diagnosis of, 695
management of, 698
prevention of, 491

Atopy, pallor with, 484, 485t
Atrial septal defect, 348, 349
Attachment
to adopted child, 290
parent-infant, 109-110
prenatal risk factors for, 84b
Attachment disorder in adopted child, 288-289, 291
Attempted suicide, 605-607, 606b
Attention Deficit Disorders Evaluation Scale, 243t
Attention deficit/hyperactivity disorder
autism and, 842
tics and, 608
Attention span of gifted child, 312
Atypical autism, 842
Atypical newborn
counseling about, 134-135
management of, 134
Audiometry, 376
Auditory canal infection, 379-385
Auditory evoked potentials
ear disorder and, 376
in preterm infant, 325
Aural diphtheria, 724t
Auscultation, respiratory, 645
Authoritative parenting style, 22, 23t
Authority, prescriptive, 5
Authority stage of parenting, 21t
Autoimmune disease, 715t-717t, 717
Automobile accident. *See* Motor vehicle accident
Automobile safety seat, 194
Autonomy
allowed by parent, 26
as core value, 69
professional, 71
Autosomal disorder, 46t, 48t
Autosomal dominant inheritance, 59t
Autosomal recessive disorder, 49t
Autosomal recessive inheritance, 59t
Avascular necrosis, 562
of femoral head, 833t
Avulsion of primary tooth, 225
Axis, foot, 548, 548f
Azathioprine, 419
Azelastine, 697, 697t
Azithromycin, 275t
AZT. *See* Zidovudine

B

Baby bottle disease, 224-225, 225f
Baby Doe law, 70
Baby food, 212b
Babysitter, in-home, 250t
Back
flexion of, 550f
neonatal assessment of, 113t, 129t
pain in, 559, 560t, 561
in pregnancy, 633
in physical examination, 102t
Baclofen, 849
Bacteria, caries caused by, 220
Bacterial conjunctivitis, 403, 404t, 406
Bacterial vaginosis
management of, 640
vulvovaginal symptoms of, 637t
Balanoposthitis, 627-628, 627t
Balloon valvuloplasty, 349

Banding, prometaphase, 54
Barbiturate, 316t
Barium study, 412
Barlow test, 117, 117f, 546, 547f
Barotrauma, 386
Barrier
    to injury prevention counseling, 206
    to tele-health/medicine, 6
Battelle Developmental Inventory, 240, 241t
Battery, 4
Becker muscular dystrophy, 856-862
Beclomethasone
    for allergic rhinitis, 697t
    for asthma, 764t
    for cystic fibrosis, 776
Bedwetting, 684-686, 685t
Bee sting, 512
Behavior
    in autism, 842
    autism and, 841-844
    bullying, 247, 248f, 248t, 249
    colic and, 445b
    discipline for, 28-29
    Down syndrome and, 855
    of gifted child, 310b-311b
    learning disabilities and, 863
    malignancy and, 822t
    of newborn, assessment of, 110, 114,
        130-131, 132t
    in preschool screening, 240, 244
    rejection, of newborn, 110b, 130b
    tics and, 607-609, 608b, 610t
Behavior therapy
    for eating disorder, 755
    for urinary incontinence, 682
Belief
    cultural differences in, 36-37, 36t
    in family assessment, 17, 18b
    parenting style and, 22
Bell-clapper deformity, 435
Beneficence, 69
Benign paroxysmal torticollis, 588b
Benign paroxysmal vertigo, 588b
Benign premature thelarche, 365-366, 365t
Benzoyl peroxide, for acne, 502t
Bereavement, 293-295
Beta-adrenergic agonist in asthma, 763
Beta-adrenergic blocking agent, 359t
Beta-hemoglobin trait, 477
Beta-hemolytic streptococcal infection,
        826-829, 827t
Beta-thalassemia
    differential diagnosis of, 473t, 475t,
        477-478
    incidence of, 471, 472
    management of, 479
Bicycle injury, 195
Bile acid malabsorption, 464t
Biliary disorder, 482
Bilirubin in neonatal hyperbilirubinemia, 147,
    150t, 480, 482, 483
Billing for services, 3-4
Bimanual examination
    of female, 612-613, 614f
    in physical examination, 104t
Binging and purging, 753
    dental disease with, 226
Biochemical assessment, nutritional, 213
Biochemical disorder, 66

Biopsy
    gastrointestinal, 411
    muscular dystrophy and, 858
    skin, 496
Biotinidase deficiency, 149t
Birth control, 271-272, 272b
    diabetes and, 781
    methods of, 273t-274t
Birth defect, 45. *See also* Congenital disorder
Birth history, 87t-88t
    of preterm infant, 323
Birthmark
    differential diagnosis of, 504, 505t, 506t
    etiology of, 504
    incidence of, 504
    management of, 504-505, 507t, 508
    risk factors for, 504
Bisacodyl, 871
Bisexual adolescent, 279
Bite, 508-513
    differential diagnosis of, 508, 509t-510t
    etiology of, 508
    incidence of, 508
    risk factors for, 508
Biting, discipline for, 28
Bitolterol, 774
Bitot's spot, 214t
Black eye, 396, 398-399
Bladder
    anomaly of, 676-677
    cystitis of, 687
    incontinence and, 679-685, 680t, 681t
    neonatal assessment of, 127t
    outlet obstruction of, 680
    spina bifida and, 871
Bladder record, 673
Bleaching, dental, 224
Bleeding. *See also* Bleeding disorder
    cancer and, 817, 824
    cystic fibrosis and, 775t
    dysfunctional uterine, 623
    as emergency, 898
    gastrointestinal, 463t, 464, 465
    gingivitis and, 224
    middle ear, 386
    nasal, 656-659, 657t-658t
    urethrorrhagia, 677, 678
    in urine, 677-679, 677b, 678t
    withdrawal, 623-624
Bleeding disorder, 787-796
    bleeding sites in, 794t-795t
    data on, 788-791, 788t, 789t, 790t
    etiology of, 787-788
    growing pains vs, 570t
    incidence of, 788
    management of, 790t, 791-793, 792t, 796
    menstrual bleeding and, 623
    risk factors for, 788
Blepharitis, 400, 401t, 402
Blindness, 389-393, 390t-391t
    injury causing, 396
Blister
    as overuse injury, 205t
    Tzanck smear for diagnosis of, 496
Blood
    gastrointestinal disorder and, 411
    lead poisoning and, 150-151, 150t, 151t,
        879, 880t
    screening of, 147, 150-151, 150t

Blood—cont'd
    in stool, 463t
    umbilical, 53t
    urethrorrhagia, 677, 678
    in urine, 677-679, 677b, 678t
Blood-borne disease
    bleeding disorder and, 793
    hepatitis, 746-747
    HIV infection, 796-815. *See also* Human
        immunodeficiency virus infection
Blood count
    musculoskeletal disorder and, 555
    in respiratory disorder, 645
Blood disorder, 468-488
    anemia, 471-480. *See also* Anemia
    cancer and, 817
    colic vs, 444
    data about, 468-471, 470t
    neonatal jaundice, 480, 481t, 482-483, 482t
    nutrition and, 468
    pallor, 483-484, 485t, 486
    petechiae and purpura, 486, 487t, 488
    prevention of Rh disease and, 468
    risk factors for, 468
    screening for, 468, 469t
    sickle cell disease, 829-838. *See also* Sickle
        cell disease
Blood gases, arterial, 342
Blood glucose, 785
Blood group incompatibility, 481t, 482
Blood pressure
    cardiovascular examination and, 342
    neonatal assessment of, 116, 118t
Blood testing
    of drug-exposed infant, 317
    of preterm infant, 325
Blood transfusion for neonatal
    jaundice, 483
Blood vessel, 102t
Blount disease, 573t, 574
Blunt trauma, abdominal, 416t
Body image in anorexia nervosa, 751
Body lice, 523, 524t, 525
Body mass index
    of adolescent, 269, 271
    as screening test, 147
Body piercing, 277
Body proportion, 119t
Body surface area in burn, 900, 900f
Boil, 496-499, 498t
Bone, fracture of. *See* Fracture
Bone age, 615
    endocrine disorder and, 362
Bone marrow failure, 476
Bone tumor, 820t-821t
Bordetella pertussis, 735-737, 736t
Borrelia burgdorferi, 728-730, 729t
Bottle caries, 224-225, 224t, 225f
Botulinum toxin in cerebral palsy, 849
Boundary dispute in stepfamily, 333
Boundary in family, 12, 12b
Bowel elimination
    cerebral palsy and, 849
    spina bifida and, 871, 872
    urinary incontinence and, 681
Brachial neuritis, 169t
Brachial plexus stretch, 556t
Brain edema, 592b
Brain lesion, 679

Brain tumor, 818t-819t
Brainstem auditory evoked potentials
  ear disorder and, 376
  in preterm infant, 325
Brazelton neonatal behavioral assessment
    scale, 131
Breast
  disorders of, 616-618, 618t-619t
  examination of, 611f, 613
  mass or change in, 616-618, 618t
  neonatal assessment of, 126t
  in pregnancy, 630b
Breast self-examination, 611f
Breastfeeding
  of drug-exposed infant, 320-321
  jaundice with, 480, 481t, 483
  of preterm infant, 327
Breath-holding, 245-247, 246b, 246t
  differential diagnosis of, 596, 597t-600t,
    598-600, 600b
Breath hydrogen test, 412
Breath sound, 126t
Breathing difficulty, 645-653
  differential diagnosis of, 646-647,
    647t-650t, 650
  etiology of, 646
  incidence of, 646
  management of, 651-653
  risk factors for, 646
Brigance Diagnostic Inventory of Early
    Development, 241t
Bronchial dilatation in cystic fibrosis, 774
Bronchiolitis
  airway obstruction in, 899t
  differential diagnosis of, 648t-650t
  management of, 652
Bronchitis
  differential diagnosis of, 648t-650t
  management of, 651-652
Bronchodilator
  asthma and, 763
  cystic fibrosis and, 777
Brudinski sign, 376b
Bruise, 525-526
  hemophilia and, 788t
Bruit, 121t
Brush, tooth, 224
Buccal cellulitis, periorbital, 531t
Buccal smear, 615
Buddhist culture, 40b
Budesonide
  for allergic rhinitis, 697t
  asthma and, 764t
Bulimia, 751-757
  amenorrhea and, 622-623
  assessment of, 752t
  data on, 752-755
  dental disease with, 226
  etiology of, 751
  incidence of, 752
  management of, 755-758
  risk factors for, 752
Bullous impetigo, 541, 541t
  chickenpox vs, 745t
  as diaper rash, 514, 515t-516t, 517
Bullying, 247, 248f, 248t, 249
Burn
  chemical, of eye, 397t
  sunburn, 491-492

Burn injury, 188t
  chemical, of eye, 396
  as emergency, 900-901, 900f, 901b
  prevention of
    in infant, 188t, 189t
    in school-aged child, 191t
    strategies for, 193b, 199-200
    in toddler, 189t
  strategies to prevent, 199-200
Burning, circular, 42b
Bursitis, sports-related, 204t
Butalbital, 590t
Butoconazole, 640

C

Café-au-lait macule, 505, 506t
Caffeine, 316t
Calcium-to-creatinine ratio, 671
  in hematuria, 678t
Calculus
  sickle cell disease and, 832t
  urinary, 677
Calgary Family Assessment Model, 10-17
  collecting data in, 16, 16f
  communication in, 16-17, 16f, 17t, 18b
  context of, 13, 13b
  diagram of, 10f
  for divorced and remarried family, 15-16
  ecomap in, 14, 15t
  engagement of family in, 11-12, 11t
  for family with adolescent, 15
  for family with young children, 14-15
  genogram in, 14
  goal of, 11
  indications for, 11
  organizing data in, 17
  planning in, 11
  structure of, 12-13, 12b, 13b
  theoretical foundations for, 10-11
Calgary Family Intervention Model, 18-19
Callus, 513-514, 513t
Calming of infant, 446b
Caloric requirement, 702t
  diabetes and, 781
  HIV infection and, 802
  for preterm infant, 327
Cambodian culture
  newborn care in, 41b
  postpartum practices in, 40b
  symptoms in, 42b
Campylobacter jejuni, 427t, 431
Canal infection, auditory, 379-385
Cancer, 815-826. *See also* Malignancy
Candidiasis
  as diaper rash, 515t-516t, 517
  differential diagnosis of, 725, 726t
  HIV and, 799
  management of, 725, 727
  oral, 447
    differential diagnosis of, 448t
    management of, 450
  vulvovaginal
    differential diagnosis of, 637t
    management of, 638, 640
Canker sore, 447
Capital femoral epiphysis, slipped, 562, 563t-
    564t, 566
Capitation, 5
Captopril, 359t

Caput succedaneum
  differential diagnosis of, 592, 593, 593t
  management of, 594
Carbamazepine, 602t-603t
Carbohydrate metabolic disorder, 66
Carbuncle, 497, 498-499, 498t
Cardiac catheterization, 342
Cardiovascular disease, 341-359. *See also* Car-
    diovascular system; Heart
  breath-holding spell and, 246b
  chest pain, 343-346, 344t
  colic vs, 444
  congenital heart, 346-350, 347t
  congenital heart disease, 346-350
  data about, 341-342
  diagnostic procedures for, 342
  health promotion and, 341
  heart murmur, 350-351, 352t, 353t
  hospitalization for, 915
  hyperlipidemia, 351-354, 355t, 356
  hypertension, 356-358, 358t, 359t
  irritability in, 713t
  risk factors for, 341
Cardiovascular system
  cancer treatment affecting, 825t
  cystic fibrosis and, 772
  diabetes and, 782t
  malnutrition and, 215t
  in physical examination, 101t
  preparticipation examination of, 549
  of preterm infant, 324
  in review of systems, 91t
  rheumatic fever and, 828
  sickle cell disease and, 830
Carditis, rheumatic fever with, 829
Carey and McDevitt questionnaire, 242t
Caries
  nursing bottle, 224-225, 224t, 225f
  prevention of, 221-222, 221t
  process of, 220-221
Case method for ethics analysis, 72-73, 72b
Cat bite, 512
Cataract, 390t, 391, 392-393
Catheterization
  cancer and, 824
  cardiac, 342
  for urinary retention, 684
Cefadroxil
  for furuncle, 498
  for pharyngitis, 666
Cefixime, 275t, 639
Cefriaxone, 275t
Ceftizoxime, 275t
Ceftriaxone
  for gonorrhea, 638, 639
  for middle ear infection, 384-385
  for urethritis, 690
Celiac disease
  diarrhea from, 431t
  differential diagnosis of, 464
  management of, 434
  symptoms of, 464t
Cellulitis
  eyelid, 400, 401t, 402
  periorbital buccal, 531t
Census data, racial, 35t
Centers for Disease Control and Prevention,
    immunization schedule of, 172t,
    173t, 174t

Central nervous system. *See* Nervous system;
  Neurologic *entries*
Central precocious puberty, 365t, 366
Cephalexin
  for furuncle, 499
  for lymphadenopathy, 717
Cephalhematoma, 592
  differential diagnosis of, 593, 593t
  management of, 594
Cephalosporin, 635
Cerebellar function, 105t
  neuropsychiatric disorder and, 581
Cerebral edema, 592b
  vomiting with, 454t
Cerebral palsy, 844b, 845-850
  differential diagnosis of, 845
  etiology of, 845
  incidence of, 845
  limp with, 562, 565t
  risk factors for, 845
  types of, 845, 846t-847t
Cerebrovascular accident in sickle cell
    disease, 831t
Certification, 3
Certified nurse midwife, 3
Cerumen, 378-379
Cervical mucus, 614-615
Cetirizine, 697t
Chalasia, 455t
Chalazion, 400, 401t, 402
Chancroid, 619, 620t, 621
Cheating, 256-257
Chemical burn
  of eye, 396, 397t
  first aid for, 198b
Chemical irritation, vulvovaginal
  differential diagnosis of, 636t
  management of, 638, 639
  symptoms, 638
Chemotherapy, 824t
  immunization and, 175
CHEOPs, 77t
Chest
  blood disorder and, 469
  cystic fibrosis and, 771-772
  Down syndrome and, 851b
  neonatal assessment of, 112t, 117, 125t
  physical abuse and, 883
  respiratory disorder and, 644-645
  sports injury to, 203t
Chest pain, 343-346, 344t
Chest syndrome, acute, 831t
Chest wall, cancer and, 823t
Chest x-ray
  cardiovascular examination and, 342
  cystic fibrosis and, 772
  in lower airway disorder, 650t
  respiratory disorder and, 645
Chewing tobacco, 226
Chickenpox, 745-746, 745t
  cancer and, 817
  oral
    differential diagnosis of, 447
    management of, 451
  vaccine for, 161t
    handling and storage of, 180t-181t
Chief complaint, 87t
Child abuse
  colic vs, 444
  prevention of, 195

Child Behavior Checklist, 243t
Child care
  as parenting concern, 249-251, 250t,
    251b, 251t
  for preterm infant, 329
Child Development Inventories, 243t
Child Welfare League of America, 300
Childbearing, cultural factors in, 40
Children of Alcoholics Screening Tool, 284
Children's Health Insurance Program, 6
Chin of newborn, 112t, 125t
Chinese culture, moxibution in, 42
Chlamydia trachomatis, 272, 275, 275t
  conjunctivitis caused by, 403, 404t
  culture for, 615
  differential diagnosis of, 637t
  management of, 638
  pneumonia caused by, 647
  vulvovaginal symptoms of, 638
Chlorpheniramine, 696t
Choking, 897-898
  by infant, 188t, 189t
  by preschool-aged child, 190t
  prevention of, 199
  strategies to prevent, 199
  by toddler, 190t
Cholangiopancreatography, endoscopic
    retrograde, 412
Cholecystitis, 413t-415t, 417
Cholecystography, 412
Cholelithiasis in sickle cell disease, 832t
Cholesterol, 353-354, 355t, 356
  screening for, 151
Chondromalacia, 205t, 558t
Chorionic gonadotropin, human, 615
Chorionic villus sampling, 53t
  Down syndrome and, 850
Chromosomal abnormality, 46t-48t
  ambiguous genitalia in, 616
  characteristics of, 64t
  short stature and, 367
  trisomy 21, 850-856. *See also* Down
    syndrome
  in Turner syndrome, 363-364
Chromosomal analysis, 55t
  in endocrine disorder, 363
Chronic arthritis, vaccine-related, 169t
Chronic disease
  anorexia nervosa, 751-757
  asthma, 757-770. *See also* Asthma
  bleeding disorder, 787-796
  cystic fibrosis, 770-778
  diabetes mellitus, 778-787
  human immunodeficiency virus infection,
    796-815
  neoplastic, 815-826. *See also* Malignancy
  rheumatic fever, 826-829, 827t
  sickle cell, 829-838
    differential diagnosis of, 473t-475t, 476-477
    growing pains vs, 570t
    incidence of, 471
Chronic lymphocytic thyroiditis, 369
Cigarette smoking, 889, 891
  cessation strategies for, 892b
  diabetes and, 781
  prenatal and neonatal effects of, 316t
Cimetidine, 458t
Ciprofloxacin
  for gonorrhea, 275t, 640
  for urinary tract infection, 689

Circular burning, 42b
Circular communication, 16-17, 16f, 18b
Circular question, 18-19
Circumcision, 251-252, 252b
Circumference, head
  abnormal, 590-595, 591b, 592b, 593t, 594b
  neonatal assessment of, 115, 120t-121t
  screening of, 147
Civilian Health and Medical Program Uni-
    formed Services, 7
Class, social
  in family assessment, 13, 13b
  parenting affected by, 23
Clavicle, 116-117
Clean-catch urine specimen, 615
Cleft lip or palate, genetics of, 50t
Click, hip, 569-570
Clindamycin, 640
Clinical Laboratory Improvement
    Amendments, 7
Clinical nurse specialist, 3
Clinical practice guidelines, 8
Cloacal anomaly, 676
Clonazepam, 602t-603t
Clonidine
  learning disability and, 865t
  for tic, 609t
Clostridium tetanus, 742-743, 743t
Clotrimazole, 638, 640
Clubfoot, 567, 567t, 568
Co-trimoxazole for acne, 502t
Coagulation disorder, 787-796. *See also* Bleed-
    ing disorder
Coagulation factor, 791, 792t
Coalition in family, 17, 18b
Coarctation of aorta, 348-349
Cobalamin, 476
Cocaine abuse, 890t
  prenatal and neonatal effects of, 316t
Cognitive development
  Piaget's stages of, 144t
  school readiness and, 238t
Cognitive function
  in cerebral palsy, 847t
  parenting affected by, 23
Coin rubbing, 42
Coitus interruptus, 273t
Colic
  differential diagnosis of, 441, 442t-443t,
    443-444
  etiology of, 441
  incidence of, 441
  irritability in, 712t
  management of, 444-447, 445b, 446b
Colitis, ulcerative, 432t, 464t
Collaboration agreement, 5
Collapse as vaccine reaction, 177
Colonoscopy, 412
Color
  skin, 119t-120t
  of stool, 462, 462t
Coma, 901-902, 901b, 902t
Combination oral contraceptive, 273t
Commendation in Calgary intervention
    model, 19
Communicating hydrocephalus, 592b
Communication. *See also* Language
  cerebral palsy and, 848, 849
  in family assessment, 16-17, 16f, 17t, 18b
  interpreter for, 42

Community issues, gay or lesbian, 307
Competence, 71
Complement in allergy, 694
Complete blood count
    in foster child, 302
    gastrointestinal disorder and, 411
    musculoskeletal disorder and, 555
    in respiratory disorder, 645
    skin disorder and, 495-496
Complex stepfamily, 331
Compound nevus, 505, 506t, 508
Computed tomography of ear, 377
Computer, tele-health/medicine and, 6
Concussion, vomiting with, 453t
Condom, 273t
Conductance regulator, cystic fibrosis trans-
        membrane, 770
Conductive hearing loss, 388
Condyloma acuminatum, 537, 538t, 540, 619,
        620t, 621
Confidentiality for adolescent, 268
Confusional migraine, 588
Congenital disorder. *See also* Genetic disorder
    anorchia, 364
    cataract, 390t, 391, 392-393
    for condition or disorder, vaginal foreign
        body, 462
    cystic fibrosis, 770-778. *See also* Cystic
        fibrosis
    failure to thrive and, 703t
    heart, 346-350, 347t
    hypothyroidism, 369, 370t
    major, 62t
    minor, 61t
    neonatal screening for, 148t-149t
    rubella, 740t
    vomiting with, 453t
Congestion, nasal, 659, 660t-661t, 662-664
    decongestant for, 642
Conjunctiva
    diphtheria and, 724t
    malnutrition and, 214t
    neonatal assessment of, 123t
Conjunctivitis, 402-407
    allergic, 695
        management of, 697
    differential diagnosis of, 403, 404t-405t
    etiology of, 402
    management of, 403-407
    risk factors for, 402
Connors ADHD/DSM-IV Scales, 243t
Consciousness, loss of, 901-902,
        901b, 902t
Consent, informed, 69
    by adolescent, 268
    failure to obtain, 4
Consequences, logical, 29, 29b
Constipation, 420-425
    cerebral palsy and, 848
    differential diagnosis of, 420, 421t-422t,
        423, 464
    Down syndrome and, 853
    etiology of, 420
    incontinence and, 681
    management of, 423-425, 423t
    in pregnancy, 632t
    risk factors for, 420
    urinary tract infection and, 687
Constitutional delay of growth, 367, 368t
Consult, duty to, 4

Contact dermatitis
    management of, 698-699
    rash of, 532
Context in family assessment, 13
Contraception, 271-272, 272b
    diabetes and, 781
    methods of, 273t-274t
    oral contraceptive, 273t-274t
        for acne, 502t, 503
Contract in eating disorder, 755
Contraction, detrusor, 679, 680, 682
Contusion
    differential diagnosis of, 571t
    sports-related, 203t
Convulsion. *See* Seizure
Cooley's anemia, 471
Coombs test, 147, 482
Coparenting in gay or lesbian family, 305-306
Coping
    eating disorder and, 757
    interventions for, 910t
    skills for, 909-910, 909b
    styles of, 909, 909b
Core value, 69-70
Corn, 513-514, 513t
Cornea
    abrasion of, 396, 397t, 398
    neonatal assessment of, 123t
Corneal light reflex, 375
Corporal punishment, 337
Corticosteroid
    for allergic rhinitis, 697, 697t
    asthma and, 762
    Crohn's disease and, 419
    cystic fibrosis and, 776, 777
    topical, 492-493, 493t
Cosmetic dentistry, 224
Cough, 653-656
    antitussive for, 643
    cystic fibrosis and, 771-772
    differential diagnosis of, 654, 760b
    management of, 654-655, 654t
    symptoms of, 654t
    whooping, 735-737, 736t
Cover-uncover test, 375
Cow's milk allergy
    colic vs, 442t-443t, 444
    diarrhea with, 464t
    management of, 446-447
Cox-2 inhibitor, 792
Coxsackievirus, 529, 530t
Crab lice, 459
Cranial nerve
    examination, 580
    eye and ear function and, 376
    malignancy and, 822t
    neuropsychiatric disorder and, 578
    in physical examination, 105t
Craniopharyngioma, 391t, 392
Cranioskeletal dysplasia, 592b
Craniosynostosis, 539-594, 593t, 595
Cream, 494
    for diaper rash, 517
    for lice, 523
Crease, 117
Creatine kinase
    in muscular dystrophy, 858
    muscular dystrophy and, 860
CRIES Scale, 77t, 115
Crisis, suicide attempt as, 605-607, 6606b

Criticizing child, 29
Crohn's disease
    diarrhea with, 432t, 464, 464t
    differential diagnosis of, 415t-416t
    management of, 419
Cromolyn
    asthma and, 764t
    cystic fibrosis and, 776
    nasal, 643, 697
Crotamiton, 742t
Croup
    airway obstruction in, 899t
    pertussis vs, 736t
Cry
    of drug-exposed infant, 320t
    neonatal assessment of, 119t
    of newborn, 132
Cryptorchidism, 632-634
Cryptosporidiosis, 428t, 732-733,
        732t, 733b
    diarrhea with, 433
    HIV and, 799
Cultural factors, 35-42
    assessment and, 38, 39t, 40-42
    cystic fibrosis and, 772
    interpreters and, 42
    magic and, 37
    multiculturalism and, 35
    opposing forces and, 37-38
    parenting affected by, 22, 24t-25t
    respiratory disorder and, 645
    in school readiness, 244
    sexuality and, 229
    for skin disorder, 496
    spirituality as, 37
    terminology of, 36
    in urinary disorder, 671
    values and beliefs, 36-37, 36b
Current Procedure Terminology, 3
Cushing syndrome, 719t, 720
Cutaneous diphtheria, 724t
Cutaneous field, radicular, 582f
Cyanotic heart disease, 346-347
    tetralogy of Fallot, 349
Cyanotic spell, breath-holding, 245-247, 246b,
        246t
Cyproheptadine, 590t
Cystic fibrosis, 770-778
    complications of, 775t
    etiology of, 770
    genetics of, 49t
    newborn screening of, 149t
    organ systems in, 770t
Cystic ovary, 623
Cystitis, 687
Cystometrogram, 674-675
Cystourethrogram, 674
Cytokine
    allergy and, 694
    asthma and, 759, 759b
Cytomegalovirus, HIV and, 799

D

Dacryocystitis, 403, 405t, 406
Dandruff, 533, 534t
Dantrolene, 849
Data
    collection of, 16
    documentation of, 17-18
Day care, 250t

DDAVP, 791, 792t
Death
  grief and, 293-295
  injury causing, 186-187, 186t
  leading causes of, 186t
  suicide prevention and, 196-197
Decoction, herbal, 444
Decongestant, 642
  for sinusitis, 663-664
  for viral rhinitis, 662
Deep tendon reflex, 582b
Deformity, 62
  torsional, 547-548, 547f, 548t
Dehydration, incontinence and, 680-681
Delavirdine, 809t-810t
Delayed puberty, 363-364, 364t
Deltoid muscle strength testing, 551f
Demineralization of tooth, 220-221
Democratic parenting style, 23t
Demulcent, 655
Dental health, 220-228
  ankyloglossia and, 227
  antibiotic prophylaxis and, 227, 227f
  bleeding disorder and, 791
  bruxism and, 227
  cancer and, 823t, 825t
  caries and
    nursing bottle, 224-225, 224t, 225f
    prevention of, 221-222, 221t
    process of, 220-221
  eating disorder affecting, 226
  nonnutritive sucking and, 226-227
  oral care and, 222-224, 223t
  prenatal factors in, 220
  sickle cell disease and, 835
  smokeless tobacco affecting, 226
  tooth development and, 220
  trauma and, 225-226
Dental injury, sports-related, 203t
Denver Articulation Screening Exam, 242t
Denver II screening tool, 240, 241t
  in Down syndrome, 852
Deoxyribonucleic acid
  analysis of, 54, 54f, 55t, 56
    cystic fibrosis and, 772-773
    for HIV infection, 799-800
    muscular dystrophy and, 858
  illustration of, 54f
Departure stage of parenting, 21t
Dependence
  drug, 75. *See also* Substance abuse
  as parenting issue, 22
Dependent edema in pregnancy, 633
Depo-Provera, 274t
Depression, 584-586, 585b
  postpartum, 133
Dermatitis
  atopic
    differential diagnosis of, 695, 725
    management of, 698
  contact
    differential diagnosis of, 695
    management of, 698-699
  diaper rash, 514, 515t-516t, 517
  heat rash vs, 520t, 521
  prevention of, 491
  seborrheic, 533, 534t, 725
Dermatoglyphics, 117
Dermatophyte, 496

Desmopressin
  bleeding disorder and, 791
  for enuresis, 686
Detrusor contraction, 679, 680, 682
Development
  of adolescent, 269
  of adopted child, 289
  asthma affecting, 761-762
  constitutional delay of, 367, 368t
  cystic fibrosis and, 773
  diabetes and, 779, 781
  fetal alcohol syndrome and, 877
  of foster child, 302
  of gifted child, 312
  HIV infection and, 801
  learning disability and, 865
  mental retardation and, 868
  muscular dystrophy and, 859
  physical abuse and, 883
  poverty and, 885-886
  of preterm infant, 325, 326t, 327, 329
  rheumatic fever and, 828
  school readiness and, 236
  of sexually abused child, 888
  sickle cell disease and, 835-836
  spina bifida and, 870
  of stepfamily, 332-333
  tooth, 220, 220t
Developmental assessment, 137-139,
    139t-145t
  in autism, 842
  in Calgary model, 14
  Down syndrome and, 852
  of foster child, 302
  guidelines for, 139, 145t
  instruments for, 137-138, 137b, 137t, 138t
  learning disabilities and, 863
  in neuropsychiatric disorder, 583t
  process of, 138-139
  purpose of, 137
  of risk factors, 138-139
  of school readiness, 240, 241t-243t, 244
Developmental care protocol for preterm
    infant, 114-115
Developmental considerations
  in grief process, 293
  in injury, 187, 188t-192t
  in pain assessment, 76t
Developmental disorder
  autism, 841-844, 844b
  cerebral palsy, 844-845, 846t-847t, 848-850
  Down syndrome, 850-856, 851b, 852t,
    854t-855t
  enuresis with, 684
  learning disability, 862-866, 863b, 864t,
    865b, 866t
  mental retardation, 867-869, 867b,
    868b, 869t
  muscular dystrophy, 856-862, 858f, 858t,
    860t, 861t
  spina bifida, 869-875, 870b, 870t
    latex allergy in, 872, 873t-874t
Developmental domain, 864t
Developmental dysplasia of hip, 562,
    565t, 566
Developmental history in muscular dystro-
    phy, 857
Developmental screening, 154-155
Deviation, eye, 393-396, 394t

Dexedrine, for tic, 610t
Dextroamphetamine, 865t
Diabetes mellitus, 778-787
  cystic fibrosis and, 775t
  data on, 779-781, 780b, 782t, 783t
  etiology of, 779
  hospitalization for, 915
  incidence of, 779
  ketoacidosis and, 454t
  management of, 781, 783-787, 784b, 786b
  risk factors for, 779
*Diagnostic and Statistical Manual of Mental
    Disorders IV-TR*
  on autism, 841
  on separation anxiety, 259b
DIAL-3 screening tool, 240
Diaper rash, 514, 515t-516t, 517-518
Diaphragm, 273t
Diarrhea
  chronic, 464t
  differential diagnosis of, 426, 427t-432t, 464
  etiology of, 425
  gastroenteritis and, 418
  incidence of, 425-426
  management of, 426, 429, 431, 433-434
  risk factors for, 426
Diazepam, 602t-603t
Dicloxacillin
  cystic fibrosis and, 774
  for diaper impetigo, 517
  for furuncle, 498
Didanosine, 807t-808t
Diet. *See* Nutrition
Difficult child, 27b
Digit, jammed, 557t
Digit sucking, 226
  as parenting concern, 265-266
Dilatation, bronchial, in cystic fibrosis, 774
Dilemma, ethical, 71-73
Diphenhydramine
  for allergic rhinitis, 696t
  for vulvovaginitis, 639
Diphtheria, 723-724, 724t
Diphtheria, tetanus, pertussis vaccine, 157
  administration of, 164t
  contraindications to, 158t, 159t
  handling and storage of, 178t, 180t-181t
  HIV infection and, 801
  rules for, 160t
Diplegia in cerebral palsy, 846t-847t
Dipstick urine test, 671t
  hearing loss and, 377
Direct fluorescent antibody test, 377
Disabled child
  dental care for, 223-224
  Education for Handicapped Children Act
    for, 7
Disaccharide malabsorption, 464t
Discharge
  ear disorder with, 379-385
    differential diagnosis of, 380, 380t-381t, 382
    etiology of, 379
    incidence of, 379-380
    management of, 382-385, 383f, 384t
    risk factors for, 380
  nipple, 616, 618t
  vaginal, 638-639
    culture of, 615
    in pregnancy, 633

Discipline
  autism and, 843
  bleeding disorder and, 790t
  cancer and, 823t
  cultural factors in, 22, 24t, 41
  cystic fibrosis and, 773
  of foster child, 302
  in HIV infection, 802
  learning disability and, 865
  mental retardation and, 868
  muscular dystrophy and, 859
  as parenting concern, 252-253
  rheumatic fever and, 828
  sickle cell disease and, 835
  in stepfamily, 333
  types of, 28-29, 28b, 29b
  violence in home and, 337
Discoloration of teeth, 224
Disease prevention, cultural factors in, 41
Disintegrative disorder, childhood, 842
Disk, herniated, 559
Diskitis, 560t, 561
Dislocation
  of hip, 546, 547f
  shoulder, 556t
Disposition of newborn, 119t
Diurnal incontinence, 679-684, 680t
Divalproex sodium, 602t-603t
Diversity, cultural, 35-42. *See also* Cultural
    factors
Diverticulum, Meckel
  colic vs, 443
  differential diagnosis of, 413t-415t, 417
Divorce, 296-299
  family assessment and, 15-16
  incidence of, 296
  risk factors for, 297
DNA, illustration of, 54f
DNA testing, 54, 55t, 56
  in cystic fibrosis, 772-773
  for HIV infection, 799-800
  muscular dystrophy and, 858
Doctrine, *respondeat superior,* 4
Documentation
  of immunization, 175
  as legal issue, 4
  of vaccine reaction, 166t-168t, 182t-183t
Dog bite, 512
Domestic violence, 335-338
  incidence of, 335
  interpersonal, 195
  interview about, 336-337
  management of, 337-338
  physical abuse, 882-884
    behavior patterns in, 130-131
  prevention strategies for, 193b, 195-196
  risk factors for, 335
  signs of, 335-336
Dominant inheritance
  autosomal, 59t
  X-linked, 60t
Dorsal rhizotomy, selective, 849
Double-outlet right ventricle, 349, 350
Down syndrome, 850-856
  clinical findings in, 850b, 851t
  data on, 852-853
  developmental milestones in, 852t
  etiology of, 850
  genetics of, 46t

Down syndrome—cont'd
  incidence of, 850
  management of, 853-856, 854t-855t
  primary care implications of, 853
  risk factors for, 852
Doxycycline
  for acne, 502t
  Chlamydia trachomatis and, 275t, 638
  Lyme disease and, 729
Dressing, wet, 494
Drinking water, fluoride in, 221-222, 221t
Driving, 276
  diabetes and, 781
Drooling in cerebral palsy, 848
Drop attack, 600
Drowning
  near, 904, 906
  prevention of
    in adolescent, 192t
    by infant, 188t, 189t
    in preschool-aged child, 190t
    in school-aged child, 191t
    strategies for, 193b, 200
    by toddler, 190t
Drug abuse, 889-894, 890t. *See also* Drug-
    exposed infant
  diabetes and, 781
  by parent, 283-286, 284b, 285b
  violence in family and, 337
Drug-exposed infant, 315-321
  complications of abuse and, 316t
  differential diagnosis for, 318
  drug history of, 316-317
  incidence of, 315
  laboratory evaluation of, 317
  management of, 318-320
  neonatal abstinence score of, 319f
  physical examination of, 317
  primary care of, 318t
  risk factors for, 315
  social history of, 315
  symptoms of, 320t
Drug history, maternal, 316-317
Drug-induced disorder
  dental, 223
  diarrhea, 426
  irritability in, 712t
  nasal bleeding, 657t
  rhinitis, 660t-661t, 662, 663
  seizure as, 596b
Drug reaction
  anaphylactic, 695
  colic vs, 444
Drug-resistant *Streptococcus pneumoniae,* 379
Dry rash, 532
Duchenne's muscular dystrophy, 49t, 856-862
  limp with, 562, 565t
Duct, nasolacrimal, obstruction of, 403, 406
Duodenal hematoma, 454t
Duty to consult, 4
Dysbetalipoproteinemia, 356
Dyscalculia, 864
Dysfunctional uterine bleeding, 623
Dysgraphia, 864
Dyslexia, 864
Dysmenorrhea
  differential diagnosis of, 414t-415t, 417, 623
  management of, 418, 625
Dysmorphin, 859

Dysmorphology, facial, 877
Dysnomia, 864
Dysplasia
  cranioskeletal, 592b
  skeleal, 367, 368t, 369
Dysplastic nevus, 506t, 508
Dyspnea. *See* Breathing difficulty
Dyspraxia, 864
Dysthymic disorder, 585
Dystrophy, muscular, 856-862
  limp with, 562, 565t

E

Ear. *See also* Ear disorder
  autism and, 842
  cancer and, 816, 825t
  cystic fibrosis and, 771
  diabetes and, 782t
  Down syndrome and, 851b, 852, 855
  endocrine disorder and, 361
  neonatal assessment of, 111t, 116, 122t
  neuropsychiatric disorder and, 580
  in physical examination, 99t-100t
  of preterm infant, 324
  respiratory disorder and, 644
  in review of systems, 91t
  sickle cell disease and, 830
Ear canal, injury to, 386
Ear disorder
  aural diphtheria and, 724t
  cerumen impaction, 378-379
  diagnosis of, 376-377
  examination for, 376
  hearing loss with, 387-389, 388b, 388t
  pain and discharge with, 379-385
    differential diagnosis of, 380,
        380t-381t, 382
    etiology of, 379
    incidence of, 379-380
    management of, 382-385, 383f, 384t
    risk factors for, 380
  prevention of, 373
  traumatic, 386-387
Early infantile autism, 842
Earwax, 378-379
Easy child, 27b
Eating disorder, 751-757
  amenorrhea and, 622-623
  assessment of, 752t
  data on, 752-755
  dental disease in, 226
  diabetes and, 779
  etiology of, 751
  incidence of, 752
  management of, 755-758
  risk factors for, 752
Ecchymosis, 398-399
Echocardiography, 342
  in Down syndrome, 853
Ecomap, 14, 15f
Ecstasy, 890t
Ectoparasite, lice, 458, 459
Ectopic pregnancy, 629t
  differential diagnosis of, 414t-415t, 417
Eczema, 695, 725
Edema
  cerebral, 592b
    vomiting with, 454t
  in pregnancy, 633

Education
  asthma, 767, 767b
  cerebral palsy and, 848
  diabetes, 781
  hearing impairment and, 389
  parent
    about newborn, 132
    on immunization, 175
    for preterm infant, 329
  on seizures, 604b
  sexuality, 229
Education for Handicapped Children Act, 7
Edward syndrome, 46t
Efavirenz, 810t-811t
Effusion, otitis media with, 379
  differential diagnosis of, 381t
  management of, 384
Elbow
  injury to, 204t, 548, 557t
  range of motion of, 552f-553f
Electroencephalography
  autism and, 842
  in neuropsychiatric disorder, 582
Electromyogram, sphincter, 675
Electromyography, 555
  in neuropsychiatric disorder, 582
Electrophoresis
  hemoglobin, 151
  sickle cell disease and, 831t
Electrophysiologic audiometry, 376
Elimination
  altered urinary, 679-684, 680t
  cerebral palsy and, 848
  Down syndrome and, 853
  in newborn, 132
  in patient history, 93t
  urinary incontinence and, 679-685
Emancipated minor, 70
Embeddedness, cultural, 36
Embryonic development, 63t
Emergency, 897
  airway obstruction, 899-900, 899t
  burn injury, 900-901, 900f
  choking, 897-898
  coma, 901-902, 901b, 902t
  fracture, 906, 906f
  frostbite, 902-903, 902b
  head injury, 903-904, 903b
  hemorrhage, 898
  hyperthermia, 904, 905t
  near drowning, 904, 906
  respiratory arrest, 898-899, 898b
  shock, 906
Emergency contraception, 274t
EMLA for pain, 79b
Emotional communication, 16, 18b
Emotional development
  of preterm infant, 328-329
  school readiness and, 238t-239t
Emotional disorder. *See also* Psychological
    entries
  in autism, 843
  of infant, 131
Enalapril, 359t
Enamel of tooth, 220-221
Encephalopathy
  HIV and, 799
  hypertensive, 454t
  in Reye syndrome, 738
  as vaccine reaction, 168t, 177

Encopresis
  diarrhea with, 426, 432t
  differential diagnosis of, 421t-422t, 423
  management of, 434
Endocrine disorder, 360-372
  amenorrhea and, 623
  anorexia and, 754
  delayed puberty, 363-364, 364t
  diagnosis of, 362-363
  irritability in, 713t
  physical examination of, 361-362
  precocious puberty, 365-366, 365t
  risk factors for, 360
  short stature, 366-367, 368t, 369
  thyroid, 369, 370t, 371
  vomiting with, 454t, 456t
Endocrine system
  cancer treatment affecting, 825t
  malnutrition and, 215t
Endoscopic retrograde cholangiopancreatog-
    raphy, 412
Endoscopy, gastrointestinal, 412
Enema
  barium, 412
  for chronic constipation, 424
Energy level of gifted child, 312
Engagement, in family assessment, 11-12, 11t
Enterobiasis, 735. *See also* Pinworm
Enuresis, nocturnal, 684-686, 685t
Environment
  allergy and, 694
  asthma and, 766-767, 767b
  behavior and, 41b
  in family assessment, 13, 13b
  of gifted child, 312-313
  of homeless youth, 279
  in infant assessment, 133-134, 133t
  injury prevention and, 193
  lead poisoning and, 879-882, 881b
  obesity and, 720
  parenting affected by, 26
  school readiness and, 235, 235b, 236
Environmental heat illness, 904, 905t
Enzyme, cystic fibrosis and, 777
Enzyme, pancreatic, 776
Enzyme-linked immunosorbent assay, 496
Epicondylitis, 204t
Epididymitis, mumps vs, 731
Epiglottitis, 646, 647t
  airway obstruction in, 899t
Epilepsy
  breath-holding spell vs, 245, 246b, 246t
  vomiting with, 455t
Epileptic aphasia, acquired, 843
Epinephrine
  for anaphylaxis, 696
  in asthma, 653
Epiphyseal injury, 906, 906f
Epiphysis
  Salter-Harris fracture of, 570
  slipped capital femoral, 562, 563t-564t, 566
Epispadias, 627, 676
Epistaxis, 656-659, 657t-658t
  hemophilia and, 788t
Equinovarus, 567, 567t, 568
Equipment for newborn, 84b
Eruption
  on skin. *See* Rash
  of tooth, 220, 220t
Erythema infectiosum, 529, 530t

Erythema multiforme
  differential diagnosis of, 449t, 450
  management of, 451-452
Erythema nodosum, 744t
Erythrocyte sedimentation rate
  gastrointestinal disorder and, 411
  musculoskeletal disorder and, 555
  skin disorder and, 496
Erythromycin
  for acne, 502t
  for *Chlamydia trachomatis,* 275t, 638
  for furuncle, 499
  for pertussis, 736
  for pharyngitis, 666
Escherichia coli, 426, 427t, 431
Esophageal manometry, 412
Esophagitis, 458
  HIV and, 799
Esophagogastroduodenoscopy, 412
Esotropia, 394t, 395
Essential hypertension, 357
Estradiol, 362
Estrogen
  amenorrhea and, 624
  endocrine disorder and, 362
Ethambutol, 744t
Ethics, 69-73
  core values and, 69-70
  dilemmas of, 71-73
  nursing values, 70-71
  practitioner integrity, 71
Ethnicity
  definition of, 36
  in family assessment, 13, 13b
  genetic evaluation and, 45
Ethnocentrism, 36
Ethosuximide, 602t-603t
European culture, 39t
Evaporated milk, 214
Evidence-based practice, 8
Evoked otoacoustic emission test, 376-377
Evoked potentials
  ear disorder and, 376
  in preterm infant, 325
Ewing's sarcoma, 820t-821t
Exanthem subitum, 738
Excellence as nursing value, 71
Exchange transfusion for neonatal
    jaundice, 483
Exercise
  for adolescent, 271
  amenorrhea and, 623
  asthma and, 762, 769t
  autism and, 843
  bleeding disorder and, 790t
  cystic fibrosis and, 773
  diabetes and, 780, 780t, 781, 783-784
  Down syndrome and, 853
  eating disorder and, 753
  fetal alcohol syndrome and, 877
  for foster child, 303
  lead poisoning and, 881
  learning disability and, 865
  mental retardation and, 868
  muscular dystrophy and, 859
  in patient history, 93t
  sickle cell disease and, 835
  stretching, 545
Exotropia, 394t, 395
Expanded role of nurse, 5

Expectorant, 643, 655
Expiratory flow rate, peak, 645
    in asthma, 653, 768t
    asthma management and, 766, 766b
Expressive functioning, 16-17, 16f, 17t, 18b
Exstrophy, bladder, 676
Extended family
    child affecting, 15
    in family assessment, 12-13
External ear canal injury, 386
External ear infection
    differential diagnosis of, 380, 380t, 381t
    etiology of, 379
    management of, 382-383
External structure in family assessment,
        12-13, 13b
Extraocular muscle, 375
Extrapyramidal cerebral palsy, 845,
        846t-847t
Extraurethral incontinence, 679, 680t, 681
    management of, 683-684
Extremity
    cancer and, 823t
    cystic fibrosis and, 772
    Down syndrome and, 851b
    examination of, 552f-555f
    fracture of, 906, 906f
    leg ulcer and, 833t
    minor anomaly of, 61t
    of newborn, 113t, 117, 128t
        preterm, 324
    physical abuse and, 883
    in physical examination, 102t
Eye
    allergic conjunctivitis and, 695, 697
    cancer and, 816
    cancer treatment affecting, 825t
    conjunctivitis of, 403-407, 404t-405t
    cystic fibrosis and, 771
    deviation in, 393-396, 394t
    diabetes and, 781, 782t
    diagnosis of disorder of, 377-378
    Down syndrome and, 851b, 852, 855
    endocrine disorder and, 361
    examination of, 375-376
    injury to, 396, 397t, 398-399
    malnutrition and, 214t
    neuropsychiatric disorder and, 580
    newborn assessment of, 112t, 116,
        122t-123t
    in physical examination, 97t
    poison in, 198b
    preparticipation examination of, 549
    of preterm infant, 324
    prevention of disorder of, 374
    red, 403-407, 404t-405t
    respiratory disorder and, 644
    in review of systems, 91t
    sickle cell disease and, 830
    spina bifida and, 870
    sports-related injury to, 203t
    vision screening and, 154
    visual impairment and, 389-393, 390t-391t
Eyelashes
    lice in, 459
    neonatal assessment of, 123t
Eyelid
    infection of, 400, 401t, 402
    injury to, 396, 397t, 398
    neonatal assessment of, 123t

F
Face
    minor anomaly of, 61t
    neonatal assessment of, 111t, 122t
    in physical examination, 97t
Faces rating scale, 77t
Facial dysmorphology, 877
Facial trauma, oral, 225
Factor, clotting, 787, 791, 792t
Failure to refer, 4
Failure to thrive, 699-703
    cerebral palsy and, 845
    differential diagnosis of, 700, 701t-702t
    etiology of, 699
    incidence of, 699
    management of, 700, 702-703, 703t
    risk factors for, 700
Fainting, 600
Fall, prevention of
    by infant, 188t, 189t
    in preschool-aged child, 190t
    strategies for, 201
    by toddler, 189t
Famciclovir, 275t
Familial adenomatous polyposis, 49t
Familial dysbetalipoproteinemia, 356
Familial short stature, 367
Family
    addictive, 283-286, 284b, 285b
    cultural assessment of, 38, 39t, 40-42
    foster, 300
    gay or lesbian, 305-307
    of preterm infant, 327
Family assessment, Calgary model of,
        10-18
Family day care, 250t
Family development in Calgary model, 14
Family history, 90t-91t
Family life cycle, 14
Family planning, 271-272, 272b
    federal grants for, 7
Fantasy in stepfamily, 332
Farm injury, 203
Fasciitis, plantar, 205t
Fatigue, pallor and, 485t
Fear
    pallor with, 484, 485t, 486
    as parenting concern, 253-254, 254t
Febrile seizure, 600, 603-604
Fecal impaction
    differential diagnosis of, 421t-422t, 423
    management of, 424-425
Federal health program, 6-8
    children's health, 6
    Civilian Health and Medical Program
        Uniformed Services, 7
    Clinical Laboratory Improvement
        Amendments, 7
    family planning, 7
    food stamps, 7
    Maternal and Child Health Services Block
        Grant, 7
    Medicaid, 6
    Public Law 94-142, 7
    Public Law 101-476, 7-8
    school lunch, 6
    Title XX block grant, 7
    WIC, 6
Federal legislation on disabled children, 869t
Fee for service, 3

Feeding. *See also* Nutrition
    blood disorder and, 469
    cerebral palsy and, 846t
    Down syndrome and, 854
    of drug-exposed infant, 320t
    formulas for, 210t-211t
    gastroenteritis and, 418
    guidelines for, 214-216, 216t
    of newborn
        assessment of, 114t
        information for parent about, 132
        maladaptive parenting and, 130
        nursing bottle caries and, 224-226, 225f
    of preterm infant, 323, 327-328, 329
Female
    androgen insensitivity syndrome in, 66
    genitalia of
        ambiguous, 616
        examination of, 104t, 612-613, 613b, 614f
        in newborn, 113t, 127t-128t
    Turner syndrome in, 66
Femoral epiphysis, slipped capital, 562, 563t-
        564t, 566
Femoral head, avascular necrosis of, 833t
Femoral hernia, 440t
Femoral torsion, internal, 566-567, 567t
Ferritin, 470t
Fertility awareness, 273t
Fetal alcohol syndrome, 877-879, 878t
    in adopted child, 288
Fetoscopy, for genetic screening, 53t
Fever, 704-710
    cancer and, 817
    differential diagnosis of, 704-705,
        706t-708t
    etiology of, 704
    febrile seizure vs, 597t
    incidence of, 704
    management of, 705, 708-710, 708t
    pharyngoconjunctival, 666t
    rheumatic, 826-829, 827t
    risk factors for, 704
    scarlet
        rash from, 529, 531t
        roseola vs, 738
    seizure with, 600
Fexofenadine, 697t
Fiber, dietary, 423t
Fibroadenoma of breast, 616
Fibrosis, cystic, 770-778. *See also* Cystic fibrosis
Fifth disease, 529, 530t
Fighting, 254-255, 255b
    logical consequences for, 29
Filiform wart, 537, 538t, 540
Finger
    jammed, 557t
    neonatal assessment of, 117, 128t-129t
    range of motion of, 553f
Finger sucking, 226
Fire ant bite, 511-512
Fire injury. *See* Burn injury
Firearm injury
    prevention of
        in adolescent, 192t
        in preschool-aged child, 190t
        in school-aged child, 191t
    suicide and, 196
    violence in home and, 337
First aid for poisoning, 198b
First-catch urine specimen, 615

Fissure, anal
  differential diagnosis of, 421t-422t, 423
  management of, 425, 461
Fistula, urinary, 679
FLACC scale, 77t
Flat wart, 537, 538t, 540
Flatfoot, 568-569, 568t
Flea bite, 511
Fleet enema, 424
Flexion, back, 550f
Flossing, 224
Flovent, 776
Flow rate, peak expiratory, 645
  in asthma, 653, 768t
  asthma management and, 766, 766b
Fluconazole, 640
Fluid therapy for diarrhea, 426, 429
Flunisolide
  for allergic rhinitis, 697t
  asthma and, 764t
  cystic fibrosis and, 776
Flunitrazepam, 890t
Fluorescein staining of eye, 378b
Fluorescence in situ hybridization, 55t
Fluoride
  age to begin, 222
  for caries prevention, 221-222, 221t
  for preterm infant, 327
Fluticasone
  for allergic rhinitis, 697t
  asthma and, 764t, 765t
Fluvoxamine, 610t
Folic acid
  deficiency of
    differential diagnosis of, 472, 473t-475t, 476
    management of, 478
  in pregnancy, 628
  sickle cell disease and, 836
Follicle, sebaceous, 499
Follicle-stimulating hormone, 362
Folliculitis
  of scalp, 533, 534t
  superficial, 497
Fontanel
  assessment of, 116, 121t
  craniosynostosis and, 593
  neuropsychiatric disorder and, 579
  sunken, 41
Food
  allergy to, 695-696
    diarrhea caused by, 429t, 433
    management of, 699
    skin testing for, 496
  cultural differences in, 37t
Food guide pyramid, 209f, 271
Food stamps, 7
Foot
  axis of, 548, 548f
  deformity of, 568-569, 568t
  neonatal assessment of, 117, 129t
  in physical examination, 102t
Forced expiratory flow, 768t
Forced vital capacity, 768t
Foreign body
  anal
    differential diagnosis of, 459, 459t
    management of, 462
  aspiration of, 897-898
    by infant, 188t, 189t
    by preschool-aged child, 190t

Foreign body—cont'd
  aspiration of—cont'd
    strategies to prevent, 199
    by toddler, 190t
  in ear, 386-387
  in eye, 396, 397t
  vaginal, 636t
    differential diagnosis of, 459, 459t
    management of, 462, 638, 639
  vomiting and, 454t
Foreskin, adhesion to, 627, 627t, 628
Form, prenatal history, 108f-109f
Formoterol, 764t
Formula
  infant, 210t-211t, 216
  ponderal index, 115
Fosphenytoin, 602t-603t
Fourth-degree burn, 901b
Fracture, 906, 906f
  facial, 225-226
  joint pain from, 570
  management of, 571-572
  orbital, 396, 397t, 399
  prevention of, in adolescent, 192t
  sports-related, 203t
  stress, 204t
  tooth, 225
  wrist, 557t
Fragile X syndrome, 47t, 66
Freckles, 505, 506t
Friendship, marital, 14-15
Frostbite, 902-903, 902b
Fructose intolerance, 454t
Full-thickness burn, 901b
Funduscopic examination, 375
Funeral, 294
Fungal infection, 725, 726t, 727
  diagnosis of, 496
  nail, 527t, 528
  tinea, 518-519
    diagnosis of, 496
Furazolidone, 732t
Furosemide, 359t
Furuncle, 497, 498-499, 498t
  of ear, 380t

G
Gabapentin, 602t-603t
Gait disturbance
  limp, 561-566, 562b, 563t-565t
  toeing-in, 566-568, 567t
Galactose malabsorption, 464t
Galactosemia, 148t
Gallbladder disease, 413t-415t
  in sickle cell disease, 832t
Gamma benzene hexachloride, 459
Gamma hydroxybutyric acid, 890t
Gardnerella vaginalis
  differential diagnosis of, 637t
  management of, 640
Gastritis, 416t
Gastroenteritis
  diarrhea caused by, 426
  differential diagnosis of, 413t-415t, 417
  etiology of, 412
  management of, 418
  painful urination with, 688t
Gastroesophageal reflux, 457-458, 457b, 458t
  asthma and, 769t
  colic vs, 443

Gastroesophageal reflux—cont'd
  cystic fibrosis and, 775t
Gastrointestinal disorder, 409-466
  abdominal pain
    differential diagnosis of, 413t-416t,
      417-418
    etiology of, 412, 417
    incidence of, 417
    management of, 418-420
    risk factors for, 417
  bleeding with, 463t, 464, 465
  breath-holding spell and, 246b
  chest pain from, 345
  colic
    differential diagnosis of, 441, 442t-443t,
      443-444
    etiology of, 441
    incidence of, 441
    management of, 444-447, 445b, 446b
  constipation, 420-425
    differential diagnosis of, 420, 421t-422t,
      423
    etiology of, 420
    management of, 423-425, 423t
    risk factors for, 420
  cystic fibrosis and, 775t
  data about, 409-410
  diarrhea, 425-434. *See also* Diarrhea
  hernia, 434-441. *See also* Hernia
  hospitalization for, 915
  infection prevention and, 409
  jaundice with, 482
  laboratory evaluation of, 410-412
  mouth sores
    differential diagnosis of, 447, 448t-449t,
      450
    etiology of, 447
    incidence of, 447
    management of, 447-452
    risk factors for, 447
  nausea and vomiting, 452-458
    differential diagnosis of, 452, 453t-455t,
      455
    etiology of, 452, 456t
    incidence of, 452
    management of, 455-458, 457b, 458b
    risk factors for, 452
  perianal itch and pain, 458-462, 459t
  risk factors for, 409
  stool change with, 462, 463t, 464-466, 464t
  vomiting with, 456t
Gastrointestinal system
  in anorexia, 754
  bleeding disorder and, 795t
  cancer treatment affecting, 825t
  cystic fibrosis and, 770t, 771
  of drug-exposed infant, 320t
  malnutrition and, 215t
  of preterm infant, 324
  in review of systems, 91t
  spina bifida and, 870
Gay parent, 305-307
Gay youth, 279
Gel, 494
Gender
  in family assessment, 12, 12b
  X-linked disorder and, 60t
Gene therapy
  in cystic fibrosis, 776
  muscular dystrophy and, 860

Generalized seizure, 600
Genetic counseling, 44, 52, 52f
Genetic disorder, 56-67
  in adolescent, 66
  allergy as, 694
  approach for, 66-67
  assessment of, 65-66
  autism, 841-844
  characteristics of, 59f-60f
  counseling for
    indications for, 45t
    process of, 52f
    purpose of, 45, 52
  cystic fibrosis, 770-778. *See also* Cystic
    fibrosis
  family history in, 57
  glucose-6-phosphate dehydrogenase defi-
    ciency, 471
  hematuria with, 677
  hemoglobin traits, 471-472
  hemophilia, 787-796
  hereditary spherocytosis
    differential diagnosis of, 473t-475t, 476
    incidence of, 471
    management of, 479
  jaundice with, 482
  management of, 66
  muscular dystrophy and, 858-861. *See also*
    Muscular dystrophy
  in newborn or infant
    approach for, 65f
    assessment of, 59-62
    classification of, 64t
    embryonic development and, 63f
    management of, 62, 65-66
    minor anomaly, 61t
    presentation of, 59-61
  pedigree and, 56f, 57, 58f
  prenatal testing for, 56
  presentation of, 65
  screening vs testing for, 52-54, 53t, 54f
  sickle cell, 829-838. *See also* Sickle cell
    disease
  spherocytosis
    differential diagnosis of, 473t-475t, 476
    incidence of, 471
  types of, 46t-51t
Genetic testing, 54, 55t, 56
  for cystic fibrosis, 772-773
  for muscular dystrophy, 858
Genetics
  definition of, 44
  muscular dystrophy and, 860
  role of, 44
Genital herpes, 275t, 276, 618-620, 620t
Genital wart, 619, 620t, 621
Genitalia
  ambiguous, 616
  endocrine disorder and, 362
  examination of, 612-613, 613b, 614f
  gastrointestinal disorder and, 410
  neonatal assessment of, 113t, 127t-128t
  physical abuse and, 883
  in physical examination, 103t-104t
Genitourinary system
  cystic fibrosis and, 772
  diabetes and, 782t
  Down syndrome and, 852
  in review of systems, 91t-92t
  spina bifida and, 870

Genogram
  of addictive family, 284
  in family assessment, 14
Genu valgum, 573-574, 573t
Genu varum, 573, 573t
German measles. *See* Rubella
Gestational age, 630t
  assessment of, 110
Giant pigmented nevus, 507t
Giardiasis, 732-733, 732b, 733t
  diarrhea with, 431t
Gifted child, 309-314
  behavioral characteristics of, 310b-311b
  data on, 309-312
  incidence of, 309
  risk factors for, 309
Gingivitis, 224
  necrotizing ulcerative
    differential diagnosis of, 447, 449t, 450
    management of, 451
  streptococcal
    differential diagnosis of, 447-448
    management of, 451
Gingivostomatitis, herpetic
  differential diagnosis of, 447, 449t
  management of, 450-451
Glasgow Coma Scale, 902t
Glasses pain rating scale, 77t
Glioma, 391t, 392, 393
Glomerulonephritis, poststreptococcal, 677
Glossopharyngeal nerve, 105t
Glucagon in diabetes, 785
Glucose
  in diabetes, 785
  malabsorption of, 464t
Glucose-6-phosphate dehydrogenase defi-
  ciency
    differential diagnosis of, 473t-475t, 476
    genetics of, 49t
    incidence of, 471
    management of, 479
Glucose tolerance, 779
Glycosylated hemoglobin, 783t
Goal
  of family assessment, 11
  of family intervention, 18
  of parenting, 22
Goal-setting in eating disorder, 756-757
Goiter, 369
Gonadal dysfunction, 363-364
Gonadotropin, human chorionic, 615
Gonadotropin-releasing hormone analog, 366
Goniometry, 555
Gonococcal conjunctivitis, 403, 404t
Gonococcal urethritis, 625, 626, 690
Gonorrhea, 272, 275, 275t
  conjunctivitis caused by, 403, 404t
  culture of, 615
  differential diagnosis of, 637t
  urethritis caused by, 625, 626
  vulvovaginal symptoms of
    in adolescence, 639-640
    in prepubsecence, 638
Goodness of fit, 26
Gower maneuver, 858, 858f
Grade retention, 240
Graves' disease, 370t, 371
Great arteries, transposition of, 349
Grief, 293-295
Groin pull, 558t

Group A beta-hemolytic streptococcus, 738
  rheumatic fever and, 826-829, 827t
Growing pains, 569, 570t
Growth
  of adolescent, 269
  asthma affecting, 761-762
  autism and, 843
  bleeding disorder and, 791
  cerebral palsy and, 848
  cystic fibrosis and, 773
  delay of, 367
  diabetes and, 779, 781
  Down syndrome and, 851b, 853
  failure to thrive and, 699-703
  fetal alcohol syndrome and, 877
  of foster child, 301-302, 302
  of gifted child, 312
  HIV infection and, 801
  lead poisoning and, 881
  learning disability and, 865
  mental retardation and, 868
  monitoring of, 146-147
  muscular dystrophy and, 859
  physical abuse and, 883
  poverty and, 885-886
  of preterm infant, 325, 329
  rheumatic fever and, 828
  school readiness and, 236
  of sexually abused child, 888
  sickle cell disease and, 835
  spina bifida and, 870
Growth factor, endocrine disorder and, 362
Growth hormone deficiency, 367, 368t, 369
  obesity in, 719t, 720
GROWTH, 361
Guaifenesin, 643
Guanfacine, for tic, 609t
Guidance. *See* Anticipatory guidance
Guidelines
  clinical practice, 8
  for developmental assessment, 139, 145t
Gums
  inflammation of, 224
  in physical examination, 98t
Gynecomastia, 616-617

H
Habit, lip, 227
Haemophilus influenzae type b, 169t
  ear infection with, 379
  meningitis and, 730
  pneumonia caused by, 647
Haemophilus influenzae type b vaccine, 161t
  administration of, 164t-165t
  contraindications to, 158t, 159t
  handling and storage of, 178t-179t
  reporting adverse event, 167t
  rules for, 161t
Hair
  neonatal assessment of, 120t, 121t
  in physical examination, 96t
Hair follicle inflammation, 497
Hair loss, 518-520, 519t, 725
Hair testing of drug-exposed infant, 317
Haitian culture
  newborn care in, 41b
  postpartum practices in, 40b
  symptoms in, 42b
Hallucinogen exposure of infant, 316t
Haloperidol, 609t

Hand
   neonatal assessment of, 117, 128t-129t
   in physical examination, 102t
   range of motion of, 553f
   sports injury to, 548, 557t
Hand-foot-mouth disease
   differential diagnosis of, 447, 448t
   management of, 451
   sore throat with, 666t
Handling of vaccine, 177, 178t-181t
Hashimoto's disease, 369, 370t
Head
   blood disorder and, 469
   cancer and, 816, 823t
   cystic fibrosis and, 771
   diabetes and, 782t
   endocrine disorder and, 361
   minor anomaly of, 61t
   neonatal assessment of, 111t, 116
   physical abuse and, 883
   in physical examination, 96t-97t
   sickle cell disease and, 830
   spina bifida and, 870
Head circumference
   abnormal, 590-595, 591b, 592b,
     593t, 594b
   neonatal assessment of, 115, 120t-121t
   neuropsychiatric disorder and, 579
   screening of, 147
Head injury
   coma in, 901-902, 901b, 902t
   ear trauma and, 386
   as emergency, 903-904, 903b
   prevention of, strategies for, 201
   sports-related, 203t
   vomiting with, 453t
Head lice, 523, 524t, 525
   differential diagnosis of, 533, 534t
Headache, 587-590, 587t, 588b, 588t, 589b,
   590t
   bleeding disorder and, 795t
   malignancy and, 822t
   vomiting with, 454t
Healing of sport-related injury, 545
Health care
   billing and reimbursement for, 3-4
   culturally congruent, 38, 39t, 40-42
Health care belief, 36-37, 36t
Health Care Financing Administration, 4
   tele-health/medicine and, 6
Health history, 86t-94t
Health maintenance organization, 5
Health People 2010, 8
Health professional shortage area, rural, 4
Hearing
   assessment of, 375
   autism and, 842
   cancer treatment affecting, 825t
   Down syndrome and, 855
   neonatal screening of, 116
   of preterm infant, 324
   in review of systems, 92t
   testing of, 153-154
Hearing loss
   assessment of, 388b
   classification of, 388b
   clinical manifestations of, 374b
   differential diagnosis of, 388
   early identification of, 374
   etiology of, 387

Hearing loss—cont'd
   incidence of, 387
   management of, 388-389
   risk factors for, 387-388
Heart
   blood disorder and, 469
   cancer and, 816
   cystic fibrosis and, 772
   Down syndrome and, 852
   endocrine disorder and, 362
   newborn assessment of, 112t
   palpation of, 342
   in physical examination, 101t
   respiratory disorder and, 644
   rheumatic fever and, 828
   sickle cell disease and, 830
Heart murmur, 350-351, 352t, 353t
Heart sounds, 126t
Heartburn in pregnancy, 632t
Heat illness, 904, 905t
   vomiting with, 455t
Heat rash, 520-521, 520t
Height
   cystic fibrosis and, 771
   diabetes and, 782t
   Down syndrome and, 852
   endocrine disorder and, 361, 362
   gastrointestinal disorder and, 410
   neuropsychiatric disorder and, 579
   of newborn, 115, 118t
   screening of, 146-147
   short stature, 366-367, 368t, 369
Helicobacter pylori, 411
Helmet, sports, 399
Hemangioma, 504, 505, 505t
Hematemesis in cystic fibrosis, 775t
Hematocrit
   blood disorder and, 470t
   cardiovascular examination and, 342
   screening of, 150
Hematologic disorder, 468-488. *See also*
   Blood disorder
Hematoma
   duodenal, 454t
   scalp, 593, 594
Hematuria, 677-679, 677b, 678t
Hemoglobin
   blood disorder and, 470t
   cardiovascular examination and, 342
   diabetes and, 783t
   screening of, 150
   sickle cell disease and, 831t
Hemoglobin H disease, 477
Hemoglobin trait, inherited
   differential diagnosis of, 473t-475t, 476-477
   incidence of, 471-472
   management of, 479-480
Hemoglobinopathy, newborn screening
   for, 148t
Hemolytic anemia, 473t-475t, 476, 479
Hemolytic disease of newborn, 482
Hemophilia, 49t, 787-796. *See also* Bleeding
   disorder
Hemoptysis in cystic fibrosis, 775t
Hemorrhage, subarachnoid, 454t. *See also*
   Bleeding
Hemorrhoid
   differential diagnosis of, 459, 459t
   incidence of, 458
   management of, 461

Hemotympanum, 386
Hemplegia in cerebral palsy, 846t-847t
Henoch-Schönlein purpura, 486, 487t, 488
   differential diagnosis of, 415t-416t, 417-418
   management of, 419
Hepatitis, 746-747, 747t
   gastrointestinal disorder and, 411
   gay or lesbian family and, 306
   testing foster child for, 302
Hepatitis A vaccine, 162t
   HIV infection and, 801
   rules for, 162t, 170
Hepatitis B vaccine
   administration of, 165t
   characteristics of, 165, 170
   contraindications to, 158t, 159t
   reporting adverse event, 167t
   rules for, 162t
Herbal decoction for colic, 444
Hereditary disease. *See* Genetic disorder
Hermaphroditism, 616
Hernia, 434-441
   development of, 439f
   differential diagnosis of, 435, 436t-438t,
     439, 441t
   etiology of, 435
   examination for, 612
   femoral, differential diagnosis of, 440t
   incidence of, 435
   inguinal
     androgen insensitivity syndrome and, 66
     development of, 439t
     differential diagnosis of, 435, 436t-438t
     management of, 439t-440t
   management of, 439-441
   risk factors for, 435
   umbilical
     differential diagnosis of, 440t
     management of, 440-441
Herniated disk, 559, 560t, 561
Heroin, 890t
Herpangina
   differential diagnosis of, 447, 448t
   management of, 451
   sore throat with, 666t
Herpes simplex virus
   conjunctivitis caused by, 403, 404t, 405t
   genital, 275t, 276, 618-620, 620t
   impetigo and, 541
Herpes zoster
   chickenpox vs, 745t
   conjunctivitis with, 407
Herpesvirus antigen direct fluorescent antibody test, 377
Herpetic gingivostomatitis
   differential diagnosis of, 447, 449t
   management of, 450-451
Herpetic whitlow, 527t, 528
Hib vaccine, 159, 159t
HIDA scan, 412
High-density lipoprotein, 354, 355t, 356
High-risk register hearing screen, 376
Hinman syndrome, 679
Hip
   developmental dysplasia of, 562, 565t, 566
   infant examination of, 546, 546f
   injury to, 558t
   neonatal assessment of, 117, 117f
   pain or clicking in, 569-570
   rotation of, 547, 547f

Hirschsprung's disease
  constipation with, 425
  diarrhea with, 426
  differential diagnosis of, 421t-422t, 423
  management of, 434
  stool of, 464
Hispanic culture, 24t-25t
  assessment of, 39t
  symptoms in, 42b
Histamine, 694
Histiocytosis, langerhans cell, 533, 534t
Histologic examination, gastrointestinal, 411
History
  blood disorder and, 469
  of drug-exposed infant, 315-316
  in endocrine disorder, 361
  family, 90t-91t
    of preterm infant, 324
  health, 86t-94t
  maternal drug, 316-317
  pain, 75-76
  prenatal, 108f-109f
  of preterm infant, 323
HIV infection, 796-815. *See also*
    Human immunodeficiency virus
    infection
Hives, 521-522, 522t, 696
Hoarseness, 668, 668t, 669
Hodgkin's lymphoma, 820t-821t
Home assessment, 133-134, 133t
Homelessness, 279, 884-886
Homicide, prevention of, 195-196
Homocystinuria, 149t
Homophobia, 306-307
Homosexual parent, 305-308
Homosexual youth, 279
Honesty as nursing value, 70
Hookworm, 734-735
Hordeolum, 400, 401t
Hormone
  antidiuretic, 684
  growth, 367, 368t, 369
  menstrual cycle and, 622
  precocious puberty and, 366
  vaginal bleeding and, 623
Hospitalization
  asthma causing, 760
  for failure to thrive, 700
  latex allergy and, 873b
  patient history of, 89t
  preparation for, 908-915, 909b, 910b,
    911t-913t, 914b
  rheumatic fever and, 828
  for suicide attempt, 606b
Hostility, parental, 26
Hot and cold theory of imbalance, 37
Human bite, 509t-510t, 511, 512
Human chorionic gonadotropin
  endocrine disorder and, 362-363
  in pregnancy testing, 615
Human immunodeficiency virus infection,
    796-815
  in adolescent, 276, 802
  categories of, 800t, 801t
  data about, 798
  discipline and, 802
  diseases indicating, 798-799
  drugs for, 803-805, 803t-813t
  etiology of, 796-797, 797f
  gay or lesbian family and, 306

Human immunodeficiency virus
    infection—cont'd
  growth and, 801
  immunization and, 801-802
  incidence of, 797-798, 797t
  management of, 803-815
  nutrition and, 802
  pain and, 803
  psychosocial issues of, 803
  risk factors for, 798
  safety and, 802
  school and, 802
  screening for, 802
  sexuality and, 802
  testing for, 799, 801
  testing foster child for, 302
Human leukocyte antigen, 555
Human papillomavirus, 275-276, 275t
Humidifier, for croup, 651
Hydralazine, 359t
Hydrocele, 439f
  differential diagnosis of, 435,
    436t-438t
Hydrocephalus
  differential diagnosis of, 592, 592b
  management of, 594
  in spina bifida, 870
Hydrochlorothiazide, 359t
Hydronephrosis, 675
Hydroxyurea, 836
Hydroxyzine
  for allergic rhinitis, 696t
  for vulvovaginitis, 635, 639
Hyocyamine sulfate, 682
Hyperbilirubinemia, 147, 150t
  management of, 150t
  neonatal, management of, 482-483, 482t
Hypercalciuria, 677, 678t
Hypercholesterolemia, 356
Hypergonadotropic hypogonadism, 363
Hyperlipidemia, 351-354, 355t, 356
Hyperoxia test, 342
Hypersensitivity, 694
  lymphadenopathy in, 715t-717t
  skin testing for, 496
Hypertension, 356-358, 358t, 359t
Hypertensive encephalopathy, vomiting
    with, 454t
Hyperthermia, 904, 905t
Hyperthyroidism, 368t, 369, 370t, 371
Hypertonicity in drug-exposed infant, 320t
Hypertriglyceridemia, 356
Hypertrophy
  of breast, 617, 618t
  diabetes and, 784
  muscular dystrophy and, 858
Hypoglycemia
  diabetes and, 779, 780t, 784, 786, 786b
  in newborn, 147
Hypogonadism, 363
Hypospadias, 627, 676
Hypothalamus in delayed puberty, 363
Hypothyroid symptoms in anorexia, 754
Hypothyroidism, 368t, 369, 370t, 371
  newborn screening for, 148t
  obesity in, 719, 719t
Hypotonia in cerebral palsy, 846t
Hypotonic-hyporesponsive collapse, 177
Hypoventilation in muscular
    dystrophy, 860

I
Ibuprofen
  for fever, 705, 708t
  for lymphadenopathy, 717
  for rash, 532
  for recurrent headache, 590t
IDEA, 7-8
Identity issues for adopted child, 291-292
Idiopathic thrombocytopenic purpura, 486,
    487t, 488
IgE-mediated reaction, 694
IgG for rubeola, 741
Iimaging, in neuropsychiatric disorder, 581
Illness
  diabetes and, 785-786
  patient history of, 89t
illness, bleeding disorder and, 791
Imaging. *See also* Radiographic evaluation
  of ear, 377
  magnetic resonance
    cardiovascular, 342
    endocrine disorder and, 362
    in neuropsychiatric disorder, 581
  in neuropsychiatric disorder, 583t
  radionuclide scan of kidney, 674
Imaging-making stage of parenting, 21t
Imipramine, 682, 686
Imiquimod, 275t
Immune system
  allergy and, 694-699
  asthma and, 759, 759b
  cancer treatment affecting, 825t
Immunization
  for adolescent, 268-269
  of adopted child, 290
  American Academy of Pediatrics recom-
    mendations for, 171t
  asthma and, 762
  benefits of, 157
  bleeding disorder and, 791
  cancer and, 823t
  chickenpox, 161t, 170, 746
  contraindications for, 157, 158t-159t
  cystic fibrosis and, 773
  diabetes and, 781
  diphtheria, 160t
  diphtheria-tetanus, 157-159, 158t
  documentation of, 175
  dosage and side effects of, 164t
  Down syndrome and, 853
  of foster child, 302
  gay or lesbian family and, 306
  Haemophilus influenzae type B, 159, 161t
  handling and storage of, 177, 178t-181t
  hepatitis A, 162t, 170
  hepatitis B, 159t, 162t, 165, 170
  HIV infection and, 801-802
  in immunocompromised child, 173, 175
  influenza, 163t, 170
  Lyme disease, 163t, 729
  measles, 741
  measles, mumps, and rubella, 159t,
    160t, 170
  meningococcal, 163t, 170
  mental retardation and, 868
  minimum age for, 174t
  mumps, 731
  muscular dystrophy and, 859
  neuropsychiatric disorder and, 576
  parent education about, 175

Immunization—cont'd
patient history of, 89t
pertussis, 736
pneumococcal, 163t, 170
polio, 158t, 161t, 164, 737
poverty and, 886
of preterm infant, 175, 323, 328
reporting adverse events and, 182f-183f
rubella, 740
rules for, 160t-163t
scheduling of, 172t, 173, 173t, 174t
screening questionnaire about, 176f
sickle cell disease and, 830, 835
spina bifida and, 870-871
standards for, 177, 177b
technique for, 175
terminology about, 157
tetanus, 160t, 743t
thimerosal in, 173
tuberculosis skin testing and, 175
varicella, 161t, 170, 746
Immunoblot test for Lyme disease, 496
Immunocompromised patient, 173, 175
Immunofluorescent antibody testing, 859
Immunoglobulin G for rubeola, 741
Immunotherapy for allergic rhinitis, 697
Impaction, fecal
cerebral palsy and, 849
differential diagnosis of, 421t-422t, 423
management of, 424-425
Impedance analysis, sonar, 376
Impetigo, 540-542, 541t
differential diagnosis of, 540-541, 541t, 725
etiology of, 540
management of, 540-541
rash of, 531t
Impingement, shoulder, 204t
In-home care, 250t
Inborn error of metabolism
pernicious anemia as, 476
vomiting with, 454t
Incest, 886-889. *See also* Sexual abuse
Incidence to service, 4
Incontinence, urinary
differential diagnosis of, 680-681, 680t, 681t
etiology of, 679-680
incidence of, 680
management of, 681-684
Indemnity insurance, 5
Independence as parenting issue, 22
Index, ponderal, of newborn, 115
Indinavir, 812t
Indirect billing, 4
Individual education plan, 7
Individual with Disabilities Education Act, 7-8
Indwelling catheter
cancer and, 824
for urinary retention, 684
Infant
anemia screening of, 469b
autism in, 841-842
blood in stool of, 463t
burn injury of, 900, 900f
caloric requirement for, 781
causes of death of, 186t
choking by, 897
colic in, 441-447
developmental counseling about, 145t
developmental milestones for, 139t

Infant—cont'd
diarrhea in, 430t
Down syndrome and, 854b
drug-exposed infant and, 315-321. *See also*
Drug-exposed infant
eczema in, 695
feeding of, 214-216, 216t
fetal alcohol syndrome in, 878
formulas for, 210t-211t
gastroenteritis in, 418
hearing assessment of, 375
hearing loss in, 374b
HIV in, 799, 801
hospitalization of, 911t
injury prevention for, 188t-189t
injury to, 188t-189t
irritability in, 710t, 711t
jitteriness in, 600
language development of, 142t
laxative for, 424, 424t
motor vehicle safety for, 194
neuropsychiatric disorder and, 576
nonnutritive sucking by, 226
nose drops in, 642
nutrition for, 214-216, 216t
oral care for, 222
pain in, 74, 76t
management of, 80t
parenting tasks and, 21t
physical development of, 140t
separation anxiety in, 909b
sexuality and, 230t
sickle cell disease and, 835
skin infection in, prevention of, 490
sleep habits in, 260
solid food for, 214, 216t
sunburn prevention for, 492
vomiting in, 456t
Infantile spasm, 599, 601
Infection, 723-748
abscess, 496-499, 498t
bleeding disorder and, 793
blood disorder and, 469
breast, 616
colic vs, 441
cough with, 655
diarrhea caused by
differential diagnosis of, 426, 427t-428t
management of, 426, 429, 431, 433
diphtheria, 723-724, 724t
ear
differential diagnosis of, 380, 380t, 381t,
382
etiology of, 379
incidence of, 379-380
management of, 382-385, 383f, 385t
risk factors for, 380
eyelid, 400, 401t, 402
failure to thrive and, 703t
fever in, 705, 706t-708t
fungal, 725, 726t, 727
gastroenteritis, 412, 413t-415t, 417
genital, 618-621, 620t
HIV, 796-815. *See also* Human immunodeficiency virus infection
as indicator of HIV infection, 798-799
influenza, 727-728, 728t
irritability in, 712t
jaundice with, 482

Infection—cont'd
laryngitis, 667-669, 668t
lice and, 523
Lyme disease, 728-730, 729t
lymphadenopathy in, 715t-717t, 717
meningitis, 730-731
mumps, 731
nail, 526-528, 527t
nasal bleeding in, 657t
oral, differential diagnosis of, 447-448
pallor and, 484
parasitic, 731-735, 732b, 732t, 734t
pertussis, 735-737, 736t
poliovirus, 737, 737t
poststreptococcal glomerulonephritis, 677
preterm infant and, 329
purpura and, 487t, 488
respiratory, irritability in, 712t
Reye syndrome with, 738
rhinitis, 659, 660t-661t
roseola, 738-739, 739t
rubella, 739-740, 740t
prenatal exposure to, 374
scabies, 741-742m 742t
scarlet fever, 738
septic arthritis
differential diagnosis of, 562, 563t-564t
management of, 565
sexually transmitted, 272, 275-276, 275t
sickle cell disease and, 833t
skin, prevention of, 490-491
sport-related injury and, 545
tetanus, 742-743, 743t
thrombocytopenia and, 486
tonsillopharyngitis
differential diagnosis of, 414t-415t, 417
management of, 419
tuberculosis, 743-744, 744t
urinary tract. *See* Urinary tract infection
vaginal bleeding and, 623
varicella zoster, 745-746, 746t
vomiting with, 453t, 456t
Infectious mononucleosis
differential diagnosis of, 448t, 450
management of, 452
sore throat with, 666t
Infertility, adoption and, 290
Inflammation
asthma and, 758-759
balanoposthitis, 627-628, 627t
cystic fibrosis and, 774
meningeal, 376b
painful urination with, 687
pelvic inflammatory disease, 635
superficial folliculitis, 497
vomiting with, 453t
Inflammatory bowel disease
diarrhea with, 426, 464
management of, 434, 465
Influence in family, 17, 18b
Influenza, 727-728, 728t
Lyme disease vs, 729t
Influenza vaccine, 163t
characteristics of, 170
handling and storage of, 178t-179t
HIV infection and, 801
Informed permission, 69
Ingestion, toxic
by adolescent, 192t

Ingestion, toxic—cont'd
  first aid for, 198b
  by infant, 188t, 189t
  by preschool-aged child, 190t
  by school-aged child, 191t
  by toddler, 190t
Ingrown toenail, 205t
Inguinal hernia
  androgen insensitivity syndrome and, 66
  development of, 439t
  differential diagnosis of, 435, 436t-438t
  management of, 439t-440t
Inhalation injury, 188t
  first aid for, 198b
  prevention of
    in adolescent, 192t
    by infant, 188t, 189t
    in preschool-aged child, 190t
    in school-aged child, 191t
    by toddler, 190t
Inhibitor in bleeding disorder, 793
Injectable contraceptive, 274t
Injury prevention, 186-207. *See also* Trauma
  to ears, 374
  environment and, 193
  to eyes, 374
  farm, 203
  strategies for, 193-199
    bicycle, skateboarding, 195
    burn injury, 199-200
    drowning, 200-201
    falls, head injury, 201
    motor vehicle accidents, 193-194
    pedestrian accidents, 194-195
    poisoning, 197, 197b, 198b
    sports-related, 201-202, 202t-205t
    suffocation and choking, 199
    suicide, 196-197
    violence-related injury, 195-196
  toxic plants and, 192t
Innocent heart murmur, 351, 352t, 353t
Insect bite, 508, 509t-510t
Insect in ear, 387
Insight of gifted child, 312
Inspection, 546-548
Inspiration-to-expiration ratio in cystic fibrosis, 772
Insulin, 780t, 784
Insurance
  managed care and, 5
  personal malpractice, 4-5
  reimbursement by, 3-4
Integrity, practitioner, 71
Integumentary system, 490-543
  hair loss and, 518-520, 519t
  nails and
    ingrown, 205t
    injury or infection of, 526-528, 527t
    neonatal assessment of, 117, 129t
  skin and. *See* Skin *entries*
Intercondylar distance, 548
Interdependent stage of parenting, 21t
Intermalleolar distance, 548
Internal femoral torsion, 566-567, 567t
Internal tibial torsion, 566
International Classification of Diseases, 3
Interpersonal violence, 195
Interpreter, 42
Interpretive stage of parenting, 21t

Interstitial pneumonitis, lymphoid, 798
Intervention, Calgary model of, 18-19
Interventive question, 18
Intervertebral disk, herniated, 559, 560t, 561
Interview about family violence, 336-337
Intoxication
  irritability in, 712t
  vomiting with, 454t
Intracranial hemorrhage, 795t
Intradermal nevus, 506t, 508
Intranasal corticosteroid, 697, 697t
Intrauterine device, 274t
Intrauterine pregnancy, 628, 629t
Intravenous pyelography, 674
Intruded tooth, 225
Intussusception
  colic vs, 443
  differential diagnosis of, 413t-415t, 417
  stool change and, 464
Inventory, neuropsychiatric symptom, 577t-580t
Ipratropium, 765t
Iron-deficiency anemia
  differential diagnosis of, 472, 473t-475t
  incidence of, 471
  irritability in, 713t
  management of, 478
  otitis media and, 384
Iron supplement
  for abnormal bleeding, 624
  for iron-deficiency anemia, 478
Irritability, 710-714
  causes of, 710t, 711, 711t
  differential diagnosis of, 712-713, 712t-713t
  infant, 441-447. *See also* Colic
  management of, 713-714
Irritable bowel syndrome
  diarrhea with, 426, 432t, 464-465, 464t
  management of, 433-434, 465
Irritant dermatitis, 514, 515t-516t, 517
Irritation
  penile, 627-628, 627t
  vaginal, 636t
  vulvovaginal, 638
Islamic culture, 40b
Isoniazid, 744t
Isotretinoin, 502t, 504
Itch, perianal, 458-459, 460t, 461

J

Jammed finger, 557t
Jaundice
  neonatal, 480-483
  in newborn
    differential diagnosis of, 480, 481t
    etiology of, 480
    incidence of, 480
    information for parent about, 132
    risk factors for, 480
Jaw fracture, 225-226
Jewish culture, 40b
Jitteriness, 600
Joint
  arthritis of
    juvenile rheumatoid, 562, 563t-564t, 565-566
    septic, 562, 563t-564t
    sports-related, 204t
    as vaccine adverse event, 169t

Joint—cont'd
  bleeding disorder and, 794t
  fluid aspiration from, 555
  in musculoskeletal examination, 546
  pain and swelling of, 570-572, 571t
  in physical examination, 102t
Joint Commission on Accreditation of Healthcare Organizations, 74
Jones criteria for rheumatic fever, 827t
Junctional nevus, 505, 506t, 508
Justice, 69
Juvenile rheumatoid arthritis, 562, 563t-564t, 565-566

K

Kangaroo care, 115
Kanner syndrome, 842
Karyotype, 615
Kasabach-Merritt syndrome, 507t
Kawasaki's disease, 345
  differential diagnosis of, 449t, 450
  irritability in, 712t
  management of, 451
  rash from, 529, 530t
Kegel exercise, 683
Kerion, 541
Kernicterus, 482
Kernig sign, 376b
Ketamine, 890t
Ketoacidosis, 454t
Kidney. *See also* Urinary disorder
  neonatal assessment of, 127t
  polycystic, 677
Klinefelter syndrome, 47t, 66
Klippel-Trénaunay-Weber syndrome, 507t
Knee injury, 548-549, 548f, 558t
Kwell, 459
Kyphosis, Scheuermann, 574-575, 575t

L

Laceration, 525-526
  renal, 677
Lachman test, 549
Lacrimal sac, 375
Lactobacillus acidophilus, 220
Lactose intolerance, 426, 432t
Lactose malabsorption, 464t
Lactulose, 424t
Lamivudine, 808t
Lamotrigine, 602t-603t
Landau-Kleffner syndrome, 843
Langerhans cell histiocytosis, 533, 534t
Language
  autism and, 841, 842
  cerebral palsy and, 848, 849
  hearing assessment and, 375
  for hospitalized child, 914t
  interpreter of, 42
  testing of, 863b
Language development, 142t
Lanugo, 120t
Laparoscopy, 555
Large head, 590, 592b, 593-595
Laryngeal diphtheria, 724t
Laryngitis, 667-669, 668t
  spasmodic, 646
Laryngotracheobronchitis, 646, 647t
Latchkey child, 255-256
Lateral stress test, 548, 549f

Latex allergy, 872, 873t-874t
Latino culture, 24t-25t
Law
  Baby Doe, 70
  on foster care, 300
Laxative, 424, 424t
  in cerebral palsy, 848
  for chronic constipation, 424-425
Lead, blood levels of, 150-151, 150t, 151t
Lead poisoning, 879-882, 880t, 881b
Learning disability, 862-866
  autism and, 842
  classification of, 864t
  data on, 862-864
  developmental domains and, 864t
  differential diagnosis of, 864-865
  etiology of, 862
  incidence of, 862
  management of, 865-866, 865b, 866b
  primary care implications of, 865
  risk factors for, 862
Learning style, 240
Leg. *See also* Extremity
  deformity of, 572-574, 573t
  neonatal assessment of, 129t
Leg-length discrepancy, 562, 565t, 566
Leg length test, 547
Leg pain, overuse causing, 204t
Leg ulcer in sickle cell disease, 833t
Legal issues
  age of minor as, 70
  on foster care, 300
  in gay or lesbian family, 305-306
  malpractice, 4-5
Legg-Calvé-Perthes disease
  differential diagnosis of, 562, 563t-564t
  management of, 566
Legislation on disabled children, 869t
Length of infant
  newborn, 115, 118t
  screening of, 147
Lens, 123t
Lesbian, 279, 305-307
Lesion, neonatal assessment of, 120t
Lethal dose, of fluoride, 222
Leukemia, 818t-819t
Leukorrhea, 636t
  differential diagnosis of, 636t
  management of, 639
    in adolescence, 639
    in prepubescence, 635
Levalbuterol, 765t
Levetiracetam, 602t-603t
Liability, 4
Lice, 522-525, 524t
  differential diagnosis of, 523, 524t, 533,
    534t
  etiology of, 523
  incidence of, 523
  management of, 523, 525
  pubic, 458, 459, 461
  risk factors for, 523
Licensure, multi-state, 3
Life cycle, family, 14
Ligamentous strain of back, 559
Light reflex testing, 375
Light therapy for neonatal jaundice,
    482-483
Limit-setting for adolescent, 276

Limp, 561-566
  differential diagnosis of, 562, 563t-565t
  etiology of, 561, 562b
  incidence of, 561
  risk factors for, 561
Lindane
  for lice, 459, 523
  for scabies, 741-742, 742t
Linear question, 18
Lip
  cleft, 50t
  neonatal assessment of, 124t
Lip habit, 227
Lipid
  diabetes and, 783t
  hyperlipidemia and, 353-354, 355t, 356
Lipodystrophy, 784
Lipomeningocele, 870
Lipoprotein, 152t
Lithium, 586
Little League elbow, 557t
Liver
  in gastrointestinal disorder, 411
  hepatitis of. *See* Hepatitis *entries*
  neonatal assessment of, 127t
Log, urination, 673
Logical consequences, 29, 29b
Lomefloxacin, 275t
Loratadine, 697t
Loss, grief and, 293-295
Loss of consciousness, 901-902, 901b, 902t
Lotion, 493-494
  for sunburn, 536
Low-density lipoprotein, 354, 355t
  classification of, 152t
Lower airway disorder, 646, 648t-650t, 650
Lower extremity. *See also* Extremity
  Down syndrome and, 851b
  examination of, 554f-555f
Loyalty issues in stepfamily, 333-334
LSD, 890t
Lubricant, 494b
  stool, 871
Lumbar puncture, 583
Lunelle, 274t, 624
Lung. *See also* Respiratory *entries*
  blood disorder and, 469
  cancer and, 816
  cystic fibrosis and, 770t, 771, 776
  maximum expansion of, 642, 742
  newborn assessment of, 113t
  in physical examination, 100t-101t
  respiratory disorder and, 644-645
  transplant of, 776
Lupus erythematosus, 725
Luteinizing hormone, 362
Lying, 256-257
Lyme disease, 728-730, 729t
  immunization against, 163t
  testing for, 496
  vaccine for, 163t
Lymph node
  gastrointestinal disorder and, 410
  in physical examination, 96t
  respiratory disorder and, 644
Lymphadenitis, 717
  mumps vs, 731
  tuberculosis vs, 744t
Lymphadenopathy, 714, 715t-717t, 717

Lymphocytic thyroiditis, 370t, 371
Lymphoid interstitial pneumonitis, 798
Lymphoma
  Hodgkin's, 820t-821t
  non-Hodgkin's, 818t-819t
Lysergic acid diethylamide, 890t

M

Macrocephaly, 529, 529b, 593
Magic, 37
Magnesium citrate, 871
Magnetic resonance imaging
  cardiovascular, 342
  endocrine disorder and, 362
  in neuropsychiatric disorder, 581
Mainstreaming, 7
Major depression, 584-586
Malabsorption, 464t, 465-466
Maladaptive parenting behavior, 130-131
Male
  gynecomastia in, 616-617
  Klinefelter syndrome in, 66
Male genitalia
  ambiguous, 616
  examination of, 613, 613f
  neonatal assessment of, 113t, 128t
  physical examination and, 103t
Malformation
  Arnold-Chiari, 870t
  definition of, 62
Malignancy, 815-826
  data about, 816-817
  differential diagnosis of, 817, 818t-821t
  etiology of, 815-816
  hospitalization for, 915
  incidence of, 816, 816t
  lymphadenopathy in, 715t-717t
  management of, 817, 824, 824t, 825t, 826
  primary care implications of, 817, 823t
  retinoblastoma, 391, 391t, 393
  risk factors for, 816
  vomiting with, 455t
  Wilms' tumor, 675
Malignant melanoma, 507t
  detection of, 492b
  prevention of, 492
  referral for, 507t
Malnutrition
  irritability in, 713t
  signs of, 214t-215t
Malpractice, 4
Malpractice insurance, 4-5
Malt soup extract, 871
Maltreatment, behavior patterns causing,
    130-131
Maltsuprex, 424t. 424
Managed care, 5
Mandible, 124t
Manometry, 412
Mantoux skin test, 153, 153t
  for foster child, 302
Maple syrup urine disease, 149t
Marijuana
  abuse of, 890t
  prenatal and neonatal effects of, 316t
Marital friendship, 14-15
Marriage
  child affecting, 14-15
  cultural factors in, 40, 40b

Marshmallowing parenting response, 29
Mass, breast, 616-618, 618t
Masturbation, 257-258
Maternal age, 45
Maternal and child health services block grant, 7
Maternal factors in rejection of newborn, 110b
Maturation of adolescent, 269
MDMA, 890t
Mean corpuscular volume, 470t
Measles, 740-741
    German, 739-740, 740t
    rash from, 530t
    as vaccine adverse event, 169t
Measles, mumps, rubella vaccine
    administration of, 164t
    characteristics of, 170
    contraindications to, 158t, 159t
    handling and storage of, 180t-181t
    HIV infection and, 801
    reporting adverse event, 166t
    rules for, 160t
Mebendazole
    for lice, 461
    for pinworms, 635, 639
Mechanical clearance of airway, 776
Meckel's diverticulum
    colic vs, 443
    differential diagnosis of, 413t-415t, 417
Meckel's scan, 412
Meconium of drug-exposed infant, 317
Media influence on sexuality, 229
Medial tress test, 548, 549f
Medicaid, 6
Medroxyprogesterone acetate, 623
Mefenamic, 624
Megaloblastic anemia, 471
Megalocephaly
    differential diagnosis of, 590, 592, 592b
    management of, 594
Melanoma
    detection of, 492b
    prevention of, 492
    referral for, 507t
Membrane, tympanic, 382, 385
Memory of gifted child, 312
Mendelian disorder, 48t-49t
Mendelian inheritance, 59t-60t
Meningeal inflammation, 376b
Meningitis
    beyond newborn period, 730-731
    colic vs, 441, 443
    febrile seizure vs, 597t
    poliomyelitis vs, 737t
    tuberculosis vs, 744t
Meningococcal immunization, 163t
    rules for, 163t, 170
Meniscal injury, 571, 571t, 572
Menometrorrhagia, 622t
Menorrhagia, 622t
Menstrual history
    bleeding disorder and, 789, 790t
    diabetes and, 779
Menstrual irregularity
    differential diagnosis of, 622-623, 622t
    etiology of, 622
    incidence of, 622
    management of, 623-625, 625t
    risk factors for, 622

Mental health assessment, of foster child, 302
Mental retardation, 867-869, 867b, 867t, 869t
    assessment of, 65
    autism and, 842
    Down syndrome and, 850-856. *See also* Down syndrome
    hypothyroidism causing, 369, 370t
6-Mercaptopurine, 419
Mesenteric artery syndrome, superior, 455t
Metabolic disorder
    irritability in, 713t
    manifestations, 65-66
    vomiting with, 454t, 456t
Metamucil, 871
Metatarsus adductus, 567-568, 567t
Metered-dose inhaler, 652-653, 766b
Methamphetamine, 890t
Methylene blue test, 675
Methylenedioxymethamphetamine, 890t
Methylphenidate, 610t
Metoprolol, 359t
Metorrhagia, 622t
Metronidazole
    Crohn's disease and, 419
    for giardiasis, 732t
    for trichomoniasis, 275t, 638
Miconazole
    for candidiasis, 638
    for vaginal candidiasis, 640
Microcephaly
    differential diagnosis of, 590, 591b
    management of, 594
Microdeletion, chromosomal, 47t
Microduplication, chromosomal, 47t
Microtrauma, 204t
Middle ear
    infection of
        differential diagnosis of, 380, 381t
        etiology of, 379
        incidence of, 379-380
        management of, 383-384, 383f
        risk factors for, 380
    injury to, 386
Migraine headache, 587, 588b, 589
    vomiting with, 454t
Milestone, developmental, 139t
    in Down syndrome, 852b
    loss of, 65
    of preterm infant, 323
Miliaria rubra, 520-521, 520t
Milk intolerance
    colic vs, 442t-443t, 444
    diarrhea from, 430t, 433
    diarrhea with, 464t
    management of, 446-447
Milk of magnesia, 424t
Mineral oil, 424t, 425
Mineral supplementation for infant, 215-216
Minnesota Preschool Development Inventory, 241t
Minocycline, 502t
Minor child, 69-70
    confidentiality for, 268
Minor trauma, 525-526
Minority, definition of, 36
Minoxidil, 359t
Miscarriage, 45
Mite, 741-742, 742t
Mitochondrial inheritance, 60t

Mitral valve prolapse, 345
Mixed cerebral palsy, 846t-847t
Mixed-headache syndrome, 588
Mixed hearing loss, 388
Mnemonic for pain assessment, 76-77
Mobility in spina bifida, 874
Molar pregnancy, 629t
Molding of neonate's head, 116
Molecular analysis, 55t
Molluscum contagiosum, 537, 538t, 539
Mometasone, 697t
Mongolian spot, 505, 506t
Monilia, 515t-516t, 517
Monitoring
    in diabetes, 785
    in HIV infection, 802
Monoamine oxidase inhibitor, 586
Mononucleosis
    differential diagnosis of, 448t, 450
    management of, 452
    sore throat with, 666t
Montelukast, 765t
Mood stabilizer, 586
Mosquito bite, 511
Mother, postpartum practices of, 40-41, 40b
Motocycle injury, 195
Motor function
    examination of, 105t
    neuropsychiatric disorder and, 578, 581, 581b
    of preterm infant, 329
Motor vehicle accident
    pedestrian, 194-195
    prevention of
        in adolescent, 192t
        in preschool-aged child, 190t
        in school-aged child, 191t
        strategies for, 193-194, 193b
Mouth
    Down syndrome and, 851b, 852
    neonatal assessment of, 112t, 116, 124t
    in physical examination, 98t
    respiratory disorder and, 644
Mouth sore
    differential diagnosis of, 447, 448t-449t, 450
    etiology of, 447
    incidence of, 447
    management of, 447-452
    risk factors for, 447
Mouthguard, 225
MPQRST, 77
Mucocutaneous lymph node syndrome, 345
Mucolytic in cystic fibrosis, 776
Mucosa
    cancer and, 824
    malnutrition and, 214t
Mucus, cervical, 614-615
Mullen Scales of Early Learning, 242t
Multi-state nurse licensure compact, 3
Multiculturalism, 35
Multifactorial genetic disorder, 64t
Mumps, 731
Munchausen syndrome by proxy, 430t, 434
Murmur, heart, 350-351, 352t, 353t
Muscle. *See also* Musculoskeletal *entries*
    bleeding disorder and, 794t
    in cerebral palsy, 846t
    detrusor, 679, 680, 682
    Down syndrome and, 851b
    extraocular, 375

Muscle—cont'd
  pelvic, 682, 683
  strength testing of, 551f
Muscle spasm, tetanus vs, 743t
Muscular dystrophy, 856-862
  data on, 857-859
  developmental status in, 858t
  etiology of, 856-857
  genetics of, 49t, 856-857
  Gower sign in, 858, 858f
  incidence of, 857
  limp with, 562, 565t
  management of, 859-862, 860t, 861t
  primary care implications of, 859
  risk factors for, 857
  signs and symptoms of, 856b
Musculoskeletal disorder, 544-575
  athletic activity and, 544-545
  back pain, 559, 560t, 561
  chest pain from, 345
  foot deformity, 568-569, 568t
  gait disturbaced caused by
    limp, 561-566, 562b, 563t-565t
    toeing-in, 566-568, 567t
  growing pains, 569, 570t
  of hip, 569-570
  joint pain and swelling, 570-572, 571t
  laboratory evaluation of, 555
  leg deformity, 572-574, 573t
  muscular dystrophy, 856-862
  physical examination for, 546-549, 546f-555f
  risk factors for, 544
  spine deformity, 573t, 574
  sports-related, 556-559, 556t-558t
Musculoskeletal system
  blood disorder and, 470, 790-791
  cancer treatment affecting, 825t
  Down syndrome and, 852
  malnutrition and, 214t-215t
  of preterm infant, 324
  in review of systems, 92t
  short stature and, 366-367, 368t, 369
  sickle cell disease and, 831t
  spina bifida and, 870
Mycobacterium avium-intracellular
    complex, 799
Mycobacterium tuberculosis, 743-744, 744t
Mycoplasma pneumonia, 418, 646,
    648t-650t, 650
Myelography, 555
Myelomeningocele, 870
Myocarditis, 345
Myoclonus, 600
Myringotomy, 377, 377b
Myths about pain, 74-75

N
Nail
  ingrown, 205t
  injury or infection of, 526-528, 527t
  neonatal assessment of, 117, 129t
Nanny, in-home, 250t
Naproxen
  for abnormal uterine bleeding, 624
  for recurrent headache, 590t
Narcotic, prenatal and neonatal effects of,
    316t
Nasal bleeding, 656-659, 657t-658t
  hemophilia and, 788t

Nasal congestion, 659, 660t-661t, 662-664
Nasal cromolyn, 697
Nasal diphtheria, 724t
Nasal obstruction
  breath-holding spell and, 246b
  clearance of, 642
Nasal spray, 643
Nasolacrimal duct obstruction, 403, 405t, 406
National Certification Board of Pediatric
    Nurse Practitioners and Nurses, 3
National Childhood Vaccine Injury Act,
    166t-168t, 177
National Commission on Family Foster
    Care, 300
National Council of State Boards of Nursing, 3
National Foster Parent Association, 300
National Institutes of Health, on neonatal
    hearing screening, 116
National School Lunch, School Breakfast, and
    Special Milk Program, 6
Native American culture
  assessment of, 39t
  newborn care in, 41b
  parenting in, 24t-25t
Natural consequences, 29, 29b
Nausea and vomiting, 452-458. *See also*
    Vomiting
Near drowning, 904, 906
Neck
  blood disorder and, 469
  cancer and, 823t
  cystic fibrosis and, 771
  Down syndrome and, 851b
  endocrine disorder and, 361
  neonatal assessment of, 112t, 116-117, 125t
  in physical examination, 100t
  range of motion of, 550f
  respiratory disorder and, 644
Necrosis
  aseptic, 562
  of femoral head, 833t
Necrotizing ulcerative gingivitis
  differential diagnosis of, 447, 449t, 450
  management of, 451
Nedocromil
  asthma and, 764t
  cystic fibrosis and, 776
Neglect, 882-884
Negligence, 4
Neisseria gonorrhoeae
  conjunctivitis caused by, 403, 404t
  culture for, 615
  urethritis caused by, 625, 626, 690
Neisseria meningitidis, 730
Nelfinavir, 813t
Neonatal Behavioral Assessment Scale, 131
Neonatal Infant Pain Scale, 77t, 115
Neonatal intensive care survivor, 114
Neonatal jaundice, 480, 481t, 482-483, 482t
Neonate. *See* Newborn *entries;* Preterm infant
Neoplastic disease, 815-826. *See also*
    Malignancy
Nephropathy, sickle cell, 832t
Nephrotic-range proteinuria, 691-692, 691t
Nerve, cranial, examination, 580
Nervous system. *See also* Neurologic *entries*
  bleeding disorder and, 469-470,
    790-791, 794t
  cancer treatment affecting, 825t

Nervous system—cont'd
  in cerebral palsy, 847t
  failure to thrive and, 703t
  fetal alcohol syndrome and, 877
  malnutrition and, 215t
  of preterm infant, 324
  respiratory disorder and, 645
  in review of systems, 92t
  rheumatic fever and, 828
  sickle cell disease and, 830
  spina bifida and, 870
Neural tube defect
  genetics of, 50t
  spina bifida, 869-876. *See also* Spina bifida
Neuritis
  brachial, 169t
  optic, 391t, 392, 393
Neuroblastoma, 818t-819t
  Wilms' tumor with, 675
Neuroendocrine system in menstrual
    cycle, 622
Neurofibromatosis, 507t
Neurologic assessment
  in endocrine disorder, 361
  learning disabilities and, 863
  of school readiness, 239t
Neurologic disorder. *See also* Neuropsychi-
    atric disorder
  alcohol-related, in adopted child, 288
  bleeding disorder and, 790-791
  in cerebral palsy, 847t
  failure to thrive and, 703t
  incontinence with, 679
  vomiting with, 456t
Neurologic examination, 104t-105t, 580-581,
    581b
Neurologic soft sign, 581
Neuromuscular disorder
  breath-holding spell and, 246b
  malignancy and, 822t
Neuromuscular system in diabetes, 782t
Neuropathic pain, 75
Neuropathy
  diabetes and, 782t
  malignancy and, 822t
Neuropsychiatric disorder, 576-610
  abnormal head circumference and, 590-
    595, 591b, 592b, 593t, 594b
  depression, 584-585, 585b
  headache, 587-590, 587t, 588b, 588t,
    589b, 590t
  laboratory evaluation in, 581-583, 583t
  neurologic examination in, 580-581, 581b,
    582b, 582f
  physical examination in, 579-580
  prevention of, 576
  risk factors for, 576
  seizure, 595-605. *See also* Seizure
  subjective data about, 576-583
  suicide, 605-607, 606b
  symptom inventory of, 577f-580f
  tics, 607-609, 608b, 609t
Nevirapine, 811t-812t
Nevus, 505, 506t, 508
New Ballard Score, 110
Newborn. *See also* Newborn assessment
  acne neonatorum and, 500, 501t
  attachment to, 109-110
  blood in stool of, 463t

Newborn—cont'd
blood screening of, 147
conjunctivitis in, 403-406, 404t-405t
cultural factors in care of, 41, 41b
drug-exposed, 315-321. *See also* Drug-exposed infant
equipment and supplies for, 84b
genetic assessment of, 59-61
genetic screening of, 52-53
gestational age of, 110
hyperbilirubinemia in, 147, 150t
injury to, 188t
jaundice in, 480, 481t, 482-483, 482t
rejection of, 110b, 130b
resuscitation of, 110
vomiting in, 456t
Newborn assessment
atypical, counseling about, 134-135
environmental, 133-134, 133t
gestational age, 110
guide for, 111t-114t
hearing, 116
neurobehavioral, 132t
pain, 115
physical, 115-130
abdomen, 126t-127t
back, 129t
blood pressure, 116
chest, 117, 125t-126t
dermatoglyphics, 117
ears, 122t
extremities, 117, 128t-129t
eyes, 116, 122t-123t
face, 116
general, 118t-119t
genitalia, 127t-128t
guide for, 111t-114t
head, 119t-122t
of head circumference, 115, 120t-121t
of height, 115, 118t
hip instability, 117
mouth, 116, 124t
nails, 117
neck and chin, 125t
nose, 123t
pain, 115
prenatal management and, 107-110, 108f-109f, 110b
preterm developmental care protocols and, 114-115
reflexes, 130t
skin, 116, 119t
techniques and measurements of, 115-117
tongue, 124t
of weight, 115, 118t
of preterm infant, 114-115
psychosocial, 130-133
Night terrors, 261-262
Nightmare, 261
Nipple
accessory, 616, 617, 618t
discharge from, 615, 616, 618t
Nitrofurantoin, 689
Nocturnal enuresis, 684-686, 685t
Non-Hodgkin's lymphoma, 818t-819t
Nonaccommodative esotropia, 395
Nonauthoritative parenting style, 22, 23t
Nonbullous impetigo, 540-541

Noncardiac chest pain, 344t
Noncommunicating hydrocele, 435
Noncommunicating hydrocephalus, 592b
Nongonococcal urethritis, 625-626
Nonmalficence, 69
Nonnutritive sucking, 226
as parenting concern, 265-266
Nonprogressive headache, 588
Nonreactive seizure, 601-603
Nonsteroidal antiinflammatory drug
for abnormal uterine bleeding, 624
asthma and, 769t
bleeding disorder and, 792
cystic fibrosis and, 776
for dysmenorrhea, 418, 625, 625t
sickle cell disease and, 836
Nonthrombocytopenic purpura, 486, 487t, 488
Nontraditional family, 28
Nonverbal communication, 16, 18b
Noonan syndrome, 360
Norplant, 274t
Nose
bleeding disorder and, 795t
cancer and, 816
cystic fibrosis and, 771
diabetes and, 782t
Down syndrome and, 851b
endocrine disorder and, 361
neonatal assessment of, 112t, 123t
in physical examination, 97t
of preterm infant, 324
respiratory disorder and, 644
in review of systems, 91t
sickle cell disease and, 830
Nose bleed, 656-659, 657t-658t
hemophilia and, 788t
Nose drops, 642, 662
Nuclear family, nontraditional, 28
Nuclear medicine, 412
Nucleoside analog reverse transcriptase inhibitor, 807t-814t
Numerical pain rating scale, 77t
Nurse anesthetist, 3
Nurse practice act, 5
Nurse practitioner
certification of, 3
duties of, 71
evidence-based practice by, 8
federal health programs and, 6-8
in grief process, 294
Healthy People 2010 and, 8
history of, 3
incidence to service and, 4
integrity of, 71
licensure of, 3
malpractice issues of, 4-5
practice guidelines for, 8
prescriptive authority of, 5
reimbursement for, 3-4
research by, 8
risk management and, 4
substance abusing family and, 285b
tele-health/medicine and, 6
utilization review and, 5
Nursing bottle caries, 224-225, 224t, 225f
Nursing Child Assessment Satellite Training, 133, 133t
Nursing value, 70-71

Nurturing of gifted child, 313b
Nurturing parenting response, 29
Nurturing stage of parenting, 21t
Nutrition
of adolescent, 269, 271
of adopted child, 289
assessment of, 208, 212-213
asthma and, 762
autism and, 843
blood disorder and, 469
cancer and, 823t
caries prevention and, 222
for disabled child, 223-224
cerebral palsy and, 845, 848, 848b
cystic fibrosis and, 773, 778
diabetes and, 780, 780t, 781, 783
Down syndrome and, 853, 854
eating disorder and, 572t, 751-757
in failure to thrive, 700
fetal alcohol syndrome and, 877
fiber and, 423t
of foster child, 303
hematologic system and, 468
HIV infection and, 802
incontinence and, 681
for infants, 214-216
lead poisoning and, 881
learning disability and, 865
muscular dystrophy and, 859
obesity and, 718-720, 720
in patient history, 92t-93t
poverty and, 886
of preterm infant, 323, 327-328
school lunch program, 6
sickle cell disease and, 835
WIC program and, 6
Nystagmus, 394t, 395, 396
Nystatin, for candidiasis, 638

O
Obesity, 718-721
in adolescent, 271
differential diagnosis of, 719-720, 719t
etiology of, 718
incidence of, 718
management of, 720
risk factors for, 718-719
Obsessive-compulsive disorder, 608
Obstruction
airway
in anaphylaxis, 695
as emergency, 899-900, 899t
stridor with, 646, 647t
bladder outlet, 680
jaundice with, 482
nasal, 659, 660t-661t, 662-664
breath-holding spell and, 246b
nasolacrimal duct, 403, 406
vomiting with, 453t, 456t
Obstructive cardiac lesion, 343-345
Occlusal service of tooth, 221
Oculomotor nerve, 105t
Odor, stool, 462, 462t
Ofloxacin
chlamydiosis, 275t
for gonorrhea, 640
Oil, 494
mineral, 424t

Ointment, 494
  for diaper rash, 517
Olfactor nerve, 105t
Oligomenorrhea, 622t
Optic disc, 123t
Optic neuritis, 391t, 392, 393
Oral candidiasis, 447
Oral care, 222-224, 223t
Oral contraceptive, 273t-274t
  for acne, 502t, 503
  amenorrhea and, 624-625
Oral hypoglycemic agent, 784-785
Oral polio vaccine, 158t
Oral rehydration therapy, 426, 429
Orbital fracture, 396, 397t, 399
Orbital infection, 400, 401t, 402
Organization, health care, 5
Orthopedic disorder in cerebral palsy, 848
Orthopedic fracture, 906, 906f
Ortolani neonatal hip test, 117, 117f, 546, 546f
Osgood-Schlatter disease, 558t
  overuse causing, 205t
Osteogenesis imperfecta, 48t
Osteoid osteoma, 559, 560t, 561
Osteomyelitis, 712t
Osteosarcoma, 820t-821t
Osterochonritis dissecans, 557t
Otitis
  differential diagnosis of, 380, 380t, 381t, 382
  incidence of, 379-380
  management of, 382-385, 383f, 385t
  risk factors for, 380
Otitis media
  colic vs, 441
  irritability in, 712t
Otoacoustic emission test, evoked, 376-377
Otoscopic examination, 376
Otoscopy, pneumatic, 153-154
Oucher scale, 77t
Outlet obstruction, bladder, 680
Ovarian failure, 624
Ovary, polycystic, 623
Overdose
  telephone management of, 198b
  vomiting with, 456t
Overfeeding
  diarrhea in infant and, 430t
  vomiting with, 456-457
Overuse injury, 204t-205t, 206t, 557
Oxcarbazepine, 602t-603t
Oxofloxacin, 275t
Oxybutynin, 682
Oxygen, retinopathy of prematurity and, 114-115
Oxygen challenge test, 342

P
PABA, 491
Pacifier, 226
PAIN, 77
Pain
  abdominal, 412-420. *See also* Abdominal pain
  algorithm for, 78f
  assessment of
    mnemonic for, 76-77
    tools for, 77t
    variables in, 77

Pain—cont'd
  back, 559, 560t, 561
  bleeding disorder and, 792
  chest, 343-346, 344t
  definition of, 75
  ear disorder with, 379-385
    differential diagnosis of, 380, 380t-381t, 382
    etiology of, 379
    incidence of, 379-380
    management of, 382-385, 383f, 384t
    risk factors for, 380
  growing, 569, 570t
  hip, 569-570
  history of, 75-76
  HIV infection and, 803
  joint, 570-572, 571t
  limp with, 562, 563t-564t
  management of, 77, 79, 79b, 80t
  myths and truths about, 74-75
  overuse injury causing, 204t
  perianal, 458-462, 459t
  procedures causing, 910, 911t-913t
  referred, to back, 559
  research on, 74
  sickle cell disease and, 830, 834, 834t, 836-837
  on urination, 686-687, 688t, 689-690
Pain assessment in newborn, 115
Painless limp, 562, 565t
Palate
  cleft, 50t
  neonatal assessment of, 116, 124t
Pallid breath-holding spell, 245
Pallor, 483-484, 485t, 486
Palpation
  chest, 125t-126t
  in musculoskeletal examination, 546
  of neonatal neck, 116-117
  rectovaginal, 613, 614f
  respiratory disorder and, 645
Palsy, cerebral, 844b, 845-850
  limp with, 562, 565t
Pancreas in cystic fibrosis, 770t
Pancreatic enzyme, 776b
Pancreatic insufficiency, 464t
Pancreatitis, 414t-415t, 417
Panner disease, 557t
Papanicolaou smear, 614, 615t
Papillomavirus infection, 275-276, 275t
Para-aminobenzoic acid, 491
Parasitic infection
  ascariasis, 733-734, 734t
  cryptosporidiosis, 732-733, 732b, 733t
  cysticercosis, 733
  diarrhea with, 428t, 431t
  giardiasis, 732-733, 732b, 733t
  HIV and, 799
  hookworm, 734-735
  pinworm, 735. *See also* Pinworm
Parent
  of adolescent, 268
  adolescent as, 278
  divorced, 296-299
  homosexual, 305-308
  of preterm infant, 328
  sexual abuse and, 888-889
  sexuality issues of, 229
Parent-child relationship, 30, 31b

Parent education
  about newborn, 132
  culture affecting, 25t
  on dental care, 223t
  on immunization, 175
  on preterm infant, 329
Parental informed permission, 69
Parenting, 20-33. *See also* Parenting concern
  adoption and, 290
  assessment of, 30-32, 30b, 31b, 32b
  consultation about, 33
  cultural factors in, 40
  discipline and, 28-29, 28b, 29b
  divorce and remarriage and, 15-16
  effective, 33
  factors affecting
    cultural, 24t-25t
    temperament, 26b, 27t
  maladaptive behavior of, 130-131
  marriage affected by, 14-15
  neuropsychiatric disorder and, 576
  of preterm infant, 325
  situations of, 28
  stages of, 20-22, 21t
  styles of, 22, 23t
  tasks of, 20
Parenting concern
  about adolescent, 276-277
  breath-holding as, 245-247, 246b, 246t
  bullying as, 247, 248f, 248t, 249
  cheating as, 256-257
  child care as, 249-251, 250t, 251b, 251t
  circumcision as, 251-252, 252b
  discipline as, 252-253
  fears as, 253-254, 254t
  fighting as, 254-255, 255b
  latchkey child as, 255-256
  lying as, 256-257
  masturbation as, 257-258
  school readiness as, 236
  separation anxiety as, 258-259, 259b
  sexuality as, 229, 276-277
  sibling rivalry as, 262-263
  sleep problems as, 260-262, 260b
  stealing as, 256-257
  stranger anxiety as, 263-264
  temper tantrums as, 264-265
  thumbsucking as, 265-266
  toilet training as, 266-267
Parents' Evaluations of Developmental Status, 243t
Paronychia, 526-528, 527t
Paroxysmal torticollis, 588b
Paroxysmal vertigo, benign, 588b
Partial anomalous pulmonary venous return, 348, 349
Partial seizure, 600
Partial-thickness burn, 901b
Paste, 494
Patau syndrome, 46t
Patellar apprehension test, 549
Patellofemoral arthralgia, 205t
Patellofemoral syndrome, 557t
Patent ductus arteriosus, 348, 349
Paternal factors in rejection of newborn, 110b
Pathologic heart murmur, 351, 352t
Patient advocacy, 70
Patient history, 87t-89t
Peabody Picture Vocabulary Test, 242t

Peak expiratory flow rate, 645, 653, 766, 766b, 768t
Pedestrian injury, 194-195
Pediatric Symptom Checklist, 243t
Pediculosis. *See* Lice
Pedigree
   information in, 57, 57f, 58f, 59
   symbols used in, 56f
Pelvic examination in blood disorder, 470
Pelvic inflammatory disease, 635
   differential diagnosis of, 414t-415t, 417, 637t
Pelvic muscle exercise, 683
Pelvic muscle relaxation, 682
Pelvis in blooding disorder, 795t
Penicillin
   diphtheria and, 723
   pharyngitis and, 665
   rheumatic fever and, 828
   syphilis and, 275t
   urethritis and, 690
Penis
   discharge from, 625-627
   examination of, 612
   hypospadias of, 676
   irritation of, 627-628, 627t
Peptic ulcer disease, 413t-415t, 417
Perception, maladaptive, 130
Percussion, chest, 126t
Percutaneous umbilical blood sampling, 53t
Perforation, tympanic membrane, 382, 385
Perianal itch, 458-459, 460t, 461
Pericarditis, 345
Perinatal transmission of HIV infection, 803
Periodontal disease, 221
Periorbital buccal cellulitis, 531t
Peripheral neuropathy, 782t
Peripheral precocious puberty, 365t, 366
Peripheral vessel, 102t
Periungual abscess, 526-528, 527t
Permethrin, 742t
Permission, informed, 69
Permissive parenting style, 23t, 26
Pernicious anemia, 476, 478
Personal malpractice insurance, 4-5
Personality, 94t
Pertussis, 735-737, 736t
Pertussis vaccine
   handling and storage of, 180t-181t
   reporting adverse event with, 166t
Pervasive developmental disorder, 842
Pes cavus, 568-569, 568t
Pes planus, 568-569, 568t
Petechiae, 486, 487t, 488
   in Langerhans cell histiocytosis, 533, 534t
pH
   esophageal, 412
   of vaginal discharge, 615
Pharyngeal diphtheria, 724t
Pharyngitis, 664-667, 665t, 666t
Pharyngoconjunctival fever, 666t
Phenobarbital
   for drug-exposed infant, 318
   for seizure, 602t-603t
Phenotypic presentation, 55t
Phenylephrine nose drops, 662
Phenylketonuria screening, 148t
Phenytoin, 602t-603t
   gingival overgrowth from, 223

Phimosis, 627, 627t, 628
Phoria, 395
Photo listing of adoptable children, 291
Photoscreening, 377
Photosensitive skin reaction, 536-537
Phototherapy for neonatal jaundice, 482-483
Phthirus pubis, 459
Physical abuse, 882-884
   behavior patterns in, 130-131
Physiologic neonatal jaundice, 480, 481t
Piaget's stages of cognitive development, 144t
Piercing, body, 277
Pigmentation, 120t
Pigmented nevus, giant, 507t
Pimozide, 609t
Pinna, 376
Pinworm
   differential diagnosis of, 459, 460t, 636t, 735
   etiology of, 735
   incidence of, 458, 735
   management of, 461, 635, 638, 735
   painful urination with, 688t
   risk factors for, 735
Piperadine, 696t
Piperazine, 461
Pit-and-fissure dental lesion, 221
Pitcher's elbow, 204t
Pituitary gland in delayed puberty, 363
Pityriasis alba, 725
Pityriasis rosea, 529, 530t
Placement of foster child, 300
Plagiocephaly, 592, 594, 595
Planning of family assessment, 11
Plant, toxic
   first aid for, 198b
   list of, 192b
Plantar fasciitis, 205t
Plantar wart, 537, 538t, 539
Plumbism, 879-882, 880t, 881b
Pneumatic otoscopy, 153-154
Pneumococcal vaccine, 163t, 801
   administration of, 165t
   characteristics of, 170
   handling and storage of, 180t-181t
   rules for, 163t
Pneumonia
   abdominal pain with, 414t-415t, 417
   airway obstruction in, 899t
   ascariasis vs, 734t
   cystic fibrosis and, 775t
   differential diagnosis of, 646-647, 648t-650t, 650
   management of, 418-419, 652
   pertussis vs, 736t
Pneumocystis carinii, 647, 798
   cancer and, 817
   drug regimen for, 804t
   prophylaxis for, 803, 803t
Pneumonitis, lymphoid interstitial, 798
Pneumoscopy, 376
Podofilox, 275t
Podophyllin, 275t
Pointer, hip, 558t
Poison ivy, 531t
Poisoning
   diarrhea with, 429t
   lead, 879-882, 880t, 881b
   by plant, 192b

Poisoning—cont'd
   prevention of, 197, 197b, 198b
      for infant, 188t, 189t
      strategies for, 193b
      by toddler, 190t
   vomiting with, 454t
Poler Chip tool, 77t
Polio vaccine
   administration of, 164t
   characteristics of, 164
   handling and storage of, 178t-179t
   reporting adverse event, 166t-167t
   rules for, 161t
Poliovirus infection, 737, 737t
   as vaccine adverse event, 169t
Polycystic kidney, 677
Polycystic ovary syndrome, 623
Polymenorrhea, 622t
Ponderal index of newborn, 115
Poorness of fit, 26
Population screening, genetic, 53
Port wine stain, 504, 505t
Position
   neonatal assessment of, 118t
   in spina bifida, 874
Positive reinforcement, 29b
Postnatal rubella, 740, 740t
Postpartum care, 40-41, 40b
Postpartum depression, 133
Poststreptococcal glomerulonephritis, 677
Postural proteinuria, 691
Postvoiding urinary residual volume, 674
Poverty, 884-886
   parenting affected by, 23
Powder, 494
Power issues in stepfamily, 333
Practice, ethics of, 69-73
Practice guidelines, 8
Practice standard
   consultation and, 4
   for immunization, 177, 177b
Practitioner, nurse. *See* Nurse practitioner
Prader-Willi syndrome, 48t
   obesity in, 719t
   signs and symptoms of, 360
Preauricular lymphadenitis, 731
Precocious puberty, 365-366, 365t
Predictive value of screening test, 146
Prednisone
   asthma and, 764t, 765t
   for inflammatory bowel disease, 465
Preferred provider organization, 5
Pregnancy
   adolescent, 277-278, 612
   antenatal care in, 630b-631b
   common complaints in, 632t-633t
   cultural factors in, 40
   differential diagnosis of, 628, 629t
   as ethical dilemma, 72-73
   HIV and, 799, 801
   in homeless youth, 279
   management of, 628, 630b-631b
   parenting tasks during, 21t
   testing for, 615
   vomiting with, 455t
Premature adrenarche, 365t, 366
Premature infant, 322-330. *See also* Preterm infant
Premature thelarche, 365-366, 365t

Premenstrual symptoms, Down syndrome and, 853
Prenatal care, 630b-631b
  of adolescent, 278
  interview in, 82-85
  management of, 107-108, 108f-109f
  neuropsychiatric disorder and, 576
  physical abuse and, 884
  prevention of eye and ear disorders, 373
Prenatal history, 87t-88t
  of preterm infant, 323
  in spina bifida, 870
Prenatal testing
  for Down syndrome, 850
  genetic, 52, 53t
  purpose of, 56
Prepubescence
  acne in, 500, 501t
  vulvovaginal symptoms in, 635, 636t-637t, 638
Preschool-aged child
  anemia screening of, 469b
  autism in, 842
  blood in stool of, 463t
  caloric requirement for, 781
  causes of death of, 186t
  death and grief and, 293
  developmental counseling about, 145t
  developmental domains of, 864t
  developmental milestones for, 139t
  Down syndrome and, 854b-855b
  fetal alcohol syndrome and, 877, 878
  hearing in, 374b, 375
  hospitalization of, 912t
  injury prevention for, 190t
  irritability in, 710t, 711t
  language development of, 142t, 143t
  laxative for, 424, 424t
  nonnutritive sucking by, 226-227
  nutrition for, 216-218
  oral care for, 222
  pain in, 76t, 80t
  parenting tasks during, 21t
  physical development of, 141t
  sexual abuse of, 887
  sexuality and, 230t-231t
  sickle cell disease and, 835-836
  skin infection in, 491
  vomiting in, 456t
Preschool screening, 235
  timing of, 240
  tools for, 240, 241t-243t
Prescriptive authority, 5
Pressure for nasal bleeding, 658
Pressure study, voiding, 675
Preterm infant, 322-330
  allergies of, 323
  behavioral assessment of, 131, 132t
  birth history of, 323
  current habits of, 323-324
  development of, 325, 326t, 327
  developmental care protocols for, 114-115
  developmental milestones of, 323
  diagnostic testing of, 324-325
  family life of, 327
  growth of, 325
  immunization and, 175, 323
  incidence of, 322
  management of, 327-330

Preterm infant—cont'd
  parent role for, 325
  physical examination of, 324
  prenatal history of, 323
  retinopathy in, 114
  review of systems of, 324
  risk factors for, 322-323
  school performance of, 324
Prevention
  of bullying, 249
  disease, cultural factors in, 41
  injury, 186-207. *See also* Injury prevention
Primidone, 602t-603t
Privilege withdrawal, 29b
Problem-solving, in family assessment, 18b
Problem-solving by family, 17
Professional autonomy, 71
Progestin, 624
Progestin-only contraceptive, 274t
Progressive headache, 588, 589
Prolactin, 362
Prolapse
  mitral valve, 345
  rectal, 775t
Prometaphase banding, 54
Propanol, 590t
Propantheline bromide, 682
Prophylaxis
  for dental procedures, 227, 227f
  headache, 590t
  for otitis media, 384
  for *Pneumocystis carinii* pneumonia, 803, 803t
  rheumatic fever and, 829
  sickle cell disease and, 836
Propranolol, 359t
Protein allergy, 431t, 433
Proteinuria, 690-692, 691t
Protozoan infection, 732-733, 732b, 733t
Provoked seizure, 601
Prune-belly syndrome, 676, 677
Pruritis, 532
Pruritis ani, 458-459, 460t, 461
Pseudoaddiction, 75
Pseudoephedrine, 683
Pseudohemophilia, 787-788
Pseudohermaphroditism, 616
Pseudomonas aeruginosa
  cystic fibrosis and, 772, 774
  ear infection with, 379
Pseudostrabismus, 394, 394t, 395
Psychoeducation test, 863b
Psychogenic disorder
  abdominal pain
    differential diagnosis of, 415t-416t
    management of, 419-420
  anorexia nervosa, 751-757
  autism, 841-844
  chest pain from, 345
  vomiting with, 455t
Psychological factors
  in anorexia nervosa. *See* Anorexia nervosa
  cystic fibrosis and, 778
  emotional maladjustment of infant, 131
  enuresis and, 684
  hearing impairment and, 389
  of preterm infant, 328-329
  separation anxiety and, 258-259, 259b

Psychosocial assessment
  in eating disorder, 753
  of foster child, 302
  of newborn, 130-133
Psychosocial factors
  HIV infection and, 803
  sickle cell disease and, 830
Psychosocial history
  bleeding disorder and, 789
  diabetes and, 779
Psychotherpy, 586
Puberty
  delayed, 363-364, 364t
  endocrine disorder and, 362
  genetic disorder apparent during, 66
  growth and maturation during, 269
  precocious, 365-366, 365t
Pubic lice, 458, 459, 461, 523, 524t, 525
Public Law 92-142, 7
Public Law 101-476, 7-8
Pulling out hair, 519-520, 519t
Pulmicort, 776
Pulmonary function test
  in asthma, 767-768, 768t
  in cystic fibrosis, 772
Pulmonary stenosis, 348
Pulmonary venous return, partial anomalous, 348
Pulse, 342
Pulse oximetry, 645
Puncture wound, 525-526
Punishment, 29b, 337. *See also* Discipline
Pupillary light reflex, 375
Pure tone audiometry, 153, 376
Purging and binging, 753
  dental disease with, 226
Purified protein derivative, 153, 153t
Purpura
  differential diagnosis of, 486, 487t, 488
  etiology of, 486
  Henoch-Schönlein, differential diagnosis of, 415t-416t, 417-418
  incidence of, 486
  management of, 488
Pus, culture of, 496
Pyelography, intravenous, 674
Pyelonephritis, 688t
Pyloric stenosis
  failure to thrive and, 703t
  vomiting with, 453t
Pyramid, food guide, 271
Pyrantel, 461
Pyrazinamide, 744t
Pyrethrin, 459

Q
Quadriplegia in cerebral palsy, 846t-847t
Question
  about adoption, 291
  in Calgary family intervention model, 18-19
  in family assessment, 16-17, 16f, 17t, 18b
Questionnaire
  on injury prevention, 194b
  for newborn behavior, 133
Questions, trigger, 31b
Quick-flick contraction, 682
Quinacrine, 732t

R

Race
  census data about, 35t
  definition of, 36
  in family assessment, 13, 13b
  genetic evaluation and, 45
Radiation, ultraviolet, 535-537, 535t
Radiation therapy, 824t
  immunization and, 175
Radicular cutaneous field, 582f
Radiographic evaluation, 552f-555f
  cystic fibrosis and, 772
  in Down syndrome, 853
  family violence and, 337
  gastrointestinal disorder and, 411-412
  of musculoskeletal disorder, 555
  in neuropsychiatric disorder, 583t
  respiratory disorder and, 645
  of violence, 337
Radionuclide scan, renal, 674
Range of motion, 550f, 552f-553f
  goniometry for, 555
  in musculoskeletal examination, 546
Ranitidine, 458t
Rank order
  in addictive family, 283
  family assessment and, 12, 12b
Rape, 886-889. *See also* Sexual abuse
Rapid urease testing, 411
Rapid–eye movement sleep, 110
Rash, 528-533
  chickenpox and, 745-746, 745t
  diaper, 514, 515t-516t, 517-518
  differential diagnosis of, 529, 530t-531t, 532
  etiology of, 529
  heat, 520-521
  hives, 521-522, 522t
  incidence of, 529
  management of, 532-533
  risk factors for, 529
  roseola, 738
Ratio
  calcium-to-creatinine, 671, 678t
  inspiration-to-expiration, 772
  upper to lower body, 361
Reactive seizure, 601
Readiness
  for school, 235-245. *See also* School
    readiness
  for toilet training, 265
Reasoning
  as discipline, 29b
  by gifted child, 312
Recessive inheritance
  autosomal, 59t
  X-linked, 60t
    hemophilia as, 787
    muscular dystrophy, 856-861
Record-keeping
  of immunizations, 175
  as legal issue, 4
  of vaccine reaction, 166t-168t, 182t-183t
Recreational injury, 195
Rectal prolapse, 775t
Rectovaginal palpation, 613, 614f
Rectum
  gastrointestinal disorder and, 410
  in physical examination, 102t
Recurrent headache, 589, 590t

Red eye, 402-407
  differential diagnosis of, 403, 404t-405t
  etiology of, 402
  management of, 403-407
  risk factors for, 402
Reduction test, hip, 546, 546f
Referred pain to back, 560t
Reflectometry, acoustic, 376
Reflex
  examination of, 105t
  light pupillary, 375
  neonatal assessment of, 113t, 130t
  neuropsychiatric disorder and, 581, 582b
Reflux
  asthma and, 769t
  cystic fibrosis and, 775t
  failure to thrive and, 703t
  gastroesophageal, 457-458, 457b, 458t
    colic vs, 443
Regional lymphadenopathy, 718
Regulator, cystic fibrosis transmembrane con-
    ductance, 770
Regurgitation, 457
Rehabilitation of athlete, 544-545
Rehydration
  diarrhea and, 426-427
  for gastroenteritis, 418
Reimbursement, 3-4
Reinforcement, 29b
Rejection of newborn, 110b, 130b
Relative based value scale, 4
Relaxation, pelvic muscle, 682
Religion, 13, 13b
Remarriage, 331-334
  in family assessment, 15-16
Renal disorder. *See also* Urinary disorder
  hearing loss in, 377
  hospitalization for, 915
  proteinuria in, 690-692
Reporting of vaccine reaction, 166t-168t, 177,
    182t-183t
Reproductive system, 611-640. *See also*
    Pregnancy
  ambiguous genitalia, 616
  breast disorder and, 616-618, 618t-619t
  cancer treatment affecting, 825t
  cystic fibrosis and, 770t, 772
  data about, 612-615, 613b, 614f, 615t
  Down syndrome and, 853
  genital infection, 618-621, 620t
  health promotion concerning, 611-612, 611f
  menstrual irregularity, 621-625, 622t, 625t
  undescended testis and, 632-634
Research
  nursing, 8
  pain, 74
Residual volume, postvoiding urinary, 674
Resin restoration, dental, 221
Resisted shoulder shrug, 551f
Respiration
  in cystic fibrosis, 771, 771b
  newborn assessment of, 118
Respiratory arrest, 898-899, 898b
Respiratory disorder, 642-643. *See also* Respi-
    ratory system
  airway maintenance and, 642-643
  airway obstruction, 899-900, 899t
    in anaphylaxis, 695
    stridor with, 646, 647t

Respiratory disorder—cont'd
  allergic, 695
  anaphylaxis, 695
  asthma, 757-770. *See also* Asthma
  breath-holding spell and, 246b
  chest pain from, 345
  cough, 653-656, 654t, 655t
  data about, 643-645
  diabetes and, 782t
  epistaxis, 656-659, 657t-658t
  infection
    diphtheria, 723-724, 724t
    influenza, 727-728, 728t
    irritability in, 712t
    laryngitis and, 667-669, 668t
    pertussis, 735-737, 736t
  muscular dystrophy and, 860
  nasal congestion, 659, 660t-661t, 662-664
  respiratory arrest, 898-899, 898b
  retinopathy of prematurity and, 114
Respiratory system
  health promotion concerning, 642-643
  newborn assessment of, 113t
  in physical examination, 100t-101t
  of preterm infant, 324, 325
  sickle cell disease and, 831t
Respondeat superior doctrine, 4
Rest for infant, 130
Restoration, dental, 221
Restrictive parenting style, 23t, 26
Resuscitation of newborn, 110
Retardation, mental, 867-869, 869t
  Down syndrome and, 850-856
Retention
  grade, 240
  urinary, 679-680, 680t, 684
Reticulocyte count
  blood disorder and, 470t
  in sickle cell disease, 831t
Retinoblastoma, 391, 391t, 393
Retinopathy
  of prematurity, 114
  sickle cell, 832t
Retractile testis, 633, 634
Retrograde cholangiopancreatography, endo-
    scopic, 412
Rett syndrome, 842
Review, utilization, 5
Review of systems
  cystic fibrosis and, 771
  eating disorder and, 753
  in patient history, 91t
  of preterm infant, 324
  in spina bifida, 870
Reye syndrome, 738
  vomiting with, 454t
Rh incompatibility
  jaundice with, 481t, 482
  prevention of, 468
Rhabdomyosarcoma, 820t-821t
Rheumatic fever, 826-829, 827t
Rheumatoid arthritis, juvenile, 562, 563t-564t,
    565-566
Rhinitis
  allergic
    asthma and, 769t
    differential diagnosis of, 658t-659t,
      659, 695
    management of, 696-697, 696t, 697t

Rhinitis—cont'd
  differential diagnosis of, 659, 660t-661t
  nasal bleeding in, 657t
Rhizotomy, selective dorsal, 849
RhoGAM, 468
Rickets, 573t, 574
Rifampin, 744t
Right ventricle, double-outlet, 349, 350
Riley Infant Pain Scale, 115
Ringworm, 725, 726t
Rinne test, 376
Risk management, 4
Risk-taking, sexual, 279
Risperidone, 609t
Ritalin, 865t
Ritonavir, 813t-814t
Rivalry, sibling, 262-263
Role
  in addictive family
    of child, 283
    of nurse, 285b
  in family assessment, 17, 18b
Rollerblading injury, 195
Roman Catholic culture, 40b
Roseola, 738-739, 739t
Rotation, hip, 547, 547f
Rotator cuff strain, 204t
Rotator cuff tear, 556t
Rotavirus, 428t
Rotavirus vaccine, 167t
Round ligament pain in pregnancy, 632t
Roundworm infestation, 733-734, 734t
Rubbing, coin, 42
Rubella, 739-740, 740t
  adverse reaction for vaccine for, 166t
  prenatal exposure to, 374
  roseola vs, 738, 739t
  testing for, 496
Rubeola, 740-741
Rule
  for immunization, 160t-163t, 170
  of nines, 900
  parenting, 28b
Runaway youth, 279
Ruptured viscus, 454t
Rural health professional shortage area, 4
Russell-Silver syndrome, 360

S
Sac, lacrimal, 375
Safety
  bleeding disorder and, 790t
  cancer and, 823t
  cerebral palsy and, 848
  diabetes and, 781
  Down syndrome and, 853
  of gifted child, 312-313
  in HIV infection, 802
  learning disability and, 865
  mental retardation and, 868
  muscular dystrophy and, 859
  poisoning and, 198b
  rheumatic fever and, 828
  sickle cell disease and, 835
  spina bifida and, 871
  in stepfamily, 333
  strategies for, 193
Safety car seat, 194
Salaam convulsions, 599

Saline nose drops, 642
Saliva, caries and, 220
Salivary gland in cystic fibrosis, 770t
Salmetrerol, 764t
Salmon patch, 504, 505t
Salmonella, diarrhea caused by, 427t, 431
Salter-Harris fracture, 570
Saqunavir, 814t
Sarcoma, 820t-821t
Sarcoptes scabiei, 741-742, 742t
Scabene, 459
Scabies, 741-742m 742t
Scalded skin syndrome, staphylococcal,
    531t, 532
Scale
  neonatal behavioral, 131
  neonatal pain, 115
  relative based value, 4
Scalp
  hematoma of, 593, 594
  neonatal assessment of, 121t-122t
  scaly, 533, 534t
Scaly scalp, 533, 534t
Scan, renal, 674
Scarlatina, 738
Scarlet fever
  rash from, 529, 531t
  roseola vs, 738, 739t
Schedule, immunization, 172t, 173, 173t,
    174t, 175
Scheuermann kyphosis, 574-575, 575t
School
  bleeding disorder and, 790t
  cancer and, 823t
  cystic fibrosis and, 773
  diabetes and, 780
  Down syndrome and, 853
  fetal alcohol syndrome and, 877
  for foster child, 302
  HIV infection and, 802
  lead poisoning and, 881
  physical abuse and, 883
  poverty and, 886
  sickle cell disease and, 835
  spina bifida and, 871
School-aged child
  anemia screening of, 469b
  autism in, 842
  blood in stool of, 463t
  bullying and, 247
  caloric requirement for, 781
  causes of death of, 186t
  death and grief and, 293
  developmental counseling about, 145t
  developmental domains of, 864t
  developmental milestones for, 139t
  diarrhea in, 432t
  Down syndrome and, 854b-855b
  fetal alcohol syndrome and, 877, 878
  hearing in, 374b, 375
  hospitalization of, 912t-913t
  injury prevention for, 191t
  irritability in, 710t, 711t
  language development of, 143t
  latchkey, 255-256
  laxative for, 424t
  learning disabilities in, 862-866
  nutrition for, 218-219
  oral care for, 222

School-aged child—cont'd
  pain in, 76t, 80t
  parenting tasks during, 21t
  physical development of, 141t
  sexual abuse of, 887
  sexuality and, 231t-232t
  sickle cell disease and, 836
  skin infection in, prevention of, 491
  vomiting in, 456t
School lunch program, 6
School readiness, 235-245
  assessment of, 236-237
  counseling about, 237
  data gathering about, 238t-239t
  developmental testing of, 240,
    241t-243t, 244
  key concepts of, 235
  neurologic determination of, 239t
  parental concerns about, 240
  as parenting concern, 236
  of preterm infant, 329
  risk factors for problems, 235, 235b
Sciatica in pregnancy, 633
Scoliosis, 574-575, 575t
  evaluation of, 548
  muscular dystrophy and, 860
Scope and standards of practice, 4, 5
Screening, 146-156
  of adolescent, 270t
  of adopted child, 289-290
  blood, 147, 148t-149t, 150t
    for disorder of, 468, 469t
  cholesterol, 151, 151t, 152t
  developmental, 154-155
  for Down syndrome, 850, 853
  follow-up of, 155-156
  of foster child, 301
  genetic, 52-54, 53t, 54f
  of gifted child, 311-312
  hearing, 153-154, 154t, 376-377
    in newborn, 116
  hemoglobin and hematocrit, 150
  for hemoglobinopathy, 151
  HIV, 802
  immunization, 176f
  integration of, 155
  lead, 150-151, 150t, 151t
  mental retardation, 867b
  muscular dystrophy, 859, 860
  neuropsychiatric, 576, 583b
  for neuropsychiatric disorder, 576
  newborn, 147, 148t-149t, 150t
  physical measurement, 146-147
  poverty and, 886
  preschool, 235
    timing of, 240
    tools for, 240, 241t-243t
  of preterm infant, 325
  principles of, 146
  purpose of, 146
  sensitivty and specificity of, 146
  sensory, 153-154, 154t
  for substance abuse, 891, 892
  TORCH, for hearing loss, 377
  tuberculosis, 152-153, 152b, 153t
  urine, 151-152
  usefulness of, 146
  vision, 154, 155t, 377-378, 378b
  vital signs, 147

Scrotum
   abnormality of, 439f
   examination of, 612
Sealant, dental, 221
Search for biological parent, 292
Sebaceous follicle, acne of, 499
Seborrheic dermatitis, 725
   diaper, 514, 515t-516t, 517
   differential diagnosis of, 533, 534t
Seckel syndrome, 360
Seizure, 595-605
   breath-holding spell vs, 245, 246b, 246t
   cerebral palsy and, 848
   classification of, 600b
   differential diagnosis of, 596, 597t-600t,
      598-600, 600b
   etiology of, 595
   hospitalization for, 915
   incidence of, 595-596, 596b
   management of, 601-604, 602t-603t, 604,
      604b
   risk factors for, 596
   as vaccine reaction, 177
Selective dorsal rhizotomy, 849
Self-esteem
   discipline and, 29, 29b
   in eating disorder, 756
Self-examination, breast, 611f
Senna, 424t. 424
   in spina bifida, 871
Senokot, 424t. 424
Sensitivity of screening test, 146
Sensorineural hearing loss, 388
Sensory function
   cerebral palsy and, 848
   neuropsychiatric disorder and, 581
   testing of, 153-154
Sensory tic, 608
Separated shoulder, 556t
Separateness as parenting issue, 22
Separation anxiety, 258-259, 259b,
      908-909, 909b
Sepsis
   colic vs, 441
   failure to thrive and, 703t
   jaundice with, 482
Septal defect, cardiac, 348
Septic arthritis
   differential diagnosis of, 562, 563t-564t
   management of, 565
Sequestration crisis, splenic, 831t
Sertraline, 610t
Serum amylase, 411
Serum ferritin assay, 470t
Sever disease, 205t
Sex chromosomal disorder, 47t
Sexual abuse, 886-889
   data on, 887-888
   etiology of, 887
   of foster child, 303
   herpes infection and, 620
   incidence of, 887
   management of, 888-889
   primary care implications of, 888
   risk factors for, 887
   in stepfamily, 333
   vaginal bleeding and, 623
Sexual orientation
   in family assessment, 12, 12b

Sexual orientation—cont'd
   homophobia and, 306-307
   homosexual parent, 305-308
   homosexual youth, 279
Sexual procacity, 366
Sexuality, 229-234
   autism and, 843
   bleeding disorder and, 790t
   cerebral palsy and, 848
   child issues about, 229
   contraception and, 271-272, 272b
      methods of, 273t-274t
   cultural issues about, 229
   cystic fibrosis and, 774
   definition of, 229
   developmental issues about, 230t-233t
   diabetes and, 781
   Down syndrome and, 853
   eating disorder and, 753, 756
   education about, 229
   fetal alcohol syndrome and, 877
   foster child and, 303
   in gay or lesbian family, 306
   of gifted child, 313
   HIV infection and, 802
   in homeless and runaway youth, 279
   learning disability and, 865
   masturbation and, 257-258
   media and, 229
   mental retardation and, 868
   muscular dystrophy and, 859
   parent issues about, 229
   poverty and, 886
   sexual abuse and, 888
   sexually transmitted disease and, 272,
      275-276, 275t
   sickle cell disease and, 835
   in stepfamily, 333
Sexually transmitted disease, 272, 275-276,
      275t, 618-621, 620t
   penile discharge with, 625-627
   prevention of, 491
   vulvovaginal symptoms and, 635-640,
      636t-637t
Shampoo, 494
   for lice, 523
   for tinea capitis, 518
Shigella, 427t, 431
Shin splints, 204t
Shock, 906
   as vaccine reaction, 177
Short stature, 366-367, 368t, 369
Shoulder
   range of motion of, 552f
   sports injury to, 556t
Shoulder impingement syndrome, 204t
Shoulder shrug, resisted, 551f
Shunt, hydrocephalus, 870
Sibling of hospitalized child, 914b
Sibling rivalry, 262-263
Sickle cell disease, 829-838
   complications of, 831t-834t
   data about, 830, 834
   differential diagnosis of, 473t-475t, 476-477
   etiology of, 829-830
   genetics of, 49t
   growing pains vs, 570t
   incidence of, 471, 830
   management of, 836-838

Sickle cell disease—cont'd
   primary care implications of, 835-836
   risk factors for, 830
   types of, 829t
Sign
   Allis, 547, 547f
   Brudinski, 376b
   Kernig, 376b
Single-gene disorder, 55t, 64t
Single parent, 28
Sinus
   cystic fibrosis and, 770t
   radiographic evaluation of, 645
   respiratory disorder and, 644
Sinusitis
   asthma and, 769t
   management of, 663-664
   nasal congestion with, 660t-661t, 662
Sixth disease, 738
Skateboarding injury, 195
Skeletal dysplasia, 367, 368t, 369
Skeletal system. *See* Musculoskeletal *entries*
Skin
   autism and, 842
   blood disorder and, 469
   cancer and, 816
   cystic fibrosis and, 771, 772
   diabetes and, 782t
   Down syndrome and, 851b, 852
   of drug-exposed infant, 320t
   endocrine disorder and, 361
   gastrointestinal disorder and, 410
   malnutrition and, 214t
   in musculoskeletal examination, 546
   neonatal assessment of, 111t, 116, 119t-120t
   neuropsychiatric disorder and, 580
   pallor of, 483-484, 485t, 486
   in physical examination, 95t-96t
   poison on, 198b
   of preterm infant, 324
   respiratory disorder and, 644
   rheumatic fever and, 828
   spina bifida and, 871
   urinary incontinence and, 682-683
Skin disorder
   abscess, 496-499, 498t
   acne, 499-500, 501t-502t, 503-504
   birthmark, 504-505, 506t, 507t, 508
   bites, 508, 509t-510t, 511-513
   candidiasis, 515t-516t, 517, 725
   corns and calluses, 513-514, 513t
   data about, 494-495
   dermatitis of. *See* Dermatitis
   hives, 521-522, 522t
   impetigo, 540-542, 541t
   laboratory evaluation of, 495-496
   minor anomaly, 61t
   minor trauma, 525-526
   rash, 528-533, 530t-531t
      diaper, 514, 515t-516t, 517-518
      differential diagnosis of, 529,
         530t-531t, 532
      heat, 520-521, 520t
      management of, 532-533
   scaly scalp, 533, 534t
   sunburn, 535-537, 536t
   terminology about, 495t
   warts, 537, 538t, 539-540
Skin testing, tuberculin, 152-153

Skinfold test, 546, 547f
Skull in Down syndrome, 851b
Sleep
　asthma and, 762
　cancer and, 823t
　fetal alcohol syndrome and, 877
　for irritable infant, 446b
　in newborn, 110
　as parenting concern, 260-262, 260b
　in patient history, 93t
　physical abuse and, 883
　poverty and, 886
　sexually abused child and, 888
　sickle cell disease and, 835
Sleep-wake cycle, of preterm infant, 329
Sleep-wake cycle of preterm infant, 323
Slipped capital femoral epiphysis, 562, 563t-
　　564t, 566
Slow-to-warm child, 27b
Small head, 590, 591b, 592-595
Smear
　buccal, 615
　papanicolaou, 614, 615t
Smoke inhalation, 188t
Smokeless tobacco, 226
Smoking, 889-890, 891
　cessation strategies for, 892b
　diabetes and, 781
　prenatal and neonatal effects of, 316t
Snake bite, 509t-510t, 511, 512-513
Snuff, 226
Social class
　in family assessment, 13, 13b
　parenting affected by, 23
Social development
　of preterm infant, 328-329
　school readiness and, 238t-239t
Social disorder, 877-894
　abuse
　　physical, 882-884
　　sexual, 886-889
　　substance, 889-894, 890t
　fetal alcohol syndrome, 877-879, 878t
　homelessness, 884-886
　lead poisoning, 879-882, 880t, 881b
　poverty, 884-886
　substance abuse, 889-894
Social history
　of drug-exposed infant, 315
　family, 91t
Social needs in hearing impairment, 389
Social security block grant, 7
Socialization, culture affecting, 25t
Socioeconomic factor, in parenting, 23
Soft tissue, bleeding disorder and, 794t
Solid food for infant, 214, 216t
Somatic pain, 75
Sonar impedance analysis, 376
Sore, mouth, 447-452
Sore throat, 664-667, 665t, 666t
Sound
　breath, 126t
　heart, 126t
Soy intolerance, 430t, 433
Spasm
　infantile, 599
　tetanus vs, 743t
Spasmodic croup, 646, 651
Spastic cerebral palsy, 845, 846t-847t
Special education, 844b, 866b

Specificity of screening test, 146
Spectinomycin, 638
Speculum examination, 612, 614f
Speech. *See* Language
Spell, breath-holding, 245-247, 246b, 246t
Spermatocele
　differential diagnosis of, 436t-437t
　incidence of, 435
　management of, 440
Spermicide, 273t
Spherocytosis, hereditary
　differential diagnosis of, 473t-475t, 476
　incidence of, 471
　management of, 479
Sphincter, urinary incontinence and, 679
Sphincter electromyogram, 675
Spider bite, 511
Spina bifida, 869-876
　Arnold-Chiari malformation in, 870t
　data on, 870-871
　differential diagnosis of, 871
　hydrocephalus and, 870t
　incidence of, 870
　latex allergy in, 872, 873t-874t
　management of, 872, 875-876
　primary care implications of, 871-872
　risk factors for, 870
　tethered cord in, 870t
Spinal cord
　spina bifida and, 869-876. *See also* Spina
　　bifida
　tethered, 870
Spinal injury, sports-related, 203t
Spindle cell nevus, 506t, 508
Spine
　back pain and, 559, 560t, 561
　deformity of, 573t, 574-575, 575t
　in musculoskeletal examination, 546
　neuropsychiatric disorder and, 580
　in physical examination, 102t
Spirituality
　cultural differences in, 37
　in family assessment, 13, 13b
Spirometry, 645
Spironolactone, 359t
Spitting up, 457
Spleen, 127t
Splenic sequestration crisis, 831t
Spondylolysis, 205t, 559, 560t, 561
Spontaneous abortion, 45
Sports, bleeding disorder and, 790t
Sports injury, 556-559, 556t-558t
　dental, 225-226
　differential diagnosis of, 556t-558t
　etiology of, 556
　evaluation of, 548-549, 548f, 549f
　eye injury prevention, 399
　incidence of, 556
　management of, 558
　overuse, 204t-205t
　prevention of, 201-202, 202t,
　　203t, 545
　risk factors for, 556-557
　shoulder, 556t
　types of, 202t, 203t
Spot, Bitot's, 214t
Sprain, 571, 571t, 572
　knee, 558t
　sports-related, 203t
　wrist, 557t

Spray, 494
　nasal, 643
Sputum in cystic fibrosis, 772
Standard
　for immunization, 177, 177b
　parental, 26
　of practice
　　consultation and, 4
　　guidelines defining, 8
　　malpractice insurance and, 5
Staphylococcal scalded skin syndrome,
　　531t, 532
Staphylococcus
　diarrhea caused by, 428t
　ear infection from, 379
Starvation, anorexia and, 753
Status epilepticus, 601
Stavudine, 808t
Stealing, 256-257
Stenosis
　aortic, 348, 349
　pyloric
　　failure to thrive and, 703t
　　vomiting with, 453t
Stepfamily
　data on, 331-332
　developmental stages of, 332-333
　incidence of, 331
　management of, 331-334,
　　333-334
　types of, 331
Stereopsis, 377
Stereotype, 36
Stevens-Johnson syndrome, 451-452
Stillbirth, 45
Stimulant, bowel, in spina bifida, 871
Stimulation of newborn, 130
Sting, 512
Stomatitis
　differential diagnosis of, 447
　management of, 451
Stool
　change in, 462, 463t, 464-466, 464t
　constipation and, 420-425. *See also*
　　Constipation diarrhea. *See*
　　Diarrhea
　newborn assessment of, 113t
　testing of, 410-411
Stool softener
　cerebral palsy and, 848
　in spina bifida, 871
Storage of vaccine, 177, 178t-181t
Strabismus, 395
Strain
　of back, 559, 560t
　differential diagnosis of, 571t
　management of, 572
　sports-related, 203t
Stranger, anxiety, 263-264
Strangulation, prevention of
　by infant, 188t, 189t
　in preschool-aged child, 190t
　by toddler, 190t
Strength
　in musculoskeletal examination, 546
　parental, 30b
Strengthening exercise, 545
Streptoccal infection, meningitis, 730
Streptococcal infection
　glomerulonephritis after, 677

Streptococcal infection—cont'd
oral
differential diagnosis of, 447
management of, 451
pharyngitis, 665-666, 665t, 666t
rheumatic fever, 826-829, 827t
scarlet fever, 738
tonsillopharyngitis
differential diagnosis of, 414t-415t, 417
management of, 419
Streptococcus mutans, 220, 225
Streptococcus pneumoniae, drug-resistant, 379
Stress, proteinuria with, 691
Stress fracture, 204t
Stress incontinence, 679, 680t, 681, 683
Stress test in sports injury, 548, 548f, 549f
Stretching exercise, 545
Stridor, 646. *See also* Breathing difficulty
Structural family assessment, 12
Sturge-Weber syndrome, 507t
Sty, 400, 401t
Style, parenting, 22, 23t
Subarachnoid hemorrhage, 454t
Subcutaneous scalp hematoma, 593, 594
Subdural hematoma, 453t
Subgaleal hematoma, 594
Submandibular lymphadenitis, 731
Substance abuse, 889-894, 890t
diabetes and, 781
by parent, 283-286, 284b, 285b
prenatal, 315-321. *See also* Drug-exposed
infant
violence in family and, 337
Substitution as discipline method, 29b
Subsystem, family, 12, 12b
Sucking, nonnutritive, 226
Sucrose malabsorption, 464t
Suffocation, prevention of
of infant, 188t, 189t
in preschool-aged child, 190t
strategies for, 199
by toddler, 190t
Suicide
differential diagnosis of, 605-606
etiology of, 605
incidence of, 605
prevention of, 196-197
risk factors for, 605
Sulfasalazine
Crohn's disease and, 419
for inflammatory bowel disease, 465
Sulfite, asthma caused by, 762
Sumatriptan, 590t
Sun exposure
pallor and, 484
prevention of, 491-492
Sunburn, 535-537, 536t
prevention of, 491-492
Sunken fontanel, 41
Superficial burn, 901b
Superficial folliculitis, 497
Superficial reflex, 582b
Superior mesenteric artery syndrome, 455t
Supplies for newborn, 84b
Support system
assessment of, 30
in grief process, 294
substance abuse and, 285
Suppressant, cough, 643

Surgery
patient history of, 89t
preparation for, 908-915, 909b, 910b, 911t-
913t, 914b
Surveillance
of preterm infant, 328
in school readiness assessment, 235
Suture, craniosynostosis and, 593
Swallowed poison, 198b
Sweat gland in cystic fibrosis, 770t
Sweat test for cystic fibrosis, 772
Swelling, joint, 570-572, 571t
Symptom inventory, neuropsychiatric,
577t-580t
Syncope, 600, 604
Synovitis, transient, 562, 565
Syphilis, 275t, 276, 619, 620t, 621
skin disorder and, 496
Systemic lupus erythematosus, 725

T
T lymphocyte
asthma and, 759, 759b
HIV infection and, 801t
Tantrum, 264-265
Tapeworm, 733
Task, parenting, 20
Tattooing, 277
Tay-Sachs disease, 49t
Teaching. *See* Education
Technetium-99m hepatoiminodiacetic acid
scan, 412
Teeth
caries in, 220
nursing bottle, 224-225, 224t, 225f
prevention of, 221-222, 221t
process of, 220-221
development of, 220
in physical examination, 98t
Teething, 712t
Tele-health/medicine, 6
Telecommunication Reform Act, 6
Telephone management
of nasal bleeding, 658
of poisoning or overdose, 198b
Temper tantrum, 264-265
Temperament
emotional maladjustment of infant and, 131
neonatal assessment of, 119t
parenting affected by, 26-28, 26b, 27b
Temperament Assessment Battery for
Children, 242t
Temperature
fever and, 704-710, 706t-708t
frostbite and, 902-903, 902b
hyperthermia and, 904, 905t
in newborn assessment, 116
Tenderness, breast, 616
Tendinitis, 204t, 205t
Tennis elbow, 204t
Tension-type headache, 588, 589
Teratogen, 64t
Terconazole, 640
Terminology, cultural, 36
Terrors, night, 261-262
Testicular torsion, 439f
differential diagnosis of, 435,
436t-438t
Testing, genetic, 54, 55t, 56

Testis
retractile, 634
undescended, 632-634
Testosterone
for delayed puberty, 364
endocrine disorder and, 362
Tetanus, 742-743, 743t
Tetanus vaccine
administration of, 164t
contraindications to, 159t
handling and storage of, 180t-181t
reporting adverse event, 166t
rules for, 160t
Tethered spinal cord, 870
Tetracycline
for acne, 502t, 503
tooth stain from, 223
for urethritis, 690
Tetralogy of Fallot, 348, 349
Thalassemia
differential diagnosis of, 473t, 475t, 477-478
incidence of, 471
management of, 479
Thelarche, premature, 365-366, 365t
Theophylline, 765t
Therapeutic abortion, 628
Thermal injury
burn, 900-901, 900f
frostbite, 902-903
hyperthermia, 904, 905t
Thimerosal, 173
Thorax, in physical examination, 100t
Throat
cancer and, 816
culture of, 645
cystic fibrosis and, 771
diabetes and, 782t
endocrine disorder and, 361
neonatal assessment of, 124t
in physical examination, 98t-99t
of preterm infant, 324
respiratory disorder and, 644
in review of systems, 91t
sickle cell disease and, 830
sore, 664-667, 665t, 666t
Thrombocytopenic purpura, 486, 487t, 488
as vaccine adverse event, 169t
Thumbsucking, 226
as parenting concern, 265-266
Thyroid disorder, 368t, 369, 370t, 371
diabetes and, 782t
in Down syndrome, 853
tests for, 362
Thyroid function test, 783t
Thyroid-stimulating hormone, 783t
Thyroxine, 783t
Tiagabine, 602t-603t
Tibial torsion, internal, 567, 567t
Tibial tubercle, apophysitis of, 205t
Tic, 607-609, 608b, 609t, 610t
Tick
bite of, 511
in ear, 387
Tick-borne disease, 728-730, 729t
Ticonazole, 640
Tincture of opium for drug-exposed infant, 319
Tinea
diagnosis of, 496
differential, 534t, 725, 726t

Tinea—cont'd
  hair loss from, 518-519
  Lyme disease vs, 729t
Tobacco, 889-890, 891
  cessation strategies for, 892b
  diabetes and, 781
  prenatal and neonatal effects of, 316t
  smokeless, 226
Tobramycin, 774
Toddler
  anemia screening of, 469b
  autism in, 842
  blood in stool of, 463t
  caloric requirement for, 781
  death of, 186t
  developmental counseling about, 145t
  developmental milestones for, 139t
  diarrhea in, 426
  Down syndrome and, 854b-855b
  fetal alcohol syndrome and, 877, 878
  hearing assessment of, 375
  hospitalization of, 911t
  injury prevention for, 189t-190t
  irritability in, 710t, 711t
  language development of, 142t
  nonnutritive sucking by, 226
  nutrition for, 216-218
  oral care for, 222
  pain in, 76t, 80t
  parenting tasks during, 21t
  physical development of, 141t
  separation anxiety in, 909b
  sexuality and, 230t
  sickle cell disease and, 835-836
  skin infection in, prevention of, 491
  vomiting in, 456t
Toe, 117, 129t
Toeing-in, 566-568, 567t
Toenail, ingrown, 205t
Toilet training, 266-267
Tolerance, drug, 75
Tone
  in cerebral palsy, 846t
  Down syndrome and, 851b
Tongue, 112t, 124t
Tongue-tie, 227
Tonsil, 124t
Tonsillar diphtheria, 724t
Tonsillopharyngitis
  differential diagnosis of, 414t-415t, 417
  management of, 419
Tooth
  development of, 220, 220t
  injury to, 225-226
Toothbrushing, 224
Toothpaste, fluoride-containing, 222
Topical drug
  for acne, 502t
  for diaper rash, 517
  guidelines for, 492
  for lice, 523
  for rash, 532
Topical fluoride, 222
Topiramate, 602t-603t
TORCH screen for hearing loss, 377
Torsion
  internal femoral, 566-567, 567t
  internal tibial, 567, 567t
  testicular, 435, 436t-438t, 439f

Torsional deformity, 547-548, 547f, 548t
Tort, 4
Torticollis, paroxysmal, 588b
Total anomalous pulmonary venous return,
    348, 349, 350
Tourette syndrome, 608, 608b
Toxic ingestion
  first aid for, 198b
  prevention of
    in adolescent, 192t
    by infant, 188t, 189t
    by preschool-aged child, 190t
    in school-aged child, 191t
Toxic plant, 192b
Toxicty, fluoride, 222
Toxoplasmosis screening, 149t
Traction alopecia, 519, 519t
Transfusion for neonatal jaundice, 483
Transgender adolescent, 279
Transient orthostatic proteinuria, 691
Transient synovitis, 562, 565
Transient urinary incontinence, 680
Transillumination, 116, 121t
Transition for preterm infant, 328
Transmembrane conductance regulator, cystic
    fibrosis, 770
Transmission of HIV infection, perinatal, 803
Transplant, lung, 776
Transposition of great arteries, 349, 350
Trapezius muscle, 551f
Trauma. *See also* Injury prevention
  abdominal, differential diagnosis of,
    415t-416t
  agent of, 187, 192
  chest pain from, 345
  child characteristics in, 187
  child development and, 188t-192t
  colic vs, 443-444
  definition of, 186
  dental, 225-226
  ear, 386-387
  eye, 396, 397t, 398-399
  eyelid, 396, 397t, 398
  irritability in, 713t
  joint pain from, 570-572, 571t
  limp caused by, 562
  meniscal, 571
  nail, 526-528, 527t
  nasal bleeding from, 657t
  overuse, 204t-205t. 206t, 557
  penile discharge from, 626
  petechiae caused by, 486, 487t, 488
  prevention of, 186-207. *See also* Injury
    prevention
  renal, 677
  vaginal bleeding and, 623
  violence and, 335-338
  vomiting with, 453t
Trench mouth, differential diagnosis of,
    447, 450
Trendelenburg test, 547, 547f
Treponema pallidum infection, 619, 620t, 621
Triamcinolone
  for allergic rhinitis, 697t
  asthma and, 764t
  cystic fibrosis and, 776
Triangle relationship, in stepfamily, 334
Trichomoniasis, 275, 275t
  culture for, 615

Trichomoniasis—cont'd
  differential diagnosis of, 637t
  management of, 638, 640
Trichophyton tonsurans, 496
Trichotillomania, 519-520, 519t
Tricyclic antidepressant, 586
Trigeminal nerve, 105t
Trigger questions, 31b
Triiodothyronine, diabetes and, 783t
Trimethoprim-sulfamethoxazole
  HIV infection and, 803
  for sinusitis, 663
  for urinary tract infection, 689
Tripelennamine, for allergic rhinitis, 696t
Trisomy, 46t
Trisomy 21, 850-856. *See also* Down syndrome
Tropia, 395
Trunk, cancer and, 823t
Tubercle, tibial, apophysitis of, 205t
Tuberculin skin testing, 152-153
Tuberculosis, 743-745, 744t
  screening for, 152b
  skin testing for, 175
  testing foster child for, 302
Tumor, 815-826. *See also* Malignancy
  melanoma, 492
  retinoblastoma, 391, 391t, 393
  vomiting with, 455t
  Wilms', 675
Turner syndrome, 47t, 66
  gonadal dysfunction in, 363-364
  signs and symptoms of, 360
Tympanic membrane perforation, 382
  management of, 385
Tympanocentesis, 377, 377b
Tympanogram, 377, 377f
Tympanometry, 153, 376
Tyrosinemia screening, 149t
Tzanck smear, 496

U
Ulcer
  aphthous, 447, 449t
  peptic, 413t-415t, 417
  sickle cell disease and, 833t
Ulcerative colitis, 432t, 464t
Ulcerative gingivitis, necrotizing
  differential diagnosis of, 447, 449t, 450
  management of, 451
Ultrasonography
  in Down syndrome, 853
  endocrine disorder and, 362
  gastrointestinal disorder and, 411-412
  for genetic screening, 53t
  musculoskeletal disorder and, 555
  of reproductive system, 615
Ultraviolet radiation, 535-537, 535t
Umbilical blood sampling, 53t
Umbilical hernia
  differential diagnosis of, 440t
  incidence of, 435
  management of, 440-441
Umbilicus, assessment of, 127t
Unconditional acceptance as nursing
    value, 70
Underweight, 755
Undescended testis, 632-634
United States Department of Agriculture food
    stamp program, 7

Universal acceptance as nursing value, 70
Unprovoked seizure, 601-603
Upper extremity. *See also* Extremity
　Down syndrome and, 851b
　of neonate, 128t-129t
Upper to lower body ratio, 361
Uremia, 454t
Urethral anomaly, 676-677
Urethritis
　in male, 625-627
　management of, 690
　painful urination with, 687, 688t
Urethrorrhagia, 677, 678
Urge incontinence, 680
　differential diagnosis of, 680-681, 681t
　etiology of, 679
　management of, 681-683
Urinalysis
　diabetes and, 783t
　of drug-exposed infant, 317
　hearing loss and, 377
　pregnancy testing and, 278
　reproductive system disorder and, 615
　in urinary disorder, 671
Urinary disorder, 670-692. *See also* Urinary tract infection
　abdominal mass with, 675-676
　of bladder and urethra, 676-677
　examination for, 671-675, 672f-673f, 674t
　health promotion concerning, 670
　hematuria in, 677-679, 677b, 678t
　incontinence, 679-684, 680t, 681t
　nocturnal enuresis, 684-686, 685t
　painful urination, 686-687, 688t, 689-690
　patient history of, 670-671
　proteinuria with, 690-692, 691t
　risk factors for, 670
Urinary retention, 679-680, 680t, 684
Urinary tract infection
　abdominal pain with, 413t-415t
　cerebral palsy and, 848
　colic vs, 441
　differential diagnosis of, 413t-415t, 417
　hematuria with, 677, 678t, 679
　incontinence with, 680
　irritability in, 712t
　management of, 418, 683
　painful urination with, 686-687, 688t
　treatment of, 689-690
Urination
　painful, 686-687, 688t, 689-690
　record of, 672f-673f, 673
　in spina bifida, 871-872
Urine
　diabetes and, 783t
　gastrointestinal disorder and, 411
　newborn assessment of, 113t
　nocturnal enuresis and, 684-686, 685t
　protein in, 690-692, 691t
　testing of, 151-152
Urodynamic testing, 674, 674t
Uroflowmetry, 674
Urography, 674
Urticaria, 521-522, 522t, 696
Uterine bleeding, dysfunctional, 623
Uterus in pregnancy, 630t
Utilization review, 5

V
Vaccine
　asthma and, 762
　HIV infection and, 801
　Lyme disease, 729
Vaginal diphtheria, 724t
Vaginal discharge, 638-639
　in pregnancy, 633
Vaginal foreign body
　differential diagnosis of, 459, 459t
　management of, 462, 638, 639
Vaginosis, bacterial
　culture for, 615
　management of, 640
Valacyclovir, 275t
Valproic acid, 602t-603t
　for recurrent headache, 590t
Value
　core, 69-70
　cultural differences in, 36-37, 36t
　nursing, 70-71
Valve disease
　aortic stenosis, 348
　mitral, 345
　pulmonary, 348
Valvuloplasty, balloon, 349
Vanillylmandelic acid test, 676
Vanishing testes syndrome, 364
Varicella, 745-746, 746t
　cancer and, 817
　oral
　　differential diagnosis of, 447, 448t
　　management of, 451
　rash from, 531t
Varicella vaccine, 161t
　administration of, 165t
　characteristics of, 170
　handling and storage of, 180t-181t
　HIV infection and, 801
　reporting adverse event, 167t
　rules for, 161t
Varicocele, 435, 438f
　differential diagnosis of, 436t-437t
　management of, 440
Vascular birthmark, 505t
Vascular hydrocephalus, 592b
Vascular nonthrombocytopenic purpura, 486, 487t, 488
Vasodilator, 359t
Vasomotor rhinitis, 660t-661t, 662, 663
Vehicular accident
　pedestrian, 194-195
　prevention of
　　in adolescent, 192t
　　in preschool-aged child, 190t
　　in school-aged child, 191t
　　strategies for, 193-194, 193b
Venereal Disease Research Laboratory test, 496
Venous return, partial anomalous pulmonary, 348
Ventricle, right, double-outlet, 349, 350
Ventricular septal defect, 348
Verbal communication, 16, 18b
Verbal skill of gifted child, 312
Vernal conjunctivitis, 403
Vernix caseosa, 120t
Verrucae, 537, 538t, 539-540
Vertical eye deviation, 395-396

Vertigo, benign paroxysmal, 588b
Very-low-density lipoprotein, 355t, 356
Vicarious liability, 4
Victim of bullying, 247, 248f, 249
Videourodynamic study, 675
Vietnamese culture
　newborn care in, 41b
　postpartum practices in, 40b
Vigabatrin, 602t-603t
Vincent's stomatitis, 447
Violence, 335-338
　incidence of, 335
　interpersonal, 195
　interview about, 336-337
　management of, 337-338
　physical abuse, 882-884
　　behavior patterns in, 130-131
　prevention strategies for, 193b, 195-196
　risk factors for, 335
　signs of, 335-336
Viral infection
　conjunctivitis, 403, 405t
　croup, 646, 647t
　　management of, 651
　culture of, 377, 615
　diarrhea caused by, 428t, 433
　exanthem caused by, 520t, 521
　of eye, 377
　genital herpes, 618-620, 620t
　hand-foot-mouth disease, 529
　　differential diagnosis of, 447, 448t
　　management of, 451
　hepatitis, 746-747, 747t
　HIV, 796-815. *See also* Human immunodeficiency virus infection
　influenza, 727-728, 728t
　laryngitis and, 667-669, 668t
　meningitis and, 730
　mumps, 731
　pharyngitis, 664-665, 665t, 666t
　poliovirus, 737, 737t
　Reye syndrome with, 738
　rhinitis
　　differential diagnosis of, 659, 660t-661t
　　management of, 662
　roseola, 738-739, 739t
　rubella, 739-740, 740t
　rubeola, 740-741
　vaginal, 615
　varicella zoster, 745-746, 745t, 746t
Visceral pain, 75
Viscus, ruptured, vomiting with, 454t
Vision
　diabetes and, 781
　Down syndrome and, 855
　of preterm infant, 325
　in review of systems, 92t
Vision screening, 154, 155t, 377-378, 378b
　early, 374
Visual analogue scale, 77t
Visual impairment, 389-393, 390t-391t
Vital signs
　diabetes and, 782t
　malignancy and, 822t
　in physical examination, 95t
　screening of, 147

Vitamin
  cystic fibrosis and, 776
  for infant, 215-216
  recommendations for, 212b
Vitamin B₁₂ deficiency
  blood disorder and, 470t
  differential diagnosis of, 472, 473t-475t, 476
  management of, 478
Vocal tic, 608
Voice change, 667-669, 668t
Voiding, timed, 682
Voiding cystourethrogram, 674
Voiding pressure study, 675
Voiding record, 672f-673f
Volume, postvoiding urinary residual, 674
Voluntary withholding of stool, 420
Vomiting, 452-458
  bulimia and, 751
  diabetes and, 785-786
  differential diagnosis of, 452, 453t-455t, 455
  etiology of, 452, 456t
  incidence of, 452
  malignancy and, 822t
  management of, 455-458, 457b, 458b
  migraine and, 588b
  in pregnancy, 632t
  in Reye syndrome, 738
  risk factors for, 452
Von Willebrand disease, 787-788
  management of, 791
  menstrual bleeding and, 623
Vulnerability, parental, 30b
Vulvovaginal symptoms, 634-640
  differential diagnosis of, 635, 636t-637t
  etiology of, 634

Vulvovaginal symptoms—cont'd
  incidence of, 634
  management of, 635, 638-640
  risk factors for, 634-635
Vulvovaginitis, nonspecific
  in adolescence, 636t, 638-639
  in prepubescence, 635, 636t

W
Wart, 537, 538t, 539-540
  genital, 619, 620t, 621
Wasp sting, 512
Wasting syndrome, HIV, 799
Water, fluoride in, 221-222, 221t
Wax, ear, 378-379
Weber test, 376
Weeping skin lesion, 532, 540-542, 541t
Weight
  cystic fibrosis and, 771
  diabetes and, 782t
  Down syndrome and, 852
  eating disorder and, 572t, 751-757
  endocrine disorder and, 361
  gastrointestinal disorder and, 410
  neuropsychiatric disorder and, 579
  of newborn, 115, 118t
  screening of, 146-147
West syndrome, 599
Western blot for Lyme disease, 496
Wet dressing, 494
Wet preparation for vaginal discharge, 615
Wheezing, 760b. *See also* Asthma; Breathing
  difficulty
White blood cell count, 645
Whitlow, herpetic, 527t, 528

Whooping cough, 735-737, 736t
WIC program, 6
Wilms' tumor, 675, 820t-821t
Withdrawal, as contraception, 273t
Withdrawal bleeding, 623-624
Withholding of stool, 420
Women, Infants, and Children program, 6
Wood's lamp examination, 496
Word Graphic pain rating scale, 77t
Worm infestation, 733-735, 734t
Wound
  culture of, 496
  puncture, 525-526
Wrist injury, 548, 557t

X
X-linked disorder
  hemophilia as, 787
  muscular dystrophy, 856-861
  types of, 49t
X-linked inheritance, 60t
Xylose test, 412
d-Xylose test, 412

Y
Yang, 37, 38b
Yersinia, 427t, 431
Yin, 37, 38b

Z
Zalcitabine, 808t
Zidovudine for HIV infection, 803t,
  808t-809t
Zonisamide, 602t-603t
Zoster, 745-746, 746t

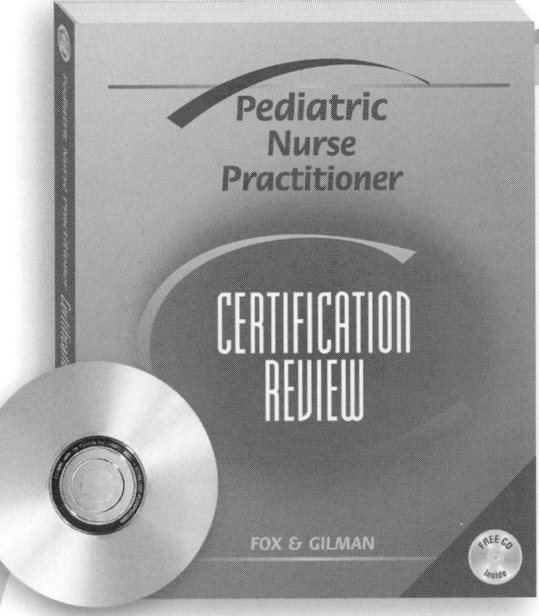
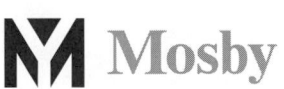

Conversions and Estimates

Temperature
To convert Celsius to Fahrenheit: $(9/5 \times \text{temperature}) + 32$
To convert Fahrenheit to Celsius: $(\text{temperature} - 32) \times 5/9$

CELSIUS	FAHRENHEIT	CELSIUS	FAHRENHEIT
34.2	93.6	38.6	101.4
34.6	94.3	39.0	102.2
35.0	95.0	39.4	102.9
35.4	95.7	39.8	103.6
35.8	96.4	40.2	104.3
36.2	97.1	40.6	105.1
36.6	97.8	41.0	105.8
37.0	98.6	41.4	106.5
37.4	99.3	41.8	107.2
37.8	100.0	42.2	108.0
38.2	100.7	42.6	108.7

From Barkin & Rosen. (1999). Emergency pediatrics: A guide to ambulatory care (5th ed.). St. Louis: Mosby.

Normal Blood Pressure for Various Ages

AGE	SYSTOLIC (MEAN ± 2 SD)	DIASTOLIC (MEAN ± 2 SD)
Newborn	80 ± 16	46 ± 16
6 months–1 year	89 ± 29	60 ± 10*
1 year	96 ± 30	66 ± 25*
2 years	99 ± 25	64 ± 25*
3 years	100 ± 25	67 ± 23*
4 years	99 ± 20	65 ± 20*
5-6 years	94 ± 14	55 ± 9
6-7 years	100 ± 15	56 ± 8
8-9 years	105 ± 16	57 ± 9
9-10 years	107 ± 16	57 ± 9
10-11 years	111 ± 17	58 ± 10
11-12 years	113 ± 18	59 ± 10
12-13 years	115 ± 19	59 ± 10
13-14 years	118 ± 19	60 ± 10

The point of muffling is shown as the diastolic pressure.
From Nelson, W.E., et al. (1999). Nelson textbook of pediatrics (16th ed.). Philadelphia: W.B. Saunders.

Mean Blood Pressure at Wrist and Ankle in Infants (Flush Technique)

AGE	BLOOD PRESSURE AT WRIST		BLOOD PRESSURE AT ANKLE	
	MEAN	RANGE	MEAN	RANGE
1-7 days	41	22-66	37	20-58
1-3 months	67	48-90	61	38-96
4-6 months	73	42-100	68	40-104
7-9 months	76	52-96	74	50-96
10-12 months	57	62-94	56	102

From Nelson, W.E., et al. (1999). Nelson textbook of pediatrics (16th ed.). Philadelphia: W.B. Saunders.

Pulse Rate at Various Ages

AGE	RANGE	AVERAGE
Newborn	70-170	120
1-11 months	80-160	120
2 years	80-130	110
4 years	80-120	100
6 years	75-115	100
8 years	70-110	90
10 years	70-110	90

	GIRLS		BOYS	
	RANGE	AVERAGE	RANGE	AVERAGE
12 years	70-110	90	65-105	85
14 years	65-105	85	60-100	80
16 years	60-100	80	55-95	75
18 years	55-95	75	50-90	70

From Nelson, W.E., et al. (1999). Nelson textbook of pediatrics (16th ed.). Philadelphia: W.B. Saunders.

Normal Respiratory Rates for Children

AGE	RATE (BREATHS/MINUTE)
Newborn	35
1-11 months	30
2 years	25
4 years	23
6 years	21
8 years	20
10 years	19
12 years	19
14 years	18
16 years	17
18 years	16-18

From Wong, D. (1999). Wong & Whaley's clinical manual of pediatric nursing (6th ed.). St. Louis: Mosby.